THE AMERICAN COLLEGE OF OBSTETRICIANS AND GYNECOLOGISTS

WOMEN'S HEALTH CARE PHYSICIANS

2001 COMPENDIUM OF SELECTED PUBLICATIONS

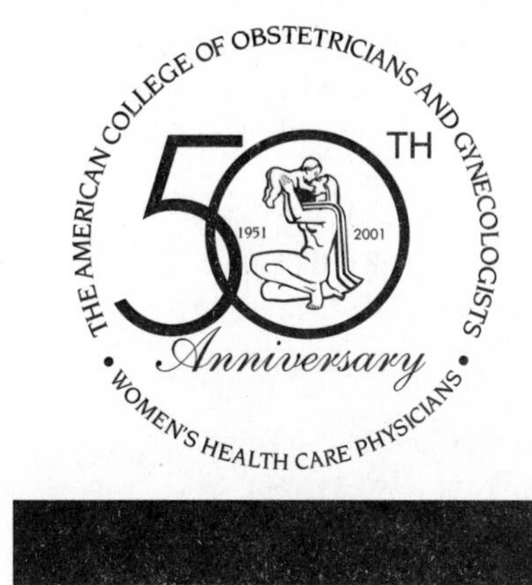

The *2001 Compendium of Selected Publications* contains current clinical practice documents published by the American College of Obstetricians and Gynecologists (ACOG) as of December 31, 2000. The information in these documents should not be viewed as establishing standards or dictating rigid rules. The guidelines are general and intended to be adapted to many different situations, taking into account the needs and resources particular to the locality, the institution, or the type of practice. Variations and innovations that improve the quality of patient care are to be encouraged rather than restricted. The purpose of these guidelines will be well served if they provide a firm basis on which local norms may be built.

The American College of Obstetricians and Gynecologists
409 12th Street, SW
PO Box 96920
Washington, DC 20090-6920

ISBN: 0-915473-65-8 12345/54321

Publications may be ordered through the ACOG Distribution Center by calling toll free 800-762-2264. To receive order forms via facsimile, call (732) 885-6364 and follow the audio instructions. Publications also may be ordered from the ACOG web site at www.acog.org.

Contents

* Title issued since publication of 2000 Compendium of Publications.

Educational and Technical Bulletins

Practice Bulletins

Foreword

The *2001 Compendium of Selected Publications* is a compilation of selected ACOG clinical practice guidelines in effect as of December 31, 2000. In this single, fully indexed volume, it is possible to refer to virtually any topic in obstetrics and gynecology that ACOG has addressed. This resource is invaluable for reference or referral to key areas in the specialty throughout the year.

The Compendium includes documents from popular ACOG series. These series are developed by committees of experts and reviewed by leaders in the specialty and the College. Each document is reviewed periodically and either reaffirmed, replaced, or withdrawn to ensure its continued appropriateness to practice. The contribution of the many groups and individuals who participated in the process is gratefully acknowledged.

Each section of the Compendium is devoted to a particular series, and the titles are listed alphabetically within that series. The contents of the Compendium reflect the changes taking place in medicine with the move toward evidence-based guidelines. Each of the following series is represented intact:

- Committee Opinions: Brief focused documents of limited scope that address clinical issues of an urgent or emergent nature or nonclinical topics in areas such as policy, economics, and social issues that relate to the practice of obstetrics and gynecology. They are consensus statements that may or may not be based on scientific evidence.

- Educational and Technical Bulletins: Educational treatises that reflect a review of a general or specific topic. Their purpose is to update the education of the practicing obstetrician–gynecologist with a concise, clinically oriented review. The topics are determined by a need process that identifies newer developments or educational concepts. Information in these bulletins is supported by satisfactory documentation.

- Practice Bulletins: Evidence-based guidelines developed to indicate a preferred method of diagnosis and management of a condition. The evidence is graded, and peer-reviewed research determines the recommendations in the document. Issues of cost are addressed in arriving at conclusions.

- Practice Patterns: Precursor to the Practice Bulletin series, the documents in this series launched ACOG's effort to develop evidence-based practice guidelines.

Also included in the Compendium are ACOG Policy Statements. As with practice guidelines, these policy statements are approved by the Executive Board and reviewed and reaffirmed periodically. The statements included are those deemed current. In addition, lists of titles of Committee Opinions and Educational and Practice Bulletins are provided to enable readers to locate specific titles by committee or category and are organized in order of publication. As a further aid, a complete subject index is provided.

New additions to the Compendium are the Scope of Practice of Obstetrics and Gynecology, which includes the ACOG Operational Mission Statement and Vision Statement, and the Code of Professional Ethics, which provides ethical foundations for professional activities in the field of obstetrics and gynecology.

As new documents are released throughout the year, which may replace existing documents in the Compendium, they will be included in a separate ACOG publications section of ACOG's official journal *Obstetrics & Gynecology*. Single copies can be obtained from the Resource Center (202-863-2518) and the series are available for sale as complete sets or subscriptions (call 800-762-2264 to order). These documents also are available to members on our web site: www.acog.org. To verify the status of documents, contact the Resource Center or check our web site.

We are making every effort to provide health professionals with current, quality information on the practice of obstetrics and gynecology. The *2001 Compendium of Selected Publications* represents still another way to disseminate material designed to promote women's health.

—Ralph W. Hale, MD, Executive Vice President

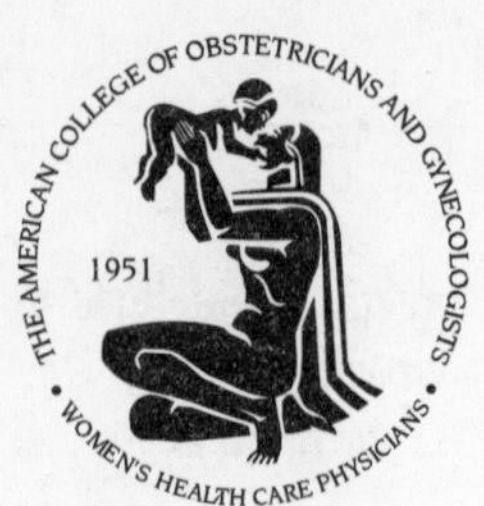

The Scope of Practice of Obstetrics and Gynecology

ACOG OPERATIONAL MISSION STATEMENT

The American College of Obstetricians and Gynecologists (ACOG) is a membership organization of obstetrician–gynecologists dedicated to the advancement of women's health through education, advocacy, practice and research.

VISION STATEMENT

Obstetrics and gynecology is a discipline dedicated to the broad, integrated medical and surgical care of women's health throughout their lifespan. The combined discipline of obstetrics and gynecology requires extensive study and understanding of reproductive physiology, including the physiologic, social, cultural, environmental and genetic factors that influence disease in women. This study and understanding of the reproductive physiology of women gives obstetricians and gynecologists a unique perspective in addressing gender-specific health care issues.

Primary and preventive counseling and education are essential and integral parts of the practice of an obstetrician–gynecologist as they advance the individual and community-based health of women of all ages.

Obstetricians and gynecologists may choose a wide or more focused scope of practice from primary ambulatory health to concentration in a particular area of specialization.

Approved by the Executive Board
May 25, 2000

THE AMERICAN COLLEGE OF OBSTETRICIANS AND GYNECOLOGISTS • WOMEN'S HEALTH CARE PHYSICIANS
409 12TH STREET, SW WASHINGTON, DC 20024-2188
MAILING ADDRESS: PO BOX 96920 WASHINGTON DC 20090-6920
202 638-5577

Code of Professional Ethics

of the American College of Obstetricians and Gynecologists

Obstetrician–gynecologists, as members of the medical profession, have ethical responsibilities not only to patients, but also to society, to other health professionals, and to themselves. The following ethical foundations for professional activities in the field of obstetrics and gynecology are the supporting structures for the Code of Conduct. The Code implements many of these foundations in the form of rules of ethical conduct. Noncompliance with the Code may affect an individual's initial or continuing Fellowship in the American College of Obstetricians and Gynecologists. In addition to the Code, certain Committee Opinions of the American College of Obstetricians and Gynecologists provide ethical guidance. Fellows are urged to read and evaluate these Committee Opinions. Opinions relevant to specific points are referenced in the Code of Conduct.

Ethical Foundations

I. The patient–physician relationship: The welfare of the patient (*beneficence*) is central to all considerations in the patient–physician relationship. Included in this relationship is the obligation of physicians to respect the rights of patients, colleagues, and other health professionals. The respect for the right of individual patients to make their own choices about their health care (*autonomy*) is fundamental. The principle of justice requires strict avoidance of discrimination on the basis of race, color, religion, national origin, or any other basis that would constitute illegal discrimination (*justice*).

II. Physician conduct and practice: The obstetrician–gynecologist should deal honestly with patients and colleagues (*veracity*). This includes not misrepresenting himself or herself through any form of communication in an untruthful, misleading, or deceptive manner. Furthermore, maintenance of medical competence through study, application, and enhancement of medical knowledge and skills is an obligation of practicing physicians. Any behavior that diminishes a physician's capability to practice, such as substance abuse, must be immediately addressed and rehabilitative services instituted. The physician should modify his or her practice until the diminished capacity has been restored to an acceptable standard to avoid harm to patients (*nonmaleficence*). All physicians are obligated to respond to evidence of question-

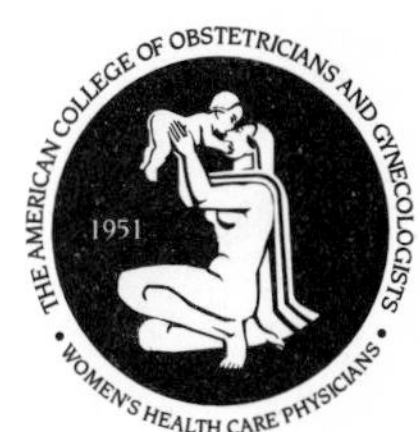

409 12th Street, SW
PO Box 96920
Washington, DC 20090-6920

able conduct or unethical behavior by other physicians through appropriate procedures established by the relevant organization.

III. Avoiding conflicts of interest: Potential conflicts of interest are inherent in the practice of medicine. Physicians are expected to recognize such situations and deal with them through public disclosure. Conflicts of interest should be resolved in accordance with the best interest of the patient, respecting a woman's autonomy to make health care decisions. The physician should be an advocate for the patient through public disclosure of conflicts of interest raised by health payor policies (managed care or others) or hospital policies.

IV. Professional relations: The obstetrician–gynecologist should respect and cooperate with other physicians, nurses, and other health-care professionals.

V. Societal responsibilities: The obstetrician–gynecologist has a continuing responsibility to society as a whole and should support and participate in activities that enhance the community. As a member of society, the obstetrician–gynecologist must respect the laws of that society. As professionals and members of medical societies, physicians are required to uphold the dignity and honor of the profession.

Code of Conduct

I. Patient–Physician Relationship

1. The patient–physician relationship is the central focus of all ethical concerns, and the welfare of the patient should form the basis of all medical judgments.

2. The obstetrician–gynecologist should serve as the patient's advocate and exercise all reasonable means to ensure that the most appropriate care is provided to the patient.

3. The patient–physician relationship has an ethical basis and is built on confidentiality, trust, and honesty. If no patient–physician relationship exists, a physician may refuse to provide care, except in emergencies. Both the patient and the obstetrician–gynecologist are free to establish or discontinue the patient–physician relationship. The obstetrician–gynecologist must adhere to all applicable legal or contractual constraints in dissolving the patient–physician relationship.

4. Sexual misconduct on the part of the obstetrician–gynecologist is an abuse of professional power and a violation of patient trust. Sexual contact or a romantic relationship between a physician and a current patient is always unethical (1).

5. The obstetrician–gynecologist has an obligation to obtain the informed consent of each patient (2, 3). In obtaining informed consent for any course of medical or surgical treatment, the obstetrician–gynecologist should present to the patient, or to the person legally responsible for the patient, in understandable terms, pertinent medical facts and recommendations consistent with good medical practice. Such information should include alternate modes of

treatment and the objectives, risks, benefits, possible complications, and anticipated results of such treatment.

6. It is unethical to prescribe, provide, or seek compensation for therapies that are of no benefit to the patient.

7. The obstetrician–gynecologist should respect the rights of patients, colleagues, and others and safeguard patient information and confidences within the limits of the law. If during the process of providing information for consent it is known that results of a particular test or other information must be given to governmental authorities or other third parties, that should be explained to the patient (4).

8. The obstetrician–gynecologist should not discriminate against patients based on race, color, national origin, religion, or on any other basis that would constitute illegal discrimination.

II. Physician Conduct and Practice

1. The obstetrician–gynecologist should recognize the boundaries of his or her particular competencies and expertise, and provide only those services and use only those techniques for which he or she is qualified by education, training, or experience.

2. The obstetrician–gynecologist should participate in continuing medical education activities to maintain current scientific and professional knowledge relevant to the medical services he or she renders. The obstetrician–gynecologist should provide medical care involving new therapies or techniques only after undertaking appropriate training and study.

3. In emerging areas of medical treatment where recognized medical guidelines do not exist, the obstetrician–gynecologist should exercise careful judgment and take appropriate precautions to protect patient welfare.

4. The obstetrician–gynecologist should not publicize or represent himself or herself in any untruthful, misleading, or deceptive manner to patients, colleagues, other health-care professionals, or the public (5).

5. The obstetrician–gynecologist who has reason to believe that he or she is infected with the human immunodeficiency virus or other serious infectious agents that might be communicated to patients should voluntarily be tested for the protection of his or her patients. In making decisions about patient-care activities, a physician infected with such an agent should adhere to the fundamental professional obligation to avoid harm to patients (6).

6. The obstetrician–gynecologist should not practice medicine while impaired by alcohol, drugs, or physical or mental disability. The obstetrician–gynecologist who experiences substance abuse problems or who is physically or emotionally impaired should seek appropriate assistance to address these problems and limit his or her practice until the impairment no longer affects the quality of patient care.

III. Conflicts of Interest

1. Potential conflicts of interest are inherent in the practice of medicine. Conflicts of interest should be resolved in accordance with the best interest of the patient, respecting a woman's autonomy to make health-care decisions. If there is concern about a possibly significant conflict of interest, the physician should disclose his or her concerns to the patient. If a conflict of interest cannot be resolved, the obstetrician–gynecologist should take steps to withdraw from the care of the patient. If conflicts of interest are unresolved, the physician should seek consultation with colleagues or an institutional ethics committee.

2. Commercial promotions of medical products and services may generate bias unrelated to product merit, creating, or appearing to create, inappropriate undue influence. The obstetrician–gynecologist should be aware of this potential conflict of interest and offer medical advice that is as accurate, balanced, complete, and devoid of bias as possible (7).

3. The obstetrician–gynecologist should prescribe drugs, devices, and other treatments based solely upon medical considerations and patient needs, regardless of any direct or indirect interests in or benefit from a pharmaceutical firm or other supplier.

4. When the obstetrician–gynecologist receives anything of substantial value, including royalties, from companies in the health-care industry, such as a manufacturer of pharmaceuticals and medical devices, this fact should be disclosed to patients and colleagues when material.

5. Financial and administrative constraints imposed by managed care may create disincentives to treatment otherwise recommended by the obstetrician–gynecologist as in the patient's best interest. Any pertinent constraints should be disclosed to the patient (8).

IV. Professional Relations

1. The obstetrician–gynecologist's relationships with other physicians, nurses, and health-care professionals should reflect fairness, honesty, and integrity, sharing a mutual respect and concern for the patient.

2. The obstetrician–gynecologist should consult, refer, or cooperate with other physicians, health-care professionals, and institutions to the extent necessary to serve the best interests of their patients.

3. The obstetrician–gynecologist should respect all laws, uphold the dignity and honor of the profession, and accept the profession's self-imposed discipline. The professional competence and conduct of obstetrician–gynecologists are best examined by professional associations, hospital peer-review committees, and state medical and/or licensing boards. These groups deserve the full participation and cooperation of the obstetrician–gynecologist.

4. The obstetrician–gynecologist should strive to address through the appropriate procedures the status of those physicians who demonstrate questionable competence, impairment, or unethical or illegal behavior. In addition, the obstetrician–gynecologist should cooperate with appropriate authorities to prevent the continuation of such behavior.

V. Societal Responsibilities

1. The obstetrician–gynecologist should support and participate in those health-care programs, practices, and activities that contribute positively, in a meaningful and cost-effective way, to the welfare of individual patients, the health-care system, or the public good.

2. Obstetrician–gynecologists who provide expert medical testimony in courts of law recognize their duty to testify truthfully. The obstetrician–gynecologist should not testify concerning matters about which he or she is not knowledgeable (9). The obstetrician–gynecologist should be prepared to have testimony, given in any judicial proceeding, subjected to peer review by an institution or professional organization to which he or she belongs. It is unethical for a physician to accept compensation that is contingent upon the outcome of litigation.

References*

1. American College of Obstetricians and Gynecologists. Sexual misconduct in the practice of obstetrics and gynecology: ethical considerations. ACOG Committee Opinion 144. Washington, DC: ACOG, 1994

2. American College of Obstetricians and Gynecologists. Ethical dimensions of informed consent. ACOG Committee Opinion 108. Washington, DC: ACOG, 1992

3. American College of Obstetricians and Gynecologists. Informed refusal. ACOG Committee Opinion 166. Washington, DC: ACOG, 1995

4. American College of Obstetricians and Gynecologists. Ethical guidance for patient testing. ACOG Committee Opinion 159. Washington, DC: ACOG, 1995

5. American College of Obstetricians and Gynecologists. Deception. ACOG Committee Opinion 87. Washington, DC: ACOG, 1990

6. American College of Obstetricians and Gynecologists. Human immunodeficiency virus infection: physicians' responsibilities. ACOG Committee Opinion 130. Washington, DC: ACOG, 1993

7. American College of Obstetricians and Gynecologists. Guidelines for relationships with industry. ACOG Committee Opinion 182. Washington, DC: ACOG, 1997

8. American College of Obstetricians and Gynecologists. Physician responsibility under managed care: patient advocacy in a changing health care environment. ACOG Committee Opinion 170. Washington, DC: ACOG, 1996

9. American College of Obstetricians and Gynecologists. Ethical issues related to expert testimony by obstetricians and gynecologists. ACOG Committee Opinion 56. Washington, DC: ACOG, 1987

*Please note that these Committee Opinions may be revised or replaced. Fellows should stay informed about relevant College Committee Opinions.

Approved by the Executive Board of the American College of Obstetricians and Gynecologists

Lists of Titles

Lists of Titles

Committee Opinions

Educational and Technical Bulletins

Practice Bulletins

Practice Patterns

Policy Statements

Index

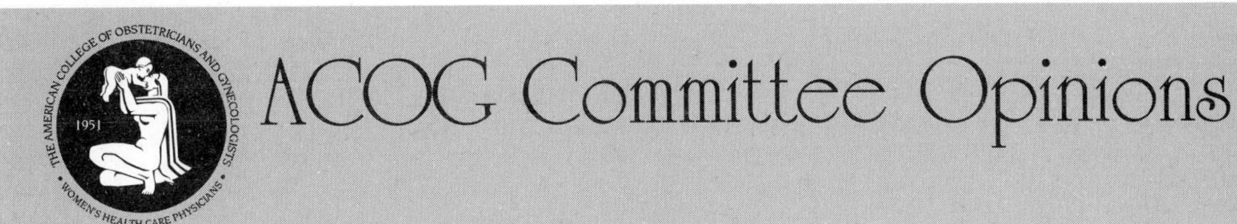

List of Titles

December 2000

Committee Opinions are intended to provide timely information on controversial issues, ethical concerns, and emerging approaches to clinical management. They represent the considered views of the sponsoring committee based on interpretation of published data in peer-reviewed journals. Committee Opinions are reviewed periodically for continued relevance or needed update. *Note:* Because individual Committee Opinions are withdrawn from and added to the series on a continuing basis, the titles listed in this index may not be identical to those contained in complete sets.

The following Committee Opinions have been withdrawn from circulation:

185 Routine Cancer Screening (replaced by Committee Opinion No. 247)
193 Physician/Patient Responsibility for Follow-Up of Diagnosis and Treatment
206 New Pap Test Screening Techniques
208 Delivery by Vacuum Extraction
229 Primary and Preventive Care: Periodic Assessments (replaced by Committee Opinion No. 246)

Number	Title	Publication Date	Reaffirmed Date
ABOG/ACOG Liaison Committee			
110	Recertification	May 1992	
Committee on Adolescent Health Care			
139	Adolescents' Right to Refuse Long-Term Contraceptives	June 1994	
154	Condom Availability for Adolescents	April 1995	
184	Hepatitis B Immunization for Adolescents	June 1997	
190	Prevention of Adolescent Suicide	October 1997	
Committee on Coding and Nomenclature			
205	Tubal Ligation with Cesarean Delivery (Obstet Gynecol Vol. 92, No. 2)	August 1998	
Committee on Ethics			
46	Endorsement of Institutional Ethics Committees	October 1985	
87	Deception	November 1990	1997
108	Ethical Dimensions of Informed Consent	May 1992	1999
129	Commercial Ventures in Medicine: Concerns About the Patenting of Procedures	November 1993	1999
130	Human Immunodeficiency Virus Infection: Physicians' Responsibilities	November 1993	
136	Preembryo Research: History, Scientific Background, and Ethical Considerations	April 1994	
144	Sexual Misconduct in the Practice of Obstetrics and Gynecology: Ethical Considerations	November 1994	1999
156	End-of-Life Decision Making: Understanding the Goals of Care	May 1995	
159	Ethical Guidance for Patient Testing	October 1995	1999
170	Physician Responsibility Under Managed Care: Patient Advocacy in a Changing Health Care Environment	April 1996	
177	Sex Selection	November 1996	2000
181	Ethical Issues in Obstetric–Gynecologic Education	April 1997	
182	Guidelines for Relationships with Industry	April 1997	
194	Obstetrician–Gynecologists' Ethical Responsibilities, Concerns, and Risks Pertaining to Adoption	November 1997	
204	Institutional Responsibility to Provide Legal Representation (Obstet Gynecol Vol. 92, No. 1)	July 1998	
213	Ethical Considerations in Research Involving Pregnant Women (Obstet Gynecol Vol. 92, No. 5)	November 1998	

Number	Title	Publication Date	Reaffirmed Date
Committee on Ethics (continued)			
214	Patient Choice and the Maternal–Fetal Relationship (Obstet Gynecol Vol. 93, No. 4)	April 1999	
215	Nonselective Embryo Reduction: Ethical Guidance for the Obstetrician–Gynecologist (Obstet Gynecol Vol. 93, No. 4)	April 1999	
216	Sterilization of Women, Including Those with Mental Disabilities (Obstet Gynecol Vol. 93, No. 4)	April 1999	
217	Ethical Issues Related to Expert Testimony by Obstetricians and Gynecologists (Obstet Gynecol Vol. 93, No. 4)	April 1999	
225	Responsibilities of Physicians Regarding Surrogate Motherhood (Obstet Gynecol Vol. 94, No. 5)	November 1999	
233	Ethical Dimensions of Seeking and Giving Consultation (Obstet Gynecol Vol. 95, No. 4)	April 2000	
Committee on Genetics			
101	Current Status of Cystic Fibrosis Carrier Screening	November 1991	1996
160	Chorionic Villus Sampling	October 1995	2000
161	Fragile X Syndrome	October 1995	2000
162	Screening for Tay–Sachs Disease	November 1995	2000
178	Genetic Evaluation of Stillbirths and Neonatal Deaths	November 1996	1998
183	Routine Storage of Umbilical Cord Blood for Potential Future Transplantation *(Joint with Committee on Obstetric Practice)*	April 1997	2000
189	Advanced Paternal Age: Risks to the Fetus	October 1997	2000
192	Genetic Screening of Gamete Donors	October 1997	1999
212	Screening for Canavan Disease (Obstet Gynecol Vol. 92, No. 5)	November 1998	2000
223	First-Trimester Screening for Fetal Anomalies with Nuchal Translucency (Obstet Gynecol Vol. 94, No. 4)	October 1999	
230	Maternal Phenylketonuria (Obstet Gynecol Vol. 95, No. 1)	January 2000	
238	Genetic Screening for Hemoglobinopathies (Obstet Gynecol Vol. 96, No. 1)	July 2000	
239	Breast–Ovarian Cancer Screening (Obstet Gynecol Vol. 96, No. 2)	August 2000	
Committee on Gynecologic Practice			
133	Colposcopy Training and Practice	March 1994	2000
146	Laparoscopically Assisted Vaginal Hysterectomy	November 1994	1999
151	Female Genital Mutilation *(Joint with Committee on International Affairs)*	January 1995	1996
152	Recommendations on Frequency of Pap Test Screening	March 1995	1998
153	Absence of Endocervical Cells on a Pap Test	March 1995	1999
164	Incidental Appendectomy	December 1995	2000
186	Role of the Obstetrician–Gynecologist in the Diagnosis and Treatment of Breast Disease	September 1997	2000
191	Length of Hospital Stay for Gynecologic Procedures	October 1997	2000
195	Role of Loop Electrosurgical Excision Procedure in the Evaluation of Abnormal Pap Test Results	November 1997	2000
203	Hepatitis Virus Infections in Obstetrician–Gynecologists (Obstet Gynecol Vol. 92, No. 1)	July 1998	1999
224	Tamoxifen and the Prevention of Breast Cancer in High-Risk Women (Obstet Gynecol Vol. 94, No. 4)	October 1999	
226	Hormone Replacement Therapy in Women with Previously Treated Breast Cancer (Obstet Gynecol Vol. 94, No. 5)	November 1999	
232	Tamoxifen and Endometrial Cancer (Obstet Gynecol Vol. 95 No. 4)	April 2000	
235	Hormone Replacement Therapy in Women Treated for Endometrial Cancer (Obstet Gynecol Vol. 95, No. 5)	May 2000	
240	Statement on Surgical Assistants (Obstet Gynecol Vol. 96, No. 2) *(Joint with Committee on Obstetric Practice)*	August 2000	
*242	Concurrent Chemoradiation in the Treatment of Cervical Cancer (Obstet Gynecol Vol. 96, No. 4)	October 2000	
*243	Performance and Interpretation of Imaging Studies by Obstetrician—Gynecologists (Obstet Gynecol Vol. 96, No. 5)	November 2000	

Number	Title	Publication Date	Reaffirmed Date
Committee on Gynecologic Practice (continued)			
*244	Androgen Treatment of Decreased Libido (Obstet Gynecol Vol. 96, No. 5)	November 2000	
*245	Mifepristone for Medical Pregnancy Termination (Obstet Gynecol Vol. 96, No. 6)	December 2000	
*246	Primary and Preventive Care: Periodic Assessments (Obstet Gynecol Vol. 96, No. 6)	December 2000	
*247	Routine Cancer Screening (Obstet Gynecol Vol. 96, No. 6)	December 2000	
Committee on Health Care for Underserved Women			
200	Mandatory Reporting of Domestic Violence (Obstet Gynecol Vol. 91, No. 3)	March 1998	
201	Cultural Competency in Health Care (Obstet Gynecol Vol. 91, No. 3)	March 1998	
202	Access to Health Care for Women with Physical Disabilities (Obstet Gynecol Vol. 91, No. 6)	June 1998	
Committee on International Affairs			
151	Female Genital Mutilation *(Joint with Committee on Gynecologic Practice)*	January 1995	1996
Committee on Obstetric Practice			
104	Anesthesia for Emergency Deliveries	March 1992	2000
105	Postpartum Tubal Sterilization	March 1992	2000
121	Obstetric Management of Patients with Spinal Cord Injury	April 1993	1999
125	Placental Pathology	July 1993	2000
138	Utility of Umbilical Cord Blood Acid–Base Assessment	April 1994	2000
149	Financial Influences on Mode of Delivery	December 1994	2000
158	Guidelines for Diagnostic Imaging During Pregnancy	September 1995	2000
163	Perinatal Care at the Threshold of Viability *(Joint with AAP Committee on Fetus and Newborn)*	November 1995	1997
167	Perinatal and Infant Mortality Statistics	December 1995	1999
172	Home Uterine Activity Monitoring	May 1996	1999
173	Prevention of Early-Onset Group B Streptococcal Disease in Newborns	June 1996	1999
174	Use and Abuse of the Apgar Score *(Joint with AAP Committee on Fetus and Newborn)*	July 1996	1999
175	Scope of Services for Uncomplicated Obstetric Care	September 1996	2000
179	Rate of Vaginal Births After Cesarean Delivery	November 1996	2000
180	New Ultrasound Output Display Standard	November 1996	2000
183	Routine Storage of Umbilical Cord Blood for Potential Future Transplantation *(Joint with Committee on Genetics)*	April 1997	2000
187	Fetal Fibronectin Preterm Labor Risk Test	September 1997	1999
196	Vitamin A Supplementation During Pregnancy	January 1998	1999
197	Inappropriate Use of the Terms Fetal Distress and Birth Asphyxia	February 1998	1999
198	Bacterial Vaginosis Screening for Prevention of Preterm Delivery	February 1998	1999
210	Antenatal Corticosteroid Therapy for Fetal Maturation (Obstet Gynecol Vol. 92, No. 4)	October 1998	
211	Anticoagulation with Low-Molecular-Weight Heparin During Pregnancy (Obstet Gynecol Vol. 92, No. 5)	November 1998	2000
220	Breastfeeding and the Risk of Hepatitis C Virus Transmission (Obstet Gynecol Vol. 94, No. 2)	August 1999	
228	Induction of Labor with Misoprostol (Obstet Gynecol Vol. 94, No. 5)	November 1999	2000
231	Pain Relief During Labor *(Joint with American Society of Anesthesiologists)* (Obstet Gynecol Vol. 95, No. 2)	February 2000	
234	Scheduled Cesarean Delivery and the Prevention of Vertical Transmission of HIV Infection (Obstet Gynecol Vol. 95, No. 5)	May 2000	
240	Statement on Surgical Assistants (Obstet Gynecol Vol. 96, No. 2) *(Joint with Committee on Gynecologic Practice)*	August 2000	
*241	Screening for Hypothyroidism (Obstet Gynecol Vol. 96, No. 3)	September 2000	
*248	Response to Searle's Drug Warning on Misoprostol (Obstet Gynecol Vol. 96, No. 6)	December 2000	

Number	Title	Publication Date	Reaffirmed Date
Committee on Practice Management			
171	Cost Containment in Medical Care	May 1996	
222	Quality of Laboratory and Imaging Services: Physician Responsibility in the Age of Managed Care *(Joint with Committee on Professional Liability)* (Obstet Gynecol Vol. 94, No. 4)	October 1999	
Committee on Primary Care			
218	Delineation of Obstetric–Gynecologic Primary Care Practice (Obstet Gynecol Vol. 93, No. 6)	June 1999	
227	Complementary and Alternative Medicine (Obstet Gynecol Vol. 94, No. 5)	November 1999	
Committee on Professional Liability			
207	Liability Implications of Recording Procedures or Treatments (Obstet Gynecol Vol. 92, No. 3)	September 1998	
221	Telecommunication in Medicine (Obstet Gynecol Vol. 94, No. 3)	September 1999	
222	Quality of Laboratory and Imaging Services: Physician Responsibility in the Age of Managed Care *(Joint with Committee on Practice Management)* (Obstet Gynecol Vol. 94, No. 4)	October 1999	
236	Coping with the Stress of Malpractice Litigation (Obstet Gynecol Vol. 95, No. 6)	June 2000	
237	Informed Refusal (Obstet Gynecol Vol. 95, No. 6)	June 2000	

Current Committee Opinions

46 87 101 104 105 108 110 121 125 129 130 133 136 138
139 144 146 149 151 152 153 154 156 158 159 160 161 162
163 164 167 170 171 172 173 174 175 177 178 179 180 181
182 183 184 186 187 189 190 191 192 194 195 196 197 198
200 201 202 203 204 205 207 210 211 212 213 214 215 216
217 218 220 221 222 223 224 225 226 227 228 230 231 232
233 234 235 236 237 238 239 240 241 242 243 244 245 246
247 248

Committee Opinions are available on a subscription basis, and complete sets may be purchased. For ordering information, contact the ACOG Distribution Center at 800-762-2264, or order online at sales.acog.com.

*Title issued since publication of last index.

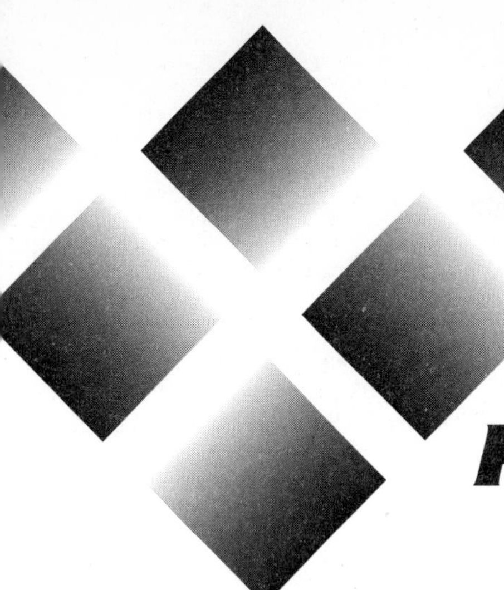

ACOG EDUCATIONAL and PRACTICE BULLETINS

LIST OF TITLES — DECEMBER 2000

Educational and Practice Bulletins provide obstetricians and gynecologists with current information on established techniques and clinical management guidelines. ACOG continuously surveys the field for advances to be incorporated in these series and monitors existing bulletins to ensure they are current. Individual bulletins are withdrawn from and added to these series on a continuing basis. Listed at the end are current Practice Patterns, which provide evidence-based guidelines.

The following titles have been withdrawn from circulation:

Educational Bulletins

159 Fetal Macrosomia (replaced by Practice Bulletin No. 22)
177 Perinatal Viral and Parasitic Infections (replaced by Practice Bulletin No. 20)

Current Bulletins

▸ 1	▸ 3	▸ 4	▸ 5	▸ 6	▸ 7	▸ 8
▸ 9	▸10	▸11	▸12	▸13	▸14	▸15
▸16	▸17	▸18	▸19	▸20	▸21	▸22
95	109	125	128	136	156	160
162	163	164	171	173	175	176
178	181	182	183	186	187	189
191	193	194	195	197	198	199
200	201	202	203	204	205	206
207	208	210	211	212	213	214
215	216	218	219	222	223	224
225	226	227	228	229	230	231
235	236	237	238	239	240	241
242	243	244	245	246	247	248
249	250	251	252	253	254	255
256	257	258	259	260		

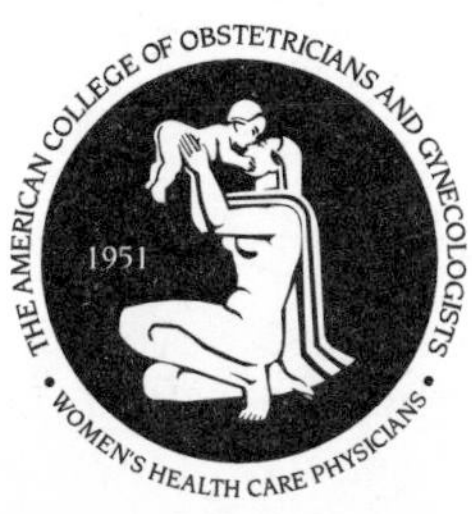

General

136 Ethical Decision-Making in Obstetrics and Gynecology (November 1989)
173 Women and Exercise (October 1992)
175 Invasive Hemodynamic Monitoring in Obstetrics and Gynecology (December 1992)
182 Depression in Women (July 1993)
194 Substance Abuse (July 1994)
199 Blood Component Therapy (November 1994)
204 Septic Shock (April 1995)
211 Sexual Dysfunction (September 1995)
229 Nutrition and Women (October 1996)
235 Hemorrhagic Shock (April 1997)
240 Smoking and Women's Health (September 1997)
242 Sexual Assault (November 1997)
249 Confidentiality in Adolescent Health Care (August 1998, Obstet Gynecol Vol. 92, No. 2)
252 Adolescent Victims of Sexual Assault (October 1998, Obstet Gynecol Vol. 92, No. 4)
254 Primary and Preventive Health Care for Female Adolescents (November 1999, Obstet Gynecol Vol. 94, No. 5)
255 Psychosocial Risk Factors: Perinatal Screening and Intervention (November 1999, Obstet Gynecol Vol. 94, No. 5)
256 Oral Contraceptives for Adolescents: Benefits and Safety (December 1999, Obstet Gynecol Vol. 94, No. 6)
257 Domestic Violence (December 1999, Obstet Gynecol Vol. 94, No. 6)
258 Breastfeeding: Maternal and Infant Aspects (July 2000, Obstet Gynecol Vol. 96, No. 1)
259 Adult Manifestations of Childhood Sexual Abuse (July 2000, Obstet Gynecol Vol. 96, No. 1)

Obstetrics

▶ 1 Premature Rupture of Membranes (June 1998, Obstet Gynecol Vol. 91, No. 6)
▶ 4 Prevention of Rh D Alloimmunization (May 1999, Obstet Gynecol Vol. 93, No. 5)
▶ 5 Vaginal Birth After Previous Cesarean Delivery (July 1999, Obstet Gynecol Vol. 94, No. 1)
▶ 6 Thrombocytopenia in Pregnancy (September 1999, Obstet Gynecol Vol. 94, No. 3)
▶ 8 Management of Herpes in Pregnancy (October 1999, Obstet Gynecol Vol. 94, No. 4)
▶ 9 Antepartum Fetal Surveillance (October 1999, Obstet Gynecol Vol. 94, No. 4)
▶ 10 Induction of Labor (November 1999, Obstet Gynecol Vol. 94, No. 5)
▶ 12 Intrauterine Growth Restriction (January 2000, Obstet Gynecol Vol. 95, No. 1)

Obstetrics *(continued)*

- ▶ 13 External Cephalic Version (February 2000, Obstet Gynecol Vol. 95, No. 2)
- ▶ 17 Operative Vaginal Delivery (June 2000, Obstet Gynecol Vol. 95, No. 6)
- ▶ 19 Thromboembolism in Pregnancy (August 2000, Obstet Gynecol Vol. 96, No. 2)
- ▶*20 Perinatal Viral and Parasitic Infections (September 2000, Obstet Gynecol Vol. 96. No. 3)
- ▶*22 Fetal Macrosomia (November 2000, Obstet Gynecol Vol. 96, No. 5)
- 95 Management of the Breech Presentation (August 1986)
- 160 Immunization During Pregnancy (October 1991)
- 163 Fetal and Neonatal Neurologic Injury (January 1992)
- 171 Rubella and Pregnancy (August 1992)
- 176 Diagnosis and Management of Fetal Death (January 1993)
- 181 Thyroid Disease in Pregnancy (June 1993)
- 187 Ultrasonography in Pregnancy (December 1993)
- 189 Exercise During Pregnancy and the Postpartum Period (February 1994)
- 195 Substance Abuse in Pregnancy (July 1994)
- 200 Diabetes and Pregnancy (December 1994)
- 205 Preconceptional Care (May 1995)
- 206 Preterm Labor (June 1995)
- 207 Fetal Heart Rate Patterns: Monitoring, Interpretation, and Management (July 1995)
- 208 Genetic Technologies (July 1995)
- 216 Umbilical Artery Blood Acid–Base Analysis (November 1995)
- 218 Dystocia and the Augmentation of Labor (December 1995)
- 219 Hypertension in Pregnancy (January 1996)
- 224 Pulmonary Disease in Pregnancy (June 1996)
- 225 Obstetric Analgesia and Anesthesia (July 1996)
- 227 Management of Isoimmunization in Pregnancy (August 1996)
- 228 Maternal Serum Screening (September 1996)
- 230 Assessment of Fetal Lung Maturity (November 1996)
- 231 Seizure Disorders in Pregnancy (December 1996)
- 236 Teratology (April 1997)
- 243 Postpartum Hemorrhage (January 1998)
- 244 Antiphospholipid Syndrome (February 1998)
- 245 Antimicrobial Therapy for Obstetric Patients (March 1998, Obstet Gynecol Vol. 91, No. 3)
- 248 Viral Hepatitis in Pregnancy (July 1998, Obstet Gynecol Vol. 92, No. 1)
- 251 Obstetric Aspects of Trauma Management (September 1998, Obstet Gynecol Vol. 92, No. 3)
- 253 Special Problems of Multiple Gestation (November 1998, Obstet Gynecol Vol. 92, No. 5)
- *260 Smoking Cessation During Pregnancy (September 2000, Obstet Gynecol Vol. 96, No. 3)

Gynecology

- ▶ 3 Medical Management of Tubal Pregnancy (December 1998, Obstet Gynecol Vol. 92, No. 6)
- ▶ 7 Prophylactic Oophorectomy (September 1999, Obstet Gynecol Vol. 94, No. 3)
- ▶ 11 Medical Management of Endometriosis (December 1999, Obstet Gynecol Vol. 94, No. 6)
- ▶ 14 Management of Anovulatory Bleeding (March 2000, Obstet Gynecol Vol. 95, No. 3)
- ▶ 15 Premenstrual Syndrome (April 2000, Obstet Gynecol Vol. 95, No. 4)
- ▶ 16 Surgical Alternatives to Hysterectomy in the Management of Leiomyomas (May 2000, Obstet Gynecol Vol. 95, No. 5)
- ▶ 18 The Use of Hormonal Contraception in Women with Coexisting Medical Conditions (July 2000, Obstet Gynecol Vol. 96, No. 1)
- ▶*21 Prevention of Deep Vein Thrombosis and Pulmonary Embolism (October 2000, Obstet Gynecol Vol. 96, No. 4)
- 109 Methods of Midtrimester Abortion (October 1987)
- 128 Amenorrhea (May 1989)
- 156 Nonmalignant Conditions of the Breast (June 1991)
- 164 The Intrauterine Device (February 1992)
- 183 Cervical Cytology: Evaluation and Management of Abnormalities (August 1993)
- 191 Hysteroscopy (April 1994)
- 193 Genital Human Papillomavirus Infections (June 1994)
- 201 Pediatric Gynecologic Disorders (January 1995)
- 210 Health Maintenance for Perimenopausal Women (August 1995)
- 212 Early Pregnancy Loss (September 1995)
- 213 Urinary Incontinence (October 1995)
- 214 Pelvic Organ Prolapse (October 1995)
- 215 Gynecologic Ultrasonography (November 1995)
- 222 Sterilization (April 1996)
- 223 Chronic Pelvic Pain (May 1996)
- 226 Vaginitis (July 1996)
- 237 Antibiotics and Gynecologic Infections (June 1997)
- 238 Lower Urinary Tract Operative Injuries (July 1997)
- 239 Operative Laparoscopy (August 1997)
- 241 Vulvar Nonneoplastic Epithelial Disorders (October 1997)

Oncology

- 162 Carcinoma of the Endometrium (December 1991)
- 178 Management of Gestational Trophoblastic Disease (March 1993)
- 186 Vulvar Cancer (November 1993)
- 250 Ovarian Cancer (August 1998, Obstet Gynecol Vol. 92, No. 2)

Reproductive Endocrinology and Fertility

- 125 Infertility (February 1989)
- 197 Managing the Anovulatory State: Medical Induction of Ovulation (September 1994)
- 198 Hormonal Contraception (October 1994)
- 202 Hyperandrogenic Chronic Anovulation (February 1995)
- 203 Evaluation and Treatment of Hirsute Women (March 1995)
- 246 Osteoporosis (April 1998, Obstet Gynecol Vol. 91, No. 4)
- 247 Hormone Replacement Therapy (May 1998, Obstet Gynecol Vol. 91, No. 5)

Practice Patterns

- 3 Emergency Oral Contraception (December 1996)
- 5 Routine Ultrasound in Low-Risk Pregnancy (August 1997)
- 6 Management of Postterm Pregnancy (October 1997)
- 7 Shoulder Dystocia (October 1997)

*Title issued since publication of last listing

▶Practice Bulletin

Practice and Educational Bulletins are available on a subscription basis, and complete sets may be purchased. For ordering information, contact the ACOG Distribution Center at 800-762-2264, or order online at sales.acog.com.

AT005

Lists of Titles

Committee Opinions

Educational and Technical Bulletins

Practice Bulletins

Practice Patterns

Policy Statements

Index

Lists of Titles

Committee Opinions

Educational and Technical Bulletins

Practice Bulletins

Practice Patterns

Policy Statements

Index

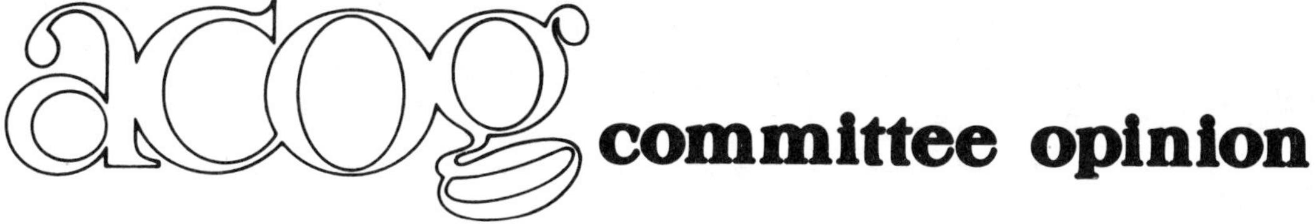

committee opinion

Committee on Gynecologic Practice Number 153—March 1995

Absence of Endocervical Cells on a Pap Test

The presence of endocervical or squamous metaplastic cells on a Pap test is regarded as evidence of adequate sampling of the transformation zone during cytologic screening of the cervix. When these cells are absent, the endocervix may not have been sampled. The Bethesda System classifies such a smear as satisfactory but limited. Studies in which these smears have been repeated immediately indicate that the discovery of premalignant lesions has been rare.

In a patient with no known risk factors, who has had three consecutive annual normal Pap tests, and whose current Pap test has no other cytologic abnormalities except absence of endocervical cells, a physician may exercise discretion and defer repeating the Pap test for 12 months.

If the patient is at increased risk (1), the physician should consider repeating the endocervical portion of the Pap test at the patient's convenience.

REFERENCE

1. American College of Obstetricians and Gynecologists. Recommendations on frequency of Pap test screening. ACOG Committee Opinion 152. Washington, DC: ACOG, 1995

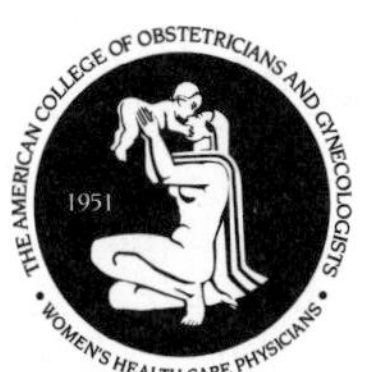

ISSN 1074-861X

The American College of Obstetricians and Gynecologists
409 12th Street, SW • Washington, DC 20024-2188

12345/98765

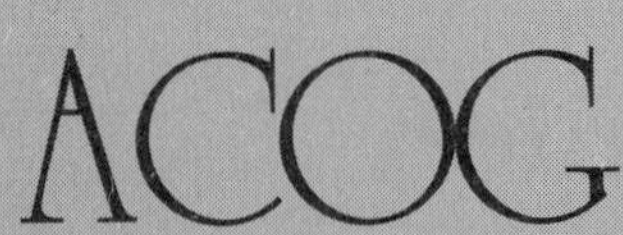

Committee on
Health Care for
Underserved Women

Committee Opinion

Number 202, June 1998

Access to Health Care for Women with Physical Disabilities

Regulations implementing the Americans with Disabilities Act of 1990 (ADA) define disability as "a physical or mental impairment that substantially limits one or more of the major life activities of an individual; a record of such impairment; or being regarded as having such an impairment" (1). Approximately 54 million Americans have disabilities, roughly 53% of whom are women. Women who are 65 years and older have the highest rate of disability (2). Neuromusculoskeletal conditions such as spinal cord injury, cerebral palsy, multiple sclerosis, and spina bifida; the large category of acquired orthopedic impairments; and osteoarthritis and osteoporosis are the most prevalent disabling conditions (3). Disorders of the special sense organs affecting vision, speech, and hearing also affect a significant number of women (see Table 1). Chronic medical illnesses often affect physical function, including the function of the reproductive system. Such illnesses include systemic lupus erythematosus, diabetes with neuropathy, and cardiovascular and peripheral vascular disease complications such as stroke and amputation.

Access to health care for individuals with disabilities often is limited. These individuals are less likely to have postsecondary education, to have household incomes greater than $15,000, or to be employed (4). A greater proportion of these individuals resides in rural areas than in metropolitan areas, which, combined with socioeconomic disadvantages, further restricts access to health care services (5). The knowledge, attitudes, and practice of physicians can be either barriers or facilitators to the availability of comprehensive health care services for women with physical disabilities.

Providers' Responsibility to Women with Special Needs

Health care providers have a societal and professional ethical responsibility to accommodate and individualize the care of women with special needs. Women with physical disabilities are often knowledgeable about their conditions and, therefore, can serve as a valuable resource to their care providers. Obstetrician–gynecologists should review the following recommendations and adopt those that will enable them to accept this responsibility.

ISSN 1074-861X

The American College of Obstetricians and Gynecologists
409 12th Street, SW
PO Box 96920
Washington, DC 20090-6920

12345/21098

Assess the environment of your medical practice site and activities, and make appropriate modifications in layout, equipment, and staff training to enhance services.

An individual may have a functional limitation, such as the inability to walk up a flight of stairs because she uses a wheelchair, as well as an activity limitation, such as the inability to obtain well-woman screening because of problems with medical office location, layout, or equipment. Title III of the ADA requires that a public accommodation operated by a private entity, including professional offices of health care providers, take steps to ensure that no individual with a disability is discriminated against on the basis of the limitation. The ADA requires the reduction of environmental barriers through both modifications of physical access and provision of auxiliary aids and services to persons with disabilities.

The ADA does not require massive reconstruction of existing facilities, nor does it require provision of aids and services if doing so would be unduly burdensome. Several resources are provided in this document to help physicians understand their responsibilities under this act. These resources also include recommendations for environmental adaptations in the office and describe techniques for gynecologic examination of women with neuromusculoskeletal conditions.

Support models of care that increase personal empowerment and self-advocacy of women with physical disabilities.

Empowerment is the process by which people can experience some measure of control over events, outcomes, and resources of value to them (6). A study of the correlates of long-term psychosocial adaptation among women with chronic physical disabilities revealed that a sense of coherence or internal resources is a more powerful predictor of positive long-term psychosocial adaptation than disability status itself (7). Women with physical disabilities are at greater risk of emotional vulnerability and lower self-esteem as a result of discrimination and social isolation.

Victimization and abuse are found to be prevalent among women with disabilities (8). Many women with physical disabilities must rely to some degree on a personal attendant or other type of caregiver. This situation can lead to exploitative relationships that are often difficult to uncover. Women who are very dependent may be reluctant to voice concerns for fear of retaliation or loss of the essential services performed by the home or personal care provider. For this and other reasons, women with disabilities need access to gynecologic examinations and interviews where concerns, injuries, and infections, including sexually transmissible infections (STIs), can be detected. Consultation with other specialists may be desirable, because it may be more complicated to advise, counsel, and intervene with patients who are in abusive situations and have physical disabilities than with nondisabled patients.

Table 1. Number of Females Limited by Disabling Conditions

Disabling Condition	Number of Females Limited by Condition
Orthopedic impairment	4,332,000
Osteoarthritis and allied disorders	3,495,000
Blindness or visual impairment	629,000
Deafness or hearing impairment	557,000
Paralysis	412,000
Osteoporosis	297,000
Speech impairment	193,000
Multiple sclerosis	161,000
Cerebral palsy	83,000
Spina bifida	25,000

LaPlante MP, Carlson D. Disability in the United States: prevalence and causes, 1992. San Francisco: Disability Statistics Rehabilitation Research and Training Center, University of California, 1996

Persons with disabilities, and women in particular, report encountering prejudicial attitudes that tend to equate physical impairment with impairment of the total person. The most significant example of this attitude is with respect to sex and sexuality. A common public and professional misconception is that women with disabilities are asexual or that their interests in sexual activity differ from those of nondisabled women. To the contrary, virtually all surveys of individuals with physical disabilities report sexual desire (in the absence of depression) comparable to that of nondisabled peers (9).

The frequency of sexual activity and behavior as well as sexual satisfaction may depend on the timing of the onset of the disability. Inadequate social development, decreased opportunity to date, difficulty finding partners, and lack of basic knowledge of sex and sexuality are more likely to be characteristics of adults whose disability began at birth (9). Parents and professionals may attempt to isolate girls with physical disabilities more frequently than boys because of concerns about sexual victimization and pregnancy.

Individuals with acquired disabilities, such as spinal cord injury or complications of stroke, report not only changes in sexual functioning after onset of the disability but also a high degree of unmet needs for counseling and explicit information to adapt to these changes during initial rehabilitation or specialized care. Health care professionals may be unaware of their own biases or lack of knowledge with regard to what some might identify as nontraditional or alternative sexual activity. The obstetrician–gynecologist cannot assume that adequate advice and care have been provided and should serve as a source for this education and service.

Acquire additional knowledge and skills through continuing medical education and use of the resources listed in this document.

To provide health care services adequately, health care professionals may need additional knowledge and skills pertaining to both clinical and access issues facing women with physical disabilities. There is a paucity of clinical research published on the health issues of women with physical disabilities; further research is needed.

Access Issues for Patients with Disabilities

Obstetrician–gynecologists who care for women with physical disabilities may need to consider specific access issues. Throughout the following discussion of these issues, two objectives are highlighted. First, physicians may need to increase their awareness of community resources for specialized and complementary services required by persons with physical disabilities. Second, they may need to maintain coordination and communication with other primary care providers and rehabilitation and disability specialists for reasons such as obtaining pertinent medical records.

In scheduling office or clinic appointments for a woman with a disability, sufficient time should be allowed for comprehensive assessment of medical and social issues. A detailed understanding of the nature of the disability requires consideration of at least the following parameters: complete menstrual, sexual, and social histories; quality of circulation with special attention to the lower extremities; degree of sensory and special sense impairments; assessment of manual dexterity; progressive or stable nature of the disability; current medication profile; and access to community resources (10).

Adolescents with Physical Disabilities

Adolescents with physical disabilities are at risk for negative general and reproductive health outcomes because of lower levels of peer integration; heightened adult orientation; low educational aspirations; and poor knowledge of parenthood, contraception, and STIs. This lack of knowledge may result from the failure of most school-based sex and family life education curricula to address disability-related issues (11). The obstetrician–gynecologist is likely to be called on to counsel adolescents on these issues. Just as in the provision of care to the nondisabled, obstetrician–gynecologists can sometimes serve as a bridge between pediatric sources of care and adult care for young women.

Family Planning and Prevention of Sexually Transmissible Infections

Women with disabilities need information on contraception and STI prevention to be provided in a nonjudgmental fashion to help individuals and their partners make appropriate choices. Working with women with physical disabilities may require more knowledge of and interaction with the partner than is often the case with nondisabled women. Such interaction is especially important to encourage successful condom use to prevent both STIs and unintended pregnancy.

Pregnancy and Parenting

Pregnancy and parenting for women with physical disabilities may have some unique medical and social aspects but are rarely precluded by the disability itself. In fact, few, if any, physical disabilities directly limit fertility. Health care professionals have the responsibility to provide appropriate reproductive health services to these women or arrange adequate consultation or referral. Nonbiased preconceptional counseling for couples in which one partner has a physical disability may decrease subsequent psychosocial and medical complications of pregnancy. Screening and provision of disability-specific information, such as folate supplementation for women who have spina bifida, is highly desirable.

Once pregnancy occurs, the patient's early contact with an obstetrician, though essential, is sometimes difficult to arrange because of general problems in gaining access to health care services. Counseling about the results of prenatal testing and options should be comprehensive and nonjudgmental. Regular consultation or referral may be required to achieve the optimum outcome, such as in cases of spinal cord injury or multiple sclerosis (12). Detailed pregnancy care plans should be developed in negotiation with managed care and other insurers to increase access to and use of prenatal care services, assure appropriate postpartum hospital length of stay, and arrange postpartum home care services, if necessary. Cesarean delivery should be done only for obstetric indications. Community resources for childbirth, breastfeeding, and parenting education should be identified early in the course of pregnancy, and timely referrals should be made for the pregnant woman and her family.

Diagnosis and management of infertility in a woman with a disability may be limited by the availability of experts sufficiently informed on needed modification of care, insurance, or payment coverage. In addition, women with physical disabilities report that providers' prejudicial attitudes also limit access to infertility services (8, 13, 14). Patients with physical disabilities who have concerns about fertility should be counseled with the same respect as nondisabled patients.

Cancer Screening

Analysis of the National Study on Women with Physical Disabilities indicated that women with physical disabilities receive Pap-test screening less regularly than their nondisabled peers partly as a result of a lack of accessible accommodations (15). As primary health care providers to women, obstetrician–gynecologists should be aware of and implement all age-appropriate cancer screening guidelines for their patients, including those with disabilities. Coordination with colleagues may facilitate the conduct of multiple examinations, such as sigmoidoscopy and colposcopy, during the same visit. Modifications to breast self-examination techniques and practice may need to be developed for a woman with a physical disability and her partner or care provider. Newer types of mammography equipment have been developed to accommodate women with mobility problems; resources of this type should be identified.

Perimenopausal Women

Menopausal and postmenopausal women represent an underserved population with regard to general gynecologic and primary care. Women with long-term or acquired physical disabilities in this stage of life require care that limits secondary complications and enhances quality of life and social interactions. Detailed analysis of cardiovascular status, risk profile for osteoporosis, and medication lists are needed for making decisions on prescribing hormone replacement therapy and choosing the formulation, when indicated. Physicians need to be fully informed on the appropriate indications for bone mineral density studies and the interpretation of results in older women and women with conditions affecting the bone.

Coordination with other primary care physicians and family members of older women with physical disabilities is essential to avoid iatrogenic complications, such as those caused by use of multiple medications.

Conclusion

Although they have special needs, persons with disabilities and their families are often very knowledgeable about the conditions and ways to negotiate complex health care delivery systems. The patients are able to participate in all aspects of medical decision-making and should be recognized as experts in their care and condition and as partners with physicians. Through ongoing communication with patients with physical disabilities and through additional training and coordination with other health care professionals, obstetrician–gynecologists can help to decrease the barriers to health care faced by these patients.

References

1. Americans with Disabilities Act of 1990. 42 U.S.C. § 12101 et seq., 28 CFR Part 36
2. McNeil JM. Americans with disabilities: 1994-1995. Current Popul Rep Series P70-61. 1–18, 1997
3. LaPlante MP. The demographics of disability. Milbank Q 1991;69 (Suppl 1/2):55–77
4. West J. The social and policy context of the Act. Milbank Q 1991;69 (Suppl 1/2):3–24
5. Lishner DM, Richardson M, Levine P, Patrick D. Access to primary health care among persons with disabilities in rural areas: a summary of the literature. J Rural Health. 1996;12:45–53
6. Fawcett SB, White GW, Balcazar FE, Suarez-Balcazar Y, Matthews RM, Paine-Andrews A, et al. A contextual-behavioral model of empowerment: case studies involving people with physical disabilities. Am J Community Psychol 1994;22:471–496
7. Dangoor N, Florian V. Women with chronic physical disabilities: correlates of their long-term psychosocial adaptation. Int J Rehabil Res 1994;17:159–168
8. Krotoski DM, Nosek MA, Turk MA. Women with physical disabilities: achieving and maintaining health and well-being. Baltimore, Maryland: Paul H. Brookes Publishing Co., 1996
9. Nosek MA, Rintala DH, Young ME, Howland CA, Foley CC, Rossi D, et al. Sexual functioning among women with physical disabilities. Arch Phys Med Rehabil 1996;77: 107–115

10. Leavesley G, Porter J. Sexuality, fertility and contraception in disability. Contraception 1982;26:417–441
11. Stevens SE, Steele CA, Jutai JW, Kalnins IV, Bortolussi JA, Biggar WD. Adolescents with physical disabilities: some psychosocial aspects of health. J Adolesc Health 1996;19:157–164
12. American College of Obstetricians and Gynecologists. Obstetric management of patients with spinal cord injury. ACOG Committee Opinion 121. Washington, DC: ACOG, 1993
13. Nosek MA, Young ME, Rintala DH, Howland CA, Foley CC, Bennet JL. Barriers to reproductive health maintenance among women with physical disabilities. J Womens Health 1995;4:505–518
14. Fiduccia BW. Multiplying choices: improving access to reproductive health services for women with disabilities. Oakland, California: Berkeley Planning Associates, 1997
15. Nosek MA, Howland CA. Breast and cervical cancer screening among women with physical disabilities. Arch Phys Med Rehabil 1997;78:S39–S44

Resources

Americans with Disabilities Act: Questions and Answers. U.S. Equal Employment Opportunity Commission and U.S. Department of Justice, Civil Rights Division. 1996. Contact: U.S. Department of Justice, ADA Information Line, (800) 514-0301, (800) 514-0383 (TDD), http://www.usdoj.gov/crt/ada/qandaeng. htm

Job Accommodation Network. (800) 526-7234 (voice and TDD)

New York State Multiple Sclerosis Consortium, Buffalo General Hospital, Department of Neurology, 100 High Street, Buffalo NY 14203. Contact: Lawrence Jacobs, MD, at (716) 889-7301

The Patient with Physical Disabilities: Issues in Gynecologic Care. A Continuing Education Monograph. The University of Texas Southwestern Medical Center at Dallas through funding from Ortho-McNeil Pharmaceutical. Contact: Regional Ortho-McNeil Pharmaceutical representative

Resourceful Woman. Contact: The Health Resource Center for Women with Disabilities, Rehabilitation Institute of Chicago, 345 East Superior Street, Room 106, Chicago IL 60611, (312) 908-7997

A Woman's Guide to Coping with Disability 1997 (second edition). Contact: Resources for Rehabilitation, 33 Bedford Street, Suite 19A, Lexington MA 02173, (617) 862-6455

United States Department of Justice: Civil Rights Division, Disability Rights Section (PO Box 66738, Washington DC 20035-6738). (800) 514-0301 or (800) 514-0383 (TDD)

U.S. Equal Employment Opportunity Commission. 1801 L Street, NW, Washington DC 20507. For ADA documents: (800) 669-3362 or (800) 800-3302 (TDD). For ADA information: (800) 669-4000 or (800) 669-6820 (TDD)

Bibliography

Beckmann CR, Gittler M, Barzansky BM, Beckmann CA. Gynecologic health care of women with disabilities. Obstet Gynecol 1989;74:75–79

Greenspoon JS, Paul RH. Paraplegia and quadriplegia: special considerations during pregnancy and labor and delivery. Am J Obstet Gynecol 1986;155:738–741

Haefner HK, Elkins TE. Contraceptive management for female adolescents with mental retardation and handicapping disabilities. Curr Opin Obstet Gynecol 1991;3:820–824

Harrison J, Glass CA, Owens RG, Soni BM. Factors associated with sexual functioning in women following spinal cord injury. Paraplegia 1995;33:687–692

Nieves J, Cosman F, Herbert J, Shen V, Lindsay R. High prevalence of vitamin D deficiency and reduced bone mass in multiple sclerosis. Neurology 1994;44:1687–1692

Rudick RA, Cohen JA, Weinstock-Guttman B, Kinkel RP, Ransohoff RM. Management of multiple sclerosis. N Engl J Med 1997;337:1604–1611

Westgren N, Hultling C, Levi R, Seiger A, Westgren M. Sexuality in women with traumatic spinal cord injury. Acta Obstet Gynecol Scand 1997;76:977–983

White MJ, Rintala DH, Hart KA, Fuhrer MJ. Sexual activities: concerns and interests of women with spinal cord injury living in the community. Am J Phys Med Rehabil 1993;72:372–378

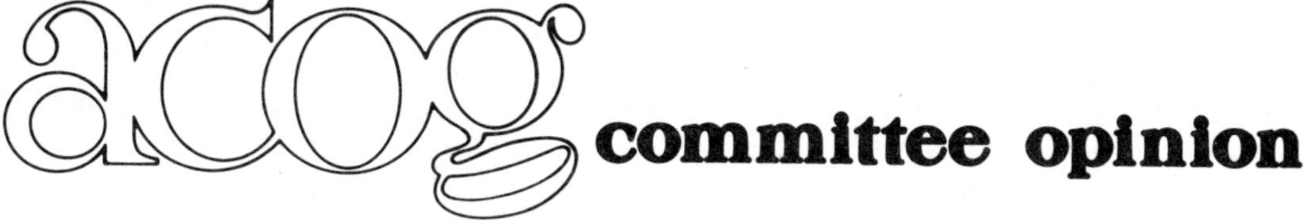

Committee on Adolescent Health Care Number 139—June 1994

Adolescents' Right to Refuse Long-Term Contraceptives

Long-acting progestin-only contraceptives are now readily available, and they are being widely promoted for use in women, including teenagers who will not or cannot use other contraceptive methods. The implantable (Norplant) and injectable (Depo-Provera) progestins are also viewed by some individuals as a method of limiting adolescent pregnancies. This raises concerns about the adolescent's right to accept or refuse a method of contraception against parental request and about the potential coercive use of such contraceptives in minors.

Parents who feel their adolescent daughter is at risk for an unintended pregnancy may request that the physician administer long-term contraceptives to their daughter against her wishes. Health care agencies, social workers, and guardians may make similar requests. The physician, however, should acknowledge that the adolescent is the patient and has the final decision and right of free choice (1, 2). Therefore, the adolescent has the right to refuse any method of contraception and to discontinue contraceptives—which includes removal of contraceptive implants—without parental notification or consent.

The physician providing care should have knowledge of his or her state laws regarding minors' rights and should also be aware that adolescents have constitutional rights to privacy and to make reproductive decisions (1). The U.S. Supreme Court first ruled over 35 years ago that the Fourteenth Amendment protects the rights of minors as well as those of adults (3). The rights of minors are subject to more limitations than the rights of adults; however, a subsequent ruling held that minors have a constitutional right to privacy that includes the right to obtain contraceptives (4). Furthermore, laws in 24 states and the District of Columbia give minors the right to make informed decisions about contraceptives without parental involvement. There are no state laws that require parental involvement for a minor to obtain medical care in connection with contraceptive services (5).

The role of the physician in providing care to an adolescent is more than that of a technician who administers a contraceptive method. In the situation in which a teenager refuses long-term contraceptives, the physician should explore thoroughly the reasons for her refusal (6). This process may help correct misinformation and allay fears. If the teenager persists in rejecting the long-term method, the physician should assist her in the selection and correct consistent use of an appropriate reliable method to prevent pregnancy. Information should also be provided on how to avoid sexually transmitted diseases, including human immunodeficiency virus infection, with both short- and long-term contraceptive methods.

The physician should also assess the reasons for the adult's request so that appropriate intervention can be instituted. If the physician determines or suspects that the disagreement between the minor and adult, especially parent or guardian, over a contraceptive choice reflects a deeper or more long-standing conflict, then the physician may make a referral to an appropriate practitioner or agency. If the parent or guardian is requesting long-term contraception for an adolescent who is incapable of giving informed consent, the decision to use long-term contraception should be based on a careful assessment. This may involve a multidisciplinary team that includes an advocate appointed for the impaired adolescent.

Finally, regardless of whether an adolescent selects or refuses a long-term contraceptive method, the physician should remain available to address related health concerns. This includes a commitment to offer continuing contraceptive care, periodic evaluation for sexually transmitted diseases, and screening via a Pap test. Physicians should encourage parents to continue to be supportive of the adolescent's growth and assist parents in guiding their daughters toward personal responsibility for their own health care (1).

REFERENCES

1. American College of Obstetricians and Gynecologists. Confidentiality in adolescent health care. ACOG Statement of Policy. Washington, DC: ACOG, 1988
2. Council on Scientific Affairs, American Medical Association. Confidential health services for adolescents. JAMA 1993;269:1420–1424
3. In re Gault, 387 US 1 (1967)
4. Carey v Population Services Intl, 431 US 678 (1977)
5. Donovan P. Our daughters' decisions: the conflict in state law on abortion and other issues. New York: The Alan Guttmacher Institute, 1992
6. Moreno JD. Treating the adolescent patient. An ethical analysis. J Adolesc Health Care 1989; 10:454–459

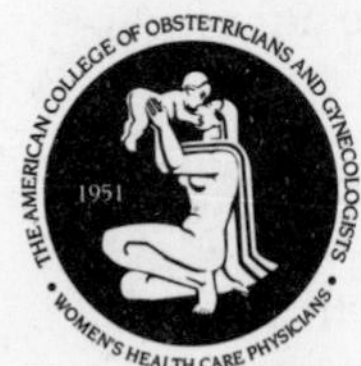

ISSN 1074-861X

The American College of Obstetricians and Gynecologists
409 12th Street, SW • Washington, DC 20024-2188

12345/87654

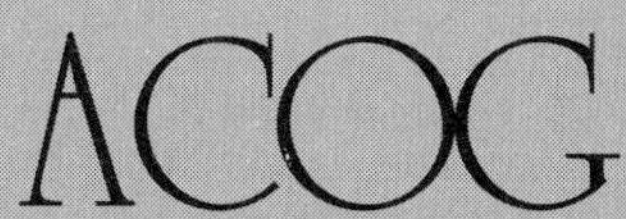

Committee Opinion

Committee on Genetics

Number 189, October 1997

Advanced Paternal Age:
Risks to the Fetus

Advanced maternal age increases the risk of having a liveborn infant with autosomal trisomies 21, 18, or 13, or with the sex chromosome aneuploidies 47,XXY or 47,XXX. Genetic counseling traditionally has been offered when a woman will be 35 years of age or older as of her estimated delivery date. With increased paternal age, however, there does not appear to be an increased risk of chromosomal anomalies in offspring. Insufficient evidence exists to provide a specific cutoff level for assessing risk in association with paternal age.

Although advancing paternal age does affect pregnancy outcome, effects on genetic disease are less completely understood. There is general agreement that advancing paternal age predisposes the fetus to mutations in autosomal dominant diseases such as neurofibromatosis, achondroplasia, Apert syndrome, and Marfan syndrome. The increased risk rises exponentially, rather than linearly, with increasing paternal age. Increasing paternal age may be associated with spontaneous germline mutations in X-linked genes that are transmitted through carrier daughters to affected grandsons. This phenomenon has been called the "grandfather effect" and may occur with several X-linked disorders, including hemophilia A and Duchenne muscular dystrophy.

Although paternal age affects autosomal dominant diseases, the exact risk for any specific disorder is small. Most of the autosomal dominant diseases affect only 1 in 5,000–10,000 individuals, so even a doubling of risk constitutes a very low overall risk. It is the collective risk of autosomal dominant diseases that constitutes the increased risk, not the risk of a particular disorder.

Currently, it is not possible to screen prenatally for all autosomal dominant and X-linked diseases in the presence of advanced paternal age. Fetal ultrasonography may detect some autosomal dominant disorders, but this technique cannot be relied upon as a screening modality. Chromosomal analysis cannot be used to detect these disorders. Only genetic counseling on an individual basis is recommended for couples to address their specific concerns if advancing paternal age is an issue.

ISSN 1074-861X

The American College of Obstetricians and Gynecologists
409 12th Street, SW
PO Box 96920
Washington, DC 20090-6920

12345/10987

Bibliography

American College of Medical Genetics. Statement on guidance for genetic counseling in advanced paternal age. Bethesda, Maryland: ACMG, 1996

Ashton GC. Mismatches in genetic markers in a large family study. Am J Hum Genet 1980;32:601–613

de Michelena MI, Burstein E, Lama JR, Vasquez JC. Paternal age as a risk factor for Down syndrome. Am J Med Genet 1993;45:679–682

Friedman JM. Genetic disease in the offspring of older fathers. Obstet Gynecol 1981;57:745–749

Hook EB. A search for a paternal-age effect upon cases of 47, +21 in which the extra chromosome is of paternal origin. Am J Hum Genet 1984;36:413–421

McIntosh GC, Olshan AF, Baird PA. Paternal age and the risk of birth defects in offspring. Epidemiology 1995;6:282–288

Olshan AF, Anath CV, Savitz DA. Intrauterine growth retardation as an endpoint in mutation epidemiology: an evaluation based on paternal age. Mutat Res 1995;344:89–94

Olshan AF, Schnitzer PG, Baird PA. Paternal age and the risk of congenital heart defects. Teratology 1994;50:80–84

Risch N, Reich EW, Wishnick MM, McCarthy JG. Spontaneous mutation and parental age in humans. Am J Hum Genet 1987;41:218-248

ACOG

Committee on Gynecologic Practice

Committee Opinion

Number 244, November 2000

Androgen Treatment of Decreased Libido

Sexual dysfunction is a complex disorder with multiple etiologies, of which psychosocial elements, chronic illness, and alcohol and other substance abuse have been implicated. Often, a specific cause cannot be defined. The prevalence of sexual dysfunction appears to increase with age. In the United States, the National Health and Social Life Survey of 1,749 women revealed that 43% experienced sexual dysfunction (1). Androgens have been proposed for some women as treatment of certain types of sexual dysfunction.

Loss of sexual drive or libido is one manifestation of sexual dysfunction. Libido appears to be influenced by both androgens and estrogens. Androgens do consistently increase libido at superphysiologic levels, but physiologic androgen replacement therapy has not been shown to consistently affect libido (2). Formulations currently available in the United States generally achieve superphysiologic serum levels at least two times the premenopausal range of values.

A relationship between libido and hormonal changes, particularly those associated with menopause, has been suspected for many years as a result of declining ovarian function. After menopause, total estrogen production decreases by approximately 80% and androgen production declines by about 50%. Of the latter, androstenedione, the primary ovarian androgen, and dehydroepiandrosterone sulfate, the principal adrenal androgen, demonstrate the greatest decline, decreasing 75% and 50%, respectively. Ovarian testosterone production is near normal during the first 5 years after menopause but declines thereafter. There is a proportionately greater reduction of circulating unbound testosterone, despite sex hormone-binding globulin decreases, which are the result of diminished estrogen production.

Available oral testosterone preparations include methyltestosterone with or without esterified estrogens, fluoxymesterone, and testosterone undecanoate. Testosterone can be administered intramuscularly as well as topically, with transdermal patches or gel. Reported side effects include hoarseness, acne, increased facial hair, clitoromegaly, hepatotoxicity, alopecia, and undesirable lipoprotein alterations. The doses in the transdermal patch are formulated specifically for male hormone replacement. Implantable testosterone pellets are available in other countries.

This document reflects emerging clinical and scientific advances as of the date issued and is subject to change. The information should not be construed as dictating an exclusive course of treatment or procedure to be followed.

ISSN 1074-861X

The American College of Obstetricians and Gynecologists
409 12th Street, SW
PO Box 96920
Washington, DC 20090-6920

12345/43210

Dehydroepiandrosterone (DHEA) also has been used for androgen replacement therapy. Benefits ascribed to DHEA include increased bone mineral density, estrogenic stimulation of vaginal cytology, and enhancement of the immune system. However, a prospective, randomized controlled trial of symptomatic, perimenopausal women who received 50 mg of DHEA supplementation for 3 months did not describe improvement in libido, mood, dysphoria, cognition, or well-being (3). Potential adverse effects of DHEA at higher doses include effects on lipoprotein levels, cortisol, glucose tolerance, and central obesity. Some DHEA products, such as those derived from the Mexican wild yam, may have virilizing effects and may be hepatotoxic. Doses should not exceed 50 mg, and even at this dose a 10% reduction in high-density lipoprotein cholesterol has been observed after 3 months of therapy (3). In addition, because the manufacture of DHEA and other supplements is not standardized, there can be uncertainty as to the identity of the active ingredient and the amount of its dose.

Diminished libido also has been treated with sildenafil citrate, and anecdotal experiences have been described. However, there have been no reported controlled trials or other studies documenting its efficacy.

Although androgen therapy has been prescribed for sexual dysfunction for many years, data regarding its safety and efficacy are incomplete and physiologic androgen replacement therapy has not been shown to consistently affect the libido. Measurement of free or total testosterone levels for diagnosis or monitoring is not clinically useful. Patients most likely to benefit from androgen therapy are young women who have undergone oophorectomy (4). Although it is possible that other women experiencing decreased libido may benefit from a trial of androgen therapy, the lack of definitive data should lead to a cautious approach. In general, lower doses of oral preparations are preferred. Appropriate monitoring for side effects, including lipoprotein alteration, should be undertaken.

References

1. Berman JR, Berman L, Goldstein I. Female sexual dysfunction: incidence, pathophysiology, evaluation, and treatment options. Urology 1999;54:385–391
2. Casson PR, Carson SA, Buster JE. Testosterone delivery systems for women: present status and future promise. Semin Reprod Endocrinol 1998;16:153–159
3. Barnhart KT, Freeman E, Grisso JA, Rader DJ, Sammel M, Kapoor S, et al. The effect of dehydroepiandrosterone supplementation to symptomatic perimenopausal women on serum endocrine profiles, lipid parameters, and health-related quality of life. J Clin Endocrinol Metab 1999;84:3896–3902
4. Sherwin BB, Gelfand MM. Differential symptom response to parenteral estrogen and/or androgen administration in the surgical menopause. Am J Obstet Gynecol 1985;151:153–160

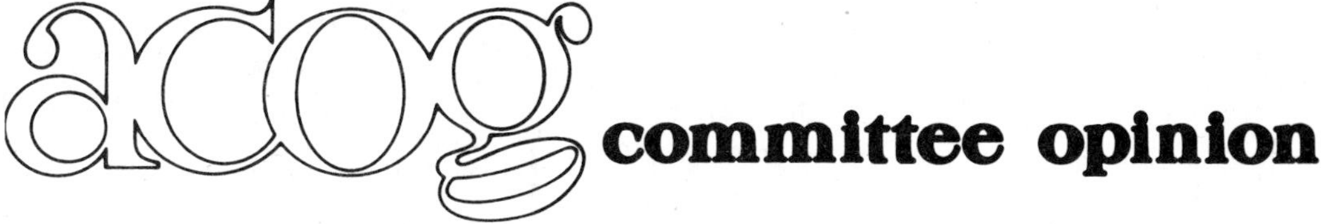

Committee on Obstetric Practice

Number 104—March 1992

Anesthesia for Emergency Deliveries

Failed intubation and pulmonary aspiration of gastric contents continue to be leading causes of maternal morbidity and mortality from anesthesia. The risk of these complications can be reduced by careful antepartum assessment to identify patients at risk, greater use of regional anesthesia when possible, and appropriate selection and preparation of patients who require general anesthesia for delivery.

ANTEPARTUM RISK ASSESSMENT

The obstetric care team should be alert to the presence of risk factors that place the parturient at increased risk for complications from emergency general or regional anesthesia. These factors include, but are not limited to, marked obesity, severe facial and neck edema, extremely short stature, a short neck, difficulty opening the mouth, a small mandible, protuberant teeth, arthritis of the neck, anatomic abnormalities of the face or mouth, a large thyroid, asthma, serious medical or obstetric complications, and a history of problems with anesthetics.

When such risk factors are identified, a physician who is credentialed to provide general and regional anesthesia should be consulted in the antepartum period to allow for joint development of a plan of management including optimal location for delivery. Strategies thereby can be developed to minimize the need for emergency induction of general anesthesia in women for whom this would be especially hazardous. For those patients at risk, consideration should be given to the planned placement in early labor of an intravenous line and an epidural or spinal catheter, with confirmation that the catheter is functional. If a patient at unusual risk of complications from anesthesia is identified (eg, prior failed intubation), strong consideration should be given to antepartum referral of the patient to allow for delivery at a hospital which can manage such anesthesia on a 24-hour basis.

EMERGENCY ANESTHESIA

The need for expeditious abdominal delivery cannot always be anticipated. When preparing for the rapid initiation of anesthesia, the maternal as well as the fetal status must be considered. Oral nonparticulate antacids should be administered immediately prior to the induction of general or major regional anesthesia to decrease the mother's risk of developing aspiration pneumonitis.

Although there are some situations in which general anesthesia is preferable to regional anesthesia, the risk of general anesthesia must be weighed against the benefit for those patients who have a greater potential for complications. Examples of circumstances in which a rapid induction of general anesthesia may be indicated include prolapsed umbilical cord with severe fetal bradycardia and active hemorrhage in a hemodynamically unstable mother.

In some cases, a nonreassuring fetal heart rate pattern is diagnosed as "fetal distress," and delivery is performed immediately. The term "fetal distress" is imprecise, nonspecific, and has little positive predictive value. The severity of the fetal heart rate abnormality should be considered when the urgency of the delivery and the type of anesthesia to be administered are determined. Cesarean deliveries that are performed for a nonreassuring fetal heart rate pattern do not necessarily preclude the use of regional anesthesia.

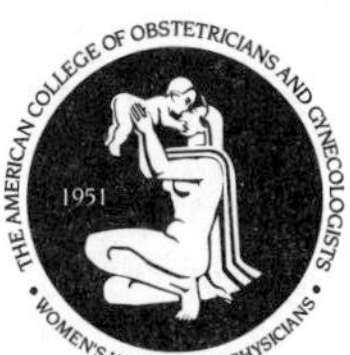

The American College of Obstetricians and Gynecologists
409 12th Street, SW • Washington, DC 20024-2188

3456/765

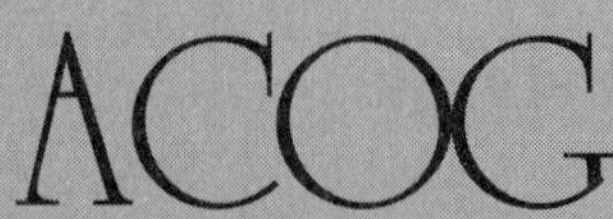

Committee on Obstetric Practice

Committee Opinion

Number 210, October 1998 *(Replaces #147, December 1994)*

Antenatal Corticosteroid Therapy for Fetal Maturation

For the past two decades, approximately 10% of all births in the United States have been preterm. Preterm birth results in approximately three fourths of all neonatal deaths not associated with congenital malformations. Moreover, neonatal morbidity is high among surviving infants born preterm, and complications such as respiratory distress syndrome (RDS), intraventricular hemorrhage, and necrotizing enterocolitis are common.

Antenatal corticosteroid therapy has been used for more than two decades in an attempt to reduce the frequency of neonatal complications, especially RDS. The beneficial effect of corticosteroids on fetal lung maturation was reported first in 1972. The type and dosage of corticosteroids, the optimal timing of treatment, and the gestational ages at which steroids are beneficial varied in early reports.

Data now have accumulated that document the benefit of corticosteroid therapy for reducing the frequency not only of RDS, but also of intraventricular hemorrhage and neonatal mortality. With regard to the type of steroids, both dexamethasone and betamethasone appear to be appropriate. These agents are virtually identical in structure and biologic activity, have a long half-life (up to 72 hours), and cross the placenta in biologically active forms. Moreover, they have little or no mineralocorticoid activity.

With regard to safety, there is no convincing scientific evidence that antenatal corticosteroid therapy increases the risk of neonatal infection or adrenal suppression. Follow-up studies of children up to 12 years of age indicate there is no apparent risk of adverse neurodevelopmental outcome associated with antenatal corticosteroids. The maternal risk of infection when corticosteroids are given to women with preterm premature rupture of membranes seems small and is outweighed by the benefit.

In 1994, the National Institute of Child Health and Human Development and the Office of Medical Applications of Research of the National Institutes of Health (NIH) convened a consensus conference sponsored by the National Heart, Lung, and Blood Institute and the National Institute of Nursing on the effects of corticosteroids for fetal maturation. It is clear that antenatal corticosteroids decrease the incidence of RDS in infants born at 29–34 weeks of gestation. Although antenatal corticosteroids do not necessarily decrease the incidence of RDS in infants born at 24–28 weeks of gestation, they reduce its severity. More importantly, antenatal corticosteroids clearly reduce mortality and the incidence of intraventricular hemorrhage in infants born at 24–28 weeks of gestation.

ISSN 1074-861X

The American College of Obstetricians and Gynecologists
409 12th Street, SW
PO Box 96920
Washington, DC 20090-6920

12345/21098

The NIH consensus panel made several recommendations for the use of antenatal corticosteroids (see box). The panel also identified several areas in which further research is needed. This includes the appropriate repeat doses and the short- and long-term benefits and risks of repeat administration of antenatal corticosteroids 7 days after the initial course.

The Committee on Obstetric Practice supports the conclusions of the NIH consensus conference. The decision to administer corticosteroids may be based either on clinical circumstances likely to result in spontaneous preterm delivery within 7 days or complications likely to lead to a decision to perform preterm delivery within 7 days. Because of the possible adverse fetal effects and possible effects on maternal immune status of repeated, weekly courses of steroids, it seems reasonable to adopt a rescue approach to therapy in the treatment of preterm labor rather than a routine readministration regimen. Following the initial course of corticosteroids, repeated doses should be given only on an as-needed basis (ie, if the woman is re-treated for threatened preterm birth).

National Institutes of Health Consensus Panel Recommendations

- The benefits of antenatal administration of corticosteroids to fetuses at risk of preterm delivery vastly outweigh the risks. These benefits include not only a reduction in the risk of RDS but also a substantial decrease in mortality and intraventricular hemorrhage.
- All women between 24 and 34 weeks of pregnancy at risk for preterm delivery are candidates for antenatal corticosteroid therapy.
- Fetal race, gender, and availability of surfactant therapy should not influence the decision to use antenatal corticosteroid therapy.
- A patient eligible for therapy with tocolytic agents also should be eligible for treatment with antenatal corticosteroids when she requires repetitive intravenous tocolytics.
- Treatment should consist of either two doses of 12 mg of betamethasone, intramuscularly, given 24 hours apart or four doses of 6 mg of dexamethasone, intramuscularly, given 12 hours apart. Optimal benefits begin 24 hours after initiation of therapy and last 7 days.
- Because treatment for less than 24 hours still can result in significant reductions in neonatal mortality, antenatal corticosteroids should be given unless immediate delivery is anticipated.
- Antenatal corticosteroid use is recommended in women with preterm premature rupture of membranes at less than 30–32 weeks of gestation in the absence of clinical chorioamnionitis because of the high risk of intraventricular hemorrhage at these early gestational ages.
- In women with complicated pregnancies for whom delivery before 34 weeks of gestation is likely, antenatal corticosteroid use is recommended unless there is evidence that corticosteroids will have an adverse effect on the mother or delivery is imminent.

Adapted from Effect of antenatal steroids for fetal maturation on perinatal outcomes. NIH Consens Statement 1994 Feb 28–Mar 2; 12(2):1–24

Bibliography

Crowley P. Corticosteroids after preterm premature rupture of membranes. Obstet Gynecol Clin North Am 1992;19:317–326

Crowley P, Chalmers I, Keirse MJ. The effects of corticosteroid administration before preterm delivery: an overview of the evidence from controlled trials. Br J Obstet Gynaecol 1990; 97:11–25

Effects of antenatal dexamethasone administration in the infant; long-term follow-up. J Pediatr 1984;104:259–267

Effect of antenatal dexamethasone administration on the prevention of respiratory distress syndrome. Am J Obstet Gynecol 1981;141:276–287

Effect of antenatal steroids for fetal maturation on perinatal outcomes. NIH Consens Statement 1994 Feb 28–Mar 2;12(2): 1–24

Gamsu HR, Mullinger BM, Donnai P, Dash CH. Antenatal administration of betamethasone to prevent respiratory distress syndrome in premature infants: report of a UK multicentre trial. Br J Obstet Gynaecol 1989;96:401–410

Garite TJ, Freeman RK, Linzey EM, Braly PS, Dorchester WL. Prospective randomized study of corticosteroids in the management of premature rupture of the membranes and the premature gestation. Am J Obstet Gynecol 1981;141:508–515

Garite TJ, Rumney PJ, Briggs GG, Harding JA, Nageotte MP, Towers CV, et al. A randomized, placebo-controlled trial of betamethasone for the prevention of respiratory distress syndrome at 24 to 28 weeks' gestation. Am J Obstet Gynecol 1992;166:646–651

Liggins GC, Howie RN. A controlled trial of antepartum glucocorticoid treatment for prevention of the respiratory distress syndrome in premature infants. Pediatrics 1972;50:515–525

Ohlsson A. Treatments of preterm premature rupture of the membranes: a meta-analysis. Am J Obstet Gynecol 1989;160: 890–906

Schmand B, Neuvel J, Smolders-de Haas H, Hoeks J, Treffers PE, Koppe JG. Psychological development of children who were treated antenatally with corticosteroids to prevent respiratory distress syndrome. Pediatrics 1990;86:58–64

Teramo K, Hallman M, Raivio KO. Maternal glucocorticoid in unplanned premature labor. Controlled study of the effects of betamethasone phosphate on the phospholipids of the gastric aspirate and on the adrenal cortical function of the newborn infant. Pediatr Res 1980;14:326–329

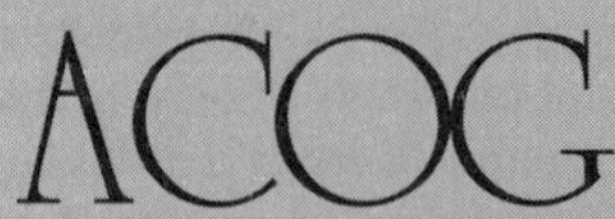

Committee on Obstetric Practice

Committee Opinion

Number 211, November 1998

Anticoagulation with Low-Molecular-Weight Heparin During Pregnancy

The use of low-molecular-weight heparin for thromboprophylaxis and treatment of venous thromboembolism has attracted attention because of its potential advantages compared with traditional unfractionated heparin. Similar to unfractionated heparin, low-molecular-weight heparin does not cross the placenta and has no teratogenic effects. However, compared with unfractionated heparin, low-molecular-weight heparin has a longer half-life and bioavailability, a more predictable dose-response relationship, and decreased risk of thrombocytopenia and hemorrhagic complications. Consequently, low-molecular-weight heparin may be administered subcutaneously in a once- or twice-daily dose, without laboratory monitoring, and dosing may be continued throughout labor and delivery or during cesarean delivery. Assessments of activated partial thromboplastin time and prothrombin time are not helpful and should not be obtained.

Experience with low-molecular-weight heparin use during pregnancy supports the following conclusions:

- Patients with venous thrombosis, pulmonary embolism, or thrombophilic disorders may be treated at least as effectively with low-molecular-weight heparin as with traditional heparin.
- The ease of administration, less frequent need for laboratory monitoring, and ability to continue anticoagulation through labor and delivery provide distinct advantages of low-molecular-weight heparin compared with unfractionated heparin. Preliminary evidence suggests that there is no greater risk of bone demineralization.
- Low-molecular-weight heparin is approximately four to six times more costly, but the ease of use in the outpatient setting and elimination of the need for laboratory monitoring (eg, activated partial thromboplastin time and prothrombin time) may compensate for the cost difference.
- There is inadequate information to recommend the use of low-molecular-weight heparin for anticoagulation in the case of a pregnant woman with a mechanical heart valve.

ISSN 1074-861X

The American College of Obstetricians and Gynecologists
409 12th Street, SW
PO Box 96920
Washington, DC 20090-6920

12345/21098

- The use of regional anesthesia may be limited by the possibility of epidural hematomas in nonpregnant individuals (1).

Reference

1. Hynson JM, Katz JA, Bueff HU. Epidural hematoma associated with enoxaparin. Anesth Analg 1996;82:1072–1075

Bibliography

Dulitzki M, Pauzner R, Langevitz P, Pras M, Many A, Schiff E. Low-molecular-weight heparin during pregnancy and delivery: preliminary experience with 41 pregnancies. Obstet Gynecol 1996;87:380–383

Horlocker TT, Wedel DJ. Spinal and epidural blockade and perioperative low molecular weight heparin: smooth sailing on the *Titanic*. Anesth Analg 1998;86:1153–1156

Hunt BJ, Doughty HA, Majumdar G, Copplestone A, Kerslake S, Buchanan N, et al. Thromboprophylaxis with low molecular weight heparin (Fragmin) in high risk pregnancies. Thromb Haemost 1997;77:39–43

Kakkar VV, Boeckl O, Boneu B, Bordenave L, Brehm OA, Brucke P, et al. Efficacy and safety of a low-molecular-weight heparin and standard unfractionated heparin for prophylaxis of postoperative venous thromboembolism: European multicenter trial. World J Surg 1997;21:2–8; discussion 8–9

Leizorovicz A. Comparison of the efficacy and safety of low molecular weight heparins and unfractionated heparin in the initial treatment of deep venous thrombosis. An updated meta-analysis. Drugs 1996;52(suppl 7):30–37

Nelson-Piercy C, Letsky EA, de Swiet M. Low-molecular-weight heparin for obstetric thromboprophylaxis: experience of sixty-nine pregnancies in sixty-one women at high risk. Am J Obstet Gynecol 1997;176:1062–1068

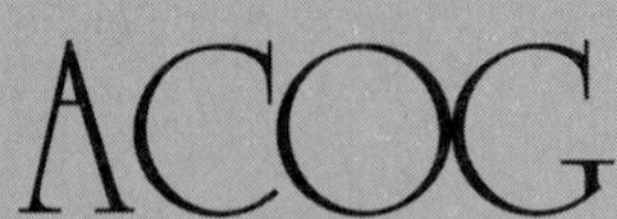

Committee on
Obstetric Practice

Committee Opinion

Number 198, February 1998

Bacterial Vaginosis Screening for Prevention of Preterm Delivery

Preterm delivery is a major contributor to neonatal morbidity and mortality, and its prevention has assumed special importance in the practice of obstetrics. Efforts to reduce spontaneous preterm deliveries have increasingly emphasized the possible causative role of infections. In particular, studies have shown an association between the presence of bacterial vaginosis (BV) and preterm delivery in high-risk populations. The possibility that BV may be a treatable cause of preterm delivery has raised hopes for a new prevention strategy. Present data, however, are still very preliminary, and only the following conclusions can be made:

- Women at high risk for preterm delivery (ie, women with a history of preterm delivery, a low prepregnant weight of <50 kg, or both) who had positive BV screening results in their second trimester and were treated with oral metronidazole had fewer preterm deliveries than women who were not treated.
- In the absence of risk factors for preterm delivery, BV has been associated with preterm delivery of low-birth-weight neonates but could not be identified as a causative factor.
- It is not clear whether the treatment of BV in a population at low risk for preterm delivery, based on a generalized screening program for asymptomatic BV, would decrease the risk of preterm delivery (ie, BV may be a marker of underlying pathology, not the pathology itself).

Given these preliminary data, it would be appropriate to adopt the following strategies for screening for and treatment of BV after the first trimester:

- Screening for BV may be considered in women at high risk for preterm labor.
- Women who have positive test results or symptoms of BV should be treated with metronidazole administered orally. Vaginal treatment appears not to be as effective in preventing preterm labor.
- Current studies do not clarify whether women who test positive and are treated or those who test negative should be rescreened periodically during pregnancy. In addition, the effect of re-treatment of persistent or recurrent BV is unclear.

ISSN 1074-861X

The American College of Obstetricians and Gynecologists
409 12th Street, SW
PO Box 96920
Washington, DC 20090-6920

12345/21098

- Routine BV screening of asymptomatic women at low risk for preterm delivery and the subsequent treatment of women with positive results cannot be endorsed based on current studies.

Bibliography

Hauth JC, Goldenberg RL, Andrews WW, DuBard MB, Copper RL. Reduced incidence of preterm delivery with metronidazole and erythromycin in women with bacterial vaginosis. N Engl J Med 1995;333:1732–1736

Hillier SL, Nugent RP, Eschenbach DA, Krohn MA, Gibbs RS, Martin DH, et al. Association between bacterial vaginosis and preterm delivery of a low-birth-weight infant. The Vaginal Infections and Prematurity Study Group. N Engl J Med 1995; 333:1737–1742

McGregor JA, French JI, Jones W, Milligan K, McKinney PJ, Patterson E, et al. Bacterial vaginosis is associated with prematurity and vaginal fluid mucinase and sialidase: results of a controlled trial of topical clindamycin cream. Am J Obstet Gynecol 1994;170:1048–1059; discussion 1059–1060

Meis PJ, Goldenberg RL, Mercer B, Moawad A, Das A, McNellis D, et al. The preterm prediction study: significance of vaginal infections. National Institute of Child Health and Human Development Maternal–Fetal Medicine Units Network. Am J Obstet Gynecol 1995;173:1231–1235

Morales WJ, Schorr S, Albritton J. Effect of metronidazole in patients with preterm birth in preceding pregnancy and bacterial vaginosis: a placebo-controlled, double-blind study. Am J Obstet Gynecol 1994;171:345–347; discussion 348–349

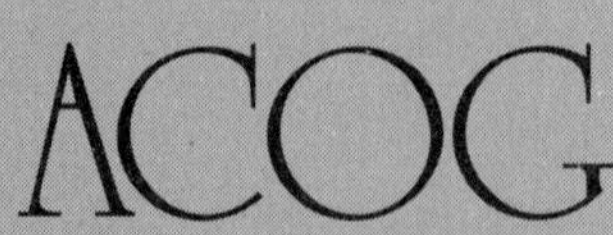

Committee on
Obstetric Practice

Committee Opinion

Number 220, August 1999

Breastfeeding and the Risk of Hepatitis C Virus Transmission

Hepatitis C virus (HCV) infection is the most common bloodborne infection in the United States. It affects 3.9 million Americans, and increasing numbers of women are being identified as hepatitis C antibody positive.

The average rate of infection for infants born to women who are HCV positive but test negative for the human immunodeficiency virus (HIV) is 5–6%. The major factor contributing to neonatal infection is the viral load of HCV ribonucleic acid in the mother at the time of birth. According to the Centers for Disease Control and Prevention, the transmission of HCV through breast milk has not been clearly documented. Studies to date evaluating the effect of breastfeeding on HCV transmission indicate that the average rate of infection is 4% in both breastfed and bottlefed infants. Therefore, it appears that breastfeeding does not appreciably increase the risk of transmitting HCV to a neonate.

Bibliography

Centers for Disease Control and Prevention. Recommendations for prevention and control of hepatitis C virus (HCV) infection and HCV-related chronic disease. MMWR Morb Mortal Wkly Rep 1998;47(RR-19):1–39

ISSN 1074-861X

The American College of Obstetricians and Gynecologists
409 12th Street, SW
PO Box 96920
Washington, DC 20090-6920

12345/32109

ACOG Committee Opinion

Committee on Genetics

Number 239, August 2000 *(Replaces No. 176, October 1996)*

Breast–Ovarian Cancer Screening

Based upon current knowledge, an estimated 5–7% of all breast and ovarian cancer is attributed to inherited mutations in two highly penetrant autosomal dominant susceptibility genes, *BRCA 1* and *BRCA 2*. In the general population, the gene frequency for *BRCA 1* and *BRCA 2* is low, occurring in approximately 1 in 800 individuals. Women who inherit either a *BRCA 1* or *BRCA 2* mutation have a 50–80% lifetime risk of breast cancer and an estimated 15–25% risk of developing ovarian cancer by age 70 years. *BRCA 1* appears to confer a higher risk of ovarian cancer than does *BRCA 2* (1, 2). *BRCA 2* is responsible for a much higher percentage of breast cancer cases in men. Mutations in *BRCA 1* and *BRCA 2* account for a substantial majority of inheritable breast cancers, while mutations in *p53*, H-*ras*, and the gene for ataxia–telangiectasia account for an additional small percentage. In the future, it is likely that other genes that contribute to the development of breast cancer will be discovered. Currently, reliance solely on genetic testing as a major predictor of breast and ovarian cancer is not supported by the science. An accurate evaluation of family history remains essential in assessing breast and ovarian cancer risk. Analysis has shown that multiple affected first- and second-degree relatives, both maternal and paternal, particularly with early onset disease, may significantly alter an individual's risk for breast and ovarian cancer (3).

BRCA 1 and *BRCA 2* are tumor suppressor genes. Women with a germline mutation in one copy of either gene have a decreased amount of the normal suppressor protein. Such individuals are at an increased risk of cancer if there is a loss of function in the normal copy of the gene. When this "second hit" occurs in a somatic cell (ie, breast cell), the result may be pathologic cell division.

Approximately 600 mutations in the *BRCA 1* gene and nearly 500 mutations of the *BRCA 2* gene have been found, of which 70–80% are thought to be disease producing. The precise biologic functions of *BRCA 1* and *BRCA 2* are still unclear.

The size of the *BRCA 1* gene, the widespread distribution of the mutations within the gene, the prevalence of different mutations in different populations, the technical problems in sequencing the entire gene, and the uncertain role of other gene pathways leading to breast–ovarian cancer in selected families make genetic testing for *BRCA 1* mutations an uncertain and incomplete science. In the future, it is possible that testing for the truncated

This opinion was developed in consultation with Francis S. Collins, MD, PhD, Director of the National Human Genome Research Institute. This document reflects emerging clinical and scientific advances as of the date issued and is subject to change. The information should not be construed as dictating an exclusive course of treatment or procedure to be followed.

ISSN 1074-861X

The American College of Obstetricians and Gynecologists
409 12th Street, SW
PO Box 96920
Washington, DC 20090-6920

12345/43210

protein product of the gene will be more practical for screening than DNA mutation analysis. Also contributing to the limitations of genetic testing for breast and ovarian cancer are the lack of understanding of the penetrance of the various mutations in diverse populations and the cost and benefit to the patient. For example, a single *BRCA 1* 185delAG mutation, previously identified in high-risk families, has been detected in approximately 1% of women of Eastern European Jewish descent. The true frequency of the mutation and implications of this finding are still uncertain, but there is a possibility that other *BRCA 1* mutations exist within the same population. For this reason, a negative test result for the *BRCA 1* 185delAG mutation alone would have little meaning in the presence of a strong family history of breast and ovarian cancer. Conversely, the interpretation of a positive test result for this mutation in the absence of a strong family history of cancer is unclear at present. Because identifying the precise mutations in a single affected relative makes looking for the same mutation in other family members easier, analysis usually begins with the DNA of an affected individual.

In selected families (multiple family members affected with breast or ovarian cancer, or a family in which a *BRCA* mutation has been discovered), *BRCA* testing may be useful. The failure to find a mutation in an individual, whose family has a known *BRCA* mutation, may reduce anxiety. The finding of a *BRCA* mutation in an individual with a strong family history for breast or ovarian cancer would allow the patient and physician to explore various management options. These might include more frequent surveillance, prophylactic surgery, such as mastectomy or oophorectomy, and trials of chemoprevention, such as oral contraceptives. Because of the problems previously described, testing of the general population is not recommended.

The Committee on Genetics of the American College of Obstetricians and Gynecologists believes that genetic testing for breast–ovarian cancer should be performed only with the individual's full informed consent. Currently, such testing continues to be best performed by investigators working under research protocols approved by an institutional review board. Individuals should be counseled before and after testing to ensure their understanding of the scope, implications, and limitations of the testing process. Counseling should include discussions of the uncertainties of applying genetic test results to the prevention and treatment of breast and ovarian cancer and the potential for genetic discrimination and loss of insurance coverage. The standard of care should emphasize genetic services, genetic information, and education and counseling, rather than the testing procedures alone. Although this document discusses DNA-based testing for inherited susceptibility to breast and ovarian cancer, the most important part of the screening process is obtaining and interpreting the family history. The National Cancer Institute Cancer Information Service (1-800-4-CANCER) can supply information about genetic services at cancer centers supported by the National Institutes of Health.

References

1. Burke W, Daly M, Garber J, Botkin J, Kahn MJ, Lynch P, et al. Recommendations for follow-up care of individuals with an inherited predisposition to cancer. II. BRCA1 and BRCA2. Cancer Genetics Studies Consortium. JAMA 1997;277:997–1003

2. Ford D, Easton DF, Bishop DT, Narod SA, Goldgar DE. Risks of cancer in BRCA1-mutation carriers. Breast Cancer Linage Consortium. Lancet 1994;343:692–695

3. Claus EB, Risch N, Thompson WD. Autosomal dominant inheritance early-onset breast cancer. Cancer 1994;73: 643–651

ACOG

Committee on Genetics

Committee Opinion

Number 160, October 1995 (*Replaces #69, November 1989*)

Chorionic Villus Sampling

Chorionic villus sampling (CVS) is a technique in which a small sample (5–40 mg) of placental tissue (chorionic villi) is obtained. Villi are derived from the same embryonic origin as the fetus; thus, the tissue reflects the genetic status of the fetus. For first-trimester prenatal diagnosis, CVS is generally performed between 10–12 weeks of gestation. It offers couples an earlier option for prenatal diagnosis of a genetic defect than mid-trimester amniocentesis. A termination performed between 17–19 weeks of gestation has greater risk than does a first-trimester termination.

Sampling may be done by transcervical CVS, transabdominal CVS, or transvaginal CVS. Because transvaginal CVS is rarely used, insufficient data are available to assess its safety. Thus, this Committee Opinion addresses only transcervical CVS and transabdominal CVS.

Transcervical CVS is performed by directing a flexible catheter with a stylet through the antiseptically prepared vagina and cervix into the placenta under direct ultrasonographic guidance. Following removal of the stylet, villi are aspirated with a syringe.

Transabdominal CVS is performed by percutaneous insertion of a needle through the anterior abdominal wall and uterine wall into the placenta under direct ultrasonographic guidance. Following removal of the stylet, villi are aspirated with a syringe. To facilitate the procedure some operators prefer to use an aspiration device to house the syringe (breast aspiration apparatus). Also, some operators prefer to use a "guide-needle" or double needle system device, which punctures the uterine wall once but permits multiple attempts at villi aspiration.

Chorionic villi may be analyzed to determine the chromosomal, enzymatic, and DNA status of the fetus. In general, CVS can be used for most of the same indications for prenatal diagnosis as genetic mid-trimester amniocentesis (1). Chorionic villi samples are particularly well suited for DNA diagnostic testing, which is also generally performed in those cases with the highest genetic risk of positive diagnosis. Chorionic villi, however, cannot be used for the prenatal diagnosis of neural tube defects, which requires analysis of amniotic fluid alpha-fetoprotein, or the fragile X syndrome. Differential methylation patterns in trophoblast as compared with the fetus limit the diagnostic utility of CVS for the diagnosis of fragile X syndrome.

ISSN 1074-861X

The American College of Obstetricians and Gynecologists
409 12th Street, SW
Washington, DC 20024-2188

12345/98765

Registry data and reports from individual centers indicate that CVS is a relatively safe and accurate technique for first-trimester prenatal diagnosis. The National Institute of Child Health and Human Development (NICHD) conducted a large-scale collaborative study involving seven centers in the United States (2). The study consisted of 2,278 women undergoing transcervical CVS and 671 in a control group undergoing mid-trimester amniocentesis. The results showed that the combined losses due to spontaneous abortion, termination of abnormal pregnancies, stillbirths, and neonatal deaths were 0.8 percentage points (95% confidence interval, -1.3% to 2.9%) higher in the CVS patients than in the control amniocentesis patients. Although this difference was not statistically significant, the data suggest some increased risk with CVS. This observation was further confirmed by findings of other collaborative studies and reports from individual centers. Cytogenetic diagnosis was obtained in 98% of the subjects and revealed a 1.8% aneuploidy rate. There were no cases of serious maternal infection (eg, septic shock) in any of the patients participating in the study. In about 1% of cases, a second prenatal diagnostic procedure (second CVS or amniocentesis) was required because of failed cytogenetic results, maternal cell contamination, or unusual cytogenetic results (eg, mosaicism) (3). The study concluded that transcervical CVS is an effective approach for early prenatal diagnosis that probably confers slightly higher risks than amniocentesis.

The results of a randomized multicenter study of transcervical CVS in Canada were similar to those reported by the NICHD collaborative study (4). The increased rate of fetal loss in the patients who had transcervical CVS was 0.6 percentage points (approximately 95% confidence intervals indicate that this difference is most unlikely to be greater than 2.7%) when compared with the rate of pregnancy loss in patients who had amniocentesis.

A subsequent NICHD randomized comparison of transcervical CVS and transabdominal CVS showed these two approaches to be equally safe (5). Among women with cytogenetically normal pregnancies who had sampling because of advanced maternal age, the rate of spontaneous fetal loss through 28 weeks of pregnancy was 2.5% in the transcervical CVS group and 2.3% in the transabdominal CVS group (difference, 0.26%; 95% confidence interval, -0.52% to 1.0%). In aggregate, data indicated that when performed by experienced operators, transcervical and transabdominal CVS did not show significantly different fetal loss rates compared with traditional midtrimester amniocentesis.

Several years ago, reports of unusual clusters of limb reduction defects in infants born to mothers following CVS raised the possibility that there might be a causal association (6–8). Subsequently, there followed a number of reports both supporting and refuting such an association. In general, the larger and more experienced CVS centers did not find any clusters similar to the initial reports.

In 1992, a workshop was convened by NICHD and the American College of Obstetricians and Gynecologists to address this concern (9). Those who attended agreed that the frequency of the syndrome of oromandibular–limb hypogenesis appeared to be more common among CVS-exposed infants. This appeared to correlate with, but may not be limited to, CVS performed earlier than 10 weeks of gestation. However, workshop participants were divided as to whether CVS performed at 10–12 weeks of gestation was associated with an increased risk for limb defects. It was recommended that further studies be done and that women being offered CVS as an option be made aware of concerns about the possible association of CVS with increased risks for limb and other defects.

Recently, a case–control study conducted by the Centers for Disease Control and Prevention (10) showed no overall increased risk of limb deficiency among infants whose mothers had undergone CVS compared with controls. However, when analyzed for specific anatomic subtypes, there was a sixfold increased risk for transverse digital deficiency with an absolute risk of approximately 1 per 3,000 births (95% confidence interval, 1 per 1,000 to 1 per 10,000). An increased risk was also found in another case–control study (11). In contrast, data from 19 centers collected through the International CVS Registry evaluating 138,000 infants born after CVS showed no significant difference in the overall frequency of limb defects, nor any difference in the pattern of limb deficiencies compared with a background population study in British Columbia (12).

In view of the preceding data, the Committee on Genetics concludes the following:

1. Transcervical CVS and transabdominal CVS, when performed at 10–12 weeks of gestation, are relatively safe and accurate procedures and may be considered acceptable alternatives to midtrimester genetic amniocentesis.
2. Until further information is available, CVS for clinical application should not be performed before 10 weeks of gestation.
3. Chorionic villus sampling requires appropriate genetic counseling before the proce-

dure, an operator experienced in performing the technique, and a laboratory experienced in processing the villus specimen and interpreting the results. Counseling should include comparing and contrasting the risks and benefits of amniocentesis and CVS.

4. Although further studies are needed to determine whether there is an increased risk of transverse digital deficiency following CVS performed at 10–12 weeks of gestation, it is prudent to counsel patients that such an outcome is possible and that the estimated risk may be in the order of 1 in 3,000 births (10).

References

1. American College of Obstetricians and Gynecologists. Antenatal diagnosis of genetic disorders. ACOG Technical Bulletin 108. Washington, DC: ACOG, September, 1987
2. Rhoads GG, Jackson LG, Schlesselman SE, de la Cruz FF, Desnick RJ, Golbus MS, et al. The safety and efficacy of chorionic villus sampling for early prenatal diagnosis of cytogenetic abnormalities. N Engl J Med 1989;320:609–617
3. Ledbetter DH, Martin AO, Verlinsky Y, Pergament E, Jackson L, Yang-Feng T, et al. Cytogenetic results of chorionic villus sampling: high success rate and diagnostic accuracy in the United States collaborative study. Am J Obstet Gynecol 1990;162:495–501
4. Multicentre randomised clinical trial of chorion villus sampling and amniocentesis. First report. Canadian Collaborative CVS-Amniocentesis Clinical Trial Group. Lancet 1989;1:1–6
5. Jackson LG, Zachary JM, Fowler SE, Desnick RJ, Golbus MS, Ledbetter DH, et al. A randomized comparison of transcervical and transabdominal chorionic-villus sampling. The U.S. National Institute of Child Health and Human Development Chorionic-Villus Sampling and Amniocentesis Study Group. N Engl J Med 1992;327: 594–598
6. Firth HV, Boyd PA, Chamberlain P, MacKenzie IZ, Lindenbaum RH, Huson SM. Limb abnormalities and chorion villus sampling. Lancet 1991;338:51
7. Burton BK, Schulz CJ, Burd LI. Limb anomalies associated with chorionic villus sampling. Obstet Gynecol 1992;79:726–730
8. Brambati B, Simoni G, Travi M, Danesino C, Tului L, Privitera O, et al. Genetic diagnosis by chorionic villus sampling before 8 gestational weeks: efficiency, reliability, and risks on 317 completed pregnancies. Prenat Diagn 1992;12:789–799
9. Holmes LB. Report of National Institute of Child Health and Human Development Workshop on Chorionic Villus Sampling and Limb and Other Defects, October 20, 1992. Teratology 1993;48:7–13
10. Olney RS, Khoury MJ, Alo CJ, Costa P, Edmonds LD, Flood TJ, et al. Increased risk for transverse digital deficiency after chorionic villus sampling—results of the United States multistate case–control study, 1988–1992. Teratology 1995;51:20–29
11. Mastroiacovo P, Botto LD. Chorionic villus sampling and transverse limb deficiencies: maternal age is not a confounder. Am J Med Genet 1994;53:182–186
12. Fishman RHB. 1994 WHO on CVS safety. Lancet 1994; 443:1420

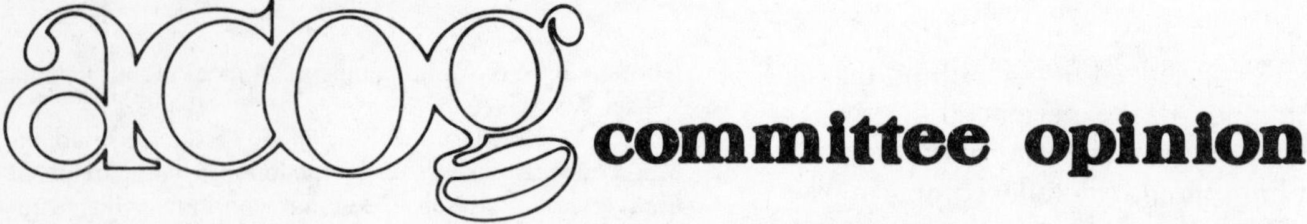

Committee on Gynecologic Practice Number 133—March 1994

Colposcopy Training and Practice

Over the past two decades, colposcopy has become the standard method for evaluating abnormal cervical cytology. When combined with the appropriate interpretation of histopathologic specimens, the technique can be used to successfully evaluate abnormal cervical cytology and aid in treatment planning. Colposcopy also is useful in the evaluation of abnormal vaginal cytology and subtle changes of the vulvar epithelium.

Ideally, training in colposcopy will occur during a 4-year obstetrics and gynecology residency. In this setting, it is possible to learn the natural history of genital intraepithelial neoplasia, review cytologic and histologic specimens, perform many examinations by colposcopy, and learn to biopsy and treat intraepithelial lesions of the cervix, vagina, and vulva.

SUGGESTED CURRICULUM CONTENT FOR COLPOSCOPY TRAINING

- Cytology and histology of the cervix
- Evaluation of Pap test results
- Indications for colposcopic examination
- Colposcopic terminology
- Normal and abnormal patterns seen on colposcopy
- Patterns seen on colposcopy and histologic correlations
- Clinical colposcopic techniques
- Biopsy of the cervix and endocervical curettage
- Documentation of findings
- Referral and follow-up
- Legal and insurance issues
- Preceptorship
- Continuing professional education

When a physician or other health care practitioner learns the technique of colposcopy in a setting other than residency, it is important that the training program include all the elements—both didactic and preceptor—that would be part of a residency program (see the box). Specifically, the health care practitioner must have sufficient didactic training to learn the natural history of intraepithelial lesions and their cytologic and histopathologic correlations.

Completion of a didactic course alone does not constitute adequate training to perform colposcopy. A period of preceptorship should always follow the didactic material. The student colposcopist should perform examinations jointly with an experienced colposcopist until the technique is well learned. All cases should be reviewed with the preceptor once the final histology and cytology have been reported and a further management plan has been developed for each patient.

The technique of colposcopy requires that the examiner recognize subtle changes in the epithelial patterns of the lower genital tract. A practicing colposcopist should be expected to perform a sufficient number of examinations on an ongoing basis to maintain colposcopic skill. It is highly desirable for the practicing colposcopist to be involved in continuing quality assurance activities to document proficiency. This should be encouraged in all settings, including clinics, hospitals, and private offices.

BIBLIOGRAPHY

Benedet JL, Anderson GH, Matisic JP, Miller DM. A quality-control program for colposcopic practice. Obstet Gynecol 1991;78:872–875

Burke L, Antonioli DA, Ducatman BS. Colposcopy. Norwalk, Connecticut: Appleton and Lange, 1991

Cartwright PS. The colposcopy clinic data system. J Reprod Med 1989;34:645–646

Coppleson M, Pixley E, Reid B. Colposcopy. 3rd ed. Springfield, Illinois: Charles C. Thomas, 1986

Homesley HD, Wolff JL, Reish RL, Jobson VW. Evaluating the acquisition of colposcopy skills in an obstetric–gynecologic residency program. J Reprod Med 1985;30:911–914

Julian TM. Teaching colposcopy. The colposcopist 1990;22(2):5–7

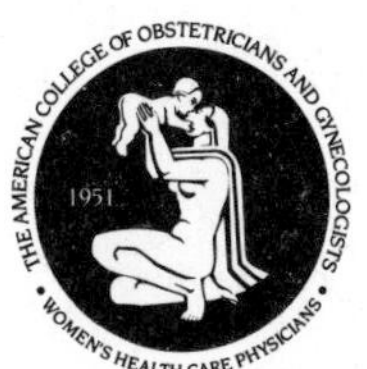

This document reflects emerging clinical and scientific advances as of the date issued and is subject to change. The information should not be construed as dictating an exclusive course of treatment or procedure to be followed.

The American College of Obstetricians and Gynecologists
409 12th Street, SW • Washington, DC 20024-2188

12345/87654

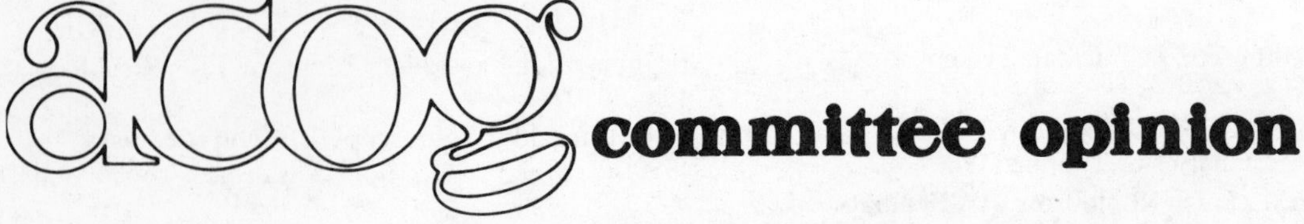

committee opinion

Committee on Ethics

Number 129—November 1993

Commercial Ventures in Medicine: Concerns About the Patenting of Procedures

New commercial ventures in medicine may threaten certain essential features of health care. Ideally, physicians should be teachers and sharers of medical information without keeping trade secrets. Physicians also have an obligation to provide advice to their patients about the most appropriate care uninfluenced by a profit motive. Patients rightfully expect safety and efficacy in the medical procedures physicians perform as well as reasonable access to such procedures. Full disclosure of research information and experience with medical procedures is necessary if safety and efficacy are to be validated or refuted by colleagues and if procedures are to be refined through the work of peers. Thus, any corporate or individual business arrangements, including patenting, licensing, and franchising, insofar as they erode these essential features of medical care, should be considered contrary to the welfare of patients and the responsibilities of physicians.

An area of contemporary and growing concern is the patenting of medical procedures. In addition to raising problems of efficacy and safety, the patenting of medical procedures may jeopardize patients' interests in the following ways: first, it delays the rapid transmission of new scientific knowledge, and second, it adds costs to a procedure that may put it out of the reach of patients who might otherwise benefit from its use. Academic physicians need to be aware of the powerful incentives placed on them by their universities to maximize extramural revenues and should urge that such policies not encourage the patenting of procedures. All physicians need to be aware of incentives to increase income in ways that may jeopardize the interests of patients.

Replaces ACOG Statement of Policy "Commercial Ventures in Medicine," July 1984

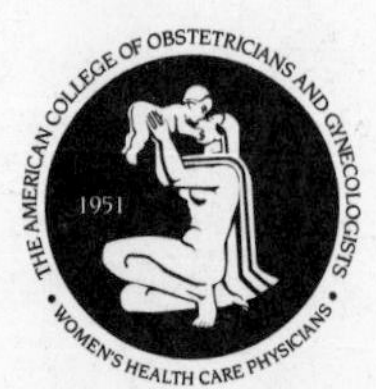

The American College of Obstetricians and Gynecologists
409 12th Street, SW • Washington, DC 20024-2188

12345/76543

ACOG

Committee on Primary Care

Committee Opinion

Number 227, November 1999

Complementary and Alternative Medicine

In 1990, 34% of adults in the United States used complementary and alternative medicine (CAM). In 1997, 42% of adults in the United States and Canada used CAM, and the use by women was 49%. This trend of increased CAM use will continue as it is reinforced and supported by continuing media attention; intense commercial efforts by providers of CAM products and services, including proprietary pharmaceutical companies; third-party reimbursement for some CAM practices and products; and the increasing over-the-counter access to CAM products in drugstores and supermarkets. The purpose of this Committee Opinion is to provide an overview of CAM, to recommend that physicians ask patients about their use of CAM, and to provide sources of additional information about the subject.

The physician, in the role of patient advocate, has an ethical responsibility to promote and protect the patient's well-being. This function includes the ability to engage in a dialogue that honors the patient's values and promotes shared decision making. Inquiring about the patient's motivation for and use of CAM and providing information on safety and effectiveness can be integral to this role.

Complementary and alternative medicine can be defined as those systems, practices, interventions, modalities, professions, therapies, applications, theories, or claims that are currently not an integral part of the dominant or conventional medical system (known as allopathy in North America). Importantly, over time some of the individual modalities do overlap with or become integrated into Western medicine. The spectrum of CAM encompasses over 350 different techniques and treatments. These can be classified into at least seven major categories:

1. *Mind–body interventions* include yoga, relaxation response techniques, meditation, t'ai chi, hypnotherapy, spirituality, support groups, and biofeedback.
2. *Alternative systems of medical practice* are exemplified by Traditional Chinese Medicine. Other systems in this category include homeopathy, ayurveda, naturopathy, chiropractic, Native-American medicine, and the various forms of acupuncture.

The Committee wishes to thank Ronald A. Chez, MD, for his assistance in the development of this opinion. This document reflects emerging clinical and scientific advances as of the date issued and is subject to change. The information should not be construed as dictating an exclusive course of treatment or procedure to be followed.

The American College of Obstetricians and Gynecologists
409 12th Street, SW
PO Box 96920
Washington, DC 20090-6920

12345/32109

3. *Pharmacologic and biologic* treatments, a diverse and large category, includes folk medicine, medicinal plants, processed blood products, and autogenous vaccines.
4. *Herbal medicine,* another large category, is the use of botanicals with pharmacologic activity. A number of these substances have formed the basis of the Western pharmacopeia. Currently, the public's attention is focused on St. John's wort for depressive disorders, echinacea for upper respiratory infections, valerian for sleep disorders, garlic for hypercholesterolemia, and ginkgo biloba for circulatory disorders.
5. *Diet and nutrition* encompass the use of vitamins, minerals, and nutritional supplements in general, and cancer and cardiovascular disease diets in particular. Treatments include megadosing, elimination of or excessive intake of certain foods, vegetarian and macrobiotic diets, and diets associated with various physicians.
6. *Manual healing methods* include massage, chiropractic and osteopathic manipulation, and biofield therapeutics (eg, Reiki, polarity, reflexology, and therapeutic touch).
7. *Bioelectromagnetic applications* include the use of magnets for musculoskeletal and neurologic pain; low-frequency thermal waves in diathermy; nonionizing, nonthermal applications such as pulsed electromagnetic waves as now used in the treatment of bone fractures; and transcutaneous electrical nerve stimulation for pain relief.

Most patients who use CAM are self-referred and do not tell their physicians they are doing so. Thus, their medical record is incomplete, and the possibility of medical risk cannot be addressed. Patients can be asked questions similar to "Have you used or have you been considering other kinds of treatment or medications for relief of your symptoms or to maintain wellness?" Follow-up questions to a positive answer can include asking when she decided to use CAM, what results she was expecting, how she chose the method, and how it has worked for her. This information can then be documented in the patient's medical record.

Safety is the critical issue when a patient asks about the merit of using a CAM product or intervention. The potential can exist for both direct and indirect risks. These risks can include patient delay in or avoidance of seeking appropriate conventional treatment, a misdiagnosis, toxic reactions from ingested substances, and interference with the mechanism of action of a prescribed drug or treatment.

Over-the-counter herbal preparations and dietary supplements, such as those marketed to relieve menopausal symptoms, may be of particular concern to the obstetrician–gynecologist. As defined in the 1994 Dietary Supplement and Health Education Act passed by Congress and as opposed to prescription items, these products are not subject to standardized manufacture, supporting clinical data, or approval or supervision by the U.S. Food and Drug Administration. Thus, there can be uncertainty as to the identity of the active ingredient and the amount of its dose. Also, the chemical composition may vary from manufacturer to manufacturer and by lot number, and there may be adulteration without this being identified on the label. Some of these problems will be addressed with the new federal regulation requiring that dietary supplement ingredients are labeled in a manner analogous to food labels, increased legislated U.S. Food and Drug Administration authority for these products, and increased attention by the Federal Trade Commission to advertised claims.

Concerns about safety can be tempered for some CAM modalities. For instance, it is unlikely that homeopathic preparations, acupuncture, biofeedback, or prayer will be associated with direct adverse side effects. In contrast, intravenous hydrogen peroxide, chelation therapy, and megadosing of supplements can be toxic and dangerous. Accordingly, when informed that the patient is using CAM, her clinician can advise if there is supporting published research, warn about real or potential dangers, ascertain if it can be continued in conjunction with conventional treatment, and monitor for positive and negative effects over time.

Some patients will request a referral to a local alternative care provider. Any such referral should be made only to a state-licensed provider and at an arm's length relationship. All states license chiropractors, but not all license other CAM providers, such as naturopaths, acupuncturists, or massage therapists. Physicians should be aware of possible liability consequences of such referrals. If the referral itself is negligent because it is inconsistent with reasonable practice, the referring physician may be exposed to liability if the patient is injured by the subsequent treatment. Also, liability may arise if the referring physician supervises the CAM care, jointly treats the patient, or knows or should have known that the CAM provider is incompetent.

It can be anticipated that patients will continue to use CAM with or without physician referral. Accompanying this use is the public's expectation that health insurance plans will reimburse for CAM treatment. A growing number of third-party payers have responded by doing so under a variety of clinical guidelines. This willingness can result in conflict between physicians and CAM providers if important operational issues are not addressed. These issues include the creation of protocols and plans of care for specific diagnoses, procedures for monitoring and follow-up with finite clinical endpoints, evidence for safety and effectiveness, and identified criteria for referral to conventional care.

Each physician can determine to what extent he or she wishes to learn more about various aspects of CAM. There are a number of ways to obtain information. Clinical studies in peer-reviewed, conventional medical journals now appear on a regular basis. In addition to continuing medical education courses, there are peer-reviewed medical journals, textbooks, and newsletters devoted to the subject. Computer databases and webpages specifically oriented to CAM now are accessible by both physicians and patients.

In the coming years, it is probable that there will be a blending of conventional medicine with various CAM therapies as evidence-based research data support clinical decision making in patient care. This comprehensive approach may become known as integrated medical care.

Bibliography

Blumenthal M, ed. The complete German Commission E Monographs. Therapeutic guide to herbal medicines. Austin, TX: American Botanical Council, 1998

Chez RA, Jonas WB, Eisenberg D. The physician and complementary and alternative medicine. In: Jonas WB, Levin JS, eds. Essentials of Complementary and Alternative Medicine. Philadelphia: Lippincott Williams & Wilkins, 1999:31–45

Jonas WB, Levin JS, eds. Essentials of complementary and alternative medicine. Philadelphia: Lippincott Williams and Wilkins, 1999

National Institutes of Health. Alternative medicine: expanding medical horizons: a report to the National Institutes of Health on alternative medical systems and practices in the United States. National Institutes of Health, Workshop on Alternative Medicine, 1995; NIH publication no. 94-066

Newall CA, Anderson LA, Phillipson JD. Herbal medicines, a guide for health-care professionals. London: Pharmaceutical Press, 1996

PDR for Herbal Medicines. Montvale, NJ: Medical Economics Co., 1998

Segen JC. Dictionary of alternative medicine. Stamford, Connecticut: Appleton & Lange, 1998

Resources

Newsletters

Complementary Medicine for the Physician, W.B. Saunders Periodicals Customer Service, 6277 Sea Harbor Drive, Orlando, FL 32887-4800, (800) 654-2452

Alternative Therapies in Women's Health, American Health Consultants, PO Box 740056, Atlanta, GA 30374, (800) 688-2421

Alternative Medicine Alert, American Health Consultants, PO Box 740056, Atlanta, GA 30374, (800) 688-2421

HerbalGram, American Botanical Council, PO Box 144345, Austin, TX 78714-4345, (800) 373-7105

Web Sites

The National Library of Medicine (http://www.ncbi.nlm.nih.gov/PubMed/)

The National Center for Complementary and Alternative Medicine (http://nccam.nih.gov/)

The NIH Office of Dietary Supplements (http://odp.od.nih.gov/ods/)

The Richard and Hinda Rosenthal Center for Complementary & Alternative Medicine (http://cpmcnet.columbia.edu/dept/rosenthal/)

The American Botanical Council (http://www.herbalgram.org/)

HealthWorld Online (http://www.healthy.net/)

Quackwatch (www.quackwatch.com)

ACOG Committee Opinion

Committee on Gynecologic Practice

Number 242, October 2000

Concurrent Chemoradiation in the Treatment of Cervical Cancer

Recently, data from several large randomized clinical trials have been published supporting the use of concurrent platinum-based chemotherapy in women who require radiation therapy for treatment of cervical cancer. The results of these well-designed studies are consistent and suggest improved local control and overall survival when cisplatin-based chemotherapy is added for women who will receive radiation therapy as either front-line or salvage therapy for cervical cancer. The risk of death from cervical cancer was reduced by 30–50% in women treated with concurrent chemoradiation. The addition of chemotherapy to radiation therapy appears to benefit women with locally advanced cervical cancer who were treated with primary radiation therapy, as well as those with early-stage disease and poor histologic prognostic factors who were treated with postoperative adjunctive radiation therapy. Toxicity was observed in association with this combination therapy but was manageable.

Based on these data, the National Cancer Institute issued a rare clinical announcement suggesting that "strong consideration should be given to the incorporation of concurrent cisplatin-based chemotherapy with radiation therapy in women who require radiation therapy for treatment of cervical cancer." The Committee on Gynecologic Practice supports this recommendation of the National Cancer Institute.

Bibliography

Keys HM, Bundy BN, Stehman FB, Muderspach LI, Chafe WE, Suggs CL 3rd, et al. Cisplatin, radiation, and adjuvant hysterectomy compared with radiation and adjuvant hysterectomy for bulky stage IB cervical carcinoma. N Engl J Med 1999;340:1154–1161 [published erratum appears in N Engl J Med 1999;341:708]

Morris M, Eifel PJ, Lu J, Grigsby PW, Levenback C, Stevens RE, et al. Pelvic radiation with concurrent chemotherapy compared with pelvic and para-aortic radiation for high-risk cervical cancer. N Engl J Med 1999;340:1137–1143

National Cancer Institute. Clinical announcement: concurrent chemoradiation for cervical cancer. February, 1999. Available at: <http://cancertrials.nci.nih.gov/types/cervical/announcement/text.html>. Retrieved June 16, 2000

ISSN 1074-861X

The American College of Obstetricians and Gynecologists
409 12th Street, SW
PO Box 96920
Washington, DC 20090-6920

12345/43210

Peters WA 3rd, Liu PY, Barrett RJ 2nd, Gordon W Jr, Stock RJ, Berek JS, et al. Concurrent chemotherapy and pelvic radiation therapy compared with pelvic radiation therapy alone as adjuvant therapy after radical surgery in high-risk early-stage cancer of the cervix. J Clin Oncol 2000;18:1606–1613

Rose PG, Bundy BN, Watkins EB, Thigpen JT, Deppe G, Maiman MA, et al. Concurrent cisplatin-based radiotherapy and chemotherapy for locally advanced cervical cancer. N Engl J Med 1999;340:1144–1153 [published erratum appears in N Engl J Med 1999;341:708]

Whitney CW, Sause W, Bundy BN, Malfetano JH, Hannigan EV, Fowler WC Jr, et al. Randomized comparison of fluorouracil plus cisplatin versus hydroxyurea as an adjunct to radiation therapy in stage IIB-IVA carcinoma of the cervix with negative para-aortic lymph nodes: a Gynecologic Oncology Group and Southwest Oncology Group study. J Clin Oncol 1999;17:1339–1348

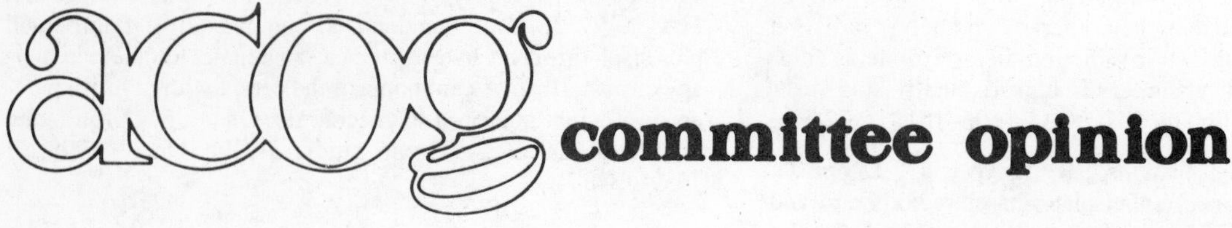

Committee on Adolescent Health Care Number 154—April 1995

Condom Availability for Adolescents

By age 19, 86% of males and 75% of females report being sexually active. In addition, 33% of unmarried males and 26% of unmarried females have experienced sexual intercourse by age 15 (1, 2). Many adolescents report having had four or more sexual partners by the time they are seniors in high school (3).

There are at least two major health consequences of unprotected intercourse among youth. First, teens have a high rate of sexually transmitted diseases (STDs). Each year, 3 million adolescents are infected with STDs, accounting for 25% of the 12 million new STDs that occur annually in the United States (4). Rates of human papillomavirus infection among sexually experienced teenage women can reach up to 50%; the rate of reported cases of infectious syphilis among adolescent women has more than doubled since the mid-1980s; sexually experienced women and men ages 15–19 have the highest rates of gonorrhea and chlamydia (4, 5). Between December 1990 and December 1992, the number of cases of acquired immunodeficiency syndrome (AIDS) among 13–24-year-olds increased by 43% (6). Second, during the last decade, 1 million teenage girls—12% of all women ages 15–19—have become pregnant each year (7).

EFFECTIVENESS OF CONDOMS IN PREVENTING SEXUALLY TRANSMITTED DISEASES AND PREGNANCY

Abstinence is the most effective way for adolescents to avoid STDs and pregnancy. Use of the latex condom should be promoted for sexually active teens because it provides protection against both STDs and unintended pregnancy. Underestimating condom efficacy weakens counseling and inappropriately discourages their use.

Condoms have been shown to be effective in preventing the transmission of herpes simplex virus, hepatitis B virus, Chlamydia trachomatis, cytomegalovirus, and human immunodeficiency virus (HIV) in laboratory studies. There is also evidence from clinical studies that condoms decrease the risks to women from herpes simplex virus, gonorrhea, and trichomonas and reduce transmission of Chlamydia, HIV, and human papillomavirus (8, 9). Natural membrane condoms are not as effective as latex condoms (8). There are inadequate data on the use of the female condom by adolescents.

It is understandable that many young women want to prevent pregnancy with a method that is completely within their control. It is important, however, to educate teenage males and females who depend upon hormonal methods of contraception about the inability of these methods to prevent STDs. Although dual use may be perceived as more difficult to maintain than reliance on a single method, condom use must be promoted in conjunction with other contraceptive methods.

Condoms are effective in preventing pregnancy. One study that compared the relative effectiveness of contraceptive methods showed that 15% of women using condoms experienced contraceptive failure during the first 12 months of use, compared with 25–26% of those using methods such as periodic abstinence or spermicide alone and with 85% of those using no method. According to the 1988 National Survey of Family Growth, contraceptive failure rates vary more by user characteristics, such as income, marital status, and age, than by method (10). Among adolescents, condom failure rates varied widely.

Condom failure rates can be attributed primarily to improper and inconsistent use rather than manufacturing defects or breakage (8, 9, 11, 12). Condom breakage rates are less than 2%, and most breakage is due to incorrect use rather than poor quality. In addition to quality assurance methods used by the manufacturer, condoms are regulated by the U.S. Food and Drug Administration and tested against standards issued by the American Society for Testing and Materials for resistance to breakage and leaks. The U.S. Food and Drug Administration has increased the percentage of batches tested, reducing the risk of the sale of defective condoms (12). The standards are designed to minimize the chance that an approved batch of condoms will contain more than 1.5% that are weak, 0.4% that leak, 2.5% that contain poor latex, or 4% that are the wrong size. If a sample fails these standards, the entire batch is rejected.

FACTORS AFFECTING CONDOM USE

Condom use by adolescents is increasing. Among sexually active 17–19-year-old males living in metropolitan areas, reported rates of condom use at most recent intercourse more than doubled between 1979 and 1988, from 21% to 58% (2). Teenage females who report condom use by their partners increased from 21% to 33% from 1982 to 1988 (13). However, condom use is not consistent. One study found that 31% of sexually active teens always used a condom, 32% used a condom sometimes, and 37% never used one (14). All age groups, including teens, can improve their use of condoms (Fig. 1).

Sexually active teens, male and female, must be taught to use condoms properly, effectively, and consistently. Successful condom use requires: using a new condom for each act of intercourse; putting it on correctly (leaving some room at the tip) prior to penetration; withdrawing while the penis is still erect, holding the condom firmly to keep it from slipping off; and using only water-based lubricants, not those that are petroleum based, like petroleum jelly and baby oil, or cooking oil with animal fat, like lard (9). In addition, young women must learn to communicate the need for condom use to their sexual partners, a skill that is not easy in practice even for older, more experienced women (15). Teens are more likely to use condoms if they (16):

- Receive comprehensive sexuality education
- Talk to their partners about the risk of STDs and AIDS
- Believe that condoms can prevent HIV infection
- Perceive peer norms as supporting condom use
- Are not embarrassed to ask a partner to use condoms
- Carry condoms with them
- Have discussed condom use with a clinician
- Have easy access to condoms

OVERCOMING BARRIERS TO CONDOM USE

Adolescents face many obstacles to obtaining and using condoms. Some of these obstacles relate to confidentiality, cost, access, transportation, embarrassment, objection by a partner, and the perception that the risks of pregnancy and infection are low (14, 17, 18). Although condoms are a widely available nonprescription item, this does not necessarily translate into ready access for adolescents. For example, in a 1988 survey of drugstores and convenience stores by teens in Washington, DC, only 13% of the stores clearly indicated where condoms were shelved. In a third of these stores, condoms were kept behind a counter, necessitating assistance from a store clerk. Furthermore, adolescent females asking for help in finding and purchasing condoms reported encountering "resistance or condemnation" 40% of the time (19).

Eliminating barriers to the use of condoms and establishing condom use as the norm for sexually active teens will help adolescents protect themselves. Instruction and availability of condoms in the schools is one appropriate means to make condoms more acceptable and accessible to adolescents. But, while programs have been implemented in some communities, proposals for school condom programs have engendered controversy in many other communities (20).

Much of the debate about condom availability programs has been ideologic; it has not focused on condom effectiveness or program effectiveness (20). For example, one major objection is that providing condoms will promote sexual activity, yet there is no evidence to indicate that this is true (21). In-depth studies of school-based clinics that dispense birth control found that making contraceptives available in school does not promote sexual activity and may, in fact, decrease it (22). Despite the controversy, a Gallup poll taken in August 1992 found that 68% of 1,316 adults surveyed thought condoms should be available in the schools, and a separate survey of 2,100 high-school seniors showed 81% felt condoms should be available in schools. Seventy-eight percent of these same students felt condom availability did not encourage sexual activity (23, 24).

SUMMARY

Although abstinence should be stressed as the certain way to prevent STDs and pregnancy, sexually

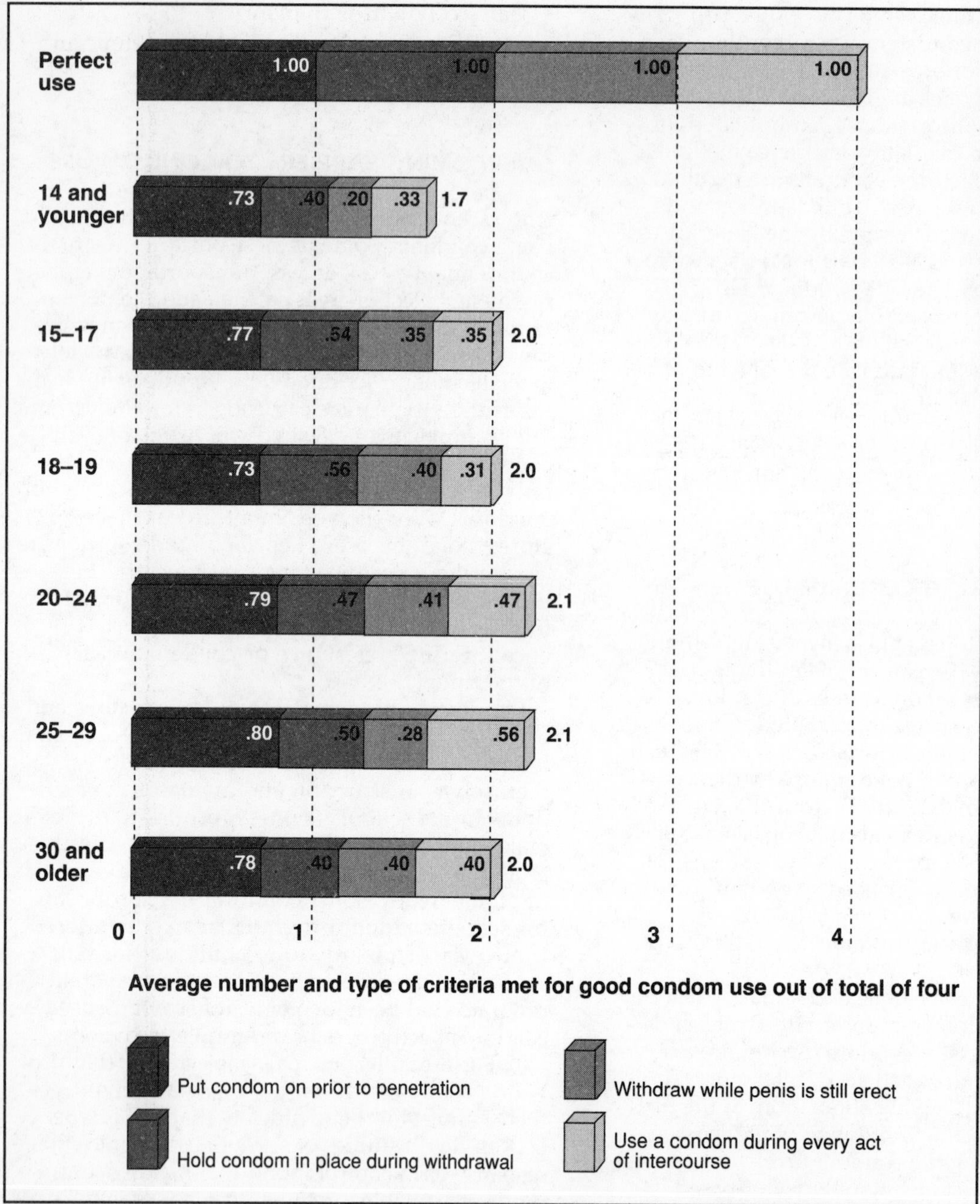

FIG. 1. Condom use needs improvement at all ages. Teenagers do almost as well as older women in trying to follow the criteria for perfect condom use. Source: Tabulations by D. Oakley of data from the University of Michigan longitudinal survey of initial clients at three family planning clinics near Detroit. February 1987–April 1989. Note: Condoms were the main contraceptive method used for any study month, and women were sexually active at least one of those months. (Reproduced with the permission of The Alan Guttmacher Institute from Sex and America's Teenagers, New York, The Alan Guttmacher Institute, 1994)

active teens, male and female, must nonetheless be taught to use condoms properly, effectively, and consistently. The latex condom should be made widely available to young people. Ideally, young persons should have access to education and counseling when contraception is dispensed.

However, condoms should be made easily available without any requirement for education. Condoms should be available not only through families, medical facilities, and commercial channels, but also through other appropriate and informed persons, without cost if possible, at sites where adolescents congregate. These sites may include schools, clubs, and other youth-serving agencies. A clear message from the medical community supporting condom use will enhance compliance.

REFERENCES

1. Centers for Disease Control. Premarital sexual experience among adolescent women—United States, 1970–1988. MMWR 1991;39:929–932
2. Sonenstein FL, Pleck JH, Ku LC. Sexual activity, condom use and AIDS awareness among adolescent males. Fam Plann Perspect 1989;21:152–158
3. Centers for Disease Control. Selected behaviors that increase risk for HIV infection among high school students—United States, 1990. MMWR 1992;41:231, 237–240
4. Centers for Disease Control and Prevention. Division of STD/HIV Prevention 1992 Annual Report. Atlanta, Georgia: CDC, 1993
5. Webster LA, Berman SM, Greenspan JR. Surveillance for gonorrhea and primary and secondary syphilis among adolescents, United States—1981–1991. MMWR 1993;42(SS-3):1–11
6. Centers for Disease Control and Prevention. CDC HIV/AIDS Surveillance Year-End Edition. U.S. cases reported through December 1992. Atlanta, Georgia: CDC, 1993
7. Henshaw SK. Teenage abortion, birth and pregnancy statistics by state, 1988. Fam Plann Perspect 1993;25: 122–126
8. Cates W Jr, Stone KM. Family planning, sexually transmitted diseases and contraceptive choice: a literature update—part I. Fam Plann Perspect 1992;24:75–84
9. Centers for Disease Control and Prevention. Update: barrier protection against HIV infection and other sexually transmitted diseases. MMWR 1993;42:589, 591–597
10. Jones EF, Forrest JD. Contraceptive failure rates based on the 1988 NSFG. Fam Plann Perspect 1992;24:12–19
11. Trussell J, Warner DL, Hatcher RA. Condom slippage and breakage rates. Fam Plann Perspect 1992;24:20–23
12. Johns Hopkins University. Condoms—now more than ever. Popul Rep H 1990;28(8):1–36
13. Mosher WD. Contraceptive practice in the United States, 1982–1988. Fam Plann Perspect 1990;22: 198–205
14. Siegel D, Lazarus N, Krasnovsky F, Durbin M, Chesney M. AIDS knowledge, attitudes, and behavior among inner city, junior high school students. J Sch Health 1991;61:160–165
15. Rickert VI, Gottlieb A, Jay S. A comparison of three clinic-based AIDS education programs on female adolescents' knowledge, attitudes, and behavior. J Adolesc Health Care 1990;11:298–303
16. Joffe A. Adolescents and condom use. Am J Dis Child 1993;147:746–754
17. Kegeles SM, Adler NE, Irwin CE Jr. Adolescents and condoms. Associations of beliefs with intentions to use. Am J Dis Child 1989;143:911–915
18. Ford K, Norris A. Urban African-American and Hispanic adolescents and young adults: who do they talk to about AIDS and condoms? What are they learning? AIDS Educ Prev 1991;3:197–206
19. Teen's survey of stores in the District of Columbia on accessibility of family methods. Washington DC: Center for Population Options Teen Council, 1988
20. Samuels SE, Smith MD, eds. Condoms in the schools. Menlo Park, California: The Henry J. Kaiser Family Foundation, 1993
21. Kirby D. Research and evaluation. In: Samuels SE, Smith MD, eds. Condoms in the schools. Menlo Park, California: The Henry J. Kaiser Family Foundation, 1993:89–109
22. Kirby D, Waszak C, Ziegler J. Six school-based clinics: their reproductive health services and impact on sexual behavior. Fam Plann Perspect 1991;23:6–16
23. Examiner News Service. Polls: most want schools to pass out condoms. San Francisco Examiner, August 28, 1992, A13
24. National Scholastic Surveys Poll, April 1992. USA Today, April 24, 1992, D1

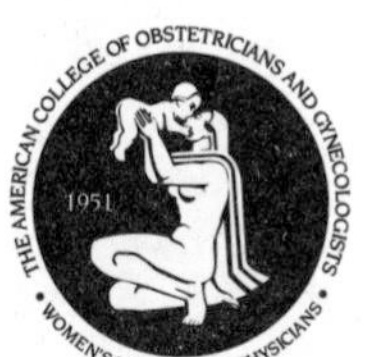

ISSN 1074-861X

The American College of Obstetricians and Gynecologists
409 12th Street, SW • Washington, DC 20024-2188

12345/98765

ACOG

Committee on
Professional Liability

Committee Opinion

Number 236, June 2000 (Replaces No. 150, December 1994)

Coping with the Stress of Malpractice Litigation

The American College of Obstetricians and Gynecologists (ACOG) has long been concerned about the psychologic and emotional impact of medical malpractice litigation on physicians, especially because 76.5% of ACOG Fellows have been sued at least once. As studies have shown, defendant physicians may experience a wide range of distressing emotions and increased stress, which can disrupt their personal lives and the lives of their families, their relationships with patients, and their medical practices. Because a medical liability case in obstetrics and gynecology takes an average of 4.2 years to resolve, this stressful period can seem interminable for all involved.

Physicians often are told by claims adjusters and defense attorneys that they should not speak to anyone regarding any aspect of the malpractice case. Nevertheless, physicians often need to express emotional responses to being sued. Literal adherence to the advice to "speak to no one" can result in isolation, increased stress, and dysfunctional behavior. Such behavior may jeopardize family relationships and may also affect the physician's ability to function professionally and to represent himself or herself appropriately and effectively during a trial. Therefore, the physician is encouraged to inform family members of the lawsuit, the allegations, the potential for publicity, and any expected testimony while maintaining confidentiality. Children should be told about the lawsuit and their questions honestly answered, commensurate with their age and ability to process the information. Open communication with family members will assist in reducing emotional isolation and self-blame.

Certainly, legal and clinical aspects of a case must be kept confidential. An exception to this rule, however, might be in the context of professional counseling. Any clinical aspects of a malpractice case that are discussed in counseling should be disclosed within the confines of a formal counselor–patient relationship to ensure the confidentiality privilege. Confidentiality may be lost if third parties are present.

Obstetrician–gynecologists should recognize that being a defendant in a medical liability lawsuit can be one of life's most stressful experiences. Although negative emotions in response to a lawsuit are normal, physicians may need help from professionals or peers to cope with this stress. State or

This document provides risk management information that is current as of the date issued and is subject to change. This document does not define a standard of care nor should it be interpreted as legal advice.

ISSN 1074-861X

The American College of Obstetricians and Gynecologists
409 12th Street, SW
PO Box 96920
Washington, DC 20090-6920

12345/43210

local medical societies and medical liability insurance carriers often sponsor support groups for defendant physicians and their families. In the absence of such services, individual professional counseling can be of great benefit.

Bibliography

Bark P, Vincent C, Olivieri L, Jones A. Impact of litigation on senior clinicians: implications for risk management. Qual Health Care 1997;6:7–13

Charles, SC. How to handle the stress of litigation. Clin Plast Surg 1999;26:69–77

Charles, SC. The doctor–patient relationship and medical malpractice litigation. Bull Menninger Clin 1993;57:195–207

Charles, SC. Psychological reactions to medical malpractice suits and the development of support groups as a response. Instr Course Lect 1988;37:289–292

Frisch PR, Charles SC, Gibbons RP, Hedeker D. Role of previous claims and specialty on the effectiveness of risk management education for office-based physicians. West J Med 1995; 163:346–350

Martin CA, Wilson JF, Fiebelman ND 3d, Gurley DN, Miller TW. Physicians' psychologic reactions to malpractice litigation. South Med J 1991;84:1300–1304

Pyskoty CE, Byrne TE, Charles SC, Frankel KJ. Malpractice litigation as a factor in choosing a medical specialty. West J Med 1990;152:309–312

ACOG

Committee on
Practice Management

Committee Opinion

Number 171, May 1996

Cost Containment in Medical Care

The quality of medical care available in the United States is unsurpassed. Physicians continually strive to identify and implement diagnostic and therapeutic advancements. The quality of and access to health care in this country has improved the quality of life and increased its duration.

The dramatic increase in health care costs over the past two decades, however, has created demands and initiatives in both the public and private sectors for curbing expenses. A variety of mechanisms have been proposed to contain costs, including reimbursement reductions and limits, practice guidelines, utilization review mechanisms, benefit reductions and limits, and increased cost sharing.

The American College of Obstetricians and Gynecologists (ACOG) fully supports and endorses the provision of cost-effective medical treatment. Physicians must be involved in the changes that are necessary to meet this goal. As the only medical specialists whose primary focus is improving women's health, we believe participation of obstetrician–gynecologists in designing, implementing, and testing cost-containment efforts is crucial. We encourage Fellows to become involved.

To assist Fellows in working with public and private health care payers and policy-making bodies, we offer the following guidance on cost containment efforts:

- Health care providers should use the most efficient and effective delivery systems and techniques available, consistent with quality medical care.
- While striving to contain health care costs, obstetrician–gynecologists must focus on their primary goal of providing quality care for all women. Physicians are expected to be, and should be, the primary advocates for the medical needs of their patients. All analyses of cost-containment proposals should begin by asking these questions: What impact will this have on the quality of women's health care? Will this be effective in appropriately containing health care costs? Will this simply shift costs to another group or individual?
- Cost constraints must be shared equitably across the health care system.
- A patient is entitled to her physician's advice on the most appropriate medical care, whether or not her insurance provides reimbursement for the recommended service, drug, or device. Physicians should be cognizant of costs in providing information on alternative modes of treatment and make a reasonable attempt to inform the patient of the relative costs

ISSN 1074-861X

The American College of Obstetricians and Gynecologists
409 12th Street, SW
P.O. Box 96920
Washington, DC 20090-6920

12345/09876

of each. Physicians should advocate the most appropriate treatment, drug, device, or test, not necessarily the newest, the most expensive, or the least expensive.

- Cost-containment measures must not discourage obtaining appropriate medical care. Care of low-income women and children is of particular concern to the College. Access to indicated medical treatment for this underserved population should be assured.
- Preventive care must be encouraged to maintain quality health care. Cost-containment measures are unacceptable if they adversely affect access to appropriate preventive services including, but not limited to, preconceptional care, prenatal care, family planning, cancer screening, and immunizations.
- Health care insurers, public and private, have the obligation to notify prospective enrollees about mechanisms, policies, and regulations that may limit their access to health care services or to specific providers. Enrollees must be informed of the procedures for appealing these decisions.
- Reduction of professional liability costs is essential to any successful cost-containment strategy. Cost-containment mechanisms that increase physician risk of liability are inappropriate.
- Cost-containment measures that result in other direct or indirect costs to the patient for appropriate, timely, and convenient care exist. If the measures are used, resultant hidden costs should be considered in calculating economic savings to the health care system. For example, if a health insurance plan does not pay for a procedure that the physician and the patient believe is necessary, and the patient pays for the procedure or it is provided at no charge, this cannot be considered a "savings," even though it is no longer a cost to the employer or the insurer.
- Cost-containment measures should not preclude or exclude allowances for the psychosocial needs of patients when determining appropriateness and duration of hospitalization or therapy.
- Managed care decisions regarding medical treatment policy must be made by qualified physicians. When possible, medical care decisions should reflect outcomes-based data contained in current literature. In the absence of such data, clinicians must have input into medical treatment decisions.
- Organizations, including medical specialty societies, that develop practice guidelines must consider the cost-effectiveness of these guidelines.

ACOG

Committee on Health Care for Underserved Women

Committee Opinion

Number 201, March 1998

Cultural Competency in Health Care

The racial and ethnic composition of the population of the United States has changed significantly during the past decade. Between 1981 and 1991 there was a 90% increase in the Asian population; a 50% increase in people of Hispanic origin; a 43% increase in Native Americans, Eskimos, and Aleuts; and a 15% increase in the African-American population. The white non-Hispanic population, however, increased by only 4%. As of August 1, 1997, Asians and Pacific Islanders comprised 3.8% of the total U.S. population, Hispanics (of any race) comprised 11%, African Americans comprised 12.7%, and Native Americans, Eskimos and Aleuts comprised 0.9% (1). In some areas of the United States, the combined number of African Americans, Hispanics, and Asians now exceeds that of whites.

Behind these figures are countless cultural differences that define and distinguish an increasingly diverse populace. Defined as ". . . the thoughts, communications, actions, customs, beliefs, values, and institutions of a racial, ethnic, religious, or social group" (2), culture is what distinguishes one group from another. Persons from similar racial and ethnic groups, countries of origin, and socioeconomic levels all have distinct cultures. Similarly, adolescents also have a separate and distinct culture. The shared systems of a given culture serve to facilitate interactions among its members. Conversely, interactions between members of differing cultures can be complicated by a lack of cultural awareness.

Culture and Health Care

During every health care encounter, the culture of the patient, the culture of the provider, and the culture of medicine converge and impact upon the patterns of health care utilization, compliance with recommended medical interventions, and health outcomes. Often, however, health care providers may not appreciate the effect of culture on either their own lives, their professional conduct, or the lives of their patients (3). When an individual's culture is at odds with that of the prevailing medical establishment, the patient's culture will generally prevail, often straining provider–patient relationships (4). Providers can minimize such situations by increasing their understanding and awareness of the culture(s) they serve. Increased sensitivity, in turn, can facilitate positive interactions with the health care delivery system and optimal health outcomes for the patients served, resulting in increased patient and provider satisfaction.

ISSN 1074-861X

The American College of Obstetricians and Gynecologists
409 12th Street, SW
PO Box 96920
Washington, DC 20090-6920

12345/21098

The Culture of Medicine

Medicine has a culture of its own, with traditional codes of conduct that have been passed on from generation to generation. This culture is pervasive within the medical profession, and it often supersedes the individual culture of the health care provider (5). The U.S. health care system has historically been dominated by traditional, middle-class values. Medical practice operates on the assumption that patients will arrive on time, will conform to physician expectations, and will not ask too many or too demanding questions (6). It is a system designed to offer diagnosis and treatment options to an individual patient who, in turn, is expected to make decisions and follow through on treatments. Furthermore, it is underpinned by the assumption that those seeking care will understand how the system works and are able and willing to comply with its stipulations.

This system and the values that shape it, however, may compromise access to care for patients from other cultures. In many health care settings, insufficient credence may be given to such cultural factors as the role of the extended family in treatment decisions, the role of spiritual or religious beliefs in health care decisions, or the role of traditional remedies for cures and relief from symptoms (7). Progress often may be measured in terms of compliance or outcomes, and the impact of the quality of interpersonal relationships involved not valued appropriately.

The physical structure of the health care system may also impose unintended cultural barriers for patients and their families. Hospitals, for example, often have detailed and complex requirements surrounding admissions, visiting hours, and meal times. Additionally, the size of many hospitals and outpatient complexes, the volume of paperwork, and the constant use of professional jargon can intimidate new immigrants, ethnic minorities, and those with little exposure to the health care system (8).

Cultural Competency

As the health care system changes and focuses increasingly on primary care and prevention, it is critical that providers develop ongoing and trusting relationships with their patients. To provide appropriate care to an increasingly diverse patient population, providers are encouraged to develop what has come to be known as *cultural competency*. This refers to "the knowledge and interpersonal skills that allow providers to understand, appreciate, and work with individuals from cultures other than their own. It involves an awareness and acceptance of cultural differences, self awareness, knowledge of a patient's culture, and adaptation of skills" (9).

Cultural competency is particularly relevant to maternity care. The birth of a child initiates another generation into a family and affords a new opportunity for cultural traditions to solidify, thus strengthening the bond between parents and child and serving to unify family members. As such, pregnancy and childbirth are often entangled in complex cultural beliefs and traditions that may be less obvious in other settings. Additionally, the perinatal period is often an immigrant family's first significant contact with the health care system. The sensitivity and understanding with which a pregnant woman and her family are treated can have a long-term impact on the family's future patterns of health care utilization.

The challenge for obstetrician–gynecologists and other prenatal care providers is to incorporate those individual family traditions that will strengthen family ties and provide a support system for the new mother and child into a medically safe birth experience. Many families from other cultures perceive technology-centered hospital births as leaving little room for the inclusion of individual family traditions and values. One way in which prenatal care providers can accommodate a pregnant woman's cultural preferences into her experience of pregnancy is through the use of a "birth plan." In a birth plan, a woman outlines the activities she would like to have take place at her child's birth, such as the people she would like to be present, her desires about clothing for the new baby, or her decision regarding the circumcision of a male infant. Every effort is then made to accommodate her wishes, as long as they fall within the guidelines of safe maternity practice. If an activity falls outside the usual guidelines of safe practice, discussion with the patient and her family can often lead to a safe substitution or compromise.

Learning from the Community

In addition to valuing diversity, providers should be sensitive to the unique needs of women in the communities they serve. Communication barriers must be examined and addressed (10). For those who do not speak English, appropriately trained interpreters should be hired, and forms, patient education materials, and signs should all be accurately translated (11). If practice resources do not allow for the hiring of additional staff, community resources should be explored and, when appropriate, used. Providers also should render services in a manner that is appropriate to the community's culture(s). This may require providers or their staff to meet with representatives from the community to discuss how the delivery of services might be modified. Health education programs jointly sponsored with community organizations and located at appropriate sites can help to demystify the health care system and familiarize women with preventive health care measures in a nonthreatening environment. Because patients interact with many people in the office and hospital, all staff should receive either cultural competency training (preferably provided by a member of the community being served) or appropriate resources for self-education.

Every health care encounter provides an opportunity to have a positive impact on patient health. By learning more about their patients' culture(s), health care providers can maximize this potential. The examples in Table 1 illustrate some of the many benefits that can be gained by learning about patients' cultures and investing in cultural competency training.

Table 1. Cultural Competency in Practice

Old Paradigm	**Cross-Cultural Competence**
An Amish woman undergoes a cesarean delivery in a hospital. After surgery the woman and her husband are interviewed by a social worker who was routinely called to see them by a nurse who noted that they had no health insurance. The social worker begins to tell them immediately how to enroll in Medicaid. They are visibly upset.	The social worker notices on rounds that the Amish couple have no health insurance and she wonders how the couple will pay their hospital bill. Before she approaches the couple she learns from the couple's physician that Amish do not believe in or accept what they consider to be welfare. When she meets with the couple she helps them plan transportation home because they do not have a car, and she assists them with reaching other members of their Amish community who, by tradition, provide financial and other assistance to their own people.
A physician addresses a 50-year-old African-American woman by her first name.	This same patient is addressed by all health care workers as Mrs. Clifford. Using first names for patients, especially for minority patients, shows disrespect.
A nurse insists that a young Hispanic mother sign a consent form for a cesarean delivery.	The entire staff involves the woman's husband and family in a discussion of the need to undergo a cesarean birth. Among many women of Hispanic heritage, it is customary to have a man give consent for treatment.
A woman misses her appointment for colposcopy. The nurses in the clinic make many attempts to reach her by telephone without success.	The hospital asks a peer health counselor to locate the patient and explain to her the reason why the colposcopy is necessary. When the peer counselor locates the patient, she discovers that the woman's phone has been disconnected because of lack of money to pay the phone bill. The woman's 5-year-old son had a high fever and diarrhea on the day of the colposcopy appointment. She had just enough money and time to get him to a pediatrician. Her son was hospitalized.
An elderly Chinese woman is asked by her doctor to go to the lab to have blood drawn for tests. She takes the lab slip but does not get the tests as ordered.	The primary care provider notes the woman's hesitation and asks her what she is worried about. She tells him that she believes that blood taken from her body will never be replenished and she is weak already. The provider spends time explaining how blood is replaced.
A woman sees a gynecologist for the first time. He is sensitive to her needs but keeps insisting that she consider using birth control. She had filled in a form saying she was sexually active. She is "not married." The woman is upset and refuses to see this gynecologist again.	The physician takes time in asking the sexual history. In asking about sexual activity, he probes gently. One question asked very openly is "Do you have sex with men, women, or both?" He then learns that she is a lesbian in a long-term committed relationship.

(continued)

Table 1. Cultural Competency in Practice *(continued)*

Old Paradigm	**Cross-Cultural Competence**
A couple is newly arrived in the United States from Afghanistan. The wife is obviously in pain. They do not speak English well, so an interpreter is found. The interpreter appears to be having some difficulty interpreting the woman's symptoms. The doctor is rushed. He cannot find any abnormalities on physical examination so he sends the patient home. She returns later with a ruptured ectopic pregnancy and is immediately admitted to the operating room.	The physician notices that the interpreter is not able to communicate well with the couple. He takes the time to discover the problem. The interpreter speaks Farsi; the couple speaks to each other in Dari, but much historical information is lost. The physician admits the patient for appropriate tests and an unruptured ectopic is diagnosed.
A young woman has recently moved to a city from a farm. She has four small children and is 4 months pregnant. She is always late for her appointments and is made to wait until everyone else is seen before she can be cared for.	The staff show concern and inquire about her difficulties. She has no one to take care of her children, so she must bring them to the prenatal clinic for her appointments. She needs to take two buses to get to the clinic, and she does not read. A peer counselor arranges for help with learning the bus route and planning her trips. She is also referred to a literacy program for help. One of her first triumphs is learning to recognize the signs on the buses. Over the course of her pregnancy, she learns to read the bus route map and schedules.

Modified from Leppert PC. Cultural competency. In: Leppert PC, Howard FM Jr, eds. Primary care for women. Philadelphia: Lippincott-Raven, 1997

Conclusion

Cultural competency is an ongoing and interactive process, based upon respect for others' beliefs and traditions. A culturally competent health care system values diversity, has the capacity for cultural self-assessment, is conscious of the dynamics inherent in any multicultural encounter, and has developed the necessary adaptations to service delivery that reflect an understanding and appreciation of cultural diversity (11). For providers of women's health care, cultural competency requires the integration of accepted and safe medical practice with the beliefs and customs of the women being served. As the cultural makeup of our nation diversifies, it is imperative that providers develop appropriate methods to ensure access to services. The first step in this process is to develop an understanding of the cultures represented in the communities served. The impact of such a step will be felt positively by both providers and their patients.

References

1. Statistical abstract of the United States: 1997. 117th ed. Washington, DC: U.S. Bureau of the Census, 1997
2. Cross TL, Bazron BJ, Dennis KW, Isaacs MR. Towards a culturally competent system of care: volume 1: a monograph on effective services for minority children who are severely emotionally disturbed. Washington, DC: CASSP Technical Assistance Center, Georgetown University Child Development Center, 1989
3. Voices of the communities: a survey of health care experiences of 22 medically underserved communities in the Seattle area. Seattle: Cross-Cultural Health Care Project, Pacific Medical Center, 1995 March
4. Leppert PC, Washington K, Partner SF. Teaching sensitivity to cultural issues in women's health care in a community hospital setting. Am J Prev Med 1996;12:69–70
5. Pachter L. Culture and clinical care. Folk illness beliefs and behaviors and their implications for health care delivery. JAMA 1994;271:690–694
6. Leppert PC. Cultural competency. In: Leppert PC, Howard FM Jr, eds. Primary care for women. Philadelphia: Lipincott-Raven, 1997:939–942
7. Kohn S. Dismantling sociocultural barriers to care. Healthcare Forum Journal 1995 May/June;30–33
8. Chapman TW. Opening doors for your patients. Trustee 1995; 48:16–20
9. Davis BJ, Voegtle KH. Culturally competent health care for adolescents: a guide for primary care providers. Chicago: American Medical Association, 1994
10. Augustyn M, Maiman LA. Psychological and sociological barriers to prenatal care. Women's Health Issues 1994;4: 20–28
11. Tawara D, Taylor MA. Getting started . . . planning, implementing and evaluating culturally competent service delivery systems for children with special health care needs and their families. Washington, DC: Maternal & Child Health, National Center for Cultural Competence, George-town University Child Development Center, 1997

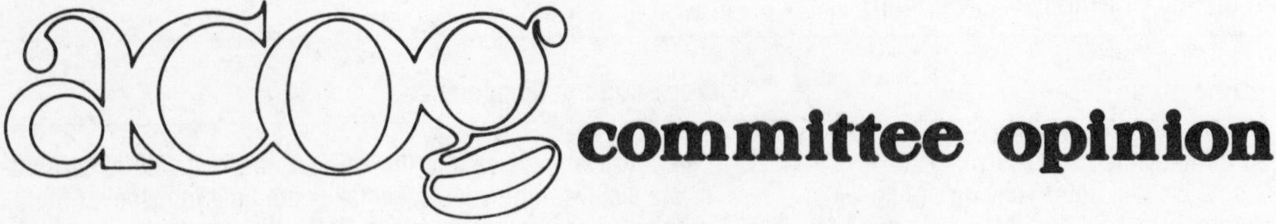

Committee on Genetics

Number 101—November 1991

Current Status of Cystic Fibrosis Carrier Screening

BACKGROUND

Cystic fibrosis (CF) is the most common serious autosomal recessive disease in North American caucasians of European ancestry. In this population, the disease frequency is about 1 in 2,500 live births and the calculated carrier frequency is about 1 in 25 individuals (1). Each offspring (male or female) of parents who are both CF carriers has a 25% chance of being affected with CF. Common clinical manifestations of CF include meconium ileus, chronic obstructive pulmonary disease leading to bronchiectasis and respiratory failure, pancreatic exocrine insufficiency with steatorrhea, liver cirrhosis, and failure to thrive. The clinical course of CF is highly variable, ranging from death in the neonatal period due to complications of meconium ileus to survival into the fifth and sixth decade; about one-half of patients can be expected to live to age 26 or longer (1).

Until the mid-1980s, families known to be at increased risk for CF could be offered only genetic counseling, using risks based on Mendelian principles. In recent years, however, a number of important scientific advances have been made. First, microvillar intestinal enzyme levels proved to be decreased in the amniotic fluid of the majority of women carrying fetuses affected with CF, although the sensitivity and specificity of this assay were less than optimal (2). Later, use of polymorphic DNA markers closely linked to the CF gene locus on chromosome 7 made possible prenatal diagnosis using either amniotic fluid cells or chorionic villi samples. This method has a very high degree of accuracy for most carrier couples. However, DNA from the relative affected was necessary for testing (3, 4). For many close relatives of CF patients (eg, siblings, aunts, and uncles), carrier testing by DNA linkage studies is informative and has a high degree of accuracy (5).

Most recently, the CF gene has been cloned and sequenced (6-8). In the U.S. caucasian population of European ancestry (excluding certain ethnic groups such as Ashkenazic Jews and Hispanics), about 75% of the mutations in CF patients correspond to a particular three-base-pair deletion. The deletion results in the loss of a phenylalanine residue at amino acid position 508 (designated ΔF508) from the 1,480-amino coding region of the CF gene. A number of other mutations in the gene have been described in CF patients.

These advances provide a basis for understanding the pathophysiology of CF and offer hope that improved therapy can be developed. They also have immediate implications for the identification of carriers of a mutant CF gene (9). Carrier screening would entail analysis of DNA from blood samples or other tissues. Such screening would allow couples to make more informed reproductive decisions with regard to the risk of CF in their offspring.

STATUS

In March 1990, the National Institutes of Health (NIH) Workshop on Population Screening for the Cystic Fibrosis Gene was convened to make suggestions regarding the introduction of CF screening into medical practice. The NIH panel concluded the following (10):

> Unlike testing in the general population, testing for carriers in families in which the disease has occurred is nearly 100% informative. This is because carrier testing can be performed with linkage analysis in addition to mutation analysis when there is a DNA sample available from an affected person in a family. Therefore, testing should be offered to all individuals and couples with a family history of CF [eg, a parent, sibling, uncle, aunt, niece, nephew, or cousin with CF]. This makes it more important than ever for pro-

> viders of medical care to obtain family histories, particularly for patients of reproductive age.
>
> [However,] there is a consensus that under the current circumstances population-based screening should not be recommended for individuals and couples with a negative family history. (Emphasis added.)

The ACOG Committee on Obstetrics: Maternal and Fetal Medicine concurs with this consensus.

Testing for the ΔF508 deletion and other additional mutations is imperfect. It will detect only one-half to two-thirds of carrier couples, depending on the specific tests performed. Furthermore, in a significant proportion of couples tested (6%), only one partner will be found to be a carrier of a CF mutation. Since the other partner may still be a carrier of an uncommon CF mutation, the risk of CF offspring may be four to six times greater in these couples than in the general population. Highly accurate prenatal diagnosis is not available to resolve this risk.

The NIH panel strongly urged that pilot programs be conducted to investigate research questions in the delivery of population-based screening for CF carriers. Issues that need to be addressed include the effectiveness of educational materials, the level of utilization of screening, laboratory aspects, counseling issues, and the beneficial and deleterious effects of screening. Of particular importance are the consequences of screening couples in which only one partner has an identified CF mutation.

The NIH panel set forth the following screening guidelines:

- Screening should be voluntary, and confidentiality must be ensured.
- Screening requires informed consent. Educational material to be used before screening should explain the hazards (eg, psychosocial effects and loss of insurability) and benefits of choosing to be tested or not to be tested.
- Providers of screening services have the obligation to ensure that adequate education and counseling are included in the program.
- Quality control of all aspects of the laboratory testing, including systematic proficiency testing, is required and should be implemented as soon as possible.
- There should be equal access to testing.

FUTURE

Since the NIH statement was released, testing for several of the most common CF mutations has increased the carrier detection rate to approximately 85%. NIH plans to fund pilot programs for CF screening. The committee recognizes that this is a rapidly evolving field and that new scientific information or technologic developments may alter this opinion in the near future. It is anticipated that population-based CF screening will be introduced into routine medical practice in the foreseeable future.

REFERENCES

1. Boat TF, Welsh MJ, Beaudet AL. Cystic fibrosis. In: Scriver CR, Beaudet AL, Sly WS, Valle D, eds. The metabolic basis of inherited disease. 6th ed. New York: McGraw-Hill, 1989, 2649–2680
2. Brock DJ, Clarke HA, Barron L. Prenatal diagnosis of cystic fibrosis by microvillar enzyme assay on a sequence of 258 pregnancies. Hum Genet 1988;78: 271–275
3. Tsui LC, Buchwald M, Barker D, Braman JC, Knolton R, Schumm JW, et al. Cystic fibrosis locus defined by a genetically linked polymorphic DNA marker. Science 1985;230: 1054–1057
4. White R, Woodward S, Leppert M, O'Connell P, Hoff M, Herbst J, et al. A closely linked genetic marker for cystic fibrosis. Nature 1985;318:382–384
5. Beaudet AL, Feldman GL, Fernbach SD, Buffone GJ, O'Brien WE. Linkage disequilibrium, cystic fibrosis, and genetic counseling. Am J Hum Genet 1989;44:319–326
6. Rommens JM, Iannuzzi MC, Kerem BS, Drumm ML, Melmer G, Dean M, et al. Identification of the cystic fibrosis gene: chromosome walking and jumping. Science 1989;245:1059–1065
7. Riordan JR, Rommens JM, Kerem BS, Alon N, Rozmahel R, Grzelczak Z, et al. Identification of the cystic fibrosis gene: cloning and characterization of complementary DNA. Science 1989;245:1066–1073
8. Kerem B, Rommens JM, Buchanan JA, Markiewicz D, Cox TK, Chakravarti A, et al. Identification of the cystic fibrosis gene: genetic analysis. Science 1989;245:1073–1080
9. Elias S, Annas GJ, Simpson JL. Carrier screening for cystic fibrosis: implications for obstetric and gynecologic practice. Am J Obstet Gynecol 1991;164:1077–1083
10. Statement from the National Institutes of Health Workshop on Population Screening for Cystic Fibrosis Gene. N Engl J Med 1990;323:70–71

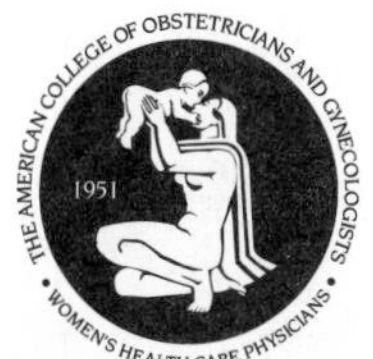

This document reflects emerging clinical and scientific advances as of the date issued and is subject to change. The information should not be construed as dictating an exclusive course of treatment or procedure to be followed.

The American College of Obstetricians and Gynecologists
409 12th Street, SW • Washington, DC 20024-2188

3456/876

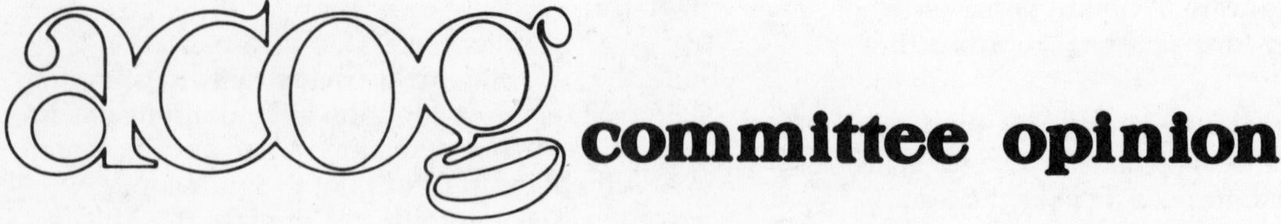

Committee on Ethics Number 87—November 1990

Deception

Deception is the deliberate misrepresentation of facts through words or actions in order to make a person believe that which is not true. Because human interaction and self-determination depend upon use of accurate information, there is a strong presumption that deception either by imparting or by withholding information is unethical.

Deception, even when intended to benefit the patient, always requires justification. The rare cases of justifiable deception are more properly discussed in the context of informed consent. The following opinion is intended to address deceptive behavior which cannot be justified. It is concerned primarily with deception as a means of abusing power in a professional relationship.

The primary duty of physicians is to apply their knowledge in a way that both promotes the health and respects the autonomy of their patients. Insofar as physicians possess greater knowledge about the intricacies of diagnosis and treatment, they have a fiduciary responsibility to patients. While professional knowledge gives physicians an advantage in the relationship, their professional commitment is to use that knowledge on behalf of patients. Unless physicians share knowledge and information, patients cannot exercise autonomy in integrating personal values and concerns. Deception for the purpose of exploiting any imbalance in the relationship in order to benefit physicians at patients' expense, economically or any other way, is unethical.

Exploitative deception can occur in the way physicians represent their expertise to patients and in the way they communicate with patients regarding medical diagnosis and treatment. The forms deception can take include explicit lying, deception by implication, and deception by omission of information that patients need to make decisions in their own regard. Examples of these kinds of deception can help to clarify their seriousness.

DECEPTION BY EXPLICIT LYING

It is unethical for a physician deliberately to misstate facts, for example, to lie about his or her credentials, experience, and/or success rates. It is also unethical to misrepresent facts about conditions or treatments that apply to the patient, such as complication rates for a procedure.

DECEPTION BY IMPLICATION

Deception by implication is a more insidious and more frequent dereliction. An example is citing national experience and success rates in infertility procedures, implying that the same data apply locally as well. Another example of unethical behavior is alarming a patient by implication about abnormal, but relatively innocuous conditions, thereby promoting excessive diagnostic procedures, unnecessary surgery or other over-treatment. Conversely, it is deceptive to imply that a condition or procedure entails fewer risks than actually exist.

DECEPTION BY OMISSION OF INFORMATION

Deception by omission can also be unethical. An example is failure to disclose options or information that might lead a patient to choose a different physician or a different mode of treatment. Similarly, failure to disclose a medical alternative that is therapeutically equal but less advantageous to the physician than a surgical intervention manipulates a patient's choice and may expose her to hazards or expense she would prefer to avoid.

Conflict of interest, or the appearance of conflict of interest, ought to be avoided insofar as possible. When unavoidable, conflict of interest that can be anticipated must be evaluated in advance and discussed with patients. If it arises in the course of diagnosis or therapy, it must then be disclosed and resolved without deception. For example, failure to disclose an interest in an imaging center or laboratory where a referral might result in financial benefit to the physician, is unethical. On the other hand deception may be involved in cases when undisclosed financial arrangements result in under-treatment of a patient. Examples of this could occur when professionals profit from inappropriately limiting care.

THE RISK OF SELF-DECEPTION

When professional prestige or financial gain is involved, self-deception is an ever-present possibility. That is, relevant information potentially detrimental to one's interests may either not be sought or may be consciously or unconsciously suppressed. To maintain professional integrity, physicians need to monitor regularly the motivations that underlie their policies on the disclosure of information to patients.

SUMMARY

Deception is the deliberate misrepresentation of facts through words or actions in order to make a person believe that which is not true. The forms deception can take include explicit lying, deception by implication, and deception by omission of information that patients need to make decisions in their own regard. Deception intended to advantage the physician economically or otherwise at the expense of the patient is unethical.

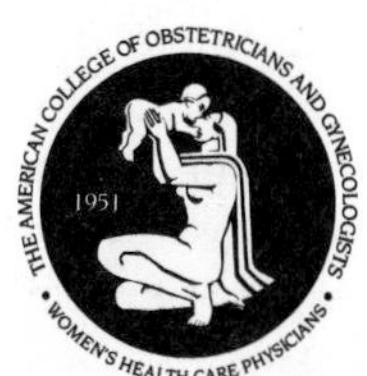

The American College of Obstetricians and Gynecologists
409 12th Street, SW • Washington, DC 20024-2188

678/21098

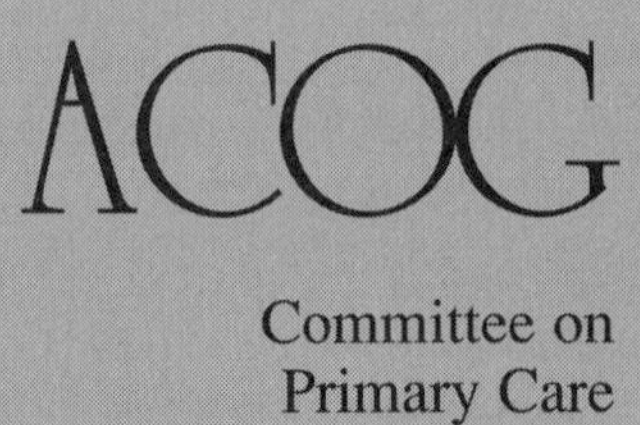

Committee on Primary Care

Committee Opinion

Number 218, June 1999

Delineation of Obstetric–Gynecologic Primary Care Practice

Obstetrician–gynecologists have a tradition of providing primary and preventive care to women. Primary care emphasizes health maintenance, preventive services, early detection of disease, availability of services, and continuity of care. The obstetrician–gynecologist often serves as a primary medical resource and counselor to the patient and her family for a wide range of medical conditions. However, all clinicians, regardless of the extent of their training, have limitations to their knowledge and skills and should seek consultation at appropriate times for the benefit of their patients in providing both reproductive and nonreproductive care.

Reproductive Care

Obstetrician–gynecologists provide comprehensive care for pregnancy and all disorders affecting the female genital system. Certain conditions affecting the reproductive organs or the process of reproduction have been recognized as requiring care beyond the scope of the typical generalist in obstetrics and gynecology. Subspecialists in obstetrics and gynecology have been educated and certified for these specific problems.

For children, care is generally provided by consultation only. For adolescents and adults, obstetrician–gynecologists provide continuing care. Care of reproductive tract disorders continues into and beyond menopause.

Nonreproductive Care

Obstetric and gynecologic training has always included the management of nonreproductive disorders that are commonly encountered during pregnancy, such as hypertension, diabetes, thyroid disease, and asthma. These disorders, as well as others, may be detected and managed by the obstetrician–gynecologist in the nonpregnant patient as well. The education of all obstetrician–gynecologists encompasses the outpatient management of many general medical conditions. Certain disorders in nonpregnant patients, especially those severe enough to require hospitalization, such as myocardial infarction, stroke, heart failure, renal failure, or fractures, are generally outside the scope of most obstetrician–gynecologists' practices.

ISSN 1074-861X

The American College of Obstetricians and Gynecologists
409 12th Street, SW
PO Box 96920
Washington, DC 20090-6920

12345/32109

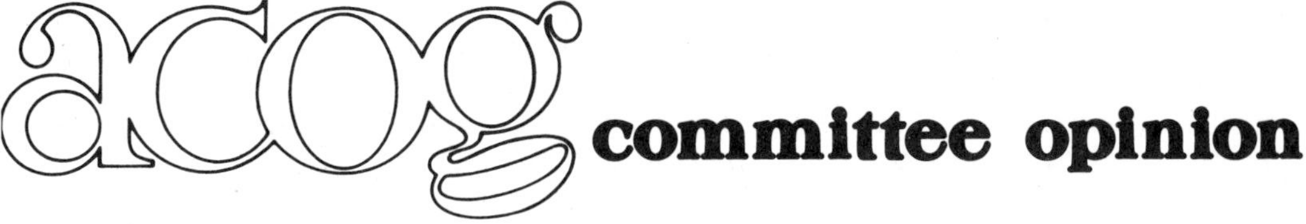

Committee on Ethics

Number 156–May 1995
(Replaces #38, June 1985)

End-of-Life Decision Making: Understanding the Goals of Care

The expressions "*withdrawal* and *withholding* of treatment" and likewise "treatment *refusal*" are reflective of an ethos that has shaped American medical research and practice for the last half century. That ethos regards the use of interventionist strategies to promote cure and prolong life as the physician's primary obligation. Consequently, any decision *not* to embrace such strategies has been construed negatively as a "withholding," a "withdrawal," or a "refusal." This statement encourages a move away from these terms and the assumptions that they embody about the aims of caregiving. It suggests a more open, collaborative approach to clinical decision making, one grounded in the *explicit* identification of the operative goals of care. In particular, this statement emphasizes the dignity, appropriateness, and ethical probity of palliation and comfort as caregiving goals. The 18th century was another era in which the duty to cure and prolong life was regarded as paramount by physicians. Medical essayist John Gregory's 1772 exhortation to his colleagues continues to be germane in this regard: "It is as much the business of a physician," he says, "to alleviate pain, and to smooth the avenues of death...as to cure diseases" (1).

This document discusses the process of communication that leads to the identification of the goals of care, and in particular to the goals that may direct end-of-life caregiving in obstetrics and gynecology. As a foundation for this discussion, the document addresses first, the ethical values that undergird medical practice, and second, legal developments that bear on end-of-life decision making.

THE ETHICAL BASES OF MEDICAL PRACTICE

The moral character of medicine is based on three values central to the healing relationship. They are patient benefit, patient self-determination, and the ethical integrity of the health care professional (2, 3).

Patient Benefit

The obligation to promote the good of the patient is a basic presumption of medical caregiving and a defining feature of the physician's ethical responsibility. To promote the patient's good is to provide care in which benefits outweigh burdens or harms. Benefits, in turn, are understood only relative to the goals that patient and physician hope to achieve through medical care.

Patient Self-Determination

The inherent value of individual autonomy or self-determination is one of the fundamental bases of democracy and of individual rights and protections in the United States. In health care, the value of individual autonomy is affirmed in the ethical and legal doctrine of informed consent (4, 5). Under this doctrine, the patient has a right to control what happens to her body. This means that 1) no treatment may be given to the patient without her consent (or, if she lacks decision-making capacity, the consent of her valid surrogate) and 2) the patient (or her surrogate) has the right to refuse unwanted medical treatment. This right is not contingent on the presence or absence of terminal illness, on the agreement of family members, or on the approval of physicians or hospital administrators.

In the medical context, physician *respect* for patient self-determination consists in an active inclusion of the patient in decisions regarding her own care. This involves frank discussion of diagnoses and prognoses, the relative risks and benefits of alternative (or no) treatments, and, based on these discussions, a mutual identification of the operative goals of care. There is a strong presumption that all information needed to make health care decisions be provided to patients (or to their surrogates). Studies suggest that most patients want to know the reality of their conditions and benefit from an honest rapport with the physician (6, 7). It is unethical for a physician to deny patients important information in order to avoid physician–patient interactions that are difficult or uncomfortable. Moreover, appropriate regard for patient autonomy involves respecting the patient's considered choice to change therapeutic modalities to better meet her current goals of care.

The Ethical Integrity of the Health Care Professional

Because physicians, like patients, are autonomous agents, they cannot be compelled to violate personal ethical or religious commitments in the service of the patient's good. If physicians have moral reservations about certain forms of caregiving, they should make that known at the outset. Although a physician is not obliged to do something that is at odds with his or her conscience, he or she must not stand in the way of a patient's desire to seek another caregiver and should, where possible, help guide the transition.

The profession of medicine is guided by its moral commitment to avoid risks to the patient that are greater than potential benefits. On this basis, physicians have a presumptive obligation *not* to provide treatments that are untested, contraindicated, or useless. For this reason, a patient's demand for care which she deems desirable is not sufficient to impose upon providers an absolute obligation to provide that care.

LEGAL DEVELOPMENTS THAT BEAR ON END-OF-LIFE DECISION MAKING

In the 1990s, there have been a number of developments in the law that bear on end-of-life decision making. First, in June 1990, in a decision on the *Cruzan* case, the United States Supreme Court affirmed that patients have a constitutionally protected right to refuse unwanted medical treatments (8). The ruling reaffirms states' authority to adopt procedural requirements for the withdrawal and withholding of life-prolonging medical interventions.

A second legal development was the passage of the federal Patient Self-Determination Act (PSDA), which went into effect December 1, 1991 (9). The PSDA requires Medicaid- and Medicare-participating health care institutions to inform all adult patients of their rights "to make decisions concerning medical care, including the right to accept or refuse medical or surgical treatment and the right to formulate an advance directive." Under the PSDA, institutions are legally required to provide this information to patients upon admission for care or upon enrollment in a health maintenance organization. The institution must note in the chart the existence of an advance directive and must respect these directives to the fullest extent under state law. Put simply, the aim of the PSDA is to empower patients to make decisions regarding their medical care.

An advance directive is the formal mechanism by which a patient may express her values regarding her future health status. It may take the form of a *proxy directive* or an *instructional directive* or both. Proxy directives, such as the durable power of attorney for health care, designate a surrogate to make medical decisions on behalf of the patient who is no longer competent to express her choices. Instructional directives, such as "living wills," focus on the types of life-sustaining treatment that a person would or would not choose in various clinical circumstances.

A patient's goals of care are very likely to change with time and differing clinical circumstances. As a static expression of the patient's wishes, an instructional directive may thus be a limited tool that could conceivably undermine a patient's most current desires. With this in mind, the patient's appointment of a proxy who knows her interests and accepts the role of surrogate decision maker may be the best way of ensuring that her wishes will be carried out.

A third related development is found in limitations on the autonomy of the pregnant woman in the area of treatment refusal. As of 1994, 36 states have statutes that explicitly forbid the withdrawal or withholding of life support from a pregnant patient regardless of her considered choice (10–12). Although it is anticipated that these restrictions will be challenged as unconstitutional, they are expressions of a belief that the therapeutic interests of the fetus limit those of the pregnant woman.

PHYSICIAN–PATIENT COMMUNICATION AND THE GOALS OF CARE

The practice of obstetrics and gynecology involves many different types of caregiving. These include but are not limited to preventive care, periodic examinations, family planning, the provision of prenatal and delivery care, medical and surgical intervention for conditions that threaten a patient's fertility, life, or quality of life, long-term care for patients with chronic illness, and palliative care for patients whose illnesses offer no chance of cure or remission. Each of these types of caregiving is linked to definable goals that not only suggest the appropriate intensity and duration of care but also entail certain treatment modalities and rule out others. Questions about the use of specific therapeutic modalities become meaningful only in relation to the goals of management for *this* particular patient (13). Goals of care in obstetrics and gynecology include:

- Relief of symptoms, pain, and suffering
- Achievement of cure or remission
- Achievement or prevention of pregnancy
- Optimization of pregnancy outcomes
- Prevention of illness in a woman or her fetus or both
- Maintenance or restoration of biological function
- Maximization of comfort
- Education of the patient about her medical condition

The operative goal or goals of care are properly identified through a process of shared and ongoing communication and decision making between the patient and physician (14). The physician is also responsible for initiating and coordinating communication with other members of the health care team so that decision making reflects the patient's entire medical condition and her identified goals of care. Explicit discussion about the goals of care is important for a number of reasons. First, assumptions about the objectives of care inevitably shape perceptions about the appropriate course of treatment. Second, these objectives may be understood differently by the patient and her caregivers. Third, unarticulated commitments to certain goals may lead to misunderstanding and conflict. Fourth, the goals of care may evolve and change in response to clinical or other factors. A comprehensive and ongoing process of communication not only advances patient self-determination but is also the basis for "preventive ethics"; that is, the establishment of a moral common ground that may prevent ethical conflict and crisis (15).

SHARED DECISION MAKING REGARDING THE END OF LIFE

The process of decision making regarding the end of life may take place under two different circumstances. In the first, decisions are made in a situation of *present* health crisis; these are immediate choices that determine actual end-of-life treatment. In the second, decisions are made that provide for possible *future* end-of-life situations; these decisions are expressed through advance directives.

Communication Regarding Immediate Health Status

An ongoing process of informed consent requires that physicians communicate information regarding the patient's health status and comparative risks and benefits of treatment (or no treatment) so that she, or if she lacks decision-making capacity, her surrogate, may determine management goals. If the patient decides that the maximization of comfort is her desired goal of care, the practitioner's responsibilities will focus on palliative strategies such as pain relief, attentive and responsive communication with the patient about her health status, and the facilitation of communication with the patient's involved family and loved ones. These components of care are essential to the physician's positive therapeutic role. For the general obstetrician–gynecologist whose patient is or has been under the care of a specialist physician, these are often the most valuable services that can be offered. The expression "nothing more can be done" is a misleading shorthand that improperly equates care with cure and, in so doing, ignores the importance of the physician's role in providing comfort to the dying patient.

In the face of end-of-life decision making, physicians trained to prize interventionist strategies must be especially careful not to impose their own conception of benefit or burden on a patient or to use coercive means to establish or achieve goals that are not shared by the patient. The obstetrician–gynecologist should recognize that the harms associated with prolonged attempts at cure may not be acceptable to the dying patient. However, neither the presence of a "Do Not Attempt Resuscitation" (DNAR/DNR) order nor specific directives regarding limitation of other treatments remove the responsibility for providing palliative care. In other words, the physician should not rely on the presence or absence of a DNAR order to make assumptions about the appropriateness of other treatment but rather should be guided by the explicitly identified goals of care.

There is considerable evidence that sociocultural and gender differences between patients and their physicians may subtly influence the style and content of physician–patient communication and the care that patients receive (16–22). Physicians who are aware of these potential problems can guard against the influence of bias in judgments concerning patient choices. Differences in ethnic, social, religious, and economic background may complicate communication, but they should not compromise care.

If the patient or surrogate and physician finally disagree on the goals that each party believes should guide care, the matter should be taken up with an ethics committee or designated ethics consultant. By using such consultation to clarify the cultural, religious, and/or personal considerations that shape their decision making, the parties may be able to resolve apparent conflict.

Communication Regarding Future Health Status: The Advance Directive

The obstetrician–gynecologist often provides the primary access that women have to the health care system. In many cases, it is the obstetrician–gynecologist who not only acts as the principal physician for female patients but also has the most contact with them. For these reasons, obstetrician–gynecologists are in an ideal position to encourage women to formulate advance directives. As an expression of the patient's values regarding care, the advance directive is not qualitatively different from a patient's articulation of general and more immediate health care decisions. As such, discussion of the advance directive should be regarded as integral to the ongoing process of communication to be initiated by the health care provider.

A good opportunity to initiate the discussion of end-of-life caregiving goals is during well-patient care, either at the time of the periodic examination or during pregnancy. Because a patient's wishes regarding care might change over time or under different conditions of illness, these discussions should include occasional reexamination of values and goals and, if necessary, updating of the advance directive. In other words, decision making should be treated as a process rather than an event (23).

To facilitate the initiation of these discussions, the patient history form could contain questions about a patient's execution of an advance directive and her designation of a surrogate or next of kin as her medical proxy. If the patient has an instructional directive or durable power of attorney or both, they should become part of her chart. If the patient does not have an advance directive, the opportunity for executing one might be provided by the social services or nursing staff of a hospital or clinical practice.

Physician–patient communication regarding advance directives should first include information on the advance directive itself: the forms it may take and its purpose as an expression of the patient's rights in the direction of her own care. Second, the physician and patient should discuss the different goals that may now guide care and those that may come into play in the case of terminal illness. It should be made clear to the patient the types of therapy that could be used to advance these different goals. Third, where applicable, physician and patient should discuss possible scenarios where the patient's own prognosis and care might adversely affect the health of her fetus. Finally, the physician should discuss with the patient the importance of consistency between her written directive and the preferences she expresses to her health care proxy or next of kin or both. In the event that a patient loses the capacity for decision making, her interests can best be served if there is as much clarity and consistency as possible regarding her wishes.

Ideally, these discussions serve an educational purpose for both patient and physician. For the physician, these discussions establish a basis for future caregiving and provide an opportunity for the candid expression of personal values regarding care. For the patient, the discussions provide the opportunity to learn about advance directives, to formulate and articulate her values regarding the goals of care and to understand the compatibility of these goals with the values of the provider.

Although it is the physician's responsibility to educate his or her patients about possible future health status and rights regarding medical care, it is the responsibility of the patient to thoughtfully assess her values and goals and to make them clearly known to those involved in her care. Again, the explicit discussion of caregiving goals provides an optimal mechanism for shared decision making.

SURROGATE DECISION MAKING

If the patient who lacks decision-making capacity has not designated a health care proxy, state law may dictate the order in which relatives should be asked to serve as surrogates. The person selected should be one who knows the patient's values and wishes and will respect them in his or her role as surrogate decision maker. If there is conflict regarding the designation of a surrogate, it may be appropriate to seek the advice of an ethics committee or consultant or, possibly, the courts.

In proxy decision making for the dying patient, surrogates and health care providers should be aware that there is documentation of gender disparity in clinical medicine and research and in court decisions surrounding the right to refuse life-sustaining treatment. In a review of "right to die" cases, it was found that courts honored the previously stated treatment decisions of men in 75% of cases, whereas they respected the prior choices of female patients in only 14% of cases (24). Given the persistence and pervasiveness of social attitudes that take women's moral choices less seriously than men's, obstetrician–gynecologists and patient surrogates must prevent these biases from undermining their care of and advocacy for female patients. Likewise, this evidence should further motivate women to make their treatment decisions as explicit as possible.

THE PREGNANT PATIENT AND END-OF-LIFE DECISIONS: PREVENTING CONFLICT

For the overwhelming majority of pregnant women, the welfare of the fetus is of the utmost concern. This concern motivates women to modify their behaviors for months at a time and to undergo the discomforts and risks of pregnancy and delivery. This maternal interest in fetal welfare has traditionally been the basis of the fundamental ethical commitment of obstetrician–gynecologists: that they are responsible for both the pregnant woman and her fetus and that they must optimize the benefits to both while minimizing the risks to each.

Within the context of obstetric care, situations may arise when a dying pregnant woman must decide between caregiving goals that emphasize palliative management for her own illness or an interventionist strategy such as cesarean delivery for the sake of her fetus. Likewise, she might be forced to decide between a curative strategy such as chemotherapy for her metastatic breast cancer and a course that poses less risk to her fetus but offers her less anticipated benefit. In either case, it is safe to assume that having been provided with all of the clinical information necessary to make her decision, she regards the choice as a difficult, possibly excruciating one and one that she wishes she did not have to make. Since the patient with a life-threatening condition identifies treatment goals by weighing obligations and concerns for her family, her fetus, and her own health and life prospects, any decision that she makes is bound to jeopardize some of the things that she cares about.

In order to make these decisions, the pregnant patient will first and foremost need the best clinical information available on the relative risks and benefits of different management strategies for her and her fetus. Different views on the moral status of the fetus generate different positions regarding the fetus as a patient and, by extension, different positions regarding the physician's obligations to the fetus. When, because of divergent beliefs on this matter, risks and benefits are valued differently by patient and physician, there is a potential for conflict. This potential highlights the importance of candid discussion of these matters in advance of a situation of conflict or crisis. The proper course for resolving conflicts that do arise is discussion of the case with an ethics committee or consultant (15, 25).

CONCLUSION

Effective communication between patient and physician is the cornerstone of the therapeutic relationship. It provides the patient with the information she needs to make her health care decisions and it provides a common ground for physician, patient, family, and other members of the health care team.

Questions about the use of specific therapeutic modalities become meaningful only in relation to the goals of management for the particular patient. Explicit identification of the operative goals of care is important, therefore, for a number of reasons: First, assumptions about the objectives of care inevitably shape perceptions about the appropriate course of treatment; second, these objectives may be understood differently by the patient and her caregivers; third, unarticulated commitments to certain goals may lead to misunderstanding and conflict; and fourth, the goals of care may evolve and change in response to clinical or other factors.

In the course of providing comprehensive care, obstetrician–gynecologists are in an ideal position to encourage women to formulate advance directives. As an expression of the patient's values regarding care, the advance directive is not qualitatively different from a patient's articulation of general and more immediate health care decisions. As such, discussion of the advance directive should be regarded as integral to the ongoing process of communication to be initiated by the health care provider.

When the maximization of comfort is the chosen therapeutic goal, the physician can continue to benefit the patient in a number of important ways by providing humane and supportive care at the end of life.

REFERENCES

1. Gregory J, Lectures and duties ref. 37. Quoted by Pernick MS. The calculus of suffering in nineteenth-century surgery. Hastings Cent Rep 1983;13(2):26–36
2. Pellegrino ED, Thomasma DC. For the patient's good: the restoration of beneficence in health care. New York: Oxford University Press, 1988
3. Beauchamp TL, Childress JF. Principles of biomedical ethics. 4th ed. New York: Oxford University Press, 1994
4. Faden RR, Beauchamp TL. A history and theory of informed consent. New York: Oxford University Press, 1986
5. American College of Obstetricians and Gynecologists. The ethical dimensions of informed consent. ACOG Committee Opinion 108. Washington, DC: ACOG, 1992

6. Edinger W, Smucker DR. Outpatients' attitudes regarding advance directives. J Fam Pract 1992;35:650–653
7. American Academy of Pediatrics, Committee on Bioethics. Guidelines on forgoing life-sustaining medical treatment. Pediatrics 1994;93:532–536
8. *Cruzan v Director of the Missouri Dept. of Health et al, 497 US 261, 262 (1990)*
9. Cate FH, Gill BA. The Patient Self-Determination Act: implementation issues and opportunities. Washington, DC: The Annenberg Washington Program, 1991
10. Stoll KD. Pregnancy exclusions in state living will and medical proxy statutes. Washington, DC: Center for Women Policy Studies, 1992
11. Choice in Dying Inc. Pregnancy restrictions in living will statutes. The Right to Die Law Digest. Third Quarter Update. New York: Choice in Dying, 1994
12. Choice in Dying Inc. Pregnancy restrictions in statutes authorizing health care agents. The Right to Die Law Digest. Third Quarter Update. New York: Choice in Dying, 1994
13. Levine RJ, Nolan KA. Do not resuscitate decisions: a policy (editorial). Conn Med 1983;47:511–512
14. Report on do not resuscitate decisions. Conn Med 1983;47:477–483
15. McCullough LB, Chervenak FA. Ethics in obstetrics and gynecology. New York: Oxford University Press, 1994
16. Eisenberg JM. Sociologic influences on decision-making by clinicians. Ann Intern Med 1979;90:957–964
17. Waitzkin H. Doctor-patient communication. Clinical implications of social scientific research. JAMA 1984;252:2441–2446
18. Levy DR. White doctors and black patients: influence of race on the doctor–patient relationship. Pediatrics 1985;75:639–643
19. Kolder VE, Gallagher J, Parsons MT. Court-ordered obstetrical interventions. N Engl J Med 1987;316:1192–1196
20. Chasnoff IJ, Landress HJ, Barrett ME. The prevalence of illicit-drug or alcohol use during pregnancy and discrepancies in mandatory reporting in Pinellas County, Florida. N Engl J Med 1990;322:1202–1206
21. Roter D, Lipkin M, Korsgaard A. Sex differences in patients' and physicians' communication during primary care medical visits. Med Care 1991;29:1083–1093
22. Lurie N, Slater J, McGovern P, Ekstrum J, Quam L, Margolis K. Preventive care for women. Does the sex of the physician matter? N Engl J Med 1993;329:478–482
23. Lidz CW, Appelbaum PS, Meisel A. Two models of implementing informed consent. Arch Intern Med 1988;148:1385–1389
24. Miles SH, August A. Courts, gender and the "right to die." Law Med Health Care 1990;18:85–95
25. American College of Obstetricians and Gynecologists. Patient choice: maternal–fetal conflict. ACOG Committee Opinion 55. Washington, DC: ACOG, 1987

SUGGESTED READING

Joint Commission on Accreditation of Healthcare Organizations. 1995 comprehensive accreditation manual for hospitals. Oakbrook Terrace, Illinois: JCAHO, 1994:66–75, 191, 397–400

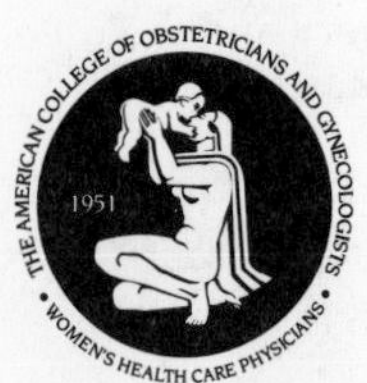

ISSN 1074-861X

The American College of Obstetricians and Gynecologists
409 12th Street, SW • Washington, DC 20024-2188

12345/98765

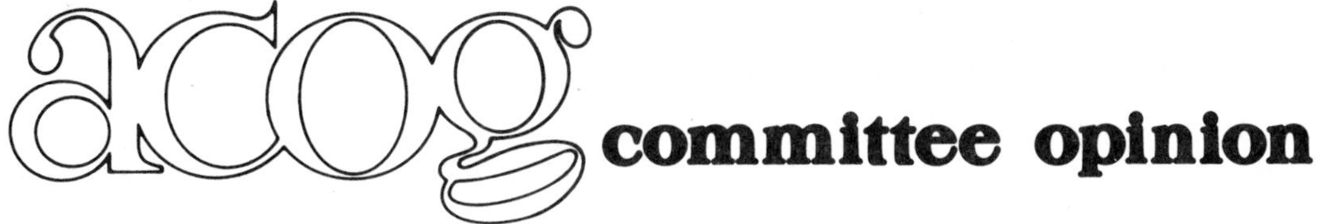

Committee on Ethics

Number 46—October 1985

Endorsement of Institutional Ethics Committees

INTRODUCTION

Changes in medical technology and social structure have moved the locus of medical intervention from the home to public institutions. Decisions once made privately and confidentially now occur under public scrutiny with wide social, economic, and ethical consequences. Although all medical care has been affected by these changes, obstetrics and gynecology has a large share of the procedures that have an impact on long-held human values. These procedures range over the entire span of life, from preconception (eg, genetic screening) to after death (eg, the delivery of an infant weeks after the brain death of its mother). Clearly, the ethical and social implications for our specialty have grown with the advent of new knowledge and technology. Continued dialogue and critical appraisal enable a dynamic society to affirm or revise its values. Patients and health care personnel need a forum for discussion and education.

To further the principle of keeping decision-making close to those most affected, the American College of Obstetricians and Gynecologists encourages the formation of institutional ethics committees, recognizing that they are only one of several alternative methods for careful consideration and review of decision-making processes. The use of institutional ethics committees is an evolving technique for helping with difficult decisions; therefore, constant reappraisal of their form and function is important. They are not meant to supplant other good techniques which have been effective in the hospital setting.

In a pluralistic society, a broad representation on the ethics committee drawn from the hospital environment and the community is ideal. Currently most committees appear to function largely as advisory rather than decision-making groups. Physicians may wish to seek counsel and reassurance when difficult decisions are required. The committee's involvement attests to the intention of physicians to act openly and in the patient's best interest while verifying the efforts of the institution to protect the rights of patients. Institutional ethics committees can play a significant role in preserving the quality of patient care by raising and maintaining the level of ethical consciousness throughout hospital programs.

FUNCTIONS OF INSTITUTIONAL ETHICS COMMITTEES

Most of our Fellows have become aware of ethics committees in the context of treatment for handicapped newborns or of withdrawal of life-sustaining therapy; however, institutional ethics committees can have much wider applications that are pertinent to our practice activities:

- To foster awareness of ethical issues and create an environment of ethical concern
- To establish educational programs regarding ethical principles, biomedical ethics literature, and relevant legal decisions
- To act as an informational resource concerning medical ethics in the institutional setting
- To offer counsel on ethical issues and problems in individual cases
- To assist and advise in formulating institutional policies by addressing ethical concerns

SERVICES OF INSTITUTIONAL ETHICS COMMITTEES

1. The initial activity should be education of the committee itself, utilizing consultants, attending seminars, reviewing the literature, and using other available resources to study rigorously the discipline of biomedical ethics. Biomedical ethics is a new discipline that consists of a complex and expanding body of knowledge, and members of institutional ethics committees should familiarize themselves with ethical principles and forms of application in order to incorporate them into use and practice. This information should then be disseminated to the hospital community.
2. Consent for or refusal of treatment should be based on medical information that is accurate, current, and offers all reasonable options. The committee should establish programs to promote this goal.

   The committee should determine that mechanisms are established to ensure, when there is doubt, that the patient has the capacity to choose. The committee should also determine that the institution has systems to identity appropriate decision-makers when the patient does not have this capacity.

3. The committee can serve to connect patients and families to social support and advocacy groups which often make new resources known, thereby increasing options to patients, families, and health care providers.
4. The committee can serve as a resource to its institution by making staff aware of state laws (such as those defining death), federal legislation (such as the law regarding medical treatment for handicapped newborns), guidelines from other institutions (such as various policies about orders not to resuscitate), and other current information not routinely encountered by the practitioner in the usual medical literature.
5. The committee can carry out review of hospital experience for the purpose of a) identifying problems that are recurrent, in order to devise useful guidelines, and b) continually evaluating the guidelines for effectiveness.
6. The committee can serve as a forum for discussion of unresolved biomedical issues, such as the application of new reproductive technologies.
7. The committee can serve as a forum for education about varying cultural, religious, or professional perspectives, e.g., religious attitudes toward autopsy, blood transfusion, and donations and reception of transplanted organs. This will help to anticipate conflicts and to accommodate or tolerate different points of view.
8. The committee may serve to advise and support primary decision-makers (patients, families, and health care professionals) when difficult decisions must be made.
9. With the ethics committee serving as a catalyst, every attempt should be made by the primary decision-makers to reach agreement about treatment; occasionally, however, this will not be possible, or the agreement will vary egregiously from accepted community and legal standards. Because their role is advisory, institutional ethics committees have no authority to make patient care decisions. However, authority exists within hospital systems to enforce hospital policies and standards and to assume appropriate legal responsibility for practices within the hospital.

PROBLEMS THAT MAY ARISE WITH INSTITUTIONAL ETHICS COMMITTEES

Ethics committees may serve to improve patient care, but there are problems which may arise:

- There is a possibility that pressures may be exerted on a competent adult or members of the family after a decision is made that is ethically defensible but not palatable to members of the committee.
- Although religious attitudes and viewpoints may be valuable and welcome for decision-makers, there is a possibility that committees or committee members may advance a particular religious or philosophical view without identifying it as such, or by misrepresenting it as medical advice. When institutions have policies based on religious beliefs that limit patient options, patients should be advised of these policies openly and as early as possible.
- There is a possibility of diffusing responsibility for decisions, so that the patient or the physician or both are confused about their respective roles and rights.
- There is a possibility of going beyond the ethical advisory capacity and infringing upon the physician's responsibilities and the patient's choices.
- There is a possibility that the committee will serve the interests of the institution or the physician rather than those of the patient.
- There is a possibility that membership on the committee will be limited to those expounding and supporting a predetermined point of view.

CONCLUSION

The use of institutional ethics committees is an evolving technique for helping with difficult decisions. Continuing appraisal of their form and function is important. Each institution must decide how the committee will articulate with the medical staff and administration. Such committees are not meant to supplant other good techniques which have been effective in the hospital setting. Because of varying values in our pluralistic society, a broad representation of disciplines, from the hospital as well as the community at large, would be ideal. Currently most committees appear to function best as an advisory, rather than a decision-making group. Legislated requirements may mandate specific duties for these committees. Institutional ethics committees can play a significant role in preserving the quality of patient care by raising and maintaining the level of ethical consciousness in the hospital community and promoting an environment of ethical concern.

BIBLIOGRAPHY

Abrams F R: Bioethical considerations for high risk pregnancy. In: Abrams R S, Wexler P (eds): Medical Care of the Pregnant Patient. Boston, Little, Brown, 1983, pp 1-12

American Hospital Association: Hospital committees on biomedical ethics (AHA Guideline). Chicago, American Hospital Association, 1984

Cranford R E, Doudera A E (eds): Institutional Ethics Committees and Health Care Decision Making. Ann Arbor, MI, Health Administration Press, 1984

Ethics: It's About Choices (a video curriculum). Denver, CO, Center for Applied Biomedical Ethics

Fost N, Cranford R E: Hospital ethics committees: Administrative aspects. JAMA 253 (18): 2687-2692, 1985

Judicial Council, American Medical Association: Guidelines for ethics committees in health care institutions. JAMA 253 (18): 2698-2699, 1985

Levine C: Questions and (some very tentative) answers about hospital ethics committees. Hastings Cent Rep 14 (3): 9-12,1984

McCormick R A: Ethics committees: Promise or Peril? Law Med Health Care 12 (4): 150-155, 1984

Randal J: Are ethics committees alive and well? Hastings Cent Rep 13 (6): 10- 12, 1983

Robertson J A: Ethics committees in hospitals: Alternative structures and responsibilities. QRB 10 (1): 6-10, 1984

Rosner F: Hospital medical ethics committees: A review of their development. JAMA 253 (18): 2693-2697, 1985

Youngner S J, Jackson D L, Coulton C, et al.: A national survey of hospital ethics committees. In: President's Commission for the Study of Ethical Problems in Medicine and Biomedical and Behavioral Research: Deciding to Forego Life-Sustaining Treatment. Washington, DC, US Government Printing Office, 1983, pp 443-449

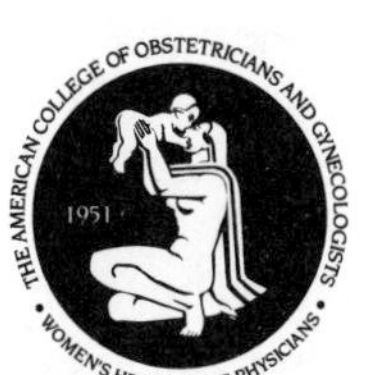

ISSN 1074-861X

The American College of Obstetricians and Gynecologists
409 12th Street, SW • Washington, DC 20024-2188

9 10/7

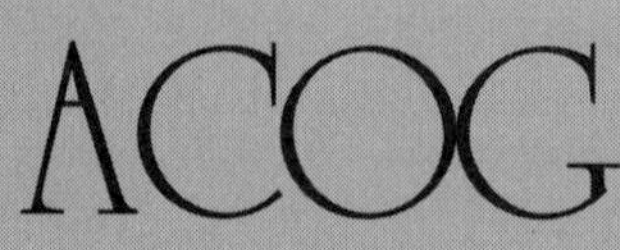

Committee on
Ethics

Committee Opinion

Number 213, November 1998

Ethical Considerations in Research Involving Pregnant Women

This Committee Opinion is designed to provide reasonable guidelines for research that involves pregnant women. In the past, investigators have been reluctant to conduct research on pregnant women because of concerns for the potential to do harm to the fetus. Although attention to the ethical principle of nonmaleficence is admirable, the resulting sense of restraint has limited the growth of knowledge in some areas of normal physiology, pathophysiology, and therapeutic approaches during pregnancy. In this Committee Opinion, the Committee on Ethics affirms both the need for such research and the obligation for researchers, institutional review boards, and others reviewing clinical research to evaluate with extreme care the potential effects of proposed research on the pregnant woman and the developing fetus (1).

Pregnant women should be presumed to be eligible for participation in clinical studies even if the research is not primarily related to pregnancy (2). Research should be encouraged to advance the management of 1) underlying medical conditions in women who become pregnant, 2) conditions of pregnancy, 3) complications of pregnancy, and 4) prenatal conditions that might threaten the health of the resulting child.

Human experimentation is a necessary part of medical research because certain information can be obtained in no other way. For example, human immunodeficiency virus (HIV) infection research using zidovudine (AZT) for pregnant women resulted in a significant reduction of the incidence of transmission of the virus to offspring (3). Such experimentation may be attended by a certain element of risk. Investigators must therefore use research design methods that employ all available means to maximize safety and to narrow risk.

Involvement in research protocols in no way diminishes the physician's responsibility to provide the most appropriate clinical management. Research objectives should not affect clinical management. For example, it is inappropriate to attempt to delay a medically indicated induction of labor solely to meet gestational age criteria for participation in a research project. The welfare of the patient and her fetus is always the primary concern. Guidelines for protection of research participants are applicable to all pregnant women, regardless of the woman's intention to complete the pregnancy (4–6). Neither physician nor patient should be expected to participate in research that is contrary to personal ethical judgment.

ISSN 1074-861X

The American College of Obstetricians and Gynecologists
409 12th Street, SW
PO Box 96920
Washington, DC 20090-6920

12345/21098

The Context: Ethics in Research

To be considered ethically justified, human research must satisfy several conditions. These include a reasonable prospect that the investigation will produce the knowledge that is being sought, a favorable balance of benefits over risks, a proven necessity to use human subjects, a system for independent monitoring of outcomes and of protection of human subjects, and a fair allocation of the burdens and benefits of research among potential subject groups (7).

Although it is important to try to distinguish ethical problems involving patient care from ethical issues related to research, a definite line cannot always be drawn between these two areas. Physicians often assume the dual role of research scientist and clinical practitioner, which may result in serious conflicts of interest. Patients may experience confusion as to whether they are, in fact, research subjects. The function of the investigator is to generate knowledge that has the potential to benefit patients in the future. But clinicians are expected to act in the best interests of their own current patients. Researchers need to recognize these potential problems, strive to resolve them before beginning specific research projects, and inform patients about potential conflicts as they seek consent for research participation.

Informed Consent

Appropriate and adequately informed consent and institutional or agency review, or both, are fundamental to the formulation of any research protocol (8). The researcher has an obligation to disclose and discuss all material risks to the woman and fetus—ones that are likely to affect the patient's decision to participate or not in the research. Research that consists of observation and recording without clinical intervention is of ethical concern only insofar as it may involve informed consent and the preservation of confidentiality.

Informed consent is an intentional and voluntary process that grants a clinician or researcher the authority to perform certain interventions. It implies the possibility of choosing not to participate in a research protocol and the right to withdraw from a study at any time. The participation of a pregnant woman in a research study is based on the expectation that she will consider carefully the best interests of the fetus as well as her own interests.

Involvement of Primary Caregivers in the Consent Process

The decision to participate in a research project that involves pregnant women requires a complex weighing of risk and benefit for mother and fetus. It is generally advantageous for the researcher to include the patient's attending obstetrician or primary caregiver in the informed consent process prior to the patient's enrollment in a study. This physician often has general knowledge of a woman's history, family, values, and lifestyle that may be helpful in the informed consent process.

The patient should be encouraged to consult her attending obstetrician independently before deciding to participate (9). When the attending physician is not initially involved in the consent process, the researcher still has an obligation to provide information about the study to the patient's primary caregiver, unless the patient has a specific objection. This information should include the requirements of the study and its possible outcomes and complications.

Both researcher and primary caregiver should avoid inappropriately inflating the patient's perception of the therapeutic benefit expected from participation in the study. Studies have shown that research subjects tend to believe, despite careful explanation of research protocols, that they will benefit from participation in the study (10). This risk of "therapeutic misconception" may be increased when the patient's own physician is involved in the consent process and especially when one physician plays both research and clinical management roles.

Research Related to Diagnosis and Therapy

Research during pregnancy requires balancing of risk and benefit for two distinct but interrelated entities—the pregnant woman and her fetus. The pregnant woman, the researcher, and the patient's obstetrician must balance potential benefit to the woman, to the fetus, and to society as a whole against the level of risk that may be incurred as a result of participation in the study. All parties concerned need to strive for clear communication about the following issues:

- *Does the research involve therapy or diagnosis that might influence the woman's or the fetus's well-being, or is the goal of the study to produce scientific results that will be likely to be useful to future patients but offer no demonstrable benefit to current subjects?* The prospective subject must be apprised if no explicit benefit is expected as a result of the study. Those studies that search for general information and are not associated with diagnostic or treatment modalities would be less likely to create the impression that the research will result in direct benefit to the participant. The researcher is still obligated to verify that the patient has understood this aspect of the study correctly.

- *Is there more than "minimal" incremental risk generated by the research?* The researcher must be able to communicate to the potential subject the incremental risks entailed in the research (beyond the level of background risk) and the probability of occurrence of adverse events. Anything more than minimal incremental risk must be weighed carefully against the potential merit of the study in considering the advisability of participation. According to applicable federal regulations, "Minimal risk means that the probability and magnitude of harm or discomfort anticipated in the research are not greater in and of themselves than those ordinarily encountered in daily life or during the performance of routine physical or psychological examinations or tests" (11).

Recommendations of the Committee on Ethics

The Committee on Ethics makes the following recommendations for research involving pregnant women. In addition, federal regulations govern conduct of all federally funded research involving pregnant women or fetuses and serve as a pattern that should be observed in the design and implementation of all research on pregnant women (5):

I. All research on pregnant women should be conducted in a manner consistent with the following ethical principles:

   A. It should conform to general scientific standards for research.

   B. Conscientious efforts should be made to avoid any financial or nonfinancial conflicts between appropriate health care and research objectives.

   C. Researchers should not offer inducements, financial or otherwise, designed to influence participation in research, beyond reasonable compensation for the pregnant woman's time and expenses. This is especially important because the pregnant woman's choices affect the fetus as well as herself.

   D. Health care needs of the individual patient should take precedence over research interests in all situations affecting clinical management.

II. Research involving diagnostic and treatment modalities for either the pregnant woman or the fetus should conform to the following:

   A. Be conducted only with the informed consent of the pregnant woman. (Currently, federal regulations require informed consent of the father, if he is available, except when the research is designed to meet the health needs of the mother [12]. Proposed regulatory revisions would eliminate the requirement for paternal consent for all research described in section D below [13]. A decision on this issue had not been reached at the time of publication.)

   B. Be evaluated for its potential impact on the fetus, and that evaluation should be communicated as part of the informed consent process.

   C. Be conducted only when the alternative modalities available within the study are considered to be one of the following:

      1. Therapeutic equivalents (clinical equipoise) (14) or

      2. Superior to the alternative of not participating in the study.

   D. Be conducted only when any incremental risk to the fetus from participation in the research is minimal or is incurred because of activities designed to meet the health needs of the woman or the fetus.

III. Research that does not have potential therapeutic value to either the pregnant woman or fetus is never appropriate if either might be placed at more than minimal risk.

Throughout the development of this Committee Opinion, there has been an attempt to strike a reasonable balance among protection of human subjects, the eligibility of pregnant women to participate in research, and the benefits that society could derive from advances in research. These potential benefits include reduction in fetal, infant, and maternal mortality and morbidity.

References

1. Robertson J. Ethical issues related to the inclusion of pregnant women in clinical trials (I). In: Mastroianni AC, Faden R, Federman D, eds. Women and health research: ethical and legal issues of including women in clinical studies. Vol 2. Washington, DC: National Academy Press, 1994:18–22
2. Mastroianni AC, Faden R, Federman D, eds. Women and health research: ethical and legal issues of including women in clinical studies. Vol 1. Washington, DC: National Academy Press, 1994:188
3. Connor EM, Sperling RS, Geber R, Kiselev P, Scott G, O'Sullivan MJ, et al. Reduction of maternal–infant transmission of human immunodeficiency virus type 1 with zidovudine treatment. Pediatric AIDS Clinical Trials Group Protocol 076 Study Group. N Engl J Med 1994;331:1173–1180
4. Department of Health, Education, and Welfare. Protection of human subjects: fetuses, pregnant women, and in vitro fertilization. Federal Register 1975;40:33256, 33552
5. Protection of Human Subjects, 45 C.F.R. Sect. 46(b) (1997)
6. Fetal Research, 42 U.S.C. Sect. 289g(b) (1996)
7. Beauchamp TL, Childress JF. Principles of biomedical ethics. 4th ed. New York: Oxford University Press, 1994:441
8. American College of Obstetricians and Gynecologists. Ethical dimensions of informed consent. ACOG Committee Opinion 108. Washington, DC: ACOG, 1992
9. Mastroianni AC, Faden R, Federman D, eds. Women and health research: ethical and legal issues of including women in clinical studies. Vol 1. Washington, DC: National Academy Press, 1994:196
10. Appelbaum PS, Roth LH, Lidz CW, Benson P, Winslade W. False hopes and best data: consent to research and the therapeutic misconception. Hastings Cent Rep 1987;17: 20–24
11. Protection of Human Subjects, 45 C.F.R. Sect. 46.102(i) (1997)
12. Protection of Human Subjects, 45 C.F.R. Sect. 46.207(b) (1997); Sect. 46.208(b) (1997)
13. Department of Health and Human Services. Protection of human subjects. Federal Register 1998;63:27794–27804
14. Beauchamp T. The intersection of research and practice. In: Goldworth A, Silverman W, Stevenson DK, Rivers R, Young EW, eds. Ethics and perinatology. New York: Oxford University Press, 1995:231–244

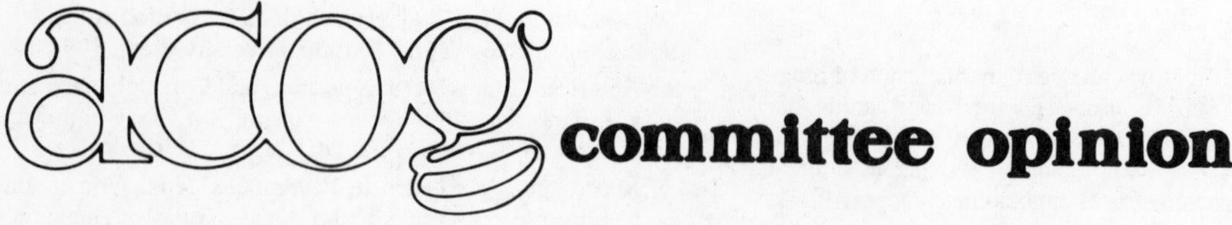

Committee on Ethics

Number 108—May 1992

Ethical Dimensions of Informed Consent

Informed consent is an ethical concept that has become integral to contemporary medical ethics and medical practice. In recognition of the ethical importance of informed consent, the Committee on Ethics affirms that:

1. Informed consent for medical treatment and for participation in medical research is an ethical requirement (which legal doctrines and requirements can in part reflect).
2. Informed consent is an expression of respect for the patient as a person; it particularly respects a patient's moral right to bodily integrity, to self-determination regarding sexuality and reproductive capacities, and to the support of the patient's freedom within caring relationships.
3. Informed consent not only ensures the protection of the patient against unwanted medical treatment, but it also makes possible the active involvement of the patient in her or his medical planning and care.
4. Freedom is maximized in relationships marked by mutuality and equality; this offers both an ethical ideal and an ethical guideline for physician–patient relationships.
5. Communication is necessary if informed consent is to be realized, and physicians can help to find ways to facilitate communication not only in individual relations with patients but also in the structured context of medical care institutions.
6. Informed consent should be looked upon as a process, a process that includes ongoing shared information and developing choices as long as one is seeking medical assistance.
7. The ethical requirement of informed consent need not conflict with physicians' overall ethical obligation to a principle of beneficence; that is, every effort should be made to incorporate a commitment to informed consent within a commitment to provide medical benefit to patients and thus to respect them as whole and embodied persons.
8. There are limits to the ethical obligation of informed consent, but a clear justification should be given for any abridgement or suspension of the general obligation.
9. Because ethical requirements and legal requirements cannot be equated, physicians should also acquaint themselves with the legal requirements of informed consent.

The application of informed consent to contexts of obstetric and gynecologic practice invites ongoing clarification of the meaning of these nine statements. What follows is an effort to provide this.

HISTORICAL BACKGROUND

In 1980, the Committee on Ethics of the American College of Obstetricians and Gynecologists (ACOG) developed a statement on informed consent.* This statement reflected what is now generally recognized as a paradigm shift in the ethical understanding of the physician–patient relationship. The 1970s had seen in the United States a marked change from a traditional almost singular focus on the benefit of the patient as the governing ethical principle of medical care to a new and dramatic emphasis on a requirement of informed consent. That is, a central and often sole concern for the medical well-being of the patient gave way to, or was at least modified to include, concern for the patient's autonomy in making medical decisions.

In the 1980s this national shift was both reinforced and challenged in medical ethics. Clinical

*This statement, "Ethical Considerations Associated with Informed Consent," was subsequently approved and issued in 1980 as a Statement of Policy by the Executive Board of ACOG. In 1989, it was withdrawn for revision by the Committee on Ethics.

experience as well as developments in ethical theory generated further questions about the practice of informed consent and the legal doctrine that promoted it. If in the 1970s informed consent was embraced as a corrective to paternalism, the 1980s exhibited a growing sense of need for shared decision-making as a corrective to the exaggerated individualism that patient autonomy had sometimes produced. At the same time, factors such as the proliferation of medical technologies, the bureaucratic and financial complexities of health care delivery systems, and the growing sophistication of the general public regarding medical limitations and possibilities continued to undergird an appreciation of the importance of patient autonomy and a demand for its safeguard in and through informed consent.

In the 1990s there are good reasons for considering once again the ethical significance and practical application of the requirement of informed consent. This is particularly true in the context of obstetric and gynecologic practice. Here medical options, public health problems, legal interventions, and political agendas have not only expanded but interconnected with one another in unprecedented ways. ACOG's concern for these matters is reflected in its more recent documents on informed consent and on particular ethical problems such as maternal–fetal conflict, sterilization, and surrogate motherhood (1–9). While a general ethical doctrine of informed consent cannot by itself resolve problems like these, it is nonetheless necessary for understanding them.

Informed consent for medical treatment and for participation in medical research is both a legal and an ethical matter. In the short 20th-century history of informed consent, statutes and regulations as well as court decisions have played an important role in the identification and sanctioning of basic duties. Judicial decisions have sometimes provided insights regarding rights of self-determination and of privacy in the medical context. Government regulations have rendered operational some of the most general norms formulated in historic ethical codes.* Yet there is little recent development in the legal doctrine of informed consent, and the most serious current questions are ethical ones before they are ones of the law. As the President's Commission reported in 1982, "Although the informed consent doctrine has substantial foundations in law, it is essentially an ethical imperative" (10). What above all bears reviewing, then, is the ethical dimension of the meaning, basis, and application of informed consent.

THE ETHICAL MEANING OF INFORMED CONSENT

The ethical concept of "informed consent" contains two major elements: *free consent* and *comprehension* (or understanding). Both of these elements together constitute an important part of a patient's "self-determination" (the taking hold of one's own life and action, determining the meaning and the possibility of what one undergoes as well as what one does).

Free consent is an intentional and voluntary act which authorizes someone else to act in certain ways. In the context of medicine, it is an act by which a person freely authorizes a medical intervention in her or his life, whether in the form of treatment or participation in research. As "consent," it implies the opposite of being coerced or unwillingly invaded by forces beyond oneself. As "free," consent implies a choice between alternatives. It includes the possibility of choosing otherwise—as the result of deliberation and/or of identification with different values and preferences. Free consent, in other words, implies the possibility of choosing this or that option or the refusal of any proposed option.

Comprehension (as an ethical element in informed consent) includes awareness and some understanding of information about one's situation and possibilities. Comprehension in this sense is necessary in order for there to be freedom in consenting. Free consent, of course, admits of degrees, and its presence is not always verifiable in concrete instances; but if it is to be operative at all in the course of medical treatment, it presupposes some level of understanding of available options.

Many people who are thoughtful about these matters have different beliefs about the actual achievement of informed consent and about human freedom. Whether and what freedom itself is has often been disputed. Despite continuing differences in underlying philosophical perspectives, however, important agreement has grown in this society about the need for informed consent and about its basic ethical significance in the context of medical practice and research. It is still important to try to clarify, however, who and what informed consent serves, and how it may be protected and fostered. This clarification cannot be achieved with-

---

*The Nuremberg Code in 1948 and the World Medical Association's Declaration of Helsinki in 1964 identified ethical restrictions for medical research on human subjects. For a history of the development of such codes and a general history of the ethical and legal concept of informed consent, see Ruth R. Faden and Tom L. Beauchamp, *A History and Theory of Informed Consent* (New York: Oxford University Press, 1986). A culminating summary of federal regulations in the United States can be found in the *Federal Register* (June 26, 1991).

out some continuing consideration of its basis and goals and the concrete contexts in which it must be realized.

THE ETHICAL BASIS AND PURPOSE OF INFORMED CONSENT

One of the important arguments for the ethical requirement of informed consent is an argument from *utility*, or from the *benefit* that can come to patients when they actively participate in decisions about their own medical care. That is, the involvement of patients in such decisions is good for their health—not only because it is a protection against treatment which patients might consider harmful, but because it contributes positively to their well-being. There are at least two presuppositions here: One is that patients know something experientially about their own medical condition that can be helpful and even necessary to the sound management of their medical care. The other is that, wherever it is possible, the active role of primary guardian of one's own health is more conducive to well-being than is a passive and submissive "sick role." The positive benefits of patient decision-making are obvious, for example, in the treatment of alcohol abuse. But the benefits of active participation in medical decisions are multifold for patients, whether they are trying to maintain their general health, or recover from illness, or conceive and deliver healthy babies, or live responsible sexual lives, or accept the limits of medical technology, or enhance whatever processes they are in that bring them to seek medical care.

Utility, however, is not the only reason for protecting and promoting patient decision-making. Indeed, the most commonly accepted foundation for informed consent is probably the principle of *respect for persons*. This principle expresses an ethical requirement to treat human persons as "ends in themselves" (that is, not to use them solely as means or instruments for someone else's purposes and goals). The logic of this requirement is based on the perception that all persons as persons have certain features or characteristics that constitute the source of an inherent dignity, a worthiness and claim to be affirmed in their own right. One of these features has come to be identified as *autonomy*—a person's capacity or at least potential for self-determination (for self-governance and freedom of choice). To be autonomous in any degree is to have the capacity to set one's own agenda—in some important way to choose one's actions and even one's attitudes, to determine the meaning of the outcome of one's life. Given this capacity in persons, it is ordinarily an ethically unacceptable violation of who and what persons are to coerce their actions or to refuse their participation in important decisions that affect their lives.

One of the important developments in ethical theory in recent years is the widespread recognition that autonomy is not the only characteristic of human persons that is a basis for the requirement of respect. Human persons, it is noted, are essentially social beings, *relational* in the structure of their personalities, their needs, and their possibilities. Given this "relationality," then, the goal of human life and the content of human well-being cannot be adequately understood only in terms of self-determination—especially if self-determination is understood individualistically and if it results in human relationships that are primarily adversarial. A sole or even central emphasis on patient autonomy in the informed consent process in the medical context risks replacing paternalism with a distanced and impersonal relationship of strangers negotiating rights and duties. If persons are to be respected and their well-being promoted, informed consent must be seen as serving a fuller notion of relationship.

Patients come to medical decisions with a history of relationships, personal and social, familial and institutional. Decisions are made in the context of these relationships, shared or not shared, as the situation allows. Above all, these decisions are made in a relationship between patient and physician (or often between patient and multiple professional caregivers).

The focus, then, for understanding both the basis and the content of informed consent must shift to include the many facets of the physician–patient relationship. Informed consent, from this point of view, is not an end, but a means. It is a means not only to the responsible participation by patients in their own medical care; it is also a means to a new form of relationship between physician (or any medical caregiver) and patient. From this perspective it is possible to see the contradictions inherent in an approach to informed consent that would, for example:

1. Lead a physician (or anyone else) to say of a patient, "I *gave* her informed consent"
2. Assume that informed consent was achieved simply by the signing of a document
3. Consider informed consent primarily as a safeguard for physicians against medical liability

It is also possible to see, from this perspective, that informed consent is not meant to undergird a patient's unlimited demand for treatment, arbitrary noncompliance with agreed upon treatment, or whimsical withdrawal from an agreed upon research protocol.

Freedom is maximized in relationships of trust; understanding is enhanced in the nuanced frameworks of conversation. Self-determination need not be either combative or submissive, but situated in relationships of mutuality of respect and, insofar as possible, equality of personal power. These kinds of professional relationships represent the preferred context for informed consent.

OBSTETRICS AND GYNECOLOGY: SPECIAL ETHICAL CONCERNS FOR INFORMED CONSENT

The practice of obstetrics and gynecology has always faced special ethical questions in the implementation of informed consent. How, for example, can the autonomy of patients best be respected when serious decisions must be made in the challenging situations of labor and delivery? What kinds of guidelines can physicians find for respecting the autonomy of adolescents, when society acknowledges this autonomy by and large only in the limited spheres of sexuality and reproduction? Do "recommendations" compromise patient autonomy in the context of genetic counseling? How much information should be given to patients about controversies surrounding specific treatments? How are beneficence requirements (regarding the well-being of the patient) to be balanced with rights of patient choice, especially in a field of medical practice where so many key decisions are irreversible? These and many other questions continue to be important for fulfilling the ethical requirement of informed consent.

Developments in the ethical doctrine of informed consent (regarding, for example, the significance that relationships have for decision-making) have helped to focus some of the concerns that are particular to the practice of obstetrics and gynecology. Where *women's* health care needs are addressed, and especially where these needs are related to women's sexuality and reproductive capacities, the issues of patient autonomy and relationality take on special significance. In other words, the gender of patients makes a difference where ethical questions of informed consent are concerned, because gender in our society has been a relevant factor in interpreting the meaning of autonomy and relationality. This is not to say that in some essential sense autonomy or relationality (or informed consent and relationships) ought to be different for women and men; indeed, quite the opposite. Rather, this alerts us to the possible inconsistencies in the application of the ethical requirement of informed consent.

While issues of gender are to be found in every area of medical practice and research,* they are particularly important in the area of obstetrics and gynecology. Of special relevance here, for example, are the insights now being articulated by women out of their experience—that is, their experience specifically in the medical setting, but also more generally in relation to their own bodies, in various patterns of relation with other persons, and in the larger societal and institutional contexts in which they live. These insights offer both a help and an ongoing challenge to the professional self-understanding and practice of obstetricians and gynecologists (whether they themselves are women or men).

Obstetrics and gynecology has in a special way seen new dimensions of informed consent emerge, and here new models for the active participation of health care recipients have been created. Some of these developments are the result of effective arguments that pregnancy and childbirth are not diseases, though they bring women importantly into relation with medical professionals. Even when women's medical needs are more precisely needs for diagnosis and treatment, their concerns to hold together the values of both autonomy and relationality have been influential in shaping not only ethical theory but also medical practice. Women themselves have questioned, for example, whether autonomy can really be protected if it is addressed in a vacuum, apart from an individual's concrete roles and relationships. But women as well as men have also recognized the ongoing importance of respect for autonomy as a requirement of moral justice in every relationship. Many women therefore continue to articulate fundamental concerns for bodily integrity and self-determination. At the same time they call for attention to the complexity of the relationships that are involved when sexuality and parenting are at issue in medical care.

The difficulties that beset the full achievement of informed consent in the practice of obstetrics and gynecology are not limited to individual and interpersonal factors. Both providers and recipients of medical care within this specialty have recognized the influence of such broad social problems as the historical imbalance of power in gender relations; the constraints on individual choice posed by complex medical technology; and the intersection of gender bias with race and class bias in the atti-

*See, for example, a recent study of court decisions on refusal of treatment regarding dying patients (Miles SH, August A. Courts, gender, and the "right to die." Law Med Health Care 1990;18(1–2 [Spring–Summer]): 85–95). The conclusion of this study is that court decisions for women patients differ from court decisions for men; that is, in general, men's previously stated wishes about "extraordinary" or "heroic" measures of treatment are taken more seriously than are women's.

tudes and actions of individuals and institutions. None of these problems makes the achievement of informed consent impossible. But, they alert us to the need to identify the conditions and limits, as well as the central requirements, of the ethical application of this doctrine.

ETHICAL APPLICATIONS OF INFORMED CONSENT

Insofar as comprehension and free consent are the basic ethical elements in informed consent, its efficacy and adequacy will depend on the fullness of their realization in patients' decisions. There are ways of assessing this and strategies for achieving it, even though—like every event of human freedom—informed consent involves a process that is not subject to precise measurement.

It is difficult to specify what consent consists in and requires, for it is difficult to describe a free decision in the abstract. Two things can be said about it in the context of informed consent to a medical intervention, however, elaborating on the conceptual elements we have already identified. The first is to describe what consent is *not*, what it is freedom *from*. Informed consent includes freedom from external coercion, manipulation, or infringement of bodily integrity. It is freedom from being acted upon by others when they have not taken account of and respected one's own preference and choice. This kind of freedom for a patient is not incompatible with a physician's giving *reasons* that favor one option over another. Medical recommendations, when they are not coercive or deceptive, do not violate the requirements of informed consent. For example, to try to convince a patient to take medication that will improve her health is not to take away her freedom (assuming that the methods of convincing are ones that respect and address, not overwhelm, her freedom). Or in another example, an attempt to persuade a woman who has tested positive for the human immunodeficiency virus that she should communicate the results of her testing to medical personnel who will be treating her infant is not in itself coercive; it need not violate her freedom.

The second thing that can be said about informed consent to a medical intervention is that while it may be an authorization of someone else's action toward one's self, it is—more profoundly—an active participation in decisions about the management of one's medical care. It is therefore (or can be) not only a "permitting" but a "doing." It can include decisions to make every effort toward a cure of a disease; or when cure is no longer a reasonable goal, to maintain functional equilibrium; or, finally, to receive medical care primarily in the form only of comfort. The variety of choices that are possible to a patient ranges, for example, from surgery to medical therapy, from diagnostic tests to hormone replacement, and from one form of contraception to another. For women in the context of obstetrics and gynecology, the choices are often ones of positive determination of this kind of assisted reproduction or that, this kind of preventive medicine or that—choices that are best described as determinations of their own actions rather than the "receiving" of care as a "patient."

Consent in this sense requires not only external freedom but the internal freedom which is a capacity for self-determination. Internal freedom includes not only freedom from inner compulsion and fear, but (as we have already observed) freedom from ignorance. Hence, consent is specified as "informed," and it depends on the further specification of what "comprehension" means.

Because comprehension requires information, it implies the disclosure of information and a sharing of interpretations of its meaning by a medical professional. The *accuracy* of disclosure, insofar as it is possible, is governed by the ethical requirement of truth-telling (11). The *adequacy* of disclosure has been judged by various criteria, including:

1. The common practice of the profession
2. The reasonable needs and expectations of the ordinary person who might be making a particular decision
3. The unique needs of an individual patient faced with a given choice*

Although these criteria have been generated in the rulings of courts, the courts themselves have not provided a unified voice as to which of these criteria should be determinative. Trends in judicial decisions in most states were for a time primarily in the direction of the "professional practice" criterion, requiring only the consistency of one physician's disclosure with the practice of disclosure by other physicians. Now the trend in many states is more clearly toward the "reasonable person" criterion, holding the medical profession to the standard of what is judged to be material to an ordinary person's decision in the given medical situation. The criterion of the subjective needs of the patient in question has been generally too difficult to implement in the legal arena, though the force of its ethical appeal is significant.

Health care providers should engage in some ethical discernment of their own as to which crite-

---

*For an overview of legal standards for disclosure, and of ethical questions that go beyond legal standards, see Ruth R. Faden and Tom L. Beauchamp, *A History and Theory of Informed Consent* (New York: Oxford University Press, 1986:30–34, 306–316).

ria are most faithful to the needs and rightful claims of patients for disclosure. All three criteria offer reminders of ethical accountability and guidelines for practice. All three can help to illuminate what needs to be shared in the usually significant categories for disclosure: diagnosis and description of the patient's medical condition; description of the proposed treatment, its nature and purpose; risks and possible complications associated with the treatment; alternative treatments or the relative merits of no treatment at all; and the probability of success of the treatment.

Listing categories of disclosure does not by itself fill out all the elements that are important to adequacy of disclosure. For example, the obligation to provide adequate information to a patient implies an obligation for physicians to be current in their own knowledge, for example, about treatments, and disease processes. And when physicians make informed consent possible for patients by giving them the knowledge they need for choice, it should be clear to patients that their continued medical care by a given physician is not contingent on their making the choice that the physician prefers (assuming the limited justifiable exceptions to this that we will note below).

Those who are most concerned with problems of informed consent insist that central to its achievement is communication—communication between physician and patient, but also communication among the many medical professionals who are involved in the care of the patient, and communication (where this is possible and appropriate) with the family of the patient. The role of documentation in a formal process of informed consent can be a help to necessary communication (depending on the methods and manner of its implementation). Yet the completion of consent forms, however legally significant, cannot substitute for the communication of disclosure, the conversation that leads to free refusal or consent (2).

To note the importance of communication for the implementation of an ethical doctrine of informed consent is, then, to underline the fact that informed consent involves a process. There is a process of communication that leads to initial consent (or refusal to consent) and that can make possible appropriate ongoing decision-making.

There are, of course, practical difficulties with ensuring the kind of communication necessary to informed consent. Limitations of time in a clinical context, patterns of authority uncritically maintained, underdeveloped professional communication skills, "language barriers" between technical discourse and ordinarily comprehensible expression, situations of stress on all sides—all of these frequently yield less than ideal circumstances for communication. Yet the ethical requirement of informed consent, no less than a requirement for good medical care, extends to a requirement for reasonable communication. The conditions for communication may be enhanced by creating institutional policies and structures that make it more possible and effective.

It is obvious that while disclosure and consent are basic ethical requirements and not only ideals, they admit of degrees. There will always be varying levels of understanding, varying degrees of internal freedom. The very matters of disclosure are of a kind that are often characterized by disagreement among professionals, uncertainty and fallibility in everyone's judgments, the results not only of scientific analysis but of medical insight and art. And the capacities of patients for comprehension and consent are more or less acute, of greater or lesser power, focused in weak or strong personal integration, compromised or not by pain, medication, or disease. Some limitations mitigate the obligation of informed consent, and some render it impossible. But any compromise or relaxation of the full ethical obligation of informed consent requires specific ethical justification.

THE LIMITS OF INFORMED CONSENT

Because informed consent admits of degrees of implementation, there are, then, limits to its achievement. These are not only the limits of fallible knowledge or imperfect communication. They are limitations in the capacity of patients for comprehension and for choice. Assessment of patient capacity is itself a complex matter, subject to mistakes and to bias. Hence, a great deal of attention has been given to criteria for determining individual capacity (and the legally defined characteristic of "competence") and for just procedures for its evaluation (12). When persons are entirely incapacitated for informed consent, the principle of respect for persons requires that they be protected. Much attention has also been given to the ways and the means of this protection. In general, decisions must be made in these situations for the patient—either by attempts to give a "substituted judgment" (a decision based on what the patient would have wanted, assuming some knowledge of what the patient's wishes would be) or by a decision made according to the "best interests" of the patient. The relative merits of these two options depend on the concrete situation of the patient and those who know and care for her.

The judgment that informed consent is impossible in some circumstances indicates a kind of limit that is different from a minimized, or partial, actualization of consent. One way to acknowledge this is to say that there are limits to the obligation to obtain informed consent at all. Another way is to identify alternative means (for example, "substituted judgment") by which the values and goals of informed consent can be preserved. Both of these ways are perhaps served by saying simply that there are exceptions to the strict rule of informed consent. These exceptions are of several kinds.

First, *impossibility* of any achievement of informed consent suspends the ethical obligation. This is exemplified in emergency situations where consent is unattainable and in other situations where a patient is not at all competent or capable of giving consent. In the practice of obstetrics and gynecology, as in any other special practice, there are situations where decisions can be based only on what is judged to be in the "best interest" of the patient—a judgment made, if possible, by family members (or a legal guardian) and medical professionals together. Yet often when a patient is not able to decide for herself (perhaps, for example, because of the amount of medication needed to control pain) a "substitute judgment" or a judgment on the basis of *prior* informed consent can be made with confidence *if* care has been taken beforehand to learn the patient's wishes. This signals the importance of early communication so that what a patient would choose in a developing situation is known—so that, indeed, it remains possible to respect the self-determination that informed consent represents.

A second way in which the rule of informed consent may be suspended is by being *overridden* by another obligation. There are a number of other ethical obligations that can in certain circumstances override or set limits to the extent of the requirement of informed consent. For example, strong claims for the *public good* (specifically, public health) may set limits to what a patient can choose or refuse. That is, the rights of others not to be harmed may sometimes take priority over an individual's right to refuse a medical procedure (as is the case in exceptional forms of mandatory medical testing and reporting). On the other hand, scarcity of personnel and equipment may in some circumstances mean that individual patients cannot have certain medical procedures "just for the choosing." Also, what is known as *therapeutic privilege* can override an obligation to disclose information and hence to obtain informed consent. "Therapeutic privilege" is the limited privilege of a physician to withhold information from a patient in the belief that this information about the patient's medical condition and options will seriously harm the patient. Concern for the patient's well-being (the obligation of beneficence) thus comes into conflict with respect for the patient's autonomy. This is a difficult notion to apply, however, and great caution must be taken in any appeal made to it. It should not, for example, be used as a justification for ignoring the needs and rights of adolescents to participate in decisions about their sexuality and their reproductive capacities. It is reasonable to argue that therapeutic privilege is almost never a basis for completely overriding the obligation of informed consent, and that when it is, it may characterize a temporary situation, one that will later allow the kind of communication conducive to the freedom of the patient.

Third, and finally,* there are limits intrinsic to the *patient–physician relationship* that keep the requirement of informed consent from ever being absolute. Physicians are moral agents or decision-makers, too, and as such retain areas of free choice—as in the freedom not to provide medical care that they deem medically or ethically irresponsible (a freedom that is sometimes called a right to "conscientious objection"). Interpretations of medical need and usefulness may lead a physician, for example, to refuse to perform surgery or prescribe medication (though the physician should provide the patient with information about her medical options). In the mutuality of the patient–physician relationship, each one is to be respected as a person and supported in her or his autonomous decisions insofar as those decisions are not, in particular circumstances, overridden by other ethical obligations. The existing imbalance of power in this relationship, however, is a reminder to physicians of their greater obligation to ensure and facilitate the informed consent of each patient. That is, differences in professional knowledge can and should be bridged precisely through efforts at communication of information. Only in this way can decisions that are truly mutual be achieved.

Acknowledging the limits of the ethical requirement of informed consent, then, clarifies but does not weaken the requirement as such. In recognition of this, the ACOG Committee on Ethics affirms the nine statements with which this document began.

---

*Sometimes another exception to the rule of informed consent is thought to occur in the rare situation when a patient effectively *waives* her right to give it. This can take the form of refusing information necessary for an informed decision, or simply refusing altogether to make any decision. However, there are two reasons for not considering this an exception with the same status as the others listed here:

1. A waiver in such instances seems to be itself an exercise of choice, and its acceptance can be part of respect for the patient's autonomy.
2. Implicit in the ethical concept of informed consent is the goal of maximizing a patient's freedoms, which means that "waivers" should not be accepted complacently without some concern for the causes of the patient's desire not to participate in the management of her care.

In any case, it should be noted that in states where informed consent forms are required, it may be necessary to meet this requirement in some legally acceptable way.

REFERENCES

1. American College of Obstetricians and Gynecologists, Department of Professional Liability. Informed consent. The assistant. Washington, DC: ACOG, 1988
2. American College of Obstetricians and Gynecologists, Department of Professional Liability. Informed consent forms. The assistant. Washington, DC: ACOG, 1988
3. American College of Obstetricians and Gynecologists. Ethical decision-making in obstetrics and gynecology. ACOG Technical Bulletin 136. Washington, DC: ACOG, 1989
4. American College of Obstetricians and Gynecologists. Patient choice: maternal-fetal conflict. ACOG Committee Opinion 55. Washington, DC: ACOG, 1987
5. American College of Obstetricians and Gynecologists. Ethical issues in pregnancy counseling. ACOG Committee Opinion 61. Washington, DC: ACOG, 1988
6. American College of Obstetricians and Gynecologists. Sterilization of women who are mentally handicapped. ACOG Committee Opinion 63. Washington, DC: ACOG, 1988
7. American College of Obstetricians and Gynecologists. Ethical considerations in sterilization. ACOG Committee Opinion 73. Washington, DC: ACOG, 1989
8. American College of Obstetricians and Gynecologists. Human immunodeficiency virus infection: physicians' responsibilities. ACOG Committee Opinion 85. Washington, DC: ACOG, 1989
9. American College of Obstetricians and Gynecologists. Ethical issues in surrogate motherhood. ACOG Committee Opinion 88. Washington, DC: ACOG, 1990
10. The President's Commission for the Study of Ethical Problems in Medicine and Biomedical Research. Making health care decisions: the ethical and legal implications of informed consent in the patient-practitioner relationship. Vol 1. (Stock no. 040-000-00459-9). Washington, DC: U.S. Government Printing Office, 1982:2
11. American College of Obstetricians and Gynecologists. Deception. ACOG Committee Opinion 87. Washington, DC: ACOG, 1990
12. The President's Commission for the Study of Ethical Problems in Medicine and Biomedical Research. Making health care decisions: the ethical and legal implications of informed consent in the patient-practitioner relationship. Vol 1. (Stock no. 040-000-00459-9). Washington, DC: U.S. Government Printing Office, 1982:Chapters 8–9

BIBLIOGRAPHY

Beauchamp TL, Childress JF. Principles of biomedical ethics. 3rd ed. New York: Oxford University Press, 1989:Chapter 1

Faden RR, Beauchamp TL. A history and theory of informed consent. New York: Oxford University Press, 1986

Katz J. The silent world of doctor and patient. New York: The Free Press, 1984

Levine RJ. Ethics and regulation of clinical research. 2nd ed. Baltimore, Maryland, and Munich, Germany: Urban and Schwarzenberg, 1986

The President's Commission for the Study of Ethical Problems in Medicine and Biomedical Research. Making health care decisions: the ethical and legal implications of informed consent in the patient-practitioner relationship. Vol 1. (Stock no. 040-000-00459-9). Washington, DC: U.S. Government Printing Office, 1982

The President's Commission for the Study of Ethical Problems in Medicine and Biomedical Research. Making health care decisions: the ethical and legal implications of informed consent in the patient-practitioner relationship. Vol 2. (Stock no. 040-000-00468-8). Washington, DC: U.S. Government Printing Office, 1982

The President's Commission for the Study of Ethical Problems in Medicine and Biomedical Research. Making health care decisions: the ethical and legal implications of informed consent in the patient-practitioner relationship. Vol 3. (Stock no. 040-000-00469-6). Washington, DC: U.S. Government Printing Office, 1982

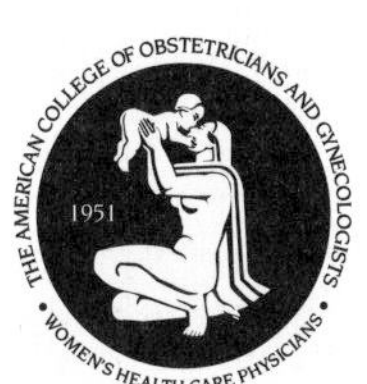

The American College of Obstetricians and Gynecologists
409 12th Street, SW • Washington, DC 20024-2188

456/7

ACOG

Committee on Ethics

Committee Opinion

Number 233, April 2000

Ethical Dimensions of Seeking and Giving Consultation

Physicians have a long history of working together and with other health care professionals to provide efficient and comprehensive care for the patients they serve. Achieving these goals requires that from time to time physicians or other care providers seek consultation from or provide consultation to their colleagues (1). The basic principles of consultation for obstetrician–gynecologists are summarized in *The Code of Professional Ethics of the American College of Obstetricians and Gynecologists* as follows (2):

- "The obstetrician–gynecologist's relationships with other physicians, nurses, and health care professionals should reflect fairness, honesty, and integrity, sharing a mutual respect and concern for the patient."
- "The obstetrician–gynecologist should consult, refer, or cooperate with other physicians, health care professionals, and institutions to the extent necessary to serve the best interests of their patients."

Although consultation usually is requested in an efficient manner that expedites patient care, situations occur in which the relationship between practitioners or between institutions and practitioners results in an inefficient, less-than-collegial consultative process that may not be in the best interest of the patient. For example, a patient and a consultant may be put at serious disadvantage when consultation is requested late in the process of care or is not accompanied by sufficient background information or the reason for consultation is not clearly stated. Conversely, those seeking consultation may be denied assistance on arbitrary grounds. The present statement outlines the purpose of consultation and referral, states the underlying ethical foundations that govern consultation and referral, and elaborates specifically the responsibilities of those who seek and those who provide consultation. This document is directed to physicians but it should be recognized that nonphysician practitioners also may be involved in consultation.

The Purpose of Consultation and Referral

Typically, a patient first seeks care from her primary caregiver (3), who should be aware that the patient's needs may go beyond his or her education,

The American College of Obstetricians and Gynecologists
409 12th Street, SW
PO Box 96920
Washington, DC 20090-6920

12345/43210

training, or experience (2, 4). Various levels of consultation may be needed to make correct diagnoses, provide technical expertise, and recommend a course of action (see box). Occasionally, consultation or referral may be indicated when a patient's request for care is in conflict with her primary caregiver's recommendations or preferences. Finally, a patient may seek consultation with another caregiver to obtain a second opinion or explore other options for care (5). In all of these types of consultation, the overriding principle is that consultation is primarily for the benefit of the patient (3).

Ethical Foundations

Ethical principles require that the consultative process be guided by the following concepts (2, 6):

- The welfare of the patient should be central to the consultant–patient relationship (beneficence)
- The patient should be fully informed about the need for consultation and participate in the selection of the consultant (autonomy)
- The patient should have access to adequate consultation regardless of her medical condition, social status, or financial situation (justice)
- Practitioners must disclose to patients any potential conflict of interest that is involved in a consultation relationship, including financial incentives or penalties or restrictive guidelines (truth-telling)

In addition, both practitioners with primary clinical responsibility and consultants must respect the rights of the patient and also the rights of their respective professional colleagues.

Responsibilities Associated With Consultation

Seeking Consultation and Requesting Referral

Consultations usually are sought when the practitioner with primary clinical responsibility recognizes a condition or situation that is beyond his or her level of expertise or available resources. Historically, this practitioner acted as an independent agent who

Definitions: Levels of Consultation

Consultation is the act of seeking assistance from another physician(s) or health care professional(s) for diagnostic studies, therapeutic interventions, or other services that may benefit the patient. There are several levels of consultation (3):

- Informal consultation
- Single-visit consultation
- Continuing collaborative care
- Transfer of primary clinical responsibility

Informal consultation, in which the consultant does not talk with or examine the patient, usually involves a simple question from the referring practitioner that is answered by the consultant. The consultant does not make an entry in the patient's medical record or charge a fee, and the referring practitioner should not attribute an opinion to the consultant. Examples of informal consultations are questions regarding the significance of an irregular blood antibody or the follow-up interval for an abnormal Pap test. Such a consultation does not establish a patient–consultant relationship.

A single-visit consultation involves examination of the patient or the patient's record and performance of diagnostic tests or therapeutic procedures. The findings, procedures, and recommendations of the consultant are recorded in the patient's medical record or provided to the practitioner with primary clinical responsibility for the patient in a written report or letter, and a fee may be charged. The subsequent care of the patient continues to be provided by the referring practitioner. Examples of such consultations are confirming the findings of a pelvic examination, performing a specific urodynamic procedure on a patient with urinary stress incontinence, and interpreting an electronic fetal monitoring tracing or imaging studies. In the latter two cases, the tracing or other output can be transmitted electronically, thus allowing for the performance of a single-visit consultation without personal contact between the patient and consultant.

Continuing collaborative care describes a relationship in which the consultant provides ongoing care in conjunction with the referring practitioner. Thus, the consultant assumes at least partial responsibility for the patient's care. An example is a high-risk obstetric patient with a medical complication of pregnancy who is periodically assessed by the consultant, while the referring practitioner is responsible for the day-to-day management of the patient.

Transfer of primary clinical responsibility to the consultant may be appropriate for management of problems outside the scope of the referring practitioner's education, training, and experience or in cases in which the patient must be transferred to another facility. Examples are the transfer of care of a patient in preterm labor from a birth center to a consultant in a perinatal center or referral of a patient with ovarian cancer to a gynecologic oncologist. In many of these situations, patients will eventually return to the care of the referring practitioner when the problem for which the consultation was sought is resolved.

decided when consultation was appropriate, determined the level of consultation, and was free to choose a particular consultant. More recently, as a result of recognition of the importance of patient autonomy, practitioners now inform patients of the need for consultation and discuss options with them. The quality of the consultation is often improved by this collaborative relationship between practitioner and patient.

Today, this practitioner–patient partnership operates under new conditions that may affect the process of consultation. Under certain types of managed care arrangements, health care guidelines and protocols may limit the freedom of the practitioner to provide complete care or to request consultation (7). These guidelines may include instructions about specific situations or medical conditions in which consultation, second opinion, or referral is mandated (8). Examples include abnormal labor that may require operative delivery or chronic uterine bleeding that may require hysterectomy. Other guidelines may require that practitioners seek consultation when patients develop signs and symptoms of severe preeclampsia or if ovarian cancer is discovered. Such arrangements and guidelines may be designed to ensure a high level of care for patients by requiring that consultants be involved appropriately in certain clinical problems.

Conversely, practitioners may find themselves in situations that create disincentives to medically appropriate consultation or that mandate use of a consultant panel that is not adequate to support appropriate patient care. The policies that lead to such situations involve potential conflicts of interest (9) and may have a negative effect on the patient's medical needs, thus limiting her autonomy and her right to informed choice. Under all conditions of practice—solo or group, fee for service or managed care contract—consultation and referral should be carried out in the patient's best interest and obtained with the patient's consent after full disclosure of limitations and potential conflicts of interest.

It is in everyone's best interest—practitioners with primary clinical responsibility, consultants, patients, and health care plans—that the criteria for consultation be mutually agreed upon in advance and stated clearly in writing. Financial incentives or penalties for consultation and referral that exist either overtly or covertly under many managed care contracts are sources of serious conflicts of interest. Practitioners must be free to inform patients of the best medical practice or options of care, even when the mandate of directed referrals under contracted care does not include these alternatives. Ethical responsibility for the patient's best interest demands that the practitioner disclose any proscriptions to serving as the patient's advocate. The practitioner has a responsibility to provide the patient with his or her best medical judgment and serve as an advocate for the patient if recommended care is denied. It then becomes the patient's responsibility to decide whether to abide by insurance plan restrictions, challenge them, or seek care outside the scope of coverage.

Giving Consultation and Accepting Referral

Physicians generally provide consultations or accept referred patients in the interest of providing excellent care for patients and promoting good relationships among colleagues. Open communication and established professional relationships facilitate effective consultation and referral. However, at times a consultant may be called on unexpectedly, inconve- niently, and sometimes inappropriately to be involved in or to assume the care of a patient. In these situations, a physician is only obligated to provide consultation or assume the care of the patient if there is a contractual agreement or a preexisting patient–physician relationship or if there is a severe medical emergency in which there is no reasonably available alternative caregiver (10). Hospital or departmental guidelines for consultation and referral may prevent such confrontations.

Practical Recommendations

Providing optimal care demands a good working relationship with a number of other physicians and health care professionals. Consultation may be needed by the practitioner with primary clinical responsibility regardless of specialty designation or level of training. Ideally, the referring practitioner–consultant relationship has been established before the need for consultation or referral arises, and the referring practitioner–consultant relationship should be an ongoing one.

One way to maximize prompt, effective consultation and collegial relationships is to have a formal consultation protocol. This may be especially advantageous for family physicians who provide obstetric or gynecologic care and for collaborative practice between the obstetrician–gynecologist and nurse practitioners, certified nurse midwives, and other health professionals. Such protocols create pathways that anticipate difficult or complex situations.

Responsibilities of the Referring Practitioner

Responsibilities of the referring practitioner can be outlined as follows:

1. The referring practitioner should request consultation in a timely manner, whenever possible before an emergency arises. A good working relationship between the referring practitioner and consultant requires shared concern for the patient's needs and a commitment to timely and clear-cut communication.
2. The referring practitioner is responsible for preparing the patient with an explanation of the reasons for consultation, the steps involved, and the names of qualified consultants.
3. The referring practitioner should provide a summary of the history, physical examination, laboratory findings, and any other information that may facilitate the consultant's evaluation and recommendations (11).
4. Whenever possible, the referring practitioner should document in the medical record the indications for the consultation and specific issues to be addressed by the consultant.
5. The level of consultation (see box) should be established by a dialogue between the referring practitioner and the consultant that results in mutual agreement.

Responsibilities of the Consultant

Responsibilities of the consultant can be outlined as follows:

1. Consultants should recognize their individual boundaries of expertise and provide only those medically accepted services and technical procedures for which they are qualified by education, training, and experience.
2. When asked to provide consultation, the consultant should do so in a timely manner and without regard to the specialty designation or qualifications of the referring practitioner. If the consultant believes that the referring practitioner is not qualified to provide an appropriate level of continuing care, the consultant should recommend to the referring practitioner and, if necessary, to the patient that the referring practitioner transfer care of the patient.
3. If a physician is asked to provide an "informal consultation" and believes an examination of the patient or her record is necessary to answer the question appropriately, that consultant may request the right to provide a formal consultation.
4. The consultant should effectively communicate findings, procedures performed, and recommendations to the referring practitioner at the earliest opportunity (5).
5. For all but informal consultations, a summary of the consultation should be included in the medical record or sent to the referring practitioner by letter or written report.
6. The extent to which the consultant will be involved in the ongoing care of the patient should be clearly established by mutual agreement of the consultant, the referring practitioner, and the patient. At times it may be appropriate for the consultant to assume primary clinical responsibility for the patient. Even if this is only a temporary circumstance, the consultant should obtain the referring practitioner's cooperation and assent whenever possible.
7. When the consultant does not have primary clinical responsibility for the patient, he or she should try to obtain concurrence for major procedures or additional consultants from the referring practitioner.
8. In all that is done, the consultant must respect the relationship between the patient and the referring practitioner, being careful not to diminish inappropriately the patient's confidence in her other caregivers (3).
9. The consultant should be cognizant of the referring practitioner's abilities. Reliance on these abilities may increase the convenience to the patient, limit transportation needs, and ulti-mately result in more cost-effective care.
10. In the rare situation in which there is clear evidence that the patient's health is likely to be harmed by a continuing level of substandard care, the consultant has an obligation to discuss with the referring practitioner the problems that have been identified, recommend appropriate medical measures, and, when necessary, inform the patient.

A complex clinical situation may call for multiple consultations. Unless authority has been transferred elsewhere, the responsibility for the patient's care should rest with the referring practitioner (3). This practitioner should remain in charge of communication with the patient and coordinate the overall care on the basis of information derived from the consultants. This will ensure a coordinated effort that remains in the patient's best interest.

References

1. American Medical Association Council on Ethical and Judicial Affairs. Code of medical ethics: current opinions with annotations. Chicago: AMA, 1998:76–77
2. American College of Obstetricians and Gynecologists. Code of professional ethics of the American College of Obstetricians and Gynecologists. Washington DC: ACOG, 1997
3. American College of Physicians Ad Hoc Committee on Medical Ethics, Kitchens LW. Ethics manual. 4th ed. Philadelphia: ACP, 1998:35
4. American College of Obstetricians and Gynecologists. Physicians working with physicians. The Assistant 8. Washington DC: ACOG, 1998
5. American Medical Association Council on Ethical and Judicial Affairs. Code of medical ethics: current opinions with annotations. Chicago: AMA, 1998:126
6. Beauchamp TL, Childress JF. Principles of biomedical ethics. 4th ed. New York: Oxford University Press, 1994
7. Wallach EE, Fox HE, Gordon T, Faden R. Symposium: managed care and ethics. Contemp Ob Gyn 1998;43: 162–176
8. Chervenak FA, McCullough LB, Chez RA. Responding to the ethical challenges posed by the business tools of managed care in the practice of obstetrics and gynecology. Am J Obstet Gynecol 1996;175:523–527
9. Cain JM, Jonsen AR. Specialists and generalists in obstetrics and gynecology: conflicts of interest in referral and an ethical alternative. Women's Health Issues 1992;2: 137–145
10. American Medical Association Council on Ethical and Judicial Affairs. Code of medical ethics: current opinions with annotations. Chicago: AMA, 1998:167
11. American College of Obstetricians and Gynecologists. Role of the obstetrician–gynecologist in the diagnosis and treatment of breast disease. ACOG Committee Opinion 186. Washington DC: ACOG, 1997

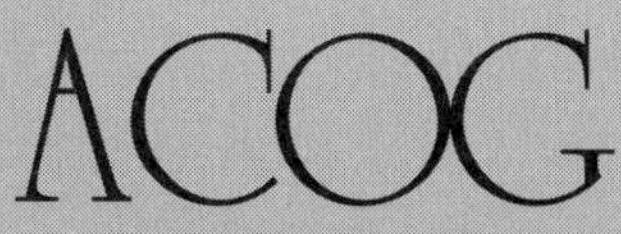

Committee
on Ethics

Committee Opinion

Number 159, October 1995

Ethical Guidance for Patient Testing

In the practice of medicine, clinical evaluation is enhanced by a broad range of tests. Recommendations to patients about testing should be based on current medical knowledge, a concern for the patient's best interests, and mutual consultation. Patient testing embodies many scientific and human ideals. From an ethical perspective, the most important principles involve a trusting patient–physician relationship, a focus on the benefits the patient may derive from testing, and an appreciation that patients make choices about their medical care.

Rapid technological development and the need to consider legal and sociocultural factors as well as medical knowledge have increased the complexity of the decision-making process. The physician is often in the position of ordering tests—human immunodeficiency virus (HIV) or genetic markers, for example—that may, unlike a urinalysis or a hemogram, have a profound nonmedical effect on the patient, her partner, her family, and society in general. This new level of complexity requires the specification of both medical and ethical guidelines for decisions about patient testing. This document provides ethical guidance for decisions about ordering tests, counseling patients, and reporting results.

Ordering Tests

- *The physician and the patient have a shared responsibility*. The quality of medical care improves when there is clear communication and mutual understanding between physician and patient. It is the responsibility of the obstetrician–gynecologist to communicate effectively and to develop skills which promote a patient–physician relationship characterized by trust and honesty. Similarly, it is the responsibility of the patient to provide information about her life style, health habits, sexual practices, and religious and cultural beliefs, when these factors may affect medical judgment. In decisions about testing, physicians should be guided by scientific knowledge. Care must be taken to avoid subjective assumptions based on bias that could affect the appropriateness of testing.
- *Testing should be performed primarily for the benefit of the patient.* Testing at the request of third parties—partners, health care providers, members of the patient's extended family, employers, or health insurers—is justifiable only when the patient or her valid proxy understands the potential risks and benefits and gives consent. Examples of this type

ISSN 1074-861X

The American College of Obstetricians and Gynecologists
409 12th Street, SW
Washington, DC 20024-2188

12345/98765

of testing include genetic tests to assist family members with reproductive decisions and HIV tests to fulfill conditions for the purchase of life insurance.

- *The decision to offer or to withhold a test should not be made solely on the basis of a physician's assumptions about the patient's expected response to test results.* Prejudgments about a patient's wishes regarding fetal abnormalities, for example, should not preclude her being offered prenatal testing. The patient should join with the physician in deciding the amount of diagnostic information appropriate for making intelligent choices about treatment options. The physician is not, however, ethically obligated to perform every test a patient requests.
- *The patient should be informed prospectively about policies regarding use of information and legal requirements.* The patient should be told what will be communicated, to whom, and the potential implications of reporting the information. If, for example, a patient is aware that a specific hospital has a policy of posting HIV test results in the medical record and access to results may be available, she may choose instead to utilize an anonymous testing procedure available through another laboratory. In some situations, reporting of results is mandated by law. Physicians should be familiar with the laws regarding mandatory testing and reporting requirements in their own jurisdictions.
- The *physician and patient should discuss concerns about cost containment and reimbursement.* The mutual goal of physician and patient should be to avoid both undertesting and overtesting. Contemporary focus on the economics of health care has created worries for both physician and patient about access to care, limitations to testing, appropriateness of utilization, and the impact of financial constraints on quality of care. Open communication about cost concerns is the best way to alleviate suspicion and to promote trust.

Pretest and Posttest Counseling

- *Testing which may have multiple medical or psychosocial consequences requires specific counseling.* The extent of counseling beneficial to each patient will vary depending on the individual and on the implications inherent in the potential test results. With simple tests like urinalysis it is sufficient to provide information about the nature and purpose of the test, and how the results will guide management. Tests which may have multiple medical or psychosocial ramifications require comprehensive explanation of the process, the goals, and the implications. Counseling is appropriate for genetic testing and maternal toxicology assays, for example, because of the potential for psychologic, social, and economic impact. Testing for HIV or genetic testing may limit future insurance coverage. A positive toxicology screen could result in the removal of children from the household.
- *Both pretest and posttest counseling facilitate women's access to appropriate health care.* Pretest counseling includes both medical considerations and issues such as the availability of emotional support while waiting for results. Posttest counseling offers an opportunity to provide access to resource networks and community-based services.
- *Referral may be needed for comprehensive counseling.* If time constraints or lack of technical expertise make it difficult to offer comprehensive counseling in a particular practice, appropriate options include either 1) referral to a specialized center for both counseling and testing, or 2) referral for counseling only, with return to the original physician for testing and medical follow-up.

Confidentiality and the Reporting of Test Results

- *Information ordinarily may not be revealed without the patient's express consent.* Maintaining confidentiality is intrinsic to respect for patient autonomy and permits the free exchange of information that is relevant to medical decision making. Situations may arise, however, in which a physician has competing obligations: on the one hand to protect the patient's confidentiality and on the other to disclose test results in order to prevent harm to a third party. In these situations, every avenue of communication should first be explored in discussions with the patient about rights and responsibilities. Consultation with an institutional ethics committee or a medical ethics specialist may be helpful in weighing benefits and harms of disclosure. Legal advice may be prudent.
- *A violation of confidentiality may be necessary in the last resort.* A violation of confidentiality may be justifiable only when legally required or when

1) there is a high probability of harm to a third party; 2) the potential harm is a serious one; 3) the information communicated can be used to prevent harm; and 4) greater good will result from breaking confidentiality than from maintaining it.

Conclusion

In addition to establishing a diagnosis, testing provides opportunities to educate, to inform, and to advise. The ethical principles of respect for autonomy (patient choice) and beneficence (concern for the patient's best interests) should guide the testing, counseling, and reporting process. Clear and ample communication fosters trust, facilitates access to services, and improves the quality of medical care.

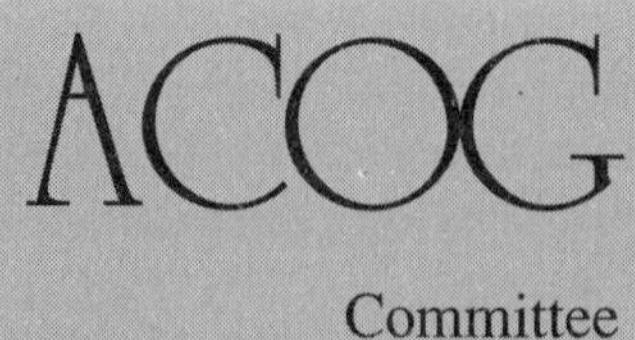

Committee on Ethics

Committee Opinion

Number 181, April 1997

Ethical Issues in Obstetric–Gynecologic Education

Education of health professionals is essential to maintain standards of competent and beneficial practice. Inherent in the education of health professionals is the problem of disparity in power and authority, including the power of teachers over students and the power of practitioners over patients (1).* It is therefore important to clarify both the professional responsibilities to those patients whose care provides educational opportunities and the responsibilities of teachers and students toward one another.

Ethical Responsibilities Toward Patients in Educational Settings

At the turn of the century, some medical educators were concerned about the needs of patients in "teaching hospitals," and they took steps to ensure that patients' rights would be protected. However, the prevailing opinion was more aptly characterized by a medical school faculty member: "Patients must clearly understand from the beginning that they are admitted for teaching purposes and that they are to be willing to submit to this when pronounced physically fit" (2). Unfortunately, this sentiment persists as an unstated presumption in some contemporary education programs. If the power inherent in the role of medical practitioner is misused in the educational setting, this misuse is likely to carry over into attitudes and relationships with future patients as well.

If health care professionals are to benefit society, they must be well educated and experienced. Acquisition of knowledge and skills in the educational process entails both benefits and risks. The benefits of health care to society provide the justification for exposure of patients to risks associated with education in clinical medicine. While the benefits generally accrue to society at large, the burdens fall primarily on individual patients, especially the economically disadvantaged. These bur-

* In this statement the term "teacher" refers to all of those in the teaching role, including medical school faculty, attending physicians, fellows, residents, interns, and, in some cases, medical students. The term "student" refers to all of those in the learning role, including fellows, residents, interns, and students. These terms are not meant to exclude other health care professionals, such as nurse midwives, nurse practitioners, and physician assistants, who may also serve in the role of teachers or students.

ISSN 1074-861X

The American College of Obstetricians and Gynecologists
409 12th Street, SW
PO Box 96920
Washington, DC 20090-6920

12345/10987

dens are inherent in situations in which patients interact with students, for example, during medical histories, physical examinations, and diagnostic and surgical procedures.

Physicians must learn new skills and techniques in a manner consistent with the ethical obligations to benefit the patient, to do no harm, and to respect a patient's right to make informed decisions about health matters. These obligations must not be unjustifiably subordinated to the need and desire to learn new skills. In consideration of society's interest in the education of physicians, all patients should be considered "teaching patients." Race or socioeconomic status should not be the basis for selection of patients for teaching.

Although patients are given the opportunity to consent to or refuse treatment by students, the obligations of the profession, the institution, and patients should be made more uniform and explicit. Professional obligations include disclosure of the risks and benefits inherent in the teaching setting and provision of adequate supervision at all levels of training. The patient has an obligation to participate in the teaching process in order to share equally in the creation of a new generation of health care providers. A situation may arise in which a patient refuses, for whatever reason, to have a student involved in her health care. Such refusals should initiate discussion and counseling. Patient choice, however, must be handled with compassion and respect.

Finally, students must hold in confidence any information about patients learned in the context of a professional relationship. They should discuss specific patient care matters only in appropriate settings, such as teaching conferences or patient-management rounds. Conversations in public places, such as hospital corridors or elevators, involving comments about patients, their families, or the care they are receiving are inappropriate (3).

Ethical Responsibilities of Teachers to Students

The relationship between teacher and student in medical education inevitably involves the problem of imbalance of power and the risk of exploitation of a student for the benefit of the teacher (1). The teacher–student relationship exists at multiple levels among faculty members, medical students, attending physicians, fellows, and residents. Complex as it may be, there is a fundamental ethical responsibility at all levels for the teacher to impart wisdom, experience, and skill for the benefit of the student, without expectation of personal service by or reward from the student.

Because so much of medicine is learned in a preceptor–student relationship, great care must be taken that the teacher does not exploit the student. An example is the teacher who expects a student to spend time that is out of proportion to the educational value involved on a research project, but gives little or no credit for such a contribution. In this regard, the behavior of teachers toward students is a powerful example of ethics in action. Students are likely to model their behavior on that of their teachers (4).

The relationship of a teacher to a student involves not only trust and confidence but also power and dependency. It is the role of the teacher to foster independence in the student while nurturing the student in the learning process. This is a complex relationship, the boundaries of which can become obscured in the intense setting of clinical preceptorship (5). For example, the long hours spent by teachers and students in relatively arduous and isolated circumstances may foster amorous relationships. Regardless of the situation, the power imbalance makes a romantic or sexual relationship between a teacher and student ethically suspect. Amorous relationships between teachers and their current students are not appropriate.

Students should not be placed in situations where they must provide care or perform procedures for which they are not qualified and not adequately supervised. To do otherwise violates an ethical responsibility to the student as well as to the patient. A healthy relationship between teachers and students allows students to request assistance or supervision without fear of humiliation or retribution. Teaching should take place in an atmosphere that fosters mutual respect.

Conduct and Responsibilities of Students Toward Their Teachers

Students have the obligation to be honest, conscientious, and respectful in their relationship with their teachers. They should act in a way that preserves the dignity of the patient and does not undermine the relationship between the patient and her physician. It is the student's responsibility to ask for assistance and supervision when it is needed. Unfettered communication between student and teacher is essential in fostering an atmosphere that will allow, even encourage, students to request help. When such communication does not occur, both education and patient care suffer.

Inherent in the teacher–student relationship is the vulnerability of the student in dealing with perceived unethical behavior or incompetent conduct of a teacher. If a student observes such behavior or conduct, the matter should be brought to the attention of the appropriate institutional authority.

Institutional Responsibilities

Institutions have ethical obligations to students, patients, and teachers. Institutions have an obligation to provide a work environment that enhances professional competence. The health care system has often exploited students at all levels of education. Students may be viewed as a source of cheap labor, especially in busy hospitals on a teaching service. Students often provide long hours of service, and the resultant neglect of the student's physical and mental health must be balanced against the provision of an effective clinical experience. Lack of sleep, heavy workloads, and increasing amounts of responsibility without commensurate levels of authority are sources of great stress in medical education, especially during residency (6–8). The potentially negative impact of such an educational experience on the student's developing attitude toward patients and the profession should be considered. The obligation to provide a good work environment includes ensuring that students and residents work reasonable hours, establishing a balance between medical education and responsibility for patient care, providing adequate ancillary and administrative support services, and, in the case of residents, providing reasonable salaries and benefits (9).

A source of substantial stress for some students and residents is the conflict between family responsibilities and the demands of medical education (10). For many students, sleep deprivation resulting from long work hours results in fatigue, irritability, and anxiety. The inability to relate with consideration or affection to a partner or spouse or to participate in any effective way with child care or other domestic responsibilities may seriously impair family relationships. Also, with increasing numbers of women in education programs, special attention must be given to the parallel demands of pregnancy and career goals. Providing ample time to sustain family relationships without adversely affecting the educational experience or imposing excessive burdens on colleagues is a daunting task, but one that must be confronted. Shared positions and more flexible time lines for completing educational requirements can be helpful in solving such problems.

Institutions should maintain a well-established reporting and review process for investigating allegations about unethical behavior or incompetent conduct. Access to such a process can facilitate fair and just relationships between students and teachers in these precarious situations.

As concerns about cost containment increase, education could become a low priority. The process of medical education may reduce the efficiency of patient care and increase costs. It is the responsibility of all physicians and institutions involved in education of health care professionals to ensure that cost-reduction efforts do not diminish the opportunities for education in clinical medicine. Institutions have an ethical responsibility to develop policy statements and guidelines for inclusion of students in patient care in ways that ensure sound medical education and high-quality medical care.

Conclusion

The effective education of students, residents, interns, fellows, and other professionals is essential if the health care professions are to benefit society. The power and authority inherent in relationships between students and patients as well as between teachers and students are important ethical concerns. Power and authority should be exercised responsibly to protect patients' dignity and welfare and to enhance the educational process.

Respect for autonomy requires that patients be informed about the extent to which students at any level are involved in their care and that patients' concerns be addressed. Students should provide only that level of care for which they are qualified and adequately supervised. Working conditions and work schedules should reflect a sensitivity for student welfare in its broadest terms. This attention to ethics will promote attitudes conducive to the compassionate and skilled treatment of patients. This emphasis should also serve as a model for the next generation of teachers.

References

1. Brody H. The healer's power. New Haven, Connecticut: Yale University Press, 1992, 12–25
2. Ludmerer KM. Learning to heal. The development of American medical education. New York, New York: Basic Books, Inc., 1985, 232–233
3. Ubel PA, Zell MM, Miller DJ, Fischer GS, Peters-Stefani D, Arnold RM. Elevator talk: observational study of inappropriate comments in a public space. Am J Med 1995; 99:190–194
4. Bosk CL. Forgive and remember. Managing medical failure. Chicago, Illinois: University of Chicago Press, 1979
5. Plaut SM. Boundary issues in teacher-student relationships. J Sex Marital Ther 1993;19:210–219

6. Butterfield PS. The stress of residency. A review of the literature. Arch Intern Med 1988;148:1428–1435
7. Stress and impairment during residency training: strategies for reduction, identification, and management. Resident Services Committee, Association of Program Directors in Internal Medicine. Ann Intern Med 1988;109:154–161
8. McCall TB. The impact of long working hours on resident physicians. N Engl J Med 1988;318:775–778
9. Asch DA, Parker RM. The Libby Zion case. One step forward or two steps backward? N Engl J Med 1988; 318:771–775
10. Green MJ. What (if anything) is wrong with residency overwork? Ann Intern Med 1995;123:512–517

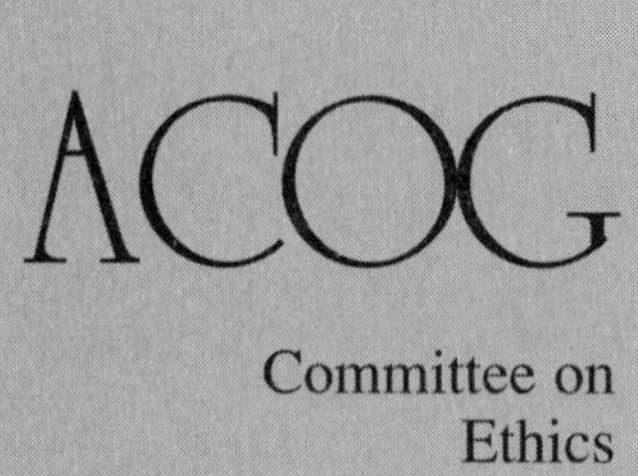

Committee on Ethics

Committee Opinion

Number 217, April 1999 (*Replaces #56, October 1987*)

Ethical Issues Related to Expert Testimony by Obstetricians and Gynecologists

The American College of Obstetricians and Gynecologists recognizes that it is the duty of obstetricians and gynecologists who testify as expert witnesses on behalf of defendants, the government, or plaintiffs to do so solely in accordance with their judgment on the merits of the case. Furthermore, the College cannot condone the participation of physicians in legal actions where their testimony will impugn performance that falls within accepted standards of practice or, conversely, will support obviously deficient practice. Because the experts articulate the standards in a given case, care must be exercised to ensure that such standards do not narrowly reflect the experts' views to the exclusion of other choices deemed acceptable by the profession. The College considers unethical any expert testimony that is misleading because the witness does not have appropriate knowledge of the standard of care for the particular condition at the relevant time or because the witness knowingly misrepresents the standard of care relevant to the case.

The Problem of Professional Liability—Reality and Perceptions

The College recognizes its responsibility, and that of its Fellows, to continue efforts to improve health care for women through every available method of quality assurance. The College also recognizes, however, that many claims of medical malpractice represent the response of a litigation-oriented society to a technologically advanced form of health care that has fostered unrealistic expectations. As technology continues to become more complex, both the benefits and risks also increase, making the complication-free practice of medicine less possible.

It therefore becomes important to distinguish between medical "maloccurrence" and medical malpractice. Medical maloccurrence is defined as a bad outcome that is unrelated to the quality of care provided. Certain medical or surgical complications can be anticipated and represent unavoidable risks of appropriate medical care. Other complications arise unpredictably and are similarly unavoidable. Still others occur as a result of decisions that

ISSN 1074-861X

The American College of Obstetricians and Gynecologists
409 12th Street, SW
PO Box 96920
Washington, DC 20090-6920

12345/32109

have been made carefully by patients and physicians with fully informed consent but appear, in retrospect, to have been a less appropriate choice among several options. Each of these situations represents a type of maloccurrence, rather than an example of malpractice, and is the result of the uncertainty inherent in all of medicine. Malpractice requires a demonstration of negligence (ie, substandard practice that causes harm). The potential for personal, professional, and financial rewards from expert testimony may encourage testimony that undermines the distinction between unavoidable maloccurrence and actual medical malpractice. It is unethical to distort or to represent a maloccurrence as an example of medical malpractice, or the converse.

The American College of Obstetricians and Gynecologists supports the concept of appropriate and prompt compensation to patients for medically related injuries. Any such response, however, should also reflect the distinction between medical maloccurrence, for which all of society should perhaps bear financial responsibility, and medical malpractice, for which health care providers should be held responsible.

Responsibility of Individual Physicians

The moral and legal duty of physicians who testify before a court of law is to do so in accordance with their expertise. This duty implies adherence to the strictest personal and professional ethics. Truthfulness is essential. Misrepresentation of one's personal clinical opinion as absolute right or wrong may be harmful to individual parties and to the profession at large. The obstetrician–gynecologist who is an expert witness should limit testimony to his or her sphere of medical expertise and should be prepared adequately. Witnesses who testify as experts should have knowledge and experience that are relevant to obstetric and gynecologic practice at the time of the occurrence and to the specific areas of clinical medicine they are discussing. The acceptance of fees that are greatly disproportionate to those customary for professional services can be construed as influencing testimony given by the witness. It is unethical for a physician to accept compensation that is contingent upon the outcome of litigation (1, 2).

The College encourages the development of policies and standards for expert testimony. Such policies should address safeguards to promote truth-telling and to encourage openness of the testimony to peer review. These policies would also encourage testimony that does not assume an advocacy or partisan role in the legal proceeding.

The following principles are offered as guidelines for the physician who assumes the role of an expert witness:

1. The physician should have experience and knowledge in the areas of clinical medicine that enable him or her to testify about the standards of care that applied at the time of the occurrence that is the subject of the legal action.
2. The physician's review of medical facts should be thorough, fair, and impartial and should not exclude any relevant information. It should not be biased to create a view favoring the plaintiff, the government, or the defendant. The goal of a physician testifying in any judicial proceeding should be to provide testimony that is complete, objective, and helpful to a just resolution of the proceeding.
3. The physician's testimony should reflect an evaluation of performance in light of generally accepted standards, neither condemning performance that falls within generally accepted practice standards nor endorsing or condoning performance that falls below these standards. Medical decisions often must be made in the absence of diagnostic and prognostic certainty.
4. The physician should make a clear distinction between medical malpractice and medical maloccurrence.
5. The physician should make every effort to assess the relationship of the alleged substandard practice to the outcome, because deviation from a practice standard is not always substandard care or causally related to a bad outcome.
6. The physician should be prepared to have testimony given in any judicial proceeding subjected to peer review by an institution or professional organization to which he or she belongs (3).

References

1. American Medical Association. Code of medical ethics: current opinions with annotations. Chicago: AMA, 1998
2. American Bar Association. Annotated model rules of professional conduct. 3rd ed. Chicago: ABA, 1996:325–333
3. American College of Obstetricians and Gynecologists. Code of professional ethics of the American College of Obstetricians and Gynecologists. Washington, DC: ACOG, 1997

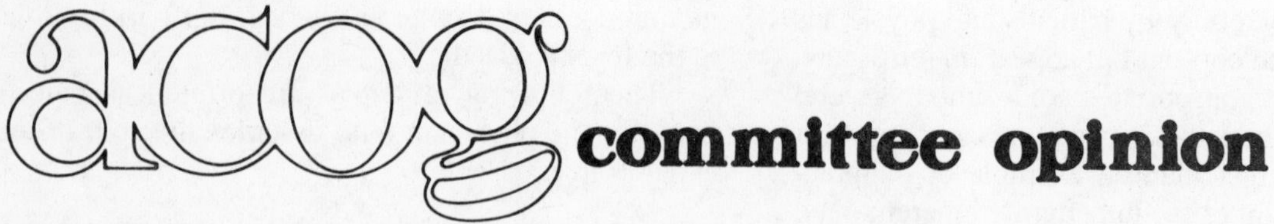

Committee on Gynecologic Practice
Committee on International Affairs

Number 151—January 1995

Female Genital Mutilation

Female genital mutilation is a practice based on cultural and traditional patterns dating back at least 2,000 years. According to the World Health Organization, approximately 80 million women have undergone these procedures. While the rationale for these procedures is lost in antiquity, the practice is still widespread in Africa, the Middle East, and Southeast Asia. The procedure is performed rarely in the United States, Canada, and western Europe; however, women who have undergone the procedure often immigrate to these countries.

There are many forms of female genital mutilation but the procedures performed most often are 1) removal of the clitoral prepuce, 2) excision of the clitoris, and 3) removal of the clitoris and labia minora and occasionally much of the labia majora, suturing the two sides together to occlude the vagina (infibulation). These procedures usually are performed prior to adolescence (between the ages of 1 week and 14 years old) by untrained individuals without benefit of sterile conditions or anesthesia.

The immediate physical effects of female genital mutilation can include infection, tetanus, shock, hemorrhage, and even death. In addition, there are long-term physical and mental disabilities, such as chronic pelvic infection, keloids, vulvar abscesses, sterility, incontinence, depression, anxiety, sexual dysfunction, and obstetric complications.

There is no scientific basis for the female genital mutilation procedure. Physicians are reminded, however, that patients who have undergone the procedure should be treated with sensitivity and compassion. The American College of Obstetricians and Gynecologists joins many other major organizations (World Health Organization, United Nations International Children's Emergency Fund, International Federation of Gynecology and Obstetrics, and the American Medical Association) in opposing all forms of medically unnecessary surgical modification of the female genitalia. Furthermore, it is recommended that the issue be addressed by promoting awareness among the public and health care workers and by developing methods for educating physicians regarding the gynecologic and obstetric care of women who have undergone this procedure.

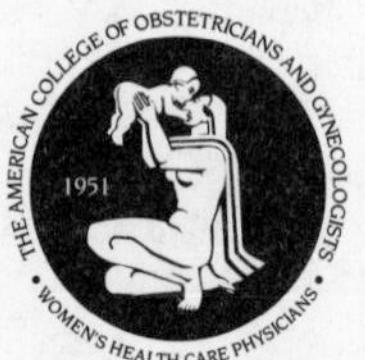

ISSN 1074-861X

The American College of Obstetricians and Gynecologists
409 12th Street, SW • Washington, DC 20024-2188

12345/98765

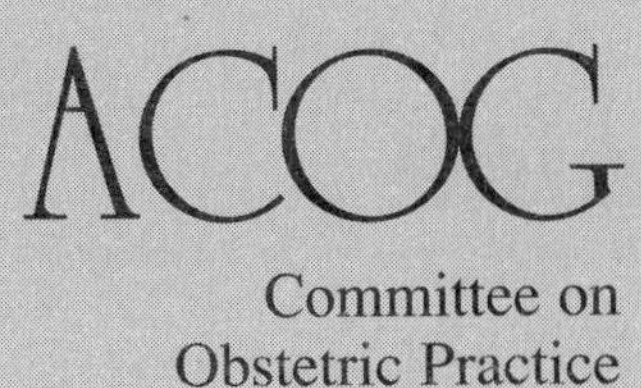

Committee on
Obstetric Practice

Committee Opinion

Number 187, September 1997

Fetal Fibronectin Preterm Labor Risk Test

The Committee on Obstetric Practice has reviewed the fetal fibronectin enzyme immunoassay kit recently approved by the Food and Drug Administration. This kit was approved as an aid in assessing the risk of preterm delivery. If the kit is to be used, the following criteria should be met:

- Amniotic membranes are intact
- Cervical dilatation is minimal (< 3 cm)
- Sampling is performed no earlier than 24 weeks, 0 days and no later than 34 weeks, 6 days of gestation

This test is not recommended for routine screening of the general obstetric population. Widespread use of the test in asymptomatic low-risk patients has the potential to add significant cost to prenatal care without proven benefit. Although a negative test appears to be useful in ruling out preterm delivery that is imminent (ie, within 2 weeks), the clinical implications of a positive result have not been evaluated fully. If the test is to be clinically useful, the results must be available from the laboratory in a timely manner.

ISSN 1074-861X

The American College of Obstetricians and Gynecologists
409 12th Street, SW
PO Box 96920
Washington, DC 20090-6920

12345/10987

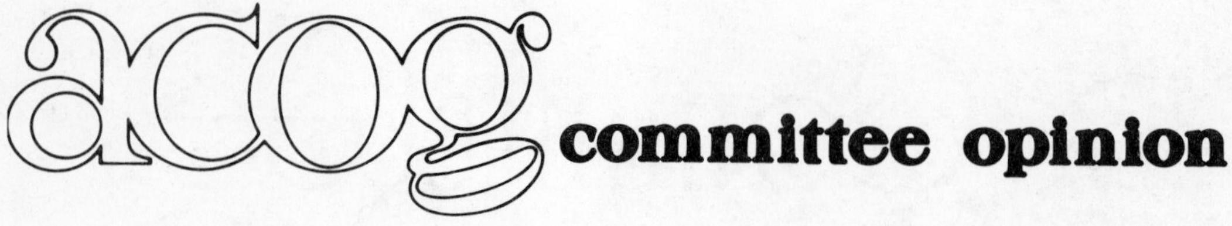

Committee on Obstetric Practice

Number 149—December 1994

Financial Influences on Mode of Delivery

Recent focus on health care costs has generated interest in developing mechanisms to change practice patterns. There is little or no evidence that the decision to perform a cesarean delivery or to offer a trial of labor is in any way motivated by a differential in payment. The Committee on Obstetric Practice does not believe that financial incentives or disincentives should be used by payers to influence physician or patient decisions relative to the mode of delivery. Decisions regarding the method of obstetric delivery should be based on standard obstetric indications and maternal–fetal safety.

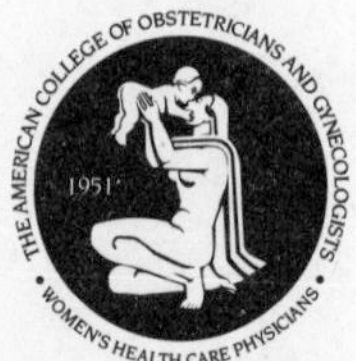

ISSN 1074-861X

The American College of Obstetricians and Gynecologists
409 12th Street, SW • Washington, DC 20024-2188

12345/87654

ACOG Committee Opinion

Committee on Genetics

Number 223, October 1999

First-Trimester Screening for Fetal Anomalies with Nuchal Translucency

This document reflects emerging clinical and scientific advances as of the date issued and is subject to change. The information should not be construed as dictating an exclusive course of treatment or procedure to be followed.

ISSN 1074-861X

The American College of Obstetricians and Gynecologists
409 12th Street, SW
PO Box 96920
Washington, DC 20090-6920

12345/32109

Maternal serum screening in the second trimester of pregnancy is the current method of screening women at low risk for carrying fetuses with neural tube defects, certain chromosome abnormalities, and other select fetal malformations. This approach detects approximately 60% of Down syndrome cases in fetuses at a screen-positive rate of 5% (1). However, first-trimester screening for chromosome abnormalities offers many potential advantages over second-trimester screening. It helps reduce maternal anxiety at an earlier gestational age and allows the patient to take advantage of first-trimester prenatal diagnosis by chorionic villus sampling. If the fetus is found to be affected, the patient may elect to terminate the pregnancy. First-trimester pregnancy termination is associated with reduced maternal morbidity.

The ultrasonographic finding of nuchal translucency (an echo-free area at the back of the fetal neck) in the first trimester of pregnancy reportedly has been associated with fetal chromosome abnormalities (2–4). The prevalence of chromosome abnormalities is reported to vary from 30% to 86% in fetuses with increased nuchal translucency. Most of the early data on nuchal translucency screening involved high-risk women undergoing first-trimester prenatal diagnosis in referral centers for indications such as advanced maternal age or family history of a chromosome abnormality.

Studies involving low-risk women in a routine clinical practice setting have produced conflicting results (5–10). These differences appear to be attributable to interobserver and intraobserver variation in nuchal translucency measurements. In addition, there is no consensus on the definition of increased nuchal translucency (3, 4, 11). In most of the reports, the nuchal translucency measurements were taken from the sagittal section of the fetus usually used to obtain the crown–rump length (2–4). This appears to be the method of choice. However, some investigators have used a transverse suboccipitobregmatic view of the fetal head to obtain the measurement (11). When measuring nuchal translucency, care should be taken to distinguish nuchal skin from the amnionic membrane. Nuchal translucency values are crown–rump length-dependent (3, 4, 11, 12).

Nuchal Translucency Screening with Maternal Serum Screening Markers

Measurement of the free beta subunit of human chorionic gonadotropin and pregnancy-associated plasma protein-A in maternal serum appears promising as a method of screening for fetal chromosome abnormalities in the first trimester (13, 14). Similar to second-trimester screening, the Down syndrome detection rate with first-trimester biochemical screening is approximately 60% with a 5% screen-positive rate (14). Ongoing research indicates that combining first-trimester maternal serum screening markers with nuchal translucency screening may allow up to an 80–90% detection rate for Down syndrome (15, 16). These preliminary data remain controversial.

Using Nuchal Translucency to Screen for Fetal Cardiac Anomalies

Prenatal detection of fetal cardiac abnormalities currently is performed during second-trimester ultrasound examination. Of fetuses with chromosome abnormalities, 50–90% have major anomalies of the heart and great vessels. It is possible that the lymphedema seen in nuchal translucency is associated with fetal cardiac abnormalities (17). It also is possible that nuchal translucency in fetuses without chromosome abnormalities is cardiogenic in nature. In fetuses with normal chromosomes and nuchal translucency, it appears that the prevalence of major cardiac abnormalities increases with nuchal translucency size (17).

Recommendations

- First-trimester screening for fetal chromosome, cardiac, and other abnormalities using the nuchal translucency marker alone or in combination with serum markers appears promising but remains investigational.
- The technique for measuring nuchal translucency and the criteria for defining increased nuchal translucency must be standardized.
- Until further studies confirm the efficacy of first-trimester nuchal translucency screening, with or without serum markers, this modality is not recommended for routine clinical use.

References

1. Haddow JE, Palomaki GE, Knight GJ, Williams J, Pulkkinen A, Canick JA, et al. Prenatal screening for Down's syndrome with use of maternal serum markers. N Engl J Med 1992;327:588–593
2. Bronshtein M, Rottem S, Yoffe N, Blumenfeld Z. First-trimester and early second-trimester diagnosis of nuchal cystic hygroma by transvaginal sonography: diverse prognosis of the septated from the nonseptated lesion. Am J Obstet Gynecol 1989;161:78–82
3. Nicolaides KH, Azar G, Byrne D, Mansur C, Marks K. Fetal nuchal translucency: ultrasound screening for chromosomal defects in first trimester of pregnancy. BMJ 1992; 304:867–869
4. Nicolaides KH, Brizot ML, Snijders RJ. Fetal nuchal translucency: ultrasound screening for fetal trisomy in the first trimester of pregnancy. Br J Obstet Gynaecol 1994; 101:782–786
5. Pajkrt E, de Graaf IM, Mol BW, van Lith JM, Bleker OP, Bilardo CM. Weekly nuchal translucency measurements in normal fetuses. Obstet Gynecol 1998;91:208–211
6. Kornman LH, Morssink LP, Beekhius JR, De Wolf BT, Heringa MP, Mantingh A. Nuchal translucency cannot be used as a screening test for chromosomal abnormalities in the first trimester of pregnancy in a routine ultrasound practice. Prenat Diagn 1996;16:797–805
7. Roberts LJ, Bewley S, Mackinson AM, Rodeck CH. First trimester fetal nuchal translucency: problems with screening the general population. 1. Br J Obstet Gynaecol 1995; 102:381–385
8. Bewley S, Roberts LJ, Mackinson AM, Rodeck CH. First trimester fetal nuchal translucency: problems with screening the general population. 2. Br J Obstet Gynaecol 1995; 102:386–388
9. Hafner E, Schuchter K, Philipp K. Screening for chromosomal abnormalities in an unselected population by fetal nuchal translucency. Ultrasound Obstet Gynecol 1995;6: 330–333
10. Hafner E, Schuchter K, Liebhart E, Philipp K. Results of routine fetal nuchal translucency measurement at weeks 10–13 in 4233 unselected pregnant women. Prenat Diagn 1998;18:29–34
11. Comas C, Martinez JM, Ojuel J, Casals E, Puerto B, Borell A, et al. First-trimester nuchal edema as a marker of aneuploidy. Ultrasound Obstet Gynecol 1995;5:26–29
12. Schuchter K, Wald N, Hackshaw AK, Hafner E, Liebhart E. The distribution of nuchal translucency at 10-13 weeks of pregnancy. Prenat Diagn 1998;18:281–286
13. Macri JN, Spencer K, Aitken D, Garver K, Buchanan PD, Muller F, et al. First-trimester free beta (hCG) screening for Down syndrome. Prenat Diagn 1993;13:557–562
14. Krantz DA, Larsen JW, Buchanan PD, Macri JN. First-trimester Down syndrome screening: free beta-human chorionic gonadotropin and pregnancy-associated plasma protein A. Am J Obstet Gynecol 1996;174:612–616
15. Orlandi F, Damiani G, Hallahan TW, Krantz DA, Macri JN. First-trimester screening for fetal aneuploidy: biochemistry and nuchal translucency. Ultrasound Obstet Gynecol 1997;10:381–386
16. Spencer K, Noble P, Snijders RJ, Nicolaides KH. First-trimester urine free beta hCG, beta core, and total oestriol in pregnancies affected by Down's syndrome: implications for first-trimester screening with nuchal translucency and serum free beta hCG. Prenat Diagn 1997;17:525–538
17. Hyett JA, Perdu M, Sharland GK, Snijders RS, Nicolaides KH. Increased nuchal translucency at 10–14 weeks of gestation as a marker for major cardiac defects. Ultrasound Obstet Gynecol 1997;10:242–246

ACOG

Committee
on Genetics

Committee Opinion

Number 161, October 1995

Fragile X Syndrome

Fragile X syndrome is the most common inherited form of mental retardation, affecting about 1 in 1,500 males and 1 in 2,500 females from a variety of ethnic backgrounds. Mental retardation ranges from borderline to severe, although most patients have moderate degrees of mental retardation. Other associated phenotypic abnormalities include autistic behaviors, macroorchidism in adult males, characteristic narrow face with a large jaw, and speech and language problems. The abnormal facial features are subtle and become more noticeable with age, making phenotypic diagnosis difficult, especially in the newborn.

Standard metaphase chromosomal analysis does not consistently demonstrate the cytogenetic abnormality in patients with fragile X syndrome. Using specific culture conditions (folate deprivation), the demonstration of a fragile site on the long (q) arm of the human X chromosome (Xq27-28) was identified in males and some females with fragile X syndrome. The syndrome was originally thought to be transmitted in a classic X-linked recessive fashion; however, the inheritance of fragile X syndrome has proven to be much more complex. Females may be affected. Nearly all males with fragile X and most carrier females who have mental retardation show the fragile site. However, about 20% of males with the mutant gene do not have mental retardation and do not demonstrate cytogenetic evidence of the fragile site. These men are referred to as transmitting males. Two thirds of carrier females are mentally normal, and only one third of these demonstrate cytogenetic findings. These variations in the expression of the fragile site complicate cytogenetic diagnosis, particularly prenatal diagnosis. Molecular diagnostic techniques have now replaced cytogenetic analysis as the diagnostic procedure of choice for the fragile X syndrome.

The molecular cloning of the fragile X mental retardation-1 gene (*FMR*-1) has helped to clarify the molecular basis of the fragile X syndrome. Nearly all of the mutations in the gene involve expansion of a triplet repeat consisting of the bases cytosine–guanine–guanine. This pattern appears to correlate with the fragile site detected by cytogenetic techniques. The number of repeats varies in unaffected individuals (Table 1). A patient with 50–200 repeats is phenotypically normal and is said to have a premutation. When greater than 200 repeats are present, the patient has a full mutation that results in phenotypic fragile X syndrome. The *FMR-1* gene nearly always becomes methylated and inactivated in these patients. The number of repeats and the status of gene methylation are

ISSN 1074-861X

The American College of Obstetricians and Gynecologists
409 12th Street, SW
Washington, DC 20024-2188

12345/98765

Table 1. Mutation in the Fragile X Mental Retardation-1 Gene

Status of Individual	Number of Triplet Repeats (Cytosine–Guanine–Guanine)
Unaffected	6–49
Premutation	50–200
Full mutation	>200

determined by using DNA-based molecular tests (ie, Southern blot analysis and polymerase chain reaction). Chorionic villus sampling may not be reliable for diagnosis because of different methylation patterns in the trophoblast as compared with the fetus. Although reliable for determining the number of triplet repeats, chorionic villus sampling may not adequately determine the methylation status of the *FMR-1* gene.

Transmission of a disease-producing mutation to a fetus depends upon the sex of the parent and the number of cytosine–guanine–guanine repeats present in the parental gene. Parents at risk for transmission of the disease are those who have either the premutation or the full DNA mutation. When a female carries the premutation and the length of the repeat exceeds 90, premutation genes are much more likely to expand and to result in the birth of an affected child. Males may transmit the premutation gene to their children, but expansion to a full mutation has not been described in the offspring of a male having the premutation gene. Empirically determined risks are available for the purposes of genetic counseling. An antibody-based test using peripheral blood is currently under investigation as a rapid approach to the screening of mentally retarded individuals and neonates for fragile X syndrome (1).

The Committee recommends the following regarding testing for fragile X syndrome:

1. DNA-based molecular analysis is the preferred method of diagnosis for fragile X syndrome and its premutations. Cytogenetic analysis should not be used for the definitive diagnosis of fragile X syndrome.
2. Testing for fragile X syndrome should be considered in any child with developmental delay of uncertain etiology or any individual with mental retardation of uncertain etiology. If there is no DNA evidence for the fragile X syndrome in an individual with mental retardation, standard chromosome analysis may also be considered in order to exclude chromosomal causes of mental retardation such as autosomal trisomies, deletions, duplications, or unbalanced translocations.
3. Patients with a family history of mental retardation or a history of fragile X mental retardation should undergo genetic evaluation to assess their risk for having an affected child.
4. Prenatal testing for fragile X syndrome by amniocentesis should be offered to known carriers of the fragile X premutation or mutation.

References

1. Willemsen R, Mohkamsing S, De Vries B, Devys D, van den Ouweland A, Mandel JL, et al. Rapid antibody test for fragile X syndrome. Lancet 1995;345:1147–1148
2. Warren ST, Nelson DL. Advances in molecular analysis of fragile X syndrome. JAMA 1994;271:536–542
3. Nussbaum RL, Ledbetter DH. The fragile X syndrome. In: Scriver CR, Beaudet AL, Sly WS, Valle D, eds. The metabolic basis of inherited disease. 6th ed. Vol I. New York: McGraw-Hill Inc, 1989:327–341
4. The American College of Medical Genetics policy statement. Fragile X syndrome: diagnostic and carrier testing. Bethesda, Maryland: Working Group of the Genetic Screening Subcommittee of the Clinical Practice Committee, ACMG, July 22, 1994, pages 1–4

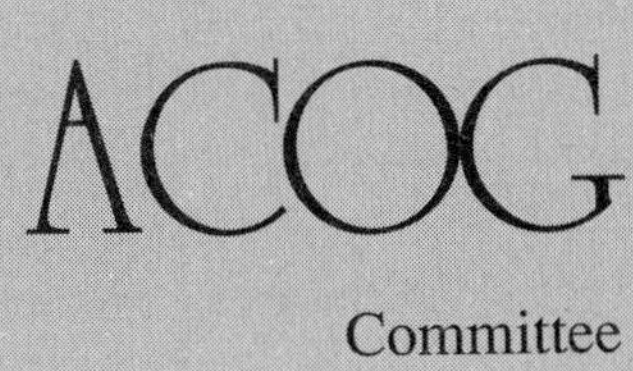

Committee
on Genetics

Committee Opinion

Number 178, November 1996

Genetic Evaluation of Stillbirths and Neonatal Deaths

In all stillbirths and neonatal deaths, autopsy findings supplemented by genetic studies may provide important information (1). This information may explain the cause of death and is particularly valuable in counseling parents about future pregnancies. Approximately 8% of stillbirths have chromosomal abnormalities, and about 20% have dysmorphic features or skeletal abnormalities (2, 3). Such findings may permit identification of a specific anomaly or syndrome, direct further investigation of the family, and allow appropriate counseling about recurrence risks.

Following a stillbirth or neonatal death, proper management includes taking a careful perinatal and family history, performing a physical examination of the fetus or infant (with documentation by description and photography if possible), and obtaining indicated laboratory studies. Chromosomal analysis of fetal blood and tissue, X-rays, examination of the placenta, autopsy, and parental counseling based on the findings should be considered. This is especially true when dysmorphic features, inconsistent growth measurements, anomalies, hydrops, or growth restriction is present or when a parent is a carrier of a balanced chromosome structural anomaly or has a mosaic chromosomal pattern. To ascertain the etiology and provide appropriate counseling to the family, clinical–pathologic correlation is best done by a team comprising obstetricians, neonatologists, pathologists, and geneticists. This knowledge should be communicated in a timely manner to the involved clinicians and to the family of the deceased infant.

When stillbirth or neonatal death occurs, the obstetric history should be reviewed, as well as the family history. Any pertinent information in the maternal or paternal pedigree should be documented and investigated further. The gestational age by last menstrual period, maternal examinations, and sonograms should be recorded for correlation with the physical examination of the neonate. Maternal data such as titers for TORCH (toxoplasmosis, other viruses, rubella, cytomegalovirus, and herpes simplex viruses) as well as other possibilities of nongenetic causes should be reviewed, but they are not the focus of this document.

The general examination of the stillborn should be done promptly, noting any dysmorphic features and obtaining body measurements including crown–rump, crown–heel, and foot lengths, as well as weight (4–6). These measurements are helpful to estimate gestational age and evaluate for intra-

ISSN 1074-861X

The American College of Obstetricians and Gynecologists
409 12th Street, SW
PO Box 96920
Washington, DC 20090-6920

12345/09876

uterine growth restriction, and foot length is especially useful before 23 weeks of gestation (4–8). Further documentation by frontal and profile photographs, with close-ups of specific abnormalities, is valuable for subsequent review and consultations. Whole body X-ray with posteroanterior and lateral views may reveal an unrecognized skeletal abnormality or further define a grossly apparent deformity. If possible, the infant should be positioned with extremities extended and the epiphyses viewed. Malformations often are present in patterns that permit classification into a particular syndrome. Syndrome identification may delineate etiologic and pathogenetic factors that could have predictive significance for recurrence risk and risk of other associated anomalies (9–11).

Gross and microscopic examination of the placenta, membranes, and umbilical cord may corroborate autopsy findings or explain apparent fetal deformity. Gross evaluation of the umbilical cord and blood vessels, membranes for amniotic bands and other anomalies, and placenta for size and condition should be performed. Samples of amniotic fluid, umbilical cord blood, or amnion may be obtained for chromosomal and any other relevant studies. Histologic study of placental samples also should be performed (11–13). Analysis of bile, vitreous humor, and urine may be helpful if umbilical cord blood is unobtainable (14, 15).

Appropriate consent must be obtained to take eye, skin, and other tissue samples, including fluid obtained by needle postmortem, as well as for autopsy. A total volume of 3 ml of umbilical cord blood should be taken into a sterile container treated with heparin for cytogenetic studies. Skin samples may be taken from any site. The skin should be washed with sterile saline, and at least 1 cm^2 with attached dermis is necessary.

If maceration is present, fascia samples are preferable to skin samples. Samples of at least 1 cm may be taken from the thigh, inguinal region, or achilles tendon, using sterile technique. Kidney, skeletal muscle, liver, and lung samples are also preferable to skin samples if an autopsy is done or proper permission is obtained. Samples of gonads may be taken if indicated.

All samples should be placed in an appropriate sterile medium from the cytogenetics laboratory if possible or in normal saline if no medium is available. The samples should be kept at room temperature, and a 1-cm tissue sample should be frozen as well. Even if a full autopsy is planned, and autopsy consent has been obtained, these specimens should be obtained as soon as possible after stillbirth or neonatal death.

When a full autopsy is performed, it should follow the guidelines for perinatal autopsy published by the College of American Pathologists or other standard references (16). However, the pathologist should be aware of the clinical history and specific interest in genetic diagnosis so that samples for cytogenetic and possible metabolic or molecular studies may be taken. The results of the autopsy, placental examination, tests, and cytogenetic studies should be discussed with the clinicians.

Final conclusions should be reached by the team of pathologists, geneticists, obstetricians, and neonatologists. The family should be counseled promptly after a consensus is reached. Counseling before the evaluation is complete or before different opinions of the various caregivers have been resolved may increase feelings of guilt or anger in parents who have experienced a perinatal death. When there is an abnormal child or a genetic defect, these feelings are often magnified. Specific testing of the parents may be offered. When no specific diagnosis is available, that information is important as well (17), and a list of diagnoses excluded may be useful in counseling the parents. Whether or not there is a specific diagnosis, compassionate counseling of the parents and sensitivity to their needs are required.

References

1. Saller DN Jr, Lesser KB, Harrel U, Rogers BB, Oyer CE. The clinical utility of the perinatal autopsy. JAMA 1995;273:663–665
2. Pauli RM, Reiser CA. Wisconsin Stillbirth Service Program: II. Analysis of diagnoses and diagnostic categories in the first 1,000 referrals. Am J Med Genet 1994;50:135–153
3. Pauli RM, Reiser CA, Lebovitz RM, Kirkpatrick SJ. Wisconsin Stillbirth Service Program: I. Establishment and assessment of a community-based program for etiologic investigation of intrauterine deaths. Am J Med Genet 1994;50:116–134
4. Reed GB, Claireaux AE, Cockburn F, eds. Diseases of the fetus and newborn: pathology, imaging, genetics, and management. London: Chapman and Hall Medical, 1995
5. Wigglesworth JS, Singer DB. Textbook of fetal and perinatal pathology. Boston: Blackwell Scientific Publications, 1991
6. Stocker JT, Dehner LP. Pediatric pathology. Philadelphia: JB Lippincott and Co, 1992
7. Naeye RL. Disorders of the placenta, fetus, and neonate: diagnosis and clinical significance. St Louis: Mosby-Year Book Inc, 1992
8. Shepard TH, Shi M, Fellingham GW, Fujinaga M, FitzSimmons JM, Fantel AG, et al. Organ weight standards for human fetuses. Pediatr Pathol 1988;8:513–524
9. Willis RA. The borderland of embryology and pathology. 2nd ed. Washington, DC: Butterworth, 1962
10. Jones KL. Smith's recognizable patterns in human malformations. 4th ed. Philadelphia: WB Saunders Co, 1988

11. Leppig KA, Werler MM, Cann CI, Cook CA, Holmes LB. Predictive value of minor anomalies. I. Association with major malformations. J Pediatr 1987;110:531–537
12. Benirschke K, Kaufman P. Pathology of the human placenta. 3rd ed. New York: Springer-Verlag, 1995
13. Genest DR. Estimating the time of death in stillborn fetuses: II. Histologic evaluation of the placenta; a study of 71 case stillborns. Obstet Gynecol 1992;80:585–592
14. Emery JL, Howat AJ, Variend S, Vawter GF. Investigation of inborn errors of metabolism in unexpected infant deaths. Lancet 1988;2(8601):29–31
15. Rashed MS, Ozand PT, Bennett MJ, Barnard JJ, Govindaraju DR, Rinaldo P. Inborn errors of metabolism diagnosed in sudden death cases by acylcarnitine analysis of postmortem bile. Clin Chem 1995;41:1109–1114
16. Valdes-Dapena MA, Huff DS. Perinatal autopsy manual. Upland, Pennsylvania: Diane Publishing, 1993
17. Rushton DI. Prognostic role of the perinatal postmortem. Br J Hosp Med 1994;52:450–454

ACOG Committee Opinion

Committee on Genetics

Number 238, July 2000 (*Replaces No. 168, February 1996*)

Genetic Screening for Hemoglobinopathies

Over the past several years, genetics research has advanced our knowledge of disease-causing mutations in the hemoglobin genes and developed tests for their precise identification. These tests can identify couples at risk for offspring with hemoglobinopathies and provide them with information to make a decision about whether to have prenatal testing. Counseling couples at increased risk for hemoglobinopathies requires a knowledge of genotype and phenotype. The ever-widening ethnic and geographic distribution of human hemoglobinopathies has made the identification of individuals at increased risk by ethnic or racial origin less reliable. Obstetrician–gynecologists who offer genetic risk assessment need to be aware of risk factors and new developments in the ability to detect mutations in carriers and identify affected fetuses.

Initiation of screening for hemoglobinopathies depends on the patient's ethnic background, medical history, family history, and red blood cell indices and on the goals of testing. In many states, screening infants for hemoglobinopathies is routine. As a result, in the future couples may know their hemoglobin genotypes when they visit an obstetrician–gynecologist. Screening of all couples of reproductive age is not recommended; however, the obstetrician–gynecologist should try to identify couples at increased risk for having offspring with a form of thalassemia or sickle cell disease. Historically, high-risk groups include people of African-American, Southeast Asian, or Mediterranean ancestry. Ethnic groups considered to be at low risk for these disorders are northern European, Japanese, Inuit (Eskimo), Native American, and individuals of Mexican and Korean descent.

A combination of laboratory tests may be necessary to provide the information required for genetic counseling of patients who are carriers of α-thalassemia, β-thalassemia, or sickle cell anemia (Fig. 1). Patients of Southeast Asian descent are at an increased risk for α-thalassemia, and patients of Mediterranean descent are at an increased risk for β-thalassemia. To ensure accurate hemoglobin identification, which is needed for genetic counseling, electrophoresis is the appropriate initial laboratory test for individuals determined to be at risk for a hemoglobin disorder. Several tests, including solubility testing such as a test for the presence of hemoglobin S (Sickledex), isoelectric focusing, and high-performance liquid chromatography (HPLC), have been used for primary screening. Solubility tests are

This document reflects emerging clinical and scientific advances as of the date issued and is subject to change. The information should not be construed as dictating an exclusive course of treatment or procedure to be followed.

ISSN 1074-861X

The American College of Obstetricians and Gynecologists
409 12th Street, SW
PO Box 96920
Washington, DC 20090-6920

12345/43210

inadequate because they fail to identify important transmissible hemoglobin gene abnormalities affecting fetal outcome. Solubility test results may be negative for individuals with an abnormal hemoglobin gene (eg, Hb C trait, β-thalassemia trait, Hb E trait, Hb B trait, Hb D trait). Many individuals with these genotypes are asymptomatic, but if their partners have sickle cell trait or other hemoglobinopathies, they may produce children with more serious hemoglobinopathies, such as Hb S/β-thalassemia and Hb SC disease. Solubility testing may be valuable, however, for rapidly screening for sickling when this information is critical for immediate patient care.

Determination of mean corpuscular volume (MCV) is recommended for patients who are at increased risk for α- or β-thalassemia. Patients who have a low MCV (<80 μ^3) may have one of the thalassemia traits and are candidates for hemoglobin electrophoresis. β-Thalassemia is associated with elevated fetal hemoglobin and elevated hemoglobin A_2 levels (>3.5%). Neither hemoglobin electrophoresis nor solubility testing will identify individuals with α-thalassemia or α-thalassemia trait; this condition can be identified only by molecular genetic testing. If the MCV is below normal, iron deficiency anemia has been excluded, and the hemoglobin electrophoresis is not consistent with β-thalassemia trait (ie, there is no elevation of hemoglobin A_2 or fetal hemoglobin), then DNA-based testing should be used to detect α-globin gene deletions characteristic of α-thalassemia. If both partners are identified as carriers of a gene for abnormal hemoglobins, counseling for DNA-based prenatal diagnostic testing should be offered.

References

1. Scriver CR, Beaudet AL, Sly WS, Valle D, eds. The metabolic and molecular basis of inherited disease. 7th ed. New York: McGraw-Hill, 1995
2. Guy G, Coady DJ, Jansen V, Snyder J, Zinberg S. alpha-Thalassemia hydrops fetalis: clinical and ultrasonographic considerations. Am J Obstet Gynecol 1985;153:500–504
3. Baysal E, Huisman TH. Detection of common deletional alpha-thalassemia-2 determinants by PCR. Am J Hematol 1994;46:208–213
4. Rimoin DL, Connor JM, Pyeritz RE, eds. Emery and Rimoin's principles and practice of medical genetics. 3rd ed. New York: Churchill Livingstone, 1997

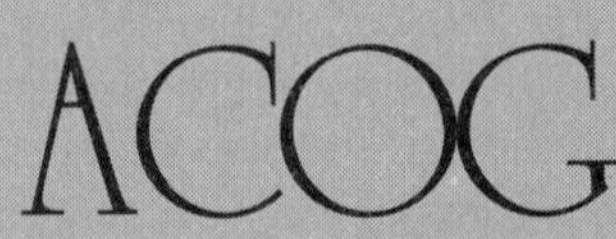

Committee on Genetics

Committee Opinion

Number 192, October 1997

Genetic Screening of Gamete Donors

When the risk to offspring is high and when prenatal diagnosis is not available or is not an acceptable alternative, the use of donor gametes is an option for couples with genetic risk factors. This is especially true if one member of the couple has a disabling autosomal dominant disorder or the couple already has a child with an autosomal recessive disorder for which prenatal diagnosis is not yet available. Even when prenatal diagnosis is available, some at-risk couples prefer gamete donation to therapeutic abortion. For others with genetic disorders that render them agonadal and infertile, gamete donation is an alternative to adoption that offers a biologic connection to the mother and control over the prenatal environment. In all such cases, gamete donation is one of the alternatives available through genetic counseling and assisted reproduction. When gamete donation is used, the Committee on Genetics recommends the clinical and genetic evaluation of all donors to avoid the transmission of heritable genetic disorders. There are other considerations when selecting a gamete donor, such as screening for infectious diseases; however, these will not be addressed in this Committee Opinion, which is limited to genetic evaluation.

Each physician should pay close attention to the number of times that a given individual in a population is used as a gamete donor. Otherwise, the rate of consanguinity might exceed that observed in the general population, and the incidence of recessive disorders might be increased. For example, if a given gamete donor is the carrier of a rare recessive mutation, excessive use of that donor might generate a cluster of similar carriers in a given locality. Over a 20- to 30-year period, this donor might generate more offspring who are homozygous for this rare autosomal recessive disorder than would otherwise have been the case. It is difficult to provide a precise number of times that a given donor can be used because one must take into consideration the population base from which the donor is selected and the catchment area that is served by the gamete donation facility. For example, to avoid inadvertent consanguinity equal to or greater than first-cousin marriages in a population of 800,000, assuming assorted mating, a single sperm donor should not be used to achieve more than 25 pregnancies (1, 2).

The most important part of the screening process is obtaining and interpreting the family history of the gamete donor in conjunction with the physical examination. A genetic questionnaire can be used as an adjunct to obtain this information. The emphasis should be on genetic information (ie, educa-

ISSN 1074-861X

The American College of Obstetricians and Gynecologists
409 12th Street, SW
PO Box 96920
Washington, DC 20090-6920

12345/10987

tion and counseling) rather than testing procedures alone. This general approach, coupled with selected testing, will help to reduce the risk of genetic diseases in this unique population of offspring.

Gamete Donors (General)

Regardless of the donor's sex, it is important to screen the donor's three-generation pedigree for any genetic disorders, perform a physical examination, and determine the donor's ethnic background. Genetic diseases in the following categories are especially important:

- Autosomal or X-linked disease with age of onset extending beyond the age of the donor (eg, Huntington's disease)
- Autosomal dominant disease with reduced penetrance or variable expressivity (eg, Marfan syndrome, neurofibromatosis)
- Autosomal recessive disease, especially if the disease has a high frequency in the population (eg, cystic fibrosis, Tay–Sachs disease)

Screening Tests

The D (Rho[D]) type of all gamete donors should be known. To minimize the small but unavoidable risk to D-negative women, this should include testing for D^u.

In addition to D typing, one should screen donors to determine their risk, on the basis of family history and ethnic background, of having offspring with the hemoglobinopathies, Tay–Sachs disease, and fragile X syndrome. However, universal screening for hemoglobinopathies is not recommended. Donors who are at increased risk for having offspring with the thalassemias should be screened initially with red-cell indices followed by hemoglobin electrophoresis. Individuals with a normal hemoglobin electrophoresis who are considered to be at risk for alpha-thalassemia require DNA analysis for precise genotyping. Patients at risk for having offspring with sickle cell disease should be screened with hemoglobin electrophoresis (3).

Donors who are of Ashkenazi Jewish, French-Canadian, or Cajun descent should be screened for Tay–Sachs carrier status. Screening of gamete donors for Tay–Sachs disease can be performed easily and rapidly using human serum.

Cystic fibrosis testing is controversial. Some have suggested that caucasian donors should be screened for cystic fibrosis because of its high carrier frequency of 1 in 25. However, general population screening of caucasians for cystic fibrosis currently is not being recommended and therefore cannot be recommended routinely for gamete donors at this time. Nevertheless, the opportunity for testing of the potential donor for cystic fibrosis may be offered as an option to the recipient of the donated gamete.

Donor Screening

A positive history in the donor or the donor's first-degree relatives (ie, parent, sibling, or offspring) of repetitive miscarriages should prompt a chromosomal analysis of the donor, regardless of the number of normal or abnormal liveborns or stillborns. Individuals who have a known balanced chromosomal rearrangement or who have previously had offspring with a chromosomal abnormality should be excluded as gamete donors.

To decrease the risk of aneuploid offspring, it is prudent to limit oocyte donors to women who are less than 35 years of age. The increased frequency of de novo mutations in sperm from older men suggests that sperm from younger men is preferable. To avoid consanguinity in gamete donation programs, the oocyte donor and the sperm donor should not be genetically related.

Embryo Recipient

Embryo recipients should be screened for antibodies against red-cell surface antigens to avoid isoimmune hemolytic disease of the fetus and newborn. Other assessments of the embryo recipient with respect to maternal health and susceptibility to disease (ie, rubella antibody titer, blood chemistries) are advisable as well.

The embryo recipient should undergo careful physical assessment to detect obstetric risk factors. This is especially critical when the indication for gamete donation is a genetic disorder in the embryo recipient that puts her at high risk (eg, gonadal dysgenesis, Marfan syndrome). In some of these genetic disorders, the embryo recipient has functional ovaries; in others, the embryo recipient is agonadal. In the former situation, the donor gamete is being used to reduce the risk of a genetically abnormal child; in the latter situation, a donor egg is essential for successful reproduction. Extrinsic, nongenetic factors that might pose a risk to the fetus or to the continuation of the pregnancy (eg, rubella antibody, uterine abnormalities) should be assessed continually. To reduce the incidence of neural tube defects, embryo recipients should receive 400 µg of folic acid per day starting 6–8 weeks prior to embryo transfer and continuing until the end of the first trimester of pregnancy.

General

Apart from a specific genetic disorder, certain gamete donors and donor–recipient combinations have cumulative or polygenic risk factors that currently cannot be easily quantitated or specified. Attempts to prevent genetic defects in gamete donors always will be imperfect, as they are in nonassisted reproduction. Due to limitations in current knowledge and technology, genetic heterogeneity, and unanticipated de novo germline mutations, unforeseen and unanticipated abnormalities cannot be prevented, despite the physician's best efforts.

References

1. deBoer A, Oosterwijk JC, Ritgers-Aris CA. Determination of a maximum number of artificial inseminations by donor children per sperm donor. Fertil Steril 1995;63:419–421
2. Curie-Cohen M. The frequency of consanguineous matings due to multiple use of donors in artificial insemination. Am J Hum Genet 1980;32:589–600
3. American College of Obstetricians and Gynecologists. Genetic screening for hemoglobinopathies. ACOG Committee Opinion 168. Washington, DC: ACOG, 1996

Bibliography

American College of Obstetricians and Gynecologists. Fragile X syndrome. ACOG Committee Opinion 161. Washington, DC: ACOG, 1995

American College of Obstetricians and Gynecologists. Hemoglobinopathies in pregnancy. ACOG Technical Bulletin 220. Washington, DC: ACOG, 1996

American College of Obstetricians and Gynecologists. Screening for Tay–Sachs disease. ACOG Committee Opinion 162. Washington, DC: ACOG, 1995

ASRM guidelines for gamete donation: 1993. Fertil Steril 1993;59(2 suppl 1):1S–9S

Barrat CL, Matson DL, Holt W. British Andrology Society guidelines for the screening of semen donors for donor insemination. Hum Reprod 1993;8:1521–1523

Curie-Cohen M, Luttrell L, Shapiro S. Current practice of artificial insemination by donor in the United States. N Engl J Med 1979;300:585–590

Findlay I, Cuckle H, Lilford RJ, Rutherford AJ, Quirke P, Lui S. Screening sperm donors for cystic fibrosis. BMJ 1995; 310:1533

Fraser FC, Forse RA. On genetic screening of donors for artificial insemination. Am J Med Genet 1981;10:399–405

Greiss MA, Terry P, Urbaniak SJ. Artificial insemination in RhD negative women. Hum Reprod 1995;10:2176

Jalbert P, Leonard C, Selva J, David G. Genetic aspects of artificial insemination with donor semen: the French CECOS Federation Guidelines. Am J Med Genet 1989;33:369–375

Modell B. Ethical aspects of genetic screening. Ann Med 1992;24:549–555

Pierce J, Reitemeier PJ, Jameton A, Maclin VM, DeJonge CJ. Should gamete donation between family members be restricted? The case of a 16-year-old donor. Hum Reprod 1995; 10:1330–1337

Smith PE. Selection against genetic defects in semen donors. Clin Genet 1984;26:87–108

Van Steirteghem AC, Pados G, Devroey P, Bonduelle M, Van Assche E, Liebaers I. Oocyte donation for genetic indications. Reprod Fertil Dev 1992;4:681–688

Wood EC. Oocyte donation—recent trends and concerns. Med J Aust 1994;160:282–284

ACOG

Committee Opinion

Committee on Obstetric Practice

Number 158, September 1995

Guidelines for Diagnostic Imaging During Pregnancy

Various imaging modalities are available for diagnosis during pregnancy. These include X-ray, ultrasonography, magnetic resonance imaging (MRI), and nuclear medicine studies. Of these, diagnostic X-ray is the most frequent cause of anxiety for both obstetrician and patient. Much of this anxiety is secondary to a general belief that any radiation exposure is harmful and will result in an anomalous fetus. This anxiety could lead to inappropriate therapeutic abortion and litigation. In fact, most diagnostic radiologic procedures are associated with little, if any, known significant fetal risks. Moreover, according to the American College of Radiology, no single diagnostic X-ray procedure results in radiation exposure to a degree that would threaten the well-being of the developing preembryo, embryo, and fetus. Thus, exposure to X-ray during pregnancy is not an indication for therapeutic abortion (1, 2).

Some women are exposed to X-rays before the diagnosis of pregnancy. Occasionally, X-ray procedures will be indicated during pregnancy for significant medical problems or trauma. To enable physicians to counsel patients appropriately, the following information is provided about the potential risks and measures that can reduce diagnostic X-ray exposure.

X-Ray Exposure

Ionizing radiation can result in the following three harmful effects: 1) cell death and teratogenic effects, 2) carcinogenesis, and 3) genetic effects or mutations in germ cells (1, 2). There is little or no information to estimate either the frequency or magnitude of adverse genetic effects on future generations.

Units traditionally used to measure the effects of X-ray include the rad and roentgen equivalent man (rem). Modern units include the gray (Gy) and sievert (Sv). The definitions of these are summarized in Table 1.

The estimated fetal exposure from some common radiologic procedures is summarized in Table 2 (3–13). A plain X-ray generally exposes the fetus to very small amounts of radiation. Commonly during pregnancy, the uterus is shielded for nonpelvic procedures. Most fluoroscopic examinations result in fetal exposure of millirads except barium enema or small bowel series. Although computed tomography pelvimetry can result in fetal exposures as high as 1.5 rad, exposure can be reduced to approximately 250 mrad (includ-

ISSN 1074-861X

The American College of Obstetricians and Gynecologists
409 12th Street, SW,
Washington, DC 20024-2188

12345/98765

Table 1. Commonly Used Measures of Radiation

Measure	Definition	Unit	Unit
Exposure	Number of ions produced by X-rays per kilogram of air	Roentgen (R)	Roentgen (R)
Dose	Amount of energy deposited per kilogram of tissue	Rad (rad)*	Gray (Gy) 1 Gy = 100 rad
Relative effective dose	Amount of energy deposited per kilogram of tissue normalized for biological effectiveness	Roentgen equivalent man (rem)*	Sievert (Sv) 1 Sv = 100 rem

* For diagnostic X-rays, 1 rad = 1 rem.

Cunningham FG, MacDonald PC, Gant NF, Leveno KJ, Gilstrap LC III. Imaging modalities during pregnancy. In: Williams obstetrics. 19th ed. Norwalk, Connecticut: Appleton & Lange, 1993:982

Table 2. Estimated Fetal Exposure From Some Common Radiologic Procedures

Procedure	Fetal Exposure
Chest X-ray (2 views)	0.02–0.07 mrad
Abdominal film (single view)	100 mrad
Intravenous pyelography	≥1 rad*
Hip film (single view)	200 mrad
Mammography	7–20 mrad
Barium enema or small bowel series	2–4 rad
CT† scan of head or chest	<1 rad
CT scan of abdomen and lumbar spine	3.5 rad
CT pelvimetry	250 mrad

* Exposure depends on the number of films.

† CT indicates computed tomography.

ing fetal gonad exposure) by using a low-exposure technique (13).

Cell Death and Teratogenic Effects

Data from animals suggest that exposure to high-dose ionizing radiation (ie, much greater than that used in diagnostic procedures) before implantation will most likely be lethal to the embryo (1). In other words, cell death is most likely an "all or none" phenomenon in early embryonic development.

A myriad of teratogenic effects has developed in animals exposed to large doses of radiation (ie, 100–200 rad). However, in humans, growth restriction, microcephaly, and mental retardation are the most common adverse effects from high-dose radiation (2, 3, 14). Based on data from atomic bomb survivors, it appears that the risk of central nervous system effects is greatest with exposure at 8–15 weeks of gestation, with no proven risk at less than 8 weeks of gestation or at greater than 25 weeks of gestation (2, 15). Thus, at 8–15 weeks of gestation, the fetus is at greatest risk for radiation-induced mental retardation, and the risk appears to be a "non-threshold linear function of dose" at doses of at least 20 rad (2, 3, 15, 16). For example, the risk of severe mental retardation in fetuses exposed to ionizing radiation is approximately 40% at 100 rad of exposure and as high as 60% at 150 rad of exposure (2, 15). It has been suggested that a threshold for this adverse effect may exist in the range of 20–40 rad (14, 15). Fortunately, even multiple diagnostic X-ray procedures rarely result in ionizing radiation exposure to this degree. In summary, fetal risks of anomalies, growth restriction, or abortions are not increased with radiation exposure of less than 5 rad, a level above the range of exposure for diagnostic procedures (1).

Carcinogenesis

The risk of carcinogenesis as a result of in utero exposure to ionizing radiation is unclear but is probably very small. It has been estimated that 1 in 2,000 children exposed to ionizing radiation in utero will develop childhood leukemia. This is increased from a background rate of approximately 1 in 3,000 (17). If elective abortion were chosen in every instance of fetal exposure to radiation, 1,999 exposed, normal fetuses would be aborted for each case of leukemia prevented (1, 4). It has been estimated that the risk of radiation-induced carcinogenesis may indeed be higher in children compared with adults but that such risks are not likely to exceed 1 in 1,000 children per rad (5). Thus, abortion should not be recommended solely on the basis of exposure to diagnostic radiation.

Ultrasonography

Ultrasonography uses sound waves and is not a form of ionizing radiation. There have been no reports of documented adverse fetal effects for diagnostic ultrasound procedures, including duplex Doppler imaging. Energy exposure from ultrasonography has been arbitrarily limited to 94mW/cm^2 by the U.S. Food and Drug Administration. There are no contraindications to ultrasound procedures during pregnancy, and this modality has largely replaced X-ray as the primary method of fetal imaging during pregnancy.

Magnetic Resonance Imaging

With MRI, magnets that alter the energy state of hydrogen protons are used instead of ionizing radiation (18). This technique could prove especially useful for diagnosis and evaluation of fetal central nervous system anomalies and growth restriction. Although there have been no documented adverse fetal effects reported, the National Radiological Protection Board arbitrarily advises against its use in the first trimester (19). However, MRI has been proven useful for evaluation of maternal pelvic masses and for evaluation of fetal growth restriction (20).

Nuclear Medicine

Nuclear studies such as pulmonary ventilation–perfusion, thyroid, bone, and renal scans are performed by "tagging" a chemical agent with a radioisotope. The fetal exposure depends on the physical and biochemical properties of the radioisotope (3).

Technetium Tc 99m is one of the most commonly used isotopes and is used for brain, bone, renal, and cardiovascular scans. In general, these latter procedures result in a uterus, embryo, or fetal exposure of less than 0.5 rad (3, 5).

One of the more common nuclear medicine studies performed during pregnancy is the ventilation–perfusion scan for suspected pulmonary embolism. Macroaggregated albumin labeled with 99^{m}Tc is used for the perfusion portion, and inhaled xenon gas (^{127}Xe or ^{133}Xe) is used for the ventilation portion. The amount of radiation to which the fetus is exposed is extremely small (approximately 50 mrad) (21).

Radioactive iodine readily crosses the placenta and can adversely affect the fetal thyroid, especially if used after 10–12 weeks of gestational age. Radioactive isotopes of iodine used for treatment of hyperthyroidism are contraindicated during pregnancy, and such therapy should be delayed until after delivery. If a diagnostic scan of the thyroid is essential, ^{123}I or 99^{m}Tc should be used in place of ^{131}I (21).

Guidelines

The following guidelines for X-ray examination or exposure during pregnancy are suggested:

1. Women should be counseled that X-ray exposure from a single diagnostic procedure does not result in harmful fetal effects. Specifically, exposure to less than 5 rad has not been associated with an increase in fetal anomalies or pregnancy loss.
2. Concern about possible effects of high-dose ionizing radiation exposure should not prevent medically indicated diagnostic X-ray procedures from being performed on the mother. During pregnancy, other imaging procedures not associated with ionizing radiation (eg, ultrasonography, MRI) should be considered instead of X-rays when possible.
3. Ultrasonography and MRI are not associated with known adverse fetal effects. However, until more information is available, MRI is not recommended for use in the first trimester.
4. Consultation with a radiologist may be helpful in calculating estimated fetal dose when multiple diagnostic X-rays are performed on a pregnant patient.
5. The use of radioactive isotopes of iodine is contraindicated for therapeutic use during pregnancy.

References

1. Brent RL. The effect of embryonic and fetal exposure to x-ray, microwaves, and ultrasound: counseling the pregnant and nonpregnant patient about these risks. Semin Oncol 1989;16:347–368
2. Hall EJ. Scientific view of low-level radiation risks. Radiographics 1991;11:509–518
3. Twickler DM, Clarke G, Cunningham FG. Diagnostic imaging in pregnancy. Supplement. Williams obstetrics. 18th ed. Norwalk, Connecticut: Appleton & Lange, June/July 1992:1–15
4. Early diagnosis of pregnancy. An invitational symposium. Comment on editorial. J Reprod Med 1974;12:6
5. Mettler FA, Guiberteau MJ. Essentials of nuclear medicine imaging. Philadelphia: WB Saunders, 1991:320–321
6. Rosenstein M. Handbook of selected organ doses for projections common in diagnostic radiology. Rockville, Maryland: Department of Health and Human Services, Food and Drug Administration, 1988; DHHS publication no. (FDA):89-8031
7. Laws PW, Rosenstein M. A somatic dose index for diagnostic radiology. Health Phys 1978;35:629–642
8. Conway BJ. Nationwide evaluation of x-ray trends: tabulation and graphical summary of surveys 1984 through 1987. Frankfort, Kentucky: Conference of Radiation Control Program Directors, Inc, 1989
9. National Council on Radiation Protection and Measurements. Exposure of the U.S. population from diagnostic medical radiation. Bethesda, Maryland: NCRPM, 1989. 26; report no. 100

10. Bednarek DR, Rudin S, Wong R, Andres ML. Reduction of fluoroscopic exposure for the air-contrast barium enema. Br J Radiol 1983;56:823–828
11. Shope TB, Gagne RM, Johnson GC. A method for describing the doses delivered by transmission x-ray computed tomography. Med Phys 1981;8:488–495
12. Ragozzino MW, Breckle R, Hill LM, Gray JE. Average fetal depth in utero: data for estimation of fetal absorbed radiation dose. Radiology 1986;158:513–515
13. Moore MM, Shearer DR. Fetal dose estimates for CT pelvimetry. Radiology 1989;171:265–267
14. Otake M, Yoshimaru H, Schull WJ. Severe mental retardation among the prenatally exposed survivors of the atomic bombing of Hiroshima and Nagasaki: a comparison of the old and new dosimetry systems. Hiroshima, Japan: Radiation Effects Research Foundation, 1987; Radiation Effects Research Foundation technical report no. 16-87
15. Committee on Biological Effects of Ionizing Radiation, Board on Radiation Effects Research Commission on Life Sciences, National Research Council. Health effects of exposure to low levels of ionizing radiation: BEIR V. Washington, DC: National Academy Press, 1990:352–370
16. Schull WJ, Otake M. Neurological deficit among the survivors exposed to the atomic bombing of Hiroshima and Nagasaki: a reassessment and new directions. In: Kriegel H, Schmahl W, Gerber GB, Stive FE, eds. Radiation risks to the developing nervous system. New York: Gustave Fischer Verlag, 1986:399–419
17. Miller RW. Epidemiological conclusions from radiation toxicity studies. In: Fry RJM, Grahn D, Griem ML, Rust JH, eds. Late effects of radiation. London: Taylor & Francis, 1970
18. Curry TS III, Dowdey JE, Murry RC Jr, eds. Christensen's physics of diagnostic radiology. 4th ed. Philadelphia: Lea & Febiger, 1990:1, 470
19. Garden AS, Griffiths RD, Weindling AM, Martin PA. Fast-scan magnetic resonance imaging in fetal visualization. Am J Obstet Gynecol 1991;164:1190–1196
20. Cunningham FG, MacDonald PC, Gant NF, Leveno KJ, Gilstrap LC III. Imaging modalities during pregnancy. In: Williams obstetrics. 19th ed. Norwalk, Connecticut: Appleton & Lange, 1993:981–989
21. Ginsberg JS, Hirsh J, Rainbow AJ, Coates G. Risks to the fetus of radiologic procedures used in the diagnosis of maternal venous thromboembolic disease. Thromb Haemost 1989;61:189–196

ACOG

Committee on Ethics

Committee Opinion

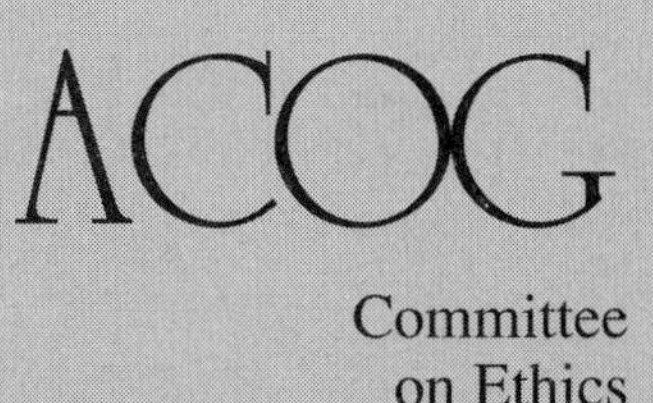

Number 182, April 1997 (*Replaces #45, October 1985*)

Guidelines for Relationships with Industry

The American College of Obstetricians and Gynecologists recognizes that the health care industry, for example, manufacturers of pharmaceuticals and medical devices, assists the College and its Fellows in pursuit of their educational goals and objectives through financial support of various medical educational programs.

In the course of such interactions, it is possible that company expenditures will generate some degree of bias or obligation unrelated to product merit, creating the actuality or the appearance of inappropriate and undue influence. When any product promotion leads to inappropriate or unbalanced medical advice or recommendations to patients, an ethical problem exists. The public holds physicians to a high standard of avoidance of conflicts of interest in decisions about patient care. Advertising or marketing practices must not influence the accuracy, completeness, or balanced presentation of medical advice to patients.

Industry–physician interactions can be divided into three major types, as characterized in the following paragraphs. Ethical implications specific to each type of interaction are discussed below.

1. *Product promotion to individual physicians by advertising, personal communication, and provision of samples.* The physician has an obligation to go beyond the information provided through advertising or other marketing strategies in selecting the best product for care of the patient.
2. *Company promotion to individual physicians and groups of physicians, such as medical specialty societies, by provision of gifts, parties, trips, and services.* Such promotional practices, whether directed toward professional groups or individual physicians, must be assumed to have as their purpose the creation both of a sense of obligation and of attitudes or practices favorable to the donor. This may result in a real or perceived conflict of interest for the recipient individual or organization. Such ethical conflicts can interfere with patient care and are not in keeping with the standards of professional conduct to which physicians are expected to adhere. The risks of ethical conflicts and adverse public opinion should be carefully weighed by any individual or group before accepting gifts, parties, trips, and services directly from industry.

ISSN 1074-861X

The American College of Obstetricians and Gynecologists
409 12th Street, SW
PO Box 96920
Washington, DC 20090-6920

12345/10987

3. *Company promotion to individual physicians and groups, including specialty societies, hospitals, and medical schools, through the support of educational activities, honorary awards, research grants, and development contracts.* Support of educational programs and the provision of awards, grants, and contracts may be accepted by the College, its districts, sections, and Fellows if such support is offered in accordance with standing guidelines of the American Medical Association and the Accreditation Council for Continuing Medical Education (1, 2) summarized below:
   a. Any gifts accepted by physicians individually should primarily entail a benefit to patients and not be of substantial value. Accordingly, textbooks, modest meals, and other gifts are appropriate if they serve a genuine educational function. Cash payments should not be accepted.
   b. Individual gifts of minimal value are permissible as long as the gifts are related to the physician's work.
   c. Subsidies to underwrite the costs of continuing medical education conferences or professional meetings can contribute to the improvement of patient care and therefore are permissible. Payments to defray the costs of a conference should not be accepted directly from the company by the physicians who are attending the conference. Funds from a commercial source should be in the form of an educational grant made payable to the accredited sponsor for the support of programs. The ultimate decision about funding arrangements for continuing medical education (CME) activities must be the responsibility of the accredited sponsor.
   d. Subsidies from industry should not be accepted directly or indirectly to pay for the costs of travel, lodging, or other personal expenses of the physicians who are attending the conferences or meetings; nor should subsidies be accepted to compensate for the physicians' time. Subsidies for hospitality should not be accepted outside of modest meals or social events that are held as part of a conference or meeting. Commercially supported social events at CME activities should not compete with, nor take precedence over, the educational events. It is appropriate for faculty at conferences or meetings to accept reasonable honoraria and to accept reimbursement for reasonable travel, lodging, and meal expenses. It is also appropriate for consultants who provide genuine services to receive reasonable compensation and to accept reimbursement for reasonable travel, lodging, and meal expenses. Token consulting or advisory arrangements cannot be used to justify the compensation of physicians for their time or their travel, lodging and other out-of-pocket expenses.
   e. Scholarship or other special funds to permit medical students, residents, and fellows to attend carefully selected educational conferences may be permissible as long as the selection of students, residents, or fellows who will receive the funds is made by the academic or training institution or by the accredited sponsor with the full concurrence of the academic or training institution.
   f. No gifts should be accepted if conditions or obligations are attached. For example, physicians should not accept gifts if they are given in relation to the physician's prescribing practices. In addition, when companies underwrite medical conferences or lectures other than their own, responsibility for and control over the selection of content, faculty, educational methods, and materials should belong to the organizers of the conferences or lectures.
   g. Accredited sponsors are responsible for the content, quality, and scientific integrity of all CME activities and materials certified for credit.
   h. Presentations must give a balanced view of all therapeutic options. Use of generic names will contribute to this impartiality. If trade names are used, those of several companies should be used rather than only those of a single company.
   i. When commercial exhibits are part of the overall program, arrangements for these should not influence planning nor interfere with the presentation of CME activities. Exhibit placement should not be a condition of support for a CME activity.

This statement is not intended to substitute for ethical judgment and responsibility, but to provide a framework for decision making for relationships between the College, its Fellows, and industry.

References

1. American Medical Association Council of Ethical and Judicial Affairs. Gifts to physicians from industry. JAMA 1991;265:501
2. Accreditation Council for Continuing Medical Education (ACCME). Standards for commercial support of continuing medical education. Chicago, Illinois: ACCME, 1992

ACOG

Committee on Adolescent Health Care

Committee Opinion

Number 184, June 1997

Hepatitis B Immunization for Adolescents

Hepatitis B virus, the only sexually transmissible infection that currently can be prevented by immunization, poses a significant health risk to adolescents (1). The Advisory Committee on Immunization Practices of the US Preventive Health Services, along with the American Academy of Pediatrics, the American Academy of Family Physicians, and the American Medical Association, issued a joint statement in 1996 recommending universal vaccination against hepatitis B for adolescents to be given at age 11–12, with immunization for older adolescents based on risk status. In addition, the American Academy of Pediatrics recommends that providers administer hepatitis B vaccine to all adolescents to whom they provide services (2).

For many adolescents, the obstetrician–gynecologist may be the only source of health care. Obstetrician–gynecologists who see adolescents in their offices or clinics need to be familiar with the necessity for hepatitis B immunization for this age group. The Committee on Adolescent Health Care recommends that all adolescent patients be screened for hepatitis B immunization status and this status noted in their chart. All adolescents who have not been previously immunized should be given hepatitis B immunization. Referral to another provider for actual immunization may be necessary if insurance or reimbursement conditions dictate.

References

1. Society for Adolescent Medicine. Position statement on hepatitis B immunization. J Adolesc Health 1995;17:256
2. Centers for Disease Control and Prevention. Immunization of adolescents: recommendations of the Advisory Committee on Immunization Practices, the American Academy of Pediatrics, the American Academy of Family Physicians, and the American Medical Association. MMWR 1996;45(RR-13):1–16

ISSN 1074-861X

The American College of Obstetricians and Gynecologists
409 12th Street, SW
PO Box 96920
Washington, DC 20090-6920

12345/10987

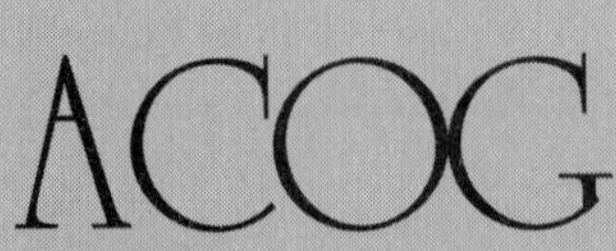

Committee on
Gynecologic Practice

Committee Opinion

Number 203, July 1998 (*Replaces #199, February 1998*)

Hepatitis Virus Infections in Obstetrician–Gynecologists

The current epidemic of human immunodeficiency virus (HIV) infection has escalated concerns about transmission from infected patients to health care workers. The concerns about HIV have increased attention to hepatitis B virus (HBV). It appears that surgeons who follow recommended infection-control procedures are at little risk of acquiring HIV while caring for HIV-infected patients (1, 2). In contrast, surgeons can readily acquire HBV from infected patients (1, 3).

The College routinely has recommended hepatitis B vaccination for obstetrician–gynecologists who are exposed to blood or blood products. Postvaccination testing for antibodies, which is recommended by the Centers for Disease Control and Prevention, can validate immunization (4). Individuals who are antibody negative after immunization should be tested for hepatitis B surface antigen to identify carriers as a result of previous HBV infection (5). The Committee on Gynecologic Practice supports the recommendation that surgeons who perform invasive procedures and who do not have evidence of immunity to HBV should know their hepatitis B surface antigen status and, if it is positive, also should know their hepatitis B e antigen status (6, 7).

The risk of acquiring hepatitis C virus (HCV) infection appears to be lower than the risk of acquiring HBV and higher than the risk of acquiring HIV (2, 3). Nonetheless, HCV is the most common cause of chronic viral hepatitis, and even chronic HCV infection symptoms typically are silent or minimal (8). Thus, surgeons who perform exposure-prone procedures should consider being tested for anti-HCV antibody and, if positive, should confirm seropositive status by documenting HCV RNA in the serum with reverse transcription polymerase chain reaction testing (8–10). Institutional and local health department rules usually are available to guide health care workers who test positive for bloodborne viruses.

ISSN 1074-861X

The American College of Obstetricians and Gynecologists
409 12th Street, SW
PO Box 96920
Washington, DC 20090-6920

12345/21098

References

1. Henderson DK. Human immunodeficiency virus infection in patients and providers. In: Wenzel RP, ed. Prevention and control of nosocomial infections. 2nd ed. Baltimore: Williams and Wilkins, 1993:42–47
2. Gerberding JL. Management of occupational exposures to blood-borne viruses. N Engl J Med 1995;332:444–451

3. Shapiro CN. Occupational risk of infection with hepatitis B and hepatitis C virus. Surg Clin N Am 1995;75:1047–1056
4. Centers for Disease Control and Prevention. Protection against viral hepatitis: recommendations of the Immunization Practices Advisory Committee. MMWR 1990;39 (RR-2):13
5. Rhodes RS. Hepatitis B virus, surgeons, and surgery. Bull Am Coll Surg 1995;80(6):32–42
6. Centers for Disease Control and Prevention. Recommendations for preventing transmission of human immunodeficiency virus and hepatitis B virus to patients du118 ring exposure-prone invasive procedures. MMWR 1991;40 (RR-8):1–9
7. American College of Surgeons. Statement on the surgeon and hepatitis B infection. Bull Am Coll Surg 1995;80(5):33–35
8. Sharara AI, Hunt CM, Hamilton JD. Update: hepatitis C. Ann Intern Med 1996;125:658–668
9. Centers for Disease Control and Prevention. Recommendations for follow-up of health-care workers after occupational exposure to hepatitis C virus. MMWR 1997;46:603–606
10. Dore GJ, Kaldor JM, McCaughan GW. Systematic review of role of polymerase chain reaction in defining infectiousness among people infected with hepatitis C virus. BMJ 1997;315:333–337

ACOG Committee Opinion

Committee on Obstetric Practice

Number 172, May 1996 (*Replaces Number 115, September 1992*)

Home Uterine Activity Monitoring

Of all neonates born alive in the United States in 1993, 7.2% weighed less than 2,500 g (1). This figure represents the highest incidence of low birth weight since 1976. The incidence of very low birth weight (births of less than 1,500 g) has also remained unchanged since 1991 with an incidence of 1.3% (1). Over the past 30 years, the incidence of neonates weighing less than 2,500 g has declined only slightly and the rate of neonates weighing less than 1,500 g has not changed substantially (2, 3).

In 1992, more than 34,000 children in the United States died in their first year of life. These deaths result in an infant mortality rate of 8.5 deaths per 1,000 live births (4). Diseases related to prematurity are a major cause. Although this is the lowest rate ever recorded in the United States, it compares unfavorably with most other Western industrialized countries. A variety of primary and secondary preventive strategies have been suggested to reduce the incidence of preterm delivery. In spite of these efforts, overall reduction in the incidence of preterm births over time has been slight.

Overview

Home uterine activity monitoring (HUAM) is a system of care to detect preterm labor. It uses a combination of the recording of uterine contractions with a tocodynamometer and daily telephone calls from a health care provider to offer patient support and advice. A recording of uterine contractions is transferred by telephone to the health care provider for rapid evaluation. The premise of HUAM is that women will have an identifiable increase in uterine contractions before the onset of preterm labor and that these prodromal uterine contractions otherwise may not be recognized by the patient. Advocates of the system propose that early identification of preterm uterine contractions will permit earlier administration of tocolytic therapy that, in turn, may be more effective than later therapy in preventing preterm births.

The ability to identify women at risk for preterm birth based on their history or risk factors is poor (5). Because many risk-scoring systems depend heavily on a history of preterm birth, the positive predictive value of risk scoring for nulliparous women is even lower than that for multiparous women. Thus, with widespread availability, HUAM may be used for many women who will not have premature labor, and some women who experience preterm labor will not receive HUAM. Widespread use could also lead to inappropri-

ISSN 1074-861X

The American College of Obstetricians and Gynecologists
409 12th Street, SW
PO Box 96920
Washington, DC 20090-6920

12345/09876

ate treatment with tocolytic agents. This treatment can result in not only adverse maternal or fetal side effects but also increased cost of obstetric care.

At least 11 randomized controlled trials examining the efficacy of HUAM have published results (Table 1). Two of these studies include data from the same patients (6, 7). In addition, there are several prospective cohort studies (8–10). The studies vary in design, criteria for inclusion of patients, and measurements of endpoints and outcomes. These differences make comparisons difficult. Furthermore, many of these studies have limitations with regard to research design, including sample size (power) or numbers of patients, which preclude reaching conclusions about the utility of HUAM. In an assessment of the work of Hill, Knuppel, and Watson, Keirse noted bias and errors sufficient to warrant dismissing their results (11). Both Grimes and Sachs have critically reviewed the literature regarding HUAM and have cautioned against widespread clinical application (12, 13). The U.S. Preventive Services Task Force performed an independent review and reached a similar conclusion (14).

Thus, the role of HUAM in the prevention of prematurity is controversial. In addition to difficulty in identifying patients who will deliver prematurely, a number of other issues should be considered: 1) accuracy and reliability of the technology, 2) the endpoint used to measure and evaluate effectiveness of HUAM, 3) effectiveness of treatment, 4) safety, and 5) a cost–benefit analysis.

Accuracy and Reliability

Criteria for the objective diagnosis of preterm labor vary among investigators and clinical settings. This variation in turn limits the precision with which preterm labor is detected by HUAM in these studies. Several investigators have attempted to measure the reliability of the home tocodynamometer (15, 16). They have reported only limited degrees of intraobserver and interobserver reliability in reading home tocodynamometry strips.

A possible benefit of HUAM might result from identification of women who will subsequently develop preterm labor. One small observational study reported that the frequency of uterine contractions increased in the 24-hour period before preterm labor developed (17). Most of the patients who developed preterm labor had more than four contractions per hour (17). No population-based studies have determined how many women have episodes of increased uterine contractions and do not go into premature labor.

Endpoints Used to Measure and Evaluate Effectiveness

The impact of HUAM on the prevention of preterm delivery is *the* important endpoint for determining the clinical utility and benefit of the technology. This impact could be established by analysis of both the entire population of patients in whom the technology is studied and controls. Unfortunately, many of the HUAM studies evaluate intermediate endpoints (eg, cervical dilatation on admission) in the subgroup of patients and controls who experience preterm labor. The results may reach statistical significance, but analyzing only the subgroup of women who experience preterm labor is a methodologic flaw and limits the value of these studies. In some of these same studies, analysis of results in the entire population does not show significant differences in the outcome of prematurity prevention.

Cervical Dilatation on Admission

Evidence supports the hypothesis that use of HUAM in pregnancies at high risk of preterm labor results in less cervical dilatation at the time of admission to the hospital for preterm labor. Morrison found that high-risk women who were monitored and who experienced preterm labor had less cervical dilatation and less effacement at the time of diagnosis of preterm labor than did controls (18). In other studies of twin pregnancies and high-risk pregnancies (19, 20), a higher percentage of monitored women presented with less advanced cervical dilatation than did women who were not monitored with HUAM. Hill's study may have included some or all of Knuppel's patients, thus limiting the conclusions that can be drawn from these findings (19, 20). Dyson was able to demonstrate a benefit from HUAM in terms of patients "favorable for suppression" of preterm labor at the time of their presentation (21), but this difference was only observed for the subgroup of women with twins. In addition, Dyson's analysis of twin data used infants rather than pregnancies as the unit of analysis; thus, Dyson artificially increased the statistical power for the twin result. Mou and Nagey also noted less cervical dilatation in high-risk pregnancies at the time of admission in preterm labor, but the latter study did not reach statistical significance (22, 23). Wapner, in a randomized control trial of HUAM without daily nursing contact in patients with a previous preterm birth, found significantly less cervical dilatation on admission in the patients who had preterm labor (24).

The Food and Drug Administration has approved the device for monitoring uterine activity and accepted cervical dilatation alone as an appropriate endpoint for the approval of this technology. It did not require proof that the device prevents premature birth and the associated neonatal morbidity and mortality, which are the most important outcomes for clinicians and patients (25). Some might argue that cervical dilatation and effacement is a subjective endpoint.

Success of Treatment of Preterm Labor

Investigators have attempted to determine the benefit of HUAM by studying its impact on the success of treatment for preterm labor. The hypothesis is that an improvement in success of treatment might be based on earlier initiation of treatment when cervical dilatation is less or before preterm labor becomes refractory to drug therapy. This approach is also limited to subgroup analysis of patients and controls with a diagnosis of preterm labor, rather than the entire study population.

Data from several of these studies suggest that treatment of preterm labor is more successful with the use of HUAM. Examining the subgroup of patients who experienced preterm labor, Morrison found that the percentage of monitored women in whom tocolysis was not effective was lower than that of women not monitored, although no statistical analysis was provided (18). Hill found a significant benefit of HUAM in preventing delivery within 48 hours in women who presented in preterm labor (19). Knuppel and Hill observed that significantly more controls failed tocolysis and delivered compared with those women who were monitored and experienced preterm labor (19, 20). In Watson's study, all of the women had preterm labor in the index pregnancy (26). In the subgroup of women who experienced recurrent preterm labor, significantly more of the controls delivered despite tocolytic treatment. Dyson also found this benefit in preterm labor with twins, although not with singleton pregnancies (21). As previously noted, the use of infants rather than pregnancies as the unit of analysis artificially increases the statistical power for the twin result. Wapner found a significant prolongation in the duration of pregnancy following treatment of preterm labor in monitored patients, and delivery was delayed by more than 48 hours in a significantly greater number of patients (24). In contrast, Iams examined the subgroup of patients who experienced preterm labor (7). He found no difference between those who were monitored and those who were not with regard to their suitability for tocolysis or the percentage of women who failed treatment.

Prevention of Preterm Delivery

A number of studies using different patient risk factors and different definitions of preterm delivery demonstrate a benefit in reducing preterm delivery but only in monitored women who had preterm labor compared with controls who had preterm labor and were not monitored (19–22, 24, 26). Reanalysis of the data from one study (19) found no significant difference in the incidence of preterm delivery when all enrolled patients are analyzed (13, 26). When the entire study population was analyzed, Wapner's study did not show a statistically significant improvement in pregnancy outcome as measured by gestational age, weight at delivery, and delivery of neonates weighing less than 2,000 g (24).

Only one of the studies that support the use of HUAM in preventing premature delivery does not depend on the analysis of subgroups of patients. In a study comparing HUAM to education and nursing contact, Morrison reported that the monitored women had a lower incidence of delivery before 37 weeks of gestation (18). Morrison also found significantly greater time elapsed from diagnosis of preterm labor to delivery in the monitored group than in controls (8.2±2.7 weeks versus 4.2±2.9 weeks). This study was not blinded and provided limited nursing contact to the control group.

In contrast, several investigators found no difference in the incidence of preterm delivery or gestational age at delivery between monitored and unmonitored women (7, 23, 27). These investigators, who did not show a benefit of HUAM, tended to analyze all women who had been randomized rather than only the subgroup of women who experienced preterm labor.

Other neonatal outcomes have been examined, such as respiratory distress syndrome, neonatal intensive care unit admissions, total length of neonatal intensive care, and total nursery days. The results regarding these other endpoints also are not consistent.

Some investigators have attempted to isolate the benefit of the components of HUAM as a system of care, specifically the health provider contact and the tocodynamometer. Because of limitations and differences in design, consistent conclusions regarding these components cannot be made. The following conclusions can be made, however:

- From a clinical point of view, use of an intermediate endpoint, such as cervical dilatation, is not justified when the endpoint—prevention of preterm delivery—can be measured.

Table 1. Summary of Randomized Clinical Trials (Reference No.) of Human Uterine Activity Monitoring*

	Morrison (18)	Iams (6,7)	Watson (26)	Knuppel (20)	Hill (19)	Dyson (21)		Mou (22)	Blondel (27)	Nagey (23)	Wapner (24)
						Singletons	Twins				
Population	High risk	High risk	Previously treated for PML	Twins	High risk	High risk	High risk	High risk	High risk and treated for PML	Previously treated for PML	High risk for PML
Experimental group	Standard HUAM	Standard HUAM	Standard HUAM	Standard HUAM	Standard HUAM	Standard HUAM	Standard HUAM	HUAM with minimal nursing care	Standard HUAM	Standard HUAM	Standard HUAM with no nursing care
Controls	Education, self-palpation, and call twice weekly	Education, maternal–fetal nurse contact	Education	Education	Education	Sham monitor	Sham monitor	Education	Home visits	Routine	High-risk care
Primary endpoint	Diagnosis of PML and prevention of PTD	PTD	PTD	Dilatation at diagnosis of PML	Dilatation at diagnosis of PML	PTD and neonatal outcome	PTD and neonatal outcome	Dilatation at diagnosis of PML and outcome	PTD	PTD	Dilatation and diagnosis of PML
Cervical dilatation	HUAM benefit[†]			HUAM benefit[†]	HUAM benefit[†]	ND	HUAM benefit[†]	HUAM benefit[†]		Trend for HUAM	HUAM benefit[†]
Delivery within 48 h					HUAM benefit[†]		HUAM benefit[†]				HUAM benefit[†]
PTD											
<32 weeks									ND[‡]	ND	
<34 weeks						ND	HUAM benefit[†]		ND[‡]	ND	
<35 weeks		ND									
<36 weeks	HUAM benefit					ND	ND		ND[‡]	ND	
<37 weeks		ND	HUAM benefit[†]	HUAM benefit[†]							
Gestational age at delivery		ND	ND			ND	HUAM benefit[†]	HUAM benefit[†]			ND
Time gained in utero	HUAM benefit[†]							HUAM benefit[†]			HUAM benefit[†]

(Continued)

Table 1. Summary of Randomized Clinical Trials (Reference No.) of Human Uterine Activity Monitoring* *(continued)*

	Morrison (18)	Iams (6,7)	Watson (26)	Knuppel (20)	Hill (19)	Dyson (21)		Mou (22)	Blondel (27)	Nagey (23)	Wapner (24)
						Singletons	Twins				
Birth weight		ND				ND	HUAM benefit†	HUAM benefit for singletons†			ND
Tocolytic failure			HUAM benefit†	HUAM benefit†	HUAM benefit†						
Incidence of LBW						ND			ND‡		ND
Incidence of VLBW		ND				ND	HUAM benefit§				
Incidence of RDS						ND					
Rate of ICN admission						ND	HUAM benefit§	HUAM benefit†			ND
Infant length of stay						ND	HUAM benefit§				ND
% requiring O_2								HUAM benefit†			
% requiring mechanical ventilation							HUAM benefit†				

*PML indicates premature labor; HUAM, home uterine activity monitoring; PTD, preterm delivery; ND, no difference; LBW, low birth weight; VLBW, very low birth weight; RDS, respiratory distress syndrome; ICN, intensive care nursery.

†Benefit was found only for the subgroup with preterm labor.

§Statistical significance may be invalidated due to counting newborns rather than deliveries in multiple gestations.

‡Power was inadequate.

- The available data do not support the effectiveness of HUAM for the prevention of preterm birth.

Effectiveness of Treatment of Preterm Labor

A system of care that is designed to provide early detection of preterm labor is of benefit only if an effective treatment of preterm labor exists. There is evidence that tocolytic therapy is of benefit, but this may be limited to prolongation of pregnancy for 48 hours following the initiation of treatment. The benefits of corticosteroids for inducing fetal pulmonary maturation have recently been reviewed (28, 29). The studies of HUAM have not been designed to determine whether benefit is derived from early detection of preterm labor that permits corticosteroid treatment.

In clinical application, oral tocolytic agents are commonly used with HUAM. They may be administered either before or after an episode of acute treatment of premature labor. A recent metaanalysis of oral tocolytic therapy fails to support a role for oral tocolytic therapy following resolution of an acute episode of preterm labor (30). The following conclusions can be made about the effectiveness of treatment:

- Any potential benefit of HUAM is limited by the effectiveness of treatment available for preterm labor.
- A benefit of HUAM derived from allowing time for corticosteroid treatment has not been evaluated.
- No apparent benefit is derived from HUAM in assisting the clinician in prescribing oral tocolytic therapy.

Risks

Use of HUAM is not invasive. Therefore, the risks are confined to interventions that might result from use of the system, such as tocolytics and corticosteroids (28, 29).

Conclusion

Well-designed, prospective, randomized clinical studies of sufficient power are still needed to establish the benefit, if any, of HUAM for the prevention of preterm delivery or for the prevention of associated adverse neonatal outcomes. Without an established benefit, cost–benefit analysis is not possible. Data are insufficient to support a benefit from HUAM in preventing preterm birth. Therefore, the American College of Obstetricians and Gynecologists does not recommend the use of this system of care. Other recently published reviews are available that do not change these conclusions (31, 32).

References

1. Ventura SJ, Martin JA, Taffel SM, Mathews TJ, Clarke SC. Advance report of final natality statistics, 1993. Monthly vital statistics report; vol 44, no. 3, suppl. Hyattsville, Maryland: National Center for Health Statistics, 1995
2. Institute of Medicine. Division of Health Promotion and Disease Prevention. Committee to Study the Prevention of Low Birthweight. Preventing low birthweight. Washington, DC: National Academy Press, 1985
3. March of Dimes Birth Defects Foundation. March of Dimes statbook: statistics for healthier mothers and babies. White Plains, New York: MODBDF, 1993
4. Kochanek DK, Hudson BL. Advance report of final mortality statistics, 1992. Monthly vital statistics report; vol 43, no. 6, suppl. Hyattsville, Maryland: National Center for Health Statistics, 1995
5. American College of Obstetricians and Gynecologists. Preterm labor. ACOG Technical Bulletin 206. Washington, DC: ACOG, 1995
6. Iams JD, Johnson FF, O'Shaughnessy RW. A prospective random trial of home uterine activity monitoring in pregnancies at increased risk of preterm labor. Am J Obstet Gynecol 1987;157:638–643
7. Iams JD, Johnson FF, O'Shaughnessy RW. A prospective random trial of home uterine activity monitoring in pregnancies at increased risk of preterm labor. Part II. Am J Obstet Gynecol 1988;159:595–603
8. Katz M, Gill PJ, Newman RB. Detection of preterm labor by ambulatory monitoring of uterine activity: a preliminary report. Obstet Gynecol 1986;68:773–778
9. Katz M, Gill PJ, Newman RB. Detection of preterm labor by ambulatory monitoring of uterine activity for the management of oral tocolysis. Am J Obstet Gynecol 1986;154:1253–1256
10. Smith JC, Floyd RC, Pittman KP, Grillo D, Roach H, Morrison JC. Reduction of preterm births in a low-income population utilizing home uterine activity monitoring. J Maternal–Fetal Investigation 1994;4:87–92
11. Keirse MJ, Van Hoven M. Reanalysis of a multireported trial on home uterine activity monitoring. Birth 1993; 20:117–122
12. Grimes DA, Schulz KF. Randomized controlled trials of home uterine activity monitoring: a review and critique. Obstet Gynecol 1992;79:137–142
13. Sachs BP, Hellerstein S, Freeman R, Frigoletto F, Hauth JC. Home monitoring of uterine activity. Does it prevent prematurity? N Engl J Med 1991;325:1374–1377
14. U.S. Preventive Services Task Force. Home uterine activity monitoring for preterm labor. Review article. JAMA 1993;270:371–376
15. Katz M, Newman RB, Gill PJ. Assessment of uterine activity in ambulatory patients at high risk of preterm labor and delivery. Am J Obstet Gynecol 1986;154:44–47
16. Scheerer LJ, Campion S, Katz M. Ambulatory tocodynamometry data interpretation: evaluating variability and reliability. Obstet Gynecol 1990;76S–79S

17. Katz M, Newman RB, Gill PJ. Assessment of uterine activity in ambulatory patients at high risk of preterm labor and delivery. Am J Obstet Gynecol 1986;154:44–47
18. Morrison JC, Martin JN Jr, Martin RW, Gookin KS, Wiser WL. Prevention of preterm birth by ambulatory assessment of uterine activity: a randomized study. Am J Obstet Gynecol 1987;156:536–543
19. Hill WC, Fleming AD, Martin RW, Hamer C, Knuppel RA, Lake MF, et al. Home uterine activity monitoring is associated with a reduction in preterm birth. Obstet Gynecol 1990;76(suppl):13S–18S
20. Knuppel RA, Lake MF, Watson DL, Welch RA, Hill WC, Fleming AD, et al. Preventing preterm birth in twin gestation: home uterine activity monitoring and perinatal nursing support. Obstet Gynecol 1990;76(suppl):24S–27S
21. Dyson DC, Crites YM, Ray DA, Armstrong MA. Prevention of preterm birth in high-risk patients: the role of education and provider contact versus home uterine monitoring. Am J Obstet Gynecol 1991;164:756–762
22. Mou SM, Sunderji SG, Gall S, How H, Patel V, Gray M, et al. Multicenter randomized clinical trial of home uterine activity monitoring for detection of preterm labor. Am J Obstet Gynecol 1991;165:858–866
23. Nagey DA, Bailey-Jones C, Herman AA. Randomized comparison of home uterine activity monitoring and routine care in patients discharged after treatment for preterm labor. Obstet Gynecol 1993;82:319–323
24. Wapner RJ, Cotton DB, Artal R, Librizzi RJ, Ross MG. A randomized multicenter trial assessing a home uterine activity monitoring device used in the absence of daily nursing contact. Am J Obstet Gynecol 1995;172:1026–1034
25. Yin L. Home monitoring for uterine activity. A response from the FDA. N Engl J Med 1991;325:1377
26. Watson DL, Welch RA, Mariona FG, Lake MF, Knuppel RA, Martin RW, et al. Management of preterm labor patients at home: does daily uterine activity monitoring and nursing support make a difference? Obstet Gynecol 1990;76(suppl):32S–35S
27. Blondel B, Breart G, Berthoux Y, Berland M, Mellier G, Rudigoz RC, et al. Home uterine activity monitoring in France; a randomized, controlled trial. Am J Obstet Gynecol 1992;167:424–429
28. American College of Obstetricians and Gynecologists. Antenatal corticosteroid therapy for fetal maturation. ACOG Committee Opinion 147. Washington, DC: ACOG, 1994
29. Effect of corticosteroids for fetal maturation on perinatal outcomes. NIH Consensus Development Panel on the Effect of Corticosteroids for Fetal Maturation of Perinatal Outcomes. JAMA 1995;273:413–418
30. Macones GA, Berlin M, Berlin JA. Efficacy of oral beta-agonist maintenance therapy in preterm labor: a meta-analysis. Obstet Gynecol 1995;85:313–317
31. The Collaborative Home Uterine Monitoring Study Group. A multicenter randomized controlled trial of home uterine monitoring: active versus sham device. Am J Obstet Gynecol 1995;173:1120–1127
32. Colton T, Kayne HL, Zhang Y, Heeren T. A metaanalysis of home uterine activity monitoring. Am J Obstet Gynecol 1995;173:1499–1505

ACOG

Committee on
Gynecologic Practice

Committee Opinion

Number 235, May 2000 (Replaces No. 126, August 1993)

Hormone Replacement Therapy in Women Treated for Endometrial Cancer

Hormone replacement therapy (HRT), which provides estrogen with or without a progestin, usually is initiated in estrogen-deficient women in an attempt to ameliorate menopausal symptoms and to provide long-term health benefits, such as reduced risk of osteoporosis, potential decreased risk of heart disease, and potential improvement of cognitive function. In women who have been treated previously for endometrial carcinoma, these benefits must be weighed against the risk of stimulating tumor growth and recurrence. Recently, numerous different HRT modalities and delivery systems have become available, including transdermal and intravaginal preparations, plant-based estrogens and progestins, as well as selective estrogen receptor modulators (SERMs), all of which are marketed as providing these short- and long-term benefits while minimizing adverse side effects and outcomes. Although retrospective studies have pointed to an absence of adverse outcomes, currently no conclusive data are available to support specific recommendations regarding the use of HRT in women previously treated for endometrial carcinoma.

In the absence of HRT, the following outcomes may be expected in women treated for endometrial cancer:

- A well-differentiated neoplasm of endometrioid cell type with superficial invasion would render an approximate 5% risk of recurrent disease.
- A moderately differentiated neoplasm of endometrioid cell type with up to one half myometrial invasion would render a 10–15% risk of recurrent disease. The risk may be as high as 50% for nonendometrioid-type tumors and serous papillary tumors.
- A poorly differentiated neoplasm, regardless of cell type, with invasion of over one half of the myometrium would render a 40–50% risk of recurrent disease.

The effect of HRT on the recurrence risk of endometrial cancer is unknown. In the absence of well-designed studies, the selection of appropriate candidates for estrogen treatment should be based on prognostic indicators, including depth of invasion, degree of differentiation, and cell type.

This document reflects emerging clinical and scientific advances as of the date issued and is subject to change. The information should not be construed as dictating an exclusive course of treatment or procedure to be followed.

ISSN 1074-861X

The American College of Obstetricians and Gynecologists
409 12th Street, SW
PO Box 96920
Washington, DC 20090-6920

12345/43210

These predictors can assist the physician in describing the risks of recurrent tumors to the patient and can assist the patient in determining the amount of risk she is willing to assume. The decision to prescribe HRT for a patient with a history of endometrial cancer should be based on the patient's perceived benefits and risks after careful counseling. The need for progestational agents in addition to estrogen is unknown at present, although progesterone supplementation after endometrial cancer therapy does not affect recurrence rate.

The introduction of SERMs may extend the options available to estrogen-deficient women. Although recent studies are encouraging, there is no information regarding the efficacy and safety of these drugs in preventing endometrial cancer or for long-term use. Raloxifene, a nonsteroidal benzothiophene approved by the U.S. Food and Drug Administration for osteoporosis prevention, has been demonstrated to exert an antiresorptive effect on bone similar to, but less effective than, that of conjugated estrogen (1). Raloxifene does not stimulate breast or endometrial tissue in postmenopausal women (2). When compared with combination estrogen and progestin, raloxifene demonstrates similar but less extensive effects on serum lipids (3). Raloxifene does not alleviate vasomotor symptoms and may be associated with symptoms of vaginal atrophy.

Because the metabolic changes of estrogen deficiency are significant, estrogen-deficient women should be given complete information, including counseling about alternative therapies, to enable them to make an informed decision. For some women, the sense of well-being afforded by the successful treatment of menopausal symptoms, the reduction of the risk of osteoporosis, and the potential provision of cardiovascular protection may outweigh the risk of stimulating tumor growth.

In summary, the area of HRT in estrogen-deficient women continues to expand at a rapid pace as newer products promise increasing benefits while minimizing adverse outcomes. Although new research appears promising, there is a clear paucity of data upon which to base specific recommendations, particularly in women who have previously been treated for endometrial carcinoma. At this time, the decision to use HRT in these women should be individualized on the basis of potential benefit and risk to the patient.

References

1. Heaney RP, Draper MW. Raloxifene and estrogen: comparative bone-remodeling kinetics. J Clin Endocrinol Metab 1997;82:3425–3429
2. Delmas PD, Bjarnason NH, Mitlak BH, Ravoux AC, Shah AS, Huster WJ, et al. Effects of raloxifene on bone mineral density, serum cholesterol concentrations, and uterine endometrium in postmenopausal women. N Engl J Med 1997;337:1641–1647
3. Walsh BW, Kuller LH, Wild RA, Paul S, Farmer M, Lawrence JB, et al. Effects of raloxifene on serum lipids and coagulation factors in healthy postmenopausal women. JAMA 1998;279:1445–1451

ACOG Committee Opinion

Committee on Gynecologic Practice

Number 226, November 1999 *(Replaces #135, April 1994)*

Hormone Replacement Therapy in Women with Previously Treated Breast Cancer

ISSN 1074-861X

The American College of Obstetricians and Gynecologists
409 12th Street, SW
PO Box 96920
Washington, DC 20090-6920

12345/32109

The use of hormone replacement therapy (estrogen with or without a progestin [HRT]) in women previously treated for breast cancer continues to be controversial. Unfortunately, reliable experimental data that would permit a definitive statement on this issue are lacking. In light of strong evidence suggesting the clinical benefits of HRT in postmenopausal women, this subject warrants review. The purpose of this Committee Opinion is to review the available evidence and its limitations and to provide recommendations for the use of HRT in women with previously treated breast cancer.

In general, recent thinking has been that the risk of recurrent disease in women previously treated for breast cancer precluded consideration of HRT. This conclusion is based on the results of both laboratory and clinical studies. Estrogen has been shown in vitro to stimulate growth of normal and malignant breast cells in tissue culture (1). This finding, together with the natural history of breast cancer, including risk factors, has led to the opinion that estrogen administration, including use of low-dose formulations, may promote breast cancer in women with active disease. In addition, the results of some early epidemiologic studies have been interpreted as evidence that HRT increases the risk of breast cancer in postmenopausal women (2–5). Finally, because an increased risk of breast cancer is associated with early menarche, late menopause, late onset of first pregnancy, and increased circulating free estrogen levels in obese women, it has been a common belief that less total endogenous estrogen exposure over a lifetime may reduce the incidence of disease. Therefore, the concern about estrogen use in women with a prior diagnosis of breast cancer has been that residual cancer may be reactivated, and mammary cells that have undergone malignant transformation may be stimulated to grow.

Hormone Replacement Therapy and Risk of Breast Cancer Development in the General Population

There is no consensus on the association of HRT with the risk of breast cancer in postmenopausal women. More than 50 epidemiologic studies have failed to demonstrate consistently or conclusively a detrimental impact of replacement estrogen use on the incidence of breast cancer.

Efforts to analyze critically the data by carefully selecting the most acceptable studies and subjecting them to meta-analysis have not clarified the situation. Overall, these studies failed to show an increased risk of postmenopausal women developing breast cancer associated with hormone replacement (6–11).

Several studies showing an increased observed risk involved both premenopausal and postmenopausal women or women using synthetic estrogen. Risk of long-term use (>15 years) cannot be calculated without extrapolation. Current users had a small increased risk that could reflect either a real increase in risk because of a promoter mechanism or an increase in detection of cases (detection bias) because of participation in a study (6–11).

In addition, data suggest the following:

- The use of progestin in combination with estrogen does not protect the user from increased breast cancer risk (10–12).
- A positive family history of breast cancer does not pose an increased risk for development of cancer in HRT users (6, 11).
- A history of benign breast disease does not increase the risk of development of breast cancer in HRT users (8, 11).

These data suggest that the question remains unanswered as to whether the risk of breast cancer is increased in postmenopausal women taking estrogen at recommended replacement doses. Lack of studies of adequate design, patient numbers, and duration of HRT preclude total reassurance that HRT is safe in these women. The ongoing Women's Health Initiative may resolve some of these issues. Quality-of-life issues and possible reduced morbidity and mortality from coronary artery disease and hip fractures must be factored in when counseling women for overall health benefits versus risks of HRT (13).

One study involved a hypothetical analysis of 10,000 50-year-old women using HRT for 25 years, with health outcomes extrapolated to age 75 (14). In this group, 574 deaths would be prevented, and women using estrogen would gain 3,951 quality-adjusted life years compared with women not using estrogen.

Pregnancy and Breast Cancer

Several studies have been performed to examine morbidity and mortality in pregnant women who develop carcinoma of the breast. Overall, the results do not indicate a reduced survival rate in these individuals despite usually greater nodal involvement (15–18). Compared with individuals who did not become pregnant, women treated for breast cancer who experience subsequent pregnancy have not been shown to consistently demonstrate either an increased or a decreased risk of recurrence (19–22).

Hormone Replacement Therapy and Risk of Breast Cancer Recurrence

Individuals with prior breast cancer are at increased risk for a second primary breast cancer, and those women with the best prognosis (stage I, small tumors with negative nodes) still have a 30% chance of recurrence in 10 years (23–26). Whether continued exposure to endogenous estrogens is instrumental in this process is unclear. There are no data that support an increased risk of breast cancer recurrence or reduction in survival rate after administration or reinstitution of HRT. Several authors have recently evaluated small groups of selected women using estrogen after being treated for breast cancer (27–30). Although the numbers studied are small, the patients usually are low risk, and the follow-up intervals are short, none of these reports showed evidence of progression or recurrence of disease and one showed fewer tumor recurrences in the HRT group. In addition, the relief of symptoms of estrogen deficiency and the possible reduced risks of osteoporosis and coronary artery disease support consideration of estrogen therapy (31). Patients included in studies are generally those who are otherwise well and may represent predominantly earlier stages of disease. Further studies involving a longer period of observation are necessary to interpret these findings adequately.

Consistent with a possible role for estrogen in recurrent breast cancer is the clinical observation that the selective estrogen receptor modulator (SERM) tamoxifen has a distinctly antiestrogenic profile in regard to its effect on the breast and reduces the rate of breast cancer recurrence (23–26). Tamoxifen now is used frequently as adjunctive therapy in the treatment of breast cancer, particularly in women whose disease is lymph-node negative, hormone-receptor positive (32). The consideration of tamoxifen with estrogen also is being explored (33). The National Surgical Adjuvant Breast and Bowel Project data showed no additional benefit of administration of tamoxifen beyond 5 years in adjunctive treatment of early breast cancer (34).

As a SERM, tamoxifen has estrogenic effects as well. These may one day lead to its use as an alternative to HRT. However, the effects of tamoxifen on preservation of bone density and coronary artery disease must be studied carefully (35). Levels of total cholesterol and low-density lipoprotein cholesterol in serum are lower in women treated with tamoxifen compared with those who are not treated, creating a similar lipid profile to that of postmenopausal women receiving HRT (36, 37). Levels of high-density lipoprotein cholesterol in women using tamoxifen may remain within the pretreatment range or decrease slightly with increased duration of use (36, 37). In addition, it has been reported that tamoxifen may be associated with a reduced calcium loss from bone and a possible reduced incidence of heart disease, although these findings have not been substantiated fully (35–37). The effects of tamoxifen versus estrogen on quality-of-life issues such as effect on genital tissues, dyspareunia, and hot flashes must be considered as well.

Somewhat worrisome is an apparent associated increase in the incidence of abnormal endometrial findings, including malignancy, in tamoxifen-treated patients (38). Although this phenomenon may be dose related or may have resulted from a preexisting endometrial abnormality, there are other features of tamoxifen therapy that point to an estrogen agonistic effect.

More recently, the SERM raloxifene, which is chemically related to tamoxifen, has been developed (39). Although its role in the treatment of breast cancer is unknown, it has offered an alternative to estrogen therapy. Its benefits are preservation of bone density and prevention of osteoporosis. It also appears to be an estrogen antagonist in the endometrium as well as in the breast (40). Its influence on lipid profile includes a slight lowering of cholesterol and low-density lipoprotein cholesterol (41). The effect of raloxifene on the central nervous system is unknown, but increased hot flashes are a documented side effect. Venous thromboembolic disease is a contradiction to its use.

Steroid Contraceptives and Breast Cancer Development

Steroid contraceptives theoretically may increase the risk of development or recurrence of breast cancer. Recent reviews of combination preparations with lower estrogen dosage (≤ 35 mcg of ethinyl estradiol) showed no evidence of a worse prognosis in a small number of women using oral contraceptive pills in the year preceding breast cancer diagnosis. Also, tumors seen in oral contraceptive users were better differentiated (42). The World Health Organization Collaborative Study of Neoplasia and Steroid Contraceptives suggested that contraceptive doses of progestins taken long term did not appear to increase the risk of breast cancer (43).

Research Limitations

Although many studies have looked at the risks of development or recurrence of breast cancer in association with HRT, steroid contraceptive use, and pregnancy, accurate interpretation of the data remains difficult.

Study parameters, such as design, medication types or dosages, patient age, or length of medication use, may vary in research in general, although such variations have been a particular problem when evaluating evidence for the role of HRT in development or recurrence of breast cancer. Similarly, numbers of study subjects and length of follow-up differ widely. The number of variables makes confounding factors possible. In addition, comparing qualitative outcomes, such as relief of menopausal symptoms and other quality-of-life issues, with numerical values (quantitative statistics) is controversial.

Interpretation of the results of studies in this review is difficult because relative risks reported are usually between 1.0 and 2.0. Such low levels of relative risk may be due to slight actual increased risk or to confounding factors or study biases.

Conclusions

There are no conclusive data to indicate an increased risk of recurrent breast cancer in postmenopausal women receiving HRT. No woman can be guaranteed protection from recurrence. Late manifestations of recurrent disease and an apparent predisposition to recurrence shown by selected subgroups of women cannot be ignored. However, the benefits of HRT are well recognized and contribute to the quality and length of life in postmenopausal women.

The following recommendations are made for postmenopausal women with previously treated breast cancer:

- The use of HRT may be considered.
- Because there are no specific data regarding particular stages or histologic types of breast cancer in which HRT may have a greater or lesser effect on breast cancer progression, caution must be exercised in all instances.
- Hormone replacement therapy should always be used in a treatment plan that includes dietary control, exercise, and, when appropriate, weight reduction and behavior modification, such as cessation of smoking and reduction of alcohol intake.

- Women with breast cancer who use HRT must continue to be monitored for recurrent disease, and, if malignancy recurs further, the use of HRT must be reevaluated.
- When the clinician explains the benefits of HRT use to the patient, this must be accompanied by a thorough explanation of the extent of current knowledge that, by necessity, will entail consultation with the patient's oncologist.

The uncertainty of this dilemma supports the need for extensive randomized, prospective trials in order to provide women with a rational and reasonable basis for therapeutic alternatives.

References

1. Thomas DB, Persing JP, Hutchinson WB. Exogenous estrogens and other risk factors for breast cancer in women with benign breast disease. J Natl Cancer Inst 1982;69: 1017–1025
2. Brinton LA, Hoover RN, Szklo M, Fraumeni JF Jr. Menopausal estrogen use and risk of breast cancer. Cancer 1981;47:2517–2522
3. Hoover R, Gray LA Sr, Cole P, MacMahon B. Menopausal estrogens and breast cancer. N Engl J Med 1976;295: 401–405
4. Ross RK, Paganini-Hill A, Gerkins VR, Mack TM, Pfeffer R, Arthur M, et al. A case-control study of menopausal estrogen therapy and breast cancer. JAMA 1980;243: 1635–1639
5. Hoover R, Glass A, Finkle WD, Azevedo D, Milne K. Conjugated estrogens and breast cancer risk in women. J Natl Cancer Inst 1981;67:815–820
6. Armstrong BK. Oestrogen therapy after the menopause—boon or bane? Med J Aust 1988;148:213–214
7. Henrich JB. The postmenopausal estrogen/breast cancer controversy. JAMA 1992;268:1900–1902
8. Dupont WD, Page DL. Menopausal estrogen replacement therapy and breast cancer. Arch Intern Med 1991;151: 67–72
9. Steinberg KK, Thacker SB, Smith SJ, Stroup DF, Zack MM, Flanders WD, et al. A meta-analysis of the effect of estrogen replacement therapy on the risk of breast cancer. JAMA 1991;265:1985–1990
10. Sillero-Arenas M, Delgado-Rodriguez M, Rodrigues-Canteras R, Bueno-Cavanillas A, Galvez-Vargas R. Menopausal hormone replacement therapy and breast cancer: a meta-analysis. Obstet Gynecol 1992;79:286–294
11. Colditz GA, Egan KM, Stampfer MJ. Hormone replacement therapy and risk of breast cancer: results from epidemiologic studies. Am J Obstet Gynecol 1993;168: 1473–1480
12. Wren BG, Eden JA. Do progestogens reduce the risk of breast cancer? A review of the evidence. Menopause 1996; 3:4–12
13. Col NF, Eckman MH, Karas RH, Pauker SG, Goldberg RJ, Ross EM, et al. Patient-specific decisions about hormone replacement therapy in postmenopausal women. JAMA 1997;277:1140–1147
14. Gorsky RD, Koplan JP, Peterson HB, Thacker SB. Relative risks and benefits of long-term estrogen replacement therapy: a decision analysis. Obstet Gynecol 1994; 83:161–166
15. Ribeiro G, Jones DA, Jones M. Carcinoma of the breast associated with pregnancy. Br J Surg 1986;73:607–609
16. Donegan WL. Breast cancer and pregnancy. Obstet Gynecol 1977;50:244–252
17. White TT, White WC. Breast cancer and pregnancy; report of 49 cases followed 5 years. Ann Surg 1956;144:384–393
18. King RM, Welch JS, Martin JK Jr, Coulam CB. Carcinoma of the breast associated with pregnancy. Surg Gynecol Obstet 1985;160:228–232
19. Cooper DR, Butterfield J. Pregnancy subsequent to mastectomy for cancer of the breast. Ann Surg 1970;171: 429–433
20. Rissanen PM. Pregnancy following treatment of mammary carcinoma. Acta Radiol Ther Phys Biol 1969;8:415–422
21. Lambe M, Hsieh C, Trichopoulos D, Ekbom A, Pavia M, Adami HO. Transient increase in the risk of breast cancer after giving birth. N Engl J Med 1994:331:5–9
22. Guinee VF, Olsson H, Moller T, Hess KR, Taylor SH, Fahey T, et al. Effect of pregnancy on prognosis for young women with breast cancer. Lancet 1994:343:1587–1589
23. Systemic treatment of early breast cancer by hormonal, cytotoxic, or immune therapy. 133 randomised trials involving 31,000 recurrences and 24,000 deaths among 75,000 women. Early Breast Cancer Trialists' Collaborative Group. Lancet 1992;339:1–15
24. Systemic treatment of early breast cancer by hormonal, cytotoxic, or immune therapy. 133 randomised trials involving 31,000 recurrences and 24,000 deaths among 75,000 women. Early Breast Cancer Trialists' Collaborative Group. Lancet 1992;339:71–85
25. Forbes JF. The control of breast cancer: the role of tamoxifen. Semin Oncol 1997;24(Suppl 1):S1-5–S1-19
26. Powles TJ. Efficacy of tamoxifen as therapy of breast cancer. Semin Oncol 1997;24(Suppl 1):S1-48–S1-54
27. DiSaia PJ, Odicino F, Grosen EA, Cowan B, Pecorelli S, Wile AG. Hormone replacement therapy in breast cancer. Lancet 1993;342:1232
28. Powles TJ, Hickish T, Casey S, O'Brien M. Hormone replacement after breast cancer. Lancet 1993;342:60–61
29. Wile AG, Opfell RW, Margileth DA. Hormone replacement therapy in previously treated breast cancer patients. Am J Surg 1993;165:372–375
30. Dhodapkar MV, Ingle JN, Ahmann DL. Estrogen replacement therapy withdrawal and regression of metastatic breast cancer. Cancer 1995;75:43–46
31. Roy JA, Sawka CA, Pritchard KI. Hormone replacement therapy in women with breast cancer. Do the risks outweigh the benefits? J Clin Oncol 1996;14:997–1006
32. Fisher B, Costantino J, Redmond C, Poisson R, Bowman D, Couture J, et al. A randomized clinical trial evaluating tamoxifen in the treatment of patients with node-negative breast cancer who have estrogen-receptor-positive tumors. N Engl J Med 1989;320:479–484
33. Powles TJ. Tamoxifen and oestrogen replacement. Lancet 1990;336:48
34. Fisher B, Costantino JP, Redmond CK, Fisher ER, Wickerham DL, Cronin WM. Endometrial cancer in tamoxifen-treated breast cancer patients: findings from the National Surgical Adjuvant Breast and Bowel Project (NSABP) B-14. J Natl Cancer Inst 1994:86:527–537

35. Love RR, Mazess RB, Barden HS, Epstein S, Newcomb PA, Jordan VC, et al. Effects of tamoxifen on bone mineral density in postmenopausal women with breast cancer. N Engl J Med 1992;326:852–856
36. Love RR, Surawicz TS, Williams EC. Antithrombin III level, fibrinogen level, and platelet count changes with adjuvant tamoxifen therapy. Arch Intern Med 1992;152: 317–320
37. Love RR, Wiebe DA, Newcombe PA, Cameron L, Leventhal H, Jordan VC, et al. Effects of tamoxifen on cardiovascular risk factors in postmenopausal women. Ann Intern Med 1991;115:860–864
38. Kedar RP, Bourne TH, Powles TJ, Collins WP, Ashley SE, Cosgrove DO, et al. Effects of tamoxifen on uterus and ovaries of postmenopausal women in a randomised breast cancer prevention trial. Lancet 1994;343:1318–1321
39. Mitlak BH, Cohen FJ. In search of optimal long-term female hormone replacement: the potential of selective estrogen receptor modulators. Horm Res 1997;48: 155–163
40. Delmas PD, Bjarnason NH, Mitlak BH, Ravoux AC, Shah AS, Huster WJ, et al. Effects of raloxifene on bone mineral density, serum cholesterol concentrations, and uterine endometrium in postmenopausal women. N Engl J Med 1997;337:1641–1647
41. Walsh BW, Kuller LH, Wild RA, Paul S, Farmer M, Lawrence JB, et al. Effects of raloxifene on serum lipids and coagulation factors in healthy postmenopausal women. JAMA 1998;279:1445–1451
42. Breast cancer and hormonal contraceptives: collaborative reanalysis of individual data on 53,297 women with breast cancer and 100,239 women without breast cancer from 54 epidemiological studies. Collaborative Group on Hormonal Factors in Breast Cancer. Lancet 1996;347:1713–1727
43. Breast cancer and depot-medroxyprogesterone acetate: a multinational study. WHO Collaborative Study of Neoplasia and Steroid Contraceptives. Lancet 1991;338:833–838

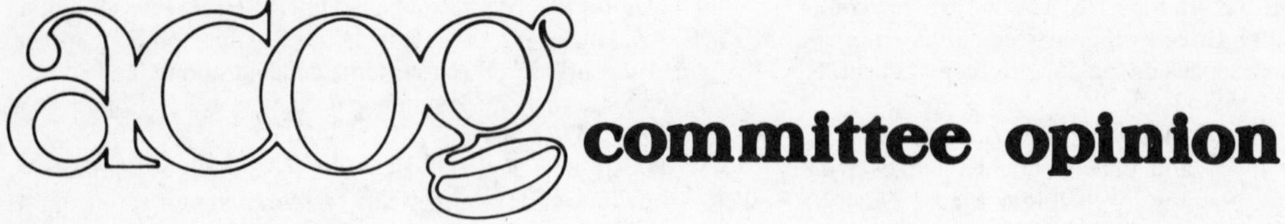

Number 130—November 1993
(Replaces #85, September 1990)

Human Immunodeficiency Virus Infection: Physicians' Responsibilities

The rate at which the incidence of infection with the human immunodeficiency virus (HIV) is increasing makes it likely that most obstetrician–gynecologists will come in contact with seropositive patients. Because of the historic variability of physician response to plague and other epidemic diseases, there is no consistent precedent to guide behavior. In the face of the acquired immunodeficiency syndrome (AIDS) epidemic, as always, physicians continue to weigh their professional obligations against their personal interests. The ethic that is evolving is founded on several important considerations.

- By voluntarily joining the medical profession, physicians commit themselves to caring for the sick. Refusal to care for a person in need compromises the essence of what it means to be a physician.
- Among the virtues to be encouraged in physicians are compassion, loyalty, courage, fairness, and a sense of altruism.
- There is a covenant implicit in the fact that society contributes to the education of physicians and, further, provides a virtual monopoly to the physicians it licenses.
- Refusal by some physicians to treat persons who are infected with HIV places an unfair burden for clinical care on their colleagues.
- In assessing personal risk, physicians should be guided by scientific and epidemiologic evidence rather than irrational fears or prejudicial attitudes toward particular societal groups. With appropriate precautions, the actual risk of a physician contracting HIV is minimal—considerably less than the risk of contracting infections such as hepatitis.

On the basis of these considerations, this committee concludes that it is unethical for an obstetrician–gynecologist to refuse to accept or continue to care for persons solely because they are or are thought to be seropositive for HIV. To avoid or delay treatment of a seropositive person is ethically equivalent to refusal of care.

Certain characteristics of the practice of obstetrics and gynecology raise issues beyond those addressed in general statements of physician responsibility.

IMPORTANCE OF EDUCATION

As primary providers of health care to women, obstetrician–gynecologists have an obligation to learn about HIV infection and its associated conditions. Education is one of the most important tasks facing society in dealing with the HIV epidemic. Obstetrician–gynecologists, in their role as providers of health care to women, have a special obligation to impart important educational information about modes of transmission of the virus, means of protection from infection, and the role of testing. They can, by their personal example and behavior, aid in allaying unreasonable public fears about casual contagion. Furthermore, they can help to promote unprejudiced professional, institutional, and societal responses to all persons infected with HIV.

HUMAN IMMUNODEFICIENCY VIRUS TESTING

Obstetrician–gynecologists should offer voluntary and confidential HIV testing to all women, with appropriate pretest and posttest counseling. To date, risk assessment instruments have not been effective in identifying all infected women. Anonymous testing through different social institutions and clinics is available and is an acceptable alternative to HIV testing in the physician's office.

Human immunodeficiency virus infection differs from most other communicable diseases in its high fatality rate, the absence of medical means for its prevention, and the lack of available curative therapy. Education of patients is one of the few ways in which spread of infection can be reduced. Pretest counseling enables the practitioner to educate the patient about HIV transmission before the psychologic impact of a positive result is felt. The physician should inform the patient of her obligation to notify those at significant risk if she is found to be infected. This counseling would include her obligation to benefit a child she delivers by disclosing her HIV status to the child's pediatrician.

The serious implications of HIV infection for a patient's future, the effect of her seropositivity on those she places at risk, and the ramifications of public disclosure of infection support the physician's obligation to obtain informed consent before HIV testing is performed on the patient or her infant. When a neonate is tested and found to be seropositive for HIV, this indicates that the mother is infected. The issues of confidentiality and risk to others should be specifically discussed before testing. Local reporting requirements and personal documentation practices should be disclosed. Respect for patient choice supports informed consent for testing by all physicians even though state and local jurisdictions differ in requirements regarding consent for testing. After testing, the physician has several obligations to the patient, the first of which is to inform the patient of her seropositive status. Following that, the physician should help ensure that comprehensive, integrated care is available. Such care might include specialists to initiate appropriate management for infectious diseases aspects of the patient's care, social institutions for nonmedical services (foster child care, ancillary domestic help) in the event that the patient progresses to debilitating symptomatic disease, and counseling groups for those infected with HIV. Finally, the physician must not only assure the patient that her medical care will continue, but also discuss issues of confidentiality. In addition, the physician may wish to inform the patient of research protocols in which she may enroll.

THE HUMAN IMMUNODEFICIENCY VIRUS-POSITIVE PATIENT

As physicians trained in both surgical and medical management of women's health problems, obstetrician–gynecologists should be aware of the ways in which decisions about which treatment options to offer may be influenced by consideration of personal risk, thereby compromising the quality of care. This awareness is particularly important when the treatment perceived as safest for the physician is one that is less safe for the woman or fetus involved or may not as appropriately address the needs and concerns of the individual woman. Disproportionate concern for physician risk may result, for example, in continuation of medical management beyond the point at which surgical intervention is indicated. It is appropriate to consider physician risk in choosing between equally effective management techniques, but patient benefit should not be compromised in an effort to protect the physician.

An individual woman's reproductive choices should be respected regardless of her HIV status. In discussing options for contraception and childbearing, the physician should make the woman aware of the risk of vertical transmission (mother to fetus) and the implications of her infection for a child she might bear as well as the potential effects of pregnancy on her own health. If she is not pregnant, a full range of contraceptive services should be made available. If the woman is pregnant, she should be provided with the information needed to decide whether to continue her pregnancy. If she chooses to continue the pregnancy, obstetric care should be provided in an effort to optimize both maternal and neonatal outcome. If an infected woman desires assistance in becoming pregnant, it is appropriate that she and her physician consider both her interest in childbearing and the potential for suffering in an infected infant before making a decision about treatment. As always, physicians should consider the medical and moral appropriateness of a given treatment when determining whether to participate.

THE HUMAN IMMUNODEFICIENCY VIRUS-NEGATIVE PATIENT

If a patient tests HIV negative, her physician needs to inform her and offer her counseling. If the patient is in a high-risk situation, she should be counseled concerning minimizing her risks.

CONFIDENTIALITY

The duty to protect a third party from infection will at times conflict with the fundamental obligation to respect the confidentiality of the physician–patient relationship. The initial strategy in such situations should include serious efforts to persuade the infected patient to disclose her status to those at risk. Convincing the patient to notify those at risk will protect others while maintaining confidentiality. Because of the importance of physician–patient confidentiality, sound justification must be sought before a breach of confidence is contemplated.

At times, despite extensive efforts on the part of the physician, the patient will remain unwilling to permit communication of information regarding

HIV infection to identifiable persons at risk. Before any breach of confidence is undertaken, the following criteria should be met:

- It should be clear that there is a high probability of harm to the uninformed individual.
- It should be clear that the potential harm is a serious one.
- It is important that the information communicated can in fact be used to prevent harm.

When a breach of confidence regarding HIV infection is contemplated, however, this evaluation of the potential harm that notification might avert must be weighed against two other significant factors:

1. There are personal risks to the individual whose confidence is breached. These include serious implications for the person's relationship with family and friends, the threat of discrimination in employment and housing, and the impact on family members.
2. Loss of patient trust may reduce the physician's ability to help the individual patient and may deter other individuals at risk who are considering testing. This latter result would have a serious negative impact on the educational efforts that lie at the heart of attempts to reduce the spread of disease.

If, on balance, a breach of confidence is deemed necessary, the physician should consider whether the goal of maintaining patient privacy would be better served by personal communication with the individual at immediate risk or by notification of local public health authorities. In some areas, provision has been made within the health department for anonymous notification of contacts.

Communication among health care professionals should always be guided by principles of confidentiality. Confidentiality should not be breached solely because of perceived risk to health care workers. Instead, health care workers should rely on strict observance of universal precautions to minimize risks.

Advances in medical treatment have led to situations in which knowledge of serostatus is important in the provision of optimal prophylactic and therapeutic care. Seropositive patients should be reminded of the health advantages of open communication with their health care team. The obstetrician has an ethical duty to counsel a pregnant woman about her obligation to give the pediatrician medical information relevant for the proper present and future care of the newborn. Knowledge of maternal HIV status is important because of the need to treat and monitor infants at risk carefully. Further, early intervention against HIV itself may be beneficial.

In general, when a seropositive patient is counseled about her condition, she will understand the advantages of making her status a part of her medical record and therefore available to those caring for her. Similarly, an informed postpartum patient will usually allow this information to be shared with those caring for her infant. If she refuses, the criteria for breach of confidentiality must be met before the pediatrician can be informed.

States and local jurisdictions vary in their regulations regarding HIV screening, reporting, disclosure, and breach of confidence. The individual physician should become familiar with the legal requirements that exist in the community.

ACCESS TO CARE

Although HIV infection occurs in all socioeconomic levels, there is a disproportionate incidence among women with limited access to health care. Seropositivity for HIV should not be a barrier to health care for women. Medical care should be provided to persons in need without regard to the circumstances of infection.

INFECTION CONTROL

It is essential that recommended infection control guidelines be followed with all patients. Such measures will help to ensure that neither health care workers nor patients are exposed to an unreasonable risk of acquired infection. The physician should take a role in seeing that the members of the health care team comply with universal precautions. Although risk cannot be avoided entirely, infection is of very low probability if precautions are taken. An effort should be made, however, to ensure that the important element of human contact is not removed from medical care in an effort to protect the provider. At no time should the implementation of universal precautions build barriers to patient–physician communication. In addition, the patient should perceive the precautions as a benefit not only to the health care team, but also to herself.

THE HUMAN IMMUNODEFICIENCY VIRUS-POSITIVE PHYSICIAN

If a physician has reason to believe that he or she is at risk of being infected, that physician should voluntarily be tested for HIV for the protection of his or her patients. The physician as a patient is entitled to the same rights to privacy and confidentiality as any other patient.

In making decisions about patient care activities, a physician who is infected with HIV should adhere to the fundamental professional obligation to avoid harm to patients. There are aspects of obstetrics and gynecology that do not involve measurable risk of transmission of infection. Some patient care activities, however, such as surgery and obstetric deliveries, may involve some potential exchange of bodily fluids.

Each infected physician must make a decision as to which procedures he or she can continue to perform safely. This decision will depend upon the physician's level of expertise, the particular surgical techniques involved, and the physician's medical condition, including mental status. The decision should be made in conjunction with such responsible individuals as his or her personal physician, the chief of the department, the hospital's director of infectious diseases, the chief of the medical staff, or with a specialized advisory panel.

Physicians who are infected with HIV should follow universal precautions, including the appropriate use of hand washing, protective barriers, and care in the use and disposal of needles and other sharp instruments. They should also comply with current guidelines for disinfection and sterilization of reusable devices used in invasive procedures.

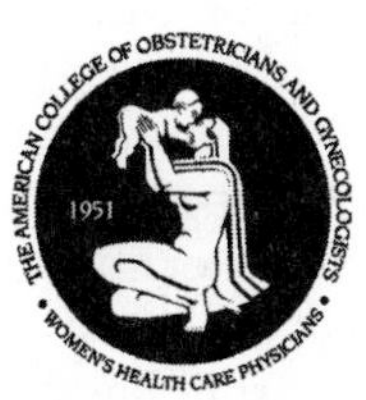

The American College of Obstetricians and Gynecologists
409 12th Street, SW • Washington, DC 20024-2188

12345/76543

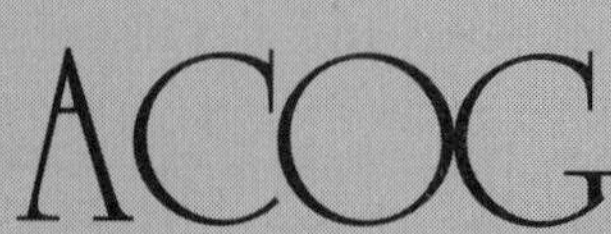

Committee on Obstetric Practice

Committee Opinion

Number 197, February 1998 (*Replaces #137, April 1994*)

Inappropriate Use of the Terms Fetal Distress and Birth Asphyxia

The Committee on Obstetric Practice is concerned about the continued use of the terms *fetal distress* as an antepartum or intrapartum diagnosis and *birth asphyxia* as a neonatal diagnosis. The Committee reaffirms that the term *fetal distress* is imprecise and nonspecific. The term has a low positive predictive value even in high-risk populations and is often associated with an infant who is in good condition at birth as determined by the Apgar score or umbilical cord blood gas analysis or both. The communication between clinicians caring for the woman and those caring for her neonate is best served by replacing the term *fetal distress* with *nonreassuring fetal status,* followed by a further description of findings (eg, repetitive variable decelerations, fetal bradycardia, and biophysical profile score of 2). Whereas *fetal distress* implies an ill fetus, *nonreassuring fetal status* describes the clinician's interpretation of data regarding fetal status (ie, the clinician is not reassured by the findings). This acknowledges the imprecision inherent in the interpre-tation of the data. Accordingly, the term *nonreassuring fetal status* is consistent with the delivery of a vigorous infant, and a good outcome does not have to be justified.

Because of the limitations of the term *fetal distress,* its use may result in inappropriate actions, such as an unnecessarily urgent delivery under general anesthesia. Fetal heart rate patterns or auscultatory findings should be considered when the degree of urgency, mode of delivery, and type of anesthesia to be given are determined. Performing a cesarean delivery for a nonreassuring fetal heart rate pattern does not necessarily preclude the use of regional anesthesia.

Effective October 1, 1998, all inclusion terms except *metabolic acidemia* will be removed from the current International Classification of Diseases (ICD) code for fetal distress. All other terms will be indexed to a new code to indicate an abnormality of the heart rate or rhythm, or they will be referenced to other more appropriate codes. A similar revision will be made to the perinatal ICD codes used by pediatricians. These changes have been made because of the waning use of *fetal distress* in clinical practice.

The term *asphyxia* should be reserved for the clinical context of damaging acidemia, hypoxia, and metabolic acidosis. The Committee strongly sup-

ISSN 1074-861X

The American College of Obstetricians and Gynecologists
409 12th Street, SW
PO Box 96920
Washington, DC 20090-6920

12345/21098

ports the concept that a neonate who has had hypoxia proximate to delivery severe enough to result in hypoxic encephalopathy will show other signs of hypoxic damage, including all of the following:

- Profound metabolic or mixed acidemia (pH <7.00) on an umbilical cord arterial blood sample, if obtained
- Persistent Apgar score of 0–3 for longer than 5 minutes
- Evidence of neonatal neurologic sequelae (eg, seizures, coma, hypotonia, and one or more of the following: cardiovascular, gastrointestinal, hematologic, pulmonary, or renal system dysfunction)

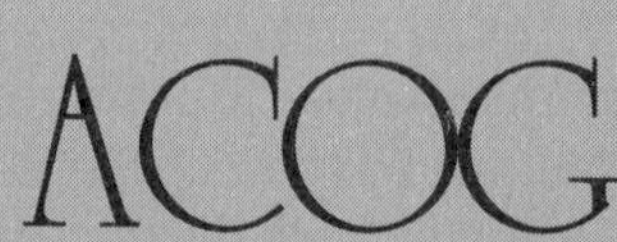

Committee on
Gynecologic Practice

Committee Opinion

Number 164, December 1995

Incidental Appendectomy

Incidental appendectomy is defined as the surgical removal of the appendix at the time of a procedure unrelated to appendiceal pathology. Routine performance of incidental appendectomy has been controversial for almost 100 years. In the past, concern focused primarily on the procedure's safety. Numerous studies attest to the safety of the procedure at the time of laparotomy, with the possible exception of an increased risk of postoperative wound infections in patients older than 65. Safety has been less well documented when the procedure is done laparoscopically.

More recently, the debate has focused on the cost–benefit issue, especially in persons at low risk for appendicitis. Throughout this century, the incidence of appendicitis and its associated morbidity and mortality have fallen precipitously. Based on the work of Addiss et al (1), the preventive value of incidental appendectomy for women was studied. With the exception of the very youngest age groups, it is clear that the preventive value of incidental appendectomy is relatively low.

Conversely, very little objective analytical data exist comparing costs. In 1987, Sugimoto and Edwards conducted a cost analysis of incidental appendectomy (2). The cost savings associated with prevented cases was well below the cost of incidental appendectomy. The authors therefore concluded that the morbidity and mortality associated with appendicitis was not significant when compared with the cost of incidental appendectomies aimed at prevention.

Although incidental appendectomy, performed by either laparotomy or laparoscopy, may only be routinely indicated in certain select groups of patients, the benefits of eliminating future emergency appendectomy and simplifying the differential diagnosis of pelvic pain may outweigh any risk or cost concerns (3–7). These subgroups include women 10–30 years of age (high-incidence group), women undergoing exploratory surgery for unexplained pelvic or right lower quadrant pain, or women in whom endometriosis is found. Other subgroups include women in whom abdominal radiation is anticipated, the mentally handicapped or those unable to provide a clear history, and women undergoing extensive surgery in whom major adhesions are anticipated postoperatively or there are other relative contraindications to abdominal surgery in the future. Patients with fixation of the appendix to the ovary or tube and patients with appendiceal calculus or fecalith should be considered for appendectomy as a definite prophylactic measure.

ISSN 1074-861X

The American College of Obstetricians and Gynecologists
409 12th Street, SW
Washington, DC 20024-2188

12345/98765

Nonemergent appendectomy is contraindicated in certain patients. These include those with known Crohn disease, an inaccessible appendix, a history of prior abdominal radiation treatment, or presence of vascular grafts or material in the abdomen and those whose medical condition is unstable at the time.

In conclusion, incidental appendectomy appears to be associated with slight if any increased risk to patients in otherwise good condition. However, except for a select group of patients, the benefit of this procedure to the patient may also be slight.

References

1. Addiss DG, Shaffer N, Fowler BS, Tauxe RV. The epidemiology of appendicitis and appendectomy in the United States. Am J Epidemiol 1990;132:910–925
2. Sugimoto T, Edwards D. Incidence and costs of incidental appendectomy as a preventive measure. Am J Public Health 1987;77:471–475
3. Grimes DA. Frontiers of operative laparoscopy: a review and critique of the evidence. Am J Obstet Gynecol 1992; 166:1062–1071
4. Luckmann R. Incidence and case fatality rates for acute appendicitis in California. A population-based study of the effects of age. Am J Epidemiol 1989;129:905–918
5. Nezhat C, Nezhat F. Incidental appendectomy during videolaseroscopy. Am J Obstet Gynecol 1991;165:559–564
6. Pelosi MA, Villalona E. Laparoscopic hysterectomy, appendectomy, and cholecystectomy. N J Med 1993;90: 207–212
7. Warren JL, Penberthy LT, Addiss DG, McBean AM. Appendectomy incidental to cholecystectomy among elderly Medicare beneficiaries. Surg Gynecol Obstet 1993; 177:288–294

ACOG

Committee on Obstetric Practice

Committee Opinion

Number 228, November 1999

Induction of Labor with Misoprostol

Induction of labor is a common obstetric intervention in the United States, occurring in up to 15% of all pregnancies. The American College of Obstetricians and Gynecologists supports induction of labor as a worthwhile therapeutic option when the benefits of expeditious delivery outweigh the risks of continuing the pregnancy (1). Prostaglandin E_2 (PGE_2), applied locally to the cervix or vagina, has been widely studied as an induction agent, and has been found to be safe and effective (2, 3). Two such agents have been approved by the U.S. Food and Drug Administration for this purpose and are commercially available as dinoprostone preparations. Recent studies have explored the effectiveness and safety of misoprostol for induction of labor. This prostaglandin E_1 analogue is less expensive, more stable, and easier to store than dinoprostone preparations. However, misoprostol currently is approved by the U.S. Food and Drug Administration for the treatment of peptic ulcer disease and not for induction of labor. Moreover, the manufacturer does not plan to pursue approval for this indication (4).

At least 19 prospective, randomized clinical trials involving more than 1,900 patients receiving doses of misoprostol ranging from 25 mcg to 200 mcg in a variety of dosage schedules have been performed. Most researchers have administered misoprostol in tablet form into the posterior fornix of the vagina, but it also has been mixed into a hydroxymethylcellulose gel or applied intracervically.

In general, misoprostol has been found to be an effective agent for the induction of labor. When compared with placebo, misoprostol use decreased oxytocin requirements and achieved higher rates of vaginal delivery within 24 hours of induction. Misoprostol also compared favorably with intracervical and intravaginal PGE_2 preparations; many studies demonstrated shorter times to delivery and reduced oxytocin requirements after misoprostol administration (5). Some studies suggest that misoprostol may reduce the rate of cesarean delivery, but further randomized clinical trials using the 25 mcg dose are required to confirm this observation (5). There have been reports of uterine rupture following misoprostol use for cervical ripening in patients with prior uterine surgery. Thus, until reassuring studies are available, misoprostol is not recommended for cervical ripening in patients who have had prior cesarean delivery or major uterine surgery (6).

When given in doses of 50 mcg or more, misoprostol use has been associated with an increased rate of uterine tachysystole (six or more uterine con-

This document reflects emerging clinical and scientific advances as of the date issued and is subject to change. The information should not be construed as dictating an exclusive course of treatment or procedure to be followed.

ISSN 1074-861X

The American College of Obstetricians and Gynecologists
409 12th Street, SW
PO Box 96920
Washington, DC 20090-6920

12345/32109

tractions in 10 minutes in consecutive 10-minute intervals) compared with either placebo or PGE_2 preparations. In two studies in which 50 mcg of misoprostol was administered intravaginally every 4 hours, researchers found increased rates of meconium passage (7) and cesarean delivery due to uterine hyperstimulation syndrome (8) when compared with dinoprostone. However, an increase in neonatal morbidity after misoprostol administration has not been documented. In trials where 25 mcg of misoprostol was administered intravaginally as frequently as every 3 hours, there did not appear to be an increase in uterine tachysystole, hyperstimulation, or meconium passage when compared with PGE_2 (9, 10). Moreover, this dosing regimen appeared to be at least as effective in inducing labor as the PGE_2 preparations.

Currently, misoprostol is available in 100 mcg and 200 mcg tablets, and the 100 mcg tablet is not scored. If misoprostol is used for cervical ripening and induction, one quarter of a 100 mcg tablet (ie, approximately 25 mcg) should be considered for the initial dose.

Given the current evidence, intravaginal misoprostol tablets appear to be effective in inducing labor in pregnant women who have unfavorable cervices. The use of higher doses (50 mcg every 6 hours) may be appropriate in some situations, although increasing the dose appears to be associated most closely with uterine tachysystole and possibly with uterine hyperstimulation and meconium staining of amniotic fluid. Further prospective trials are required to define an optimal dosing regimen for misoprostol. However, misoprostol is not recommended for patients with prior uterine surgery (11). Patients undergoing such therapy should receive fetal heart rate and uterine activity monitoring in a hospital setting until further studies evaluate and confirm the safety of outpatient therapy.

References

1. American College of Obstetricians and Gynecologists. Induction of labor. ACOG Practice Bulletin. Washington, DC: ACOG, 1999
2. Brindley BA, Sokol RJ. Induction and augmentation of labor: basis and methods for current practice. Obstet Gynecol Surv 1988;43:730–743
3. Rayburn WF. Prostaglandin E_2 gel for cervical ripening and induction of labor: a critical analysis. Am J Obstet Gynecol 1989;160:529–534
4. Bauer TA, Brown D, Chai LK. Vaginal misoprostol for term labor induction. Ann Pharmacother 1997;31: 1391–1393
5. Sanchez-Ramos L, Kaunitz AM, Wears RL, Delke I, Gaudier FL. Misoprostol for cervical ripening and labor induction: a meta-analysis. Obstet Gynecol 1997;89: 633–642
6. Hofmeyr GJ. Vaginal misoprostol for cervical ripening and labour induction in late pregnancy. The Cochrane Library 1999; Issue 2:1–18 (Meta-analysis)
7. Wing DA, Jones MM, Rahall A, Goodwin TM, Paul RH. A comparison of misoprostol and prostaglandin E_2 gel for preinduction cervical ripening and labor induction. Am J Obstet Gynecol 1995;172:1804–1810
8. Buser D, Mora G, Arias F. A randomized comparison between misoprostol and dinoprostone for cervical ripening and labor induction in patients with unfavorable cervices. Obstet Gynecol 1997;89:581–585
9. Wing DA, Paul RH. A comparison of different dosing regimens of vaginally administered misoprostol for preinduction cervical ripening and labor induction. Am J Obstet Gynecol 1996;175:158–164
10. Wing DA, Ortiz-Omphroy G, Paul RH. A comparison of intermittent vaginal administration of misoprostol with continuous dinoprostone for cervical ripening and labor induction. Am J Obstet Gynecol 1997;177:612–618
11. Wing DA, Lovett K, Paul RH. Disruption of prior uterine incision following misoprostol for labor induction in women with previous cesarean section. Obstet Gynecol 1998;91:828–830

ACOG

Committee Opinion

Committee on Professional Liability

Number 237, June 2000 *(Replaces No. 166, December 1995)*

Informed Refusal

Informed refusal is a relatively recent concept of law regarding patient–physician relations, and it has developed in conjunction with the law of informed consent. Almost universally, informed-consent laws have been liberalized in recent years from the relatively paternalistic "professional or reasonable physician" standard to the "materiality or patient viewpoint" standard. In the professional or reasonable physician standard, a physician must disclose to a patient the risks and benefits that are customarily disclosed by the medical community for that treatment, test, or procedure. In the materiality or patient viewpoint standard, a physician must disclose to the patient the risks and benefits that a reasonable person in the patient's position would want to know in order to make an informed decision. As the perspective for evaluating the level of disclosure of risks and benefits in informed consent has changed, it has become clear that patients are entitled to participate with their physicians in a process of shared decision making with regard to medical procedures, tests, or treatments (1).

Once a patient has been informed of the material risks and benefits involved with a treatment, test, or procedure, that patient has the right to exercise full autonomy in deciding whether to undergo the treatment, test, or procedure or whether to make a choice among a variety of treatments, tests, or procedures. In the exercise of that autonomy, the informed patient also has the right to refuse to undergo any of these treatments, tests, or procedures. This election by the patient to forgo a treatment, test, or procedure that has been offered or recommended by the physician constitutes informed refusal.

Documentation always has been an important component of informed consent. Performing an operative procedure on a patient without the patient's permission can constitute "battery" under common law. In most circumstances this is a criminal act, and documentation of the patient's consent is protection against liability. In many instances, the documentation is an informed-consent form signed by the patient, but in some situations a notation in the patient's medical record is sufficient and appropriate.

Documentation rarely has been an important component of informed refusal in the past but has become more important in the present health care environment. Managed care and increased patient autonomy are two factors that warrant a reexamination of the need for documentation of informed refusal. The widespread implementation of managed care and utilization review has created a conflict between cost containment and medical necessity.

This document provides risk management information that is current as of the date issued and is subject to change. This document does not define a standard of care nor should it be interpreted as legal advice.

ISSN 1074-861X

The American College of Obstetricians and Gynecologists
409 12th Street, SW
PO Box 96920
Washington, DC 20090-6920

12345/43210

It is not uncommon for a physician to recommend a treatment, test, or procedure to a patient that will not be paid for by a third-party insurance carrier, in whole or in part. Legal precedents have established that an attending physician should act as a patient advocate in such coverage disputes and attempt to convince the managed care organization that coverage is warranted. In spite of that obligation, however, there will be many situations in which physician advocacy will not prevail and coverage will be denied. In such circumstances, a physician should discuss with the patient whether she wishes to pay for the treatment, test, or procedure personally or seek alternative funding. If the patient then refuses to undergo the treatment, test, or procedure for economic reasons, the physician should document that informed refusal in the patient's medical record. In some situations the physician might want to obtain a written statement from the patient, acknowledging that the risk of refusal was fully explained.

The increased respect accorded individual patient autonomy in medical decision making has given rise to other circumstances when documentation of an informed refusal is appropriate. In spite of a physician's medical advice or recommendation, a patient who is informed of the material risks and benefits of a particular treatment, test, or procedure may elect to forgo all or some of these or may decline a procedure or test that might be recommended or become necessary during treatment. Such a refusal may be based on religious beliefs, personal preference, or comfort.

Whenever a patient refuses a treatment, test, or procedure, a physician should document the informed refusal in the patient's medical record and include the following information:

- The patient's refusal to consent to a treatment, test, or procedure
- The reasons stated by the patient for refusal
- Documentation that the need for the treatment, test, or procedure has been explained
- A statement that the consequences of the refusal, including possible jeopardy to health or life, have been described to the patient

Reference

1. American College of Obstetricians and Gynecologists. Ethical dimensions of informed consent. ACOG Committee Opinion 108. Washington, DC: ACOG, 1992

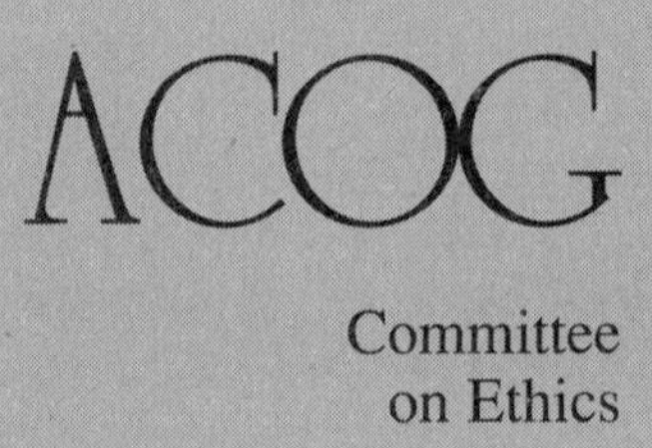

Committee Opinion

Number 204, July 1998

Institutional Responsibility to Provide Legal Representation

The *Code of Professional Ethics of the American College of Obstetricians and Gynecologists* states, "The obstetrician–gynecologist should strive to address through the appropriate procedures the status of those physicians who demonstrate questionable competence, impairment, or unethical or illegal behavior. In addition, the obstetrician–gynecologist should cooperate with appropriate authorities to prevent the continuation of such behavior" (1).

Academic institutions, professional corporations, hospitals, and other health care organizations should have policies and procedures by which alleged violations of professional behavior can be reported and investigated. Also, it is necessary for these institutions to adopt policies on legal representation and indemnification for their employees or others acting in an official capacity who, in discharging their obligations relative to unethical or illegal behavior of individuals, are exposed to potential costly legal actions.

The American College of Obstetricians and Gynecologists agrees with the position of the American Association of University Professors in their 1995 statement, "Institutional Responsibility for Faculty Liability," that institutions should ensure effective legal and other necessary representation and full indemnification for any faculty member named or included in lawsuits or other legal proceedings arising from an act or omission in the discharge of institutional or professional duties (2).

References

1. American College of Obstetricians and Gynecologists. Code of professional ethics of the American College of Obstetricians and Gynecologists. Washington, DC: ACOG, 1997
2. American Association of University Professors. American Association of University Professors policy documents and reports. Washington, DC: AAUP, 1995:102

ISSN 1074-861X

The American College of Obstetricians and Gynecologists
409 12th Street, SW
PO Box 96920
Washington, DC 20090-6920

12345/21098

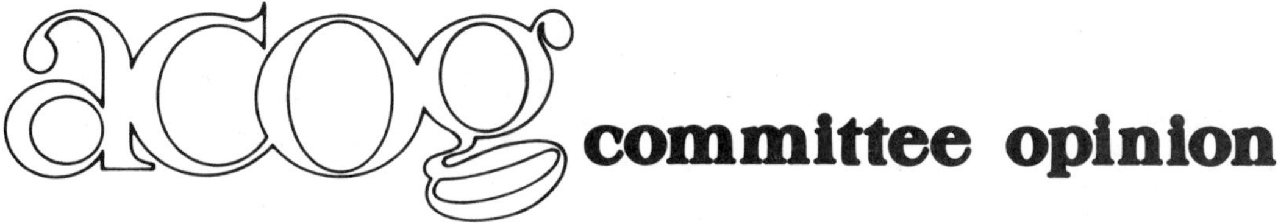

Committee on Gynecologic Practice

Number 146—November 1994

Laparoscopically Assisted Vaginal Hysterectomy

Use of a laparoscope to assist in the performance of a vaginal hysterectomy in cases that might otherwise require an abdominal hysterectomy is an established technique. Specific procedures that can be completed by laparoscopically assisted vaginal hysterectomy include the following:

- Lysis of adhesions
- Treatment of pelvic endometriosis
- Ligation of infundibulopelvic ligaments for ovarian removal

The benefits of laparoscopically assisted vaginal hysterectomy must be weighed against the potential increased hazard and expense of undertaking two distinct operative procedures, each with its own associated risks.

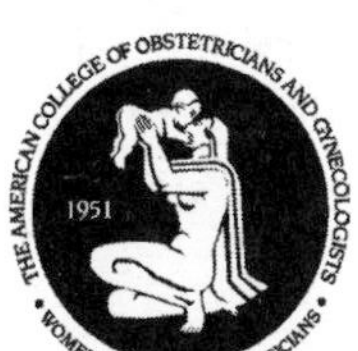

ISSN 1074-861X

The American College of Obstetricians and Gynecologists
409 12th Street, SW • Washington, DC 20024-2188

2345/8765

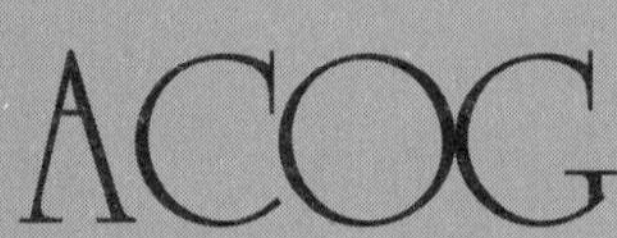

Committee on
Gynecologic Practice

Committee Opinion

Number 191, October 1997 (*Replaces #134, March 1994*)

Length of Hospital Stay for Gynecologic Procedures

The American College of Obstetricians and Gynecologists is concerned about the compromise in quality of care that can occur as a result of the "cost-saving" measure of reducing length of hospital stay. Length-of-stay normative data record the average stay in hospital days for a given gynecologic procedure and reflect generally recognized practice across geographic areas. These data have changed radically in the past several years and are continuing to change.

Length-of-stay determinants are based upon a range of individual factors, such as concurrent disease process, severity of illness, intensity of care required, and therapeutic approach. Although standard protocols or predetermined number of days for length of stay can offer general guidance, individual patient characteristics, physician judgment, and physician–patient consultation always should determine length of stay in individual cases.

After gynecologic surgery, a patient's readiness for release from the hospital should be based on positive discharge criteria. These criteria generally include (but are not limited to)

- Stable vital signs
- No evidence of untreated infections
- Adequate oral intake
- Satisfactory bowel and urinary tract function

Before discharge, instructions regarding diet, medications, wound and drainage device care, activity, and follow-up should be communicated to the patient or her caregivers. The patient or her caregivers should understand the instructions and be able to provide ongoing care and monitor recovery as needed.

ISSN 1074-861X

The American College of Obstetricians and Gynecologists
409 12th Street, SW
PO Box 96920
Washington, DC 20090-6920

12345/10987

ACOG

Committee on Professional Liability

Committee Opinion

Number 207, September 1998

Liability Implications of Recording Procedures or Treatments

The widespread use of recording technology has affected the practice of obstetrics and gynecology. Within the health care setting, all images, even those that are noninvasive, should be obtained primarily for clinical indications. Although there is no consensus on whether a recording of a procedure is part of the medical record, there are liability issues to consider.

Written consent from the patient or guardian and the involved health care personnel should be obtained when using electronic recording media for telemedicine, educational purposes (such as laparoscopic videotapes), or any other reason. The written consent should indicate the specific purposes for which the images may be used.

Each institution should develop policies concerning the recording of routine and emergency procedures by health care personnel as well as the recording of deliveries by third parties or family members. These policies should be discussed before the procedure or soon after the physician–patient relationship has been established.

Recording solely for the purpose of patient memorabilia or marketing is not without liability, and each institution should weigh these competing concerns. The Committee on Professional Liability strongly discourages any recording of medical and surgical procedures for patient memorabilia. If an institution allows such recording, however, the written consent of the patient and health care personnel should be obtained in advance, and the institution's ability to retain the original and provide a copy to the patient should be clarified.

ISSN 1074-861X

The American College of Obstetricians and Gynecologists
409 12th Street, SW
PO Box 96920
Washington, DC 20090-6920

12345/21098

ACOG Committee Opinion

Committee on Health Care for Underserved Women

Number 200, March 1998

Mandatory Reporting of Domestic Violence

Domestic violence—also known as intimate partner violence—can be defined as a pattern of assaultive and coercive behaviors, including physical, sexual, and psychologic attacks, as well as economic coercion used against current or former intimate partners (1). Nearly 5 million women are victims of violent incidents each year. Approximately 75% of all lone-offender violence against women was perpetrated by offenders whom the victim knew; 29% was reported to be perpetrated by current or former spouses or boyfriends. In 1992, more than 1,400 women were killed by their husband, ex-husband, or boyfriend (2). Race or ethnicity is not associated with increased risk of victimization (3). Intimate partner abuse may also affect other family members. Fifty percent of the men who abuse their partners also abuse their children. Violence may begin or escalate during pregnancy (4). Research indicates that violence during pregnancy may be a more prevalent problem than pregnancy-induced hypertension, gestational diabetes, or placenta previa, conditions for which pregnant women are routinely screened (5). The American College of Obstetricians and Gynecologists has published a comprehensive overview of domestic violence that details the role of the physician in identification and intervention (6).

There is no standard response to victims of domestic violence. The availability of services for victims of domestic violence varies from community to community and may include emergency shelters, legal advocacy, telephone hotlines with crisis counseling, support groups, court-ordered restraining orders, and mandatory arrest of the perpetrator. Various national efforts also exist, including a 24-hour national toll-free telephone hotline (1-800-799-SAFE; 1-800-787-3224 [TDD]).

Some jurisdictions have policies in place that allow for the arrest and prosecution of suspected perpetrators of domestic violence regardless of a victim's willingness to press charges or testify in court. These "pro-arrest" and "no-drop" policies may reduce the risk of retaliation by the perpetrator because the victim herself does not have to take the lead in pursuing a legal remedy.

Background on Mandatory Reporting of Domestic Violence

Almost all states require physicians to report injuries sustained by gun, knife, or other deadly weapon, primarily to detect criminal activity. A number of

ISSN 1074-861X

The American College of Obstetricians and Gynecologists
409 12th Street, SW
PO Box 96920
Washington, DC 20090-6920

12345/21098

states also require the reporting of injuries resulting from acts of violence or nonaccidental acts. In many instances, these laws may require the reporting of injuries resulting from domestic violence. Additionally, in an attempt to respond more directly to violence against women, some states have enacted specific requirements that explicitly direct health care providers to report suspected or confirmed acts of domestic violence. However, no uniform approach to reporting domestic violence exists among these states. The laws vary in terms of the definition of domestic violence, who is required to report the incident, and how and to whom it is to be reported. Most of the state laws regarding mandatory reporting of domestic violence provide physicians with immunity from civil or criminal liability if good faith is employed when filing a report (7). Physicians should be familiar with all laws pertaining to the reporting of domestic violence and should contact state officials to learn under what conditions and to whom reports of domestic violence should be made.

Examples of two very different approaches taken with respect to mandatory reporting follow. In Kentucky, any person, including a physician, who has a reasonable cause to suspect that an adult has suffered abuse must report the abuse to the state's health and human resources agency. Once contacted, the agency must notify the police, investigate the complaint, and provide protective services where necessary unless the woman refuses these services. California law, on the other hand, requires health practitioners to file reports with local law enforcement officials when any person suffers from any wound caused by a firearm or when the injury is the result of assaultive or abusive conduct, including abuse by spouse or cohabitant (7).

Support for Mandatory Reporting

Supporters of mandatory reporting of domestic violence underscore the fact that intimate partner violence is a crime. They acknowledge that the power imbalance endemic to many abusive relationships often prevents or deters the abused person from seeking available legal remedies. Supporters believe that mandatory reporting helps identify battered women so that services and protection can be provided before violence recurs. They believe if reporting is required, then physicians and others may be prompted to implement universal screening in part to avoid penalties and liability issues. The need for more accurate data on the incidence of domestic violence is often noted by supporters of reporting requirements.

Opposition to Mandatory Reporting

Opponents of mandatory reporting statutes argue that there are no data to support the benefits of enactment of these laws and that, while well intentioned, they may place the woman at greater risk of retaliation by the perpetrator (7–10). Most state laws do not include provisions that permit the victim to "veto" the filing of a report of domestic violence by someone other than the victim, even though the reason cited most often by women who do not report domestic violence crimes is a fear of reprisal by their abusive partner (7, 11, 12). A court order of protection or restraining order is not a guarantee against reprisal by the abusive partner. The battered woman herself is often in the best position to determine when law enforcement or social services are desirable. Unlike child abuse and elder abuse laws that are intended to provide protection to individuals deemed incompetent to do so for themselves, laws requiring the mandatory reporting of domestic violence are applied to women who are usually considered legally competent adults. Mandatory reporting laws, then, diminish the ability of a woman to exercise self-determination, thereby damaging her self-esteem further.

Moreover, reporting requirements presuppose the availability of resources to help an abused woman establish a new life for herself and her children. Opponents underscore the inadequacy of resources available to protect victims once they have been identified, as well as waiting lists for support services (7, 13).

Mandatory reporting by physicians of suspected or confirmed abuse of a patient may have additional unintended consequences, such as 1) deterring a woman from confiding in her physician or from seeking care; 2) inhibiting providers from screening patients for abuse; 3) impairing a woman's ability to plan and negotiate a safe exit for herself and her children; and 4) threatening the essential tenet of physician–patient confidentiality.

Conclusion—Mandatory Reporting Not Yet Justified

Given the lack of data to support the benefits of mandatory reporting laws and the inadequate infrastructure of services for victims of violence, the benefits of this approach remain questionable. Such statutes should not be implemented without provisions that provide women with the ability to override or veto reporting requirements. Before supporting further implementation of mandatory reporting laws by states, a comprehensive evaluation of the effects of existing mandatory reporting laws is needed. Particular attention should be given to analyzing their effect upon the use and availability of support services, the frequency of physician screening, and the incidence of domestic violence.

As physicians who treat women exclusively, obstetrician–gynecologists should recognize domestic violence through screening and provide appropriate referrals on behalf of their abused patients. Additionally, the obstetrician–gynecologist is in a unique position to provide such assistance because of the special nature of the patient–physician relationship. The American College of Obstetricians and Gynecologists, therefore, reaffirms its long-standing commitment to the safety of domestic violence victims and their children, as well as to a comprehensive response to the problem of domestic violence.

References

1. Warshaw C, Ganley AL, Salber PR. Improving the health care response to domestic violence: a resource manual for health care providers. San Francisco: The Family Violence Prevention Fund, 1995
2. Bachman R, Saltzman LE. Violence against women: estimates from the redesigned survey. Washington, DC: Bureau of Justice Statistics, U.S. Department of Justice, 1995 August; publication no. NCJ-154348
3. Craven D. Female victims of violent crime. Washington, DC: Bureau of Justice Statistics, U.S. Department of Justice, 1996 December; publication no. NCJ-162602
4. American College of Obstetricians and Gynecologists. Domestic violence: the role of the physician in identification, intervention, and prevention. Washington, DC: ACOG, 1995
5. Gazmararian JA, Lazorick S, Spitz A, Ballard TJ, Saltzman LE, Marks JS. Prevalence of violence against pregnant women. JAMA 1996;275:1915–1920
6. American College of Obstetricians and Gynecologists. Domestic violence. Technical Bulletin 209. Washington, DC: ACOG, 1995
7. Hyman A, Schillinger D, Lo B. Laws mandating reporting of domestic violence: do they promote patient well-being. JAMA 1995;273:1781–1787
8. AMA opposes mandatory medical reporting. Domestic Violence Report 1997;3:1, 7
9. Chez RA, Jones RF III. Treating battered women: the medicolegal aspects. OBG Management 1996;6:29–30
10. Hyman A, Chez RA. Mandatory reporting of domestic violence by health care providers: a misguided approach. Womens Health Issues 1995;5:208–213
11. Brookoff D, O'Brien KK, Cook CS, Thompson TD, Williams C. Characteristics of participants in domestic violence. JAMA 1997;277:1369–1373
12. Rodriguez MA, Quiroga SS, Bauer HM. Breaking the silence. Battered women's perspectives on medical care. Arch Fam Med 1996;5:153–158
13. Schornstein SL. Domestic violence and health care: what every professional needs to know. Thousand Oaks, California: Sage Publications, 1997

ACOG

Committee on Genetics

Committee Opinion

Number 230, January 2000

Maternal Phenylketonuria

Phenylketonuria (PKU) is an autosomal recessive disorder of phenylalanine metabolism that, if untreated, can cause severe mental retardation. Phenylketonuria is caused by a deficiency of the enzyme phenylalanine hydroxylase. Children of women with PKU will carry at least one abnormal gene, which is inherited from their homozygous affected mother. Even though the fetus is unlikely to be affected, approximately 1 in 120 children will inherit an abnormal phenylalanine hydroxylase gene from both parents and also have PKU. The remainder of children are carriers and should receive genetic counseling in the future. Phenylalanine crosses the placenta by an active transport process that results in a fetal-to-maternal plasma phenylalanine ratio of 1.5. This results in higher levels of phenylalanine in fetal blood than would be expected based on maternal blood levels.

Routine screening for PKU in newborns and early dietary therapy with a phenylalanine-restricted diet have markedly reduced mental retardation in affected individuals. As a result of these advances in the detection and treatment of PKU, there are large numbers of young adults with PKU who received early dietary treatment for this disorder and have IQs in the normal or near-normal range. The failure of young women with PKU to adhere to dietary restrictions has led to a new public health challenge. The heterozygous fetus is metabolically normal. However, these metabolically normal fetuses of women with PKU who are on an unrestricted diet may develop microcephaly, low birth weight, heart defects, and mental retardation due to maternal hyperphenylalaninemia. Children of women with PKU on unrestricted diets are at a 92% risk for mental retardation, a 73% risk for microcephaly, and a 12% risk for congenital heart defects (1).

In the United States, approximately 3,000 women of reproductive age are affected with PKU. Evidence indicates that women with PKU will benefit from remaining on a phenylalanine-free diet throughout their lives. Many of these women are not currently on phenylalanine-restricted diets, which require the consumption of phenylalanine-free products and supplements that many women find unpalatable. Unless these women are identified and placed on an appropriate diet before and during pregnancy, they are at risk for having children affected with PKU. It has been suggested that dietary control should be implemented at least 3 months prior to conception to help prevent fetal structural defects, including cardiac defects (2). If phenylalanine levels are normalized by 8 weeks of gestation, there is evidence to suggest a reduction in intrauterine growth restriction (3).

This document reflects emerging clinical and scientific advances as of the date issued and is subject to change. The information should not be construed as dictating an exclusive course of treatment or procedure to be followed.

ISSN 1074-861X

The American College of Obstetricians and Gynecologists
409 12th Street, SW
PO Box 96920
Washington, DC 20090-6920

12345/43210

Conclusions and Recommendations

1. All women with PKU should be strongly encouraged to receive family planning and preconceptional counseling.
2. Women with PKU should begin dietary phenylalanine restriction prior to conception (4).
3. Ideally, pregnant women with PKU should be managed in consultation with practitioners from experienced PKU centers.

References

1. Lenke RR, Levy HL. Maternal phenylketonuria and hyperphenylalaninemia. An international survey of the outcome of untreated and treated pregnancies. N Engl J Med 1980; 303:1202–1208
2. Waisbren SE, Hamilton BD, St. James PJ, Shiloh S, Levy HL. Psychosocial factors in maternal phenylketonuria: women's adherence to medical recommendations. Am J Public Health 1995;85:1636–1641
3. Koch R, Friedman E, Azen C, Hanley W, Levy H, Matalon R, et al. The international collaborative study of maternal phenylketonuria status report 1998. MRDD Res Rev 1999;5:117–121
4. Levy HL, Waisbren SE, Lobbregt D, Allred E, Schuler A, Trefz FK, et al. Maternal mild hyperphenylalaninaemia: an international survey of offspring outcome. Lancet 1994; 344: 1589–1594

Bibliography

Koch R, Levy HL, Matalon R, Rouse B, Haney WB, Trefz F, et al. The international collaborative study of maternal phenylketonuria: status report 1994. Acta Paediatr Suppl 1994;407: 111–119

Levy HL, Waisbren SE. Effects of untreated maternal phenylketonuria and hyperphenylalaninemia on the fetus. N Engl J Med 1983;309:1269–1274

Lipson A, Beuhler B, Bartley J, Walsh D, Yu J, O'Halloran M, et al. Maternal hyperphenylalaninemia fetal effects. J Pediatr 1984;104:216–220

Luke B, Keith LG. The challenge of maternal phenylketonuria screening and treatment. J Reprod Med 1990;35:667–673

MacCready RA. Admissions of phenylketonuric patients to residential institutions before and after screening programs of the newborn infant. J Pediatr 1974;85:383–385

Platt LD, Koch R, Azen C, Hanley WB, Levy HL, Matalon R, et al. Maternal phenylketonuria collaborative study, obstetric aspects and outcome: the first 6 years. Am J Obstet Gynecol 1992;166:1150–1162

ACOG

Committee on Gynecologic Practice

Committee Opinion

Number 245, December 2000

Mifepristone for Medical Pregnancy Termination

Mifepristone (RU-486), an antiprogestin, has been approved by the U.S. Food and Drug Administration (FDA) for use in combination with the prostaglandin misoprostol as a medical method for terminating intrauterine pregnancy up to 49 days from the first day of the last menstrual period.

This method has been well-tested and extensively used. Since 1988, almost 500,000 women in 20 countries have used mifepristone in combination with one of several prostaglandins to terminate intrauterine pregnancies (1). This method is very effective: studies indicate one dose of mifepristone, when combined with one dose of misoprostol 2 days later, is 92–99% successful in terminating intrauterine pregnancies up to 49 days from the first day of the last menstrual period (2). Accurate dating of gestational age is essential to reduce complications and increase efficacy. Failures include an ongoing pregnancy rate of 1% or less and a rate of incomplete abortion requiring surgical intervention of 5% or less (2).

This regimen appears to be as safe as surgical abortion performed under the safest conditions (3). It is usually well-tolerated and has been reported to be acceptable by the majority of women using it (1). Vaginal bleeding, a natural consequence of the abortion process, occurs in all women using mifepristone. Other common effects include abdominal pain, nausea, vomiting, and diarrhea. Hospitalization, surgical intervention, and intravenous-fluid administration for these effects are rarely needed, but 24-hour availability of a clinician is required for assessment of potential complications. Careful clinical follow-up is necessary to ensure that termination is complete. Because of potential teratogenicity with this regimen, patients should be counseled appropriately.

Contraindications include chronic adrenal failure, severe asthma, long-term glucocorticoid therapy, an intrauterine device (IUD) in place, inherited porphyrias, and a history of allergy to mifepristone, misoprostol, or other prostaglandin. Mifepristone should be used cautiously in women with complicated diabetes mellitus, severe anemia, and hemorrhagic disorders, and in those receiving anticoagulant treatment (4). Mifepristone is ineffective in the termination of ectopic pregnancies and is less effective in the termination of intrauterine pregnancies after 49 days from the first day of the last menstrual period.

This document reflects emerging clinical and scientific advances as of the date issued and is subject to change. The information should not be construed as dictating an exclusive course of treatment or procedure to be followed.

ISSN 1074-861X

The American College of Obstetricians and Gynecologists
409 12th Street, SW
PO Box 96920
Washington, DC 20090-6920

12345/43210

The FDA has approved mifepristone for distribution to physicians only. Under terms of the approval, the protocol requires three office visits, and the drug may be administered only in a clinic, medical office, or hospital, by or under the supervision of a physician who meets the following qualifications. Physicians must be able to:

- Assess the gestational age of an embryo and diagnose ectopic pregnancies
- Provide surgical intervention in cases of incomplete abortion or severe bleeding, or have made plans to provide such care through others
- Assure patient access to medical facilities equipped to provide blood transfusions and resuscitation, if necessary

Physicians will indicate that they meet these qualifications by signing and returning a prescriber's agreement to the distributor. The physician also is required to have patients read a medication guide and sign a patient agreement provided by the distributor. Physicians must notify the distributor of any ongoing pregnancy and report any hospitalization, transfusion, or other serious events.

Additional information regarding mifepristone is available on the FDA web site at <www.fda.gov/cder> or by contacting the FDA at <druginfo@cder.fda.gov> or (301) 827-4570. The distributor of mifepristone also provides a web site at <www.earlyoptionpill.com> and can be contacted by phone toll free at 877-432-7596.

In conclusion, approval of mifepristone for use in combination with misoprostol provides women with an effective and safe alternative to surgical abortion for very early intrauterine pregnancy termination.

References

1. Virgo KS, Carr TR, Hile A, Virgo JM, Sullivan GM, Kaikati JG. Medical versus surgical abortion: a survey of knowledge and attitudes among abortion clinic patients. Womens Health Issues 1999;9:143–154
2. Spitz IM, Bardin CW, Benton L, Robbins A. Early pregnancy termination with mifepristone and misoprostol in the United States. N Engl J Med 1998;338:1241–1247
3. Spitz IM, Bardin CW. Mifepristone (RU 486)—a modulator of progestin and glucocorticoid action. N Engl J Med 1993:329:404–412
4. Christin-Maitre S, Bouchard P, Spitz IM. Medical termination of pregnancy. N Engl J Med 2000;342:946–956

ACOG

Committee on Obstetric Practice

Committee Opinion

Number 180, November 1996

New Ultrasound Output Display Standard

Ultrasonography is the most commonly used method of imaging in pregnancy. The potential for bioeffects of ultrasonography can be estimated by measuring the acoustic output. No independently confirmed adverse effects on the fetus resulting from prenatal diagnostic ultrasound exposure have been reported to date. Nevertheless, obstetricians who perform ultrasonography should be familiar with current safety standards of the equipment with regard to acoustic output. Recently, the U.S. Food and Drug Administration, together with the American Institute of Ultrasound in Medicine, the American College of Obstetricians and Gynecologists, the National Electrical Manufacturers Association, and several other organizations, has developed standards for the display directly on the ultrasound screen of meaningful information about the acoustic output of ultrasound equipment. It is important for obstetricians who use ultrasonography to be familiar with this new standard and to ensure that recommended limits of acoustic output are not exceeded.

The two measurements of acoustic output that may be displayed are the thermal index (TI) and the mechanical index (MI). They are defined as follows:

- TI—A calculated estimate of temperature rise due to ultrasound absorption
- MI—A relative measure of the compressive and decompressive mechanical effects of ultrasound pulses

For applicable devices, at least one of the two measurements must be displayed on the screen at all times. Some equipment will display both. If only one is shown, it will be the MI for imaging and the TI for Doppler studies.

Thermal Index

If the value of the TI is below 1.0, temperature changes are not a concern. Values higher than 1.0, however, could result in significant temperature changes, even with only a few minutes of exposure.

Change in tissue temperature is affected by many factors, including the type of tissue being insonated, the duration and area of exposure, and the

ISSN 1074-861X

The American College of Obstetricians and Gynecologists
409 12th Street, SW
PO Box 96920
Washington, DC 20090-6920

12345/09876

blood flow to the area. Measurable temperature changes in insonated tissues are possible, particularly at soft tissue–bone interfaces. Significant thermal effects of imaging ultrasonography are highly unlikely not only because of the relatively large area insonated but also because much more time of the duty cycle of the machine is spent receiving returning echoes than creating pulses of energy. On the other hand, pulsed Doppler ultrasonography uses long energy pulses that are highly focused on a small area of tissue and could result in greater thermal change.

Some equipment may allow the user to display various subsets of the TI. Currently available subsets are TIS (TI, soft tissue; appropriate for first-trimester fetal examinations), TIB (TI, bone; appropriate for second- and third-trimester fetal examinations), or TIC (TI, cranial; used only for transcranial Doppler).

Mechanical Index

The MI is calculated as the peak rarefactional pressure of the ultrasound pulse divided by the square root of the transducer center frequency. An MI value below 1 is not of concern regarding potential bioeffects on the fetus.

The potential mechanical bioeffect of most concern is cavitation, or the formation of microbubbles in tissue due to cyclic compressive and decompressive effects of the sound wave emitted by the transducer. The amount of energy reaching the fetus depends on the thickness of intervening tissues and the attenuation of energy within the tissues. The latter relates to how much energy is absorbed versus how much is scattered in different directions.

Acoustic Output Regulations

In the past, the Food and Drug Administration limited acoustic output for the fetal application to 94 mW/cm^2 spatial peak temporal average. Manufacturers of ultrasound equipment are only required to limit the power outputs of their machines to 720 mW/cm^2 spatial peak temporal average and to display the TI or MI if these indices can exceed 1. Ultrasound machines in which TI or MI cannot exceed 1 are not required to display these indices.

Appropriate Use of Fetal Ultrasonography

Many ultrasound machines are designed for multiple uses and can have power outputs above the limits placed by the Food and Drug Administration. Even "fetal presets" may exceed these limits in some configurations, including color Doppler or power Doppler mode. Thus, obstetricians could be using equipment with acoustic outputs that are set at levels above those that are considered acceptable for fetal exposure.

The appropriate use of fetal ultrasonography includes performing examinations only when there is diagnostic information to be obtained. Attention should be directed to the acoustic output and the length of the examination. The display of TI or MI or both provides information about the actual acoustic output of the instrument being operated. Awareness of the TI or MI by the sonologist can be used to minimize fetal exposure to acoustic output, while obtaining the needed diagnostic information. In general, the lowest possible output settings that will allow obtaining adequate imaging should be used. This is known as the ALARA (as low as reasonably achievable) principle. Other controls, such as the gain, which amplifies returning echoes, can be adjusted to enhance the images obtained without increasing the acoustic output. Use of the TI and MI allows the sonologist to implement the ALARA principle more effectively than has been possible previously.

Bibliography

American Institute of Ultrasound in Medicine. Bioeffects and safety of diagnostic ultrasound. Laurel, Maryland: AIUM, 1993

American Institute of Ultrasound in Medicine. Medical ultrasound safety. Laurel, Maryland: AIUM, 1994

American Institute of Ultrasound in Medicine. Standard for real-time display of thermal and mechanical acoustic output indices on diagnostic ultrasound equipment. Laurel, Maryland: AIUM, 1992

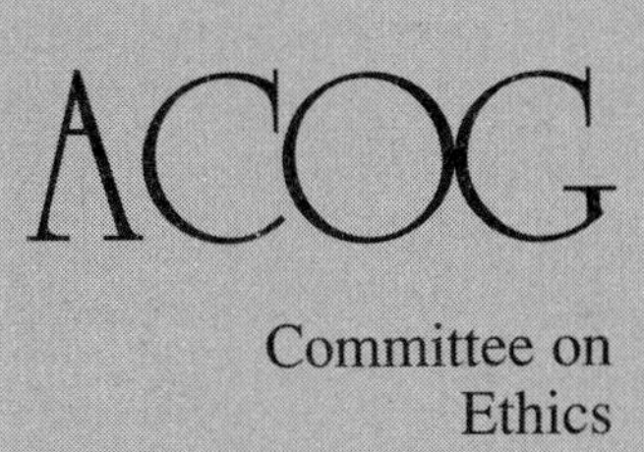

Committee on Ethics

Committee Opinion

Number 215, April 1999 (*Replaces #94, April 1991*)

Nonselective Embryo Reduction: Ethical Guidance for the Obstetrician–Gynecologist

The ethical issues surrounding the use and consequences of reproductive technologies are highly complex, and no one position reflects the variety of opinions within the College membership. This document is designed to review the ethical issues involved in nonselective embryo reduction. For the purposes of this statement, nonselective embryo reduction is defined as a first-trimester procedure for termination of any one or more embryos in a multiembryo pregnancy, in order to increase the chances of survival of the remaining embryos (1).

To many, the ethical issues involved in nonselective embryo reduction are somewhat different from the issues involved in abortion, as discussed in the Analysis section later in this Committee Opinion. Although no physician need participate in any activity that he or she finds morally unacceptable, all physicians should be aware of the medical and ethical issues in these complex situations and be prepared to respond in a professional, ethical manner to patient requests for information and procedures.

Background

Spontaneous occurrences of multiembryo pregnancy have always been a medical problem. More recently, the use of potent ovulation-inducing drugs and the development of assisted reproductive technologies (ART), such as in vitro fertilization, gamete intrafallopian transfer, and zygote intrafallopian transfer, have been effective in the treatment of infertility (2). Thousands of patients previously unable to have children have been assisted to achieve conception. In a small percentage of these patients, the resultant pregnancy has involved more than two embryos, thereby creating potentially serious problems (2–7). There is widespread agreement that the risks of perinatal mortality and morbidity and maternal morbidity increase with embryo number (8). Recent reports have shown improving outcomes with multiembryo pregnancies, but risks are still significant (9, 10).

ISSN 1074-861X

The American College of Obstetricians and Gynecologists
409 12th Street, SW
PO Box 96920
Washington, DC 20090-6920

12345/32109

Prevention

The first approach to this problem is or should be prevention. It might be argued that the problem is best remedied by discontinuing technologic assistance to reproduction. On the one hand, this approach discounts the major benefits that ART offers to patients and suggests an unwarranted coercive restriction on parental choice and autonomy. On the other hand, the association of an increased rate of multiple pregnancy with infertility treatment deserves serious attention. Some multiembryo gestations will inevitably occur despite the best of intentions, knowledge, skill, and equipment, but it is essential that those providing infertility treatment exercise a high degree of diligence to minimize the problem.

In ovulation induction, the pressure to maximize success rates may affect the decision to give or withhold human chorionic gonadotropin (hCG) at midcycle in cycles in which ultrasound imaging demonstrates the presence of many mature follicles, each capable of releasing an ovum. If an hCG injection is withheld, the patient will have spent considerable time, energy, emotion, and money for a nonovulatory cycle. Yet, if hCG is given and ovulation is triggered, multiembryo pregnancy of high order may result.

In ART, there are similar pressures. Some programs, for example, maintain flexible upper limits for the number of embryos to be transferred in any one cycle (11–13). As the number of embryos transferred increases, program success rates may rise, but so does the risk of multiembryo pregnancy.

The physician who makes decisions about circumstances for triggering ovulation or guidelines for embryo transfer must, as in any medical situation, place the best interests of the patient and the future child or children at the center of the risk–benefit equation. For this reason, in England, where ART is centrally regulated, a decision has been made to permit no more than three embryos to be transferred in any one cycle, even in cases in which advanced maternal age suggests that success would be unlikely if this limit were observed.

In the absence of regulation in the United States, the decision is left to individual physicians and programs. In almost all cases, it is preferable to terminate a cycle or limit the number of embryos to be transferred in order to prevent a situation in which patient(s) and physician will have to consider embryo reduction. The Practice Committee of the American Society for Reproductive Medicine has issued a report suggesting age- and diagnosis-dependent guidelines for limiting the number of embryos to be transferred. These guidelines limit risk while allowing individualization of patient care for optimal results (14). Nonselective embryo reduction should be viewed as a response to an unforeseen and unavoidable contingency, not a routinely accepted treatment for an iatrogenic problem.

Counseling

As with all medical care, counseling for treatment of infertility should incorporate discussions of risks, benefits, and treatment alternatives, including the option for no treatment. Counseling should be considered an ongoing process, beginning before treatment decisions are made and continuing throughout the patient's care. The risks of certain treatments of infertility include, but are not limited to, the occurrence of multiple gestation, with its associated risks of spontaneous abortion, premature labor and delivery, and neonatal mortality and morbidity. The informed consent process must include information about the potential for multiembryo pregnancy and associated maternal risks, such as prolonged hospitalization, antepartum bleeding, postpartum hemorrhage, hypertensive diseases of pregnancy, and an increased rate of cesarean delivery.

It also is the responsibility of the physician to inform patients that embryo reduction as a response to multiembryo pregnancy has inherent medical risks to the remaining embryos, such as a reported pregnancy loss of 7.6% for triplet to twin reduction in a large multicenter sample (15). Reports of lower birthweights for twins reduced from triplets also are of concern (16, 17). Patients should not be given the impression that multiembryo pregnancy is without problems because embryo reduction is available.

Patients struggle with the ethical and emotional issues of embryo reduction. In two postdelivery informational surveys of couples who had undergone nonselective reduction (18, 19), more than half of the small samples of respondents reported that they did not understand the procedure or its consequences fully at the time of embryo reduction (20). A significant proportion reported still feeling guilt (19, 20), even though they believed the procedure was necessary. Many infertility patients have unrealistic ideas about outcomes for high-order multiple pregnancies (20–22) that leave them unprepared for feelings of loss and grief at the time of a reduction procedure. However, in studies that utilized standard psychologic tests to assess the emotional state of patients after nonselective reduction, serious long-term psychologic sequelae were not identified; depression scores for women who did not carry to term after reduction were similar to scores for a control group of women who experienced a spontaneous abortion but no reduction (23, 24).

The report that 93% of patients who decided to proceed with reduction would make that decision again despite their experience of stress and sadness is somewhat reassuring, but the number of patients studied, either by self-report survey or by standard psychologic measures, was quite small (24). The ethical issues that this option involves should be discussed with patients before the initiation of any treatment that could increase the risk of multiembryo pregnancy. Although patients should be encouraged to examine their feelings about these risks and options at the onset, the counseling process should encourage them to continue this assessment at appropriate points in the treatment process (25).

Options

In the presence of already established multiembryo pregnancies, the options are inevitably difficult. No choice is without harmful consequences, and potential benefits must be carefully weighed against the potential harms. There are three options:

1. Abort all the embryos.
2. Attempt to carry all the embryos to term.
3. Terminate some of the embryos.

First, the entire multiembryo pregnancy can be aborted. However, for some patients, abortion is not an acceptable option. For other patients who may have achieved pregnancy after lengthy infertility treatment, this option may be considered the least desirable.

Second, an attempt can be made to carry all the embryos to term. However, the risks of perinatal and maternal morbidity and mortality increase directly with embryo number (8). There are significant risks of losing all the embryos or having some survive with permanent impairment. The assessment of "significant risk" varies among patients and physicians and is therefore not amenable to uniform definition. Physicians should respect each patient's conclusions about which risks are acceptable and which are too high.

Third, when multiembryo pregnancies have occurred, the increased risks have led physicians to reduce the number of embryos in an attempt to benefit those remaining. The technique brings about the demise of some embryos with the intent to allow continuance of the pregnancy, resulting in the delivery of a smaller number of babies with lower risks of prematurity, morbidity, and mortality. Although this procedure is successful in a majority of instances, it raises some unsettling ethical concerns. There is a complex interrelationship between the intention to reduce the morbidity of a smaller number of surviving embryos and the intentional sacrifice of others that demands an ethical as well as medical assessment of the relative benefits and risks of nonselective embryo reduction. What follows is an attempt to outline such an assessment, with the understanding that each case ultimately must be examined individually on its own merits.

Analysis

There are differences between the ethical analyses involved in multiembryo reduction and elective abortion because the intent is different. A woman has an elective abortion because, for many complex and varied reasons, she does not wish or feels unable to have a child. In contrast, an infertility patient with a multiembryo pregnancy undergoes reduction precisely because she does wish to bear a child. The patient and her physician may conclude that embryo reduction is the preferred way to continue her pregnancy. For some persons, the primary intention justifying embryo reduction may be the life and well-being of the embryos that survive and continue to develop. For others, it is unethical to terminate an apparently healthy embryo, even for the sake of the survival or well-being of other embryos in the pregnancy.

Some individuals who believe that abortion is generally unacceptable find nonselective embryo reduction to be justified ethically when the risks of carrying the pregnancy are considerable and could be reduced if the number of embryos were fewer. Varying degrees of risk will be interpreted differently by individual patients. It is reasonable to assume that with advances in maternal–fetal and neonatal medicine, the number of fetuses that one attempts to leave may change gradually over time. The issues of patient choice and physician participation and consultation need to be analyzed on a case-by-case basis.

In Summary

Although physicians may choose not to participate in nonselective embryo reduction, they should be knowledgeable about this procedure and be prepared to react in a professional and ethical manner to patient requests for information or services or both. The first approach to the problem of multiple gestation should be prevention. Although embryo reduction will be ethically acceptable to many as a response to an unforeseen and unavoidable contingency, in almost all cases it is preferable to terminate a cycle or limit the number of embryos to be transferred in order to prevent a situation in which the patient and physician need to consider an embryo reduction. Counseling for treatment of infertility should include the risks of multiple gestation, and the ethical issues surrounding embryo reduction should be discussed with patients before the initiation of any treatment that could increase the risk of multiembryo pregnancy.

References

1. Berkowitz RL, Lynch L. Selective reduction: an unfortunate misnomer. Obstet Gynecol 1990;75:873–874
2. Centers for Disease Control and Prevention. 1995 assisted reproductive technology success rates: national summary and fertility clinic reports. Atlanta: CDC, 1998
3. Evans MI, Fletcher JC, Zador IE, Newton BW, Quigg MH, Struyk CD. Selective first trimester termination in octuplet and quadruplet pregnancies: clinical and ethical issues. Obstet Gynecol 1988;71:289–296
4. Berkowitz RL, Lynch L, Chitkara U, Wilkins IA, Mehalek KE, Alvarez E. Selective reduction of multifetal pregnancies in the first trimester. N Engl J Med 1988;318:1043–1047
5. Wapner RJ, Davis GH, Johnson A, Weinblatt VJ, Fischer RL, Jackson LG, et al. Selective reduction of multifetal pregnancies. Lancet 1990;335:90–93
6. Lynch L, Berkowitz RL, Chitkara U, Alvarez M. First trimester transabdominal multiple pregnancy reduction: a report of 85 cases. Obstet Gynecol 1990;75:735–738
7. Evans MI, May M, Drugan A, Fletcher JC, Johnson MP, Sokol RJ. Selective termination: clinical experience and residual risks. Am J Obstet Gynecol 1990;162:1568–1572; discussion 1572–1575
8. Petrikovsky BM, Vintzileos AM. Management and outcome of multiple pregnancies of higher fetal order: literature review. Obstet Gynecol Surv 1989;44:578–584
9. Newman RB, Hamer C, Miller MC. Outpatient triplet management: a contemporary review. Am J Obstet Gynecol 1989;161:547–553; discussion 553–555
10. Collins MS, Bleyl JA. Seventy-one quadruplet pregnancies: management and outcome. Am J Obstet Gynecol 1990;162: 1384–1391; discussion 1391–1392
11. Qasim SM, Karacan M, Corsan G, Shelden R, Stillman RJ. High order oocyte transfer in gamete intrafallopian transfer patients 40 or more years of age. Fertil Steril 1995;64: 107–110
12. Widra EA, Ginoff PR, Smotrich DB, Stillman RJ. Achieving multiple order embryo transfer identifies women over 40 years of age with improved in vitro fertilization outcomes. Fertil Steril 1996;65:103–108
13. Martin PM, Welch HG. Probabilities for singleton and multiple pregnancies after in vitro fertilization. Fertil Steril 1998;70:478–481
14. American Society for Reproductive Medicine. Guidelines on number of embryos transferred. Birmingham, Alabama: ASRM, 1998
15. Evans MI, Dommergues M, Wapner RJ, Goldberg JD, Lynch L, Zador IE, et al. International, collaborative experience of 1789 patients having multifetal pregnancy reduction: a plateauing of risks and outcomes. J Soc Gynecol Investig 1996;3:23–26
16. Silver RK, Helfland BT, Russell TL, Ragin A, Scholl JS, MacGregor SN. Multifetal reduction increases the risk of preterm delivery and fetal growth restriction in twins: a case control study. Fertil Steril 1997;67:30–33
17. Groutz AS, Yovel I, Amit A, Yaron Y, Azem F, Lessing JB. Pregnancy outcome after multifetal pregnancy reduction to twins compared with spontaneously conceived twins. Hum Reprod 1996;11:1334–1336
18. Kanhai HH, de Haan M, van Zanten LA, Geerinck-Vercammen C, van der Ploeg HM, Gravenhorst JB. Follow-up of pregnancies, infants and families after multifetal pregnancy reduction. Fertil Steril 1994;62:955–959
19. Vauthier-Brouzes D, Lefebvre G. Selective reduction in multifetal pregnancies: technical and psychological aspects. Fertil Steril 1992;57:1012–1016
20. Garel M, Starck C, Blondel B, Lefebvre G, Vauthier-Brouzes D, Zorn JR. Psychological effects of embryonal reduction: from the decision making to four months after delivery. J Gynecol Obstet Biol Reprod (Paris) 1995;24:119–126
21. Gleicher N, Campbell DP, Chan CL, Karande V, Rao R, Balin M, et al. The desire for multiple births in couples with infertility problems contradicts present practice patterns. Hum Reprod 1995;10:1079–1084
22. Goldfarb J, Kinzer DJ, Boyle M, Kjurit D. Attitudes of in vitro fertilization and intrauterine insemination couples toward multiple gestation pregnancy and multifetal pregnancy reduction. Fertil Steril 1996;65:815–820
23. McKinney M, Downey J, Timor-Trisch I. The psychological effects of multifetal pregnancy reduction. Fertil Steril 1995;64:51–61
24. Schreiner-Engel P, Walther VN, Mindes J, Lynch L, Berkowitz RI. First trimester multifetal pregnancy reduction: acute and persistent psychological reactions. Am J Obstet Gynecol 1995;172:541–547
25. Zaner RM, Boehm FH, Hill GA. Selective termination in multiple pregnancies: ethical consideration. Fertil Steril 1990;54:203–205

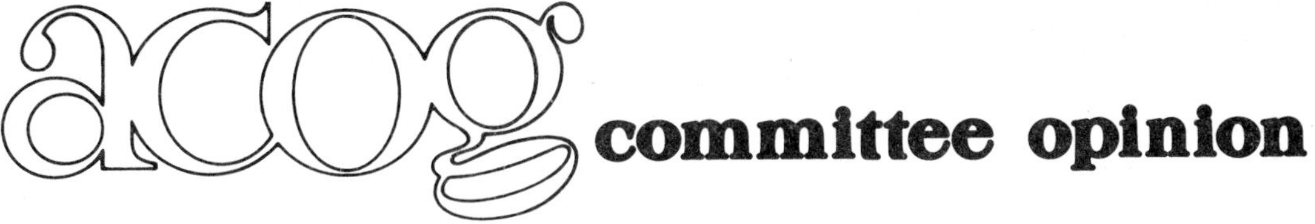

Committee on Obstetrics: Maternal and Fetal Medicine

Number 121—April 1993
(*Replaces #83, May 1990)*

Obstetric Management of Patients with Spinal Cord Injury

Approximately 11,000 new spinal cord injuries (SCIs) are reported per year in the United States. More than 50% occur in persons between 15 and 25 years of age, and women constitute approximately 15% of these cases. Effective rehabilitation and modern reproductive technology may increase the number of these patients considering pregnancy. It is important that obstetricians caring for patients with SCI acquaint themselves with problems related to SCI that may occur throughout pregnancy.

Ideally, women with SCI should have an appropriate preconceptional evaluation. Both partners should be interviewed together, and they should be counseled regarding the anticipated course and outcome of pregnancy. Chronic medical conditions and the woman's adaptation to her disability must be evaluated. Baseline pulmonary and renal function studies may be appropriate if not performed previously. Family planning should be discussed. It should be recognized that fertility in these patients is usually not affected by their condition.

Experience has shown that women with complete transverse lesions, including those who are quadriplegic, can give birth vaginally; cesarean delivery is rarely necessary except for obstetric indications. Knowledge of the patient's lesion and the clinical course of her pregnancy may help predict problems that may arise during childbirth. Common problems are anemia (which occurs in 63% of women with SCI), urinary tract infections (which occur in 80%), and pressure sores (which occur in 26%). Patients with high thoracic or cervical lesions may require ventilatory support during late pregnancy or labor.

POTENTIAL COMPLICATIONS

Special problems in patients with SCI include the difficulty of ascertaining labor, urinary tract infections, and autonomic dysreflexia. These potential complications place the pregnancy at risk, and management and general supportive care should be provided accordingly. Collaboration among all personnel providing care to the patient is desirable.

Ascertainment of Labor

Women with spinal cord transection above the T-10 segment may have painless labor. In a patient with total transection at a lower thoracic level, labor pain may be so reduced as to make the patient unaware of uterine contractions, especially during sleep. However, symptoms under the control of the sympathetic nervous system (eg, abdominal or leg spasms, shortness of breath) concurrent with uterine contractions may make patients aware of labor. All patients with SCI are at increased risk for an unattended delivery. Patients should be instructed in uterine palpation techniques to detect contractions at home; the use of home tocodynamometry may be considered. If increasing uterine activity is ascertained, the cervix should be examined. Cervical examinations starting in the late second or early third trimester may be helpful to confirm the status of the cervical effacement and dilatation. However, any vaginal examination must be performed with appropriate precautions in patients at risk for autonomic dysreflexia. If a change in cervical effacement or dilatation or both is detected, hospitalization should be considered. Preterm labor may be managed using traditional therapy. Transferring patients at risk for preterm birth to a tertiary care center should be considered.

Urinary Tract Infections

When urinary tract infection is present, suppressive antibiotic therapy, as well as treatment for concomitant yeast vaginitis, may be appropriate in selected patients. The decision to use antibiotic prophylaxis and the choice of agents are best made in collaboration with the patient's principal physician. This decision may be influenced by whether the patient performs intermittent self-catheterization or whether she has an indwelling catheter. It is important to monitor the patient for signs and symptoms of an ascending urinary tract infection and treat any such infection promptly.

Autonomic Dysreflexia

Of the patients with SCI at or above the T-5 segment, 85% are subject to autonomic dysreflexia syndrome, a serious and potentially life-threatening complication. This condition is attributed to a loss of hypothalamic control over sympathetic spinal reflexes and occurs in patients with viable cord segments distal to the level of injury. It can occur in patients with incomplete transections. In susceptible patients, afferent stimuli from a hollow viscus (eg, the bladder, bowel, or uterus) and from the skin below the level of the lesion or of the genital areas ascend in the spinothalamic tracts and posterior columns. This causes reflex sympathetic activation, unmodified by the supraspinal centers. The resultant catecholamine release and vasoconstriction lead to hypertension associated with headache, bradycardia, cardiac arrhythmia, sweating, flushing, tingling, nasal congestion, and, occasionally, respiratory distress. Uteroplacental vasoconstriction may result in fetal hypoxemia.

It is important to avoid unnecessary stimuli that can lead to autonomic dysreflexia. It may be caused by distension of the vagina, bladder, or bowel or may be provoked by a simple manipulation such as changing a urinary catheter. Constipation should be treated with increased dietary fiber and stool softeners. During labor, the symptoms of autonomic dysreflexia are commonly synchronous with uterine contractions and abate with uterine relaxation, ceasing after placental expulsion. The severity of the syndrome during labor ranges from annoying symptoms to hypertensive encephalopathy, cerebrovascular accidents, intraventricular and retinal hemorrhages, and death. Therefore, continual monitoring of cardiac rhythm and blood pressure during labor is mandatory in all patients at risk for autonomic dysreflexia.

Although patients with SCI may perceive no pain in labor, anesthesia should be used to prevent autonomic dysreflexia. Spinal or epidural anesthesia extending to the T-10 level is the most reliable method of preventing autonomic dysreflexia by blocking stimuli that arise from pelvic organs. Thus, antepartum consultation with an anesthesiologist and the establishment of a plan for induction of epidural or spinal anesthesia at the onset of labor is highly desirable in susceptible patients. If autonomic dysreflexia occurs before a regional anesthetic is available or occurs despite regional anesthesia, hypertension may be treated with antihypertensive agents that have a rapid onset and offset (eg, sodium nitroprusside or nitroglycerin), ganglionic blocking agents (eg, trimethaphan), adrenergic blocking agents (eg, guanethidine), or a direct vasodilator (eg, hydralazine).

If there is evidence of autonomic dysreflexia during the second stage of labor, delivery can be expedited by forceps or vacuum extraction with adequate anesthesia. If dysreflexia during labor cannot be controlled by any means, cesarean delivery may be necessary. Adequate anesthesia is needed for cesarean delivery in all patients with SCI.

GENERAL SUPPORT

In patients with SCI there is an increased risk for decubitus ulcers. Patients should be made aware of the importance of appropriate padding and frequent position changes throughout pregnancy. These patients tend to gain excessive weight, which may increase the difficulty of moving and transporting them. Muscle-strengthening exercises may be recommended for the upper extremities of nonquadriplegic patients. For all patients, elevation of legs and range-of-motion exercises may be implemented as pregnancy advances. The possibility of increased need for social support services should be addressed. The time allotted for office examination of these patients may need to be increased, and office personnel should be prepared to offer greater assistance than is needed by other patients.

BIBLIOGRAPHY

American Society of Anesthesiologists. Standards for basic intra-operative monitoring. In: ASA standards, guidelines and statements. Park Ridge, Illinois: ASA, 1991:6–7

Cohen BS, Hilton EB. Spinal cord disorders and pregnancy. In: Goldstein PJ, ed. Neurological disorders of pregnancy. Mount Kisco, New York: Futura, 1992

Craig DI. The adaptation to pregnancy of spinal cord injured women. Rehabil Nurs 1990;15:6–9

Paonessa K, Fernand R. Spinal cord injury and pregnancy. Spine 1991;16:596–598

Porter SS. Anesthetic management of the patient with spinal cord injury. Kans Med 1988;89:299–304

Verduyn WH. Spinal cord injured women, pregnancy and delivery. Paraplegia 1986;24:231–240

Wanner MB, Rageth CJ, Zach GA. Pregnancy and autonomic hyperreflexia in patients with spinal cord lesions. Paraplegia 1987;25:482–490

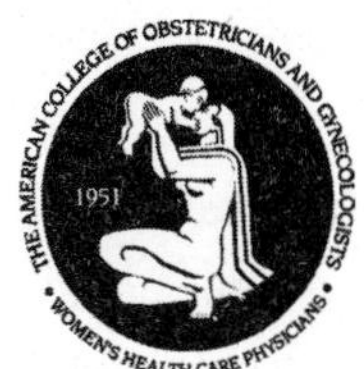

This document reflects emerging clinical and scientific advances as of the date issued and is subject to change. The information should not be construed as dictating an exclusive course of treatment or procedure to be followed.

The American College of Obstetricians and Gynecologists
409 12th Street, SW • Washington, DC 20024-2188

12345/76543

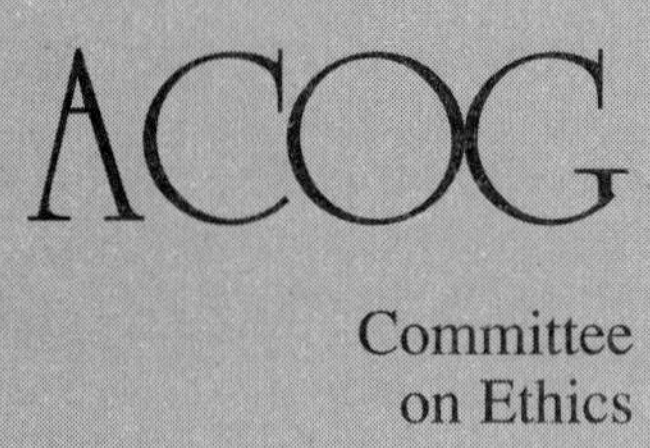

Committee on Ethics

Committee Opinion

Number 194, November 1997

Obstetrician–Gynecologists' Ethical Responsibilities, Concerns, and Risks Pertaining to Adoption

Adoption is a commonly used alternative strategy for family building. Although adoption is not a medical event per se, obstetrician–gynecologists may find themselves at the center of adoption issues because of their expertise in the assessment and management of infertility, pregnancy, and childbirth. There are several specific roles that the obstetrician–gynecologist may be asked to assume in regard to adoption. Physicians commonly provide information, advice, and counsel, and they refer birth parents and prospective adoptive parents to adoption agencies. They also may be asked to link or match pregnant women with families desiring adoption. Frequently, they are asked to provide information about prospective parents to adoption agencies. In each of these roles, it is important that obstetrician–gynecologists consider the rights, responsibilities, and safety of all concerned parties: the child, the birth parents, the prospective adoptive parents, and themselves.

Six principles had traditionally guided adoption practices in this century (1):

1. Consent of the birth mother was a necessary precondition for adoption, whereas presumed waiver of consent by absent birth fathers has been routine.
2. The purpose of adoption was to serve the child's best interests by placement with suitable adoptive parents.
3. Adoption practices were based on the principle of gratuitous transfer, and financial transactions suggestive of purchase of a child were prohibited.
4. Relationships with adoptive parents were expected to substitute entirely for relationships with biologic parents.
5. Relinquishing birth mothers and adopting parents were assured that their confidentiality and anonymity would be protected.
6. Adoptive relationships were presumed to be permanent once they were finalized in court.

ISSN 1074-861X

The American College of Obstetricians and Gynecologists
409 12th Street, SW
PO Box 96920
Washington, DC 20090-6920

12345/10987

These principles are currently undergoing redefinition and reconsideration. Physicians should be aware of new trends in adoption practices:

1. There is increased emphasis on the rights of biologic fathers and reluctance to use a waiver process to release a child for adoption when the biologic father can not be located.
2. Concepts of *suitability of adoptive parents* and *the best interests of the child* are undergoing reconsideration.
3. The present environment of competition for adoptive infants may lead to inducements in the form of subsidies for medical care and other support, making the gratuitous nature of adoption less clear and free of financial conflict.
4. Proponents of openness in adoption argue that adoption should include complementary relationships with birth parents.
5. It is no longer possible to guarantee absolute confidentiality to either birth or adoptive parents.
6. Adoption can no longer be considered to be permanent in every case, because situations have arisen in which adoptive relationships were terminated *after* a final adoption decree has been granted—by adoptive parents, by biologic parents, or by adopted children.

The resulting lack of clarity about both ethical issues and legal consequences may create a potentially hazardous situation for physicians. In the following sections, the different roles that the obstetrician–gynecologist may be asked to play in adoption are described. Ethical concerns are discussed and safeguards proposed.

Education

The physician's role in education is to ensure that adoption is introduced into the description of alternatives for women with unwanted pregnancies and for potential adoptive parents. Physicians have a responsibility to provide information about adoption to all patients with unwanted pregnancies, and to all patients with infertility concerns (2). Fact sheets distributed by the American Society for Reproductive Medicine support this educational role (3). Physicians have an obligation to present alternatives fairly, regardless of personal values and beliefs. They should not advocate for or against relinquishment or adoption. Nor should they avoid discussing these issues when they are appropriate to the patient's situation. This position is consistent with the right of adults to the information required to make fully informed decisions. It is also consistent with the ethical obligation to promote what is good for the patient. These obligations can be met, for some patients, by placing literature about adoption in the waiting room, thereby validating adoption as a legitimate, respected choice. A lengthy counseling session, in which the risks and benefits of adoption are weighed against other alternatives, may be indicated for other patients.

Physicians may have both positive and negative personal biases about adoption for various reasons. For example, physicians who have chosen the adoption alternative as their own method of family building may present this option either positively or negatively, depending on their individual experiences. Physicians would do well to disclose their potential sources of bias, and take special care to uphold the principle of respect for patient autonomy.

Physicians should also ensure that financial incentives do not bias the presentation of information about adoption. For example, physicians must be especially careful to offer information about adoption to patients with established infertility, because money accrues to a gynecologist from the treatment of infertile patients, and these fees may cease with a decision to adopt rather than pursue further treatment.

Advice and Counseling

The physician's role in advising and counseling patients is to assist those for whom adoption may be appropriate in making a decision that is right for them. Patients often turn to a physician and say, "Doctor, what do you think I ought to do?" Women experiencing unwanted pregnancy or infertility are vulnerable, facing confusing and painful situations. The physician is a caregiver, trained to solve problems and help people feel better. The temptation to advocate for a specific position can be great. It may seem to the physician that the obvious solution for a young woman who is unemployed is to relinquish her child, or for an infertile couple who are reasonable candidates for in vitro fertilization to pursue that option before considering adoption.

It is appropriate for physicians to give advice on medical matters. This is an essential part of the physician–patient relationship, and an expert role for which physicians are trained. Patients count on the guidance of physicians for medical decisions. Adoption, however, is only tangentially a medical matter, and few physicians are expert in this field. Furthermore, for the physician, the particular encounter with an individual patient or couple, no matter how compelling, occurs only during a finite point in time. The patients will be living with the lifelong consequences of these decisions. Therefore, physicians who provide advice and counsel, unless they are truly expert in the field of adoption, should guard against advocating for a particular action. The best counsel will permit the involved parties to explore their options fully and make a decision that arises out of their own beliefs, values, needs, and circumstances.

Referrals

The physician's role in referrals is to identify appropriate resources. Physicians may often best fulfill their obligations to patients through referral to other professionals who have the appropriate skills and expertise to address the difficult issues raised by adoption. For example, referral to a mental health professional for short-term counseling provides an opportunity for both birth and prospective adoptive parents to explore their emotional reactions and the ways that different alternatives may affect their lives. Some patients may feel more comfortable having a discussion of this type with someone who is not involved with their ongoing medical care.

When an obstetrician–gynecologist makes a medical referral, there is an ethical obligation to investigate the skills and credentials of the consultant. The same responsibility for protecting the patient's best interests pertains to psychologic and social referral resources. As a starting point, there are many sources of information available to assist physicians in developing their own lists of referral alternatives (see "Resources"). In addition, local hospitals maintain referral rosters.

Screening

When authorized by patients, the physician's role in screening is to provide appropriate information to screening agencies regarding patients' qualifications as prospective parents for an adoptive child. Physicians are often asked by patients to fill out forms requesting information about their mental, psychologic, and medical suitability as prospective adoptive parents. Physicians are bound by ethical precepts to be truthful, to act in their patients' best interests, and to protect the patient's confidentiality. Adoption agencies, on the other hand, give precedence to the needs and interests of adoptive children.

Adversarial situations may arise. A patient may request, for example, that a physician not reveal to the agency the extent of her chronic illness and its potential effect on her life expectancy. Although a physician may wish to advocate for a patient, there is an obligation to be truthful and to let patients know what can and what can not be said.

Many agency forms request the treating physician to certify that the individual or couple is fit to parent. If the physician of record believes that he or she does not have enough information to make a judgment, the agency may count that as evidence against the couple. The physician must be honest and speak accurately to the information that is available. The best approach is for the physician to disclose to the patient what he or she plans to write, followed by frank discussion with the patient of the potential impact of the report.

Limits to the Physician's Role

If asked to serve as a broker in an independent adoption, the physician's role is to refer the patient to an appropriate agency or adoption resource. Among all the roles that physicians play in adoption, that of broker is perhaps the most hazardous because of ethical issues related to undue influence, competing obligations, and lack of expertise.

Although both birth parents and prospective adoptive parents generally view the adoption agreement as a binding promise, patients may find themselves unable or unwilling to fulfill that promise after delivery of the child. The pregnant woman who agreed to relinquish her child may have done so in good will with the best knowledge available to her at that time. She may not know what that promise really means or if she can really do what she agreed to until she has given birth to this child, held it, and experienced the extent of loss. The couple who agreed to accept a child may regret that decision and feel unable to keep their part of this agreement if, for example, this child is born with serious medical problems. For these and similar reasons, no private adoption agreement is legally binding prior to the birth of the child.

If a physician has acted as a broker and the adoption agreement falls through, he or she will be aware of the loss suffered by the other party, may feel responsible, and may be tempted to use the power of the patient–physician relationship to influence the patient to fulfill the original promise. The physician's ability to provide current or future medical care for this patient may be compromised by these events.

Brokering adoptions is properly the role of an independent authority or agency, which is in a position to protect the interests of all involved parties—the child, the birth parents, and the adoptive parents. For these reasons, many hospitals have bylaws prohibiting staff physicians from direct involvement as adoption brokers. Physicians should avoid matching prospective adoptive parents with women who have unwanted pregnancies and should instead refer patients to agencies or other adoption resources, when available. Physicians should receive only the usual compensation for medical and counseling services. Referral fees and other arrangements for financial gain beyond usual fees for clinical services are inappropriate.

When the physician is also a prospective adoptive parent, there may be a temptation to adopt a baby from one of his or her own patients. This arrangement is unethical. It contravenes principles of fairness to other potential parents and takes advantage of the patient's highly vulnerable situation.

Summary

The adoption field is evolving and the issues are complex. Obstetrician–gynecologists can play helpful and effective roles in adoption as educators and advisers. Adoption should be presented fairly, along with other options, to all those who might benefit. Physicians can be excellent sources of information, can assist in weighing risks and benefits, and can provide emotional support. When authorized by patients to fill out forms for adoption agencies, physicians should do so truthfully, with full disclosure to patients of what they intend to say.

Physicians should involve themselves in counseling and screening roles with great care because potential exists for unintended misuse of the physician–patient relationship. Patient confidentiality, patient autonomy, and the principle of the patient's best interest may be compromised by subtle or blatant conflicts of interest. Physicians are advised to delegate to an independent authority all responsibility for matching pregnant women with prospective adoptive parents.

References

1. Hollinger JH. Adoption law. Future Child 1993;3:43–61
2. Kaunitz AM, Grimes DA, Kaunitz KK. A physician's guide to adoption. JAMA 1987;258:3537–3541
3. American Society for Reproductive Medicine. Fact sheet: adoption. Birmingham, Alabama: ASRM, 1996

Resources

Perspectives Press (PO Box 90318, Indianapolis, IN 46290-0318; telephone: 317-872-3055) concentrates on issues related to adoption.

Posner J, Gulianelli J. Adoption resource guide: a national directory of licensed agencies. Washington, DC: Child Welfare League of America, 1990

Resolve (1310 Broadway, Somerville, MA 02144-1731; telephone: 617-623-0744), the organization for infertile couples, maintains a directory of nationally and locally recognized and accredited organizations and individuals who provide adoption support.

ACOG
Committee on
Obstetric Practice

American Society of
Anesthesiologists
Committee on
Obstetric Anesthesia

Committee Opinion

Number 231, February 2000 *(Replaces #118, January 1993)*

Pain Relief During Labor

Labor results in severe pain for many women. There is no other circumstance where it is considered acceptable for a person to experience untreated severe pain, amenable to safe intervention, while under a physician's care. In the absence of a medical contraindication, maternal request is a sufficient medical indication for pain relief during labor. Pain management should be provided whenever medically indicated.

Nonetheless, the American Society of Anesthesiologists (ASA) and the American College of Obstetricians and Gynecologists (ACOG) have received reports that some third-party payers have denied reimbursement for regional analgesia and anesthesia during labor unless a physician has documented the presence of a "medical indication" for regional analgesia and anesthesia. Of the various pharmacologic methods used for pain relief during labor and delivery, regional analgesia techniques—epidural, spinal, and combined spinal epidural—are the most flexible, effective, and least depressing to the central nervous system, allowing for an alert participating mother and an alert neonate. It is the position of ACOG and ASA that third-party payers who provide reimbursement for obstetric services should not deny reimbursement for regional analgesia and anesthesia because of an absence of other "medical indications."

This document reflects emerging clinical and scientific advances as of the date issued and is subject to change. The information should not be construed as dictating an exclusive course of treatment or procedure to be followed.

ISSN 1074-861X

The American College of Obstetricians and Gynecologists
409 12th Street, SW
PO Box 96920
Washington, DC 20090-6920

12345/43210

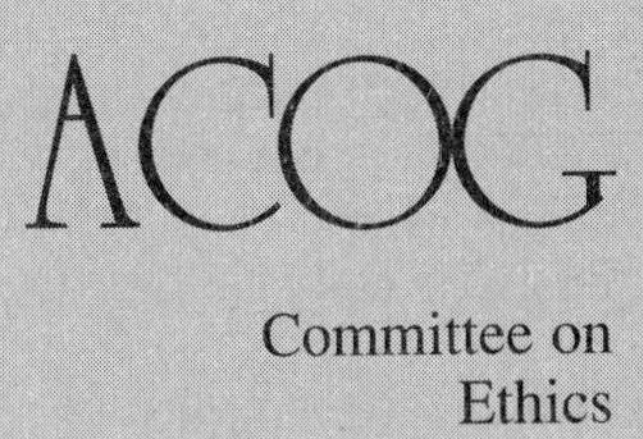

Committee on Ethics

Committee Opinion

Number 214, April 1999 (*Replaces #55, October 1987*)

Patient Choice and the Maternal–Fetal Relationship

The maternal–fetal relationship is unique in medicine because of the complete physiologic dependence of the fetus upon the pregnant woman and because both the fetus and the woman are regarded as patients of the obstetrician. Moreover, therapeutic access to the fetus occurs through the body and person of the pregnant woman, who may experience negative effects from interventions designed to benefit the fetus. The welfare of the fetus is of the utmost importance to almost all pregnant women. However, there are two areas in which maternal and fetal interest can be divergent: 1) the pregnant woman may refuse a diagnostic procedure, medical therapy, or a surgical procedure intended to enhance or preserve fetal well-being; and 2) the pregnant woman's behavior may be deleterious to the fetus.

Medicine aims to foster the greatest benefit with the least risk. Risks and benefits, however, may be valued differently by the pregnant woman and the obstetrician, creating the potential for disagreement. When the fetus may be in danger, the woman often is asked to consent to diagnostic procedures or therapy for the sole or primary benefit of the fetus. Examples of this are a cesarean delivery for fetal indications, intrauterine fetal transfusion for isoimmunization, or zidovudine to prevent the perinatal transmission of human immunodeficiency virus (HIV) infection. Also, a pregnant woman may be entreated to modify her behavior in the interest of fetal well-being and almost always in her own interest as well. For example, the obstetrician may suggest a smoking cessation program or modifications of diet for diabetes or phenylketonuria. The obstetrician's response to a patient's unwillingness to cooperate with medical advice in these situations should be to convey clearly the reasons for the recommendations to the pregnant woman, examine the barriers to change along with her, and encourage the development of health-promoting behavior. The obstetrician should be aware of state and local laws and regulations that may require reporting certain maternal behaviors to designated authorities.

In interactions with a woman who appears to resist following medical advice that might improve her health or that of her fetus, the obstetrician must keep in mind that medical knowledge has limitations and medical judgment

ISSN 1074-861X

The American College of Obstetricians and Gynecologists
409 12th Street, SW
PO Box 96920
Washington, DC 20090-6920

12345/32109

is fallible. Existing methods for detection of nonreassuring fetal status are not always reliable indicators of poor outcome, and there is often insufficient evidence for risk determination or risk–benefit evaluation for the fetus. In addition, expected benefits for the fetus cannot always be achieved. Similarly, in situations such as cesarean delivery, in which there is statistically a low degree of maternal risk, occasional serious maternal complications may occur. Because of the inability to determine with certainty when a situation is harmful to the fetus and to guarantee that the pregnant woman will not be harmed by the medical intervention, great care should be exercised to present a balanced evaluation of expected outcomes for both parties. The obstetrician's recommendations must be made in clear, understandable terms, taking into consideration the patient's age, educational level, cultural background, and language ability. Family members, friends of the patient, social workers, religious counselors, interpreters, and other caregivers may help the patient clarify her position if she chooses to confide in them. Consultation with an institutional ethics committee or other institutional resource may provide a useful forum for discussion and potential resolution of the problem.

The pregnant woman may decide that the risk of a recommended treatment is greater than she wishes to accept, or she may doubt the benefit of the treatment for either herself or the fetus. When a competent patient chooses not to comply with the recommended treatment after all reasonable attempts to explain and persuade have been exhausted, the obstetrician has three choices. One choice is to respect the patient's autonomy and not proceed with the recommended intervention regardless of the consequences. A second is to offer the patient the option of obtaining medical care from another individual before an emergency situation arises that might put the pregnant woman and the caregiver in unresolvable conflict. A caregiver would exercise this alternative if unwilling to comply with a patient's expressed decision about medical intervention or nonintervention, because of the caregiver's opinion that such actions might adversely affect the fetus. Patients should be encouraged to discuss fully their concerns and choices early in the course of prenatal care so that appropriate action may be taken before a crisis occurs. A third option, exercised on rare occasions, is to request involvement of the court. The choice among these unpleasant options will depend upon the urgency of the clinical circumstances, the potential consequences for both the pregnant woman and the fetus, and the reliability of predictions of such consequences.

Three ethical principles are involved in choosing among these options: 1) autonomy, or the right of the pregnant woman to choose or refuse recommended treatment; 2) beneficence, or the obligation of the physician to promote the pregnant woman's well-being as well as that of the fetus; and 3) the pregnant woman's beneficence-based obligation to promote the welfare of her fetus. Abiding by the patient's autonomous decision will provide the best care for the pregnant woman and the fetus in most circumstances. In the event of an emergency, when there is insufficient time to obtain either transfer of care or judicial review of a pregnant woman's refusal, the obstetrician must respect the patient's autonomy, continue to care for the pregnant woman, and not intervene against the patient's wishes, regardless of the consequences. Such action may subordinate the caregiver's personal ethic to his or her professional obligation to respect the patient's autonomy.

When health care providers contemplate going to court for authorization of intervention that is against the pregnant patient's wishes, the following four conditions must be met:

- There is high probability of serious harm to the fetus in respecting the patient's decision.
- There is high probability that the recommended treatment will prevent or substantially reduce harm to the fetus.
- There are no comparably effective, less-intrusive options to prevent harm to the fetus.
- There is high probability that the recommended treatment also benefits the pregnant woman or that the risks to the pregnant woman are relatively small.

These criteria must be weighed against the following factors:

- A woman is wronged and may be harmed, whether physically, psychologically, or spiritually, when her autonomy is violated.
- The patient's subsequent loss of trust in the health care system may reduce the health care provider's ability to help her and may deter others from seeking care.
- There may be other social costs associated with this violation of individual liberty.

Even in the presence of a court order authorizing intervention, the use of physical force against a resistant, competent woman is not justified. The use of force will substantially increase the risk to the mother, thereby diminishing the ethical justification of such therapy.

Conclusions

1. The maternal–fetal relationship is unique, because it involves the pregnant woman's autonomy concerning her health, the obstetrician's beneficence-based obligations to enhance the health of the pregnant woman and the fetus, and the pregnant woman's beneficence-based responsibility to promote the welfare of her fetus. Every reasonable effort should be made to protect the fetus, but the pregnant woman's autonomy should be respected.
2. The vast majority of pregnant women are willing to assume significant risk for the welfare of the fetus. Problems arise when potentially beneficial advice is rejected. The role of the obstetrician should be one of an informed educator and counselor, weighing the risks and benefits to both patients as well as realizing that tests, judgments, and decisions are fallible. Consultation with others, including an institutional ethics committee, should be sought when appropriate to aid the pregnant woman and obstetrician in resolving the conflict. The use of the courts to resolve these conflicts is warranted only in extraordinary circumstances.
3. Obstetricians should refrain from performing procedures that are unwanted by a pregnant woman. The use of judicial authority to implement treatment regimens in order to protect the fetus violates the pregnant woman's autonomy and should be avoided unless the four stringent criteria specified in this Committee Opinion are met. In addition to wronging the pregnant woman, appeal to judicial authority may lead to undesirable societal consequences, such as the criminalization of noncompliance with medical recommendations.

Bibliography

Draper H. Women, forced caesareans and antenatal responsibilities. J Med Ethics 1996;22:327–333

Johnsen D. A new threat to pregnant women's autonomy. Hastings Cent Rep 1987;17(4):33–40

Murray TH. Moral obligations to the not-yet-born child. In: The worth of a child. Berkeley: The University of California Press, 1996:96–114

Robertson JA. Legal issues in fetal therapy. Semin Perinatol 1985;9:136–142

Robertson JA, Schulman JD. Pregnancy and prenatal harm to offspring: the case of mothers with PKU. Hastings Cen Rep 1987;17(4):23–33

Tauer CA. Lives at stake. How to respond to a woman's refusal of cesarean surgery when she risks losing her child or her life. Health Prog 1992;73:18–27

ACOG Committee Opinion

Committee on Gynecologic Practice

Number 243, November 2000

Performance and Interpretation of Imaging Studies by Obstetrician–Gynecologists

Obstetrician–gynecologists are experienced in diagnostic imaging methods and receive privileges to perform and interpret imaging studies on the basis of their training, experience, and demonstrated current competence. Obstetrician–gynecologists can perform the immediate and timely interpretation of imaging studies, correlate these studies with clinical findings, counsel the patient, and assume the responsibility for determining the treatment of the patient.

Education and Training

By virtue of their education and experience, obstetrician–gynecologists are qualified to perform the imaging studies that are a necessary and integral part of obstetric–gynecologic care. Training in diagnostic imaging is a part of obstetric–gynecologic residencies, and questions related to this field are a part of the certifying examinations of the American Board of Obstetrics and Gynecology. For example, the performance and interpretation of ultrasound images are required components of obstetric and gynecologic residency training and are monitored by the Residency Review Committee for Obstetrics and Gynecology. In addition to interpreting images in descriptive terms, obstetrician–gynecologists add functional, anatomical, and clinical assessments, resulting in patient-specific information. It is the obstetric–gynecologic interpretation of the images, in concert with the history and physical examination, that determines the course of treatment and carries with it the responsibility for patient care. A written report, signed by the interpreting physician, should be considered an integral part of the performance and interpretation of an imaging study.

Timeliness

For optimal patient care, imaging studies should be performed and interpreted in a timely manner. Many obstetric–gynecologic imaging procedures are performed when the patient is in the obstetrician–gynecologist's office or in

ISSN 1074-861X

The American College of Obstetricians and Gynecologists
409 12th Street, SW
PO Box 96920
Washington, DC 20090-6920

12345/43210

the labor and delivery suite so that judgments can be made, without delay, at the time of clinical decision making.

Appropriate management of certain obstetric–gynecologic emergencies, such as suspected ectopic pregnancy, requires timely performance and interpretation of imaging studies. In many cases, the obstetrician–gynecologist is the most appropriate physician to provide these services.

Conclusion

The responsibility for obstetric–gynecologic patient care rests with the treating obstetrician–gynecologist and may include the immediate performance and interpretation of diagnostic imaging studies. Obstetrician–gynecologists are qualified to perform and interpret obstetric–gynecologic imaging studies. The American College of Obstetricians and Gynecologists believes that obstetrician–gynecologists are entitled to adequate compensation for the cost and work involved in providing these services. Any policy that prohibits obstetrician–gynecologists from performing and interpreting imaging studies of which they are competent interferes with the patient's access to optimal care. Such a policy is likely to ultimately increase the cost of providing such services and substantially increases the risk of less than optimal outcomes in those patients requiring timely management of obstetric–gynecologic emergencies.

ACOG

Committee on Obstetric Practice

Committee Opinion

Number 167, December 1995

Perinatal and Infant Mortality Statistics

Perinatal and infant mortality statistics are important indicators of the quality of health care and the health status of the population. Comparisons of these statistics are often used for political purposes, as well as for policy and program development and the allocation of resources. Reporting and classification differences, however, can invalidate comparisons of perinatal and infant mortality rates. United States perinatal and infant mortality statistics are often compared unfavorably with those of other industrial countries, partly because of these discrepancies (1). Perhaps more important, within the United States, comparisons among states and localities can be equally unreliable for the same reasons.

Problems with the Current Statistical Data

With the advent of modern obstetric techniques, blood banking, antibiotics, neonatal intensive care nurseries, and perinatal regionalization, the incidence of infant mortality has greatly decreased. In the United States, the remaining infant mortality tends to occur mostly in very low birth weight infants and in infants with congenital anomalies. Fifty percent of all infant deaths occur within the first week of life, with 50% of these occurring in the first 24 hours. Any inconsistency in data collection regarding very low birth weight fetuses and infants who survive only briefly can markedly alter the infant mortality statistics.

Although standard definitions (2, 3) have been promulgated and widely acknowledged, variations in data collection practices persist. Some problems make fetal and infant mortality statistics difficult to compare among states and countries:

- The reporting of infant mortality is usually based on local interpretation of definitions and guidelines for data collection and on local legal requirements and can differ markedly among states and countries. A particular problem occurs when infant deaths are misclassified as fetal deaths and therefore are not included in the calculation of infant mortality rates.
- Improved neonatal intensive care allows providers to attempt to salvage an extremely high-risk fetus that might otherwise die in utero. Often, these are very low birth weight infants, who have mortality rates of up to 40%. A

ISSN 1074-861X

The American College of Obstetricians and Gynecologists
409 12th Street, SW
Washington, DC 20024-2188

2345/987

misleading, technologically driven increase may thus be introduced into infant mortality rates when more advanced or aggressive health care delivery systems exist for neonatal care.

- Despite well-known methodologic shortcomings, many states and countries continue to use gestational age criteria, which are often less objective and accurate than birth weight in determining whether to report a fetal death.
- Most states and countries require certain fetal deaths (formerly termed *stillbirths*) to be reported, but lower limits of the requirement vary (eg, only deaths of fetuses more than 20 or 28 weeks of gestation or of fetuses weighing more than 350 g). These variations in the lower limit may impede accurate comparisons among various jurisdictions.
- The number of days of the neonatal period used in calculating perinatal mortality statistics varies from 7 days of life to 28 days of life, often without clear identification of the period being used.
- Perinatal and infant mortality rates are commonly used to measure quality and to allocate resources for maternal and child health programs. This may provide an incentive to use definitions that serve these interests.

Recommendations

Obstetric units should adopt a method for recording each perinatal event by specific birth weight (rather than ranges), actual hours or days of life in the case of live births, and gestational age of the fetus or infant as determined by crown–rump length or first-trimester ultrasonography. These data can then be aggregated into categories that are appropriate and useful. In this way, various reporting requirements can be met without additional data collection, but statistical analysis can be based on valid comparisons of consistent data.

The following standard definitions should be used to refer to live birth, fetal death, and induced abortion:

- A live birth is one that shows any evidence of life at delivery. Evidence includes beating of the heart or movement of voluntary muscles. However, heartbeats are to be distinguished from transient cardiac contractions; respirations are to be distinguished from fleeting respiratory efforts or gasps (3).
- A fetal death (formerly termed *stillbirth*) is a fetus who shows no sign of life at delivery (2, 3).
- Induced abortion is the purposeful interruption of an intrauterine pregnancy with the intention other than to produce a liveborn infant. This definition excludes management of prolonged retention of products of conception following fetal death (3).

To simplify and standardize the reporting periods for perinatal events, the following time periods are recommended:

- The perinatal period is from 22 weeks of gestation (or 500 g) through 28 completed days of life.
- The neonatal period is from birth through 28 completed days of life (1).
- The early neonatal period is the first 7 days of life; the late neonatal period is from 8 days through 28 completed days of life (1).
- During the first 24 hours after delivery, age at death is expressed in hours. After the first 24 hours, age at death is expressed in completed days of life (1).

It is recognized that obstetric units must continue to make reports that meet the requirements of the jurisdiction in which they are located. However, the consistent use of these simplified and standardized reporting periods by obstetrician–gynecologists and obstetric units for all other purposes is recommended to encourage their adoption by statistical and legislative bodies.

For purposes of comparison among states in the United States, perinatal statistics should be computed using only deaths of fetuses and infants weighing 500 g or more at delivery (1). On an international basis, perinatal statistics should be computed using only deaths of fetuses and infants weighing 1,000 g or more at delivery (1). All perinatal mortality statistics should be computed excluding induced abortions (2).

References

1. Sachs BP, Fretts RC, Gardner R, Hellerstein S, Wampler NS, Wise PH. The impact of extreme prematurity and congenital anomalies on the interpretation of international comparisons of infant mortality. Obstet Gynecol 1995;85:941–946
2. World Health Organization. Strengthening of Epidemiological and Statistical Services Unit. The international conference for the tenth revision of the International Classification of Diseases. World Health Stat Rep 1990;43: 204–245
3. American Academy of Pediatrics, American College of Obstetricians and Gynecologists. Guidelines for perinatal care. 3rd ed. Elk Grove Village, Illinois: AAP; Washington, DC: ACOG, 1992

Bibliography

Alberman E, Botting B. Trends in prevalence and survival of very low birthweight infants, England and Wales: 1983-7. Arch Dis Child 1991;66:1304–1308

Agdestein S. Perinatal and infant mortality: trends and risk factors in Norway 1967-1990. Acta Obstet Gynecol Scand Suppl 1994;160:1–30

Blondel B, Grandjea H, Kaminski M, Breat G, Pontonnier G, Sureau C. Criteria for registering births. Lancet 1991;337:981

Cartlidge PHT, Stewart JH. Effect of changing the stillbirth definition on evaluation of perinatal mortality rates. Lancet 1995;346:486-488

Carver JD, McDermott RJ, Jacobson HN, Sherin KM, Kanarek K, Pimentel B, et al. Infant mortality statistics do not adequately reflect the impact of short gestation. Pediatrics 1993;92: 229–232

United Nations Department for Economic and Social Information and Policy Analysis. 1992 demographic yearbook, 44th issue. New York: United Nations, 1994

Doornbos JP, Nordbeck HJ, Treffers PE. The reliability of perinatal mortality statistics in The Netherlands. Am J Obstet Gynecol 1987;156:1183–1187

Fenton AC, Field DJ, Mason E, Clarke M. Attitudes to viability of preterm infants and their effect on figures for perinatal mortality. BMJ 1990;300:434–436

Field DJ, Smith H, Mason E, Milner AD. Is perinatal mortality still a good indicator of perinatal care? Paediatr Perinat Epidemiol 1988;2:213–219

Gourbin C, Masuy-Stroobant G. Are live and stillbirths comparable all over Europe? Legal definitions and vital registration data processing. Working paper 170. Belgium: Institut de Demographie Louvaine la Neuve, January 1993

Howell EM, Blondel B. International infant mortality rates: bias from reporting differences. Am J Public Health 1994;84: 850–852

Keirse MJ. Perinatal mortality rates do not contain what they purport to contain. Lancet 1984;1:1166–1169

Lee S, Paneth N, Gartner LM, Pearlman M. The very low-birthweight rate: principal predictor of neonatal mortality in industrialized populations. J Pediatr 1980;97:759–764

Mugford M. A comparison of reported differences in definitions of vital events and statistics. World Health Stat Q 1983;36: 201–212

Wegman ME. Annual summary of vital statistics—1993. Pediatrics 1994;94:792–803

World health statistics report. World Health Stat Rep 1976;29: 416–477

Wilcox A, Skjaerven R, Buekens P, Kiely J. Birth weight and perinatal mortality. A comparison of the United States and Norway. JAMA 1995;273:709–711

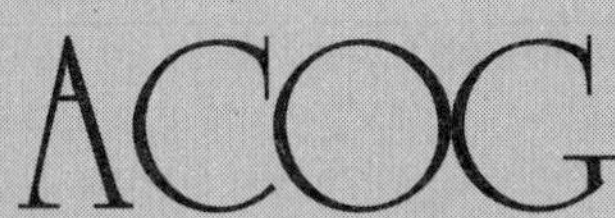

Committee on
Obstetric Practice

American Academy
of Pediatrics
Committee on
Fetus and Newborn

Committee Opinion

Number 163, November 1995

Perinatal Care at the Threshold of Viability

The survival rate for infants born prematurely has changed over the last two decades and is likely to change in the future. Currently, the birth of an infant at or before 25 weeks of gestation or weighing less than 750 g presents a variety of complex medical, social, and ethical decisions. Although the prevalence of such births is low, the impact on the infants, their families, the health care system, and society is profound.

The survival of infants born from 23 to 25 weeks of gestation increases with each additional week of gestation. However, the overall neonatal survival rate for infants born during this early gestational period remains less than 40% (1, 2). Of those who survive, about 40% have moderate or serious disabilities, and many have neurobehavioral dysfunction and poor school performance (3, 4). Many require prolonged intensive care and long-term care (2). The commitment for all aspects of care may be extensive, multidisciplinary, lifelong, and costly. Because the families bear the emotional and financial consequences of the birth of an extremely low birth weight infant, it is essential to inform the prospective parents regarding the expectations for infant outcome and the risks and benefits of various approaches to care.

Counseling Regarding Potential Fetal Outcomes

Most parents are unfamiliar with the complexities of care required for an extremely premature infant, both in the intensive care unit and after discharge from the hospital. Therefore, it is often necessary to provide the information in small segments at frequent intervals to allow the parents to comprehend the messages. The family can benefit from a clear explanation of the various supportive procedures that will likely be necessary in the infant's first days of life. Family members should also be provided with an overview of the potential complications of prolonged intensive care. Finally, they should be informed of the range of survival rates and of the rates of long-term disabilities that can be expected. In compiling such information, practitioners should consider data reported in the current literature as well as outcomes based on local experience; they should allow for some error in the best estimate of gestational age and fetal weight.

Neonatal survival rates experienced over the last decade in different neonatal units are provided in Table 1. These rates do not represent ultimate survival rates, as deaths may occur in the postneonatal period. The prevalence

ISSN 1074-861X

The American College of Obstetricians and Gynecologists
409 12th Street, SW
Washington, DC 20024-2188

12345/98765

Table 1. Neonatal Survival by Gestational Age and Birth Weight

Factor	Mean (%) Survival Rates (Range) Reported for*	
	1987–1988	1989–1990
Age (wk)		
23	23 (0–33)	15 (0–29)
24	34 (10–57)	54 (27–100)
25	54 (30–72)	59 (47–74)
Weight (g)		
501–600	21 (0–44)	20 (0–33)
601–700	33 (9–50)	41 (25–56)
701–800	53 (31–73)	65 (38–83)

* Rates were reported by the National Institute of Child Health and Human Development neonatal centers.

Data from Hack M, Horbar JD, Malloy MH, Tyson JE, Wright E, Wright L. Very low birth weight outcomes of the National Institute of Child Health and Human Development Neonatal Network. Pediatrics 1991;87:587–597 and Hack M, Wright LL, Shankaran S, Tyson JE, Horbar JD, Bauer CR, et al. Very-low-birth-weight outcomes of the National Institute of Child Health and Human Development Neonatal Network, November 1989 to October 1990. Am J Obstet Gynecol 1995;172:457–464

of a number of morbidities common to these extremely premature infants is shown in Table 2.

It is difficult to counsel parents regarding long-term disabilities because outcomes are only now being reported for neonates born since the use of surfactant became common and who have survived to school age. Recent experience suggests that almost half of the surviving children who weigh less than 750 g at birth experience moderate or severe disability, including blindness and cerebral palsy, and require special education. Many infants have more than one disability. Families should be counseled that, despite the high rate of overall disability, many of these children are educable and can function within their family unit.

The estimation of gestational age before premature delivery forms the main basis for subsequent decision making. Clinical assessment to determine gestational age is usually appropriate for the woman with regular menstrual cycles and a known last menstrual period that was confirmed by an early examination. Fetal measurements derived through the use of ultrasonography at the time of anticipated delivery should not be used to alter estimated gestational age unless there is a discrepancy of 2 weeks or more between the age derived by menstrual dating and the age derived sonographically or the woman is uncertain about the date of her last menstrual period. Ultrasonography may provide useful information regarding the presence or absence of fetal malformations that may alter the prognosis. The accuracy of sonographic measurements and the ability to ascertain malformations, however, may be reduced in the presence of oligohydramnios, such as occurs with ruptured membranes.

Even in ideal circumstances, the 95% confidence limits for a formula-based estimate of fetal weight are ±15% to 20% (5). Thus, an infant estimated to weigh 600 g may have an actual birth weight of less than 500 g or more than 700 g. Even relatively small discrepancies of 1 or 2 weeks in gestational age or 100–200 g in birth weight may have major implications for survival and long-term morbidity. This underscores the importance of counseling about the range of possible outcomes. Furthermore, multiple gestation increases the difficulty of accurate gestational age assessment, and the prognosis for one infant ultimately may differ from that of the other(s).

Ideally, the obstetric and neonatal physicians, primary care physicians, and neonatal nurses should confer before recommendations are made to the parents. The range of possible outcomes and management options can then be outlined for the patient and her family. If maternal transport may be needed, the obstetrician should be knowledgable about the available regional resources and be prepared to provide basic information to the parents if the specific clinical circumstances warrant. More detailed counseling can then be accomplished at the receiving unit. Additional medical opinions and input from other

Table 2. Serious Morbidities in Infants With Birth Weight <750 g Experienced by the NICHD Neonatal Centers, 1989–1990*

Condition	Frequency (%)	Range (%)
Respiratory distress syndrome	86	80–100
Ventilator support at 28 days†	72	23–100
Chronic lung disease‡	35	8–82
Necrotizing enterocolitis	9	2–19
Septicemia	34	13–50
Grade III intraventricular hemorrhage	13	5–20
Grade IV intraventricular hemorrhage	17	0–24
Seizures	10	2–14
Periventricular leukomalacia	11	7–20

* NICHD indicates the National Institute of Child Health and Human Development.

† Data are for infants alive at 28 days.

‡ Data are for survivors.

Data from Hack M, Wright LL, Shankaran S, Tyson JE, Horbar JD, Bauer CR, et al. Very-low-birth-weight outcomes of the National Institute of Child Health and Human Development Neonatal Network, November 1989 to October 1990. Am J Obstet Gynecol 1995;172: 457–464

important sources such as clergy, social workers, and the institution's bioethics committee may be offered to the parents. Counseling should be sensitive to cultural and ethnic diversity, and a skilled translator should be available for parents whose primary language differs from the language of the care providers. It should be emphasized that the prognosis for the newborn may change after birth since a more accurate assessment of the newborn's gestational age and condition may be made at that time.

Counseling Regarding the Risks and Benefits of Management Options

Obstetric Management

Decisions regarding obstetric management must be made by the parents and their physicians if the neonate's prognosis is uncertain; the decisions must be documented in the obstetric records. Some decisions, such as the choice of cesarean birth, can result in increased risk of morbidity to the woman.

Few studies have been done to evaluate the influence of obstetric management on the outcome of infants at the threshold of viability. Furthermore, literature on this subject is largely retrospective and often lacks sufficient data regarding potential confounding variables. Despite these limitations, study results have consistently failed to document benefits of cesarean delivery for extremely premature infants (6–10). It has even been difficult to document improved outcome with cesarean birth for infants in the breech position who are extremely premature (7, 8). Furthermore, injuries to the infant can occur during a difficult cesarean birth.

Physicians should avoid characterizing managements of uncertain benefit as "doing everything possible." Rather, they should hold discussions with the family regarding available data and provide an explanation of the risks incurred by management options, including route of delivery. In the case of cesarean delivery, risks to the woman include not only those incurred during the perioperative period but also long-term implications for childbearing since a vertical uterine incision is often used. A vertical uterine incision at these gestational ages may extend into the upper segment and would preclude the option of vaginal birth in future pregnancy. Counseling regarding management decisions such as whether to effect maternal transport should include a discussion of the potential disadvantages of separating the mother from supportive family members and familiar caregivers when benefit for the mother or baby is uncertain.

Parents should be encouraged to actively participate in discussion regarding maternal transport and other management decisions. Counseling about management options and potential outcome allows the family to more easily choose a course of action that is both medically appropriate and consistent with their own personal values and goals. Whenever possible, a nondirective approach needs to be used; in some circumstances, however, directive counseling may be appropriate (11). Counseling may result in the family choosing a noninterventive approach to delivery and management. Because the benefits of different types of obstetric management have not been delineated, families should be supported in such decisions.

Neonatal Management

Ethical decisions regarding the extent of resuscitative efforts and subsequent support of the neonate are complex (12–14). Parents should understand that decisions about neonatal management made before delivery may be altered depending on the condition of the neonate at birth, the postnatal gestational age assessment, and the infant's response to resuscitative and stabilization measures. Recommendations regarding the extent of continuing support depend on frequent reevaluations of the infant's condition and prognosis.

When a decision is made not to resuscitate the infant or to discontinue resuscitation, the family should be treated with dignity and compassion. This should include the acknowledgment of the birth of the infant. Humane and compassionate care must be provided to the infant, including careful handling, maintaining a neutral thermal environment, and gentle monitoring of vital signs.

When medical support is discontinued or death is inevitable, time should be allowed for the parents and other family members to hold, touch, and interact with the infant if they desire to do so, both before and after the infant has died. Naming the infant and obtaining a photograph may be important to the parents, and a crib card and name band should be provided. Birth weight and other measurements should be provided to the family as well. Clergy and other family and friends should be allowed access to the infant in a setting that maintains the dignity of both the family and infant.

Support should be provided to the family by physicians, nurses, and other staff beyond the time of the infant's death. Perinatal loss support groups, intermittent contact by phone, and a later conference with the family to review the medical events surrounding the infant's death and to evaluate the grieving response of the parents may be considered.

Summary

The survival rate for infants at the threshold of viability has been improving. However, there are insufficient data regarding the cost(s) of initial and ongoing care of these infants and the long-term outcome of survivors. Furthermore, there has been little study of the impact of obstetric management on the survival rates of extremely low birth weight infants and on long-term morbidities. Continued research on these issues is imperative, and physicians need to remain informed of changing statistics.

References

1. Hack M, Horbar JD, Malloy MH, Tyson JE, Wright E, Wright L. Very low birth weight outcomes of the National Institute of Child Health and Human Development Neonatal Network. Pediatrics 1991;87:587–597
2. Hack M, Wright LL, Shankaran S, Tyson JE, Horbar JD, Bauer CR, et al. Very-low-birth-weight outcomes of the National Institute of Child Health and Human Development Neonatal Network, November 1989 to October 1990. Am J Obstet Gynecol 1995;172:457–464
3. Ehrenhaft PM, Wagner JL, Herdman RC. Changing prognosis for very low birth weight infants. Obstet Gynecol 1989;74:528–535
4. Hack M, Taylor HG, Klein N, Eiben R, Schatschneider C, Mercuri-Minich N. School-age outcomes in children with birth weights under 750 g. N Engl J Med 1994;331: 753–759
5. Hadlock FP, Harrist RB, Sharman RS, Deter RL, Park SK. Estimation of fetal weight with the use of head, body, and femur measurements—a prospective study. Am J Obstet Gynecol 1985;151:333–337
6. Hack M, Fanaroff AA. Outcomes of extremely-low-birth-weight infants between 1982 and 1988. N Engl J Med 1989;321:1642–1647
7. Malloy MH, Rhoads GG, Schramm W, Land G. Increasing cesarean section rates in very low-birth weight infants. Effect on outcome. JAMA 1989;262:1475–1478
8. Malloy MH, Onstad L, Wright E. The effect of cesarean delivery on birth outcome in very low birth weight infants. National Institute of Child Health and Human Development Neonatal Research Network. Obstet Gynecol 1991;77:498-503
9. Worthington D, Davis LE, Grausz JP, Sobocinski K. Factors influencing survival and morbidity with very low birth weight delivery. Obstet Gynecol 1983;62:550–555
10. Kitchen W, Ford GW, Doyle LW, Rickards AL, Lissenden JV, Pepperell RJ, et al. Cesarean section or vaginal delivery at 24 to 28 weeks' gestation: comparison of survival and neonatal and two-year morbidity. Obstet Gynecol 1985;66: 149–157
11. American College of Obstetricians and Gynecologists. Ethical decision-making in obstetrics and gynecology. ACOG Technical Bulletin 136. Washington, DC: ACOG, 1989
12. Rhoden NK. Treating Baby Doe: the ethics of uncertainty. Hastings Cent Rep 1986;16(4):34–42
13. Lantos JD, Meadow W, Miles SH, Ekwo E, Paton J, Hageman JR, et al. Providing and forgoing resuscitative therapy for babies of very low birth weight. J Clin Ethics 1992;3:283–287
14. Allen MC, Donohue PK, Dusman AE. The limit of viability—neonatal outcome of infants born at 22 to 25 weeks' gestation. N Engl J Med 1993;329:1597–1601

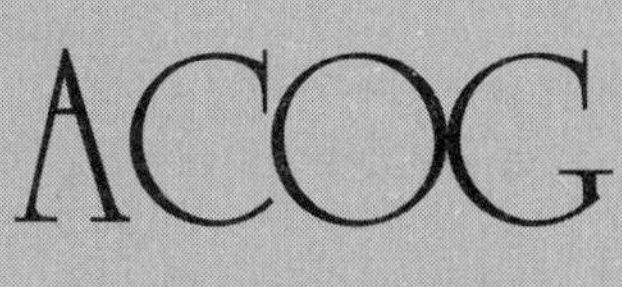

Committee on Ethics

Committee Opinion

Number 170, April 1996

Physician Responsibility Under Managed Care:

Patient Advocacy in a Changing Health Care Environment

With the rise of managed care, health care financing and delivery in the United States have entered a period of profound transformation. The changes raise important ethical questions regarding the values that should guide the broad formulation of health policy, the benefits packages of third party payers, and decisions at the bedside. The most pressing of these questions concern the potential conflict between the traditional values of patient benefit and autonomy and the ascendant values of economic self-interest, profit-taking, and economic efficiency. A central ethical concern at the heart of this transformation is to what degree, if at all, new health care financing and delivery schemes inappropriately influence clinical decision making and threaten patients' health interests.

Financial incentives have always had the potential to influence health care providers. Within the traditional ethos of medicine, however, these interests have been a source of concern insofar as they may come into conflict with the professional obligation to benefit the patient. Under managed care, the locus of authority and decision making has, in many instances, shifted from the physician–patient relationship to health care system administrators and employer groups for whom patient health may be a purely financial concern. Now, the contract that carries primacy is often the one between the employer and the managed care organization, not the implicit contract between physician and patient. As a result, those with growing influence over patient care have, unlike health care professionals, no ethos of accountability to the patient's interests. It is in this context that obstetrician–gynecologists and patients are increasingly reporting limitations on testing, treatment, length of hospital stay, and coverage of home health services, when they believe these limitations have a negative impact on women's health and well-being.

As administrative control increasingly influences clinical judgment and supplants the physician–patient relationship, certain fundamental ethical values are endangered. These include *fiduciary beneficence*—the health care provider's obligation to act for the benefit of the patient—and *patient autonomy*—the right of the patient to make informed decisions regarding her care. Other values at stake in the shift to managed care are *medicine as a social*

ISSN 1074-861X

The American College of Obstetricians and Gynecologists
409 12th Street, SW
P.O. Box 96920
Washington, DC 20090-6920

12345/09876

good—the obligation of society to preserve and promote the health of its members and to facilitate advances in medical knowledge, education, and training—and *justice*—the extent to which an adequate level of health care is made equally available and accessible to all.

This document examines how these values operate within the context of managed care. It 1) raises ethical questions regarding physicians' responses to the incentives that structure managed care and capitation strategies; 2) delineates the obligations of physicians and third party payers to disclose financial and other restrictions on care; and 3) describes the physician's responsibility as a patient advocate within a restrictive environment. It raises these questions with particular reference to women's health issues.

Fiduciary Beneficence

The patient's vulnerability in illness and the physician's implicit promise to help are the bases of the physician's obligation to act for the benefit of the patient (1). These essential features of the healing relationship give rise to the obligation of fidelity and ground the physician's role as patient advocate. Cost-containment strategies associated with managed care may compromise the way physicians work to benefit their patients and thus may directly challenge these foundational professional obligations.

Patient Autonomy

The inherent value of individual autonomy (self-determination) serves as one of the keystones of democracy and of individual rights and protections in the United States. In health care, the value of autonomy is affirmed in the doctrine of informed consent. Now widely acknowledged as central in health care decision making, this concept asserts the patient's right to be informed of the potential risks and benefits associated with treatment options and to decide on the acceptable level of risk she will bear (2–4). To the extent that physicians, whether working in fee-for-service or managed care systems, fail to disclose the financial restrictions and incentives that influence treatment decisions, they undermine the patient's right to make informed decisions about her care.

Managed Care: Constraints and Incentives in Health Care Decision Making

No matter how care is financed, individual and institutional providers should make available the most efficient and effective services consistent with quality patient care (5). Managed care offers the potential of cost savings in the delivery of health care through, for example, economies of scale and standardization of certain care patterns. Because physician decision making determines 80% of health care expenditures in the United States (6), most plans seek to control costs by modifying physician behavior (7). Efforts to modify decision making take the form of various constraints and incentives. As for constraints, managed care plans may restrict outright the physician's freedom to make referrals and to prescribe certain medications and diagnostic tests (8). Managed care plans may also dictate the length of hospital stay, the general treatment plan, and time spent with patients during office visits. Unless flexibly applied, these attempts to standardize caregiving threaten to overlook any nonstandard needs of the individual patient.

Economic incentives designed to modify physician behavior typically take two forms. On the one hand, physicians may be offered bonuses or other monetary rewards for treatment decisions that result in cost savings for the plan. On the other hand, physicians whose advocacy for the patient does not conform to the economic objectives of a plan must bear the financial risk of costs over covered amounts, risk being fired or dropped from a plan, or pass uncovered costs back to the patient. In addition, "economic credentialing"—the economic assessment of physician performance—may be used as the basis of a plan's decision to include or exclude particular providers.

Disclosure of Financial Restrictions on Care: Obligations of Physicians and Third Party Payers

As reflected in the doctrine of informed consent, respect for patient autonomy requires that the physician disclose to the patient information regarding the risks and benefits associated with proposed care. In managed care, patient risk may be increased by the financial objectives of a third party payer. Thus, physicians are obliged to disclose financial considerations that may jeopardize patients' health interests. In the face of financial conflicts of interest, the obligation of truth-telling should be paramount.

In this regard, honest, comprehensible disclosure on the part of third party payers is essential in fostering a constructive, nonadversarial relationship between payers and patients and payers and practitioners. The recent market-oriented conception of the patient as an "informed consumer"—implied in the terms "client" or "subscriber"—is inappropriate on a number of counts. First, patients rarely have the expertise to recognize which interventions are required to meet their health needs or which are being withheld. Second, patient choice may not be free; rather, it may be compromised by illness. Third, unlike other service arrangements, the provider of health services has a *prima facie* obligation to *enhance* the patient's decision-making capacity through the provision of information in the informed consent process and/or through medical means that, for example, restore consciousness. Fourth, given the link between health care insurance and employment, patients often have limited, if any, choice of which health care plans to enter* (9). Fifth, most market transactions operate under the ethos of "caveat emptor" (let the buyer beware). However, the health care professional's implicit promise to act in the patient's interests gives patients the right to expect that their health will be paramount when they seek medical services. For these reasons, health care plans must clearly state—both at the time of plan enrollment and also at the time that treatment decisions occur—their restrictions on services (10, 11). Some provider contracts may specifically forbid physicians to disclose the existence of services not covered by the plan (12). Because such restrictions directly conflict with the physician's obligations of truth-telling and respect for patient self-determination, these contractual proscriptions should be prohibited.

If a physician believes, based on clinical evidence, that a patient's health interests are jeopardized by the policies, coverage limits, or utilization restrictions of a plan, his or her role as the patient's advocate demands that an appeal be made to the plan or medical director. Advocacy, or intercession on behalf of the patient, may also involve a special request to a pharmaceutical company for discounted pharmaceuticals when coverage for more expensive but necessary drugs has been denied.

Physician advocacy does not, however, extend to deceptive practices even though the subterfuge is intended to benefit the patient. For example, physicians may be tempted to add a covered diagnostic category to patient information so that the patient may receive treatment that is believed to be necessary but is not covered. However well-intentioned, such strategies do nothing to challenge or correct egregious policies, and they introduce dishonesty into the healing relationship.

As payers increasingly dictate the permissible economic impacts of health care decision making, physicians increasingly will be challenged to guard patients' health interests in the face of competing concerns. To ensure that a plan's policies do not threaten patient welfare, obstetrician–gynecologists should become actively involved with the policy-making boards of managed care plans in which they participate and should contribute to the quality improvement processes that result in plan guidelines.

Implications for Women and Women's Health Care

The shift to managed care has important implications for women. First, many of the cost-cutting strategies that influence the visible and measured cost of managed care may be based on hidden costs to women (13). For example, decreased lengths of stay for the elderly and children are often compensated for by increased at-home care provided by women as caregivers (14). Similarly, the added inconveniences of the gatekeeper referral system and the need, in some systems, to go to many different sites for diagnostic tests may place a disproportionate burden on patients or on women who are principally responsible for helping loved ones obtain needed health care.

Second, a patient's enrollment in a managed care plan that does not include her current obstetrician–gynecologist or other familiar providers may result in discontinuity of care and the loss of established relationships of trust.

Third, managed care plans may prohibit obstetrician–gynecologists from making referrals for such services as surgical consultation following abnormal mammography or dermatology consultation for enigmatic skin disorders. Women who have relied on their obstetrician–gynecologists for referrals may find their access to specialized services impeded.

Fourth, as already noted, by constraining clinical judgment, managed care policies may preclude the effective individualization of care and thereby increase the risk of patient morbidity. For example, policies that dictate the duration of inpatient postpartum stays may not permit retaining the mother and baby in the hospital when additional observation or nursing care seem prudent (15). Similarly, populations such as the elderly, adolescents, and the very sick may have needs that require more than the standard amount of time allotted for consultation. Flexibility, not zealous standardization, seems most likely to best serve patients' interests.

Fifth, many managed care plans also attempt to cut costs by excluding the sickest or most burdensome populations from coverage (16, 17). Currently, it is estimated that approximately 20% of women aged 15–44 lack health insurance (18). Of poor wom-

*About one half of insured employees have no choice among alternate plans. Further, a decline in employer-provided coverage has left more people uninsured.

en ages 18–64, 33% are uninsured (19). According to the Office of Technology Assessment, the uninsured are three times more likely than the insured to have inadequate care and poor health outcomes (20). The American College of Obstetricians and Gynecologists supports strong social policy committed to the value of justice in access to and allocation of health care. It does not support plans that encourage perpetuating limits on access to care for women burdened by poverty, unemployment, or language or transportation barriers (21).

Justice and the Limits of Fiduciary Beneficence

Whatever the future face of health care reform, methods of cost containment will remain a central concern. Inevitably, this raises questions regarding the just distribution of fiscal and material resources within plans.

In situations where resources are limited, the physician's obligation to the individual patient may come into tension with the fair and equitable treatment of all persons covered within a plan. In such cases, treatment decisions will hinge on the interpretation of what constitutes "appropriate" and "costworthy" care (22). From the point of view of patient benefit and the obligation of fidelity, determinations of clinical appropriateness should be made in consultation with the patient and on the basis of sound evidence and judgment, not on the basis of resource rationing. By contrast, justice and community welfare call for assessing which services and outcomes are "cost-worthy" within the constraints of a global budget for health care. When the obligations of beneficence and justice conflict, the following steps should be taken to preserve trust between providers and patients:

- Decisions to ration community health care resources for the purpose of just allocation should be made explicitly within a public forum, not at the bedside.
- The needs of all patients, not financial loss or gain, should be the primary basis of allocation decisions. Patients should be fully informed not only of services available within a plan but also of potentially beneficial services that are not available because of cost or other allocation constraints.

Medicine as a Social Good

Medical knowledge is not proprietary. It is gained only through the contributions of society and individual patients. For example, medical education and research are heavily subsidized by federal and state taxes. Also, patients contribute to medical knowledge by serving as subjects in publicly funded research projects and by permitting a portion of their care to be provided by physicians and nurses in training. In the arena of public health, where the fruits of biomedical science are applied broadly and without regard to an individual's ability to pay, our society endorses the view that medical knowledge belongs to the entire community. Medical knowledge should not, therefore, be owned as private property, but must be "held in trust" for individual patients and the good of society (23).

As managed care entities have increased their share of the health care market, the opportunities for education and training of providers have diminished. However, because managed care organizations depend on medical knowledge to operate, they have a responsibility to foster the education of health care providers within their institutions. Society cannot support health care arrangements that profit from the availability of medical knowledge but do nothing to ensure its continuance through research, education, and training.

Conclusion

Many cost-containment strategies associated with managed care directly challenge the ethical values of beneficence, autonomy, justice, and medicine as a social good. If cost containment and economic efficiency are to be morally legitimate goals—goals that enhance rather than undermine the quality of health care—they must be placed in the service of the broader goals of patient welfare and social justice. Non–health-related goals, such as shareholder profit, physician bonuses, and extravagant executive or physician salaries, appear to compromise these fundamental values and thus find little justification within the ethics of medicine. The following points are intended to aid obstetrician–gynecologists and institutional providers in fostering these values in the changing system of health care financing and delivery:

- Trust between physicians and patients—an essential element of the healing relationship—can be jeopardized by deception, discrimination, and financial conflicts of interest. Trust can be maintained and fostered by patient advocacy and honest disclosure of financial or other considerations that either are or appear to be at odds with the patient's health interests.

- Physicians should inform patients of the best treatment options whether or not these options are covered by the patient's plan.
- When treatment that a physician judges to be beneficial is excluded from coverage, the physician has a duty to act as an advocate for coverage on the patient's behalf.
- Third party payers have an obligation to inform patients and providers in a clear and comprehensive way of coverage exclusions and limitations in their plans.
- Third party payers have an obligation to justify to both physician and patient the denial of coverage for beneficial services.
- Plans must not penalize physicians for carrying out their fiduciary duty as patient advocates.
- Obstetrician–gynecologists should become actively involved with the policy-making boards of managed care plans in which they participate and should contribute to the quality improvement processes that result in plan guidelines.
- Physicians should refuse to participate in managed care arrangements with policies that are deemed unethical.
- Physicians and institutions should continue to contribute uncompensated care to those who have no other access to needed services. An equitable solution to the problem of limited access, however, will depend on public policy. Obstetrician–gynecologists should support mechanisms to achieve universal access to benefit poor women, women of color, and other populations who now have inadequate obstetric–gynecologic services.

Managed care organizations that profit from their activities should recognize a social obligation to support medical education, research, and care of the indigent, to enhance the overall health of our population in a cost-effective manner.

References

1. Pellegrino ED, Thomasma DC. For the patient's good: the restoration of beneficence in health care. New York: Oxford University Press, 1988
2. Faden RR, Beauchamp TL. A history and theory of informed consent. New York: Oxford University Press, 1986
3. American College of Obstetricians and Gynecologists. The ethical dimensions of informed consent. ACOG Committee Opinion 108. Washington, DC: ACOG, 1992
4. American College of Obstetricians and Gynecologists. End-of-life decision making: understanding the goals of care. ACOG Committee Opinion 156. Washington, DC: ACOG, 1995
5. Council on Ethical and Judicial Affairs, American Medical Association. Ethical issues in managed care. JAMA 1995;273:330–335
6. Morreim EH. Balancing act: the new medical ethics of medicine's new economics. Boston: Kluwer, Academic, 1991: 31
7. Woodstock Theological Center. Seminar in business ethics, Ethical considerations in the business aspects of health care. Washington, DC: Georgetown University Press, 1995
8. Rodwin MA. Conflicts in managed care. N Engl J Med 1995;332:604–607
9. Starr P. Look who's talking health care reform now. New York Times Magazine, September 3, 1995: 42–43
10. Mechanic D. Trust and informed consent to rationing. Milbank Q 1994; 72(2):217–23
11. Rodwin MA. Medicine, money and morals: physicians' conflicts of interest. New York: Oxford University Press, 1993
12. Kassirer JP. Managed care and the morality of the marketplace. N Engl J Med 1995;333:50–52
13. American Association of Retired Persons. A national survey of caregivers: a final report. Washington, DC: AARP, 1988
14. Osterkamp L. Family caregivers: America's primary long-term care resource. Aging 1988;358:1–5
15. American Academy of Pediatrics Committee on Child Health Financing. Guiding principles for managed care arrangements for the health care of infants, children, adolescents, and young adults. Pediatrics 1995;95:613–615
16. Relman AS. The new medical-industrial complex. N Engl J Med 1980;303:963–970
17. Luft HS, Miller RH. Patient selection in a competitive health care system. Health Affairs, Summer 1988:97–119
18. Women's Research and Education Institute. Women's health care costs and experiences. Washington, DC: WREI, 1994
19. Collins KS, Rowland D, Salganicoff A, Chait E. Assessing and improving women's health. Washington, DC: WREI, 1994
20. U.S. Congress, Office of Technology Assessment. Does health insurance make a difference? Washington, DC: US Government Printing Office, 1992
21. American College of Obstetricians and Gynecologists. Statement of policy: access to women's health care. Washington, DC: ACOG, July 1988
22. Sharpe VA, Faden AI. Appropriateness in patient care: a new conceptual framework. Milbank Q 1996;74(1):1–24
23. Pellegrino ED. Is health care rationing ethically defensible in our country today? In: Hamner JE III, ed. The 1991 distinguished visiting professorship lectures. Memphis: University of Tennessee, 1992

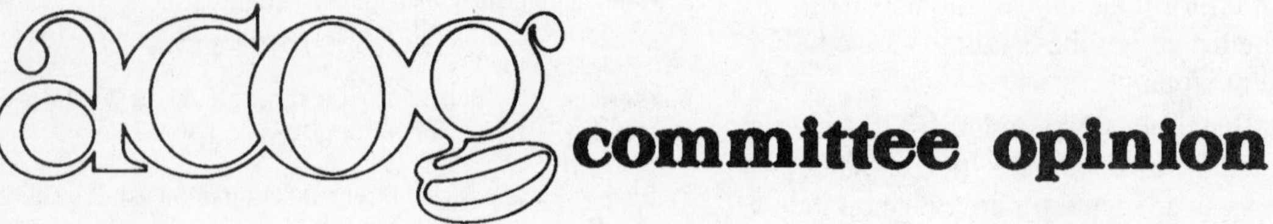

Committee on Obstetrics: Maternal and Fetal Medicine

Number 125—July 1993
(Replaces #102, December 1991)

Placental Pathology

Recently, there has been heightened interest in clinical–pathologic correlation between placental abnormalities and adverse pregnancy outcome. When a skilled and systematic examination of the umbilical cord, membranes, and placenta is performed on properly prepared specimens, insight into antepartum pathophysiology may be gained under certain circumstances.

In most of these instances, such as chorioamnionitis, the diagnosis already will have been made on clinical grounds, with the placental examination providing confirmation. In other cases of poor outcome, a disorder that was not suspected clinically may be revealed by placental pathology. Examples of pathologic findings and the disorders they suggest include the microabscesses of listeriosis and amnion nodosum suggesting long-standing oligohydramnios. The underlying pathophysiology of these lesions has been confirmed by laboratory testing or consistent and specific clinical associations.

The significance of other findings, such as villous edema, hemorrhagic endovasculitis, and chronic villitis, has not been as well delineated. These lesions, among others, have been variously reported to correlate with poor short-term and long-term neonatal outcome. The paucity of properly designed studies of adequate size with appropriate outcome parameters has prevented universal agreement as to positive predictive values, underlying pathophysiology, or even the consistency of clinical correlations with these findings. Furthermore, the distribution of pathologists with the expertise to interpret more subtle placental findings is uneven from region to region. Although a protocol for obtaining routine placental pathologic examination under certain obstetric and neonatal conditions has been recommended (1), there are few data to support the clinical utility of this approach.

In addition to the issue of positive and negative predictive values of the spectrum of placental findings, there are practical concerns regarding examination of the placenta. In some instances, a neonatal problem may not be ascertained until days or weeks after birth, when the placenta is no longer available. Different approaches have been recommended to address this problem, including routinely examining all placentas, securing a small section from each placenta in a fixed state for an indefinite period, and saving all placentas unfixed at 4°C for 1 week before discarding. However, routine determinations of placental pathology are not feasible on either a cost or manpower basis, and a small portion of placenta obtained at random would be unlikely to provide useful information. The practice of saving all placentas for 1 week after delivery would permit ascertaining most neonatal problems in which pathologic examination of the placenta may be appropriate, but the effectiveness of this approach has not been proven.

In conclusion, an examination of the umbilical cord, membranes, and placenta may assist the obstetric care provider in clinical–pathologic correlation when there is an adverse perinatal outcome. However, the scientific basis for clinical correlation with placental pathology is still evolving, and the benefit of securing specimens on a routine basis is as yet unproven. Continued research and education in this field should be encouraged. Research should be designed with the goal of defining clinical indications for placental examination. In contrast, pathologic examination of the stillborn fetus and placenta is always potentially informative. Obstetric providers should be persistent in seeking consent from parents for autopsy examinations.

REFERENCE

1. College of American Pathologists Conference XIX. The examination of the placenta: patient care and risk management. Arch Pathol Lab Med 1991;115: 641–732

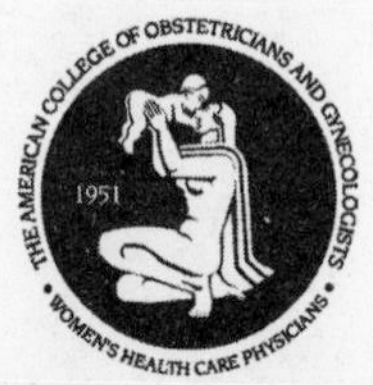

This document reflects emerging clinical and scientific advances as of the date issued and is subject to change. The information should not be construed as dictating an exclusive course of treatment or procedure to be followed.

The American College of Obstetricians and Gynecologists
409 12th Street, SW • Washington, DC 20024-2188

12345/76543

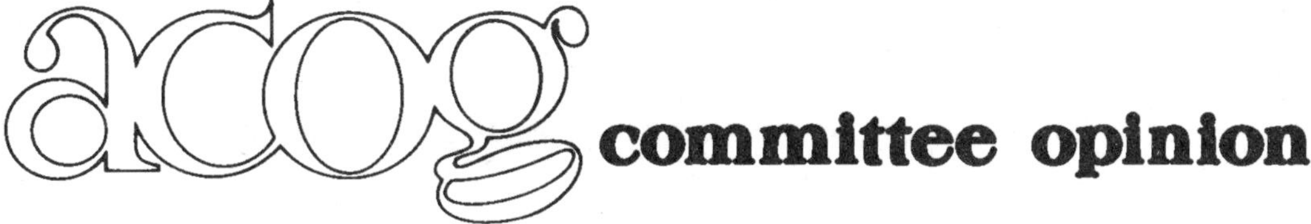

Committee on Obstetric Practice

Number 105—March 1992
(Replaces #50, February 1987)

Postpartum Tubal Sterilization

Many factors influence the decision about choice of method and timing of sterilization. For many women, postpartum tubal ligation offers a convenient and appropriate method. Assuming maternal and neonatal well-being as well as adequate medical and nursing resources, it is reasonable to proceed with tubal sterilization following a vaginal delivery.

Despite increased availability of regional analgesia for pain relief during labor, most candidates for postpartum tubal sterilization will not have received a major anesthetic for a normal delivery. When a continuous analgesic technique (ie, lumbar epidural or continuous spinal) has been used, if the same catheter is still functional it can offer a safe route for administration of anesthesia for the surgical procedure. Nevertheless, a major anesthetic (regional or general) should only be initiated after careful evaluation by the anesthesia service. Since the parturient may have an increased risk of regurgitation and aspiration of acidic gastric contents, many anesthesiologists prefer to wait a period of time following delivery in order to allow for increased gastric emptying. Postpartum sterilization is an elective procedure, and one should not proceed unless conditions are safe.

All patients requesting sterilization will have signed consent forms on a timely basis in accordance with local regulation and hospital policy. Appropriate counseling regarding risks of failure, permanency of the procedure, physical risks, and potential psychosocial reactions to the procedure shall have taken place well in advance of delivery. Last-minute patient ambivalence is not unusual and may indicate an advantage of deferring to an ambulatory procedure following the puerperium.

When a woman has had prior or concurrent psychologic difficulties, the risks and benefits of early postpartum sterilization must be carefully considered. In patients who have had medical or obstetric complications during their pregnancy or who have cardiovascular, respiratory, infectious, or metabolic abnormalities during the peripartum period (such as serious anemia, hypovolemia, upper respiratory infections, or hypertension), the procedure should be deferred unless there are overriding medical indications for proceeding. Major physiologic changes occur at delivery in all parturients. In particular, cardiovascular stability of the patient should be ensured.

In addition to such maternal considerations, special attention must also be paid to situations in which neonatal outcome is in doubt. Both infant survival and long-term well-being may ultimately influence a decision with respect to desire for a subsequent pregnancy.

Furthermore, consideration of overall number of patients in relationship to available staffing of the labor–delivery suite is also relevant. An elective procedure such as tubal ligation should not be attempted at a time when it might compromise other aspects of patient care. Thus, the decision to proceed with anesthesia and surgery should not only be a joint one between anesthesiologist and obstetrician, but one which also appropriately involves the patient and nursing and pediatric personnel.

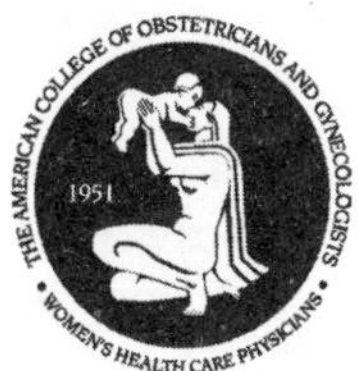

The American College of Obstetricians and Gynecologists
409 12th Street, SW • Washington, DC 20024-2188

3456/765

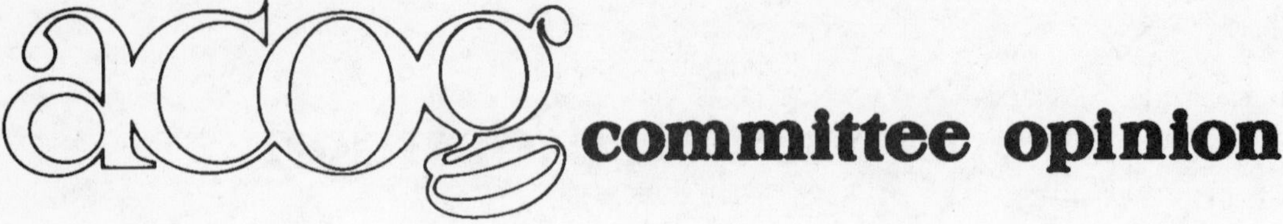

Committee on Ethics

Number 136—April 1994

Preembryo Research: History, Scientific Background, and Ethical Considerations

Research on the **preembryo*** has been surrounded with ethical questions for many years. These questions remain important because of the potential benefits to be gained from the research and the ongoing urgency of the ethical concerns both for and against it. This document does not assume the resolution of all debate on these questions; it acknowledges the diversity of ethical opinions among the members of the American College of Obstetricians and Gynecologists (ACOG) as among others in society at large. Positions range from complete rejection of all human preembryo research to approval of generating preembryos solely for research. Even among those who accept preembryo research on ethical grounds, there is disagreement about the conditions under which it may be carried out ethically. This document aims to present relevant considerations from the findings of contemporary embryology and to propose ethical guidelines for research.

HISTORICAL PERSPECTIVE: RESTRICTIONS AND POLICIES

In 1974, the U.S. Congress established the National Commission for the Protection of Human Subjects of Biomedical and Behavioral Research. The commission recommended and the government adopted guidelines for National Institutes of Health (NIH) funding of fetal research. In 1975, a federal regulation was adopted stating that "No application or proposal involving human in vitro fertilization may be funded by the Department [now Health and Human Services] or any component thereof until the application or proposal has been reviewed by the Ethical Advisory Board and the Board has rendered advice as to its acceptability from an ethical standpoint." (1). Consequently, a national Ethics Advisory Board (EAB) was established to review in vitro fertilization (IVF) research protocols and certain protocols for fetal research. In May 1978, the EAB agreed to review the ethics, legality, safety, efficacy, and scientific merit of IVF research receiving NIH support. In a May 4, 1979, report, the EAB agreed that "the human embryo is entitled to profound respect; but this respect does not necessarily encompass the full legal and moral rights attributed to persons." (2). The EAB statement supported research on the safety and efficacy of IVF and embryo transfer techniques to be used for the treatment of infertility. The EAB recommended allowing the use of **gametes** of informed and consenting **donors** in order to study the safety and efficacy of clinical IVF, provided that developing human cells not be sustained longer than 14 days in vitro. These recommendations have yet to be approved by the Secretary of Health and Human Services. In 1980, the EAB ceased to exist because of the Administration's unwillingness to appoint new members. Thus, until now, no federal support of IVF research has been permitted.

Despite the moratorium on federal funding for IVF research in the United States, private and university-based research has proceeded in the context of infertility treatment. The American Fertility Society (AFS) Committee on Ethics recognized the ethical dilemmas implicit in IVF research and recommended specific guidelines for conducting such research. The AFS noted that the preembryonic stage is considered to last until 14 days after **fertilization**. The AFS Committee on Ethics, in its 1986 and 1990 reports, recommended that human preembryos not be maintained for research beyond the 14th day after fertilization (3, 4). A 14-day limit was also recognized by the EAB in 1979, the Waller

*Terms defined in the glossary are shown in bold print.

Commission Report (Victoria, Australia) in 1984 (5), and the Warnock Committee Report (Great Britain) in 1984 (6).

In the absence of a national consensus, the climate in the United States has been influenced by these generally prudent and conservative recommendations. In 1991, the National Advisory Board on Ethics in Reproduction was established within the private sector. Among its goals, according to the board's statement of purpose, are providing a forum for public discussion and reviewing "such issues as in vitro fertilization research, research with early human embryos, research on preimplantation genetic diagnosis, and fetal tissue transplantation research."

Efforts to move forward with human preembryo research, then, have almost always been accompanied by a recognition of the need to deliberate about ethical problems and guidelines. Deliberations in this regard have often included a weighing of the importance of the research in relation to its risks to individuals and society and in relation to varying perceptions of the moral status of the preembryo.

THE BENEFITS AND RISKS OF HUMAN PREEMBRYO RESEARCH

Potential Benefits

The goals and objectives of preembryo research are numerous, varied, and—at least in some cases—relatively uncontroversial. They include, for example, the following:

- Increasing knowledge about embryogenesis and embryopathy
- Developing a better understanding of the biology of human **implantation**
- Understanding better the causes of spontaneous abortion
- Developing more effective or simpler forms of contraception
- Improving methods of IVF treatment for both male and female infertility
- Developing preembryo biopsy techniques for a preimplantation diagnosis of genetic or chromosomal abnormalities by new technologies such as DNA amplification
- Improving the technique of **microinjection** of **spermatozoa** directly into eggs

Risks of Harm

In all research, the value of the knowledge to be gained must be balanced with the risk of harm that is incurred. In the case of preembryo research, there are three areas of potential harm. First, some preembryo research, such as in vitro testing and genetic therapy, can be scientifically validated and clinically beneficial only if there is subsequent transfer of the preembryo to a woman's uterus in an attempt to achieve pregnancy. While such research may enhance the prospects for a normal, successful pregnancy, it may also reduce them. Second, preembryo research may be performed in a way that risks infringement of the rights of sperm and **oocyte** donors. Third, the harm that is of central concern to many, however, is the potential harm to the preembryo itself—not only damage but sometimes destruction, and the possible subjection of the preembryo to research that is not aimed at its own benefit. Allied to this is a concern that the manipulation of preembryos will diminish societal respect for human life in general. It is this third area of potential harms that has motivated the attention of national ethics advisory committees and commissions to the question of the moral status of the preembryo. As more and more biologic information has become available, it has shaped judgments regarding the degree of moral weight to be given to a preembryo. Since this information is relevant to many of the ethical questions surrounding preembryo research, it is useful to begin with the knowledge now available about the biologic processes involved.

FERTILIZATION AND PREEMBRYONIC DEVELOPMENT STAGES

The process out of which a human preembryo emerges is complex (Fig. 1) (7–11). The current scientific description of this process uses terms that are morally neutral and extremely helpful for identifying the biologic entity with which this document is concerned. Thus, for example, the preembryo refers to an entity in a stage of development that begins after fertilization and ends approximately 14 days later with the appearance of the **primitive streak** (that is, the band of cells at the caudal end of the **embryonic disc** from which the **embryo** develops). The characteristics of the preembryo, insofar as they are known, are understandable only within the details of the process that precedes the preembryo and the process of which it is itself a part. Hence, it is necessary to add some details to the description of fertilization and the early development that follows fertilization.

Fertilization

Fertilization is a complex biochemical process and sequence of events that takes approximately 24 hours after penetration of the oocyte by the sperm (12). It usually occurs in the fallopian tube at the end nearest the ovary. It begins with contact of the

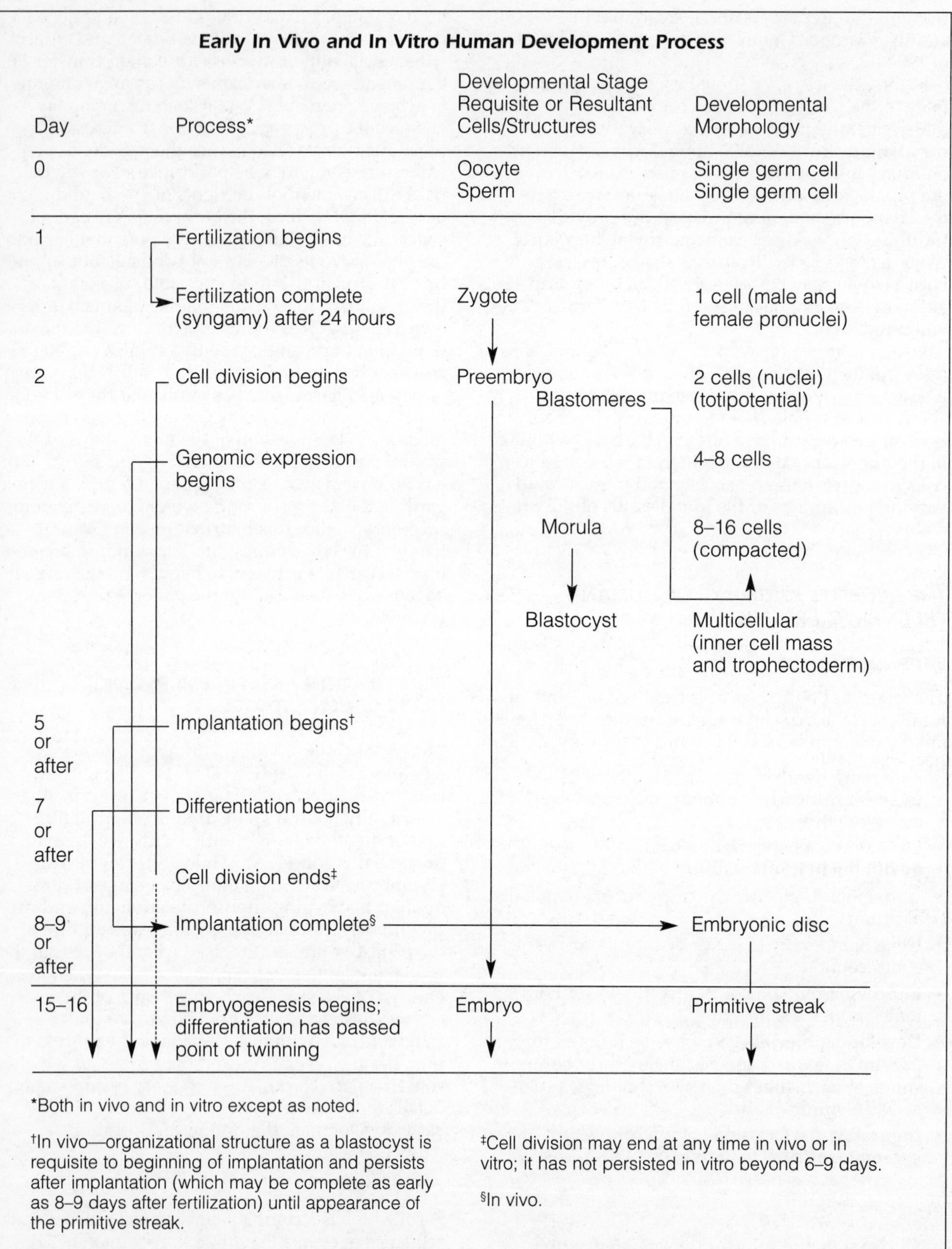

Early In Vivo and In Vitro Human Development Process
Day
Process*
Developmental Stage Requisite or Resultant Cells/Structures
Developmental Morphology
0
Oocyte
Sperm
Single germ cell
Single germ cell
1
Fertilization begins
Fertilization complete (syngamy) after 24 hours
Zygote
1 cell (male and female pronuclei)
2
Cell division begins
Preembryo
Blastomeres
2 cells (nuclei) (totipotential)
Genomic expression begins
4–8 cells
Morula
8–16 cells (compacted)
Blastocyst
Multicellular (inner cell mass and trophectoderm)
5 or after
Implantation begins†
7 or after
Differentiation begins
Cell division ends‡
8–9 or after
Implantation complete§
Embryonic disc
15–16
Embryogenesis begins; differentiation has passed point of twinning
Embryo
Primitive streak
*Both in vivo and in vitro except as noted.
†In vivo—organizational structure as a blastocyst is requisite to beginning of implantation and persists after implantation (which may be complete as early as 8–9 days after fertilization) until appearance of the primitive streak.
‡Cell division may end at any time in vivo or in vitro; it has not persisted in vitro beyond 6–9 days.
§In vivo.

FIG. 1. *Early in vivo and in vitro human development process.*

male and female gametes, continues with the gradual penetration of the sperm into the various layers of the oocyte, and is completed when the **pronuclei** of the sperm and oocyte lose their nuclear membranes and fuse to form a new cell called the **zygote**. Paternal and maternal genetic contributions during the fertilization process are from separate pronuclei; as separate entities, they can be experimentally removed from the process. The last stage of the mingling process is called **syngamy**. In this stage, the male and female **haploid** chromosome sets finally fuse, following the breakdown of their pronuclear membranes, into a zygote, a **diploid** cell with 46 chromosomes.

Early Preembryonic Development

After syngamy, the zygote undergoes mitotic cell division as it moves down the fallopian tube toward the uterus. The first division takes approximately 20 hours. A series of mitotic divisions then leads to the development of the preembryo. The newly divided cells are called **blastomeres**. From 1 to 3 days after syngamy, there is a division into two cells, then four cells. Approximately 3 days after syngamy, the developing entity reaches the eight-cell stage, and from 4 to 5 days, the eight- to sixteen-cell stages. Blastomeres form cellular aggregates of distinct, **totipotent**, undifferentiated cells that, during several early cell divisions, retain the capacity to develop independently into normal preembryos. Single blastomeres are distinct until after the eight- to sixteen-cell stages when changes occur in their membranes and cytoplasms that allow them to adhere more tightly to one another during the process of compaction to form the **morula**.

Several interesting observations can be made about the earliest stages of cell division. For example, with the first three and possibly four cell divisions (during the first 1 to 4 days after syngamy), there is no fusion between the individual cells. What exists is a loose collection of distinct totipotent cells (blastomeres) held together by the zona pellucida. Therefore, there is as yet no designation of an individual cell to become a specific entity or a particular part of an entity. In addition, early events such as chromosomal condensation and pronuclear formation may be controlled by factors within the oocyte cytoplasm prior to fertilization. Messenger RNA from the oocyte, along with oocyte organelles, supports the nutritional, synthetic, and energetic requirements of the preembryo. The function of the new genes of the preembryo cannot be detected until the four- to eight-cell stage, even though the 46 chromosomes of the developing entity (23 from the oocyte and 23 from the sperm) have associated at syngamy. Experimental evidence suggests that expression of the paternal genome does occur around the eight-cell stage (13, 14). Thus, the single- and two-cell stages of human development appear to be regulated by information derived from the oocyte (not from the fused gametes). Activation of gene function of the preembryo first occurs between the four- and eight-cell stages of development (36–72 hours after fertilization). Also, though the number of cells of the developing entity increases from two to four to eight, and so forth, the blastomeres produced at each cycle of division become progressively smaller; the size of the preembryo does not therefore increase at these stages. It remains essentially the size of the fertilized oocyte.

From 4 to 5 days after syngamy, the compacted morula develops into a **blastocyst**, which is a cellular aggregate with a central cavity, a **trophectoderm**, and a distinct **inner cell mass**. The multicellular blastocyst, now within the uterus, remains unattached in the uterine cavity fluid for approximately 48 hours. After this (now 5–7 days after syngamy), the process of implantation begins.

Implantation

As the blastocyst is in the process of attaching to the uterine wall, the cells increase in number and organize into two layers of cells. Implantation progresses as the outer cell layer of the blastocyst, the trophectoderm, invades the uterine wall and erodes blood vessels and glands. Having begun 5 or more days after fertilization with the attachment of the blastocyst to the endometrial lining of the uterus, implantation is completed when the blastocyst is fully embedded in the endometrium several days later. The extra-embryonic outer cell layer establishes a complex interaction with maternal uterine tissues to allow implantation to continue, and these cells give rise to the placenta and membranes. The inner cell mass is the progenitor of all the cells and cell types of the future embryo. But, at this time, these cells are not yet totally differentiated in terms of their determination to specific cells or organs of the embryo.

The term *preembryo*, then, includes the developmental stages from the first cell division of the zygote through the morula and the blastocyst. By approximately the 14th day after the end of the process of fertilization, all cells, depending on their position, will have become parts of the placenta and membranes or the embryo. The "embryo" stage, therefore, begins approximately 16 days after the beginning of the fertilization process and continues until the end of 8 weeks after fertilization, when organogenesis is complete.

ETHICAL RELEVANCE OF SCIENTIFIC INFORMATION

Scientific information alone cannot resolve questions about the moral status of the preembryo. Scientists themselves sometimes disagree in interpreting available data, and science is not the sole arbiter in debates about values. Nonetheless, embedded in scientific descriptions of the processes of preembryonic development are at least two factors that may influence the evaluation of the moral status of the preembryo—and, hence, the ethical arguments concerning preembryo research. These two factors, taken into account by national committees and commissions that have identified a 14-day limit for research on human preembryos, are the lack of individuation of the developing entity during that period and the natural failure of a high percentage of zygotes to develop into embryos.

Individuation or Singleness

From what is known of developing preembryos, their final individuation as entities with a concrete potential to become human persons is only accomplished with development of the primitive streak about 14 days after the completion of the fertilization process (15–17). Several factors are relevant to this observation. First, fertilization is not a momentary event but a 2-day process. Second, once fertilization is completed, there is an entity with a new genotype. But this entity is not, at its earliest stages, capable of expression (ie, **transcription**) of the new genotype, being regulated instead by information from the oocyte for continued growth and development. Third, relevant animal research has demonstrated that in the initial stages of preembryonic development a) up to at least the eight-cell stage, one or more blastomeres can be removed from the aggregate and the remainder can still produce a complete adult; b) individual blastomeres can be removed and develop into a complete individual; and c) cells derived from two preembryos of different genetic origin can aggregate into one larger mass and develop into one individual called a **chimera**. Fourth, and perhaps most notable, from the earliest stages of cell division all the way to the complete formation of the primitive streak, the preembryo is capable of dividing into more than one entity. Twinning may occur during the development of the inner cell mass, or, even later, the primitive streak may split and form two centers that organize the development of separate preembryos. Such splits and separations may be incomplete, resulting in the formation of conjoined twins. Hence, division and recombination may occur up to 14 days after fertilization. Only after this period of time has **differentiation** of embryonic cells advanced to the point that separation can no longer result in two or more individuals.

The evidence that there is, for approximately 14 days after fertilization is complete, not yet an individuated human entity determined for development as a single being is arguably relevant to an assessment of the moral status of the preembryo. It can yield a conclusion that the human preembryo does not possess the biologic individuality necessary for a concrete potentiality to become a human person, even though it does possess a unique human genotype. The preembryo can thus be considered valuable but not at the same level as a human person.

Spontaneous Early Preembryo Loss

Not unrelated to the issue of lack of individuation is the evidence that there is a naturally high percentage of loss of preembryos. That is, in unassisted human reproduction, the development and spontaneous loss of preembryos is a frequent occurrence (18–21). Traditionally, the generally accepted findings have been that 10–15% of clinically recognized pregnancies terminate in spontaneous abortion. Recent data based on the use of highly sensitive assays for human chorionic gonadotropin indicate that a significant number of losses occur subclinically. Research has shown that up to 60% of fertilizations do not survive long enough to result in a missed menstrual period. Approximately half of chemically detected pregnancies are lost during the first postovulatory week. This high rate of early losses may be due to errors in gametogenesis, defects in the fertilization process, developmental abnormalities after fertilization, or a delay in implantation secondary to altered tubal transport time. Whatever the reasons, natural reproduction occurs in such a way that over half (some estimates range as high as 78%) of fertilizations do not result in live births. According to available data, in vivo pregnancy loss is highest in the first 14 days after fertilization, precisely the same developmental period in which in vitro preembryo research would be taking place.

Successful fertilization and early cell division stages of the preembryo require a complex biochemical environment that can be artificially provided in the laboratory for some species. Investigators have not sustained viable in vitro human preembryos beyond 6–9 days after fertilization. Up to the point at which the in vitro human preembryo ceases to demonstrate cell division, the developmental changes that occur and the chances of loss are similar to those during in vivo development.

The high rate of loss of preembryos during in vivo development may undergird the conclusion that the moral status of preembryos is to be differentiated from that of embryos. The ACOG Committee on Ethics notes this, though it regards considerations of lack of settled individuality in the preembryo as a more significant basis for this conclusion.

ETHICAL CONSIDERATIONS

The context for the ethical recommendations and commentary that follow is the clinical situation in which prospective parents seek assistance in their goals of pregnancy and childbearing. In this context of treatment for infertility, some preembryos not ultimately dedicated to the goal of pregnancy may become available for research. Though generated for procreation, they become "spare" preembryos, and they may then (through their use in research) serve a secondary purpose of overcoming human problems of procreation in general.

The ethical question of whether preembryos should be generated solely for the purpose of scientific research is not explicitly addressed by these guidelines. Without the further ethical analysis required to evaluate this possibility, the ACOG Committee on Ethics takes only the position that it is preferable to use "spare" preembryos rather than to generate preembryos specifically for research. Reasons for this position include a concern not to place women at unnecessary risk during the required ovulation induction process and a preference for a process that is less vulnerable to the commercialization of gametes.

Guidelines

The ACOG Committee on Ethics recommends the following guidelines for clinical and laboratory research on the preembryo. Some of these guidelines parallel general ethical guidelines for research on human subjects, but some are particular to the case of research on human preembryos (22).

Research on the human preembryo may be conducted under the following conditions:

1. Research is conducted only by scientifically qualified persons and in settings that include appropriate and adequate resources and protections.
2. The question to be explored is scientifically valid in the sense that it takes into account scientific work to date.
3. The information sought offers potential scientific and clinical benefit relative to the growth and development of the preembryo or embryo.
4. The research objectives cannot be met through research on animals or on nonfertilized gametes.
5. The design of the research and each of its procedures is clearly formulated in a research protocol that is submitted to a specially appointed independent committee such as an Institutional Review Board (IRB) for evaluation, guidance, and approval. The protocol includes provision for detailed records of the study.
6. The research will be concluded at the earliest possible developmental stage of the preembryo.
7. Any preembryo that has undergone research will be transferred to a uterus only if the research was related to the preembryo's preparation for placement and there is reasonable scientific confidence in its normal development.
8. The research protocol does not involve the purchase or sale of preembryos.
9. Potential donors of gametes are adequately informed of the goals, methods, anticipated benefits, and potential hazards of research. Each potential donor is informed that she or he is at liberty to refuse participation in the research and to withdraw from the research.
10. Gamete donors are provided with the opportunity to determine, with adequate information and freedom, the disposition of preembryos. This presupposes an explicit policy on the part of the researchers and their sponsoring institutions—a policy that articulates options and that provides for informed donor choice.

Ethical Commentary on Guidelines

Because some of the guidelines express standard ethical and scientific requirements for research, they need no comment. Others, however, call for further clarification or support. Underlying all of the guidelines is the ethical position that if preembryo research is to be justifiable, it must be guided by a particular application of ethical standards parallel to those for research on human subjects. This position itself can now be more clearly focused along with clarifications of particular guidelines.

Guideline 4: Creating a Preliminary Knowledge Base for Human Research

Guideline 4 expresses the reasonable ethical maxim that human research should be engaged in only when alternative means of developing knowledge are inadequate. Whenever possible, animal models or cell and tissue culture systems should be used to advance the understanding of human biology. However, direct extrapolation of results from in vitro animal preembryo studies to humans can be misleading. Unfertilized oocytes also do not offer the same opportunities for knowledge of growth processes as do preembryos.

Guidelines 6–8: Limits to Preembryo Research

The ACOG Committee on Ethics takes the position that human preembryo research can be justified under certain conditions. This position is based on an interpretation of the moral status of the preembryo as a living entity with a human genetic code, deserving of some form of respect in itself and not solely for its usefulness in research. But this position also recognizes the value of the preembryo as relative, in the sense that it does not require the degree of protection and absolute respect that is accorded to human persons. In other words, the preembryo is human—not simply like other human tissue (for it is genetically unique and has human potential), but it is also not a human person, and does not as yet have within itself a determinate potential to become an individual human person (it lacks settled unity and individuality, and it evidences a high level of natural loss before implantation). On this interpretation, risks of harm to the preembryo in research can be justified, but not without limits. Preembryos, for example, ought not to be subjected to frivolous or poorly designed research programs; each succeeding developmental stage requires stronger justifications for doing research involving risk of harm; if the preembryos are designated for transfer to a uterus, the goals of successful pregnancy are given priority; the real and symbolic values of the preembryo are not negated or trivialized by treating them as commodities.

Guidelines 9–10: Donation and Consent

While informed consent of participants is a basic requirement in all human research, particular issues in decisions about preembryo research deserve elaboration. Among the most urgent of these issues is what to do with those preembryos that are not transferred to a uterus or are transferred only after research or a storage interval.

In order to enhance the probability that adequate numbers of normally developing preembryos will result, more oocytes are usually fertilized in vitro than will be transferred to the woman. If the number of resulting normally developing preembryos exceeds expectations, questions arise regarding the disposition of unused preembryos. Possible options may include **cryopreservation** of preembryos for the couple's future use, donation of preembryos to a recipient who is unable to produce usable oocytes or whose genetic background makes it inadvisable for her to use her own oocytes, donation of preembryos for research, and disposal of preembryos.

The appropriate individuals to exercise responsible decision-making regarding the disposition of preembryos are the persons who provide the gametes. Their informed consent is required before preembryos are used in research. The gamete donors in IVF should presumptively have an equal say in the use of their preembryos; therefore, the preembryos should not be used for research without the consent of both parties. If research is to be done on a preembryo that is to be transferred to a third party, this person and the persons who plan to rear the potential child (if different from the gamete donors) should also give informed consent.

Each IVF program should develop policies regarding the options of transfer, storage, donation, research, and discard. These policies should cover the disposition of gametes and of both normally developing preembryos and preembryos with a preimplantation diagnosis of genetic disease. They should include provision for counseling gamete providers and for fullest possible implementation of informed consent. Policies should be developed in light of ethical and legal considerations, and they should cover eventualities such as informing gamete providers of what will be done with preembryos in the absence of a written statement of the gamete providers' wishes.

Couples considering IVF therapy should be fully informed of the options available to them and of the policies of the IVF program. Their choices should be made in circumstances free of financial or other coercion. Full information should therefore include assurance that consent to donation of preembryos for research is not a condition for receiving services and that fee scales are not contingent upon consent to research. Gamete providers should also be made aware of the possible need for further choices in the future (eg, when cryopreservation is involved, passing time may alter circumstances and affect choices).

CONCLUSION

The ACOG Committee on Ethics has offered a position that approves preembryo research but limits it according to ethical guidelines. This position advocates treatment of the preembryo with respect but not the same level of respect as is given to human persons. It is a position that will be acceptable even to those who accord full respect to embryos and fetuses but not to those who believe that full respect ought to be extended to the gamete, zygote, and preembryo throughout the process of fertilization and beyond. In arriving at its position, the ACOG Committee on Ethics considered scientific and clinical information relevant to ethical analysis, though it recognizes the role of both scientific and ethical interpretation of what cannot be simply incontrovertible "facts."

The ACOG Committee on Ethics once again acknowledges that no single position can encompass the variety of opinions within the membership of ACOG, and it affirms that no physician should be required to participate in preembryo research if he or she finds it morally objectionable. Nonetheless, it is important to public discourse and to the practice of responsible medicine that physicians become aware of the medical and ethical issues involved in the complex area of preembryo research. To advance this discourse, it is helpful for physicians to reflect on and share the basis of their own views and to recognize and explore the ethical perspectives of their patients and colleagues.

GLOSSARY

Blastocyst: A stage in early human development that follows from the formation of the morula. The blastocyst is a sphere of cells containing a fluid-filled cavity forming about 4 days after fertilization and prior to the beginning of the process of implantation.

Blastomere: Each of the cells derived from the first and subsequent cell divisions of the zygote.

Chimera: An organism composed of cells derived from an aggregation of cells originating from two different genotypes. Such an aggregation is possible up to the eight-cell stage.

Cryopreservation: Storage by freezing.

Differentiation: The process of acquiring individual characteristics, as occurs in progressive diversification of cells and tissues of the developing preembryo and embryo.

Diploid: A cell having two chromosome sets, usually one maternal and one paternal, twice the haploid number (in humans, 46).

Donor: A person providing either sperm or ova.

Embryo: The stage in human development starting from about 2 weeks after fertilization, with organization around a single primitive streak, and continuing until the end of the eighth week after fertilization when all major structures are represented.

Embryonic disc: The group of cells from which the embryo will develop, usually visible at the end of the first week of development after fertilization in humans.

Fertilization: The process which renders gametes capable of further development; it begins when the sperm contacts the plasma membrane of the oocyte and ends with the formation of the zygote.

Gamete: A mature reproductive cell, usually haploid in chromosome number (eg, sperm or ovum).

Haploid: The chromosome number of a normal gamete (sperm or ovum). In humans, the haploid number is 23, representing one member of each chromosome pair.

Implantation: Attachment of the blastocyst to the endometrial lining of the uterus and subsequent embedding in the endometrium. Implantation begins at about 5–7 days after fertilization and may be complete as early as 8–9 days after fertilization.

Inner cell mass: The centrally located cells within the blastocyst; these cells will develop into the embryo.

Microinjection (of sperm): Injection of one or more sperm under the outer covering of the oocyte for fertilization.

Morula: A compact sphere of 16 blastomeres that forms at about 3–4 days after fertilization.

Oocyte: An immature female reproductive cell, one that has not completed the maturing process to form an ovum (gamete).

Ovum: The mature female germ cell after penetration of the sperm during fertilization and completion of the second meiotic division.

Preembryo: The developing cells produced by the division of the zygote until the formation of the embryo proper at the appearance of the primitive streak about 14 days after fertilization.

Primitive streak: The initial band of cells from which the embryo begins to develop, located at the caudal end of the embryonic disc. The primitive streak is present at about 15 days after fertilization.

Pronuclei: The egg and sperm nuclei after penetration of the sperm into the egg during fertilization.

Spermatozoa: Mature male germ cells (gametes).

Syngamy: The final stage of the fertilization process in which the haploid chromosome sets from the male and female gametes come together following breakdown of the pronuclear membranes to form the zygote.

Totipotent: Able to differentiate along any line; the capacity of a cell or group of cells to produce all of the products of conception—the extra-embryonic membrane and tissue, the embryo, and, subsequently, the fetus.

Transcription: Transfer of genetic code information from one kind of nucleic acid to another.

Trophectoderm: Peripheral cells of the blastocyst that form the membrane sac surrounding the embryo.

Zygote: The single cell formed by the union of the male and female haploid gametes at syngamy.

REFERENCES

1. U.S. Department of Health and Human Services. National Institutes of Health. Office for Protection from Research Risks. Protection of human subjects. 45 CFR §46.204 (d)
2. U.S. Department of Health, Education, and Welfare. Ethics Advisory Board. Report and conclusions: HEW support of research involving human in vitro fertiliza-

tion and embryo transfer. Washington, DC: Department of Health, Education, and Welfare, Ethics Advisory Board, 1979:101

3. American Fertility Society. Ethics Committee. Research on preembryos: justifications and limitations. Fertil Steril 1986;46(1 Suppl):56S–57S
4. American Fertility Society. Ethics Committee. Research on preembryos: justifications and limitations. Fertil Steril 1990;53(2 Suppl):62S–63S
5. Australia. Victoria. Committee to Consider the Social, Ethical and Legal Issues Arising from In Vitro Fertilization. Report on the disposition of embryos produced by in vitro fertilization. Melbourne, Australia: The Committee, 1984:47
6. Great Britain Department of Health and Social Security. Report of the Committee on Inquiry into human fertilization and embryology. London: Her Majesty's Stationery Office, 1984:66
7. Dimmick JE, Kalousek DK, eds. Developmental pathology of the embryo and fetus. Philadelphia: JB Lippincott, 1992:1–4
8. Moore KL, Persaud TVN. The developing human: clinically oriented embryology. 5th ed. Philadelphia: WB Saunders, 1993:29–34
9. Sadler TW. Langman's medical embryology. 6th ed. Baltimore: Williams and Wilkins, 1990:30–33
10. Jones HW Jr, Schrader C. And just what is a preembryo? Fertil Steril 1989;52:189–191
11. Grobstein C. The early development of human embryos. J Med Philos 1985;10:213–236
12. Veeck LL. Fertilization and early embryonic development. Curr Opin Obstet Gynecol 1992;4:702–711
13. Braude P, Bolton V, Stephen M. Human gene expression first occurs between the four- and eight-cell stages of preimplantation development. Nature 1988;332:459–461
14. O'Farrell PH, Edgar BA, Lakich D, Lehner CF. Directing cell division during development. Science 1989;246: 635–640
15. McCormick RA. Who or what is the preembryo? Kennedy Institute of Ethics Journal 1991;1(1):1–15
16. Grobstein C. Science and the unborn. New York: Basic Books, 1988:21–39
17. Society of Obstetricians and Gynaecologists of Canada Committee Report. Ethical considerations of the new reproductive technologies: III. Considerations on the status of human gametes and preembryos. J SOGC 1992;14(6):84–85
18. Chard T. Frequency of implantation and early pregnancy loss in natural cycles. Baillières Clin Obstet Gynaecol 1991;5(1):179–189
19. Wilcox AJ, Weinberg CR, Wehman RE, Armstrong EG, Canfield RE, Nisula BC. Measuring early pregnancy loss: laboratory and field methods. Fertil Steril 1985;44:366–374
20. Wilcox AJ, Weinberg CR, O'Connor JF, Baird DD, Schlatterer JP. Incidence of early loss of pregnancy. N Engl J Med 1988;319:189–194
21. Edmonds DK, Lindsay KS, Miller JF, Williamson E, Wood PJ. Early embryonic mortality in women. Fertil Steril 1982;38:447–453
22. Beauchamp TL, Walters L, eds. Research involving human subjects. In: Contemporary issues in bioethics. 2nd ed. Belmont, California: Wadsworth Publishing Co, 1982:503–568

BIBLIOGRAPHY

American College of Obstetricians and Gynecologists. Ethical issues in human in vitro fertilization and embryo placement. ACOG Committee Opinion 47. Washington DC: ACOG, 1986

American Fertility Society. Ethics Committee. Ethical considerations of the new reproductive technologies. Fertil Steril 1990;53(6[2 Suppl]):62s–63s

Australia. Victoria. Committee to Consider the Social, Ethical and Legal Issues Arising from In Vitro Fertilization. Report on the disposition of embryos produced by in vitro fertilization. Melbourne, Australia: The Committee, 1984

Great Britain Department of Health and Social Security. Report of the Committee on Inquiry into human fertilization and embryology. London: Her Majesty's Stationery Office, 1984

Grobstein C. Science and the unborn. New York: Basic Books, 1988

Seppälä M. Factors of importance for implantation. Baillières Clin Obstet Gynaecol 1991;5(1):1–252

Singer P, Kuhse H, Buckle S, Dawson K, Kaimba P, eds. Embryo experimentation. New York: Cambridge University Press, 1990

U.S. Department of Health, Education, and Welfare. Ethics Advisory Board. Report and conclusions: HEW support of research involving human in vitro fertilization and embryo transfer; and appendix. Washington, DC: Department of Health, Education, and Welfare, Ethics Advisory Board, 1979

U.S. Department of Health and Human Services. National Institutes of Health. Office for Protection from Research Risks. Protection of human subjects. 45 CFR 46

Walters L. Ethics and new reproductive technologies: an international review of committee statements. Hastings Cent Rep 1987;17(3 [Suppl]):3–9

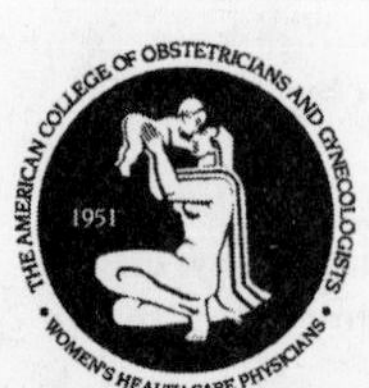

The American College of Obstetricians and Gynecologists
409 12th Street, SW • Washington, DC 20024-2188

12345/87654

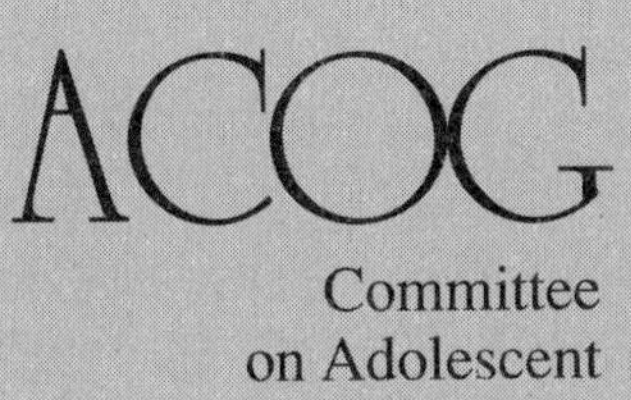

Committee on Adolescent Health Care

Committee Opinion

Number 190, October 1997

Prevention of Adolescent Suicide

The rate of adolescent suicide in the United States has tripled over the past 40 years (1). After accidents and homicide, suicide is the third leading cause of death in those aged 15–24 years and accounts for 13.7% (4,849) of all deaths in this group (2). Between 1952 and 1992, the rate of suicide among persons aged 15–19 years increased 386%; among persons aged 10–14 years, the rate increased 567% (2). Between 1980 and 1992, the rate of suicide for these same groups increased 28.3% and 120%, respectively (1). Although suicide rates among adolescent males exceed rates for females by nearly six to one, it is widely believed that females *attempt* suicide more frequently (3). No official national effort has been made to gather data on attempted suicides, primarily because surveillance of nonfatal suicide attempts is difficult and no well-developed surveillance system exists. Estimates of the ratio between attempted and completed suicides for young persons range from 50:1 to 200:1 (2, 4).

Methods of Suicide

Drug ingestion is the most frequent method of attempted suicide, particularly among adolescent females (5); the most common method of completed suicide among all adolescents is by firearms. The lethality of attempted suicide is high and increasing because of a corresponding increase in the use of firearms by suicidal adolescents. Between 1980 and 1992, firearms accounted for 81% of the increase in overall suicide rates for 15–19-year-olds; in 1992, they accounted for 64.9% of suicides among persons aged 25 years and younger (1). Although this method is preferred by males and contributes to their higher rate of completed suicides, most adolescent females who complete suicide also do so with a firearm. One factor that may explain the prominent role of firearms in adolescent suicide is the rise in gun ownership. Half of U.S. households now contain a gun.

Risk Factors

Risk factors for suicide include the presence of a mental disorder, especially major depressive disorder, bipolar disorder, conduct disorder, or psychosis; substance abuse; or family history of suicide. Particularly vulnerable are sexually abused youth, delinquents, gay and lesbian youth, runaways, and any adolescent living in nontraditional settings such as juvenile detention centers, prisons, halfway houses, or group homes. Because very high-achieving ado-

ISSN 1074-861X

The American College of Obstetricians and Gynecologists
409 12th Street, SW
PO Box 96920
Washington, DC 20090-6920

12345/10987

lescents, who may have personalities of rigid perfectionism, and impulsive youth also are at increased risk of suicide, "problem teens" are not the only group that clinicians need to evaluate for suicide potential. Stressors such as loss of a loved one through death, divorce, or breakup of a relationship; school problems; and interpersonal or family conflict are common precipitants. It is important to recognize that stressors the adult perceives as trivial may be very significant to the adolescent, precipitating a threat to self-worth and suicidal behavior. Family disorder, particularly family violence, is also an important risk factor because it lessens the likelihood of appropriate supportive responses to an adolescent crisis (5).

Although pregnancy has been suggested as a risk factor for suicide among adolescent girls, it is not. In fact, fewer than expected suicides, adjusted for age, occur during or following teen pregnancy. Divorced teen females, however, are at increased risk for suicide. It has been suggested that women of any age do not fully anticipate the economic and other hardships associated with divorce and are thus ill-prepared for the depression and role conflict that may follow the dissolution of their marriages (6). Media coverage of suicide, both fictional and nonfictional, can serve as a trigger for vulnerable teens to act on suicidal thoughts, as can exposure to a recent suicide or suicide attempt in the community ("cluster suicides") (7).

Depression is associated very strongly with suicide. The defining symptoms of depression are depressed mood, diminished interest or pleasure, and one or more of the following other symptoms: weight loss when not dieting or weight gain; insomnia or hypersomnia; fatigue or loss of energy; and indecisiveness or diminished ability to think or concentrate (8). Depression in adolescents, however, may not have the same clinical manifestations as in adults and may present as

- Isolation from family or friends
- Irritability or unusually argumentative and temperamental behavior
- Hyperactivity
- Delinquency
- School failure
- Repeated accidents or injuries

Sexual acting-out also may be a symptom of depression and may cause the adolescent to come to the attention of the obstetrician–gynecologist. Physical illness and consequent functional impairment (eg, inability to participate in school activities due to illness) have been found to contribute to suicidal behavior among adolescents (9). Although certain circumstances or events may seem to make depression more "understandable," they in no way lessen the importance of depression as a suicide risk factor.

Risk Assessment and Prevention

Obstetrician–gynecologists have a front-line opportunity for the primary prevention of adolescent suicide. Adolescents contemplating suicide rarely offer that information as a presenting complaint. Often, however, they feel relieved to have the subject broached. Accordingly, clinicians should ask directly about suicidal thoughts or fantasies. Most nonsuicidal patients will recognize an inquiry as indicative of concern and will not be offended. This subject may be addressed as part of background questioning in the context of family, school, and relationships. Questions should be asked in a nonjudgmental, direct, and nonthreatening manner:

1. "Sometimes patients I've seen dealing with similar issues/problems get very down and start to question life itself. Does this happen to you?"
2. "Have you ever thought about suicide?"
3. "Are you thinking about suicide now?"
4. "Do you have a plan for committing suicide?"
5. If yes, "What is your plan for committing suicide?"
6. "Have you ever attempted suicide?"

A positive response indicates the need for further questioning and an assessment of risk factors that could increase the suicide potential.

The degree of risk at any particular encounter should, to the extent possible, be fully assessed, and any response or intervention should be based on the level of risk. Significant insight is gained into the intent of the suicidal thought by analyzing the method and location of a planned suicide. Ingesting over-the-counter drugs in a location where the individual is likely to be discovered suggests a gesture that is looking for a response, whereas planning to use a firearm indicates strong intent on the part of the individual to accomplish the suicide (5, 10).

Low Risk

A low-risk profile is one where there is ambivalence about wanting to die, no history of prior attempts, no alcohol or drug abuse, and no suicide plan. Additionally, this teen will have good family or peer support, will experience suicidal thoughts that are mild and transient, and will exhibit receptivity to getting help. This patient should be encouraged to enlist the assistance of family and significant others, consider counseling, and see a health professional weekly until the crisis is resolved.

Moderate Risk

A moderate-risk situation is one in which there is a psychiatric history or a history of suicide attempts. If this patient uses drugs or alcohol, their effects may increase the risk of suicide. These patients may have more persistent thoughts of death or suicide, but their plans are only vaguely formulated or incompatible with methods available to them. Involvement of families and mental health practitioners is critical. Although this situation calls for expedient linkage with a mental health professional, other health professionals can assist in this process. If depression is diagnosed and antidepressants are considered, referral to a psychiatrist or a provider with additional training may be appropriate.

High Risk

Evidence of high risk for suicide can include psychotic thinking, depression, or unremitting crisis, particularly when an adolescent has formulated a clear suicide plan and has the means to carry it out (such as a household firearm the patient intends to use) or when the ability to regulate behavior is compromised (eg, by substance use). Risk is especially high when the adolescent is cut off from or rejects resources or family support. If an adolescent appears at high risk for suicide, immediate referral to a mental health clinician for surveillance, psychiatric evaluation, and psychotherapeutic intervention is indicated. If psychiatric evaluation is not immediately available, referral to a hospital emergency department for possible admission to protect the patient from self-harm may be indicated.

Conclusion

Counseling techniques for the suicidal adolescent should emphasize that the patient's current emotional state is temporary and treatable, offering alternatives to deal with the problem (5, 10). "No-suicide" contracts in which the adolescent pledges not to attempt suicide often are helpful but should not be relied upon to prevent a suicide (11). Teens frequently request that their suicidal thoughts not be revealed. It is important to avoid being sworn to secrecy or making promises that cannot be kept because suicidal intent is not information that can be kept confidential. Moreover, it is imperative that, where applicable, the family of an adolescent at risk be advised immediately to make firearms in the home inaccessible and to remove all medications from the medicine chest.

Physicians have an important role in addressing the problem of adolescent suicide. The rising rate of adolescent suicide mandates an increasing awareness of depressive disorders, anxiety disorders, and chemical dependence in this population. Physicians should be prepared to assess suicide risk and, when necessary, provide immediate counseling or referral to mental health clinicians. Each patient encounter may be the only opportunity for intervention and may be, in fact, life saving.

References

1. Suicide among children, adolescents, and young adults—United States, 1980–1992. MMWR 1995;44:289–291
2. Gardner P, Hudson BL. Advance report of final mortality statistics, 1993. Monthly Vital Statistics Report; vol 44, no 7 (suppl 1). Hyattsville, Maryland: National Center for Health Statistics, 1996
3. National Institutes of Mental Health, suicide facts. Bethesda, Maryland: National Institute of Mental Health, June 1996
4. Sells CW, Blum RW. Morbidity and mortality among US adolescents: an overview of data and trends. Am J Publ Health 1996;86:513–519
5. Berman AL, Jobes DA. Adolescent suicide. Assessment and intervention. Washington, DC: American Psychological Association, 1991
6. Stack S. New microlevel data on the impact of divorce on suicide. 1959–1980: a test of two theories. J Marriage Fam 1990;52:119–127
7. Gould MS, Shaffer D. The impact of suicide in television movies. Evidence of imitation. N Engl J Med 1986;315: 690–694
8. American Psychiatric Association. Diagnostic and statistical manual of mental disorders (DSM-IV). 4th ed. Washington, DC: American Psychiatric Association, 1994
9. Lewinsohn P, Rohde P, Seeley JR. Adolescent suicidal ideation and attempts: prevalence, risk factors, and clinical implications. Clin Psychol Sci Pract 1996;3:25–46
10. Tishler CL. Adolescent suicide. Assessment of risk, prevention, and treatment. Adolesc Med 1992;3:51–59
11. Jacobs D. The no-suicide contract. Forum 1992;18:9

ACOG Committee Opinion

Committee on Obstetric Practice

Number 173, June 1996

Prevention of Early-Onset Group B Streptococcal Disease in Newborns

During the past two decades, group B streptococci (GBS), or *Streptococcus agalactiae*, has emerged as an important cause of perinatal morbidity and mortality. The gram-positive organism can colonize the lower gastrointestinal tract, and secondary spread to the genitourinary tract is common. Between 10 to 30% of pregnant women are colonized with GBS in the vaginal or rectal areas (1–4). The organism may cause urinary tract infection, amnionitis, endometritis, and wound infection in women who are pregnant or recently delivered. Recently, a multistate active surveillance system in a population of 10 million persons found that 6% of early-onset GBS infections resulted in death (5). Morbidity due to overwhelming sepsis and to neurologic sequelae of meningitis is also clinically important but more difficult to estimate.

Vertical transmission of GBS during labor or delivery may result in invasive infection in the newborn during the first week of life. This is known as early-onset GBS infection and constitutes approximately 80% of GBS disease in the newborn. Late-onset GBS disease in the newborn may be the result of vertical transmission or of nosocomial or community-acquired infection. Invasive GBS disease in the newborn is characterized primarily by sepsis, pneumonia, or meningitis. Annually, approximately 7,600 episodes of GBS sepsis occur in newborns (a rate of 1.8/1,000 live births) in the United States and result in about 310 deaths among infants less than 90 days of age, a case–fatality rate of 5–20% (5–7).

Factors Associated with Early-Onset Disease

A number of obstetric factors have been associated with an increased likelihood of early-onset GBS disease in the newborn (8). These include prenatal cultures colonized with GBS, premature deliveries, prolonged rupture of membranes, or intrapartum fever. The incidence of GBS disease is also higher among infants born to African–American mothers (5, 9) and to mothers less than 20 years of age (9–10). Also more likely to be infected are neonates born to mothers with a history of birth of an infant with GBS disease (11–13), heavy colonization such as that seen with GBS bacteriuria (14–18), and low levels of anti-GBS capsular antibody (19). An apparent increased risk in twins may be attributable to the increased frequency of prematurity and of low birth weight with multiple gestations (20–21).

ISSN 1074-861X

The American College of Obstetricians and Gynecologists
409 12th Street, SW
PO Box 96920
Washington, DC 20090-6920

12345/09876

Ideally, GBS disease would be prevented by active immunization of the mother and newborn. As yet, vaccines have not been developed for clinical use. Therefore, the primary strategy for preventing GBS disease is chemoprophylaxis using antibiotics. Several strategies have been recommended for the prevention of early-onset GBS, including intrapartum chemoprophylaxis that is based on risk factors such as GBS carriers identified by culture during pregnancy and certain intrapartum complications.

Several studies of colonized women who were treated during the third trimester found that a wide range of patients (20–70%) remained colonized at term (22–24). In one study of 20 colonized women treated in the third trimester, however, none of the 19 who were reexamined at term by culture remained colonized (25). Similarly, immediate postnatal treatment with antibiotics has not been shown to be effective in reducing overall mortality from infection (26–28). In one study, this finding was related partly to higher mortality resulting from penicillin-resistant pathogens (27). Because GBS infection may be acquired in utero, the administration of antimicrobial agents to the newborn, while important in the treatment of infection, will not always prevent early-onset GBS disease.

Intrapartum administration of antibiotics to the mother (during labor or after rupture of the membranes, but before delivery) has been demonstrated to reduce early-onset neonatal GBS disease. Several investigators have found that antibiotics administered intrapartum to all women determined to be colonized by prenatal cultures has reduced the incidence of early-onset disease (29–32). Others have found a benefit of selective administration of intrapartum antibiotics to colonized women on the basis of the development of other intrapartum risk factors such as premature labor, prolonged rupture of membranes, and intrapartum fever (33–34). Studies focused specifically on prophylactic treatment on the basis of prolonged rupture of membranes (35) and heavy genital colonization (36–37) have also been reported. A recent metaanalysis of seven trials studied groups of women, all of whom were carriers or were carriers with additional obstetric risk factors (38). They estimated a 30-fold reduction in early-onset GBS disease with the administration of intrapartum chemoprophylaxis.

Appropriate culture technique requires obtaining a swab from the lower vagina (introitus) and perianal area and using selective broth media. Obtaining the culture does not require visualization of the cervix with a speculum. Use of prenatal cultures remote from term to identify women who are colonized with GBS at delivery is controversial. Many of the aforementioned studies primarily have used cultures taken early in the third trimester. In one study, 7.4% of women who had negative cultures at 26–28 weeks of gestation were found to carry GBS at delivery, and a single positive culture during pregnancy had a 67% predictive value at delivery (4). The estimated sensitivity and specificity were 70.0% and 90.4%, respectively. Among 26 women who delivered within 5 weeks after a culture was obtained, there were no false-positive or false-negative culture results (4). In another study of 16 infants who developed early-onset GBS disease, 14 (88%) were born to mothers who had positive prenatal cultures (34). Larger studies evaluating the sensitivity, specificity, and predictive value of a positive culture close to delivery are urgently needed.

Strategies for Antibiotic Prophylaxis

Different strategies for selecting women to receive intrapartum antibiotic prophylaxis of early-onset GBS disease in newborns have been proposed. Boyer and Gotoff, on the basis of findings of their own studies, recommend 26–28-week cultures followed by intrapartum antibiotic prophylaxis for those women identified as GBS carriers who subsequently had rupture of membranes greater than 12 hours, onset of labor or rupture of membranes at less than 37 weeks of gestation, or intrapartum fever (39). They estimate that this strategy will result in intrapartum treatment of approximately 3.4% of women and prevent one half of early-onset GBS disease in newborns. These figures will vary, depending on differences in populations for whom care is being provided. In 1992, this approach was endorsed in a statement issued by the American Academy of Pediatrics (40). The statement extended intrapartum risk factors to include multiple gestation in a GBS carrier and previous birth of an infant with GBS disease.

In contrast, the American College of Obstetricians and Gynecologists (ACOG) has supported use of intrapartum antibiotic prophylaxis based on the clinical risk factors of preterm labor (less than 37 weeks), preterm premature rupture of membranes (preterm PROM) (less than 37 weeks), rupture of membranes greater than 18 hours, previous birth of a child with GBS disease, or maternal fever during labor (greater than or equal to 38°C or 100.4°F). The ACOG criterion of greater than 18 hours of rupture of membranes was selected on the basis of an observational study by Boyer et al demonstrating a statistically significant increase in attack rate of GBS with rupture of membranes more than 18 hours (4). The strategy supported by ACOG did not incorporate the use of cultures because of several concerns. These included the potential acquisition of GBS following a negative culture in patients who might later develop an intrapartum risk factor and concern about the predictive value of positive cultures remote from term.

Rouse et al reported a decision analysis of 19 different strategies for the prevention of early-onset neonatal GBS sepsis (41). In the absence of randomized clinical trials, this type of analysis allows consideration of which strategies may be reasonable for clinical use and further study. The difference in approaches for the prevention of early-onset GBS disease has caused considerable controversy and confusion among providers of obstetric care as to the most appropriate strategy to use in clinical practice (42–43). This confusion has occurred because the ideal strategy for prevention of early-onset GBS in clinical practice has not been scientifically determined. No clinical trials comparing these different strategies have been conducted. To compare the efficacy of the strategies using antepartum culture and selective intrapartum prophylaxis with intrapartum prophylaxis based on clinical risk factors alone, estimates are that at least 100,000 pregnant women would need to be studied in each arm of a randomized prospective trial (44). It is, therefore, unlikely that a study will resolve the controversy. However, either of these two strategies is expected to reduce the occurrence of early-onset GBS disease significantly. Nevertheless, it should be noted that neither will prevent all early-onset GBS disease.

Recently, the Centers for Disease Control and Prevention (CDC) issued recommendations for the active prevention of GBS (43). The ACOG Committee on Obstetric Practice concurs with those recommendations. The recommendations relevant to maternal care are listed in the appendix. Important differences from previous recommendations include the following:

- The use of *either* a strategy based on late prenatal culture (35–37 weeks) as the primary risk determinant *or* a strategy based solely on clinical risk factors
- The offer, when the culture-based strategy is used, of intrapartum antibiotic prophylaxis to all women who have a positive culture, irrespective of intrapartum risk factors
- The use of penicillin as an alternative to ampicillin for prophylaxis

In addition, CDC provides a sample empiric-care algorithm for management of newborns born to mothers who received intrapartum antimicrobial prophylaxis for GBS disease (not included in the appendix).

Commentary

The Committee supports the recommendation that obstetric providers adopt a strategy for the prevention of early-onset GBS disease in the newborn. This strategy should be based on intrapartum administration of antibiotic agents to patients at increased risk of delivering an infant who develops GBS disease. Risk may be based solely on clinical risk factors or late prenatal cultures for GBS. The Committee concurs with the specific drugs, dosage, and routes of administration recommended by CDC (see appendix). Patients should be informed of the GBS prevention strategy used. This may be accomplished by providing patient information materials such as the patient information pamphlet produced by ACOG.

If the strategy adopted by the provider is based solely on clinical risk factors, some patients may request that GBS cultures be done. Such requests from informed patients should be honored by obtaining culture at 35–37 weeks of gestation as recommended by CDC (45). Cultures taken remote from term, particularly during early pregnancy, may have less predictive value for carrier status at delivery and are *not* recommended, nor is antepartum treatment for GBS carriers.

Irrespective of the strategy adopted by the obstetric provider, all women who have had a previous infant with GBS disease or who have had GBS bacteriuria during the current pregnancy should be offered intrapartum chemoprophylaxis.

Neither the strategy using late prenatal culture (35–37 weeks of gestation) as the primary indicator of risk nor the strategy based on intrapartum risk factors alone has been evaluated extensively in clinical practice or compared by randomized controlled trials. Approximately 4% of neonates born to women who are carriers and who have intrapartum clinical risk factors are expected to have GBS disease. By comparison, 0.5% (1 in 200) of neonates born to women who are carriers but have no other risk factors are expected to have GBS disease. When a strategy is used that incorporates late prenatal cultures and offers of intrapartum chemoprophylaxis to women who are carriers but have no other risk factors, most of these women can be expected to accept intrapartum treatment. Using a number of assumptions, Rouse and colleagues have estimated that this strategy will result in intrapartum treatment of 26.7% of women and prevent 86% of early-onset GBS in the newborn (41). Similarly, using a number of assumptions, a strategy based solely on intrapartum risk factors could result in intrapartum treatment of 18.3% of women and prevent 68.8% of early-onset GBS in the newborn (41). Because these are estimates, they will need further validation and comparison in clinical practice.

The Committee is concerned that with implementation of these strategies, the widespread use of intrapartum prophylaxis (eg, up to 18.3% or 26.7% of women) will lead to emergence of resistant pathogens. Also, the benefit of GBS prevention must be weighed against the risk to the mother and the fetus of maternal allergic reactions during labor. Although the risk of fatal anaphylaxis has been estimated at 1 per 100,000, the risk of less severe anaphylactic or allergic reactions to the laboring mother and fetus are important (46–47). The Committee agrees with CDC that local responsible health agencies should establish surveillance systems to monitor the incidence of early-onset neonatal GBS disease, the emergence of infection in mothers and newborns that is caused by resistant organisms, and other complications of widespread maternal antibiotic administration such as severe allergic reactions.

Comparative scientific evidence is insufficient for the Committee to determine criteria for the provider or obstetric service to use in selecting one of the two recommended strategies. In considering which strategy to adopt, practitioners and obstetric services may wish to consider a number of factors that may affect the implementation or effectiveness of one strategy or the other in their patient population. These may include, but not be limited to, GBS carrier rates in the population served, the frequency of obstetric complications that are associated with an increased risk of early-onset GBS disease in the newborn (eg, prematurity, preterm PROM, and fever in labor), and practical considerations regarding implementation. Information system technology now available theoretically could significantly enhance access to culture results. The potential benefits of information technology, however, have not yet been fully realized in actual clinical practice. Lack of prompt availability of culture results may render use of late prenatal cultures impractical in some settings.

Irrespective of the strategy adopted, the Committee believes that if the results of late prenatal cultures are not available, intrapartum prophylaxis should be offered only on the basis of the presence of intrapartum risk factors for early-onset GBS disease. This is consistent with CDC recommendations.

The Committee lacks sufficient evidence for recommending a course of management, specifically predelivery antibiotic prophylaxis for prevention of early onset GBS disease in newborns, for women with positive GBS culture results who have elective cesarean delivery with intact membranes. Evidence is also insufficient to recommend a single course of management when a woman has preterm PROM at less than 37 weeks of gestation. Culture for GBS should be obtained in all women with preterm PROM. Following culture, antibiotic prophylaxis may be withheld. Antibiotics should be started if positive culture results are obtained or if labor begins before culture results are available. An acceptable alternative approach is to initiate prophylactic antibiotics until culture results are available. Treatment can be discontinued if the culture is negative for GBS. The appropriate duration of treatment for patients who have preterm PROM and positive GBS cultures has not been determined.

References

1. Anthony BF, Okada DM, Hobel CJ. Epidemiology of group B streptococcus: longitudinal observations during pregnancy. J Infect Dis 1978;137:524–530
2. Regan JA, Klebanoff MA, Nugent RP. The epidemiology of group B streptococcal colonization in pregnancy. Vaginal Infections and Prematurity Study Group. Obstet Gynecol 1991;77:604–610
3. Dillon HC Jr, Gray E, Pass MA, Gray BM. Anorectal and vaginal carriage of group B streptococci during pregnancy. J Infect Dis 1982;145:794–799
4. Boyer KM, Gadzala CA, Kelly PD, Burd LI, Gotoff SP. Selective intrapartum chemoprophylaxis of neonatal group B streptococcal early-onset disease. II. Predictive value of prenatal cultures. J Infect Dis 1983;148:802–809
5. Zangwill KM, Schuchat A, Wenger JD. Group B streptococcal disease in the United States, 1990: report from a multistate active surveillance system. MMWR 41(6): 25–32
6. Baker CJ, Edwards MS. Group B streptococcal infections. In: Remington JS, Klein JO, eds. Infectious diseases of the fetus and newborn infant. 4th ed. Philadelphia: WB Saunders, 1995:980–1054
7. Weisman LE, Stoll BJ, Cruess DF, Hall RT, Merenstein GB, Hemming VG. Early-onset group B streptococcal sepsis: a current assessment. J Pediatr 1992;121:428–433
8. Boyer KM, Gotoff SP. Strategies for chemoprophylaxis of GBS early-onset infections. Antibiot Chemother 1985;35: 267–280
9. Schuchat A, Oxtoby M, Cochi S, Sikes RK, Hightower A, Plikaytis B, et al. Population-based risk factors for neonatal group B streptococcal disease: results of a cohort study in metropolitan Atlanta. J Infect Dis 1990;162:672–677
10. Schuchat A, Deaver-Robinson K, Plikaytis BD, Zangwill KM, Mohle-Boetani J, Wenger JD. Multistate case-control study of maternal risk factors for neonatal group B streptococcal disease. The Active Surveillance Group. Pediatr Infect Dis J 1994;13:623–629
11. Carstensen H, Christensen KK, Grennert L, Persson K, Polberger S. Early-onset neonatal group B streptococcal septicaemia in siblings. J Infect 1988;17:201–204
12. Faxelius G, Bremme K, Kvist-Christensen K, Christensen P, Ringertz S. Neonatal septicemia due to group B streptococcal–perinatal risk factors and outcome of subsequent pregnancies. J Perinat Med 1988;16:423–430

13. Christensen KK, Dahlander K, Linden V, Svenningsen N, Christensen P. Obstetrical care in future pregnancies after fetal loss in group B streptococcal septicemia. A prevention program based on bacteriological and immunological follow-up. Eur J Obstet Gynecol Reprod Biol 1981;12: 143–150
14. Pass MA, Gray BM, Khare S, Dillon HC Jr. Prospective studies of group B streptococcal infections in infants. J Pediatr 1979;95:437–443
15. Wood EG, Dillon HC Jr. A prospective study of group B streptococcal bacteriuria in pregnancy. Am J Obstet Gynecol 1981;140:515–520
16. Moller M, Thomsen AC, Borch K, Dinesen K, Zdravkovic M. Rupture of fetal membranes and premature delivery associated with group B streptococci in urine of pregnant women. Lancet 1984;2(8394):69–70
17. Liston TE, Harris RE, Foshee S, Null DM Jr. Relationship of neonatal pneumonia to maternal urinary and neonatal isolates of group B streptococci. South Med J 1979;72: 1410–1412
18. Persson K, Christensen KK, Christensen P, Forsgren A, Jorgensen C, Persson PH. Asymptomatic bacteriuria during pregnancy with special reference to group B streptococci. Scand J Infect Dis 1985;17:195–199
19. Baker CJ, Kasper DL. Correlation of maternal antibody deficiency with susceptibility to neonatal group B streptococcal infection. N Engl J Med 1976;294:753–756
20. Pass MA, Khare S, Dillon HC Jr. Twin pregnancies: incidence of group B streptococcal colonization and disease. J Pediatr 1980;97:635–637
21. Edwards MS, Jackson CV, Baker CJ. Increased risk of group B streptococcal disease in twins. JAMA 1981;245: 2044–2046
22. Hall RT, Barnes W, Krishnan L, Harris DJ, Rhodes PG, Fayez J. Antibiotic treatment of parturient women colonized with group B streptococci. Am J Obstet Gynecol 1976;124:630–634
23. Gardner SE, Yow MD, Leeds LJ, Thompson PK, Mason EO Jr, Clark DJ. Failure of penicillin to eradicate group B streptococcal colonization in the pregnant woman. A couple study. Am J Obstet Gynecol 1979;135:1062–1065
24. Lewin EB, Amstey MS. Natural history of group B streptococcus colonization and its therapy during pregnancy. Am J Obstet Gynecol 1981;139:512–515
25. Merenstein GB, Todd WA, Brown G, Yost CC, Luzier T. Group B beta-hemolytic streptococcus: randomized controlled treatment study at term. Obstet Gynecol 1980;55: 315–318
26. Pyati SP, Pildes RS, Jacobs NM, Ramamurthy RS, Heh TF, Raval DS, et al. Penicillin in infants weighing two kilograms or less with early-onset group B streptococcal disease. N Engl J Med 1983;308:1383–1389
27. Siegel JD, McCracken GH Jr, Threlkeld N, Milvenan B, Rosenfeld CR. Single dose penicillin prophylaxis against neonatal group B streptococcal infections. A controlled trial in 18,738 newborn infants. N Engl J Med 1980;303: 769–775
28. Siegel JD, McCracken GH Jr, Threlkeld N, DePasse BM, Rosenfeld CR. Single-dose penicillin prophylaxis of neonatal group B streptococcal disease. Lancet 1982; 1(8287):1426–1430
29. Matorras R, Garcia-Perea A, Omenaca F, Diez-Enciso M, Madero R, Usandizaga JA. Intrapartum chemoprophylaxis of early-onset group B streptococcal disease. Eur J Obstet Gynecol Reprod Biol 1991;40:57–62
30. Lim DV, Morales WJ, Walsh AF, Kazanis D. Reduction of morbidity and mortality rates for neonatal group B streptococcal disease through early diagnosis and chemoprophylaxis. J Clin Microbiol 1986;23:489–492
31. Allardice JG, Baskett TF, Seshia MM, Bowman N, Malazdrowicz R. Perinatal group B streptococcal colonization and infection. Am J Obstet Gynecol 1982;142:617–620
32. Garland SM, Fliegner JR. Group B streptococcus (GBS) and neonatal infections: the case for intrapartum chemoprophylaxis. Aust N Z J Obstet Gynaecol 1991;31:119–122
33. Boyer KM, Gadzala CA, Burd LI, Fisher DE, Paton JB, Gotoff SP. Selective intrapartum chemoprophylaxis of neonatal group B streptococcal early-onset disease. I. Epidemiologic rationale. J Infect Dis 1983;148:795–801
34. Boyer KM, Gotoff SP. Antimicrobial prophylaxis of neonatal group B streptococcal sepsis. Clin Perinatol 1988;15: 831–850
35. Morales WJ, Lim D. Reduction of group B streptococcal maternal and neonatal infections in preterm pregnancies with premature rupture of membranes through a rapid identification test. Am J Obstet Gynecol 1987;157:13–16
36. Morales WJ, Lim DV, Walsh AF. Prevention of neonatal group B streptococcal sepsis by the use of a rapid screening test and selective intrapartum chemoprophylaxis. Am J Obstet Gynecol 1986;155:979–983
37. Tuppurainen N, Hallman M. Prevention of neonatal group B streptococcal disease: intrapartum detection and chemoprophylaxis of heavily colonized parturients. Obstet Gynecol 1989;73:583–587
38. Allen UD, Navas L, King SM. Effectiveness of intrapartum penicillin prophylaxis in preventing early-onset group B streptococcal infection: results of a meta-analysis. Can Med Assoc J 1993;149:1659–1665
39. Boyer KM, Gotoff SP. Prevention of early-onset neonatal group B streptococcal disease with selective intrapartum chemoprophylaxis. N Engl J Med 1986;314:1665–1669
40. American Academy of Pediatrics Committee on Infectious Diseases and Committee on Fetus and Newborn. Guidelines for prevention of group B streptococcal (GBS) infection by chemoprophylaxis. Pediatrics 1992;90:775–778
41. Rouse DJ, Goldenberg RL, Cliver SP, Cutter GR, Mennemeyer ST, Fargason CA Jr. Strategies for the prevention of early-onset neonatal group B streptococcal sepsis: a decision analysis. Obstet Gynecol 1994;83:483–494
42. Towers CV. Group B streptococcus: the US controversy. Lancet 1995;346:197–199
43. Centers for Disease Control and Prevention. Prevention of perinatal group B streptococcal disease: a public health perspective. MMWR 1996;45(RR-7):1–24
44. Landon MB, Harger J, McNellis D, Mercer B, Thom EA. Prevention of neonatal group B streptococcal infection. Obstet Gynecol 1994;84:460–462
45. American College of Obstetricians and Gynecologists. Ethical guidance for patient testing. ACOG Committee Opinion 159. Washington DC: ACOG, 1995
46. Schwartz B, Schuchat A, Oxtoby MJ, Cochi SL, Hightower A, Broome CV. Invasive group B streptococcal disease in adults. A population-based study in metropolitan Atlanta. JAMA 1991;266:1112–1114

47. Gilman AG, Rall TW, Nies AS, Taylor P. Goodman and Gilman's the pharmacological basis of therapeutics. 8th ed. New York: Pergamon Press, 1990

Appendix

CDC Recommendations for GBS Prophylaxis*

1. Obstetric care practitioners, in conjunction with supporting laboratories and labor and delivery facilities, should adopt a strategy for the prevention of early-onset GBS disease in neonates. Patients should be informed regarding the GBS prevention strategy available to them. Individual patient requests regarding GBS cultures should be honored. Insurance coverage for obstetrical care should include payment for GBS cultures.
2. Regardless of the preventive strategy used, women should be managed as follows:
   a) Treat women found to have symptomatic or asymptomatic GBS bacteriuria during pregnancy at the time of diagnosis. Because such women are usually heavily colonized with GBS, they should receive intrapartum chemoprophylaxis.
   b) Give intrapartum chemoprophylaxis to women with a history of previously giving birth to an infant with GBS disease; prenatal screening is not necessary.
3. Until further data become available to define the most effective prevention strategy, the following strategies are appropriate:
   a) Screen all pregnant women at 35–37 weeks gestation for anogenital GBS colonization (Fig. 1). Patients should be informed of screening results and of potential benefits and risks of intrapartum chemoprophylaxis for GBS carriers. Information systems should be developed and monitored to assure that prenatal culture results are available at the time and place of delivery. Offer intrapartum chemoprophylaxis to all pregnant women identified as GBS carriers by culture at 35–37 weeks.
      i) If the result of GBS cultures is not known at the time of labor, intrapartum chemoprophylaxis should be administered if one of the following is present: gestation < 37 weeks, duration of membrane rupture ≥ 18 hours, or temperature ≥ 38°C (100.4°F).
      ii) Use culture techniques that maximize the likelihood of GBS recovery. Since lower vaginal and rectal cultures are recommended, cultures should not be collected by speculum examination. The optimal method for GBS screening is collection of a single standard culture swab or two separate swabs of the distal vagina and anorectum. Swabs may be placed in a transport medium (eg, Amies) if the microbiology laboratory is offsite. The sample should be identified for the laboratory as specifically for GBS culture. Specimens should be inoculated into selective broth medium (either SBM broth or Lim broth), followed by overnight incubation and then subculture onto solid blood agar medium. In this screening culture, there is no need for the laboratory to culture for other organisms.
      iii) Laboratories should report results to the anticipated site of delivery as well as to the health care provider who ordered the test. Ideally, laboratories that perform GBS cultures will assure clinicians 24-hour, 7-day-a-week access to culture results.
      iv) Oral antimicrobial agents should not be used to treat women who are found to be colonized with GBS during prenatal screening. Such treatment is not effective in eliminating carriage or preventing neonatal disease.
   b) A chemoprophylaxis strategy based only on the presence of intrapartum risk factors (eg, gestation < 37 weeks, duration of membrane rupture ≥ 18 hours, or temperature ≥ 38°C) is an acceptable alternative (Fig. 2).
4. For intrapartum chemoprophylaxis, use intravenous penicillin G (5 million units initially and then 2.5 million units every 4 hours) until delivery. Intravenous ampicillin (2 g initially and then 1 g every 4 hours until delivery) is an acceptable alternative to penicillin G, but penicillin G is preferred since it has a narrow spectrum and is therefore less likely to select for antibiotic-resistant organisms. Clindamycin or erythromycin may be

* Centers for Disease Control and Prevention. Prevention of perinatal group B streptococcal disease: a public health perspective. MMWR 1996;45(RR-7):1–24

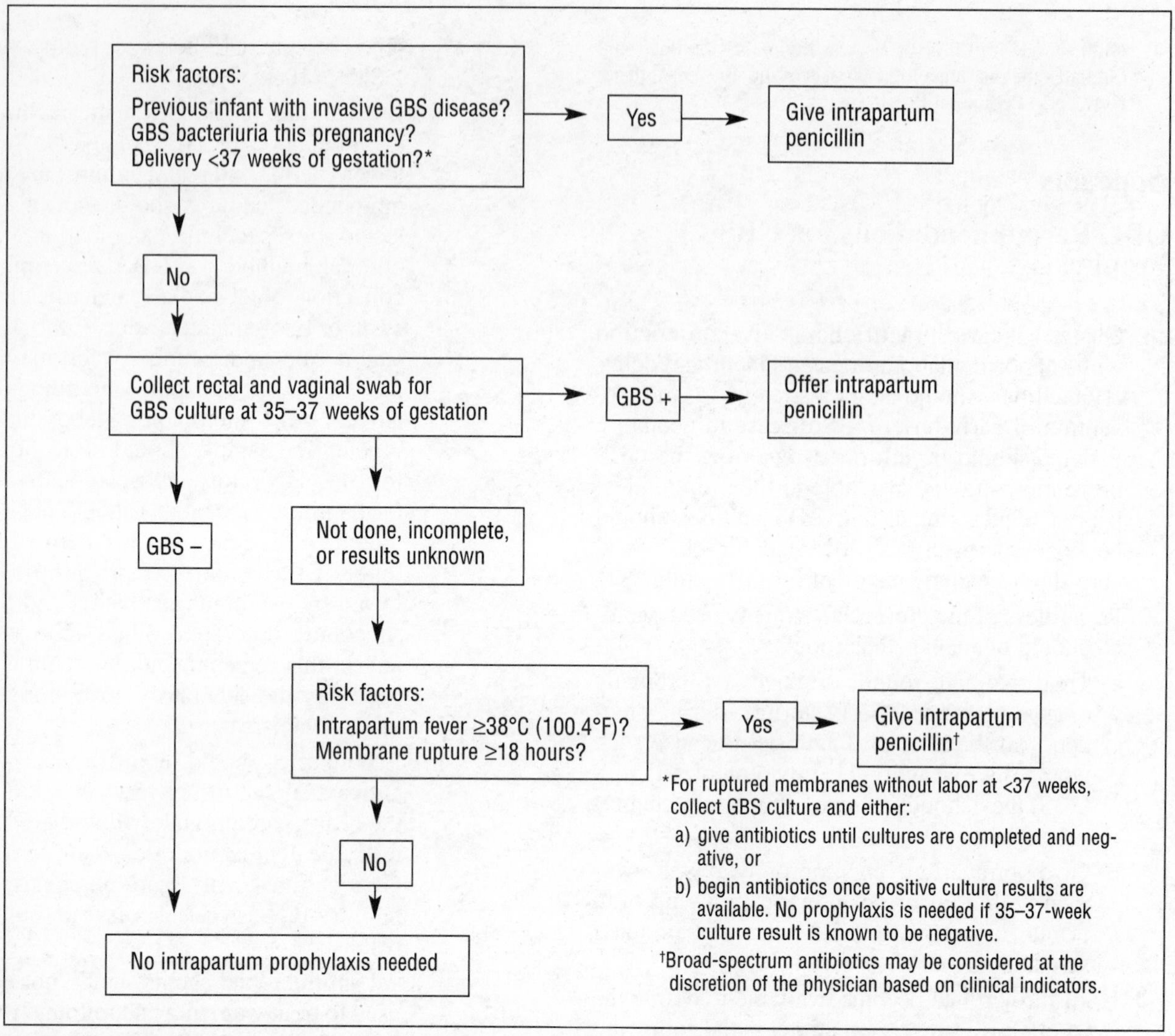

Risk factors:
Previous infant with invasive GBS disease?
GBS bacteriuria this pregnancy?
Delivery <37 weeks of gestation?*
Yes
Give intrapartum penicillin
No
Collect rectal and vaginal swab for GBS culture at 35–37 weeks of gestation
GBS +
Offer intrapartum penicillin
GBS –
Not done, incomplete, or results unknown
Risk factors:
Intrapartum fever ≥38°C (100.4°F)?
Membrane rupture ≥18 hours?
Yes
Give intrapartum penicillin†
No
No intrapartum prophylaxis needed
*For ruptured membranes without labor at <37 weeks, collect GBS culture and either:
a) give antibiotics until cultures are completed and negative, or
b) begin antibiotics once positive culture results are available. No prophylaxis is needed if 35–37-week culture result is known to be negative.
†Broad-spectrum antibiotics may be considered at the discretion of the physician based on clinical indicators.

Fig. 1. Prevention strategy for early-onset group B streptococci (GBS) disease using prenatal screening at 35–37 weeks. (Centers for Disease Control and Prevention. Prevention of perinatal group B streptococcal disease: a public health perspective. MMWR 1996;45[RR-7]:1–24)

One or more of the following risk factors:
• Previous infant with invasive GBS disease?
• GBS bacteriuria this pregnancy?
• Delivery < 37 weeks of gestation?*
• Duration of ruptured membrane ≥18 hours?
• Temperature ≥38°C (100.4°F)?
Yes
Give intrapartum penicillin†
No
No intrapartum prophylaxis needed
*For ruptured membranes without labor at <37 weeks, collect GBS culture and either:
a) give antibiotics until cultures are completed and negative, or
b) begin antibiotics once positive culture results are available
†Broad-spectrum antibiotics may be considered at the discretion of the physician based on clinical indicators.

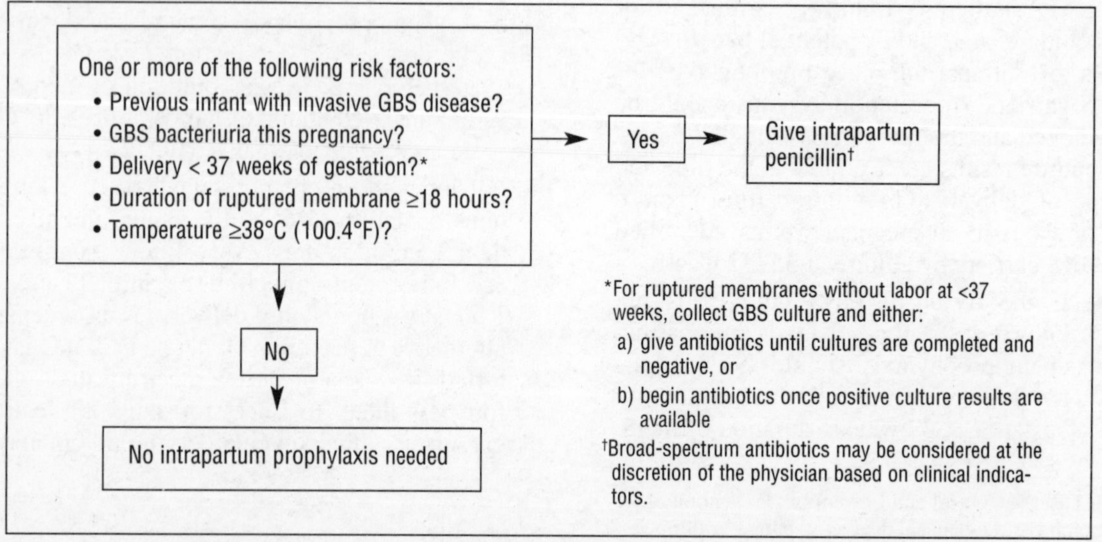

Fig. 2. Prevention strategy for early-onset group B streptococci (GBS) disease using risk factors. (Centers for Disease Control and Prevention. Prevention of perinatal group B streptococcal disease: a public health perspective. MMWR 1996;45[RR-7]:1–24)

used for women allergic to penicillin, although the efficacy of these drugs for GBS prevention has not be assessed.

(Women with a clinical diagnosis of chorioamnionitis who are receiving other treatment regimens that include agents active against GBS, such as ampicillin or clindamycin, do not need penicillin G added to the regimen)....

6. Local health agencies, in conjunction with appropriate groups of hospitals, should consider establishing surveillance to monitor the incidence of neonatal GBS disease, occurrence of adverse reactions to chemoprophylaxis, and the emergence of perinatal infections due to penicillin-resistant organisms.

Investigations designed to evaluate and compare these and other strategies are urgently needed. Such studies will require the participation of multiple institutions and should evaluate outcomes, including perinatal GBS infections, adverse reactions to chemoprophylaxis, and perinatal infections due to penicillin-resistant organisms. Characterization of protocol failures is also important.

ACOG Committee Opinion

Committee on Gynecologic Practice

Number 246, December 2000 (Replaces No. 229, December 1999)

Primary and Preventive Care: Periodic Assessments

This document reflects emerging clinical and scientific advances as of the date issued and is subject to change. The information should not be construed as dictating an exclusive course of treatment or procedure to be followed.

ISSN 1074-861X

The American College of Obstetricians and Gynecologists
409 12th Street, SW
PO Box 96920
Washington, DC 20090-6920

12345/43210

The following charts are updated versions of those previously published by the American College of Obstetricians and Gynecologists (ACOG) in *Guidelines for Women's Health Care* (1996); Primary Care Review No. 1, "Primary and Preventive Care" (1997); and Committee Opinion No. 229. This version replaces those previous versions. The policies and recommendations of ACOG committees regarding specific aspects of the health care of women have been incorporated; they may differ from the recommendations of other groups. Except as noted, these recommendations are for nonpregnant women.

Periodic assessments provide an excellent opportunity to counsel patients about preventive care. These assessments, yearly or as appropriate (unless otherwise noted), should include screening, evaluation, and counseling based on age and risk factors. Personal behavioral characteristics are important aspects of a woman's health. Positive behaviors, such as exercise, should be reinforced. The following guidelines indicate routine assessments for women based on age groups and risk factors (Table 1) and list leading causes of death and morbidity for each age group identified by various sources (see box). It is recognized that variations may be required to adjust to the needs of a specific individual. For example, certain risk factors may influence additional assessments and interventions. Physicians should be alert to high-risk factors (indicated by an asterisk and further elucidated in Table 1). During evaluation, the patient should be made aware of high-risk conditions that require targeted screening or treatment.

The material in these charts is based heavily on evidence of effectiveness and cost-effectiveness. It should be recognized, however, that making these determinations is both complex and inexact in the present environment. Nonetheless, the progress that has been made is encouraging, and the goal is desirable and of great importance. Although there will be differences of opinion regarding some specific recommendations, the major benefit to be derived should not be lost in debating those issues.

Periodic Assessment
Ages 13–18 Years

Screening

History

Reason for visit

Health status: medical, surgical, family

Dietary/nutrition assessment

Physical activity

Use of complementary and alternative medicine

Tobacco, alcohol, other drug use

Abuse/neglect

Sexual practices

Physical Examination

Height

Weight

Blood pressure

Secondary sexual characteristics (Tanner staging)

Pelvic examination (yearly when sexually active or beginning at age 18 years)

Skin*

Laboratory Testing

Periodic

Pap testing (yearly when sexually active or beginning at age 18 years)

*High-Risk Groups**

Hemoglobin level assessment

Bacteriuria testing

Sexually transmitted disease testing

Human immunodeficiency virus testing

Genetic testing/counseling

Rubella titer assessment

Tuberculosis skin testing

Lipid profile assessment

Fasting glucose testing

Cholesterol testing

Hepatitis C virus testing

Colorectal cancer screening†

Evaluation and Counseling

Sexuality

Development

High-risk behaviors

Preventing unwanted/unintended pregnancy

—Postponing sexual involvement

—Contraceptive options

Sexually transmitted diseases

—Partner selection

—Barrier protection

Fitness and Nutrition

Dietary/nutrition assessment (including eating disorders)

Exercise: discussion of program

Folic acid supplementation (0.4 mg/d)

Calcium intake

Psychosocial Evaluation

Interpersonal/family relationships

Sexual identity

Personal goal development

Behavioral/learning disorders

Abuse/neglect

Satisfactory school experience

Peer relationships

Cardiovascular Risk Factors

Family history

Hypertension

Dyslipidemia

Obesity

Diabetes mellitus

Health/Risk Behaviors

Hygiene (including dental); fluoride supplementation

Injury prevention

—Safety belts and helmets

—Recreational hazards

—Firearms

—Hearing

Skin exposure to ultraviolet rays

Suicide: depressive symptoms

Tobacco, alcohol, other drug use

Immunizations

Periodic

Tetanus–diphtheria booster (once between ages 11 years and 16 years)

Hepatitis B vaccine (one series for those not previously immunized)

*High-Risk Groups**

Influenza vaccine

Hepatitis A vaccine

Pneumococcal vaccine

Measles–mumps–rubella vaccine

Varicella vaccine

Leading Causes of Death‡

1. Motor vehicle accidents
2. Homicide
3. Suicide
4. Cancer
5. All other accidents and adverse effects
6. Diseases of the heart
7. Congenital anomalies
8. Chronic obstructive pulmonary diseases

Leading Causes of Morbidity‡

Acne

Asthma

Chlamydia

Depression

Dermatitis

Headaches

Infective, viral, and parasitic diseases

Influenza

Injuries

Nose, throat, ear, and upper respiratory infections

Sexual assault

Sexually transmitted diseases

Urinary tract infections

*See Table 1.

†Only for those with a family history of familial adenomatous polyposis or 8 years after the start of pancolitis. For a more detailed discussion of colorectal cancer screening, see Byers T, Levin B, Rothenberger D, Dodd GD, Smith RA. American Cancer Society guidelines for screening and surveillance for early detection of colorectal polyps and cancer: update 1997. American Cancer Society Detection and Treatment Advisory Group on Colorectal Cancer. CA Cancer J Clin 1997;47:154–160.

‡See box.

Periodic Assessment
Ages 19–39 Years

Screening

History
- Reason for visit
- Health status: medical, surgical, family
- Dietary/nutrition assessment
- Physical activity
- Use of complementary and alternative medicine
- Tobacco, alcohol, other drug use
- Abuse/neglect
- Sexual practices
- Urinary and fecal incontinence

Physical Examination
- Height
- Weight
- Blood pressure
- Neck: adenopathy, thyroid
- Breasts
- Abdomen
- Pelvic examination
- Skin*

Laboratory Testing
- *Periodic*
  - Pap testing (physician and patient discretion after three consecutive normal tests if low risk)
- *High-Risk Groups**
  - Hemoglobin level assessment
  - Bacteriuria testing
  - Mammography
  - Fasting glucose testing
  - Cholesterol testing
  - Sexually transmitted disease testing
  - Human immunodeficiency virus testing
  - Genetic testing/counseling
  - Rubella titer assessment
  - Tuberculosis skin testing
  - Lipid profile assessment
  - Thyroid-stimulating hormone testing
  - Hepatitis C virus testing
  - Colorectal cancer screening

Evaluation and Counseling

Sexuality
- High-risk behaviors
- Contraceptive options for prevention of unwanted pregnancy
- Preconceptional and genetic counseling for desired pregnancy
- Sexually transmitted diseases
- —Partner selection
- —Barrier protection
- Sexual function

Fitness and Nutrition
- Dietary/nutrition assessment
- Exercise: discussion of program
- Folic acid supplementation (0.4 mg/d)
- Calcium intake

Psychosocial Evaluation
- Interpersonal/family relationships
- Domestic violence
- Work satisfaction
- Lifestyle/stress
- Sleep disorders

Cardiovascular Risk Factors
- Family history
- Hypertension
- Dyslipidemia
- Obesity
- Diabetes mellitus
- Lifestyle

Health/Risk Behaviors
- Hygiene (including dental)
- Injury prevention
- —Safety belts and helmets
- —Occupational hazards
- —Recreational hazards
- —Firearms
- —Hearing
- Breast self-examination
- Chemoprophylaxis for breast cancer (for high-risk women ages 35 years or older)†
- Skin exposure to ultraviolet rays
- Suicide: depressive symptoms
- Tobacco, alcohol, other drug use

Immunizations

- *Periodic*
  - Tetanus–diphtheria booster (every 10 years)
- *High-Risk Groups**
  - Measles–mumps–rubella vaccine
  - Hepatitis A vaccine
  - Hepatitis B vaccine
  - Influenza vaccine
  - Pneumococcal vaccine
  - Varicella vaccine

Leading Causes of Death‡
1. Accidents and adverse effects
2. Cancer
3. Human immunodeficiency virus infection
4. Diseases of the heart
5. Homicide
6. Suicide
7. Cerebrovascular diseases
8. Chronic liver disease and cirrhosis

Leading Causes of Morbidity‡
- Asthma
- Back symptoms
- Breast disease
- Deformity or orthopedic impairment
- Depression
- Diabetes
- Gynecologic disorders
- Headache/migraines
- Hypertension
- Infective, viral, and parasitic diseases
- Influenza
- Injuries
- Nose, throat, ear, and upper respiratory infections
- Sexual assault/domestic violence
- Sexually transmitted diseases
- Skin rash/dermatitis
- Substance abuse
- Urinary tract infections
- Vaginitis

*See Table 1.

†The decision to use tamoxifen should be individualized. For a more detailed discussion of risk assessment and chemoprevention therapy, see American College of Obstetricians and Gynecologists. Tamoxifen and the prevention of breast cancer in high-risk women. ACOG Committee Opinion 224. Washington, DC: ACOG, 1999.

‡See box.

Periodic Assessment
Ages 40–64 Years

Screening

History

Reason for visit

Health status: medical, surgical, family

Dietary/nutrition assessment

Physical activity

Use of complementary and alternative medicine

Tobacco, alcohol, other drug use

Abuse/neglect

Sexual practices

Urinary and fecal incontinence

Physical Examination

Height

Weight

Blood pressure

Oral cavity

Neck: adenopathy, thyroid

Breasts, axillae

Abdomen

Pelvic examination

Skin*

Laboratory Testing

Periodic

Pap testing (physician and patient discretion after three consecutive normal tests if low risk)

Mammography (every 1–2 years until age 50 years; yearly beginning at age 50 years)

Cholesterol testing (every 5 years beginning at age 45 years)

Yearly fecal occult blood testing plus flexible sigmoidoscopy every 5 years *or* colonoscopy every 10 years *or* double contrast barium enema (DCBE) every 5–10 years, with digital rectal examination performed at the time of each screening sigmoidoscopy, colonoscopy, or DCBE (beginning at age 50 years)

Fasting glucose testing (every 3 years after age 45 years)

*High-Risk Groups**

Hemoglobin level assessment

Bacteriuria testing

Fasting glucose testing

Sexually transmitted disease testing

Human immunodeficiency virus testing

Tuberculosis skin testing

Lipid profile assessment

Thyroid-stimulating hormone testing

Hepatitis C virus testing

Colorectal cancer screening

Evaluation and Counseling

Sexuality†

High-risk behaviors

Contraceptive options for prevention of unwanted pregnancy

Sexually transmitted diseases

—Partner selection

—Barrier protection

Sexual functioning

Fitness and Nutrition

Dietary/nutrition assessment

Exercise: discussion of program

Folic acid supplementation (0.4 mg/d before age 50 years)

Calcium intake

Psychosocial Evaluation

Family relationships

Domestic violence

Work satisfaction

Retirement planning

Lifestyle/stress

Sleep disorders

Cardiovascular Risk Factors

Family history

Hypertension

Dyslipidemia

Obesity

Diabetes mellitus

Lifestyle

Health/Risk Behaviors

Hygiene (including dental)

Hormone replacement therapy

Injury prevention

—Safety belts and helmets

—Occupational hazards

—Recreational hazards

—Sports involvement

—Firearms

—Hearing

Breast self-examination

Chemoprophylaxis for breast cancer (for high-risk women)‡

Skin exposure to ultraviolet rays

Suicide: depressive symptoms

Tobacco, alcohol, other drug use

Immunizations

Periodic

Influenza vaccine (annually beginning at age 50 years)

Tetanus–diphtheria booster (every 10 years)

*High-Risk Groups**

Measles–mumps–rubella vaccine

Hepatitis A vaccine

Hepatitis B vaccine

Influenza vaccine

Pneumococcal vaccine

Varicella vaccine

Leading Causes of Death§

1. Cancer
2. Diseases of the heart
3. Cerebrovascular diseases
4. Accidents and adverse effects
5. Chronic obstructive pulmonary disease
6. Diabetes mellitus
7. Chronic liver disease and cirrhosis
8. Pneumonia and influenza

Leading Causes of Morbidity§

Arthritis/osteoarthritis

Asthma

Back symptoms

Breast disease

Cardiovascular disease

Carpal tunnel syndrome

Deformity or orthopedic impairment

Depression

Diabetes

Headache

Hypertension

Infective, viral, and parasitic diseases

Influenza

Injuries

Menopause

Nose, throat, and upper respiratory infections

Obesity

Skin conditions/dermatitis

Substance abuse

Urinary tract infections

Urinary tract (other conditions, including urinary incontinence)

Vision impairment

*See Table 1.

†Preconceptional and genetic counseling is appropriate for certain women in this age group.

‡The decision to use tamoxifen should be individualized. For a more detailed discussion of risk assessment and chemoprevention therapy, see American College of Obstetricians and Gynecologists. Tamoxifen and the prevention of breast cancer in high-risk women. ACOG Committee Opinion 224. Washington, DC: ACOG, 1999.

§See box.

Periodic Assessment
Ages 65 Years and Older

Screening

History

- Reason for visit
- Health status: medical, surgical, family
- Dietary/nutrition assessment
- Physical activity
- Use of complementary and alternative medicine
- Tobacco, alcohol, other drug use, and concurrent medication use
- Abuse/neglect
- Sexual practices
- Urinary and fecal incontinence

Physical Examination

- Height
- Weight
- Blood pressure
- Oral cavity
- Neck: adenopathy, thyroid
- Breasts, axillae
- Abdomen
- Pelvic examination
- Skin*

Laboratory Testing

Periodic

- Pap testing (physician and patient discretion after three consecutive normal tests if low risk)
- Urinalysis
- Mammography
- Cholesterol testing (every 3–5 years before age 75 years)
- Yearly fecal occult blood testing plus flexible sigmoidoscopy every 5 years *or* colonoscopy every 10 years *or* double contrast barium enema (DCBE) every 5–10 years, with digital rectal examination performed at the time of each screening sigmoidoscopy, colonoscopy, or DCBE
- Fasting glucose testing (every 3 years)

*High-Risk Groups**

- Hemoglobin level assessment
- Sexually transmitted disease testing
- Human immunodeficiency virus testing
- Tuberculosis skin testing
- Lipid profile assessment
- Thyroid-stimulating hormone testing
- Hepatitis C virus testing
- Colorectal cancer screening

Evaluation and Counseling

Sexuality

- Sexual functioning
- Sexual behaviors
- Sexually transmitted diseases
- —Partner selection
- —Barrier protection

Fitness and Nutrition

- Dietary/nutrition assessment
- Exercise: discussion of program
- Calcium intake

Psychosocial Evaluation

- Neglect/abuse
- Lifestyle/stress
- Depression/sleep disorders
- Family relationships
- Work/retirement satisfaction

Cardiovascular Risk Factors

- Hypertension
- Dyslipidemia
- Obesity
- Diabetes mellitus
- Sedentary lifestyle

Health/Risk Behaviors

- Hygiene (general and dental)
- Hormone replacement therapy
- Injury prevention
- —Safety belts and helmets
- —Prevention of falls
- —Occupational hazards
- —Recreational hazards
- —Firearms
- Visual acuity/glaucoma
- Hearing
- Breast self-examination
- Chemoprophylaxis for breast cancer (for high-risk women)†
- Skin exposure to ultraviolet rays
- Suicide: depressive symptoms
- Tobacco, alcohol, other drug use

Immunizations

Periodic

- Tetanus–diphtheria booster (every 10 years)
- Influenza vaccine (annually)
- Pneumococcal vaccine (once)

*High-Risk Groups**

- Hepatitis A vaccine
- Hepatitis B vaccine
- Varicella vaccine

Leading Causes of Death‡

1. Diseases of the heart
2. Cancer
3. Cerebrovascular diseases
4. Chronic obstructive pulmonary diseases
5. Pneumonia and influenza
6. Diabetes mellitus
7. Accidents and adverse effects
8. Alzheimer's disease

Leading Causes of Morbidity‡

- Arthritis/osteoarthritis
- Back symptoms
- Breast cancer
- Chronic obstructive pulmonary diseases
- Cardiovascular disease
- Deformity or orthopedic impairment
- Degeneration of macula retinae and posterior pole
- Diabetes
- Hearing and vision impairment
- Hypertension
- Hypothyroidism and other thyroid disease
- Influenza
- Nose, throat, and upper respiratory infections
- Osteoporosis
- Skin lesions/dermatoses/dermatitis
- Urinary tract infections
- Urinary tract (other conditions, including urinary incontinence)
- Vertigo

*See Table 1.

†The decision to use tamoxifen should be individualized. For a more detailed discussion of risk assessment and chemoprevention therapy, see American College of Obstetricians and Gynecologists. Tamoxifen and the prevention of breast cancer in high-risk women. ACOG Committee Opinion 224. Washington, DC: ACOG, 1999.

‡See box.

Table 1. High-Risk Factors

Intervention	High-Risk Factor
Bacteriuria testing	Diabetes mellitus
Cholesterol testing	Familial lipid disorders; family history of premature coronary heart disease; history of coronary heart disease
Colorectal cancer screening*	Colorectal cancer or adenomatous polyps in first-degree relative younger than 60 years or in two or more first-degree relatives of any ages; family history of familial adenomatous polyposis or hereditary nonpolyposis colon cancer; history of colorectal cancer, adenomatous polyps, or inflammatory bowel disease
Fasting glucose testing	Obesity; first-degree relative with diabetes mellitus; member of a high-risk ethnic population (eg, African American, Hispanic, Native American, Asian, Pacific Islander); have delivered a baby weighing more than 9 lb or history of gestational diabetes mellitus; hypertensive; high-density lipoprotein cholesterol level of at least 35 mg/dL; triglyceride level of at least 250 mg/dL; history of impaired glucose tolerance or impaired fasting glucose
Fluoride supplementation	Live in area with inadequate water fluoridation (<0.7 ppm)
Genetic testing/counseling	Exposure to teratogens; considering pregnancy at age 35 years or older; patient, partner, or family member with history of genetic disorder or birth defect; African, Acadian, Eastern European Jewish, Mediterranean, or Southeast Asian ancestry
Hemoglobin level assessment	Caribbean, Latin American, Asian, Mediterranean, or African ancestry; history of excessive menstrual flow
Hepatitis A vaccination	International travelers; illegal drug users; people who work with nonhuman primates; chronic liver disease; clotting-factor disorders; sex partners of bisexual men; measles, mumps, and rubella nonimmune persons; food-service workers; health-care workers; day-care workers
Hepatitis B vaccination	Intravenous drug users and their sexual contacts; recipients of clotting factor concentrates; occupational exposure to blood or blood products; patients and workers in dialysis units; persons with chronic renal or hepatic disease; household or sexual contact with hepatitis B virus carriers; history of sexual activity with multiple partners; history of sexual activity with sexually active homosexual or bisexual men; international travelers; residents and staff of institutions for the developmentally disabled and of correctional institutions
Hepatitis C virus (HCV) testing	History of injecting illegal drugs; recipients of clotting factor concentrates before 1987; chronic (long-term) hemodialysis; persistently abnormal alanine aminotransferase levels; recipient of blood from a donor who later tested positive for HCV infection; recipient of blood or blood-component transfusion or organ transplant before July 1992; occupational percutaneous or mucosal exposure to HCV-positive blood
Human immunodeficiency virus (HIV) testing	Seeking treatment for sexually transmitted diseases; drug use by injection; history of prostitution; past or present sexual partner who is HIV positive or bisexual or injects drugs; long-term residence or birth in an area with high prevalence of HIV infection; history of transfusion from 1978 to 1985; invasive cervical cancer; pregnancy. Offer to women seeking preconceptional care.
Influenza vaccination	Anyone who wishes to reduce the chance of becoming ill with influenza; resident in long-term care facility; chronic cardiopulmonary disorders; metabolic diseases (eg, diabetes mellitus, hemoglobinopathies, immunosuppression, renal dysfunction); health-care workers; day-care workers; pregnant women who will be in the second or third trimester during the epidemic season. Pregnant women with medical problems should be offered vaccination before the influenza season regardless of stage of pregnancy.
Lipid profile assessment	Elevated cholesterol level; history of parent or sibling with blood cholesterol of at least 240 mg/dL; first-degree relative with premature (<55 years of age for men, <65 years of age for women) coronary heart disease; diabetes mellitus; smoking habit
Mammography	Women who have had breast cancer or who have a first-degree relative (ie, mother, sister, or daughter) or multiple other relatives who have a history of premenopausal breast or breast and ovarian cancer

Table 1. High-Risk Factors *(continued)*

Intervention	High-Risk Factor
Measles–mumps–rubella (MMR) vaccination	Adults born in 1957 or later should be offered vaccination (one dose of MMR) if there is no proof of immunity or documentation of a dose given after first birthday; persons vaccinated in 1963–1967 should be offered revaccination (2 doses); health-care workers, students entering college, international travelers, and rubella-negative postpartum patients should be offered a second dose.
Pneumococcal vaccination	Chronic illness such as cardiovascular disease, pulmonary disease, diabetes mellitus, alcoholism, chronic liver disease, cerebrospinal fluid leaks, functional or anatomic asplenia; exposure to an environment where pneumococcal outbreaks have occurred; immunocompromised patients (eg, HIV infection, hematologic or solid malignancies, chemotherapy, steroid therapy); pregnant patients with chronic illness. Revaccination after 5 years may be appropriate for certain high-risk groups.
Rubella titer assessment	Childbearing age and no evidence of immunity
Sexually transmitted disease (STD) testing	History of multiple sexual partners or a sexual partner with multiple contacts, sexual contact with persons with culture-proven STD, history of repeated episodes of STDs, attendance at clinics for STDs; routine screening for chlamydial and gonorrheal infection for all sexually active adolescents and other asymptomatic women at high risk for infection
Skin examination	Increased recreational or occupational exposure to sunlight; family or personal history of skin cancer; clinical evidence of precursor lesions
Thyroid-stimulating hormone testing	Strong family history of thyroid disease; autoimmune disease (evidence of subclinical hypothyroidism may be related to unfavorable lipid profiles)
Tuberculosis skin testing	Human immunodeficiency virus infection; close contact with persons known or suspected to have tuberculosis; medical risk factors known to increase risk of disease if infected; born in country with high tuberculosis prevalence; medically underserved; low income; alcoholism; intravenous drug use; resident of long-term care facility (eg, correctional institutions, mental institutions, nursing homes and facilities); health professional working in high-risk health care facilities
Varicella vaccination	All susceptible adults and adolescents, including health-care workers; household contacts of immunocompromised individuals; teachers; day-care workers; residents and staff of institutional settings, colleges, prisons, or military installations; international travelers; nonpregnant women of childbearing age

*For a more detailed discussion of colorectal cancer screening, see Byers T, Levin B, Rothenberger D, Dodd GD, Smith RA. American Cancer Society guidelines for screening and surveillance for early detection of colorectal polyps and cancer: update 1997. American Cancer Society Detection and Treatment Advisory Group on Colorectal Cancer. CA Cancer J Clin 1997;47:154–160.

Sources of Leading Causes of Mortality and Morbidity

Leading causes of mortality are provided by the Mortality Statistics Branch at the National Center for Health Statistics. Data are from 1996, the most recent year for which final data are available. The causes are ranked.

Leading causes of morbidity are unranked estimates based on information from the following sources:

- National Health Interview Survey, 1994
- National Ambulatory Medical Care Survey, 1996
- National Hospital Discharge Survey, 1996
- U.S. Department of Justice National Crime Victimization Survey
- U.S. Centers for Disease Control and Prevention Sexually Transmitted Disease Surveillance, 1996
- U.S. Centers for Disease Control and Prevention HIV/AIDS Surveillance Report, 1997
- National Nursing Home Survey, 1995

ACOG

Committee on Practice Management

Committee on Professional Liability

Committee Opinion

Number 222, October 1999

Quality of Laboratory and Imaging Services: Physician Responsibility in the Age of Managed Care

With the expansion of managed care, obstetrician–gynecologists find it necessary to work with multiple laboratories for the processing of pap tests and other laboratory and imaging studies. The use of specific laboratory or imaging services may be dictated by the patient's health plan if reimbursement is to be expected. When dealing with numerous laboratories, the physician often lacks firsthand knowledge of a particular laboratory's quality assurance programs or test-result reporting processes. Similar problems may occur when dealing with imaging services. Physicians might be placed at increased medical–legal risk if they find these services to be substandard and yet are unable to refer a patient to alternate services covered by her health plan.

The Committee on Practice Management and the Committee on Professional Liability make the following recommendations to Fellows to help protect their patients and practices from adverse consequences due to substandard pap test and other laboratory and imaging reporting processes and performance:

1. Create office tracking systems for appropriate laboratory and imaging studies. These systems could include patient name; date of office visit; name of laboratory or imaging service; type of test or study; date the specimen is sent to the laboratory site or date the patient is referred to the imaging service; date the results are returned; the results; date the results are relayed to the patient, by whom, and in what way; and date of follow-up appointment. These systems could be either in the form of a paper medical record log or computerized.
2. All laboratory results should be reported to the physician in a timely manner. Physicians should request that laboratory and imaging services send a monthly list of patients' abnormal results that can be cross-checked with office tracking systems to ensure appropriate patient notification and follow-up.

This document provides risk management information that is current as of the date issued and is subject to change. This document does not define a standard of care nor should it be interpreted as legal advice.

ISSN 1074-861X

The American College of Obstetricians and Gynecologists
409 12th Street, SW
PO Box 96920
Washington, DC 20090-6920

12345/32109

3. Document complaints regarding laboratory or imaging quality and service. Problems with laboratory quality or service should be documented in a letter (with patients' names omitted) copied to the laboratory director, the managed care organization (MCO), and the appropriate state regulatory authority. If there is an inadequate response, consider sending a copy to the patient. Keep a file of these letters to share with the appropriate MCO's quality monitoring personnel and for regulatory or accrediting agencies. With respect to problematic laboratories, the patient's safety and quality medical care should take precedence. (For further information, refer to Committee Opinion number 193, "Physician/Patient Responsibility for Follow-Up of Diagnosis and Treatment," and Committee Opinion number 166, "Informed Refusal.")

Although these recommendations may be time consuming to physicians and staff, appropriate handling and reporting of laboratory and imaging results, as well as quality laboratory and imaging services, are important to the provision of quality health care to our patients. Attention to this issue also minimizes medical–legal risk to the physician.

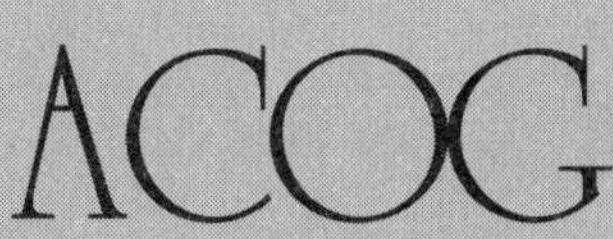

Committee on
Obstetric Practice

Committee Opinion

Number 179, November 1996

Rate of Vaginal Births After Cesarean Delivery

Currently, about 24% of the births in the United States are cesarean births. One third of the cesarean births are repeat cesarean deliveries. The safety of vaginal birth after a previous low transverse cesarean delivery and when established criteria are met has been demonstrated in many studies. In August 1995, the American College of Obstetricians and Gynecologists published an evidence-based guideline for vaginal birth after cesarean delivery (VBAC) in its ACOG Practice Pattern.

The literature evaluating VBAC generally focuses on the criteria for, the safety of, and the success rate of trial of labor after cesarean delivery. The success rate usually has been quoted as 60-80%, depending on selection criteria and other variables. Given the current focus on cost-containment in health care, the VBAC rate is a commonly used measure of obstetric practice by hospital quality assessment and improvement committees, insurers, and government agencies.

To facilitate an accurate comparison of VBAC rates between providers and between institutions, the Committee on Obstetric Practice believes it is important to use standardized definitions that are based on numbers that are readily available. Although there are some women who have absolute contraindications for a trial of labor after cesarean delivery, it may be difficult to identify this group accurately. It is a small number, however, and will not affect the VBAC rate substantially. For this reason, women who are not candidates for a trial of labor after cesarean delivery are included here in the denominator when the VBAC rate is calculated. The committee proposes that two rates related to VBAC be defined as follows:

$$\text{VBAC Rate} = \frac{\text{No. of VBACs}}{\text{No. of women with prior cesarean deliveries}} \times 100$$

$$\text{Success Rate (of trial of labor after cesarean delivery)} = \frac{\text{No. of VBACs}}{\text{No. of women who had trial of labor after cesarean delivery}} \times 100$$

ISSN 1074-861X

The American College of Obstetricians and Gynecologists
409 12th Street, SW
PO Box 96920
Washington, DC 20090-6920

2345/0987

The number of women with prior cesarean deliveries includes women who were candidates for a trial of labor after cesarean delivery but declined and women who were not candidates for a trial of labor after cesarean.

Clearly, these rates are interrelated. However, calculation and use of the rates defined here allow a more accurate comparison of practice between providers and between institutions.

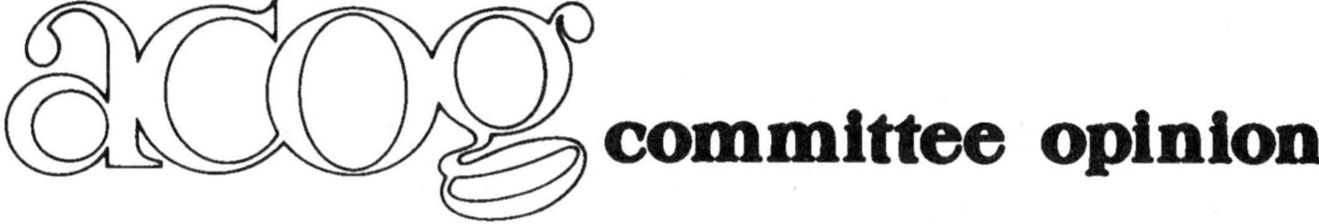

ABOG/ACOG Liaison Committee

Number 110—May 1992

Recertification

The American Board of Obstetrics and Gynecology, Inc. (Board) and The American College of Obstetricians and Gynecologists (College) have the common objective of assisting obstetrician–gynecologists in maintaining clinical competence of the specialist.

The College is responsible for continuing education of the obstetrician–gynecologist, using a wide range of educational approaches, including self assessment and recording of continuing medical education accomplishments. The College also assists measurement of clinical performance at the hospital level through programs of quality assurance and voluntary peer review. The Board is responsible for a periodic method of assessment of the individual physician's competence, measured against his or her peers by predetermined standards. Such periodic assessment should include both measurements of current cognitive knowledge and clinical practice review.

All Diplomates of the Board certified in the year 1986 or later are issued a certificate limited to 10 years. Certification renewal is required at or before the 10-year interval to maintain certification. The first such examinations and practice reviews will be given by the Board in 1994. Those Diplomates of the Board certified in 1985 or earlier were issued a certificate without time limitation. A process of voluntary recertification is available for such specialists. This serves as an accolade, rather than as a defined requirement.

Fellowship in the College requires, among other criteria, "successful completion of an examination in obstetrics and gynecology." The examination requirement may be satisfied by a number of examinations around the world, but for United States graduates it is almost always the examination of the American Board of Obstetrics and Gynecology, Inc. The Fellowship requirement is met for all Fellows by successful completion of the appropriate initial examination and, by action of the Executive Board, Fellowship continues regardless of subsequent recertification.

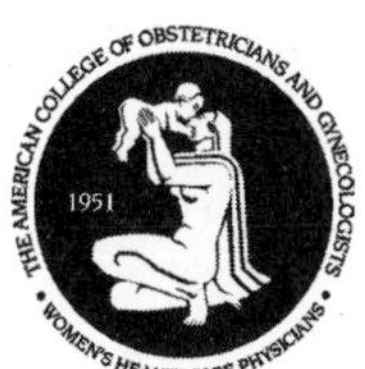

The American College of Obstetricians and Gynecologists
409 12th Street, SW • Washington, DC 20024-2188

456/87

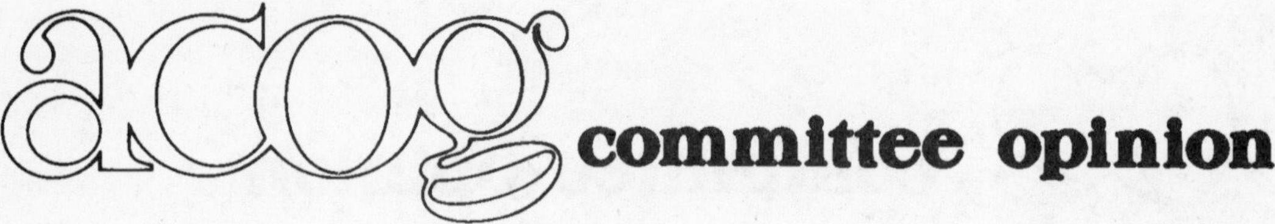

Committee on Gynecologic Practice Number 152—March 1995

Recommendations on Frequency of Pap Test Screening

The College's current recommendations on the frequency of Pap test screening are:

> All women who are or who have been sexually active or who have reached age 18 should undergo an annual Pap test and pelvic examination. After a woman has had three or more consecutive, satisfactory annual examinations with normal findings, the Pap test may be performed less frequently in a low-risk woman at the discretion of her physician.

The recognized problems of the high number of false-negative results and failure of patients to return at regular intervals raise questions about the safety of screening every 3 years as recommended by the American Cancer Society. Recent proposals for health care financing have suggested that Pap test screening may be done even less frequently or may be eliminated altogether in certain groups of women. Theoretical models may show this strategy to be cost-saving; however, a reduction in the frequency of Pap test screening in England has been accompanied by an increased incidence of cervical cancer cases and deaths from cervical carcinoma. In contrast, the Canadian province of British Columbia has had a continuing reduction in morbidity and mortality from invasive squamous cell cancers of the cervix, which is directly attributable to the province's 30-year history of performing annual Pap tests.

Certain high-risk factors have been associated with the development of cervical intraepithelial neoplasia and cervical carcinoma. The College recommends that when one or more of these risk factors is present, more frequent Pap tests may be required. High-risk factors include:

- Women who have had multiple sexual partners or whose male sexual partners have had multiple partners
- Women who began sexual intercourse at an early age
- Women whose male sexual partners have had other sexual partners with cervical cancer
- Women with current or prior human papillomavirus infection or condylomata or both
- Women with current or prior herpes simplex virus infections
- Women who are infected with the human immunodeficiency virus (HIV)
- Women with a history of other sexually transmitted diseases
- Women who are immunosuppressed (such as those who have received renal transplants)
- Smokers and abusers of other substances, including alcohol
- Women who have a history of cervical dysplasia or cervical cancer or endometrial, vaginal, or vulvar cancer
- Women of lower socioeconomic status*

The cost-effectiveness of cytologic screening for vaginal neoplasia after removal of the cervix for benign disease has not been demonstrated. Nonetheless, periodic cytologic evaluation of the vagina in such cases, based on the above risk factors, is warranted.

Physicians are encouraged to consider these risk factors when determining the frequency of Pap test screening. Annual health maintenance physical examinations and pelvic examinations continue to be encouraged even for women who appear to be at low risk for developing cervical intraepithelial neoplasia or cervical cancer. Many women may not be aware of previous or other sexual contacts of their partner, and they may be unknowingly at high risk.

*Low socioeconomic status appears to be a surrogate for a number of closely related risk factors that place these women at greater risk for cervical cancer.

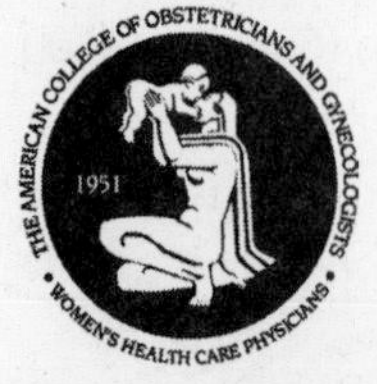

ISSN 1074-861X

This document reflects emerging clinical and scientific advances as of the date issued and is subject to change. The information should not be construed as dictating an exclusive course of treatment or procedure to be followed.

The American College of Obstetricians and Gynecologists
409 12th Street, SW • Washington, DC 20024-2188

12345/98765

ACOG

Committee on Ethics

Committee Opinion

Number 225, November 1999 (Replaces #88, November 1990)

Responsibilities of Physicians Regarding Surrogate Motherhood

Although the practice of surrogate motherhood has become more common since ACOG issued previous statements on this subject in 1983 and 1990, it continues to be controversial. On the one hand, there are those who believe that surrogacy should be permitted because such arrangements can be beneficial to all parties, and to prohibit them would limit the autonomy of infertile couples and of actual and potential surrogates. On the other hand, there are those who believe that the risks outweigh the benefits or that because of shifting emotions and attitudes toward the fetus during gestation, it is not possible for a pregnant woman to give truly informed consent to relinquish an infant until after birth has occurred (1).

Many issues related to surrogate motherhood have not been resolved, and considerable disagreement persists within the medical profession, the medical ethics community, state legislatures, the courts, and the general public. Similarly, no one position reflects the variety of opinions on surrogacy within the College membership. While recognizing these differences of opinion, this document will focus on the ethical responsibilities of obstetrician–gynecologists who choose to participate in surrogacy arrangements on a variety of levels, including caring for the pregnant woman and her fetus.

The first part of the document provides an overview of public policy issues, descriptions of the types of surrogacy, arguments supporting and opposing surrogacy arrangements, and particular concerns related to payment and commercialization. The second part offers ethical recommendations to physicians who are involved in counseling infertile couples or potential surrogate mothers, who provide obstetric services for pregnant surrogates, or who offer assisted reproductive techniques using surrogacy. The ethical obligations of the physician will vary depending on the type and level of his or her involvement in the surrogacy arrangement.

General Issues

Public Policy

In most states, the practice of surrogate motherhood is not clearly covered under existing law. Among the states that have statutes, most either prohibit surrogacy contracts or make them void and unenforceable. Some of the states that prohibit surrogacy arrangements ban them under all circumstances, whereas others ban them only if compensation is involved. A few states

ISSN 1074-861X

The American College of Obstetricians and Gynecologists
409 12th Street, SW
PO Box 96920
Washington, DC 20090-6920

12345/32109

specifically allow surrogacy contracts provided that certain conditions are met (2, 3).

When a court is asked to decide a dispute regarding parental rights or custody of a child born as a result of a surrogacy arrangement, existing statutes may not prove adequate because of the complexity of the problem. Courts faced with such decisions have given preference to different factors: the best interest of the child, the rights of the birth mother (as in adoption situations), the genetic link between the child and his or her genetic parents, and the intent of the couple who entered into a surrogacy contract in order to become parents. Often two or more of these factors conflict with each other, and there is no consensus in the legal or ethical communities as to which ought to have priority (2–7).

The obstetrician–gynecologist who facilitates surrogacy arrangements should be aware of any statutes or court cases in the state in which he or she practices. In counseling individuals seeking a child through surrogacy or a woman who is considering becoming a surrogate, the physician should encourage them to consider the possible consequences of a surrogacy arrangement, including potential legal complications.

Types of Surrogacy

Surrogacy can be either "traditional" or "gestational." Besides these two types of surrogacy, other variations related to the source of the genetic material are possible. Eggs, sperm, or both may be donated, thereby altering the "commissioning couple's" relationship to the child.

In traditional surrogacy, the would-be parents are a husband and wife (the commissioning couple). The couple reaches an agreement with a woman (the "surrogate mother") who will be artificially inseminated with sperm provided by the husband of the commissioning couple. Thus, the genetic and gestational mother of any resultant child is the surrogate mother, and the genetic father is the husband of the commissioning couple. The commissioning couple intend to be the "social" or "rearing" parents of the child. Although this document refers to a married commissioning couple, individuals and nontraditional couples also may seek surrogacy services.

In gestational surrogacy, in vitro fertilization and embryo transfer are combined with surrogate parenting arrangements. In this case, it is possible for both the husband and the wife of the commissioning couple to be the genetic parents of the child, and the surrogate fulfills only the role of gestational mother. This type of arrangement originally was called surrogate gestational motherhood, and now the carrying woman is called the "gestational carrier" or "gestational surrogate."

The different types of relationships that are possible—genetic (either, both, or neither commissioning parent), gestational (the surrogate), and social or rearing (the commissioning couple)—give rise to both conceptual problems about the nature of parenthood and legal problems as to who ought to be considered the parents responsible for the child.

Major Arguments for and Against Surrogate Parenthood Arrangements

Surrogate parenthood can allow a couple to have a child when they would otherwise be unable to do so except by adoption, due to inability to achieve pregnancy or medical contraindications to pregnancy for the commissioning woman. Adoption, however, does not provide a genetic link to the child, an important consideration for some prospective parents. Surrogate parenthood is chosen by some prospective parents because of a desire for genetic linkage or for practical reasons, such as the scarcity of adoptable children.

Arguments based on reproductive liberty also support surrogate parenthood arrangements. In the United States, the freedom to decide whether and when to conceive or bear a child is a highly protected right. Thus, some have argued that commissioning couples and surrogate mothers ought to be free to cooperate in procreating, at least in cases of medical need and where care is taken to avoid harming others, especially the prospective child. Furthermore, the surrogate mother may derive satisfaction from helping the commissioning couple. Some women become surrogates primarily for altruistic reasons and see their services as a gift.

The primary arguments against surrogate motherhood are based on the harms that the practice may be thought to produce—harms to the child that is born, harms to the surrogate herself, harms to her existing children if she has children, and harms to society as a whole. It is surely harmful to any child to be the object of a custody dispute. In addition, the rejection of an infant—for example, a disabled infant's rejection by both commissioning parents and surrogate mother—is a significant harm. If an existing relationship is used to coerce relatives or close friends to become surrogate mothers, that coercion is a harm resulting from the practice of surrogate motherhood. The existing children of a surrogate mother may be harmed if her pregnancy and relinquishment result in high levels of stress for the surrogate or her family. These children and society as a whole may be harmed by the perception that reproduction is trivialized by transactions that translate women's reproductive capacities and the infants that result into commodities to be bought and sold. Depersonalization of a pregnant woman as a "vehicle" for the genetic perpetuation of other individuals may harm not only surrogate mothers but also the status of women as a whole. There is also a concern that redefining concepts of motherhood may threaten traditional understandings of parenting and family.

Children are much more vulnerable than adults. Harms to children who have no choice in the matter are more serious, from an ethical standpoint, than harms to adults who make a choice that they later regret. Further, a distinction should be drawn between harms that inevitably, or almost invariably, are associated with a practice and harms that perhaps could be avoided through advance planning, appropriate counseling, or oversight mechanisms.

Few studies provide data about harms and benefits resulting from surrogate parenting arrangements. Speculative discussion about possible outcomes does not provide a solid foundation for ethical conclusions and clinical guidelines. It is important to know whether these outcomes actually occur and, if so, how frequently. Studies that will provide more data of this type are needed (8, 9).

In summary, there are strong arguments both for and against the practice of surrogate parenthood. Physicians will be on both sides of this debate. If, after careful consideration of the arguments, a physician chooses to facilitate or recommend surrogacy arrangements, then all precautions should be taken to prevent medical, psychologic, and legal harms to the commissioning couple, the potential surrogate, and the prospective child.

Payment to the Surrogate Mother

Perhaps no topic related to surrogate motherhood is more contentious than compensation of the surrogate mother by the commissioning couple (10). Payment to surrogates often is substantial because of the duration and complexity of involvement. As noted earlier, some states specifically prohibit surrogacy contracts that involve payment. Several questions about payment for surrogacy should be raised:

For what is payment made? Although there is debate on this point, it is clear that payment must not be made contingent on the delivery of an "acceptable product"—a live-born, healthy child. Rather, payment should be construed as compensation for the surrogate mother's time and effort, her initiating and carrying the pregnancy, her giving birth to an infant, her acceptance of the risks of pregnancy and childbirth, and her possible loss of employment opportunities.

Why is payment offered or requested? In many surrogate parenthood arrangements among close friends or relatives, there is no payment for the services of the surrogate. Rather, the surrogate may provide her services as an act of altruism, and the commissioning couple will be asked to reimburse her only for out-of-pocket expenses connected with the pregnancy. However, most women are understandably reluctant to undertake the burdens and risks of pregnancy on behalf of strangers without some kind of compensation for their time, effort, and risk.

Is payment likely to lead to the exploitation of potential surrogates? Surrogacy arrangements often take place between parties with unequal power, education, and economic status (11). Unless independent legal representation and mental health counseling are mandated, women serving as surrogates may be particularly vulnerable to being treated as commodities. If a payment offered to a candidate for surrogacy is too low, it may be said to exploit her by not providing adequate compensation; if the payment is too high, it may be said to exploit her by being irresistible and coercive. Opponents of surrogate motherhood also have argued that if a fee must be paid to the surrogate mother, only affluent couples will be able to become commissioning couples. This access barrier exists, however, for most services related to infertility, for certain other medical procedures, and for adoption, and thus is not specific to surrogacy agreements.

Responsibilities of Obstetrician–Gynecologists

Ethical recommendations will focus on four categories of physician involvement: advising couples who are considering surrogacy, counseling potential surrogate mothers, providing obstetric services for pregnant surrogates, and offering assisted reproductive techniques related to surrogacy. Although the obligations of the physician will vary depending on the type and level of his or her involvement, in all cases the physician should carefully examine all relevant issues, including medical, ethical, legal, and psychologic aspects.

Commissioning parents and surrogate mothers have both divergent and common interests. Because of these divergent interests, one professional person or agency (eg, physician, attorney, or psychologist) should not represent the interests of both major parties in surrogate parenting arrangements. The physician who treats the commissioning couple should not have the surrogate mother as an obstetric patient, because conflicts of interest may arise that would not allow the physician to serve all parties properly.

Responsibilities of Physicians to Couples Considering Surrogacy

When approached by a couple considering surrogacy, the physician should, as in all other aspects of medical care, be certain that there will be a full discussion of ethical and legal issues as well as medical risks, benefits, and alternatives, many of which have been addressed in this statement. An obstetrician–gynecologist who is not familiar with these issues should refer the couple for appropriate counseling. Additional recommendations for advising couples considering surrogacy are as follows:

1. Because of the risks inherent in surrogacy arrangements, such arrangements should be considered only in the case of infertility or health-related needs, not for convenience alone.
2. A physician may justifiably decline to participate in initiating surrogate motherhood arrangements for personal, ethical, or medical reasons.
3. If a physician decides to become involved in facilitating surrogate motherhood arrangements, he or she should follow these guidelines:
   - The physician should be assured that appropriate procedures are used to screen the commissioning couple and the surrogate. Such screening should include appropriate fertility studies, medical screening, and psychologic assessment.
   - Mental health counseling should be provided prior to initiation of a pregnancy 1) to permit the potential surrogate and the commissioning couple to explore the range of outcomes and possible long-term effects and 2) to consider possible psychologic risks to and vulnerabilities of both parties and the prospective child.
   - It is preferable that surrogate parenting arrangements be overseen by private nonprofit agencies with credentials similar to those of adoption agencies. However, many existing agencies are entrepreneurial and for-profit (9). A physician making a referral to an agency must have assurance that the agency is medically and ethically reputable and that it is committed to protecting the interests of all parties involved.
   - The physician should receive only usual compensation for medical services. Referral fees and other arrangements for financial gain beyond usual fees for medical services are inappropriate.
   - The physician should not refer patients to surrogacy programs in which the financial arrangements are likely to exploit any of the parties.
4. The obstetrician–gynecologist should urge the commissioning couple to discuss preconditions and possible contingencies with the surrogate or her representative and to agree in advance on the response to them. These include, but may not be limited to, the expected health-related behaviors of the surrogate; the prenatal diagnosis of a genetic or chromosomal abnormality; the inability or unwillingness of the surrogate to carry the pregnancy to term; the death of a member of the commissioning couple or the dissolution of the couple's marriage during the pregnancy; the birth of an infant with a disability; a decision by the surrogate mother to abrogate the contract and to contest custody of an infant conceived through the sperm of the commissioning husband; or, in the case of gestational surrogacy, the option of registering the commissioning couple as the legal parents.
5. The obstetrician–gynecologist should urge the parties involved to record in writing the preconditions and contingency plans on which they have agreed in order to make explicit the intentions of the parties, to facilitate later recollection of these intentions, and to help promote the interests of the future child. In the preparation of this agreement, both parties should be encouraged to have independent legal representation.
6. Whatever compensation is provided to the surrogate mother should be paid solely on the basis of her time and effort, her initiating and carrying the pregnancy, her acceptance of the risks of pregnancy and childbirth, and her possible loss of employment opportunities. Compensation must not be contingent on a successful delivery or on the health of the child.
7. Where possible, obstetrician–gynecologists should cooperate with and participate in research intended to provide data on outcomes of surrogacy arrangements.

Responsibilities of Physicians to Potential Surrogates

When approached by a patient considering becoming a surrogate mother, the physician should, as in all other aspects of medical care, be certain that there will be a full discussion of ethical and legal issues and medical risks and benefits, many of which have been addressed in this statement. In particular, the physician should be sure that preconditions and contingencies, such as those outlined in the previous section, have been thoroughly considered and that the potential surrogate recognizes the importance of having explicit written precondition and contingency agreements. In the preparation of this agreement, both parties should be encouraged to have independent legal representation. Additional recommendations for counseling and providing other services for potential surrogate mothers are as follows:

1. In order to avoid conflict of interest, the physician should not facilitate a woman's becoming a surrogate mother for a couple whom the physician also is treating.
2. The physician should ensure that appropriate procedures are used to screen and counsel both the commissioning couple and the surrogate. Referral for mental health counseling should be provided prior to initiation of a pregnancy 1) to permit the potential surrogate to explore the range of outcomes and possible long-term effects and 2) to evaluate her psychologic risks and vulnerabilities as well as the possible effects of surrogacy on her existing relationships and on any existing children.
3. A physician who provides examinations and performs procedures for an agency that arranges surrogacy contracts should be aware of the policies of the agency and should decline involvement with any agency whose policies are not consistent with the ethical recommendations of this document and those of other professional organizations related to reproductive medicine, such as the American Society for Reproductive Medicine (formerly known as the American Fertility Society) (8, 9).
4. Whatever compensation is provided to the surrogate mother should be paid solely on the basis of her time and effort, her initiating and carrying the pregnancy, her acceptance of the risks of pregnancy and childbirth, and her possible loss of employment opportunities. Compensation must not be contingent on a successful delivery or on the health of the child.
5. The physician should not facilitate surrogacy arrangements in which the financial or other arrangements are likely to exploit any of the parties. A physician who agrees to provide medical care in clearly exploitative circumstances becomes a party to that exploitation. The physician is therefore obliged to become informed about the financial and other arrangements between the surrogate and commissioning parents in order to make ethical decisions about providing medical care.

Responsibilities of Physicians to Pregnant Surrogates

When a pregnant surrogate seeks medical care for an established pregnancy, the obstetrician should explore with the surrogate her understanding of her contract with the commissioning couple and any provisions of it that may affect her care. If the physician believes that provisions of the contract may conflict with his or her professional judgment, the physician may refuse to accept the patient under those terms. Once accepted as a patient, she should be cared for as any other obstetric patient, regardless of the method of conception, or referred to an obstetrician who will provide that care. Additional recommendations regarding the provision of obstetric services to surrogates are as follows:

1. The obstetrician's professional obligation is to support the well-being of the pregnant woman and her fetus, to support the pregnant woman's goals for the pregnancy, and to provide the appropriate standard of care regardless of the patient's plans to keep or relinquish the future child. If a physician's discomfort with surrogacy arrangements might interfere with that obligation, the patient should be referred to another obstetrician.
2. The pregnant surrogate should be the sole source of consent regarding clinical intervention and management of the pregnancy, labor, and delivery.
3. Agreements the surrogate has made with the commissioning couple regarding her care and behavior during pregnancy and delivery should not affect the physician's care of the patient. The obstetrician must make recommendations that are in the best interests of the pregnant woman and her fetus, regardless of prior agreements between her and the commissioning couple.
4. Confidentiality between the physician and the pregnant patient should be maintained. The com-

missioning couple may have access to the patient's medical information only with her explicit consent.

5. Obstetrician–gynecologists are encouraged to assist in the development of hospital policies to address labor, delivery, postpartum, and neonatal care in situations in which surrogacy arrangements exist.

Responsibilities of Infertility Specialists and Reproductive Endocrinologists to Commissioning Couples and Surrogates

In providing medical services related to surrogate motherhood arrangements, infertility specialists and reproductive endocrinologists should follow the recommendations in the two previous sections. In particular, these specialists should ensure that appropriate procedures are used to screen the commissioning couple and the surrogate and that mental health counseling is provided to all parties prior to initiation of a pregnancy. Additional recommendations regarding the provision of assisted reproductive techniques are as follows:

1. A physician who performs artificial insemination for traditional surrogacy or in vitro fertilization for gestational surrogacy necessarily will have to deal with both the commissioning couple and the surrogate. However, the couple and the surrogate should have independent counseling and independent legal representation, and the surrogate should obtain obstetric care from a physician who is not involved with the commissioning couple.
2. A physician who provides examinations and performs procedures for an agency that arranges surrogacy contracts should be aware of the policies of the agency and should decline involvement with any agency whose policies are not consistent with the ethical recommendations of this document and those of other professional organizations related to reproductive medicine (8, 9).
3. Specialists in infertility and reproductive endocrinology are encouraged to participate in research that is intended to provide data on the outcomes of surrogacy arrangements.

Summary

The obstetrician–gynecologist has an ethical responsibility to review the risks and benefits of surrogate parenthood fully and fairly with couples who are considering surrogacy arrangements. The obstetrician who is consulted by a pregnant woman who has made surrogacy arrangements owes her the same care as any pregnant woman and must respect her right to be the sole source of consent for all matters regarding prenatal care and delivery. The gynecologist or specialist in reproductive endocrinology who performs procedures required for surrogacy should be guided by the same ethical principles aimed at safeguarding the well-being of all participants, including the future child.

References

1. Lederman RP. Psychosocial adaptation in pregnancy: assessment of seven dimensions of maternal development. New York: Springer, 1996
2. Brandel A. Legislating surrogacy: a partial answer to feminist criticism. Maryland Law Rev 1995;54:488–527
3. Dolgin JL. Defining the family: law, technology, and reproduction in an uneasy age. New York: New York University Press, 1997
4. Andrews LB. Alternative modes of reproduction: position paper. In: Cohen S, Taub N, eds. Reproductive laws for the 1990s. Clifton, New Jersey: Humana Press, 1989:361–403
5. Serratelli A. Surrogate motherhood contracts: should the British or Canadian model fill the U.S. legislative vacuum? George Washington J Intl Law Econ 1993;26:633–674
6. Field M. Reproductive technologies and surrogacy: legal issues. Creighton Law Rev 1992;25:1589–1598
7. New York State Task Force on Life and the Law. Assisted reproductive technologies: analysis and recommendations for public policy. New York State Task Force, April 1998
8. Ethics Committee, American Fertility Society. Surrogate gestational mothers: women who gestate a genetically unrelated embryo. In: Ethical considerations of assisted reproductive technologies. Fertil Steril 1994;62 (suppl 1):67S–70S
9. Ethics Committee, American Fertility Society. Surrogate mothers. In: Ethical considerations of assisted reproductive technologies. Fertil Steril 1994;62 (suppl 1):71S–77S
10. Moody-Adams MM. On surrogacy: morality, markets, and motherhood. Public Affairs Q 1991;5:175–190
11. Harrison M. Financial incentives for surrogacy. Womens Health Issues 1991;1:145–147

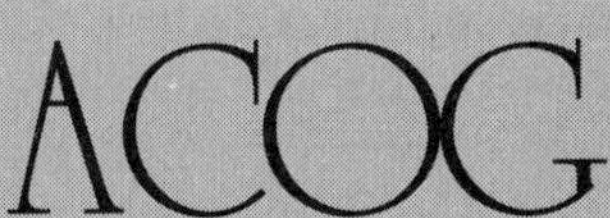

Committee on Gynecologic Practice

Committee Opinion

Number 195, November 1997

Role of Loop Electrosurgical Excision Procedure in the Evaluation of Abnormal Pap Test Results

Traditionally, the evaluation of abnormal Pap test results has been done by colposcopy and directed biopsy and endocervical curettage. Once invasive cancer has been ruled out and a biopsy diagnosis of cervical intraepithelial neoplasia (CIN) has been made, treatment options might include observation, cryotherapy, laser vaporization, cone biopsy, or hysterectomy. More recently, the loop electrosurgical excision procedure (LEEP) has allowed the clinician to combine diagnosis and treatment using a relatively simple outpatient procedure done under local anesthesia. Unlike colposcopically directed biopsies, the loop excision specimen usually includes the entire transformation zone, which potentially reduces the risk of missing invasive cancer.

Loop diathermy uses a relatively inexpensive, low-current, high-frequency electrical generator and thin stainless steel or tungsten wires of various shapes and sizes to excise lesions of the transformation zone. This technique was originally described by Prendiville et al, who modified an earlier small wire loop used by Cartier (1). Other names for LEEP are large loop excision of the transformation zone (LLETZ) or loop excision of the transformation zone (LETZ).

This technique has the advantages of providing a tissue specimen for pathologic confirmation of the diagnosis, technical ease of performance, inexpensive equipment, and the ability to perform the procedure in an outpatient setting in either an office or clinic. Complications of LEEP include bleeding and infection, but they are relatively uncommon. The potential long-term sequelae of LEEP are cervical stenosis and cervical incompetence. Although several studies suggest that these risks are minimal (2), long-term evaluation of large groups of patients treated with LEEP are not yet available.

The clinician should have a broad understanding of the natural history and pathophysiology of CIN and human papillomavirus (HPV) to obtain the best results with minimum morbidity, to make management decisions, and to provide adequate and effective patient counseling. Good colposcopic skills are also necessary to identify those lesions appropriate for excision. Good

ISSN 1074-861X

The American College of Obstetricians and Gynecologists
409 12th Street, SW
PO Box 96920
Washington, DC 20090-6920

12345/10987

surgical skill and experience are necessary to minimize complications and manage them should they occur.

In patients in whom atypical squamous cells of undetermined significance or low-grade lesions have been identified by Pap test, the appropriate sequence of diagnostic biopsy and treatment is not clear. Excision of the entire transformation zone may represent overtreatment for metaplasia, inflammation, repair, and even focal HPV changes or mild dysplasia (CIN I). Most cases of atypical squamous cells of undetermined significance and many cases of low-grade intraepithelial neoplasia of the cervix regress spontaneously. In patients who will adhere to follow-up, early cervical neoplasia (mild dysplasia, CIN I, low-grade squamous intraepithelial neoplasia) may be monitored without treatment. It should be recognized, however, that approximately 15% of these lesions may progress. Standard colposcopically directed biopsy with close follow-up, given the recurrent nature of HPV and its prevalence in the population, will reduce morbidity and costs of treatment. In most circumstances, LEEP should be reserved for cases that persist, progress, or recur after other conservative measures have been attempted and for patients thought to be unreliable for follow-up.

Women with high-grade squamous intraepithelial lesions are the most appropriate candidates for LEEP. Most patients with histologically positive margins can be followed by cytologic and colposcopic assessment safely, as long as invasive cancer is not suspected. Several large studies have identified a number of patients with occult invasive cancer found on the LEEP specimen although colposcopy with directed biopsy showed only CIN (3, 4). In those women in whom microinvasive cancer or glandular lesions are suspected, the necessity for a large enough biopsy sample to ensure an adequate diagnosis safely and satisfactorily precludes LEEP in the opinion of many experts (5). Thermal damage occurs at the margins during LEEP and may obscure precise histologic detail.

Some clinicians recommend an immediate "see-and-treat" approach in which women with abnormal Pap test results undergo colposcopic evaluation and LEEP at the same visit. They propose that this reduces the cost and the risk of patient noncompliance in returning for treatment. However, the use of LEEP for low-grade lesions and the see-and-treat approach remains controversial and awaits the results of further studies.

References

1. Prendiville W, Cullimore J, Norman S. Large loop excision of the transformation zone (LLETZ). A new method of management for women with cervical intraepithelial neoplasia. Br J Obstet Gynaecol 1989;96:1054–1060
2. Haffenden DK, Bigrigg A, Codling BW, Read MD. Pregnancy following large loop excision of the transformation zone. Br J Obstet Gynaecol 1993;100:1059–1060
3. Bigrigg MA, Codling BW, Pearson P, Read MD, Swingler GR. Colposcopic diagnosis and treatment of cervical dysplasia at a single clinic visit. Lancet 1990;336:229–231
4. Luesley DM, Cullimore J, Redman CWE, Lawton FG, Emens JM, Rollason TP, et al. Loop diathermy excision of the cervical transformation zone in patients with abnormal cervical smears. BMJ 1990;300:1690–1693
5. Gold M, Dunton CJ, Murray J, Macones G, Hanau C, Carlson JA Jr. Loop electrocautery excisional procedure: therapeutic effectiveness as an ablation and a conization equivalent. Gynecol Oncol 1996;61:241–244

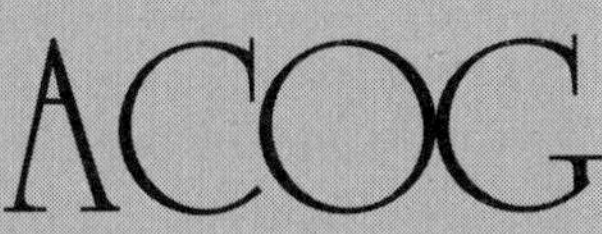

Committee Opinion

Committee on
Gynecologic Practice

Number 186, September 1997 (*Replaces #140, June 1994*)

Role of the Obstetrician–Gynecologist in the Diagnosis and Treatment of Breast Disease

Obstetrician–gynecologists are in a favorable position to diagnose breast disease in their patients. The American College of Obstetricians and Gynecologists (ACOG) has adopted the goals of assisting in educating obstetrician–gynecologists in the diagnosis and treatment of benign breast disease and in reducing mortality from breast cancer. As an initial step toward these goals, ACOG has developed the following guidelines for the early diagnosis of breast disease:

1. Breast examination by visual inspection and palpation should be an integral part of initial obstetric and all complete gynecologic examinations.
2. Patients should be instructed in the technique of life-long periodic self-examination of the breast and informed of the importance of self-examination.
3. Patients should be encouraged to undergo screening by mammography in accordance with ACOG guidelines. Earlier or more frequent screening is recommended for women who have had breast cancer or who have a first-degree relative (ie, mother, sister, or daughter) or multiple other relatives who have a history of premenopausal breast or breast and ovarian cancer.
4. Obstetrician–gynecologists should perform diagnostic procedures when indicated.
5. When indicated, referrals should be made to physicians who specialize in the diagnosis and treatment of the type of breast disease that is suspected.
6. Institutions that credential physicians to perform breast surgery should apply the same criteria for clinical competence to obstetrician–gynecologists as to other physicians requesting to obtain or maintain such privileges.
7. A persistent palpable breast mass requires evaluation. Mammography alone is not sufficient to rule out malignant pathology in a patient with a palpable breast mass. Ultrasonography or magnified mammographic imaging of the breast containing the mass may provide additional information and may identify cystic structures or variations in normal breast architecture that account for the palpable abnormality.

ISSN 1074-861X

The American College of Obstetricians and Gynecologists
409 12th Street, SW
PO Box 96920
Washington, DC 20090-6920

12345/10987

When cyst aspiration is performed, the fluid may be discarded if it is clear (transparent and not bloody) and the mass disappears. Otherwise, the patient should be considered a candidate for a breast biopsy.

Solid masses usually require histologic diagnosis. Fine-needle aspiration or stereotactic needle biopsy may be an alternative to open breast biopsy in some cases. If breast cancer or a specific benign condition is not detected by fine-needle aspiration or needle core biopsy, open biopsy is necessary. Because the incidence of breast cancer is extremely low in patients younger than 20 years of age, patients in this age group who have solid masses that appear to be benign when examined by ultrasonography can be monitored without biopsy at the discretion of the physician. These guidelines apply both to pregnant and to nonpregnant women.

8. When a patient is referred to another physician for management of a breast disorder, following are the responsibilities of the obstetrician–gynecologist:

   - Explain to the patient that she needs further care
   - Provide names of qualified physicians from whom the patient can receive care
   - Answer the patient's questions
   - Document these steps and include a detailed description of the clinical findings in the medical record

The American College of Obstetricians and Gynecologists encourages both basic and clinical research into the etiology, early diagnosis, and treatment of all breast disease. Postgraduate education, including residency training programs in obstetrics and gynecology and continuing medical education, should include education in the early diagnosis and management of all forms of breast disease. Obstetrician–gynecologists also should take advantage of opportunities to educate other physicians involved in the health care of women about the diagnosis and treatment of breast disease.

Bibliography

American College of Obstetricians and Gynecologists. Nonmalignant conditions of the breast. ACOG Technical Bulletin 156. Washington, DC: ACOG, 1991

American College of Obstetricians and Gynecologists. Carcinoma of the breast. ACOG Technical Bulletin 158. Washington, DC: ACOG, 1991

American College of Obstetricians and Gynecologists. Guidelines for women's health care. Washington, DC: ACOG, 1996

American College of Obstetricians and Gynecologists. Routine cancer screening. ACOG Committee Opinion 185. Washington, DC: ACOG, 1997

Brenner RJ, Fajardo L, Fisher PR, Dershaw DD, Evans WP, Bassett L, et al. Percutaneous core biopsy of the breast: effect of operator experience and number of samples on diagnostic accuracy. AJR Am J Roentgenol 1996;166:341–346

Mainiero MB, Philpotts LE, Lee CH, Lange RC, Carter D, Tocino I. Stereotaxic core needle biopsy of breast microcalcifications: correlation of target accuracy and diagnosis with lesion size. Radiology 1996;198:665–669

Mitnick JS, Vazquez MF, Feiner HD, Pressman P, Roses DF. Mammographically detected breast lesions: clinical importance of cytologic atypia in stereotaxic fine-needle aspiration biopsy samples. Radiology 1996;198:319–322

ACOG

Committee on Gynecologic Practice

Committee Opinion

Number 247, December 2000 *(Replaces No. 185, September 1997)*

Routine Cancer Screening

General Health Counseling and Cancer Evaluation

For many women, the obstetrician–gynecologist is the only physician who provides them with regular health care. Therefore, the obstetrician–gynecologist should be able to provide cancer evaluation and counseling. Evaluation of risk for cancer includes questions about high-risk habits, assessment of family history of cancer, and review of symptoms pertinent to each organ system. The estimated number of women who would develop various types of cancer and the number of women estimated to die from the disease are shown in Table 1.

The Committee on Gynecologic Practice recommends that every woman undergo examination of the pelvis and breast annually, beginning at age 18 years or earlier if she is sexually active. The examination also may include the skin, lymph nodes, thyroid gland, oral cavity, anus, and rectum to detect signs of premalignant or malignant conditions. Cancer screening components currently recommended by the Committee on Gynecologic Practice, taking into consideration the recommendations of major nationally recognized experts, are summarized in Table 2. Although these guidelines apply specifically to routine cancer screening, other ACOG publications containing recommendations for high-risk groups are included in the bibliography.

Cervical Cancer

The Pap test, unlike most screening tests, is used principally to diagnose preinvasive lesions that, when treated, will result in a decrease in the incidence of and deaths from invasive cancer. The Pap test appears to have accomplished that goal.

The results of screening studies indicate that since the Pap test was introduced, the number of advanced lesions has decreased, whereas the number of early invasive lesions, as well as cervical intraepithelial neoplasia, has increased. Because of a large amount of strong indirect evidence of the effectiveness of the Pap test, it would be unethical to conduct randomized clinical trials to confirm its utility.

In the United States, 90% of women aged 18 years or older have had at least one Pap test, and more than 60% have had a Pap test within 3 years (1). Considering that cervical cancer has not been eradicated, that the incidence of cervical intraepithelial neoplasia appears to have increased over the past

This document reflects emerging clinical and scientific advances as of the date issued and is subject to change. The information should not be construed as dictating an exclusive course of treatment or procedure to be followed.

ISSN 1074-861X

The American College of Obstetricians and Gynecologists
409 12th Street, SW
PO Box 96920
Washington, DC 20090-6920

Table 1. Estimated Number of Women Who Will Develop or Die from Various Types of Cancer in 2000

Type of Cancer	No. of New Cases	No. of Deaths
Cervical	12,800	4,600
Breast	182,800	40,800
Lung	74,600	67,600
Endometrial	36,100	6,500
Ovarian	23,100	14,000
Colorectal	66,600	28,500

Data from American Cancer Society. Cancer facts and figures—2000. Atlanta: ACS, 2000

decade, that the Pap test has an appreciable false-negative rate, and that women tend to extend screening intervals, the guidelines recommending annual cervical cytology screening for most women are prudent and warranted if early precursors to cervical cancer are to be detected and successfully treated.

Breast Cancer

Breast cancer is the second leading cause of death due to cancer in women (2). One in eight women will develop breast cancer during her lifetime. At present, mammography is the only screening method available to detect subclinical, or occult, breast cancer—the stage at which cancer is least likely to have spread to regional nodes and beyond.

Any recommendations concerning screening must be based on the current understanding of the risk/benefit ratio. Evidence from reports from the Breast Cancer Detection Demonstration Project of the American Cancer Society, as well as from numerous other studies, indicates that there is a decrease in mortality for all women when appropriate screening by mammography is instituted and carried out by qualified personnel.

Randomized, controlled trials have clearly demonstrated a decreased death rate from breast cancer in women who were offered mammography between the ages of 50 years and 69 years. Even among this group of women, however, less than 40% have had a mammogram in the past year.

The benefit of mammography in women ages 40–49 years is less clear. In 1993, the National Cancer Institute considered the evidence showing the benefits of screening by mammography in women 40–49 years of age and, finding it equivocal, subsequently withdrew its recommendation for routine screening of women in this age group. However, because of inadequate numbers of patients studied and length of follow-up, ACOG did not believe there were sufficient data to warrant a change in its current screening recommendations. As a result, ACOG continues to recommend offering screening by mammography every 1–2 years to women ages 40–49 years

Table 2. Suggested Cancer Screening Guidelines

Topic	Guideline
General health counseling and cancer evaluation	All women should have a general health evaluation annually or as appropriate, which should include evaluation for cancer and examination to detect signs of premalignant or malignant conditions.
Breast cancer	Mammography should be performed every 1–2 years for women 40–49 years of age and then annually thereafter.
Cervical cancer	All women who are or who have been sexually active or who have reached 18 years of age should undergo an annual Pap test and pelvic examination. After a woman has had three or more consecutive, satisfactory, annual cytologic examinations with normal findings, the Pap test may be performed less frequently on a low-risk woman at the discretion of her physician.
Endometrial cancer	Screening all women for endometrial cancer and its precursors is neither cost-effective nor warranted.
Ovarian cancer	No techniques that have proved to be effective in reducing the disease-specific mortality of ovarian cancer are currently available.
Colorectal cancer	Beginning at age 50 years one of three screening options should be selected: yearly fecal occult blood testing plus flexible sigmoidoscopy every 5 years *or* colonoscopy every 10 years *or* double contrast barium enema (DCBE) every 5–10 years. A digital rectal examination should be performed at the time of each screening sigmoidoscopy, colonoscopy, or DCBE.
Lung cancer	No available techniques are currently suitable for routine screening.

and annually to women older than 50 years. In 1997, the National Institutes of Health convened the consensus development conference "Breast Cancer Screening for Women Ages 40–49." It declined to recommend routine screening in this age group, instead advising that each woman, in consultation with her physician, decide whether to undergo screening.

Although data regarding women ages 70 years and older are insufficient to make a definitive recommendation about screening in this age group, the incidence of breast cancer does increase with age. Therefore, ACOG continues to recommend annual screening in this age group.

Clinicians should encourage screening by mammography for those women for whom benefit clearly has been established. The safety and effectiveness of mammography have been demonstrated. However, it is recognized that mammography is the most costly of all screening modalities. Dedicated equipment is essential, and considerable skill and experience are required to interpret the films. It is important, therefore, to determine the most prudent use of resources.

Lung Cancer

Among women, there has been a steady overall increase in the number of deaths from lung cancer, which now surpasses that from breast cancer; lung cancer is the major cause of cancer death in women (2). The only effective way to reduce mortality is to promote smoking cessation.

Endometrial Cancer

Endometrial cancer is the most common gynecologic cancer in women ages 45 years and older. The significant increase in the prevalence of endometrial cancer observed in the 1980s was attributed primarily to the increasing longevity of postmenopausal women, the more frequent use of unopposed estrogen replacement therapy, and the refinement of criteria for diagnosing early endometrial adenocarcinoma. In the early 1990s, there appears to have been a stabilization of the incidence of the disease. The reasons for this are unclear but may be related to the increased use of progesterone with estrogen replacement therapy.

The cost-effectiveness of screening asymptomatic women for endometrial cancer and its precursors is very low; therefore, endometrial assessment is unwarranted. Endometrial sampling is not required before or during estrogen–progestin therapy unless unexpected bleeding occurs. The Pap test has insufficient sensitivity to be used as a screening technique for endometrial cancer.

Ovarian Cancer

One woman in 70 will develop ovarian cancer during her lifetime (3). Ovarian cancer is the leading cause of death from gynecologic cancer. More women die from ovarian cancer than from cervical and endometrial cancers combined. Measuring CA 125 levels in serum and ultrasonography have not been shown to be effective in population-based screening for ovarian cancer.

Colorectal Cancer

The incidence of colorectal cancer increases with age. Because colorectal cancer is a significant risk to women, it is suggested that routine evaluation take place.

Future Screening Studies

The Prostate, Lung, Colorectal and Ovarian Cancer Screening Trial, a study sponsored by the National Institutes of Health/National Cancer Institute, is designed to identify effective ways to reduce cancer deaths in older Americans. Women participating in this study will have serial bimanual examinations, transvaginal ultrasonography, and CA 125 screening.

References

1. Trends in cancer screening—United States, 1987 and 1992. MMWR Morb Mortal Wkly Rep 1996;45:57–61
2. American Cancer Society. Cancer facts and figures—2000. Atlanta: ACS, 2000
3. Ovarian cancer: screening, treatment, and followup. NIH Consens Statement 1994 Apr 5–7;12(3):1–30

Bibliography

Cervical Cancer

American College of Obstetricians and Gynecologists. Recommendations on frequency of Pap test screening. ACOG Committee Opinion 152. Washington, DC: ACOG, 1995

Bearman DM, MacMillan JP, Creasman WT. Papanicolaou smear history of patients developing cervical cancer: an assessment of screening protocols. Obstet Gynecol 1987;69:151–155 [erratum in Obstet Gynecol 1987;69:660]

Cervical cancer screening programs: summary of the 1982 Canadian task force report. Can Med Assoc J 1982;127:581–589

Eddy DM. Screening for cervical cancer. Ann Intern Med 1990; 113:214–226

Johannesson G, Geirsson G, Day N. The effect of mass screening in Iceland, 1965–74, on the incidence and mortality of cervical carcinoma. Int J Cancer 1978;21:418–425

Mandelblatt J, Schechter C, Fahs M, Muller C. Clinical implications of screening for cervical cancer under Medicare. The natural history of cervical cancer in the elderly: what do we know? What do we need to know? Am J Obstet Gynecol 1991;164:644–651

Richart RM. Screening. The next century. Cancer 1995;76: 1919–1927

Screening for squamous cervical cancer: duration of low risk after negative results of cervical cytology and its implication for screening policies. IARC Working Group on evaluation of cervical cancer screening programmes. Br Med J (Clin Res Ed) 1986;293:659–664

Shy K, Chu J, Mandelson M, Greer B, Figge D. Papanicolaou smear screening interval and risk of cervical cancer. Obstet Gynecol 1989;74:838–843

Wilkinson EJ. Pap smears and screening for cervical neoplasia. Clin Obstet Gynecol 1990;33:817–825

Breast Cancer

American College of Obstetricians and Gynecologists. Role of the obstetrician–gynecologist in the diagnosis and treatment of breast disease. ACOG Committee Opinion 186. Washington, DC: ACOG, 1997

Bailar JC 3d. Mammography before age 50 years? JAMA 1988; 259:1548–1549

Baines CJ. The Canadian National Breast Screening Study. Why? What next? And so what? Cancer 1995;76:2107–2112

Bassett LW, Hendrick RE, Bassford TL, Butler PF, Carter D, DeBor M, et al. Quality determinants of mammography. Clinical Practice Guideline No. 13. Rockville, Maryland: Agency for Health Care Policy and Research, Public Health Service, U.S. Department of Health and Human Services, 1994; AHCPR publication no. 95-0632

Champion VL. Strategies to increase mammography utilization. Med Care 1994;32:118–129

Champion VL. The relationship of selected variables to breast cancer detection behaviors in women 35 and older. Oncol Nurs Forum 1991;18:733–739

Dawson DA, Thompson GB. Breast cancer risk factors and screening: United States, 1987. Vital Health Stat [10]1990;172: iii–iv, 1–60

Eddy DM, Hasselblad V, McGivney W, Hendee W. The value of mammography screening in women under age 50 years. JAMA 1988;259:1512–1519

Feig SA. Mammographic screening of women aged 40–49 years. Benefit, risk, and cost considerations. Cancer 1995;76:2097–2106

Feig SA. Mammography screening: published guidelines and actual practice. Recent Results Cancer Res 1987;105:78–84

Howard J. Using mammography for cancer control: an unrealized potential. CA Cancer J Clin 1987;37:33–48

Solin LJ, Fox K, August DA, Dershaw DD, Rebbeck TR, Weber BL, et al. Breast cancer. In: Hoskins WJ, Perez CA, Young RC, eds. Principles and practice of gynecologic oncology. 2nd ed. Philadelphia: Lippincott–Raven, 1997:1079–1142

Moskowitz M. Breast cancer: age specific growth rates and screening strategies. Radiology 1986;161:37–41

Screening mammography: a missed clinical opportunity? Results of the NCI Breast Cancer Screening Consortium and National Health Interview Survey Studies. JAMA 1990;264:54–58

Seidman H, Gelb SK, Silverberg E, LaVerda N, Lubera JA. Survival experience in the Breast Cancer Detection Demonstration Project. CA Cancer J Clin 1987;37:258–290

Shapiro S, Venet W, Strax P, Venet L, Roeser R. Ten- to fourteen-year effect of screening on breast cancer mortality. J Natl Cancer Inst 1982;69:349–355

Sickles EA, Kopans DB. Mammographic screening for women aged 40 to 49 years: the primary care practitioner's dilemma. Ann Intern Med 1995;122:534–538

Smart CR. The role of mammography in the prevention of mortality from breast cancer. Cancer Prev 1990;June 1–16

Tabar L, Fagerberg G, Chen HH, Duffy SW, Smart CR, Gad A, et al. Efficacy of breast cancer screening by age. New results from the Swedish Two-County Trial. Cancer 1995;75:2507–2517

Tabar L, Fagerberg G, Duffy SW, Day NE, Gad A, Grontoft O. Update of the Swedish two-county program of mammographic screening for breast cancer. Radiol Clin North Am 1992;30: 187–210

Use of mammography—United States, 1990. MMWR Morb Mortal Wkly Rep 1990;39:621, 627–630

Woolf SH. United States Preventive Services Task Force recommendations on breast cancer screening. Cancer 1992;69: 1913–1918

Wright CJ. Breast cancer screening: a different look at the evidence. Surgery 1986;100:594–598

Zapka JG, Hosmer D, Costanza ME, Harris DR, Stoddard A. Changes in mammography use: economic, need, and service factors. Am J Public Health 1992;82:1345–1351

Zapka JG, Stoddard A, Maul L, Costanza ME. Internal adherence to mammography screening guidelines. Med Care 1991;29:697–707

Lung Cancer

Berlin NI, Buncher CR, Fontana RS, Frost JK, Melamed MR. The National Cancer Institute Cooperative Early Lung Cancer Detection Program. Results of the initial screen (prevalence). Early lung cancer detection: introduction. Am Rev Respir Dis 1984;130:545–549

Epstein DM. The role of radiologic screening in lung cancer. Radiol Clin North Am 1990;28:489–495

Endometrial Cancer

American College of Obstetricians and Gynecologists. Tamoxifen and endometrial cancer. ACOG Committee Opinion 232. Washington, DC: ACOG, 2000

Chambers JT, Chambers SK. Endometrial sampling: When? Where? Why? With what? Clin Obstet Gynecol 1992;35:28–39

Ciotti MC. Screening for gynecologic and colorectal cancer: is it adequate? Womens Health Issues 1992;2:83–92; discussion 92–93

Ferenczy A, Mutter G. Endometrial hyperplasia and neoplasia: definition, diagnosis, and management principles. In: Sciarra JJ, ed. Gynecology and obstetrics. Vol 4. Philadelphia: Lippincott Williams & Wilkins, 2000:1–15

Greenwood SM, Wright DJ. Evaluation of the office endometrial biopsy in the detection of endometrial carcinoma and atypical hyperplasia. Cancer 1979;43:1474–1478

Koss LG. Diagnosis of early endometrial cancer and precancerous states. Ann Clin Lab Sci 1979;9:189–194

Koss LG, Schreiber K, Moussouris H, Oberlander SG. Endometrial carcinoma and its precursors: detection and screening. Clin Obstet Gynecol 1982;25:49–61

Koss LG, Schreiber K, Oberlander SG, Moussouris HF, Lesser M. Detection of endometrial carcinoma and hyperplasia in asymptomatic women. Obstet Gynecol 1984;64:1–11

Pritchard KI. Screening for endometrial cancer: is it effective? Ann Intern Med 1989;110:177–179

Reagan JW. Can screening for endometrial cancer be justified? Acta Cytol 1980;24:87–89

Stovall TG, Photopulos GJ, Poston WM, Ling FW, Sandles LG. Pipelle endometrial sampling in patients with known endometrial carcinoma. Obstet Gynecol 1991;77:954–956

Vuopala S. Diagnostic accuracy and clinical applicability of cytological and histological methods for investigating endometrial carcinoma. Acta Obstet Gynecol Scand Suppl 1977;70:1–72

Zucker PK, Kasdon EJ, Feldstein ML. The validity of Pap smear parameters as predictors of endometrial pathology in menopausal women. Cancer 1985;56:2256–2263

Ovarian Cancer

Bast RC Jr, Klug TL, St John E, Jenison E, Niloff JM, Lazarus H, et al. A radio-immunoassay using a monoclonal antibody to monitor the course of epithelial ovarian cancer. N Engl J Med 1983;309:883–887

Berek JS, Bast RC Jr. Ovarian cancer screening. The use of serial complementary tumor markers to improve sensitivity and specificity for early detection. Cancer 1995;76:2092–2096

Berek JS, Knapp RC, Malkasian GD, Lavin PT, Whitney C, Niloff JM, et al. CA 125 serum levels correlated with second-look operations among ovarian cancer patients. Obstet Gynecol 1986;67:685–689

Bourne TH, Whitehead MI, Campbell S, Royston P, Bhan V, Collins WP. Ultrasound screening for familial ovarian cancer. Gynecol Oncol 1991;43:92–97

Campbell S, Bhan V, Royston P, Whitehead MI, Collins WP. Transabdominal ultrasound screening for early ovarian cancer. BMJ 1989;299:1363–1367

Jacobs I, Stabile I, Bridges J, Kemsley P, Reynolds C, Grudzinskas J, et al. Multimodal approach to screening for ovarian cancer. Lancet 1988;1(8580):268–271

Jacobs I, Davies AP, Bridges J, Stabile I, Fay T, Lower A, et al. Prevalence screening for ovarian cancer in postmenopausal women by CA 125 measurement and ultrasonography. BMJ 1993;306:1030–1034

Skates SJ, Xu FJ, Yu YH, Sjovall K, Einhorn N, Chang Y, et al. Toward an optimal algorithm for ovarian cancer screening with longitudinal tumor markers. Cancer 1995;76:2004–2010

van Nagell JR Jr, DePriest PD, Puls LE, Donaldson ES, Gallion HH, Pavlik EJ, et al. Ovarian cancer screening in asymptomatic postmenopausal women by transvaginal sonography. Cancer 1991;68:458–462

van Nagell JR Jr, Gallion HH, Pavlik EJ, DePriest PD. Ovarian cancer screening. Cancer 1995;76:2086–2091

Colorectal Cancer

Byers T, Levin B, Rothenberger D, Dodd GD, Smith RA. American Cancer Society guidelines for screening and surveillance for early detection of colorectal polyps and cancer: update 1997. American Cancer Society Detection and Treatment Advisory Group on Colorectal Cancer. CA Cancer J Clin 1997; 47:154–160

Hardcastle JD, Chamberlain JO, Robinson MH, Moss SM, Amar SS, Balfour TW, et al. Randomised controlled trial of faecal-occult-blood screening for colorectal cancer. Lancet 1996; 348:1472–1477

Kronborg O, Fenger C, Olsen J, Jorgensen OD, Sondergaard O. Randomised study of screening for colorectal cancer with faecal-occult-blood test. Lancet 1996;348:1467–1471

Lang CA, Ransohoff DF. Fecal occult blood screening for colorectal cancer. Is mortality reduced by chance selection for screening colonoscopy? JAMA 1994;271:1011–1013

Mandel JS, Bond JH, Church TR, Snover DC, Bradley GM, Schuman LM, et al. Reducing mortality from colorectal cancer by screening for fecal occult blood: Minnesota Colon Cancer Control Study. N Engl J Med 1993;328:1365–1371 [erratum in N Engl J Med 1993;329:672]

Newcomb PA, Norfleet RG, Storer BE, Surawicz TS, Marcus PM. Screening sigmoidoscopy and colorectal cancer mortality. J Natl Cancer Inst 1992;84:1572–1575

Selby JV, Friedman GD, Quesenberry CP Jr, Weiss NS. A case-control study of screening sigmoidoscopy and mortality from colorectal cancer. N Engl J Med 1992;326:653–657

U.S. Preventive Services Task Force. Guide to clinical preventive services. 2nd ed. Baltimore: Williams & Wilkins, 1996

Winawer SJ, Fletcher RH, Miller L, Godlee F, Stolar MH, Malrow CD, et al. Colorectal cancer screening: clinical guidelines and rationale. Gastroenterology 1997;112:594–642 [errata in Gastroenterology 1997;112:1060 and 1998;114:625]

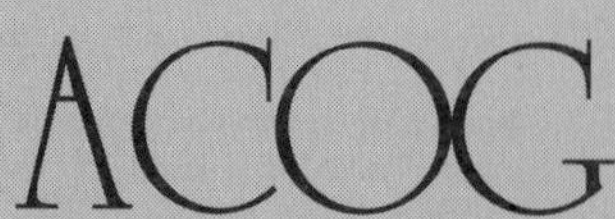

Committee on Obstetric Practice

Committee on Genetics

Committee Opinion

Number 183, April 1997

Routine Storage of Umbilical Cord Blood for Potential Future Transplantation

Reconstitution of the bone marrow can be a life-saving procedure in the treatment of hematologic disease (eg, Fanconi anemia) or advanced malignancy. The necessary hematopoietic stem and progenitor cells are usually obtained from allogeneic or autologous bone marrow. If autologous marrow is not an option, then a human leukocyte antigen (HLA)-identical sibling is the donor most likely to result in successful engraftment and minimization of the risk of graft-versus-host (GVH) disease. Most people do not have an HLA-identical sibling available, and they must look outside of their families. There is a national registry of potential bone marrow donors, but finding an identical match and convincing that individual to undergo the unpleasant donation procedure is not always easy. Many individuals who could potentially benefit from transplantation die while awaiting donors.

A recently recognized potential source for hematopoietic stem and progenitor cells is human fetal cord blood. Early results from more than 200 transplants of human cord stem cells, primarily to treat childhood malignancies, seem very encouraging for several reasons. There appears to be a relatively high success rate for the procedure even in the face of HLA mismatches at one or more loci. There also appears to be a somewhat lower risk for GVH disease than that which is true for traditional bone marrow transplantation. These encouraging preliminary reports have generated considerable enthusiasm because the 4 million births per year in the United States would appear to provide a large reservoir of genetically diverse, potentially transplantable specimens. Large volumes of cord blood are now being "wasted" as "discarded human material" that could theoretically be easily collected, typed, screened for infections, and banked cryogenically for transplantation.

The use of this technology raises a number of scientific, legal, and ethical issues that need to be addressed:

- Should cord blood specimens be collected and banked centrally for allogeneic transplantation in a system analogous to the way that we now handle blood, or would parents be well-advised to bank their own child's cord blood at birth for potential future autologous use should it ever be necessary?

ISSN 1074-861X

The American College of Obstetricians and Gynecologists
409 12th Street, SW
PO Box 96920
Washington, DC 20090-6920

12345/10987

- What is the probability that any individual will ever need his or her own cord blood for transplantation? If that need does arise 18 years later, what is the probability that a specimen stored for 18 years will still be viable?
- Most transplants to date have been done in babies and young children. More cells are needed to reconstitute the bone marrow of persons of larger size. What percentage of cord blood specimens will have adequate numbers of cells to reconstitute the bone marrow of adults?
- Are cord blood stem and progenitor cells more efficient at reconstituting marrow than are cells obtained from adult marrow? Would fewer cells on a per-kilogram body weight basis be as effective?
- Could the number of stem and progenitor cells in a specimen of cord blood be expanded in vitro to provide enough cells for a reliable reconstitution of the bone marrow of persons of adult size?
- If the apparently lower incidence of GVH disease compared with adult marrow sources is real, it may represent reduced immunocompetence of cord stem and progenitor cells. This may be disadvantageous in treating patients with cancer. It may also permit a higher incidence of second primary cancers in transplant survivors.
- As many as 38% of cord blood specimens may be contaminated with maternal cells. What effect will this contamination with adult cells that are (presumably) immunocompetent have upon graft success rate?
- In the future, there may be other medical approaches to manage these diseases.
- Should this technology continue to show promise, and the decision is made to establish cord blood banks, should cord blood continue to be regarded as "discarded human material?"
- Could cord blood be collected routinely at deliveries without consent?
- All specimens would need to be tested for infectious and selected genetic diseases before use. Should parents be informed if their child's specimen tests positive for an infection (eg, human immunodeficiency virus) or genetic disease?
- If nonpaternity is discovered in the course of testing, should that be disclosed to the mother, father, or child?
- Physicians should resist the pressures of marketing, and they should evaluate thoroughly the potential benefits and risks—emotional as well as physical—of all new medical interventions.

Privately owned for-profit companies have been established to bank cord blood samples for potential future use by those individuals or their family members. There is a significant cost associated with the initial specimen processing (approximately $1,500) and an annual storage fee (approximately $100). Given the low probability of needing a stem cell transplant (which has been estimated at between 1 in 1,000 and 1 in 200,000 by age 18) and the other uncertainties regarding success rates with increasing body mass and time in storage, is this a "good" investment? In view of the apparent success rate, despite HLA mismatch, will there be an advantage to receiving one's own banked cells, or could one do just as well with someone else's cord blood? Once banked, to whom do the cells there belong? Do they belong to the parents who paid the fees or the child from whom they came? Do the parents have the right to give them away or sell them, or should they be held for the person from whom they came until he or she reaches the age of majority? If the cells are to be used for someone other than the person from whom they came, must both parents agree or is consent from one adequate? What happens if the parents disagree?

There are clearly many questions about this technology that remain to be answered. Some are relatively simple, such as the success rate of the procedure for various diseases and at various body weights. These simply await a larger number of cases. Some will be more difficult, such as the viability of cells in long-term storage; these questions will take time to answer. The most difficult will be the moral, ethical, and social questions, which need extensive public discussion and may never all be resolved to everyone's satisfaction. Until there is a fuller understanding of all of these issues, we must proceed with considerable circumspection. Parents should not be sold this service without a realistic assessment of their likely return on their investment. Commercial cord blood banks should not represent the service they sell as "doing everything possible" to ensure the health of children. Parents and grandparents should not be made to feel guilty if they are not eager or able to invest these considerable sums in such a highly speculative venture.

Bibliography

Broxmeyer HE. Questions to be answered regarding umbilical cord blood hematopoietic stem and progenitor cells and their use in transplantation. Transfusion 1995;35:694-702

Kurtzberg J, Laughlin M, Graham ML, Smith C, Olson JF, Halperin EC, et al. Placental blood as a source of hematopoietic stem cells for transplantation into unrelated recipients. N Engl J Med 1996;335:157-166

Laporte JP, Gorin NC, Rubinstein P, Lesage S, Portnoi MF, Barbu V, et al. Cord-blood transplantation from an unrelated donor in an adult with chronic myelogenous leukemia. N Engl J Med 1996;335:167-170

Marshall E. Clinical promise, ethical quandary. Science 1996;271:586-588

Rubinstein P, Rosenfield RE, Adamson JW, Stevens CE. Stored placental blood for unrelated bone marrow reconstitution. Blood 1993;81:1679-1690

Scaradavou A, Carrier C, Mollen N, Stevens C, Rubenstein P. Detection of maternal DNA in placental/umbilical cord blood by locus-specific amplification of the noninherited maternal HLA gene. Blood 1996;88:1494-1500

Silberstein LE, Jefferies LC. Placental-blood banking—a new frontier in transfusion medicine. N Engl J Med 1996;335:199-201

Wagner JE, Rosenthal J, Sweetman R, Shu XO, Davies SM, Ramsay NK, et al. Successful transplantation of HLA-matched and HLA-mismatched umbilical cord blood from unrelated donors: analysis of engraftment and acute graft-versus-host disease. Blood 1996:88:795-802

ACOG Committee Opinion

Committee on Obstetric Practice

Number 234, May 2000 (*Replaces No. 219, August 1999*)

Scheduled Cesarean Delivery and the Prevention of Vertical Transmission of HIV Infection

This document reflects emerging clinical and scientific advances as of the date issued and is subject to change. The information should not be construed as dictating an exclusive course of treatment or procedure to be followed.

ISSN 1074-861X

The American College of Obstetricians and Gynecologists
409 12th Street, SW
PO Box 96920
Washington, DC 20090-6920

12345/43210

Prevention of transmission of the human immunodeficiency virus (HIV) from mother to fetus or newborn (vertical transmission) is a major goal in the care of pregnant women infected with HIV. An important advance in this regard was the demonstration that treatment of the mother with zidovudine (ZDV) during pregnancy and labor and of the neonate for the first 6 weeks after birth could reduce the transmission rate from 25% to 8% (1).

Continuing research into vertical transmission of HIV suggests that a substantial number of cases occur as the result of fetal exposure to the virus during labor and delivery; the precise mechanisms are not known. Transmission could occur by transplacental maternal–fetal microtransfusion of blood contaminated with the virus during uterine contractions or by exposure to the virus in maternal cervicovaginal secretions and blood at delivery. Data also indicate that the risk of vertical transmission is proportional to the concentration of virus in maternal plasma (viral load). At very low concentrations of virus in maternal plasma (viral load less than 1,000 copies per milliliter), the observed incidence of vertical transmission among 141 mother–infant pairs was 0 with a 95% upper confidence bound of about 2% (2, 3).

In theory, the risk of vertical transmission in mothers with high viral loads could be reduced by performing cesarean deliveries before the onset of labor and before rupture of membranes (termed *scheduled cesarean delivery* in this document). Early studies of the relationship between the mode of delivery and the risk of vertical transmission yielded inconsistent results. Data from two prospective cohort studies (4, 5), an international randomized trial (6), and a meta-analysis of individual patient data from 15 prospective cohort studies, including more than 7,800 mother–child pairs (7), indicate that there is a significant relationship between the mode of delivery and vertical transmission of HIV. This body of evidence, accumulated mostly before the use of highly active antiretroviral therapy (HAART) and without any data regarding maternal viral load, indicates that scheduled cesarean delivery reduces the likelihood of vertical transmission of HIV compared with either unscheduled cesarean delivery or vaginal delivery. This finding holds true whether or not the patient is receiving ZDV therapy. Whether cesarean delivery offers any benefit to women on HAART or to women with low or undetectable maternal viral loads is unknown. Data are insufficient to address the question of how long after the onset of labor or rupture of membranes the benefit is lost. It is clear that maternal morbidity is greater with cesarean delivery than with vaginal delivery, as is true for women not infected with HIV (8–10). Increases in postpartum morbidity seem to be greatest among women infected with HIV who have low CD4 cell counts (9).

Although many issues remain unresolved because of insufficient data, there is consensus that the following should be recommended:

- Patients should be counseled that in the absence of antiretroviral therapy, the risk of vertical transmission is approximately 25%. With ZDV therapy, the risk is reduced to 5–8%. When care includes both ZDV therapy and scheduled cesarean delivery, the risk is approximately 2%. A similar risk of 2% or less is seen among women with viral loads of less than 1,000 copies per milliliter, even without the systematic use of scheduled cesarean delivery. No combination of therapies can guarantee that a newborn will not become infected (a 0% transmission rate).
- Women infected with HIV, whose viral loads are greater than 1,000 copies per milliliter, should be counseled regarding the potential benefit of scheduled cesarean delivery to further reduce the risk of vertical transmission of HIV beyond that achievable with antiretroviral therapy alone.
- Neonates of women at highest risk for vertical transmission, with relatively high plasma viral loads, are most likely to benefit from scheduled cesarean delivery. Data are insufficient to demonstrate a benefit for neonates of women with plasma viral loads of less than 1,000 copies per milliliter. The available data indicate no reduction in the transmission rate if cesarean delivery is performed after the onset of labor or rupture of membranes. The decision regarding the route of delivery must be individualized in these circumstances.
- The patient's autonomy in making the decision regarding route of delivery must be respected. A patient's informed decision to undergo vaginal delivery must be honored, with cesarean delivery performed only for other accepted indications and with patient consent.
- Patients should receive antiretroviral chemotherapy during pregnancy according to currently accepted guidelines for adults (11). This should not be interrupted around the time of cesarean delivery. For those patients receiving ZDV, adequate levels of the drug in the blood should be achieved if the infusion is begun 3 hours preoperatively (1), according to the dosing schedule recommended by the Centers for Disease Control and Prevention (www.cdc.gov/hiv/treatment).
- Because morbidity is increased in HIV-infected women undergoing cesarean delivery, physicians should consider using prophylactic antibiotics during all such cesarean deliveries.
- The American College of Obstetricians and Gynecologists generally recommends that scheduled cesarean deliveries not be performed before 39 completed weeks of gestation. In women with HIV infection, however, delivery at 38 completed weeks of gestation is recommended to reduce the likelihood of onset of labor or rupture of membranes before delivery.
- Best clinical estimates of gestational age should be used for planning cesarean delivery. Amniocentesis to determine fetal lung maturity in pregnant women infected with HIV should be avoided whenever possible.
- Current recommendations for adults indicate that plasma viral load should be determined at baseline and then every 3 months or following changes in therapy (11). Plasma viral load should be monitored, according to these guidelines, during pregnancy as well. The patient's most recently determined viral load should be used to direct counseling regarding mode of delivery.
- Preoperative maternal health status affects the degree of risk of maternal morbidity associated with cesarean delivery. All women should be clearly informed of the risks associated with cesarean delivery. Ultimately, the decision to perform a cesarean delivery must be individualized in each case according to circumstances.

A skin-penetrating injury (eg, needlestick or scalpel laceration) is a risk to care providers during all deliveries, vaginal or cesarean. This risk is not greater during cesarean delivery, although there generally are more health care personnel present and, thus, at risk during a cesarean delivery than during a vaginal delivery (12). Appropriate care and precautions against such injuries always should be taken, but these concerns should not affect decisions regarding route of delivery (13).

In summary, cesarean delivery performed before the onset of labor and before rupture of membranes effectively reduces the risk of vertical transmission of HIV infection. Scheduled cesarean delivery should be discussed and recommended for women with viral loads greater than 1,000 copies per milliliter whether or not they are taking antiretroviral therapy. As with all complex clinical decisions, the choice of delivery must be individualized. Discussion of the option of scheduled cesarean delivery should begin as early as possible in pregnancy with every pregnant woman with HIV infection to give her an adequate opportunity to consider the choice and plan for the procedure. The risks, which are greater for the mother, must be balanced with the benefits expected for the neonate. The patient's autonomy must be respected when making the decision to perform a cesarean delivery, because the potential for maternal morbidity is significant.

References

1. Connor EM, Sperling RS, Gelber R, Kiselev P, Scott G, O'Sullivan MJ, et al. Reduction of maternal-infant transmission of human immunodeficiency virus type 1 with zidovudine treatment. Pediatric AIDS Clinical Trials Group Protocol 076 Study Group. N Engl J Med 1994;331:1173–1180
2. Mofenson LM, Lambert JS, Stiehm ER, Bethel J, Meyer WA 3rd, Whitehouse J, et al. Risk factors for perinatal transmission of human immunodeficiency virus type 1 in women treated with zidovudine. Pediatric AIDS Clinical Trials Group Study 185 Team. N Engl J Med 1999;341:385–393
3. Garcia PM, Kalish LA, Pitt J, Minkoff H, Quinn T, Burchett SK, et al. Maternal levels of plasma human immunodeficiency virus type 1 RNA and the risk of perinatal transmission. Women and Infants Transmission Study Group. N Engl J Med 1999;341:394–402
4. Kind C, Rudin C, Siegrist CA, Wyler CA, Biedermann K, Lauper U, et al. Prevention of vertical HIV transmission: additive protective effect of elective cesarean section and zidovudine prophylaxis. AIDS 1998;12:205–210
5. Mandelbrot L, Le Chenadec J, Berrebi A, Bongain A, Benifla JL, Delfraissy JF, et al. Perinatal HIV-1 transmission: interaction between zidovudine prophylaxis and mode of delivery in the French Perinatal Cohort. JAMA 1998;280:55–60
6. The European Mode of Delivery Collaboration. Elective caesarean-section versus vaginal delivery in prevention of vertical HIV-1 transmission: a randomized clinical trial. Lancet 1999;353:1035–1039
7. The International Perinatal HIV Group. The mode of delivery and the risk of vertical transmission of human immunodeficiency virus type 1: a meta-analysis of 15 prospective cohort studies. N Engl J Med 1999;340:977–987
8. Nielsen TF, Hakegaard KH. Postoperative cesarean section morbidity: a prospective study. Am J Obstet Gynecol 1983; 146:911–915
9. Semprini AE, Castagna C, Ravizza M, Fiore S, Savasi V, Muggiasca ML, et al. The incidence of complications after cesarean section in 156 HIV-positive women. AIDS 1996; 9:913–917
10. Bulterys M, Chao A, Dushimimana A, Saah A. Fatal complications after cesarean section in HIV-infected women. AIDS 1996;10:923–924
11. Centers for Disease Control and Prevention. Report of the NIH Panel to define principles of therapy of HIV infection and guidelines for the use of antiretroviral agents in HIV-infected adults and adolescents. MMWR Morb Mortal Wkly Rep 1998;47(RR-5):1–82
12. Duff P, Robertson AW, Read JA. Single-dose cefazolin versus cefonicid for antibiotic prophylaxis in cesarean delivery. Obstet Gynecol 1987;70:718–721
13. Centers for Disease Control. Update: universal precautions for prevention of transmission of human immunodeficiency virus, hepatitis B virus, and other bloodborne pathogens in health-care settings. MMWR Morb Mortal Wkly Rep 1988;37:377–382;387–388

Bibliography

Rodman JH, Robbins BL, Flynn PM, Fridland A. A systematic and cellular model for zidovudine plasma concentrations and intracellular phosphorylation in patients. J Infect Dis 1996;174: 490–499

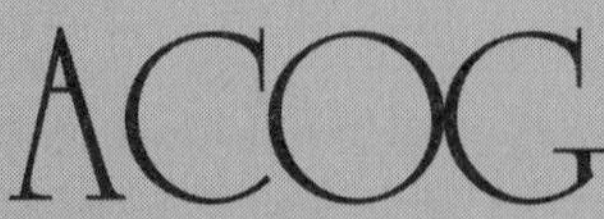

Committee Opinion

Committee on Obstetric Practice

Number 175, September 1996 (*Replaces # 79, January 1990*)

Scope of Services for Uncomplicated Obstetric Care

Total obstetric care comprises services normally provided in uncomplicated obstetric care. These include antepartum care, intrapartum care, and postpartum care.

Antepartum Care

1. First prenatal visit with initial history and physical examination
2. The frequency of follow-up visits is determined by the individual needs of the woman and the assessment of her risks. Generally, a woman with an uncomplicated pregnancy is examined every 4 weeks for the first 28 weeks of gestation, every 2–3 weeks until 36 weeks of gestation, and weekly thereafter, although flexibility is desirable.

Intrapartum Care

1. Supervision of uncomplicated labor
2. Uncomplicated vaginal delivery

Postpartum Care

1. Hospital
2. Office (routine, uncomplicated—42 days)

ISSN 1074-861X

The American College of Obstetricians and Gynecologists
409 12th Street, SW
PO Box 96920
Washington, DC 20090-6920

12345/09876

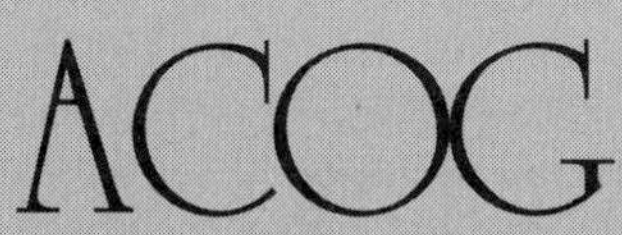

Committee on Genetics

Committee Opinion

Number 212, November 1998

Screening for Canavan Disease

Canavan disease is a severe progressive genetic disorder of the central nervous system. The clinical features of Canavan disease usually appear after the first few months of life and include developmental delay, macrocephaly, hypotonia, and poor head control. As the disease progresses, seizures, optic atrophy, gastrointestinal reflux, and deterioration of swallowing develop. Most children with Canavan disease die in the first decade of life. Presently, there is no cure or effective therapy for Canavan disease.

Canavan disease is caused by a deficiency of the enzyme aspartoacylase, which leads to increased excretion of its substrate, *N*-acetylaspartic acid (NAA). A diagnosis of Canavan disease is established by determining an increased level of urinary NAA by organic acid analysis. These abnormally high levels of NAA lead to demyelination and spongy degeneration of the brain, which cause the neurologic features of Canavan disease.

As in Tay–Sachs disease, Canavan disease is inherited as an autosomal recessive condition and is more prevalent among individuals of Eastern European Jewish (Ashkenazi) background. It is estimated that the carrier frequency in the Ashkenazi Jewish population is approximately 1 per 40. Thus, the risk for an affected offspring in this population approximates 1 in 6,400 births. Unlike Tay–Sachs disease, however, there do not appear to be other high-risk ethnic populations, although Canavan disease has been reported in individuals of non-Ashkenazi Jewish background.

Molecular studies have revealed two specific mutations in the aspartoacylase gene on chromosome 17. These account for approximately 97% of the mutations causing Canavan disease in the Ashkenazi Jewish population. One is a mutation in codon 285 of the aspartoacylase gene, and the other is a mutation in codon 231. Screening of Ashkenazi Jewish individuals can be performed by analyzing for these two mutations. In non-Jewish persons, the mutations may be different and more diverse. The most common mutation is in codon 305, which has been noted in approximately 36% of the 70 identified alleles from unrelated non-Jewish individuals.

Carrier screening for Canavan disease requires molecular diagnostic methods. Simple enzymatic assays, as commonly used in Tay–Sachs screening, cannot be used for Canavan disease because the activity of the deficient enzyme, aspartoacylase, is not detectable in blood. Testing for the three most common Canavan disease mutations will identify about 97% of Ashkenazi Jewish carriers and 40–50% of non-Jewish carriers.

ISSN 1074-861X

The American College of Obstetricians and Gynecologists
409 12th Street, SW
PO Box 96920
Washington, DC 20090-6920

12345/21098

When both parents are carriers of identifiable Canavan disease mutations, prenatal diagnosis by chorionic villus sampling (CVS) or amniocentesis can be accomplished using DNA analysis. In couples where one or both members have unknown mutations, biochemical analysis of NAA levels in the amniotic fluid can be used reliably. Elevated NAA levels can be used to detect an affected fetus. The analysis should be done in a laboratory that has personnel who have expertise in performing this test. Enzyme analysis of aspartoacylase in cultured fetal cells from CVS or amniocentesis is not reliable.

Based on the preceding information, the Committee on Genetics makes the following recommendations:

1. Ideally, molecular carrier screening for Canavan disease should be offered preconceptionally if both members of the couple are of Ashkenazi Jewish genetic background. This screening could be combined with screening for Tay–Sachs disease because both disorders are more common in this group. Many specialized laboratories already offer screening for both diseases. Those with a family history consistent with Canavan disease also should be offered screening, which should be voluntary; informed consent and assurance of confidentiality are required. If potential carriers have not been screened preconceptionally, screening may be offered during early pregnancy.
2. If only one partner is of high risk (of Ashkenazi Jewish descent or with a family history consistent with Canavan disease), this partner should be screened first. Ideally, this should be performed preconceptionally. If it is determined that the high-risk partner is a carrier, the other partner should be offered screening. The couple, however, must be informed of the limitations of testing. If the woman is already pregnant, it may be necessary to screen both partners simultaneously so that results are obtained in a timely fashion and to ensure that all options are available for the couple.
3. If it is determined by DNA-based analysis that both partners are carriers of Canavan disease, prenatal diagnosis should be offered either by CVS or amniocentesis, using DNA-based testing of the fetal cells.

Bibliography

American College of Medical Genetics Board of Directors. Position statement on carrier testing for Canavan disease. Bethesda, Maryland: January 10, 1998

American College of Obstetricians and Gynecologists. Screening for Tay–Sachs disease. ACOG Committee Opinion 162. Washington, DC: ACOG, 1995

Bennett MJ, Gibson KM, Sherwood WG, Divry P, Rolland MO, Elpeleg ON, et al. Reliable prenatal diagnosis of Canavan disease (aspartoacylase deficiency): comparison of enzymatic and metabolite analysis. J Inherit Metab Dis 1993;16:831–836

Kaul R, Gao GP, Matalon M, Aloya M, Su Q, Jin M, et al. Identification and expression of eight novel mutations among non-Jewish patients with Canavan disease. Am J Hum Genet 1996;59:95–102

Kronn D, Oddoux C, Philips J, Ostrer H. Prevalence of Canavan disease heterozygotes in the New York metropolitan Ashkenazi Jewish population. Am J Hum Genet 1995;57:1250–1252

Matalon R. Canavan disease: diagnosis and molecular analysis. Genetic Testing 1997;1:21–25

Matalon R, Michals K, Kaul R. Canavan disease: from spongy degeneration to molecular analysis. J Pediatr 1995;127:511–517

ACOG

Committee on Obstetric Practice

Committee Opinion

Number 241, September 2000

Screening for Hypothyroidism

Thyroid hormone is critical to normal development of the human fetal brain. The fetal thyroid gland does not begin to function until early in the second trimester. There is evidence that first-trimester fetal thyroid hormone needs are met by transplacental passage of maternal thyroid hormone and that maternal first-trimester hypothyroidism is associated with poor infant psychomotor development (1).

An observational study has drawn considerable attention to the subject of maternal hypothyroidism (2), which has resulted in calls for universal screening for maternal hypothyroidism from some professional organizations. The researchers screened maternal serum samples—obtained in the second trimester for purposes of maternal serum alpha-fetoprotein screening for neural tube defects—for elevated thyroid-stimulating hormone levels. They then compared the results of neuropsychologic testing, performed on 62 children, 8 years of age, of hypothyroid women with that of 124 children of matched euthyroid women. They found a small (4-point) but statistically significant difference in performance between the groups, which favored the children of euthyroid women. Also, they found that the children of known hypothyroid women who were taking thyroid hormone replacement therapy performed better than the children of untreated women even though the thyroid hormone replacement therapy was not adequate. Among the children of the untreated women, 19% had full-scale IQ scores below 85 compared with only 5% of the children of euthyroid women.

It is important to acknowledge the limitations of our current understanding of this issue. The data available are observational. There are no intervention trials to demonstrate the efficacy of screening and treatment to improve neuropsychologic performance in children of hypothyroid women. The available data are consistent with the possibility that first-trimester maternal hypothyroidism is associated with suboptimal fetal brain development. Even if proven to be true, it is possible that screening for hypothyroidism as early as the initial prenatal visit in the first trimester may be too late to obviate the potential deficiency in fetal brain development. It is possible that screening and intervention may need to occur before pregnancy to be successful.

It is premature to call for universal screening for hypothyroidism during pregnancy. Although it would be reasonable to screen for hypothyroidism as part of prepregnancy counseling and evaluation and prenatal laboratory studies, there is no clear evidence of the efficacy of this intervention.

ISSN 1074-861X

The American College of Obstetricians and Gynecologists
409 12th Street, SW
PO Box 96920
Washington, DC 20090-6920

12345/43210

References

1. Pop VJ, Kuijpens JL, van Baar AL, Verkerk G, van Son MM, de Vijlder JJ, et al. Low maternal free thyroxine concentrations during early pregnancy are associated with impaired psychomotor development in infancy. Clin Endocrinol 1999;50:149–155
2. Haddow JE, Palomaki GE, Allan WC, Williams JR, Knight GJ, Gagnon MA, et al. Maternal thyroid deficiency during pregnancy and subsequent neuropsychological development of the child. N Engl J Med 1999;341:549–555

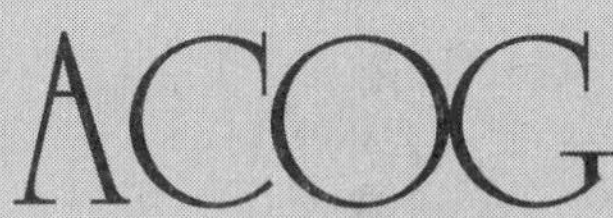

Committee on Genetics

Committee Opinion

Number 162, November 1995 *(Replaces #93, March 1991)*

Screening for Tay–Sachs Disease

Tay–Sachs Disease (TSD) is a lysosomal storage disease in which GM_2 gangliosides accumulate throughout the body. The accumulation of these gangliosides in the central nervous system results in a severe progressive neurologic disease with death in early childhood.

The enzyme hexosaminidase occurs in two principal forms, Hex-A and Hex-B. Hex-A is composed of one α- and one β-subunit, whereas Hex-B is composed of two β-subunits. Tay–Sachs disease is caused by a deficiency of Hex-A, whereas Sandhoff disease is caused by a deficiency of both Hex-A and Hex-B. Both of these diseases are transmitted in an autosomal recessive fashion. Laboratories report Hex-A levels as a percentage of total hexosaminidase activity. Hex-A is almost completely absent in patients with classical TSD. Hex-A comprises 0.5% of total hexosaminidase activity in the late infantile type and 2–4% in the adult form activity. The percentage of Hex-A activity in carriers is usually less than 55% of total activity, whereas Hex-A activity in non-carriers is generally more than 60% of total activity. Tay–Sachs disease can be diagnosed prenatally by measuring hexosaminidase activity in samples obtained by amniocentesis or by chorionic villus sampling.

The frequency of TSD carriers in Jews of Eastern European descent (Ashkenazi) is about 1 in 30; the carrier rate for non-Jewish groups is estimated at 1 in 300. It has been determined that people of French–Canadian and Cajun descent also have a greater carrier frequency than the general population.

Carrier screening using serum is inaccurate when performed in women who are pregnant or taking oral contraceptives. If the serum test is used, many pregnant women will be misclassified as carriers. If testing is to be done in women who are pregnant or taking oral contraceptives, leukocyte testing must be used.

Molecular analyses of the α-subunit gene for TSD have been reported in both Jewish and non-Jewish populations. Three mutations comprise more than 90% of mutant genes in Ashkenazi Jewish persons. Other less common mutations are often seen in non-Jewish carriers. Molecular analysis may be required in some of these patients.

When the serum test is inconclusive, biochemical analysis should be performed on leukocytes from peripheral blood. DNA analysis is reserved for those couples who consistently have ambiguous enzymatic tests in both

ISSN 1074-861X

The American College of Obstetricians and Gynecologists
409 12th Street, SW
Washington, DC 20024-2188

12345/98765

serum and leukocytes and for individuals who are suspected to have a rare pseudodeficiency condition.

Pseudodeficiency refers to a state in which asymptomatic individuals have a low amount of Hex-A activity when tested with conventional artificial substrate. However, these normal but Hex-A–minus individuals are able to catalyze the breakdown of natural substrate GM_2 ganglioside. Pseudodeficiency mutations comprise about one third of the mutations identified in non-Jewish individuals. Because some of these individuals are compound heterozygotes for a Tay–Sachs mutation and a pseudodeficiency allele, the delineation of their precise genotype for reproductive purposes usually requires further biochemical assessment complemented with DNA analysis.

Based on the preceding information, the Committee on Genetics makes the following recommendations:

1. Ideally, serum screening for TSD should be offered before pregnancy if both members of a couple are Ashkenazi Jews or of French–Canadian or Cajun descent. Those with a family history consistent with TSD should also be screened.
2. When one member of a couple is at high risk (ie, Ashkenazi Jew, of French–Canadian or Cajun descent, or has a family history consistent with TSD) but the other partner is not, the high-risk partner should be screened. This is particularly important if there is uncertainty about ancestry or if there is a family history consistent with TSD. If the high-risk partner is determined to be a carrier, the other partner should also be screened. If the woman is already pregnant, it may be necessary to screen both partners simultaneously so that results are obtained in a timely fashion and to ensure that all options are available to the couple.
3. Ambiguous screening tests or positive screening tests in individuals not at high risk should be confirmed by molecular analysis for the most common mutations. This will detect patients who carry genes associated with mild disease or pseudodeficiency states.
4. If TSD screening is performed in women who are pregnant or on oral contraceptives, leukocyte testing must be used.
5. If both partners are determined to be carriers of TSD, genetic counseling and prenatal diagnosis should be offered (1).

Reference

1. American College of Obstetricians and Gynecologists. Antenatal diagnosis of genetic disorders. ACOG Technical Bulletin 108. Washington, DC: ACOG, 1987

Bibliography

Kaback M, Lim-Steele J, Dabholkar D, Brown D, Levy N, Zeiger K. Tay-Sachs disease—carrier screening, prenatal diagnosis, and the molecular era. An international perspective, 1970 to 1993. The International TSD Data Collection Network. JAMA 1993;270:2307–2315

Prence EM, Natowicz MR, Zalewski I. Unusual thermolability properties of leukocyte beta-hexosaminidase: implications in screening for carriers of Tay-Sachs disease. Clin Chem 1993; 39:1811–1814

Triggs-Raine BL, Feigenbaum AS, Natowicz M, Skomorowski MA, Schuster SM, Clarke JT, et al. Screening for carriers of Tay-Sachs disease among Ashkenazi Jews. A comparison of DNA-based and enzyme-based tests. N Engl J Med 1990; 32:6–12

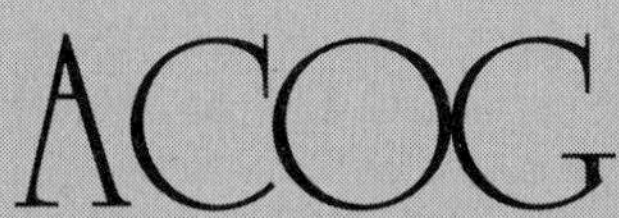

Committee
on Ethics

Committee Opinion

Number 177, November 1996

Sex Selection

Sex selection is the practice of using medical techniques to choose the sex of offspring. Patients may request sex selection for different reasons. Medical indications include the prevention of sex-linked genetic disorders. In addition, there are a variety of social, economic, cultural, and personal reasons for selecting the sex of children. In cultures in which males are more highly valued than females, sex selection has been practiced in order to ensure that offspring will be male.

Currently, reliable techniques for selecting sex are limited to postfertilization methods. Postfertilization methods include techniques used during pregnancy as well as techniques used in assisted reproduction prior to the transfer of preembryos (1).

This Committee Opinion discusses various ethical considerations and arguments relevant to sex selection. It also provides recommendations for health professionals who may be asked to participate in sex selection.

Indications

The principal medical indication for sex selection is known or suspected risk of sex-linked genetic disorders. For example, 50% of males born to women who carry the gene for hemophilia will have this condition. By identifying the sex of the preembryo or fetus, a woman can learn whether or not the 50% risk of hemophilia applies, and she can receive appropriate prenatal counseling. To ensure that surviving offspring will not have this condition, some women at risk for transmitting hemophilia choose to abort male fetuses or choose not to transfer male preembryos. Where the marker or gene for a sex-linked genetic disorder is known, selection on the basis of direct identification of affected offspring, rather than on the basis of sex, is possible. Direct identification has the advantage of avoiding the possibility of aborting or deciding not to transfer healthy offspring. Despite increased ability to identify genes and markers, in certain situations, sex determination is the only current method of identifying preembryos or fetuses potentially affected with sex-linked disorders (2).

Inevitably, identification of sex occurs whenever karyotyping is performed. When medical indications for genetic karyotyping do not require information about sex chromosomes, the prospective parent(s) may elect not to be told the sex of the fetus.

ISSN 1074-861X

The American College of Obstetricians and Gynecologists
409 12th Street, SW
PO Box 96920
Washington, DC 20090-6920

12345/09876

Other reasons sex selection is requested are personal, social, or cultural in nature. For example, prospective parent(s) may prefer that an only or first-born child be of a certain sex or may desire a balance of sexes in the completed family (3).

Methods

There are a variety of techniques for sex identification and selection. These include techniques used before fertilization, after fertilization but prior to preembryo transfer, and, most frequently, after implantation.

Prefertilization

Techniques for sex selection prior to fertilization include timing sexual intercourse and using various methods for separating X-bearing and Y-bearing sperm (4–11). No current techniques for prefertilization sex selection have been shown to be reliable.

Postfertilization, Pretransfer

Assisted reproductive technologies, such as in vitro fertilization and zygote intrafallopian transfer, make possible biopsy of one or more cells from a developing preembryo at the cleavage or blastocyst stage (12). Sex selection is therefore possible in conjunction with these reproductive technologies.

Postimplantation

After implantation of a fertilized egg, karyotyping of fetal cells will provide information about fetal sex. This presents patients with the option of terminating pregnancies for the purpose of sex selection.

Ethical Positions of Other Organizations

Many organizations have issued statements concerning the ethics of provider participation in sex selection. The ethics committee of the American Society for Reproductive Medicine (formerly, the American Fertility Society) maintains that couples should be free to use sex selection, but that providers should use "moral suasion" to encourage couples to allow sex determination to be resolved by chance even when advanced reproductive technologies are used and sex selection before preembryo transfer is therefore possible (13).

Both the President's Commission for the Study of Ethical Problems in Medicine and Biomedical and Behavioral Research and the Programme of Action adopted by the United Nations International Conference on Population and Development oppose the use of sex selection techniques for any nonmedical reason (14, 15). The latter group urges governments of all nations "to take necessary measures to prevent... prenatal sex selection."

The International Federation of Gynecology and Obstetrics rejects sex selection when it is used as a tool for sex discrimination. It supports sex selection when used to avoid sex-linked genetic disorders (16).

Discussion

Medical Testing Not Expressly for the Purpose of Sex Selection

Providers may participate unknowingly in sex selection when information about the sex of a fetus results from a medical procedure performed for some other purpose. For example, when a procedure is done to rule out fetal disorders, the sex of a fetus may become known and may be used for sex selection without the provider's awareness.

The Committee on Ethics maintains that when a medical procedure is done for a purpose other than obtaining information about the sex of a fetus but will reveal the fetus's sex, this information should not be withheld from the pregnant woman who requests it. This is because this information legally and ethically belongs to the patient (17–19). As a consequence, it might be difficult for providers to avoid the possibility of unwittingly participating in sex selection. To minimize the possibility that they will unknowingly participate in sex selection, physicians should foster open communication with patients aimed at clarifying patients' goals. Although providers may not ethically withhold medical information from patients who request it, they are not obligated to perform an abortion, or other medical procedure, to select fetal sex. Physicians should explicitly inform patients, in advance when possible, if they are unwilling to perform specific medical procedures that patients might request.

Medical Testing Expressly for the Purpose of Sex Selection

With regard to medical procedures performed for the express purpose of selecting the sex of a fetus, the following three potential ethical positions are outlined to facilitate discussion:

1. *Position 1: Never participate in sex selection.* Providers may never ethically perform medical procedures with the intended purpose of sex selection.

2. *Position 2: Participate in sex selection when medically indicated.* Providers may ethically perform medical procedures with the intended purpose of preventing sex-linked genetic disorders.
3. *Position 3: Participate in sex selection whenever requested.* Providers may ethically perform medical procedures for the purpose of sex selection whenever the patient requests such procedures.

The committee rejects, as too restrictive, the position that sex selection techniques are always unethical (Position 1). The committee supports, as ethically permissible, the practice of offering patients procedures for the purpose of preventing serious sex-linked genetic diseases (Position 2). For example, it supports offering patients using assisted reproductive techniques the option of preembryo biopsy for identification of male sex chromosomes if patients are at risk for transmitting Duchenne muscular dystrophy. This position is consistent with the stance of equality between the sexes as it does not imply that the sex of a child itself makes that child more or less valuable.

The committee rejects the position that sex selection should be performed on demand (Position 3), because this position may reflect and encourage sex discrimination. In most societies where sex selection is widely practiced, families prefer male offspring. While this preference sometimes has an economic rationale, such as the financial support or physical labor male offspring traditionally provide or the financial liability associated with female offspring, it also reflects the belief that males are inherently more valuable than females. There exists a relationship between women's social, legal, and economic status and the tendency of women and men to prefer sons: in general, son-preference increases as women's social status declines (20). Where systematic preferences for a particular sex dominate, this suggests the need to address underlying inequalities between the sexes.

The committee shares the concern expressed by the President's Commission for the Study of Ethical Problems in Medicine and Biomedical and Behavioral Research, the United Nations, and the International Federation of Gynecology and Obstetrics that sex selection can be motivated by and reinforce the devaluation of women. The committee supports the ethical principle of equality between the sexes.

Some argue that sex selection techniques are ethically justified when used for reasons other than disease prevention. For example, sex selection may be requested to achieve a "balance" in a family in which all current children are the same sex and a child of the opposite sex is desired. To achieve this goal, couples may request 1) transferring preembryos of only one sex in assisted reproduction; 2) reducing, based on sex, the number of fetuses in a multifetal pregnancy; or 3) aborting fetuses who are not of the desired sex. In these situations, individual parents may consistently judge sex selection to be an important personal or family goal, and at the same time reject the idea that children of one sex are *inherently* more valuable than children of another sex.

Although this stance is, in principle, consistent with the principle of equality between the sexes, it nonetheless raises ethical concerns. First, it is often impossible to ascertain patients' true motives for requesting sex selection procedures. For example, patients who wanted to abort female fetuses because they valued male offspring more than female offspring, or because they wanted first-born children to be male, would be unlikely to espouse such beliefs openly if they thought this would lead physicians to deny their requests. Second, even when sex selection is requested for nonsexist reasons, the very idea of preferring a child of a particular sex may be interpreted as condoning sexist values and, hence, create a climate in which sex discrimination can more easily flourish. The committee concludes that nonmedical uses of sex selection techniques have the potential to undermine equality between the sexes; moreover, this ethical objection arises irrespective of the stage of development of the preembryo or fetus.

Conclusion

The committee accepts, as ethically permissible, the practice of sex selection to prevent sex-linked genetic disorders. The committee opposes meeting requests for sex selection that are based on the belief that offspring of a certain sex are inherently more valuable. The committee opposes meeting requests for sex selection for personal and family reasons due to the concern that such requests may ultimately support sexist practices.

Medical techniques intended for other purposes have the potential of being used by patients for sex selection without the provider's knowledge or consent. Because patients are entitled to obtain personal medical information, including information about the sex of their fetus, it will sometimes be impossible for health professionals to avoid unwitting participation in sex selection.

In this document, the committee has sought to assist physicians and other health care providers facing requests from patients for sex selection by calling attention to relevant ethical considerations, affirming the value of equality between the sexes, and emphasizing that individual providers are never ethically required to participate in sex selection.

References

1. American College of Obstetricians and Gynecologists. Preembryo research: history, scientific background, and ethical considerations. ACOG Committee Opinion 136. Washington, DC: ACOG, 1994
2. Winston RML, Handyside AH. New challenges in human in vitro fertilization. Science 1993;260:932–936
3. Young R. The ethics of selecting for fetal sex. Ballieres Clin Obstet Gynaecol 1991;5:575–591
4. Gray RH. Natural family planning and sex selection: fact or fiction? Am J Obstet Gynecol 1991;165:1982–1984
5. Shushan A, Schenker JG. Prenatal sex determination and selection. Hum Reprod 1993;8:1545–1549
6. Pyrzak R. Separation of X- and Y-bearing human spermatozoa using albumin gradients. Hum Reprod 1994;9: 1788–1790
7. Check JH, Zavos PM, Katsoff D, Kiefer D. Effects of Percoll discontinuous density gradients vs Spermprep II vs Sephadex G-50 gel infiltration on semen parameters. Arch Androl 1993;31:69–73
8. Martin RH. Human sex pre-selection by sperm manipulation. Hum Reprod 1994;9:1790–1791
9. Check JH, Kastoff D. A prospective study to evaluate the efficacy of modified swim-up preparation for male sex selection. Hum Reprod 1993;8:211–214
10. Check JH, Katsoff D, Kozak J, Lurie D. Effect of swim-up, Percoll, and Sephadex sperm separation methods on the hypo-osmotic swelling test. Hum Reprod 1992;7: 109–111
11. Wang HX, Flaherty SP, Swann NJ, Matthews CD. Discontinuous Percoll gradients enrich X-bearing human spermatozoa. Hum Reprod 1994;9:1265–1270
12. Hardy K, Martin KL, Leese HJ, Winston RM, Handyside AH. Human preimplantation development in vitro fertilization is not adversely affected by biopsy at the 8-cell stage. Hum Reprod 1990;5:708–714
13. American Fertility Society Ethics Committee. Ethical considerations of assisted reproductive technologies. Fertil Steril 1994;62:5(1 suppl):1S–126S
14. President's Commission for the Study of Ethical Problems in Medicine and Biomedical and Behavioral Research. Screening and counseling for genetic conditions. Washington, DC: Government Printing Office, 1983
15. United Nations. Population and development, vol 1: programme of action adopted at the International Conference on Population and Development (Cairo, 5–13 September 1994). New York: United Nations, 1995:20–21
16. International Federation of Gynecology and Obstetrics. Recommendations on ethical issues in obstetrics and gynecology. London: FIGO, 1994:9
17. Jonsen AR, Siegler M, Winslade WJ. Clinical ethics: a practical approach to ethical decisions in clinical medicine. 3rd ed. New York : McGraw-Hill Inc, 1992:40–42, 52–54, 64
18. American Hospital Association Institutional Practices Committee. A patient's bill of rights. In: Management advisories to the American Hospital Association. AHA: Chicago, 1990
19. American Medical Association Council on Ethical and Judicial Affairs. American Medical Association code of medical ethics. Current opinions with annotations. Chicago: AMA, 1994:118
20. Warren MA. Gendercide: the implications of sex selection. Totowa, New Jersey: Rowman and Allanheld, 1985:13

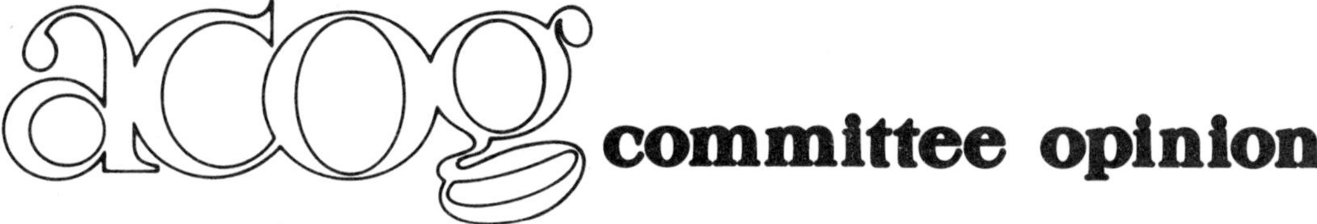

Committee on Ethics Number 144—November 1994

Sexual Misconduct in the Practice of Obstetrics and Gynecology: Ethical Considerations

The privilege of caring for patients, often over a long period of time, can yield considerable professional satisfaction. The obstetrician–gynecologist may fill many roles for patients: as primary physician, technology expert, prevention specialist, counselor, and confidante. Privy to both birth and death, obstetrician–gynecologists assist women as they pass through adolescence; grow into maturity; make choices about sexuality, partnership, and family; experience the sorrows of reproductive loss, infertility, and illness; and adapt to the transitions of midlife and aging. The practice of obstetrics and gynecology includes interaction at times of intense emotion and vulnerability for the patient and involves both sensitive physical examinations and medically necessary disclosure of especially private information about symptoms and experiences. The relationship between physician and patient, therefore, requires a high level of trust and professional responsibility.

Trust of this sort cannot be maintained without a basic understanding of the limits and responsibilities of the professional's role. Physician sexual misconduct is an example of abuse of limits and failure of responsibility. The valued human experience of the physician–patient relationship is damaged when there is either confusion regarding professional goals and behavior or clear lack of integrity that allows sexual exploitation and harm.

Sexual misconduct is of particular concern in today's environment of shifting roles for women and men, greater sexual freedom, and critical evaluation of power relations in society (1–4). Prohibitions against sexual contact between patient and physician are not new, however; they can be found in the earliest guidelines in western antiquity. From the beginning, physicians were enjoined to "do no harm" and specifically avoid sexual contact with patients (5). In the intervening centuries, as the study of medical ethics has evolved, attention has been focused on respect for individual rights, the problem of unequal power in relationships between professionals and patients, and the potential for abuse of that power (6).

In this context, the American Medical Association's Council on Ethical and Judicial Affairs developed a report, "Sexual Misconduct in the Practice of Medicine," condemning sexual relations between physicians and current patients (7). It raises serious questions about the ethics of romantic relationships with former patients. It is summarized as follows:

> Sexual contact that occurs concurrent with the physician–patient relationship constitutes sexual misconduct. Sexual or romantic interactions between physicians and patients detract from the goals of the physician–patient relationship, may exploit the vulnerability of the patient, may obscure the physician's objective judgment concerning the patient's health care, and ultimately may be detrimental to the patient's well-being (8).

The Council provides clear guidelines (7):

- Mere mutual consent is rejected as a justification for sexual relations with patients since the disparity in power, status, vulnerability, and need make it difficult for a patient to give meaningful consent to sexual contact or sexual relations.
- Sexual contact or a romantic relationship concurrent with the physician–patient relationship is unethical.
- Sexual contact or a romantic relationship with a former patient may be unethical under certain circumstances. The relevant standard is the potential for misuse of physician power and exploitation of patient emotions derived from the former relationship.

- Education on ethical issues involved in sexual misconduct should be included throughout all levels of medical training.
- Physicians have a responsibility to report offending colleagues to disciplinary boards.

The Society of Obstetricians and Gynaecologists of Canada has adopted a similar statement that "acknowledges and deplores the fact that incidents of physicians abusing patients do occur" and finds that "these incidents can include 'sexual impropriety' due to poor clinical skills, chauvinism, or abuse of the power relationship or outright systematic sexual abuse." The Society of Obstetricians and Gynaecologists of Canada also supports the right to "informed, safe, and gender-sensitive" care and recommends "prompt treatment of the victims of abuse" and "identification, discipline, and, where possible, rehabilitation of the perpetrators" (9).

Although much discussion of sexual misconduct by physicians in the past decade has centered around the particular vulnerability that exists within the psychiatrist–patient relationship (10), sexual contact between patients and obstetrician–gynecologists has also been documented. Physicians themselves acknowledge that there is a problem, but the extent of the problem is difficult to determine because information relies on self-reporting, which carries the potential for bias in response.

The Committee on Ethics of the American College of Obstetricians and Gynecologists endorses the ethical principles expressed by the American Medical Association and the Society of Obstetricians and Gynaecologists of Canada and affirms the following:

- Sexual contact or a romantic relationship between a physician and a current patient is always unethical.
- Sexual contact or a romantic relationship between a physician and a former patient may also be unethical. Potential risks to both parties should be considered carefully. Such risks may stem from length of time and intensity of the previous professional relationship; age differences; the length of time since cessation of the professional relationship; the former patient's residual feelings of dependency, obligation, or gratitude; the patient's vulnerability to manipulation as a result of private information disclosed during treatment; or physician vulnerability if a relationship initiated with a former patient breaks down.
- Physicians should be careful not to mix roles that are ordinarily in conflict. For example, they should not perform breast or pelvic examinations on their own minor children unless an urgent indication exists. Children and adolescents are particularly vulnerable to emotional conflict and damage to their developing sense of identity and sexuality when roles and role boundaries with trusted adults are confused. It is essential to ensure the young person's privacy and prevent subtly coercive violations from occurring.
- The request by either a patient or a physician to have a chaperon present during a physical examination should be accommodated irrespective of the physician's gender. Local practices and expectations differ with regard to the use of chaperons, but the presence of a third person in the examination room can confer benefits for both patient and physician, regardless of the gender of the chaperon. Chaperons can provide reassurance to the patient about the professional context and content of the exam and the intention of the physician and offer witness to the actual events taking place should there be any misunderstanding. The presence of a third party in the room may, however, cause some embarrassment to the patient and limit her willingness to talk openly with the physician because of concerns about confidentiality. If a chaperon is present, the physician should provide a separate opportunity for private conversation. If the chaperon is an employee of the practice, the physician must establish clear rules about respect for privacy and confidentiality. In addition, some patients (especially, but not limited to, adolescents) may consider the presence of a family member as an intrusion. Family members should not be used as chaperons unless specifically requested by the patient.
- Examinations should be performed with only the necessary amount of physical contact required to obtain data for diagnosis and treatment. Appropriate explanation should accompany all examination procedures.
- Physicians should avoid sexual innuendo and sexually provocative remarks.
- When a physician has questions and concerns about his or her sexual feelings and behavior, he or she should seek advice from mentors or appropriate professional organizations (11).
- It is important for physicians to self-monitor for any early indications that the barrier between normal sexual feelings and inappropriate behavior is not being maintained (12). These indicators might include special scheduling, seeing a patient outside of normal office hours or outside the office, driving a patient home, or making sexually explicit comments about patients.
- Physicians involved in medical education should actively work to include as part of the basic curriculum information about both doctor and patient vulnerability, avoidance of sexually offensive or denigrating language, risk factors for sexual misconduct, and procedures for reporting and rehabilitation.

- Physicians aware of instances of sexual misconduct on the part of any health professional have an obligation to report such situations to appropriate authorities such as institutional committee chairs, department chairs, peer review organizations, supervisors, or professional licensing boards.
- Physicians with administrative responsibilities in hospitals, other medical institutions, and licensing boards should develop clear and public guidelines for reporting instances of sexual misconduct, prompt investigation of all complaints, and appropriate disciplinary and remedial action.

In conclusion, sexual misconduct on the part of physicians is an abuse of professional power and a violation of patient trust. It jeopardizes the well-being of patients and carries an immense potential for harm. The ethical prohibition against physician sexual misconduct is ancient and forceful, and its application to contemporary medical practice is essential.

REFERENCES

1. Kardener SH, Fuller M, Mensh IN. A survey of physicians' attitudes and practices regarding erotic and nonerotic contact with patients. Am J Psychiatry 1973; 130:1077–1081
2. Wilbers D, Veenstra G, van de Wiel HB, Schultz WC. Sexual contact in the doctor–patient relationship in The Netherlands. BMJ 1992;304: 1531–1534
3. Gartrell NK, Milliken N, Goodson WH 3d, Thiemann S, Lo B. Physician–patient sexual contact. Prevalence and problems. West J Med 1992;157:139–143
4. Johnson SH. Judicial review of disciplinary action for sexual misconduct in the practice of medicine. JAMA 1993;270:1596–1600
5. Campbell ML. The oath: an investigation of the injunction prohibiting physician–patient sexual relations. Perspect Biol Med 1989;32:300–308
6. Beauchamp TL, Childress JF. Principles of biomedical ethics. 3rd ed. New York: Oxford University Press, 1989
7. Council on Ethical and Judicial Affairs, American Medical Association. Sexual misconduct in the practice of medicine. JAMA 1991;266:2741–2745
8. Council on Ethical and Judicial Affairs, American Medical Association. Code of medical ethics: current opinions with annotations. Chicago: American Medical Association, 1994:120–121
9. Society of Obstetricians and Gynaecologists of Canada. SOGC resolution on sexual abuse by physicians. JSOGC 1992;14:96
10. Gabbard GO, ed. Sexual exploitation in professional relationships. Washington, DC: American Psychiatric Press, 1989
11. Abel GG, Barrett DH, Gardos PS. Sexual misconduct by physicians. J Med Assoc Ga 1992;81:237–246
12. Searight HR, Campbell DC. Physician–patient sexual contact: ethical and legal issues and clinical guidelines. J Fam Pract 1993;36:647–653

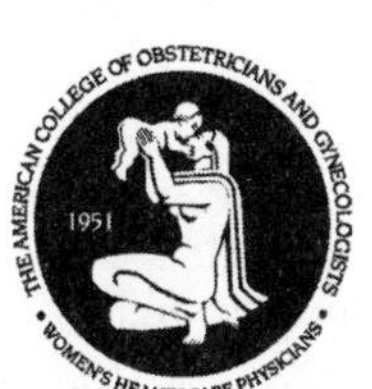

ISSN 1074-861X

The American College of Obstetricians and Gynecologists
409 12th Street, SW • Washington, DC 20024-2188

12345/87654

ACOG

Committee on Gynecologic Practice

Committee on Obstetric Practice

Committee Opinion

Number 240, August 2000 *(Replaces No. 145, November 1994)*

Statement on Surgical Assistants

Competent surgical assistants should be available for all major obstetric and gynecologic operations. In many cases, the complexity of the surgery or the patient's condition will require the assistance of one or more physicians to provide safe, quality care. Often, the complexity of a given surgical procedure cannot be determined prospectively. Procedures including, but not limited to, operative laparoscopy, major abdominal and vaginal surgery, and cesarean delivery may warrant the assistance of another physician to optimize safe surgical care.

The primary surgeon's judgment and prerogative in determining the number and qualifications of surgical assistants should not be overruled by public or private third-party payers. Surgical assistants should be appropriately compensated.

ISSN 1074-861X

The American College of Obstetricians and Gynecologists
409 12th Street, SW
PO Box 96920
Washington, DC 20090-6920

12345/43210

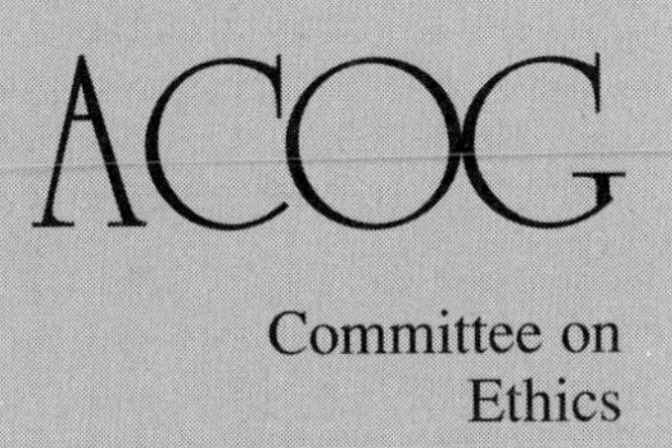

Committee on Ethics

Committee Opinion

Number 216, April 1999

(*Replaces #63, September 1988, and #73, September 1989*)

Sterilization of Women, Including Those with Mental Disabilities

Sterilization, like any other surgical procedure, must be carried out under the general ethical principles of patient autonomy and beneficence. Special ethical considerations are imposed by the unique attributes of sterilization. The procedure usually is done not for medical indications, but electively for family planning. It may have a significant impact on individuals other than the patient, especially her partner. It is intended to be permanent, although techniques are available to attempt reversal or circumvention of sterility. Finally, sterilization affects procreation, and therefore, may conflict with the moral beliefs of the patient, her family, or the physician. When the patient has diminished mental abilities or chronic mental illness, even more stringent ethical constraints apply.

General Ethical Principles

Under the principle of autonomy, patients have the right to seek, accept, or refuse care. Sterilization is for many a social choice rather than purely a medical issue, but all patient-related activities engaged in by physicians are subject to the same ethical guidelines. Patients sometimes request a physician's counsel in deciding whether to request sterilization. Physicians should be cautious in giving advice and making recommendations that go beyond health-related issues, even though nonmedical factors might be the most compelling for the patient. On the one hand, it may be difficult for the physician to address nonmedical issues without bias. Also, the physician may not have a full understanding of the patient's situation. On the other hand, it would be entirely appropriate for the physician to assist the patient in exploring and articulating the reasons for her decision.

Although a woman's request for sterilization may conflict with the physician's medical judgment or moral beliefs, the patient's values must be respected. In such cases, the physician has an obligation to inform the patient of his or her professional recommendation and the medical reasons for it. The physician remains responsible for his or her actions and is not obligated to act

ISSN 1074-861X

The American College of Obstetricians and Gynecologists
409 12th Street, SW
PO Box 96920
Washington, DC 20090-6920

12345/32109

in violation of personal principles of conscience, but the patient should be informed of such principles if she inquires. If the patient continues to desire sterilization, the physician has the obligation to refer her to another caregiver or at least to inform her that sterilization services may be available elsewhere. The physician's values, sense of societal goals, and racial, ethnic, or socioeconomic issues should not be the basis of a recommendation to undergo sterilization.

Sterilization requires the patient's informed consent, for ethical and medical–legal reasons. The physician performing the procedure has the responsibility of ensuring that the patient is properly counseled concerning the risks and benefits of sterilization and its alternatives. The procedure's intended permanence should be stressed, as well as the possibility of future regret. An estimate of the procedure's failure rate and risk of ectopic pregnancy should be provided. A variety of patient education materials are available to assist in preoperative counseling, but it is essential for the patient to be given the opportunity to discuss all relevant issues with her physician and to ask questions.

The physician should be familiar with any laws and regulations that may constrain sterilization, such as limitations on the patient's age and requirements for the consent process. The physician should inform the patient that insurance coverage for sterilization is variable so she can discuss this issue with her insurer.

Specific Ethical Issues

Because sterilization may have important effects on persons other than the patient, women requesting sterilization should be encouraged to discuss the issues with their families, especially with their sexual partners. In many cases, it is preferable for the male partner to be sterilized. It may be helpful for the physician to counsel the partner directly, with the patient's consent.

Hysterectomy solely for the purpose of sterilization is inappropriate. The risks and cost of the procedure are disproportionate to the benefit, given the available alternatives.

Women may be vulnerable to various forms of coercion in their medical decision making. For example, the withholding of other medical care by linking it to the patient's consent to undergo sterilization is ethically unacceptable. Laws, regulations, and reimbursement restrictions concerning sterilization have been created to protect vulnerable individuals, including those with mental disabilities, from abuse. However, sterilization should not be denied to individuals simply because they also may be vulnerable to coercion. Physicians caring for patients who request or require procedures that result in sterilization may find themselves in a dilemma when legal and reimbursement restrictions interfere with a patient's choice of treatment. Rigid timing and age requirements can restrict access to good health care and result in unnecessary risk (1). Physicians are encouraged to seek legal or ethical consultation or both whenever necessary in their efforts to provide care that is most appropriate in individual situations.

At a public policy level, the medical profession has an opportunity to be a voice of reason and compassion, pointing out when legislative and regulatory measures intended to be safeguards interfere with patient choice and appropriate medical care.

Special Considerations Concerning Patients with Mental Disabilities

As used in this document, the term *women with mental disabilities* refers to individuals whose ability to participate in the informed consent process is, or might be, limited and whose autonomy is, or might be, thereby impaired. Such individuals constitute a heterogeneous group, including those with varying degrees of presumably irreversible "mental retardation," as well as those with varying types and degrees of "chronic mental illness." Some of these illnesses are reversible to varying degrees and for varying periods. The concept of "chronically and variably impaired autonomy" has been proposed to describe such situations (2).

Physicians who perform sterilizations must be aware of widely differing federal, state, and local laws and regulations, which have arisen in reaction to a long and unhappy history of sterilization of "unfit" persons in the United States and elsewhere. The potential remains for serious abuses and injustices. Persons who are objectively capable of parenting but who may be simplistically labeled as incapacitated may be deprived of their procreative rights, or conversely persons for whom pregnancy is a serious burden or harm may be denied opportunity for a full range of contraceptive options. For example, federal funds may not be used for the sterilization of "mentally incompetent" or "institutionalized" persons (1). Physicians should always have the maximum respect for patient autonomy, and the presence of a mental disability does not, in itself, justify either sterilization or its denial.

Determination of Ability to Give Informed Consent

Before carrying out any surgical procedure, the physician has the important responsibility of ascertaining the patient's capacity to provide informed consent. It may be difficult to be sure that patients with normal intellectual function understand the complexities of some situations; when the patient has a mental disability, the task is more difficult and the responsibility is more challenging.

Evaluating a mentally impaired person's ability to provide informed consent is seldom straightforward (3). For example, although degrees of mental retardation have been defined according to IQ, there is no direct relationship between such diagnostic categories and the capacity to consent. Among the issues that may need to be considered in the assessment are the patient's language and culture, the quality of information provided (clarity, completeness, lack of bias), the setting of counseling (privacy, comfort), and possible fluctuations in the patient's comprehension. Such fluctuations may result from various stressors and medications. Multiple interviews over an adequate period may be required. Obtaining the assistance of professionals trained in communicating with mentally disabled persons is essential. These professionals may include special educators, psychologists, nurses, attorneys familiar with disability law, and physicians accustomed to working with mentally disabled persons.

The process of evaluating a person's ability to give informed consent may be set forth in laws of the jurisdiction involved, and legal requirements for the determination of competence vary greatly. The concept of legal competence is quite complex. Standards for the definition of competence may vary with the specific purpose (eg, marriage, making a will, consenting or refusing life-saving treatment or, as in the case of sterilization, consenting to elective surgery).

Court approval of sterilization may be required by law or may be necessary in difficult cases because of disagreement among the patient's caregivers and consultants. In most jurisdictions, court action is not required to carry out a sterilization procedure if there is agreement among these consultants that a nonminor is capable of consenting. Certain jurisdictions may not recognize guardian consent for sterilization of minors with mental disabilities under any circumstances. Whether or not recourse to the courts is necessary, every effort should be made to conduct the determination of competence fairly and to preserve autonomy.

Ethical Issues When the Patient Cannot Give Informed Consent

When the patient has been determined to be irreversibly incapable of participating in all or part of the informed consent process, others must make beneficence-based decisions regarding medical treatment. Such a determination is relatively uncommon. Even in these situations, it is often possible and highly desirable to obtain at least the patient's assent. The initial premise should be that nonvoluntary sterilization generally is not ethically acceptable because of the violation of privacy, bodily integrity, and reproductive rights that it may represent.

Physicians and other caregivers should avoid paternalistic decisions in all cases in which the individual may be capable of participating to some degree in decisions regarding her care. The following recommendations are based in part on those of McCullough et al (2). They do not apply to mentally impaired individuals who can participate in the consent process.

For patients with chronically and variably impaired autonomy, initial efforts should be directed toward restoring decision-making ability by such means as adjustment of medication and avoiding stressors. This may allow the patient to exercise full autonomy. For cases in which these efforts fail, recommended guidelines include the following:

- Efforts should be made to conform to the patient's expressed values and beliefs regarding reproduction. Such information may be available from interviewing the patient, her family, caregivers, and others in her environment. If possible, alternatives (including no action) consistent with her beliefs should be presented to decision makers.
- Physicians should be aware of the possibility of undue pressure from family members whose interests, no matter how legitimate, may not be the same as the patient's. When appropriate, the patient should have the opportunity to be interviewed without family members present.
- Noninvasive modalities, such as socialization training, sexual abuse avoidance training, family counselling, and sexuality education, should be considered as alternatives to medical contraception or sterilization.
- Consideration should be given to the degree of certainty of various adverse outcomes. For example, given the patient's living circumstances, how likely is it that she might be sexually exploited? Given available knowledge concerning her reproductive potential (ovulatory status, tubal patency),

how likely is it that she will become pregnant? How likely are adverse medical or social consequences from a pregnancy? Because it is uncommon for such risks to be reliably predictable, it may be preferable to recommend a reversible long-term form of contraception, such as the intrauterine device, long-term injectable progestin, or long-acting subdermal progestin implants, instead of sterilization. In most cases, the chosen method of contraception should be the least restrictive in preserving future reproductive options. This is especially true when a major factor in the request for sterilization is concern about burdens for others. At the same time, risks and inconveniences of contraception over a long period, as compared with a single, relatively simple and definitive surgical procedure, should not be ignored.

- The well-being of a child potentially conceived also should receive consideration.

Summary

Sterilization is an elective procedure with permanent and far-reaching consequences. Physicians who perform sterilization have ethical responsibilities of the highest order to counsel patients fully and without bias. Physicians must assess thoroughly the capacity of patients with impaired mental abilities to participate fully in the informed consent process. When this capacity is limited, the physician must consult with the patient's other caregivers in reaching a decision, based on the patient's best interests, and preserve her autonomy to the maximum extent possible. In difficult cases, a hospital ethics committee may provide useful perspectives.

References

1. 42 U.S.C. § 50.201–210 (1997)
2. McCullough LB, Coverdale J, Bayer T, Chervenak FA. Ethically justified guidelines for family planning interventions to prevent pregnancy in female patients with chronic mental illness. Am J Obstet Gynecol 1992;167:19–25
3. Appelbaum PS, Grisso T. Assessing patients' capacities to consent to treatment. N Engl J Med 1988;319:1635–1638

ACOG Committee Opinion

Committee on Gynecologic Practice

Number 232, April 2000 *(Replaces No. 169, February 1996)*

Tamoxifen and Endometrial Cancer

Tamoxifen, a nonsteroidal antiestrogen agent, is used widely as adjunctive therapy for women with breast cancer. Its efficacy has been recognized by the U.S. Food and Drug Administration, which has approved tamoxifen for the following indications:

- Adjuvant treatment of breast cancer
- Metastatic breast cancer
- Reduction in breast cancer incidence in high-risk women

As the use of tamoxifen to treat both patients with breast cancer and women at risk for the disease becomes more widespread, gynecologists will be consulted more frequently for advice on the proper follow-up of these individuals. Unfortunately, data from prospective trials are insufficient to give definitive guidelines. The purpose of this Committee Opinion is to recommend care to prevent and detect endometrial cancer in women taking tamoxifen.

Tamoxifen is one of a class of agents known as selective estrogen receptor modulators (SERMs). Although the primary therapeutic effect of tamoxifen is derived from its antiestrogenic properties, this agent also has modest estrogenic activity. In standard dosages, tamoxifen may be associated with endometrial proliferation, hyperplasia, polyp formation, and invasive carcinoma.

Most studies have found the increased relative risk of developing endometrial cancer while taking tamoxifen to be two to three times higher than that of an age-matched population (1–3). The level of risk of endometrial cancer in women treated with tamoxifen is dose and time dependent. Studies suggest that the stage, grade, histology, or biology of tumors that develop in individuals treated with tamoxifen (20 mg/d) is no different from those that arise in the general population (3, 4). However, some reports have indicated that women treated with a higher dosage of tamoxifen (40 mg/d) are more prone to develop more biologically aggressive tumors (5).

The rate of endometrial cancer occurrence among tamoxifen users who were administered 20 mg/d in the National Surgical Adjuvant Breast and Bowel Project (NSABP) was 1.6 per 1,000 patient years, compared with 0.2 per 1,000 patient years among control patients taking placebo (3). In this study, the 5-year disease-free survival rate from breast cancer was 38% higher in the tamoxifen group than in the placebo group, suggesting that the small risk of developing endometrial cancer is outweighed by the significant survival benefit provided by tamoxifen therapy for women with breast cancer (3).

This document reflects emerging clinical and scientific advances as of the date issued and is subject to change. The information should not be construed as dictating an exclusive course of treatment or procedure to be followed.

ISSN 1074-861X

The American College of Obstetricians and Gynecologists
409 12th Street, SW
PO Box 96920
Washington, DC 20090-6920

12345/43210

The survival advantage with 5 years of tamoxifen therapy continued with long-term follow-up, but extending the duration of tamoxifen use to 10 years failed to improve the survival benefit gained from 5 years of tamoxifen use (6).

The association between tamoxifen treatment and endometrial cancer is being scrutinized because data support a chemopreventive role for tamoxifen in women at high risk for developing breast cancer. The NSABP prevention trial (P-1) data suggest their risk for both invasive and noninvasive breast cancer is reduced markedly with tamoxifen prophylaxis. In this trial, the risk ratio for developing endometrial cancer was 2.53 in women using tamoxifen compared with women receiving a placebo (7). The Pilot Breast Cancer Prevention Trial showed that 39% of healthy postmenopausal women who were administered tamoxifen at a dosage of 20 mg/d had a histologically abnormal endometrium, compared with 10% of the placebo-treated control group (8). However, no case of endometrial cancer was identified in this small cohort of 111 postmenopausal women.

Several approaches are being explored for screening asymptomatic women using tamoxifen for abnormal endometrial proliferation or endometrial cancer. Correlation may be poor between ultrasonographic measurements of endometrial thickness and abnormal pathology in asymptomatic tamoxifen users because of tamoxifen-induced subepithelial stromal hypertrophy (9). In asymptomatic women using tamoxifen, screening for endometrial cancer with routine transvaginal ultrasonography, endometrial biopsy, or both has not been shown to be effective (10–13).

Although the concurrent use of progestin reduces the risk of endometrial hyperplasia and cancer in patients receiving unopposed estrogen, the impact of progestin on the course of breast cancer and on the endometrium of women receiving tamoxifen is not known. Therefore, such use cannot be advocated as a means of lowering risk in women taking tamoxifen.

On the basis of these data, the committee recommends the following:

- Women taking tamoxifen should be monitored closely for symptoms of endometrial hyperplasia or cancer and should have a gynecologic examination at least once every year.
- Women taking tamoxifen should be educated about the risks of endometrial proliferation, endometrial hyperplasia, and endometrial cancer. Women should be encouraged to promptly report any abnormal vaginal symptoms, including bloody discharge, spotting, staining, or leukorrhea.
- Any abnormal vaginal bleeding, bloody vaginal discharge, staining, or spotting should be investigated.
- Because screening tests have not been effective in increasing the early detection of endometrial cancer in women using tamoxifen and may lead to more invasive and costly diagnostic procedures, they are not recommended.
- Tamoxifen use should be limited to 5 years' duration because a benefit beyond this time has not been documented.
- If atypical endometrial hyperplasia develops, appropriate gynecologic management should be instituted, and the use of tamoxifen should be reassessed. If tamoxifen therapy must be continued, hysterectomy should be considered in women with atypical endometrial hyperplasia. Tamoxifen use may be reinstituted following hysterectomy for endometrial carcinoma in consultation with the physician responsible for the woman's breast care.

References

1. Sismondi P, Biglia N, Volpi E, Giai M, de Grandis T. Tamoxifen and endometrial cancer. Ann N Y Acad Sci 1994;734:310–321
2. Bissett D, Davis JA, George WD. Gynaecological monitoring during tamoxifen therapy. Lancet 1994;344:1244
3. Fisher B, Costantino JP, Redmond CK, Fisher ER, Wickerham DL, Cronin WM. Endometrial cancer in tamoxifen-treated breast cancer patients: findings from the National Surgical Adjuvant Breast and Bowel Project (NSABP) B-14. J Natl Cancer Inst 1994;86:527–537
4. Barakat RR, Wong G, Curtin JP, Vlamis V, Hoskins WJ. Tamoxifen use in breast cancer patients who subsequently develop corpus cancer is not associated with a higher incidence of adverse histologic features. Gynecol Oncol 1994;55:164–168
5. Magriples U, Naftolin F, Schwartz PE, Carcangiu ML. High-grade endometrial carcinoma in tamoxifen-treated breast cancer patients. J Clin Oncol 1993;11:485–490
6. Fisher B, Dignam J, Bryant J, DeCillis A, Wickerham DL, Wolmark N, et al. Five versus more than five years of tamoxifen therapy for breast cancer patients with negative lymph nodes and estrogen receptor-positive tumors. J Natl Cancer Inst 1996;88:1529–1542
7. Fisher B, Costantino JP, Wickerham DL, Redmond CK, Kavanah M, Cronin WM, et al. Tamoxifen for prevention of breast cancer: report of the National Surgical Adjuvant Breast and Bowel Project P-1 Study. J Natl Cancer Inst 1998;90:1371–1388
8. Kedar RP, Bourne TH, Powles TJ, Collins WP, Ashley SE, Cosgrove DO, et al. Effects of tamoxifen on uterus and ovaries of postmenopausal women in a randomised breast cancer prevention trial. Lancet 1994;343:1318–1321

9. Achiron R, Lipitz S, Sivan E, Goldenberg M, Horovitz A, Frenkel Y, et al. Changes mimicking endometrial neoplasia in postmenopausal, tamoxifen-treated women with breast cancer: a transvaginal Doppler study. Ultrasound Obstet Gynecol 1995;6:116–120
10. Bertelli G, Venturini M, Del Mastro L, Garrone O, Cosso M, Gustavino C, et al. Tamoxifen and the endometrium: findings of pelvic ultrasound examination and endometrial biopsy in asymptomatic breast cancer patients. Breast Cancer Res Treat 1998;47:41–46
11. Cecchini S, Ciatto S, Bonardi R, Mazzotta A, Grazzini G, Pacini P, et al. Screening by ultrasonography for endometrial carcinoma in postmenopausal breast cancer patients under adjuvant tamoxifen. Gynecol Oncol 1996;60: 409–411
12. Love CD, Muir BB, Scrimgeour JB, Leonard RC, Dillon P, Dixon JM. Investigation of endometrial abnormalities in asymptomatic women treated with tamoxifen and an evaluation of the role of endometrial screening. J Clin Oncol 1999;17:2050–2054
13. Seoud M, Shamseddine A, Khalil A, Salem Z, Saghir N, Bikhazi K, et al. Tamoxifen and endometrial pathologies: a prospective study. Gynecol Oncol 1999;75:15–19

ACOG

Committee on Gynecologic Practice

Committee Opinion

Number 224, October 1999

Tamoxifen and the Prevention of Breast Cancer in High-Risk Women

Breast cancer is a significant health problem for women in the United States. It is estimated that, in 1999, there will be 175,000 new cases of breast cancer in women and approximately 43,300 deaths as a result of the disease (1). Although gains have been made in the diagnosis and treatment of breast cancer, there has been very little success in its prevention. Recently, the Breast Cancer Prevention Trial (BCPT), initiated in 1992 by the National Surgical Adjuvant Breast and Bowel Project and funded by the National Cancer Institute, was completed. This study showed that tamoxifen administration to women at high risk of developing breast cancer was associated with a 49% reduction in the occurrence of primary disease (2).

Tamoxifen is a nonsteroidal compound with both antiestrogenic and estrogenic effects on select tissues (3, 4). The ability of tamoxifen to retard or arrest the growth of breast cancer tumor cells (antiestrogenic action) eventually led to its study as a breast cancer treatment (5–7). For the past 25 years, the drug has been used as a chemotherapeutic agent for women with advanced stages of breast cancer (8–10). In 1985, the U.S. Food and Drug Administration (FDA) recommended its use as an adjuvant or additional therapy in women receiving primary surgical or radiation treatment for early stage breast cancer (11–15). Therefore, tamoxifen has been used to treat 1) postmenopausal women with advanced or metastatic breast cancer, 2) postmenopausal women with resected node-positive disease, and 3) both premenopausal and postmenopausal women with resected node-negative disease. Subsequent follow-up studies have demonstrated that tamoxifen is effective at reducing the recurrence risk of breast cancer and prolonging survival in treated patients (15–17).

Tamoxifen's possible usefulness in preventing breast cancer was suggested by several observations. First, studies showed that tamoxifen-treated patients had a statistically significant lower incidence of contralateral breast cancer (16, 17). Second, in vitro and in vivo animal studies showed that tamoxifen blocked the initiation and progression of tumors and inhibited the growth of cancer cells by several mechanisms (5–7). Third, a great deal of information was known about the pharmacodynamics, metabolism, and antitumor effects of tamoxifen in animals and humans (18–21).

ISSN 1074-861X

The American College of Obstetricians and Gynecologists
409 12th Street, SW
PO Box 96920
Washington, DC 20090-6920

12345/32109

These observations resulted in the creation of the BCPT, a large, multicenter prospective breast cancer prevention study involving 13,388 women. This study was designed as a double-blind, randomized, placebo-controlled trial to test the ability of tamoxifen to reduce the incidence of breast cancer in a high-risk population, which was composed of women older than 60 years and those between 35 and 59 years of age with an increased predicted risk of breast cancer. The predicted risk was derived from a computerized program that considered a combination of variables, including number of first-degree relatives with breast cancer, nulliparity, age at first delivery, number of breast biopsies, age at menarche, and history of previous lobular carcinoma in situ (22).

The results showed that high-risk women receiving tamoxifen had a 49% reduction in the incidence of breast cancer, compared with the placebo control group. Additionally, the incidence of noninvasive in situ breast cancer was decreased by half in the treatment group. The results were so conclusive that the independent auditor (Endpoint Review, Safety Monitoring, and Advisory Committee) recommended that the National Surgical Adjuvant Breast and Bowel Project terminate the study earlier than planned. This recommendation was adopted based on the belief that any additional information from continuing the study would be outweighed by the benefit of providing therapy to women in the placebo group and other women at increased risk.

However, it must be recognized that tamoxifen was not without significant side effects. The incidence of endometrial cancers doubled in the treatment group. All endometrial cancers were stage I, except for one stage IV cancer in the placebo group, and no deaths were reported. In addition, there was a threefold increase in the number of pulmonary emboli and a 50% increase in the number of deep venous thrombi in the treatment group compared with the control group. There was an increased relative risk of cataract formation and surgery for cataracts of 1.14 and 1.57, respectively.

Following the announcement of the BCPT results, two related studies were published that showed that the incidence of breast cancer was not decreased in tamoxifen-treated women compared with those receiving a placebo. However, there were significant methodologic differences between these studies and the BCPT. One study was conducted for 5 years and involved 5,408 women 35–70 years of age who had undergone hysterectomy (23). These women were not selected for high risk of breast cancer and, in fact, represented a low- to normal-risk population. Because of these differences in experimental design, the findings of this report do not necessarily contradict those of the BCPT. The other study occurred over 6 years and included only 2,471 women 30–70 years of age with a family history of breast cancer, thereby excluding nongenetic risk factors (24). An explanation for the disparity in results between this study and the BCPT was not readily apparent. The authors suggested that genetic differences associated with the study subjects' family histories may have affected the preventive effect of tamoxifen.

In a recent decision, the FDA granted approval of tamoxifen for the purpose of reducing the incidence of breast cancer in women at high risk for breast cancer. "High risk" is defined as women at least 35 years of age with a 5-year predicted risk of breast cancer of at least 1.67%, as calculated by the Gail model. The FDA also approved tamoxifen for the reduction of contralateral breast cancer risk in patients receiving adjuvant tamoxifen therapy for breast cancer. The FDA emphasized that patients should be informed about tamoxifen's adverse effects, including increased risk of endometrial cancer, deep vein thrombosis, pulmonary embolism, and cataracts, in addition to tamoxifen's potential benefits. The FDA Advisory Committee also emphasized that the effects of long-term treatment with tamoxifen are unknown because follow-up data are limited to 5 years.

In summary, the BCPT results are encouraging and provide an opportunity for chemoprevention in women at high risk for the development of breast cancer. However, several issues remain under consideration. For example, there are insufficient data on the long-term use of tamoxifen and subsequent occurrence of and death from breast cancer. Research addressing the associated increased risk of endometrial cancer, vascular morbidity, and potential mortality must continue. Finally, the role of tamoxifen in women at low or normal risk for breast cancer and in those individuals with genetic mutations of *BRCA1* or *BRCA2* should be defined. Some of these concerns may be addressed by continued surveillance of women receiving tamoxifen over an extended period, whereas other issues will warrant additional studies in the future.

Researchers from the National Cancer Institute and the National Surgical Adjuvant Breast and Bowel Project have developed a computer-based tool to allow clinicians to project a woman's individualized estimate of breast cancer risk. The Breast Cancer Risk Assessment Tool, currently available through a pilot program, is a computer disk that a woman and her health care professional can use to estimate her chances of developing breast cancer based on several established risk factors. The disk is available at no charge, in PC-compatible and Macintosh computer formats. To order, call the National Cancer Institute's Cancer Information Service at 1-800-422-6237 or visit the National Cancer Institute's cancer trials web site at http://cancertrials.nci.nih.gov/.

The obstetrician–gynecologist has the unique opportunity to inform high-risk patients of the need for breast cancer screening and the availability of chemopreventive therapy. However, the decision to use tamoxifen to reduce the risk of breast cancer should be individualized. Because a key factor to be considered is the woman's risk of breast cancer, it is important that clinicians take a thorough history to assess her risk adequately. Other factors to be considered include potential tamoxifen-associated side effects and risks, patient preference, clinician judgment, and clinician ability to monitor for and manage tamoxifen-related side effects, referring as necessary.

References

1. Landis SH, Murray T, Bolden S, Wingo PA. Cancer statistics, 1999. CA Cancer J Clin 1999;49:8–31
2. Fisher B, Costantino JP, Wickerham DL, Redmond CK, Kavanah M, Cronin WM, et al. Tamoxifen for prevention of breast cancer: report of the National Surgical Adjuvant Breast and Bowel Project P-1 Study. J Natl Cancer Inst 1998;90:1371–1388
3. Love RR. Antiestrogens as chemopreventive agents in breast cancer: promise and issues in evaluation. Prev Med 1989;18:661–671
4. Jordan VC. Tamoxifen: toxicities and drug resistance during the treatment and prevention of breast cancer. Annu Rev Pharmacol Toxicol 1995;35:195–211
5. Terenius L. Effect of anti-oestrogens on initiation of mammary cancer in the female rat. Eur J Cancer 1971;7:65–70
6. Jordan VC. Effect of tamoxifen (ICI 46,474) on initiation and growth of DMBA-induced rat mammary carcinomata. Eur J Cancer 1976;12:419–424
7. Jordan VC, Allen KE. Evaluation of the antitumour activity of the non-steroidal antioestrogen monohydroxytamoxifen in the DMBA-induced rat mammary carcinoma model. Eur J Cancer 1980;16:239–251
8. Heuson JC. Current overview of EORTC clinical trials with tamoxifen. Cancer Treat Rep 1976;60:1463–1466
9. Mouridsen H, Palshof T, Patterson J, Battersby L. Tamoxifen in advanced breast cancer. Cancer Treat Rev 1978;5:131–141
10. Legha SS, Buzdar AU, Hortobagyi GN, Wiseman C, Benjamin RS, Blumenschein GR. Tamoxifen. Use in treatment of metastatic breast cancer refractory to combination chemotherapy. JAMA 1979;242:49–52
11. Controlled trial of tamoxifen as adjuvant agent in management of early breast cancer. Interim analysis at four years by Nolvadex Adjuvant Trial Organisation. Lancet 1983;1: 257–261
12. Controlled trial of tamoxifen as single adjuvant agent in management of early breast cancer. Analysis at six years by Nolvadex Adjuvant Trial Organisation. Lancet 1985;1: 836–840
13. Fisher B, Redmond C, Brown A, Fisher ER, Wolmark N, Bowman D, et al. Adjuvant chemotherapy with and without tamoxifen in the treatment of primary breast cancer: 5-year results from the National Surgical Adjuvant Breast and Bowel Project Trial. J Clin Oncol 1986;4:459–471
14. Adjuvant tamoxifen in the management of operable breast cancer: the Scottish Trial. Report from the Breast Cancer Trials Committee, Scottish Cancer Trials Office (MRC), Edinburgh. Lancet 1987;2:171–175
15. Fisher B, Costantino J, Redmond C, Poisson R, Bowman D, Couture J, et al. A randomized clinical trial evaluating tamoxifen in the treatment of patients with node-negative breast cancer who have estrogen-receptor-positive tumors. N Engl J Med 1989;320:479–484
16. Cyclophosphamide and tamoxifen as adjuvant therapies in the management of breast cancer. CRC Adjuvant Breast Trial Working Party. Br J Cancer 1988;57:604–607
17. Rutqvist LE, Cedermark B, Glas U, Mattsson A, Skoog L, Somell A, et al. Contralateral primary tumors in breast cancer patients in a randomized trial of adjuvant tamoxifen therapy. J Natl Cancer Inst 1991;83:1299–1306
18. Furr BJ, Patterson JS, Richardson DN, Slater SR, Wakeling AE. Tamoxifen. Pharmacol Biochem Prop Drug Subst 1979;2:355–399
19. Adam HK. Pharmacokinetic studies with Nolvadex. Rev Endocr Relat Cancer 1981;9:131–143
20. Wakeling AE, Valcaccia B, Newboult E, Green LR. Non-steroidal antioestrogens-receptor binding and biological response in rat uterus, rat mammary carcinoma and human breast cancer cells. J Steroid Biochem Mol Biol 1984;20: 111–120
21. Jordan VC, Fritz NF, Tormey DC. Long-term adjuvant therapy with tamoxifen: effects on sex hormone binding globulin and antithrombin III. Cancer Res 1987; 47:4517–4519
22. Gail MH, Brinton LA, Byar DP, Corle DK, Green SB, Schairer C, et al. Projecting individualized probabilities of developing breast cancer for white females who are being examined annually. J Natl Cancer Inst 1989;81:1879–1886
23. Veronesi U, Maisonneuve P, Costa A, Sacchini V, Maltoni C, Robertson C, et al. Prevention of breast cancer with tamoxifen: preliminary findings from the Italian randomised trial among hysterectomised women. Italian Tamoxifen Prevention Study. Lancet 1998;352:93–97
24. Powles T, Eeles R, Ashley S, Easton D, Chang J, Dowsett M, et al. Interim analysis of the incidence of breast cancer in the Royal Marsden Hospital tamoxifen randomised chemoprevention trial. Lancet 1998;352:98–101

ACOG

Committee on
Professional Liability

Committee Opinion

Number 221, September 1999

Telecommunication in Medicine

Telemedicine is defined as the provision of medical services by means of telecommunication and computer systems. Medical consultations, diagnostic imaging and laboratory studies, as well as real-time physician examinations and consultations (eg, electronic fetal heart rate monitoring, fetal ultrasound examination, and echocardiography) can be transmitted electronically to an off-site physician–consultant who can participate in diagnostic and treatment decisions. The ability to transmit this information through telecommunication systems can offer access to additional health care resources, thereby enhancing local medical services.

The purpose of this Committee Opinion is to alert physicians to certain professional liability concerns created by the use of telemedicine.

- Informed consent, which specifies the purpose for which a particular telemedicine technique is to be used, must be obtained from the patient. Some states require a written informed consent. All of the usual requirements for informed consent are operative.
- Confidentiality can be compromised when medical information is transferred through telecommunication systems. This may be of little concern, for example, in the real-time transmission of an electronic fetal heart recording. However, a medical history might contain information so sensitive that the patient may feel that the risk of losing confidentiality outweighs the sought-after benefit. Reasonable precautions should be taken to achieve computer and telecommunication security, and patients must be educated to understand that no physician or institution can guarantee complete security of electronically transmitted data.
- The standards of care for medical practice apply with equal force and vitality to telemedicine if a patient–physician relationship is deemed to exist. If a patient receives professional advice or treatment, even gratuitously, there is *prima facie* evidence that a patient–physician relationship exists. Such a relationship could become the basis of liability.
- A license is required to practice medicine within a particular state. Some states require licensure of any physician providing medical advice to a patient located in that state, even when the physician is providing the telemedicine services from another state in which he or she is licensed. Physicians who practice telemedicine across state lines should be aware of applicable state licensure requirements.

This document provides risk management information that is current as of the date issued and is subject to change. This document does not define a standard of care nor should it be interpreted as legal advice.

ISSN 1074-861X

The American College of Obstetricians and Gynecologists
409 12th Street, SW
PO Box 96920
Washington, DC 20090-6920

12345/32109

Advances in computer and related telecommunication technologies allow local, state, national, and international dissemination of medical information, thereby benefiting patients, physicians, and the entire population. As with many new technologies, however, some degree of risk accompanies the benefit. In applying telemedicine to the diagnosis and treatment of patients, it is important that both patients and physicians have a clear understanding of the risks and benefits of the technology within the context of specific clinical circumstances. It also is important that physicians understand the potential for exposure to liability arising out of patient–physician telemedicine relationships.

ACOG

Committee on Coding and Nomenclature

Committee Opinion

Number 205, August 1998

Tubal Ligation with Cesarean Delivery

Tubal ligation at the time of cesarean delivery requires significant additional physician work even though the technical work of the procedure is brief. Informed consent by the patient requires considerably more counseling by the physician regarding potential risks and benefits of this procedure than is necessary with alternative means of sterilization and contraception. Also, many states require completion of special informed consent documents in addition to the customary consent forms required by hospitals. These forms must be completed before scheduling the procedure.

Patients have the right to change their minds. Thus, it is important to reconfirm the patient's decision shortly before the operation.

Tubal ligation with cesarean delivery involves removal of a segment of fallopian tube, which is sent for histologic confirmation. With most cesarean deliveries, tissue is not evaluated by a pathologist. Accordingly, it is important for the surgeon to verify the pathology report, which adds an additional component to post-service work.

The risk of professional liability for operative complications is increased with this procedure. This risk is low, but real. Furthermore, sterilization failure occurs in about 1 in 100 cases even though the operation was performed properly. This failure also carries a liability risk.

Because tubal ligation is a discrete extra service, it should be coded accordingly: 59510 or 59618—routine obstetric care including antepartum care, cesarean delivery, and postpartum care—and 58611—ligation or transection of fallopian tube(s) done at the time of cesarean delivery or intra-abdominal surgery.

ISSN 1074-861X

The American College of Obstetricians and Gynecologists
409 12th Street, SW
PO Box 96920
Washington, DC 20090-6920

12345/21098

ACOG
Committee on Obstetric Practice

American Academy of Pediatrics
Committee on Fetus and Newborn

Committee Opinion

Number 174, July 1996 (*Replaces #49, November 1986*)

Use and Abuse of the Apgar Score

The Apgar score, devised in 1952 by Dr. Virginia Apgar, is a quick method of assessing the clinical status of the newborn infant (1, 2). Ease of scoring has led to its use in many studies of outcome. However, its misuse has led to an erroneous definition of asphyxia. Intrapartum asphyxia implies fetal hypercarbia and hypoxemia, which if prolonged will result in eventual metabolic acidemia. Because the intrapartum disruption of uterine or fetal blood flow is rarely, if ever, absolute, *asphyxia* is an imprecise, general term. Terms such as *hypercarbia, hypoxia,* and *metabolic, respiratory,* or *lactic acidemia* are more precise, both for immediate assessment of the newborn and for retrospective assessment of intrapartum management. Although the Apgar score continues to provide a convenient "shorthand" for reporting the status of the newborn and the effectiveness of resuscitation, the purpose of this statement is to place the Apgar score in its proper perspective.

The Apgar score comprises five components: heart rate, respiratory effort, muscle tone, reflex irritability, and color, each of which is given a score of 0, 1, or 2 (Table 1). Reliable Apgar scores require assessment of individual components of the score by trained personnel.

Factors That May Affect the Apgar Score

Although rarely stated, it is important to recognize that elements of the Apgar score such as tone, color, and reflex irritability are partially dependent on the physiologic maturity of the infant. The healthy premature infant with no evidence of anoxic insult, acidemia, or cerebral depression may thus receive a low score only because of immaturity (3, 4).

A number of maternal medications and infant conditions may influence Apgar scores, including, but not limited to, neuromuscular or cerebral malformations that may decrease tone and respiratory effort. Cardiorespiratory conditions may also decrease the infant's heart rate, respiration, and tone. Infection may interfere with tone, color, and response to resuscitative efforts. Additional information is required to interpret Apgar scores properly in infants receiving resuscitation. Thus, to equate the presence of a low Apgar score solely with asphyxia or hypoxia represents a misuse of the score.

ISSN 1074-861X

The American College of Obstetricians and Gynecologists
409 12th Street, SW
PO Box 96920
Washington, DC 20090-6920

12345/09876

Table 1. Apgar Score: Five Components and Score Definitions

	Score		
Component	**0**	**1**	**2**
Heart rate	Absent	Slow (<100 beats/min)	>100 beats/min
Respirations	Absent	Weak cry, hypoventilation	Good, strong cry
Muscle tone	Limp	Some flexion	Active motion
Reflex irritability	No response	Grimace	Cry or active withdrawal
Color	Blue or pale	Body pink, extremities blue	Completely pink

Adapted from Apgar V, Holaday DA, James LS, Weisbrot IM, Berrien C. Evaluation of the newborn infant: second report. JAMA 1958;168:1985–1988

Apgar Score and Subsequent Disability

A low 1-minute Apgar score does not correlate with the infant's future outcome. The 5-minute Apgar score, and particularly the change in the score between 1 and 5 minutes, is a useful index of the effectiveness of resuscitation efforts. However, even a 5-minute score of 0–3, although possibly a result of hypoxia, is limited as an indicator of the severity of the problem and correlates poorly with future neurologic outcome (5, 6). An Apgar score of 0–3 at 5 minutes is associated with an increased risk of cerebral palsy in term infants, but this increase is only from 0.3% to 1% (5, 6). A 5-minute Apgar score of 7–10 is considered "normal." Scores of 4, 5, and 6 are intermediate and are not markers of high levels of risk of later neurologic dysfunction. As previously mentioned, such scores are affected by physiologic immaturity, medication, the presence of congenital malformations, and other factors.

Because Apgar scores at 1 and 5 minutes correlate poorly with either cause or outcome, the scores alone should not be considered evidence of or a consequence of substantial asphyxia. Therefore, a low 5-minute Apgar score alone does not demonstrate that later development of cerebral palsy was caused by perinatal asphyxia.

Correlation of the Apgar score with future neurologic outcome increases when the score remains 0–3 at 10, 15, and 20 minutes but still does not indicate the cause of future disability (5, 7). The term *asphyxia* in a clinical context should be reserved to describe a combination of damaging acidemia, hypoxia, and metabolic acidosis. A neonate who has had "asphyxia" proximate to delivery that is severe enough to result in acute neurologic injury should demonstrate all of the following:

- Profound metabolic or mixed acidemia (pH <7.00) on an umbilical cord arterial blood sample, if obtained
- An Apgar score of 0–3 for longer than 5 minutes
- Neonatal neurologic manifestations (eg, seizures, coma, or hypotonia)
- Multisystem organ dysfunction (eg, cardiovascular, gastrointestinal, hematologic, pulmonary, or renal system)

The Apgar score alone cannot establish hypoxia as the cause of cerebral palsy. A term infant with an Apgar score of 0–3 at 5 minutes whose 10-minute score improved to 4 or higher has a 99% chance of not having cerebral palsy at 7 years of age (5). Conversely, 75% of children with cerebral palsy had normal Apgar scores at birth (5).

Cerebral palsy is the only neurologic deficit clearly linked to perinatal asphyxia. Although mental retardation and epilepsy may accompany cerebral palsy, there is no evidence that they are caused by perinatal asphyxia unless cerebral palsy is also present, and even then a relationship is in doubt (8, 9).

Conclusion

Apgar scores are useful in assessing the condition of the infant at birth. Their use in other settings, such as collection of a child's Apgar score upon entry to school, is inappropriate. Low Apgar scores may be indicative of a number of maternal and infant factors. Apgar scores alone should not be used as evidence that neurologic damage was caused by hypoxia that results in neurologic damage or by inappropriate intrapartum management. In the infant who later is found to have cerebral palsy, low 1-minute or 5-minute Apgar scores are not sufficient evidence that the damage was due to hypoxia or inappropriate intrapartum management. Hypoxia as a cause of acute neurologic injury and adverse neurologic outcome occurs in infants who demonstrate the four perinatal findings listed in this Committee Opinion and in whom other possible causes of neurologic damage have been excluded. In the absence of such evidence, subsequent neurologic deficiencies cannot be ascribed to perinatal asphyxia or hypoxia (10, 11).

References

1. Apgar V. A proposal for a new method of evaluation of the newborn infant. Curr Res Anesth Analg 1953;32:260–267
2. Apgar V, Holaday DA, James LS, Weisbrot IM, Berrien C. Evaluation of the newborn infant: second report. JAMA 1958;168:1985–1988
3. Catlin EA, Carpenter MW, Brann BS IV, Mayfield SR, Shaul PW, Goldstein M, et al. The Apgar score revisited: influence of gestational age. J Pediatr 1986;109:865–868
4. Amon E, Sibai BM, Anderson GD, Mabie WC. Obstetric variables predicting survival of the immature newborn (less than or equal to 1000 gm): a five-year experience in a single perinatal center. Am J Obstet Gynecol 1987;156: 1380–1389
5. Nelson KB, Ellenberg JH. Apgar scores as predictors of chronic neurologic disability. Pediatrics 1981;68:36–44
6. Stanley FJ. Cerebral palsy trends: implications for perinatal care. Acta Obstet Gynecol Scand 1994;73:5–9
7. Freeman JM, Nelson KB. Intrapartum asphyxia and cerebral palsy. Pediatrics 1988;82:240–249
8. Levene MI, Sands C, Grindulis H, Moore JR. Comparison of two methods of predicting outcome in perinatal asphyxia. Lancet 1986;1:67–69
9. Paneth N. The causes of cerebral palsy: recent evidence. Clin Invest Med 1993;16:95–102
10. Brann AW Jr, Dykes FD. The effects of intrauterine asphyxia on the full-term neonate. Clin Perinatol 1977;4: 149–161
11. Nelson KB, Leviton A. How much of neonatal encephalopathy is due to birth asphyxia? Am J Dis Child 1991;145: 1325–1331

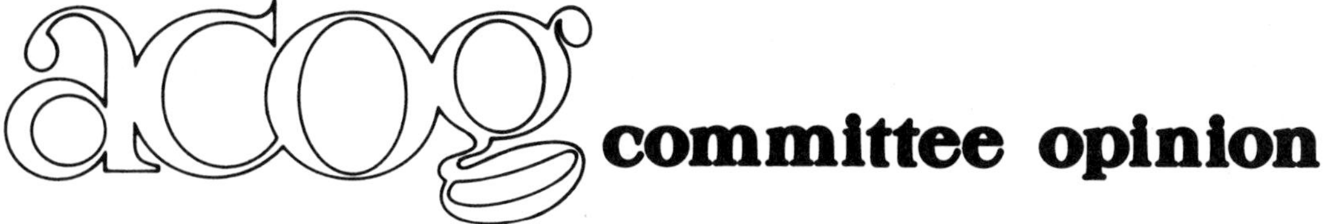

Committee on Obstetric Practice

Number 138—April 1994
(Replaces #91, February 1991)

Utility of Umbilical Cord Blood Acid–Base Assessment

Despite new neonatal and obstetric technologies, the rate of cerebral palsy in term infants (1–2 cases per 1,000 births) has not been reduced over the past 20 years in Western industrialized countries. The persistent misuse of the term birth asphyxia, with the misperception that it accounts for a significant portion of infants with cerebral palsy, continues to exist, despite the fact that there is no evidence to support this misperception. A number of clinical and experimental reports confirm that only severe and prolonged hypoxia is associated with an increased risk of subsequent neurologic dysfunction. This level of hypoxia is very uncommon with birthing conditions in the United States and modern industrialized countries. When prolonged and severe hypoxia occurs, it is often followed by death or the prolonged requirement for life support systems. Most survivors develop normally.

The American College of Obstetricians and Gynecologists and the American Academy of Pediatrics have challenged the use of the Apgar score to define birth asphyxia. Umbilical cord blood acid–base assessment is a more objective measure of the acid–base status of a newborn than is the Apgar score. The exact lower limits of newborn pH (metabolic acidemia) and depression (low 5-minute Apgar score) that are predictive of subsequent neurologic dysfunction have not been determined. However, some studies have reported a significantly increased incidence of newborn morbidity associated with acidemia in term newborns with an umbilical artery pH of less than 7.00 and a 5-minute Apgar score of 3 or less and in whom the acidemia has a metabolic component. Again, most infants with this severe degree of acidemia will develop normally.

Intrapartum asphyxia implies fetal hypercarbia and hypoxemia, which, if prolonged, will result in metabolic acidemia. Because the intrapartum disruption of uterine or fetal blood flow is rarely, if ever, absolute, asphyxia is an imprecise, general term and should be reserved for the clinical context of damaging acidemia, hypoxia, and metabolic acidosis. Terms such as hypercarbia, hypoxia, metabolic acidemia, and respiratory or lactic acidemia are more precise, both for immediate assessment of the newborn and for retrospective assessment of intrapartum management.

Although fetal acidemia has been defined as an umbilical arterial blood pH of less than 7.20, this level is arbitrarily high. In normal uncomplicated pregnancies, the lower range of umbilical arterial blood pH has been reported as 7.10–7.15. Although the precise value that is required to define acidemia is not known, umbilical arterial blood pH values of less than 7.00 more realistically represent clinically significant acidosis. It should be noted that acidemia by itself is not sufficient evidence to establish that a hypoxic injury has occurred. A neonate who has had severe hypoxia proximate to delivery that is severe enough to result in hypoxic encephalopathy will show other evidence of hypoxic damage, including all of the following:

- Profound metabolic or mixed acidemia (pH less than 7.00) on an umbilical cord arterial blood sample, if obtained
- Persistent Apgar score of 0–3 for 5 minutes or longer
- Evidence of neonatal neurologic sequelae (eg, seizures, coma, prolonged hypotonia, and one or more of the following: cardiovascular, gastrointestinal, hematologic, pulmonary, or renal system dysfunction)

TECHNIQUE

Immediately after delivery of the neonate, a segment of umbilical cord should be doubly clamped, divided, and placed on the delivery table pending assignment of the 5-minute Apgar score. Values from the umbilical artery provide the most accurate information regarding fetal and newborn acid–base status. A clamped segment of cord is stable for pH and blood gas assessment for at least 60 minutes, and a cord blood sample in a syringe flushed with heparin is stable for up to 60 minutes. If the 5-minute Apgar score is satisfactory and the infant appears stable and vigorous, the segment of umbilical cord can be discarded. If a serious abnormality that arose in the delivery process or a problem with the neonate's condition or both persist at or beyond the first 5 minutes, blood can be drawn from the cord segment and sent to a laboratory for blood gas analysis. It should be noted that, occasionally, it may be difficult to obtain an adequate cord arterial blood sample.

CONCLUSION

In the depressed newborn, the documentation of umbilical blood acid–base measurements provides an objective fetal assessment and, if levels are within the normal range, can exclude intrapartum hypoxia as a proximate cause of neonatal depression. This knowledge may aid practitioners in their assessment of the depressed newborn.

BIBLIOGRAPHY

Dennis J, Johnson A, Mutch L, Yudkin P, Johnson P. Acid base status at birth and neurodevelopment at four and one-half years. Am J Obstet Gynecol 1989;161:213–220

Dorland's illustrated medical dictionary. 27th ed. Philadelphia: WB Saunders, 1988

Duerbeck NB, Chaffin DG, Seeds JW. A practical approach to umbilical artery pH and blood gas determinations. Obstet Gynecol 1992;79:959–962

Fee SC, Malee K, Deddish R, Minogue JP, Socol ML. Severe acidosis and subsequent neurologic status. Am J Obstet Gynecol 1990;162:802–806

Freeman JM, ed. Prenatal and perinatal factors associated with brain disorders. Washington, DC: U.S. Government Printing Office, 1985; NIH publication no. 85-1149

Freeman JM, Nelson KB. Intrapartum asphyxia and cerebral palsy. Pediatrics 1988;82:240–249

Gilstrap LC 3rd, Leveno KJ, Burris J, Williams ML, Little BB. Diagnosis of birth asphyxia on the basis of fetal pH, Apgar score and newborn cerebral dysfunction. Am J Obstet Gynecol 1989;161:825–830

Goldenberg RL, Huddleston JF, Nelson KG. Apgar scores and umbilical artery pH in preterm newborn infants. Am J Obstet Gynecol 1984;149:651–654

Nelson KB, Ellenberg JH. Antecedents of cerebral palsy multivariate analysis of risk. N Engl J Med 1986;315:81–86

Riley RJ, Johnson JW. Collecting and analyzing cord blood gases. Clin Obstet Gynecol 1993;36:13–23

Ruth VJ, Raivio KO. Perinatal brain damage: predictive value of metabolic acidosis and the Apgar score. BMJ 1988;297:24–27

Thorp JA, Sampson JE, Parisi VM, Creasy RK. Routine umbilical cord blood gas determinations? Am J Obstet Gynecol 1989;161:600–605

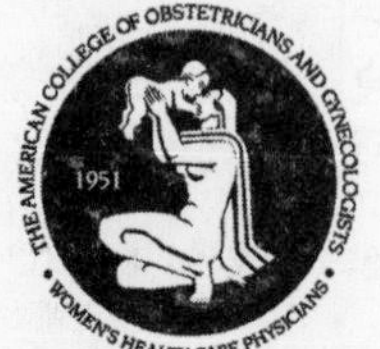

The American College of Obstetricians and Gynecologists
409 12th Street, SW • Washington, DC 20024-2188

12345/87654

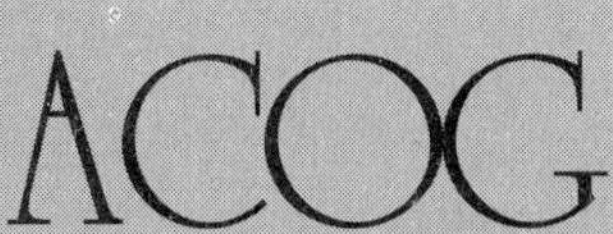

Committee on Obstetric Practice

Committee Opinion

Number 196, January 1998 (*Replaces #157, September 1995*)

Vitamin A Supplementation During Pregnancy

Vitamin A is essential to normal reproduction, and its deficiency is a serious worldwide problem. An increasing awareness of its important contribution to adequate nutrition recently has led to the use of vitamin A supplements by many women. Vitamin A deficiency is rare in the United States, however, and most women in the United States have adequate stores of the vitamin in their livers. Therefore, it is important that obstetrician–gynecologists recognize the possible health risks of excessive use of vitamin A supplements before conception or during early pregnancy.

A small number of case reports suggest an association between the use of high doses of vitamin A (retinol and retinyl esters) during pregnancy and birth defects. These malformations are similar to those produced by the vitamin A derivative isotretinoin (13-*cis*-retinoic acid [Accutane]), which is a proven teratogen in both humans and animals. The minimum human teratogenic dose of vitamin A is not known, but it is probably at least 25,000–50,000 IU daily. A recent report suggests that it may be as little as 10,000 IU (1). Use of beta-carotene, the precursor of vitamin A found in fruits and vegetables, has not been shown to produce vitamin A toxicity.

Recently, there has been concern regarding the very high levels of vitamin A in animal (calf, cattle, pork, and chicken) livers. Measurements of 80,000 IU or more of vitamin A per 100-g serving of calf liver have been recorded in Europe. The teratogenic risk posed by this dietary source of potentially large quantities of vitamin A is uncertain. The levels of vitamin A in animal livers available in retail markets in the United States appear to be below those in Europe and to be in the nontoxic range.

The National Research Council's Committee on Dietary Allowances advocates a recommended dietary allowance of 800 retinol equivalents per day for nonpregnant women of childbearing age; this is not increased during pregnancy. The recommended dietary allowance is equivalent to 2,700 IU of vitamin A obtained from a supplement as retinol or 4,800 μg of beta-carotene.

Dietary intake of vitamin A in the United States appears to be adequate to meet the needs of most pregnant women throughout gestation. Therefore, routine supplementation during pregnancy is not recommended. In cases in which the dietary intake of vitamin A may not be adequate (for example, in

ISSN 1074-861X

The American College of Obstetricians and Gynecologists
409 12th Street, SW
PO Box 96920
Washington, DC 20090-6920

12345/21098

strict vegetarians), dietary intake should be supplemented. Carefully supervised supplementation also may be desirable for some pregnant women, such as recent emigrants from countries where vitamin A deficiency is endemic.

Supplementation with 5,000 IU of vitamin A per day should be considered the maximum intake before and during pregnancy. This is well below the probable minimum human teratogenic dose. Prenatal multivitamins in common use contain 5,000 IU or less of vitamin A, but vitamin tablets containing 25,000 IU or more of vitamin A are available as over-the-counter preparations. Pregnant women or those planning to become pregnant who use high doses of vitamin A supplements (retinol and retinyl esters) should be cautioned about the potential teratogenicity.

Reference

1. Rothman KJ, Moore LL, Singer MR, Nguyen US, Mannino S, Milunsky A. Teratogenicity of high vitamin A intake. N Engl J Med 1995;333:1369–1373

Educational and Technical Bulletins

Lists of Titles

Committee Opinions

Educational and Technical Bulletins

Practice Bulletins

Practice Patterns

Policy Statements

Index

ACOG EDUCATIONAL BULLETIN

Number 252, October 1998

Adolescent Victims of Sexual Assault

Rape is one of the most frequently committed violent crimes in America, and it is one of the most costly to society (1). The National Institute of Justice estimates that one million women in the United States are the victims of rape each year (1). This is substantially higher than some published estimates because of underreporting (2). The National Crime Victimization Survey indicates that approximately 30% of rapes are reported to the police (3), 50% of rape victims tell no one, and only 5% visit a rape crisis center (4). Contrary to the popular, yet inaccurate, notion of rape involving an assailant unknown to the victim, most rape victims know their attacker (3). Many victims are adolescent females and children. In a survey of 11 states and the District of Columbia, 50% of the females who had been raped were under the age of 18, and 16% were under the age of 12 (5). Similarly, the National Victim Center (6) and the Department of Justice (5) report that adolescents have the highest reported rates of sexual assault, more than 50–60% of all cases. Despite the fact that rape constitutes a threat to the health and future of young women in the United States, it has failed to capture national attention as a major public health issue (7).

This Educational Bulletin was developed under the direction of the Committee on Adolescent Health Care of the American College of Obstetricians and Gynecologists as an aid to obstetricians and gynecologists. This document is not to be construed as establishing a standard of practice or dictating an exclusive course of treatment. Rather, it is intended as an educational tool that presents current information on obstetric–gynecologic issues.

Definitions

The legal term *rape* has traditionally referred to forced vaginal penetration of a woman by a male assailant. Many states have now abandoned this concept in favor of the gender-neutral term *sexual assault*. The legal definition of criminal sexual assault is any genital, oral, or anal penetration by a part of the accused's body or by an object, using force or without the victim's consent (7). Criminal sexual assault, or rape, is often further stratified to include *acquaintance rape, date rape, statutory rape, child sexual abuse,* and *incest*. Such terms generally describe the age of the victim and her relationship to the abuser. Despite these various classifications of rape, it is important to remember that all are acts of rape.

Acquaintance rape refers to those sexual assaults committed by someone known to the victim, frequently a date, teacher, employer, or family member. Instances in which the perpetrator is related to the victim generally

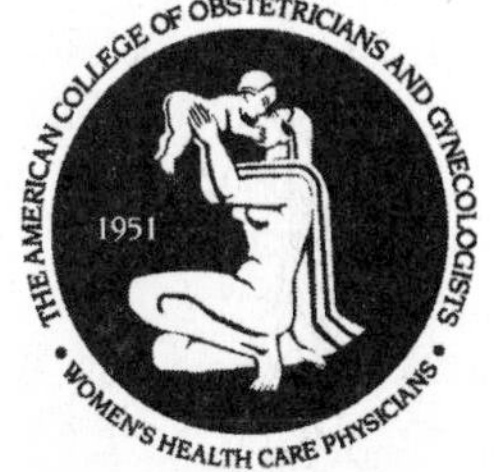

Replaces Committee Opinion Number 122, May 1993

are defined as incest. Although incest refers to sexual intercourse among family members, or those legally barred from marriage (8), this definition has been conceptually broadened to also include step-relatives and parental figures living in the home.

Date rape, which is a subset of acquaintance rape, generally refers to forced or unwanted sexual activity that occurs within a dating relationship. For a significant number of adolescents, however, the classic one-on-one date is no longer the social norm. Instead, an adolescent female may be more likely to socialize with a group at a dance, a party, or another unsupervised group activity. As such, she may not respond accurately to questions regarding date rape. The classic date rape, however, remains a significant problem on college campuses.

Statutory rape refers to sexual intercourse with a female under a specified age (9). All 50 states and the District of Columbia have laws criminalizing statutory rape. Such laws typically base the severity of the crime on the age of the adolescent victim and the age difference between the adolescent and her assailant. The age at which an adolescent may consent to sexual intercourse varies by state and ranges from 14 to 18 years of age; however, the consent of an adolescent younger than this range is legally irrelevant because she is defined as being incapable of consenting.

Sexual assault occurring in childhood also is defined by most states as child abuse. The National Center on Child Abuse and Neglect defines childhood sexual abuse as "contact or interaction between a child and an adult when the child is being used for the sexual stimulation of that adult or another person" (10). Childhood sexual abuse may be committed by another minor when that person is either significantly older than the victim (often defined as more than 5 years) or when the abuser is in a position of power or control over the child (10).

Prevalence

It is difficult to establish conclusively the prevalence of sexual assault in the adolescent population because victims may be particularly reluctant to report the sexual assault. Embarrassment, fear of retribution, feelings of guilt, and lack of knowledge of their rights are frequently cited reasons for not disclosing victimization. The adolescent victim also may feel that she in some way contributed to the act, or she may not identify what has happened to her as rape because her experience does not fit the popular concept of rape (11). For example, sexual intercourse between younger girls and older men, or when the male is in a position of relative authority over the adolescent victim, may not fit the stereotypical image of rape, but such encounters should not automatically be considered consensual. Instead, they should be considered for inclusion in any assessment of the prevalence of adolescent sexual assault.

More than 75% of adolescent rapes are committed by an acquaintance of the victim; less than 25% are committed by a stranger (6, 12). Studies conducted in high schools and colleges throughout the country indicate that a substantial number of adolescents have experienced some form of sexual assault in dating relationships. The Sexual Experience Survey, administered in 1985 to 6,159 women and men enrolled in 32 higher-education institutions across the United States, revealed that since age 14, 27.5% of college women had experienced an act that meets the legal definition of rape and 7.7% of college men had committed such an act (13). The vast majority of sexual assaults on campuses are committed by boyfriends, friends, or acquaintances of the victims, with more than 50% occurring on dates (14). Acquaintance rape among younger adolescents is frequently incestuous. Using the expanded definition of incest, the United States Bureau of Justice Statistics reports that 20% of rape victims aged 12 to 17 years were attacked by family members (5).

Adolescent Perceptions of Violence

Many teens have not yet developed the necessary skills to recognize and avoid potentially dangerous dating or social situations. Some adolescents may have a distorted perception of violence and may fail to recognize a partner's behavior as violent. Some adolescents also may believe that violence is acceptable in certain situations. Also, adolescent males and females may bring different expectations to dating situations and attribute different meanings to the same behaviors. Adolescent males may be likely to interpret certain behaviors by females as an indication of sexual intent even though she had no such intention (8). In a study that questioned adolescents about their attitudes toward violence, 32% of the young women believed forced sex was acceptable if the couple had been dating a long time, 31% believed it acceptable if the woman agreed to have sex with her partner but later changed her mind, and 27% believed it acceptable if the woman "led him on." Of the young men in the study, 54% believed that forced sex was acceptable if the young woman said "yes" even though she later changed her mind; 40% believed that forced sex was acceptable if the man spent a lot of money on the date (15).

Alcohol, marijuana, and cocaine are frequently used in instances of acquaintance and date rape. These and other illicit substances can distort an adolescent's perception of, and susceptibility to, violence. Because these drugs may be consumed voluntarily, there has been concern that intoxicated individuals may be viewed as having encouraged the sexual advances. In those instances of rape where alcohol or illegal substances are involved, prosecution should still be encouraged.

Recent media accounts have focused on flunitrazepam (Rohypnol) and gamma hydroxbutyrate, the so-called "date-rape drugs," which can be slipped surreptitiously into a victim's drink. The misuse of these sedating substances, as well as other benzodiazepines, is particularly onerous because they can inhibit temporarily a person's ability to remain conscious and may cause periods of impaired memory. The Drug-Induced Rape Prevention and Punishment Act of 1996 increases penalties for those who use controlled substances to commit rape (16).

Identification of the Adolescent Sexual Assault Victim

It is the responsibility of the obstetrician–gynecologist, as a health care provider for adolescents, to be knowledgeable about sexual victimization and its consequences. The physician evaluating the victim of sexual assault in the acute phase should provide medical and counseling services, inform the victim of her rights, refer her to legal assistance, and help her develop prevention strategies to avoid future victimization (17). Often, however, the adolescent victim may not visit the obstetrician–gynecologist until significant time has elapsed, and her visit may be for reasons unrelated to the assault. Physical signs of the assault may not be present, and the patient often does not initiate a discussion about her situation. Therefore, the health care provider must recognize certain behavioral signs as well as the physical health problems that often result from sexual assault (see the boxes).

A review of emerging and existing data suggests an association between a history of nonvoluntary sexual activity and any of the following behaviors among adolescents: early initiation of voluntary sexual activity, unintended pregnancy, poor use of contraceptives, and involvement with a significantly older man (defined as at least 5 years older) (18–25). Adolescents with a history of prior sexual abuse may have difficulty setting boundaries regarding sexual limits, may feel powerless to stop sexual aggression, and may be confused about normal dating and sexual behavior (26). One study estimated that approximately 74% of women who had sexual intercourse before age 14 and 60% of those who had sex before age 15 reported having sex involuntarily at some earlier point in their lives (27). Additionally, recent analyses of the 1988 National Maternal and Infant Health Survey indicate that 24% of births to 17 year olds, 27% of births to 16 year olds, and 40% of births to 14 year olds were fathered by men at least 5 years older (26).

Intervention and Prevention

Although health care providers have learned to screen adolescents for anxiety, depression, substance abuse, and sexually transmissible infections, screening for sexual

Behavioral and Psychologic Sequelae That May Suggest a History of Sexual Assault

Teen pregnancy

Poor contraceptive use

Substance abuse (drug and alcohol)

Human immunodeficiency virus/acquired immunodeficiency syndrome (HIV/AIDS)-related risky health behaviors

Prostitution

Multiple sexual partners

Sexual dysfunction

Problems with interpersonal and sexual relations

Poor self-esteem

Depression

Somatization

Eating disorders/obesity

Insomnia and nightmares

Suicidal attempts

Psychiatric admissions

Posttraumatic stress disorder

Anxiety

School failure

Physical Health Problems That May Suggest a History of Sexual Assault

Chronic abdominal pain

Gastrointestinal tract symptoms (irritable bowel syndrome and other gastrointestinal symptoms)

Chronic pelvic pain

Vulvodynia and dyspareunia

Breast pain

Gynecologic infections

Sexually transmissible infections

Chronic headache

Musculoskeletal complaints

Multiple physical complaints

victimization may prove to be more difficult. Often, victims will minimize or deny their experiences. They may feel guilty about what has happened to them or they may feel in some way responsible (11). As part of the routine screening for a history of violence, all teens should be asked direct questions regarding their past sexual experiences (7). The health care provider may ask questions such as:

- Have you ever had sex?
- When was your first sexual experience?
- Did you choose to have sex?
- Has anyone forced you to have sex?
- Would you like to tell me what happened or ask any questions?

Additionally, providers should be prepared to pose additional questions, based upon the responses elicited. Because of the way some adolescents perceive violence, providers who suspect that a patient may be a victim of sexual assault should approach the subject with sensitivity. During this discussion, it also is essential to observe nonverbal communication that may indicate a need for further questioning. The practitioner who is knowledgeable about sexual assault and is aware of community resources for support will be more open to disclosures by patients and better able to deal with these difficult discussions.

Once the patient reveals that an assault has occurred, she should be allowed to describe the experience at a comfortable pace and in her own words (28). Sufficient time should be provided for this discussion. It is important that health care providers know the assault and rape laws in their state so that they can comply with any legal requirements. Victims of acquaintance rape of any age have the same legal rights as those who have been raped by a stranger (17).

In all 50 states and the District of Columbia, physicians are mandated to report child abuse to a child protective service agency in the area or to the local police department; in most states, child abuse includes sexual assault against children and adolescents (7). Nearly half of the states further require physicians to report victims of statutory rape (29). Physicians who fail to report sexual assaults against children may be subject to fines and incarceration periods of as long as 1 year. Reporting, however, should be done in a sensitive manner and must preserve the safety of the adolescent victim.

The physician should encourage the patient to talk about what has happened and express her feelings. Most victims go through the three stages of rape trauma syndrome: 1) trauma (fear of being alone, fear of men, sexual problems, depression); 2) denial (not wanting to talk about it); and 3) resolution (dealing with fears and feelings, regaining a sense of control over life) (30). These reactions may take years to resolve, and they do not necessarily occur in this order. For these reasons, it is important that providers in primary care settings be aware of the long-term consequences of sexual assault as previously outlined. A counseling referral to mental health professionals trained in the treatment of sexual assault victims is frequently helpful, although not every patient will be receptive. Periodic referrals may be more helpful than referring only once.

Health care providers also should provide the patient with strategies to prevent sexual assault. Educational materials targeted at adolescents can reinforce guidance and risk-reduction counseling. Prevention messages for adolescents include the following (7):

- You have the right to say no to sexual activity.
- You have the right to set sexual limits and insist that your partner honor them.
- Be assertive.
- Stay sober and watch out for dates or anyone else who tries to get you drunk or high.
- Recognize and avoid situations that may put you at risk for unwanted sexual activity.
- Never leave a party with someone you don't know well.
- Trust your feelings and intuitions. If it feels wrong, it probably is.
- Communicate with your friends and dates about sexual assault and educate them if necessary.
- No one should be raped or otherwise forced, coerced, or pressured into engaging in any unwanted sexual behavior.

Summary

Acquaintance rape and date rape are widespread problems among adolescents. Clinicians are faced with the challenging responsibility of identifying victims and providing effective interventional and preventive counseling. Recognizing the behavioral signals exhibited by victims and understanding adolescents' attitudes toward violence can help the health care provider to screen patients for current or past assaults. All adolescents need to be empowered with preventive strategies to avoid future violence in their relationships. Obstetrician–gynecologists must work with other health care and legal professionals to develop approaches to help adolescents. The prevalence of adolescent victimization warrants routine screening and effective counseling strategies by all obstetrician–gynecologists.

References

1. National Institute of Justice. The extent and costs of crime victimization: a new look. Washington, DC: U.S. Department of Justice, 1996
2. Dupre AR, Hampton HL, Morrison H, Meeks GR. Sexual assault. Obstet Gynecol Surv 1993;48:640–648
3. Bureau of Justice Statistics. Criminal victimization 1994. Washington, DC: U.S. Department of Justice, 1996; publication no. NCJ-158022
4. Koss MP, Harvey MR. The rape victim: clinical and community interventions. Newbury Park, California: Sage Publications, 1991
5. Langan PA, Harlow CW. Bureau of Justice Statistics: child rape victims, 1992 crime data brief. Washington, DC: U.S. Department of Justice, 1994; publication no. NCJ-147001
6. National Victim Center. Rape in America: a report to the nation. Arlington, Virginia: NVC, 1992
7. American Medical Association. Strategies for the treatment and prevention of sexual assault. Chicago: AMA, 1995
8. Hibbard R, Orr DP. Incest and sexual abuse. Semin Adolesc Med 1985;1:153–164
9. Donovan P. Can statutory rape laws be effective in preventing adolescent teen pregnancy? Fam Plann Perspect 1997; 29:30–34, 40
10. National Center on Child Abuse and Neglect. Child sexual abuse: incest, assault and sexual exploitation. Washington, DC: U.S. Government Printing Office, 1981
11. The Commonwealth Fund. In their own words: adolescent girls discuss health and health care issues. New York: Louis Harris and Associates, 1997
12. Heise LL. Reproductive freedom and violence against women: where are the intersections. J Law Med Ethics 1993;21:206–216
13. Koss MP, Gidycz CA, Wisniewski N. The scope of rape: incidence and prevalence of sexual aggression and victimization in a national standard of higher education students. J Consult Clin Psychol 1987;55:162–170
14. Abbey A. Acquaintance rape and alcohol consumption on college campuses: how are they linked? J Am Coll Health 1991;39:165–169
15. Parrot A. Acquaintance rape among adolescents: identifying risk groups and intervention strategies. J Soc Work Hum Sex 1989;8:47–61
16. Drug-Induced Rape Prevention and Punishment Act of 1996, Pub. L. No. 104-305, 110 Stat. 3807 (Oct. 13, 1996)
17. American College of Obstetricians and Gynecologists. Sexual assault. ACOG Technical Bulletin 242. Washington, DC: ACOG, 1997
18. Boyer D, Fine D. Sexual abuse as a factor in adolescent pregnancy and child maltreatment. Fam Plann Perspect 1992;24:4–11
19. Moore KA, Nord CW, Peterson JL. Nonvoluntary sexual activity among adolescents. Fam Plann Perspect 1989;21: 110–114
20. Katz S, Mazur M. Understanding the rape victim: a synthesis of research findings. New York: John Wiley, 1979
21. Smith MD, Besharov DJ, Gardiner KN, Hoff T. Early sexual experiences: how voluntary? How violent? Menlo Park, California: Henry J. Kaiser Foundation, 1996
22. Taylor D, Chavez G, Chabra A, Boggess J. Risk factors for adult paternity in births to adolescents. Obstet Gynecol 1997;89:199–205
23. Ventura SJ, Martin JA, Curtin SC, Mathews TJ. Report of final natality statistics, 1996. Monthly vital statistics report; vol 46, no. 11 (suppl). Hyattsville, Maryland: National Center for Health Statistics, 1998
24. Landry DJ, Forrest JD. How old are U.S. fathers? Fam Plann Perspect 1995;27:159–161, 165
25. Lindberg LD, Sonenstein FL, Ku L, Martinez G. Age difference between minors who give birth and their adult partners. Fam Plann Perspect 1997;29:61–66
26. Small SA, Kerns D. Unwanted sexual activity among peers during early and middle adolescence: incidence and risk factors. J Marriage Fam 1993;55:941–952
27. Alan Guttmacher Institute. Sex and America's teenagers. New York: AGI, 1994
28. Koval JE. Violence in dating relationships. J Pediatr Health Care 1989;3:298–304
29. Elstein SG, Davis N. Sexual relationships between adult males and young teen girls: exploring the legal and social responses. Chicago: American Bar Association, 1997
30. Hughes J, Sandler BR. "Friends" raping friends: could it happen to you? Washington, DC: Association of American Colleges, 1987

ISSN 1074-8628

The American College of Obstetricians and Gynecologists
409 12th Street, SW
PO Box 96920
Washington, DC 20090-6920

12345/21098

ACOG EDUCATIONAL BULLETIN

Number 259, July 2000

Adult Manifestations of Childhood Sexual Abuse

Obstetricians and gynecologists encounter patients with a wide array of symptoms that may be associated with a history of childhood sexual abuse. Frequently, the underlying cause of these symptoms is not recognized by the physician and, in many cases, by the patient. For some survivors of childhood sexual abuse (CSA), there is minimal compromise to their adult functioning. Others will have myriad psychologic, physical, and behavioral symptoms as a result of their abuse (1). Adult CSA survivors have disproportionately high use of health care services, more severe symptoms with more complex patterns of presentation, and often somatic symptoms that do not respond to routine treatment (2–4). These issues can create frustration for women and treatment challenges for their physicians. An understanding of the magnitude and impact of childhood sexual abuse, along with knowledge about screening and intervention methods, can help obstetricians and gynecologists offer appropriate care and support to patients with such histories.

This Educational Bulletin was developed under the direction of the Committee on Health Care for Underserved Women of the American College of Obstetricians and Gynecologists as an aid to obstetricians and gynecologists. This document is not to be construed as establishing a standard of practice or dictating an exclusive course of treatment. Rather, it is intended as an educational tool that presents current information on obstetric–gynecologic issues.

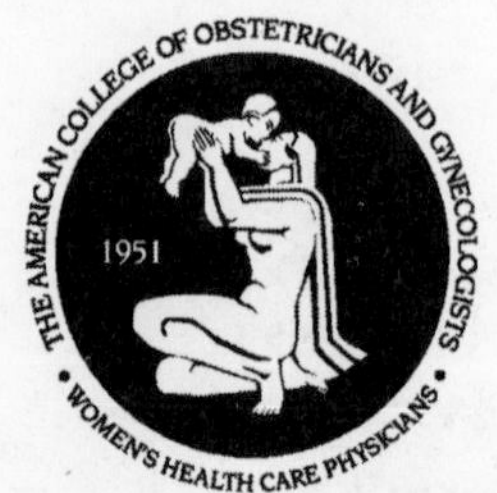

Definitions

Childhood sexual abuse can be defined as any exposure to sexual acts imposed on children who inherently lack the emotional, maturational, and cognitive development to understand or to consent to such acts. These acts do not always involve sexual intercourse or physical force; rather, they involve manipulation and trickery. Authority and power enable the perpetrator to coerce the child into compliance. Characteristics and motivations of perpetrators of childhood sexual abuse vary: some may act out sexually to exert dominance over another individual; others may initiate the abuse for their own sexual gratification (5, 6).

Although specific legal definitions may vary among states, there is widespread agreement that abusive sexual contact can include breast and genital fondling, oral and anal sex, and vaginal intercourse. Definitions have been expanded to include noncontact events such as coercion to watch sexual acts or posing in child pornography (7).

Prevalence

The prevalence of childhood sexual abuse in the United States is unknown. Because of the shame and stigma associated with abuse, many victims never disclose such experiences. Incest was once thought to be so rare that its occurrence was inconsequential. However, in the past 25 years there has been increased recognition that incest and other forms of childhood sexual abuse occur with alarming frequency (8). Researchers have found that victims come from all cultural, racial, and economic groups (9).

Current estimates of incest and other childhood sexual abuse range from 12% to 40% depending on settings and population. Most studies have found that among women, approximately 20%—or 1 in 5—have experienced childhood sexual abuse (9). Consistent with this range, studies have revealed that:

- Among girls who had sex before they were 13 years old, 22% reported that first sex was nonvoluntary (10).
- Twelve percent of girls in grades 9 through 12 reported they had been sexually abused; 7% of girls in grades 5 through 8 also reported sexual abuse. Of all the girls who experienced sexual abuse, 65% reported the abuse occurred more than once, 57% reported the abuser was a family member, and 53% reported the abuse occurred at home (11).
- Approximately 40% of the women surveyed in a primary care setting had experienced some form of childhood sexual contact; of those, 1 in 6 had been raped as a child (12).
- A national telephone survey on violence against women conducted by the National Institute of Justice and the Centers for Disease Control and Prevention found that 18% of 8,000 women surveyed had experienced a completed or attempted rape at some time in their lives. Of this number, 22% were younger than 12 years and 32% were between 12 and 17 years old when they were first raped (9).

Sequelae

Although there is no single syndrome that is universally present in adult survivors of childhood sexual abuse, there is an extensive body of research that documents adverse short- and long-term effects of such abuse. To appropriately treat and manage survivors of CSA, it is useful to understand that survivors' symptoms or behavioral sequelae often represent coping strategies employed in response to abnormal, traumatic events. These coping mechanisms are used for protection during the abuse or later to guard against feelings of overwhelming helplessness and terror. Although some of these coping strategies may eventually lead to health problems, if symptoms are evaluated outside their original context, survivors may be misdiagnosed or mislabeled (see box) (5).

In addition to the psychologic distress that may potentiate survivors' symptoms, there is evidence that abuse may result in biophysical changes. For example, one study found that, after controlling for history of psychiatric disturbance, adult survivors had lowered thresholds for pain (13). It also has been suggested that chronic or traumatic stimulation (especially in the pelvic or abdominal region) heightens sensitivity, resulting in per-

Common Symptoms in Adult Survivors of Childhood Sexual Abuse

Physical Presentations
- Chronic pelvic pain
- Gastrointestinal symptoms/distress
- Musculoskeletal complaints
- Obesity, eating disorders
- Insomnia, sleep disorders
- Pseudocyesis
- Sexual dysfunction
- Asthma, respiratory ailments
- Addiction
- Chronic headache
- Chronic back pain

Psychologic and Behavioral Presentations
- Depression and anxiety
- Posttraumatic stress disorder symptoms
- Dissociative states
- Repeated self-injury
- Suicide attempts
- Lying, stealing, truancy, running away
- Poor contraceptive practices
- Compulsive sexual behaviors
- Sexual dysfunction
- Somatizing disorders
- Eating disorders
- Poor adherence to medical recommendations
- Intolerance of or constant search for intimacy
- Expectation of early death

sistent pain such as abdominal and pelvic pain or other bowel symptoms (14, 15).

Although responses to sexual abuse vary, there is remarkable consistency in mental health symptoms, especially depression and anxiety. These mental health symptoms may be found alone or more often in tandem with physical and behavioral symptoms. More extreme symptoms are associated with abuse onset at an early age, extended or frequent abuse, incest by a parent, or use of force (4). Responses may be mitigated by such factors as inherent resiliency or supportive responses from individuals who are important to the victim (4). Even without therapeutic intervention, some survivors maintain the outward appearance of being unaffected by their abuse. Most, however, experience pervasive and deleterious consequences (4).

The primary aftereffects of childhood sexual abuse have been divided into seven distinct, but overlapping categories (16):

1. Emotional reactions
2. Symptoms of posttraumatic stress disorder (PTSD)
3. Self-perceptions
4. Physical and biomedical effects
5. Sexual effects
6. Interpersonal effects
7. Social functioning

Responses can be greatly variable and idiosyncratic within the seven categories. Also, survivors may fluctuate between being highly symptomatic and relatively symptom free. Health care providers should be aware that such variability is normal. Some common life events that may "trigger" the return of physical or psychologic symptoms for a CSA survivor who, until such time, functions well are listed in the box (4).

Common Life Event Symptom Triggers for CSA Survivors

Pregnancy or birth of a child

Illness or death of parent or perpetrator

Divorce of parents

Age of survivor's child the same as onset of abuse

Key "anniversary" dates or holidays

Family reunions

Illness or injury of a child

Hospitalization or medical workup

Workplace situation that mirrors a relationship with abuser

Home relocation, especially to geographic area where abuse occurred

Viewing movies or television shows with abuse content

Emotional Reactions

Emotional sequelae are the most frequently reported aftereffects by adult survivors. Depression, anxiety, and anger are the most reported emotional responses to childhood sexual abuse. Adults with a history of sexual abuse may have as much as a fourfold greater lifetime risk for major depression than individuals not abused as children (17). A recent study found that 46% of abused girls had depressive symptoms; 54% of the abused girls reported suicidal ideation (11). Among abuse survivors, anxiety disorder is 10 times more likely to be diagnosed than among nonabused individuals (18). The anxiety may be especially pronounced in intimate or close relationships or when interacting with authority figures. Fear, shame, humiliation, guilt and self-blame, grief, and urges to hurt oneself are often mentioned. All these emotions may have behavioral, somatic, and relational manifestations (5, 17).

Symptoms of Posttraumatic Stress

Adult survivors of childhood sexual abuse frequently have symptoms of PTSD. Responses tend to fall into two categories that may alternate or parallel each other: 1) intrusive or re-experiencing symptoms, and 2) numbing or denial symptoms (16). Especially prominent are the intrusive PTSD-related nightmares or flashbacks—sudden, intrusive sensory experiences, which often involve visual, auditory, olfactory, and tactile sensations reminiscent of the original assault. These nightmares or flashbacks are experienced as though they were occurring in the present rather than as a memory of a past event. Triggers of flashbacks may include sexual stimuli or interactions, gynecologic or pelvic examinations, abusive behavior by other adults, disclosure of one's abuse experiences to others, or reading or viewing sexual or violent media content (17).

Dissociative disorders have been linked to sexual abuse and are believed to be complex posttraumatic conditions used to numb or deny the incident(s). Survivors may experience amnesia, the partial or total loss of memory. Derealization or depersonalization may result in a survivor separating her mind from her body and her emotions. The survivor may experience the sensation of floating in space while observing her physical body. No emotional pain is connected with this observation. Physicians may observe a patient "zoning out." Dissociative identity disorder allows an individual to separate a group of related psychologic activities or memories into autonomously functioning units, as in the generation of multiple personalities (16, 19). Although dissociative defenses may effectively numb the memory or help the patient deny the experience of the abuse, it also may interfere with self-protection. Such patients may seek care for conditions related to secondary interpersonal violence, such as rape (18).

Self-Perceptions

The development of a sense of self is thought to be one of the earliest developmental tasks of young children. It typically unfolds in the context of early relationships (16, 17). The development of a positive self-perception is adversely affected by the following traumatic factors of abuse (16):

- Traumatic sexualization or the introduction of premature and coerced sexual involvement with an adult
- Powerlessness or the exploitation of a child's vulnerability to those in authority
- Betrayal by an adult who breaks the trust of the relationship, especially if the abuse was committed by a parent
- Stigmatization or the sense of shame and belief that the individual is fundamentally defective, which is internalized by the child and often carried throughout life

In an attempt to make sense of sexual abuse, most children develop the belief that something about them caused the abuse to happen or that they somehow deserved to be abused (16). As adults, survivors of CSA may maintain the image of the abuser as good while they view themselves as bad. These images, therefore, perpetuate the notion that they were deserving of the abuse and are not entitled to assistance and rescue. Such beliefs frequently result in high-risk or self-destructive behaviors and in engaging in abusive relationships.

The closer the relationship between child and perpetrator, the greater the extent of the trauma caused by childhood sexual abuse (16, 17). If the trust and protection ascribed to primary care givers such as parents or guardians is violated by mistreatment, a child's sense of self is badly damaged and the world becomes viewed as unsafe. Without basic trust, individuals lack the ability to cope, causing them to overreact to stress or painful events (17). The establishment of personal boundaries is essential for psychologic stability, allowing an individual to interact with another person without sacrificing his or her own identity, values, or preferences. Individuals with a history of sexual violence may not have had the opportunity to establish a secure sense of self. Adults molested early in life have more problems in understanding or relating to others independent of their experiences or needs, and they may not be able to perceive or experience their own internal states independent of the reactions or demands of others (20). Many such individuals may exhibit "loose boundaries," where they are overly compliant. Conversely, they may have excessively "rigid boundaries," where they are hostile or threatened.

Physical and Biomedical Effects

One review of the literature on the sequelae of adult survivors of childhood sexual abuse summarized the biomedical sequelae of childhood sexual abuse as having the following manifestations (21):

- Chronic or diffuse pain, either the result of trauma or conversion symptoms representative of the abuse
- Symptoms of anxiety or depression
- Eating and substance abuse disorders
- Self-neglect

It is common for survivors of CSA to exhibit physical symptoms in areas that were sexually traumatized (16). Some examples of chronic and diffuse pain in sexual abuse survivors are listed in the the box.

Eating disorders, especially obesity and bulimia, have been linked to a past history of sexual abuse. A recent survey found that girls reporting physical or sexual abuse were almost three times as likely to binge and purge as those who said they had not been abused (32% versus 12%) (11). The abused girls were also likely to binge and purge frequently. One in six abused girls reported such behavior more than once per week, and 13% of the abused girls said they did so daily.

Substance abuse often is the result of the survivor's attempt to either self-medicate the symptoms of sexual abuse or to avoid memories about the abuse. Self-neglect, including neglect of basic needs such as sleep, rest, and food, can result in exacerbation of existing medical problems as well as predisposition to medical problems. The survivor can have dental problems as a result of dental phobia related to trauma involving the oral cavity, and will often avoid preventive health examinations out of fear of physicians (21).

In addition to physical problems that develop from the abuse, adverse health consequences frequently are associated with many of the behaviors commonly

Examples of Chronic and Diffuse Pain in Sexual Abuse Survivors*

Headaches
- Migraine
- Temporomandibular joint syndrome
- Muscle tension

Genitourinary pain
- Chronic pain
- Rectal discomfort
- Hemorrhoids
- Constipation
- Diarrhea
- Irritable bowel syndrome
- Spastic colon

Gastrointestinal problems
- Gagging
- Nausea, vomiting
- Choking

Conversion symptoms
- Fainting
- Vertigo
- Seizures
- Muscle tension/spasms
- Joint pain
- Tinnitus
- Respiratory problems
  - Asthma
  - Shortness of breath

*May be suggestive of the abuse or somatic signs of depression.

employed, consciously or unconsciously, as coping devises. Furthermore, risky coping behaviors, such as smoking and alcohol or drug use may be employed chronically because they are perceived to be effective in relieving symptoms. According to a recent study, adults abused as children are (22):

- Twice as likely to smoke
- Nearly twice as likely to be severely obese
- Nearly twice as likely to be physically inactive
- Nearly five times more likely to have a history of alcohol abuse
- Nearly four times as likely to abuse illicit drugs
- Seven times more likely to have injected drugs
- Three times more likely to have had 50 or more intercourse partners
- Nearly twice as likely to have had a sexually transmitted disease (STD)

Sexual Effects

Disturbances in sexual identity and sexual functioning are prominent in studies of incest survivors (23). Women sexually abused in childhood may develop gender and sexual identities that emphasize self-worth based on sexuality. Moreover, they may unconsciously attempt to re-create sexual situations in order to control and change the outcome. Attempts at this "trauma mastery," coupled with inadequate personal boundaries and low self-esteem, may help to explain CSA survivors' increased risk for engaging in unsafe sexual behaviors that have negative health consequences, such as STDs and unintended pregnancy. One study found that, compared with their nonabused pregnant counterparts, sexually abused teens began intercourse earlier, were more likely to have used drugs and alcohol, and were less likely to use contraception (24).

The pronounced sexual dysfunction in adult survivors of incest has been described as "the most obvious example of conditioned, abuse-related fear" (17). Because of the association between sexual stimuli and invasion or pain, many adults abused as children report fear or anxiety-related difficulties during sexual contact.

For adult survivors, the most frequently reported chronic sexual problems include fear of intimate relationships, feelings of repulsion or lack of enjoyment, flashbacks during sexual activity, dysfunctions of desire and arousal, and primary or secondary anorgasmia. Compulsive promiscuity and prostitution also may be present because survivors often confuse sexuality with nurturing behavior (21). There is no evidence that a history of childhood sexual abuse is related to sexual orientation.

Interpersonal Effects

For incest survivors the ability to have emotionally healthy relationships with others may be profoundly damaged. Many survivors have relationships that are unstable and include patterns of excessive self-sufficiency, withdrawal, and hostility. Others may assume the care taking of others, extreme dependence, overcompliance, learned helplessness, and nonassertion (16).

The inability of CSA survivors to separate themselves from others may manifest as problems with defining their boundaries and individual rights when faced with the needs and demands of others. Such problems are frequently associated with great difficulties in interpersonal relationships, including gullibility, inadequate self-protectiveness, and likelihood of being victimized or abused by others (17).

Deleterious and troubling sequelae to childhood sexual abuse include the apparent vulnerability of women with such histories to be repeatedly victimized later in life, often on multiple occasions, by individuals who may or may not be known to them. This tendency to be victimized repeatedly may be the result of a general vulnerability in dangerous situations and to exploitation by untrustworthy people. Childhood abuse seems to have the effect of making adult women less skilled at self-protection and more apt to accept being victimized by others (25).

Social Functioning

The social functioning of CSA survivors varies considerably. Survivors' social functioning can range from exceptional and overfunctioning to greatly deficient and deviant, exhibiting such behaviors as delinquency, prostitution, dangerous sexual practices (including sadomasochism, indiscriminate sexual activity, and sexual abuse of others), and substance abuse. Overfunctioning is often an attempt to palliate the profound low self-esteem that survivors have and to channel their anxiety. Conversely, researchers suggest that some of the most marginally functional and disenfranchised members of society, such as the chronically mentally ill and the homeless, may have histories of sexual abuse at the core of their problems (16).

As previously discussed, not all survivors will have the same symptoms or symptoms of equal severity. A recent literature review of factors that moderate and mediate the effects of childhood sexual abuse found that heightened adult distress results from:

- Molestation at an especially early age
- Extended and frequent abuse
- Incest by a biologic parent
- The presence of force
- Greater number of perpetrators

The most pronounced psychologic problems also are predicted by the presence of other concomitant forms of child maltreatment, including physical and psychologic abuse or neglect, and subsequent victimization in adulthood (17).

For most survivors, childhood sexual abuse frequently occurs in conjunction with other forms of child abuse or household dysfunction. For example, a survey was administered to members of a large health maintenance organization to determine exposure to several categories of adverse childhood experiences, including physical or sexual abuse, violence against mother, or living with household members who were substance abusers. The risk of long-term adverse consequences increased dramatically as the number of adverse experiences increased for an individual. The study revealed that 65% of the individuals reporting childhood sexual abuse also reported one other type of adverse experience; 41% reported two additional adverse experiences (22).

Effects on Reproductive Health and Pregnancy

Gynecologic problems, including chronic pelvic pain, dyspareunia, vaginismus, and nonspecific vaginitis, are common complaints of adult survivors of childhood sexual abuse (6, 21, 26–28). Disturbances in sexual interest and sexual functioning are widely reported and range from sexual inhibition to compulsive sexuality (6, 21, 29, 30).

Disturbances of desire, arousal, and orgasm are among the inhibitory aftereffects of childhood sexual abuse and likely result from the association between sexual activity, violation, and pain. Conversely, compulsive sexuality, promiscuity, and prostitution also may occur (21). Childhood sexual abuse is significantly associated with prostitution (30, 31). Early adolescent or unintended pregnancy also is suggestive of a history of sexual abuse (31). This may be the direct result of incest or a result of promiscuity without the use of contraceptives, a sign of impaired self-care (21, 24). The incidence of STDs also is higher in childhood sexual abuse survivors, and adolescent and adult survivors of childhood sexual abuse are at greater risk of human immunodeficiency virus (HIV) infection than those without such histories (12, 32). Survivors may be less likely to have regular Pap tests and may seek little or no prenatal care (33, 34).

Vaginal examinations may be associated with terror and pain for abuse survivors. Additionally, feelings of vulnerability in the lithotomy position, being connected to intravenous lines and labor monitors, and being examined by relative strangers in the delivery room may leave the survivor vulnerable to re-experiencing past feelings of powerlessness, violation, and fear. The physical pain of labor and delivery also may trigger memories of past abuse with or without conscious memory of or connection to the earlier abuse (4, 5, 35–37).

Pregnancy and delivery may be an especially difficult time for survivors for a variety of reasons. Pregnancy may trigger memories of abuse. In some cases, women with no prior conscious memories of their abuse may begin to experience emotions, dreams, or partial memories that are troubling. With all of the attendant changes in a woman's body and her lifestyle, coping mechanisms that had previously kept the abusive history from her memory may now fail, and what she had once repressed comes to the surface (36, 37). Pregnant women reporting a history of childhood sexual abuse are significantly more likely than those without such history to report suicidal ideation and depression (13, 19, 38). Pregnant adolescents also have been found to be more likely to report substance abuse during pregnancy and to give birth to significantly smaller and less mature infants (39). Smoking was common among pregnant survivors of childhood sexual abuse (40). There are no consistent data regarding adverse pregnancy outcome for women with histories of childhood sexual abuse.

Issues Affecting Memory

Recently, there has been controversy over the issue of delayed recall of childhood sexual abuse. Although most emotionally laden events are stored in memory along with their accompanying effects, traumatic memory is different (4). Proponents of "false memory syndrome" contend that experiments and studies on memory prove that false memories can be readily implanted. Currently, research results are divided on this issue. It is not incumbent upon the obstetrician–gynecologist to make a determination of the veracity of "recovered memories." Rather, a prudent obstetrician–gynecologist should be a supportive ally for all patients and should consult with a mental health practitioner with experience working with sexual abuse issues. Not every mental health practitioner has such expertise.

Screening

With recognition of the extent of family violence, medical groups have issued recommendations for screening all patients (especially women) for histories of abuse (4). Patients overwhelmingly favor universal inquiry about sexual assault (41). At the same time, they report a reluctance to initiate a discussion of this subject. Following are some basic guidelines:

1. Make the question "natural." As physicians ask patients about possible sexual abuse, they will develop increased comfort with the process. They should be aware of their body language and avoid a guarded or closed posture. Over time, they will ask about sexual abuse as routinely as they ask about menstrual cycles.
2. Normalize the experience. As physicians learn to ask questions in a natural way, they may want to offer explanatory statements like: "About 1 woman in 5 was sexually abused as a child. Because these experiences can have an impact on health and well-being, I ask all of my patients about unwanted touching or sexual experiences in childhood."
3. Give the patient control over disclosure. Ask every patient about childhood abuse and rape trauma, but let her control what she says and when she says it. She will be the best judge of how to keep her emotional defenses intact.
   - If the physician suspects abuse, but the patient chooses not to disclose it, she can be assured that the physician is a resource for her if she ever needs to discuss such issues. Patients very commonly bring up the subject three to four visits later, especially if they have developed trust and want assistance.
   - If the patient says "yes," it is important to ask whether she has ever talked with anyone about the abuse or rape. Many women will have dealt with the issues in another forum. Asking whether any parts of the breast or pelvic examination cause her emotional discomfort should also be posed at this time.
   - If the patient has never talked with anyone about her abuse or rape, this is likely to be a very emotional time for her. Revelations often are accompanied by much anguish. Sitting quietly through this period can be difficult, but is very important. Excessive reassurance negates the pain of her experience. Detached self-protection or anger directed toward the perpetrator limits her ability to work through her emotional pain. If the physical portion of the examination has not yet been done, it should be postponed until another visit. If she is in an examination gown, allowing her to compose and dress herself may help her to regain some control. This is a good time to ask if she wishes to see a therapist. If the patient appears overtly depressed, the physician should ask about suicidal ideas, intentions, or attempts in the past.

Even when questions are carefully phrased and the assessment has been conducted in a caring and sensitive manner, some patients with histories of abuse will not disclose their experiences. Survivors may need to test the physician's trustworthiness with such information. In other instances, repression does not allow survivors access to such memories at the time of the physician's questioning. Despite the possibility that survivors will not be able to respond positively to the physician's questions, they will be made aware that the physician is someone who considers such information essential to comprehensive health care (8). It has been suggested that not inquiring about sexual abuse gives tacit support to the survivor's belief that abuse does not matter, that it does not have long-term effects, and that it is a subject that is not to be discussed (42).

If screening does not occur and the patient appears to tolerate pelvic examinations or other procedures, the obstetrician–gynecologist may mistakenly assume that the patient does not have a history of abuse. Instead, many survivors may not be able to express discomfort or fear and may silently experience a great deal of distress (42). Given the frequency of childhood sexual abuse and its many deleterious sequelae across the life span, patients should be screened for such histories periodically. Evaluating only those women who have symptoms that create a high index of suspicion will likely result in many abuse survivors being undetected (43).

Intervention

Once it is known that a patient is a survivor of childhood sexual abuse, there are a number of ways that the obstetrician–gynecologist can offer support. This includes the use of empowering messages and counseling referrals.

Positive Messages

Some positive and healing responses to the disclosure of abuse include letting the patient know that (21, 42, 44):

- She is the victim of abuse. She is in no way to blame. The perpetrator is always at fault.
- It took a great deal of courage for her to disclose the abuse.
- She has been heard and believed.
- Her symptoms "make sense" given what she has experienced.
- She has the right to say "no" or "stop" during any examination or procedure. She can and should set limits for herself. She has the right to control who touches her body and when and how. Physicians should ask permission to begin an examination.
- She also has the right to maintain her silence on the issue.

Counseling Referrals

Traumatized patients generally benefit from mental health care. Survivors who have disclosed abuse should be asked if they have ever talked to anyone about their experiences. For patients who have not sought such care, the obstetrician–gynecologist can be a powerful ally in the patient's healing by offering support and referral. Not every mental health professional is experienced in working with CSA survivors. Every effort should be made to refer them to professionals with significant experience in abuse-related issues.

Physicians may begin compiling a list of experts with experience in abuse. Contacting state boards of psychology or medicine often can be beneficial in locating therapists who are skilled in treating victims of such trauma. Veterans' centers, battered women's shelters, and rape crisis centers are often familiar with therapists and programs that treat various types of trauma, as are many university-based counseling programs. Because of the relationship between trauma histories and alcohol and drug abuse, therapists should be skilled in working with individuals who have dual diagnoses (43). Obstetrician–gynecologists should become familiar with appropriate crisis hotlines that may operate in their communities.

When referring patients to other professionals, it is especially helpful to identify a specific purpose. For example, saying "I would like Dr. Hill to assess you to determine if your past abuse is contributing to your current health problems" is more effective than telling the survivor that her symptoms are all "psychologic" and that she should see a therapist (44). It is important to secure the patient's express authorization prior to speaking to the therapist when collaborative practice between the obstetrician–gynecologist and therapist is warranted.

It is important to help the patient not feel abandoned or rejected when a counseling referral is made. If it is appropriate, the physician should emphasize his or her ongoing involvement in the patient's case. If the therapist or agency that the patient is being referred to is known personally by the physician, the patient will feel more confident about the referral. The obstetrician–gynecologist also should reassure the survivor that she is reacting in normal, predictable ways for someone who has survived such abuse (44).

Avoiding Retraumatization

Obstetrician–gynecologists must be sensitive to the possibility of retraumatizing adult survivors of childhood sexual abuse during health care procedures. The risk for retraumatization is present during such care because many procedures involve touch, are invasive, and are performed by authority figures in positions of control or power. All procedures need to be thoroughly explained in advance, and whenever possible the patient should be allowed to suggest ways that the procedure can be done to lessen her fear. This may mean allowing the patient to invite friends or family members to be present (16).

Pelvic, rectal, vaginal ultrasound, and breast examinations may be particularly traumatic for sexual abuse survivors, and it is important for providers to give survivors as much control as possible. Techniques to increase the patient's comfort include: talking her through the steps, maintaining eye contact, allowing her to control the pace, allowing her to see more (eg, use of a mirror in pelvic examinations) or having her assist during her examination (ie, putting her hand over the physician's to guide the examination) (4, 42). It is always important to ask permission to touch the patient, especially during the examinations previously mentioned.

Summary

Obstetrician–gynecologists will regularly provide care for women who are survivors of childhood sexual abuse. To ensure that patients receive appropriate care, whether or not they have disclosed a history of abuse, obstetricians and gynecologists should screen women for such histories.

Long-term effects of childhood sexual abuse are varied, complex, and often devastating for survivors. Symptoms that once served as effective survival strategies eventually may result in significant physical or mental health problems. An understanding of and appreciation for the long-term effects of abuse are essential in developing a differential diagnosis, formulating treatment strategies, and providing patient care.

References

1. McCauley J, Kern DE, Kolodner K, Schroeder AF, DeChant HK, Ryden J, et al. Clinical characteristics of women with a history of childhood abuse: unhealed wounds. JAMA 1997;277:1362–1368
2. Koss MP, Koss PG, Woodruff WJ. Deleterious effects of criminal victimization on women's health and medical utilization. Arch Intern Med 1991;151:342–347
3. Drossman DA, Leserman J, Nachman G, Li ZM, Gluck H, Toomey TC, et al. Sexual and physical abuse in women with functional or organic gastrointestinal disorders. Ann Intern Med 1990;113:828–833
4. American Medical Association. Diagnostic and treatment guidelines on mental health effects of family violence. Chicago: AMA, 1995
5. Hendricks-Matthews M. Long-term consequences of childhood sexual abuse. In: Rosenfeld J, Alley N, Acheson LS, Admire JB, eds. Women's health in primary care. Baltimore: Williams & Wilkins, 1997:267–276
6. Britton H, Hansen K. Sexual abuse. Clin Obstet Gynecol 1997;40:226–240
7. Maltz W. Adult survivors of incest: how to help them overcome the trauma. Med Aspects Hum Sex 1990;24:42–47
8. Hendricks-Matthews MK. Caring for victims of childhood sexual abuse. J Fam Pract 1992;35:501–502
9. Tjaden P, Thoennes N. Prevalence, incidence, and consequences of violence against women: findings from the National Violence Against Women Survey. Research in Brief. Washington, DC: U.S. Dept of Justice, Office of Justice Programs, November 1998, NCJ 172837
10. Moore KA, Driscoll A. Partners, predators, peers, protectors: males and teen pregnancy. New data analysis of the 1995 National Survey of Family Growth. In: Not just for girls: the roles of boys and men in teen pregnancy. Washington, DC: The National Campaign to Prevent Teen Pregnancy, 1997: 7–12
11. Schoen C, Davis K, Collins KS, Greenberg L, Des Roches C, Abrams M. The Commonwealth Fund survey of the health of adolescent girls. New York: The Commonwealth Fund, 1997
12. Walker EA, Torkelson N, Katon WJ, Koss MP. The prevalence rate of sexual trauma in a primary care clinic. J Am Board Fam Pract 1993;6:465–471
13. Scarinci IC, McDonald-Haile J, Bradley LA, Richter JE. Altered pain perception and psychosocial features among women with gastrointestinal disorders and history of abuse: a preliminary model. Am J Med 1994:97:108–118
14. Cervero F, Janig W. Visceral nociceptors: a new world order? Trends Neurosci 1992;15:374–378
15. Drossman DA. Physical and sexual abuse and gastrointestinal illness: what is the link? Am J Med 1994;97: 105–107
16. Courtois CA. Adult survivors of sexual abuse. Prim Care 1993;20:433–446
17. Briere JN, Elliott DM. Immediate and long-term impacts of child sexual abuse. Future Child 1994;4(2):54–69
18. Kaplan SJ. Family violence: a clinical and legal guide. Washington, DC: American Psychiatric Press, 1996
19. Anderson G, Yasenik L, Ross CA. Dissociative experiences and disorders among women who identify themselves as sexual abuse survivors. Child Abuse Negl 1993; 17:677–686
20. Cole PM, Putnam FW. Effect of incest on self and social functioning: a developmental psychopathology perspective. J Consult Clin Psychol 1992;60:174–183
21. Wahlen SD. Adult survivors of childhood sexual abuse. In: Hendricks-Matthews M, ed. Violence education: toward a solution. Kansas City, Missouri: Society of Teachers of Family Medicine, 1992:89–102
22. Felitti VJ, Anda RF, Nordenberg D, Williamson DF, Spitz AM, Edwards V, et al. Relationship of childhood abuse

and household dysfunction to many of the leading causes of death in adults. The Adverse Childhood Experiences (ACE) Study. Am J Prev Med 1998;4:245–258

23. Putnam FW. Disturbances of "self" in victims of childhood sexual abuse. In: Kluft RP, ed. Incest-related syndromes of adult psychopathology. Washington, DC: American Psychiatric Press, 1990:113–131

24. Boyer D, Fine D. Sexual abuse as a factor in adolescent pregnancy and child maltreatment. Fam Plann Perspec 1992;24:4–11, 19

25. Rieker PP, Carmen EH. The victim-to-patient process: the disconfirmation and transformation of abuse. Am J Orthopsychiatry 1986;56:360–370

26. Harrop-Griffiths J, Katon W, Walker E, Holm L, Russo J, Hickok L. The association between chronic pelvic pain, psychiatric diagnosis, and childhood sexual abuse. Obstet Gynecol 1988;71:589–594

27. Reiter RC, Shakerin LR, Gambone JC, Milburn AK. Correlation between sexual abuse and somatization in women with somatic and nonsomatic chronic pelvic pain. Am J Obstet Gynecol 1991;165:104–109

28. Toomey TC, Hernandez JT, Gittelman DF, Hulka JF. Relationship of sexual and physical abuse to pain and psychological assessment variables in chronic pelvic pain patients. Pain 1993;53:105–109

29. Luster T, Small SA. Sexual abuse history and number of sex partners among female adolescents. Fam Plann Perspect 1997;29:204–211

30. Windom CS, Kuhns JB. Childhood victimization and subsequent risk for promiscuity, prostitution, and teenage pregnancy: a prospective study. Am J Public Health 1996; 86:1607–1612

31. Bachmann GA, Moeller TP, Bennett J. Childhood sexual abuse and the consequences in adult women. Obstet Gynecol 1988;71:631–642

32. Lodico MA, DiClemente RJ. The association between childhood sexual abuse and prevalence of HIV-related risk behaviors. Clin Pediatr 1994;33:498–502

33. Springs FE, Friedrich WN. Health risk behaviors and medical sequelae of childhood sexual abuse. Mayo Clin Proc 1992;67:527–532

34. Burian J. Helping survivors of sexual abuse through labor. MCN Am J Matern Child Nurs 1995;20:252–256

35. Grant LJ. Effects of childhood sexual abuse: issues for obstetric caregivers. Birth 1992;19:220–221

36. Waymire V. A triggering time. Childbirth may recall sexual abuse memories. AWHONN Lifelines 1997;1:47–50

37. Rhodes N, Hutchinson S. Labor experiences of childhood sexual abuse survivors. Birth 1994;21:213–220

38. Farber EW, Herbert SE, Reviere SL. Childhood abuse and suicidality in obstetrics patients in a hospital-based urban prenatal clinic. Gen Hosp Psychiatry 1996;18:56–60

39. Stevens-Simon C, McAnarney ER. Childhood victimization: relationship to adolescent pregnancy outcome. Child Abuse Negl 1994;18:569–575

40. Grimstad H, Schei B. Pregnancy and delivery for women with a history of child sexual abuse. Child Abuse Negl 1999;23:81–90

41. Friedman LS, Samet JH, Roberts MS, Hudlin M, Hans P. Inquiry about victimization experiences. A survey of patient preferences and physician practices. Arch Intern Med 1992;152:1186–1190

42. Holz KA. A practical approach to clients who are survivors of childhood sexual abuse. J Nurse Midwifery 1994;39: 13–18

43. Hendricks-Matthews MK. Recognition of sexual abuse. J Am Board Fam Pract 1993;6:511–513

44. Laws A. Sexual abuse history and women's medical problems. J Gen Intern Med 1993;8:441–443

The American College of
Obstetricians and Gynecologists
409 12th Street, SW
PO Box 96920
Washington, DC 20090-6920

12345/43210

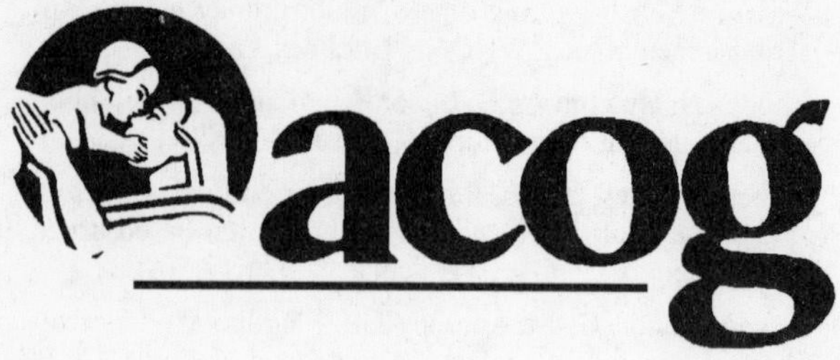

Number 128—May 1989

Technical Bulletin

An Educational Aid to Obstetrician–Gynecologists

Amenorrhea

Amenorrhea indicates failure of the hypothalamic–pituitary–gonadal axis to induce cyclic changes in the endometrium that normally result in menses. Amenorrhea may also result from the absence of end organs or from obstruction of the outflow tract. Thus, amenorrhea may result from an abnormality at any level of the reproductive tract. The duration of amenorrhea that is considered pathologic is arbitrary; any woman who has concerns, however, should be evaluated.

Amenorrhea has been defined as 1) the absence of menstruation for 3 or more months in women with past menses (referred to as secondary amenorrhea) or 2) the absence of menarche by the age of 16 years in girls who have never menstruated (referred to as primary amenorrhea). Although it is traditional to categorize amenorrhea as primary or secondary, this distinction is artificial and should not be considered in the evaluation of the amenorrheic woman. Similarly, the term "postpill amenorrhea," used to refer to women who do not menstruate within 3 months of discontinuing oral contraceptives, conveys nothing about the cause of the amenorrhea and should not alter the evaluation.

Amenorrhea is not a diagnosis in itself. Affected individuals should be investigated to determine the etiology. Although amenorrhea is physiologic in prepubertal girls, during pregnancy and lactation, and after menopause, it should be regarded as pathologic when it is present at any other time during the normal reproductive years. Nonphysiologic amenorrhea is estimated to occur in 5% of women of reproductive age. In general, menses occur at intervals of 28 ± 3 days in two-thirds of women, with a normal range of 18–40 days (1).

Etiologies

After pregnancy has been excluded, it is useful to divide the causes of amenorrhea into three categories (see box):

1. *Anatomic causes* are those that preclude menstrual bleeding, including abnormal differentiation of the genital tract and intrauterine adhesions (synechiae).
2. *Ovarian failure* includes disorders in which the ovaries are devoid of germ cells and those in which the germ cells do not respond appropriately to follicle-stimulating hormone (FSH).
3. *Endocrine imbalances* resulting in chronic anovulation are present in women who fail to ovulate spontaneously but in whom ovulation can be induced with appropriate therapy. This category is the most common form of amenorrhea and includes individuals with hypothalamic or pituitary dysfunction, adrenal and thyroid disorders, and inappropriate steroid feedback, such as polycystic ovarian syndrome (PCO).

Diagnosis

History and Physical Examination

The most important aspect of the clinical evaluation is the history and physical examination. In taking a history, the physician should establish the timing of pubertal milestones. Life style, employment, dietary and exercise habits, use of medications or drugs, environmental and psychologic stress, and any family history of amenorrhea or genetic anomalies are important. Previous pelvic surgery should be noted. Evidence of increased androgen, including acne, hirsutism, temporal balding, deepening of the voice, increased muscle mass, and decreased breast size should be sought, as should historical evidence of decreased estrogen, including hot flushes, night sweats, and dyspareunia. Any history of galactorrhea or symptoms of other endocrinopathies should be elicited. The physiologic response of the patient to her own gonadal steroids results in a clinical bioassay. For example, breast development indicates exposure to estrogens, whereas the presence of pubic and axillary hair indicates exposure to androgens.

During the physical examination, special attention should be directed to evaluating the following:

- Body dimensions and habitus
- Distribution and extent of terminal androgen-stimulated body hair

Causes of Amenorrhea*

I. Anatomic causes
- A. Pregnancy
- B. Intrauterine adhesions (Asherman syndrome)
- C. Disorders of sexual differentiation
  1. Distal genital tract obstruction (müllerian agenesis and dysgenesis)
  2. Gonadal dysgenesis
  3. Ambiguity of external genitalia (male and female pseudohermaphroditism)
- D. Gestational trophoblastic disease

II. Ovarian failure
- A. Menopause
- B. Physical causes
  1. Surgical extirpation of the gonads
  2. Irradiation of the gonads
  3. Chemotherapeutic agents
  4. Viral agents
  5. Cigarette smoking
- C. Chromosomal abnormalities
  1. Gonadal dysgenesis (X0, XX, mosaics)
  2. Trisomy X with or without chromosomal mosaicism
- D. Autoimmune disorders
  1. Polyglandular
  2. Isolated ovarian failure
  3. Congenital thymic aplasia
- E. Enzymatic defects
  1. 17α-hydroxylase deficiency
  2. Galactosemia
- F. Idiopathic

III. Endocrine imbalances
- A. Central origin
  1. Hypothalamic chronic anovulation (functional amenorrhea)
     - a. Anorexia nervosa and bulimia
     - b. Simple weight loss, diet, or malnutrition
     - c. Exercise-associated amenorrhea
     - d. Psychogenic amenorrhea
     - e. Pseudocyesis
     - f. Systemic illnesses
  2. Forms of isolated gonadotropin deficiency (including Kallman syndrome)
  3. Hypopituitarism
     - a. Hypothalamic–pituitary damage from any of several causes
     - b. Idiopathic
  4. Hyperprolactinemic chronic anovulation (galactorrhea–amenorrhea) of multiple etiologies
- B. Inappropriate peripheral feedback
  1. Functional androgen excess of adrenal and/or ovarian origin (including polycystic ovarian syndrome)
  2. Neoplasms producing androgens or estrogens
  3. Neoplasms producing chorionic gonadotropin
  4. Liver and renal disease
  5. Obesity
- C. Other endocrine disorders
  1. Thyroid dysfunction
  2. Adrenal hyperfunction

* Modified from The Merck Manual of Diagnosis and Therapy, edition 15, pp 1691–1694, edited by Robert Berkow. Copyright 1987 by Merck & Co., Inc. Used with permission.

- Extent of breast development by Tanner staging (2) and the presence or absence of any breast secretions
- External and internal genitalia, with emphasis on evidence of exposure to androgens and estrogens

Asynchronous pubertal development with significant breast development in the absence of a normal amount of pubic and axillary hair, together with a blind ending or absent vagina, suggests androgen insensitivity syndrome (testicular feminization). The diagnosis can be confirmed by karyotype or by the measurement of peripheral testosterone concentrations, which are generally in the normal adult male range.

Any abnormality of the genital outflow tract should be identified during the examination, but diagnosis of the specific disorder may prove difficult and require additional testing. Disorders of the genital tract accompanied by normal external genitalia and other secondary sex characteristics are found in women with normal ovarian function who have anomalies of müllerian duct derivatives, including imperforate hymen, vaginal and uterine aplasia, and vaginal septa. Obstruction to the normal efflux of menstrual blood can result in hematocolpos and hematometra. Although a bulging perineum and a pelvic mass are commonly present, differentiating vaginal agenesis from a vaginal septum or an imperforate hymen may be very difficult. The occurrence of intermittent abdominal pain may suggest intraabdominal bleeding.

The existence of intrauterine synechiae or adhesions (Asherman syndrome) should be considered in women who develop oligomenorrhea or amenorrhea following pregnancy-related curettage or endometritis. Tuberculous endometritis may also cause such intrauterine scarring. This diagnosis can be confirmed by hysterosalpingography or hysteroscopy.

Although it may prove difficult to differentiate chronic anovulation from ovarian failure without additional laboratory testing, it is generally possible to form strong clinical impressions about the etiology of the amenorrhea. Menopausal symptoms, especially hot flushes or dyspareunia, are suggestive of ovarian failure. The degree of development of secondary sex characteristics should be noted, as previously stated. For example, the presence of excess body hair or galactorrhea may suggest increased androgen activity or hyperprolactinemia. Signs and symptoms of adrenal or thyroid dysfunction may be important as well.

Current evidence indicates that hypothalamic chronic anovulation is a heterogeneous group of disorders with similar manifestations (3). Emotional and physical stresses, diet, body composition, exercise, environment, and other aspects of the life style of the individual contribute to the amenorrhea to various degrees. The diagnosis of hypothalamic chronic anovulation is a diagnosis of exclusion, suggested by the history and findings and confirmed by laboratory testing.

Individuals with amenorrhea and significant weight loss may have anorexia nervosa or bulimia or both. Kallman syndrome (isolated gonadotropin deficiency or familial hypogonadotropic hypogonadism) should be considered in young women who present with primary amenorrhea and absent to minimal sexual development. Associated findings may include anosmia or hyposmia, color blindness, and cleft lip and cleft palate. Hypopituitarism, in which the clinical presentation depends on the age of onset, the etiology, and the nutritional status of the patient, may be obvious or so subtle as to defy diagnosis without sophisticated endocrine testing. The possibility of hypopituitarism should be evaluated if secondary sex characteristics fail to develop or progress after puberty is initiated. Endocrine testing will be required to establish these diagnoses.

Polycystic ovarian syndrome (PCO), or chronic hyperandrogenemic anovulation, is a heterogeneous disorder in which clinical and biochemical variability exists. Anovulation may occur because of inappropriate feedback signals to the hypothalamic–pituitary unit and may be characterized by luteinizing hormone (LH)-dependent excess androgen production (3). Affected women generally present with amenorrhea, hirsutism, and obesity from puberty, but they may also present with irregular and profuse uterine bleeding and be neither hirsute nor obese. Patients are invariably feminized and rarely present with overt virilization. Because it appears that excess androgen from any source can lead to the typical findings of PCO, laboratory assessment is essential even if the clinical presentation seemingly makes the diagnosis apparent.

Administration of exogenous progestin is frequently recommended, both as a clinical aid to diagnosis and to evaluate the biological levels of estrogen. This will also determine with certainty whether the outflow tract is intact. Either progesterone in oil (100–200 mg intramuscularly) or medroxyprogesterone acetate (5–10 mg orally daily for 5–10 days) can be given. Any genital bleeding within 10 days of the completion of these regimens indicates a positive test. Such a positive result makes the diagnosis of Asherman syndrome unlikely (though still possible) and suggests (but does not prove) chronic anovulation, rather than hypothalamic-pituitary insufficiency or ovarian failure. If the test is negative (suggesting low levels of endogenous estrogen), then estrogen and a progestin together (eg, oral conjugated estrogen, 2.5 mg daily for 25 days, together with oral medroxyprogesterone acetate, 5–10 mg for the last 10 days of estrogen therapy) should induce bleeding if the endometrium is normal. It is important to recognize that, although progestin challenge may be helpful in evaluating amenorrheic women, the results are not always definitive. Progestin challenge should not be used as the sole diagnostic test by which amenorrheic women are evaluated.

Laboratory Evaluation

If pregnancy and anatomic causes of amenorrhea have been excluded and an evaluation for possible chromosomal abnormalities and sexual ambiguity has been performed, the laboratory evaluation should focus on distinguishing ovarian failure and endocrine causes of chronic anovulation. Measurements of basal concentrations of LH, FSH, prolactin, and thyroid-stimulating hormone (TSH) will confirm the clinical impression in all amenorrheic women (3). Measurement of peripheral tetraiodothyronine or triiodothyronine may also be warranted.

Although elevated levels of TSH indicate primary hypothyroidism, basal levels of prolactin may or may not be elevated because of the increased secretion of thyrotropin-releasing hormone. Primary hypothyroidism may be associated with amenorrhea even in individuals in whom tetraiodothyronine and triiodothyronine levels are within the normal range (4). Sellar radiographs may indicate pituitary gland enlargement in primary hypothyroidism because of hyperplasia of the pituitary thyrotrophs. If the diagnosis of primary hypothyroidism is in doubt, an abnormally large increase in TSH levels in response to exogenous thyrotropin-releasing hormone (200–500 μg intravenously) will confirm the clinical impression.

If the basal prolactin level is elevated (greater than 20 ng/ml) on initial testing, the drug and medication history should be reviewed and the measurement repeated with the patient in the relaxed, fasting state, because prolactin levels may be increased by nonspecific stimuli such as stress, exercise, anxiety, sleep, and food ingestion. If thyroid function is normal and prolactin levels are elevated, then radiographic evaluation of the sella turcica is indicated to rule out a pituitary adenoma or empty-sella syndrome. Formal visual-field and extensive pituitary function testing, as well as endocrine consultation, are indicated whenever a pituitary neoplasm is 10 mm or greater in diameter on radiograph or there is clinical or radiographic evidence of suprasellar extension.

Increased FSH levels (generally greater than 40 mIU/ml) indicate ovarian failure. A karyotype performed in hypergonadotropic women under age 30 may identify those with gonadal dysgenesis or mosaicism in whom a Y chromosome is present. Because of the association of autoimmune endocrine disturbances with premature ovarian failure, thyroid antibodies should be measured to rule out thyroiditis, circulating levels of calcium and phosphorus should be determined to eliminate hypoparathyroidism, at least random cortisol should be measured to eliminate the possibility of hypoadrenalism, and circulating glucose levels should be evaluated to rule out diabetes mellitus. Additional screening tests to eliminate autoimmune dysfunction (eg, sedimentation rate, antinuclear antibody, complete blood count with differential, rheumatoid factor, total serum protein, and albumin/globulin ratio) may be indicated as well. Measurement of basal circulating LH, FSH, and estradiol levels on more than one occasion may help in determining whether any functional oocytes remain in the ovary. If the estradiol concentration is greater than 50 pg/ml or if the level of LH is significantly greater than that of FSH (in terms of milliunits per milliliter) in any sample, then viable oocytes probably still exist. Irregular uterine bleeding or withdrawal bleeding in response to exogenous progestin also provides good evidence of endogenous estrogen production, indicating probable follicular activity. Women are occasionally identified who present with intermittent menstruation, signs and symptoms of hypoestrogenism, and hypergonadotropinism. Because pregnancies have occurred in women who had ovarian biopsies devoid of oocytes, ovarian biopsy is not recommended in order to establish this diagnosis.

If basal prolactin, TSH, and FSH levels are within the normal ranges or even low, then further evaluation is dependent on the clinical presentation. Total circulating testosterone levels should be determined in selected circumstances, because not all hyperandrogenic women are hirsute. Although slightly increased levels of testosterone, and perhaps of dehydroepiandrosterone sulfate (DHEA-S) as well, imply PCO, circulating androgen levels are sometimes normal in women with PCO because of alterations in the metabolic clearance rates of androgens and in concentrations of sex hormone-binding globulin. Increased circulating levels of LH (>20 mIU/ml) or an LH/FSH ratio of greater than 2.5 may also aid in diagnosing PCO. Although the use of pelvic ultrasound is increasing, the diagnosis of PCO is not made by this modality. Polycystic ovaries may be normal or increased in size and may or may not appear cystic on ultrasound.

In women with evidence of hirsutism or virilization, both total testosterone and DHEA-S levels should be determined. These measurements are made to eliminate a serious cause for the hirsutism. Total testosterone levels of 200 ng/ml or greater or DHEA-S levels of greater than 7.0 μg/dl should lead to investigation for an androgen-secreting neoplasm, more likely of ovarian origin in the former and of adrenal origin in the latter circumstance (5). There is no need to measure unbound or free circulating testosterone levels, because the appearance of the patient indicates increased androgen activity.

Some estimate of cortisol secretion is indicated in women with amenorrhea who present with any stigmata of Cushing syndrome. The measurement of the basal circulating level of 17-hydroxyprogesterone or of the 24-hour excretion of pregnanetriol in urine is warranted if 21-hydroxylase deficiency is suspected because of virilization rather than feminization occurring precociously or at the expected age of puberty in a phenotypic and genotypic female. Some degree of sexual ambiguity may be present as well.

Therapy

Rational and appropriate management can be instituted only after the etiology of the amenorrhea has been determined.

Abnormalities of the Outflow Tract

Outflow tract obstruction associated with a normal uterus should be treated surgically when diagnosed to prevent tubal damage resulting from endometriosis and adhesions caused by intraabdominal menstrual blood. Adolescent patients who have no vagina should undergo vaginoplasty (McIndoe procedure) or use dilators of increasing size (Frank method) on a daily basis when regular sexual activity is anticipated. Intrauterine synechiae are most easily treated by hysteroscopic lysis, and the use of estrogen may help regeneration of the endometrium; restoration of normal menses occurs in approximately 90% of patients. Of those women achieving a subsequent pregnancy, about 80% have had term deliveries (6).

Hypergonadotropic Amenorrhea (Premature Ovarian Failure)

Women with the diagnosis of hypergonadotropic amenorrhea should have a karyotype performed, since the presence of a Y chromosome on karyotype requires laparotomy and excision of gonadal tissue to prevent the 25% incidence of malignancy that occurs. Genetic evaluation is generally considered unnecessary in women with elevated gonadotropin levels who become amenorrheic after the age of 30, because no gonadal neoplasms have been reported in these older women. Women with associated autoimmune (often endocrine) disorders should be treated appropriately.

Even in affected women with evidence of intermittent ovarian function, hormone replacement therapy is indicated to prevent accelerated bone loss and to treat the intermittent signs and symptoms of hypoestrogenism. Because virtually all women diagnosed with ovarian failure who have conceived do so while on estrogen therapy, affected women should be cautioned to have a pregnancy test if withdrawal bleeding does not occur during any month or if they develop signs and symptoms suggesting pregnancy. Contraception should be used by those women who do not wish pregnancy but who are sexually active, because pregnancy may occur in up to 10% of individuals (7, 8). Although rare pregnancies in women with premature ovarian failure have been reported following ovulation induction with human menopausal gonadotropin (hMG)–human chorionic gonadotropin (hCG), the extremely low likelihood of success should lead the physician to discourage patients from undergoing such therapy. Oocyte donation with embryo transfer now offers the greatest possibility for pregnancy in women desiring fertility.

Hypothalamic Chronic Anovulation

As noted, hypothalamic chronic anovulation is characterized by low to normal levels of gonadotropins, as well as by relative hypoestrogenism. Psychologic counseling or a change in life style may be effective in inducing ovulation in affected individuals (9). For women desiring pregnancy, ovulation may be induced with clomiphene citrate (50–100 mg per day orally for 5 days). If ineffective, individualized treatment with hMG–hCG or with pulsatile gonadotropin-releasing hormone (GnRH) may be necessary. Hypoestrogenic patients who do not desire pregnancy should be treated with exogenous estrogen to prevent osteoporosis. Appropriate therapy is similar to that prescribed for menopausal women (10), except that doses of estrogen twice as great must sometimes be employed to alleviate symptoms in these younger women. Alternatively, low-dose oral contraceptive agents can be administered to sexually active individuals. Patients should be informed that amenorrhea may still be present after therapy is discontinued. Women who decline hormone therapy can be encouraged to have spinal bone density evaluated by periodic computerized tomography (CT) scan or dual-photon absorptiometry to determine whether bone loss is accelerated. Adequate calcium ingestion should also be encouraged in all affected women, regardless of whether hormone therapy is utilized. Available data indicate that hypoestrogenic women must ingest more calcium to achieve a positive calcium balance than do women receiving estrogen.

Pituitary Dysfunction

Following appropriate therapy of any pituitary lesion, ovulation can be induced with hMG–hCG (if the pituitary no longer produces gonadotropins) in women desiring pregnancy. Hormone replacement therapy and calcium supplementation as already outlined are indicated for women not desiring pregnancy.

Hyperprolactinemic Chronic Anovulation

The treatment of hyperprolactinemia is controversial. Therapy with the dopamine agonist bromocriptine (Parlodel) is generally recommended today for individuals with microadenomas (less than 10 mm in diameter) and for those with no radiographic evidence of a pituitary lesion. Normoprolactinemia or return of ovulatory menses can be expected in 80–90% of patients.

The risk of progression from microadenoma to macroadenoma (≥0 mm in diameter) appears to be less than 5%. Thus, the patient with a microadenoma who does not desire fertility has no pressing need for any therapy. Patients in whom observation is the only therapy probably should have bone density measured at periodic intervals. Calcium supplementation should be encouraged in all hyperprolactinemic women. Women without radiologic evidence of a neoplasm may be treated with bromocriptine or observed, depending upon their desire for fertility.

Current therapy for macroadenomas is even more controversial. The surgical "cure" rate for macroadenomas following transsphenoidal resection is only 10–40%. As a result, the majority of endocrinologists favor initial therapy with bromocriptine for at least 6 months after thorough endocrine and visual-field testing (11). Surgery can be performed later in patients who have little response to bromocriptine or cannot tolerate it. Whether surgery should be considered for removal of a shrunken tumor during bromocriptine therapy is not established. Such patients could be continued on bromocriptine indefinitely, treated by surgery or irradiation, or managed with a combination of these approaches. Comparative results permitting rational selection of therapy currently do not exist. When bromocriptine is discontinued, tumor size quickly returns to pretreatment size in most cases. Caution must therefore be used in discontinuing therapy.

Polycystic Ovarian Syndrome

Appropriate therapy demands that potential etiologies of this heterogeneous group of disorders, including neoplasms and systemic illnesses, be excluded (3). Aside from treating infertility, the aims of therapy in women with PCO are to control hirsutism and to prevent endometrial hyperplasia from unopposed estrogen secretion. Therapy must be individualized according to the needs and desires of each patient. The need for endometrial biopsy before initiating any therapy should always be considered because of the increased risk of endometrial hyperplasia and carcinoma in these patients.

In the anovulatory woman with PCO who is not hirsute and does not desire pregnancy, therapy with an intermittent progestin (eg, medroxyprogesterone acetate, 5–10 mg orally for 10–14 days) or oral contraceptive agents (if she is under 40 years of age, does not smoke, and has no other significant risk factors) should be given to reduce the risk of endometrial hyperplasia and carcinoma. The need for effective barrier contraception in sexually active women choosing progestin therapy should be stressed, because ovulation may occur occasionally in women with PCO.

Therapy for hirsute women with PCO who do not desire pregnancy is complex and is similar to that for ovulatory hirsute women (5). Since no pharmacologic agent is ideal or completely effective, the use of physical adjuncts (bleaching, electrolysis, plucking, waxing, and depilation) may be encouraged.

Oral contraceptive agents provide initial therapy for affected women with mild hirsutism and provide protection from endometrial hyperplasia as well. For patients in whom oral contraceptives are contraindicated or not desired, continuous suppression with oral progestin (eg, medroxyprogesterone acetate, 5–10 mg daily) can be utilized. Side effects of progestins include mastodynia, bloating, and depression. The pharmacologic therapy of hirsutism is discussed in detail elsewhere (5).

In women with PCO who desire pregnancy, clomiphene citrate is the first choice with which to induce ovulation because of its simplicity and high success rate (with an ovulation rate of 75% and a pregnancy rate of 35–40%). Other potential methods of ovulation induction include use of hMG–hCG, human purified FSH and hCG, pulsatile GnRH, and ovarian wedge resection or laparoscopic follicular puncture. None of the other approaches to therapy is more successful than clomiphene, although recent data suggest that unresponsive women may ovulate if first suppressed with a GnRH analog (12). Moreover, wedge resections should be performed very rarely today and only in patients in whom all other therapies fail, in whom there is a question of an ovarian tumor because of ovarian size or high circulating androgen levels, or in whom fertility is not an issue because pelvic adhesions may result following surgery. Laparoscopic follicular puncture may represent a surgical alternative with less chance of resulting pelvic adhesions, but available data as to the efficacy of this procedure are scarce (13). Thus, medical therapy remains the therapy of choice for PCO.

REFERENCES

1. Treloar AE, Boynton RE, Benn BG, et al: Variation of the human menstrual cycle through reproductive life. Int J Fertil 12(1):77–126, 1967
2. Marshall WA, Tanner JM: Variations in patterns of pubertal changes in girls. Arch Dis Child 44(235):291–303, 1969
3. Rebar RW: The ovaries. In: Wyngaarden JB, Smith LH Jr (eds): Cecil Textbook of Medicine, 18 ed. Philadelphia, WB Saunders Company, 1988, 1425–1446
4. Miller MM, Rebar RW: Successful treatment of infertility with thyroid replacement in a clinically euthyroid patient with galactorrhea–amenorrhea syndrome. Clin Decis Obstet Gynecol 1(1):1–4, 1987
5. American College of Obstetricians and Gynecologists: Evaluation and Treatment of Hirsute Women (ACOG Technical Bulletin 103). Washington DC, ACOG, 1987
6. Siegler AM, Valle RF: Therapeutic hysteroscopic procedures. Fertil Steril 50(5):685–701, 1988
7. Aiman J, Smentek C: Premature ovarian failure. Obstet Gynecol 66(1):9–14, 1985
8. Rebar RW, Erickson GF, Coulam CB: Premature ovarian failure. In: Gondos B, Riddick DH (eds): Pathology of Infertility. New York, Thieme Medical Publishers Inc, 1987, pp 123–141
9. Yen SSC: Chronic anovulation due to CNS-hypothalamic–pituitary dysfunction. In: Yen SSC, Jaffe RB (eds): Reproductive Endocrinology: Physiology, Pathophysiology and Clinical Management, 2 ed. Philadelphia, WB Saunders Company, 1986, pp 441–545
10. American College of Obstetricians and Gynecologists: Estrogen Replacement Therapy (ACOG Technical Bulletin 93). Washington DC, ACOG, 1986
11. Molitch ME, Elton RL, Blackwell RE, et al: Bromocriptine as primary therapy for prolactin-secreting macroadenomas: Results of a prospective multicenter study. J Clin Endocrinol Metab 60(4):698–705, 1985
12. Filicori M, Campaniello E, Michelacci L, et al: Gonadotropin-releasing hormone (GnRH) analog suppression renders polycystic ovarian disease patients more susceptible to ovulation induction with pulsatile GnRH. J Clin Endocrinol Metab 66(2):327–333, 1988
13. Greenblatt E, Casper RF: Endocrine changes after laparoscopic ovarian cautery in polycystic ovarian syndrome. Am J Obstet Gynecol 156(2):279–285, 1987

This Technical Bulletin was developed under the direction of the Committee on Technical Bulletins of the American College of Obstetricians and Gynecologists as an educational aid to obstetricians and gynecologists. The committee wishes to thank Robert W. Rebar, MD, for his assistance in the development of this bulletin. This Technical Bulletin does not define a standard of care, nor is it intended to dictate an exclusive course of management. It presents recognized methods and techniques of clinical practice for consideration by obstetrician–gynecologists for incorporation into their practices. Variations of practice taking into account the needs of the individual patient, resources, and limitations unique to the institution or type of practice may be appropriate.

Reviewed February 1994

THE AMERICAN COLLEGE OF OBSTETRICIANS AND GYNECOLOGISTS
409 12th Street, SW
Washington, DC 20024-2188

6789/87

ACOG EDUCATIONAL BULLETIN

Number 237, June 1997

Antibiotics and Gynecologic Infections

Various antibiotic agents are used to prevent and treat infection. The causes of gynecologic infection are numerous and fall into two broad categories: those attributable to sexually transmissible organisms and those caused by endogenous vaginal flora. To use antibiotics properly in the prevention and treatment of gynecologic infections, physicians should be aware of the variety of bacteria that constitute the endogenous vaginal flora. Indiscriminate use of antibiotics leads to resistant bacteria and exposes patients to the risk of adverse effects (Table 1).

This Educational Bulletin was developed under the direction of the Committee on Educational Bulletins of the American College of Obstetricians and Gynecologists as an aid to obstetricians and gynecologists. The College wishes to thank David L. Hemsell, MD, for his assistance in the development of this bulletin. This document is not to be construed as establishing a standard of practice or dictating an exclusive course of treatment. Rather, it is intended as an educational tool that presents current information on obstetric–gynecologic issues.

Prophylaxis

Prophylaxis can reduce significantly the incidence of surgical site infection. Prophylactic use of antibiotics is indicated only for those patients who are not infected at the time of an operative or invasive procedure that is associated with a significant risk of infection. Antibiotic prophylaxis reduces the risk of pelvic infection in patients undergoing either abdominal or vaginal hysterectomy. Patients undergoing other procedures also may benefit from antibiotic prophylaxis, although data are limited.

Hysterectomy

The infections most likely to develop in a patient undergoing a hysterectomy are pelvic or cuff cellulitis and pelvic abscess. These infections arise via contamination of the surgical area by the patient's vaginal flora. The vaginal flora can be viewed as part of a larger vaginal ecosystem that consists of many gram-positive and gram-negative, aerobic and anaerobic (facultative and obligate) bacteria.

In a balanced vaginal ecosystem, *Lactobacillus acidophilus* is the dominant bacterium. When the vaginal ecosystem is balanced and the patient is undergoing pelvic surgery, the risk of postoperative pelvic infection is minimal. A single dose of antibiotic, administered prophylactically, usually can prevent infection (1). When the vaginal ecosystem is unbalanced, however, antibiotic prophylaxis is more likely to fail in the patient undergoing surgery. Even three doses of antibiotic may be insufficient to maintain serum and tis-

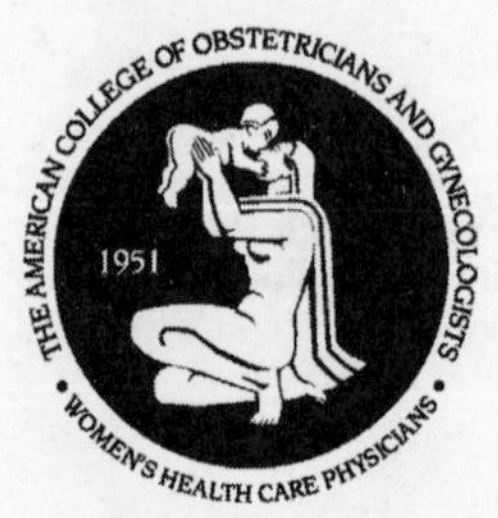

Replaces Number 153, March 1991

Table 1. Potential Adverse Reactions of Specific Antibiotics

Antibiotic	Reaction	Comments
Penicillins	Allergy	Allergy occurs in 10%, incidence lower with oral use than with intravenous use
	Anaphylactic reaction	Occurs in 1:7,000–1:125,000, with mortality in 1:50,000–1:60,000 treatment courses[1]; desensitization can be performed
	Nausea, vomiting, pain, diarrhea	More common with oral administration
	Renal dysfunction, irritability, confusion, hallucination, seizures, coma	Occurs with intravenous administration
	Hemolytic anemia, granulocytopenia, hypokalemia, increased levels of transaminases, sodium overload, interstitial cystitis, renal failure	
Cephalosporins	Allergy	Occurs in up to 3%, more common in patients with known penicillin allergy
	Fever	
	Disulfiramlike reaction after alcohol use	Results from methylthiotetrazole side chain
	Bleeding complications	May be due to effect on vitamin K metabolism
Vancomycin	Toxicity	Rare
	Ototoxicity	
	"Red man" or "red neck" syndrome (pruritic and erythematous rash involving face, neck, and upper torso; hypotension)	Related to histamine release; can be prevented by infusing over 1 hour
	Thrombophlebitis at site of injection	Occurs in approximately 13%
	Hypersensitivity reactions, neutropenia, nephrotoxicity	Patients can be desensitized rapidly if severe hypersensitivity reactions occur[2]
Clindamycin	Pseudomembranous colitis	Most clinically significant; caused by an overgrowth of *Clostridium difficile*; has been reported with a variety of antibiotics
	Nausea, anorexia, vomiting, abnormal liver function, allergic reactions, neuromuscular blockade	
Metronidazole	Nausea, metallic taste, disulfiram reaction	
	Peripheral neuropathy, seizures	More common with higher dosing (>3 g/d)
Fluoroquinolones	Rash	Not uncommon
	Dyspepsia, nausea, vomiting, diarrhea, headache, dizziness, restlessness, insomnia, hallucinations	Occurs in 4–8% of patients
	Seizures, anaphylaxis	May occur but are rare; seizures reported in patients also taking nonsteroidal antiinflammatory agents
	Increases in serum concentration, accentuation of caffeine side effects	In patients also taking theophylline
	Tendon rupture	Reports are increasing[3,4]
Carbapenems	Gastrointestinal disturbances, rashes, fever	Most common side effects
	Seizures	Especially with doses ≥2 g; risk factors are renal insufficiency, history of seizure activity, increased age, and central nervous system lesions
Trimethoprim–sulfamethoxazole	Anorexia, nausea, vomiting, pruritus, erythema	
Macrolides*	Gastrointestinal disturbances, including pain Significant drug interactions possible with warfarin, digoxin, ergotamine, triazolam, some antihistamines (eg, terfenadine), and drugs metabolized by the cytochrome P-450 system	

*Macrolides include erythromycin, clarithromycin, and azithromycin.

[1] Wendell GD Jr, Stark BJ, Jamison RB, Molina RD, Sullivan TJ. Penicillin allergy and desensitization in serious infections during pregnancy. N Engl J Med 1985;312:1229–1232

[2] Amaan ST, Reents T. Severe hypersensitivity reactions to vancomycin can be rapidly desensitized. Infectious Diseases in Clinical Practice 1994;3:366–367

[3] Szarfman A, Chen M, Blum M. More on fluoroquinolone antibiotics and tendon rupture (letter). N Engl J Med 1995;332:193

[4] Pierfitte C, Gillet P, Royer RJ. More on fluoroquinolone antibiotics and tendon rupture (letter). N Engl J Med 1995;332:193

sue levels for an adequate period to overcome the bacterial population (inoculum) (2). If a condition such as bacterial vaginosis is diagnosed preoperatively, it can be treated with either clindamycin (2% vaginal cream) or metronidazole (0.75% intravaginal gel). Following treatment, the patient should be a suitable candidate for antibiotic prophylaxis at the time of surgery.

Antibiotics that can be used for prophylaxis before a hysterectomy are the first-, second-, and third-generation cephalosporins (eg, cefazolin, cefotetan, cefoxitin, ceftizoxime) (Table 2) and the penicillins (eg, ampicillin, mezlocillin, penicillin, piperacillin) (Table 3). The choice of agent should be based on efficacy in the institution and cost. It is important to monitor infection rates within each institution to determine the effectiveness of the prophylactic agent being used and the types of infections that develop. An increasing infection rate would indicate either serious breaks in sterile technique or loss of effectiveness of the prophylactic agent.

A prophylactic agent should be given as a single dose prior to most operative procedures. If the operation lasts 3 hours or longer, or if blood loss exceeds 1,500 mL, a second dose may be beneficial. There are two reasons for using this regimen: (1) during this period, patients have significant urine output, and these antibiotics are actively secreted by the kidney; and (2) if there is a considerable loss of blood volume, the antibiotic concentration would be reduced significantly.

Although antibiotic prophylaxis has significant benefits, there is a disadvantage as well. Multiple cephalosporin doses lead to the emergence of resistant strains of bacteria, especially *Enterococcus faecalis, Escherichia coli,* and *Bacteroides fragilis,* whereas penicillins tend to select for resistant strains of gram-negative facultative bacteria. If the patient who develops a pelvic infection after hysterectomy with prophylaxis fails to respond to initial antibiotic therapy, the presence of a resistant bacterium should be considered. Patients who are allergic to penicillins or cephalosporins can be given clindamycin, doxycycline, or metronidazole.

Table 2. Classification of Cephalosporins

Classification	Products
First generation	Cefazolin Cephalexin Cefadroxil
Second generation	Cefotetan Cefoxitin
Third generation	Cefotaxime Ceftizoxime Ceftriaxone

Table 3. The Penicillin Family

Type of Penicillin	Product
Natural	Penicillin G, penicillin V
Penicillinase-resistant	Cloxacillin, dicloxacillin, oxacillin, methicillin, nafcillin
Aminopenicillins	Ampicillin, amoxicillin, bacampicillin
Carboxypenicillins	Carbenicillin, ticarcillin
Ureidopenicillins	Azlocillin, mezlocillin, piperacillin
Combination with β-lactamases	Amoxicillin + clavulanic acid Ampicillin + sulbactam Piperacillin + tazobactam Ticarcillin + clavulanic acid

Elective Abortion

Patients undergoing elective abortion are at risk for postabortal endometritis. The organisms most likely to cause postabortal endometritis are *Neisseria gonorrhoeae, Chlamydia trachomatis,* and *Streptococcus agalactiae*. Doxycycline, ofloxacin, and ceftriaxone are active against these bacteria and, in a high-risk population, can be used for the prevention of postabortal endometritis. Patients taking ceftriaxone and azithromycin are receiving a therapeutic regimen for cervical infection secondary to *N gonorrhoeae* and *C trachomatis*.

Insertion of an Intrauterine Device

In a prospective, randomized clinical trial, a single oral dose of 200 mg of doxycycline significantly decreased the number of unscheduled postinsertion visits for pain, discharge, or bleeding but not the infection rate, which was 1.3% (1.9% with placebo) (3). One study showed that moving the time of insertion from during menses to within 2 days of predicted ovulation eliminated inflammatory-type reactions (4). This may be taken into consideration in determining the timing of insertion.

Other Procedures

Procedures in which operative site tissue is not exposed to lower genital tract flora (eg, laparoscopy, ovarian cystectomy) probably do not warrant antibiotic prophylaxis. No prospective clinical trials have evaluated prophylaxis in patients undergoing hysterosalpingography, although prophylaxis has been recommended since the late 1970s. In 90% of patients, bacteria were carried with the injected dye first into the endometrial cavity by transvaginal or transcervical transport and then into a previously sterile peritoneal cavity (5). One report showed a significant decrease in febrile morbidity and length of hospital stays associated with antibiotic prophylaxis in patients undergoing suprapubic urethropexy (6). Intraperitoneal irrigation with antibiotics is not recommended for use during infertility-related surgery because it may be associated with crystallization and adhesion formation (7).

Procedures in Women at Risk for Bacterial Endocarditis

As many as 75% of patients who develop endocarditis after undergoing a surgical procedure have preexisting cardiac abnormalities. Patients at highest risk are those who have prosthetic heart valves or other surgically repaired intracardiac lesions with a residual hemodynamic abnormality such as aortic or mitral valve regurgitation or stenosis. Congenital abnormalities such as patent ductus arteriosus, ventricular septal defect, coarctation of the aorta, and cyanotic disease also are associated with increased risk. Mitral valve prolapse with regurgitation poses an intermediate risk. Patients without regurgitation are at a much lower or negligible risk of bacterial endocarditis, as are those who have a pacemaker, coronary disease, arteriosclerotic plaque, or an isolated atrial septal defect. In the absence of infection at the surgical site, endocarditis prophylaxis usually is not warranted for such patients undergoing urethral catheterization, dilation and curettage, removal of an intrauterine device, tubal sterilization, or laparoscopy (8).

Prophylaxis should be given to women at increased risk for endocarditis who undergo hysterectomy or incision and drainage of an abscess or infected area, as well as women who have a urinary tract infection who undergo catheterization or genitourinary tract surgery. The regimen recommended by the American Heart Association for women at increased risk and for those undergoing genitourinary procedures as described above is ampicillin, 2 g intravenously (IV) or intramuscularly (IM), plus gentamicin, 1.5 mg/kg one half hour before the procedure (not to exceed 80 mg), followed by amoxicillin, 1.5 g orally 6 hours after initial dose, or alternatively, a repeat of the initial intravenous or intramuscular ampicillin and gentamicin 8 hours later (8). This combination is effective against those bacteria most likely to cause endocarditis following pelvic surgery. Patients allergic to penicillin should receive vancomycin 1 g IV administered slowly over 1 hour before the operative procedure instead of ampicillin, plus gentamicin 1.5 mg/kg IM or IV (not to exceed 80 mg). This regimen may be repeated 8 hours later. Patients undergoing minor genitourinary procedures may be given amoxicillin, 3 g orally 1 hour before the procedure, and 1.5 g 6 hours later (9).

Bowel Preparation

Mechanical and parenteral bowel preparation should be administered to patients undergoing pelvic surgery if the colon may be involved in the operative procedure. A 3-day mechanical preparation has largely been replaced by the use of chilled oral polyethylene glycol electrolyte solution taken the day before the scheduled surgery at the rate of 1 L/h or until the rectal effluent is clear. Administration should not be continued for more than 4 hours, and the total volume taken should not exceed 4 L of solution. A parenteral dose of the usual hysterectomy prophylactic antibiotic (eg, an agent effective against anaerobic organisms such as cefoxitin [2 g], ceftizoxime [1 g], or cefotetan [1 g]) would normally be given. Ampicillin/sulbactam (3 g) is another good choice because of antienterococcal activity.

Treatment of Postoperative Pelvic Infections

The most common cause of postoperative pelvic infection is the patient's own vaginal flora. Patients undergoing vaginal or abdominal hysterectomy may develop a vaginal cuff hematoma. This hematoma can easily become infected because it is usually colonized by the vaginal flora. Patients who have had a postoperative infection diagnosed should undergo pelvic examination to detect the presence of an abscess or hematoma that may be easily drained. Antibiotic therapy should be instituted empirically.

Empiric therapy for pelvic or cuff cellulitis is usually begun with a single agent with broad antimicrobial activity (Table 4). Regardless of which agent is chosen, studies have shown that the initial broad-spectrum antibiotic will cure the infection in 80–90% of the patients. Failures usually result from the presence of an infected mass, which may require drainage, or resistant gram-positive aerobic or gram-negative facultative anaerobic bacterium. Failure rarely is due to the presence of resistant

Table 4. Some Broad-Spectrum Antibiotics for Treating Postoperative Pelvic Infection

Class	Product
Cephalosporins	Cefotetan, cefoxitin, ceftizoxime
Penicillins	Ampicillin + sulbactam Piperacillin + tazobactam Ticarcillin + clavulanic acid
Carbapenem	Imipenem, meropenem
Combinations	Clindamycin + gentamicin ± ampicillin Metronidazole + gentamicin + ampicillin

obligate anaerobes. It should be considered, however, that an obligate anaerobe is likely to be involved in the infectious process.

In those instances in which a patient fails to improve with a therapeutic course of antibiotic therapy, results of the genital culture may be helpful. If an aerobic or facultative anaerobic bacterium is present, growth should be obvious within 48 hours and the organism can be tested by Gram stain. If the organism is gram positive, it is likely to be an enterococcus, especially if a cephalosporin was used for prophylaxis or treatment or if clindamycin plus gentamicin was used for treatment. None of these regimens provides coverage for enterococci. If the patient currently is receiving a cephalosporin and there is no evidence of bacteremia, ampicillin may be added to the regimen. If the patient is receiving clindamycin and gentamicin, ampicillin should be added. The combination of ampicillin plus gentamicin provides excellent synergistic activity against enterococci and is suitable for bacteremic patients. If the patient is receiving an expanded-spectrum penicillin, an aminoglycoside should be added to provide synergistic activity. However, if the patient is receiving ticarcillin/clavulanic acid, the antibiotic should be changed to metronidazole, aminoglycoside, and ampicillin.

If the bacterial culture reveals the presence of an aerobic gram-negative rod, it is likely to be either *Enterobacter* species or another gram-negative, resistant, facultative bacterium. An aminoglycoside should be added; if gentamicin is being administered, it should be discontinued and amikacin initiated.

When aminoglycosides are given every 8 hours, determinations of aminoglycoside serum trough and peak levels should be obtained in selected circumstances (such as prolonged therapy, obesity, bacteremia, and renal dysfunction). Although ototoxicity or nephrotoxicity still can occur with such monitoring, it should reduce the risk of adverse events and enable the physician to administer an appropriate therapeutic dose. Determination of serum trough and peak levels will prevent subtherapeutic dosing if a gram-negative facultative anaerobic bacterium is the cause of infection. Recently, administering gentamicin every 24 hours intravenously (5–7 mg/kg, infused over 1 hour) to patients with normal renal function has been established because it obviates the need for both peak and trough levels and is less toxic and more effective (10, 11).

Pelvic Inflammatory Disease

Pelvic inflammatory disease can be viewed as a spectrum of disease beginning with cervicitis and progressing to endometritis, with eventual involvement of the fallopian tubes. Progressive infection may result in the development of a pyosalpinx or tuboovarian abscess. The goal of antimicrobial therapy is to prevent damage to the fallopian tube. Once the fallopian tube becomes damaged, the patient is at risk for ectopic pregnancy or infertility. Severe infection may result in end-stage pelvic inflammatory disease and development of a pyosalpinx or tuboovarian abscess that may lead to the patient undergoing a hysterectomy with bilateral salpingo-oophorectomy.

Cervicitis

Patients at risk or who are suspected of having cervicitis should be evaluated and treated for both *N gonorrhoeae* and *C trachomatis,* because the coinfection rate may be as high as 60%. Sexual contacts should be treated. Because of the relatively high rates of coinfection of human immunodeficiency virus (HIV) and hepatitis B virus with gonorrhea and chlamydia, testing for these infections should be considered.

One of the following regimens may be used for treating cervicitis in nonpregnant women (12):

- Ceftriaxone, 125 mg IM, *plus* doxycycline, 100 mg orally twice daily for 7 days
- Ofloxacin, 400 mg orally, *plus* doxycycline, 100 mg orally twice daily for 7 days
- Ceftriaxone, 125 mg IM, *plus* azithromycin, 1 g orally

Endometritis

Patients with endometritis usually present with one of the following complaints:

- Intermenstrual bleeding
- Bleeding at inappropriate times while taking oral contraceptives
- Recent onset of dyspareunia
- Vague, crampy lower abdominal pain

The diagnosis can be established by performing an endometrial biopsy and processing the tissue specimen for both microbiologic and histologic studies. The presence of plasma cells is indicative of the presence of endometritis. The involvement of anaerobic bacteria should be considered at this stage of the infection. Treatment for *N gonorrhoeae* and *C trachomatis* can be instituted prior to obtaining results.

One of the following antibiotic regimens is recommended for the outpatient treatment of endometritis (12):

- Cefoxitin 2 g IM, *plus* probenecid, 1 g orally, *plus* doxycycline, 100 mg orally twice daily for 14 days
- Ceftriaxone 250 mg IM, *plus* doxycycline, 100 mg orally twice daily for 14 days

- Ofloxacin, 400 mg orally twice daily for 14 days, *plus either* clindamycin, 450 mg orally four times a day for 14 days, *or* metronidazole, 500 mg orally twice a day for 14 days

Although no data specifically address the question of antibiotic treatment for endometritis, it is logical to extrapolate regimens from studies concerning the treatment of pelvic inflammatory disease, postoperative pelvic infection, and postpartum endometritis. The concepts and the basic microbial etiology are the same.

Salpingitis

The most common causes of acute salpingitis are *N gonorrhoeae* and *C trachomatis*. When treating acute salpingitis or salpingitis of prolonged duration, however, other bacteria, especially the gram-positive and gram-negative bacteria that commonly inhabit the lower genital tract, should be considered. Other predisposing factors to take into account include the use of invasive instrumentation and the patient's age (eg, if the patient is in the age group in which diverticulitis should be evaluated). If one considers factors other than sexually transmissible infections, nongonococcal, nonchlamydial etiology becomes significant. Therefore, antibiotic regimens also should include coverage for the gram-positive and gram-negative bacteria (13). Outpatient regimens for women with salpingitis are the same as those for women with endometritis.

One of the following antibiotic regimens is recommended for the inpatient treatment of acute and complex pelvic inflammatory disease (12):

- Cefoxitin, 2 g IV every 6 hours, *or* cefotetan, 2 g IV every 12 hours, *plus* doxycycline, 100 mg IV or orally every 12 hours. This regimen should be continued for at least 48 hours after the patient demonstrates substantial clinical improvement, after which doxycycline, 100 mg orally twice daily should be continued for a total of 14 days.
- Clindamycin, 900 mg IV every 8 hours, *plus* a loading dose of gentamicin, 2 mg/kg of body weight IV or IM, followed by a maintenance dose of 1.5 mg/kg every 8 hours. This regimen should be continued for at least 48 hours after the patient demonstrates substantial clinical improvement, then followed with doxycycline, 100 mg orally twice daily or clindamycin, 450 mg orally 4 times a day to complete a total of 14 days of therapy.

Use of the expanded-spectrum penicillins provides excellent coverage against gram-positive and gram-negative bacteria, including penicillinase-producing *N gonorrhoeae*. The presence of a β-lactamase inhibitor (sulbactam, tazobactam, and clavulanic acid) broadens the spectrum of activity of the parent penicillin to include β-lactamase–producing strains of many bacteria. These penicillins have been shown to be active against *C trachomatis*. The combination of clindamycin plus gentamicin is active against gonorrhea and *C trachomatis*.

Most patients with a tuboovarian complex or abscess are treated successfully with antibiotics. Studies have shown that a single agent with a broad spectrum of activity is adequate in treating patients. Successful antimicrobial treatment depends on the stage of development of the abscess and the status of the patient. If the abscess has a thick wall and is multiloculated, surgical intervention may be necessary. This can be provided by interventional radiology. If the patient has signs of sepsis, triple antibiotic therapy (ie, ampicillin plus metronidazole plus gentamicin) is indicated to provide broad-spectrum coverage.

Bacterial Vaginosis

Bacterial vaginosis is an overgrowth of facultative and obligate anaerobic bacteria derived from the patient's own endogenous vaginal flora. Therefore, the intent of treatment is not to eradicate these bacteria but to reduce their numbers and allow for the lactobacilli to become dominant. This, in turn, will restore the pH to the normal range between 3.8 and 4.2 in adult women. Treatment regimens for bacterial vaginosis include the following (12, 14):

- Clindamycin cream, 2%, one full applicator (5 g) intravaginally at bedtime for 7 days *or* 300 mg orally twice daily for 7 days
- Metronidazole gel, 0.75%, one full applicator (5 g) intravaginally twice daily for 5 days *or* 500 mg orally twice daily for 7 days

Lower Urinary Tract Infection

Lower urinary tract infections can be categorized as acute uncomplicated cystitis, acute complicated cystitis, or recurrent cystitis. Dysuria may reflect not only cystitis, but also acute urethritis caused by sexually transmitted pathogens such as *Trichomonas vaginalis, N gonorrhoeae,* and *C trachomatis,* and possibly by nonsexually transmitted bacteria such as *Mycoplasma hominis* and *Ureaplasma urealyticum*. Microscopic pyuria or positive leukocyte esterase or nitrite tests may be considered as presumptive confirmatory tests for bacterial cystitis. Culture is usually unnecessary when treating an adult patient for initial infection. *Escherichia coli* is responsible for approximately 80% and *Staphylococcus saprophyticus* for 5–15% of the cases of acute uncomplicated cystitis. Most risk factors are related to sexual activity or hypoestrogenism. Postmenopausal women not receiving estrogen replacement therapy are at increased risk for urinary tract infection. Estrogen administration appears to prevent recurrent infection (15).

Uncomplicated cystitis can be successfully treated with a 3-day antibiotic regimen, which has been shown to be as efficacious as 7–10-day therapeutic regimens (16). The benefits of short-course therapy are fewer side effects, lower cost, and better compliance. Three-day regimens are more effective than single-dose therapy, which tends to fail because the causative bacterium (typically *Escherichia coli*) is not eradicated from the periurethral, vestibular, and rectal flora (16). The following 3-day regimens should be taken orally every 12 hours:

- Trimethoprim, 100 mg
- Trimethoprim–sulfamethoxazole, 160/800 mg
- Nitrofurantoin, 100 mg

The use of quinolones should be reserved for isolation of a resistant strain that is sensitive only to these agents. Therefore, the quinolones should be used for treating resistant strains, treatment failures, recurrent infection, or infection in patients who are allergic to other antimicrobial agents (17, 18). A 3-day course of trimethoprim–sulfamethoxazole is more effective and less expensive than most 3-day regimens because of its ability to eradicate *Escherichia coli* from the urethra.

Complicated lower urinary tract infections are typically caused by bacteria resistant to a variety of antibiotics or bacteria found in patients with metabolic, anatomic, or functional abnormalities. They also develop in women who have had symptoms of infection for more than a week. *Escherichia coli* is the pathogen most frequently recovered (35%), but other enterobacteriaceae (eg, *Proteus, Klebsiella, Pseudomonas, Enterobacter*) account for a similar percentage, followed by *Enterococcus faecalis* (16%) and *Staphylococcus* species (16%). Patients with complicated cystitis appear to be cured most efficiently by 10–14-day regimens with one of the quinolones.

The cause of recurrent cystitis should be documented by culture. Such patients may be candidates for continuous or postcoital prophylaxis with nitrofurantoin, trimethoprim, trimethoprim–sulfamethoxazole (19), or cephalexin (20). In young patients, the possibility of an anatomic anomaly should be explored.

Upper Urinary Tract Infection

Uncomplicated pyelonephritis is caused predominantly by *Escherichia coli*. Women who do not have evidence of sepsis can be treated on an ambulatory basis with a 14-day course of either trimethoprim–sulfamethoxazole (160/800 mg orally) every 12 hours or an oral quinolone. Women with evidence of sepsis require hospitalization for treatment over 2–3 days with one of the following preparations:

- Trimethoprim–sulfamethoxazole, 160/800 mg IV every 12 hours
- Ceftriaxone, 1–2 g IV every 24 hours
- Gentamicin, 1 mg/kg of body weight IV every 8 hours with or without ampicillin, 1 g every 6 hours
- Ofloxacin *or* ciprofloxacin, 200–400 mg IV every 12 hours

Once the patient can tolerate oral nourishment and there is indication of improvement, oral therapy should be started and continued until a 14-day course has been completed.

Summary

Because most gynecologic procedures are elective, the opportunity exists to identify patients at increased risk for postoperative site infection. Sexually transmissible species and altered vaginal flora can be treated. Operative site infections are usually polymicrobial, and most respond to single-agent, broad-spectrum antibacterial agents. Transvaginal drainage of a cuff abscess or an infected hematoma after hysterectomy, or interventional radiology drainage of a pyosalpinx/tuboovarian abscess may be necessary in addition to antibiotic therapy.

References

1. Mittendorf R, Aronson MP, Berry RE, Williams MA, Kupelnick B, Klickstein A, et al. Avoiding serious infections associated with abdominal hysterectomy: a meta-analysis of antibiotic prophylaxis. Am J Obstet Gynecol 1993;169:1119–1124 (Level III)

2. Shapiro M, Munoz A, Tager IB, Schoenbaum SC, Polk BF. Risk factors for infection at the operative site after abdominal or vaginal hysterectomy. N Engl J Med 1982;307:1661–1666 (Level II-2)

3. Sinei SKA, Schulz KF, Lamptey PR, Grimes DA, Mati JKG, Rosenthal SM, et al. Preventing IUCD-related pelvic infection: the efficacy of prophylactic doxycycline at insertion. Br J Obstet Gynaecol 1990;97:412–419 (Level I)

4. Jovanovic R, Barone CM, Van Natta FC, Congema E. Preventing infection related to insertion of an intrauterine device. J Reprod Med 1988;33:347–352 (Level I)

5. Pyper RJD, Ahmet Z, Houang ET. Bacteriological contamination during laparoscopy with dye injection. Br J Obstet Gynaecol 1988;95:367–371 (Level III)

6. Bhatia NN, Karram MM, Bergman A. Role of antibiotic prophylaxis in retropubic surgery for stress urinary incontinence. Obstet Gynecol 1989;74:637–639 (Level I)

7. Cartwright PS, Pittaway DE, Jones HW III, Entman SS. The use of prophylactic antibiotics in obstetrics and gynecology: a review. Obstet Gynecol Surv 1984;39:537–554 (Level III)

8. Dajani AS, Bisno AL, Chung KJ, Durack DT, Freed M, Gerber MA, et al. Prevention of bacterial endocarditis: recommendations by the American Heart Association. JAMA 1990;264:2919–2922 (Level III)

9. Rust OA, Magann EF. Prophylaxis for subacute bacterial endocarditis in obstetrics and gynecology. Prim Care Update Ob/Gyns 1994;1:183–187 (Level III)

10. Del Priore G, Jackson-Stone M, Shim EK, Garfinkel J, Eichmann MA, Frederiksen MC. A comparison of once-daily and 8-hour gentamicin dosing in the treatment of postpartum endometritis. Obstet Gynecol 1996;87:994–1000 (Level I)

11. Belliveau PP, Nicolau DP, Nightingale CH, Quintiliani R. Once-daily gentamicin: experience in one hundred eighteen patients with postpartum endometritis. J Infect Dis Pharmacotherapy 1995;1:11–18 (Level III)

12. Centers for Disease Control and Prevention. 1993 Sexually transmitted diseases treatment guidelines. MMWR 1993;42 (RR-14):1–102 (Level III)

13. American College of Obstetricians and Gynecologists. Gonorrhea and chlamydial infections. ACOG Technical Bulletin 190. Washington, DC: ACOG, 1994 (Level III)

14. American College of Obstetricians and Gynecologists. Vaginitis. ACOG Technical Bulletin 226. Washington, DC: ACOG, 1996 (Level III)

15. Raz R, Stamm WE. A controlled trial of intravaginal estriol in postmenopausal women with recurrent urinary tract infections. N Engl J Med 1993;329:753–756 (Level I)

16. Hooton TM, Winter C, Tiu F, Stamm WE. Randomized comparative trial and cost analysis of 3-day antimicrobial regimens for treatment of acute cystitis in women. JAMA 1995;273:41–45 (Level II-2)

17. Stamm WE, Hooton TM. Management of urinary tract infections in adults. N Engl J Med 1993;329:1328–1334 (Level III)

18. Kunin CM. Urinary tract infections in females. Clin Infect Dis 1994;18:1–12 (Level III)

19. Stapleton A, Latham RH, Johnson C, Stamm WE. Postcoital antimicrobial prophylaxis for recurrent urinary tract infection: a randomized, double-blind, placebo-controlled trial. JAMA 1990;264:703–706 (Level I)

20. Pfau A, Sacks TG. Effective postcoital quinolone prophylaxis of recurrent urinary tract infections in women. J Urol 1994;152:136–138 (Level II-2)

The references in this bulletin are graded according to the method outlined by the U.S. Preventive Services Task Force:

- I Evidence obtained from at least one properly designed randomized controlled trial
- II-1 Evidence obtained from well-designed controlled trials without randomization
- II-2 Evidence obtained from well-designed cohort or case–control analytic studies, preferably from more than one center or research group
- II-3 Evidence obtained from multiple time series, with or without intervention, or dramatic results in uncontrolled experiments
- III Opinions of respected authorities, based on clinical experience, descriptive studies, or reports of expert committees

Other publications from ACOG:

- **Committee Opinions**, focused updates on emerging areas
- **Practice Patterns**, evidence-based guidelines
- **Criteria Sets**, baseline guidelines for review of diagnostic and management procedures

ISSN 1074-8628

The American College of Obstetricians and Gynecologists
409 12th Street, SW
PO Box 96920
Washington, DC 20090-6920

12345/10987

ACOG EDUCATIONAL BULLETIN

Number 245, March 1998

Antimicrobial Therapy for Obstetric Patients

Antimicrobial agents are among the most frequently used drugs in pregnant patients. In addition to their common uses in nonpregnant individuals, antimicrobial agents may be used to treat infections specific to pregnancy, to treat the fetus, or to provide prophylaxis against adverse obstetric outcomes. Although several antibiotics have the potential for undesirable maternal, fetal, or neonatal effects, these drugs mostly are well tolerated, and relatively few are contraindicated during pregnancy (Table 1). In general, treatment should not be altered substantially because of pregnancy. The use of antibiotics to reduce maternal and neonatal infectious morbidity in patients with premature rupture of membranes has been controversial. The management of this condition, which is an important aspect of antimicrobial therapy in the obstetric patient, is beyond the scope of this document.

This Educational Bulletin was developed under the direction of the Committee on Educational Bulletins of the American College of Obstetricians and Gynecologists as an aid to obstetricians and gynecologists. The College wishes to thank Lindsay S. Alger, MD, for her assistance in the development of this bulletin. This document is not to be construed as establishing a standard of practice or dictating an exclusive course of treatment. Rather, it is intended as an educational tool that presents current information on obstetric–gynecologic issues.

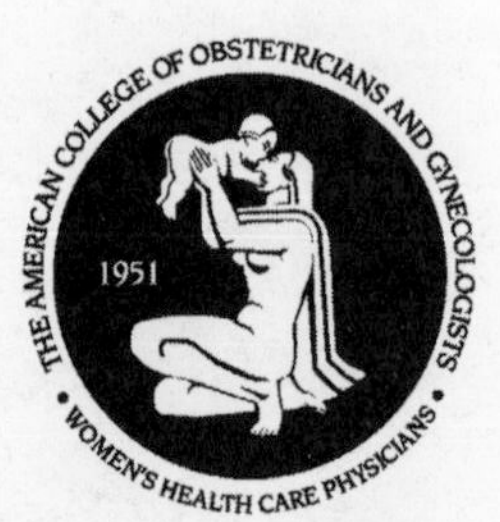

General Guidelines

As the modifications for antimicrobial therapy and the choices of therapies expand, one must consider several principles to gain maximal benefit. In general, the narrowest spectrum of antimicrobial should be chosen so as to limit the emergence of resistant organisms. Although efficacy and safety of a given antimicrobial regimen are paramount, costs should also be considered, including costs to the patient.

Modifications in drug dosage and frequency of administration may be necessary during pregnancy because of the expanded maternal blood volume, increased glomerular filtration rate, increased hepatic metabolism, and sequestration of the drug in the fetal compartment. Overall, maternal drug levels are generally 10–50% lower in late pregnancy and in the immediate postpartum period than in nonpregnant women (1). For agents excreted primarily via the kidney, doses at the upper end of the recommended range are appropriate.

All antibiotics cross the placenta and enter the fetal circulation to some degree. Passage is affected by the duration of pregnancy and the protein-binding capacity of the drug; greater transfer occurs with advancing gestational age and with agents that are minimally protein bound. Thus, ampicillin

Replaces Number 117, June 1988

Table 1. Commonly Used Antibiotics

Agent	Risk Category*	Fetal Effects	Maternal Effects†	Excretion Route	Half Life T 1/2 (h)‡
Considered safe					
Natural penicillins (eg, penicillin G)	B	None known	Allergic	Renal	0.5
Aminopenicillins (eg, ampicillin)	B	None known	Allergic, rash 5–7%	Renal	1
Antistaphylococcal (eg, nafcillin)	B	None known	Allergic	Renal, hepatic	0.5
Antipseudomonal (eg, ticarcillin)	B	None known	Allergic	Renal	1.2
Extended spectrum (eg, piperacillin)	B	None known	Allergic	Renal	1.0
Cephalosporins (1st, 2nd, 3rd, 4th generations)	B	None known	Allergic, bleeding if methylthiotetrazole side chain	Renal, hepatic	0.5–8
Erythromycin (base, stearate, or ethylsuccinate)	B	None known	GI upset, allergic	Hepatic	2–4
Clindamycin	B	None known	Pseudomembranous colitis	Hepatic	2.4
Spectinomycin	B	None known	Allergic	Renal	2.0
Probably safe—use with caution					
Azithromycin	B	None known	Occasional GI symptoms	Hepatic	68
Aztreonam	B	None known	Rashes, elevated serum transaminases	Renal	2
Gentamicin	C	None known, but ototoxicity reported with other aminoglycosides	Increased neuromuscular blockade	Renal	2
Imipenem-cilastatin	C	None known	Allergic, rarely seizures	Renal	1
Metronidazole	B	None known	GI; reversible neuropathy, intolerance to alcohol	Renal	8
Nitrofurantoin	B	None known	Hemolysis if G6PD deficient; neuropathy	Renal	0.3–1
Sulfonamides	B; D at term	Hemolysis if G6PD deficient; avoid at term	Allergic	Renal	Variable
Trimethoprim	C	Folate antagonism, possibly teratogenic; avoid in first trimester	Allergic	Renal	11
Vancomycin	C	None known	Allergic; rarely, hearing loss; hypotension if given too rapidly	Renal	6
Contraindicated					
Tetracyclines	D	Discoloration of decidual teeth; inhibition of bone growth	GI symptoms, hepatotoxicity, renal failure	Renal	8–19
Fluoroquinolones	C	Insufficient information in humans; arthropathy when given to immature animals	Rare	Renal, hepatic	4–8
Streptomycin, kanamycin	D	Eighth cranial nerve damage	Ototoxicity, nephrotoxicity	Renal	2–3
Erythromycin estolate	B	None known	Hepatoxicity	Hepatic	2–4

*Risk categories are as assigned in: Briggs GG, Freeman RK, Yaffe SJ. Drugs in pregnancy and lactation. Baltimore: Williams & Wilkins, 1994.
†GI indicates gastrointestinal; G6PD indicates glucose-6-phosphate dehydrogenase.
‡T 1/2 indicates half-life in nonpregnant individuals. T 1/2 varies with gestational age. Data during pregnancy are generally unavailable.

(20% bound) achieves high levels in the fetus, whereas dicloxacillin sodium (98% bound) does not (1). After the first intravenous dose, most antibiotics peak in concentration in cord blood within 30–60 minutes of the maternal serum peak. However, there is a delay of as much as several hours before significant levels are achieved in amniotic fluid because entry into the fluid depends upon fetal urinary excretion of the antibiotic. Consequently, after fetal death, therapeutic levels cannot be achieved in the amniotic cavity, and chorioamnionitis will be difficult to treat in this setting (2).

All antibiotics are excreted into breast milk to varying degrees, but adverse effects on the neonate rarely are encountered. Relatively small amounts are present in breast milk, and the neonatal intestinal tract absorbs only a portion of the ingested drug. Hence, levels achieved in the neonate usually are very low or negligible. For example, the American Academy of Pediatrics considers tetracycline compatible with breastfeeding because neonatal serum levels are undetectable (3). Theoretical concerns regarding alteration of bowel flora, allergic reactions, and interference with interpretation of neonatal culture results in the breastfed infant have not been substantiated. Certain agents (eg, sulfonamides) may be potentially toxic in specific situations such as prematurity or hereditary glucose-6-phosphate dehydrogenase deficiency; in general, however, breastfeeding need not be discontinued during maternal antibiotic therapy.

Pharmaceutical companies and funding agencies have been reluctant to support research on antibiotic therapy in pregnant women because of concerns regarding adverse fetal effects. For many drugs (eg, azithromycin, acyclovir, and the newer cephalosporins), there are no known or theoretical risks to the fetus, and there are reports of uneventful use during pregnancy. However, controlled trials during pregnancy are of insufficient size or number to determine the safety of these agents with certainty. For other drugs, theoretical risks exist but no untoward effects have been reported in humans. For example, despite many years of use of sulfonamides, there are no reported cases of neonatal kernicterus resulting from prenatal exposure at any gestational age. Use of gentamicin or tobramycin has not resulted in hearing loss in neonates, although this has been reported with kanamycin and streptomycin (4, 5). Similarly, hemolytic anemia in the newborn as a result of in utero exposure to nitrofurantoin has not been reported, nor has an increase in birth defects or subsequent cancer been documented after antenatal metronidazole use (6). It is reasonable to use these antibiotics when they offer specific advantages over alternative agents.

Until more information becomes available, some potentially useful drugs should be avoided during pregnancy because the associated risks are unknown. The entire group of quinolone antibiotics is considered contraindicated in pregnancy because of reports of arthropathy associated with their use in young animals. Although there have been no reports of adverse effects in children in studies conducted in Europe, there are almost no data regarding use in pregnant women.

Information on the newer extended-spectrum penicillins and second-, third-, and fourth-generation cephalosporins is not extensive, but these antibiotics most likely are safe to use in pregnant women. Although there are no situations in which these agents are clearly the drug of choice for therapy, they have several advantages. They may be used as single agents, are generally very well tolerated, cross the placenta well, and have very good reported success rates in the treatment of moderately severe polymicrobial infections. None of these agents has been demonstrated to be more effective than others in its class or to the combination of clindamycin with an aminoglycoside. None of these agents has a sufficient spectrum of activity to warrant use as a single agent in the treatment of some especially serious obstetric infections.

Infections Related to Pregnancy

The most commonly encountered infections specific to pregnancy and the puerperium are usually the result of ascending contamination of the uterine cavity and its contents by the lower genital tract flora. Many female pelvic infections, such as postcesarean endometritis, involve a mixture of aerobic and anaerobic organisms, which may include the following:

- Anaerobes: *Peptostreptococcus species, Prevotella bivia* and *Prevotella disiens, Bacteroides fragilis* group, *Porphyromonas asaccharolyticus, Fusobacterium* species, *Clostridium* species, *Mobiluncus* species
- Aerobes: Groups A, B, and D streptococci, enterococci, *Escherichia coli, Klebsiella* species, *Proteus* species, *Staphylococcus aureus, Gardnerella vaginalis*
- Other: Genital mycoplasmas, *Chlamydia trachomatis, Neisseria gonorrhoeae*

In most situations, antibiotic therapy is initiated empirically on the basis of a clinical diagnosis without the benefit of culture results. Amniotic fluid obtained by amniocentesis or by aspiration from an intrauterine pressure catheter can be sent for Gram stain and aerobic and anaerobic cultures, but patients usually will already have responded to an appropriate empiric regimen before the culture results become available. Anaerobes are notoriously difficult organisms to isolate, and most hospital laboratories are unable to replicate the specialized techniques of research laboratories dedicated to this activity. Hence, anaerobic culture results are frequently disappointing and unreliable. It is also very difficult to obtain an accurate postpartum endometrial specimen for culture without introducing contamination by the lower genital tract, even when using double-lumen techniques. Thus, genital tract cultures are of questionable benefit and may not be cost-effective. However, endometrial and blood cultures may prove useful for directing antibiotic selection for those patients who fail to respond to initial therapy or in whom staphylococci are isolated. Cervical cultures to assess for chlamydial infection or gonorrhea also are appropriate.

Intraamniotic Infection

Intraamniotic infection may complicate both preterm and term deliveries. Prompt intrapartum initiation of broad-spectrum antibiotic therapy for such infections results in better maternal and fetal outcomes than when therapy is delayed until after delivery (7). Neonatal bacteremia and pneumonia as well as maternal febrile morbidity and duration of hospitalization are all reduced. Initiation of treatment, even in advanced labor, should not be delayed by concern that it will mask neonatal infection.

Appropriate antimicrobial agents should not only provide coverage for the wide variety of organisms associated with intraamniotic infection and neonatal infection but also cross the placenta sufficiently well that therapeutic levels can be achieved in the fetus. The most extensively tested regimens are a combination of ampicillin, 2 g intravenously (IV) every 4–6 hours or penicillin, 5 million U every 4–6 hours plus an aminoglycoside such as gentamicin, 1.5 mg/kg IV every 8 hours. Although some recent investigations have supported the use of single daily dosing of aminoglycosides for postpartum infections and infections in gynecologic patients, presently data are insufficient to confirm the safety of the single-dose regimen in pregnant women.

This combination has excellent activity against group B streptococci (GBS) and *E coli,* the two major causes of neonatal sepsis. Bactericidal concentrations of antibiotics in the fetus, membranes, and amniotic fluid can be achieved rapidly after infusion and allow an infected woman to continue labor without adversely affecting neonatal outcome. Although it is desirable to expedite delivery judiciously in the presence of intraamniotic infection, cesarean delivery should be reserved for obstetric indications (8).

Although anaerobes are infrequently isolated from the newborn, they play a prominent role in the pathogenesis of postcesarean endometritis. Thus, for those patients receiving ampicillin and gentamicin who require cesarean delivery, clindamycin (900 mg IV every 8 hours) or metronidazole (500 mg every 12 hours) should be added immediately after cord clamping (9). Alternatively, extended-spectrum cephalosporins and penicillins such as cefotetan, ampicillin/sulbactam, ticarcillin with or without clavulanic acid, piperacillin with or without tazobactam, and ceftizoxime provide good coverage for most organisms causing intraamniotic infection and can be continued postoperatively should a cesarean delivery be necessary. Although there is less information regarding the efficacy of these agents, they have been used successfully as single agents. Therapy should be continued postoperatively until the patient has been afebrile and asymptomatic for approximately 24–48 hours. In contrast, after vaginal delivery most patients will defervesce promptly, and antibiotics may be discontinued shortly thereafter.

Postpartum Endometritis

Postpartum endometritis has a similar pathophysiology to that of chorioamnionitis, involves similar microorganisms, and often is preceded by clinical or subclinical intraamniotic infection. Anaerobic pathogens play a major role in endometritis following cesarean delivery and are isolated from 40–60% of properly collected and cultured specimens.

Prophylaxis

Short-course antibiotic prophylaxis in women undergoing nonelective cesarean delivery reduces both endometritis and wound infections. Although few studies have directly addressed cost savings, the use of prophylactic antibiotics in this setting appears to be cost-effective (10, 11). The preferred agent is a first-generation cephalosporin such as cefazolin, 1 g IV, or ampicillin, 1–2 g IV. Cefazolin has the advantage of a longer half-life and produces fewer allergic reactions than other antibiotics, but it may be more likely to allow the emergence of enterococci in cases of prophylaxis failure. Newer, extended-spectrum cephalosporins are no more effective, are associated with increased recovery of enterococci, and are more expensive (12). Pseudomembranous colitis is more common after cefoxitin administration than after other prophylactic antibiotics (13).

The agent used for prophylaxis should not be used to treat a subsequent infection should one develop. Therefore, extended-spectrum agents should not be used for prophylaxis, but should be reserved for treatment. Antibiotic choices for prophylaxis are limited in patients with documented immediate hypersensitivity reactions to penicillin. A single dose of clindamycin, 900 mg, with gentamicin, 1.5 mg/kg, is a reasonable selection.

For a regimen to be considered prophylaxis rather than treatment, no more than three doses should be given. Single-dose prophylaxis usually is sufficient and, in several studies, has had efficacy similar to that of two- or three-dose regimens. Because prophylaxis is equally effective given before or after cord clamping, it should be initiated immediately after cord clamping unless GBS is present. Routine prophylaxis for elective cesarean delivery is controversial. Prophylaxis is not recommended routinely in low-risk patients because of the concerns about adverse side effects, bacteriologic shifts toward resistant organisms, and relaxation of standard infection-control measures and proper operative technique.

Treatment

Women in whom endometritis develops after vaginal delivery typically respond to the traditional regimen of a penicillin plus an aminoglycoside, despite the somewhat limited anaerobic spectrum of this combination. Women with endometritis following vaginal delivery are much more likely to have infection secondary to a single pathogen, such as *Streptococcus*.

However, after cesarean delivery, more than 25% of patients experiencing endometritis will fail to respond unless an agent that provides good anaerobic coverage is used (14). To date, no regimen has been found to be superior to the standard regimen of gentamicin, 1.5 mg/kg, admixed with clindamycin, 900 mg, in the same intravenous solution, administered every 8 hours. In specific circumstances, such as with septic shock or when enterococcal infection is suspected, the addition of ampicillin may be warranted. Reported cure rates range from 90% to 97%. This three-times-daily dosing schedule also is economical. Once-daily gentamicin dosing has gained favor recently for treating pregnant and nonpregnant individuals because of its efficacy, reduced toxicity, and economy (15). Aztreonam, with its similar antimicrobial spectrum, may be substituted for gentamicin but is much more expensive; it is generally reserved for women with impaired renal function. Gentamicin peak and trough levels usually are not required for patients with normal renal function because eighth cranial nerve damage and nephrotoxicity have not been reported in patients receiving normal doses for less than 1 week. If a patient does not respond after 48–72 hours of therapy, a peak level can be useful in ensuring that adequate serum levels are being achieved. Pseudomembranous colitis may develop infrequently after intravenous administration of clindamycin, but it has been associated with the use of many other antibiotics as well.

Several alternative antibiotic regimens for the treatment of endometritis have been evaluated recently, but most of the trials have been small. The extended-spectrum penicillins and cephalosporins can be used as single agents for endometritis after vaginal or cesarean delivery in patients who are not severely ill. In addition to ease of administration, therapeutic serum levels can be achieved without individualized dosing. Regimens reported as equivalent to gentamicin plus clindamycin include cefotetan, cefoxitin, ceftizoxime, cefotaxime, piperacillin with or without tazobactam, and ampicillin/sulbactam. Most of these agents must be administered 4–6 times per day, but the long half-life of cefotetan permits twice-daily dosing. Cefotetan is therapeutically equivalent to cefoxitin. The carbapenem combination of imipenem and cilastatin also is effective. This drug has the broadest spectrum of in vitro activity of any β-lactam antibiotic; however, because of this unusual spectrum, it should be reserved for special situations involving resistant organisms or im-munocompromised women. Intravenous therapy of all regimens should be continued until the patient has been afebrile and asymptomatic for 24–48 hours (16). This completes therapy, and the patient may then be discharged without oral antibiotics unless she has had a staphylococcal bacteremia. This condition requires an extended course of intravenous and oral therapy with an agent providing specific antistaphylococcal activity.

Approximately 10% of patients will not be cured with initial therapy. Women who do not respond within 48–72 hours often have another source of fever, such as a wound infection, drug-induced fever, septic thrombophlebitis, infected bladder-flap hematoma, or a nongenital site of infection. However, in about 20% of treatment failures, the lack of response is due to resistant organisms. For example, neither the cephalosporins nor the combination of gentamicin with clindamycin is effective against enterococci, a genus that is particularly likely to emerge in patients in whom cephalosporin prophylaxis failed at cesarean delivery. Most women from whom enterococci are isolated will respond to regimens that do not provide specific coverage for this organism (17); however, when gentamicin plus clindamycin is ineffective, the clinician should consider adding ampicillin or penicillin to provide synergy with gentamicin against the enterococcus. The substitution of metronidazole for clindamycin may be effective against resistant gram-negative anaerobes. If an abscess is suspected, aztreonam may be substituted for gentamicin because it remains active in an anaerobic environment, unlike the aminoglycosides (18). Should an extended-spectrum penicillin or cephalosporin fail as initial therapy, the regimen may be changed to the combination of ampicillin or penicillin plus gentamicin, and clindamycin (or metronidazole) (19).

Bacterial Endocarditis

Endocarditis, a potentially life-threatening disease, may develop in individuals with underlying structural cardiac defects that have been exposed to bacteremia. The likelihood that endocarditis will develop following a procedure is related to the degree of risk associated with the patient's underlying cardiac condition, the type of bacteria involved, and the risk of bacteremia as a result of the procedure. Women with a history of endocarditis or who have prosthetic heart valves, complex cyanotic congenital heart disease, or surgically constructed systemic pulmonary shunts are at high risk. Examples of patients at moderate risk include those with uncorrected ventricular septal defects, coarctation of the aorta, hypertrophic cardiomyopathy, and mitral valve prolapse if associated with mitral regurgitation (demonstrated by Doppler or a murmur).

Infrequently, bacteremia follows uncomplicated vaginal delivery; documented cases of endocarditis are rare. Therefore, the American Heart Association does not recommend prophylaxis for cesarean delivery or normal vaginal delivery with the possible exception of high-risk patients for whom it is optional (20). If this option is selected in the delivery setting, prophylaxis should be directed primarily against enterococci. The recommended regimen is ampicillin, 2.0 g intramuscularly (IM) or IV plus gentamicin, 1.5 mg/kg (not to exceed 120 mg) within 30 minutes of delivery, followed in 6 hours by ampicillin, 1.0 g IM or IV, or amoxicillin, 1.0 g orally. If the patient is allergic to ampicillin, vancomycin (1.0 g IV over 1–2 hours completed within 30 minutes of delivery) is substituted and no postdelivery dose is given. Patients who are febrile at delivery and, therefore, already potentially bacteremic, should receive prophylaxis.

Common Infections in Obstetric Patients

Sexually Transmissible Infections

Chlamydia

The most common sexually transmitted bacterial organism in the United States is *C trachomatis*. It has been associated with preterm delivery and preterm premature rupture of membranes. Pregnant patients may be treated with one of the following:

- Erythromycin base, 500 mg, or erythromycin ethylsuccinate, 800 mg orally four times daily for 7 days (if poorly tolerated, the dose may be halved and given over 14 days)
- Amoxicillin, 500 mg orally three times daily for 7 days
- Azithromycin, 1 g orally as one dose

Azithromycin, with its prolonged tissue half-life of 2–4 days, is the only agent that can successfully treat chlamydia in a single dose. Although the safety and efficacy of azithromycin in pregnancy are not as well established as those of the other regimens, theoretically this agent, like other macrolides, should be safe (21). In addition, it has fewer side effects, compliance can be ensured, and retesting for cure is not required. As of the date of publication, the 1-g powder formulation of azithromycin is about one third of the cost of the capsule formulation.

Gonorrhea

Current treatment guidelines for *N gonorrhoeae* reflect the increasing frequency of resistant strains and the excellent therapeutic reserve of low doses of ceftriaxone. Recommended treatment regimens include one of the following:

- Ceftriaxone, 125 mg IM in a single dose
- Cefixime, 400 mg orally in a single dose
- Spectinomycin, 2 g IM in a single dose (for patients who cannot tolerate a cephalosporin)

Ceftriaxone is effective for treatment of gonorrhea at all sites, including the pharynx. Because cefixime is given orally, it may result in improved compliance, particularly when treating adolescent partners. Unlike former treatments, none of these regimens requires probenecid. In addition, a treatment regimen for chlamydia as outlined previously should be administered because of the likelihood of coinfection.

Syphilis

Pregnant patients with syphilis should be treated with the penicillin regimen appropriate for the applicable stage of syphilis in nonpregnant individuals. Thus, for cases of early syphilis, benzathine penicillin G, 2.4 million U, is administered IM in a single dose. Some experts recommend a second dose 1 week after the initial dose, particularly for women in the third trimester or those who have secondary syphilis. For late-stage syphilis (more than 1 year of duration), treatment is 2.4 million U IM once a week for 3 successive weeks. Neurosyphilis should be treated according to the guidelines of the Centers for Disease Control and Prevention. There are no satisfactory alternatives to penicillin that will permit safe and effective treatment of the fetus as well. Women who are allergic to penicillin (preferably confirmed by skin testing) can be treated with penicillin after oral desensitization where appropriate resuscitation and backup facilities are available (Table 2). A single oral test dose is sufficient before subsequent injections if they are repeated within 1–2 weeks of the initial desensitization (22).

Vaginal Trichomoniasis

Oral metronidazole is the only approved treatment for *Trichomonas vaginalis*. Recent evidence of a possible relationship between vaginal trichomoniasis and adverse pregnancy outcomes (premature rupture of membranes and preterm delivery) has led to more aggressive diagnosis and treatment in pregnancy. Metronidazole is not recommended in the first trimester of pregnancy; after the first trimester, patients may be treated with 2 g orally in a single dose (23).

Bacterial Vaginosis

Bacterial vaginosis, although not strictly classified as a sexually transmissible infection, is the most common cause of vaginal discharge or malodor. Historically, treatment during pregnancy has been reserved for those women who are symptomatic. However, recent studies

Table 2. Oral-Desensitization Protocol Used in 13 Pregnant Women with Allergies to Penicillin*

Dose†	Penicillin V Suspension (U/mL)	Amount‡ mL	Amount‡ U	Cumulative Dose (U)
1	1,000	0.1	100	100
2	1,000	0.2	200	300
3	1,000	0.4	400	700
4	1,000	0.8	800	1,500
5	1,000	1.6	1,600	3,100
6	1,000	3.2	3,200	6,300
7	1,000	6.4	6,400	12,700
8	10,000	1.2	12,000	24,700
9	10,000	2.4	24,000	48,700
10	10,000	4.8	48,000	96,700
11	80,000	1.0	80,000	176,700
12	80,000	2.0	160,000	336,700
13	80,000	4.0	320,000	656,700
14	80,000	8.0	640,000	1,296,700

*Observation period: 30 minutes before parenteral administration of penicillin.

†Interval between doses, 15 minutes; elapsed time, 3 hours and 45 minutes; cumulative dose, 1.3 million U.

‡The specific amount of drug was diluted in approximately 30 mL of water and then given orally.

Modified from Wendel GD Jr, Stark BJ, Jamison RB, Molina RD, Sullivan TJ. Penicillin allergy and desensitization in serious infections during pregnancy. N Engl J Med 1985;312: 1230.

suggest that treatment of bacterial vaginosis may reduce rates of preterm delivery for certain high-risk women. In a randomized trial, women with a history of preterm delivery or a prepregnancy weight of less than 50 kg were screened for bacterial vaginosis, then treated with oral metronidazole and erythromycin. There was a significant decrease in preterm birth in those women who tested positive for bacterial vaginosis and were treated in the second trimester. However, there is no evidence to suggest that screening and treatment of bacterial vaginosis in all women (including those without the aforementioned risk factors) is beneficial to prevent adverse pregnancy outcome (24).

In the first trimester, symptomatic bacterial vaginosis can be treated with clindamycin cream, 2%, one full applicator (5 g) intravaginally at bedtime for 7 days or 300 mg orally twice daily for 7 days; however, clindamycin cream is recommended instead of the oral regimen because it limits fetal exposure to the medication. After the first trimester, metronidazole, 250 mg orally three times daily or 500 mg orally twice daily for 7 days can be used for treatment (23). The three times daily dosing minimizes exposure to the fetus but may result in poorer compliance. Alternatively, metronidazole, 2 g orally in a single dose or clindamycin, 300 mg orally twice daily for 7 days can be used. Although intravaginal therapies are effective in the treatment of bacterial vaginosis, they do not reduce preterm delivery (25).

Herpes

Little progress has been made in knowledge of the use of acyclovir for herpes infection in pregnancy. Orally administered acyclovir crosses the placenta well, with a mean maternal/infant plasma ratio at term of 1.3:1 (26). Prospective data from more than 850 women (578 first-trimester exposures) show no increase in spontaneous abortions or birth defects. There also are no reports of adverse effects from using acyclovir in preterm neonates. However, information on long-term effects is lacking. Pregnant women with primary genital herpes (particularly in the third trimester) have a high rate of major complications, including premature labor, intrauterine growth restriction, congenital infection, and persistent genital viral shedding later in pregnancy. Use of acyclovir for primary infection must be decided upon on an individual risk-to-benefit basis after appropriately counseling the patient. Rarely, infection may become disseminated and life threatening; in this situation, acyclovir, 5–10 mg/kg of body weight IV every 8 hours for 5–7 days, or until clinical resolution, is clearly indicated. Oral acyclovir suppression has been used successfully near term to prevent the need for a cesarean delivery after a first episode of genital herpes (27). Currently, there is insufficient information to make recommendations regarding the use of acyclovir for recurrent episodes or for suppression throughout pregnancy. Use has generally been avoided, but in certain situations such as frequent recurrences or when genital herpes recurs in the presence of ruptured membranes remote from term, acyclovir therapy may be appropriate with informed consent.

Urinary Tract Infections

Infection of the urinary tract is the most common medical complication of pregnancy. Although infection is not more frequent than in nonpregnant women, it is more likely to become symptomatic and progress to pyelonephritis as a result of anatomic and physiologic changes occurring in pregnancy. Of additional concern is the association of low birth weight and preterm delivery with untreated bacteriuria, confirmed by a meta-analysis of published reports (28). In this analysis, eradication of bacteriuria improved outcomes.

Asymptomatic bacteriuria occurs in 2–9% of pregnant women. Treatment usually is considered when 25,000–100,000 colony-forming units per milliliter of a single pathogenic organism are found in a clean-catch, midstream urine specimen. All pregnant women should be screened for asymptomatic bacteriuria early in pregnancy, and infected women should be treated. The outcome of positive test results obtained by the dipstick technique should be confirmed by cultures.

Escherichia coli is the organism isolated in more than 80% of cases. Other aerobic, gram-negative rods (eg, *Klebsiella–Enterobacter* and *Proteus* species) and gram-positive cocci (mainly enterococci and GBS) also may be found. Antibiotic sensitivity test results normally will be available to the physician at the time of diagnosis, and an appropriate oral agent may be selected (avoiding the tetracycline and quinolone groups) (Table 3).

Single-dose treatment has been studied in pregnant patients and is successful in most, but overall, it is associated with a higher failure rate than when longer courses are used (29). A 3-day course of antibiotics should be sufficient to treat an otherwise healthy woman (30). It is not the duration of therapy that is of primary importance, but the documentation of successful treatment by obtaining a follow-up culture approximately 10 days after completion of therapy. A positive repeat culture showing the same organism will necessitate a longer subsequent course of antibiotics and possibly long-term suppressive therapy.

Women with symptomatic cystitis and no evidence of upper urinary tract disease also can be treated with one of the 3-day oral antibiotic regimens in Table 3, with appropriate follow-up. In this situation, treatment often is initiated before culture results are available, but the same organisms as found in asymptomatic bacteriuria are involved. Because *E coli* is again the most commonly isolated microorganism and is resistant to ampicillin in more than one third of isolates, ampicillin or amoxicillin should not be used empirically.

Table 3. Antimicrobial Treatment of Asymptomatic Bacteriuria or Acute Cystitis

Agent	Dosage*
Trimethoprim–sulfamethoxazole	160/180 mg, po, every 12 h for 3 d
Nitrofurantoin macrocrystals	50–100 mg, po, every 6 h for 3 d
Nitrofurantoin monohydrate/macrocrystals	100 mg, po, every 12 h for 3 d
Cephalexin	250–500 mg, po, every 6 h for 3 d
If antibiotic sensitivities are available:	
Ampicillin	250–500 mg, po, every 6 h for 3 d
Amoxicillin	250–500 mg, po, every 8 h for 3 d
Trimethoprim	200 mg, po, every 12 h for 3 d
Sulfisoxazole	2 g loading dose, then 1 g every 6 h for 3 d

*po indicates by mouth.

Acute pyelonephritis traditionally has been treated with hospitalization and intravenous antibiotics. Effective regimens include:

- Ampicillin 1–2 g every 6 hours, plus gentamicin, 1.5 mg/kg every 8 hours
- Ceftriaxone, 1–2 g every 24 hours; *or*
- Trimethoprim–sulfamethoxazole, 160/800 mg every 12 hours

Gentamicin also may be used alone in most women. However, in seriously ill patients, it is preferable to initiate therapy with both ampicillin and gentamicin; once culture results are available, ampicillin can be discontinued if it is not required. Trimethoprim–sulfamethoxazole should not be used empirically as a single agent in geographic areas where *E coli* resistance is common. Aztreonam and imipenem–cilastatin should be reserved for resistant pathogens or for women who do not tolerate first-line agents. Intravenous therapy usually is continued until the patient is afebrile and symptomatically improved, followed by outpatient oral antibiotics to complete 10 days of therapy.

Nonpregnant patients with pyelonephritis have been treated successfully as outpatients with various combinations of intravenous, intramuscular, and oral antibiotic therapies (31, 32). This reduces cost and is less disruptive to the patient and her family. Recent studies have supported a similar approach in pregnant populations, but information is not extensive (33–35). Some form of home health care should be provided for women treated as outpatients because the complications of acute pyelonephritis during pregnancy may be severe and life threatening. Women who have signs and symptoms of sepsis should be hospitalized.

Women treated for pyelonephritis require antibiotic suppression and periodic rescreening for the remainder of pregnancy to prevent a recurrence. In addition, all other women treated for urinary tract infections should have periodic rescreening for infection with cultures or urine dipstick for nitrites or leukocyte esterase. If infection recurs, patients should be retreated and then placed on chronic suppression. Nitrofurantoin, 50–100 mg each night before bedtime, is effective and, because of its unusual mechanism of action, does not promote the development of resistant organisms. Alternatively, sulfisoxazole, 500 mg at bedtime, may be used.

Summary

Antimicrobial agents can be of great benefit to both the pregnant woman and her fetus. As the list of antimicrobial agents and options for treatment continue to broaden, one must remember that appropriate use of these drugs requires special knowledge of adverse fetal effects, altered kinetics, and the causes of various infections. Of equal importance is the knowledge of when antibiotics should not be used. A useful resource for the expanding repertoire of antimicrobial agents and current treatment options is the Centers for Disease Control and Prevention web site at www.cdc.gov.

References

1. Chow AW, Jewesson PJ. Pharmacokinetics and safety of antimicrobial agents during pregnancy. Rev Infect Dis 1985;7:287–313
2. Bray RE, Boe RW, Johnson WL. Transfer of ampicillin into fetus and amniotic fluid from maternal plasma in late pregnancy. Am J Obstet Gynecol 1966;96:938–942
3. Committee on Drugs, American Academy of Pediatrics. The transfer of drugs and other chemicals into human milk. Pediatrics 1994;93:137–150
4. Donald PR, Sellars SL. Streptomycin ototoxicity in the unborn child. S Afr Med J 1981;60:316–318
5. Jones HC. Intrauterine ototoxicity: a case report and review of literature. J Natl Med Assoc 1973;65:201–203
6. Burtin P, Taddio A, Ariburnu O, Einarson TR, Koren G. Safety of metronidazole in pregnancy: a metaanalysis. Am J Obstet Gynecol 1995;172:525–529
7. Gibbs RS, Dinsmoor MJ, Newton ER, Ramamurthy RS. A randomized trial of intrapartum versus immediate postpartum treatment of women with intra-amniotic infection. Obstet Gynecol 1988;72:823–828
8. Hauth JC, Gilstrap LC, Hankins GDV, Connor KD. Term maternal and neonatal complications of acute chorioamnionitis. Obstet Gynecol 1985;66:59–62
9. Earl P, Sisson PR, Ingham HR. Twelve-hourly dosage schedule for oral and intravenous metronidazole. J Antimicrob Chemother 1989;23:619–621
10. Ford LC, Hammil HA, Lebherz TB. Cost-effective use of antibiotic prophylaxis for cesarean section. Am J Obstet Gynecol 1987;157:506–510
11. Iams JD, Chawla A. Patient costs in the prevention and treatment of post–cesarean section infection. Am J Obstet Gynecol 1984;149:363–366
12. Carlson C, Duff P. Antibiotic prophylaxis for cesarean delivery: is an extended-spectrum agent necessary? Obstet Gynecol 1990;76:343–346
13. Block BS, Mercer LJ, Ismail MA, Moawad AH. Clostridium dificile-associated diarrhea follows perioperative prophylaxis with cefoxitin. Am J Obstet Gynecol 1985;153:835–838
14. diZerega G, Yonekura L, Roy S, Nakamura RM, Ledger WJ. A comparison of clindamycin-gentamicin and penicillin-gentamicin in the treatment of post-cesarean section endometritis. Am J Obstet Gynecol 1979;134:238–242
15. Del Priore G, Jackson-Stone M, Shim EK, Garfinkel J, Eichmann MA, Frederiksen MC. A comparison of once-daily and 8-hour gentamicin dosing in the treatment of postpartum endometritis. Obstet Gynecol 1996;87: 994–1000
16. Dinsmoor MJ, Newton ER, Gibbs RS. A randomized, double-blind, placebo-controlled trial of oral antibiotic therapy following intravenous antibiotic therapy for postpartum endometritis. Obstet Gynecol 1991;77:60–62
17. Walmer D, Walmer KR, Gibbs RS. Enterococci in post-cesarean endometritis. Obstet Gynecol 1988;71:159–162
18. Stutman HR. Clinical experience with aztreonam. Pediatr Infect Dis J 1989;8:S109–S112
19. Duff P. Antibiotic selection for infections in obstetric patients. Semin Perinatol 1993;17:367–378
20. Dajani AS, Taubert KA, Wilson W, Bolger AF, Bayer A, Ferrieri P, et al. Prevention of bacterial endocarditis: recommendations by the American Heart Association. JAMA 1997;277:1794–1801
21. Bush MR, Rosa C. Azithromycin and erythromycin in the treatment of cervical chlamydial infection during pregnancy. Obstet Gynecol 1994;84:61–63
22. Wendel GD Jr, Stark BJ, Jamison RB, Molina RD, Sullivan TJ. Penicillin allergy and desensitization in serious infections during pregnancy. N Engl J Med 1985;312;1229–1232
23. Centers for Disease Control and Prevention. 1998 Guidelines for treatment of sexually transmitted diseases. MMWR 1998;47(RR-1):1–116
24. Hauth JC, Goldenberg RL, Andrews WW, DuBard MB, Copper RL. Reduced incidence of preterm delivery with metronidazole and erythromycin in women with bacterial vaginosis. N Engl J Med 1995;333:1732–1736
25. Joesoef MR, Hillier SL, Wiknjosastro G, Sumampouw H, Linnan M, Norojono W, et al. Intravaginal clindamycin treatment for bacterial vaginosis: effects on preterm delivery and low birth weight. Am J Obstet Gynecol 1995;173:1527–1531
26. Frenkel LM, Brown ZA, Bryson YJ, Corey L, Unadkat JD, Hensleigh PA, et al. Pharmacokinetics of acyclovir in the term human pregnancy and neonate. Am J Obstet Gynecol 1991;164:569–576
27. Scott LL, Sanchez PJ, Jackson GL, Zeray F, Wendel G Jr. Acyclovir suppression to prevent cesarean delivery after first-episode genital herpes. Obstet Gynecol 1996;87:69–73
28. Romero R, Oyarzun E, Mazor M, Sirtori M, Hobbins JC, Bracken M. Meta-analysis of the relationship between asymptomatic bacteriuria and preterm delivery/low birth weight. Obstet Gynecol 1989;73:576–582
29. Powers RD. New directions in the diagnosis and therapy of urinary tract infections. Am J Obstet Gynecol 1991;164:1387–1389
30. Stamm WE, Hooton TM. Management of urinary tract infections in adults. N Engl J Med 1993;329:1328–1334
31. Pinson AG, Philbrick JT, Lindbeck GH, Schorling JB. Oral antibiotic therapy for acute pyelonephritis: a methodologic review of the literature. Gen Intern Med 1992;7:544–553
32. Safrin S, Siegel D, Black D. Pyelonephritis in adult women: inpatient versus outpatient therapy. Am J Med 1988;85:793–798
33. Angel JL, O'Brien WF, Finan MA, Morales WJ, Lake M, Knuppel RA. Acute pyelonephritis in pregnancy: a prospective study of oral versus intravenous antibiotic therapy. Obstet Gynecol 1990;76:28–32

34. Millar LK, Wing DA, Paul RH, Grimes DA. Outpatient treatment of pyelonephritis in pregnancy: a randomized controlled trial. Obstet Gynecol 1995;86:560–564

35. Sanchez-Ramos L, McAlpine KJ, Adair D, Kaunitz AM, Delke I, Briones DK. Pyelonephritis in pregnancy: once-a-day ceftiaxone versus multiple doses of cefazolin. Am J Obstet Gynecol 1995;172:129–133

ISSN 1074-8628

The American College of Obstetricians and Gynecologists
409 12th Street, SW
PO Box 96920
Washington, DC 20090-6920

12345/21098

ACOG EDUCATIONAL BULLETIN

Number 244, February 1998

Antiphospholipid Syndrome

Antiphospholipid syndrome is an autoimmune condition characterized by the presence of certain clinical features and moderate-to-high levels of circulating antiphospholipid antibodies. The most specific clinical features are thrombotic events (venous or arterial), autoimmune thrombocytopenia, and fetal loss (Table 1) (1–3). Other clinical features include transient ischemic attacks, amaurosis fugax, Coombs-positive hemolytic anemia, and a dermatologic condition known as livedo reticularis. "Primary" antiphospholipid syndrome occurs in patients with no other recognized autoimmune disease and is probably the most common presentation of antiphospholipid syndrome recognized by obstetrician–gynecologists. "Secondary" antiphospholipid syndrome is diagnosed when the patient has another underlying autoimmune disease such as systemic lupus erythematosus (SLE). Antiphospholipid syndrome may be seen in children, adolescents, and adults and is more prevalent in females than males.

This Educational Bulletin was developed under the direction of the Committee on Educational Bulletins of the American College of Obstetricians and Gynecologists as an aid to obstetricians and gynecologists. The College wishes to thank D. Ware Branch, Jr, MD, and Robert M. Silver, MD, for their assistance in the development of this bulletin. This document is not to be construed as establishing a standard of practice or dictating an exclusive course of treatment. Rather, it is intended as an educational tool that presents current information on obstetric–gynecologic issues.

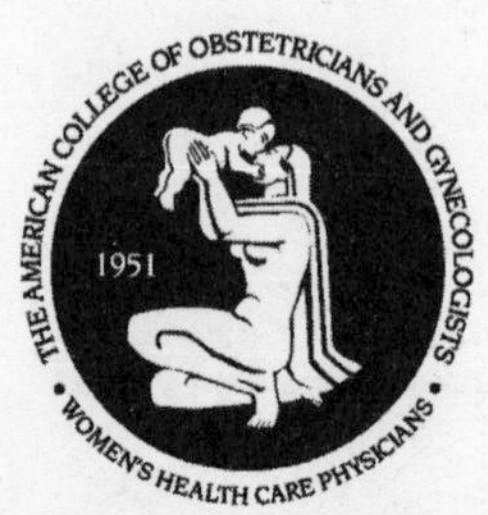

Antiphospholipid Antibodies

Two antiphospholipid antibodies for which assays are widely available are lupus anticoagulant and anticardiolipin antibodies. The lupus anticoagulant antibody was first described in 1952 (4) and was subsequently named "lupus anticoagulant" because it was initially recognized in patients with SLE and because it prolongs clotting in vitro. Paradoxically, lupus anticoagulant (and anticardiolipin) is associated with clinical thrombosis, not bleeding. Anticardiolipin antibodies were first identified as autoantibodies in 1983 (5) using a solid phase immunoassay with the phospholipid cardiolipin as the antigen. In the assays for both lupus anticoagulant and anticardiolipin antibodies, the antiphospholipid autoantibodies bind moieties on negatively charged phospholipids or moieties formed by the interaction of negatively charged phospholipids with other lipids, phospholipids, or proteins. Some investigators have found that lupus anticoagulant and anticardiolipin antibodies may be separated in the laboratory, suggesting that they are different

Table 1. Clinical and Laboratory Criteria for the Diagnosis of Antiphospholipid Syndrome*

Criterion	Definition
Clinical	
Fetal loss	Three or more spontaneous abortions with no more than one live birth, or unexplained second- or third-trimester fetal death
Thrombosis	Unexplained venous or arterial thrombosis, including stroke and arterial insufficiency due to arterial thrombosis
Autoimmune thrombocytopenia	Other causes of thrombocytopenia excluded
Other features	Otherwise unexplained transient ischemic attacks or amaurosis fugax, livedo reticularis, Coombs-positive hemolytic anemia, chorea, and chorea gravidarum
Laboratory	
Lupus anticoagulant	Detected by phospholipid-dependent clotting assays, without correction with normal plasma, and confirmed by demonstration of phospholipid dependency
Anticardiolipin antibodies	IgG isotype >15–20 GPL units (medium-to-high positive) detected in standardized assay using standard serum calibrators†

*Antiphospholipid syndrome is diagnosed when the patient has (1) at least one clinical feature *and* (2) lupus anticoagulant or medium-to-high positive immunoglobulin G anticardiolipin antibodies or both. Because antiphospholipid antibodies may appear transiently following infection, positive tests should be confirmed 8 or more weeks after initial testing.

†IgM and IgA isotypes are of uncertain significance and should not be used to diagnose antiphospholipid syndrome unless patient also has lupus anticoagulant or IgG anticardiolipin antibodies (GPL units).

immunoglobulins (6–8). Others believe that these antibodies are the same immunoglobulins being detected by different methods (9). Despite this controversy, lupus anticoagulant and anticardiolipin antibodies are associated with the same set of clinical problems and are therefore likely members of the same "family" of autoantibodies. Most patients with antiphospholipid syndrome have lupus anticoagulant and anticardiolipin antibodies. However, some patients with antiphospholipid syndrome have either lupus anticoagulant or anticardiolipin antibodies, but not both. Thus, tests for both antibodies should be performed to confirm the diagnosis of antiphospholipid syndrome.

The laboratory testing for antiphospholipid antibodies remains somewhat confusing for clinicians. Part of the difficulty is that some laboratories offering antiphospholipid antibody testing use assays that are not standardized or operate with inadequate quality control analysis of results (10, 11). Underlying this problem is the fact that reliable testing for antiphospholipid antibodies is difficult. Whenever possible, clinicians should identify and use a reliable laboratory with a special interest in antiphospholipid antibody testing.

Tests for Antiphospholipid Antibodies

Indications for testing for antiphospholipid antibodies are shown in the box. Only individuals with these clinical features should be tested because the presence of antiphospholipid antibodies in the absence of these features is of uncertain significance. In contrast to the reporting of anticardiolipin antibodies, which involves accepted international units, lupus anticoagulant is considered present or absent and is not quantified by current methodology.

Indications for Testing for Antiphospholipid Antibodies

Obstetric
- Otherwise unexplained fetal death or stillbirth
- Recurrent pregnancy loss (three or more spontaneous abortions with no more than one live birth, or unexplained second- or third-trimester fetal death)
- Severe pregnancy-induced hypertension <34 weeks of gestation
- Severe fetal growth restriction or other evidence of uteroplacental insufficiency in the second or early third trimester

Medical
- Nontraumatic thrombosis or thromboembolism (venous or arterial)
- Stroke, especially in individuals <50–55 years of age
- Autoimmune thrombocytopenia
- Transient ischemic attacks or amaurosis fugax, especially in individuals <50–55 years of age
- Livedo reticularis
- Hemolytic anemia
- Systemic lupus erythematosus
- False-positive serologic test for syphilis

Lupus Anticoagulant

Lupus anticoagulant is detected in plasma by using a sequence of phospholipid-dependent coagulation assays such as the activated partial thromboplastin time, dilute Russell viper venom time, or kaolin clotting time. In these assays, lupus anticoagulant binds to phospholipids or moieties formed by the interaction of phospholipids and clotting factors, thus interfering with the clotting cascade and delaying the time to clot formation. The result is a prolonged clotting time. In vivo, phospholipids play a dual role, facilitating both thrombotic and antithrombotic mechanisms. Though not certain, it is likely that lupus anticoagulant predisposes to clotting in vivo by interfering predominantly with the antithrombotic role of phospholipids. Lupus anticoagulant is one of the most common reasons for a prolonged activated partial thromboplastin time that does not correct with mixture of normal pooled plasma.

Anticardiolipin Antibodies

Anticardiolipin antibodies are detected by conventional immunoassays. Laboratories should use the standardized method (12) or a modified assay known to produce similar results. Standard positive serum calibrators are available from the Antiphospholipid Standardization Laboratory in Atlanta, Georgia, and should be used in each assay. Results are measured as GPL (IgG aCL), MPL (IgM aCL), or APL (IgA aCL) units and reported in semiquantitative terms as *negative*, *low-positive*, *medium-positive*, or *high-positive* (12). Most patients with antiphospholipid syndrome have medium-to-high positive anticardiolipin antibodies of IgG isotype. Low-positive results and isolated IgM aCL results (ie, IgM positive, but lupus anticoagulant negative and IgG aCL negative) are of questionable clinical significance and should not be regarded as diagnostic of antiphospholipid syndrome (13). Isolated IgA aCL results also are of uncertain clinical significance and are not diagnostic of antiphospholipid syndrome. Antiphospholipid syndrome is diagnosed when the patient has lupus anticoagulant, IgG aCL in medium-to-high levels, or both, on two occasions at least several weeks apart (1, 3).

Other Phospholipid-Binding Antibodies

Several investigators have found that anticardiolipin antibodies actually bind to β_2-glycoprotein I or a complex formed by this glycoprotein and cardiolipin (14). At present, however, tests for antibodies to β_2-glycoprotein I are still in development and are not approved for clinical use. Other antiphospholipid antibodies that may be detected include antibodies binding to phospholipid antigens other than cardiolipin (phosphatidylserine, phosphatidylethanolamine, phosphatidylinositol, phosphatidylglycerol, phosphatidylcholine, and phosphatidic acid). Although tests for such antibodies may have merit in diagnosing antiphospholipid syndrome, their status is uncertain.

Clinical Features of Antiphospholipid Syndrome

Obstetric Features

The relationship between antiphospholipid syndrome and fetal loss has been reviewed recently (15). Several important points deserve emphasis. First, positive test results for IgG or IgM aCL antibodies may be found in up to 20% of women with recurrent pregnancy loss (16–23), but many positive results are low level or only IgM isotype and therefore are not diagnostic of antiphospholipid syndrome (13). Second, antiphospholipid syndrome may present with either recurrent embryonic pregnancy loss (24) or death of the fetus at or beyond 10 weeks of gestation (25). The latter presentation may be more specific for antiphospholipid syndrome. Third, studies of general unselected populations show that lupus anticoagulant and medium-to-high positive levels of anticardiolipin antibodies (IgG or IgM) may be found in 2–4% of otherwise normal individuals (26). However, only 0.2% of IgG results are in the medium- or high-positive range.

It also is clear that sporadic miscarriage or early fetal death infrequently is associated with antiphospholipid antibodies (27, 28), a finding that is not surprising because antiphospholipid syndrome is rare. However, antiphospholipid antibodies are found in 10–15% of women with fetal deaths at or beyond 20 weeks of gestation (29, 30). The importance of identifying antiphospholipid syndrome lies not in its prevalence, but in its implications for the individual patient and its status as a potentially treatable cause of pregnancy loss.

In addition to fetal loss, other obstetric complications in women with antiphospholipid syndrome include pregnancy-induced hypertension (PIH), uteroplacental insufficiency, and preterm birth. The reported rates of these conditions vary considerably between studies, probably as a result of the differences in clinical and laboratory criteria used in patient selection (31). An unusually high rate of PIH has been noted in patients with well-characterized antiphospholipid syndrome (31–35), and PIH is a major contributor to the high rate of preterm delivery in this condition. The rate of PIH is not markedly diminished by treatment with low-dose aspirin, glucocorticoids, or heparin. In the two largest series of pregnant women with well-characterized antiphospholipid syndrome, 48% and 18%, respectively, developed PIH (31, 34).

Several studies with conflicting results have attempted to determine the rate of antiphospholipid antibodies among patients with PIH. In two studies of patients with PIH, including those with mild PIH and PIH near term, investigators did not find a relationship between antiphospholipid antibodies and PIH (1, 36). However, in four other studies, 11.7–17% of women with PIH had significant levels of antiphospholipid antibodies (37–40). In two of these studies, only patients with early-onset, severe PIH were studied (37, 39). A relationship between antiphospholipid antibodies and PIH has been confirmed by two prospective studies of unselected obstetric patients (41, 42), but not by another (43). The weight of evidence supports testing women with early-onset (<34 weeks of gestation), severe PIH for antiphospholipid antibodies. Routinely testing for antiphospholipid antibodies in women with mild or near-term PIH is not justified.

Women with antiphospholipid syndrome are at a substantial risk for placental insufficiency, which is manifested by fetal growth restriction and fetal compromise (31–34). The rate of fetal growth restriction is approximately 30% among pregnant women with well characterized antiphospholipid syndrome (31, 34). Even in women with IgG or IgM aCL antibodies, but no lupus anticoagulant, the rate of fetal growth restriction among live-born infants approaches 15% (44).

Antiphospholipid antibodies also may contribute to the overall rate of fetal growth restriction. One group of investigators found that 24% of mothers delivered of growth-restricted infants had medium- or high-positive tests for anticardiolipin antibodies, which was significantly more than controls (45). In a prospective study, 12% of women testing positive for IgG aCL antibodies had small-for-gestational age infants compared with 2% of women testing negative (42). However, in two other prospective studies, investigators did not find a relationship between antiphospholipid antibodies and fetal growth restriction (41, 43). Based on this controversy, routine testing of women with fetal growth restriction for antiphospholipid syndrome is not warranted. Instead, only those women who have severe fetal growth restriction or other evidence of uteroplacental insufficiency in the second or early third trimester should be tested for antiphospholipid antibodies.

Nonreassuring fetal heart rate patterns are relatively common in pregnant women with antiphospholipid syndrome (31–35). In the two largest studies of women treated for antiphospholipid syndrome, half of all pregnancies with successful outcomes were complicated by abnormal fetal heart rate tracings resulting in delivery (31, 34). However, as with fetal growth restriction, prospective studies do not confirm a significant relationship between nonreassuring fetal heart rate patterns and antiphospholipid antibodies in unselected patients. Thus, a nonreassuring fetal heart rate pattern is not an indication for antiphospholipid testing unless other clinical features suggest antiphospholipid syndrome.

Preterm deliveries, usually secondary to PIH and placental insufficiency (31–35), occur in approximately one third of pregnant women with antiphospholipid syndrome (31, 34). One investigator found preterm birth in 13% of 31 women with either IgG or IgM aCL antibodies, but not with lupus anticoagulant (44). In another study, 12% of 60 women testing positive for IgG aCL antibodies alone were delivered preterm as compared with 4% of those testing negative (42).

Nonobstetric Medical Problems

Thrombosis

Numerous studies confirm a link between antiphospholipid antibodies and thrombosis (5, 46, 47). Venous thrombosis accounts for about 65–70% of such episodes. The lower extremities are the most common site of involvement, but thrombosis can occur in any part of the vascular system. In particular, the diagnosis of antiphospholipid syndrome should be considered in women with venous thrombosis in unusual sites, such as the portal, mesenteric, splenic, subclavian, and cerebral veins. Antiphospholipid antibodies are detected in approximately 2% of patients with non-traumatic venous thrombosis (48), a rate similar to that of several inherited conditions of hypercoagulability such as antithrombin III deficiency and protein C deficiency. Women with nontraumatic thrombosis should be tested for antiphospholipid antibodies, as well as inherited predispositions such as activated protein C resistance, antithrombin III deficiency, and deficiencies of protein C and protein S.

Antiphospholipid antibodies also are associated with arterial thrombosis and appear to be a predisposing factor in 4–6% of cases of stroke in otherwise healthy patients under age 50 (49–51). The region of the middle cerebral artery is most commonly involved. Some events are due to thromboembolism as opposed to in situ central nervous system arterial thrombosis. As with venous thrombosis, arterial thrombosis in individuals with antiphospholipid syndrome may occur in relatively unusual locations, such as the retinal artery, subclavian or brachial artery, and digital arteries. Antiphospholipid antibodies also are associated with transient ischemic attacks and amaurosis fugax (13, 52).

Women with antiphospholipid syndrome, even those without a prior thrombotic event, are at risk for thrombosis. In a historic cohort study, investigators found that 22% of women with antiphospholipid syndrome had venous thrombosis, and 6.9% had a cerebrovascular incident over a median follow-up period of 60 months (13). Retrospective analyses of women with antiphospholipid syndrome and a history of thrombosis indicate that a very high proportion of initial thrombotic episodes occur in relationship to pregnancy or the use of combination oral contraceptives (31, 53). This observation was confirmed in the historic cohort study; in the follow-up period, 24% of thrombotic events occurred during pregnancy or the postpartum period (52). In two prospective studies of pregnancies in women with well-characterized antiphospholipid syndrome, the rates of thrombosis or stroke were 5% (31) and 12% (34). These observations suggest that women with documented antiphospholipid syndrome should not take estrogen–progestin combination oral contraceptives. Also, the risk of pregnancy-associated thrombosis in women with well-characterized antiphospholipid syndrome is substantial enough to warrant consideration of anticoagulant prophylaxis during pregnancy and the postpartum period, depending on individual circumstances.

Patients with antiphospholipid syndrome and prior thrombotic events are at very high risk for recurrent thromboses (54–57). In one study, 69% of patients with antiphospholipid syndrome and prior thrombosis had one or more recurrent thrombotic episodes; the median interval to recurrent thrombosis was only 12 months (55). Treatment with high-intensity warfarin was more effective than other therapies or no therapy in preventing recurrent thrombosis.

Thrombocytopenia

Thrombocytopenia also has been strongly associated with antiphospholipid antibodies (1, 2, 58). Anticardiolipin antibodies have been shown to correlate independently with the development of thrombocytopenia in patients with underlying connective tissue disease (1, 58). Thrombocytopenia occurs in up to 40% of individuals with primary antiphospholipid syndrome (2). The risk of thrombocytopenia is similar for patients with primary and secondary antiphospholipid syndrome (52, 59).

Thrombocytopenia associated with antiphospholipid syndrome can be difficult to distinguish from that due to other causes, and the distinction between this disorder and immune thrombocytopenic purpura (ITP [formerly known as idiopathic thrombocytopenia purpura]) is blurred. In fact, anticardiolipin antibodies have been detected in the sera of patients with ITP (60). Laboratory evidence suggests that platelet antigens associated with thrombocytopenia and antiphospholipid syndrome are different from those found in ITP (61). Unfortunately, there are no tests available to distinguish between these disorders, and antiplatelet antibodies detected in ITP also are present in some patients with antiphospholipid syndrome (61). Other causes of thrombocytopenia such as disseminated intravascular coagulation, human immunodeficiency virus (HIV) infection, drug-induced thrombocytopenia, thrombotic thrombocytopenia, gestational thrombocytopenia, PIH, and laboratory error also must be considered.

Other Associations

Because the reagents used in the Venereal Disease Research Laboratory and rapid plasma reagin tests contain cardiolipin, some patients with lupus anticoagulant or anticardiolipin antibodies also will have biologic false-positive serologic test results for syphilis (31). Also, individuals with positive serologic test results for syphilis (true-positive or false-positive) may have anticardiolipin (62). Syphilis must be excluded using appropriate methods. Women with biologic false-positive serologic test results for syphilis should be evaluated for lupus anticoagulant and anticardiolipin antibodies.

Livedo reticularis is the most widely recognized cutaneous condition linked to antiphospholipid syndrome (1, 2, 63, 64). It appears as a reticulated network of reddish blue discoloration especially evident on the extremities and intensified by exposure to cold. It is caused by dilation of the blood vessels and stagnation of blood in the capillaries or larger arterioles resulting from intravascular obstruction to flow. Other cutaneous manifestations associated with antiphospholipid syndrome include digital cyanosis, digital gangrene, and leg ulcers like those resulting from pyoderma. Antiphospholipid antibodies have been associated with a positive Coombs test and autoimmune hemolytic anemia (65, 66).

There are a number of neurologic manifestations associated with antiphospholipid syndrome. The most widely recognized is cerebrovascular stroke. Others include transient ischemic attacks, amaurosis fugax, chorea and chorea gravidarum, migraine headaches, multiinfarct dementia, and transverse myelitis. Amaurosis fugax, a condition characterized by transient, monocular visual field deficits usually lasting from a few seconds to a few minutes, is probably due to small-vessel thrombosis, thromboembolism, or spasm.

Management

Management of antiphospholipid syndrome in women should include both obstetric care and medical care. Recommended management regimens are shown in Table 2.

Obstetric Care

Patients with antiphospholipid syndrome should undergo preconceptional assessment and counseling. A detailed medical and obstetric history should be obtained, and the presence of relevant levels of antiphospholipid antibodies (ie, lupus anticoagulant, medium-to-high levels of anticardiolipin antibodies, or both) should be confirmed. The patient should be informed of potential maternal and obstetric problems, including fetal loss, thrombosis or stroke, PIH, fetal growth restriction, and preterm delivery. In those women who also have SLE, issues related to exacerbation of SLE also should be discussed. All patients with antiphospholipid syndrome should be assessed for evidence of anemia and thrombocytopenia, because both may occur in association with this syn-

Table 2. Proposed Managements for Women with Antiphospholipid Antibodies

Feature	Management*	
	Pregnant†	Nonpregnant‡
Antiphospholipid Syndrome (APS)		
APS with prior fetal death or recurrent pregnancy loss	Heparin in prophylactic doses (15,000–20,000 U of unfractionated heparin or equivalent per day) administered subcutaneously in divided doses and low-dose aspirin daily Calcium and vitamin D supplementation	Optimal management uncertain; options include no treatment or daily treatment with low-dose aspirin
APS with prior thrombosis or stroke	Heparin to achieve full anticoagulation *or* Heparin in prophylactic doses (15,000–20,000 U of unfractionated heparin or equivalent per day) administered subcutaneously in divided doses *plus* Low-dose aspirin daily Calcium and vitamin D supplementation	Warfarin administered daily in doses to maintain international normalized ratio ≥3:0
APS without prior pregnancy loss or thrombosis	Optimal management uncertain; options include no treatment, daily treatment with low-dose aspirin, daily treatment with prophylactic doses of heparin and low-dose aspirin	Optimal management uncertain. Options include no treatment or daily treatment with low-dose aspirin
Antiphospholipid Antibodies Without APS		
Lupus anticoagulant (LA) or medium-to-high-positive IgG aCL	Optimal management uncertain; options include no treatment, daily treatment with low-dose aspirin, daily treatment with prophylactic doses of heparin and low-dose aspirin	Optimal management uncertain. Options include no treatment or daily treatment with low-dose aspirin
Low levels of IgG aCL, only IgM aCL, only IgA aCL without LA, antiphospholipid antibodies other than LA, or aCL	Optimal management uncertain; options include no treatment or daily treatment with low-dose aspirin	Optimal management uncertain. Options include no treatment or daily treatment with low-dose aspirin

*The medications shown should not be used in the presence of contraindications.
†Close obstetric monitoring of mother and fetus is necessary in all cases.
‡The patient should be counseled in all cases regarding symptoms of thrombosis and thromboembolism.

drome. Evaluation for underlying renal disease may be useful.

A pregnant woman with antiphospholipid syndrome should be examined frequently and educated about the signs or symptoms of thrombosis or thromboembolism, severe PIH, or decreased fetal movement. Once the diagnosis of antiphospholipid syndrome is confirmed, serial antiphospholipid antibody determinations are not useful.

A primary goal of the antenatal visits after 20 weeks of gestation for patients with antiphospholipid syndrome is the detection of hypertension or proteinuria or both. Because of the risk of uteroplacental insufficiency, fetal ultrasonography should be performed every 4–6 weeks starting at 18–20 weeks of gestation. In patients with otherwise uncomplicated antiphospholipid syndrome, fetal surveillance should be started at 30–32 weeks of gestation. Earlier and more frequent ultrasonography and fetal testing is indicated in patients with poor obstetric histories, evidence of PIH, or evidence of fetal growth restriction. In selected cases, fetal surveillance as early as 24–25 weeks may be justified (67).

In an attempt to improve pregnancy outcome, a number of medications and regimens have been used to treat pregnant women with antiphospholipid syndrome who have experienced pregnancy loss (Table 2). In a randomized trial, prednisone and heparin were found to be of similar efficacy for achieving successful fetal outcome (68). However, because heparin-treated patients had fewer serious side effects and obstetric complications, heparin is the preferred treatment. Most physicians prefer a thromboprophylactic dose of 15,000–20,000 U of unfractionated sodium heparin per day administered subcutaneously in two or three divided doses in women with antiphospholipid syndrome (31, 68, 69). In otherwise normal women with recurrent embryonic loss, but not thrombosis, as little as 10,000–15,000 U of heparin per day during pregnancy improves fetal outcome (44, 70). Low-molecular-weight heparin may be used in pregnancy, and it will likely replace unfractionated sodium heparin in the treatment of antiphospholipid syndrome.

It is important to counsel the patient regarding potential adverse effects of heparin. Heparin-induced osteoporosis with fracture occurs in 1–2% of women in whom full anticoagulation has been achieved during pregnancy (71). In an attempt to avoid severe osteoporosis, women treated with heparin should be encouraged to take supplemental calcium (1,500 mg calcium carbonate) and vitamin D daily. It is prudent to encourage axial skeleton weight-bearing exercise such as walking. Warfarin may be substituted for heparin during the postpartum period to limit further risk of heparin-induced osteoporosis and fracture.

Heparin also is associated with an uncommon idiosyncratic thrombocytopenia known as heparin-induced thrombocytopenia. This complication is immune mediated and usually has its onset 3–15 days after initiation of therapy. The frequency is difficult to determine, but it probably occurs in less than 5% of patients treated with heparin, with most cases being relatively mild. A more severe form of heparin-induced thrombocytopenia, paradoxically involving venous and arterial thromboses, may occur in up to 0.5% of patients treated with unfractionated sodium heparin. It has recently been shown that low-molecular-weight heparin is much less likely to be associated with heparin-induced thrombocytopenia (72), a major safety advantage over unfractionated sodium heparin.

The use of high-dose intravenous immune globulin has generated interest because of anecdotal reports of successful pregnancy outcomes (73–77). However, all but one also were treated with prednisone, heparin, or low-dose aspirin. The reported cases appear to involve more severe cases of antiphospholipid-related pregnancy loss in which other therapies had failed. Definitive evidence of the efficacy of high-dose immune globulin will be necessary before this treatment can be recommended. A prospective, randomized trial is currently being conducted.

Patients with antiphospholipid syndrome who do not have a history of thrombosis appear to have a risk of developing thrombosis during pregnancy (31, 34), and prophylaxis should be considered (16). If used, prophylaxis should be continued for about 6–8 weeks postpartum. Warfarin may be substituted for heparin during the postpartum period to limit further risk of heparin-induced osteoporosis and fracture.

Nonobstetric Care

Women with antiphospholipid syndrome are at substantial risk of developing other medical problems related to the disease. Nearly one half of women with antiphospholipid syndrome develop thrombosis, stroke, transient ischemic attacks, amaurosis fugax, new-onset SLE, or new-onset autoimmune thrombocytopenia over a median follow-up interval of 5 years (13). Thus, women with antiphospholipid syndrome require careful and close medical follow-up with a team of specialists with expertise in the management of antiphospholipid syndrome. Given the maternal and fetal risks associated with pregnancy, women with antiphospholipid syndrome should avoid unintended pregnancy.

Patients who have had prior thrombotic events are particularly prone to have recurrent thromboses. The annual risk of new thrombosis is approximately 33% for untreated patients and 20% for patients treated with low-dose aspirin alone (78). Long-term anticoagulation with warfarin to maintain the international normalized ratio of at least 3:0 is advisable for patients with antiphospholipid syndrome who have had a prior thrombotic event. In patients treated with warfarin, the risk of hemorrhage is 2–5% per year. In women taking warfarin, dysfunctional uterine bleeding and ovarian hemorrhage associated with ovulation pose unique and difficult problems. Suppression of ovulation may be beneficial, but hormonal formulations containing estrogen, including estrogen–progestin combination oral contraceptives, are contraindicated. Immunosuppressive agents should be reserved for the treatment of symptoms of SLE in patients with secondary antiphospholipid syndrome. Pending the results of further studies, women with antiphospholipid syndrome who have not had a prior thrombotic event should receive either no treatment or daily low-dose aspirin. However, such patients should receive thromboprophylaxis for thrombogenic circumstances such as abdominal or orthopedic surgery.

Summary

Antiphospholipid syndrome is a recently recognized autoimmune condition that may present with fetal loss, thrombosis, or autoimmune thrombocytopenia. Women with these clinical features should be tested for lupus anticoagulant and anticardiolipin antibodies; most patients with antiphospholipid syndrome will be found to have both lupus anticoagulant and IgG aCL antibodies. Tests for other antiphospholipid antibodies are not yet standardized, leaving the interpretation of results open to question.

Women with antiphospholipid syndrome should be treated during pregnancy with thromboprophylactic doses of heparin and low-dose aspirin. It is incumbent upon the obstetrician to be aware of the adverse effects of heparin. Close obstetric care is indicated in all cases because of an increased risk of PIH, fetal growth restriction, and a nonreassuring fetal heart rate pattern. Nonpregnant women with antiphospholipid syndrome are at increased risk for developing thrombosis, transient ischemic attacks, new-onset SLE, or new-onset autoimmune thrombocytopenia; thus, close medical follow-up is indicated. In women with antiphospholipid syndrome and one or more prior thrombotic events, lifelong anticoagulation with warfarin is advisable to avoid recurrent thrombosis.

References

1. Alarcon-Segovia D, Deleze M, Oria CV, Sanchez-Guerrero J, Gomez-Pacheco L, Cabiedes J, et al. Antiphospholipid antibodies and the antiphospholipid syndrome in systemic lupus erythematosus:a prospective analysis of 500 consecutive patients. Medicine 1989;68:353–365
2. Asherson RA, Khamashta MA, Ordi-Ros J, Derksen RHWM, Machin SJ, Barquinero J, et al. The "primary" anti-phospholipid syndrome: major clinical and serological features. Medicine 1989;68:366–374
3. Harris EN. Syndrome of the black swan. Br J Rheumatol 1987;26:324–326
4. Conley CL, Hartman RC. A hemorrhagic disorder caused by circulating anticoagulant in patients with disseminated lupus erythematosus. J Clin Invest 1952;31:621–622
5. Harris EN, Gharavi AE, Boey ML, Patel BM, Mackworth-Young CG, Loizou S, et al. Anti-cardiolipin antibodies: detection by radioimmunoassay and association with thrombosis in systemic lupus erythematosus. Lancet 1983;2: 1211–1214
6. Chamley LW, Pattison NS, McKay EJ. Separation of lupus anticoagulant from anticardiolipin antibodies by ion-exchange and gel filtration chromatography. Haemostasis 1991;21:25–29
7. Exner T, Sahman N, Trudinger B. Separation of anticardiolipin antibodies from lupus anticoagulant on a phospholipid-coated polystyrene column. Biochem Biophys Res Commun 1988;155:1001–1007
8. McNeil HP, Chesterman CN, Krillis SA. Binding specificity of lupus anticoagulants and anticardiolipin antibodies. Thromb Res 1988;52:609–619
9. Pierangeli SS, Harris EN, Gharavi AE, Goldsmith G, Branch DW, Dean WL. Are immunoglobulins with lupus anticoagulant activity specific for phospholipids? Br J Haematol 1993;85:124–132
10. Coulam CB, McIntyre JA, Wagenknecht D, Rote N. Interlaboratory inconsistencies in detection of anticardiolipin antibodies. Lancet 1990;335:865
11. Peaceman AM, Silver RK, MacGregor SN, Socol ML. Interlaboratory variation in antiphospholipid antibody testing. Am J Obstet Gynecol 1992;166:1780–1787
12. Harris EN. The second international anti-cardiolipin standardization workshop/The Kingston antiphospholipid antibody study (KAPS) group. Am J Clin Pathol 1990;94: 476–484
13. Silver RM, Porter TF, van Leeuween I, Jeng G, Scott JR, Branch DW. Anticardiolipin antibodies: clinical consequences of "low titers." Obstet Gynecol 1996;87:494–500
14. Krilis SA, Sheng YH, Kandiah DA. The role of β_2-glycoprotein I in the antiphospholid syndrome. Lupus 1996;5:150–152
15. American College of Obstetricians and Gynecologists. Early pregnancy loss. ACOG Technical Bulletin 212. Washington, DC: ACOG, 1995
16. Branch DW, Silver RM, Pierangeli S, van Leeuwen I, Harris EN. Antiphospholipid antibodies other than lupus anticoagulant and anticardiolipin antibodies in women with recurrent pregnancy loss, fertile controls, and antiphospholipid syndrome. Obstet Gynecol 1997;89:549–555
17. MacLean MA, Cumming GP, McCall F, Walker ID, Walker JJ. The prevalence of lupus anticoagulant and anticardiolipin antibodies in women with a history of first trimester miscarriages. Br J Obstet Gynaecol 1994;101:103–110
18. Out HJ, Bruinse HW, Christiaens GCML, van Vliet M, Meilof JF, de Groot PG, et al. Prevalence of antiphospholipid antibodies in patients with fetal loss. Ann Rheum Dis 1991;50:553–557
19. Parazzini F, Acaia B, Faden D, Lovotti M, Marelli G. Cortelazzo S. Antiphospholipid antibodies and recurrent abortion. Obstet Gynecol 1991;77:854–858
20. Parke AL, Wilson D, Maier D. The prevalence of anti-phospholipid antibodies in women with recurrent spontaneous abortion, women with successful pregnancies, and women who have never been pregnant. Arthritis Rheum 1991;34:1231–1235
21. Petri M, Golbus M, Anderson R, Whiting-O'Keefe Q, Corash L, Hellmann D. Antinuclear antibody, lupus anticoagulant, and anticardiolipin antibody in women with idiopathic habitual abortion. A controlled prospective study of forty-four women. Arthritis Rheum 1987;30:601–606
22. Plouffe L Jr, White EW, Tho SP, Sweet CS, Layman LC, Whitman GF, et al. Etiologic factors of recurrent abortion and subsequent reproductive performance of couples: have we made any progress in 10 years? Am J Obstet Gynecol 1992;167:313–321
23. Yetman DL, Kutteh WH. Antiphospholipid antibody panels and recurrent pregnancy loss: prevalence of anticardiolipin antibodies compared with other antiphospholipid antibodies. Fertil Steril 1996;66:540–546
24. Rai RS, Clifford K, Cohen H, Regan L. High prospective fetal loss rate in untreated pregnancies of women with recurrent miscarriage and antiphospholipid antibodies. Hum Reprod 1995;10:3301–3304
25. Oshiro BT, Silver RM, Scott JR, Yu H, Branch DW. Antiphospholipid antibodies and fetal death. Obstet Gynecol 1996;87:489–493
26. Harris EN, Spinnato JA. Should anticardiolipin tests be performed in otherwise healthy pregnant women? Am J Obstet Gynecol 1991;165:1272–1277

27. Haddow JE, Rote NS, Dostal-Johnson D, Palomaki GE, Pulkkinen AJ, Knight GJ. Lack of an association between late fetal death and antiphospholipid antibody measurements in the second trimester. Am J Obstet Gynecol 1991; 165:1308–1312

28. Infante-Rivard C, David M, Gauthier R, Rivard G-E. Lupus anticoagulants, anticardiolipin antibodies, and fetal loss. A case control study. N Engl J Med 1991;325:1063– 1066

29. Ahlenius I, Floberg J, Thomassen P. Sixty-six cases of intrauterine fetal death: a prospective study with an extensive test protocol. Acta Obstet Gynecol Scand 1995;74: 109–117

30. Bocciolone L, Meroni P, Parazzini F, Tincani A, Radici E, Tarantini M, et al. Antiphospholipid antibodies and risk of intrauterine late fetal death. Acta Obstet Gynecol Scand 1994;73:389–392

31. Branch DW, Silver RM, Blackwell JL, Reading JC, Scott JR. Outcome of treated pregnancies in women with antiphospholipid syndrome: an update of the Utah experience. Obstet Gynecol 1992;80:614–620

32. Branch DW, Scott JR, Kochenour NK, Hershgold E. Obstetric complications associated with lupus anticoagulant. N Engl J Med 1985;313:1322–1326

33. Caruso A, De Carolis S, Ferrazzani S, Valesini G, Caforio L, Manusco S. Pregnancy outcome in relation to uterine artery flow velocity waveforms and clinical characteristics in women with antiphospholipid syndrome. Obstet Gynecol 1993;82:970–976

34. Lima F, Khamashta MA, Buchanan NMM, Kerslake S, Hunt BJ, Hughes GRV. A study of sixty pregnancies in patients with the antiphospholipid syndrome. Clin Exp Rheumatol 1996;14:131–136

35. Lockshin MD, Druzin ML, Goei S, Qamar T, Magid MS, Jovanovic L, Ferenc M. Antibody to cardiolipin as a predictor of fetal distress or death in pregnant patients with systemic lupus erythematosus. N Engl J Med 1985;313: 152–156

36. Scott RAH. Anti-cardiolipin antibodies and pre-eclampsia. Br J Obstet Gynaecol 1987;94:604–605

37. Branch DW, Andres R, Digre KB, Rote NS, Scott JR. The association of antiphospholipid antibodies with severe preeclampsia. Obstet Gynecol 1989;73:541–545

38. Milliez J, Lelong F, Bayani N, Jannet D, El Medjadi M, Latrous H, et al. The prevalence of autoantibodies during third-trimester pregnancy complicated by hypertension or idiopathic fetal growth retardation. Am J Obstet Gynecol 1991;165:51–56

39. Moodley J, Bhoola V, Duursma J, Pudfin D, Byrne S, Kenoyer DG. The association of antiphospholipid antibodies with severe early-onset pre-eclampsia. S Afr Med J 1995;85:105–107

40. Sletnes KE, Wislof F, Moe N, Dale PO. Antiphospholipid antibodies in pre-eclamptic women: relation to growth retardation and neonatal outcome. Acta Obstet Gynecol Scand 1992;71:112–117

41. Pattison NS, Chamley LW, McKay EJ, Liggins GC, Butler WS. Antiphospholipid antibodies in pregnancy: prevalence and clinical associations. Br J Obstet Gynaecol 1993; 100: 909–913

42. Yasuda M, Takakuwa K, Tokunaga A, Tanaka K. Prospective studies of the association between anticardiolipin antibody and outcome of pregnancy. Obstet Gynecol 1995; 86:555–559

43. Lynch A, Marlar R, Murphy J, Davila G, Santos M, Rutledge J, et al. Antiphospholipid antibodies in predicting adverse pregnancy outcome. A prospective study. Ann Intern Med 1994;120:470–475

44. Kutteh WH. Antiphospholipid antibody-associated recurrent pregnancy loss: treatment with heparin and low-dose aspirin is superior to low-dose aspirin alone. Am J Obstet Gynecol 1996;174:1584–1589

45. Polzin WJ, Kopelman JN, Robinson RD, Read JA, Brady K. The association of antiphospholipid antibodies with pregnancy complicated by fetal growth restriction. Obstet Gynecol 1991;78:1108–1111

46. Bowie EJW, Thompson JH Jr, Pascuzzi CA, Owen CA Jr. Thrombosis in systemic lupus erythematosus despite circulating anticoagulants. J Lab Clin Med 1963;62:416–431

47. Lechner K, Pabinger-Fasching I. Lupus anticoagulants and thrombosis. A study of 25 cases and review of the literature. Haemostas 1985;15:254–262

48. Malm J, Laurell M, Nilsson IM, Dahlback B. Thromboembolic disease—critical evaluation of laboratory investigation. Thromb Haemost 1992;68:7–13

49. Brey RL, Hart RG, Sherman DG, Tegeler CH. Antiphospholipid antibodies and cerebral ischemia in young people. Neurology 1990;40:1190–1196

50. Ferro D, Quintarelli C, Rasura M, Antionini G, Violi F. Lupus anticoagulant and the fibrinolytic system in young patients with stroke. Stroke 1993;24:368–370

51. Hart RG, Miller VT, Coull BM, Bril V. Cerebral infarction associated with lupus anticoagulants—preliminary report. Stroke 1984;15:114–118

52. Silver RM, Draper ML, Scott JR, Lyon JL, Reading J, Branch DW. Clinical consequences of antiphospholipid antibodies: an historic cohort study. Obstet Gynecol 1994; 83:372–377

53. Branch DW, Scott JR. Clinical implication of anti-phospholipid antibodies: the Utah experience. In Harris EN, Exner T, Hughes GRV, Asherson RA, eds. Phospholipid-binding antibodies. Boca Raton, Florida: CRC Press, 1990:335–346

54. Derksen RHWM, de Groot PG, Kater L, Nieuwenhuis HK. Patients with antiphospholipid antibodies and venous thrombosis should receive a long term anticoagulant treatment. Ann Rheum Dis 1993;52:689–692

55. Khamashta MA, Cuadrado MJ, Mujic F, Taub NA, Hunt BJ, Hughes GRV. The management of thrombosis in the antiphospholipid-antibody syndrome. N Engl J Med 1995; 332:993–997

56. Levine SR, Brey RL, Joseph CLM, Havstad S. Risk of recurrent thromboembolic events in patients with focal cerebral ischemia and antiphospholipid antibodies. Stroke 1992;23 (suppl I):I-29–I-32

57. Rosove MH, Brewer PMC. Antiphospholipid thrombosis: clinical course after the first thrombotic event in 70 patients. Ann Intern Med 1992;117:303–308

58. Harris EN, Asherson RA, Gharavi AE, Morgan SH, Derue G, Hughes GRV. Thrombocytopenia in SLE and related autoimmune disorders: association with anticardiolipin antibody. Br J Haematol 1985;59:227–230

59. Italian Registry of Antiphospholipid Antibodies. Thrombosis and thrombocytopenia in antiphospholipid syndrome (idiopathic and secondary to SLE): first report from the Italian registry. Haematologica 1993;78:313–318

60. Harris EN, Gharavi AE, Hedge U, Derue G, Morgan SH, Englert H, et al. Anticardiolipin antibodies in autoimmune thrombocytopenia purpura. Br J Haematol 1985;59:231–234

61. Fabris F, Steffan A, Cordiano I, Borzini P, Luzzatto G, Randi ML, et al. Specific antiplatelet autoantibodies in patients with antiphospholipid antibodies and thrombocytopenia. Eur J Haematol 1994;53:232–236

62. Harris EN, Gharavi AE, Wasley GD, Hughes GRV. Use of an enzyme-linked immunosorbent assay and of inhibition studies to distinguish between antibodies to cardiolipin from patients with syphilis or autoimmune disorders. J Infect Dis 1988;157:23–31

63. Asherson RA, Mayou SC, Merry P, Black MM, Hughes GRV. The spectrum of livedo reticularis and anticardiolipin antibodies. Br J Dermatol 1989;120:215–221

64. Grob JJ, Bonerandi JJ. Thrombotic skin disease as a marker of the anticardiolipin syndrome: livedo vasculitis and distal gangrene associated with abnormal serum antiphospholipid activity. J Am Acad Dermatol 1989;20:1063–1069

65. Deleze M, Oria CV, Alarcon-Segovia D. Occurrence of both hemolytic anemia and thrombocytopenic purpura (Evan's syndrome) in systemic lupus erythematosus. Relationship to antiphospholipid antibodies. J Rheumatol 1988;15:611–615

66. Hazeltine M, Rauch J, Danoff D. Antiphospholipid antibodies in systemic lupus erythematosus: evidence of an association with positive Coombs' and hypocomplementemia. J Rheumatol 1988;15:80–86

67. Druzin ML, Lockshin M, Edersheim TG, Hutson JM, Krauss AL, Kogut E. Second trimester fetal monitoring and preterm delivery in pregnancies with systemic lupus erythematosus and/or circulating anticoagulant. Am J Obstet Gynecol 1987;157:1503–1510

68. Cowchock FS, Reece EA, Balaban D, Branch DW, Plouffe L. Repeated fetal losses associated with antiphospholipid antibodies: a collaborative randomized trial comparing prednisone to low-dose heparin treatment. Am J Obstet Gynecol 1992;166:1318–1323

69. Rosove MH, Tabsh K, Wasserstrum N, Howard P, Hahn BH, Kalunian KC. Heparin therapy for pregnant women with lupus anticoagulant or anticardiolipin antibodies. Obstet Gynecol 1990;75:630–634

70. Rai RS, Cohen H, Dave M, Regan L. Randomized controlled trial of aspirin and aspirin plus heparin in pregnant women with recurrent miscarriage associated with phospholipid antibodies (or antiphospholipid antibodies). BMJ 1997;314:253–257

71. Dahlman TC. Osteoporotic fractures and the recurrence of thromboembolism during pregnancy and the puerperium in 184 women undergoing thromboprophylaxis with heparin. Am J Obstet Gynecol 1993;168:1265–1270

72. Warkentin TE, Levine MN, Hirsh J, Horsewood P, Roberts RS, Gent M, et al. Heparin-induced thrombocytopia in patients treated with low-molecular-weight heparin or unfractionated heparin. N Engl J Med 1995;332:1330–1335

73. Kaaja R, Julkunen H, Ammala P, Palosuo T, Kurki P. Intravenous immunoglobulin treatment of pregnant patients with recurrent pregnancy losses associated with antiphospholipid antibodies. Acta Obstet Gynecol Scand 1993;72:63–66

74. Katz VL, Thorp JM Jr, Watson WJ, Fowler L, Heine RP. Human immunoglobulin therapy for preeclampsia associated with lupus anticoagulant and anticardiolipin antibody. Obstet Gynecol 1990;76:986–987

75. Scott JR, Branch DW, Kochenour NK, Ward K. Intravenous immunoglobulin treatment of pregnant patients with recurrent pregnancy loss caused by antiphospholipid antibodies and Rh immunization. Am J Obstet Gynecol 1988;159:1055–1056

76. Spinnato JA, Clark AL, Pierangeli SS, Harris EN. Intravenous immunoglobulin therapy for the antiphospholipid syndrome in pregnancy. Am J Obstet Gynecol 1995;172: 690–694

77. Wapner RJ, Cowchock FS, Shapiro SS. Successful treatment in two women with antiphospholipid antibodies and refractory pregnancy losses with intravenous immunoglobulin infusions. Am J Obstet Gynecol 1989;161:1271–1272

78. Lockshin MD. Answers to the antiphospholipid-antibody syndrome? N Engl J Med 1995;332:1025–1027

ISSN 1074-8628

The American College of Obstetricians and Gynecologists
409 12th Street, SW
PO Box 96920
Washington, DC 20090-6920

12345/21098

ACOG EDUCATIONAL BULLETIN

Number 230, November 1996

Assessment of Fetal Lung Maturity

Approximately 300,000–500,000 of the deliveries in the United States each year are preterm. Preterm birth causes significant neonatal morbidity and mortality, which are often due to difficulty in providing oxygen transfer to an immature neonatal pulmonary system (1).

The pulmonary system is among the last of the fetal organ systems to become functionally mature. Thus, pulmonary maturity has been assumed to connote adequate maturation in other fetal systems. This assumption may not be true in fetuses relatively remote from term (2). Documentation of fetal pulmonary maturity should not be used as the sole indication for delivery of a preterm infant. Although preterm delivery may be indicated in many situations, delivery of fetuses with immature pulmonary systems should be avoided when possible.

Direct methods of assessing fetal pulmonary maturity have been available for more than 20 years, and a number of new tests have been introduced (3, 4). Proper use of these tests can aid the clinician in determining the optimal time for delivery.

This Educational Bulletin was developed under the direction of the Committee on Educational Bulletins of the American College of Obstetricians and Gynecologists as an aid to obstetricians and gynecologists. The College wishes to thank William N. P. Herbert, MD, for his assistance in the development of this bulletin. This document is not to be construed as establishing a standard of practice or dictating an exclusive course of treatment. Rather, it is intended as an educational tool that presents current information on obstetric–gynecologic issues.

Indications for Assessing Maturity

Fetal pulmonary maturity should be confirmed before elective delivery at less than 39 weeks of gestation unless fetal maturity can be inferred from any of the following criteria:

- Fetal heart tones have been documented for 20 weeks by nonelectronic fetoscope or for 30 weeks by Doppler.
- It has been 36 weeks since a serum or urine human chorionic gonadotropin pregnancy test was found to be positive by a reliable laboratory.
- Ultrasound measurement of the crown–rump length at 6–11 weeks of gestation supports a gestational age equal to or greater than 39 weeks.
- Ultrasound measurement at 12–20 weeks of gestation supports a clinically determined gestational age of 39 weeks or greater.

If any of the aforementioned criteria confirms a gestational age of 39 weeks or more in a patient with normal menstrual cycles (no oral contraceptive use immediately prior to conception), it is appropriate to schedule delivery at 39 weeks

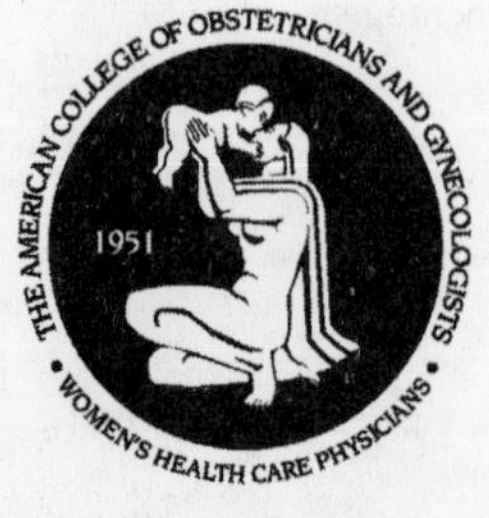

of gestation or beyond in accordance with menstrual dates. Ultrasonography may be considered confirmatory of menstrual dates if there is a gestational age agreement within 1 week by crown–rump measurements obtained at 6–11 weeks of gestation or within 10 days by an average of multiple measurements obtained between 12–20 weeks of gestation. Unless circumstances preclude continued expectant management, awaiting the onset of spontaneous labor is another option for some patients (5).

Amniocentesis for fetal pulmonary assessment is rarely warranted before 33 weeks of gestation because test results confirming lung maturity are unlikely. Confirmation of a mature fetal pulmonary system does not preclude consideration of the fetal risk of intraventricular hemorrhage and necrotizing enterocolitis.

Physiology and Pathophysiology

Fetal Lung Development

Knowledge of the development of the fetal pulmonary system and the evolution of surfactant production is helpful in understanding the tests performed for fetal lung maturity. The development of the fetal pulmonary system begins about 3 weeks after conception and continues for about 8 years after birth. The pulmonary tree development begins in the glandular period, which ends at about 16 weeks of gestation. During the canalicular period (16–24 weeks of gestation), early bronchioles develop and the epithelium vascularizes and differentiates. The alveolar (or terminal sac) period is the last stage of pulmonary development, which extends from about 24 weeks of gestation well into childhood. Bronchiolar division during this period leads to the development of thin spherical saccules, known as alveoli, that are lined by type II pneumocytes. The concomitant proliferation of capillaries around these alveoli makes effective gas exchange possible after delivery.

The type II pneumocytes produce intracellular stores, or "packages," of phospholipids called lamellar bodies, which can be released into the alveolar spaces. Surfactant is the name given to this group of "surface-active" phospholipid compounds that can reduce the surface tension within the alveolar spaces following delivery. Low surface tension within the alveoli allows these sacs to remain expanded during respiratory activity permitting continuous and maximally effective gas exchange. As a result of in utero "respiratory" activity, these substances enter the amniotic fluid cavity, where they can be measured.

The most prominent of these surfactant compounds is lecithin (phosphotidylcholine). The phospholipid compound phosphatidylglycerol (PG) appears later, and documentation of its presence is the basis of several of the commonly used tests for fetal lung maturity. Other phospholipids (phosphatidylinositol, phosphatidylethanolamine), a variety of proteins, and cholesterol contribute to this group of surface-active substances within the lung as well.

Respiratory Distress Syndrome

A deficiency in the quantity of surfactant in premature infants leads to higher surface tension within the alveoli, which can cause alveolar collapse and make gas exchange more difficult. Impaired gas exchange can result in neonatal hypoxia, with further worsening of pulmonary status manifested by acidosis and increased shunting within the lungs. Signs of respiratory distress syndrome (RDS) include neonatal tachypnea, grunting, retractions, and cyanosis, often occuring within several hours of birth. Radiography of the infant's chest revealing atelectasis, air bronchograms, and a diffuse reticulogranular infiltrate is suggestive of RDS.

Other complications associated with RDS include necrotizing enterocolitis, patent ductus arteriosus, intraventricular hemorrhage, and infection, which can result in long-term disability or death. Some survivors of RDS will suffer long-term pulmonary sequelae in the form of bronchopulmonary dysplasia (6). The Centers for Disease Control and Prevention reports that 2,000 of the 20,000–30,000 infants who develop RDS each year will die (7). Despite the positive impact of antepartum corticosteroid therapy and neonatal administration of surfactant compounds, RDS continues to be a significant cause of neonatal morbidity and mortality.

Classification of Fetal Maturity Tests

Fetal pulmonary testing can be categorized as either indirect or direct measures of fetal lung maturation. Indirect tests do not measure pulmonary function per se but rather evaluate the age or size of the fetus. From these parameters, maturity can be inferred and neonatal respiratory function predicted. Such methods include obstetric estimation of gestational age (menstrual history, first appearance of fetal heart tones, and physical examination), ultrasound examination (identification or evaluation of gestational sac, crown–rump length, biparietal diameter, etc), and the rarely used amniotic fluid analysis for fetal fat cells or creatinine.

Direct tests of fetal maturity measure either the concentration of particular components of pulmonary surfactant (biochemical tests) or the surface-active effects of these phospholipids (biophysical tests). Biochemical tests include determining the lecithin–sphingomyelin ratio (L/S) and identifying PG. Biophysical tests include the foam stability index (FSI) and fluorescence polarization. Although these tests differ in their techniques, all predict pulmonary maturity (the absence of RDS) with much greater certainty than they predict pulmonary immaturity (the presence of RDS) (3) (Table 1).

Tests of Fetal Maturity

Lecithin–Sphingomyelin Ratio

The first widely accepted direct test for assessment of fetal pulmonary status was the L/S ratio (8). This test evaluates a change in the relative amounts of lecithin (phosphatidylcholine) and sphingomyelin (a sphingolipid of unknown origin) in amniotic fluid samples as gestational age increases. Until about 32–33 weeks of gestation, the concentrations of these two substances are quite similar; thereafter, the concentration of lecithin increases significantly compared with the relatively constant concentration of sphingomyelin. In the absence of complications, the densitometric ratio of these two components reaches 2.0 at about 35 weeks of gestation. Infants delivered after attaining an L/S ratio of 2.0 or higher rarely develop RDS. This value of 2.0 has become the commonly accepted standard value indicating maturity in the fetus of a nondiabetic woman. However, correlation with clinical outcome in individual centers should precede acceptance of this threshold for pulmonary maturity, as variations within and between laboratories can be considerable. The predictive value of a negative result (value less than 2.0) is quite low.

Determination of the L/S ratio involves thin-layer chromatography after organic solvent extraction. Commercial versions of this test are available. Identification of lecithin and sphingomyelin is accomplished by using any one of a number of different staining procedures, with planimetry or densitometry used to compare the relative amounts of lecithin and sphingomyelin. This methodology is quite cumbersome and labor intensive despite numerous modifications to the original technique.

As with many tests of fetal maturity, blood and meconium can interfere with test interpretation (4). Plasma is rich in lipids that can be difficult to distinguish from phospholipids in surfactant. A bloody amniotic fluid sample may be difficult to interpret. The L/S ratio in plasma is similar to the maturity threshold (2.0) found in amniotic fluid. Theoretically, L/S values significantly lower or higher than 2.0 should be reliable, but caution is advised in relying on results from bloody amniotic fluid samples. Likewise, the mucoid nature of meconium may obscure the thin-layer chromatography pattern and interfere with the accuracy of the L/S values. Moreover, with some L/S procedures, a heme derivative in meconium may resemble PG on the thin-layer chromatography plate.

Since amniotic fluid contains enzymes, improper storage conditions can affect the L/S ratio (9). An amniotic fluid sample should be centrifuged shortly after it is obtained. If the determination is not performed immediately or if the sample is transported to an outside laboratory, the specimen should be frozen, preferably at –20°C (9). The L/S ratio decreases if an uncentrifuged sample either remains at room temperature for at least 1 hour or is cooled but not frozen for more than 12 hours. Failure to properly handle the amniotic fluid specimen can result in invalid conclusions and difficulty in interpretation of the results.

Phosphatidylglycerol

Phosphatidylglycerol is a minor constituent of surfactant that generally appears in sufficient quantity to be measured several weeks after the increase in lecithin concentration (10). Because PG enhances the spread of phospholipids on the alveolar surface, its presence indicates a more advanced state of fetal pulmonary maturity.

Phosphatidylglycerol determination can be accomplished by thin-layer chromatography, either alone or as an extension of L/S ratio testing. In addition, a slide-agglutination test has been developed using antisera specific for PG.

An advantage of PG determination in assessing fetal maturity is the fact that it is not generally affected by blood, meconium, or other contaminants. This characteristic allows PG determination by using vaginal pool samples from patients who have experienced spontaneous rupture of membranes. A disadvantage of using PG for assessing fetal maturity is its relatively late appearance in pregnancy. Compared with results of other tests, an "immature" result (negative PG) is associated with a greater proportion of patients who will deliver infants who do not develop RDS (11).

"Shake" Test and Foam Stability Index

Prediction of pulmonary maturity based on the ability of pulmonary surfactant to generate and maintain a stable foam in the presence of ethanol was first reported in 1972 (12). In this biophysical test, the addition of ethanol to amniotic fluid eliminates foam formation caused by "nonsurfactant" substances in the amniotic fluid. The generation of a stable ring of foam by shaking amniotic fluid and ethanol in a test tube demonstrates the presence of surface-active material in the amniotic fluid. Serial dilutions with ethanol allow determination of the concentration of surfactant.

This procedure has been modified and named the FSI, which uses a series of test tubes containing successively greater amounts of 95% ethanol in an attempt to quantitate surface-active properties over a wider range of concentrations (13). In effect, a single cut-off point of 47 or 48 or greater is used to indicate fetal maturity. A commercial version of this test is available. Amniotic fluid should not be placed in a siliconized collection tube if the "shake" test or FSI is used, as stable foam will result from this contamination. The presence of blood or meconium in samples interferes with the results of these tests as well.

Table 1. Commonly Used Direct Tests of Fetal Maturity

Test*	Technique	Time/Ease of Testing†	Threshold	Typical Predictive Value (%)		Relative Cost	Notes
				Mature	Immature		
Lecithin/sphingomyelin ratio	Thin-layer chromatography	4+	2.0–3.5	95–100	33–50	High	Many variations in technique; laboratory variation significant
Phosphatidylglycerol	Thin-layer chromatography	4+	"Present" (usually means >3% of total phospholipid)	95–100	23–53	High	Not affected by blood, meconium; vaginal pool samples satisfactory
	Antisera	1+	0.5 = low positive 2.0 = high positive	95–100	23–53	Commercial version—moderate	Not affected by blood, meconium; vaginal pool samples satisfactory
Foam stability index	Ethanol added to amniotic fluid, solution shaken, presence of stable bubbles at meniscus noted	2+	≥47 or 48	95	51	Laboratory—low Commercial version—moderate	Affected by blood, meconium, vaginal pool debris, silicone-coated test tubes
Fluorescence polarization	Fluorescence polarization	1+	≥55 mg/g of albumin‡	96–100	47–61	Moderate	Minimal intraassay and interassay variability; simple testing procedure
Optical density (OD) at 650 nm	Spectrophotometric reading	1+	OD ≥0.15	98	13	Low	Simple technique
Lamellar body counts	Counts using commercial hematology counter	2+	30,000–40,000 (still investigational)	97–98	29–35	Low	Promising technique

*Commercial versions are available for all tests except optical density and lamellar body counts.

†Range in complexity: 1+ indicates procedure is simple, is available all the time, requires only short procedure time, and personnel effort is not intensive; 4+ indicates procedure is complex or difficult, time consuming, and therefore, frequently not available at all times.

‡The manufacturer has reformulated the product and revised the testing procedure. Currently, the threshold for maturity is 55; with the original assay it was 70.

Fluorescence Polarization

Fetal maturity testing using fluorescence polarization is based on competitive binding of a fluorescent probe to albumin and surfactant. When the probe is bound to albumin, net polarization values are high; when bound to surfactant, polarization values are low. In amniotic fluid samples, the fluorescence polarization measured by an automated analyzer reflects the ratio of surfactant to albumin, a value that correlates with lung maturity. Recent modifications of this concept provide a simple, automated, rapid test that is widely available and varies minimally between laboratories. In the recently modified commercial version of this assay, the ratio indicating maturity is at or above 55 mg of surfactant per gram of albumin in the nondiabetic patient. Preliminary use of this test in patients with diabetes is promising (14).

This assay compares favorably with other direct tests (15, 16), but blood and meconium contamination interfere with its interpretation. Sufficient testing on amniotic fluid samples obtained vaginally has not been done.

Optical Density at 650 nm

Measuring optical absorbance of amniotic fluid at a wavelength of 650 nm is a rapid indirect biophysical test for fetal maturity. It is based on the concept that the opalescence of mature amniotic fluid is due to an increasing number of lamellar bodies, which scatter light. After centrifugation, amniotic fluid samples are analyzed on a spectrophotometer, an instrument commonly available in hospital laboratories. An optical density reading of absorbancy of 0.15 or greater is used as the indicator of pulmonary maturity. It is a simple procedure that compares favorably with other methods of fetal maturity assessment (3, 17). The degree of centrifugation and presence of blood and meconium can alter the validity of this method.

Lamellar Body Counts

Lamellar bodies represent packages of surfactant that are extruded into the alveoli from within type II pneumocytes. The similarity of lamellar body size to platelet size permits the use of a standard hematologic counter to determine lamellar body concentrations. Values of approximately 30,000–50,000/μL appear to indicate pulmonary maturity; however, alterations in technique and determinations on different commercial hematology counters yield varying results for maturity assessment (3, 17, 18). Neither bilirubin nor meconium interferes with this test, but erythrocytes lower the lamellar body number density.

Other Amniotic Fluid Tests of Maturity

Other direct and indirect tests of fetal pulmonary status have been introduced. Direct enzymatic assays have been developed for lecithin, sphingomyelin, and PG, but their use in predicting respiratory outcome has not been evaluated adequately. The lack of commercial kits and preparation costs limit use of these assays. Surfactant proteins (apoproteins) are nonphospholipid markers of fetal maturity that have been investigated for use in maturity assessment. Immunoassay for the presence of the surfactant apoproteins SP-A and SP-B in amniotic fluid has permitted such evaluation, but further investigations are necessary to clarify the usefulness of this approach.

Imaging

Ultrasonography has replaced radiographic techniques for assessing fetal age. A biparietal diameter of 9.2 cm or more, a femur length of 7.3 cm or more, the presence and size of epiphyseal ossification centers, placental grading (classification based on chorionic convolutions and calcifications), and other imaging determinations have been evaluated as means to assess maturity (19–21). Some fetuses at term, however mature, may lack these findings, and some fetuses with these characteristics may be immature (eg, maternal diabetes complicated by macrosomia). In general, ultrasound assessment of gestational age (indirectly evaluating for maturity) in the third trimester is inferior to the other methods available.

Effect of Associated Conditions on Fetal Lung Maturity

Accelerated fetal lung maturity has been reported to occur with a number of obstetric conditions, including hypertensive disorders, hemoglobinopathies, narcotics addiction, intrauterine growth restriction, classes of diabetes that are long-standing or associated with complications, premature rupture of membranes, multiple gestation, and smoking. Conversely, a delay in fetal lung maturation has been reported in patients with certain other classes of diabetes, nonhypertensive renal disease, and isoimmunization. For virtually all of these conditions, however, conflicting results concerning their effect on pulmonary maturation and testing have been reported.

Fetal lung maturity in patients with diabetes is the condition that has been studied most extensively, yet consensus is still lacking. While some have reported altered maturity test results and an increased rate of RDS in newborns of diabetic patients, others have reported no difference in either test results or clinical outcome. Causes other than deficient surfactant may be responsible for some cases of respiratory distress (22).

Other Considerations

Administration of corticosteroids to pregnant women at risk for preterm delivery has been shown to be effective in decreasing the prevalence, severity, and complications of RDS (23). Corticosteroids accelerate pulmonary maturity by stimulation of both the synthesis and release of surfactant from the type II pneumocytes into the alveolar spaces. In general, fetal maturity test results measured soon after steroid administration are affected minimally. This is probably due in part to the time interval required between steroid administration and the synthesis and release of the surface-active materials into the alveolar spaces and subsequently into the amniotic fluid.

Amniotic fluid present in the vagina following spontaneous rupture of membranes can be used for fetal maturity assessment. As noted, PG is not present in other tissue fluids and, for this reason, has particular importance in assessing maturity in patients from whom vaginal pool specimens can be obtained. Unfortunately, PG is often absent in preterm patients with fetal pulmonary maturity and may be present in others who are not mature because of bacterial contamination. There is no consensus on the utility of other tests using vaginal samples.

Comparison Among Tests

Various characteristics of commonly used tests to assess fetal maturity are compared in Table 1. Although the L/S ratio was the first direct test used to assess fetal maturity, other tests perform equally well and, because of technical aspects of the testing procedure for L/S ratio determination, have become more widely used. Regardless of the test used, the predictive value of all mature results is over 95%. That is, if the result of any test indicates maturity, the likelihood that RDS will be diagnosed in a delivered infant is less than 5%. Conversely, all available tests share a relatively poor predictive value in assessing the likelihood of the presence of RDS. The predictive values for RDS of immature test results range from approximately 30% to 60%. Other test characteristics, including cost, ease of test performance, availability, and reproducibility, are important factors in selecting maturity tests.

Testing Strategies

With the introduction of newer tests for fetal maturity assessment, it has become a common practice to order multiple tests routinely for the assessment of fetal maturity. Results are often reported as a "lung profile" or "pulmonary profile." Since a mature result on any one of the commonly used tests of fetal lung maturity is strongly predictive of the absence of RDS, the practice of multiple testing on a routine basis should be questioned. Little additional information will be gained by the performance of multiple assays. When multiple tests are performed, discordant results are sometimes found, which is not surprising because these tests measure various components or aspects of maturity by different means. Obviously, costs are increased when multiple tests are obtained.

Because of the strong predictive value of a single mature result, the strategy of ordering tests individually, but within a defined protocol, is logical. This so-called "cascade" (24) or "sequential" (25) testing involves the performance of a rapid, inexpensive test initially, with a subsequent test ordered only if the result of the initial test is immature. Such a practice can provide clinicians with around-the-clock availability of a test for fetal maturity and yet maximizes laboratory efficiency by decreasing the overall number of tests performed. The testing sequence should be determined jointly between clinicians and laboratory personnel.

Women with diabetes are thought by some to have altered fetal lung maturation or fetal maturity test results or both; thus, some practitioners approach the assessment of these women differently from that of women who do not have diabetes. In the woman whose diabetes is well controlled, awaiting the appearance of PG may be justified, as its presence seems to provide the strongest evidence of pulmonary maturity. However, it must be remembered that PG may be absent in approximately 20% of women with gestational or overt diabetes at a gestational age as late as 38–39 weeks (26). In a recent multicenter study, only 2 of 13 patients with a mature fluorescence polarization test and absent PG delivered infants who developed RDS. Neither required intubation or prolonged oxygen therapy (14). Other strategies for managing patients with diabetes include delaying delivery until two separate tests (eg, FSI, L/S) indicate fetal lung maturity or using a higher threshold for maturity on which to proceed with delivery.

Regardless of which method of fetal lung maturity assessment is chosen, it should be emphasized that no mature result from one test or a group of tests can completely eliminate the risk of RDS or other neonatal complications (2). The risk of adverse outcome with delivery on the basis of lung maturity assessment must be weighed against the potential risk of untoward outcome by permitting the pregnancy to continue in utero.

References

1. Parilla BV, Dooley SL, Jansen RD, Socol ML. Iatrogenic respiratory distress syndrome following elective repeat cesarean delivery. Obstet Gynecol 1993;81:392–395 (Level III)

2. Wigton TR, Tamura RK, Wickstrom E, Atkins V, Deddish R, Socol ML. Neonatal morbidity after preterm delivery in the presence of documented lung maturity. Am J Obstet Gynecol 1993;169:951–955 (Level II-3)

3. Dubin SB. The laboratory assessment of fetal lung maturity. Am J Clin Pathol 1992;97:836–849 (Level III)

4. Spillman T, Cotton DB. Current perspectives in assessment of fetal pulmonary surfactant status with amniotic fluid. Crit Rev Clin Lab Sci 1989;27:341–389 (Level III)

5. American College of Obstetricians and Gynecologists. Fetal maturity assessment prior to elective repeat cesarean delivery. ACOG Committee Opinion 98. Washington, DC: ACOG, 1991 (Level III)

6. Whitsett JA, Pryhuber GS, Rice WR, Warner BB, Wert SE. Acute respiratory disorders. In: Avery GB, Fletcher MA, MacDonald MG, eds. Neonatology pathophysiology and management of the newborn. Philadelphia: JB Lippincott Company 1994;429–452 (Level III)

7. National Center for Health Statistics. Births, marriages, divorces, and deaths for 1993. Monthly vital statistics report; vol 42, no. 12. Hyattsville, Maryland: Public Health Service, 1994 (Level III)

8. Gluck L, Kulovich MV, Borer RC Jr, Brenner PH, Anderson GG, Spellacy WN. Diagnosis of respiratory distress by amniocentesis. Am J Obstet Gynecol 1971;109: 440–445 (Level II-3)

9. Blumenfeld TA. Clinical laboratory tests for fetal lung maturity. Pathol Annu 1975;10:21–36 (Level III)

10. Hallman M, Kulovich M, Kirkpatrick E, Sugarman RG, Gluck L. Phosphatidylinositol and phosphatidylglycerol in amniotic fluid: indices of lung maturity. Am J Obstet Gynecol 1976;125:613–617 (Level II-3)

11. Lewis DF, Towers CV, Major CA, Asrat T, Nageotte MP, Freeman RK, et al. Use of amniostat-FLM in detecting the presence of phosphatidylglycerol in vaginal pool samples in preterm premature rupture of membranes. Am J Obstet Gynecol 1993;169:573–576 (Level II-3)

12. Clements JA, Platzker ACG, Tierney DF, Hobel CJ, Creasy RK, Margolis AJ, et al. Assessment of the risk of the respiratory-distress syndrome by a rapid test for surfactant in amniotic fluid. N Engl J Med 1972;286:1077–1081 (Level II-3)

13. Sher G, Statland BE, Freer DE, Kraybill EN. Assessing fetal lung maturation by the foam stability index test. Obstet Gynecol 1978;52:673–677 (Level II-3)

14. Livingston EG, Herbert WNP, Hage ML, Chapman JF, Stubbs TM. Use of the TDx-FLM assay in evaluating fetal lung maturity in an insulin-dependent diabetic population. Obstet Gynecol 1995;86:826–829 (Level III)

15. Herbert WNP, Chapman JF, Schnoor MM. Role of the TDx FLM assay in fetal lung maturity. Am J Obstet Gynecol 1993;168:808–812 (Level II-3)

16. Hagen E, Link JC, Arias F. A comparison of the accuracy of the TDx-FLM assay, lecithin–sphingomyelin ratio, and phosphatidylglycerol in the prediction of neonatal respiratory distress syndrome. Obstet Gynecol 1993;82:1004–1008 (Level II-3)

17. Ashwood ER, Palmer SE, Taylor JS, Pingree SS. Lamellar body counts for rapid fetal lung maturity testing. Obstet Gynecol 1993;81:619–624 (Level II-3)

18. Delance CR, Bowie LJ, Dohnal JC, Farrell EE, Neerhof MG. Amniotic fluid lamellar body count: a rapid and reliable fetal lung maturity test. Obstet Gynecol 1995;86:235–239 (Level II-2)

19. Mahony BS, Bowie JD, Killam AP, Kay HH, Cooper C. Epiphyseal ossification centers in the assessment of fetal maturity: sonographic correlation with the amniocentesis lung profile. Radiology 1986;159:521–524 (Level II-3)

20. Goldstein I, Lockwood C, Belanger K, Hobbins J. Ultrasonographic assessment of gestational age with the distal, femoral and proximal tibial ossification centers in the third trimester. Am J Obstet Gynecol 1988;158:127–130 (Level II-3)

21. Tahilramaney MP, Platt LD, Golde SH. Use of femur length measured by ultrasonography to predict fetal maturity. J Perinatol 1991;11:157–160 (Level II-3)

22. Kjos SL, Walther FJ, Montoro M, Paul RH, Diaz F, Stabler M. Prevalence and etiology of respiratory distress in infants of diabetic mothers: predictive value of fetal lung maturation tests. Am J Obstet Gynecol 1990;163:898–903 (Level II-3)

23. Effect of corticosteroids for fetal maturation on perinatal outcomes. NIH Consens Statement 1994 Feb 28–Mar 2; 12(2):1–24 (Level III)

24. Garite TJ, Freeman RK, Nageotte MP. Fetal maturity cascade: a rapid and cost-effective method for fetal lung maturity testing. Obstet Gynecol 1986;67:619–622 (Level II-3)

25. Herbert WNP, Chapman JF. Clinical and economic considerations associated with testing for fetal lung maturity. Am J Obstet Gynecol 1986;155:820–823 (Level II-3)

26. Ojomo EO, Coustan DR. Absence of evidence of pulmonary maturity at amniocentesis in term infants of diabetic mothers. Am J Obstet Gynecol 1990;163:954–957 (Level II-3)

The references in this bulletin are graded according to the method outlined by the U.S. Preventive Services Task Force:

- I Evidence obtained from at least one properly designed randomized controlled trial
- II-1 Evidence obtained from well-designed controlled trials without randomization
- II-2 Evidence obtained from well-designed cohort or case–control analytic studies, preferably from more than one center or research group
- II-3 Evidence obtained from multiple time series, with or without intervention, or dramatic results in uncontrolled experiments
- III Opinions of respected authorities, based on clinical experience, descriptive studies, or reports of expert committees

Other publications from ACOG:

- **Committee Opinions**, focused updates on emerging areas
- **Practice Patterns**, evidence-based guidelines
- **Criteria Sets**, baseline guidelines for review of diagnostic and management procedures

ISSN 1074-8628

The American College of Obstetricians and Gynecologists
409 12th Street, SW
PO Box 96920
Washington, DC 20090-6920

12345/09876

Number 199—November 1994
(Replaces #78, July 1984)

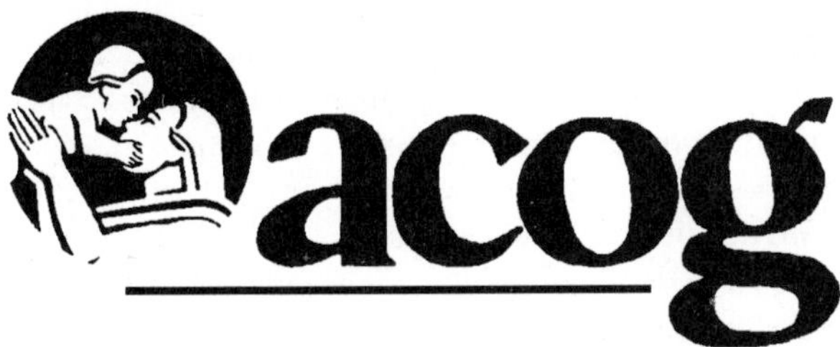

Technical Bulletin

An Educational Aid to Obstetrician–Gynecologists

Blood Component Therapy

Technologic advances have made it possible to separate a unit of whole blood into its various components. Thus, each donated unit can yield erythrocytes (red blood cells, or RBCs) plus one or two other components, such as platelets, cryoprecipitate, or fresh frozen plasma (FFP). Advances in the use of blood components have made whole blood transfusions necessary much less frequently. The use of blood components, rather than whole blood, is usually a better treatment option because it provides only the specific component needed. Furthermore, the use of blood components helps to conserve blood resources, because the various components from a single unit of donated blood can be used to treat several patients.

Technique

Blood Bank

The development of plastic bags has made component therapy possible. The bags are manufactured as closed, connected containers, thus allowing the various blood components to be separated by differential centrifugation without risk of bacterial contamination.

Blood components are available in virtually all blood centers throughout the United States, and 70–90% of donated units can be separated into one or more components. The blood components used most widely are listed in Table 1.

TABLE 1. INDICATIONS FOR ADMINISTRATION OF VARIOUS BLOOD PRODUCTS

Product	Content	Acceptable Indication	Unacceptable Indication
Red blood cells	Red cells	To increase oxygen-carrying capacity in anemic women For orthostatic hypotension secondary to blood loss	For volume expansion In place of a hematinic To enhance wound healing To improve general well-being
Platelet concentrates	Platelets	To control or prevent bleeding associated with deficiencies in platelet number or function	In patients with immune thrombocytopenic purpura (unless bleeding is life threatening) Prophylactically with massive blood transfusion
Fresh frozen plasma	Plasma, clotting factors	To increase the level of clotting factors in patients with demonstrated deficiency	For volume expansion As a nutritional supplement Prophylactically with massive blood transfusion
Cryoprecipitate	Factors I, V, VIII, XIII, von Willebrand factor, fibronectin	To increase the level of clotting factors in patients with demonstrated deficiency of fibrinogen, factor VIII, factor XIII, fibronectin, or von Willebrand factor	Prophylactically with massive blood transfusion

Administration

Correct identification of each unit of blood is critical. Physicians and nurses should exercise extreme care in identifying blood products when transfusion is initiated. A second individual should check the identification of each unit before it is transfused.

Warming blood components is rarely needed. However, if the rate of administration exceeds 50 ml/kg/h, the risk of developing transfusion-induced cardiac hypothermia increases. The presence of cold agglutinin disease is another indication for warming. When blood components must be warmed, an in-line blood warmer equipped with a monitoring system should be used. Both coil-in-water and electric bag-warming devices are available.

All blood products should be administered through a filter designed to remove debris. Standard filters are incorporated into straight and Y-type blood administration sets. Leukocyte-depleting filters, which remove 99.9% of the leukocytes, are also available. The use of leukocyte filters may prevent febrile, nonhemolytic transfusion reactions and also lower the risk of cytomegalovirus infections. If an RBC leukocyte-depleting filter is used for platelet transfusion, most of the platelets also will be removed.

Only normal saline should be infused through the same line as blood or blood components. Crystalloid solutions other than 0.9% saline may cause agglutination or hemolysis or both, and calcium-containing solutions will cause the blood to clot in the tubing. Medications should not be added to a unit of blood or blood product because it is difficult to know in advance if a drug will interact with a component. Also, if a reaction should occur, it is difficult to assess whether it is drug or transfusion related. Finally, if the transfusion is stopped, the patient will not receive the full dose of medication.

Components

Erythrocytes

Erythrocytes are available both as packed RBCs and whole blood. The only indication for the administration of RBCs is to increase oxygen-carrying capacity in anemic patients (1) and orthostatic hypotension secondary to blood loss (Table 1). Oxygen-carrying capacity is met for most women by a hemoglobin (Hgb) of 7 g/dl (a hematocrit [Hct] of approximately 21%) or less when the intravascular volume produces adequate perfusion. Transfusion with RBCs may be appropriate when the Hgb level is 7–10 g/dl if there is ongoing, active bleeding; during surgery, if there are signs or symptoms of decreased oxygen-carrying capacity (chronic lung or cardiovascular disease); in cases of decreased erythropoiesis; or when autologous blood will be used. Each unit of transfused RBCs will increase the Hgb by approximately 1 g/dl (and increase Hct by 1–3%) in a 70-kg (154-lb) woman.

When the etiology of anemia indicates that the anemia can be treated (eg, iron, folate, or vitamin B_{12} deficiency), specific replacement therapy should be used before transfusion is considered.

With the availability of component therapy, the need for and availability of whole blood has decreased. For almost all types of hemorrhagic shock, packed RBCs and volume expansion with crystalloid solutions (normal saline and lactated Ringer's injection) serve as adequate substitutes for whole blood. Packed RBCs are the treatment of choice for acute hemorrhage. Packed RBCs and FFP combined in a ratio of 4 to 1 yields very satisfactory results. When the total blood loss exceeds 25% of the blood volume, it is appropriate to administer whole blood. However, packed RBCs and FFP are very effective if only components are available.

Packed RBCs and whole blood are prepared in volumes of 200–250 ml and 450 ml, respectively, and contain citrate–phosphate–dextrose or citrate–phosphate–dextrose adenine-1 as a preservative. The shelf life is 21–35 days when citrate–phosphate–dextrose is used and 35 days with citrate–phosphate–dextrose adenine-1. Packed RBCs usually have an Hct of 70%, and thus this product has a relatively high viscosity. If rapid infusion is required, the packed cells should be mixed with 200 ml of normal saline through a Y infusion set immediately before administration. When stored for more than 24 hours, both products have few platelets and granulocytes and decreased levels of the labile plasma coagulation factors.

It may be advantageous to freeze RBCs if the blood type is rare or if many units will be required for an autologous donation. Frozen RBCs are prepared by adding glycerol to blood that is less than 5 days old. The RBCs are then frozen and stored at -80°C for up to 3 years. When needed, the cells are thawed and washed. Because of the time required to thaw and wash frozen cells, this product is not available on an emergency basis. Also, because of the open technique used during washing, the cells must be discarded if not used within 24 hours.

Platelet Concentrates

Platelet transfusions are administered to control or prevent bleeding associated with a deficiency in either the number or function of platelets (2). Prophylactic platelet transfusion may be indicated for women with platelet counts less than 20×10^9/L (20,000/mm^3). Transfusion also may be indicated for platelet counts of 10×10^9/L to 50×10^9/L (10,000–50,000/mm^3) if an operative procedure is planned, if there is active bleeding, or if massive transfusion is anticipated. When the count is greater than 50×10^9/L (50,000/mm^3) and an operative procedure is planned, prophylactic transfusion is unlikely to be beneficial, except when there is systemic bleeding or bleeding because of additional coagulation defects, sepsis, or platelet dysfunction related to medication or disease.

Platelets are prepared in a volume of 40 ml containing 55×10^9 platelets and have a shelf life of 3–5 days at 20–24°C. Small amounts of RBCs are present in platelet concentrates, and if ABO and CDE (Rh) type-specific platelets are not available, a D-negative woman can be sensitized by D-positive platelets. Under these circumstances, sensitization can be prevented by administration of anti-D prophylaxis. One 300-μg dose of D (Rho [D]) immune globulin is needed for every 15 ml of RBCs. A pooled unit of four volumes of platelets could have as much as 2 ml of RBCs, so one dose (or a minidose) should suffice. Similarly, platelet concentrates contain leukocytes and should be irradiated if they are to be used in immunocompromised patients.

One unit of platelet concentrate will usually increase the count of a 70-kg (154-lb) woman by 5×10^9/L to 10×10^9/L (5,000–10,000/mm^3). Thus, the usual dosage is one unit per 10 kg of body weight. The increase will be smaller if the patient has disseminated intravascular coagulation, thrombotic thrombocytopenic purpura, sepsis, hypersplenism, or the presence of anti-platelet antibodies. Platelets should always be administered through a blood filter.

Single-donor platelets (apheresis platelets) can be prepared. A 2–3-hour apheresis gives the same number of platelets as six to eight units of random donor blood. This technique is usually reserved for patients in whom antiplatelet antibodies are present and a donor matched for human leukocyte antigens has been identified.

Platelet transfusions should not be used prophylactically with massive blood transfusion. A massive transfusion is the replacement of one or more blood volumes within 24 hours (10 units in a 70-kg [154-lb] person). The addition of specific coagulation factors (I, V, and VIII) should be based on clinical and laboratory observations. Testing of prothrombin time, partial thromboplastin time, and thrombin time should be performed after the administration of every 5–10 units of blood. Additional components should be ordered on the basis of the values observed. Usually, platelets and FFP will correct the abnormalities encountered.

Fresh Frozen Plasma

Fresh frozen plasma should only be administered when patients have a demonstrated clotting factor deficiency or when a specific factor concentrate is not available (3). It is especially useful in treating multiple factor deficiency as seen with liver disease, disseminated intravascular coagulation, massive transfusion, and sodium warfarin administration. It is also useful in treating antithrombin III deficiency, thrombotic thrombocytopenic purpura, and hemolytic uremic syndrome.

Fresh frozen plasma is prepared in a volume of 200–250 ml; each unit contains one unit of each coagulation factor and will increase any clotting factor by 2–3% in a 70-kg (154-lb) woman. It should only be used to increase clotting factors in patients with a demonstrated deficiency of factor II, V, VII, IX, X, or XI or multifactor deficiency such as that seen in liver disease or disseminated intravascular coagulation. As infection-free single-factor products become available, they will be preferable to FFP. If the prothrombin time or partial thromboplastin time is less than 1.5 times normal (usually more than 55–60 seconds), FFP is rarely indicated. The usual starting dose is two bags of FFP. It should not be used for volume expansion, as a nutritional supplement, or prophylactically with massive blood transfusion. Alternative colloid solutions for volume expansion are albumin, hydroxyethyl starch, dextran, and purified protein fractions. Fresh frozen plasma is useful under circumstances of massive blood loss when coagulation studies are not available.

As is true for platelet transfusion, coagulation studies including a prothrombin time and partial thromboplastin time should be obtained after the administration of every 5–10 units of blood. Additional component therapy should be administered on the basis of the results observed.

Cryoprecipitate

Cryoprecipitate is concentrated from FFP into a volume of 10–15 ml. The precipitate contains factor VIII, von Willebrand factor, fibrinogen, factor XIII, and fibronectin and is indicated for the treatment of demonstrated deficiencies of one of these factors (4). It also allows for the replacement of specific clotting factors without administering large volumes of fluid. For hypofibrinogenemia, a dose of one bag of cryoprecipitate per 5 kg of body weight will bring the fibrinogen level above 100 mg/dl. Additional doses depend on the rate of fibrinogen degradation and should be based on periodic measurements of the fibrinogen level. For von Willebrand disease, the standard dosage is one bag of cryoprecipitate per 10 kg of body weight daily. As with FFP, it should not be used prophylactically in cases of massive blood transfusion. If a coagulopathy is present and laboratory studies are not yet available, FFP should be used empirically.

Adverse Effects

Infection, alloimmunization, and transfusion reaction are the major complications associated with the transfusion of blood components. Table 2 summarizes the current

TABLE 2. CURRENT ESTIMATE OF TRANSFUSION RISKS*

Complication	Risk/Unit Transfused
Infection	
Hepatitis B	1:50,000
Hepatitis C	1:3,300
HIV-1, -2	1:150,000–1:1,000,000
HTLV-I, -II	1:50,000
Fatal transfusion reaction	1:100,000

*HIV indicates human immunodeficiency virus; HTLV, human T cell-lymphotropic virus.

level of risk (5, 6). A relationship has been demonstrated among risk, the number of units transfused, and the geographic location of donors. While hepatitis and human immunodeficiency virus (HIV) are of greatest concern, a variety of other infections can be blood borne. However, the risk of a transfusion-acquired infection for blood-borne infections other than hepatitis and HIV is less than 1:1,000,000. Cytomegalovirus infection is a significant threat only to immunocompromised individuals. Because of the fetal immune status, cytomegalovirus-negative blood should be used for all intrauterine transfusions and all transfusions of undelivered parturients. Additional, less serious effects include allergic reactions, febrile reactions, and circulatory overload.

An acute, hemolytic reaction occurs once for every 6,000 units transfused and carries a mortality rate of about 1:17 (7). Most acute hemolytic reactions are secondary to ABO incompatibility, which leads to intravascular hemolysis. Classic signs and symptoms include chills, fever, chest and flank pain, nausea, cardiovascular collapse, and the development of disseminated intravascular coagulation. Febrile nonhemolytic reactions are usually due to recipient antibodies against leukocyte and platelet antigens. Most patients respond to antipyretic medication, but use of leukocyte-reduced components may be required if repeated febrile reactions occur. Hemolytic reactions also occur with other blood groups such as Kidd (Jk^a), Duffy (Fy^a), and Kell. These are usually extravascular and are associated with fever, anemia, hyperbilirubinemia, and a positive direct Coombs antiglobulin test. Many of these reactions will be delayed, occurring approximately 7–10 days after blood administration.

Use of Autologous Blood

Autologous transfusion is the collection and reinfusion of the patient's own blood. Since most planned surgical procedures do not result in the loss of large amounts of blood, autologous strategies are not appropriate for all patients. Three techniques of autologous transfusion are available: preoperative autologous blood donation, intraoperative blood salvage, and acute normovolemic hemodilution (8).

Preoperative Autologous Blood Donation

If a patient is likely to require transfusion during or after surgery or delivery, a preoperative donation may be appropriate. Blood should be donated at least 2 weeks prior to surgery or delivery, and the patient must have an adequate RBC mass (Hgb of 11 g/dl or more or Hct of 34% or more). If large amounts of blood will be required and time allows, frozen cells can be used.

Several studies have demonstrated the safety of autologous donation during pregnancy (9, 10). However, so few parturients require transfusion during or after delivery that routine donation should not be encouraged. Placenta previa is one obstetric condition for which autologous donation may be appropriate (11, 12). The minimum criteria for donation are an Hgb of 11.0 g/dl and an Hct of 34%.

Many patients can donate as frequently as every 3 days, although once a week is more common. The patient should be given a therapeutic dose of oral iron (ferrous sulfate, ferrous gluconate, or ferrous fumarate) prior to and during donation. The risks of autologous donation are minor; vasovagal reactions occur in about 2–5% of all donors.

The indications for autologous transfusion are the same as those for RBC transfusion. Unused autologous units may be destroyed or released to the homologous blood pool depending on local and U.S. Food and Drug Administration policy. Even when transferred to the homologous pool, autologous blood has little impact on the overall blood supply, and transferability should not be used as a rationale for encouraging patients to donate autologous units if there is little likelihood that transfusion will be needed.

Intraoperative Blood Salvage

Intraoperative blood salvage is the sterile collection and reinfusion of shed blood. Contraindications include infection and contamination with malignant cells. The safety of intraoperative salvage in situations such as ruptured ectopic pregnancy and cesarean delivery has yet to be established.

Intraoperative salvage is usually accomplished with a semicontinuous flow centrifugation device that washes cells as they are collected. Disposable suction systems are also available for collecting and anticoagulating cells. The RBCs are collected in sterile plastic bags, washed and concentrated by standard blood banking techniques outside the operating room, and then reinfused by gravity. Semiautomatic systems that also wash the RBCs before reinfusion are also available. Proper and safe use of these instruments requires a trained operator who has no other responsibility in the operating room.

Acute Normovolemic Hemodilution

Acute normovolemic hemodilution is the removal of blood immediately before or after the induction of anesthesia. Crystalloid solution is administered simultaneously to maintain normovolemia. At the end of surgery, the patient's RBCs are reinfused. The procedure is usually performed by an anesthesiologist; the number of units removed is determined by the anticipated blood loss and the patient's size.

Because patients have a lower Hct during surgery, fewer RBCs are lost. Additional suggested benefits include the availability of fresh whole blood and decreased blood viscosity leading to better tissue perfusion and oxygenation. Additional studies are required to document the safety and benefits of this procedure.

Summary

Component therapy is the standard method for most transfusion needs and has made the use of whole blood rarely necessary. By giving only the specific component that is needed, blood component therapy usually provides better treatment. Because blood and blood products are in short supply and most carry some risk of infection, the National Institutes of Health guidelines for the use of each component should be followed closely. When significant blood loss is anticipated, autologous predonation should be considered and discussed with the patient.

REFERENCES

1. National Institutes of Health. Office of Medical Applications of Research. Perioperative red blood cell transfusion. JAMA 1988;260:2700–2703
2. National Institutes of Health. Office of Medical Applications of Research. Platelet transfusion therapy. JAMA 1987;257:1777–1780
3. National Institutes of Health. Office of Medical Applications of Research. Fresh–frozen plasma: indications and risks. JAMA 1985;253:551–553
4. Ness PM, Perkins HA. Cryoprecipitate as a reliable source of fibrinogen replacement. JAMA 1979;241:1690–1691
5. Dodd RY. Will blood products be free of infectious agents? In: Nance SJ, ed. Transfusion medicine in the 1990s. Arlington, Virginia: American Association of Blood Banks, 1990:223–251
6. Cumming PD, Wallace EL, Schorr JB, Dodd RY. Exposure of patients to human immunodeficiency virus through the transfusion of blood components that test anti-body-negative. N Engl J Med 1989;321:941–946
7. Sazama K. Reports of 355 transfusion-associated deaths: 1976 through 1985. Transfusion 1990;30:583–590
8. National Heart, Lung, and Blood Institute. National Blood Resource Education Program Expert Panel. The use of autologous blood. JAMA 1990;263:414–417
9. Kruskall MS. Controversies in transfusion medicine: the safety and utility of autologous donation by pregnant patients: pro. Transfusion 1990;30:694–695
10. McVay PA, Hoag RW, Hoag MS, Toy PTCY. Safety and use of autologous blood donation during the third trimester of pregnancy. Am J Obstet Gynecol 1989;160:1479–1488
11. Combs CA, Murphy EL, Laros RK Jr. Factors associated with postpartum hemorrhage with vaginal birth. Obstet Gynecol 1991;77:69–76
12. Combs CA, Murphy EL, Laros RK Jr. Factors associated with hemorrhage in cesarean deliveries. Obstet Gynecol 1991;77:77–82

SUGGESTED READING

College of American Pathologists. Practice parameter for the use of fresh–frozen plasma, cryoprecipitate, and platelets. JAMA 1994;271:777–781

Stehling L, Simon TL. The red blood cell transfusion trigger. Physiology and clinical studies. Arch Pathol Lab Med 1994;118:429–434

This Technical Bulletin was developed under the direction of the Committee on Technical Bulletins of the American College of Obstetricians and Gynecologists as an educational aid to obstetricians and gynecologists. The committee wishes to thank Russell K. Laros, Jr, MD, for his assistance in the development of this bulletin. This Technical Bulletin does not define a standard of care, nor is it intended to dictate an exclusive course of management. It presents recognized methods and techniques of clinical practice for consideration by obstetrician–gynecologists for incorporation into their practices. Variations of practice taking into account the needs of the individual patient, resources, and limitations unique to the institution or type of practice may be appropriate.
ISSN 1074-8628

THE AMERICAN COLLEGE OF OBSTETRICIANS AND GYNECOLOGISTS
409 12th Street, SW
Washington, DC 20024-2188

12345/87654

ACOG EDUCATIONAL BULLETIN

Number 258, July 2000

Breastfeeding: Maternal and Infant Aspects

Breastfeeding rates decreased significantly in the past half century as formula feeding gained popularity. In 1971, only 24.7% of mothers left the hospital breastfeeding. Recently, breastfeeding initiation rates have been increasing, reaching 64.3% in 1998, according to the Mothers' Survey (Ross Products Division, Abbott Laboratories, Inc., Columbus, Ohio). These increases reflect a growing awareness of the advantages of breast milk over formula. Improvement in breastfeeding initiation rates, however, has been uneven, as women attempt to overcome practical obstacles.

Evidence continues to mount regarding the value of breastfeeding for both women and their infants. Human milk provides developmental, nutritional, and immunologic benefits to the infant that cannot be duplicated by formula feeding. Breastfeeding also provides significant benefits to women. It is critical that women be prepared to make an informed choice in deciding what is best for them, their families, and their babies. Obstetrician–gynecologists and other health professionals caring for pregnant women should regularly impart accurate information about breastfeeding to expectant mothers and be prepared to support them should any problems arise while breastfeeding.

This document will focus primarily on breastfeeding by healthy mothers with healthy infants born at term. Human milk and breastfeeding are recommended for premature newborns and mother–infant pairs with other special needs; however, specific information in this regard is beyond the scope of this document.

This Educational Bulletin was developed under the direction of the Committees on Health Care for Underserved Women and Obstetric Practice of the American College of Obstetricians and Gynecologists. The college wishes to thank John T. Queenan, MD, for his assistance in the development of this bulletin. This document is not to be construed as establishing a standard of practice or dictating an exclusive course of treatment. Rather, it is intended as an educational tool that presents current information on obstetric–gynecologic issues.

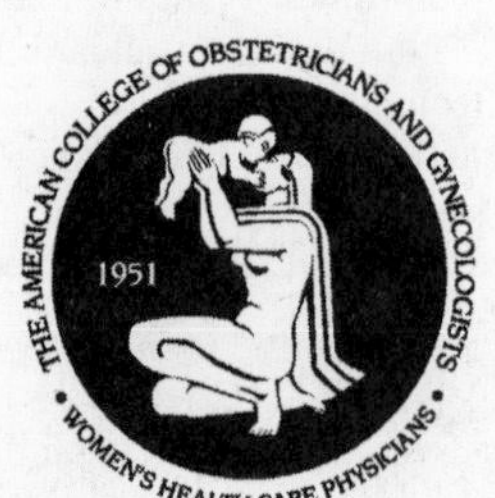

Benefits of Breastfeeding

Research in the United States and throughout the world indicates that breastfeeding and human milk provide benefits to infants, women, families, and society. These studies have been done in a variety of settings, resulting in information derived from culturally and economically diverse populations.

Infants

The benefits of breastfeeding for the infant have been established in the following areas. Human milk provides species-specific and age-specific nutrients for the infant (1). Colostrum, the fluid secreted immediately following the infant's birth, conveys a high level of immune protection, particularly secretory immunoglobulin A (IgA). During the first 4–7 days following delivery, protein and mineral concentrations decrease and water, fat, and lactose increase. Milk composition continues to change to match infant nutritional needs. In addition to the right balance of nutrients and immunologic factors, human milk contains factors that act as biologic signals for promoting cellular growth and differentiation. It also contains multiple substances with antimicrobial properties, which protect against infection (1, 2). Human milk alone, however, may not provide adequate iron for premature newborns, infants whose mothers have low iron stores, and infants older than 6 months.

In 1997, the American Academy of Pediatrics (AAP) published a policy statement, "Breastfeeeding and the Use of Human Milk" (3). The statement was developed by the AAP Work Group on Breastfeeding, which evaluated the research literature on relationships between breastfeeding and infant health and development. The statement's summary paragraph (see the box below) on established infant protective effects, as well as positive associations (which require further study), is well referenced. Obstetrician–gynecologists who review these sources of evidence for infant benefit will be better prepared to care for the women in their practices.

Women

The benefits of breastfeeding for women are well documented. During the immediate postpartum period, the oxytocin released during milk let-down causes increased uterine contractions and lessens maternal blood loss (4). Evidence exists that the hormones of lactation (oxytocin and prolactin) contribute to feelings of relaxation and attachment (5). Breastfeeding is associated with a decreased risk of developing ovarian and premenopausal breast cancer (6, 7). Breastfeeding also delays postpartum ovulation, supporting birth spacing (8–10). Although breastfeeding causes some bone demineralization, studies indicate that "catch-up" remineralization occurs following weaning; some studies also show a lower incidence of osteoporosis and hip fracture after menopause (11, 12). The incidence of pregnancy-induced long-term obesity also is reduced (13).

There are psychologic benefits as well. A woman who breastfeeds her baby is able to take advantage of the natural dynamics of nurturing and bonding.

Research on Established and Potential Protective Effects of Human Milk and Breastfeeding on Infants

Research in the United States, Canada, Europe and other developed countries, among predominantly middle-class populations, provides strong evidence that human milk feeding decreases the incidence and/or severity of diarrhea, lower respiratory infection, otitis media, bacteremia, bacterial meningitis, botulism, urinary tract infection, and necrotizing enterocolitis. There are a number of studies that show a possible protective effect of human milk feeding against sudden infant death syndrome, insulin-dependent diabetes mellitus, Crohn's disease, ulcerative colitis, lymphoma, allergic diseases, and other chronic digestive diseases. Breastfeeding has also been related to possible enhancement of cognitive development.

American Academy of Pediatrics, Work Group on Breastfeeding. Breastfeeding and the use of human milk. Pediatrics 100;1997: 1035–1039 (Paragraph includes 39 citations.)

Families and Society

Studies indicate that the breastfed child has fewer illnesses and, therefore, fewer visits to the doctor and hospital (14). This translates into less absenteeism from work for the mother and lower medical expenses. The improvement in work productivity may be significant for society as well, because women now constitute a large portion of the workforce. More than 60% of all women return to outside employment during the first year following birth of a child.

Breastfeeding, while demanding maternal time and attention, can save individual families and society considerable money compared with formula feeding (15). On a national scale, disposal of formula cans, bottles, and bottle liners may be an ecologic consideration.

Obstacles to Breastfeeding

Women need to know that breastfeeding, like other aspects of having a new baby, may be demanding as well as rewarding. They should be assured that they will have support and that there are options for problem solving and for addressing the practical obstacles they may face. Some women will decide the challenges outweigh the benefits for themselves and their babies, given the overall circumstances of their lives. However, physicians and other health professionals should recognize the potential effectiveness of applying their knowledge and skills to encourage and support women in initiating and continuing breastfeeding.

Modern society creates some of the obstacles to breastfeeding. Short hospital stays make the teaching of breastfeeding a challenge. Lack of spousal or partner support and family custom may discourage breastfeeding. Having to return to work is an obstacle, which is being diminished for some women as more employers learn that encouraging breastfeeding as a policy improves employee morale and decreases absenteeism (16, 17). An unfriendly social environment may make it difficult to breastfeed in public. The effect of these obstacles can be mitigated by educating the families, employers, and society. All share in the benefits and, through positive attitudes and workplace and public policies, also can support women who are willing to breastfeed.

Who Can Breastfeed

Breastfeeding is a natural function; nearly every woman can breastfeed her child. Mother and newborn can more easily learn the basics and how to deal with the challenges if they have skilled and experienced support. Mothers who have cesarean deliveries should be reassured that they can breastfeed their newborns as well as those women having vaginal deliveries. Specific infections such as endometritis or mastitis are not contraindications to breastfeeding.

Women with structural problems such as hypoplastic or tubular breasts may have difficulty producing sufficient milk. True inverted nipples are rare but generally preclude nursing; most women with nipples that appear flat or inverted can breastfeed, given appropriate assistance in the early days of lactation. Pumping for a minute or two before offering the breast to the newborn has been shown to facilitate latch-on (1). Lactation is not possible for women who have had breast surgery involving the complete severing of the lactiferous ducts. However, some women may breastfeed after reduction mammoplasty or augmentation mammoplasty with implants, and most women can breastfeed after breast biopsies.

Mothers with premature infants also can breastfeed. A mother's milk has specific properties that match the needs of her premature newborn. However, nutrition requirements for the premature newborn are different and require special attention. Some babies with cleft lips or palate may be able to breastfeed. The soft breast tissue may fill the defect and enable the infant to develop a seal. Sometimes a palatal obturator allows the infant to breastfeed and not aspirate milk. A newborn that is premature or has other special needs may benefit from breastfeeding but requires individual evaluation by appropriate experts.

Who Should Not Breastfeed

Although it is true that most women can breastfeed, there are exceptions. These exceptions should be understood by all clinicians so that a patient's frustration and disappointment can be minimized. The number of contraindications is small (18). Women who should not breastfeed are those who:

- Take street drugs or do not control alcohol use
- Have an infant with galactosemia
- Are infected with the human immunodeficiency virus (HIV)
- Have active, untreated tuberculosis
- Take certain medications
- Are undergoing treatment for breast cancer (1)

Women who use illegal drugs should not breastfeed because it is unknown which agent or how much of the agent the infant will be exposed to. Alcohol is a toxin, so a breastfeeding woman should minimize or avoid it, and a mother who drinks significant amounts of alcohol should not breastfeed (2).

Infants with galactosemia should neither breastfeed, because this will exacerbate the condition, nor consume any formula containing lactose (eg, cows' milk). They need special lactose-free formula.

Some infections contraindicate breastfeeding; others require precautions. Approaches to breastfeeding vary according to the infection and the environment. Comprehensive information about breastfeeding in relation to the following common maternal infections and others is available for further reference (1). Women in the United States who have HIV infections should not breastfeed because breast milk can carry HIV and pass the infection to the infant. In some countries with high infant mortality rates, however, the benefits of breastfeeding in providing nutrition and preventing infections may still outweigh the risks of transmitting HIV.

If a woman has active pulmonary tuberculosis, the repeated and prolonged close contact involved in feeding exposes the infant to risk of airborne infection. Therefore the woman should neither breastfeed nor bottle feed her newborn until she has been appropriately treated for at least 2 weeks and is otherwise considered to be noncontagious. The infant can be given the mother's expressed breast milk because it does not contain *Mycobacterium tuberculosis* (1).

Similarly, if a woman has varicella, she should be isolated from the infant and neither breastfeed nor bottle feed while she is clinically infectious. Once the infant has received varicella-zoster immune globulin (1), the woman can provide expressed breast milk for the infant if there are no skin lesions on the breasts. An immunocompetent woman who develops herpes zoster infection (shingles) can continue breastfeeding if lesions are covered and are not on the breast. Maternal antibodies delivered through the placenta and breast milk will prevent the disease or diminish its severity. An infant may be given varicella-zoster immune globulin in these circumstances as an added precaution (1).

Breastfeeding also is contraindicated in women who have active herpes simplex infections on the breast until the lesion is cleared. In women with cytomegalovirus infection, both the virus and maternal antibodies are present in breast milk. Because of the antibodies, otherwise healthy infants born at term with congenital or acquired cytomegalovirus infections usually do better if they are breastfed. A study of infants who developed infections during breastfeeding found the infants also developed an immune response, did not develop the disease, and rarely manifested symptoms (18).

Hepatitis infections do not preclude breastfeeding. With appropriate immunoprophylaxis, including hepatitis B immune globulin (HBIG) and hepatitis vaccine, breastfeeding of babies born to women positive for hepatitis B surface antigen poses no additional risk for the transmission of hepatitis B virus (19). If a woman has acute hepatitis A infection, her infant can breastfeed after receiving immune serum globulin and vaccine (1). The average rate of hepatitis C virus (HCV) infection reported in infants born to HCV-positive women is 4% for both breastfed and bottle-fed infants. Therefore maternal HCV is not considered a contraindication to breastfeeding (20).

Many medications are compatible with breastfeeding. The AAP Committee on Drugs reviewed the current data on the transfer of drugs and other chemicals in human milk. The committee classified drugs for safety in breastfeeding on a scale of 1 (contraindicated) to 6 (compatible) (21). Generally, breastfeeding is contraindicated for women taking antineoplastic, thyrotoxic, and immunosuppressive agents (Table 1) (19). Medications with relative contraindications may sometimes be used cautiously by timing doses to immediately follow a feeding.

Table 1. Medications Contraindicated During Breastfeeding

Medication	Reason
Bromocriptine	Suppresses lactation; may be hazardous to the mother
Cocaine	Cocaine intoxication
Cyclophosphamide	Possible immune suppression; unknown effect on growth or association with carcinogenesis; neutropenia
Cyclosporine	Possible immune suppression; unknown effect on growth or association with carcinogenesis
Doxorubicin*	Possible immune suppression; unknown effect on growth or association with carcinogenesis
Ergotamine	Vomiting, diarrhea, convulsions (at doses used in migraine medications)
Lithium	One third to one half of therapeutic blood concentration in infants
Methotrexate	Possible immune suppression; unknown effect on growth or association with carcinogenesis; neutropenia
Phencyclidine	Potent hallucinogen
Phenindione	Anticoagulant; increased prothrombin and partial thromboplastin time in one infant; not used in United States
Radioactive iodine and other radiolabeled elements	Contraindications to breastfeeding for various periods

*Medication is concentrated in human milk.

American Academy of Pediatrics, American College of Obstetricians and Gynecologists. Guidelines for perinatal care. 4th ed. Elk Grove Village, Illinois: AAP; Washington, DC: ACOG, 1997

Education on Breastfeeding

Teaching the pregnant woman and her partner about childbirth and breastfeeding is an integral part of good prenatal care. Other family members who could support breastfeeding may be included. Education can occur in the physician's office or clinic. Alternatively, hospitals and other organizations provide education for pregnant women and their partners. The advice and encouragement of the obstetrician–gynecologist are critical in making the decision to breastfeed. Other health professionals such as pediatricians, nurses, and certified lactation specialists play an important role, as do mother-to-mother groups and other lay organizations. The health benefits of breastfeeding warrant efforts in professional cooperation and coordination among all health care workers to educate and encourage women and their families to choose breastfeeding. Patient education materials can reinforce the message (see the boxes, "Patient Education Materials" and "References for Health Care Workers and Patients Seeking In-depth Information").

Some women who choose to breastfeed were breastfed themselves or had a sibling who was breastfed, which established it as normal behavior in their household. These women would probably benefit from some education and reinforcement concerning breastfeeding. Women whose family and friends have not shared breastfeeding experiences also approach pregnancy with a desire to do what is healthiest for their babies. Guidance and consideration of life situations are important in helping these women and their families make a decision about feeding their infants. Information about the benefits and challenges of breastfeeding compared with the use of formula will help them make good decisions. The obstetrician–gynecologist often

Patient Education Materials

Breast-feeding your baby. Patient Education Pamphlet AP029. Washington, DC: American College of Obstetricians and Gynecologists, 1997

Breastfeeding: loving support for a bright future. Q & A. Physicians' breastfeeding support kit. Tampa, Florida: Best Start Social Marketing, 1998

Working & breastfeeding. Can you do it? Yes, you can! Alexandria, Virginia: National Healthy Mothers, Healthy Babies Coalition, 1997

Ten steps to support parents' choice to breastfeed their baby. American Academy of Pediatrics Task Force on Breastfeeding. Elk Grove Village, Illinois: AAP, 1999

References for Health Care Workers and Patients Seeking In-depth Information

American Academy of Pediatrics and the American College of Obstetricians and Gynecologists. Guidelines for perinatal care. 4th ed. Elk Grove Village, Illinois: AAP, and Washington, DC: ACOG, 1997

American Academy of Pediatrics Committee on Drugs. The transfer of drugs and other chemicals into human milk. Pediatrics 1994;93:137–150.

American Academy of Pediatrics, Work Group on Breastfeeding. Breastfeeding and the use of human milk. Pediatrics 1997;100:1035–1039

ABM News and Views. The Newsletter of The Academy of Breastfeeding Medicine. Lenexa, Kansas: ABM

Lawrence RA. A review of the medical benefits and contraindications to breastfeeding in the United States. Maternal and Child Health Technical Information Bulletin. Arlington, Virginia: National Center for Education in Maternal and Child Health, 1997

Lawrence RA, Lawrence RM. Breastfeeding: a guide for the medical profession. 5th ed. St. Louis, Missouri: Mosby, 1999

U.S. Department of Health and Human Services, Health Resources & Services Administration, Maternal and Child Health Bureau, U.S. Department of Agriculture, Food and Nutrition Service. Physicians' breastfeeding support kit. Tampa, Florida: Best Start Social Marketing, 1998

can allay a woman's anxieties and suggest solutions or resources to make breastfeeding a practical choice for her and her family.

Periodic Gynecologic Examinations

Obstetrician–gynecologists can begin to educate women who have their reproductive lives ahead of them by mentioning breastfeeding during the breast examination portion of routine gynecologic visits, if appropriate. Women whose anatomy appears to be normal can be told that if they decide to have a baby, there are no structural impediments to breastfeeding.

First Obstetric Visit

The initial prenatal visit is the optimal time to encourage or reinforce the decision to breastfeed. It is also an ideal time to let the patient know the advantages of breastfeeding over formula feeding. Most patients seek information and guidance from their doctors. The importance of the physician's recommendation should never be underestimated. If a woman has not yet made a decision to breastfeed, this and subsequent visits may provide an opportunity for her to do so. During the breast examination, the physician can perform a breastfeeding-specific examination and answer any questions about the usual pattern of changes in the breasts during pregnancy and breastfeeding. If there are no structural problems, the woman can be reassured about her ability to breastfeed. If her nipples appear to be inverted, she should know that appearance is not necessarily prognostic and she may be able to breastfeed, but that techniques to assist in nipple eversion are not recommended during pregnancy because of the potential for stimulating contractions.

Antenatal Breastfeeding Instruction

In the past, when hospital stays were longer, women could receive fairly adequate education about breastfeeding before discharge. Today, with shorter hospital stays, it is imperative that pregnant women come to the hospital for delivery with a good foundation of knowledge gained during the antepartum period. Prenatal education groups have been shown to be particularly effective in increasing duration of breastfeeding (22). Education in the hospital can then focus on operational aspects of breastfeeding such as latch-on and feeding techniques.

The woman who is appropriately counseled on breastfeeding options and chooses not to breastfeed should be reassured that her milk production will abate during the first few days after delivery. Hormone treatment to stop milk production is no longer recommended. She should be treated with a well-fitted support bra, analgesics, and ice packs to relieve the pain. She also can be assured that if she changes her mind, she may still be able to initiate breastfeeding within the first few days.

Hospital Stay

Shortened hospital stays for childbirth have made the teaching of breastfeeding difficult. Certain protocols and practices, however, will increase rates of successful breastfeeding (see the box, "Ten Hospital Practices to Encourage and Support Breastfeeding") (23).

Delivery

The immediate postpartum period should allow the woman and her newborn to experience optimal bonding with immediate physical contact, preferably skin to skin. The initial feeding should occur as soon after birth as possible, preferably in the first hour when the baby is awake, alert, and ready to suck. Newborn eye prophylaxis, weighing, measuring, and other such examinations can be done after the feeding. Such procedures usually can be performed later in the woman's room.

Rooming-In

Today, all hospitals should make trained personnel available to provide breastfeeding support and should offer 24-hour rooming-in to maximize the interaction between the woman and her newborn. Separation of a breastfeeding woman and newborn should be avoided whenever possible. Most newborn care and procedures, including bathing, blood drawing, physical examinations, and administration of medication and phototherapy, can be performed in the mother's room. In this way, mother and baby can benefit together from the nursing care available (3).

The rooming-in experience allows a woman and her newborn to start the adjustment to a breastfeeding routine. Normally a newborn will show signs of hunger, such as increased alertness or activity, mouthing, or rooting. Crying is a late sign of hunger. Newborns should be nursed approximately 8–12 times every 24 hours until satiety; time at breast varies but may be 10 to 15 minutes on each breast (3).

Instruction

Hospital personnel should have adequate time allotted to each patient, no matter when the delivery occurs, and provide a specific program on practical aspects of breastfeeding that women master before discharge. Trained staff should assess breastfeeding behavior of the woman and newborn during the first 24–48 hours after birth for correct nursing positions, latch-on, and adequacy of newborn swallowing. They also should ensure that the woman is skilled in the technique of manual expression of milk (3).

Before discharge the woman should be educated about age-appropriate elimination patterns of her newborn during the first week after birth. At least six urinations per day and three to four stools per day are to be expected by 5–7 days of age. She can be shown how to keep simple records for the first few weeks, noting the frequency and length of feedings and the number of stools and wet diapers, for discussion with her care providers. She should understand expected patterns of newborn weight loss and gain (3). Before gaining, the breastfeeding newborn may lose 5–7% of birth weight in the first week. When the loss is greater than 5–7% or reaches that level in the first 3 days, a clinician should evaluate the breastfeeding process to address any problems before they become serious. A loss of up to 10% is the maximum acceptable. Follow-up should confirm that the newborn is beginning to regain weight after the first week (1).

Ten Hospital Practices to Encourage and Support Breastfeeding*

- Maintain a written breastfeeding policy that is communicated to all health care staff.
- Train all pertinent health care staff in skills necessary to implement this policy.
- Inform all pregnant women about the benefits of breastfeeding.
- Offer all mothers the opportunity to initiate breastfeeding within 1 hour of birth.
- Show breastfeeding mothers how to breastfeed and how to maintain lactation even if they are separated from their infants.
- Give breastfeeding infants only breast milk unless medically indicated.
- Facilitate rooming-in; encourage all mothers and infants to remain together during their hospital stay.
- Encourage unrestricted breastfeeding when baby exhibits hunger cues or signals or on request of mother.
- Encourage exclusive suckling at the breast by providing no pacifiers or artificial nipples.
- Refer mothers to established breastfeeding and mother's support groups and services, and foster the establishment of those services when they are not available.

*The 1994 report of the Healthy Mothers, Healthy Babies National Coalition Expert Work Group recommended that the UNICEF-WHO Baby Friendly Hospital Initiative be adapted for use in the United States as the United States Breastfeeding Health Initiative, using the adapted 10 steps above.

Randolph L, Cooper L, Fonseca-Becker F, York M, McIntosh M. Baby Friendly Hospital Initiative feasibility study: final report. Healthy Mothers, Healthy Babies National Coalition Expert Work Group. Alexandria, Virginia: HMHB, 1994

Latch-On

Breastfeeding should not be painful, but minor discomfort is common during the first 2 weeks. Painful breastfeeding almost always results from poor positioning or latch-on, which should be immediately corrected. ACOG's "Breast-feeding Your Baby" pamphlet is an example of a resource that can be used to help women with positioning and latch-on (24). Discomfort may occur temporarily as the woman's milk supply is beginning to be established. Any significant pain or tenderness should be assessed promptly by a physician.

Latch-on is one of the most important steps to successful breastfeeding. There are several helpful approaches, including gently stroking the newborn's lower lip with the nipple to get the baby to open his or her mouth wide, or gently pulling the newborn's chin down. The newborn should take a large amount of breast into his or her mouth, generally an inch or more of the areola with the nipple pointing toward the soft palate. The mother may hold her breast to facilitate this position, using a hand position comfortable for her. The nipple and the areola elongate into a teat, and the baby's tongue should be slightly cupped beneath it. The mother should adopt a comfortable position and draw the baby to the breast. The newborn should be held close, facing the mother, with his chin and the tip of his nose touching but not completely occluded by the breast. Usually, it is wise to alternate the breast used to initiate the feeding and to equalize the time spent at each breast over the day. The mother can break the suction by gently inserting her finger in the newborn's mouth before taking him off the breast.

Home

All breastfeeding women and their babies who are discharged from the hospital in less than 48 hours after delivery should be seen by a pediatrician or other knowledgeable health care practitioner when the baby is 2–4 days old. This is important in order to evaluate health status of the newborn (eg, weight, hydration, and hyperbilirubinemia) at this critical age, as well as to observe the woman and newborn during breastfeeding (3).

Women can be reassured that eating a well-balanced diet generally will provide the nutrients their infants need. On average, it is estimated that women will need approximately 500 kcal per day more than nonpregnant and nonlactating recommended levels, and the additional maternal food intake generally will provide additional needed vitamins and minerals (with the possible exceptions of calcium and zinc). Women of childbearing age need to maintain a calcium intake of 1,000 mg per day at all times, including during pregnancy and lactation (1,300 for adolescents through 18 years of age). Dietary intake is the preferred source of all needed nutrients. However, many women breastfeed on a lower calorie intake level than suggested, consuming bodily stores instead. This will result in gradual weight loss and is not likely to affect breastfeeding, but further questions may need to be asked about sources of magnesium, vitamin B_6, folate, calcium, and zinc (2, 25, 26). Corrective measures can be suggested for improving nutrient intakes of women with restrictive eating patterns (2). Women should be encouraged to drink plenty of fluids to satisfy their thirst and maintain adequate hydration. They need not avoid certain foods (spicy or strong flavored) because of breastfeeding unless the infant seems to react negatively to specific foods.

The spouse or partner can play a vital support role for the breastfeeding woman by encouraging her, bringing the newborn to her for feeding, changing the newborn, and holding the newborn. Couples may find that caring for a baby can complicate their own relationship, including a desired resumption of sexual intercourse. They may be encouraged to discuss emotional adjustments to their new family status as well as physical problems of soreness, fatigue, and vaginal dryness secondary to lactation. When a woman is ready to resume sexual intercourse, prelubricated latex condoms can be recommended to prevent infection and ease vaginal dryness.

Phone-In Resource

The departure of a woman and her newborn from the hospital can be a joyous but daunting experience. The family is now responsible for the care and feeding of the newborn. Whether or not they have a support system at home, a phone-in resource is needed for ongoing instruction and advice. The obstetrician–gynecologist's office, the place where the woman has received most of her care, should be that resource or at least provide links to other resources in the community, such as lactation specialists and support groups.

Contraception

Women should be encouraged to consider their future plans for additional childbearing during prenatal care and be given information and services that will help them meet their goals. This is especially important for a woman who breastfeeds, because there are fewer variables in her nutrition status if the next pregnancy is delayed until she has completed breastfeeding.

In nonbreastfeeding women, the average time to first ovulation is 45 days (range, 25–72 days) (27). Many women resume intercourse well before they return for their postpartum checkup, thus some women are at risk of becoming pregnant.

For breastfeeding women, however, the situation is different. Exclusive breastfeeding helps prevent pregnancy for the first 6 months after delivery, but should be relied on only temporarily and when it meets carefully observed criteria of the lactational amenorrhea method (LAM) (see "Lactational Amenorrhea Method").

Nonhormonal Methods

If a breastfeeding woman needs or wants more protection from pregnancy, options are available that do not affect breastfeeding or pose even a theoretical risk to the infant. *She should first consider the nonhormonal methods such as copper intrauterine contraceptive devices, condoms, or other barrier methods* (see the box, "ACOG Recommendations for Nonhormonal Contraception for Breastfeeding Women"). Condoms have additional, noncontraceptive advantages. Female sterilization or vasectomy may be considered by couples desiring permanent methods of birth control (27).

Hormonal Methods

Hormonal contraception offers effective protection from becoming pregnant. Several factors should be considered before prescribing hormonal contraception for the lactating woman. Contradictory lines of thought have resulted in conflicting recommendations that have been put forward by generally authoritative sources. The ACOG recommendations represent a more practical approach to the woman's needs, based on relevant research.

Progestin-Only Contraceptives

Progestin-only contraceptives, including progestin-only tablets (minipills), depot medroxyprogesterone acetate (DMPA), and levonorgestrel implants, do not affect the quality of breast milk and may slightly increase the volume of milk and duration of breastfeeding compared with nonhormonal methods (28–32). Accordingly, progestin-only methods are the hormonal contraceptives of choice for breastfeeding women. Nonetheless, some authorities have recommended delays of various lengths before introduction of progestin-only contraceptives on the basis of two sets of theoretical concerns:

- The normal 2–3-day postdelivery decrease of progesterone is part of the process that initiates lactation. There is theoretical concern that giving progestins in the first few days before lactation is established could interfere with optimal lactation. Note that DMPA enters the milk at approximately the same level found in the woman's blood; by contrast norgestrel and norethindrone enter the milk at only one tenth the level in the woman's blood. The injectable route of administration also may result in a comparatively high initial dose (27).
- Progestin methods carry a theoretical risk to the newborn because of exposure to exogenous steroids at a time when the newborn's system is very immature in its ability to metabolize drugs. Because of this concern, research studies presented to the FDA for drug approval investigated only the effects of these methods administered several weeks after birth. Because documentation of experience with earlier initiation was not presented to the FDA, package inserts recommend initiation of progestin-only oral contraceptives at 6 weeks for women who are exclusively breastfeeding and at 3 weeks for those who are breastfeeding with supplementation. Most authorities recommend introduction of long-acting progestin-only injectables or implants 6 weeks after delivery for breastfeeding women (27, 33, 34).

To balance these conservative recommendations, it is important to understand that the few studies that included early administration of progestin-only methods—oral contraceptives at 1 week postpartum (35, 36) and injectable medroxyprogesterone acetate at 2 days (37) and 7 days (38)—found no adverse effects on the newborn or on breastfeeding. In the absence of evidence that earlier introduction of progestin-only contraceptives has adverse effects on the newborn and on breastfeeding, the labeling for progestin-only oral contraceptives focuses instead on what is known about fertility after childbirth. Taking only biologic factors into account, contraception is not needed in the first 3 weeks postpartum because of a delay in return of ovulation in all women. And this delay is extended for women who breastfeed exclusively. An implied prohibi-

ACOG Recommendations for Nonhormonal Contraception for Breastfeeding Women

Exclusive breastfeeding up to 6 months meeting lactational amenorrhea method criteria (see "Lactational Amenorrhea Method")

Additional protection if desired

- Prelubricated latex condoms
- Other barrier methods
- Copper intrauterine contraceptive devices
- Male or female sterilization if permanent contraception is desired

tion on earlier administration is more in the nature of a pragmatic rather than a scientific resolution of the question. From the perspective of routine clinical practice, it would appear reasonable to apply the same rationale, even though conservative, to the initiation of DMPA and implants in postpartum breastfeeding women. However, the package labeling for these methods has the effect of being even more conservative as noted, outlining a 6-week start for all breastfeeding women, with no flexibility. Sometimes, however, there are practical reasons a breastfeeding woman may consider initiating hormonal contraception while in the hospital or shortly after. For example, there may be uncertainty about opportunities for follow-up visits. The breastfeeding woman and her physician can then weigh the reasons for early use of these contraceptives against potential disadvantages, make an appropriate decision, and continue to evaluate the woman's individual breastfeeding experience if hormonal contraceptives are chosen.

Combination Estrogen–Progestin Contraceptives

The postpartum patient has a hypercoagulable state that predisposes her to venous thrombosis (39). The use of estrogen-containing contraceptives during this phase of approximately 3 weeks after childbirth could contribute to this state. Furthermore, estrogen–progestin contraceptives have been shown to reduce the quantity and quality of breast milk. The World Health Organization recommends that the breastfeeding woman wait at least 6 months after childbirth to start using them (33). Labeling required by the FDA for combined oral contraceptives states, "If possible, the nursing mother should be advised not to use oral contraceptives but to use other forms of contraception until she has completely weaned her child" (34). These conservative approaches emanate for the most part from earlier combination oral contraceptive studies using higher doses of estrogens. Low-dose tablets (35 μg or lower) probably have a lesser effect on quality and quantity of breast milk. Effects are variable and if there are strong reasons the woman wishes to start combined estrogen–progestin contraceptive use earlier, she should understand and weigh the potential disadvantages. If estrogen–progestin contraceptives are prescribed, they should not be started before 6 weeks postpartum, and the physician should continue to evaluate the woman's individual breastfeeding experience.

The summary recommendations given in the box, "ACOG Recommendations for Hormonal Contraception If Used by Breastfeeding Women," with regard to progestin-only methods are based on the conservative timing outlined in labeling. Exceptions may be considered for earlier use on an individual basis. With combined estrogen–progestin contraceptives, a minimum 6-week delay is prudent because practical obstacles in developing successful breastfeeding techniques are likely to be resolved by 6 weeks. Most women experience reduced milk volume as a result of estrogen ingestion; this may be dealt with more easily after breastfeeding skills and patterns are established, should combined contraceptives be chosen despite this disadvantage. FDA labeling, however, is more conservative than the summary recommendation offered for combined estrogen–progestin contraceptives here. As noted earlier, prelubricated condoms are a good interim contraceptive choice and will address vaginal dryness associated with breastfeeding as well as help prevent infection.

Lactational Amenorrhea Method

Women who breastfeed can make use of the natural contraceptive effect of lactation. The LAM is most appropriate for women who plan to fully breastfeed 6 months or longer. If the baby is fed only mother's milk or is given supplemental nonbreast-milk feedings only to a minor extent and the woman has not experienced her first postpartum menses, then breastfeeding provides more than 98% protection from pregnancy in the first 6 months following delivery (27, 40, 41). Four prospective clinical trials of the contraceptive effect of LAM demonstrated cumulative 6-month life-table, perfect-use pregnancy rates of 0.5%, 0.6%, 1.0%, and 1.5% among women who relied solely on it. Women should be advised that for significant fertility impact, intervals between feedings should not exceed 4 hours during the day or 6 hours at night (Fig. 1). Supplemental feedings should not exceed 5–10% of the total (42–46). For example, more than one supplemental feeding out of every 10 might increase the

ACOG Recommendations for Hormonal Contraception If Used by Breastfeeding Women

- Progestin-only oral contraceptives prescribed or dispensed at discharge from the hospital to be started 2–3 weeks postpartum (eg, the first Sunday after the newborn is 2 weeks old)
- Depot medroxyprogesterone acetate initiated at 6 weeks postpartum*
- Hormonal implants inserted at 6 weeks postpartum*
- Combined estrogen–progestin contraceptives, if prescribed, should not be started before 6 weeks postpartum, and only when lactation is well established and the infant's nutritional status well-monitored

*There are certain clinical situations in which earlier initiation might be considered.

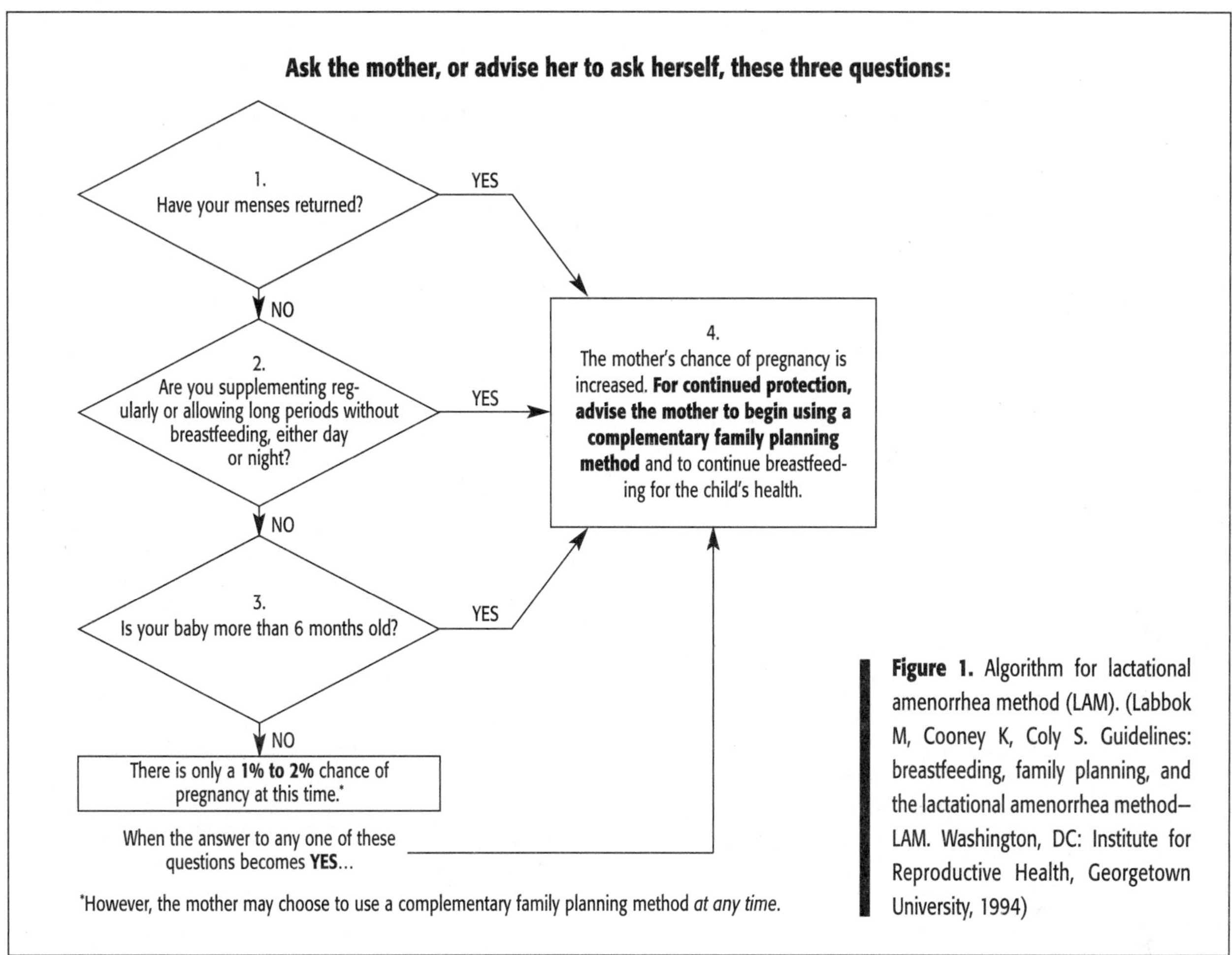

Ask the mother, or advise her to ask herself, these three questions:
1. Have your menses returned?
YES
NO
2. Are you supplementing regularly or allowing long periods without breastfeeding, either day or night?
YES
NO
3. Is your baby more than 6 months old?
YES
NO
4. The mother's chance of pregnancy is increased. For continued protection, advise the mother to begin using a complementary family planning method and to continue breastfeeding for the child's health.
There is only a 1% to 2% chance of pregnancy at this time.*
When the answer to any one of these questions becomes YES...
*However, the mother may choose to use a complementary family planning method at any time.

Figure 1. Algorithm for lactational amenorrhea method (LAM). (Labbok M, Cooney K, Coly S. Guidelines: breastfeeding, family planning, and the lactational amenorrhea method—LAM. Washington, DC: Institute for Reproductive Health, Georgetown University, 1994)

likelihood of returning fertility. Feeding practices other than direct breastfeeding, insofar as they may reduce the vigor and frequency of suckling and the maternal neuroendocrine response, increase the probability of returning ovulation (47). If there is uncertainty regarding the extent to which a given woman is breastfeeding, it would be prudent to recommend additional contraception.

Maintaining Milk Supply

Regular breastfeeding generally ensures adequate milk supply. As the baby grows and requires more milk, the woman's supply, which is demand driven, increases to accommodate the baby's needs.

Bottle Supplements and Pacifiers

The use of pacifiers and supplemental bottle feeding have been considered deterrents to sustained breastfeeding. Studies do not provide clear evidence that bottle feeding and pacifiers directly interfere with breastfeeding. A recent prospective cohort study indicated that pacifier use in the first 6 weeks was independently associated with declines in the duration of full and overall breastfeeding in the long term, but not short term (during the first 3 months of life). Women who introduced pacifiers early tended to breastfeed fewer times per day. The authors suggested that maternal behavior, such as extending intervals between feedings and decisions to begin weaning, may lead to introduction of pacifiers. They suggested that pacifier use, through an association with infrequent breastfeeding, may mediate (rather than cause) the declines observed in breastfeeding duration (48). It is important to help mothers understand that substituting for or delaying breastfeedings may ultimately reduce milk supply because of the reduction in stimulation of milk production that depends on infant suckling. Another study found that fluid supplements offered by bottle with or without the use of pacifiers during the first 5 days of life were not associated with a lower frequency or shorter duration of breastfeeding during the first 6 months of life (49).

Interruption of Breastfeeding

Separation of mother and infant should be avoided whenever possible, especially during the early establishment of lactation (first 3 weeks). If it is known in advance that hospitalization or a trip, for example, will require the mother to be separated from the infant for more than a day, careful planning can ensure that the ability to breastfeed will be preserved and breast milk will be available for the infant. During the separation, regular pumping of the breasts should be sufficient to maintain the milk supply. The milk may be saved for feeding the infant. When the separation is because of hospitalization, the milk should be discarded if it is judged to contain anesthetic or contraindicated medications. When the mother and infant are reunited, the reestablishment of normal breastfeeding generally progresses well.

Positioning and Latch-On for Breastfeeding

When observing an infant being breastfed, take note of the following:

- Position of mother, body language, and tension. Pillows may provide support for arms or infant.
- Position of infant. Ventral surface should be to mother's ventral surface, with lower arm, if not swaddled, around mother's thorax. Infant cannot swallow if head has to turn to breast, and grasp of areola will be poor. Infant's head should be in crook of arm and moved toward breast by arm movement.
- Position of mother's hand on breast not in way of proper grasp by infant
- Position of infant's lips on areola about 1–1½ inches (2.5–3.7 cm) from base of nipple
- Lower lip not folded in so that infant does not suck it; lips flanged
- Actual events around presenting breast and assisting infant to latch on
- Response of infant to lower lip stimulus by opening mouth wide
- Motion of masseter muscle during suckling and sounds of swallowing
- Mother comfortable with no breast pain

Lawrence RA, Lawrence RM. Breastfeeding: a guide for the medical profession. 5th ed. St. Louis, Missouri: Mosby, 1999

Sore Nipples

Having sore nipples is a common problem for the breastfeeding woman. It usually results from poor positioning or latch-on (see box, "Positioning and Latch-On for Breastfeeding"). The first-line treatment should be counseling about these basic techniques (24). Purified lanolin cream and breast shells (to protect the nipples from friction between feedings) may be initiated to facilitate healing (50).

Mastitis

Mastitis occurs in 1–2% of breastfeeding women (51). It most commonly occurs between the first and fifth weeks postpartum but may be seen any time throughout the first year (52). Mastitis is manifested by a sore, reddened area on one breast and often is accompanied by chills, fever, and malaise. A segment of the breast becomes hard and erythematous, the fever can be as high as 40ºC, and the mother feels ill.

The differential diagnosis includes clogged milk duct, marked engorgement, and a rare condition, inflammatory breast carcinoma. Clogged milk ducts present as localized tender masses. They respond to warm wet compresses and manually massaging the loculated milk towards the nipple. Breast engorgement is always bilateral with generalized involvement. It occurs most commonly in the first 2 weeks postpartum. The major feature that differentiates it from inflammatory breast cancer is the knowledge of previous negative breast examination results during the pregnancy. If examination results have been normal, breast engorgement is the more likely diagnosis (51). Inflammatory breast cancer is a lethal form of breast cancer. It presents as unilateral erythema, heat, and induration that is more diffuse and recurrent (53).

The most common causative agent in mastitis is *Staphylococcus aureus,* occurring in 40% of cases (54). It is also the most common cause of abscess. Other common organisms in mastitis are *Hemophilus influenzae* and *H parainfluenzae, Escherichia coli, Enterococcus faecalis, Klebsiella pneumoniae, Enterobacter cloacae, Serratia marcescens,* and *Pseudomonas pickettii* (53).

The condition usually can be treated successfully with narrow-spectrum antibiotic therapy (first choice for women who are not allergic is dicloxacillin, 500 mg four times daily), hydration, bedrest, and acetaminophen. The mother should continue to breastfeed or express the milk from both breasts because it is important to empty the affected breast. In some cases, the woman may be advised to discard the milk until she has been treated for 24 hours.

If mastitis is not treated aggressively, an abscess may develop. Treatment is successful in curing mastitis if started early; the most common cause of recurrent mastitis is inadequate treatment. Delayed administration of antibiotics is associated with an increased incidence of breast abscess. Many staphylococcal infections are caused by organisms sensitive to penicillin or a cephalosporin. Dicloxacillin may be started empirically (55). Women who are allergic to penicillin may be given erythromycin. If the infection is caused by resistant, penicillinase-producing staphylococci, an antibiotic such as vancomycin or cefotetan should be given and continued until 2 days after the infection subsides, a minimum of 10 –14 days.

Abscess

Abscess is diagnosed by a palpable mass or failure to defervesce within 48–72 hours of antibiotic therapy. Generally, abscesses are treated with incision and drainage. Multiple abscesses may require multiple incisions, with a finger inserted to break down the locules. Breast milk should be discarded for the first 24 hours after surgery, with breastfeeding resuming thereafter if there is no drainage into the breast milk (1). Recently, ultrasonographically guided needle aspiration was shown to be successful in treating abscesses in 18 of 19 women (56).

Working Mothers and Time Away

Over half of mothers are employed outside the home. In some situations, the mother is able to feed her infant at work, but this is not common. Health professionals can help the mother consider the method by which she plans to feed her infant when she returns to work. Employers are increasingly supportive of accommodating the needs of their breastfeeding employees (16). If a woman wants to continue to breastfeed or breast-milk feed, she should plan to pump her breasts to maintain her milk supply and to provide stored milk for the caregiver to feed the infant in her absence. A mother can be reassured that continuing breastfeeding and use of breast milk to whatever degree she finds possible will benefit her infant.

Expressing Milk

Several methods are available to collect milk. Health professionals should ensure that breastfeeding women can successfully express milk by hand. Because use of a breast pump is more efficient, rental or purchase of a pump can be considered. In general, electric pumps are more efficient than hand pumps. Pumping both breasts simultaneously is more effective and saves time.

On occasion, women have to educate employers about the necessity of time and location to pump breasts during the workday. The influence of the physician in creating a better environment should not be underestimated. A physician's letter or phone call to the employer explaining how simple but vital the breastfeeding employee's needs are can be effective.

Storage of Milk

Breast milk can be stored in the refrigerator or on ice in glass or plastic containers. The use of refrigerated milk within 2 days is recommended, which is well before appreciable bacterial growth usually occurs. Breast milk intended for longer storage should be frozen as soon as possible and kept at the lowest and most constant temperatures available; for example, a deep freezer is preferable to a refrigerator freezer with a self-defrost cycle. Milk should be dated and used in date order to avoid loss of beneficial properties over time. Frozen milk can be thawed quickly under running water or gradually in the refrigerator. It should not be left out at room temperature for more than 4–8 hours, exposed to very hot water, or put in the microwave. Once the milk has thawed, it can be kept in the refrigerator for 24 hours (1, 57).

Breastfeeding Expectations in Daily Life

Despite sporadic instances of authorities forbidding breastfeeding in public, there is an increased level of acceptance of breastfeeding nationally. Supportive laws and policies are becoming the trend. Recently, breastfeeding mothers have had increasing success in leading active lives. Couples commonly take their babies with them to meetings, outings, restaurants, and while traveling. Women can be skillful at unobtrusively feeding their babies in public. There are many baby-friendly restaurants that welcome families and have a positive approach to breastfeeding.

Physicians' offices and other health facilities should welcome and encourage breastfeeding by providing educational material and an atmosphere receptive to breastfeeding women. All staff members should be aware of the value and importance of breastfeeding and understand that their contacts with patients can help them decide to breastfeed and encourage them to continue (see the box, "Office Tips").

Formula companies try to attract the interest of pregnant women with gift packs. Care providers should be aware that the giving of gift packs with formula to breastfeeding women is commonly a deterrent to continuation of breastfeeding (58, 59). A professional recommendation of the care and feeding products in the gift pack is implied. Physicians may conclude that noncommercial educational alternatives or gift packs without health-related items are preferable.

Office Tips

- Make ACOG Patient Education Pamphlets and other patient education materials available in waiting and examination rooms.
- Offer a call-in telephone number for advice–yours or another health care resource available in the community or hospital of birth.
- Provide information about and phone numbers of lactation consultants, such as La Leche League, in your community.
- Show videos on breastfeeding; if women's health videos normally play in waiting room, include those on breastfeeding so all patients see them, not just pregnant or breastfeeding patients.
- Provide seating, such as pillows and a rocking chair for women with infants, that keeps breastfeeding in mind.
- Have pumps and an appropriate room for employees and patients. If in a medical office complex with other practices, make its availability known to other employees (they may be your patients) or collaborate in setting up a room elsewhere in the building.
- Identify a staff member interested in being a special resource on breastfeeding in the office and facilitate further training for the individual in order to assist you, other staff, and patients.
- Develop breastfeeding statistics for your practice and encourage staff by showing changes over time on displays in staff areas.
- Ask about hospital policies and practices and offer to help with staff training and patient orientation materials.
- Find out about breastfeeding skills, interests, and services of family physician and pediatric colleagues in the community. Encourage women and parents to choose a supportive caregiver for the infant and meet with him or her during pregnancy.

How Long to Breastfeed

During the first 6 months of life, exclusive breastfeeding is the preferred feeding approach for the healthy infant born at term. It provides optimal nutrients for growth and development of the infant. The ACOG recommends that exclusive breastfeeding be continued until the infant is about 6 months old. A longer breastfeeding experience is, of course, beneficial. The professional objectives are to encourage and enable as many women as possible to breastfeed and to help them continue as long as possible.

Gradual introduction of iron-enriched solid foods in the second half of the first year should complement the breast milk diet (3). The AAP recommends that breastfeeding continue for at least 12 months, and thereafter for as long as is mutually desired (3). "Vitamin D and iron may need to be given before 6 months of age in selected groups of infants (vitamin D for infants whose mothers are vitamin D-deficient or those infants not exposed to adequate sunlight, iron for those who have low iron stores or anemia)" (3).

Weaning

The weaning process should be gradual. Eliminating a feeding every 2–3 days will achieve a comfortable transition for the infant and prevent engorgement in the mother. An infant weaned before 12 months should receive iron-fortified infant formula rather than cows' milk (3). If an infant is less than 9 months, weaning can be accomplished by substituting a bottle or cup for a breastfeeding. If an infant is 9 months or older, he or she may use a cup and substitute other foods for breastfeeding.

Abrupt weaning can be difficult for the mother and the baby. When this is necessary, certain measures can be helpful. The mother should wear a support bra. She does not need to restrict fluids. She may manually express sufficient milk to relieve the engorgement, but not so much that more milk production is stimulated. Cool compresses will reduce engorgement. Hormonal therapy is not recommended.

Weaning creates a hormonal milieu conducive to remineralization of bone and maternal replenishment. This may be a consideration favoring delay of the next pregnancy until the mother has completed breastfeeding.

Breast Cancer Detection

Because of normal changes in the breasts during pregnancy and lactation, cancer detection by palpation becomes more difficult. Breast self-examination is recommended, as it is for all women; however, in general, significant changes are difficult to distinguish from the normal changes in the breast during breastfeeding. Any suspicious lesion should be investigated. Studies indicate there are delays in diagnosis of breast cancer during pregnancy and lactation, including greater intervals between palpation of a lesion and diagnosis. These delays result in an increased risk of metastatic disease at diagnosis and a reduced chance of diagnosis at stage I (60). If a mass or other abnormality is detected during lactation, it should be fully evaluated, including biopsy, if indicated. Breastfeeding can continue during the evaluation. During lactation, mammograms are less reliable because of the associated increase in breast tissue density, which may make the test more difficult to interpret (53).

With these difficulties in detection during pregnancy and lactation as a backdrop, clinical breast examinations of women who may become pregnant are especially important. In addition, increasing age is one of many risk factors for breast cancer. Women are having babies in their late 30s and early 40s, and screening may be difficult during a 1- or 2-year period of pregnancy and lactation. This may influence some women who would not otherwise be candidates for mammography to consider it with their physicians as part of the total clinical evaluation before pregnancy.

Healthy People 2010

The goal set by the U.S. Public Health Service for *Healthy People 2010* is to "increase the proportion of mothers who breastfeed their babies" with specific targets for breastfeeding of 75% in the early postpartum period, 50% at 6 months, and 25% at 12 months (61). These are basically the same levels that were called for in *Healthy People 2000* except that the 12-month target has been added. Significant progress has been made from the rates of the early 90s. By 1998, the most recent year for which data are available, the proportion of mothers choosing to breastfeed reached a high of 64.3% after a concerted effort on the part of health professionals and support people. The highest breastfeeding rates are among college-educated women, those older than the age of 30, those living in the Mountain or Pacific census regions, and those not enrolled in WIC (Special Supplemental Nutrition Program for Women, Infants, and Children). Breastfeeding initiation rates are lowest among black women, women younger than 20 years old, women enrolled in WIC, those who did not complete high school, and those living in the East South Central census region (Mothers' Survey, Ross Products Division, Abbott Laboratories, Inc., Columbus, Ohio).

Some concentrated educational efforts also have had a statistical impact in specific populations (62). Women enrolled in WIC, because of increased breastfeeding support, are among those with the most rapid increases in rates of breastfeeding, although their rates remain well below national averages. Between 1990 and 1998, the most rapidly increasing initiation rate was among black women, the demographic group with the lowest breastfeeding rate (44.9% in-hospital compared with 64.3% nationally) in 1998 despite this increase (Mothers' Survey).

In 1998, the breastfeeding rate at 6 months reached 28.6%, the highest rate in the nearly 30 years such data have been collected. The highest 6-month rates are among mothers with the same demographic and socioeconomic characteristics as those who have the highest in-hospital breastfeeding rates. Younger women, black women, WIC participants, women in the East South Central census region, and women who are employed full time outside the home have the lowest 6-month breastfeeding rates (Mothers' Survey).

With the cooperation of many dedicated caregivers, it appears that the 2010 goals may be achievable. However, even if 75% of women initiate breastfeeding, two thirds of them will need to continue breastfeeding, to reach the proposed 6-month target of 50% of all women breastfeeding. Obstetrician–gynecologists should ensure that women have the correct information to make an informed decision and, together with pediatricians, they should ensure that each woman has the help and support necessary to continue to breastfeed successfully (63). The combined efforts of all health care providers will be necessary to meet this goal.

References

1. Lawrence RA, Lawrence RM. Breastfeeding: a guide for the medical profession. 5th ed. St. Louis, Missouri: Mosby, 1999
2. Institute of Medicine. Subcommittee on Nutrition During Lactation, Committee on Nutritional Status During Pregnancy and Lactation, Food and Nutrition Board. Nutrition during lactation. Washington, DC: National Academy Press, 1991
3. American Academy of Pediatrics, Work Group on Breastfeeding. Breastfeeding and the use of human milk. Pediatrics 1997;100:1035–1039
4. Chua S, Arulkumaran S, Lim I, Selamat N, Ratham SS. Influence of breastfeeding and nipple stimulation on postpartum uterine activity. Br J Obstet Gynaecol 1994;101:804–805
5. Carter CS, Altemus M. Integrative functions of lactational hormones in social behavior and stress management. Ann N Y Acad Sci 1997;807:164–174
6. Rosenblatt KA, Thomas DB. Lactation and the risk of epithelial ovarian cancer. The WHO Collaborative Study of Neoplasia and Steroid Contraceptives. Int J Epidemiol 1993;22:192–197
7. Newcomb PA, Storer BE, Longnecker MP, Mittendorf R, Greenberg ER, Clapp RW, et al. Lactation and a reduced risk of premenopausal breast cancer. N Engl J Med 1994;330:81–87
8. Kennedy KI, Visness CM. Contraceptive efficacy of lactational amenorrhoea. Lancet 1992;339:227–230
9. Gray RH, Campbell OM, Apelo R, Eslami SS, Zacur H, Ramos RM, et al. Risk of ovulation during lactation. Lancet 1990;335:25–29
10. Labbok MH, Colie C. Puerperium and breast-feeding. Curr Opin Obstet Gynecol 1992;4:818–825

11. Melton LJ 3d, Bryant SC, Wahner HW, O'Fallon WM, Malkasian GD, Judd HL, et al. Influence of breastfeeding and other reproductive factors on bone mass later in life. Osteoporos Int 1993;3:76–83

12. Cumming RG, Klineberg RJ. Breastfeeding and other reproductive factors and the risk of hip fractures in elderly women. Int J Epidemiol 1993;22:684–691

13. Dewey KG, Heinig MJ, Nommsen LA. Maternal weight-loss patterns during prolonged lactation. Am J Clin Nutr 1993;58:162–166

14. Ball TM, Wright AL. Health care costs of formula-feeding in the first year of life. Pediatrics 1999;103:870–876

15. Montgomery DL, Splett PL. Economic benefit of breast-feeding infants enrolled in WIC. J Am Diet Assoc 1997; 97:379–385

16. Jacobson M, Kolarek MH, Newton B. Business, babies and the bottom line: corporate innovations and best practices in maternal and child health. Washington, DC: Washington Business Group on Health, 1996

17. Cohen R, Mrtek MB, Mrtek RG. Comparison of maternal absenteeism and infant illness rates among breast-feeding and formula-feeding women in two corporations. Am J Health Promot 1995;10:148–153

18. Lawrence RA. A review of the medical benefits and contraindications to breastfeeding in the United States. Maternal and Child Health Technical Information Bulletin. Arlington, Virginia: National Center for Education in Maternal and Child Health, 1997

19. American Academy of Pediatrics, American College of Obstetricians and Gynecologists. Guidelines for perinatal care. 4th ed. Elk Grove Village, Illinois: AAP; Washington, DC: ACOG, 1997

20. Recommendations for prevention and control of hepatitis C virus (HCV) infection and HCV-related chronic disease. Centers for Disease Control and Prevention. MMWR Morb Mortal Wkly Rep 1998;47(RR-19):1–39

21. American Academy of Pediatrics Committee on Drugs. The transfer of drugs and other chemicals into human milk. Pediatrics 1994;93:137–150

22. Pugin E, Valdes V, Labbok MH, Perez A, Aravena R. Does prenatal breastfeeding skills group education increase the effectiveness of a comprehensive breastfeeding promotion program? J Hum Lact 1996;12(1):15–19

23. Randolph L, Cooper L, Fonseca-Becker F, York M, McIntosh M. Baby friendly hospital initiative feasibility study: final report. Healthy Mothers Healthy Babies National Coalition Expert Work Group. Alexandria, Virginia: HMHB, 1994

24. American College of Obstetricians and Gynecologists. Breast-feeding your baby. ACOG Patient Education Pamphlet AP029. Washington, DC: ACOG, 1997

25. Institute of Medicine. Standing Committee on the Scientific Evaluation of Dietary Reference Intakes, Food and Nutrition Board. Dietary reference intakes for calcium, phosphorus, magnesium, vitamin D, and fluoride. Washington, DC: National Academy Press, 1997

26. Institute of Medicine. Committee on Nutritional Status During Pregnancy and Lactation, Food and Nutrition Board. Nutrition services in perinatal care. 2nd ed. Washington, DC: National Academy Press, 1992

27. Hatcher RA, Trussell J, Stewart F, Cates W Jr, Stewart GK, Guest F, et al. Contraceptive technology. 17th rev. ed. New York: Ardent Media, Inc, 1998

28. Tankeyoon M, Dusitsin N, Chalapati S, Koetsawang S, Saibiang S, Sas M, et al. Effects of hormonal contraceptives on milk volume and infant growth. WHO Special Programme of Research, Development, and Research Training in Human Reproduction, Task Force on Oral Contraceptives. Contraception 1984;30:505–522

29. World Health Organization (WHO) Task Force on Oral Contraceptives. Effects of hormonal contraceptives on milk composition and infant growth. Stud Fam Plann 1988;19:361–369

30. Speroff L, Darney P. A clinical guide for contraception. 2nd ed. Baltimore, Maryland: Williams & Wilkins, 1996

31. Abdulla KA, Elwan SI, Salem HS, Shaaban MM. Effect of early postpartum use of the contraceptive implants, NORPLANT, on the serum levels of immunoglobulins of the mothers and their breastfed infants. Contraception 1985; 32:261–266

32. Shaaban MM, Salem HT, Abdullah KA. Influence of levonorgestrel contraceptive implants, NORPLANT, initiated early postpartum upon lactation and infant growth. Contraception 1985;32:623–635

33. World Health Organization. Division of Family and Reproductive Health. Improving access to quality care in family planning: medical eligibility criteria for contraceptive use. Geneva: WHO, 1996

34. Physicians' Desk Reference. 53rd ed. Montvale, New Jersey: Medical Economics, Inc, 1999

35. McCann MF, Moggia AV, Higgins JE, Potts M, Becker C. The effects of a progestin-only oral contraceptive (levonorgestrel 0.03 mg) on breast-feeding. Contraception 1989;40:635–648

36. Moggia AV, Harris GS, Dunson TR, Diaz R, Moggia MS, Ferrer MA, et al. A comparative study of a progestin-only oral contraceptive versus non-hormonal methods in lactating women in Buenos Aires, Argentina. Contraception 1991;44:31–43

37. Guiloff E, Ibarra-Polo A, Zañartu J, Toscanini C, Mischler TW, Gómez-Rogers C. Effect of contraception on lactation. Am J Obstet Gynecol 1974;118:42–45

38. Karim M, Ammar R, el Mahgoub S, el Ganzoury B, Fikri F, Abdou I. Injected progestogen and lactation. BMJ 1971; 1:200–203

39. WHO Task Force on Oral Contraceptives. Contraception during the postpartum period and during lactation: the effects on women's health. Int J Gynaecol Obstet 1987;25 (suppl):13–26

40. Kennedy KI, Rivera R, McNeilly AS. Consensus statement on the use of breastfeeding as a family planning method. Contraception 1989;39:477–496

41. World Health Organization. Task Force on Methods for the Natural Regulation of Fertility. The WHO multinational study of breast-feeding and lactational amenorrhea. III. Pregnancy during breast-feeding. Fertil Steril 1999;72;431–440

42. Perez A, Labbok MH, Queenan JT. Clinical study of the lactational amenorrhoea method for family planning. Lancet 1992;339:968–970

43. Ramos R, Kennedy KI, Visness CM. Effectiveness of lactational amenorrhea in prevention of pregnancy in Manila, the Philippines: non-comparative prospective trial. BMJ 1996;313:909–912

44. Labbok MH, Hight-Laukaran V, Peterson AE, Fletcher V, von Hertzen H, Van Look PF. Multicenter study of the Lactational Amenorrhea Method (LAM): I. Efficacy, duration and implications for clinical application. Contraception 1997;55:327–336

45. Kazi A, Kennedy KI, Visness CM, Khan T. Effectiveness of the lactational amenorrhea method in Pakistan. Fertil Steril 1995;64:717–723

46. Labbok M, Cooney K, Coly S. Guidelines: breastfeeding, family planning, and the lactational amenorrhea method—LAM. Washington, DC: Institute for Reproductive Health, Georgetown University, 1994

47. Campbell OM, Gray RH. Characteristics and determinants of postpartum ovarian function in women in the United States. Am J Obstet Gynecol 1993;169:55–60

48. Howard CR, Howard FM, Lanphear B, deBlieck EA, Eberly S, Lawrence RA. The effects of early pacifier use on breastfeeding duration. Pediatrics 1999;103:E33

49. Schubiger G, Schwarz U, Tonz O. UNICEF/WHO baby-friendly hospital initiative: does the use of bottles and pacifiers in the neonatal nursery prevent successful breastfeeding? Neonatal Study Group. Eur J Pediatr 1997;156:874–877

50. Brent N, Rudy SJ, Redd B, Rudy TE, Roth LA. Sore nipples in breast-feeding women: a clinical trial of wound dressings vs conventional care. Arch Pediatr Adolesc Med 1998;152:1077–1082

51. Stehman FB. Infections and inflammations of the breast. In: Hindle WH, ed. Breast disease for gynecologists. Norwalk, Connecticut: Appleton & Lange, 1990:151

52. Niebyl JR, Spence MR, Parmley TH. Sporadic (nonepidemic) puerperal mastitis. J Reprod Med 1978;20: 97–100

53. Hankins GD, Clark SL, Cunningham FG, Gilstrap LC III. Breast disease during pregnancy and lactation. In: Hankins GD, Clark SL, Cunningham FG, Gilstrap LC III, eds. Operative obstetrics. Norwalk, Connecticut: Appleton & Lange, 1995:667–694

54. Matheson I, Aursnes I, Horgen M, Aabo O, Melby K. Bacteriological findings and clinical symptoms in relation to clinical outcome in puerperal mastitis. Acta Obstet Gynecol Scand 1988;67:723–726

55. Hindle WH. Other benign breast problems. Clin Obstet Gynecol 1994;37:916–924

56. Karstrup S, Solvig J, Nolsoe CP, Nilsson P, Khattar S, Loren I, et al. Acute puerperal breast abscesses: US-guided drainage. Radiology 1993;188:807–809

57. Arnold LDW. Recommendations for collection, storage and handling of a mother's milk for her own infant in the hospital setting. 3rd ed. Denver: Human Milk Banking Association of North America, 1999

58. Howard C, Howard F, Lawrence R, Andresen E, DeBlieck E, Weitzman M. Office prenatal formula advertising and its effect on breast-feeding patterns. Obstet Gynecol 2000;95:296–303

59. Pérez-Escamilla R, Pollitt E, Lönnerdal B, Dewey KG. Infant feeding policies in maternity wards and their effect on breast-feeding success: an analytical overview. Am J Public Health 1994;84:89–97

60. Zemlickis D, Lishner M, Degendorfer P, Panzarella T, Burke B, Sutcliffe SB, et al. Maternal and fetal outcome after breast cancer in pregnancy. Am J Obstet Gynecol 1992;166:781–787

61. Healthy people 2010, volume II. Washington, DC: U.S. Department of Health and Human Services, 2000: 16-46–16-48

62. Ryan AS. The resurgence of breastfeeding in the United States. Pediatrics 1997;99:E12

63. Freed GL, Clark SJ, Cefalo RC, Sorenson JR. Breast-feeding education of obstetrics-gynecology residents and practitioners. Am J Obstet Gynecol 1995;173:1607–1613

The American College of
Obstetricians and Gynecologists
409 12th Street, SW
PO Box 96920
Washington, DC 20090-6920

12345/43210

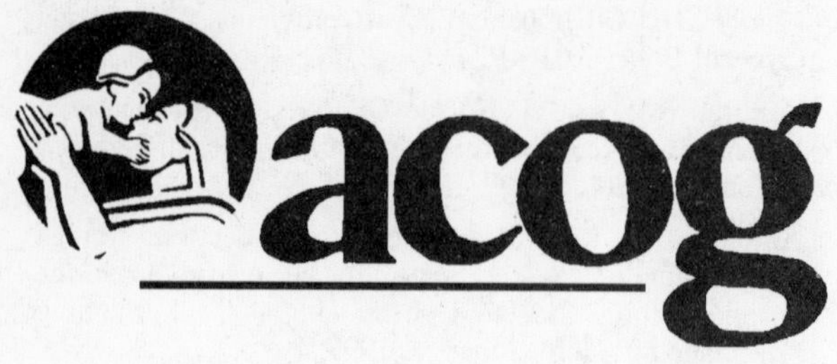

Number 162—December 1991
(Replaces #76, March 1984)

Technical Bulletin

An Educational Aid to Obstetrician–Gynecologists

Carcinoma of the Endometrium

Carcinoma of the endometrium is the most common gynecologic malignancy in the United States. The incidence of endometrial cancer has increased over the past 50 years as a result of the longer life expectancy of women, improved methods of diagnosis, and an increased frequency of certain predisposing conditions. Although the incidence appears to have stabilized in recent years, about 2–3% of women in the United States will develop cancer of the endometrium at some point during their lives. Several factors have been identified that may substantially increase this risk.

Risk Factors

Adenocarcinoma of the endometrium is predominantly a disease of postmenopausal women. When endometrial cancer develops before age 40, it occurs most often in women who are either obese or chronically anovulatory (1). As a general rule, endometrial cancer in young women or in women taking estrogen has a better prognosis than in older women and women not taking estrogens.

The principal factor that predisposes women to the development of endometrial cancer is chronic, unopposed exposure to estrogen, whether endogenous or exogenous. Factors conferring this risk are:

- Endogenous factors:
  - —Early menarche
  - —Late menopause
  - —Obesity
  - —Chronic anovulation
  - —Estrogen-secreting ovarian tumors
- Exogenous factors: Ingestion of unopposed estrogen

Other factors that have been associated with endometrial cancer risk include pelvic radiation therapy (2), hypertension, and diabetes mellitus; the data suggesting the latter two relationships, however, are inconclusive and are more likely related to obesity. Women who have had breast or ovarian cancer also have a higher-than-average risk for developing endometrial cancer, whereas high parity, smoking, and the use of combination oral contraceptives are associated with a reduction in this risk (2, 3).

The probability for developing endometrial cancer correlates directly with the dose and duration of unopposed estrogen use, and the increased risk persists after discontinuation of estrogen (4). Adequate progestin therapy can substantially reduce or nullify the increased risk associated with the use of local or systemic estrogen replacement therapy and may reduce the risk below the background incidence. Nevertheless, when a physician considers prescribing estrogens to achieve beneficial effects on menopausal symptoms, genital tissues, bone mineral metabolism, and coronary atherosclerosis, the patient should be informed of the potential risk of developing endometrial hyperplasia or cancer, as well as the measures required to monitor these conditions.

Diagnosis

At present, there are no effective screening methods to detect endometrial cancer. Specifically, routine endometrial sampling has not been shown to be cost-effective in asymptomatic patients (5).

The presenting symptom of endometrial cancer is usually abnormal uterine bleeding occurring after the menopause. Endometrial cancer should be suspected in postmenopausal women who have any bleeding and in perimenopausal women who have menstrual abnormalities characterized by an increased menstrual flow, a decreased menstrual interval, or intermenstrual bleeding. A routine Pap smear cannot be relied upon to indicate the presence of endometrial cancer or hyperplasia. However, endometrial cancer should be suspected when atypical endometrial cells are found in the Pap smear of a nonpregnant woman of any age or when normal endometrial cells are found in a postmenopausal woman not taking estrogens (6).

The outpatient evaluation of women suspected to have endometrial cancer includes the following components:

- Careful inspection of the vulva, anus, vagina, and cervix
- Pap smear taken from the ectocervix and endocervix
- Bimanual rectovaginal palpation of the uterus, parametria, adnexa, cervix, vagina, and rectum for nodules, masses, induration, and lack of mobility
- Endometrial biopsy and endocervical curettage in postmenopausal women with vaginal bleeding or perimenopausal women with a menstrual abnormality as described previously
- Biopsy of any suspicious genital lesion
- Test for occult blood in stool

An office biopsy, when possible, to evaluate the endometrium for neoplasia in symptomatic women may eliminate the need for most dilation and curettage (D&C) procedures, which are usually done under general anesthesia. Consequently, much of the added cost, the potential for complications, and the inconvenience of day hospital care are avoided without affecting outcome. The accuracy of office endometrial biopsy under optimal conditions approaches that of D&C (7). Paracervical block may be used for endometrial biopsy, if necessary. Endocervical curettage is an essential part of the evaluation of postmenopausal bleeding because an endocervical carcinoma could be missed by the endometrial biopsy.

If the endometrial biopsy and endocervical curettage can be performed adequately and no significant abnormality is detected, no further evaluation is needed. If high-risk factors coexist and the cause of the bleeding remains undiagnosed, a fractional D&C should be considered. A fractional curettage is also indicated when atypical hyperplasia is diagnosed or in cases in which endometrial sampling is inadequate. Hysteroscopy may also be helpful to evaluate the endometrium further if there is reason to suspect that a lesion (eg, a polyp or submucosal myoma) may have been missed, such as in the case of recurrent bleeding (8).

If endometrial cancer is diagnosed, further information is needed to assess the status of the tumor as completely as possible and to provide a data base for treatment planning. In addition to the results of the gynecologic examination that has already been performed (especially with regard to involvement of the cervix, vagina, parametria, and adnexa), the peripheral (supraclavicular, inguinal) lymph nodes should be palpated and a careful abdominal examination performed. The histologic type and grade, as well as evidence for invasion of cervical stroma, may be determined from the endometrial biopsy and endocervical curettage. Cervical involvement is diagnosed by the presence of stromal invasion as evidenced on endocervical curettage (9).

Other studies to be done include:

- Two-view chest X-ray
- Routine laboratory studies:
  —Serum electrolytes
  —Complete blood count
  —Renal and hepatic function tests
  —Urinalysis

Other studies that may be performed, based on the patient's age and risk factors, include sigmoidoscopy and barium enema, intravenous pyelogram, or colonoscopy. In some cases, such as when a high-grade cancer is found (eg, grade 2 or 3 adenocarcinoma, papillary serous carcinoma, or clear cell carcinoma), serum CA 125 assay (10) and computed tomography or magnetic resonance imaging of the abdomen and pelvis may be helpful, but these studies are not warranted on a routine basis.

Preoperatively, the histologic grade, cell type, and, possibly, hormone receptor status of the tumor can provide information about the prognosis in the absence of clinically obvious metastasis. Evidence for local extension or metastasis is obtained from the physical examination (extension to the cervix or vagina; parametrial disease; abdominal mass; enlargement of the adnexa, groin, or supraclavicular node), an elevated serum CA 125 value (10), and chest X-ray. Another important prognostic factor of endometrial cancer is myometrial invasion, which is most often determined in the hysterectomy specimen. If it is necessary to determine this prognostic factor without surgery, both ultrasound and magnetic resonance imaging of the uterus may be helpful and are reported to have 80% or greater reliability in determining the depth of myometrial invasion in endometrial cancer (11, 12).

Management

The staging system established by the International Federation of Gynecology and Obstetrics (FIGO) for endometrial cancer has been clinical from its inception; that is, the stage was determined on the basis of information obtainable prior to surgery. The usual survival rates reported for this staging system are 85% for stage I, 60% for stage II, 30% for stage III, and 10% for stage IV. This system is still used in the unusual case of the patient who is not a candidate for surgery because of advanced disease or severe medical problems. The new FIGO staging system (see box) is based on surgical and pathologic evaluation and provides for a more precise assessment of the extent of the cancer and the prognostic features of the tumor itself. This surgical staging system, which was adopted in 1988, recognizes the large body of data on surgical staging that has been developed during the past 20 years. These data delineate the relationships among histology, grade, myometrial invasion, and the probability for extrauterine spread, especially pelvic and aortic lymph node metastases (13–15). The new system also reflects the generally accepted evidence that most patients with endometrial cancer do not need adjuvant radiation therapy, that preoperative radiation therapy can obscure important surgical–pathologic information about the cancer, and that postoperative radiation is as effective as preoperative radiation in reducing the risk for local or regional recurrence (16–19). During the past decade, there has been a shift to surgical–pathologic staging at the time of abdominal hysterectomy, with individualized postoperative adjuvant therapy based on the surgical–pathologic findings.

The treatment of endometrial carcinoma varies in the extreme. The roles of preoperative versus postoperative radiation and intracavitary therapy versus external beam therapy are among the most prominent areas of dispute. The following commentary presents a reasonable treatment plan based on the recent surgical–pathologic staging data and reported treatment results. Some centers continue to use preoperative intracavitary therapy in all or in selected patients with stage I disease (eg, those with grade 3 tumors), while others employ postoperative therapy either routinely or in selected patients. If preoperative intracavitary therapy is used, it is recommended that hysterectomy be performed within 3 days to determine the extent of tumor growth within the uterus. Although the FIGO 1988 staging system implies that pelvic and aortic node biopsy should be done, this is an area of controversy and is estimated to be of low clinical value in 30–40% of patients.

Surgical staging as defined by FIGO (1988) for patients with endometrial carcinoma that is apparently confined to the uterus requires the following:

FIGO Staging for Carcinoma of the Corpus Uteri

Stage IA G123	Tumor limited to endometrium
Stage IB G123	Invasion to less than one-half the myometrium
Stage IC G123	Invasion to more than one-half the myometrium
Stage IIA G123	Endocervical glandular involvement only
Stage IIB G123	Cervical stromal invasion
Stage IIIA G123	Tumor invades serosa and/or adnexa, and/or positive peritoneal cytology
Stage IIIB G123	Vaginal metastases
Stage IIIC G123	Metastases to pelvic and/or paraaortic lymph nodes
Stage IVA G123	Tumor invasion of bladder and/or bowel mucosa
Stage IVB	Distant metastases including intraabdominal and/or inguinal lymph nodes

Histopathology—degree of differentiation:

Cases of carcinoma of the corpus should be classified (or graded) according to the degree of histologic differentiation, as follows:

G1 = 5% or less of a nonsquamous or nonmorular solid growth pattern

G2 = 6–50% of a nonsquamous or nonmorular solid growth pattern

G3 = more than 50% of a nonsquamous or nonmorular solid growth pattern

Notes on pathological grading:

1) Notable nuclear atypia, inappropriate for the architectural grade, raises the grade of a grade 1 or grade 2 tumor by 1.
2) In serous adenocarcinomas, clear-cell adenocarcinomas, and squamous cell carcinomas, nuclear grading takes precedence.
3) Adenocarcinomas with squamous differentiation are graded according to the nuclear grade of the glandular component.

Rules related to staging:

1) Because corpus cancer is now staged surgically, procedures previously used for determination of stages are no longer applicable, such as the findings from fractional D&C to differentiate between stage I and stage II.
2) It is appreciated that there may be a small number of patients with corpus cancer who will be treated primarily with radiation therapy. If that is the case, the clinical staging adopted by FIGO in 1971 would still apply, but designation of that staging system would be noted.
3) Ideally, width of the myometrium should be measured along with the width of tumor invasion.

International Federation of Gynecology and Obstetrics. Annual report on the results of treatment in gynecologic cancer. Int J Gynecol Obstet 1989;28:189–190

- Abdominal approach
- Peritoneal cytology
- Careful inspection and palpation of the abdominal and pelvic organs, including the diaphragm, liver, omentum, retroperitoneal nodes (aortic and pelvic), and pelvic peritoneum
- Total hysterectomy and bilateral adnexectomy
- Biopsy of pelvic and aortic nodes

There is disagreement concerning the requirement for lymph node biopsy for all patients with stage I endometrial cancer. The incidence of pelvic and aortic node metastasis is related to tumor differentiation and depth of invasion of the myometrium. Patients with grade 1 or 2 tumors with superficial invasion are at low risk for node metastasis and may be spared the risks associated with node biopsy (Tables 1 and 2). Pelvic and aortic node sampling is suggested for all patients with suspicious nodes encountered at surgery, those with grade 3 tumors, and those with tumors of any grade with invasion into the middle third of the myometrium or into the cervix. If necessary, a frozen section can be performed to help guide the need for lymph node biopsy (20). Patients with papillary serous adenocarcinomas are at increased risk for extrapelvic metastases, and partial omentectomy, in addition to standard staging, is recommended.

Postoperatively, patients can be selected for treatment based on risk of recurrence. Risk groups are determined by using data analyzed in the large prospective study conducted by the Gynecologic Oncology Group (14). In this study, myometrial invasion was divided into thirds rather than halves; thus, it varies slightly from the FIGO staging system.

Low-risk patients are identified as those with grade 1 or 2 tumors confined to the fundus with superficial (inner one-third) or no myometrial invasion. These patients require no further therapy, as their disease-free survival rate is 96% (21).

Intermediate-risk patients are those with grade 1 or 2 tumors with middle one-third invasion and no extrauterine spread. There are no prospective, randomized studies to demonstrate that postoperative therapy improves survival rates in these patients; however, it appears that it improves local/regional control (14). Postoperative radiation therapy may be delivered by whole-pelvis radiation or by intracavitary vaginal brachytherapy.

High-risk patients are those with adnexal spread, pelvic node metastasis, outer one-third myometrial invasion, cervical invasion, or grade 3 tumors with any invasion. These patients may benefit from adjuvant postoperative whole-pelvis radiotherapy using 4,000–5,000 cGy. If metastasis to the aortic nodes is found, extended-field radiation therapy is recommended in the absence of other distant metastases, since 40% of these patients can be expected to survive 5 years or longer (14, 22).

Patients who have endometrial carcinoma with microscopic involvement of the endocervix at fractional curettage can undergo surgery initially, as for patients with endometrial carcinoma in whom an endocervical curettage is negative. When there is clinical involvement of the cervix, however, as demonstrated by gross disease or enlargement, the proper treatment is either radical hysterectomy with pelvic lymphadenectomy and aortic lymph node sampling, or preoperative radiation followed by extrafascial hysterectomy and aortic lymph node biopsy.

The management of patients with positive peritoneal cytology is controversial (23). Since peritoneal cytology is difficult to interpret, obtaining a second opinion is a good policy. In general, however, if there are abundant malignant cells, the prognosis is seriously affected and aggressive treatment is indicated. In most instances, there will be other high-risk features requiring pelvic irradiation. Thus, intraperitoneal ^{32}P is not usually suited to treat this group of patients, since the rate of complications with these two treatments combined is excessive. Whole-abdomen radiotherapy, chemotherapy, or progestin therapy

TABLE 1. GRADE, DEPTH OF INVASION, AND PELVIC NODE METASTASIS OF ENDOMETRIAL CARCINOMA

Depth of Myometrial Invasion	Histologic Grade G1 (n = 180)	G2 (n = 288)	G3 (n = 153)
Endometrium only (n = 86)	0 (0%)	1 (3%)	0 (0%)
Inner third (n = 281)	3 (3%)	7 (5%)	5 (9%)
Middle third (n = 115)	0 (0%)	6 (9%)	1 (4%)
Outer third (n = 139)	2 (11%)	11 (19%)	22 (34%)

(Creasman WT, Morrow CP, Bundy BN, Homesley HD, Graham JE, Heller PB. Surgical pathologic spread patterns of endometrial cancer: a Gynecologic Oncology Group study. Cancer 1987;60(8 suppl):2035–2041)

TABLE 2. GRADE, DEPTH OF INVASION, AND AORTIC NODE METASTASIS OF ENDOMETRIAL CARCINOMA

Depth of Myometrial Invasion	Histologic Grade G1 (n = 180)	G2 (n = 288)	G3 (n = 153)
Endometrium only (n = 86)	0 (0%)	1 (3%)	0 (0%)
Inner third (n = 281)	1 (1%)	5 (4%)	2 (4%)
Middle third (n = 115)	1 (5%)	0 (0%)	0 (0%)
Outer third (n = 139)	1 (6%)	8 (14%)	15 (23%)

(Creasman WT, Morrow CP, Bundy BN, Homesley HD, Graham JE, Heller PB. Surgical pathologic spread patterns of endometrial cancer: a Gynecologic Oncology Group study. Cancer 1987;60(8 suppl):2035–2041)

combined with pelvic and aortic radiation therapy are treatment modalities that may be selected in specific situations (14, 24–25).

Perhaps 10% of women with clinical stage I endometrial carcinoma are medically inoperable because of serious cardiopulmonary disease or morbid obesity. In these cases, even vaginal hysterectomy may not be feasible or safe. Radiation therapy is often curative in this situation and should be administered. The best results are achieved with external beam and intracavitary treatment, although either can be used alone. The expected 5-year survival rate in patients with stage I disease treated by radiation alone is about 50% (26). Because of the risk of persistent tumor growth within the uterus, a dilation and curettage performed about 3 months after therapy is recommended. If residual cancer is found, the contraindications to surgery should be reassessed.

A minority of women with endometrial carcinoma will have advanced disease at diagnosis. For these women, treatment should be individualized with progestin therapy (medroxyprogesterone acetate or megestrol acetate) or chemotherapy (doxorubicin, cisplatin, and cyclophosphamide). Long-term control of endometrial cancer by both hormone therapy and chemotherapy has been reported, but such a good result is exceptional (27, 28).

Patients with recurrent carcinoma following surgery should be considered for radiotherapy. Those in whom disease recurs following both surgery and radiotherapy may be treated with chemotherapy or progestin therapy as described previously. Estrogen receptor and progesterone receptor levels may be used to select therapy.

There are no definitive data to support specific recommendations regarding the use of estrogen in women previously treated for endometrial cancer. If the patient is free of tumor, estrogen replacement therapy cannot result in recurrence. If cancer is present, however, estrogen replacement therapy may result in an earlier recurrence. The physician should counsel the patient concerning her risk of recurrence based on known risk factors to enable her to make an informed decision (29). Since 76% of recurrences will be evident by 3 years (30), those women who are free of disease beyond 3 years may be treated with estrogen replacement therapy. When estrogen is prescribed, progestin should also be given.

REFERENCES

1. Gallup DG, Stock RJ. Adenocarcinoma of the endometrium in women 40 years of age or younger. Obstet Gynecol 1984;64:417–420

2. Davies JL, Rosenshein NB, Antunes CMF, Stolley PD. A review of the risk factors for endometrial carcinoma. Obstet Gynecol Surv 1981;36:107–116

3. Lesko SM, Rosenberg L, Kaufman DW, Helmrich SP, Miller DR, Strom B, et al. Cigarette smoking and the risk of endometrial cancer. N Engl J Med 1985;313:593–596

4. Paganini-Hill A, Ross RK, Henderson BE. Endometrial cancer and patterns of use of oestrogen replacement therapy: a cohort study. Br J Cancer 1989;59:445–447

5. American College of Obstetricians and Gynecologists. Report of Task Force on Routine Cancer Screening. ACOG Committee Opinion 68. Washington, DC: ACOG, 1989

6. Mencaglia L, Valle RF, Perino A, Keith LG. Early detection of endometrial carcinoma and its precursors. Curr Prob Obstet Gynecol Fertil 1988;11(5):173–202

7. Grimes DA. Diagnostic dilation and curettage: a reappraisal. Am J Obstet Gynecol 1982;142:1–6

8. Gimpelson RJ, Rappold HO. A comparative study between panoramic hysteroscopy with directed biopsies and dilation and curettage: a review of 276 cases. Am J Obstet Gynecol 1988;158:489–492

9. Chen SS, Lee L. Reappraisal of endocervical curettage in predicting cervical involvement by endometrial carcinoma. J Repro Med 1986;31(1):50–52

10. Duk JM, Aalders JG, Fleuren GJ, de Bruijn HW. CA 125: a useful marker in endometrial carcinoma. Am J Obstet Gynecol 1986;115:1097–1102

11. Cacciatore B, Lehtovirta P, Wahlstrom T, Ylostalo P. Preoperative sonographic evaluation of endometrial cancer. Am J Obstet Gynecol 1989;160:133–137

12. Chen SS, Rumancik WM, Spiegel G. Magnetic resonance imaging in stage I endometrial carcinoma. Obstet Gynecol 1990;75:274–277

13. Boronow RC, Morrow CP, Creasman WT, Disaia PJ, Silverberg SG, Miller A. Surgical staging in endometrial cancer: clinical-pathologic findings of a prospective study. Obstet Gynecol 1984;63:825–832

14. Morrow CP, Bundy BN, Kurman RJ, Creasman WT, Heller P, Homesley HD, et al. Relationship between surgical–pathological risk factors and outcome in clinical stages I and II carcinoma of the endometrium: a Gynecologic Oncology Group study. Gynecol Oncol 1991;40:55–65

15. Creasman WT, Morrow CP, Bundy BN, Homesley HD, Graham JE, Heller PB. Surgical pathologic spread patterns of endometrial cancer: a Gynecologic Oncology Group study. Cancer 1987;60(8 suppl):2035–2041

16. Boronow RC. Endometrial cancer: the emergence of therapeutic individualization. In: Taymor ML, Nelson JH Jr, eds. Progress in gynecology. Vol VII. New York: Grune & Stratton, 1983

17. Eifel PJ, Ross J, Hendrickson M, Cox RS, Kempson R, Martinez A. Adenocarcinoma of the endometrium: analysis of 256 cases with disease limited to the uterine corpus: treatment comparisons. Cancer 1983;52:1026–1031

18. Aalders J, Abeler V, Kolstad P, Onsrud M. Postoperative external irradiation and prognostic parameters in stage I endometrial carcinoma: clinical and histopathologic study of 540 patients. Obstet Gynecol 1980;56:419–426

19. Chung CK, Stryker JA, Nahhas WA, Mortel R. The role of adjunctive radiotherapy for stage I endometrial carcinoma: preoperative vs postoperative irradiation. Int J Radiat Oncol Biol Phys 1981;7:1429–1435

20. Daniel AG, Peters WA III. Accuracy of office and operating room curettage in the grading of endometrial carcinoma. Obstet Gynecol 1988;71:612–614

21. Hording U, Hansen U. Stage I endometrial carcinoma: a review of 140 patients primarily treated by surgery only. Gynecol Oncol 1985;22:51–58

22. Potish RA, Twiggs LB, Adcock LL, Savage JE, Levitt SH, Prem KA. Paraaortic lymph node radiotherapy in cancer of the uterine corpus. Obstet Gynecol 1985;65:251–256

23. Harouny VR, Sutton GP, Clark SA, Geisler HE, Stehman FB, Ehrlich CE. The importance of peritoneal cytology in endometrial carcinoma. Obstet Gynecol 1988;72:394–398

24. Turner DA, Gershenson DM, Atkinson N, Sneige N, Wharton AT. The prognostic significance of peritoneal cytology for stage I endometrial cancer. Obstet Gynecol 1989;74:775–780

25. Martinez A, Schray M, Podratz K, Stanhope R, Malkasian G. Postoperative whole abdomino-pelvic irradiation for patients with high risk endometrial cancer. Int J Radiat Oncol Biol Phys 1989;17:371– 377

26. Varia M, Rosenman J, Halle J, Walton L, Currie J, Fowler W. Primary radiation therapy for medically inoperable patients with endometrial carcinoma—stages I–II. Int J Radiat Oncol Biol Phys 1987;13:11–15

27. Hancock KC, Freedman RS, Edwards CL, Rutledge FN. Use of cisplatin, doxorubicin, and cyclosphosphamide to treat advanced and recurrent adenocarcinoma of the endometrium. Cancer Treat Rep 1986;70:789–791

28. Podratz KC, O'Brien PC, Malkasian GD Jr, Decker DG, Jeffries JA, Edmonson JH. Effects of progestational agents in treatment of endometrial carcinoma. Obstet Gynecol 1985;66:106–110

29. American College of Obstetricians and Gynecologists. Estrogen replacement therapy and endometrial cancer. ACOG Committee Opinion 80. Washington, DC: ACOG, 1990

30. Aalders J, Abeler V, Kolstad P. Recurrent adenocarcinoma of the endometrium: a clinical and histopathological study of 379 patients. Gynecol Oncol 1984;17:85–103

This Technical Bulletin was developed under the direction of the Committee on Technical Bulletins of the American College of Obstetricians and Gynecologists as an educational aid to obstetricians and gynecologists. The committee wishes to thank C. Paul Morrow, MD, for his assistance in the development of this bulletin. This Technical Bulletin does not define a standard of care, nor is it intended to dictate an exclusive course of management. It presents recognized methods and techniques of clinical practice for consideration by obstetrician–gynecologists for incorporation into their practices. Variations of practice taking into account the needs of the individual patient, resources, and limitations unique to the institution or type of practice may be appropriate.

Reviewed May 1993

THE AMERICAN COLLEGE OF OBSTETRICIANS AND GYNECOLOGISTS
409 12th Street, SW
Washington, DC 20024-2188

4567/98

Number 183—August 1993
(Replaces #81, October 1984)

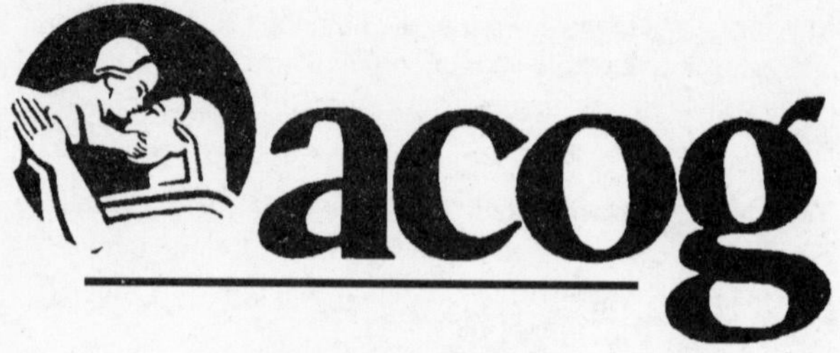

Technical Bulletin
An Educational Aid to Obstetrician–Gynecologists

Cervical Cytology: Evaluation and Management of Abnormalities

Despite the significant decrease in the incidence of and mortality from invasive cervical carcinoma in the United States, there is evidence that the rate of decline is leveling off, and the rate may even be rising slightly in young women (1). Since cervical cytology screening continues to be the mainstay in the early detection of this neoplasm, this Technical Bulletin will review the current status of cervical cytology in the light of current recommendations for the frequency of screening, improvements in the methodology of specimen collection, and recent changes in the diagnostic terminology used to report cervical and vaginal cytologic diagnoses. In view of the persuasive evidence that has been advanced implicating human papillomavirus (HPV) in the etiology of preinvasive and invasive cervical neoplasms, the role of HPV detection is discussed (2). Finally, the diagnostic evaluation and guidelines for management and therapy of cervical cytologic abnormalities will be summarized.

Frequency of Cytologic Screening

In 1988, a consensus recommendation was developed by the American College of Obstetricians and Gynecologists, the American Cancer Society, the National Cancer Institute, the American Medical Association, the American Nurses' Association, the American Academy of Family Physicians, and the American Medical Women's Association. The recommendation suggested that all women who are or who have been sexually active or who have reached age 18 years of age should have an annual cervical smear and pelvic examination (3). It was further recommended that after a woman had three or more consecutive, satisfactory, normal annual examinations, the cervical smear could be performed less frequently at the discretion of her physician. The U.S. Preventive Services Task Force recommended in 1989 that the time interval between smears should be 1–3 years, depending on the presence of risk factors for cervical cancer (4). The risk of an abnormality occurring within 3–5 years after three consecutive negative annual smears is minimal in low-risk patients.

Women who are at increased risk for preinvasive lesions of the cervix include those who are infected with HPV (5, 6) or human immunodeficiency virus (HIV) (7) and those who smoke cigarettes (8). Because having multiple sexual partners increases the likelihood of exposure to human papillomavirus and HIV, it could also be considered a risk factor. Women with any of these risk factors should have cervical smears performed annually.

The cost-effectiveness of cytologic screening for vaginal neoplasia after removal of the cervix for benign disease has not been demonstrated. In consideration of the low risk of preinvasive vaginal lesions or invasive cancer, however, periodic cytologic evaluation of the vagina, based on the patient's risk factors, is suggested.

Following treatment of preinvasive lesions of the cervix or vagina, patients should undergo cytologic evaluation at frequent intervals, every 3–4 months if feasible, for approximately 1 year and then annually thereafter (9). For invasive lesions, evaluation should occur every 3–4 months for approximately 2 years and then every 6 months (10). Close follow-up of these women is necessary because those treated for squamous cell carcinoma of the cervix are at increased risk of developing preinvasive or invasive squamous neoplasms elsewhere in the lower genital tract.

Technique of Cytologic Screening

One of the major factors that accounts for false-negative smears is sampling error. A cellular sample from the endocervical canal obtained with an endocervical brush and a scraping of the portio, to include the entire transformation zone, provides a reliable sample. In the past, endocervical samples have been obtained either by aspiration of cervical mucus with a bulb syringe or with a cotton-tipped applicator. Recent studies have shown that the use of an endocervical brush can increase the yield of endocervical cells by sevenfold (11). Preliminary findings suggest that the brush can be used during pregnancy (12). If the brush is used in pregnancy, it is important that the patient be informed that slight spotting may occur immediately after the procedure but that this is not thought to jeopardize the pregnancy. Providers should use the technique that is most reliable for them in terms of identifying CIN, providing adequate cytologic specimens, and limiting false-negatives and false-positives.

A single slide combining both the endocervical and ectocervical samples or two separate slides from the ectocervix and endocervix can be used. The most important consideration is rapid fixation; it should be appreciated that cellular samples, particular those from the endocervical canal, can become air dried in a matter of seconds, underscoring the need for prompt fixation. Important steps in obtaining an adequate sample include the following:

- Cells should be collected prior to the bimanual examination.
- Care should be taken to avoid contaminating the sample with lubricant.
- If testing for sexually transmitted diseases is indicated, the Pap smear should be taken first, followed by tests for gonococcus and chlamydia.
- Ideally, the entire portio should be visible when the smear is obtained.
- Vaginal discharge, when present in large amounts, should be carefully removed before obtaining the smear so as not to disturb the epithelium. Small amounts of blood will not interfere with cytologic evaluation, but large amounts, as occurring during menses, preclude cytologic sampling. If the patient has no signs or symptoms of a cervical disorder, consideration may be given to treating the vaginitis first.
- The portio sample should be obtained first and then the endocervical sample because of the frequency of bleeding from the endocervix when the brush is used and the drying factor.
- The endocervical canal is best sampled by gently rotating a brush. Excessive manipulation should be avoided to prevent bleeding.
- The collected material should be applied uniformly to the slide, without clumping, and should be rapidly fixed to avoid air drying.
- If spray fixatives are used, the spray should be held at least 10 inches away from the slide to prevent dispersal and destruction of the cells by the propellant.
- For diethylstilbestrol-exposed patients, some providers take smears circumferentially from the upper two thirds of the vagina in addition to evaluating the cervix.

Reporting of Cytologic Diagnosis

Since December 1988, multidisciplinary workshops have been convened by the National Cancer Institute to address the "diagnostic chaos" that existed in cervical cytology reporting. The classification that was developed was designated the Bethesda System for Reporting Cervical/Vaginal Cytologic Diagnoses (13). The Bethesda system (TBS) eliminates the numerical Papanicolaou class designations, requires an evaluation of specimen adequacy as an integral part of the diagnostic report, and uses new terms that can be correlated with the histologic diagnosis (see box).

Since TBS represents a significant departure from the previously used classification, the following discussion elaborates on the rationale of TBS terminology with respect to 1) atypical squamous cells of undetermined significance (ASCUS); 2) the inclusion of changes associated with HPV (ie, koilocytosis) along with cervical intraepithelial neoplasia (CIN) 1 within the category of low-grade squamous intraepithelial lesion (LSIL); and 3) the use of only two terms, LSIL and high-grade squamous intraepithelial lesion (HSIL), to encompass the spectrum of squamous cell carcinoma precursors, in lieu of four degrees of dysplasia/carcinoma in situ (CIS) (mild, moderate, severe, CIS) or the three grades of CIN (CIN 1, 2, 3).

Atypical Squamous Cells of Undetermined Significance

In the past, the terms *inflammatory atypia* and *atypia* were overused to refer to anything from benign reactive changes to preinvasive cellular changes. With such diagnoses, gynecologists have been uncertain as to the appropriate follow-up. The Bethesda system directs the cytopathologist to be more specific in the use of the term *atypia*. Cellular changes thought to be purely reactive in nature are described as such and are not included under the category of ASCUS. In TBS, *atypia* is limited to those cases in which the cytologic findings are of uncertain significance. Relatively few cytology specimens should be reported as ASCUS, as laboratories will be encouraged to avoid this designation when a more precise diagnosis is appropriate. Any questions about the significance of specimens reported as ASCUS should be resolved through communication with the laboratory.

Cellular Changes Associated with Human Papillomavirus and Low-Grade Squamous Intraepithelial Lesion

Koilocytosis is a term that has been used in various and imprecise ways. *Koilocytosis* is a descriptive, not a diagnostic, term that should be applied to squamous cells showing both cytoplasmic vacuolization and nuclear abnormalities characterized by enlargement, hyperchroma-

The Bethesda System for Reporting Cervical/Vaginal Cytologic Diagnoses

Format of the Report:

a. A statement on Adequacy of the Specimen for Evaluation
b. A General Categorization which may be used to assist with clerical triage (optional)
c. The Descriptive Diagnosis

Adequacy of the Specimen

Satisfactory for evaluation
Satisfactory for evaluation but limited by . . . (specify reason)
Unsatisfactory for evaluation . . . (specify reason)

General Categorization (Optional)

Within normal limits
Benign cellular changes: See descriptive diagnoses
Epithelial cell abnormality: See descriptive diagnoses

Descriptive Diagnoses

Benign cellular changes
- Infection
  - *Trichomonas vaginalis*
  - Fungal organisms morphologically consistent with *Candida* spp
  - Predominance of coccobacilli consistent with shift in vaginal flora
  - Bacteria morphologically consistent with *Actinomyces* spp
  - Cellular changes associated with herpes simplex virus
  - Other

Reactive changes
- Reactive cellular changes associated with:
  - Inflammation (includes typical repair)
  - Atrophy with inflammation ("atrophic vaginitis")
  - Radiation
  - Intrauterine contraceptive device (IUD)
- Other

Epithelial Cell Abnormalities
- Squamous Cell
  - Atypical squamous cells of undetermined significance: Qualify*
  - Low-grade squamous intraepithelial lesion encompassing:
    - HPV†
    - Mild dysplasia/CIN 1
  - High-grade squamous intraepithelial lesion encompassing:
    - Moderate and severe dysplasia
    - CIS/CIN 2 and CIN 3
  - Squamous cell carcinoma
- Glandular Cell
  - Endometrial cells, cytologically benign, in a postmenopausal woman
  - Atypical glandular cells of undetermined significance: Qualify*
  - Endocervical adenocarcinoma
  - Endometrial adenocarcinoma
  - Extrauterine adenocarcinoma
  - Adenocarcinoma, not otherwise specified (NOS)

Other malignant neoplasms: Specify

Hormonal evaluation (applied to vaginal smears only)
- Hormonal pattern compatible with age and history
- Hormonal pattern incompatible with age and history: Specify
- Hormonal evaluation not possible due to: Specify

*Atypical squamous or glandular cells of undetermined significance should be further qualified as to whether a reactive or a premalignant/malignant process is favored.

†Cellular changes of human papillomavirus (HPV)—previously termed koilocytosis atypia, or condylomatous atypia—are included in the category of low-grade squamous intraepithelial lesion.

sia, and wrinkling (14). Cytoplasmic vacuolization in the absence of these nuclear alterations does not qualify as koilocytosis. This latter change can be found in normally glycogenated squamous epithelium or in association with various types of inflammation, notably that due to *Trichomonas*.

The Bethesda system incorporates cellular changes associated with HPV (ie, koilocytosis and CIN 1) within the category of LSIL because the natural history, distribution of various HPV types, and morphologic features of both of these lesions—and thus their treatment—are similar. First, long-term follow-up studies have shown that lesions classified as "koilocytosis" and mild dysplasia progress to high-grade intraepithelial neoplasia at similar rates (15–17). Second, a recent pathologic and molecular virologic analysis has demonstrated a similar heterogeneous distribution of low- and high-risk HPV types in both koilocytosis and CIN 1 (18–20). Third, studies evaluating the dysplasia/CIS or CIN terminology have repeatedly demonstrated a lack of interobserver and intraobserver reproducibility (21). The greatest lack of reproducibility is between koilocytosis and CIN 1 (22). Thus, the distinction between koilocytosis and CIN 1 is blurred on the basis of clinical behavior, molecular virologic findings, and morphologic features. The forthcoming World Health Organization (WHO) Histologic Classification of Cervical Neoplasms also combines koilocytosis and CIN 1 into one category.

High-Grade Squamous Intraepithelial Lesion

The Bethesda system combines moderate dysplasia with severe dysplasia and CIS into a single category (HSIL) for several reasons. First, separating moderate dysplasia from severe dysplasia and severe dysplasia from CIS has been shown to be irreproducible (21, 22). Second, from a clinical standpoint, no useful purpose is served by this separation; moderate dysplasia is not usually managed differently from severe dysplasia and CIS. Third, combining moderate dysplasia with severe dysplasia and CIS will reduce discordance between the cytology and the biopsy reports by reducing the possible categories from three to one. Since the management of cervical lesions is based on correlation of the cytologic and histologic findings, greater concordance will reduce the morbidity, anxiety, and cost to the patient of repeated examinations.

Human Papillomavirus Detection in Diagnosis and Management

With highly sensitive molecular techniques, HPV DNA can be detected in over 90% of preinvasive and invasive squamous neoplasms of the cervix (23). Although 70% of invasive squamous carcinomas contain HPV types 16 or 18, these HPV types can also be detected in many patients with LSIL. Prevalence rates vary for women with normal cytology according to the population studied and the HPV detection method used but generally range from 10–50%, with a mean of 25–30% when sensitive techniques are used (24). It has been estimated that 10–20 million women between the ages of 18–50 years in the United States have detectable HPV DNA in the cervix when sensitive assays are used, and each year there are approximately 16,000 incident cases of cervical cancer. It is therefore clear that HPV testing lacks the specificity necessary to be a useful screening test for cervical cancer or its precursors, since the vast majority of women with HPV DNA detected from cervical lavages would be cytologically normal.

Finally, the natural history of HPV infection, especially in cytologically normal women, is not currently known. Preliminary results from a large cohort study suggest that HPV testing with identification of specific HPV types may be of value in the triage of certain subsets of patients, such as those with LSIL or ASCUS and older women. The utility of HPV testing in conjunction with cytology, however, must be evaluated prospectively in a clinical trial before it can be recommended for routine clinical use.

Diagnostic Procedures

The evaluation of the cervix following an abnormal cytology report includes visual inspection of the cervix and vagina, repeat cytology, colposcopic examination with directed biopsies, endocervical curettage (ECC), and bimanual pelvic examination. This approach minimizes the need for diagnostic and therapeutic cervical conization and permits individualized treatment. Occasionally, cervical conization and dilation and fractional curettage are necessary. The first objective is to rule out the presence of invasive carcinoma. Once this has been accomplished, the objectives are to determine the grade and distribution of the intraepithelial lesion.

Colposcopically Directed Biopsies

Following the liberal application of a solution of 3–5% acetic acid, the cervix is inspected to detect abnormal areas (white epithelium, punctation, mosaic cells, atypical vessels). Punch biopsies of the abnormal areas are obtained under direct vision with the colposcope. If necessary, hemostatic agents such as Monsel solution (ferric subsulfate) or silver nitrate may be applied to the biopsy site. The accuracy of directed biopsies has been reported to vary from 85–95%. If the physician is not experienced in grading lesions colposcopically, it is important to obtain samples of all the areas involved and mark the location of the specimen.

Endocervical Curettage

Most colposcopists advocate routine ECC except during pregnancy. The ECC should be performed under direct colposcopic visualization; otherwise, a positive ECC may not necessarily indicate a lesion in the endocervical canal but may represent inadvertent detection of a lesion on the ectocervix near the external os.

Conization of the Cervix

A cone specimen suitable for histologic evaluation can be obtained by surgery (cold knife cone), laser, or loop electrode excision procedure. With the latter two methods, a certain degree of "cautery effect, which may interfere with histologic evaluation of the surgical margins, is unavoidable, but with proper technique, this should be minimal. An ECC performed immediately after the conization provides additional tissue for microscopic assessment.

Diagnostic conization is indicated in the following instances:

- An intraepithelial lesion or microinvasive carcinoma is present in the endocervical curettings.
- Cytologic assessment indicates an abnormality that is not consistent with the tissue diagnosis.
- The entire transformation zone is not visible.
- Microinvasive carcinoma is diagnosed by directed biopsy.
- Cytologic or biopsy evidence of premalignant or malignant glandular epithelium is detected.

Recent data indicate that the use of colposcopy has reduced the incidence of conization to approximately 5–20% of patients with atypical cytology. Conization is not generally indicated as an initial diagnostic procedure.

Endometrial Sampling of Atypical Glandular Cells

Women with atypical glandular cells of endocervical origin should undergo biopsy and ECC directed by colposcopy. If preinvasive or invasive adenocarcinoma is suspected from these studies, diagnostic conization is indicated. Abnormal endometrial cells on cytology should be investigated by endometrial biopsy, fractional dilation and curettage, or hysteroscopy to exclude the possibility of endometrial adenocarcinoma. If no abnormalities are detected with diagnostic dilation and curettage, the possibility of extrauterine sites of malignancy should be considered (ie, ovary, fallopian tube, gastrointestinal tract, breast).

Guidelines for Management

Unfortunately, TBS terminology was not "pretested" before introduction. Thus, the implications of some reports are not known. A long-term research project is needed to develop guidelines for the management of patients with abnormal cytology reports and is under consideration by the National Cancer Institute. Until this research is completed, interim guidelines for patient management have been proposed by the National Cancer Institute which are similar to those outlined below.

Atypical Squamous Cells of Undetermined Significance

In TBS, the term *atypia* is reserved for abnormalities that do not qualify as squamous intraepithelial lesions or reactive changes. These cellular changes are therefore truly of undetermined significance. The prognosis of patients with an ASCUS report can vary depending on the cytopathologist or laboratory. Thus, the clinician is encouraged to either have good communication and understanding with the cytopathologist or monitor a number of patients with this diagnosis in order to substantiate the clinical implications of an ASCUS report from that laboratory. If little or no intraepithelial neoplasia is found in these patients, the need for colposcopic examination is minimized. On the other hand, if the practitioner finds many patients with ASCUS cytology reports have moderate or severe dysplasia or intraepithelial neoplasia, colposcopic evaluation of this group of patients is indicated.

When a patient can be relied upon to return for repeat cytologic examinations at scheduled intervals (usually not more frequent than every 6 months), she can be followed by cytology alone. If a patient receives two or more ASCUS reports, she should undergo colposcopic evaluation. When patient compliance with follow-up recommendations is uncertain, initial colposcopic examination should be considered.

Low-Grade Squamous Intraepithelial Lesion

Most cytology specimens demonstrating LSIL represent processes that will spontaneously revert to normal without therapy. However, a few women in this category will have a lesion that will progress. At a minimum, patients with a smear indicating LSIL should have cervical smears repeated at intervals of approximately 4–6 months and should have colposcopic evaluation performed if an abnormality persists. Because of the high rate of false-negative results in cervical cytology, physicians may perform colposcopic examination after the initial LSIL smear to determine whether a lesion is present.

Following histologic confirmation, if the entire lesion is visualized and the limits of the transformation zone are seen, the lesion can be ablated or excised or the patient can be monitored with no treatment. Management depends to a large degree on the desire and compliance of the patient. Since approximately 15% of these lesions progress to HSIL (17), ablation or excision is a reasonable treatment. On the other hand, since approximately 60% of these lesions regress spontaneously (17), follow-up is an appropriate form of management for a compliant patient when indicated. An LSIL that is limited to the endocervical canal can be closely followed with repeat smears obtained with a cytobrush and an ECC without resorting to a cone biopsy or other treatment. If follow-up and no ablation or excision is selected and the lesion persists for a year, treatment is indicated.

High-Grade Squamous Intraepithelial Lesions

Any woman with a cytology specimen suggesting the presence of HSIL (moderate or severe dysplasia, CIN 2 or 3, or CIS) should undergo colposcopic examination and directed biopsy. Following colposcopically directed biopsy and determination of the distribution of the lesion, ablative therapy aimed at destruction or removal of the entire transformation zone usually should be performed. This management can be undertaken only if the entire lesion and limits of the transformation zone are seen and results of ECC are negative. Conization may be appropriate as outlined above.

Squamous Intraepithelial Lesions in Pregnancy

Pregnant patients with squamous intraepithelial lesions may be monitored during pregnancy by frequent smears and colposcopic examination with biopsies as indicated by abnormal smears, followed by reassessment of the cervix and definitive therapy after delivery.

The patient whose biopsy indicates a possibility of early stromal invasion or microinvasion (stage IA) requires excision of the affected area to rule out invasive cancer (stage IB). Following excision, treatment of pregnant patients with microinvasion may be postponed until after delivery.

It is important that the pathologist and gynecologist communicate frequently. This should include evaluating the appropriateness of patient care and the adequacy of the cytologic smear, tissue diagnosis, and laboratory quality control. When a problem cannot be safely resolved by the physician, proper consultation should be sought.

Therapy

Before treatment is instituted, it is important that the histologic diagnosis be accurate and that the extent of the lesion be determined. A variety of ablative techniques have been employed in the treatment of squamous intraepithelial lesions, including surgical excision, cryosurgery, laser vaporization procedures, and, more recently, loop electrode excision procedure. Most of these techniques can be performed in an outpatient setting, which is one of the main objectives in the management of this disease. Since all therapeutic modalities carry an inherent recurrence rate of up to 10%, cytologic follow-up at approximately 3-month intervals for 1 year is necessary. After invasive cancer has been ruled out, ambulatory therapy is appropriate when the following conditions exist:

- The lesion is located on the ectocervix.
- There is no involvement of the endocervix as determined by colposcopic examination and ECC.

Local Excision

Local excision may be accomplished by excision or punch biopsy removal of the entire lesion area. Completeness of excision should be checked by colposcopic examination.

Cryocautery

Cryocautery using nitrous oxide or carbon dioxide as a refrigerant may be used to treat lesions which can be completely covered by the probe and which do not extend into the canal. A double-freeze technique is helpful to extend 4–5 mm beyond the edge of the probe. Lubricant applied to the tip prior to freezing provides a better interface. Mild cramping occurs during treatment, and vaginal discharge ensues for at least 4 weeks.

Carbon Dioxide Laser Vaporization

Laser vaporization is used for the treatment of lesions which are too large for a cryocautery probe, which extend into the endocervical canal, or which have deep gland involvement. These lesions are not as effectively treated by cryosurgery because of its more limited depth of destruction. Tissue should be vaporized to a depth adequate to ensure that the bases of the deepest endocervical crypts are destroyed. A depth of 7 mm from the surface will be effective for over 99% of patients (25). This procedure is usually carried out with a power density of approximately 1,000 W/cm^2.

Vaporization of the cervix usually causes only minor cramps and can be performed with local infiltration of the cervix, with a paracervical block, or without anesthesia. Posttreatment discharge may be present for 5–10 days. Following laser therapy, the squamocolumnar junction returns to the level of the external os in most patients. This facilitates follow-up with colposcopic examination.

Loop Electrode Excision Procedure

In the past, electrocautery was used for removal of small, well-defined local lesions but failed to provide tissue for histologic evaluation. Recently, thin wire loop electrodes that permit excision of the entire transformation zone have been developed. Following local infiltration of the cervix with xylocaine and a dilute solution of a vasoconstrictor and application of Lugol solution to facilitate visualization of the area to be removed, an appropriate loop size is used to excise the transformation zone to a depth of 7–8 mm extending 4–5 mm beyond the affected area. Following removal of the specimen, the base of the excised area is cauterized and a hemostatic agent such as Monsel solution or silver nitrate is applied. This technique provides a tissue specimen suitable for histologic evaluation and may be used as a diagnostic and treatment procedure.

After treatment, patients experience mild discharge for 5–10 days. This procedure is comparatively new; long-term follow-up and large trials have not been done. Complications are expected to be similar to those of cervical conization but may be less frequent.

Hysterectomy

Some patients with HSIL may be candidates for hysterectomy. It may also be appropriate for those with recurrent HSIL or those who have lesions that cannot be treated adequately with local therapies (26).

Summary

As a result of rapidly evolving technology, advances in the understanding of the pathogenesis of cervical neoplasia, and the introduction of TBS terminology, we stand at a crossroads in the screening and management of this disease. This bulletin reflects management considered appropriate at this time. A number of key issues as indicated above must be addressed before more specific guidelines can be incorporated into routine clinical practice. Until data from clinical trials evaluating these new methods are available, the gynecologist is best advised to manage patients using the guidelines in this Technical Bulletin.

REFERENCES

1. Devesa SS, Silverman DT, Young JL Jr, Pollack ES, Brown CC, Horm JW, et al. Cancer incidence and mortality trends among whites in the United States, 1947-84. J Natl Cancer Inst 1987:79:701–770
2. Ambros RA, Kurman RJ. Current concepts in the relationship of human papillomavirus infection to the pathogenesis and classification of precancerous squamous lesions of the uterine cervix. Semin Diagn Pathol 1990;7:158–172
3. Fink DJ. Change in American Cancer Society Checkup Guidelines for detection of cervical cancer. CA 1988; 38:127–128
4. U.S. Preventive Services Task Force. Screening for cervical cancer. In: Guide to clinical preventive services: an assessment of the effectiveness of 169 interventions. Baltimore: Williams and Wilkins, 1989:57–62
5. Muñoz N, Bosch FX. Epidemiology of cervical cancer. In: Muñoz N, Bosch FX, Jensen OM, eds. Human papillomavirus and cervical cancer. Lyon, France: International Agency for Research on Cancer (WHO), 1989:9–39
6. Schiffman MH. Recent progress in defining the epidemiology of human papillomavirus infection and cervical neoplasia. J Natl Cancer Inst 1992;84:394–398
7. Maiman M, Fruchter RG, Serur E, Remy JC, Feuer G, Boyce J. Human immunodeficiency virus infection and cervical neoplasia. Gynecol Oncol 1990;38:377–382
8. Winklestein W. Smoking and cervical cancer—current status: a review. Am J Epidemiol 1990;131:945–957
9. Ferenczy A, Winkler B. Cervical intraepithelial neoplasia and condyloma. In: Kurman RJ, ed. Blaustein's pathology of the female genital tract. 3rd ed. New York: Springer Verlag, 1987:177–217
10. Ferenczy A, Winkler B. Carcinoma and metastatic tumors of the cervix. In: Kurman RJ, ed. Blaustein's pathology of the female genital tract. 3rd ed. New York: Springer Verlag, 1987:218–256
11. Taylor PT Jr, Andersen WA, Barber SR, Covell JL, Smith EB, Underwood PB Jr. The screening Papanicolaou smear: contribution of the endocervical brush. Obstet Gynecol 1987;70:734–738
12. Orr JW Jr, Barrett JM, Orr PF, Holloway RW, Holimon JL. The efficacy and safety of the cytobrush during pregnancy. Gynecol Oncol 1992;44:260–262
13. National Cancer Institute Workshop. The 1988 Bethesda system for reporting cervical/vaginal cytological diagnoses. JAMA 1989;262:931–934
14. Kurman RJ, Malkasian GD Jr, Sedlis A, Solomon D. From Papanicolau to Bethesda: the rationale for a new cervical cytologic classification. Obstet Gynecol 1991;77:779–782
15. Nash JD, Burke TW, Hoskins WJ. Biologic course of cervical human papillomavirus infection. Obstet Gynecol 1987;69: 160–162
16. Montz FJ, Monk BJ, Fowler JM, Nguyen L. Natural history of the minimally abnormal Papanicolau smear. Obstet Gynecol 1992;80:385–388
17. Nasiell K, Roger V, Nasiell M. Behavior of mild cervical dysplasia during long-term follow-up. Obstet Gynecol 1986;67: 665–669
18. Willett GD, Kurman RJ, Reid R, Greenberg M, Jenson AB, Lorincz AT. Correlation of the histologic appearance of intraepithelial neoplasia of the cervix with human papillomavirus types. Emphasis on low grade lesions including so-called flat condyloma. Int J Gynecol Pathol 1989;8:18–25
19. Lorincz AT, Reid R, Jenson AB, Greenberg MD, Lancaster W, Kurman RJ. Human papillomavirus infection of the cervix: relative risk associations of 15 common anogenital types. Obstet Gynecol 1992;79:328–337
20. Lungu O, Sun XW, Felix J, Richart RM, Silverstein S, Wright TC Jr. Relationship of human papillomavirus type to grade of cervical intraepithelial neoplasia. JAMA 1992;267:2493–2496
21. Ismail SM, Colclough AB, Dinnen JS, Eakins D, Evans DMD, Gradwell E, et al. Reporting cervical intra-epithelial neoplasia (CIN): intra- and interpathologist variation and factors associated with disagreement. Histopathology 1990;16:371–376
22. Sherman ME, Schiffman MH, Erozan YS, Wacholder S, Kurman RJ. The Bethesda system. A proposal for reporting abnormal cervical smears based on the reproducibility of cytopathologic diagnoses. Arch Pathol Lab Med 1992;116: 1155–1158
23. Lorincz AT, Temple GF, Kurman RJ, Jenson AB, Lancaster WD. Oncogenic association of specific human papillomavirus types with cervical neoplasia. J Natl Cancer Inst 1987;79: 671–677
24. Bauer HM, Ting Y, Greer CE, Chambers JC, Tashiro CJ, Chimera J, et al. Genital human papillomavirus infection in female university students as determined by a PCR-based method. JAMA 1991;265:472–477
25. Anderson MC, Hartley RB. Cervical crypt involvement by intraepithelial neoplasia. Obstet Gynecol 1980; 55:546–550
26. DiSaia PJ, Creasman WT, eds. Preinvasive disease of the cervix, vagina and vulva. In: Clinical gynecologic oncology. 3rd ed. St Louis: CV Mosby Co, 1989:1–44

This Technical Bulletin was developed under the direction of the Committee on Technical Bulletins of the American College of Obstetricians and Gynecologists as an educational aid to obstetricians and gynecologists. The committee wishes to thank Robert J. Kurman, MD, for his assistance in the development of this bulletin. This Technical Bulletin does not define a standard of care, nor is it intended to dictate an exclusive course of management. It presents recognized methods and techniques of clinical practice for consideration by obstetrician–gynecologists for incorporation into their practices. Variations of practice taking into account the needs of the individual patient, resources, and limitations unique to the institution or type of practice may be appropriate.

Reviewed February 1995

THE AMERICAN COLLEGE OF OBSTETRICIANS AND GYNECOLOGISTS
409 12th Street, SW
Washington, DC 20024-2188

45/765

Number 223—May 1996
(Replaces #129, June 1989)

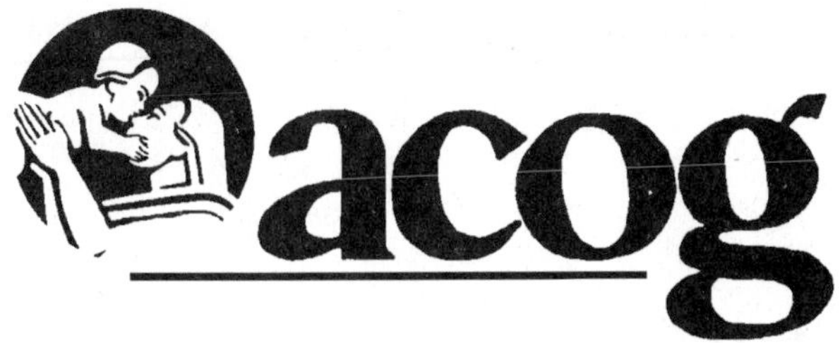

Technical Bulletin

An Educational Aid to Obstetrician–Gynecologists

Chronic Pelvic Pain

Chronic pain is often accompanied by poorly defined symptoms and a sense of failure by both doctor and patient. When confronted with such pain, the practitioner may feel daunted by the process of establishing the cause. In spite of the challenge inherent to the management of chronic pain, it is reasonable to anticipate a positive outcome. Obstetricians and gynecologists are often confronted with patients who have chronic pelvic pain, which may or may not have a gynecologic cause. Pain that is not gynecologic in origin may require a different approach and possible referral.

Evolution of Pain

Under most circumstances, "pain" involves four phases:

1. Nociception: the origination and detection of a neurologic signal based on a noxious event
2. Pain: the recognition of the signal or event
3. Suffering: affective responses to the event
4. Pain behavior: adaptive changes (functional or dysfunctional) made based on the pain.

The physiologic (or pathophysiologic) processes that evoke the perception of pain are few: thermal (heat or cold), mechanical (stretch, distension, or muscular contraction), and chemical irritation (including the liberation of histamines, bradykinin, prostaglandins, serotonin, acetylcholine, acids, proteolytic enzymes and potassium ions released by ischemia, necrosis, or inflammation). The stimulus that creates pain is somewhat tissue specific; for example, thermal injury to the skin is painful, but thermal injury to the bowel is not. The cause of chronic pain may be grouped into three categories: structural (ongoing processes such as arthritis or cancer), psychophysiologic (such as continuing muscle spasm causing pain after the original insult has passed), and somatic (as is found among those who internalize stresses and express them in the form of pain).

Localization of the source of pain is often difficult or inaccurate, especially in the case of visceral pain that is transmitted via slow pain fibers (generally characterized as burning or aching in nature). This pain does not generally arise from highly localized processes or damage. Instead, it arises from conditions that affect a wider area, such as inflammation or ischemia. Fast pain fibers transmit pain that is sharp and moderately well localized and mediate pain sensation from the parietal, but not visceral, peritoneum. Like slow fibers, fast pain fibers do not adapt to a stimulus, but rather continue to generate the pain signal for as long as the stimulus is present. Because the visceral and parietal pain fibers travel through different routes, the perception of pain may be interpreted as arising from, or referred to, different areas of the body. For example, in patients with appendicitis, the aching pain of visceral sensation is localized to the periumbilical area, while the sharp pain of parietal peritoneal irritation is felt directly over the right lower quadrant.

Acute pain and pain of less than 3 months' duration are most likely to be associated with identifiable pathophysiologic processes. The diagnosis and management of this type of pain is generally straightforward; in some cases, however, specific diagnosis may be deferred while emergency treatment is provided. Most subacute (3–6 months' duration) and chronic (greater than 6 months' duration) pain states begin with a nociceptive event or process, although that event may go unrecognized or unremembered.

Evaluation Strategies

Pain of any duration is assessed by history and physical examination. The technique of assessment is similar, regardless of the duration of the pain. Laboratory and diagnostic studies also may be helpful depending on the clinical findings.

History

The history provides descriptions of the nature, intensity, and distribution of the pain. Nuances of characteristics and location of pain are important, although imprecise localization is typical with intraabdominal processes. Radiation of the pain or coexisting pain in other locations should be assessed. The temporal patterns of the pain (onset, duration, changes, cyclicity) and any factors that modify the pain, such as posture, meals, bowel movements, voiding, menstruation, intercourse, or medications, should be determined. Associated symptoms, such as anorexia, constipation, or fatigue should be evaluated. Previous surgeries, pelvic infections, infertility, or obstetric experiences may be significant. For patients of reproductive age, the timing and characteristics of their last menstrual period, the presence of nonmenstrual vaginal bleeding or discharge, and the method of contraception used, if any, should be established. The role of the pain in the patient's life, as well as life situations and events that affect the pain, should be explored. The possibility of physical or sexual abuse should be considered, and the patient should be questioned directly about this possibility.

The history should also include a review of gastrointestinal, urologic, and musculoskeletal functions, including the relationship between these systems and the patient's pain. Coexisting symptoms, such as frequent headaches, nonrestoring sleep, diffuse tender points, and fatigue, may be suggestive of systemic disorders such as fibromyalgia.

The history and the patient's affect may suggest depression or other mood disorders. These will compound the effect of any pain experienced and complicate the diagnosis and management of chronic pain. Thus, the patient should be asked about a history of mental illness, with or without treatment.

Physical Evaluation

The physical evaluation of a patient with pelvic pain should begin with a general physical and neurologic assessment. The patient should be asked to indicate the location of the pain. If she uses a single finger to indicate the location, it is more likely that the pain has a discrete source than if she uses a sweeping motion of the whole hand. Site identification may be aided by simple drawings (1).

The physical examination of the abdomen should begin with inspection for deformity, erythema, or edema; the presence of scars, hernias, or distension should be noted. The presence and characteristics of bowel sounds are important when gastrointestinal processes are suspected. Palpation should include the epigastrium, flanks, midback and low back, and inguinal areas.

In addition to performing a comprehensive gynecologic examination, the physician should focus specific attention on pain reproduction during the physical examination. The patient should be fully informed of what will take place, and her cooperation should be enlisted. Useful adjuncts include isolating pain by using either the vaginal or abdominal hand. Systematic palpation of the external genitalia may be aided with a cotton-tipped swab. Hyperesthesia may be present despite normal vulvar skin.

Alternatively, internal discomfort may be exacerbated by insertion of a speculum or midline placement of the examining hand. Women may also experience pain from trigger points (areas overlying muscles that induce spasms and pain) in the myofascial layers of the pelvic sidewall or pelvic floor. The obturator internus and levator ani are common sites for myofascial trigger points and should be specifically palpated. Direct visceral palpation and mobilization that reproduces the pain does not necessarily signify that removal of that organ will provide pain relief. Although endometriosis may be suspected based on the physical examination, extirpative surgery should not be considered until a definitive diagnosis is established with further evaluation. Episodic, organ-specific pain symptoms may not necessarily be reproduced during the physical examination.

Postural and musculoskeletal alterations must be considered. Assessment includes viewing the patient's spine while she is sitting, standing, and walking. When a patient bends at the waist, a previously overlooked scoliosis may become apparent. Assessment of discrepancies in the patient's leg length, range of motion of joints, and muscle strength may reveal an unexpected source of pain referred to the pelvis or lower abdomen. An attempt should be made to elicit trigger points. Neurologic testing, encompassing touch and reflex testing, should also be performed.

Laboratory Studies

Laboratory studies should be dependent on the history and physical examination and should be tailored to the patient. The individual's signs and symptoms may indicate the need for cultures, serum chemistry and electrolyte evaluations, or specific enzyme tests. A red cell sedimentation test may be of help in detecting chronic disease states.

Diagnostic Studies

Ultrasonography and other imaging technologies have a limited place in the evaluation of chronic pelvic pain. In selected patients with chronic pain, ultrasonography may be useful to supplement an inadequate or inconclusive pelvic examination. Further imaging studies should be directed by the patient's signs and symptoms.

Specialized diagnostic studies based on the patient's symptoms and the presumptive diagnosis may require consultation with other specialists in anesthesiology, orthopedics, neurology, or gastroenterology. A physical medicine consultation may be especially helpful in the evaluation of musculoskeletal processes, such as nerve entrapment, myofascial trigger points, or neurologic disorders. Assessment of the urinary tract may be warranted.

In selected cases, diagnostic laparoscopy may be helpful in the evaluation and treatment of patients experiencing chronic pelvic pain (2, 3). Laparoscopy is of greatest value when the pelvic examination is abnormal or when initial therapy fails. Hysteroscopy is of little value in the evaluation of chronic pain.

Depression and sleep disorders are common in patients with chronic pelvic pain. They complicate both diagnosis and effective therapy. Psychologic factors should be considered and explored, but they do not rule out an organic cause for the pain. The Beck Depression Inventory may be used as a screening test for depression (4). More involved psychologic instruments, such as the Minnesota Multiphasic Personality Inventory and the Eysenck Personality Questionnaire, have limited utility.

Other contributing factors in the patient's life, both past and present, should be sought to explain the pain. Domestic discord, physical or sexual abuse, rape or incest, parental loss or divorce, a disturbing or abusive family background, alcohol or drug abuse, intense fear of pregnancy, or other stresses may all be expressed in the form of pain. When carried to the extreme, internalization of stresses expressed as physical symptoms is referred to as somatization or Briquet disorder.

Gynecologic Pelvic Pain

There are no symptoms that uniquely identify genitourinary structures as the source of a patient's pain. Even the relationship of recurrent pain to menstruation or the presence of dyspareunia are no more than suggestive. For this reason, all patients require a thorough and wide-ranging evaluation that includes assessments of other organ systems and structures in addition to genitourinary structures (see box).

The characteristics of symptoms that arise from genitourinary organs range from cramps to sharp pain; the pain is felt in the lower abdomen in the midline and occasionally radiates to the back. Bladder or ureteral pain may

Causes of Chronic Pelvic Pain

- Gynecologic
  - Extrauterine
    - Adhesions
    - Chronic ectopic pregnancy
    - Chronic pelvic infection
    - Endometriosis
    - Residual ovary syndrome
  - Uterine
    - Adenomyosis
    - Chronic endometritis
    - Leiomyomata
    - Intrauterine contraceptive device
    - Pelvic congestion
    - Pelvic support defects
    - Polyps
- Urologic
  - Chronic urinary tract infection
  - Detrusor overactivity
  - Interstitial cystitis
  - Stone
  - Suburethral diverticulitis
  - Urethral syndrome
- Gastrointestinal
  - Cholelithiasis
  - Chronic appendicitis
  - Constipation
  - Diverticular disease
  - Enterocolitis
  - Gastric/duodenal ulcer
  - Inflammatory bowel disease (Crohn disease, ulcerative colitis)
  - Irritable bowel syndrome
  - Neoplasia
- Musculoskeletal
  - Coccydynia
  - Disk problems
  - Degenerative joint disease
  - Fibromyositis
  - Hernias
  - Herpes zoster (shingles)
  - Low back pain
  - Levator ani syndrome (spasm of pelvic floor)
  - Myofascial pain (trigger points, spasms)
  - Nerve entrapment syndromes
  - Osteoporosis (fractures)
  - Pain posture
  - Scoliosis/lordosis/kyphosis
  - Strains/sprains
- Other
  - Abuse (physical or sexual, prior or current)
  - Heavy metal poisoning (lead, mercury)
  - Hyperparathyroidism
  - Porphyria
  - Psychiatric disorders (depression, bipolar disorders, inadequate personality disorder)
  - Psychosocial stress (marital discord, work stress)
  - Sickle cell disease
  - Sleep disturbances
  - Somatiform disorders
  - Substance use (especially cocaine)
  - Sympathetic dystrophy
  - Tabes dorsalis (third-degree syphilis)

radiate to the vagina or groin. Both the characteristics and location attributed to the pain depend on the underlying process.

The genitourinary systems are frequently inappropriately blamed for chronic pelvic pain syndromes (eg, a small stable adnexal cyst should not be a source of chronic pain). Endometriosis, with its attendant scarring and chemical irritation, is thought to cause pelvic heaviness and dyspareunia, though some studies find the prevalence of endometriosis is the same in women with and without pain, raising questions about causality (3, 5).

The urinary system may play a role. Interstitial cystitis, chronic cystitis, urethritis, and urethral syndromes all may create symptoms of chronic pelvic pain.

Other possible causes of chronic pain are conditions such as pelvic vascular congestion and adhesive disease (6). These conditions are more likely to present as dyspareunia or pain during bowel movements; the direct tie to chronic pain is conjectural and difficult to justify based on basic mechanisms of pain.

When gynecologic or urinary tract processes are the source of chronic complaints, the symptoms generally will be felt toward the midline or, in the case of adnexal pathology, the side of the lesion. Dyspareunia, in these cases, is sufficiently common that its absence suggests the need for a wider ranging differential diagnosis.

Cyclic pelvic pain and dysmenorrhea represent a special subset of chronic pain syndromes. While the association of cyclic pain with the menstrual cycle implies a causal relationship with the genital tract or the ovaries, this is not always the case.

Dyspareunia may result from any number of factors, ranging from anatomic to psychosocial. It is seldom the result of a single, simple factor. In addition to routine inquiries, the patient should be asked about sexual function in general. Specific information about sexual activities, such as the places, positions, partners, and forms of expression that do or do not engender discomfort, should be investigated. Questions about when the discomfort begins and how long it lasts should be included. The results of previous attempts to deal with the problem—by the patient or other physicians—should be discussed to provide further insight into possible causes. A thorough history of other pain symptoms should also be obtained to identify processes that may arise elsewhere but are felt as sexual pain.

Patients with deep, internal, or "thrust" dyspareunia often express a feeling that something is "being bumped into" during sexual activity. Any pelvic pathology may be responsible for this discomfort, but abnormalities such as endometriosis, pelvic adhesions, pelvic relaxation or malposition (retroversion), adnexal pathology or prolapse, or uterine fibroids are the most likely causes. Interstitial cystitis may cause dyspareunia before it proceeds to chronic, unremitting pain. Inflammatory bowel conditions may cause tenderness at the apex of the vagina and lead to dyspareunia.

Nongynecologic Pelvic Pain

Because of the commonality of innervation, lower abdominal symptoms may arise from most pelvic or abdominal structures, as well as from musculoskeletal elements that make up the back and abdominal walls. Pain may be referred to the abdomen by any number of processes. In some cases, no pathology will be detected as a cause for the pain.

Gastrointestinal Causes

Gastrointestinal disorders are common sources of chronic pelvic pain. The most common is irritable bowel syndrome (IBS), which may be responsible for as much as one half of all cases of chronic pelvic pain (7, 8). The pain of IBS is usually colicky in character and associated with a sensation of rectal fullness or incomplete emptying; it is improved with bowel movement but is intensified by meals. The pain is often worse at or around the time of menstruation and may be associated with dyspareunia. The symptoms of IBS often wax and wane but remain present for cycles that last from weeks to months, often paralleling physical or emotional stress. Although in some cases pain is the only symptom of IBS, constipation, frequently with intermittent diarrhea, is common. As is true with other chronic pain syndromes, women with IBS have been characterized as having an increased prevalence of somatiform disorders. When IBS is suspected, bulk-forming agents, anxiolytics, and low doses of antidepressants are recommended. Anticholinergics are not generally recommended because of their lack of effectiveness at doses that do not cause significant side effects.

The inflammation of the bowel with Crohn disease or ulcerative colitis causes visceral pain even in the absence of obstruction or perforation. Most patients report poorly localized pain and diarrhea as in IBS, though the fever and bloody stool that are common in inflammatory bowel disease are not a part of IBS. The widely separated nature of Crohn disease lesions, which often involves both the large and small bowel, results in diffuse and nonspecific symptoms and findings. When the small bowel is involved, pain is often located in the periumbilical region or right lower quadrant. Colon involvement may cause pain in either or both lower quadrants. Patients with ulcerative colitis are less likely to have acute pain. Cramping that is relieved by voluminous, often bloody diarrhea is typical of ulcerative colitis.

In older patients, diverticular disease can be a source of significant morbidity. Bleeding, perforation, and abscess formation may occur, but abdominal pain and diarrhea are more common and mimic IBS. The pain is usually in the left lower quadrant and improves with bowel movements and the passage of flatus.

Physical examination in patients with gastrointestinal disease often provides indeterminate findings. Patients with IBS may have diffuse tenderness over the entire abdomen, with greater sensitivity over the sigmoid. When such left lower quadrant tenderness is present without signs of inflammation, it is highly suggestive of IBS. When inflammation is present, especially with a mass, diverticulitis should be suspected. Anorectal findings of fistulae or abscesses suggest inflammatory bowel disease, while masses forewarn the possibility of neoplasm or endometriosis. Excessive discomfort during rectal examination is common in patients with IBS.

Musculoskeletal Causes

Herniation of a disk, spondylolisthesis, exaggerated lumbar lordosis, or "pain postures" that induce abnormal stresses on muscles or ligaments (such as the chronic pelvic tilt brought on by carrying a child on one hip) may all cause ongoing pelvic pain. Pain over the distribution of a single nerve root or peripheral nerve may be found when herniation of a disk occurs, following surgery, in conditions such as arthritis, or in obese patients in whom soft tissue or weight-induced posture change may cause impingement on the nerve.

Musculoskeletal pain frequently radiates to areas quite distant from the source of the nociceptive signal. A trigger point may be identified that induces or reproduces the pain. Trigger points may be found throughout the body but are most common in the abdominal wall, back, and, when pelvic pain is reported, the pelvic floor (9, 10).

Therapy

The general principles of pain management are outlined in the box. Whenever possible, therapy should be directed toward resolving the underlying condition. However, it is not always necessary or possible to establish a diagnosis prior to proceeding with treatment.

Pharmacologic Therapy

Analgesic treatment can be given to address discomfort while therapy directed toward the underlying cause is instituted. Processes that involve inflammation and prostaglandin release will respond well to nonsteroidal antiinflammatory drug (NSAID) therapy. Processes that do not involve prostaglandins require the use of centrally acting analgesics, adjunctive medications, or less common modalities, such as transcutaneous electrical nerve stimulation.

When central analgesics are used, they should be commensurate with the degree of discomfort involved. Mild analgesics such as aspirin, acetaminophen, pro-

Pain Management Principles

Use positive reinforcement and support.

- Placebos should not be used to assess pain.
- The placebo effect should be used to supplement other therapy through positive reinforcement.

Assess psychologic factors early in the evaluation process.

- Coexisting depression or sleep disorders should be sought.
- The diagnosis of "psychogenic pain" should not be a diagnosis of exclusion. Rather, it should be made only when there are clear indications for it.

Treat the underlying disorder whenever possible.

- Pain receptors do not adapt, and under some circumstances actually lower their thresholds causing hyperalgesia.

Treat the pain promptly and continue on a regular basis.

- Treatment that effectively suppresses pain or that is not based on the need to reexperience pain gives the best results (eg, patient-controlled analgesia for postoperative patients). Frequent, scheduled follow-ups are better than "as needed" visits.

Consider use of multiple treatment modalities in synergy.

- Different methods of treatment work by way of different routes (eg, relaxation techniques, transcutaneous electrical nerve stimulation, physical therapy, vocational rehabilitation, biofeedback).
- The nuances of the treatments used should be understood (eg, site of action, half-life, administration routes available, interactions).
- Combinations of medications that increase sedation without enhancing analgesia should be avoided.

Use narcotic drugs with caution.

- Tolerance and dependence may occur with long-term use.
- Narcotics should not be withheld if other therapies are ineffective.

poxyphene, and NSAIDs may be appropriate for mild pain. One or more of these agents should be tried, beginning with the mildest (mild analgesics or NSAIDs), then progressing to centrally acting drugs and serotonin uptake inhibitors.

Stronger pain, especially pain that does not respond to this initial escalating series of treatments, warrants stronger agents, such as narcotics (Table 1). Brief use of these agents is generally well tolerated and does not present a significant potential for abuse. Undertreatment of pain is more likely to lead to chronic pain states and drug-seeking behavior than early, aggressive, time-limited, effective therapies. Drug abuse and dependence are more likely when care is fragmented, episodic (such as through frequent emergency room visits), or provided by multiple physicians. In long-term opiate users, tolerance and physical dependence may occur, but these effects should be distinguished from psychologic dependence. If abuse or drug-seeking behavior is suspected, agents such as methadone can provide analgesia with less addictive euphoria and have no significant street value for the purpose of resale. The use of combinations of medications (such as NSAIDs and opiates) may increase analgesic potency, but care must be exercised to avoid compounding side effects.

When the definitive therapy is not practical or available, modifications of the menstrual cycle may be indicated in individuals with cyclic menstrual pain. This may be accomplished through menstrual suppression. If suppression of the menstrual cycle fails to provide improvement, it is unlikely that surgical removal of the reproductive organs will provide any better results.

In using any pharmacologic therapy, care must be taken to avoid secondary gains that may contribute to, or worsen, the psychosocial aspects of the problem. When the patient takes an active responsibility for relieving the pain, positive adaptive behaviors increase, allowing somatic and psychosocial factors to be separated from other causes and minimized. Even in patients in whom somatiform disorders are diagnosed, intercurrent physical illness should be considered, as should drug or alcohol dependence. If the latter are detected, appropriate detoxification should be instituted.

Medications should be given on a regular basis, not "as needed." The appointment schedule and medication dosage should be maintained on a regular basis. Office visits may be less frequent and shorter as the severity of symptoms declines, but both the patient and physician should understand the long-term nature of the illness and its treatment.

Adjunctive treatment with antidepressants or sleeping aids may be appropriate. Such treatment may improve coping skills or may directly influence the perception of pain through the induced actions of serotonin or enkephalins. Amitriptyline in doses as low as 25–50 mg at bedtime may be of help in improving sleep patterns and reducing the severity of chronic pain complaints. In patients with guarding, splinting, or reactive muscle spasms, the use of a muscle relaxant may prove useful.

Surgical Therapy

Surgical therapy for chronic pain is limited to the treatment of surgically correctable etiologies. Even in those patients with surgically correctable conditions, both the physician and the patient must understand the possibility (if not the probability) that the pain may be unchanged, or even worsened, by the procedure, and that other nonsurgical therapies may still be applicable (11).

Even greater reserve must be exercised in patients who have already undergone exploratory or "therapeutic" surgery without relief. Further surgery is even less likely to result in improvements. Other causes, including disease affecting other organ systems and psychosocial factors, must be evaluated. These patients are best served by a multidisciplinary approach.

Many procedures have been proposed to interrupt the neural pathways that transmit "pain" in the pelvis. These range from laparoscopic uterosacral nerve ablation to presacral neurectomy. Short-term favorable results are often claimed for dysmenorrhea (12), but variable long-term effects for other chronic pain and the high rate of complications associated with some procedures severely limit the applicability of these techniques (13–16).

Because of an uncertain role for endometriosis and pelvic adhesions in the creation of chronic pelvic pain, the appropriate place for surgical therapy of these conditions in chronic pain patients is uncertain (17–20). Hysterectomy or oophorectomy is often carried out "for pelvic pain," but studies show that long-term success is often disappointing when this is the only indication (21). If significant pathology is not detected by using laparoscopy, hysterectomy for chronic pelvic pain is warranted if the pain has persisted for more than 6 months, does not respond to analgesics (including antiinflammatory agents), and impairs the patient's normal function. Prior to the procedure, trials of other therapy should be undertaken, other possible sources of pelvic pain should be eliminated, and the absence of cervical malignancy should be confirmed. It may be prudent to ensure that the patient has had the opportunity for psychosocial evaluation before extirpative surgery is undertaken because hysterectomy may not cure the pain (22).

Multidisciplinary Diagnosis and Management

Some of the greatest successes reported in the diagnosis and management of chronic pain states have come from multidisciplinary approaches (23–28). This is consistent with the biopsychosocial model of pain development in

TABLE 1. Narcotics Commonly Used for the Treatment of Chronic Pelvic Pain

Drug	Dosage	Comments
Intermediate Potency		
Propoxyphene	65 mg orally every 3–4 h	Related to methadone; may accumulate with repetitive doses; overdose may cause convulsions
Codeine	15–60 mg orally every 4–6 h 30–60 mg IM* every 4–6 h	Well absorbed orally
Oxycodone	5–30 mg orally every 4–6 h 5–10 mg IM every 4–6 h	Short acting; fewer side effects than codeine; may be combined with other agents
Pentazocine	50–150 mg orally every 4–6 h 30–60 mg IM every 4 h	Mixed agonist/antagonist; may cause withdrawal in narcotic-dependent patients
High Potency		
Meperidine	50–150 mg orally every 3–4 h 50–100 mg IM every 2–4 h	Has toxic metabolites; not for use in patients on monoamine oxidase inhibitors or those with renal dysfunction; 75% of oral dose lost in feces; not recommended for chronic use
Butorphanol tartrate	2 mg IM every 3–4 h	Mixed agonist/antagonist; may cause withdrawal in narcotic-dependent patients; has dose ceiling
Denocine	10 mg IM every 3–6 h	Mixed agonist/antagonist; may cause withdrawal in narcotic-dependent patients; has dose ceiling
Nalbuphine hydrocholoride	10 mg IM every 3–6 h	Mixed agonist/antagonist; may cause withdrawal in narcotic-dependent patients; has dose ceiling
Morphine	30–60 mg orally every 3–4 h 90–120 mg orally every 12 h 10 mg IM every 3–4 h	Controlled release form allows twice-daily dosing
Hydromorphone	2–6 mg orally every 3–4 h 1–2 mg IM every 4–6 h	Short-acting narcotic
Methadone	10–20 mg orally every 3–4 h 2.5–10 mg IM every 3–4 h	Long-acting oral method; used for maintenance treatment of addicts; little abuse potential
Levorphanol	4 mg orally every 6–8 h 2 mg IM every 6–8 h	Long-acting; good oral absorption; similar to methadone
Oxymorphone	1 mg IM every 3–4 h Rectal suppositories, 5 mg every 4–6 h	
Fentanyl	Transdermally, 25–50 mg/h	Used only for long-term therapy (eg, cancer pain)

* IM indicates intramuscular dose; best reserved for short-term therapy.

which the expression of pain depends heavily on multiple physical, psychologic, and social factors. This approach can help patients by teaching methods for improving coping mechanisms or relaxation techniques; providing biofeedback; providing depression therapy, psychotherapy, or marital or sexual counseling; administering nerve blocks; developing exercise programs; or providing hypnosis or other services directed to the needs of the individual patient.

Physical therapy and exercise programs may be of great help in patients with pain that is related to musculoskeletal components. Massage and tactile stimulation in the area of pain can suppress pain signals. The application of heat or cold, when not otherwise contraindicated, may provide relief for some patients. The use of transcutaneous electrical nerve stimulation therapy can provide excellent pain relief for some patients without the side effects associated with pharmacologic agents. Nerve blocks and trigger point injections maybe of significant help in selected patients.

Summary

Although treating patients with chronic pelvic pain may pose a challenge, such patients can often be treated successfully. Effective modalities are available to lessen the impact of the pain and offer the reasonable expectation of return to normal function.

REFERENCES

1. Smith RP, Metheny WP, Nolan TE. A tool for the assessment of chronic pelvic pain. J Psychosom Obstet Gynaecol 1992;13:281–286
2. Lundberg WI, Wall JE, Mathers JE. Laparoscopy in the evaluation of pelvic pain. Obstet Gynecol 1973;42: 872–876
3. Kresch AJ, Seifer DB, Sachs LB, Baresse I. Laparoscopy in 100 women with chronic pelvic pain. Obstet Gynecol 1984;64:672–674
4. Williamson HA Jr, Williamson MT. The Beck Depression Inventory: normative data and problems with generalizability. Fam Med 1989;21:58–60
5. Cunanan RG, Couren NG, Lippes J. Laparoscopic findings in patients with pelvic pain. Am J Obstet Gynecol 1983; 146:589
6. Rapkin AJ. Adhesions and pelvic pain: a retrospective study. Obstet Gynecol 1986;68:13–15
7. Hogston P. Irritable bowel syndrome as a cause of chronic pain in women attending a gynecology clinic. BMJ 1987;294:934–935
8. Longstreth GF, Preskill DB, Youkeles L. Irritable bowel syndrome in women having diagnostic laparoscopy or hysterectomy: relation to gynecologic features and outcome. Dig Dis Sci 1990;35:1285–1290
9. Applegate WV. Abdominal cutaneous nerve entrapment syndrome. Surgery 1972;71:118–124
10. Slocumb JC. Neurological factors in chronic pelvic pain: trigger points and the abdominal pelvic pain syndrome. Am J Obstet Gynecol 1984;149:536–543
11. Carleson KJ, Miller BA, Fowler FJ Jr. The Maine Women's Health Study. II. Outcomes of nonsurgical management of leiomyomas, abnormal bleeding, and chronic pelvic pain. Obstet Gynecol 1994;83:566–572
12. Black WT Jr. Use of presacral sympathectomy in the treatment of dysmenorrhea: a second look after twenty-five years. Am J Obstet Gynecol 1964;89:16–22
13. Lee RB, Stone K, Magelssen D, Belts RP, Benson WL. Presacral neurectomy for chronic pelvic pain. Obstet Gynecol 1986;68:517–521
14. Lichten EM. Three years experience with LUNA: outpatient laser laparoscopic treatment of dysmenorrhea. Am J Gynecol Health 1989;5:144–147
15. Lichten EM, Bombard J. Surgical treatment of primary dysmenorrhea with laparoscopic uterine nerve ablation. J Reprod Med 1987;32:37–41
16. Parsons LH, Stovall TG. Surgical management of chronic pelvic pain. Obstet Gynecol Clin North Am 1993;20: 765–778
17. Fukaya T, Hoshiai H, Yajima A. Is pelvic endometriosis always associated with chronic pain? A retrospective study of 618 cases diagnosed by laparoscopy. Am J Obstet Gynecol 1993;169:719–722
18. Steege JF, Stout AL. Resolution of chronic pelvic pain after laparoscopic lysis. Am J Obstet Gynecol 1991;165: 278–283
19. Roseff SJ, Murphy AA. Laparoscopy in the diagnosis and therapy of chronic pelvic pain. Clin Obstet Gynecol 1990;33:137–144
20. Soellner W, Huter O, Wurm B, Kanter J, Rumplmair W. Longitudinal follow-up of chronic pelvic pain and occurrence of new symptoms 5 to 7 years after laparoscopy. Am J Obstet Gynecol 1993:168:1645
21. Stovall TG, Ling FW, Crawford DA. Hysterectomy for chronic pelvic pain of presumed uterine etiology. Obstet Gynecol 1990;75:676–679
22. American College of Obstetricians and Gynecologists. Guidelines for women's health care. Washington, DC: ACOG, 1996
23. Flor H, Fydrich T, Turk DC. Efficacy of multidisciplinary pain treatment centers: A meta-analytic review. Pain 1992;49:221–230
24. Gambone JC, Reiter RC. Nonsurgical management of chronic pelvic pain: a multidisciplinary approach. Clin Obstet Gynecol 1990;33:205–211
25. Malone MD, Strube MJ. Meta-analysis of non-medical treatments for chronic pain. Pain 1988;34:231–244
26. Maruta T, Swanson DW, McHardy MJ. Three year follow-up of patients with chronic pain who were treated in a multidisciplinary pain management center. Pain 1990;41: 47–53
27. Peters AA, van Dorst E, Jellis B, van Zuuren E, Hermans J, Trimbos JB. A randomized clinical trial to compare two different approaches in women with chronic pelvic pain. Obstet Gynecol 1991;77:740–744
28. Rapkin AJ, Kames LD. The pain management approach to chronic pelvic pain. J Reprod Med 1987;32:323–327

SUGGESTED READING

American Fertility Society. Management of endometriosis in the presence of pelvic pain. Fertil Steril 1993;60:952–955

Beck AT. Beck Depression Inventory. San Antonio, Texas: Psychological Corporation, 1993

Bonica JJ, ed. The management of pain. 2nd ed. Philadelphia: Lea & Febiger, 1990

DiGregorio GJ, Barbieri EJ, Ferko AP, Sterling GH, Camp JF, Prout MF. Handbook of pain management. 4th ed. West Chester, Pennsylvania: Medical Surveillance Inc, 1994

Ford CV. The somatizing disorders. Psychosomatics 1986;27: 327–331

Hillis SD, Marchbanks PA, Peterson HB. The effectiveness of hysterectomy for chronic pelvic pain. Obstet Gynecol 1995;86:941–945

International Association for the Study of Pain. Classification of chronic pain, descriptions of chronic pain syndromes and definitions of pain terms. Pain 1986;3(suppl):S1–S225

Jacox A, Carr DB, Payne R, Berde CB, Breitbart W, Cain JM, et al. Management of cancer pain. Clinical Practice Guideline no. 9. AHCPR Publication No. 94-0592. Rockville, Maryland: Agency for Health Care Policy and Research, U.S. Department of Health and Human Services, Public Health Service, March 1994

King PM, Myers CA, Ling FW, Rosenthal RH. Musculoskeletal factors in chronic pelvic pain. J Psychosom Obstet Gynaecol 1991;12(suppl):87–98

Ling FW, ed. Contemporary management of chronic pelvic pain. Obstet Gynecol Clin North Am 1993;20:627–853

Loeser JD, Egan KJ, eds. Managing the chronic pain patient: theory and practice at the University of Washington Multidisciplinary Pain Center. New York: Raven Press, 1989

Rachlin ES, ed. Myofascial pain and fibromyalgia: trigger point management. St Louis: Mosby, 1994

Rapkin AJ, Kames LD, Darke LL, Stampler FM, Naliboff BD. History of physical and sexual abuse in women with chronic pelvic pain. Obstet Gynecol 1990;76:92–96

Rapkin AJ, Reading AE. Chronic pelvic pain. Curr Probl Obstet Gynecol Fertil 1991;14:102–104

Reiter RC. Occult somatic pathology in women with chronic pelvic pain. Clin Obstet Gynecol 1990;33:154–160

Summitt RL, Ling FW. Urethral syndrome presenting as chronic pelvic pain. J Psychosom Obstet Gynaecol 1991;12(suppl):77–86

Travell JG. Chronic myofascial pain syndromes: mysteries of the history. Adv Pain Res Ther 1990;17:129–138

Walker EA, Katon WJ, Jemelka R, Alfrey H, Bowers M, Stenchever MA. The prevalence of chronic pelvic pain and irritable bowel syndrome in two university clinics. J Psychosom Obstet Gynaecol 1991;12(suppl):65–75

This Technical Bulletin was developed under the direction of the Committee on Technical Bulletins of the American College of Obstetricians and Gynecologists as an educational aid to obstetricians and gynecologists. The committee wishes to thank Roger P. Smith, MD, for his assistance in the development of this bulletin. This Technical Bulletin does not define a standard of care, nor is it intended to dictate an exclusive course of management. It presents recognized methods and techniques of clinical practice for consideration by obstetrician–gynecologists for incorporation into their practices. Variations of practice taking into account the needs of the individual patient, resources, and limitations unique to the institution or type of practice may be appropriate.
ISSN 1074-8628

THE AMERICAN COLLEGE OF OBSTETRICIANS AND GYNECOLOGISTS
409 12th Street, SW
PO Box 96920
Washington, DC 20090-6920

12345/09876

ACOG EDUCATIONAL BULLETIN

Number 249, August 1998

Confidentiality in Adolescent Health Care

Adolescents are a relatively healthy subgroup of the U.S. population. Much of their behavior, however, puts them at substantial risk for poor health. Behaviorally related morbidities include alcohol and substance abuse, sexually transmissible infections (STIs), human immunodeficiency virus (HIV), pregnancy, depression, injury, violence, and suicide. Because these behaviors can jeopardize an adolescent's development, future opportunities, and even life, any barriers to needed health care services should be identified and removed.

Most adolescents underuse existing health care services (1). A major obstacle to the delivery of health care to adolescents is concern about confidentiality. Confidentiality refers to the privileged and private nature of information shared during a health care encounter (2). Although ensuring confidentiality is relatively simple when providing services to adults, providing the same degree of confidentiality for adolescents can be less straightforward. The legal status of a minor and requirements for parental consent before the provision of medical services often encumber the physician–patient relationship.

Confidentiality also may be compromised by economic considerations because few adolescents have the financial resources to pay for medical services and, therefore, may need parental or adult help in arranging payment. Although a few states allow adolescents to qualify for Medicaid on the basis of their own incomes, the majority of states consider family income and assets when determining eligibility. To supply such information, adolescents may need to consult with family members. Explanation of Benefits forms issued by indemnity insurers, managed care organizations, and Medicaid are sent to parent policyholders, which also can compromise the confidentiality of information and, therefore, a minor's access to health care services.

To overcome barriers to confidentiality imposed by legal and economic constraints, physicians should discuss confidentiality with both the adolescent girl and, where appropriate, her parent(s) or guardian(s). Clinicians should be familiar with current state and local statutes on the rights of minors to consent to health care services, as well as those laws that affect confidentiality. It also is important to involve and inform office staff about those policies and procedures that facilitate and ensure confidentiality. Finally, physicians

This Educational Bulletin was developed under the direction of the Committee on Adolescent Health Care of the American College of Obstetricians and Gynecologists as an aid to obstetricians and gynecologists. This document is not to be construed as establishing a standard of practice or dictating an exclusive course of treatment. Rather, it is intended as an educational tool that presents current information on obstetric–gynecologic issues.

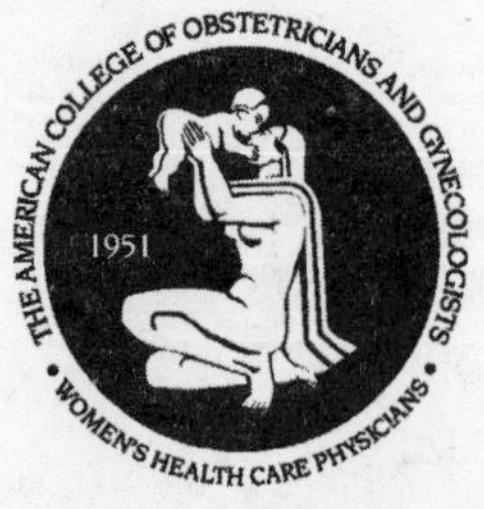

should work with the political process to eliminate laws unduly restrictive of confidential health services for adolescents (1).

Addressing Confidentiality

Parents should be counseled that it is appropriate for the maturing adolescent girl to assume increasing responsibility for her health and health care. Adolescence is a period of significant change and maturation, and learning to make appropriate health care decisions is a major developmental task. Physicians can assist in this process by providing an environment in which adolescents can discuss candidly their concerns. Adolescents are more likely to develop trusting relationships with their health care providers when the issue of confidentiality has been addressed. A confidential relationship, in turn, facilitates the open disclosure of health histories and risky behaviors. The health and behavioral issues of adolescent patients can then be addressed with nonjudgmental counseling and medical intervention.

Physicians should stress to parents that they share a common goal—the health and well-being of the minor patient. The mutual trust that follows from this common goal will enhance and support the adolescent–physician relationship. The involvement of a concerned adult can contribute to the health and success of an adolescent. Providers should encourage and, when appropriate, facilitate communication between a minor and her parent(s) (3).

Parents and adolescents should be informed, both separately and together, that they each have a private and privileged relationship with the provider. Additionally, they should be informed of any restrictions on the confidential nature of that relationship. For instance, the physician should explain that if the patient discloses any risk of bodily harm to herself or others (4), confidentiality will be breached. Furthermore, state laws may mandate the reporting of physical or sexual abuse of minors.

Legal Issues

Because the legal status of minors differs from that of adults, physicians who treat minors should be aware of laws that affect the provision of services. The following information is an introduction to the laws that address the medical treatment of minors. Providers of care to adolescents are encouraged to familiarize themselves with state statutes to determine which services mandate confidentiality. When necessary, they should seek appropriate legal advice.

All states require consent for the medical treatment of a minor from a person legally entitled to authorize such care. Although this usually will be a parent, other guardians such as foster parents, juvenile courts, social workers, and probation officers may, in certain instances, provide the necessary consent.

There are, however, exceptions to this requirement for consent. Generally, where such exceptions apply, minors have the right to prevent physicians from disclosing information about the care they receive. First, in an emergency situation, when immediate treatment is necessary to safeguard the life or health of a minor, parental consent is assumed (5). Second, "emancipated minors" generally are held to be capable of consenting to medical treatment. Such minors may include those who are married, those who are members of the Armed Forces, those who live apart from their parents and are financially self-supporting, and those who are themselves the parent of a child (1). Third, all states have statutes allowing minors to consent to at least some specific health care services, such as contraceptive services, prenatal care and delivery services, STI services, HIV testing and treatment, treatment of drug and alcohol abuse, and mental health treatment (6). These laws may specify the age at which minors can begin to consent to such care.

In addition, courts increasingly recognize the growing independence of adolescents and the seriousness of their health care needs. Through case law, the right of a "mature minor" to consent to some forms of medical care without prior parental consent has been established. A mature minor is defined as an adolescent younger than the age of majority who, although living at home as a dependent, demonstrates the cognitive maturity to give informed consent (2). The age of majority has been set at 18 years in most states. The ability to consent will be influenced by the minor's developmental maturity, prior experience with illness, the gravity of the current illness, and the risks of proposed therapy (7). Although the mature-minor doctrine has been written into law in only a few states, during the past several decades there have been no reported decisions holding a physician liable solely for failing to obtain parental consent when nonnegligent care was provided to a mature minor (typically at least age 15) who had given informed consent (8). When dealing with high-risk health concerns such as contraception, pregnancy, STIs, and mental health, most states have concluded that the need for confidential services outweighs parental rights of notification. When deciding whether or not to accept a mature minor as a patient, individual providers should evaluate their personal views. If a provider's views on confidentiality restrict the provision of services to a minor, the patient should be referred.

A minor's right to obtain an abortion without parental consent or notification is one area in which the rights of a minor have been statutorily restricted. As of 1997, 29 states have adopted either mandatory parental consent or mandatory parental notification laws. An additional nine states have parental involvement laws that are either enjoined or unenforceable (9). In states where parental consent or notification is required for the termination of a minor's pregnancy, a judicial bypass system must be provided. Such a system allows minors to seek consent from the court in lieu of a parent or guardian. Further-more, the U.S. Supreme Court has ruled that if a minor chooses this option, the judge must consent to the procedure if he or she has determined the adolescent to be a "mature minor, or if termination of the pregnancy is in the minor's best interest" (10).

A Model Office Visit

Physicians should develop office procedures that safeguard their adolescent patients' rights. Furthermore, every member of the office staff must be aware of these procedures and their role in preserving confidentiality. Outlined in Table 1 and described as follows is an initial office visit process that works well when an adolescent girl is accompanied by her parent(s) or guardian(s).

1. The physician initially sees the parent and adolescent patient together to explain the structure of the visit. The reason for the visit and the patient's medical and family history are then reviewed. It is important to direct questions to, and maintain eye contact with, the adolescent patient during this discussion, deferring to the parent or guardian only when supplemental information or clarification is needed.

   The issue of confidentiality also should be discussed. Physicians should inform both the adolescent and her parent of the scope of the minor's authority to consent to medical care; physicians also should reassure them that family communication is encouraged and facilitated, and that no attempt is being made to undermine good parent–child relationships.

   An adjunct to this discussion may be a simple written agreement (see box). Such a document recognizes the adolescent's emerging autonomy and at the same time promotes communication between parent(s) and child. It must be stressed that the agreement is not legally binding. It does, however, acknowledge the importance of confidentiality and outline the expectations of the new adolescent patient–parent–physician relationship. Parents also may be reminded that medical protocols may require pregnancy testing and screens for STIs when the adolescent has gynecologic concerns or complaints.

2. The parent(s) or guardian(s) should then be excused from the room. This allows for a confidential discussion between the physician and the patient about her health-related behaviors and concerns. Discussions of sexuality, substance abuse, alcohol, smoking, eating disorders, violence, depression, relationships, and school performance can be facilitated by adopting an open, relaxed, and non-judgmental attitude. At this point it is important to distinguish between judging the behavior and judging the individual. Although certain behaviors can clearly be judged as negative or inappropriate, the adolescent patient should not be judged as "bad."

   Disclosures made during the discussion will determine the need for a physical examination. Should this be necessary, the patient should be provided with a description of this process and asked if she would like her parent or other individual present.

3. While the patient prepares for examination, a confidential meeting with the parent(s) or guardian(s) often proves beneficial. Parents may express specific concerns regarding their daughter's health, and physicians can provide them with a brief overview of adolescent development. Such a meeting often helps to relieve any anxiety parents feel in their new "passive" role. Physicians should reassure parents that they will encourage the adolescent to include her parents in important health decisions.

Table 1. An Adolescent Office Visit That Supports Confidentiality

In Consultation With:	The Physician Should:
Patient and Parent(s) or Guardian(s)	Outline structure of visit Obtain general medical and family history Discuss confidentiality
Patient	Obtain health history, including risk-taking behaviors Address patient concerns Provide health guidance Address billing issues
Parent	Address parental concerns Provide guidance about adolescent development
Patient*	Perform physical examination, as indicated
Patient	Summarize findings and recommendations Determine parental involvement Determine method of notification of laboratory results
Patient and Parent(s) or Guardian(s)	Summarize findings and recommendations, as appropriate Address billing issues

*Parent may be present, at patient's discretion

4. Upon completion of the physical examination, consultation with the patient should address physical findings and diagnosis and treatment options, if needed. Once a mutually agreed-upon treatment plan is established, the adolescent is encouraged to include her parent in treatment planning. Depending on the adolescent's level of maturity, the nature of the medical problem, the clinician's medical judgment, and legal constraints, parental involvement may be more or less strongly advised and facilitated. A method for reporting confidential laboratory results to the adolescent should be established at this time. If the adolescent agrees to parental input, and a conflict in treatment planning develops once the parents are involved, the physician often will have to take the role of arbitrator. Such a conflict may be resolved by determining if the adolescent has the legal right to consent to the services in question.
5. At the conclusion of the meeting, the patient, her parent, and the physician meet again. During this meeting findings and recommendations are discussed, if appropriate. Any remaining concerns also can be addressed.
6. Finally, a claim is filed. Most office visits can be coded to ensure adolescent confidentiality. Laboratory billing for pregnancy testing and STIs, however, remains problematic. Many laboratories do not offer alternative codes. Also, insurance companies and HMOs may not reimburse for indicated routine screening, such as chlamydia, which may result in an itemized bill being sent to the parent(s). The disclaimer that "these tests are necessary in medical protocols" may be sufficient to satisfy the concerns of some parents. To ensure confidentiality, however, some adolescents may choose to pay for these tests without parental involvement. Some practitioners offer a reduced rate for these tests or refer patients to agencies that charge on a sliding scale according to income. Office personnel should be cognizant of the issues of confidentiality with billing, reviewing claims with parents, and reporting laboratory results.

Patient preferences or special circumstances (eg, reading level, learning disabilities) may necessitate a modification of the initial office visit process, and physicians should allow additional time for separate patient and parent interviews. Although this process may take more time than an adult patient visit, in the long run it should result in fewer telephone calls from parents who do not fully understand their changing role in their adolescent daughter's health care or the nature of confidential services for minors.

Confidential Agreement

Parent

I, ___________________ (parent or guardian), allow my daughter, _______________ (patient), to enter a confidential patient–physician relationship. I understand that my daughter can make independent health care decisions, but that my input and involvement will be encouraged.

My daughter has permission to schedule appointments and receive confidential reports from this office. I further understand that various laboratory tests may be necessary in medical protocols and accept responsibility for physician charges and laboratory fees.

______________________________ ______________________________

Parent or Guardian Physician

Patient

I, ______________________________________ (patient), am entering a confidential physician–patient relationship with ____________________________ (physician). I will make an effort to communicate with my parent(s) about issues concerning my health. I accept the personal responsibility of being honest and will follow the health care recommendations my physician and I establish.

______________________________ ______________________________

Patient Physician

Conclusion

Confidential health services promote the health and well-being of all adolescents. Legal requirements and economic constraints, however, impose significant barriers to confidential health services for adolescents. Both minors and providers consistently identify concerns about the lack of confidentiality as a major obstacle to minors obtaining needed health care. Overcoming the obstacles imposed by such constraints is not difficult. Providers should broach discussions of confidentiality with minor patients and their parents or guardians, familiarize themselves with current state and local statutes affecting confidentiality, and develop office procedures aimed at maintaining confidentiality. Family communication is the desired goal, and health care providers are able to assist in this effort. Confidential care does not preclude working toward this goal. By showing concern both for a parent's desire to be involved in a daughter's health care decisions and for the minor's growing need for autonomy, physicians can aid in a minor's healthy transition from childhood to adulthood.

References

1. ACOG Statement of Policy. Confidentiality in adolescent health care. Washington, DC: American College of Obstetricians and Gynecologists, 1988.
2. American Medical Association. AMA guidelines for adolescent preventative services (GAPS). Baltimore: Williams & Wilkins, 1994:1–12
3. McCabe MA, Rushton CH, Glover J, Murray MG, Leikin S. Implications for the patient self-determination act: guidelines for involving adolescents in medical decision making. J Adolesc Health 1996;19:319–324
4. Gans JE. Policy compendium on confidential health services for adolescents. Chicago: American Medical Association, 1993
5. Donovan P. Our daughters' decisions: the conflict in state law on abortion and other issues. New York: Alan Guttmacher Institute,1992:4–35
6. Holder A. Disclosure and consent problems in pediatrics. Law Medicine and Health Care 1988;16:219–228
7. Council on Scientific Affairs, American Medical Association. Confidential health services for adolescents. JAMA 1993;269:1420–1424
8. English A, Matthews M, Extavour K, Palamountain C, Yang J. State minor consent statutes: a summary. Cincinnati, Ohio: Center for Continuing Education in Adolescent Health, 1995
9. Turnbull WR. Teens' ability to consent to reproductive health care commonly recognized at state level. State Reprod Health Monit 1997;8:3–8
10. American Academy of Pediatrics, Committee on Adolescence. The adolescent's right to confidential care when considering abortion. Pediatrics 1996;97:746–751

ISSN 1074-8628

The American College of Obstetricians and Gynecologists
409 12th Street, SW
PO Box 96920
Washington, DC 20090-6920

12345/21098

Number 182—July 1993

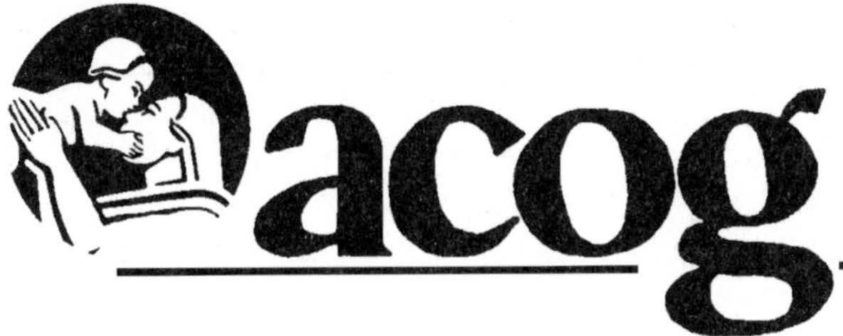

Technical Bulletin

An Educational Aid to Obstetrician–Gynecologists

Depression in Women

Mood disorders, particularly depression, are among the most common psychiatric illnesses in women. The expectancy of developing depression during one's lifetime is approximately 20% for women, in contrast to 10% for men (1), and is most common among women of reproductive age, with a prevalence of 8–10% (2). Major depressive episodes occur two times more frequently in women than men (1).

The rates of depressive disorders increase during adolescence, and the increase is greater for girls than boys (3). Although the onset of depression can occur at any age, 50% of patients have the onset between 20 and 50, the mean being about 40 years of age (1).

The high rates of depression in women are not due simply to biological differences between the sexes, but also to specific social, economic, and emotional factors that are unique to the experience of being female in contemporary society (4). In addition, depression can be overdiagnosed in women who have experienced grief reactions. Clinical symptoms in both entities are similar, but grief reaction is generally self-limited and self-esteem is preserved, whereas depression involves a general loss of self-esteem that is long term and requires treatment.

It is estimated that only 20–25% of those who meet the criteria for major depression receive appropriate treatment (4). The obstetrician–gynecologist should be cognizant of the various factors that influence the presentation, diagnosis, and treatment of depression in women. This awareness will enable the obstetrician–gynecologist to differentiate clinical depression from more transient emotional disturbances, such as those related to the natural grieving process, and determine the need for intervention.

Patients should be made aware that major depression is a medical condition that can be treated successfully. In many cases, the diagnosis and treatment of major depression can be accomplished successfully by primary care practitioners (5). This document is intended as a resource for understanding the disorder and its management.

Role Factors

Women's lives, regardless of age, are affected to various degrees by the roles they assume. Whereas past generations of women planned and organized their lives primarily to meet family-related goals, most American women today are involved in some combination of paid employment and homemaking. Seventy percent of women in the work force have children under 18 years of age (6). Successfully blending and fulfilling these multiple roles and demands can be a source of considerable frustration, particularly for those women who are responsible for the sole support, both financial and emotional, of their children, often without adequate resources. Such a situation imposes stress that can place women at risk for depression. Other important factors that contribute to the prevalence of the diagnosis of depression in women are female roles in which life conditions encourage passivity, devaluation, and a sense of helplessness; the readiness with which women report negative symptoms; and the higher likelihood that they will seek help for depression (7).

Clinical Manifestations

Mood refers to the internal emotional state of an individual. Affect is the external expression of emotional experiences. A normal individual experiences a wide range of moods, displays an equally wide range of affective expression, and feels in control of these mood states (1). A sad mood is a normal reaction to disappointments or losses; it is not to be confused with major depression. Depressive disorders are a group of clinical conditions characterized by a disturbance of mood, a loss of sense of control, and intense mental, emotional, and physical anguish. Depression disrupts family, job, and social functioning (5).

Depression can be unipolar, with depressive episodes that last at least 2 weeks and often longer, or bipolar, which is characterized by discrete episodes of depression and mania between which the patient may feel perfectly normal. Dysthymic disorders feature a low-grade, persistent depressed mood and associated symptoms for at least 2 years, during which time a major depressive episode has not occurred.

Specific criteria are diagnostic of depression (see the box), and those who have depression will demonstrate at least five of these symptoms. Women with mania may demonstrate expansiveness, flight of ideas, decreased sleep, heightened self-esteem, and grandiose ideas. Patients with depression are often, but not always, sad. Other symptoms and signs of depression include changes in activity level, cognitive abilities, speech, abnormalities in sleep, appetite, sexual activity, or other biological rhythms.

Diagnostic Criteria for Major Depressive Episode

At least five of the following symptoms have been present during the same two week period and represent a change from previous functioning; at least one of the symptoms is either 1) depressed mood, or 2) loss of interest or pleasure. (Do not include symptoms that are clearly due to a physical condition, mood-incongruent delusions or hallucinations, incoherence, or marked loosening of associations.)

1. Depressed mood (or can be irritable mood in children or adolescents) most of the day, nearly every day, as indicated either by subjective account or observation by others
2. Markedly diminished interest or pleasure in all, or almost all, activities most of the day, nearly every day (as indicated either by subjective account or observation by others of apathy most of the time)
3. Significant weight loss or weight gain when not dieting (eg, more than 5% of body weight in a month), or decrease or increase in appetite nearly every day (in children, consider failure to make expected weight gains)
4. Insomnia or hypersomnia nearly every day
5. Psychomotor agitation or retardation nearly every day (observable by others, not merely subjective feelings of restlessness or being slowed down)
6. Fatigue or loss of energy nearly every day
7. Feelings of worthlessness or excessive or inappropriate guilt (which may be delusional) nearly every day (not merely self-reproach or guilt about being sick)
8. Diminished ability to think or concentrate, or indecisiveness, nearly every day (either by subjective account or as observed by others)
9. Recurrent thoughts of death (not just fear of dying), recurrent suicidal ideation without a specific plan, or a suicide attempt or a specific plan for committing suicide.

(American Psychiatric Association. Diagnostic and statistical manual of mental disorders. 3rd ed. Washington, DC: APA, 1987)

Predisposing Factors

A number of factors may predispose women to depression (4):

- Earlier childhood loss such as death or prolonged illness of a parent
- Physical or sexual abuse, including that by a spouse or partner (domestic violence)
- Socioeconomic deprivation
- Genetic predisposition
- Life style stress of multiple roles

These risk factors can cause an exaggeration or prolongation of depressive symptoms. For example, a spontaneous abortion or diagnosis of early endometriosis in a young, otherwise healthy woman may not be appreciated by the obstetrician–gynecologist to represent a significant emotional insult. If predisposing risk factors are not addressed, they may result in a prolonged depressive episode.

A life cycle perspective appears to be one of the keys to understanding depression in women. Relationships between a history of major depression and reproductive events, menstrual cycle mood changes, and postpartum depression are likely to be important predictors of psychologic morbidity. For example, women at risk for postpartum depression are more likely to have a history of major depression, premenstrual syndrome, and depression during the antenatal period (4). Other conditions in obstetrics and gynecology may also precipitate or contribute to depression in women. These include the lack of opportunity to achieve pregnancy or motherhood as a result of single status or infertility (8–10) and reproductive failure or loss (11).

Perinatal Loss

Women who have experienced perinatal loss are vulnerable to an acute grief reaction or adjustment disorder which can be misdiagnosed as major depression. Such women may experience problems with sleep, loss of appetite, fatigue, apathy, or difficulty with normal daily activities. However, in contrast to clinical depression, self-esteem is preserved. Depressive symptoms in such circumstances are more likely a manifestation of perinatal loss than of primary depression (12). Intervention specific to the management of acute grief that focuses on perinatal loss can be particularly helpful in such circumstances. The opportunity to see, hold, and name the baby, in addition to receiving photographs, is important to the grieving process; an autopsy and a memorial service should also be offered such families (12). Parental contact with the infant may facilitate the resolution of bereavement (13). Ongoing support from the obstetrician and medical staff for the patient and family may be more beneficial than antidepressant medication or psychiatric referral. If the mood disturbance is intense or long-standing, psychiatric consultation is important (11). Follow-up visits should be scheduled at approximately 6 weeks, 3 months, and 6 months to determine whether symptoms are decreasing.

Infertility

Infertility patients have been found to report higher levels of subjective distress than control groups of age-matched women. However, their self-esteem remains normal, and they do not demonstrate a higher prevalence of major depression (8). The most emotionally difficult events are those associated with repeated failed attempts at conception, particularly following complex interventions such as the assisted reproductive technologies (10). The physician should be sensitive to the stress the patient and her partner are experiencing and refer for appropriate intervention. Psychologic counseling may be helpful, particularly when repeated interventions have been attempted or when treatment has proven unsuccessful and termination of medical care is planned. Group treatment can be successful in reducing symptoms and facilitating coping.

Pregnancy

Pregnancy has the potential to change a woman's perceptions of herself, her own mother, and the father of the child as she assumes a new role. For an adult woman, the experience can stimulate genuine developmental change and adaptation. Even when pregnancy has been anticipated and uneventful and the outcome successful, depressive symptoms may surface following delivery. The obstetrician–gynecologist must be able to differentiate between self-limited postpartum blues and more significant depressive symptoms, which are present in approximately 8–10% of women (14).

Major clinical depression has been thought to be more common following childbirth than during other periods of a woman's life. However, current studies do not substantiate this belief (15). Women at risk for significant postpartum depression are more likely to have a family history of depression, a previous postpartum depression, or significant adjustment problems with childbirth. It has been demonstrated that women who have a planned pregnancy in a secure environment, enjoy a supportive relationship with their partner, and have manageable levels of life stress are less likely to experience postpartum depression.

Postpartum adjustment for a woman involves a major psychologic shift from viewing herself as a woman who is pregnant to viewing herself as a new mother. Anticipation, excitement, and joy may be mixed with a sense of sadness, anger, and loss of a simpler life style and a marital relationship uncomplicated by parenthood. The process of adjustment comes into play as a new mother must cope with the loss of the idealized baby she carried during pregnancy and adjust to the realities and demands of her new infant. Postpartum blues and the increased vulnerability for depressive symptoms during this period are most likely precipitated by this major emotional upheaval and developmental shift and possibly by the significant endocrine changes that occur at this time.

Menopause and Aging

Research has increased understanding of the developmental changes associated with the menopausal and postmenopausal years (16). During this period, losses and decline in health can demand new adaptations and psychologic adjustments. Epidemiologic studies of the prevalence of depression in women have dispelled the notion of an increase in depression at the time of menopause or so-called involutional melancholia (2, 17–19). The complex experience of menopause and midlife adjustment disorders must be considered within their social, cultural, and psychologic contexts.

Aging involves additional and unexpected losses. Children mature and leave home, and a spouse may be lost through death or divorce or be seriously incapacitated through illness. In addition, physical changes in women may result in unfulfilled reproductive aspirations or goals, the need to confront lost youth, or a general decline in health and vitality. Hysterectomy, with or without oophorectomy, may offer relief for some women from menstrual disorders, worries of pregnancy, and genital tract cancer; it may also raise concerns about premature aging or a loss of sexuality and femininity in both premenopausal and postmenopausal women. Depression, per se, does not appear to increase following hysterectomy or oophorectomy (20, 21). However, unrecognized depression, as expressed in chronic pelvic pain, may lead to unwarranted hysterectomy (19).

Cancers of the breast and genital tract become more prevalent with advancing age. The successful adjustment to living with chronic illness, uncertainties about developing cancer, or aging in general depends upon the woman's past history of depression, her emotional resources, and the extended family and community support available to her (22).

Although depression in midlife is less common than during the reproductive years, aging and illness associated with advancing years brings an increased frequency of psychologic distress, depression, and even suicide (23). Psychiatric admissions increase after age 65 to affect 1 in every 16 (13). Hopelessness out of proportion to the circumstances of the elderly patient may be an indication of serious depression. Successful adjustment to old age occurs through the continued use of previously successful patterns of mastery, the integration of the past, and the acquisition of wisdom and acceptance of physical limitations in the final phase of life.

Diagnosis, Intervention, and Management

Warning Signs

Depression may present primarily as a disturbance of mood or affect or indirectly as somatic complaints, such as chronic fatigue (24). The following are common complaints presented to the obstetrician–gynecologist that may indicate an unrecognized or underlying depression:

- Chronic, clinically unconfirmed vulvovaginitis; idiopathic vulvodynia; and chronic vaginal pain and burning
- Chronic pelvic and genitourinary tract pain (25)
- Exaggerated or prolonged depressive symptoms following common ob/gyn events or procedures, such as miscarriage, stillbirth or prematurity, infertility, hysterectomy, mastectomy, and menopause
- Reports of severe, incapacitating premenstrual syndrome
- Multiple somatic complaints that include dysmenorrhea, dyspareunia, and sexual dysfunction

Approximately 10–15% or more of major depressive conditions are caused by general medical illnesses or other conditions such as substance abuse, concurrent medication, eating disorders or other nonmood psychiatric disorders, or grief reaction (5).

Careful diagnosis is critical in the treatment of depression. Because their symptoms are not recognized or are blamed on personal weakness, patients with depressive disorders often do not receive appropriate treatment.

Various somatic manifestations of chronic depression may present without apparent cause or may be associated with such life crises as financial difficulties, parent–child problems, marital conflict, job loss, or relocation. Family situations can have an effect on depression. In unhappy marriages, women are three times as likely as men to be depressed (4). Mothers of young children are highly vulnerable to depression; the more children in the home, the more depression is reported (4). High rates of depression are commonly found in victims of interpersonal violence. In a study of 60 battered women, depressive illness was the most common diagnostic category (26).

The obstetrician–gynecologist may find it useful to use a simple depression screening scale, such as the Beck Depression Inventory, to identify patients suspected of having significant depression (27). The Beck Inventory is a group of 21 statements designed to evaluate the feelings of the individual over the last week. The statements relate to the signs and symptoms of depression. It is a self-administered questionnaire. The higher the score, the more likely the patient is depressed.

Risk Factors for Suicide

Women attempt suicide more frequently than men, but young men outnumber young women in numbers of completed suicides. Suicide is more likely in white or elderly women who have an underlying affective disorder or general medical illnesses, experience feelings of hopelessness, live alone, have a history of attempting suicide or abusing substances, or have a family history of substance abuse or suicide. Women who have mentioned suicide are also at risk. When women attempt suicide in their reproductive years, it is more likely in postpartum, premenstrual, and seasonal periods. Early psychiatric intervention and continuous outpatient contact with this group of patients is essential to prevent suicide.

Intervention

In assessing and treating women's depression, it is essential to understand issues of gender, predisposing childhood, family and reproductive-related risk factors within social, marital, or interpersonal contexts.

Generally, medical illnesses or substance use that may be associated with depression should be treated first. If depression persists, it should be treated.

The choice of treatment for depression is based on the history of the illness and the severity of the major depressive episode. A patient with severe depression manifests almost all of the symptoms of depression, and this almost always interferes with her daily activities. Patients with moderate depression have some symptoms and are often unable to complete activities; those with mild depression also have some symptoms and feel that it requires extra effort to do what they need to do. Various forms of psychotherapy, pharmacotherapy (antidepressants), electroconvulsive therapy (ECT), and phototherapy are used individually or in combination to treat significant depression.

Psychotherapy should be considered for patients whose depression is mild to moderate. It is also helpful for those who have had an incomplete response to medication or for whom medication is contraindicated or unacceptable. Psychotherapy has been reported to benefit 45–60% of depressed patients and appears to be equal in efficacy to pharmacotherapy in treating mild to moderate depression (5).

During psychotherapy, problems are discussed and resolved through the emotional support, insight, and understanding gained from the patient–therapist relationship. Depressed women tend to think negatively about themselves, the world, and their future. They expect to fail and often make faulty inferences about the behaviors and comments of others. These maladaptive beliefs and negative thought patterns may be corrected through psychotherapy, thereby promoting realistic thinking and enhancing behavior and mood. Focusing on these underlying issues allows the therapist to help a woman better understand her feelings and her illness and be more independent and autonomous in her life.

Medical therapy should be considered for patients with severe, chronic, or recurrent depression; with psychotic or melancholic symptoms; or with a family history of depression. Of patients who take antidepressants, 50–65% experience marked improvement or complete remission of their depressive symptoms (5).

Categories of medications prescribed for depressive disorders are antidepressants such as tricyclic and heterocyclic antidepressants, selective serotonin reuptake inhibitors, and monoamine oxidase (MAO) inhibitors (Table 1). The choice of agent is based on the symptoms and its efficacy in treating those symptoms.

With cyclic antidepressants, symptoms sometimes can be alleviated in weeks, depending on which medication is prescribed. They alleviate such symptoms as:

- Loss of appetite and weight
- Decreased perception of pleasurable activities
- Loss of energy
- Psychomotor retardation
- Suicidal thoughts
- Thought patterns dominated by hopelessness
- Helplessness and excessive guilt

The MAO inhibitors are more likely to be used in women with the following symptoms:

- Increased appetite
- Excessive sleepiness
- High levels of anxiety
- Phobic or obsessive–compulsive tendencies

All medications have side effects, and antidepressants are no exception. Common adverse effects of antidepressant medications are listed in Table 2. Antidepressants should not be prescribed by those who are not familiar with their mechanisms and side effects. In the pregnant woman, pros and cons of antidepressant use should be weighed carefully to avoid potential teratogenic effects on the fetus. As delayed cardiac conduction and disturbance in rhythm are also known to occur, baseline electrocardiography with periodic monitoring of the QRS complex is recommended for elderly women.

Some antidepressants, especially the selective serotonin reuptake inhibitors, have minimal anticholinergic side effects and effect on weight gain. Alprazolam can lead to tolerance in a very small group of women. Frequent requests for refills by the patient, "lost prescriptions," or withdrawal symptoms should alert the physician to abuse or dependence.

Maintenance on medication is indicated for women with recurrent forms of depression, particularly bipolar depression and recurring episodes of major depression. Continuous treatment can offer essentially normal functioning to those whose lives might otherwise be impaired significantly.

A combination of pharmacotherapy and psychotherapy may be more effective for patients who have severe or recurrent depression, an incomplete therapeutic response to either medication or psychotherapy, marked difficulty adhering to therapy, or need for symptom reduction (addressed by medication) and resolution of psychologic or social problems (addressed by psychotherapy). It has been reported to benefit 50–65% of patients (5).

With the availability of psychoactive drugs, the use of ECT has come to play a less important role in treating major depression. Nonetheless, ECT remains a very effective treatment for major depression and mania, particularly in women who are severely depressed, are at high risk for suicide, or do not respond to medical therapy. This is more common in elderly women, particularly when they are malnourished or cannot tolerate medications because of heart disease or other medical problems.

Phototherapy involves exposure several hours each day to special lighting conditions which approximate three times the brightness of ordinary, artificial room light. Phototherapy may prove helpful to women with seasonal affective disorder, a condition associated with decreased exposure to sunlight. Criteria for the diagnosis include depression during the winter, often with elevated moods during the summer.

Referral and Follow-Up

It is advantageous for the obstetrician–gynecologist to develop a close working relationship with a psychiatrist who is available for consultation. Early intervention provides the greatest chance of successful treatment.

It is beneficial for women with significant predisposing factors to remain in contact with the consulting psychiatrist even after acute depressive problems are resolved. If the depression is situational, as in the case of domestic violence, referral to a mental health professional who specializes in this area may be considered. Self-

TABLE 1. PHARMACOLOGY OF ANTIDEPRESSANT MEDICATIONS

Drug	Therapeutic Dosage Range (mg/d)	Average (Range) of Elimination Half-Lives (h)*	Potentially Fatal Drug Interactions
Tricyclics			
Amitriptyline (Elavil, Endep)	75–300	24 (16–46)	Antiarrhythmics, MAO inhibitors
Clomipramine (Anafranil)	75–300	24 (20–40)	Antiarrhythmics, MAO inhibitors
Desipramine (Norpramin, Pertofrane	75–300	18 (12–50)	Antiarrhythmics, MAO inhibitors
Doxepin (Adapin, Sinequan)	75–300	17 (10–47)	Antiarrhythmics, MAO inhibitors
Imipramine (Janimine, Tofranil)	75–300	22 (12–34)	Antiarrhythmics, MAO inhibitors
Nortriptyline (Aventyl, Pamelor)	40–200	26 (18–88)	Antiarrhythmics, MAO inhibitors
Protriptyline (Vivactil)	20–60	76 (54–124)	Antiarrhythmics, MAO inhibitors
Trimipramine (Surmontil)	75–300	12 (8–30)	Antiarrhythmics, MAO inhibitors
Heterocyclics			
Amoxapine (Asendin)	100–600	10 (8–14)	MAO inhibitors
Bupropion (Wellbutrin)	225–450	14 (8–24)	MAO inhibitors (possibly)
Maprotiline (Ludiomil)	100–225	43 (27–58)	MAO inhibitors
Trazodone (Desyrel)	150–600	8 (4–14)	—
Selective Serotonin Reuptake Inhibitors			
Fluoxetine (Prozac)	10–40	168 (72–360)†	MAO inhibitors
Paroxetine (Paxil)	20–50	24 (3–65)	MAO inhibitors‡
Sertraline (Zoloft)	50–150	24 (10–30)	MAO inhibitors‡
Monoamine Oxidase Inhibitors (MAO Inhibitors)§			
Isocarboxazid (Marplan)	30–50	Unknown	For all 3 MAO inhibitors: vasoconstrictors,‖ decongestants,‖ meperidine, and possibly other narcotics
Phenelzine (Nardil)	45–90	2 (1.5–4.0)	
Tranylcypromine (Parnate)	20–60	2 (1.5–3.0)	

*Half-lives are affected by age, sex, race, concurrent medications, and length of drug exposure.

†Includes both fluoxetine and norfluoxetine.

‡By extrapolation from fluoxetine data.

§MAO inhibition lasts longer (7 days) than drug half-life.

‖Including pseudoephedrine, phenylephrine, phenylpropanolamine, epinephrine, norepinephrine, and others.

(Depression Guideline Panel. Depression in primary care: detection, diagnosis, and treatment. Quick reference guide for clinicians, No. 5. Rockville, Maryland: U.S. Department of Health and Human Services, Public Health Service, Agency for Health Care Policy and Research, 1993:15; AHCPR publication no. 93-0552)

help and support groups are especially helpful in educating women about depression and decreasing the feeling of being alone.

Summary

Depression is a common, often overlooked, illness in women that should be recognized and treated. The obstetrician–gynecologist should be aware of factors that contribute to the high prevalence of depression in women, and particular attention should be given to family and work roles, victimization, early childhood loss of parent, personality variables, and reproductive-related events such as pregnancy, childbirth, and menopause. It is also important to distinguish between a grief reaction and major depression. Grief occurs secondary to losses such as abortion, miscarriage, stillbirth, or infertility and is generally self-limiting; self-esteem is preserved. In major depression, changes in sleeping patterns, appetite, energy, and mood persist, along with loss of self-esteem.

TABLE 2. SIDE-EFFECT PROFILES OF ANTIDEPRESSANT MEDICATIONS

	Side Effect*						
	Central Nervous System			Cardiovascular		Other	
Drug	Anticholinergic†	Drowsiness	Insomnia/ Agitation	Orthostatic Hypotension	Cardiac Arrhythmia	Gastrointestinal Distress	Weight Gain (over 6 kg)
Amitriptyline	4+	4+	0	4+	3+	0	4+
Desipramine	1+	1+	1+	2+	2+	0	1+
Doxepin	3+	4+	0	2+	2+	0	3+
Imipramine	3+	3+	1+	4+	3+	1+	3+
Nortriptyline	1+	1+	0	2+	2+	0	1+
Protriptyline	2+	1+	1+	2+	2+	0	0
Trimipramine	1+	4+	0	2+	2+	0	3+
Amoxapine	2+	2+	2+	2+	3+	0	1+
Maprotiline	2+	4+	0	0	1+	0	2+
Trazodone	0	4+	0	1+	1+	1+	1+
Bupropion	0	0	2+	0	1+	1+	0
Fluoxetine	0	0	2+	0	0	3+	0
Paroxetine	0	0	2+	0	0	3+	0
Sertraline	0	0	2+	0	0	3+	0
Monoamine Oxidase Inhibitors	1	1+	2+	2+	0	1+	2+

*Numerals indicate the likelihood of side effect occuring ranging from 0 for absent or rare to 4+ for relatively common.

†Dry mouth, blurred vision, urinary hesitancy, constipation

(Depression Guideline Panel. Depression in primary care: detection, diagnosis, and treatment. Quick reference guide for clinicians, No. 5. Rockville, Maryland: U.S. Department of Health and Human Services, Public Health Service, Agency for Health Care Policy and Research, 1993:14; AHCPR publication no. 93-0553)

As a part of patient education, it should be emphasized that depression is a medical illness and not a character defect or weakness and that in most cases it can be treated effectively. However, the risk of recurrence is significant; patients should be alert to early signs and symptoms of recurrence and seek treatment. Antidepressants that are well tolerated are now available, and appropriate use of these medications, along with psychotherapy as needed, will provide effective treatment for most patients.

REFERENCES

1. Kaplan HI, Sadock BJ. Mood disorders. In: Clinical psychiatry. Baltimore, Maryland: Williams and Wilkins, 1988
2. Myers JK, Weissman MM, Tischler GL, Holzer CE III, Leaf PJ, Orvaschel H, et al. Six-month prevalence of psychiatric disorders in three communities: 1980 to 1982. Arch Gen Psychiatry 1984;41:959–967
3. Kandel DB, Davies M. Epidemiology of depressive mood in adolescents. An empirical study. Arch Gen Psychiatry 1982;39:1205–1212
4. McGrath E, Ketia GP, Strickland BR, Russo NF. Women and depression: risk factors and treatment issues. Washington, DC: American Psychological Association, 1990
5. Depression Guideline Panel. Depression in primary care: detection, diagnosis, and treatment. Quick reference guide for clinicians, No. 5. Rockville, Maryland: U.S. Department of Health and Human Services, Public Health Service, Agency for Health Care Policy and Research, 1993; AHCPR publication no. 93-0552
6. McBride AB. Women's Mental Health Research Agenda: multiple roles. Women's Mental Health Occasional Paper Series. Rockville, Maryland: National Institute of Mental Health, 1988
7. Notman MT. Depression in women. Psychoanalytic concepts. Psychiatr Clin North Am 1989;12:221–230
8. Downey J, Yingling S, McKinney M, Husami N, Jewelewicz R, Maidman J. Mood disorders, psychiatric symptoms, and distress in women presenting for infertility evaluation. Fertil Steril 1989;52:425–432
9. Wright J, Duchesne C, Sabourin S, Bissonnette F, Benoit J, Girard Y. Psychosocial distress and infertility: men and women respond differently. Fertil Steril 1991;55:100–108
10. Kopitzke EJ, Berg BJ, Wilson JF, Owens D. Physical and emotional stress associated with components of the infertility investigation: perspectives of professionals and patients. Fertil Steril 1991;55:1137–1143
11. Kirkley-Best E, Kellner KR. The forgotten grief: a review of the psychology of stillbirth. Am J Orthopsychiatr 1982;52:420–429

12. Kellner KR, Donnelly WH, Gould SD. Parental behavior after perinatal death: lack of predictive demographic and obstetric variables. Obstet Gynecol 1984;63:809–814

13. Graham MA, Thompson SC, Estrada M, Yonekura ML. Factors affecting psychological adjustment to a fetal death. Am J Obstet Gynecol 1987;157:254–257

14. O'Hara MW. Postpartum mental disorders. In: Sciarra JJ, ed. Gynecology and obstetrics. Vol 6. Philadelphia: JB Lippincott, 1991;1–17

15. O'Hara MW. Social support, life events, and depression during pregnancy and the puerperium. Arch Gen Psychiatry 1986;43:569–573

16. Notman MT. Menopause and adult development. Ann NY Acad Sci 1990;592:149–155

17. Youngs DD. Some misconceptions concerning the menopause. Obstet Gynecol 1990;75:881–883

18. Hunter MS. Emotional well-being, sexual behaviour and hormone replacement therapy. Maturitas 1990;12:299–314

19. Stovall TG, Ling FW, Crawford DA. Hysterectomy for chronic pelvic pain of presumed uterine etiology. Obstet Gynecol 1990;75:676–679

20. Gath D, Cooper P, Day A. Hysterectomy and psychiatric disorder: I. Levels of psychiatric morbidity before and after hysterectomy. Br J Psychiatry 1982;140:335–342

21. Gath D, Cooper P, Bond A, Edmonds G. Hysterectomy and psychiatric disorder: II. Demographic psychiatric and physical factors in relation to psychiatric outcome. Br J Psychiatry 1982;140:343–350

22. Rodin G, Voshart K. Depression in the medically ill: an overview. Am J Psychiatry 1986;143:696–705

23. Rich CL, Warsradt GM, Nemiroff RA, Fowler RC, Young D. Suicide, stressors, and the life cycle. Am J Psychiatry 1991;148:524–527

24. Kendell RE. Chronic fatigue, viruses, and depression. Lancet 1991;337:160–162

25. Walker E, Katon W, Harrop-Griffiths J, Holm L, Russo J, Hickok LR. Relationship of chronic pelvic pain to psychiatric diagnoses and childhood sexual abuse. Am J Psychiatry 1988;145:75–80

26. Hilberman E, Munson K. Sixty battered women. Victimology Int J 1977–1978; 2:460–470

27. Beck AT, Ward CH, Mendelson M, Mock J, Erbaugh JK. An inventory for measuring depression. Arch Gen Psychiatry 1961;4:561–571

SUGGESTED READING

American College of Obstetricians and Gynecologists. Postpartum depression. ACOG Patient Education Pamphlet AP091. Washington, DC: ACOG, 1990

American Medical Association. Diagnostic and treatment guidelines on domestic violence. Chicago: AMA, 1992

Sargent M. Depressive illnesses: treatments bring new hope. U.S. Department of Health and Human Services, National Institute of Mental Health. Publication no. (ADM) 89–1491, 1989

Stotland NL. Psychiatric aspects of reproductive technology. Washington, DC: American Psychiatric Press, Inc, 1990

This Technical Bulletin was developed under the direction of the Committee on Technical Bulletins of the American College of Obstetricians and Gynecologists as an educational aid to obstetricians and gynecologists. The committee wishes to thank David D. Youngs, MD; Lilian Gonsalves, MD; Malkah T. Notman, MD; and Kenneth R. Kellner, MD, PhD, for their assistance in the development of this bulletin. This Technical Bulletin does not define a standard of care, nor is it intended to dictate an exclusive course of management. It presents recognized methods and techniques of clinical practice for consideration by obstetrician–gynecologists for incorporation into their practices. Variations of practice taking into account the needs of the individual patient, resources, and limitations unique to the institution or type of practice may be appropriate.

THE AMERICAN COLLEGE OF OBSTETRICIANS AND GYNECOLOGISTS
409 12th Street, SW
Washington, DC 20024-2188

2345/765

Number 200—December 1994
(Replaces #92, May 1986)

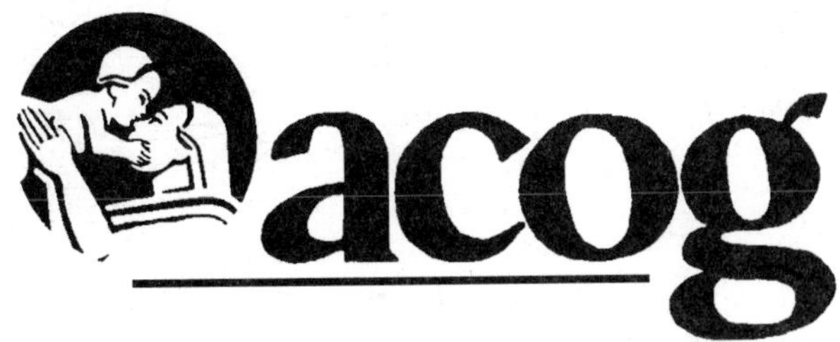

Technical Bulletin

An Educational Aid to Obstetrician–Gynecologists

Diabetes and Pregnancy

Diabetes mellitus is the most common medical complication of pregnancy. Approximately 2–3% of pregnancies are affected by diabetes; 90% of these cases represent gestational diabetes mellitus (GDM). With the implementation of treatment programs emphasizing normalization of maternal glucose levels and better techniques to assess fetal well-being and maturity, fetal and neonatal mortality have now become uncommon events in those pregnancies complicated by diabetes mellitus. When diabetic women receive optimal care prior to and during gestation, the perinatal mortality rate is nearly equivalent to that observed in normal pregnancies.

Classification

Diabetes is classified as Type I (insulin-dependent) or Type II (non-insulin-dependent) according to whether the patient requires exogenous insulin injection to avoid ketoacidosis. Patients with Type II diabetes may require insulin for glucose regulation but do not become ketotic if insulin is discontinued. Type I diabetes is frequently associated with certain human leukocyte antigen haplotypes and the presence of antiislet cell antibodies, whereas Type II is not.

The Priscilla White classification system, which is based on age of onset and duration of diabetes as well as the presence of certain vascular complications in the pregnant woman, was derived in order to estimate the degree of microvascular disease present and thus to provide a prognosis for pregnancy outcome and to help determine the timing of planned delivery. Improvements in fetal assessment, neonatal care, and metabolic management of the pregnant woman have rendered the White classification less helpful. A simple classification, based on the presence or absence of good maternal metabolic control and the presence or absence of maternal diabetic vasculopathy, is more helpful. Gestational diabetes is carbohydrate intolerance first recognized during pregnancy. If the abnormality persists after delivery, the patient's diagnosis is revised to Type I or Type II diabetes or impaired glucose tolerance (Table 1).

Pregestational Diabetes

Women with established diabetes should receive preconceptional counseling. The fourfold increase in the incidence of major congenital malformations in the offspring of women with pregestational diabetes has been related to poor control of diabetes during embryogenesis (Table 2). Several large studies document a significant reduction in fetal malformation rate in women whose diabetes is tightly controlled or who seek early specialized prenatal care during the period of organogenesis (1–4).

Counseling a woman with diabetes and formulating a plan of management require assessment of both maternal and fetal risks. While it is well known that the 5–10% of patients with underlying vascular disease are at increased risk for preeclampsia, fetal growth retardation, and, thus, preterm delivery, the quality of maternal glucose control must also be considered in assessing risk for any pregnant woman with diabetes. Several studies have failed to demonstrate a permanent worsening of diabetic renal disease

Table 1. POSTPARTUM EVALUATION FOR CARBOHYDRATE INTOLERANCE

	Plasma glucose level* (mg/dl) in		
Time Tested	No Diabetes	Impaired Glucose Tolerance	Diabetes Mellitus
Fasting	<115	<140	≥140†
$^1/_2$, 1, 1$^1/_2$ h	All <200	1 value ≥ 200	1 value ≥ 200
2 h	<140	140–199	≥ 200

*Values are based on a 2-h, 75-g oral glucose tolerance test.

†Fasting plasma glucose determinations of ≥ 140 on two occasions establish the diagnosis.

Table 2. CONGENITAL MALFORMATIONS IN INFANTS OF DIABETIC MOTHERS

Anomaly	Ratio of Incidences*	Gestational Age After Ovulation (wk)
Caudal regression	252	3
Spina bifida, hydrocephalus or other central nervous system defect	2	4
Anencephalus	3	4
Heart anomalies	4	
Transposition of great vessels		5
Ventricular septal defect		6
Atrial septal defect		6
Anal/rectal atresia	3	6
Renal anomalies	5	
Agenesis	6	5
Cystic kidney	4	5
Ureter duplex	23	5
Situs inversus	84	4

* This ratio is derived from Kucera's equation:

$$\frac{\text{Number of cases of this anomaly in diabetic group} \div \text{total diabetic group}}{\text{Number of cases of this anomaly in control group} \div \text{total control group}}$$

Mills J, Baker L, Goldman AS. Malformations in infants of diabetic mothers occur before the seventh gestational week. Implications for treatment. Diabetes 1979;28:292–293

as a result of pregnancy (5). In contrast, pregnancy has been tentatively associated with a greater than twofold risk for the progression of diabetic retinopathy (6), although the study could not distinguish between the effects of pregnancy and those of the sudden institution of rigorous metabolic control, which has itself been linked to transient worsening of retinopathy (7, 8). Progression to proliferative retinopathy during pregnancy rarely occurs in women without any retinal disease or those with background changes. However, proliferative retinopathy may lead to vision loss if untreated and thus should be monitored closely and managed with photocoagulation as appropriate (9).

Measurement of glycosylated hemoglobin, including hemoglobin A_{1C}, can be used to assess prior control of diabetes and also to guide plans for pregnancy. An ideal threshold for preconceptional glycosylated hemoglobin has not been uniformly established. However, the available data suggest that a periconceptional hemoglobin A_{1C} level in the normal range (which varies among laboratories) is associated with a rate of fetal anomalies approaching that seen in nondiabetic women and that the most significant risk of malformations occurs in women with levels exceeding 10%. Maternal status should be determined before pregnancy by means of a history, physical examination, ophthalmologic evaluation, and 24-hour urine collection for measurement of creatinine clearance and protein excretion. If this evaluation has not been accomplished before pregnancy, it should be done as early in pregnancy as possible.

Metabolic Control

Maternal hyperglycemia leads to fetal hyperglycemia and fetal hyperinsulinemia, a combination which may cause fetal macrosomia and fetal death as well as delayed pulmonary maturation. Therefore, diabetic women should attempt to achieve and maintain euglycemia throughout pregnancy. The patient should monitor her glucose levels using a portable glucose reflectance meter and record the results in a log book. Glucose should be measured several times daily; however, there is not universal agreement as to the exact timing. Some recommend a schedule of fasting and preprandial (before each meal) testing, while others use fasting and postprandial (1 or 2 hours after each meal) measurements.

In normal pregnancies, maternal plasma glucose levels rarely exceed an average of 100 mg/dl, ranging from fasting levels of 60–90 mg/dl to 1-hour and 2-hour postprandial levels of 140 mg/dl or less and 120 mg/dl or less, respectively. Normalization of maternal blood glucose levels reduces fetal mortality and neonatal morbidity. The following ranges of plasma glucose levels should be the therapeutic objectives in pregnancies complicated by diabetes mellitus:

- Fasting: 60–90 mg/dl
- Before lunch, dinner, or bedtime snack: 60–105 mg/dl
- After meals: (1 hour) no higher than 130–140 mg/dl
(2 hours) no higher than 120 mg/dl
- From 2 AM to 6 AM: 60–90 mg/dl

Although specific recommendations for the nutritional management of diabetes during pregnancy are lacking, some authorities have suggested the following guidelines. For women of medium height and normal weight, for example, the average caloric intake should range from 2,200 to 2,400 kcal, with protein accounting for 12–20% of total energy intake, carbohydrate for 50–60%, and fat making up the remainder (10). Caloric intake may be less in the first trimester. Approximately 25% of the calories should be consumed at breakfast, 30% at lunch, 30% at dinner, and 15% as a bedtime snack. Caloric intake should be established based on prepregnancy weight measured in terms of body mass index (BMI) and weight gain (11). Nutritional counseling is usually prescribed in early pregnancy with follow-up visits as necessary.

Control of maternal glycemia usually can be achieved with multiple daily injections of insulin and adjustment of dietary intake. Oral hypoglycemic agents are not used during pregnancy, as these drugs may reach the fetus and produce fetal hyperinsulinemia. Most patients require a combination of both intermediate-acting and short-acting (regular) human insulin in the morning and evening. An alternative regimen for the evening is to administer separate injections of short-acting insulin at dinnertime and intermediate-acting insulin at bedtime to reduce the frequency of nocturnal hypoglycemia. Finally, some patients respond well to an injection of long-acting insulin at bedtime or before breakfast or both plus short-acting insulin before each meal. Patients and their families should be instructed on the treatment of hypoglycemia, including the use of glucagon.

Compliant patients who fail to maintain adequate control despite multiple insulin injections and dietary adjustment may be candidates for continuous subcutaneous insulin infusion pump therapy. The risk of nocturnal hypoglycemia is increased in pregnancy, and, therefore, great care should be taken in selecting patients for this therapy. While the pump may be valuable for a small group of women with diabetes mellitus, it has not been demonstrated to be superior to multiple insulin injections (12). However, women who have maintained good glycemic control using the pump prior to pregnancy can generally maintain glycemic control using this therapy during pregnancy.

Outpatient care, with frequent visits and phone contacts, can help ensure that optimal glucose control is achieved. For some women, hospitalization may be required early in gestation for improvement of blood glucose control and intensive education. Most diabetic women can be treated as outpatients during the final weeks of pregnancy (13). Self-monitoring of blood glucose and outpatient fetal testing have significantly reduced the need for antepartum hospital admission. Nonetheless, hospitalization should be strongly considered for women whose diabetes is poorly controlled and those with other complications, such as vascular disease or hypertension, which may affect fetal growth, or preeclampsia. If benign retinopathy has been identified early in gestation, repeat examinations should be performed in each trimester. Proliferative retinopathy requires more frequent follow-up or therapy or both.

Fetal Evaluation

Ultrasonography has been shown to be an extremely valuable tool in evaluating fetal growth, estimating weight, and detecting hydramnios and some malformations. A determination of maternal serum alpha-fetoprotein levels at 16–20 weeks of gestation should be used in association with an ultrasound study at 18–20 weeks in an attempt to detect neural tube defects and other anomalies. Since maternal serum alpha-fetoprotein values may be lower in pregnancies complicated by diabetes, interpretation may need to be altered accordingly (14). One study suggests that fetal echocardiography performed at 20–22 weeks of gestation may be a useful adjunctive procedure when cardiac anomalies are suspected (15).

During the third trimester, when fetal death is most likely to occur, a program of fetal surveillance should be initiated. The primary value of such surveillance is to allow the clinician to delay delivery safely in order for the fetus to mature (16). Abnormal results of fetal monitoring and testing are rare in patients whose diabetes has been well controlled and those without vascular disease or hypertension. Maternal monitoring of fetal activity is often used as an adjunct to some form of biophysical testing. The timing and frequency of biophysical surveillance, including the nonstress test, biophysical profile, or contraction stress test, depend on the degree of risk present. For example, in a pregnancy complicated by severe nephropathy, such testing may be initiated at 28 weeks. However, testing may be started considerably later in gestation for a patient whose condition has been well controlled, who does not have vascular disease, and whose fetus demonstrates normal growth on several ultrasound examinations. Other reasons to increase fetal surveillance include ketoacidosis, pyelonephritis, preeclampsia, and poor patient compliance (Pedersen's prognostically bad signs in pregnancy) (17).

Delivery Considerations

Improved glycemic control and better methods of antepartum fetal surveillance have obviated the need for elective preterm delivery to avoid fetal death (18). The timing of delivery should be determined by a combination of maternal and fetal risk factors. If a patient has maintained excellent glycemic control and all parameters of fetal surveillance have remained normal, she may await the spontaneous onset of labor. For patients at highest risk, such as those with vascular disease, poor metabolic control, problems with compliance, or a previous stillbirth, the timing of delivery should be based on clinical factors, with the goal being to reach documented pulmonary maturity. Significant maternal hypertension, fetal growth delay, or worsening retinopathy may mandate preterm delivery. Prior to elective delivery, patients with poor or undocumented metabolic control or those at less than 39 weeks of gestation by accurate gestational dating should undergo amniocentesis to document fetal pulmonary maturity (19).

Laboratory standards for the lecithin/sphingomyelin (L/S) ratio and its predictive relationship to respiratory distress syndrome may differ and should be defined by each hospital laboratory. With a mature L/S ratio, a low incidence of respiratory distress syndrome can be expected in women whose pregnancies are complicated by well-controlled diabetes, even in the absence of phosphatidylglycerol (20). If chemical tests do not confirm lung maturity, delivery may be postponed and a repeat amniocentesis based on the initial L/S value and other clinical factors may be planned.

When antepartum testing is nonreassuring and tests indicate lung maturity, the fetus should be delivered. If amniotic fluid analysis does not confirm maturity, the risks to the fetus of remaining in utero should be weighed against the risks of premature delivery.

If premature labor occurs in a pregnancy complicated by diabetes, tocolytic therapy with parenteral β-sympathomimetic agents is best avoided. These medications may significantly worsen maternal glucose control, causing ketoacidosis in some cases. For this reason, magnesium sulfate is the preferred intravenous tocolytic agent for women with diabetes mellitus. Corticosteroids to promote fetal lung maturity should also be used with caution. Glucose levels should be monitored closely, and intravenous insulin administration may be needed.

Because neonatal hypoglycemia is related to intrapartum maternal hyperglycemia, it is important to maintain euglycemia. Continuous infusion of both insulin and glucose has proven valuable to control maternal glucose levels during labor and delivery (21). In patients with well-controlled diabetes who are scheduled for elective induction of labor, the usual dose of insulin is given at bedtime, and morning insulin is withheld. Once active labor begins, a constant infusion of dextrose is given to supply caloric needs (Table 3). Short-acting insulin is added if the patient becomes hyperglycemic. Capillary glucose values are determined at the bedside every 1–2 hours. If rapid intravenous infusion of fluid is necessary, dextrose should be avoided because of the risk of fetal acidemia (22).

The optimal route of delivery for the diabetic patient remains controversial. Cephalopelvic disproportion and shoulder dystocia accompanied by traumatic birth injury are more likely with vaginal delivery of large infants of diabetic women (23). The risk of such complications rises exponentially when birth weight exceeds 4,000 g. Excessive fat deposition on the shoulders and trunk makes the risk of birth injury greater for the fetus of a woman with diabetes when compared with a fetus of similar birthweight whose mother does not have diabetes (24). While ultrasonography can be used to assess fetal size at term, errors in the estimation of fetal weight may be significant. If a large fetus is suspected, midpelvic operative delivery should be avoided, particularly in the presence of a prolonged second stage of labor (25). Although controversy remains as to the estimated weight at which an elective cesarean delivery should be performed to avoid birth trauma, a suspected birthweight in excess of 4,500 g is a reasonable threshold (26).

Table 3. LOW-DOSAGE CONSTANT INSULIN INFUSION FOR THE INTRAPARTUM PERIOD*

Blood Glucose (mg/100 ml)	Insulin Dosage (U/h)	Fluids (125 ml/h)
<100	0	Dextrose/Lactated Ringer's injection
100–140	1.0	Dextrose/Lactated Ringer's injection
141–180	1.5	Normal saline
181–220	2.0	Normal saline
>220	2.5	Normal saline

*Dilution is 25 U of regular insulin in 250 ml of normal saline with 25 ml flushed through line administered intravenously. A finger stick glucose test is performed every 1–2 hours. The insulin pump and intravenous solution are adjusted accordingly.

Adapted from Hollingsworth DR, Moore TR. Diabetes and pregnancy. In: Creasy RK, Resnik R. Maternal–fetal medicine: principles and practices. Philadelphia: WB Saunders, 1989:975

Elective cesarean delivery should be scheduled for early morning. The usual morning insulin dose is withheld, and glucose levels are monitored frequently. After delivery, intravenous dextrose is given and glucose levels are checked every 4–6 hours. To avoid maternal hypoglycemia, the antepartum objective of tight metabolic control is relaxed. Short-acting insulin is administered only for significant hyperglycemia, for example, levels above 200 mg/dl. Once the patient begins a regular diet, subcutaneous insulin can be reinstituted at dosages substantially lower than those given in the third trimester. It is helpful if the pregestational dose is known.

Selecting a method of contraception postpartum is an important consideration for the diabetic woman that requires a careful review of the patient's history and complete gynecologic examination with counseling at the postpartum follow-up visit. Because there are no inherent risks to the use of a diaphragm or other barrier methods, these are commonly recommended interim methods of contraception for the insulin-dependent patient.

While combination oral contraceptives (OCs) are a most effective reversible method of contraception, there is controversy regarding their use in women with overt diabetes. A retrospective study documented five cardiovascular complications in 136 diabetic women using primarily low-dose OCs (27). In contrast, a cross-sectional study of 384 insulin-dependent women failed to demonstrate an association between OC use and progression of vascular complications (28). The use of low-dose OCs in diabetic women should probably be restricted to patients without vasculopathy or additional risk factors, such as a strong family history of ischemic heart disease. The lowest dose of estrogen and progesterone should be prescribed. Patients should have their blood pressure monitored after the first cycle and quarterly and their baseline and follow-up lipid levels determined as well.

Screening and Diagnosis of Gestational Diabetes

Gestational diabetes mellitus has been characterized as the onset or recognition of glucose intolerance during pregnancy (29). Patients with GDM have about a 50% likelihood of developing diabetes mellitus within 20 years (30). The detection and treatment of GDM may reduce the risks for several adverse perinatal outcomes including excessive fetal growth and birth trauma, fetal death, and neonatal morbidity, including hypoglycemia and hyperbilirubinemia. These observations, however, have been derived primarily from retrospective clinical data.

Traditionally, obstetricians have relied on historical and clinical risk factors to identify those patients most likely to develop GDM. However, in some populations, almost half of all patients with GDM lack specific risk factors (31). Although there is evidence that the frequency of GDM increases with maternal age, use of arbitrary age cutoffs to select patients for screening will result in a significant proportion of these cases being overlooked (31).

In the past, selective screening of women age 30 and older has been recommended, and some advocate universal screening. There are no data to support the benefit of screening, however, and further studies are needed on which to base a recommendation.

Whereas selective screening for GDM (ie, screening women with traditional risk factors) may be appropriate in some clinical settings such as teen clinics, universal screening may be more appropriate in other settings. Examples of the latter include populations with a high background prevalence of Type II diabetes and practices consisting predominantly of women who have risk factors for GDM. In these settings, the effort expended to perform risk factor analysis for each patient may not be warranted if as a result only a minority of patients are spared from screening. This is particularly true given the limited sensitivity of GDM screening based on risk factors alone. Conversely, in certain Native American populations, the prevalence of GDM is so high that pregnant women in these populations can be considered to have a positive screen. They may proceed directly to diagnostic testing.

Screening for GDM is performed with a 50-g oral glucose load followed by a glucose determination 1 hour later (29). Screening should be performed between 24 and 28 weeks of gestation. Patients with risk factors, such as a previous history of GDM, may benefit from earlier screening. If screening in early pregnancy yields a normal result, subsequent testing should be performed at 24–28 weeks. Patients whose plasma glucose levels equal or exceed 140 mg/dl should be evaluated with a diagnostic 3-hour glucose tolerance test (GTT).

Sensitivity (the proportion of patients correctly identified as having GDM) of the 50-g screen is improved if the test is performed when the patient is in a fasting state, but fasting is not required (32). The sensitivity of screening may be improved by using thresholds lower than 140 mg/dl, but specificity (the proportion of patients correctly identified as not having GDM) may be decreased. For example, a threshold of 140 mg/dl may identify 90% of cases of GDM and require that 15% of all patients screened have a GTT. A threshold of 130 mg/dl may identify almost all cases of GDM, but 25% of women screened will require a GTT.

The normal values for a 100-g diagnostic GTT are listed in Table 4. (Other glucose challenges have been used in specific populations.) These plasma values represent a theoretical conversion of O'Sullivan's thresholds in whole blood. Some clinicians prefer to use other modifications of these data (33, 34). In each case, two abnormal glucose values are required to diagnose GDM.

In some series, women with one abnormal value on the diagnostic 3-hour GTT have been found to be at increased risk for fetal macrosomia (35). When such women undergo a repeat test, one third will subsequently demonstrate GDM. Further data are needed to establish whether repeat testing or treatment in such women is justified (36).

Table 4. DETECTION OF GESTATIONAL DIABETES

Test	Plasma Glucose Level (mg/dl)*	
Screening		
50-g, 1 h screen	130–140	
Diagnostic	**O'Sullivan Criteria (30)†**	
100-g oral glucose tolerance test‡	NDDG Conversion (44)†	Carpenter Conversion (33)†
Fasting	105	95
1 h	190	180
2 h	165	155
3 h	145	140

*Result is upper limit of normal.

†Data are reported in the references shown in parentheses.

‡Diagnosis of gestational diabetes is made when any two values are met or exceeded.

Management of Gestational Diabetes

Women with GDM generally do not require hospitalization for dietary instruction and management. Following the diagnosis, patients should be placed on a diet such as that prescribed for preexisting diabetes in pregnancy. Proposed daily caloric requirements for treatment of GDM are presented in Table 5. Significant caloric restriction to 1,200–1,800 kcal/d has been studied in overweight women with GDM (37). While maternal weight gain and fetal macrosomia may be decreased, the safety of this approach has not been established, and thus it is not recommended.

Continued monitoring is necessary in patients with GDM to determine whether glucose levels are well controlled by diet or, if not, to determine the need for insulin therapy. Fasting and postprandial glucose levels should be monitored at least weekly. Some clinicians prefer daily self-monitoring of glucose to better ascertain the level of glycemic control achieved by dietary therapy (38).

Insulin therapy is recommended when standard dietary management does not consistently maintain the fasting plasma glucose at less than 105 mg/dl or the 2-hour postprandial plasma glucose at less than 120 mg/dl (29). Patients who require insulin should monitor their glucose levels daily. It should be recognized that the level of glycemia necessary to reduce fetal and neonatal complications in GDM pregnancies has not been established. Treatment with insulin at lower fasting and postprandial thresholds may reduce the risk of fetal macrosomia (39). Treatment based on daily self-monitoring may also reduce macrosomia (38).

Women with GDM who maintain an active life style should be encouraged to continue a program of exercise approved for pregnancy (40, 41). Preliminary studies suggest that initiation of regular upper-extremity exercise in previously sedentary women with GDM may improve glycemic control (40).

Table 5. DIETARY STRATEGIES FOR WOMEN WITH GESTATIONAL DIABETES: DAILY CALORIC REQUIREMENTS

Current Weight in Relation to Ideal Body Weight	Daily Caloric Intake (kcal/kg)*
<80%	35–40
80–120%	30
120–150%	24
>150%	12–15

*Caloric content is expressed for present pregnant weight.

Adapted from Mulford MI, Jovanovic-Peterson L, Peterson CM. Alternative therapies for the management of gestational diabetes. Clin Perinatol 1993;20:630

Patients with GDM whose condition is well controlled are at low risk for fetal death. Those whose condition is not well controlled or who require insulin therapy should be managed in the same manner as those with pregestational diabetes. In women with well-controlled gestational diabetes, there is no consensus regarding the criteria for initiation and timing of fetal testing. Some clinicians recommend weekly biophysical fetal testing as early as 34 weeks of gestation (42), while others do not begin testing until 40 weeks of gestation (43). More intensive biophysical fetal testing has been recommended by some in at least three groups of patients with GDM: those who require insulin, those with hypertension, and those with a history of previous stillbirth (43). In most cases, women with GDM may be managed expectantly as long as fasting and postprandial glucose values remain normal. As with patients with pregestational diabetes, ultrasonography, despite its limitations, may be used to estimate fetal size and aid in the choice of timing and route of delivery.

Because women with GDM are at increased risk for overt diabetes, follow-up testing is recommended during the first few months following delivery and thereafter on a yearly basis. The 2-hour, 75-g oral GTT is used (44). Diabetes is diagnosed if the fasting plasma glucose is greater than or equal to 140 mg/dl or two postglucose challenge measurements meet or exceed 200 mg/dl. Impaired glucose tolerance may also be identified by the 75-g oral GTT (Table 1). In cases in which a complete oral GTT cannot be performed easily, a fasting threshold of 115 mg/dl can be used as a cutoff point for performing a full oral GTT (45).

Contraception is also an important consideration for the woman who has had GDM. Low-dose OCs may be used safely by women who experienced GDM who do not have other risk factors. The rate of subsequent diabetes in OC users is approximately 15–20% after 1 year of follow up. This rate is not significantly different from that of those who did not use OCs (17%) (46). No adverse effects on levels of total cholesterol, low-density lipoproteins, high-density lipoproteins, or triglycerides have been observed in women who experienced GDM and use low-dose OCs, although serial measurements of these parameters have been recommended (47).

REFERENCES

1. Kitzmiller JL, Gavin LA, Gin GD, Jovanovic-Peterson L, Main EK, Zigrang WD. Preconception care of diabetes. Glycemic control prevents congenital anomalies. JAMA 1991;265:731–736

2. Lucas MJ, Leveno KJ, Williams ML, Raskin P, Whalley PJ. Early pregnancy glycosylated hemoglobin, severity of diabetes, and fetal malformations. Am J Obstet Gynecol 1989;161:426–431

3. Miller E, Hare JW, Cloherty JP, Dunn PJ, Gleason RE, Soeldner JS, et al. Elevated maternal hemoglobin A_{1c} in early pregnancy and major congenital anomalies in infants of diabetic mothers. N Engl J Med 1981;304:1331–1334

4. Mills JL, Knopp RH, Simpson JL, Jovanovic-Peterson L, Metzger BE, Holmes LB, et al. Lack of relation of increased malformation rates in infants of diabetic mothers to glycemic control during organogenesis. N Engl J Med 1988;318:671–676

5. Reece EA, Coustan DR, Hayslett JP, Holford T, Coulehan J, O'Connor TZ, et al. Diabetic nephropathy: pregnancy performance and fetomaternal outcome. Am J Obstet Gynecol 1988;159:56–66

6. Klein BEK, Moss SE, Klein R. Effect of pregnancy on progression of diabetic retinopathy. Diabetes Care 1990; 13:34–40

7. Van Ballegooie E, Hooymans JMM, Timmerman Z, Reitsma WD, Sluiter WJ, Schweitzer NMJ, et al. Rapid deterioration of diabetic retinopathy during treatment with continuous subcutaneous insulin infusion. Diabetes Care 1984;7:236–242

8. Dahl-Jørgensen K, Brinchmann-Hansen O, Hanssen KF, Sandvik L, Aagenæs Ø, Aker Diabetes Group. Rapid tightening of blood glucose control leads to transient deterioration of retinopathy in insulin-dependent diabetes mellitus: the Oslo study. BMJ 1985;290:811–815

9. Sunness JS. The pregnant woman's eye. Surv Ophthalmol 1988;32:219–238

10. Ney D, Hollingsworth DR. Nutritional management of pregnancy complicated by diabetes: historical perspective. Diabetes Care 1981;4:647–655

11. Institute of Medicine. Nutrition during pregnancy. Part I. Weight gain. Washington, DC: National Academy Press, 1990

12. Coustan DR, Reece EA, Sherwin RS, Rudolf MCJ, Bates SE, Sockin SM, et al. A randomized clinical trial of the insulin pump vs intensive conventional therapy in diabetic pregnancies. JAMA 1986;255:631–636

13. Landon MB, Gabbe SG, Piana R, Mennuti MT, Main EK. Neonatal morbidity in pregnancy complicated by diabetes mellitus: predictive value of maternal glycemic profiles. Am J Obstet Gynecol 1987;156:1089–1095

14. Martin AO, Dempsey LM, Minogue J, Liu K, Keller J, Tamura R, et al. Maternal serum α-fetoprotein levels in pregnancies complicated by diabetes: implications for screening programs. Am J Obstet Gynecol 1990;163: 1209–1216

15. Shields LE, Gan EA, Murphy HF, Sahn DJ, Moore TR. The prognostic value of hemoglobin A1c in predicting fetal heart disease in diabetic pregnancies. Obstet Gynecol 1993;81:954–957

16. Landon MB, Gabbe SG. Antepartum fetal surveillance and delivery timing in diabetic pregnancies. Clin Diabetes 1990;8:33–46

17. Pedersen J, Mølsted-Pedersen L, Andersen B. Assessors of fetal perinatal mortality in diabetic pregnancy. Analysis of 1,332 pregnancies in the Copenhagen series, 1946–1972. Diabetes 1974;23:302–305

18. Cousins L. Pregnancy complications among diabetic women: review 1965–1985. Obstet Gynecol Surv 1987;42:140–149

19. American College of Obstetricians and Gynecologists. Fetal maturity assessment prior to elective repeat cesarean delivery. ACOG Committee Opinion 98. Washington, DC: ACOG, 1991

20. Kjos SL, Walther FJ, Montoro M, Paul RH, Diaz F, Stabler M. Prevalence and etiology of respiratory distress in infants of diabetic mothers: predictive value of fetal lung maturation tests. Am J Obstet Gynecol 1990; 163:898–903

21. Jovanovic L, Peterson CM. Management of the pregnant, insulin-dependent diabetic woman. Diabetes Care 1980;3: 63–68

22. Kenepp NB, Kumar S, Shelley WC, Stanley CA, Gabbe SG, Gutsche BB. Fetal and neonatal hazards of maternal hydration with 5% dextrose before caesarean section. Lancet 1982;1:1150–1152

23. Acker DB, Sachs BP, Friedman EA. Risk factors for shoulder dystocia. Obstet Gynecol 1985;66:762–768

24. Modanlou HD, Komatsu G, Dorchester W, Freeman RK, Bosu SK. Large-for-gestational-age neonates: anthropometric reasons for shoulder dystocia. Obstet Gynecol 1982;60:417–423

25. Benedetti TJ, Gabbe SG. Shoulder dystocia: a complication of fetal macrosomia and prolonged second stage of labor with midpelvic delivery. Obstet Gynecol 1978; 52:526–529

26. American College of Obstetricians and Gynecologists. Fetal macrosomia. ACOG Technical Bulletin 159. Washington, DC: ACOG, 1991

27. Steel JM, Duncan LJP. Serious complications of oral contraception in insulin-dependent diabetics. Contraception 1978;17:291–295

28. Klein BEK, Moss SE, Klein R. Oral contraceptives in women with diabetes. Diabetes Care 1990;13:895–898

29. Metzger BE. Summary and recommendations of the Third International Workshop-Conference on Gestational Diabetes Mellitus. Diabetes 1991;40(Suppl 2):197–201

30. O'Sullivan JB. Body weight and subsequent diabetes mellitus. JAMA 1982;248:949–952

31. Coustan DR, Nelson C, Carpenter MW, Carr SR, Rotondo L, Widness JA. Maternal age and screening for gestational diabetes: a population-based study. Obstet Gynecol 1989;73:557–561

32. Coustan DR, Widness JA, Carpenter MW, Rotondo L, Pratt DC, Oh W. Should the fifty-gram, one-hour plasma glucose screening test for gestational diabetes be administered in the fasting or fed state? Am J Obstet Gynecol 1986;154:1031–1035

33. Carpenter MW, Coustan DR. Criteria for screening tests for gestational diabetes. Am J Obstet Gynecol 1982; 144:768–773

34. Sacks DA, Abu-Fadil S, Greenspoon JS, Fotheringham N. Do the current standards for glucose tolerance testing in

pregnancy represent a valid conversion of O'Sullivan's original criteria? Am J Obstet Gynecol 1989;161:638–641

35. Langer O, Anyaegbunam A, Brustman L, Divon M. Management of women with one abnormal oral glucose tolerance test value reduces adverse outcome in pregnancy. Am J Obstet Gynecol 1989;161:593–599

36. Neiger R, Coustan DR. The role of repeat glucose tolerance tests in the diagnosis of gestational diabetes. Am J Obstet Gynecol 1991;165:787–790

37. Dornhorst A, Nicholls JSD, Probst F, Paterson CM, Hollier KL, Elkeles RS, et al. Calorie restriction for treatment of gestational diabetes. Diabetes 1991;40(Suppl 2):161–164

38. Goldberg JD, Franklin B, Lasser D, Jornsay DL, Hausknecht RU, Ginsberg-Fellner F, et al. Gestational diabetes: impact of home glucose monitoring on neonatal birth weight. Am J Obstet Gynecol 1986;154:546–550

39. Langer O, Berkus M, Brustman L, Anyaegbunam A, Mazze R. Rationale for insulin management in gestational diabetes mellitus. Diabetes 1991;40(Suppl 2):186–190

40. Jovanovic-Peterson L, Peterson CM. Is exercise safe or useful for gestational diabetic women? Diabetes 1991; 40(Suppl 2);179–181

41. Bung P, Artal R, Khodiguian N, Kjos S. Exercise in gestational diabetes. An optional therapeutic approach? Diabetes 1991;40(Suppl 2):182–185

42. Girz BA, Divon MY, Merkatz IR. Sudden fetal death in women with well-controlled, intensively monitored gestational diabetes. J Perinatol 1992;12:229–233

43. Landon MB, Gabbe SG. Antepartum fetal surveillance in gestational diabetes mellitus. Diabetes 1985;34(Suppl 2):50–54

44. National Diabetes Data Group. Classification and diagnosis of diabetes mellitus and other categories of glucose intolerance. Diabetes 1979;28:1039–1057

45. American Diabetes Association. Position statement: screening for diabetes. Diabetes Care 1989;12:588–590

46. Kjos SL, Shoupe D, Douyan S, Friedman RL, Bernstein GS, Mestman JH, et al. Effect of low-dose oral contraceptives on carbohydrate and lipid metabolism in women with recent gestational diabetes: results of a controlled, randomized, prospective study. Am J Obstet Gynecol 1990; 163:1822–1827

47. Kjos SL. Contraception in the diabetic woman. Clin Perinatol 1993;20:649–661

This Technical Bulletin was developed under the direction of the Committee on Technical Bulletins of the American College of Obstetricians and Gynecologists as an educational aid to obstetricians and gynecologists. The committee wishes to thank Mark B. Landon, MD, and Steven G. Gabbe, MD, for their assistance in the development of this bulletin. This Technical Bulletin does not define a standard of care, nor is it intended to dictate an exclusive course of management. It presents recognized methods and techniques of clinical practice for consideration by obstetrician–gynecologists for incorporation into their practices. Variations of practice taking into account the needs of the individual patient, resources, and limitations unique to the institution or type of practice may be appropriate.

ISSN 1074-8628

THE AMERICAN COLLEGE OF OBSTETRICIANS AND GYNECOLOGISTS
409 12th Street, SW
Washington, DC 20024-2188

12345/87654

Number 176—January 1993
(Replaces #98, November 1986)

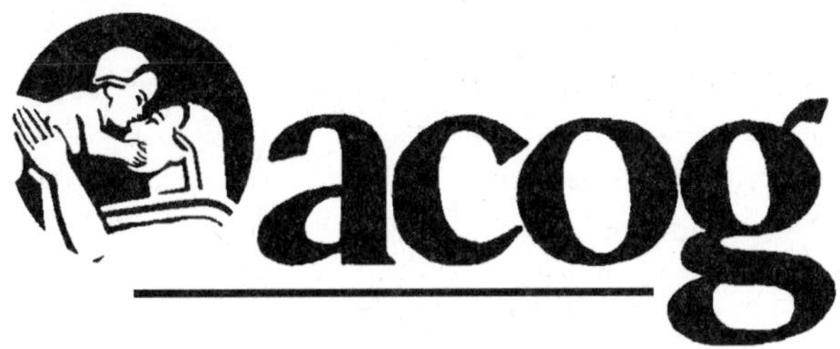

Technical Bulletin

An Educational Aid to Obstetrician–Gynecologists

Diagnosis and Management of Fetal Death

The World Health Organization defines fetal death as death prior to complete expulsion or extraction from the mother, regardless of the duration of pregnancy. "Standard Terminology for Reporting of Reproductive Health Statistics in the United States" supplements this all-inclusive definition by providing recommendations for reporting and tabulating vital events (1). The National Center for Health Statistics is moving forward with implementation of these recommendations through its own and state models. The goal is for each jurisdiction to report data that are at least as detailed as were reported in 1986, when the "Standard Terminology" was agreed upon. At present, most (but not all) states require reporting of fetal death after 20 weeks of gestation, with or without a weight designation (see the box). Many other countries include only fetal deaths occurring after 28 weeks of gestation, adding further difficulty in comparing vital statistics. Thus, when fetal death rates or ratios are presented, it is essential that the reporting requirements and tabulation methods used be stated clearly. For purposes of quality assurance outcome review, birth weight (eg, 500 g) is a useful clinical indicator.

Current Reporting Requirements

The following general fetal death reporting requirements are as of March 1991 (1):

20 weeks or more of gestation
Alabama
Alaska
Arizona*
California
Connecticut
Delaware
Florida
Guam
Illinois
Indiana
Iowa
Maryland*
Minnesota
Montana
Nebraska
Nevada
New Jersey
North Carolina
North Dakota
Ohio
Oklahoma
Oregon*
Puerto Rico
Texas
Utah
Vermont*
Washington
West Virginia
Wyoming

20 weeks or more of gestation or birth weight of 500 g or more
District of Columbia

20 weeks or more of gestation or birth weight of 350 g or more
Idaho
Kentucky
Louisiana
Massachusetts
Mississippi
Missouri
New Hampshire
South Carolina
Wisconsin

Birth weight in excess of 350 g
Kansas

20 weeks or more of gestation or birth weight of 400 g or more
Michigan

Birth weight of 500 g or more
New Mexico
South Dakota
Tennessee*

16 weeks or more of gestation
Pennsylvania

All products of human conception
American Samoa
Arkansas
Colorado
Georgia
Hawaii
Maine
New York
Northern Mariana Islands
Rhode Island
Virginia
Virgin Islands

*Specific modifiers apply

Epidemiologic Considerations

Customarily, the fetal death rate is expressed as the number of fetal deaths per 1,000 total births. In the United States, the fetal death rate has declined by more than half over the past 50 years. The decrease has been more or less progressive. For example, over the period of 1945–1988, the fetal death rate among white women declined from slightly more than 21 to 6 per 1,000 total births, whereas that among other races decreased from 42 to 11 per 1,000 births (2). Thus, a distinct racial difference persists, although it may be narrowing.

As of 1988, the fetal death rate in the United States among all races was 7.5 per 1,000 total births, representing approximately half of perinatal mortality (ie, fetal plus neonatal deaths) (2). Characteristics consistently associated with an increased risk of fetal death include maternal age (both high and low), unmarried status, male fetal sex, and multiple gestation.

A number of maternal, placental, and fetal conditions are known to be associated with fetal death (3). In some instances, such as in prolapse of the umbilical cord, the mechanism is obvious, whereas in others it is less clear. Among the maternal diseases associated with increased risk to the fetus are chronic hypertension, preeclampsia, metabolic diseases (especially uncontrolled diabetes mellitus), and certain viral and bacterial infections. D isoimmunization was formerly a common cause of fetal death, but its frequency has diminished markedly. Cord and placental complications (previa, abruption) account for a certain number of fetal deaths; however, in many cases this is difficult to prove and is a presumptive diagnosis made after other causes have been excluded. Up to 35% of fetal deaths are associated with the presence of a congenital malformation.

Clinical Considerations

Diagnosis

Fetal death is usually suspected by the gravida when fetal movements cease. The physician is unable to hear fetal heart tones. Formerly, various radiographic signs confirmed fetal death; now, real-time ultrasound is used to confirm the absence of cardiac activity. In experienced hands, real-time ultrasound is 100% accurate in this regard.

When the question of fetal death arises during labor, a fetal monitor can be applied to the presenting part. Maternal cardiac electrical activity can be transmitted through a dead fetus, however, so the rate and rhythm on the tracing should be compared with those of the mother. When fetal death is suspected, ultrasound should be used when possible to resolve the issue.

Natural History

Overall, 80–90% of patients enter spontaneous labor within 2 weeks of fetal death (4). This interval, called the "latency period," can vary in individual cases. In general, the latency period is inversely proportional to the duration of the gestation when the demise occurred. The latency period seems to vary somewhat with the cause of fetal death. For example, erythroblastosis fetalis tends to be associated with a longer latency period than are other causes of fetal death.

The consumptive coagulopathy associated with prolonged retention of a dead fetus presumably results from release of tissue thromboplastin from the fetus into the maternal circulation (5). Although factors V and VIII, fibrinogen, prothrombin, and platelets are all consumed, plasma fibrinogen is the most useful clinical index to screen for subclinical disseminated intravascular coagulation. A coagulopathy will be seen in about one fourth of women who retain a dead fetus for longer than 4 weeks, and the proportion increases progressively thereafter. Since the process is gradual, weekly measurements of plasma fibrinogen should be adequate to detect an abnormality before a clinically significant coagulopathy develops. The plasma fibrinogen level during normal gestation averages 450 mg/dl, but a clinically significant coagulopathy does not occur until levels fall to less than 100 mg/dl.

Delivery

Most women find the prospect of carrying a dead fetus distressing and, in some cases, repugnant and want the pregnancy terminated as soon as possible. Since a coagulopathy rarely develops prior to the spontaneous onset of labor, the indication for pregnancy termination usually reflects psychologic and emotional considerations.

Vaginal prostaglandin E_2 (PGE_2) suppositories are a popular and efficient means of inducing labor in cases of fetal death. If labor is to be induced, the patient should be informed that she will experience strong contractions at decreasing intervals, as well as side effects from the induction. Vomiting, diarrhea, and pyrexia are quite common but usually can be controlled pharmacologically. Consideration may be given to the prophylactic use of antiemetic, antipyretic, and antidiarrheal agents. The customary dosage of PGE_2 is one 20-mg suppository inserted vaginally every 4 hours until uterine contractions are sufficient to promote progressive cervical dilation. Although the package insert for dinoprostone vaginal suppositories (Prostin E_2) lists "missed abortion or intrauterine fetal death up to 28 weeks gestational age" as an indication, some authors have reported safe use in the third trimester (6).

Intravenous oxytocin is a time-honored and safe method for inducing labor; it is less effective when used well before term. Large, prolonged doses are often required, and water intoxication may become a risk. When oxytocin is required for more than 12 hours, consideration should be given to using only electrolyte-containing solutions and limiting total fluid intake. Laminaria or similar osmotic dilators placed in the cervix may be a useful adjunct prior to oxytocin or vaginal PGE_2 induction.

Some authors have reported the use of high-dose oxytocin when the gestational age is less than 24 weeks. After exclusion of sensitivity to oxytocin at usual and customary doses and exclusion of preexisting hyponatremia, oxytocin is then given at high concentrations. One regimen described using approximately 300 mU per minute (200 units of oxytocin in 500 ml of 5% dextrose lactated Ringer solution or 5% dextrose and half normal saline at 50 ml per hour). In this setting, 5% dextrose and water has been associated with hyponatremia. Electrolytes should be checked before beginning oxytocin and should be repeated every 24 hours or if signs or symptoms of water intoxication occur. Attention should be paid to fluid intake and urinary output (7). Failure to respond to oxytocin or prostaglandins should lead to an evaluation of the possibility of an abdominal pregnancy.

Although sometimes difficult for a patient to accept, expectant management is the ideal treatment in many cases, particularly near term when spontaneous labor is likely soon to ensue. In the presence of a complicating medical condition such as cardiac disease, in which prostaglandins are contraindicated and in which fluid management is critical, awaiting spontaneous labor while monitoring coagulation indices seems preferable. Hospital and community support systems can be used to give the patient a contact person during the difficult waiting period.

Seeking the Cause

Discovery of the cause of fetal death typically occupies the full attention of the patient, her family, and the physician. If the cause can be identified, the process of psychologic and emotional adaptation may be facilitated, particularly for patients who blame themselves. Moreover, a substantial proportion of deaths occur because of conditions that carry a risk of recurrence, and recognition of the cause is essential for counseling regarding subsequent pregnancies. A formal algorithm for evaluation of fetal death helps ensure that details are not missed and that there is an orderly, systematic search for the cause (Fig. 1). Such a checklist approach delineates the roles of various health care providers. The information is then collated and presented in a counseling session 2 to 3 months postpartum. Such a systematic approach reduces the number of cases ascribed to "unknown etiology." The way in which the information is obtained and used may vary based on local resources. It should be collected by the individual most qualified to perform the evaluation. In addition to placing a copy of the information in the patient's medical record, consideration should be given to giving the mother a duplicate copy. These data may be critical if she moves or seeks prenatal care with another provider in a subsequent pregnancy.

Routine prenatal care includes a number of tests that should be reviewed in an effort to identify the cause of fetal death or any predisposing condition. Blood pressure records should be examined carefully; positive serologies and tests for glucose intolerance and isoimmunization should be rechecked. At the time of delivery, the important events of the delivery and the appearance of the fetus, umbilical cord, and placenta should be carefully described in the records.

Parental involvement in the development of a protocol for investigation of a fetal death is essential. The nature, purpose, and especially the cost of each of the tests under consideration should be explained to the parents and their concurrence obtained; some of the tests (eg, karyotyping) can be quite expensive.

Autopsy

A carefully performed autopsy is the single most useful step in identifying the cause of fetal death (8). Special expertise in the area of perinatal pathology or genetics may be helpful. Gross and microscopic examination of the placenta should be included (9). Radiographs and gross photographs may also be useful (10).

Genetic Analysis

The frequency of chromosomal abnormalities in unselected stillbirths is 5–6%, which is about 10 times that in live births (11). The potential value of chromosomal studies should be considered in all cases of fetal death. Abnormal karyotypes are more likely to be found when there is a history of recurrent pregnancy losses or abnormal offspring or when the current pregnancy has malformations, growth retardation, or stigmata of aneuploidy.

The success of cytogenetic analysis decreases with the duration of latency. When the death is recent, appropriate specimens for karyotype determination include fetal blood, skin, fascia lata, or patellar tendon. When, as is often the case, it is anticipated that autolysis will interfere with successful cytogenetic analysis (eg, prolonged latency), amniocentesis for culture of amniocytes offers the best likelihood of success (12).

Application of recombinant DNA technology to DNA obtained from fetal tissues shows promise for prenatal diagnosis. Hybridization to labeled viral oligonucleotides currently enables the diagnosis of some intrauterine infections (13). Comparisons with samples of paternal and sibling DNA may allow the diagnosis of germinal and somatic cell mutations resulting in fetal death, types of mutations which are not discernible through

Fig. 1. Assessment of fetal death (courtesy Medical College of Virginia, Richmond).

Physician Responsibilities	Nursing Responsibilities
______ Review of prenatal records and laboratory results ______ Maternal testing All patients ☐ Random glucose ☐ CBC with platelet count ☐ Antibody screen ☐ VDRL ☐ Kleihauer-Betke ☐ Urine toxicology screen Selected patients ☐ Thyroid function testing ☐ CMV titer (IgM, acute and convalescent IgG) ☐ Lupus anticoagulant/anticardiolipin antibody ______ Genetic w/u indicated _____/contacted _____ ______ Confirm completion of stillbirth/fetal examination (page ii) and placement on mother's chart Consents obtained: ______ Autopsy ______ Others (eg, photographs) ______ ______ ______ Placenta sent to pathology ______ Fetal death/stillborn autopsy form (page iii) completed ______ Additional studies: ______ Photographs ______ Viral cultures ______ X-rays ______ Bacterial cultures ______ Others ______	Saw baby: ☐ Mother ☐ Father ☐ Other Held baby: ☐ Mother ☐ Father ☐ Other Baby's name ______ ______ Keepsakes given to family by hospital: ☐ Commemorative card ☐ Footprints ☐ Photo ☐ Blanket ☐ Bracelet ☐ Tape measure ☐ Baptismal card/blessing card ☐ Referral to support organization ☐ Lock of hair ☐ Booklets (specify) ______ ______ ______ ______ Unit chosen: ☐ Ob ☐ Gyn Resources: ☐ Social Services ☐ Chaplain ☐ Community Support Groups ☐ Mental Health ☐ Burial options explained Option chosen ______ ☐ Grief process explained to: ☐ Mother ☐ Father ☐ Other ☐ Address/telephone number on in-patient admission record verified for follow-up call Comments ______ ______ ______ ______ ______

(*Continued*)

Fetal Death/Stillborn Examination Page ii

Key: +, present; –, absent; ?, unsure

Date ____________

Weight ________ Head Circumference ________ Crown–heel length (stretched) ________

General ________ Macerated ________ Intact ________

Other (describe) ________________

Head

____ Normal
____ Hydrocephalic
____ Scalp defects
____ Anencephalic
____ Abnormal skull shape
____ Collapsed
Other (describe) ________

Eyes

____ Normal
____ Close together
____ Far apart
____ Straight
____ Up slanting
____ Down slanting
____ Abnormally small
____ Abnormally large
____ Epicanthus
Other (describe) ________

Nose

____ Normal
Other (describe) ________

Mouth

____ Normal
____ Cleft palate
____ Cleft lip
____ Large tongue
____ Small chin
Other (describe) ________

Ears

____ Normal
____ Lowset (top below eyes)
____ Tags
____ Pits
____ Symmetric
Other (describe) ________

Neck

____ Normal
____ Excess skin

Neck *(continued)*

____ Cystic mass
Other (describe) ________

Chest

____ Normal
____ Asymmetric
____ Small
Other (describe) ________

Abdomen

____ Normal
____ Distension
____ Omphalocele
____ Gastroschisis
____ Hernia
____ 3-vessel cord
Other (describe) ________

Back

____ Normal
____ Spina bifida (defect level____)
____ Scoliosis
____ Kyphosis
Other (describe) ________

Limbs

Length: nl, short, long
Form: nl, symmetric missing parts
Position: nl, abnl

Arms	*Length*	*Form*	*Position*
Right	______	______	______
Left	______	______	______

Legs	*Length*	*Form*	*Position*
Right	______	______	______
Left	______	______	______

Hands

Right

____ Fingers (#)
____ Webbing/syndactyly
____ Transverse crease
Other (describe) ________

Hands *(continued)*

Left

____ Fingers (#)
____ Webbing/syndactyly
____ Transverse crease
Other (describe) ________

Feet

Right

____ Toes (#)
____ Webbing
____ Wide space between toes 1-2
Other (describe) ________

Left

____ Toes (#)
____ Webbing
____ Wide space between toes 1-2
Other (describe) ________

Nails

____ Normal
____ Small (which ones?________)
Other (describe) ________

Genitalia

____ Normal
____ Imperforate anus
____ Ambiguous genitalia (describe)
____

Male

____ Hypospadias
____ Chordee
____ Undescended testes
Other (describe) ________

Female

____ Normal urethral opening
____ Clitoromegaly
Other (describe) ________

(*Continued*)

Fetal Death/Stillborn Autopsy Page iii

To accompany body to morgue: Fill in as completely as possible

Date ____________

Medical Record # ________________________

Mother ________________________

Fetus ________________________

Name ________________________

LMP __________

Estimated gestational age __________ Weeks

Gravida_____ Para____ A____ Living Children_____

Ultrasound dx ________________________

Placenta examination ________________________

Cord examination ________________________

Cytogenetics obtained:

Blood: ☐ Yes ☐ No

Skin: ☐ Yes ☐ No

Alpha-fetoprotein ________________________

Prenatal assessment ________________________

Labor:

Spontaneous ________________________

Induced ________________________

Delivery:

Date________ Time ______

Vaginal ________________________

Cesarean ________________________

Pregnancy complications ________________________

Delivery complications ________________________

Indication(s) for pathologic examination ________________________

Special requests for gross and microscopic evaluation

____

Attending clinician ________________________

Phone number ________________________

karyotyping (14). Presently, however, these technologies are largely restricted to research purposes and are not generally available.

Fetal–Maternal Hemorrhage

The incidence of transplacental passage of erythrocytes from fetus to mother varies, but the volume is typically small (≤ 0.1 ml). Under usual circumstances, the only clinical consequence is isoimmunization in D-negative patients. In rare instances, however, fetal–maternal hemorrhage may be massive and sufficient to cause fetal death. This phenomenon has been reported in 10–15% of otherwise unexplained fetal deaths and in 3–5% of all fetal deaths (15, 16).

The standard method of testing for fetal erythrocytes in the maternal circulation is Kleihauer–Betke staining of a peripheral blood smear. This test is based on the different acid elution characteristics of fetal and adult hemoglobin. The proportion of erythrocytes containing fetal hemoglobin is multiplied by the estimated maternal blood volume with corrections for differences in maternal and fetal red blood cell counts, yielding the volume of fetal–maternal hemorrhage. Theoretically, the test should be done before labor, but testing during the puerperium is satisfactory (16).

Phospholipid Antibodies

An association has been found between the presence of antibodies that bind to anionic phospholipids and the occurrence of spontaneous abortion and fetal death. This effect presumably is mediated through an increased tendency for coagulation (17, 18). Originally described in patients with systemic lupus erythematosus and termed the "lupus anticoagulant," this heterogeneous group of antibodies also includes those that react with cardiolipin and other negatively charged phospholipids. Both lupus anticoagulant and anti-cardiolipin antibodies exist in immunoglobulin G and immunoglobulin M forms. These antibodies are found frequently in patients with lupus erythematosus and other autoimmune diseases, but they may also occur without apparent disease. The association between lupus anticoagulant and pregnancy loss appears strong (19). Antiphospholipid antibodies in the absence of lupus anticoagulant have been less well studied and their significance remains unclear (20).

Infections

Intraamniotic infection usually results from bacteria that ascend from the vagina and cervix. Severe forms can produce fetal death. This condition is usually obvious because of maternal signs and symptoms. Some infections, however, cause few maternal signs and therefore should be included in the differential diagnosis of unexplained fetal death. A histologic examination of the fetus, placenta, and cord is the best available aid in making the diagnosis.

Infection with *Listeria monocytogenes* carries a substantial risk to the fetus and newborn. In a well-studied outbreak in Los Angeles County in which the source was contaminated, unpasteurized cheese, nearly all of the deaths reflected perinatal infection (21). Fetal listeriosis usually occurs through the transplacental route, although ascending infection may occur as well. Because listeriosis is often asymptomatic in adults or may cause only a mild flulike syndrome, an infectious cause may not be obvious. Special stains and cultures of the placenta are necessary to make the diagnosis.

Counseling and Emotional Support

Formerly it was believed that grieving in cases of fetal death was minimal because there had not been any opportunity for attachment. It is now recognized that parents experiencing perinatal loss usually go through a grief process that is similar to that experienced with the death of an older child. The classic grief reaction of shock, guilt, anger, disorientation, and reorganization occurs in some way in all parents experiencing such a loss, and it is the role of the health care team to help guide them through the process.

It is essential that all providers be sensitive to the parents and communicate in an empathetic and appropriate manner. Care is best provided by staff who are skilled in postpartum care, understand the grieving process, and are able to meet the needs of parents experiencing perinatal loss (10). Statements such as "Don't worry, you'll have another baby," should be avoided. Parents often express a need to talk about the experience. Literature on perinatal death may decrease the feelings of isolation, and community support groups become helpful after the first month.

A number of choices must be made by the parents shortly after birth; whether to see the baby, to hold or touch the baby, or to name him or her, and what to do with the remains are among the decisions to be made. Research has indicated that responses to these questions are highly variable and dependent on demographic and obstetric characteristics (22). Parents may change their minds, and arrangements should be made to accommodate this (23). The assistance of nursing and social services personnel and clergy can be enlisted to aid in preparation of the body and viewing of the baby. Prudent individualization is the key.

Investigation of the possible causes of the event, whether or not a cause is found, is important in helping the parents adapt. If the cause is found, or at least if there has been a thorough investigation, adaptation is facilitated. Arrangements should be made for a follow-up visit to monitor grief reaction, review the details of the evaluation and discuss what is known about the cause of death, answer questions, and make recommendations for a future pregnancy. Such a visit is usually with the primary obstetrician, the midwife (if involved), and any family member or friend whom the mother wishes to have in attendance with her. If nurses or social workers from the hospital have been working with the family, they should be included whenever possible.

REFERENCES

1. American Academy of Pediatrics, American College of Obstetricians and Gynecologists. Guidelines for perinatal care. 3rd ed. Elk Grove Village, Illinois: AAP; Washington, DC: ACOG, 1992:253–270
2. National Center for Health Statistics. Vital statistics of the United States, 1988, Vol II, Mortality, Part A. DHHS Pub. No. (PHS) 91-1101. Washington, DC: U.S. Government Printing Office, 1991
3. Pitkin RM. Fetal death: diagnosis and management. Am J Obstet Gynecol 1987;157:583–589
4. Goldstein DP, Reid DE. Circulatory fibrinolytic activity—a precursor of hypofibrinogemia following fetal death in utero. Obstet Gynecol 1963;22:174–180
5. Weiner AE, Reid DE, Roby CC, Diamond KK. Coagulation defects with intrauterine death from Rh isosensitization. Am J Obstet Gynecol 1950;60:1015–1022
6. Kent DR, Goldstein AI, Linzey EM. Safety and efficacy of vaginal prostaglandin E_2 suppositories in the management of third-trimester fetal demise. J Repro Med 1984;29:101–102
7. Toaff R, Ayalon D, Gogol G. Clinical use of high concentration oxytocin drip. Obstet Gynecol 1971;37:112–120
8. Mueller RJ, Sybert VP, Johnson J, Brown ZA, Chen WJ. Evaluation of a protocol for post-mortem examination of stillbirths. N Engl J Med 1983;309:586–590
9. Rayburn W, Sander C, Barr M Jr, Rygiel R. The stillborn fetus: placental histologic examination in determining a cause. Obstet Gynecol 1985;65:637–641
10. American Academy of Pediatrics, American College of Obstetricians and Gynecologists. Guidelines for perinatal care. 3rd ed. Elk Grove Village, Illinois: AAP; Washington, DC: ACOG, 1992:215–221
11. Boué A, Boué J. Chromosomal abnormalities associated with fetal malformations. In: Schrimgeout J, ed. Towards the prevention of fetal malformation. Edinburgh: Edinburgh University Press, 1978:49–65
12. Brady K, Duff P, Harlass FE, Reid S. The role of amniotic fluid cytogenetic analysis in the evaluation of recent fetal death. Am J Perinatol 1991;8:68–70
13. Sahakian V, Weiner CP, Naides SJ, Williamson RA, Scharosch LL. Intrauterine transfusion treatment of nonimmune hydrops fetalis secondary to human parvovirus B19 infection. Am J Obstet Gynecol 1991;164:1090–1091
14. Kovacs BW, Shahbahrami B, Comings DE. Studies of human germinal mutations by deoxyribonucleic acid hybridization. Am J Obstet Gynecol 1989;160:798–804
15. Laube DW, Schauberger CW. Fetomaternal bleeding as a cause for "unexplained" fetal death. Obstet Gynecol 1982;60:649–651
16. Owen J, Stedman CM, Tucker TL. Comparison of predelivery versus postdelivery Kleihauer–Betke stains in cases of fetal death. Am J Obstet Gynecol 1989; 161:663–666
17. Branch DW, Scott JR, Kochenour NK, Hershgold E. Obstetric complications associated with the lupus anticoagulant. N Engl J Med 1985;313:1322–1326
18. Branch DW, Dudley DJ, Mitchell MD, Creighton KA, Abbott TM, Hammond EH, et al. Immunoglobulin G fractions from patients with antiphospholipid antibodies cause fetal death in BALB/c mice: a model for autoimmune fetal loss. Am J Obstet Gynecol 1990;163:210–216
19. Scott JR, Rote NS, Branch DW. Immunologic aspects of recurrent abortion and fetal death. Obstet Gynecol 1987;70:645–656
20. Harris EN, Spinnato JA. Should anticardiolipin tests be performed in otherwise healthy pregnant women? Am J Obstet Gynecol 1991;165:1272–1277
21. Linnan MJ, Mascola L, Lou XD, Goulet V, May S, Salminen C, et al. Epidemic listeriosis associated with Mexican-style cheese. N Engl J Med 1988;319:823–828
22. Kellner KR, Donnelly WH, Gould SD. Parental behavior after perinatal death: lack of predictive demographic and obstetric variables. Obstet Gynecol 1984;63:809–814
23. American College of Obstetricians and Gynecologists. Grief related to perinatal death. ACOG Technical Bulletin 86. Washington, DC: ACOG, 1985

This Technical Bulletin was developed under the direction of the Committee on Technical Bulletins of the American College of Obstetricians and Gynecologists as an educational aid to obstetricians and gynecologists. The committee wishes to thank Roy M. Pitkin, MD, for his assistance in the development of this bulletin. This Technical Bulletin does not define a standard of care, nor is it intended to dictate an exclusive course of management. It presents recognized methods and techniques of clinical practice for consideration by obstetrician–gynecologists for incorporation into their practices. Variations of practice taking into account the needs of the individual patient, resources, and limitations unique to the institution or type of practice may be appropriate.

THE AMERICAN COLLEGE OF OBSTETRICIANS AND GYNECOLOGISTS
409 12th Street, SW, Washington, DC 20024-2188

12345/76543

ACOG EDUCATIONAL BULLETIN

Number 257, December 1999

Domestic Violence

Domestic or intimate partner violence is a widespread problem that disproportionately burdens women and affects all age, racial, and socioeconomic groups. In the United States, it is a major cause of physical injuries, mental illness, and homelessness among women. In addition to the individual lives affected by domestic violence, it is a societal problem with tremendous public health and economic implications.

Although there is no single definition of domestic violence that satisfies medical, social, and criminal justice purposes, the term "domestic violence" typically refers to violence perpetrated against adolescent and adult females within the context of family or intimate relationships. Although the victim of domestic violence may be male or female, the cases overwhelmingly involve female victims (1). Domestic violence crosses all racial, ethnic, religious, educational, and socioeconomic lines and usually is a progressive phenomenon with psychologic and physical components that tend to occur in a predictable cycle (Fig. 1) (2). Violent acts may include threats, throwing objects, pushing, kicking, hitting, beating, sexual assault, threatening with a weapon, or using a weapon. Domestic violence frequently includes verbal abuse, intimidation, progressive social isolation, and deprivation of things such as food, money, transportation, or access to health care (2). Domestic violence often occurs within a framework of family violence that can include child abuse, elder abuse, or abuse of adults who are disabled.

During the past two decades, domestic violence has been increasingly recognized as a major public health problem. Guidelines for screening, diagnosis, and treatment have been developed and disseminated by numerous medical professional organizations (2–7). In 1993, the National Center for Injury Prevention and Control was established within the Centers for Disease Control and Prevention to apply a public health approach in developing strategies to prevent interpersonal violence and its consequences. The 1994 Violence Against Women Act (PL 103-322) was the first comprehensive policy established by the federal government to counteract violence against women by providing grant funding, establishing legal protection for victims, and supporting interdisciplinary programs that develop effective policies, protocols, and services to prevent violent crimes against women.

This Educational Bulletin was developed under the direction of the Committee on Underserved Women of the American College of Obstetricians and Gynecologists as an aid to obstetricians and gynecologists. This document is not to be construed as establishing a standard of practice or dictating an exclusive course of treatment. Rather, it is intended as an educational tool that presents current information on obstetric–gynecologic issues.

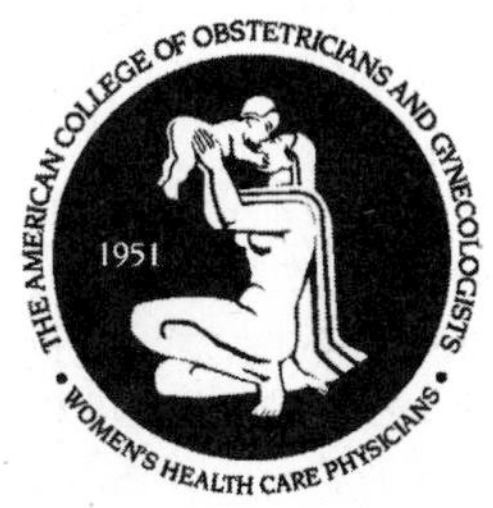

Replaces Number 209, August 1995

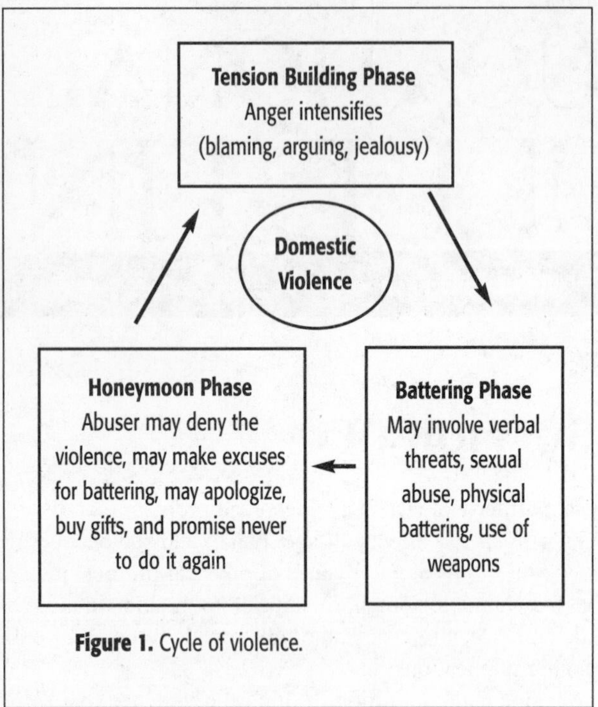

Figure 1. Cycle of violence.

Epidemiology

The true extent of domestic violence is difficult to ascertain. Early epidemiologic studies resulted in inconsistent findings due to variations in definitions, the populations sampled, and survey methodology. Recent efforts to standardize definitions have produced results that can be generalized to the American public and have identified more consistent findings (8). Nevertheless, estimates of domestic violence rates are most likely understated because many victims will not disclose their personal experiences of violence.

Among prevalence studies, violence is defined in two categories: severe and total. Severe violence includes acts that can inflict serious injury such as kicking, hitting, choking, and threats or use of a weapon. Total violence includes severe violence as well as less physically injurious acts such as throwing objects, shoving, and pushing (9). Every year, 2–4% of American women in an ongoing relationship experience at least one episode of severe violence; that percentage increases to 8–12% when total violence is considered (6). Furthermore, about one third of female victims experienced violence more than once during the preceding 6 months. These findings indicate that in the United States, nearly 5 million adult women experience domestic violence each year with 1.7 million experiencing severe abuse (10).

According to the Department of Justice, violence by an intimate partner accounts for about 21% of all the violent crime experienced by women. Among female murder victims, about 30% are killed by an intimate partner (11).

The Impact

A major cause of physical injuries among women is domestic violence (1, 10, 11). When injuries occur, they often are severe and repetitive and most commonly involve the head, face, breasts, or abdomen (2). In pregnancy, injuries commonly involve the abdomen and breasts. Emergency department data indicates that up to one third of women seen for injuries in the emergency setting may have symptoms related to abuse, although most will not report the abuse to health care providers or to law enforcement officers (12). Instead, these women may only offer vague somatic complaints and may be frequent users of health care (13). If an injury is acknowledged, the patient's explanation often is inconsistent with the injury, or there may be a significant delay between when the injury occurred and when medical attention was sought.

A growing body of research describes long-term physical and psychologic consequences as a result of ongoing or past violence (10). The stress of living in an ongoing abusive relationship may contribute to problems such as chronic headaches, chronic pelvic pain, sleep and appetite disturbances, sexual dysfunction, abdominal complaints, palpitations, and chronic vaginitis. Mental health symptoms associated with domestic violence include feelings of inadequacy and self-blame, depression, substance abuse, mood and anxiety disorders, and suicide attempts. Compared with nonvictims, women with a history of domestic violence also perceive themselves as having poorer health (8, 10).

The societal and economic impact of domestic violence is profound. Economic losses related to adult domestic violence, including medical costs, other tangible losses, and quality of life losses are estimated at $67 billion each year (14). In 1994, hospitals recognized that nearly a quarter million hospital visits are the result of domestic violence (14), and it is well established that only a fraction of domestic violence cases seen in hospital emergency rooms are recognized or documented as such.

Screening and Identification

Despite the medical community's increasing recognition of the problem of violence against women, many barriers to screening all patients still remain (15, 16). Lack of recognition of the widespread prevalence of the problem appears to be one of the principle barriers. Physicians also identify barriers to screening related to time constraints, fear of offending the patient, and a feeling of powerlessness in the area of treatment (17). Although physicians have expressed concern about offending their patients by asking about domestic or sexual violence, 78% of patients favor universal inquiry about physical assault and 68% favor universal inquiry about sexual assault (16). More importantly, about 90% of female patients in a primary care population believe that physicians can help with problems related to abuse. Because of the prevalence of violence, being female is a significant enough risk factor to warrant screening every patient at periodic intervals, such as annual examinations and new patient visits. Research suggests that the use of abuse assessment questions on standard medical records may increase screening and documentation (18).

The relevance of screening for domestic violence in primary care settings and in emergency settings has been well established. In emergency rooms, up to 24% of women seen for any reason have been battered (19), and up to 35% of women presenting with injuries have been battered (12, 20). Many of these women present repeatedly with injuries but are never recognized as battered women. Among all pregnant women, 0.9–21% experience domestic violence, although most will not volunteer this information (21). Asking each patient directly about prior or ongoing victimization increases the likelihood of disclosure (22).

Specific measures can be taken to improve identification and facilitate disclosure of domestic violence. A prefacing statement followed by a few simple, direct questions will identify most women with a history of abuse or assault. The introduction or preface should establish that screening is universal. A simple phrase such as, "I would like to ask you a few questions about physical, sexual, and emotional trauma because we know that these are common and affect women's health," demonstrates knowledge and sensitivity and provides context for the inquiry. The screening assessment should follow with direct questioning. Disclosure rates will be higher if the questions use behaviorally specific descriptions rather than the terms "abuse," "domestic violence," or "rape." Some examples of behaviorally specific phrasing are shown in the box.

Abuse victims often are accompanied to health care appointments by the perpetrator, who may appear overprotective or overbearing. Because partner control is a key factor in violence and abuse, it is essential to ask the patient questions in private, apart from the male partner and apart from children, family, or friends. It is especially important to avoid using a family member or friend as an interpreter when asking questions about violence.

Most perpetrators do not lash out at others, even at those they believe can jeopardize their control over their victim. However, infrequently the physician and clinical staff may become targets of verbal attacks or threats by an enraged perpetrator. Law enforcement officials increasingly recognize the need for prompt response should this be necessary. Also, they may be helpful in devising security plans for your office and staff.

If the patient has no history of prior abuse or assault, universal screening establishes that the problem of intimate violence is medically relevant. If the patient subsequently experiences some form of interpersonal violence, she may be more likely to report it and receive medical attention. In the event of a positive response, it is important to remember that the patient may have been living with the violence for a significant period, but this disclosure may be the first time she has discussed the problem openly. It is important to assess the nature and extent of the abuse because most victims have experienced multiple episodes of violence, and about one third have experienced violence in other relationships (1, 8, 11).

Intervention

If universal screening is employed, positive responses will be encountered. In order to avoid delays in a busy office setting, it is useful to have a protocol for responding that is easily implemented, and uses available resources. In the office setting, the most effective and efficient strategy for providing assistance to a woman who has disclosed abuse involves acknowledging the trauma, providing education and support, and offering referrals to community support services. A summary of

Behaviorally Specific Phrasing for Screening Questions

- Has anyone close to you ever threatened to hurt you?
- Has anyone ever hit, kicked, choked, or hurt you physically?
- Has anyone, including your partner, ever forced you to have sex?
- Are you ever afraid of your partner?

the physician's responsibility in addressing domestic violence is shown in the box. The physician must be prepared to discuss the abuse with the woman and establish a plan to deal with medical needs, psychosocial needs, and emergent issues. When past or ongoing victimization is identified, an important step is to acknowledge the trauma and reinforce the fact that the patient is not to blame. Many victims of domestic violence have trouble believing that they are not responsible for the abuse. Providing educational materials about domestic or intimate partner violence and its consequences can sometimes help victims take action toward ending the violence. Displaying and providing educational materials on domestic violence is an important intervention that demonstrates to women that their physicians' offices are both a resource and a safe place should they encounter future abuse or choose to disclose victimization.

Once domestic violence is identified and acknowledged, the next step is to assess immediate safety. If the violence in the woman's home has escalated to the point where she is afraid for her safety, she should be offered shelter. This can be accomplished by directly contacting or referring her to social work services, homeless shelters, or community services for battered women. Shelters do get filled, however, and although it can be more difficult to arrange, sometimes hospital admission can be provided until other arrangements are made. If the patient is not in need of immediate shelter, she should be advised that shelter is available if needed in the future. She should be provided with information on community resources and referred for continued assistance and support. In particularly distressed women, an assessment for suicide risk may be indicated. Obviously, in acute crisis situations that involve serious risks to the life of the victim, her children, or others, crisis intervention resources should be utilized. These instances are rare in the office setting but occur more commonly in emergency settings.

Another important step in addressing ongoing violence is to help the victim establish a safety plan; ACOG distributes pocket cards with suggested steps that can be very helpful (see the box for suggested steps for making an exit plan). These cards or other resource materials can be handed directly to the patient or left in patient restrooms where a woman can pick it up without concern of being seen by an accompanying partner. Reinforce the availability of help from the physician's office and from other resources when she is ready to leave or is in imminent danger. Physicians should recognize, however, that many women may attempt to leave a violent relationship several times before leaving it permanently.

The Physician's Responsibility in Addressing Domestic Violence

- Implement universal screening
- Acknowledge the trauma
- Assess immediate safety
- Help establish a safety plan
- Review options
- Offer educational materials
- Offer list of community and local resources
- Provide referrals
- Document interactions
- Provide ongoing support at subsequent visits

Making an Exit Plan

Making a decision to leave an abusive relationship can be very difficult. It may take time for you to feel ready. Call a woman's shelter; someone there can help with a safety plan–you don't have to give anyone your name.

If you are ready to leave:

- Pack a bag in advance and leave it at a neighbor's house. Include cash or credit cards and extra clothes for you and your children. Take a favorite toy or plaything.
- Hide an extra set of car and house keys outside of your house in case you have to leave quickly.
- Take important papers such as:
  - –Birth certificates for you and your children
  - –Health insurance cards and medicine
  - –Deed or lease to your house or apartment
  - –Checkbook and extra checks
  - –Social security number or green card/work permit
  - –Court papers or orders
  - –Driver's license or photo identification
  - –Pay stubs

Talking to your doctor about abuse isn't easy, but it can help. When you're ready, your doctor will listen.

Referrals

Psychologic and social assistance is best provided by services that are "trauma specific," meaning the providers are experienced in treating victims of intimate partner abuse. Most agencies for battered women and rape crisis centers have expertise in dealing with all forms of violence against women. A list of resources should be readily available in medical offices and hospital emergency departments. The list should include telephone numbers for police departments, emergency departments, shelters for battered women, counseling services, and advocacy agencies that can provide legal, financial, and emotional support. ACOG's web site (www.acog.org) lists state and local resources. Additional information often can be found in the telephone book.

Documentation

Accurate documentation following domestic violence screening is no different than any other recording of interaction with patients and has no different medical–legal implications. However, it can be an important part of being able to assist victims in putting an end to the violence. Although most abused women endure multiple episodes of violence before ever attempting to leave the situation or seek legal action, medical record documentation can help validate the recurrent nature of the problem and provide important supportive evidence in the courtroom. Such documentation, however, has resulted in discrimination against abused women for health, life, and disability insurance. The possibility of discrimination should not deter physicians from documenting abuse in the medical record. As recently as 1995, more than half of health insurers were using domestic violence documentation to make insurance coverage decisions (23). Since that time, model state legislation has been developed and promoted to end this problem. Currently, over half of the states have passed legislation or rulings that prohibit insurance discrimination against victims of domestic violence (23).

When documenting positive responses to screening questions, it is advantageous to use direct quotations of the patient's explanation of her injuries. Photographs may be taken after consent is granted and added to the patient's chart (2). Because perpetrators often retaliate when they suspect disclosure of abuse, every effort should be made to maintain confidentiality, especially regarding telephone calls or when materials, such as bills, are sent to the patient. Office staff must be informed about the importance of confidentiality when there is any contact with the patient's home.

Special Populations

Children of Abuse Victims

The presence of violence between intimate partners also affects the children in the household. Studies demonstrate that child abuse occurs in 33–77% of families in which there is abuse of adults (5). Among women who are being abused, 28% have demonstrated abusive behavior toward their children while living in the violent environment (24). Even if not directly victimized by violence, children growing up in violent homes demonstrate increased risk-taking behaviors and are at increased risk for becoming future victims or perpetrators of interpersonal violence (25). Children from abusive homes demonstrate higher levels of conduct problems, emotional problems, and lower levels of social functioning (26). Adolescent exposure to domestic violence is associated with anger, depression, anxiety, and posttraumatic stress (24). Children in violent homes should be evaluated by a professional who can assess the child's behavioral patterns and help the child address the emotional impact of the violence. Referrals to such resources are essential, because the victim may not be willing or able to do so on her own, especially if she fears removal of the child more than the violence.

Adolescents

Adolescents are at risk for physical and sexual abuse from two distinct groups: parents and dating partners. Many adolescents lack skills that help them recognize and avoid violent dating situations, and some even believe that violence in a dating relationship is justifiable in certain situations (27). Adolescence is a time when young women are establishing patterns of behaviors in relationships. It is an important opportunity to identify and address dating violence and family violence, or to provide anticipatory guidance that will assist the adolescent in recognizing and avoiding violence in the future. Prevention efforts and education are important for both female and male adolescent populations.

Abuse During Pregnancy

Abuse during pregnancy affects both maternal and fetal well being. The prevalence of violence during pregnancy ranges from 1% to 20% with most studies identifying rates between 4% and 8% (21). Higher rates are identified when screening occurs more than once during the pregnancy (28, 29). The perpetrator usually is a current or former intimate partner, and among younger pregnant women in particular, may also be a parent or other family member. Pregnancy complications such as poor maternal weight gain, infection, anemia, and second- and third-trimester bleeding occur more commonly among pregnant women who are battered. Some evidence suggests that the pattern of violence may escalate during pregnancy (30, 31, 32), and it may become even more prevalent in the postpartum period than during pregnancy (31). Violence may occur more frequently in pregnancy than other conditions for which routine screening is done, such as gestational diabetes and preeclampsia (27). Regular contact with medical providers increases the likelihood of disclosure, therefore, the pregnancy offers a unique opportunity to screen and identify partner and family violence. Screening all patients at various times during the pregnancy is important because some women do not disclose abuse the first time they are asked. Screening should occur at the first prenatal visit, at least once per trimester, and at the postpartum checkup.

Elder Abuse

Elder abuse refers to acts of omission or commission that result in harm or threatened harm to the health or welfare of an older adult (persons older than 60 years). Federal definitions of elder abuse, neglect, and exploitation appeared for the first time in the 1987 Amendments to the Older Americans Act (PL 100-175). These definitions were provided in the law only as guidelines for identifying the problem. For enforcement purposes, most states have laws that address elder abuse, although state definitions vary considerably from one jurisdiction to another. Additionally, researchers have used many different definitions to study the problem. In general, there are three basic categories of elder abuse: (1) domestic elder abuse, (2) institutional elder abuse, and (3) self-neglect or self-abuse.

The exact incidence of elder abuse is unknown (33). Approximately 1 out of 14 elder mistreatment cases is reported to a public agency (33). A recent incidence survey revealed that approximately 450,000 elderly persons in domestic settings were abused or neglected (34). Exploitation, psychologic abuse, and neglect are common components of elder abuse. In almost 90% of elder abuse and neglect incidents with a known perpetrator, the perpetrator is a family member, and two thirds of the perpetrators are adult children or spouses (34).

Theoretic risk factors for elder abuse and neglect include the following: 1) transgenerational learned behaviors; 2) psychopathology of the care taker (alcoholism, drug addiction, and financial dependency); 3) medical, functional, or cognitive disability of the elderly that contributes to dependence and vulnerability; and 4) stress (economic, lack of support, or physical dependency of the elder person) (33).

Few physicians are fully aware of the variations of domestic violence that include abuse in the elderly. Fear, intimidation, and lack of opportunity may retard the disclosure of the problem to medical personnel or authorities. The Diagnostic and Treatment Guidelines on Elder Abuse and Neglect of the American Medical Association emphasize that health professionals may ignore signs and symptoms of elder mistreatment because they are unaware of the extent of the problem and are uncomfortable with the responsibility of further assessment and action (33, 35–37). Resolution of this problem through education could stimulate early recognition and definitive interventions.

Physicians or other health care workers who provide acute or chronic medical care to the older adult may see the older adult on a regular basis and have unique opportunities for screening and assessment. Additionally, an opportunity for screening and recognition exists during all health-related encounters of older individuals, such as routine gynecologic examinations. Incorporating screening related to elder abuse and neglect into these encounters will increase identification of abuse. Physicians should assess patients for elder abuse and respond as they would to domestic violence in general.

Other At-Risk Populations

Other at-risk individuals include adults aged 18–65 years with physical or mental disabilities. As with elder abuse, abuse of vulnerable adults may include physical, psychologic, or financial abuse, neglect, or exploitation. The abuse may result from intentional or unintentional harm to the victim. Unintentional mistreatment includes mistreatment due to ignorance, inexperience, or lack of ability to provide appropriate care.

Legal Issues

A basic understanding of legal measures and legal considerations can enhance a physician's ability to counsel and assist women in violent relationships. Because laws vary widely between states, familiarity with local laws and policies is critical. In all states, physicians are required by law to report suspected child abuse, and most states require reports of suspected abuse (36, 38). Mandatory reporting of domestic violence is required by some states, but this remains a controversial issue especially with regard to issues of patient safety and confidentiality (39). Information regarding state reporting requirements are available through state medical associations, local domestic violence programs, or the state attorney general's office. Table 1 summarizes basic components of legal remedies that generally are available to battered women in the United States (39).

Summary

Many physicians, especially in the current managed care environment, are concerned that abuse screening and disclosure will require inordinate amounts of time, but with an established protocol and referral system this important problem can be managed. Screening all patients is the key to identifying abuse. With disclosure of ongoing domestic violence, the physician's responsibility should include acknowledgment of abuse, making a safety assessment, assisting with a safety plan, providing appropriate referrals, documentation, and continued support. For disclosure of past violence, the responsibilities are similar but generally do not require immediate intervention. Women with a history of past victimization need to have that history identified and acknowledged and may need referral to other professionals to assist with the resolution of their trauma-related issues. Regardless of the types of victimization a woman has experienced, providing a safe setting in which she can discuss the problem and receive support is an important part of her recovery. Through these measures, the health care team can help abused women take the first steps toward ending the violence and achieving a healthy recovery.

Table 1. Summary of Legal Measure

Legal Measure	Description	Important Considerations
Criminal justice intervention	Reporting a crime such as battery, rape, threats, harassment, kidnapping, property destruction, forcible entry of a residence, assault with a weapon	Follow-up that occurs depends on local laws. Prosecution policies and judicial practices may vary widely from region to region. Victim needs a good understanding of her legal rights and responsibilities.
Civil protection orders (ie, restraining order, eviction order, monetary compensation order, orders to forbid contact)	A petition filed with the court to obtain immediate but temporary protection. These can be obtained without notice to the abuser until after the order is granted. A more permanent order can be obtained through another hearing at a later date.	The protected person must keep a copy of the order with her at all times. The Violence Against Women Act provides that restraining orders issued by courts of one state are upheld across all state lines. Survivors who have children should be advised to seek legal consultation regarding custody and visitation orders.
Divorce and support actions	Specific measures accomplished through the court system to award child and spousal support or an order to distribute the marital property.	May be useful for women who are struggling to gain independence for themselves and their children apart from the batterer
Immigration remedies	Specific legal measures that enable immigrant battered women to apply for permanent legal status without requiring assistance from an abusive partner	Domestic violence and immigration assistance programs can be very helpful, particularly for women who are at extreme disadvantage because of language barriers, legal status, and inability to gain access to social, legal, and health services.
Civil action	Victims may sue abusers under civil law tort actions such as infliction of emotional distress, false imprisonment, trespass, invasion of privacy	Legal counsel recommended to thoroughly explore options and their implications

References

1. Bachman R, Saltzman LE. Violence against women: estimates from the redesigned survey. Bureau of Justice Statistics Special Report. Washington, DC: U.S. Department of Justice, 1995; NCJ-154348
2. American Medical Association. Diagnostic and treatment guidelines on domestic violence. Chicago, Illinois: AMA, 1992
3. American College of Obstetricians and Gynecologists. Domestic violence. ACOG Technical Bulletin 209. Washington, DC: ACOG, 1995
4. Adolescent assault victim needs: a review of issues and a model protocol. American Academy of Pediatrics Task Force on Adolescent Assault Victims Needs. Pediatrics 1996;98:991–1001
5. The role of the pediatrician in recognizing and intervening on behalf of abused women. American Academy of Pediatrics Committee on Child Abuse and Neglect. Pediatrics 1998;101:1091–1092
6. Family violence: an AAFP white paper. The AAFP Commission on Special Issues and Clinical Interests. Am Fam Physician 1994;50:1636–1640, 1644–1646
7. Joint Commission on Accreditation of Health Care Organizations. 1999 hospital accreditation standards. Oakbrook Terrace, Illinois: JCAHO, 1999
8. Wilt S, Olsen S. Prevalence of domestic violence in the United States. J Am Med Womens Assoc 1996; 51:77–82
9. Straus MA. Measuring intrafamily conflict and violence: the conflict tactics (CT) scales. J Marriage Fam 1979; 41:75–88
10. Addressing domestic violence and its consequences. Policy Report of the Commonwealth Fund Commission on Women's Health. New York; The Commonwealth Fund, February 1998
11. Greenfield LA, Rand MR, Craven D, Klaus PA, Perkins CA, Ringel C, et al. Violence by intimates: analysis of data on crimes by current or former spouses, boyfriends, and girlfriends. Bureau of Justice Statistics Factbook. Washington, DC: U.S. Department of Justice, 1998; NCJ-167237
12. Abbott J, Johnson R, Koziol-McLain J, Lowenstein SR. Domestic violence against women. Incidence and prevalence in an emergency department population. JAMA 1995;273:1763–1767
13. Koss MP, Heslet L. Somatic consequences of violence against women. Arch Fam Med 1992;1:53–59
14. Miller TR, Cohen MA, Wiersema B. Victim costs and consequences: A new look. Washington, DC: National Institute of Justice, U.S. Department of Justice, 1996 January; NCJ-155282
15. Chambliss LR, Bay RC, Jones RF 3rd. Domestic violence: an educational imperative? Am J Obstet Gynecol 1995;172:1035–1038
16. Friedman LS, Samet JG, Roberts MS, Hudlin M, Hans P. Inquiry about victimization experiences. A survey of patient preferences and physician practices. Arch Intern Med 1992;152:1186–1190
17. Sugg NK, Inui T. Primary care physicians' response to domestic violence. Opening Pandora's box. JAMA 1992; 267:3157–3160
18. McFarlane J, Wiist WH. Documentation of abuse to pregnant women: a medical chart audit in public health clinics. J Womens Health 1996;5:137–142
19. Goldberg WG, Tomlanovich MC. Domestic violence victims in the emergency department; new findings. JAMA 1984;251:3259–3264
20. McLeer SV, Anwar R. A study of battered women presenting in an emergency department. Am J Public Health 1989;79:65–66
21. Gazmararian JA, Lazorick S, Spitz AM, Ballard TJ, Saltzman LE, Marks JS. Prevalence of violence against pregnant women. JAMA 1996;275:1915–1920
22. McFarlane J, Christoffel K, Bateman L, Miller V, Bullock L. Assessing for abuse: self-report versus nurse interview. Public Health Nurs 1991;8:245
23. Fromson T, Durborow N. Insurance discrimination against victims of domestic violence. Philadelphia: Pennsylvania Coalition Against Domestic Violence and the Women's Law Project, 1998
24. Walker LE. The battered woman syndrome. New York: Springer, 1984
25. Singer MI, Anglin TM, Song LY, Lunghofer L. Adolescents' exposure to violence and associated symptoms of psychological trauma. JAMA 1995;273:477–482
26. Fantuzzo JW, DePaola LM, Lambert L, Martino T, Anderson G, Sutton S. Effects of interparental violence on the psychological adjustment and competencies of young children. J Consult Clin Psychol 1991;59: 258–265
27. Parrot A. Acquaintance rape among adolescents: identifying risk groups and intervention strategies. J Soc Work Hum Sex 1989;8:47–61
28. McFarlane J, Parker B, Soeken K, Bullock L. Assessing for abuse during pregnancy. Severity and frequency of injuries and associated entry into prenatal care. JAMA 1992;267:3176–3178
29. Parker B, McFarlane J, Soeken K. Abuse during pregnancy: effects on maternal complications and birth weight in adult and teenage women. Obstet Gynecol 1994;84: 323–328
30. Berenson AB, San Miguel VV, Wilkinson GS. Prevalence of physical and sexual assault in pregnant adolescents. J Adolesc Health 1992;13:466–469
31. Helton AS, McFarlane J, Anderson ET. Battered and pregnant: a prevalence study. Am J Public Health 1987;77: 1337–1339
32. Stewart DE, Cecutti A. Physical abuse in pregnancy. CMAJ 1993;149:1257–1263
33. American Medical Association. Diagnostic and treatment guidelines on elder abuse and neglect. Chicago, Illinois: AMA, 1992
34. National Center on Elder Abuse. The national elder abuse incidence study. Final report. Administration for Children

and Families and the Administration on Aging, September 1998

35. Elder abuse, neglect and family violence: a guide for health care professionals. Wisconsin Coalition Against Domestic Violence. State of Wisconsin Department of Health & Family Services, 1997; PSL-3077

36. Ehrlich P, Anetzberger G. Survey of state public health departments on procedures for reporting elder abuse. Public Health Rep 1991;106:151–154

37. Pillemer K, Suittor JJ. Violence and violent feelings: what causes them among family caregivers? J Gerontol 1992; 47:S165–S172

38. American College of Obstetricians and Gynecologists. Mandatory reporting of domestic violence. Committee Opinion 200. Washington, DC: ACOG, 1998

39. Hyman A. Domestic violence: legal considerations for health care practitioners and institutions. J Am Med Womens Assoc 1996;51:101–105

ISSN 1074-8628

The American College of Obstetricians and Gynecologists
409 12th Street, SW
PO Box 96920
Washington, DC 20090-6920

12345/32109

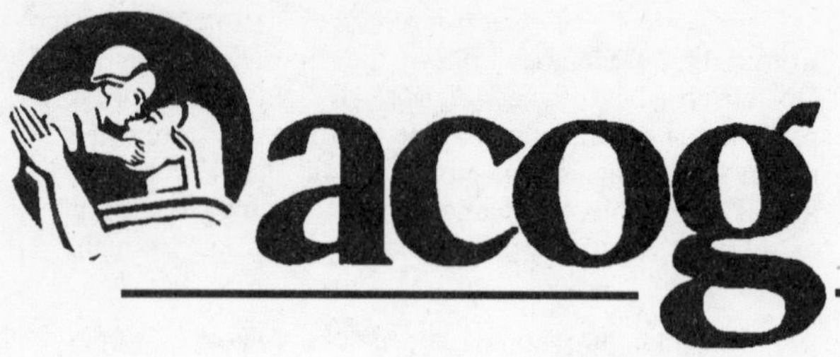

Number 218—December 1995
(Replaces #137, December 1989,
and #157, July 1991)

Technical Bulletin

An Educational Aid to Obstetrician–Gynecologists

Dystocia and the Augmentation of Labor

The dramatic increase in the number of cesarean births among U.S. women in the past 25 years is due mainly to the number of repeat cesarean deliveries and cesarean deliveries performed for dystocia. Dystocia is the most common indication for primary cesarean delivery, accounting for more than three times as many primary cesarean births as either "nonreassuring fetal status" or malpresentations (1). Reducing the rate of cesarean deliveries for dystocia would therefore decrease the overall rate of cesarean birth quite substantially.

Central to the management of dystocia is augmentation of labor, that is, correcting ineffective uterine contractions. Despite vast experience with labor augmentation, considerable variability in practice exists regarding criteria for initiating oxytocin and for the oxytocin dosage regimen prescribed. The purpose of this Technical Bulletin is to describe an approach to the diagnosis and management of dystocia, including a range of acceptable methods of augmentation of labor.

Normal Labor

Labor commences when uterine contractions of sufficient frequency, intensity, and duration result in effacement and dilation of the cervix. The first stage of labor has been divided into a latent and an active phase (Fig. 1). During the latent phase, uterine contractions typically are infrequent and irregular and often result in only modest discomfort; however, they do result in gradual effacement and dilation of the cervix. Although the onset of the latent phase of labor is often difficult to define precisely, a prolonged latent phase is considered as one exceeding 20 hours in the nullipara and 14 hours in the multipara (2).

The active phase of labor is characterized both by an increased rate of cervical dilation and, ultimately, by descent of the presenting fetal part. The beginning of the active phase of labor is signaled by an abrupt change in the slope of the curve that results when cervical dilatation is plotted against time; this generally occurs when the cervix reaches 3–4 cm of dilatation. The active phase of labor has been further subdivided into an acceleration phase, a phase of maximum slope, and a deceleration phase.

The second stage of labor is usually brief, averaging 20 minutes for parous women and 50 minutes for nulliparous women. Older studies demonstrated increased perinatal and maternal morbidity associated with a second stage of labor in excess of 2 hours. Consequently, 2 hours became the accepted point at which a prolonged second stage of labor was diagnosed in nulliparous patients, with 3 hours considered abnormal if epidural anesthesia was used. For multiparous patients, the definition of a prolonged second stage of labor was 1 or 2 hours depending on the use of epidural anesthesia. Other data, however, have shown the duration of the second stage of labor to be unrelated to perinatal outcome in the absence of a nonreassuring fetal heart rate pattern or traumatic delivery as long as progress occurs, however slowly (3).

Abnormal Labor

Dystocia is defined as difficult labor or childbirth. It can result from abnormalities primarily involving the cervix and uterus, the fetus, the maternal pelvis, or combinations of these factors.

The term cephalopelvic disproportion has been used to describe a disparity between the size of the maternal pelvis and the fetal head that precludes vaginal delivery. This condition can rarely be diagnosed with certainty; in fact, it is often given as an indication for operative delivery when the true abnormality is malposition of the fetal head (ie, asynclitism or extension of the fetal head that presents bony diameters too great to allow passage through the maternal pelvis). Similarly, the term failure to progress is imprecise and has been used to include lack of progressive cervical dilation or lack of descent of the fetal

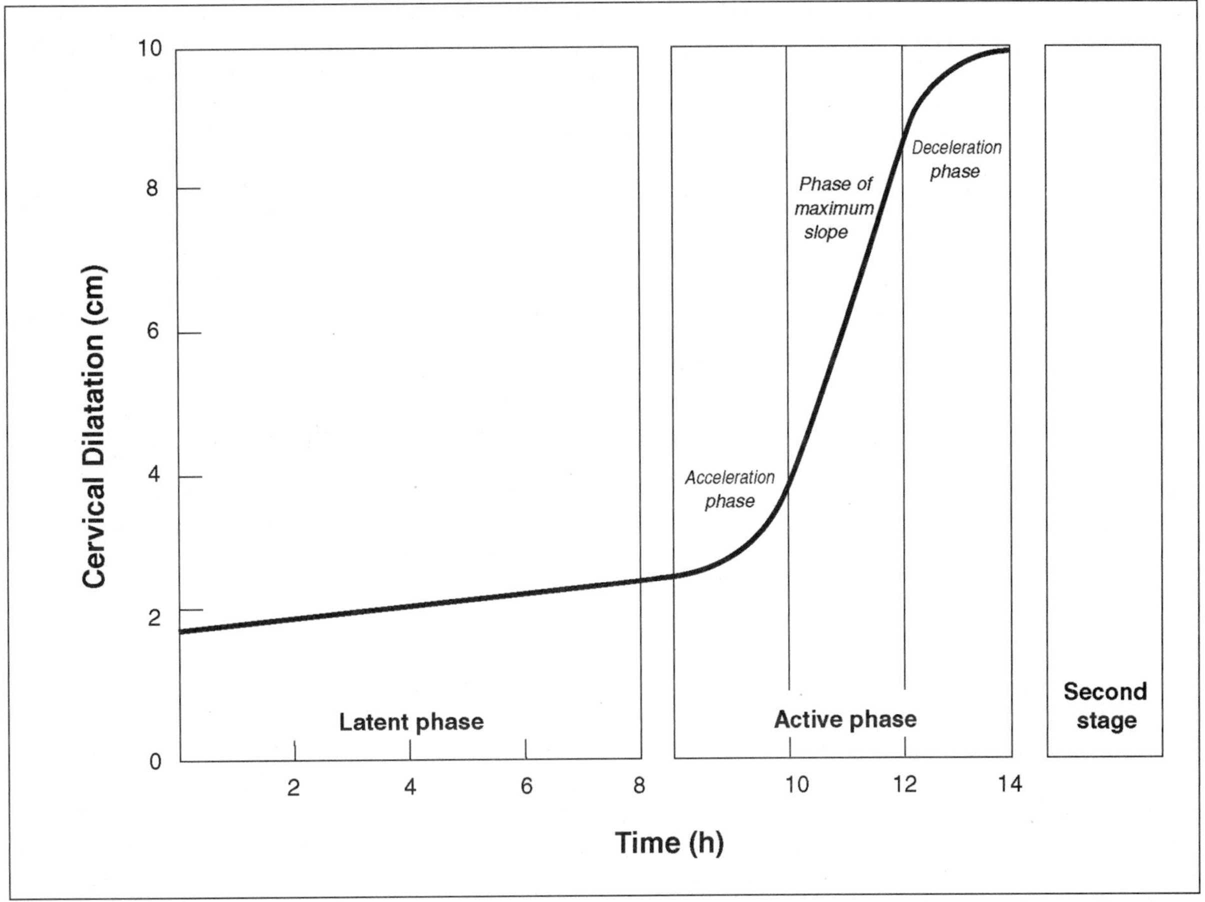

FIG. 1. Composite graph of cervical dilatation for nulliparous women. The first stage is divided into a Flat latent phase and a rapidly progressive active phase. (Modified from Friedman EA. Labor: clinical evaluation and management. 2nd ed. New York: Appleton–Century–Crofts, 1978)

head or both. Often, the diagnosis of failure to progress is made before the active phase of labor and before an adequate trial of labor has been achieved.

A more practical classification is to categorize labor abnormalities as either slower-than-normal (protraction disorders) or complete cessation of progress (arrest disorder) (2). These disorders require the parturient to have entered the active phase of labor. A prolonged latent phase of labor is not indicative of dystocia as this diagnosis cannot be made in the latent phase of labor. Criteria for diagnosis are listed in Table 1.

Abnormalities of the first stage of labor complicate 8–11% of all cephalic deliveries (4). Second-stage abnormalities may be at least as common. Identification of an abnormal labor and institution of the proper management for dystocia require assessment of the *powers* (uterine contractility and expulsive effort), the *passenger* (the fetus), and the *passage* (the pelvis).

TABLE 1. ABNORMAL LABOR PATTERNS AND DIAGNOSTIC CRITERIA

Labor Pattern	Nulligravida	Multipara
Protraction disorders		
Dilation	<1.2 cm/h	<1.5 cm/h
Descent	<1.0 cm/h	<2.0 cm/h
Arrest disorders		
Dilation	>2 h	>2 h
Descent	>1 h	>1 h

Powers

Assessment of powers during the active phase of the first stage of labor involves the investigation of uterine contractility. The minimal contractile pattern of 95% of women in spontaneous labor consists of three to five contractions in a 10-minute window (5). Uterine activity may be quantified by palpation, external tocodynamometry, or internal uterine pressure sensors.

Several methods of quantifying uterine activity with internal monitors have been described (6–10). In a retrospective report of induction of labor with oxytocin, 91% of women achieved at least 200–224 Montevideo units (the strength of contractions in millimeters of mercury multiplied by the frequency per 10 minutes), and 40% achieved at least 300 Montevideo units (11). Accordingly, it has been suggested that before the arrest disorder can be diagnosed in the first stage of labor the following criteria should be met: 1) the latent phase is completed (ie, cervical dilatation is a minimum of 4 cm), and 2) a uterine contraction pattern exceeds 200 Montevideo units for 2 hours without cervical change. However, there is no convincing evidence to demonstrate a reduction in the rate of cesarean deliveries or improvement in perinatal outcome attributable to the use of the sophisticated measurements of uterine activity as compared with external tocodynamometry.

In assessing the optimal uterine contraction pattern, the effects of anesthesia should be considered. One randomized study suggested that epidural bupivacaine analgesia administered before 5 cm of dilatation prolonged the first stage of labor and increased the incidence of cesarean delivery in nulliparous women (12). An increased incidence of malpresentations and operative vaginal delivery has also been reported with the use of epidural anesthesia (13). Two randomized trials compared early versus late administration of epidural anesthesia. The early administration group consisted of nulliparous women who were in spontaneous labor or who were receiving intravenous oxytocin for induction or augmentation of early labor. The late administration group consisted of similar women who received intravenous nalbuphine followed by late administration of epidural analgesia (14, 15). These studies demonstrated that early administration of epidural analgesia (ie, before 3 and 5 cm of cervical dilatation) did not prolong labor or increase the incidence of cesarean delivery.

Passenger

Assessment of the passenger—the fetus—in cephalic presentation consists of estimating fetal weight, position, and attitude and judging their respective roles in dystocia. Estimations of fetal size, even those obtained by ultrasonography, are frequently inaccurate, especially in fetuses weighing more than 4–4.5 kg. Consequently, with cephalic presentation in the first stage of labor, excluding obvious pelvic deformity, the diagnosis of dystocia first requires progression into the active phase of labor and adequate uterine contractile forces.

Although in some cases the relationship between the size of the fetus and the adequacy of the pelvis may appear appropriate on physical examination, poor progress of labor may occur as a result of the influence of excessive degrees of asynclitism or extension of the fetal head, thereby presenting an unusually large diameter to the pelvis. When the presenting part is at +2 station or below in the second stage of labor, abnormalities of fetal head position or asynclitism can be approached either manually or by forceps application and rotation, depending on the experience and skills of the physician. With traction, the vacuum extractor may also result in spontaneous rotation. When a positional dystocia cannot be corrected manually or with instruments or when personnel with such skills are not available, cesarean delivery is appropriate. Such instrument-assisted vaginal deliveries after a prolonged second stage should be preceded by careful assessment, especially in a fetus with suspected macrosomia, because of the increased risk of shoulder dystocia (16, 17).

Fetal anomalies such as hydrocephaly, encephalocele, and soft tissue tumors may obstruct labor. Fetal imaging should be considered when malpresentation or anomalies are suspected based on vaginal or abdominal examination or when the presenting fetal part is persistently high. Further management is dictated by the location and size of the specific anomaly as well as the ultimate prognosis for the fetus.

Passage

Inefficient uterine action should be corrected before attributing dystocia to a pelvic problem. With rare exceptions, the bony pelvis is not the factor that limits vaginal delivery of a fetus in cephalic presentation. Although grossly misshapen pelves may infrequently result from severe malnutrition or trauma, radiographic pelvimetry is of limited value in managing most cephalic presentations. Moreover, X-rays provide no information regarding soft tissue resistance. On the other hand, clinical pelvimetry can be useful to qualitatively identify the general architectural features of the pelvis and assist in the performance of operative vaginal delivery. For example, the deeply engaged head with occiput posterior and a narrow maternal pubic arch may best be delivered without rotation.

Extrinsic Factors

A number of extrinsic factors may influence the likelihood of cesarean birth. Social support and childbirth preparation classes may lead to a reduction in fear, pain, and anxiety (18). Consequently, whether through an effect on uterine activity or other means, operative delivery appears to be decreased. Although some studies suggest that epidural anesthesia may predispose to desultory labor and fetal malpresentations, others have refuted this. Prospective randomized trials of electronic fetal monitoring versus intermittent auscultation have not identified a decline in operative deliveries with electronic monitoring. To the contrary, electronic monitoring has been associated with a comparable or even a higher incidence of abdominal deliveries without improvement in neonatal outcome (19–22). Explanations for the increase in cesarean births include the restrictive postures and activity for parturients and the overinterpretation of fetal heart rate patterns. Many practitioners feel that changes in maternal position may be helpful in aiding descent and rotations in fetuses with occiput transverse or occiput posterior positions (23–25).

Labor Augmentation

Uterine hypocontractility should be augmented only after both the maternal pelvis and fetal presentation have been assessed. Contraindications to augmentation are similar to those for labor induction and may include placenta or vasa previa, umbilical cord presentation, prior classical uterine incision, active genital herpes infection, pelvic structural deformities, or invasive cervical cancer.

Amniotomy has been used for years to augment labor; however, whether amniotomy confers more benefit than harm has been a matter of debate (26). In the latent phase of labor or once the diagnosis of dystocia secondary to uterine hypocontractility is made in the active phase of labor, it may be reasonable to perform amniotomy, initiate oxytocin therapy, or both. A theoretical advantage of amniotomy includes correction of hypocontractility without the need for oxytocin; on the other hand, administration of oxytocin with intact membranes may be protective against infectious morbidity (27). A randomized trial of elective amniotomy on admission to the labor and delivery suite for patients with cervical dilatation of 4–6 cm found that this procedure shortened the active phase of labor and decreased the need for oxytocin augmentation. A greater number of mild and moderate variable decelerations were observed in patients who had amniotomy as compared with control patients, but the incidence of severe abnormal fetal heart rate patterns or operative intervention was not increased (28). In another randomized trial of elective amniotomy in nulliparous patients, rupture of membranes was associated with a shortened duration of labor, but the rate of cesarean delivery was not reduced (29).

Oxytocin

Oxytocin is an octapeptide whose pharmacokinetics are still incompletely understood. The mean in vitro half-life of oxytocin has been reported to be 3–5 minutes (30), and this is consistent with the observation that oxytocin-induced hyperstimulation usually resolves quickly with discontinuation of the oxytocin infusion. Investigators have pointed out that the half-life may vary with the infusion rate (31) and have found that the interval to reach a steady-state concentration of oxytocin in plasma is between 20 and 40 minutes (32).

Clinically, the response to oxytocin depends on preexisting uterine activity, uterine sensitivity, gestational age, and cervical status. One study identified cervical dilatation, parity, and gestational age as clinical variables related to the maximum dose of oxytocin required for labor augmentation (33). However, despite analysis of nearly 2,000 cases of augmented labors, individual variability precluded the ability to predict confidently the dosage of oxytocin needed to successfully augment a given patient's labor.

The goal of oxytocin administration is to effect uterine activity that is sufficient to produce cervical change and fetal descent while avoiding uterine hyperstimulation and fetal compromise. Minimally effective uterine activity has been defined as three contractions per 10 minutes averaging greater than 25 mm Hg above baseline. However, adequate labor describes a wide range of uterine activity, as previously noted. The amplitude of each contraction may vary from 25 to 75 mm Hg, and contractions may occur for a total of 2–4.5 minutes in every 10-minute window achieving from 95 to 395 Montevideo units. Typically, a goal of a maximum of five contractions in a 10-minute period with resultant cervical dilatation is considered adequate. As a general guideline, hyperstimulation may be defined as a persistent pattern of more than five contractions in 10 minutes, contractions lasting 2 minutes or more, or contractions of normal duration occurring within 1 minute of each other.

Oxytocin should be administered when a patient is progressing slowly through the latent phase of labor or has a protraction or arrest disorder of labor, when a hypotonic uterine contraction pattern is identified, and when there are no maternal or fetal contraindications. A physician or qualified nurse should perform an examination in reasonable proximity to the initiation of oxytocin infusion. Oxytocin is usually diluted (10 units USP) in 1,000 ml of a balanced salt solution administered via a controlled infusion device. To avoid bolus administration, the infusion should be inserted as a secondary line into the main intravenous line close to the venous puncture site. Personnel who are familiar with the effects of oxytocin and who are able to identify both maternal and fetal complications should be in attendance during the administration of oxytocin. The resting uterine tone and frequency and duration of uterine contractions should be monitored appropriately, either by electronic monitoring or palpation. Fetal well-being should be assessed electronically or by auscultation and recorded every 15 minutes during the first stage of labor and every 5 minutes during the second stage of labor. A physician who has privileges to perform cesarean delivery should be readily available.

Adverse effects of oxytocin are primarily dose related. The most common adverse effect is fetal heart rate deceleration associated with uterine hyperstimulation. Decreasing the oxytocin dose rather than stopping it may correct the abnormal pattern yet prevent an unwarranted delay in delivery. Additional measures may include changing the patient's position and administering oxygen or more intravenous fluid. If it is necessary to discontinue oxytocin, it may be restarted once fetal heart rate and uterine activity return to acceptable levels. When restarting the oxytocin, it may be necessary to lower the dose and lengthen the interval between increases. If oxytocin-induced uterine hyperstimulation does not respond to conservative measures, intravenous terbutaline (0.125–0.25 mg) or magnesium sulfate (2–6 g in 10–20% dilution) may be used for uterine relaxation (34, 35).

Numerous protocols for oxytocin augmentation of labor varying with respect to the initial dose, incremental dose increases, and intervals between dose increases have been studied, and a few are listed in Table 2. Low-dose oxytocin regimens were developed based on the knowledge that it takes oxytocin up to 40 minutes to reach steady-state concentration in maternal serum. Low-dose regimens have been reported to be associated with a lower incidence of uterine hyperstimulation. In Ireland and the United States, high-dose protocols have been applied. In the United States, these protocols were in response to rising cesarean delivery rates and have been credited with shortening time in labor and reducing the number of cesarean deliveries for dystocia. Thus, there are advantages and disadvantages of using high- and low-dose oxytocin regimens. Any of the oxytocin regimens outlined in Table 2, as well as many others, are appropriate for labor stimulation provided proper precautions are met (5, 11, 32, 36, 37).

Active Management

A system of labor management for nulliparous women, termed active management of labor, has been developed and practiced in Ireland. The active management of labor has been associated with a cesarean delivery rate of 4.8% (36). This approach is beginning to gain acceptance in the United States. Although many American obstetricians have focused on the use of a high-dose oxytocin regimen as a means to reduce the high cesarean delivery rate, it is important to emphasize that high-dose oxytocin is just one part of the active management of labor. In fact, many women who undergo active management of labor do not even receive oxytocin.

Active management of labor is confined to nulliparous women with singleton, cephalic presentations at term who show no evidence of fetal compromise. Active management of labor, as developed and practiced in Ireland, involves several distinct entities:

- Patient education
- Strict criteria for the diagnosis of labor
- Strict criteria for the determination of abnormal progress in labor
- High-dose oxytocin infusion
- The presence of a personal nurse in labor
- Strict criteria for interpretation of fetal compromise
- Peer review of operative deliveries

Women are instructed during pregnancy as to the signs and symptoms of labor, and they are encouraged to go to the hospital early in labor. Confirmation of labor depends on the presence of regular, painful uterine contractions and one of the following: passage of a mucus plug, complete effacement, or spontaneous rupture of membranes. Patients not meeting the criteria of labor are not admitted to the labor suite. For patients in labor with intact membranes, artificial rupture of membranes is performed within the first hour of admission. A vaginal examination is performed hourly, and oxytocin infusion is begun if there has not been at least 1 cm of dilation since the last examination. Thus, the active management of labor does not differentiate latent phase and active phase of labor, and the diagnosis and treatment of a protraction disorder requires only 1 hour without progress in labor.

According to the active management protocol, oxytocin infusion is begun with 6 mU/min and increased by 6 mU/min every 15 minutes to a maximum of about 40 mU/min to achieve a labor pattern of no more than seven uterine contractions per 15 minutes (36). As practiced in Ireland, a nurse attends each woman in labor, and the

TABLE 2. LABOR STIMULATION WITH OXYTOCIN: EXAMPLES OF LOW-DOSE AND HIGH-DOSE REGIMENS

Regimen	Starting Dose (mU/min)	Incremental Increase	Dosage Interval (mU/min)	Maximum Dose (min) (mU/min)
Low-Dose	0.5–1	1	30–40	20
	1–2	2	15	40
High-Dose	≈ 6	≈ 6	15	≈ 40
	6	6*, 3, 1	20–40	42

* The incremental increase is reduced to 3 mU/min in presence of hyperstimulation and reduced to 1 mU/min with recurrent hyperstimulation.

Data from references 5, 11, 32, 36, and 37.

fetus is monitored by intermittent auscultation. Electronic monitors are restricted to cases in which fetal blood sampling is deemed necessary, such as when meconium is present or an abnormal heart rate is auscultated. Fetal compromise is mainly diagnosed by fetal scalp pH sampling, not the interpretation of continuous electronic fetal heart rate tracings. Cesarean delivery is performed if delivery has not occurred or is not imminent 12 hours after admission or, rarely, for fetal compromise.

The Irish experience with active management of labor includes a low cesarean delivery rate without untoward events. In the United States, a randomized trial of the active management of labor (that did not include one-on-one nursing care or peer review of operative deliveries but did include electronic fetal monitoring) as compared with a traditional approach to labor management was associated with decreases in cesarean births, length of labor, and infectious morbidity (38). It is important to emphasize that this disciplined approach to labor management involves several distinct facets in addition to the higher doses of oxytocin. It is uncertain which of these is responsible for the low cesarean delivery rate. In a subsequent American investigation, active management of labor did not reduce the rate of cesarean delivery in nulliparous women but was associated with shorter labors and less maternal fever (39). Interestingly, the cesarean delivery rate with the active management of labor in Ireland has doubled, and this change has been attributed to more widespread use of epidural analgesia (40).

Summary

The diagnosis of dystocia is currently a leading indication for cesarean delivery in the United States. Efforts to identify abnormal labor and correct abnormal contraction patterns, fetal malposition, and inadequate expulsive efforts may help eliminate many cesarean deliveries without compromising the outcome for either mother or fetus. Cesarean deliveries for dystocia should not be performed in the latent phase of labor or in the active phase of labor unless adequate uterine activity has been achieved. Cesarean deliveries in the second stage of labor may be reduced if, after reevaluation of the fetus and pelvis, there is potential for correction of uterine forces with oxytocin, correction of malposition, operative vaginal delivery, or safe continued observation. Use of either a low-dose or high-dose oxytocin regimen is appropriate for augmentation of labor. Regardless of the regimen used, oxytocin should be administered by trained personnel capable of responding to complications. A physician who has privileges to perform cesarean delivery should be readily available.

REFERENCES

1. Shiono PH, McNellis D, Rhoads GG. Reasons for the rising cesarean delivery rates: 1978–1984. Obstet Gynecol 1987;69:696–700
2. Friedman EA, ed. Labor: clinical evaluation and management. 2nd ed. New York: Appleton-Century-Crofts, 1978
3. Cohen WR. Influence of the duration of second stage labor on perinatal outcome and puerperal morbidity. Obstet Gynecol 1977;49:266–269
4. Cohen WR, Friedman EA, Acker DB, eds. Management of labor. 2nd ed. Rockville, Maryland: Aspen Publishers, 1988
5. Seitchik J, Castillo M. Oxytocin augmentation of dysfunctional labor. II. Uterine activity data. Am J Obstet Gynecol 1983;145:526–529
6. Caldeyro-Barcia R, Poseiro JJ. Oxytocin and contractility of the pregnant human uterus. Ann N Y Acad Sci 1959;75:813–830
7. El-Sahwi S, Gaafar AA, Toppozada HK. A new unit for evaluation of uterine activity. Am J Obstet Gynecol 1967;98:900–903
8. Hon EH, Paul RH. Quantitation of uterine activity. Obstet Gynecol 1973;42:368–370
9. Steer PJ. The measurement and control of uterine contractions. In: Beard RW, Campbell S, eds. The current status of fetal heart rate monitoring and ultrasound in obstetrics. London: Royal College of Obstetricians and Gynaecologists, 1977:48–70
10. Phillips GF, Calder AA. Units for the evaluation of uterine contractility. Br J Obstet Gynaecol 1987;94:236–241
11. Hauth JC, Hankins GDV, Gilstrap LC III, Strickland DM, Vance P. Uterine contraction pressures with oxytocin induction/augmentation. Obstet Gynecol 1986;68:305–309
12. Thorp JA, Hu DH, Albin RM, McNitt J, Meyer BA, Cohen GR, et al. The effect of intrapartum epidural analgesia on nulliparous labor: A randomized, controlled, prospective trial. Am J Obstet Gynecol 1993;169:851-858
13. Thorp JA, Parisi VM, Boylan PC, Johnston DA. The effect of continuous epidural analgesia on cesarean section for dystocia in nulliparous women. Am J Obstet Gynecol 1989;161:670–675
14. Chestnut DH, Vincent RD Jr, McGrath JM, Choi WW, Bates JN. Does early administration of epidural analgesia affect obstetric outcome in nulliparous women who are receiving intravenous oxytocin? Anesthesiology 1994;80: 1193–1200
15. Chestnut DH, McGrath JM, Vincent RD Jr, Penning DH, Choi WW, Bates JN, et al. Does early administration of epidural analgesia affect obstetric outcome in nulliparous women who are in spontaneous labor? Anesthesiology 1994;80:1201–1208
16. Benedetti TJ, Gabbe SG. Shoulder dystocia: a complication of fetal macrosomia and prolonged second stage of labor with midpelvic delivery. Obstet Gynecol 1978; 52:526–529

17. American College of Obstetricians and Gynecologists. Fetal macrosomia. ACOG Technical Bulletin 159. Washington, DC: ACOG, 1991

18. Sosa R, Kennell J, Klaus M, Robertson S, Urrutia J. The effect of a supportive companion on perinatal problems, length of labor, and mother–infant interaction. New Engl J Med 1980;303:597–600

19. Kelso IM, Parsons RJ, Lawrence GF, Arora SS, Edmonds DK, Cooke ID. An assessment of continuous fetal heart rate monitoring in labor: a randomized trial. Am J Obstet Gynecol 1978;131:526–532

20. Haverkamp AD, Orleans M, Langendoerfer S, McFee J, Murphy J, Thompson HE. A controlled trial of the differential effects of intrapartum fetal monitoring. Am J Obstet Gynecol 1979;134:399–412

21. Macdonald D, Grant A, Sheriden-Pereira M, Boylan P, Chalmers I. The Dublin randomized controlled trial of intrapartum fetal heart rate monitoring. Am J Obstet Gynecol 1985;152:524–539

22. Luthy DA, Shy KK, van Belle G, Larson EB, Hughes JP, Benedetti TJ, et al. A randomized trial of electronic fetal monitoring in preterm labor. Obstet Gynecol 1987;69: 687–695

23. Fenwick L, Simkin P. Maternal positioning to prevent or alleviate dystocia in labor. Clin Obstet Gynecol 1987; 30:83–89

24. Johnson N, Johnson VA, Gupta JK. Maternal positions during labor. Obstet Gynecol Surv 1991;46:428–434

25. Gardosi J, Sylvester S, B-Lynch C. Alternative positions in the second stage of labour: a randomized controlled trial. Br J Obstet Gynaecol 1989;96:1290–1296

26. Keirse MJNC. Augmentation of labour. In: Chalmers I, Enkin M, Keirse MJNC, eds. Effective care in pregnancy and childbirth. Vol 2. Childbirth, parts VI–X. Oxford: Oxford University Press, 1989

27. Rouse DJ, McCullough C, Wren AL, Owen J, Hauth JC. Active-phase labor arrest: a randomized trial of chorioamnion management. Obstet Gynecol 1994;83:937–940

28. Garite TJ, Porto M, Carlson NJ, Rumney PJ, Reimbold PA. The influence of elective amniotomy on fetal heart rate patterns and the course of labor in term patients: a randomized study. Am J Obstet Gynecol 1993;168:1827–1832

29. Fraser WD, Marcoux S, Moutquin J-M, Christen A, and the Canadian Early Amniotomy Study Group. Effect of early amniotomy on the risk of dystocia in nulliparous women. N Engl J Med 1993;328:1145–1149

30. Rydén G, Sjöholm I. The metabolism of oxytocin in pregnant and non–pregnant women. Acta Obstet Gynecol Scand 1971;50:37

31. Seitchik J, Amico JA, Castillo M. Oxytocin augmentation of dysfunctional labor. V. An alternative oxytocin regimen. Am J Obstet Gynecol 1985;151:757–761

32. Seitchik J, Amico J, Robinson AG, Castillo M. Oxytocin augmentation of dysfunctional labor. IV. Oxytocin pharmacokinetics. Am J Obstet Gynecol 1984;150:225–228

33. Satin AJ, Leveno KJ, Sherman ML, McIntire DD. Factors affecting the dose response to oxytocin for labor stimulation. Am J Obstet Gynecol 1992;166:1260–1261

34. Reece EA, Chervenak FA, Romero R, Hobbins JC. Magnesium sulfate in the management of acute intrapartum fetal distress. Am J Obstet Gynecol 1984;148:104–107

35. Patriarco MS, Viechnicki BM, Hutchinson TA, Klasko SK, Yeh S-Y. A study on intrauterine fetal resuscitation with terbutaline. Am J Obstet Gynecol 1987;157:384–387

36. O'Driscoll K, Foley M, MacDonald D. Active management of labor as an alternative to cesarean section for dystocia. Obstet Gynecol 1984;63:485–490

37. Satin AJ, Leveno KJ, Sherman ML, Brewster DS, Cunningham FG. High- versus low-dose oxytocin for labor stimulation. Obstet Gynecol 1992;80:111–116

38. López-Zeno JA, Peaceman AM, Adashek JA, Socol ML. A controlled trial of a program for the active management of labor. N Engl J Med 1992;326:450–454

39. Frigoletto FD Jr, Lieberman E, Lang JM, Cohen A, Barss V, Ringer S, et al. A clinical trial of active management of labor. N Engl J Med 1995;333:745–750

40. Boylan P, Robson M, McParland P. Active management of labor 1963–1993. Am J Obstet Gynecol 1993;168:295

This Technical Bulletin was developed under the direction of the Committee on Technical Bulletins of the American College of Obstetricians and Gynecologists as an educational aid to obstetricians and gynecologists. The committee wishes to thank Andrew J. Satin, MD, for his assistance in the development of this bulletin. The opinions expressed in this manuscript are those of the author and not necessarily those of the United States Air Force or the Department of Defense. This Technical Bulletin does not define a standard of care, nor is it intended to dictate an exclusive course of management. It presents recognized methods and techniques of clinical practice for consideration by obstetrician–gynecologists for incorporation into their practices. Variations of practice taking into account the needs of the individual patient, resources, and limitations unique to the institution or type of practice may be appropriate.

ISSN 1074-8628

THE AMERICAN COLLEGE OF OBSTETRICIANS AND GYNECOLOGISTS
409 12th Street, SW
Washington, DC 20024-2188

2345/9876

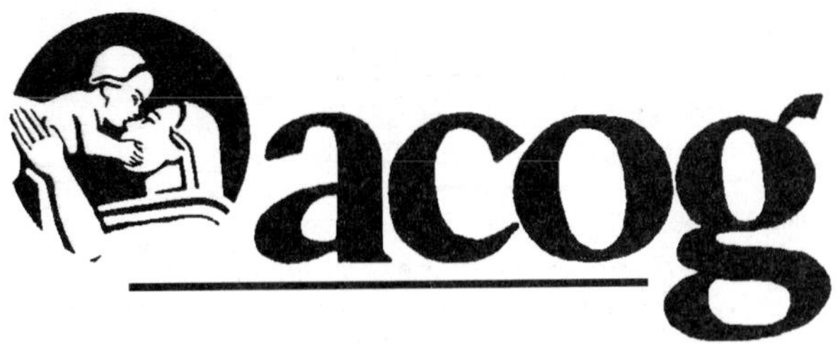

Number 212—September 1995

Technical Bulletin

An Educational Aid to Obstetrician–Gynecologists

Early Pregnancy Loss

Approximately 50–75% of pregnancies end in spontaneous abortion (1). Most of these pregnancy losses are unrecognized because they occur before or at the time of the next expected menses (2). Approximately 15–20% of clinically diagnosed pregnancies are lost in the first or early second trimester. Early pregnancy loss is usually a sporadic event, and the subsequent pregnancy usually results in a live birth.

Recurrent abortion has been traditionally defined as the loss of three or more consecutive pregnancies and occurs in 0.5–1% of pregnant women. Retrospective and prospective studies show that women with two successive spontaneous abortions have a recurrence risk of 25–45% (3–7). However, the risk of abortion is influenced by the obstetric history, and the prognosis for a successful pregnancy is probably increased by 10–20% in women with at least one previous live birth (3). The risk of abortion after two successive abortions is clinically similar to the risk of recurrence among women with three or more consecutive abortions (8–10). Thus, depending on the patient's age and wishes, patients with two or more spontaneous abortions are candidates for an evaluation. Because management for recurrent abortions differs from that of sporadic abortions, different approaches are needed.

Sporadic Pregnancy Loss

Abnormalities in embryonic growth and development cause most preclinical pregnancy losses. Half of preimplantation embryos and one third of implanted embryos are morphologically abnormal (11). These embryos are probably cytogenetically abnormal and presumably are destined to be aborted before or soon after the next expected menses.

Abnormalities in embryonic growth and development also cause most recognized pregnancy losses. Nearly one fifth of specimens from losses occurring in the first half of pregnancy and one third of those occurring at or before 8 weeks of gestation are anembryonic (blighted ovum); that is, the abortus specimen consists of an intact or ruptured gestational sac with no apparent embryo, yolk sac, or umbilical cord (11). Identifiable embryos or fetuses are found in 50–60% of first-trimester or early second-trimester abortus specimens, but only one half of these appear normal. The remainder of the embryos and fetuses are dysmorphic, growth impaired, or too macerated for examination.

Overall, 30–50% of sporadic spontaneous abortions are cytogenetically abnormal. Karyotypic abnormalities drop from a high of approximately 50% at 8–11 weeks of gestation to approximately 30% at 16–19 weeks of gestation (12).

Infections appear to be associated with some first-trimester and early second-trimester pregnancy losses. However, a causal relationship between infections and recurrent abortion has not been established. Bacteria such as *Treponema pallidum*, *Borrelia burgdorferi*, *Chlamydia trachomatis*, *Neisseria gonorrhoeae*, *Streptococcus agalactiae*, and *Listeria monocytogenes* have been identified in specimens from first-trimester or early second-trimester spontaneous abortions. Viruses also have been identified in specimens from early pregnancy loss.

The antineoplastic agents aminopterin and methotrexate have been found to cause abortion when administered at therapeutic doses. Certain drugs and chemical agents have been associated with spontaneous abortion, such as anesthetic gases, chloroquine, oral hypoglycemic agents, arsenic, heavy metals, ethanol, caffeine, and cigarette smoking. Studies of the association of some of these agents (eg, anesthetic gases) with abortion have shown conflicting results. A causal relationship between exposure and abortion has not been established for many of these agents. It is questionable whether any of these is an abortifacient at typical levels of exposure. The contention that exposure to video display terminals for more than 20 h/wk is related to spontaneous abortion has been refuted (13, 14).

Evaluation of the woman is not recommended for a single first-trimester or early second-trimester spontaneous abortion if the woman is otherwise healthy. Pathologic evaluation of abortus tissue is recommended in some cases to confirm an intrauterine pregnancy and to exclude trophoblastic disease or ectopic gestation. The patient should be reassured that most spontaneous abortions are the inevitable consequence of morphologic or cytogenetic abnormalities of the embryo or fetus. Prospective studies have demonstrated that approximately 80–90% of women who have had a single early spontaneous abortion deliver a viable infant in the next pregnancy (4, 7, 15). The chance of a successful pregnancy is probably higher for women who previously have had one or more live births. The rate of successful outcome per recognized pregnancy is also influenced by the maternal age. Approximately 85–90% of pregnancies result in live births in women 20–30 years of age. The live birth rate begins to decline after age 33–35 years. By age 40, the live birth rate is reduced to approximately 70% (16).

Recurrent Early Pregnancy Loss

Recurrent early pregnancy loss can be a difficult and frustrating problem for patients and physicians. None of the traditional etiologies nor their suggested treatments are unequivocally established by well-designed studies. For couples with recurrent pregnancy loss, it is reasonable to offer a basic evaluation as outlined in the box. In up to 50% of couples with recurrent pregnancy loss, however, an evaluation will not identify a cause. Informative and supportive counseling appears to play an important role and may lead to the best pregnancy outcomes (17, 18). The live birth rate in couples with unexplained recurrent pregnancy loss who undertake an untreated subsequent pregnancy is 52–61% (19). Such couples should be counseled about these rates.

Factors to Be Considered in the Assessment of Recurrent Early Pregnancy Loss

History

- Pattern, trimester, and characteristics of prior pregnancy losses
- Exposure to environmental toxins and drugs
- Gynecologic or obstetric infections
- Features associated with antiphospholipid syndrome (ie, thrombosis, autoimmune phenomena, false-positive tests for syphilis)
- Genetic relationship between reproductive partners (consanguinity)
- Family history of recurrent spontaneous abortion or syndrome associated with embryonic or fetal loss
- Previous diagnostic tests and treatments

Physical

- General physical, including gynecologic, examination

Tests to Be Considered

- Endocrine evaluation
- Hysterosalpingography
- Parental karyotypes
- Endometrial biopsy
- Identification of lupus anticoagulant and anticardiolipin antibodies

The sequence of testing should take into consideration the cost, clinical circumstances, and indications. If other tests are negative, consider performing hysteroscopy.

Luteal Phase Defect

It is well recognized that corpus luteum progesterone is necessary for successful implantation and the maintenance of early pregnancy. The luteal phase defect (LPD) is considered by some investigators to be the cause of recurrent early pregnancy loss in approximately one quarter of patients (20, 21). There remains, however, no unequivocal evidence that LPD is a cause of recurrent loss, and studies performed to date have not included concurrently tested controls. Including women appropriately diagnosed with luteal phase defects in a control group would be ethically difficult to carry out.

The diagnosis of LPD must be made with a full-thickness endometrial biopsy obtained from the lateral wall of the uterus beginning at the top of the fundus and histologically dated according to Noyes and Hertig. The endometrium is considered out-of-phase when the histological dating lags behind the menstrual dating by 3 days or more. There is considerable interobserver variation in the interpretation of the biopsies, and 6–7% of normal fertile women will have an out-of-phase histology on a single biopsy (22). It would seem, therefore, that the diagnosis of LPD should be made by using two out-of-phase biopsies in consecutive cycles.

Uncontrolled studies indicate that patients with recurrent pregnancy loss and LPD are very likely to achieve term pregnancy when treated with supplemental progesterone (23, 24), and this therapy is widely accepted. In contrast, a metaanalysis of randomized controlled trials found that progesterone therapy was ineffective (25).

Uterine Abnormalities

About 10–15% of women with recurrent first-trimester abortions have congenital uterine abnormalities (23, 26, 27). The most common malformations reported to be associated with pregnancy loss are variations of the double uterus (bicornuate, septate, didelphic). Severe uterine synechiae (Asherman syndrome), uterine abnormalities associated with in utero exposure to diethylstilbestrol, and submucosal leiomyomata also may be associated with spontaneous abortion. It is theorized that pregnancy loss in patients with uterine abnormalities may be due to space constraints or inadequate placentation resulting from poorly vascularized endometrium.

Uterine abnormalities can be diagnosed by hysterosalpingography, ultrasonography, hysteroscopy, and, as indicated, laparoscopy. During hysterosalpingography, cervical traction should be applied to straighten the uterus so that a complete view of the uterus can be obtained. Initially, only a small amount of radiopaque contrast material should be injected so that subtle defects are not overlooked.

Corrective surgery may be a reasonable treatment option if other causes of recurrent early pregnancy loss have been excluded. Although there are no well-designed, controlled trials to prove that correcting uterine abnormalities results in successful pregnancy, approximately 70–85% of patients who have had recurrent pregnancy loss who undergo surgical correction of a bicornuate or septate uterus deliver viable infants in their next pregnancy (28–30) (Table 1).

Infections

Although certain infections are associated with spontaneous abortion, no infectious agent has been proven to cause recurrent pregnancy loss. One group of investigators found that women with recurrent spontaneous abortion have a significantly higher rate of endometrial colonization with *Ureaplasma urealyticum* when compared with controls (31). This suggests that endometrial colonization with mycoplasmas may play a role in abortion, but it requires confirmation before endometrial culture can be recommended clinically.

Toxoplasma gondii and some viruses (eg, rubella, herpes simplex virus, cytomegalovirus, measles virus, and coxsackievirus) have been linked to abortion. However, none has been convincingly associated with recurrent pregnancy loss. Thus, serologic testing (ie, TORCH [toxoplasmosis, other viruses, rubella, cytomegalovirus, herpes simplex virus] titers) or cultures for these organisms should be guided by the patient's history. New molecular genetic techniques may help clarify the role of bacterial, parasitic, and viral colonization or infection in causing recurrent abortion.

TABLE 1. PREGNANCY OUTCOME ASSOCIATED WITH REPRODUCTIVE TRACT ANOMALIES*

Anomaly	Term Pregnancy Outcome
Transverse vaginal septum	50%
Absence of cervix	Rare pregnancy
Rudimentary horn	64–85% (normal horn)
Unicollis	69%
Septate uterus	15% (78% after repair)
Bicornuate uterus	10% (84% after repair)
Didelphic uterus	57%

*Data are based on case series with limited number of patients.

Adapted from Rock JA, Schlaff WD. The obstetric consequences of uterovaginal anomalies. Fertil Steril 1985;43:681–692. Reproduced with permission of the publisher, The American Fertility Society.

Genetic Abnormalities

Parental Structural Chromosome Abnormalities

Genetically balanced structural chromosome rearrangements are present in approximately 2–3% of couples with recurrent abortion. The rate is slightly higher in couples with a history of anomalous infants or stillborns (32), but the fact that a couple may have phenotypically normal offspring does not exclude the possibility of a parental chromosome abnormality.

When obtained, parental karyotypes may demonstrate no chromosome abnormality. In such cases, a structural chromosome rearrangement predisposing to recurrent abortions can be excluded. However, couples with abnormal karyotypes should receive genetic counseling and may require future prenatal diagnosis.

Balanced translocations account for the largest proportion of karyotypic abnormalities in couples with recurrent pregnancy loss. The most common type of structural abnormality found in couples with recurrent abortion involves the exchange of chromatin between two nonhomologous chromosomes (reciprocal translocation) or the addition of part of one chromosome to another nonhomologous chromosome (simple translocation). Robertsonian translocations, which involve the fusion of acrocentric chromosomes (chromosomes 13, 14, 15, 21, or 22), also occur among couples with recurrent abortion. Chromosome inversions or ring chromosomes also may be found, though they are rare.

The vast majority of parental balanced translocations can result in chromosomally normal conceptions, balanced carrier conceptions, or chromosomally abnormal conceptions. The risk of the last is related to many variables, including the specific type of abnormality and whether the male or female partner is the carrier. Since most reciprocal or simple translocations are unique, the rate of adverse reproductive outcome will be specific for the family in question. The risks for miscarriage or chromosomally abnormal offspring may be estimable if there is sufficient family history of abnormal outcomes. The overall risk of miscarriage in couples with reciprocal or simple translocations is approximately 25–50%, and the overall risk of an offspring carrying an unbalanced translocation is approximately 10%.

The 11:22 reciprocal translocation is frequent enough that empirical data are available for counseling. This translocation predisposes to 3:1 malsegregation in meiosis I, with a subsequent high risk of chromosome abnormalities in conceptuses.

In the situation of a parent with a 14:21 Robertsonian translocation, theoretically half of all conceptions would be incompatible with fetal viability (ie, monosomy 14, monosomy 21, or trisomy 14), one third would be phenotypically normal, and one sixth would have trisomy 21. Similar theoretical proportions exist for a 13:14 Robertsonian translocation. Fortunately, the observed risk of adverse reproductive outcome is much lower. For a 14:21 translocation, the risk of having a liveborn infant with Down syndrome is 10–15% if the female reproductive partner is the carrier and only 2% if the male is the carrier. For a 13:14 translocation, the observed risk of delivering an infant with trisomy 13 is only 1%. The observed risk of miscarriage for these translocations is approximately 25%. Certain rare Robertsonian translocations (eg, 21:21 translocation) are incompatible with a chromosomally normal offspring.

Though uncommon among couples with recurrent miscarriage, pericentric inversions may be found in couples with recurrent abortion. Paracentric inversions, though theoretically a cause of recurrent abortion, are exceedingly rare. The inv(9)(p11q13) inversion of the centromeric region of chromosome 9 deserves special mention. It is a normal chromosomal variant found in 1–3% of the population and is not associated with adverse reproductive risk. The finding of a balanced structural chromosome rearrangement, such as a translocation or pericentric inversion, may be an indication for prenatal cytogenetic diagnosis in future pregnancies.

Chromosome Abnormalities of the Conceptus

Analyses of karyotypes in consecutive abortions suggest that recurrent aneuploidy in the conceptus may be a cause of recurrent pregnancy loss. In one compilation of data, the karyotype of the second successive spontaneous abortion was abnormal in nearly 70% of cases in which aneuploidy was found in the first abortus but in only 20% of cases in which the first abortus was chromosomally normal (33). However, this observation may have been due to the age of the mothers rather than to a nonrandom event in predisposed couples (34). The subject remains controversial, and routine cytogenetic testing of abortus specimens is not indicated at this time.

Molecular Genetic Abnormalities of the Conceptus

In the past decade, the importance of single-gene mutations as a cause for a number of human diseases has been brought to light by the development of techniques for DNA analysis. The potential mechanisms by which such a defect might result in pregnancy loss are innumerable. As yet, recurrent abortions of fetuses affected by certain X-linked dominant conditions with high lethality in males represent the only examples of single gene mutations causing recurrent abortion in humans.

Metabolic and Hormonal Disorders

Maternal metabolic and endocrinologic disorders have been implicated as causes of recurrent pregnancy loss. It is plausible that any disease that results in moderate-to-severe systemic metabolic derangements might result in pregnancy loss. There is no evidence from controlled trials, however, that asymptomatic metabolic or endocrinologic disorders cause recurrent pregnancy loss (23, 26, 27).

Immunologic Factors

Autoimmune Disorders

Antiphospholipid syndrome (APS) is an autoimmune disorder characterized by the presence of significant levels of antiphospholipid antibodies and one or more clinical features, including pregnancy loss, thrombosis, or autoimmune thrombocytopenia. Antiphospholipid syndrome may occur as a secondary condition in patients with underlying autoimmune disease (eg, systemic lupus erythematosus) or as a primary condition in women with no other recognizable autoimmune disease.

The two pertinent antiphospholipid antibodies are lupus anticoagulant and anticardiolipin. In spite of an impressive effort at standardization, anticardiolipin antibody results vary considerably, and false-positive or low-positive test results are common. Therefore, anticardiolipin antibody testing should be performed using standards available from the Antiphospholipid Standardization Laboratory in Louisville, Kentucky, and reported in semi-quantitative terms (negative, low-positive, medium-positive, high-positive). Low-positive results are of questionable significance; patients with APS virtually always have medium- or high-positive results. Whether or not other antiphospholipid antibodies (eg, antiphosphatidylserine) are independently associated with pregnancy loss remains controversial.

Antiphospholipid syndrome is the cause of pregnancy loss in no more than 5–10% of women with recurrent pregnancy loss (35–38). Women with a previous fetal death (39, 40) and high levels of anticardiolipin immunoglobulin G antibodies (40) are at the greatest risk of fetal loss in subsequent pregnancies.

Glucocorticoids, heparin, low-dose aspirin, intravenous immune globulin, or some combination of these medications have been used to treat pregnant women in an attempt to improve pregnancy outcomes among women with APS and pregnancy loss. Direct comparison of these studies is virtually impossible because of differences in patient selection and treatments (39). The two most widely used treatment regimens have been 1) a combination of prednisone and low-dose aspirin or 2) heparin, with or without low-dose aspirin. Successful pregnancy outcomes have been reported in approximately 55–85% of treated cases. The efficacy of these treatments remains controversial because none of the studies to date has included appropriate controls. Some women with antiphospholipid antibodies have had successful pregnancies without specific medical treatment, but there is currently no way to identify these patients prospectively. When such treatment is being considered, heparin or heparin and aspirin may be the preferred choice because of the risk of side effects with prednisone.

Women with APS who become pregnant appear to be at high risk for maternal and fetal complications regardless of treatment. One study found that half developed preeclampsia and half developed "fetal distress" that required delivery (39). Nearly one third of live-born infants were small for gestational age, and over one third were delivered at or before 32 weeks of gestation. Finally, 5% of pregnancies were complicated by maternal thrombosis, including one case of stroke. Pregnancies in women with APS demand close maternal and fetal surveillance.

Some investigators have proposed that a subclinical autoimmune condition(s) might be associated with recurrent pregnancy loss, and several have found that some women with recurrent pregnancy loss have detectable antinuclear antibodies (ANAs). However, the proportion of patients with unexplained recurrent abortion and positive ANAs is not statistically different from that of appropriate controls (41, 42). Other autoantibodies also have been associated with spontaneous abortion, including anti-SSA, thyroid autoantibodies, and positive results in auto-antibody profiles. However, these studies were not convincing or require confirmation of their significance in women with recurrent spontaneous abortion. The currently available data do not support testing women with recurrent pregnancy loss for ANAs or autoantibodies other than antiphospholipid antibodies. Moreover, there is no reasonable recommendation as to how best to treat patients found to have positive tests.

Allogeneic Factors

The term *alloimmune* refers to immunologic differences between individuals of the same species. Familiar allogeneic traits in humans include the ABO and Rh blood groups and major histocompatibility antigen systems. Allogeneic factors have been proposed as the cause of otherwise unexplained recurrent pregnancy loss in a fashion similar to allograft rejection organ transplantation. However, there is no direct scientific evidence that alloimmune factors play a role in human pregnancy loss.

Some reproductive immunologists believe that allogeneic similarities between the male and female reproductive partners might be associated with recurrent pregnancy loss. Several groups have reported a tendency for reproductive partners with unexplained recurrent pregnancy loss to share human leukocyte antigens, for the female partner to fail to produce serum blocking factors, or for the female partner to fail to produce antileukocytotoxic antibodies against paternal leukocytes (43). Other investigators have refuted the significance of each of these factors, and none of these tests provides results that predict the subsequent pregnancy outcome in treated or untreated recurrent spontaneous abortion patients (44, 45). It is doubtful that these relatively expensive tests are necessary in the clinical evaluation of couples with recurrent pregnancy loss.

A number of immunotherapeutic regimens are being used empirically in couples with otherwise unexplained pregnancy loss. The most widely used regimen involves immunizing the female partner with the male partner's leukocytes. Two recent metaanalyses found a clinically marginal but statistically significant benefit to leukocyte immunizations in the prevention of recurrent pregnancy loss (19). There is, however, no consensus regarding patient selection or the dose, route, or timing of immunizations. A randomized, multicenter trial sponsored by the National Institutes of Health is currently under way to determine the efficacy of leukocyte immunotherapy. Since no clear picture has emerged regarding the value of immunotherapy, maternal immunization with paternal leukocytes should be considered experimental, and a cautious approach is recommended.

Conclusions

Presently, it is reasonable to evaluate patients with recurrent pregnancy loss for the traditionally accepted causes outlined in this bulletin. Couples in which one partner is found to have a chromosome abnormality should be counseled regarding the recurrence risk for spontaneous abortions and be offered prenatal genetic studies in all future pregnancies to detect possible unbalanced chromosome abnormalities in the fetus. Treatment for LPD is relatively inexpensive and appears to carry negligible risk to mother or conceptus, though there is no proof in randomized, controlled trials of treatment efficacy. Depending on the type of structural uterine abnormalities, corrective surgery may be a reasonable treatment option after other possible causes of recurrent pregnancy loss have been excluded. Women with APS should be counseled regarding the potential for a successful pregnancy and the risks of maternal and fetal complications. Treatment with heparin or heparin and low-dose aspirin may be considered in women with APS, but the efficacy of such treatment in preventing pregnancy loss is unproven and the medications pose certain risks to the mother.

It may be useful to discuss alleged alloimmune causes of pregnancy loss with couples with unexplained recurrent pregnancy loss, but the proposed treatments for this condition are relatively expensive and of uncertain efficacy and safety. They cannot be recommended outside of an experimental protocol.

Couples with otherwise unexplained recurrent pregnancy loss should be counseled regarding the potential for successful pregnancy. They should be informed of the rate of successful pregnancy that can be expected without treatment.

Recurrent abortion is a frustrating problem for the patient and the physician. In at least 50% of cases, no etiology is found. In other cases, such as with a parental structural chromosome abnormality, the cause of the recurrent miscarriage cannot be remedied. The physician should be equipped to carry out indicated diagnostic evaluations, provide accurate prognostic information, and discuss experimental or controversial treatments with these often anxious and vulnerable patients. Above all, the physician should offer a sympathetic approach that encourages appropriate evaluation and management.

REFERENCES

1. Boklage CE. Survival probability of human conceptions from fertilization to term. Int J Fertil 1990;35:75–94
2. Wilcox AJ, Weinberg CR, O'Connor JF, Baird DD, Schlatterer JP, Canfield RE, et al. Incidence of early loss of pregnancy. N Engl J Med 1988;319:189–194
3. Warburton D, Fraser FC. Spontaneous abortion risks in man: data from reproductive histories collected in a medical genetics unit. Hum Genet 1964;16:1–25
4. Boué J, Boué A, Lazar P. Retrospective and prospective epidemiological studies of 1500 karyotyped spontaneous human abortions. Teratology 1975;12:11–26
5. Poland BJ, Miller JR, Jones DC, Trimble BK. Reproductive counseling in patients who have had a spontaneous abortion. Am J Obstet Gynecol 1977;127:685–691
6. FitzSimmons J, Jackson D, Wapner R, Jackson L. Subsequent reproductive outcome in couples with repeated pregnancy loss. Am J Med Genet 1983;16:583–587
7. Regan L. A prospective study of spontaneous abortion. In: Beard RW, Sharp F, eds. Early pregnancy loss. London: Springer-Verlag, 1988:23–37
8. Mowbray JF, Gibbings C, Liddell H, Reginald PW, Underwood JL, Beard RW. Controlled trial of treatment of recurrent spontaneous abortion by immunization with paternal cells. Lancet 1985;1:941–943
9. Ho H-N, Gill TJ III, Hsieh H-J, Jiang J-J, Lee T-Y, Hsieh C-Y. Immunotherapy for recurrent spontaneous abortions in a Chinese population. Am J Reprod Immunol 1991;25:10–15
10. Cauchi MN, Lim D, Young DE, Kloss M, Pepperell RJ. Treatment of recurrent aborters by immunization with paternal cells–controlled trial. Am J Reprod Immunol 1991;25:16–17
11. Fantel AG, Shepard TH. Morphological analysis of spontaneous abortuses. In: Bennett MJ, Edmonds DK, eds. Spontaneous and recurrent abortion. Oxford: Blackwell Scientific Publications, 1987:8–28
12. Kline J, Stein Z. Epidemiology of chromosomal anomalies in spontaneous abortion: prevalence, manifestation and determinants. In: Bennett MJ, Edmonds DK, eds. Spontaneous and recurrent abortion. Oxford: Blackwell Scientific Publications, 1987:29–50
13. Blackwell R, Chang A. Video display terminals and pregnancy. A review. Br J Obstet Gynaecol 1988;95:446–453
14. Schnorr TM, Grajewski BA, Hornung RW, Thun MJ, Egeland GM, Murray WE, et al. Video display terminals and the risk of spontaneous abortion. N Engl J Med 1991;324:727–733
15. Lauritsen JG. Aetiology of spontaneous abortion. A cytogenetic and epidemiological study of 288 abortuses and their parents. Acta Obstet Gynecol Scand Suppl 1976;52:1–29
16. Stein Z, Kline J, Susser E, Shrout P, Warburton D, Susser M. Maternal age and spontaneous abortion. In: Porter IH, Hook EB, eds. Human embryonic and fetal death. New York: Academic Press, 1980:107–126
17. Tupper C, Weil RJ. The problem of spontaneous abortion. Am J Obstet Gynecol 1962;83:421–429
18. Stray-Pedersen B, Stray-Pedersen S. Recurrent abortion: the role of psychotherapy. In: Beard RW, Sharp F, eds. Early pregnancy loss. London: Springer-Verlag, 1988:433–440
19. Coulam CB, Clark DA, Collins J, Scott JR, Schlesselman JJ. A worldwide collaborative observational study and meta-analysis on allogenic leukocyte immunotherapy for recurrent spontaneous abortion. Am J Reprod Immunol 1994;23:55–72
20. Byrne J, Warburton D, Kline J, Blanc W, Stein Z. Morphology of early fetal deaths and their chromosomal characteristics. Teratology 1985;32:297–315
21. Daya S, Ward S, Burrows E. Progesterone profiles in luteal phase defect cycles and outcome of progesterone treatment in patients with recurrent spontaneous abortion. Am J Obstet Gynecol 1988;158:225–232
22. Davis OK, Berkeley AS, Naus GJ, Cholst IN, Freedman KS. The incidence of luteal phase defect in normal, fertile

women, determined by serial endometrial biopsy. Fertil Steril 1989;51:582–586

23. Tho PT, Byrd JR, McDonough PG. Etiologies and subsequent reproductive performance of 100 couples with recurrent abortion. Fertil Steril 1979;32:389–395
24. Jones GS. The luteal phase defect. Fertil Steril 1976; 27:351–356
25. Goldstein P, Berrier J, Rosen S, Sacks HS, Chalmers TC. A meta-analysis of randomized control trials of progestational agents in pregnancy. Br J Obstet Gynaecol 1989;96: 265–274
26. Harger JH, Archer DF, Marchese SG, Muracca-Clemens M, Garver KL. Etiology of recurrent pregnancy losses and outcome of subsequent pregnancies. Obstet Gynecol 1983;62:574–581
27. Stray-Pedersen B, Stray-Pedersen S. Etiologic factors and subsequent reproductive performance in 195 couples with a prior history of habitual abortion. Am J Obstet Gynecol 1984;148:140–146
28. Rock JA, Murphy AA. Anatomic abnormalities. Clin Obstet Gynecol 1986;29:886–911
29. DeCherney AH, Russell JB, Graebe RA, Polan ML. Resectoscopic management of müllerian fusion defects. Fertil Steril 1986;45:726–728
30. March CM, Israel R. Hysteroscopic management of recurrent abortion caused by septate uterus. Am J Obstet Gynecol 1987;156:834–842
31. Stray-Pedersen B, Lorentzen-Stry A. Uterine toxoplasma infections and repeated abortions. Am J Obstet Gynecol 1977;128:716–721
32. Simpson JL, Elias S, Meyers CM, Ober C, Martin AO. Translocations are infrequent among couples having repeated spontaneous abortions but no other abnormal pregnancies. Fertil Steril 1989;51:811–814
33. Hassold TJ. A cytogenetic study of repeated spontaneous abortions. Am J Hum Genet 1980;32:723–730
34. Warburton D, Kline J, Stein Z, Hutzler M, Chin A, Hassold T. Does the karyotype of a spontaneous abortion predict the karyotype of a subsequent abortion?—Evidence from 273 women with two karyotyped spontaneous abortions. Am J Hum Genet 1987;41:465–483
35. Branch DW, Scott JR. Clinical implications of anti-phospholipid antibodies: the Utah experience. In: Harris EN, Exner T, Hughes GRV, Asherson RA, eds. Phospholipid-binding antibodies. Boca Raton, Florida: CRC Press, 1991:335–346
36. Out HJ, Bruinse HW, Christiaens GCML, van Vliet M, Meilof JF, de Groot PG, et al. Prevalence of antiphospholipid antibodies in patients with fetal loss. Ann Rheum Dis 1991;50:553–557
37. Parazzini F, Acaia B, Faden D, Lovotti M, Marelli G, Cortelazzo S. Antiphospholipid antibodies and recurrent abortion. Obstet Gynecol 1991;77:854–858
38. Parke AL, Wilson D, Maier D. The prevalence of anti-phospholipid antibodies in women with recurrent spontaneous abortion, women with successful pregnancies, and women who have never been pregnant. Arthritis Rheum 1991;34:1231–1235
39. Branch DW, Silver RM, Blackwell JL, Reading JC, Scott JR. Outcome of treated pregnancies in women with antiphospholipid syndrome: an update of the Utah experience. Obstet Gynecol 1992;80:614–620
40. Lockshin MD, Druzin ML, Qamar T. Prednisone does not prevent recurrent fetal death in women with antiphospholipid antibody. Am J Obstet Gynecol 1989; 160:439–443
41. Cowchock S, Smith JB, Gocial B. Antibodies to phospholipids and nuclear antigens in patients with repeated abortions. Am J Obstet Gynecol 1986;155:1002–1010
42. Maier DB, Parke A. Subclinical autoimmunity in recurrent aborters. Fertil Steril 1989;51:280–285
43. Branch DW. Immunologic aspects of pregnancy loss: alloimmune and autoimmune considerations. In: Reece EA, Hobbins JC, Mahoney MJ, Petrie RH, eds. Medicine of the fetus and mother. Philadelphia: JB Lippincott Co, 1992:217–233
44. Cowchock FS, Smith JB. Predictors for live birth after unexplained spontaneous abortions: correlations between immunologic test results, obstetric histories, and outcome of next pregnancy without treatment. Am J Obstet Gynecol 1992;167:1208–1212
45. Coulam CB. Immunologic tests in the evaluation of reproductive disorders: a critical review. Am J Obstet Gynecol 1992;167:1844–1851

This Technical Bulletin was developed under the direction of the Committee on Technical Bulletins of the American College of Obstetricians and Gynecologists as an educational aid to obstetricians and gynecologists. The committee wishes to thank D. Ware Branch, MD, for his assistance in the development of this bulletin. This Technical Bulletin does not define a standard of care, nor is it intended to dictate an exclusive course of management. It presents recognized methods and techniques of clinical practice for consideration by obstetrician–gynecologists for incorporation into their practices. Variations of practice taking into account the needs of the individual patient, resources, and limitations unique to the institution or type of practice may be appropriate.
ISSN 1074-8628

THE AMERICAN COLLEGE OF OBSTETRICIANS AND GYNECOLOGISTS
409 12th Street, SW
Washington, DC 20024-2188

12345/98765

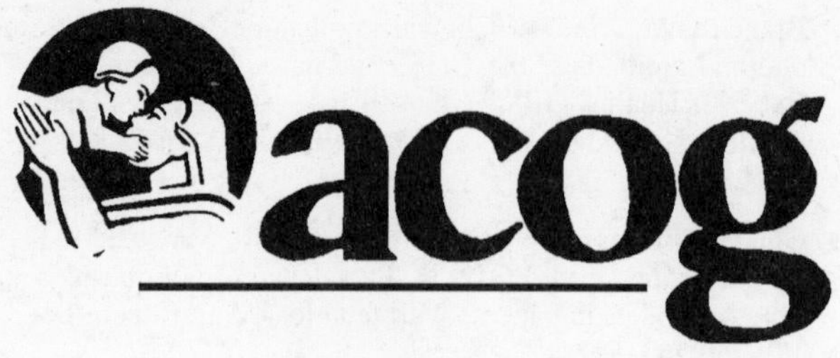

Number 136—November 1989

Technical Bulletin

An Educational Aid to Obstetrician–Gynecologists

Ethical Decision-Making in Obstetrics and Gynecology

Recent growth in scientific technology has expanded the possibilities available for the management of various medical conditions. It has also expanded medicine's ability to affect the processes of human birth, life, and death. In no specialty is this more apparent than in the field of obstetrics and gynecology. The capabilities for technically assisted reproduction, fetal surgery, and interventions at the end of life raise questions that cannot be addressed with medical knowledge alone. Good decisions in these areas depend upon a thoughtful consideration of the values, desires, and goals of those involved. Physicians, as a result of their formal medical education, become astute in making decisions based on medical indications. It is also important for them to acquire skill in addressing decisions involving competing values or diverging personal goals.

The President's Commission for the Study of Ethical Problems in Medicine has made clear that "the primary responsibility for ensuring that morally justified decisions are made lies with the physician" (1). Before an ethical approach to confronting difficult problems can be achieved, however, certain fundamental issues must be addressed (2):

1. The physician should have an understanding of the structure of his or her own value system and of the ways in which personal judgments about right and wrong, good and bad, influence decisions in various areas of life.
2. The physician should have a general background of knowledge in the discipline of ethics.
3. The process by which a physician makes and implements ethical decisions should be systematic and logically consistent.

Values, Morals, and Ethics

Each individual, as a result of a variety of life experiences, acquires a personal sense as to what is of value. Certain objects, relationships, and outcomes are regarded as more desirable than others. These values serve as a prism through which information is reflected before it is interpreted and applied to life's decisions. Values also serve as a foundation for the rules by which individuals govern their own actions.

Morals can be described as common conceptions of what is right or wrong, of what ought or ought not be done. In confronting simple daily decisions, these conceptions of right and wrong, ideally based on a sound system of values and principles, will usually serve the individual well in seeking a reasonable resolution. When questions begin to require value-based judgments from a number of parties with competing goals or divergent viewpoints, personal determinations about right and wrong become inadequate for reaching a resolution. A logical and disciplined approach to complex problems is necessary if sound decisions are to be made. Ethics can provide such an approach.

Ethics is the formal study of moral behavior in which moral obligations are analyzed in terms of recognized ethical principles. After critical reflection, an attempt is made to determine which of a number of commonly held moral assumptions are justifiable. Ethics as a discipline has evolved from this critical analysis and discussion of moral issues over many centuries of civilization. Important contributions have been made by such prominent historical figures in moral philosophy as Plato, Aristotle, Thomas Aquinas, Immanuel Kant, and John Stuart Mill.

An ethical dilemma may arise when value-based justifications can be found to support two or more opposing courses of action. Fundamental principles that dictate how individuals ought to think and behave may appear to support competing approaches to a question. On initial examination, the two arguments may appear equally compelling. For example, a physician faced with a woman refusing surgical treatment of a large pelvic mass will feel torn between the obligation to promote what appear to be the patient's best medical interests and the duty to respect her personal choice to refuse therapy.

Ethical conflict may also arise because of a lack of consensus among decision-makers about the values on which judgments are to be based. A major source of such ethical conflict is the personal beliefs or the policies that the physician or the institution brings to the decision-making process. These personal beliefs and institutional policies must be understood and recognized before an objective analysis can be undertaken. For instance, an individual physician may support a woman in her desire to obtain treatment for her infertility, while another, the "gatekeeper" at her health maintenance organization, may be more concerned with providing cost-effective health care for a large number of people.

In applying moral rules and principles to human action, the discipline of ethics does not identify any particular moral view as the correct one. It serves instead as a frame-work for systematically analyzing different moral points of view. In carrying out this analysis, one attempts to achieve a rational justification for one course of action over another, based on consideration of recognized principles and accepted values.

Ethical Principles

As the ethical analysis of a problem is carried out, principles are frequently invoked as justification for the rules that govern actions. Conflicting obligations in health care can often be clarified when the principles underlying them are identified and understood. The principles most often referred to in discussions about ethics include autonomy, beneficence, and justice (3).

Autonomy

Autonomy is defined literally as self-rule. A person is free to establish personal norms of conduct and to voluntarily choose a course of action based on a set of consistent personal values and the principles derived from them. This freedom imposes on others an obligation of noninterference. Autonomy is considered by some to be almost absolute unless it infringes on the personal freedom of others. Other views impose narrower limits on individual autonomy.

Respect for autonomy plays an important role in many areas of medical practice. Although a physician may consider a particular course of treatment to be best for a patient, he or she may agree to a somewhat different therapy at the patient's request. As another example, a physician who advises a woman with a history of life-threatening peripartum cardiomyopathy to avoid future pregnancy is prevented, out of respect for her autonomy, from taking further steps to interfere with her reproductive choice.

Beneficence

Beneficence is the obligation to promote the well-being of others. The related principle of nonmaleficence obliges one to avoid doing harm. With roots in the Hippocratic tradition, beneficence and nonmaleficence are fundamental to the ethic of medicine. The application of these principles consists of balancing benefits and harms. The concept of "harms" in this context includes intentional harms as well as those harms that can be anticipated to arise despite the best intentions (eg, unwanted side effects of medication or complications of surgical treatment). These principles, therefore, are the source of a physician's obligation to act with due care.

Beneficence underlies a physician's obligation to promote the well-being of a woman with salpingitis by recommending intravenous antibiotic therapy. In balancing beneficence with autonomy, one attempts to define a patient's "best interests" as objectively as possible. An effort to override patient autonomy in order to promote what the physician perceives as a patient's best interests is called "paternalism."

Justice

Justice is the right of individuals to claim what is due them based on certain personal properties or characteristics. Some theories of justice determine distribution of benefits and burdens based on specific properties, using criteria such as need, effort, contribution, or merit. Other theories specify that all benefits and burdens be distributed equally. It is important that the criteria used are selected in a manner consistent with accepted moral rules and principles and that they are relevant to the benefits and burdens being assigned. In this society, for example, race, sex, and religion are not considered to be morally legitimate criteria for the distribution of benefits such as employment and housing. Justice generates an obligation to treat equally those who are alike according to whatever criteria are selected. No person should receive unequal treatment unless it is demonstrated that he or she differs from others in a way that is relevant to the treatment in question.

At times, constraints such as scarcity of resources force moral judgments about competing claims made by those who appear equal based on previously used criteria. Different criteria must then be chosen on the basis of which the distribution of benefits can then be effected. Selection of these criteria is in itself a moral decision. A common scenario involves a critically ill patient and an intensive care unit (ICU) that is filled to capacity. All the patients in the ICU were initially felt to merit the degree of care provided there. When a scarcity of beds arises, however, new criteria must be identified in order to decide who most "deserves" a bed. Discussions in such situations often focus on the likelihood of successful recovery and the risk to the patient of transfer into a less intensive setting.

Ethical Concepts

Several ethical norms can be derived from these fundamental ethical principles. These norms or concepts are important because they apply to many of the decisions made in obstetrics and gynecology. An understanding of these concepts will increase the likelihood that the decisions made will be consistent with accepted ethical principles.

Informed Consent

Informed consent may be defined as "the willing and uncoerced acceptance of a medical intervention by a patient after adequate disclosure by the physician of the nature of the intervention, its risks and benefits, as well as of alternatives with their risks and benefits" (4). The primary purpose of the consent process is the protection of patient autonomy. By encouraging an ongoing and open communication of relevant information, the physician enables the patient to exercise personal choice. This sort of communication is central to the physician–patient relationship.

It is important to acknowledge that a patient's right to make her own decisions about medical issues extends to the right to refuse recommended medical treatment. This freedom to accept or refuse treatment is supported legally as well as ethically. For example, Judge Benjamin Cardozo stated in 1914 that "every human being of adult years and sound mind has a right to determine what shall be done with his own body" (5).

At times, a patient's capacity to comprehend and process the medical information presented to her may be in doubt. The physician should, through consultation and further discussion with the patient, attempt to clarify the patient's capacity to provide consent. If a patient is unable to provide consent, a substitute decision-maker should be sought.

Honesty

The principle of autonomy requires that a patient be given complete and truthful information about her medical condition and about any proposed treatment. Only with such information is she able to exercise her right to make choices about health care. If complete information is not available, existing uncertainty should be shared with the patient. It is inappropriate for a physician to assume that he or she is better able to assess what the patient would want to know than is the patient herself. In general, a patient benefits from a full understanding of her medical condition, its prognosis, and the treatment available. The perception that a physician has concealed the truth or has engaged in deception will weaken patient trust and undermine the physician–patient relationship. Thus, the norm of honesty can be based on the principle of beneficence as well as on the principle of autonomy.

Confidentiality

A patient's right to make decisions about health care includes a right to decide how and to whom personal medical information will be communicated. The principle of autonomy underlies a physician's duty to respect patient privacy. In addition, the patient benefits from protection of her right to confidentiality. As is the case with dishonesty, breaches of confidentiality threaten the patient's trust in the physician and may destroy the physician–patient relationship.

Situations may arise in which maintaining patient confidentiality results in harm to a third party. For example, a patient may refuse to inform her husband of a sexually transmitted disease that she acquired during an extramarital relationship. Her physician then faces an ethical dilemma: the obligation to respect the patient's autonomy comes into conflict with the obligation to avoid harm to others who are at risk. An examination of the competing principles and of the claims arising from them will aid the physician in reaching a decision about which course of action to take. In general, the duty to maintain confidentiality takes precedence over other obligations.

Decision-Making Relationships

The nature of the relationships between parties involved in health care decisions has an important impact on the decisions that are made. The goals and values of the individuals involved may not be in agreement. A decision intended to benefit one party may result in relative harm to another. An understanding of the relationship between the parties involved in an ethical dilemma is essential to any attempts at reaching a well-considered solution.

The Physician–Patient Relationship

The way in which principles are weighed in examining ethical questions will depend on how the physician–patient relationship and the goals of medicine are defined. Central to this definition is the decision of whether a patient's interests are best defined from the perspective of medicine or from the perspective of the patient. The value systems of those addressing an ethical question will further influence the way in which competing principles or norms are weighed and may be the source of conflict.

In general, physicians consider beneficence to be a very important obligation. Working from a medical orientation, they tend to value physical well-being very highly and therefore select actions to promote it. Personal and economic "discomfort" may be viewed by some physicians as reasonable burdens to bear in seeking improved physical health. The beneficence-dominated model of the physician–patient relationship seeks to promote the patient's best interests as defined from a medical perspective. According to this model, the goals and values of medicine are of primary importance in deciding what is best for a patient. The physician operating under this model may act in a paternalistic fashion by disregarding patient preferences in order to promote what he or she perceives to be in the patient's best interests.

In contrast, a model based on autonomy, one that seeks to promote the patient's best interests as defined by that patient, will be most likely to ensure that the patient's own beliefs and values underlie any decision that is made. The patient may not conceive of "good" in the same way as the physician does. Healing may not be her most important goal, or the costs of achieving good health may seem too high. In making decisions about medical treatment, some individuals will place family concerns or adherence to religious beliefs ahead of the pursuit of physical health. Ethical conflict may be decreased if the physician is able to determine the goals of treatment according to the values of the patient. In rare instances, a physician may feel morally unable to cooperate in pursuing the medical goals of a particular patient. In such a case, appropriate alternatives for care should be recommended.

Maternal–Fetal Relationships

In the care of the obstetric patient, the traditional physician–patient relationship expands to include the fetus. The physician retains an obligation to respect the autonomy of the pregnant woman while promoting her medical well-being. In addition, the physician must assume an obligation of beneficence toward a second patient, the fetus. The weight that this obligation is given in comparison with previously established obligations to the woman is central to many ethical dilemmas in the practice of obstetrics.

The physician may interpret the best interests of the fetus either according to the viewpoint and values of the pregnant woman, in an effort to respect her autonomy, or according to the physician's own viewpoint and values as a medical doctor. Both perspectives can make valuable contributions to the decision-making process. Often, the woman and the physician are in agreement as to the benefit sought for both the woman and the fetus. At times, however, the woman's conclusions as to relative risks and benefits differ significantly from those of her physician. Because of respect for her autonomy, a woman is considered the source of consent for the fetus she carries. Her concept of benefit for the fetus will generally determine the treatment selected. In most situations, pregnant women are willing to go to great lengths to promote the well-being of their future children.

Rarely, a particularly difficult situation arises when a pregnant woman neglects her obligation to benefit her fetus by refusing life-saving treatment or by engaging in behavior that is hazardous to the health of the fetus. The obstetrician should make an effort, through discussion and consultation, to make the woman aware of the implications of her actions for the health of the fetus. Although it may be agreed that a pregnant woman has fundamental obligations toward her fetus, no other party, including the state, should override her autonomy in order to enforce those obligations (6).

Relationships with Third Parties

Although the concerns of the patient and her physician usually determine what medical choices are made, the interests of third parties must sometimes be considered. Claims made by these parties are often grounded in recognized principles or norms. Although most physicians feel a strong obligation to respect the confidentiality of their patients, they may also wonder to what extent the duty of beneficence extends to third parties at risk. Such a dilemma may arise when the physician's knowledge about a patient includes information about genetic or infectious diseases that pose a risk to others.

In the obstetric setting, a father may make the claim that a woman should undergo treatment for the benefit of the fetus. This claim might be grounded in his own autonomy as well as in his desire to benefit the fetus (and thereby his future child). Although obstetric decisions remain primarily the concern of the pregnant woman and her physician, a physician may be faced with a third party making claims that have a degree of merit.

Goals of health care institutions differ at times from those of the individual physician and patient. Concerns over financial solvency may be in conflict with the need to provide adequate distribution of care. While individuals working within institutions or employed by other health care providers may adopt the values of those institutions to some degree, conflicts can arise among an individual's personal or professional values and adopted institutional policies. For example, there may be pressure to cut costs by restricting some procedures in order to ensure that all patients receive a basic level of care. While the physician may understand the rationale behind an institution's policy or decision, he or she will be frustrated by thwarted attempts to secure a certain level of health care. The potential for conflict may be offset if institutional values are clearly communicated to those expected to respect them.

In most situations, medical decisions will be made by individual patients with the advice and recommendations of their physicians. At times, however, individuals or institutions who are not strictly party to the patient–physician relationship will make claims that also have merit. Whether these claims should ever be decisive when a difficult problem is addressed will depend on a close examination of the ethical principles involved in the case at hand.

Guidelines for Decision-Making

Often more than one course of action may be morally justifiable based on an examination of basic principles. At times, no course of action will seem acceptable, because each may result in significant harms. Nevertheless, one of the available options must be selected and its choice supported with ethical reasoning. Attempts to resolve such difficulties can be aided by a rational analysis of the various factors involved. In addition, the involvement of individuals with a variety of backgrounds and perspectives can be useful when ethical questions are being addressed. Consultation with those from related services or with a hospital ethics committee can be very helpful in ensuring that all viewpoints and possibilities are considered as a decision is made (7).

It is important for the individual physician to develop a decision-making scheme that can be consistently applied when ethical dilemmas are faced. An approach consisting of a series of logical steps can aid the practitioner in approaching an ethical problem. Several useful schemes have been proposed (2, 4, 8, 9), elements of which are incorporated here.

1. *Identify the decision-makers*. The first step in addressing any question is to answer the question "Whose decision is it?" In general, the ultimate decision-making power rests with the patient.
   a. At times the patient's ability to make a decision is not clear. A person's capacity to make a decision depends on that person's ability to understand information and use it, based on a coherent system of values, to come to a decision about a course of action. In contrast, competence and incompetence are legal determinations that may or may not truly reflect functional capacity. Assessment of a patient's capacity to make decisions must at times be made by professionals with expertise in making such determinations. Decisions about competence can be made only in a court of law.
   b. If a patient is thought to be incapable of making a decision or has been found legally incompetent, a surrogate decision-maker must be identified. This person should be in a position to act for and to promote the best interests of the patient. The physician does not automatically become the decision-maker. Traditionally, family members have been called upon to render proxy decisions. In some situations, the court may be called upon to appoint a guardian. The physician, however, has an obligation to assist those representing the patient in examining the issues and reaching a resolution.
   c. Two primary criteria exist according to which proxy decisions are made. In the case where information is available that reveals what a patient would have chosen in like circumstances were she still able to express self-will, a substituted judgment can be offered. This process comes as close as possible to respecting the autonomy of the person involved. In some jurisdictions, this concept has been formalized by the living will or by the durable power of attorney. If a substituted judgment is not possible because prior statements from the patient are not available, the proxy decision-maker should make the decision that will promote the best interests of the patient. Whatever information is available about the patient will help to define what that person would have considered "good."
   d. In the obstetric setting, a pregnant woman is generally considered the appropriate decision-maker for the fetus she is carrying.
2. *Collect data, establish facts*.
   a. It is important to be aware that decisions about what may or may not be relevant or important to a case are based on personal values. One should remain as objective as possible when collecting the basic information on which a decision will be based.
   b. Use consultants to ensure that all available information about the diagnosis and prognosis has been obtained.
3. *Identify all major options*.
   a. Make an effort to identify all major options, even those that may initially appear to be morally unreasonable.
   b. Use consultation to ensure that all major options have been considered.
4. *Evaluate options according to the values and principles involved*.
   a. Start by gathering information about the values of the involved parties, trying to get a sense of the perspective and values each is bringing to the discussion. The values of the decision-maker will be the most important as decision-making proceeds.
   b. Decide whether any of the options violate ethical principles that all agree are important. Eliminate those options that, after analysis, are found to be morally unacceptable by all parties.
   c. Reexamine the remaining options according to the interests and values of each party. Some alternatives may be successfully combined.

d. Weigh the ethical consequences of each option—of the action itself and of the foreseeable outcomes.

5. *Identify ethical conflicts and try to set priorities.*
   a. Try to define the problem in terms of the ethical principles involved, eg, wanting to treat a woman's carcinoma (beneficence) versus respecting her desire not to spend her remaining time in pain and in the hospital (autonomy, nonmaleficence).
   b. Weigh the principles underlying each of the arguments made. Does one of the principles appear more important than others as the conflict is examined? Does one proposed course of action therefore seem to have more merit than the others?
   c. Consider respected opinions about similar cases and decide to what extent they can be useful in addressing the current problem. Look for morally relevant differences and similarities between this and other cases. Usually, it will be found that the basic dilemma at hand is not a new one and that points considered by others in resolving past dilemmas can be useful.
6. *Select the option that can be best justified.* Try to arrive at a rational resolution to the problem, one that can be justified to others in terms of ethical principles with universal appeal.
7. *Reevaluate the decision after it is acted upon.* Repeat the evaluation of the major options in light of information gained during the implementation of the decision. Was the best possible decision made? What lessons can be learned from the discussion and resolution of the problem?

Summary

As physicians become more familiar with the discipline of medical ethics, with its fundamental principles and its associated concepts or norms, they will be less troubled when faced with clinical decisions requiring not only expert medical judgement but also insight into the ways in which personal values and goals affect the choices made. By approaching complex ethical situations in a logical and organized fashion, the physician increases the likelihood that all relevant factors will be considered. Close examination of competing principles or conflicting obligations will often tip the balance and allow a resolution. Crystal-clear solutions to difficult ethical dilemmas, however, are rarely achieved. What can be sought in examining a particular case is a point at which, in light of the values and goals of the individuals involved, some agreement as to the relative weight of competing principles can be reached and a decision made.

REFERENCES

1. President's Commission for the Study of Ethical Problems in Medicine and Biomedical and Behavioral Research. Deciding to forego life-sustaining treatment: a report on the ethical, medical, and legal issues in treatment decisions. Washington, DC: U.S. Government Printing Office, 1983
2. Pellegrino ED. The anatomy of clinical–ethical judgements in perinatology and neonatology: a substantive and procedural framework. Semin Perinatol 1987;11(3): 202–209
3. Beauchamp TL, Childress JF. Principles of biomedical ethics. 3rd ed. New York: Oxford University Press, 1989
4. Jonsen AR, Siegler M, Winslade WJ. Clinical ethics: a practical approach to ethical decisions in clinical medicine. 2nd ed. New York: Macmillan, 1986
5. Schloendorff v Society of New York Hospitals, 211 NY 125, 126; 105 NE 92, 93 (1914)
6. American College of Obstetricians and Gynecologists. Patient choice: maternal–fetal conflict. ACOG Committee Opinion 55. Washington, DC: ACOG, 1987
7. American College of Obstetricians and Gynecologists. Endorsement of institutional ethics committees. ACOG Committee Opinion 46. Washington, DC: ACOG, 1985
8. Kanoti GA. Ethics and medical–ethical decisions. Crit Care Clin 1986;2(1):3–12
9. Abrams FR. Bioethical considerations for high-risk pregnancy. In: Abrams RS, Wexler P, eds. Medical care of the pregnant patient, Boston: Little, Brown, 1983:1–12

RESOURCES

Organizations

Kennedy Institute of Ethics, Georgetown University, Washington, DC 20057 (site of the National Reference Center for Bioethics Literature, 1-800-MED-ETHX)

The Hastings Center, 255 Elm Road, Briarcliffe Manor, NY 10510; (914) 762-8500

Society for Health and Human Values, 6728 Old McLean Village Drive, McLean, VA 22101; (703) 556-9222

Online Data Bases

BIOETHICSLINE, searchable through the MEDLARS network. For information, contact the National Library of Medicine, 1-800-638-8480

MEDLINE, searchable through most medical libraries

Bibliographies

The Hastings Center's Bibliography of Ethics, Biomedicine and Professional Responsibility. Frederick, MD: University Publications of America, 1984

Walters L, Kahn TJ, eds. Bibliography of bioethics. Washington, DC: Kennedy Institute of Ethics (issued annually)

Journals

American Journal of Law and Medicine
Bioethics
Hastings Center Report
Journal of Medical Ethics
Journal of Medicine and Philosophy

Books and Special Publications

Beauchamp TL, Childress JF. Principles of biomedical ethics. 3rd ed. New York: Oxford University Press, 1989

Beauchamp TL, McCullough LB. Medical ethics: the moral responsibilities of physicians. Englewood Cliffs, New Jersey: Prentice-Hall, 1984

Beauchamp TL, Walters L. Contemporary issues in bioethics. 3rd ed. Belmont, California: Wadsworth Publishing Co., 1989

Elias S, Annas GJ. Reproductive genetics and the law. Chicago: Year Book Medical Publishers, 1987

Engelhardt HT. The foundations of bioethics. New York: Oxford University Press, 1986

Ethics Committee of the American Fertility Society. Ethical considerations of the new reproductive technologies. Fertil Steril 1986;46(suppl 1)

Hastings Center. Guidelines on the termination of life-sustaining treatment and the care of the dying. Bloomington, Indiana: Indiana University Press, 1987

Jonsen AR, Siegler M, Winslade WJ. Clinical ethics: a practical approach to ethical decisions in clinical medicine. 2nd ed. New York: Macmillan, 1986

Reich WT, ed. Encyclopedia of bioethics. New York: Free Press, 1978

President's Commission Reports

Published by the President's Commission for the Study of Ethical Problems in Medicine and Biomedical and Behavioral Research. Available from the U.S. Government Printing Office, Washington, DC 20402; (202) 783-3238, and in many libraries. Reports issued include the following:

- Deciding to Forego Life-Sustaining Treatment, 1983
- Making Health Care Decisions, 1982–83
- Screening and Counseling for Genetic Conditions, 1983
- Securing Access to Health Care, 1983
- Summing Up: The Ethical and Legal Problems in Medicine and Biomedical and Behavioral Research, 1983

ACOG Committee on Ethics

Committee Opinions are available through the College. Subjects addressed include informed consent, sterilization, maternal–fetal conflict, withholding and withdrawing life-sustaining therapy, in vitro fertilization, abortion, surrogacy, sterilization of mentally handicapped women, expert testimony, relationships with industry and commercial ventures, and pregnancy counseling.

This Technical Bulletin was developed under the direction of the Committee on Technical Bulletins of the American College of Obstetricians and Gynecologists as an educational aid to obstetricians and gynecologists. The committee wishes to thank Elena A. Gates, MD, for her assistance in the development of this bulletin. This Technical Bulletin does not define a standard of care, nor is it intended to dictate an exclusive course of management. It presents recognized methods and techniques of clinical practice for consideration by obstetrician–gynecologists for incorporation into their practices. Variations of practice taking into account the needs of the individual patient, resources, and limitations unique to the institution or type of practice may be appropriate.

THE AMERICAN COLLEGE OF OBSTETRICIANS AND GYNECOLOGISTS
409 12th Street, SW
Washington, DC 20024-2188

6789/98

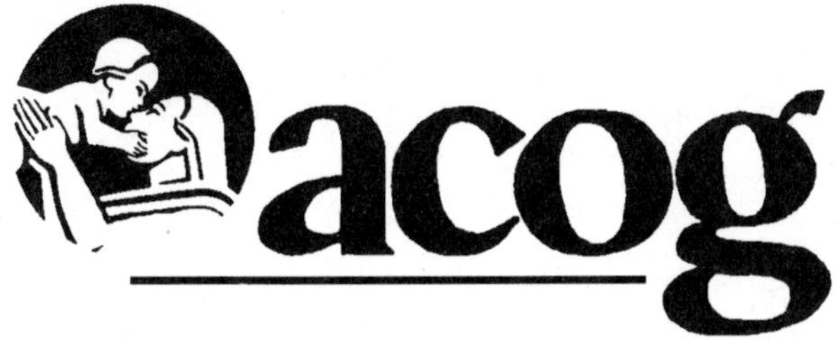

Number 203—March 1995
(Replaces #103, April 1987)

Technical Bulletin

An Educational Aid to Obstetrician–Gynecologists

Evaluation and Treatment of Hirsute Women

Hirsutism is androgen-stimulated excessive hair growth. It generally occurs in the midline. The term *virilization* includes hirsutism accompanied by recession of the temporal hairline, deepening of the voice, loss of female body contour, development of a male-type pubic hair pattern, enlargement of the clitoris, or some or all of the above. True hirsutism must be distinguished from hypertrichosis, which is the presence of increased terminal hairs on the extremities in the absence of excess androgen.

Hirsutism can signal significant metabolic alterations that should be recognized and targeted for management once the risks and benefits of treatment have been considered. Associated abnormal menstrual function requires appropriate evaluation because of the propensity of a patient with polycystic ovary syndrome (PCO) to develop endometrial cancer at an early age (1). The significance of hirsutism must be considered on two levels. First, as a sign of exaggerated androgen activity, hirsutism should arouse suspicion of a potentially hormonally active tumor. Ovarian and adrenal androgen-secreting tumors, however, are rare. In most cases, hirsutism signals a dysfunction of androgen secretion. Second, when abnormal hair production is not directly attributable to a specific lesion, the benefit of the cosmetic effect of therapy for the patient must be considered.

Physiology

There are two kinds of hair on the body: vellus hairs, which are short, fine, nonpigmented hairs that have not responded to hormones, and terminal hairs, which are long, coarse, pigmented, and, in certain areas of the body, responsive to hormonal influence. The terminal hairs undergo a defined growth cycle that includes a growing phase (anagen), an involutional phase (catagen), and a resting phase (telogen). The number of hairs per unit area of skin is fixed by heredity, and follicle units are developed during early embryogenesis. Because the number and distribution of pilosebaceous units are largely controlled by genetic factors, hirsutism in women occurs more often in some ethnic or racial groups than in others.

An understanding of the factors that control hair growth is necessary to diagnose and treat patients with hirsutism. The endocrinologic factors that influence the pilosebaceous unit (sebaceous gland and the hair follicle) include the following:

- Rate and amount of androgen secretion
- Concentration of sex hormone-binding globulin (SHBG)
- Peripheral conversion of weak androgens to potent androgens (ie, metabolism of androgens)
- Sensitivity of the pilosebaceous unit to androgens

In general, the sebaceous gland is more sensitive to androgens than is the hair follicle. Hyperstimulation of the sebaceous gland accompanied by bacterial infection results in acne and, rarely, hidradenitis suppurativa. Androgenic stimulation of the hair follicle can transform some vellus hairs into terminal hairs. Once the conversion from vellus to terminal hair takes place, the terminal hair grows and sheds cyclically. This cycle is partially independent of hormonal stimulation or control.

A certain amount of androgenic stimulation is expected in the normal woman. The increased rate of production of androgens that occurs at puberty induces acne and the appearance of terminal hair on the extremities, axilla, and pubis. Pronounced androgenization results in virilization.

The ovary secretes the androgens androstenedione (0.8–1.6 mg/d) and dehydroepiandrosterone (0.3–3.0 mg/d), whereas the adrenal gland secretes primarily dehydroepiandrosterone and its sulfate (DHEAS) (6–8 mg/d) and androstenedione (0.8–1.6 mg/d) (2). Testosterone is secreted in approximately equal quantities by the ovary and adrenal gland and is also converted from androgen precursors in the periphery. When it is present in excessive concentrations, the source frequently involves the ovary and the adrenal gland.

Therefore, simultaneous determinations of testosterone, androstenedione, and DHEAS concentrations in serum may provide some clue to the source of excessive androgen. For example, if the concentrations of testosterone and androstenedione in serum are elevated while that of DHEAS is normal, it is likely that the ovaries, not the adrenal gland, are the major source. Many clinicians do not measure androstenedione because concentrations fluctuate widely even in normal women. From a clinical standpoint, it is not usually necessary to perform elaborate testing in hirsute women to determine the source of androgen secretion. During states of estrogen deficiency (eg, menopause), altered estrogen/androgen ratios may result in mild hirsutism.

Etiology

On the basis of factors known to control hair growth, the etiology of hirsutism can be ascribed to abnormalities that result in the following:

- Altered androgen metabolism
- Increased androgen production
- Decreased androgen binding in the circulation
- Exogenous androgen ingestion

Altered Androgen Metabolism

Among the most common types of hirsutism is idiopathic. Idiopathic hirsutism appears to be caused by an increased conversion of testosterone to dihydrotestosterone (DHT) locally in the skin and not by an increase in the number of androgen receptors (3).

Increased Androgen Production

The adrenal glands and the ovaries are the only sex steroid-secreting glands in adult women. There are two mechanisms by which these glands produce excess androgen: 1) hypersecretion of precursors that are converted to testosterone at other sites and 2) direct secretion of testosterone or conversion to DHT by 5α-reductase (3). Either DHT or its metabolites or both are believed to be the active forms of testosterone in many androgen-sensitive tissues. Pathologic conditions of the ovaries and the adrenal glands that result in increased androgen production can vary from malignant tumors to benign alterations in steroid metabolism.

Adrenal Glands

Adrenal abnormalities that result in excessive androgen production are relatively uncommon, although dysfunctional excess androgen secretion is common. Disorders include virilizing congenital adrenal hyperplasia, Cushing syndrome, and androgen-secreting neoplasms. Virilizing congenital adrenal hyperplasia is most commonly caused by a deficiency of steroid 21-hydroxylase or, much less commonly, 11-hydroxylase or 3β-hydroxy-Δ^5-steroid dehydrogenase. In Cushing syndrome, adrenal androgen overproduction occurs in association with hypersecretion of cortisol. Androgen-secreting neoplasms are exceedingly rare.

In addition, the adrenal gland is enriched with prolactin receptors; patients with hyperprolactinemia might experience excessive stimulation of adrenal androgen biosynthesis (4). Although up to 40% of patients with hyperprolactinemia and a macroadenoma may have increased secretion of androgens from the adrenal gland, peripheral action of androgens is limited by the blocking action of prolactin on the conversion of testosterone to DHT and its metabolites. As a result, hirsutism is relatively uncommon and, if present, mild in hyperprolactinemic patients.

Ovaries

The most common cause of excessive androgen production is PCO, which is often characterized by menstrual aberration and variable degrees of excessive androgen, often dating from puberty. Hyperthecosis may represent the most severe form of PCO and may result in hirsutism and virilization.

Insulin resistance also may be associated with excessive androgen effect. Many patients with PCO are now known to demonstrate insulin resistance regardless of whether they are obese. Hyperandrogenism, insulin resistance, and acanthosis nigricans (a velvet, pigmented skin lesion located in intertriginous regions) are common in hyperandrogenic patients. The physician should be alert to the presence of significant metabolic abnormalities (dyslipidemia, hyperuricemia, carbohydrate intolerance, diabetes mellitus, hypertension, or hypercoagulation). Acanthosis nigricans is common in hirsute women. It is most commonly seen on the vulva (5) and may be seen in a variety of benign and malignant conditions.

Any ovarian neoplasm (primary or metastatic) can stimulate the stroma and cause excessive androgen production. About 5–6% of ovarian tumors have functional activity (6), and most of the functioning neoplasms are of the sex-cord stromal type. This type of neoplasm includes Sertoli–Leydig cell tumors, granulosa cell tumors, and gynandroblastomas.

Decreased Androgen Binding in the Circulation

Almost all androgens in the circulation are bound to SHBG or albumin. Only the free androgen is biologically active. In general, estrogens increase and androgens decrease hepatic synthesis of SHBG. Thus, a relative increase in free testosterone may lead to hirsutism, as may estrogen deficiency.

Exogenous Androgens

Adding androgens to estrogen replacement therapy has been associated with hirsutism and frank virilization. Androgen-containing creams used for the treatment of vulvar dystrophies also have been associated with symptoms of excessive androgen, as has danazol, used for the treatment of endometriosis (7). Oral contraceptives that contain norgestrel have been implicated in the development of symptoms of mild androgen excess (7). The use of anabolic steroids, alone or in combination, can cause hirsutism.

Evaluation

Women with excessive hair growth should be evaluated. The initial history and physical examination will often give a clue as to the cause. An effort should be made to document objectively the extent of the findings by a detailed description or photographs. Any evidence of virilization should be noted. One common method for objectively assessing the severity of hirsutism is the Ferriman–Gallwey system (8). Perhaps more practical is the approach of Bardin and Lipsett, which assigns scores of 1+ each for upper lip, chin, and temporal hair and 4+ for a complete beard (9).

Laboratory Studies

The purpose of laboratory evaluation is to rule out androgen-producing tumors. Several laboratory tests are available for this purpose, and some are more helpful than others. The basic laboratory studies should include determinations of total testosterone and DHEAS (Fig. 1). Concentrations of total testosterone in serum correlate poorly with the degree of hirsutism or virilization. A determination of testosterone concentration in serum is important, however, because values greater than 200 ng/dl are usually found in the presence of a tumor. Measurement of DHEAS in plasma provides a means of assessing adrenal function. A DHEAS concentration of greater than 700 μg/dl (greater than two times normal) is usually present with an adrenal androgen-secreting tumor.

Several notable exceptions to the algorithm shown in Fig. 1 should be considered: Cushing syndrome, hyperprolactinemia, and adult-onset congenital adrenal hyperplasia. Cushing syndrome may be manifested by truncal obesity, purple striae over the abdomen, buffalo hump, hypertension, easy bruisability, or some combination of these symptoms. In patients with physical signs of cortisol excess, an overnight suppression test with dexamethasone should be performed as follows. After the patient ingests 1 mg of dexamethasone orally at 11 PM, a blood sample should be obtained to measure the 8-AM cortisol value. It should be less than 5 μg/dl. Alternatively, urine may be collected for a 24-hour period, and measurements of free cortical and creatinine clearance can be obtained. False-

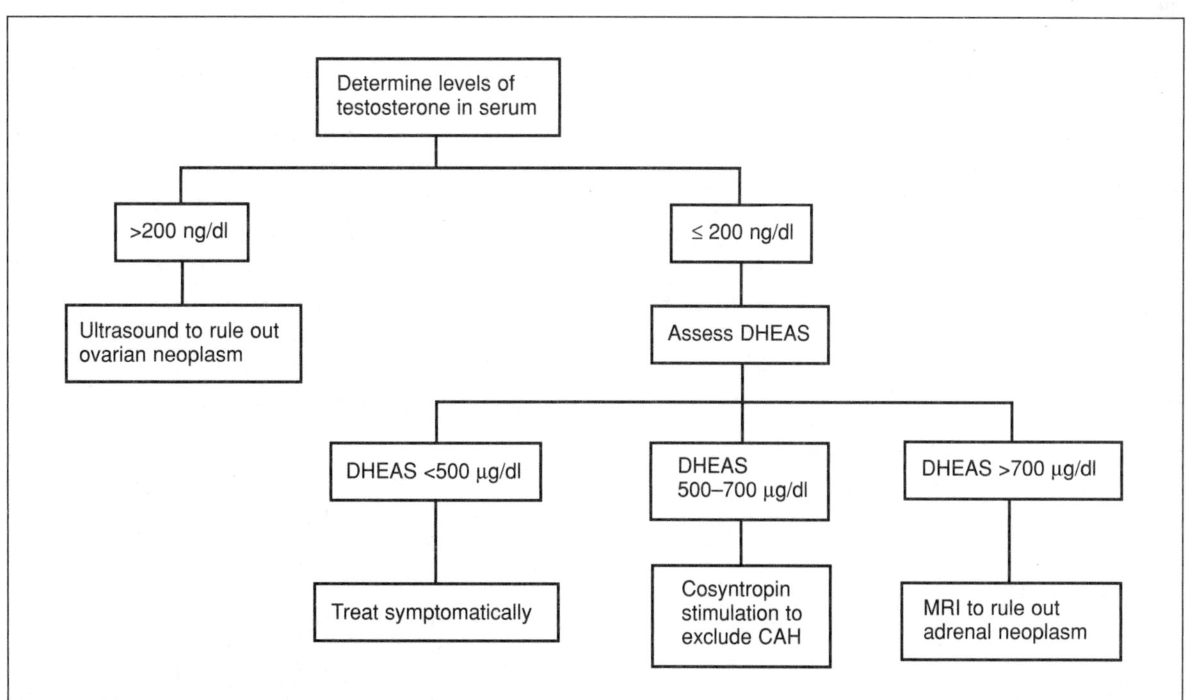

FIG. 1. Laboratory assessment for the diagnosis of hirsutism. Abbreviations: DHEAS indicates dehydroepiandrosterone sulfate; CAH, congenital adrenal hyperplasia; MRI, magnetic resonance imaging.

positive results may occur in obese patients and patients suffering from depression or anorexia nervosa. More extensive evaluation may be warranted in these patients.

Hyperprolactinemia is a rare cause of hirsutism. When it is suggested by amenorrhea or galactorrhea, serum levels of prolactin should be determined.

The third exception to the algorithm is nonclassical adrenal 21-hydroxylase deficiency. Measurements of 17α-hydroxyprogesterone levels both in the basal state and following corticotropin stimulation (ACTH [cosyntropin] stimulation) may be warranted in hirsute women of certain racial groups (Ashkenazi Jews and Eskimos) and in others in whom the incidence of nonclassical 21-hydroxylase deficiency is increased. Women at increased risk include those with severe hirsutism since puberty or a strong family history of hirsutism, those who are shorter than other family members, and those with evidence of defeminization (eg, decrease in breast size). The cost-effectiveness of routine ACTH stimulation in other than high-risk populations has not been demonstrated clearly, especially in view of the fact that large series have demonstrated nonclassical 21-hydroxylase deficiency in only 2–5% of hirsute women (10, 11). Many clinicians screen for this disorder by using an 8-AM 17α-hydroxyprogesterone determination. Values of greater than 4 ng/ml diagnose the condition; it must be remembered, however, that 17α-hydroxyprogesterone is normally elevated in the early luteal phase of ovulatory women and in some forms of PCO. Values of less than 2 ng/ml suggest that nonclassical 21-hydroxylase deficiency is highly unlikely, and values between 2 and 4 ng/ml may be followed up by an ACTH stimulation test (12).

Other Diagnostic Procedures

Several additional diagnostic tests have been suggested as being potentially useful in localizing the site of excess androgen production. They include selective ovarian and adrenal vein catheterization and iodocholesterol scanning. With the availability of ultrasonography to evaluate the ovaries and magnetic resonance image scanning to assess the adrenal glands, these tests are rarely, if ever, indicated.

Measurement of 3α-androstanediol glucuronide in serum has been suggested to determine whether there is increased metabolism of testosterone in hair follicles. Clinical usefulness of this test, however, has not been established.

Because metabolic problems are very common in hirsute patients and because hirsute women often have clusters of risk factors for coronary vascular disease, lipoprotein lipid profiles and evaluations for altered insulin sensitivity and carbohydrate metabolism are in order, particularly for obese hirsute patients (13, 14). Primary cardiovascular and diabetes risk prevention should be practiced once risk factors are recognized.

Treatment

Hirsutism is a sign and not a specific disease. Once an androgen-producing tumor, Cushing syndrome, and congenital adrenal hyperplasia have been ruled out, treatment should focus on the patient's wishes. She should be alerted that her condition is chronic but can be controlled. The patient should be told at the outset that successful treatment will take several months to become apparent because of the physiology of hair growth. Options for treatment include medical therapy and cosmetic-based temporary and permanent hair removal. Temporary methods of hair removal do not alter the rate of hair growth.

The success of medical treatment depends on the severity of the symptoms. Medical treatment is generally successful in limiting new hair growth but does not affect existing hair, which should be controlled by mechanical depilatory methods. The mainstay of medical therapy is low-dose combination oral contraceptives, which effectively suppress ovarian function and reduce ovarian androgen secretion. Moreover, the estrogen in oral contraceptives stimulates hepatic synthesis of SHBG and results in greater binding of testosterone, thus limiting its bioavailability. Oral contraceptives decrease plasma ACTH and thus also reduce adrenal androgen secretion (15). Symptomatic postmenopausal patients may benefit from hormone replacement therapy.

A number of other medications also have been shown to have value in the treatment of patients with hirsutism. Spironolactone, a medication approved by the U.S. Food and Drug Administration for the treatment of hypertension, inhibits a number of enzymes important in androgen synthesis and action. It appears to compete directly at the androgen-receptor level. A daily dose of 100–200 mg is often effective in causing a repression of hirsutism as measured by the diameter and density of hair follicles and in the rate of facial hair growth (16). Other than initial diuresis, late mastodynia, and irregular menses, side effects are minimal. Because ovulation may occur with androgen suppression and because the effects of spironolactone on a developing fetus are unknown, effective contraception is needed. Low-dose combination oral contraceptives and spironolactone are commonly prescribed together. Creams that contain spironolactone or its active metabolite canrenone are now undergoing testing and appear to be effective in treating localized hirsutism.

Long-acting gonadotropin-releasing hormone analogues (both agonists and antagonists) suppress gonadotropin secretion and produce a "medical oophorectomy." Studies are under way to determine how effective these agents are in treating ovarian hyperandrogenism and hirsutism.

Because in most cases of hirsutism the problem is ovarian, routine use of glucocorticoids to achieve adrenal suppression is not warranted in the treatment of hirsutism. Glucocorticoids are sometimes effective when used for mixed sources of hyperandrogenism. However, glucocorticoids have not been shown to be more effective than other agents used to treat hirsutism, and adrenal suppression is potentially serious. For anovulatory women who have slightly elevated levels of DHEAS, glucocorticoids (dexamethasone, 0.25–0.5 mg orally at bedtime) may be effective in inducing ovulation when added to clomiphene citrate. Routine treatment with glucocorticoids is indicated only in patients with a documented deficiency of 21-hydroxylase, 11β-hydroxylase, or 3β-hydroxysteroid dehydrogenase-isomerase.

Cyproterone acetate, a potent progestational agent as well as an antiandrogen, is used throughout the world in a number of cyclic regimens with ethinyl estradiol so that regular withdrawal bleeding occurs. It has not been approved for use in the United States. Significant side effects include decreased libido and mental depression. It appears to control hirsutism in 50–75% of women, but there is no evidence that cyproterone is any more effective than spironolactone in this regard.

The antifungal agent ketoconazole also blocks androgen synthesis and may be effective, but there are concerns about its side effects. Studies are also under way to examine the effectiveness and safety of other 5α-reductase inhibitors such as flutamide.

Surgical removal of the ovaries is rarely warranted in the treatment of ovarian hyperandrogenism. Perhaps the only circumstance in which it may be warranted is in patients with severe hirsutism clearly ovarian in origin who have completed childbearing and whose condition is resistant to the various medical therapies available.

REFERENCES

1. Dahlgren E, Friberg L-G, Johansson S, Lindström B, Odén A, Samsioe G, et al. Endometrial carcinoma; ovarian dysfunction—a risk factor in young women. Eur J Obstet Gynecol Reprod Biol 1991;41:143–150
2. Biberoglu K, Behrman SJ. Hirsutism: diagnostic approach and stimulation-suppression dynamics of androgens in the female. Int J Fertil 1982;27:146–152
3. Horton R, Hawks D, Lobo R. 3α, 17β-androstanediol glucuronide in plasma: a marker of androgen action in idiopathic hirsutism. J Clin Invest 1982;69:1203–1206
4. Glickman SP, Rosenfield RL, Bergenstal RM, Helke J. Multiple androgenic abnormalities, including elevated free testosterone, in hyperprolactinemic women. J Clin Endocrinol Metab 1982;55:251–257
5. Grasinger CC, Wild RA, Parker IJ. Vulvar acanthosis nigricans: a marker for insulin resistance in hirsute women. Fertil Steril 1993;59:583–586
6. Norris HJ, Chorlton I. Functioning tumors of the ovary. Clin Obstet Gynecol 1974;17(1):189–228
7. Bates GW, Cornwell CE. Iatrogenic causes of hirsutism. Clin Obstet Gynecol 1991;34:848–851
8. Ferriman D, Gallwey JD. Clinical assessment of body hair growth in women. J Clin Endocrinol Metab 1961;21:1440–1447
9. Bardin CW, Lipsett MB. Testosterone and androstenedione blood production rates in normal women and women with idiopathic hirsutism or polycystic ovaries. J Clin Invest 1967;46:891–902
10. Lobo RA, Goebelsmann U. Adult manifestation of congenital adrenal hyperplasia due to incomplete 21-hydroxylase deficiency mimicking polycystic ovarian disease. Am J Obstet Gynecol 1980;138:720–726
11. Chrousos GP, Loriaux DL, Mann DL, Cutler GB Jr. Late-onset 21-hydroxylase deficiency mimicking idiopathic hirsutism or polycystic ovarian disease. Ann Intern Med 1982;96:143–148
12. Siegel SF, Finegold DN, Lanes R, Lee PA. ACTH stimulation tests and plasma dehydroepiandrosterone sulfate levels in women with hirsutism. N Engl J Med 1990;323:849–854
13. Wild RA, Painter PC, Coulson PB, Carruth KB, Ranney GB. Lipoprotein lipid concentrations and cardiovascular risk in women with polycystic ovary syndrome. J Clin Endocrinol Metab 1985;61:946–951
14. Wild RA, Grubb B, Hartz A, VanNort JJ, Bachman W, Bartholomew M. Clinical signs of androgen excess as risk factors for coronary artery disease. Fertil Steril 1990;54:255–259
15. Wild RA, Umstot ES, Andersen RN, Givens JR. Adrenal function in hirsutism. II. Effect of an oral contraceptive. J Clin Endocrinol Metab 1982;54:676–681
16. Cumming DC, Yang JC, Rebar RW, Yen SSC. Treatment of hirsutism with spironolactone. JAMA 1982;247:1295–1298

SUGGESTED READING

Yen SSC. Chronic anovulation caused by peripheral endocrine disorders. In: Yen SSC, Jaffe RB, eds. Reproductive endocrinology: physiology, pathophysiology, and clinical management. 3rd ed. Philadelphia: WB Saunders Co, 1991;576–630

This Technical Bulletin was developed under the direction of the Committee on Technical Bulletins of the American College of Obstetricians and Gynecologists as an educational aid to obstetricians and gynecologists. The committee wishes to thank Robert A. Wild, MD, for his assistance in the development of this bulletin. This Technical Bulletin does not define a standard of care, nor is it intended to dictate an exclusive course of management. It presents recognized methods and techniques of clinical practice for consideration by obstetrician–gynecologists for incorporation into their practices. Variations of practice taking into account the needs of the individual patient, resources, and limitations unique to the institution or type of practice may be appropriate.

ISSN 1074-8628

THE AMERICAN COLLEGE OF OBSTETRICIANS AND GYNECOLOGISTS
409 12th Street, SW
Washington, DC 20024-2188

12345/98765

Number 189—February 1994

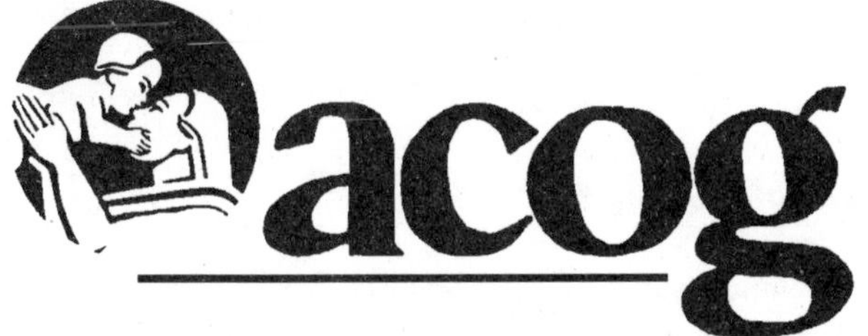

Technical Bulletin

An Educational Aid to Obstetrician–Gynecologists

Exercise During Pregnancy and the Postpartum Period

Physical fitness and active recreation are integral parts of the life styles of many women. In the absence of obstetric or medical complications, pregnant women who engage in a moderate level of physical activity can maintain cardiorespiratory and muscular fitness throughout pregnancy and the postpartum period. Pregnancy-related physiologic changes, however, may interfere with the ability to engage safely in some forms of physical activities. The obstetrician is in a position to advise the pregnant patient of such physical limitations and to explain the available information regarding the effects of exercise during pregnancy as well as uncertainties in the current state of knowledge.

The American College of Obstetricians and Gynecologists has issued guidelines for women who exercise, most of which also apply to exercise during pregnancy (1). This Technical Bulletin will outline specific recommendations and concerns unique for pregnant women and their physiologic bases.

Cardiovascular Changes

Pregnancy induces profound alterations in maternal hemodynamics. Such changes include an increase in blood volume, cardiac output, and resting pulse and a decrease in systemic vascular resistance (2–4). Hemodynamic changes are also significantly influenced by body position during pregnancy (5). Cardiac output in third-trimester pregnancy is maximal with the subject in the left or right lateral recumbent position. In contrast, after the first trimester, the supine position results in relative obstruction of venous return by the enlarging uterus and a significant decrease in cardiac output. In some women, such decreases in cardiac output may be symptomatic, resulting in supine hypotensive syndrome. In addition, during pregnancy, motionless standing is associated with an even greater decrease in cardiac output than that seen in the supine position (5).

Conflicting evidence exists concerning maternal heart rate response to steady-state aerobic exercise during pregnancy; both blunted and normal responses to weight-bearing and non-weight-bearing exercise have been reported (6, 7). The responses of both stroke volume and cardiac output to steady-state exercise, however, are significantly increased (6, 7). Exercise during pregnancy also induces a greater degree of hemoconcentration than does exercise in the nonpregnant state (7). ST segment depression has been noted in 12% of patients in response to strenuous bicycle exercise both before and during pregnancy, without apparent clinical sequelae (8). Because this depression has had no adverse clinical sequelae, it appears to be related to heart rate, not ischemia, and is similar to those effects observed with tocolytic therapy with beta-mimetics (9).

Respiratory Changes

During pregnancy, minute ventilation increases by almost 50%, largely as a result of increased tidal volume (10, 11). This results in an increase in arterial oxygen tension to 106–108 mm Hg in the first trimester, decreasing to a mean of 101–106 mm Hg by the third trimester (12). There is an associated increase in oxygen uptake, and a 10–20% increase in baseline oxygen consumption. Physiologic dead space during pregnancy remains unchanged (11, 13, 14). During treadmill exercise in pregnancy, arteriovenous O_2 difference is decreased (6). Comparative physiologic studies in pregnancy between weight-bearing and non-weight-bearing exercise indicate further hyperventilation during strenuous exercise in the latter (15).

Because of the increased resting oxygen requirements and the increased work of breathing brought about by physical effects of the enlarged uterus on the diaphragm, there is decreased oxygen available for the performance of aerobic exercise during pregnancy. Thus, both subjective workload and maximum exercise performance are decreased (10, 16). However, in some fit women, there do not appear to be associated changes in maximum aerobic power or acid–base balance during exercise in pregnancy when compared with the nonpregnant state (2, 13, 17).

Mechanical Changes

The enlargement of the uterus and breasts that occurs during normal pregnancy results in a shift in the physical center of gravity in the pregnant woman. Because balance may be affected, such changes must be kept in mind when considering physical activity in which balance is an important concern or in which loss of balance may prove dangerous (2). While, theoretically, hormonal influences may result in generalized increases in joint laxity, predisposing the pregnant woman to mechanical trauma or sprains, this hypothesis has been substantiated by objective data only with regard to the metacarpophalangeal joints (18).

Thermoregulatory Changes

Both basal metabolic rate and heat production increase during pregnancy (19). Moderate aerobic exercise is associated with significant increases in core body temperature in nonpregnant individuals (2). In one study of nonpregnant women exercising at 70% of maximal effort on a treadmill for 20 minutes, the core body temperature rose by an average of 1.5°C.

Data regarding the effects of exercise on core temperature during pregnancy are limited (2). Fit individuals are known to thermoregulate their core temperature more efficiently. Fetal temperature remains approximately 1°C above that of the mother. In studies of pregnant animals, an increase in maternal core body temperature during embryogenesis exceeding 1.5°C has been observed to cause cessation of neuronal mitotic cell growth in the ependymal layer of the developing brain (20). Such findings have suggested a possible maternal threshold for human teratogenesis of 39.2°C, possibly accounting for observed increases in congenital anomalies associated with hot tub use in early pregnancy (20, 21). It appears that in fit women, during pregnancy, the peak rectal temperature following exercise at an intensity of 64% of maximum oxygen consumption decreases by 0.3°C at 8 weeks and falls further at a rate of 0.1°C per month through 37 weeks of gestation (22). Thus, the magnitude of exercise-associated thermal stress for the embryo and fetus may be reduced by maternal physiologic adaptation to pregnancy. Indeed, there has been no demonstrated increase in neural tube or other birth defects among pregnancies of women who continue to perform even vigorous exercise during early pregnancy (2, 16).

Metabolic Changes

Approximately 300 extra kilocalories per day are required to meet the metabolic needs of pregnancy (2, 15, 16). This caloric requirement is increased further in pregnant women who exercise regularly. Such concerns do not appear to be significant for most exercising pregnant women. Pregnant women have lower fasting blood glucose levels than do nonpregnant women. In addition, pregnant women utilize carbohydrates during exercise at a greater rate than do their nonpregnant counterparts (23). Thus, hypoglycemia is more likely to occur both during a resting, fasting state and during exercise in pregnancy. On the cellular level, exercise induces substrate mobilization, while pregnancy is associated with increased tissue storage of fat. These opposing physiologic events could theoretically limit fetal substrate availability (16). Thus, adequate carbohydrate intake for exercising pregnant patients is essential. In fact, the use of exercise to treat or prevent hyperglycemia in pregnancies complicated by gestational diabetes or insulin-dependent diabetes is currently being investigated (24, 25).

Fetal Response

Exercise induces significant increases in levels of both epinephrine and serum norepinephrine (2, 26). While epinephrine tends to inhibit uterine activity, norepinephrine increases both the amplitude and frequency of spontaneous uterine contractions. These changes do not necessarily negate one another, and the increased levels of norepinephrine have the potential to cause significant uterine activity or to precipitate preterm labor in individuals at risk for this complication. Although one study found an association between strenuous physical work and an increased incidence of preterm birth, effects of recreational exercise were not examined (27). In a second study, there was a trend toward a decrease in preterm birth among women who exercised (28). It appears that in the majority of healthy pregnant women without additional risk factors for preterm labor, exercise does not increase either baseline uterine activity or the incidence of preterm labor or delivery (29, 30).

During exercise at moderate intensity, overall visceral–splanchnic blood flow diminishes by 50% (31). A specific 20–25% decrease in myometrial clearance of labelled sodium was noted in nonpregnant women during short-term, low-intensity bicycle ergometry (32). During pregnancy, however, the increase in blood volume and resting cardiac output and the reduction in systemic vascular resistance may reduce the magnitude of such shunting. Such adverse effects of splanchnic shunting may also be minimized by an increase in oxygen and substrate extraction, which under normal conditions averages only 25–30% of capacity (16). Although changes in uterine blood flow in pregnancy have been studied during exercise using Doppler wave form analysis, the results have been conflicting and no definite conclusions can be drawn in this regard (33, 34).

Several studies have suggested a decrease in birth weight among offspring of women performing heavy work in the standing position during pregnancy (35, 36). A similar decrease in birth weight has been demonstrated in some studies among offspring of women who exercise at high intensities throughout pregnancy (37). This reduction in birth weight averaged 300–350 g and appeared to reflect primarily a decrease in subcutaneous fat in the newborn (37). Intrauterine growth retardation and other deleterious short- or long-term effects of decreased fetal weight have not been documented.

Vigorous maternal exercise is associated with a 5–15-beats-per-minute increase in fetal heart rate (2, 16, 38). Although brief periods of fetal bradycardia have been described anecdotally, such alterations may be motion-induced artifacts associated with Doppler (2). One study using ultrasound to observe fetal heart rate during and after maternal exercise noted fetal bradycardia in less than 1% of patients during exercise. Fetal bradycardia was observed in 19% of patients within 3 minutes after cessation of maximal exercise, but in only 1% after submaximal exercise (39). The investigators concluded that brief submaximal maternal exercise (up to approximately 70% of maternal aerobic power) does not affect fetal heart rate. Adverse fetal effects related to exercise-induced fetal heart rate changes have not been demonstrated in humans (2, 40).

Developing an Exercise Program

Most women who perform regular weight-bearing exercise prior to pregnancy note a progressive decline in performance beginning in early pregnancy (16). In one study involving runners, aerobic dancers, and cross-country skiers, 60% noted significantly decreased exercise performance in early pregnancy, and over 50% had voluntarily stopped exercise completely by the third trimester (41). Only 10% of patients had maintained their performance at or near preconceptional levels throughout pregnancy (42). In another study of well-conditioned runners, overall performance decreased by approximately 10% in early pregnancy followed by a gradual decline to roughly 50% of preconceptional levels by the early third trimester (43). Aerobic capacity, however, was not the only reason for the decline in exercise performance, as many women implicated early pregnancy fatigue, nausea, vomiting, and maternal morphologic changes, especially in the third trimester. Other studies, however, suggest that women who began various forms of non-weight-bearing exercise (cycling or swimming) in early pregnancy were able to maintain a high-intensity, moderate-duration regimen of exercise training throughout the third trimester (41, 44). Thus, the maternal adaptation to both physiologic and morphologic changes appears to favor non-weight-bearing exercise over weight-bearing exercise during pregnancy (15).

Most of the guidelines for designing a general fitness program in women outlined previously by the American College of Obstetricians and Gynecologists also apply to pregnant women (1). An exercise prescription in pregnancy should be individualized and should include a health assessment. However, the physiologic changes occurring during pregnancy described here should lead obstetricians and pregnant women to consider several modifications of these general guidelines. It must be emphasized that none of these recommendations has a firm basis in prospective, randomized, clinical trials. These guidelines follow from a critical analysis of the available physiologic data regarding exercise and pregnancy and represent reasonable extrapolations from such knowledge.

Recommendations for Exercise in Pregnancy and Postpartum

There are no data in humans to indicate that pregnant women should limit exercise intensity and lower target heart rates because of potential adverse effects. For women who do not have any additional risk factors for adverse maternal or perinatal outcome, the following recommendations may be made:

1. During pregnancy, women can continue to exercise and derive health benefits even from mild-to-moderate exercise routines. Regular exercise (at least three times per week) is preferable to intermittent activity.
2. Women should avoid exercise in the supine position after the first trimester. Such a position is associated with decreased cardiac output in most pregnant women; because the remaining cardiac output will be preferentially distributed away from splanchnic beds (including the uterus) during vigorous exercise, such regimens are best avoided during pregnancy. Prolonged periods of motionless standing should also be avoided.
3. Women should be aware of the decreased oxygen available for aerobic exercise during pregnancy. They should be encouraged to modify the intensity of their exercise according to maternal symptoms. Pregnant women should stop exercising when fatigued and not exercise to exhaustion. Weight-bearing exercises may under some circumstances be continued at intensities

similar to those prior to pregnancy throughout pregnancy. Non-weight-bearing exercises such as cycling or swimming will minimize the risk of injury and facilitate the continuation of exercise during pregnancy.

4. Morphologic changes in pregnancy should serve as a relative contraindication to types of exercise in which loss of balance could be detrimental to maternal or fetal well-being, especially in the third trimester. Further, any type of exercise involving the potential for even mild abdominal trauma should be avoided.
5. Pregnancy requires an additional 300 kcal/d in order to maintain metabolic homeostasis. Thus, women who exercise during pregnancy should be particularly careful to ensure an adequate diet.
6. Pregnant women who exercise in the first trimester should augment heat dissipation by ensuring adequate hydration, appropriate clothing, and optimal environmental surroundings during exercise.
7. Many of the physiologic and morphologic changes of pregnancy persist 4–6 weeks postpartum. Thus, prepregnancy exercise routines should be resumed gradually based on a woman's physical capability.

Contraindications to Exercise

The aforementioned recommendations are intended for women who do not have any additional risk factors for adverse maternal or perinatal outcome. A number of medical or obstetric conditions may lead the obstetrician to recommend modifications of these principles. The following conditions should be considered contraindications to exercise during pregnancy:

- Pregnancy-induced hypertension
- Preterm rupture of membranes
- Preterm labor during the prior or current pregnancy or both
- Incompetent cervix/cerclage
- Persistent second- or third-trimester bleeding
- Intrauterine growth retardation

In addition, women with certain other medical or obstetric conditions, including chronic hypertension or active thyroid, cardiac, vascular, or pulmonary disease, should be evaluated carefully in order to determine whether an exercise program is appropriate.

Summary

In the absence of either obstetric or medical complications, pregnant women can continue to exercise and derive related benefits. Women who have achieved cardiovascular fitness prior to pregnancy should be able to safely maintain that level of fitness throughout pregnancy and the postpartum period. Depending on the individual's needs and the physiologic changes associated with pregnancy, women may have to modify their specific exercise regimens. Despite findings that suggest lower birth weights among offspring of women who continue to exercise vigorously throughout pregnancy, there currently are no data to confirm that, with the specific exceptions mentioned here, exercise during pregnancy has any deleterious effects on the fetus. While maternal fitness and sense of well-being may be enhanced by exercise, no level of exercise during pregnancy has been conclusively demonstrated to be beneficial in improving perinatal outcome.

REFERENCES

1. American College of Obstetricians and Gynecologists. Women and exercise. ACOG Technical Bulletin 173. Washington, DC: ACOG, 1992
2. Artal Mittelmark R, Wiswell RA, Drinkwater BL, eds. Exercise in pregnancy. 2nd ed. Baltimore: Williams and Wilkins, 1991
3. Clark SL, Cotton DB, Lee W, Bishop C, Hill T, Southwick J, et al. Central hemodynamic assessment of normal term pregnancy. Am J Obstet Gynecol 1989;161:1439–1442
4. Wolfe LA, Ohtake PJ, Mottola MF, McGrath MJ. Physiological interactions between pregnancy and aerobic exercise. Exerc Sport Sci Rev 1989;17:295–351
5. Clark SL, Cotton DB, Pivarnik JM, Lee W, Hankins GDV, Benedetti TJ, et al. Position change and central hemodynamic profile during normal third-trimester pregnancy and post partum. Am J Obstet Gynecol 1991;164:883–887
6. Pivarnik JM, Lee W, Clark SL, Cotton DB, Spillman HT, Miller JF. Cardiac output responses of primigravid women during exercise determined by the direct Fick technique. Obstet Gynecol 1990;75:954–959
7. McMurray RG, Hackney AC, Katz VL, Gall M, Watson WJ. Pregnancy-induced changes in the maximal physiological responses during swimming. J Appl Physiol 1991; 71:1454–1459
8. van Doorn MB, Lotgering FK, Struijk PC, Pool J, Wallenburg HCS. Maternal and fetal cardiovascular responses to strenuous bicycle exercise. Am J Obstet Gynecol 1992;166;854–859
9. Hendricks SK, Keroes J, Katz M. Electrocardiographic changes associated with ritodrine-induced maternal tachycardia and hypokalemia. Am J Obstet Gynecol 1986;154:921–923
10. Artal R, Wiswell R, Romem Y, Dorey F. Pulmonary responses to exercise in pregnancy. Am J Obstet Gynecol 1986;154:378–383
11. Prowse CM, Gaensler EA. Respiratory and acid–base changes during pregnancy. Anesthesiology 1965;26:381– 392
12. Templeton A, Kelman GR. Maternal blood-gases, $(PA_{O}^{2}—Pa_{O}^{2})$, physiological shunt and *VD/VT* in normal pregnancy. Br J Anaesth 1976;48:1001–1004
13. Pivarnik JM, Lee W, Spillman T, Clark SL, Cotton DB, Miller JF. Maternal respiration and blood gases during aerobic exercise performed at moderate altitude. Med Sci Sports Exerc 1992;24:868–872
14. Sady SP, Carpenter MW, Thompson PD, Sady MA, Haydon B, Coustan DR. Cardiovascular response to cycle exercise during and after pregnancy. J Appl Physiol 1989;66:336–341

15. Artal R, Masaki DI, Khodiguian N, Romem Y, Rutherford SE, Wiswell RA. Exercise prescription in pregnancy: weight-bearing versus non-weight-bearing exercise. Am J Obstet Gynecol 1989; 161:1464–1469

16. Clapp JF III. Exercise in pregnancy: a brief clinical review. Fetal Med Rev 1990;2:89–101

17. Lotgering FK, Van Doorn MB, Struijk PC, Pool J, Wallenburg HCS. Maximal aerobic exercise in pregnant women: heart rate, O_2 consumption, CO_2 production, and ventilation. J Appl Physiol 1991;70:1016–1023

18. Calguneri M, Bird HA, Wright V. Changes in joint laxity occurring during pregnancy. Ann Rheum Dis 1982; 41:126–128

19. Hytten FE. Nutrition. In: Hytten FE, Chamberlain G, eds. Clinical physiology in obstetrics. Oxford: Blackwell, 1980

20. Edwards MJ. Hyperthermia as a teratogen: a review of experimental studies and their clinical significance. Teratogenesis Carcinog Mutagen 1986;6:563–582

21. Milunsky A, Ulcickas M, Rothman KJ, Willett W, Jick SS, Jick H. Maternal heat exposure and neural tube defects. JAMA 1992;268:882–885

22. Clapp JF III. The changing thermal response to endurance exercise during pregnancy. Am J Obstet Gynecol 1991;165: 1684–1689

23. Clapp JF III, Seaward BL, Sleamaker RH, Hiser J. Maternal physiologic adaptations to early human pregnancy. Am J Obstet Gynecol 1988;159:1456–1460

24. Jovanovic-Peterson L, Durak EP, Peterson CM. Randomized trial of diet versus diet plus cardiovascular conditioning on glucose levels in gestational diabetes. Am J Obstet Gynecol 1989;161:415–419

25. Bung P, Bung C, Artal R, Khodiguian N, Fallenstein F, Spätling L. Therapeutic exercise for insulin-requiring gestational diabetics: effects on the fetus—results of a randomized prospective longitudinal study. J Perinat Med 1993;21:125–137

26. Artal R, Platt LD, Sperling M, Kammula RK, Jilek J, Nakamura R. Exercise in pregnancy. I. Maternal cardiovascular and metabolic responses in normal pregnancy. Am J Obstet Gynecol 1981; 140:123–127

27. Papiernik E, Kaminski M. Multifactorial study of the risk of prematurity at 32 weeks of gestation. I. A study of the frequency of 30 predictive characteristics. J Perinat Med 1974;2:30–36

28. Berkowitz GS, Kelsey JL, Holford TR, Berkowitz RL. Physical activity and the risk of spontaneous preterm delivery. J Reprod Med 1983;28:581–588

29. Veille J-C, Hohimer AR, Burry K, Speroff L. The effect of exercise on uterine activity in the last eight weeks of pregnancy. Am J Obstet Gynecol 1985;151:727–730

30. Katz VL, McMurray R, Berry MJ, Cefalo RC. Fetal and uterine responses to immersion and exercise. Obstet Gynecol 1988;72:225–230

31. Rowell LB. Human cardiovascular adjustments to exercise and thermal stress. Physiol Rev 1974;54:75–159

32. Morris N, Osborn SB, Wright HP, Hart A. Effective uterine bloodflow during exercise in normal and pre-eclamptic pregnancies. Lancet 1956;2:481–484

33. Hackett GA, Cohen-Overbeek T, Campbell S. The effect of exercise on uteroplacental Doppler waveforms in normal and complicated pregnancies. Obstet Gynecol 1992;79:919–923

34. Erkkola RU, Pirhonen JP, Kivijärvi AK. Flow velocity waveforms in uterine and umbilical arteries during sub-maximal bicycle exercise in normal pregnancy. Obstet Gynecol 1992;79:611–615

35. Naeye RL, Peters EC. Working during pregnancy: effects on the fetus. Pediatrics 1982;69:724–727

36. Tafari N, Naeye RL, Gobezie A. Effects of maternal undernutrition and heavy physical work during pregnancy on birth weight. Br J Obstet Gynaecol 1980;87:222–226

37. Clapp JF III, Capeless EL. Neonatal morphometrics after endurance exercise during pregnancy. Am J Obstet Gynecol 1990;163:1805–1811

38. Artal R, Rutherford S, Romen Y, Kammula RK, Dorey F, Wiswell RA. Fetal heart rate responses to maternal exercise. Am J Obstet Gynecol 1986;155:729–733

39. Carpenter MW, Sady SP, Hoegsberg B, Sady MA, Haydon B, Cullinane EM, et al. Fetal heart rate response to maternal exertion. JAMA 1988;259:3006–3009

40. Paolone AM, Shangold M, Paul D, Minnitti J, Weiner S. Fetal heart rate measurement during maternal exercise—avoidance of artifact. Med Sci Sports Exerc 1987;19:605–609

41. Collings CA, Curet LB, Mullin JP. Maternal and fetal responses to a maternal aerobic exercise program. Am J Obstet Gynecol 1983;145:702–707

42. Clapp JF III, Dickstein S. Endurance exercise and pregnancy outcome. Med Sci Sports Exerc 1984;16:556–562

43. Clapp JF III. The effects of maternal exercise on early pregnancy outcome. Am J Obstet Gynecol 1989;161:1453– 1457

44. Sibley L, Ruhling RO, Cameron-Foster J, Christensen C, Bolen T. Swimming and physical fitness during pregnancy. J Nurse-Midwif 1981;26:3–12

This Technical Bulletin was developed under the direction of the Committee on Technical Bulletins of the American College of Obstetricians and Gynecologists as an educational aid to obstetricians and gynecologists. The committee wishes to thank Raul Artal, MD, for his assistance in the development of this bulletin. This Technical Bulletin does not define a standard of care, nor is it intended to dictate an exclusive course of management. It presents recognized methods and techniques of clinical practice for consideration by obstetrician–gynecologists for incorporation into their practices. Variations of practice taking into account the needs of the individual patient, resources, and limitations unique to the institution or type of practice may be appropriate.

THE AMERICAN COLLEGE OF OBSTETRICIANS AND GYNECOLOGISTS
409 12th Street, SW
Washington, DC 20024-2188

12345/87654

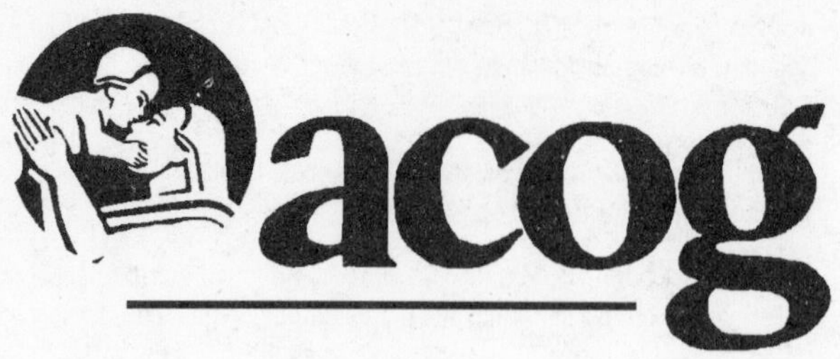

Number 163—January 1992

Technical Bulletin

An Educational Aid to Obstetrician–Gynecologists

Fetal and Neonatal Neurologic Injury

Cerebral palsy is defined as a chronic neuromuscular disability characterized by aberrant control of movement or posture appearing early in life and not the result of recognized progressive disease (1). It may be accompanied by a seizure disorder or mental retardation or both. Epilepsy or mental retardation is seldom associated with perinatal asphyxia in the absence of cerebral palsy (2, 3).

Definition

Perinatal asphyxia is an imprecise term, but long usage prevents its abandonment. Perinatal asphyxia in a contemporary context implies severe metabolic acidemia; the severity and associated factors necessary to cause damage are not precisely determined. Unless pH is less than 7.00 and is accompanied by a significant metabolic component, and there is an abnormal newborn course as described later in this bulletin, there is not a substantial increase in the risk of bad outcome. If all these factors are present, perinatal asphyxia is high on the differential diagnosis. However, metabolic acidosis, neonatal depression (including low Apgar scores), and neonatal neurologic and systemic symptoms may have causes other than asphyxia.

Factors Associated with Cerebral Palsy

Much is known about the factors associated with cerebral palsy, but the association of two events does not prove cause and effect. The largest study of risk factors associated with cerebral palsy did not confirm a strong relationship between perinatal asphyxia and cerebral palsy (4). For example, only 40 (21%) of 189 children with cerebral palsy in the Collaborative Perinatal Project had even one clinical marker of asphyxia (low fetal heart rate, low 5-minute Apgar score, time to first cry >5 minutes), and only 17 of those 40 did not have an alternative explanation for the cerebral palsy. Factors identified by multivariate analyses to be more frequent than expected in babies with cerebral palsy were maternal mental retardation, albuminuria during pregnancy, breech presentation (but not vaginal breech delivery), neonatal seizures, and a major non-central nervous system malformation. Gestational age of less than 32 weeks was strongly predictive of cerebral palsy. Of note is the fact that only 37% of the cases of cerebral palsy occurred in the 5% of infants with the highest risk. Thus, the authors concluded that the causes of most cases of cerebral palsy are unknown (4).

Perinatal Asphyxia as a Cause for Cerebral Palsy

Asphyxia around the time of labor and delivery can be a cause of cerebral palsy, but the asphyxia must be nearly lethal to be considered a possible cause. It has been estimated that about 10% of cerebral palsy in term infants is associated with perinatal asphyxia, but it is erroneous to believe that the observed asphyxia caused the cerebral palsy in all cases (5). Alternative explanations for the association include the possibility that the asphyxia was incidental in a child with existing brain damage (about 90% of children with cerebral palsy were not asphyxiated at birth), or that signs attributed to asphyxia were induced by an abnormality of the fetal brain, or that fetal weakness and motor abnormalities increased the risk of malpresentation or other complications of labor.

Role of Electronic Fetal Monitoring in Prevention of Cerebral Palsy

Because electronic fetal monitoring (EFM) was thought to be the most accurate method of recognizing early fetal asphyxia, and because EFM changes reflective of fetal asphyxia were thought to precede any fetal brain damage, it seemed reasonable to presume that the use of EFM would reduce the risk of cerebral palsy (6). However, it subsequently was established that EFM does not reduce the risk of cerebral palsy when compared with frequent intermittent auscultation (7–9). There are at least two possible explanations for this unexpected finding: 1) perinatal asphyxia may be a cause of cerebral palsy too uncommonly to be detectable by epidemiologic tools, or 2) EFM is a poor predictor of fetal asphyxia.

Actually, both of these explanations may be correct. If most cases of cerebral palsy are due to factors other than asphyxia, only extremely large epidemiologic studies could identify the small subgroup caused by asphyxia. Moreover, there is convincing evidence that nonreassuring EFM tracings are only fair predictors of fetal asphyxia (10). Although there is a relatively widespread opinion that persistent late decelerations, severe variable decelerations (variously defined), and prolonged bradycardia (the time interval required is frequently not defined) constitute possible fetal distress, there is no agreement on how quickly the nonreassuring pattern must be terminated or how other abnormalities of the EFM tracing affect the decision.

A neurologically abnormal fetus may be especially likely to have nonreassuring fetal heart rate patterns that may be attributed to asphyxia. At least 13 studies have reported a greatly increased risk of such patterns in the presence of hydrocephalus, decerebration, trisomy 18, and other abnormalities (11). Electronic fetal monitoring abnormalities that precede delivery of the abnormal child are not consistent, but loss of beat-to-beat variability, late decelerations, a sinusoidal pattern, tachycardia, and bradycardia have been described. In many cases, severe acidosis has been absent. Thus, EFM patterns that have been thought to reflect fetal distress may reflect intrinsic fetal abnormality and not necessarily acidosis.

Relationship Between Neonatal Acidosis and Cerebral Palsy

Because changes in cord blood gases have been used as an indicator of perinatal asphyxia and cerebral palsy was thought to be caused by asphyxia, it was reasonable to expect that there would be a strong association between neonatal metabolic acidosis and cerebral palsy. However, no close association has been observed. In one study (12), a birth cohort of over 900 children in whom umbilical artery blood gases were measured were followed to 1 year of age. At 1 year, none of the four children who had cerebral palsy had shown severe acidemia at birth. In another study, umbilical artery blood gases were recorded in 15,528 neonates; 142 (0.91%) were acidotic (pH <7.05, base deficit >10 mEq/L) (13). Nine of the 110 acidotic term infants were neurologically abnormal in the nursery and some had very low pH values, but none of the seven who were followed in the neurodevelopmental clinic demonstrated a major abnormality. Fourteen of the 32 acidotic preterm neonates showed neurologic abnormalities in the nursery, but none of the eight who were followed subsequently demonstrated a major abnormality. Another study examined 203 children at 4 years of age in whom umbilical artery blood gas analysis had been performed. No association was found between acidosis (pH ≤ 7.10, base deficit >12 mmol/L) and developmental outcome (14). Thus it is apparent that documented metabolic acidosis in the fetus or neonate who develops cerebral palsy should not a priori imply a cause-and-effect relationship.

In assessing a possible relationship between perinatal asphyxia and neurologic deficit in an individual patient, all of the following criteria must be present before a plausible link can be made (15):

- Profound umbilical artery metabolic or mixed acidemia (pH <7.00)
- Persistence of an Apgar score of 0–3 for longer than 5 minutes
- Neonatal neurologic sequelae, eg, seizures, coma, hypotonia
- Multiorgan system dysfunction, eg, cardiovascular, gastrointestinal, hematologic, pulmonary, or renal

These criteria require some amplification, especially as to details of the clinical course of the severely asphyxiated neonate who subsequently develops cerebral palsy. Unfortunately, there is no clear-cut way to determine when intrapartum asphyxia is severe enough to cause cerebral palsy. Certainly, epidemiologic studies have not shown that the use of EFM reduces the rate of cerebral palsy (9). Meconium-stained amniotic fluid, which in the past was considered by some to be a classic indicator of asphyxia, does not add to the accuracy of recognizing fetal distress (16). A low Apgar score alone does not establish the presence of asphyxia exclusive of other causes of "neonatal depression," but a very low Apgar score (0–3) at 10 minutes was found to be a powerful predictor of cerebral palsy (1). Indeed, 34% of infants weighing over 2,500 g at birth with an Apgar score of 0–3 at 10 minutes died, and 17% of the survivors developed cerebral palsy.

Fetal asphyxia causes a redistribution of blood from nonvital organs (the kidney) to vital organs (the brain, heart, and adrenal gland). The severely asphyxiated neonate will therefore demonstrate evidence of asphyxial effects in other organs, such as the kidneys, lungs, gut, and heart. Without such evidence, it is unreasonable to postulate an asphyxial effect on the brain (13, 17). The neurologic course in a neonate sufficiently asphyxiated to account for later cerebral palsy will be very abnormal, with a cluster of events that includes a low Apgar score; continuing disturbances of tone, consciousness, and feeding; and seizures in the subsequent hours and days (18). Neuroimaging studies in such infants commonly show cerebral edema (19, 20).

Unless all of these characteristics are present and other potential causes have been eliminated, a plausible link between any observed asphyxia and subsequent cerebral palsy is lacking. Caution is advised in making this connection, because, as discussed previously, a preexisting brain lesion may cause a similar clinical picture.

Quality of Intrapartum Obstetric Care and Cerebral Palsy

Because some cases of cerebral palsy do result from intrapartum asphyxia, it would be helpful to determine whether inadequate obstetric reaction to asphyxia caused the neurologic damage. In a case-control study of cerebral palsy from Oxford, the investigators did not identify a single instance of cerebral palsy in which there had been a delayed reaction to evidence of fetal asphyxia (21). The quality of obstetric care was studied in a group of term infants with early neonatal seizures and compared with that in a group of controls (22). While a delayed reaction to asphyxia was more common in children with seizures, cerebral palsy did not occur more often in children in the seizure group who received inadequate intrapartum care than in those who had appropriate intrapartum care. Similarly, it was reported that a large percentage of term infants with seizures developed cerebral palsy, but an inadequate response to an abnormal EFM tracing did not explain the cerebral palsy (23). Finally, a group of children with ominous EFM tracings, many of whom seemed questionably neurologically normal in the early months, were followed (24). In follow-up studies done at 6–9 years of age, only one child was found to have neurologic damage, apparently owing to an inherited metabolic disorder. All of these observations suggest that obstetric management of asphyxia is seldom responsible for cerebral palsy.

Birth Trauma as a Cause of Cerebral Palsy

Birth trauma apparently plays a minimal role in the development of cerebral palsy. The Collaborative Perinatal Project showed no relationship between cerebral palsy and arrested labor, use of oxytocin, or prolonged labor (25). Breech presentation was related to cerebral palsy, but vaginal breech delivery was not (4). Cerebral palsy sometimes develops following large cerebral or posterior fossa hemorrhages in term neonates. Many, but not all, of these brain hemorrhages seem to be associated with birth trauma and sometimes with a difficult forceps delivery (26). Some of these children die in the neonatal period and, of those who survive, only a few show evidence of cerebral palsy. In such cases, the neonatal neurologic course is a stormy one that is usually associated with seizures and apneic spells, bloody spinal fluid, and evidence of a large hemorrhage on imaging studies. Similarly, trauma plays little role in cerebral palsy that develops in the child who is delivered preterm. It is of note that no change in the incidence of neurologic deficit has been noted over the years during which the use of obstetric forceps has decreased and the rate of cesarean delivery has increased (27).

Preterm Birth and Cerebral Palsy

About 25–30% of cases of cerebral palsy are identified in children who were delivered preterm, and this proportion appears to be increasing as very-low-birth-weight infants survive in greater numbers. Periventricular hemorrhage and necrosis of periventricular white matter are common pathologic findings in these infants. Many studies support the suggestion that intrapartum asphyxia is not often the mechanism for this association. Persistently low Apgar scores at 10–20 minutes of age correlate strongly with cerebral palsy in term infants, but very few preterm infants survive such lengthy depression (1). The use of EFM compared with frequent intermittent auscultation in a carefully controlled study of preterm deliveries did not demonstrate a decreased incidence of cerebral palsy in the EFM group (7). Finally, it was reported that birth asphyxia was not significantly associated with cerebral palsy in infants weighing less than 1,500 g (5).

There are a number of factors that appear to increase the risk for cerebral palsy. For example, chorioamnionitis and congenital malformations are more common in preterm infants who develop cerebral palsy. Current evidence, however, suggests that method of delivery, low Apgar scores, and acidosis play minimal roles (28).

Conclusion

In Western industrialized countries, the rate of cerebral palsy in term infants (1–2/1,000) has not changed in the past 20 years, despite new neonatal and obstetric technologies. However, a continuing misperception that birth asphyxia accounts for a significant portion of infants with cerebral palsy continues to exist, despite the fact that there is no evidence to support this impression. A number of clinical and experimental reports confirm that only severe and prolonged asphyxia is associated with an increased risk of subsequent neurologic dysfunction.

Such asphyxia is very uncommon in birthing conditions in the United States and modern industrialized countries. When prolonged and severe asphyxia does occur, it is often followed by death or the prolonged requirement for life support systems. The majority of infants who survive severe birth asphyxia are later clinically normal.

REFERENCES

1. Nelson KB, Ellenberg JH. Apgar scores as predictors of chronic neurologic disability. Pediatrics 1981;68;36–44
2. Nelson KB, Ellenberg JH. The asymptomatic newborn and risk of cerebral palsy. Am J Dis Child 1987;141:1333–1335
3. Freeman JM, Nelson KB. Intrapartum asphyxia and cerebral palsy. Pediatrics 1988;82:240–249
4. Nelson KB, Ellenberg JH. Antecedents of cerebral palsy. Multivariate analysis of risk. N Engl J Med 1986;315: 81–86
5. Blair E, Stanley FJ. Intrapartum asphyxia: a rare cause of cerebral palsy. J Pediatr 1988;112:515–519
6. Quilligan EJ, Paul RH. Fetal monitoring: is it worth it? Obstet Gynecol 1975;45:96–100
7. Shy KK, Luthy DA, Bennett FC, Whitfield M, Larson EB, van Belle G, et al. Effects of electronic fetal heart-rate-monitoring, as compared with periodic auscultation, on the neurologic development of premature infants. N Engl J Med 1990;322:588–593
8. Freeman R. Intrapartum fetal monitoring—a disappointing story. N Engl J Med 1990;322:624–626
9. McDonald D, Grant A, Sheridan-Pereira M, Boylan P, Chalmers I. The Dublin randomized control trial of intrapartum fetal heart rate monitoring. Am J Obstet Gynecol 1985;152:524–539
10. Banta H, Thacker S. Assessing the costs and benefits of electronic fetal monitoring. Obstet Gynecol Surv 1979;34: 627
11. Niswander KR. EFM and brain damage in term and post-term infants. Contemp Ob/Gyn 1991;36(February 15, 1991):39–50
12. Ruth VJ, Raivio KO. Perinatal brain damage: predictive value of metabolic acidosis and the Apgar score. BMJ 1988;297(6640):24–27
13. Fee S, Malee K, Deddish R, Minogue JP, Socol ML. Severe acidosis and subsequent neurologic status. Am J Obstet Gynecol 1990;162:802–806
14. Dennis J, Johnson A, Mutch L, Yudkin P, Johnson P. Acid-base status at birth and neurodevelopmental outcome at four and one-half years. Am J Obstet Gynecol 1989;161:213–220
15. Nelson KB. Perspective on the role of perinatal asphyxia in neurologic outcome: its role in developmental deficits in children. Can Med Assoc J 1989;141(4[Suppl]):3–10
16. Steer PJ, Eigbe F, Lissauer TJ, Beard RW. Interrelationships among abnormal cardiotocograms in labor, meconium staining of the amniotic fluid, arterial cord blood pH, and Apgar scores. Obstet Gynecol 1989;74:715–721
17. Perlman JM, Tack ED. Renal injury in the asphyxiated newborn infant: relationship to neurologic outcome. J Pediatr 1988;113:875–879
18. Ellenberg JH, Nelson KB. Cluster of perinatal events identifying infants at high risk for death or disability. J Pediatr 1988;113:546–552
19. Lupton BA, Hill A, Roland EH, Whitfield MF, Flodmark O. Brain swelling in the asphyxiated term newborn: pathogenesis and outcome. Pediatrics 1988;82:139–146
20. Myers RE. Four patterns of perinatal brain damage and their conditions of occurrence in primates. Adv Neurol 1975;10:223–234
21. Niswander K, Henson G, Elbourne D, Chalmers I, Redman C, MacFarlane A, et al. Adverse outcome of pregnancy and the quality of obstetric care. Lancet 1984;2:287–831
22. Minchom P, Niswander K, Chalmers I, Dauncey M, Newcombe R, Elbourne D, et al. Antecedents and outcome of very early neonatal seizures in infants born at or near term. Br J Obstet Gynaecol 1987;94:431–439
23. Keegan KA Jr, Waffarn F, Quilligan EJ. Obstetric characteristics and fetal heart rate patterns of infants who convulse during the newborn period. Am J Obstet Gynecol 1985;153:732–737
24. Painter MJ, Scott M, Hirsch RP, O'Donoghue P, Depp R. Fetal heart rate patterns during labor: neurologic and cognitive development at six to nine years of age. Am J Obstet Gynecol 1988;159:854–858
25. Nelson KB, Ellenberg JH. Antecedents of cerebral palsy. Univariate analysis of risks. Am J Dis Child 1985;139: 1031–1038
26. Fenichel GM, Webster DL, Wong WK. Intracranial hemorrhage in the term newborn. Arch Neurol 1984;41:30–34
27. Hensleigh PA, Fainstat T, Spencer R. Perinatal events and cerebral palsy. Am J Obstet Gynecol 1986;154:978–981
28. Beverley DW, Chance GW, Coates CF. Intraventricular hemorrhage—timing of occurrence and relationship of perinatal events. Br J Obstet Gynaecol 1984;91:1007–1013

This Technical Bulletin was developed under the direction of the Committee on Technical Bulletins of the American College of Obstetricians and Gynecologists as an educational aid to obstetricians and gynecologists. The committee wishes to thank Kenneth R. Niswander, MD, and Karin Nelson, MD, for their assistance in the development of this bulletin. This Technical Bulletin does not define a standard of care, nor is it intended to dictate an exclusive course of management. It presents recognized methods and techniques of clinical practice for consideration by obstetrician–gynecologists for incorporation into their practices. Variations of practice taking into account the needs of the individual patient, resources, and limitations unique to the institution or type of practice may be appropriate.

Reviewed June 1993
THE AMERICAN COLLEGE OF OBSTETRICIANS AND GYNECOLOGISTS
409 12th Street, SW
Washington, DC 20024-2188

34567/87654

Number 207—July 1995
(Replaces #132, September 1989)

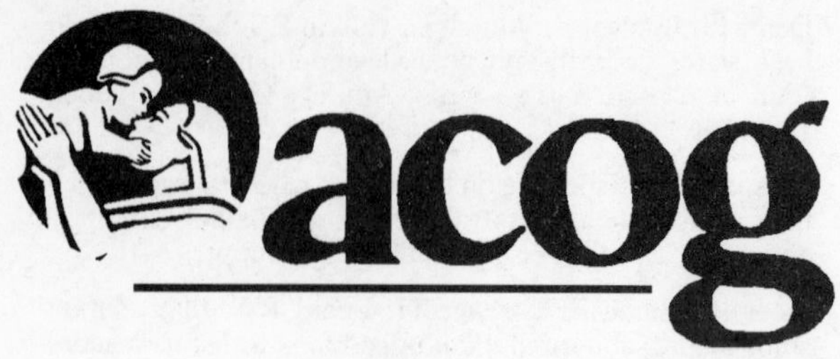

Technical Bulletin

An Educational Aid to Obstetrician–Gynecologists

Fetal Heart Rate Patterns: Monitoring, Interpretation, and Management

Intrapartum fetal heart rate (FHR) monitoring can help the physician identify and interpret changes in FHR patterns that may be associated with such fetal conditions as hypoxia, umbilical cord compression, tachycardia, and acidosis. The ability to interpret FHR patterns and understand their correlation with the fetus' condition allows the physician to institute management techniques, including maternal oxygenation, amnioinfusion, and tocolytic therapy. Current data indicate that FHR monitoring is equally effective whether done electronically or by auscultation.

Intrapartum fetal assessment by FHR monitoring is only one parameter of fetal well-being. It involves evaluation of the pattern as well as the rate, but it is not a substitute for informed clinical judgment.

Transient and repetitive episodes of hypoxemia and hypoxia, even at the level of the central nervous system (CNS), are extremely common during normal labor and are generally well tolerated by the fetus. Further, a progressive intrapartum decline in baseline fetal oxygenation and pH is virtually universal; levels of acidemia that would be ominous in an infant or adult are commonly seen in normal newborns. Only when hypoxia and resultant metabolic acidemia reach extreme levels is the fetus at risk for long-term neurologic impairment (1).

For the purposes of this bulletin, the following definitions will be used:

Hypoxemia:	Decreased oxygen content in blood
Hypoxia:	Decreased level of oxygen in tissue
Acidemia:	Increased concentration of hydrogen ions in the blood
Acidosis:	Increased concentration of hydrogen ions in tissue
Asphyxia:	Hypoxia with metabolic acidosis

Physiologic Basis

The fetus is well adapted to extracting oxygen from the maternal circulation even with the additional stress of normal labor and delivery. However, alterations in the fetoplacental unit resulting from labor or intrapartum complications may subject the fetus to decreased oxygenation, leading to potential damage to any susceptible organ systems or even fetal death.

Oxygen delivery is critically dependent on uterine blood flow. Uterine contractions decrease placental blood flow and result in intermittent episodes of decreased oxygen delivery. Normally, the fetus tolerates contractions without difficulty, but if the frequency, duration, or strength of contractions becomes excessive, fetal hypoxemia may result. Maternal position and the use of conduction anesthesia can also alter uterine blood flow and oxygen delivery during labor. Finally, labor may be complicated by conditions such as preeclampsia, abruptio placentae, chorioamnionitis, and other pathologic situations that can further alter blood flow and oxygen exchange within the placenta.

The umbilical cord is particularly vulnerable during labor because it can prolapse once membranes rupture or become compressed either through cord entanglement or secondary to oligohydramnios. While umbilical cord compression is common during labor, prolonged compression is infrequent but can seriously disrupt oxygen delivery and carbon dioxide removal and lead to acidosis or death.

Some fetuses are unusually susceptible to the effects of intrapartum hypoxemia, such as fetuses with growth retardation and those who are delivered prematurely. In these circumstances, hypoxia tends to progress more rapidly and is more likely to cause or aggravate metabolic acidemia which, in extreme cases, correlates with poor long-term outcome. In severe cases, such hypoxia may lead to death (2, 3).

Experimentally induced hypoxia has been associated with consistent, predictable changes in the FHR (4). The fetal CNS is susceptible to hypoxia. Since the FHR and its alterations are most directly under CNS control through sympathetic and parasympathetic reflexes, alterations in the FHR can be sensitive indicators of fetal hypoxia (4, 5).

In some instances of decreased oxygenation, the pattern of the FHR change can identify the mechanism. Umbilical cord compression or, occasionally, head compression coincides with variable decelerations (6). These are defined as slowing of the FHR with abrupt onset and return and are frequently preceded and followed by small accelerations of the FHR. These decelerations vary in depth, duration, and shape on the tracing but generally coincide in timing and duration with the compression of the cord which, in turn, usually coincides with the timing of the uterine contractions.

Uterine contractions that result in decreases in fetal oxygenation exceeding that usually seen in labor may result in delayed or late decelerations. These are U-shaped decelerations of gradual onset and gradual return that are usually shallow (10–30 beats per minute [bpm]) and that reach their nadir after the peak of the contraction. In milder cases, they can be a reflex and the result of CNS hypoxia; in more severe cases, it has been postulated that they may be the result of direct myocardial depression.

Early decelerations are shallow and symmetrical with a pattern similar to that of late decelerations but reach their nadir at the same time as the peak of the contraction. They are seen in the active phase of labor, albeit infrequently. They are benign changes caused by fetal head compression.

Changes in the baseline FHR may also indicate the response of the fetus to an episode of hypoxia. Two specific parameters of the baseline FHR are important: rate and variability. The FHR at term usually ranges from 120–160 bpm. The initial response of the FHR to intermittent hypoxia is deceleration, but baseline tachycardia may develop if the hypoxia is prolonged and severe. Tachycardia also may be associated with conditions other than hypoxia (such as maternal fever, intraamniotic infection, and congenital heart disease). The presence of variability—or variation of successive beats in the FHR—is a useful indicator of fetal CNS integrity. In the absence of maternal sedation or extreme prematurity, decreasing variability—or flattening of the FHR baseline—may serve as a barometer of the fetal response to hypoxia. Because this is presumed to be a CNS response, in most situations, decelerations of the FHR will precede the loss of variability, indicating the cause of neurologic depression. Many other factors, such as a fetal sleep cycle or medications, may decrease the activity of the CNS and the variability of the FHR. The development of decreased variability in the absence of decelerations is unlikely to be due to hypoxia (7).

Accelerations are common periodic changes in labor and are nearly always associated with fetal movement. These changes are virtually always reassuring and almost always confirm that the fetus is not acidotic at that time (8).

Guidelines for Performing Fetal Heart Rate Monitoring

The FHR may be evaluated by auscultation or by electronic monitoring. Auscultation is usually performed with a DeLee stethoscope or a Doppler ultrasound device.

Continuous FHR and contraction monitoring may be performed externally or internally. Most external monitors use a Doppler device with computerized logic to interpret and count the Doppler signals. Internal FHR monitoring is accomplished with a fetal electrode, which is a spiral wire placed directly on the fetal scalp or other presenting part. This method records the fetal electrocardiogram. In either case, the FHR is recorded continuously on the upper portion of a paper strip and every beat-to-beat interval is recorded as a rate. The lower portion of the strip records uterine contractions, which also may be monitored externally or internally. The most common paper speed in the United States is 3 cm/min.

Well-controlled studies have shown that intermittent auscultation of the FHR is equivalent to continuous electronic monitoring in assessing fetal condition when performed at specific intervals with a 1:1 nurse-to-patient ratio (9–14).

The intensity of FHR monitoring used during labor should be based on risk factors. When intensified monitoring is undertaken, such as when risk factors are present during labor, the fetal heart rate should be assessed according to the following guidelines:

- During the active phase of the first stage of labor: If auscultation is used the FHR should be evaluated and recorded at least every 15 minutes after a uterine contraction. If continuous electronic monitoring is used, the tracing should be evaluated at least every 15 minutes.
- During the second stage of labor: With auscultation, the FHR should be evaluated and recorded at least every 5 minutes. When electronic monitoring is used, FHR should also be evaluated at least every 5 minutes.

There are no comparative data indicating the optimal frequency at which intermittent auscultation should be performed in the absence of risk factors. One method is to evaluate and record the fetal heart rate at least every 30 minutes in the active phase of the first stage of labor and at least every 15 minutes in the second stage of labor.

With either auscultation or electronic monitoring, documentation of the evaluation is required. Auscultated FHR should be recorded in the chart after each observation. With electronic FHR monitoring, the monitor strip should be carefully labeled and the complete strip is usually retained, as with other medical records. Computer storage of fetal monitor records on devices such as laser discs which do not permit overwriting or revision appears to be a reasonable alternative, as do various methods of microfilm recording.

Documentation may consist of narrative notes or the use of comprehensive flow sheets detailing the periodic assessment. Specific responses to an abnormal FHR pattern such as further diagnostic procedures or therapeutic interventions also should be documented, as should the nature, date, and time of other pertinent events (eg, administration of medication or anesthesia).

Risks and Benefits

Currently, neither the most effective method of FHR monitoring nor the specific frequency or duration of monitoring to ensure optimal perinatal outcome has been identified by a significant body of scientific evidence. With the advent and liberal use of electronic FHR monitoring in the 1970s, there was great hope that intrapartum fetal death and morbidity associated with intrapartum asphyxia could be virtually eliminated. Retrospective studies of electronic FHR monitoring in both high- and low-risk populations were encouraging. A review of 11 studies including almost 40,000 electronically monitored patients and nearly 100,000 historical controls suggested a reduction in the intrapartum fetal death rate from 1.76/1,000 births in controls to 0.54/1,000 births in monitored patients (15). Similar reductions in neonatal death rates were also observed.

Subsequently, seven randomized, controlled trials have compared continuous electronic FHR monitoring with intermittent auscultation in both high- and low-risk patients; no differences in intrapartum fetal death rates were found (9–14, 16). It is significant that the intermittent auscultation groups in all but one of the seven studies had a dedicated 1:1 nurse-to-patient ratio. Nurses auscultated the FHR at least every 15 minutes in the first stage of labor and every 5 minutes in the second stage. If only the results of the studies with this intensity of FHR auscultation are included, the intrapartum fetal death rate in auscultated women was only 0.5/1,000. This rate is nearly identical to those seen with electronic FHR monitoring in both prospective, randomized, controlled trials and retrospective, controlled studies (9–14).

In contrast, the most recently published randomized, controlled trial did show a significant reduction in perinatal deaths due to asphyxia in the electronically monitored group (17). It is not clear why this single study is so discordant with the others, but it does provide some promise that further studies may yet elucidate the real value of electronic FHR monitoring.

Likewise, a substantial body of evidence disproves the hypothesis that electronic fetal monitoring would reduce long-term neurologic impairment and cerebral palsy in newborns so monitored. Electronic FHR monitoring has been no more effective in reducing the rates of low Apgar scores at birth and long-term neurologic morbidity than has intensive intrapartum auscultative monitoring (as described here). One study did suggest that electronic FHR monitoring may decrease the rate of seizures in the newborn (14); however, this reduction did not persist into late childhood. On the other hand, another study showed a significant increase in cerebral palsy among premature infants monitored electronically during labor (18).

Certainly a correlation exists between abnormal FHR patterns and neurologic depression at birth; similarly, neonatal depression is correlated to some extent with adverse long-term neurologic outcome. It must be emphasized, however, that this correlation occurs only with prolonged and severe intrapartum fetal compromise. Indeed, the various methods of intrapartum fetal assessment currently used are not effective in predicting or preventing adverse long-term neurologic outcomes. Management of nonreassuring FHR patterns does not appear to affect the risk of subsequent cerebral palsy (19). This is due to the facts that neurologic abnormalities infrequently result from subtle events occurring during labor and delivery and, conversely, that most hypoxic and asphyxic episodes do not result in irreversible neurologic damage (19, 20).

The primary risk of electronic FHR monitoring is a potential increase in the cesarean delivery rate. This effect has been observed in both retrospective trials and the majority of prospective, randomized, controlled trials. More accurate interpretation of FHR monitoring, the use of fetal scalp blood pH monitoring, and possibly, the use of acoustic or scalp stimulation to elicit FHR accelerations can lead tomoreprecisediagnosis of the condition of the fetus and, by inference, may lead to a decrease in the cesarean delivery rate. The use of amnioinfusion has also been shown in randomized, controlled trials to lower the cesarean delivery rate for those patients with FHR patterns consistent with umbilical cord compression (21–23).

Interpretation and Management

A normal FHR pattern is reassuring and, when obtained by careful auscultation or electronic monitoring, is nearly always associated with a newborn who is vigorous at birth. Therefore, the terminology of *reassuring* implies that in the absence of patterns defined as nonreassuring, the fetus can be assumed—with a great deal of reliability—to have normal oxygen and acid–base status.

Conversely, nonreassuring patterns are quite nonspecific and cannot reliably predict whether a fetus will be well oxygenated, depressed, or acidotic. However, factors other than hypoxia may lead to a nonreassuring FHR. In addition, an abnormal FHR pattern associated with hypoxia may neither depict the severity of hypoxia nor predict how it will progress if labor is allowed to proceed.

The term *fetal distress*, while imprecise and inaccurate, has been applied so commonly to abnormal FHR patterns in labor that it is difficult to abandon. It is more helpful clinically to describe the fetal heart rate patterns in terms of type and severity, and to outline a management plan accordingly.

Interpretation of Fetal Heart Rate Patterns

The initial FHR pattern should be carefully evaluated for the presence or absence of accelerations, decelerations, and abnormalities of the baseline. In one study, the first 30 minutes of electronic FHR monitoring identified about 50% of all fetuses for whom cesarean delivery will be required for a nonreassuring FHR pattern or "fetal distress" (24). While the progression of decelerations will usually explain changes in the baseline later in labor, abnormalities of the baseline on admission, such as fetal tachycardia or loss of variability, are the most difficult to interpret, as data regarding previous changes are lacking.

Periodic changes in FHR are common in labor; they occur in response to contractions or fetal movement and include accelerations and decelerations. Variable decelerations are the most common decelerations seen in labor and indicate umbilical cord compression; they are generally associated with a favorable outcome (25). Only when they become persistent, progressively deeper, and longer lasting are they considered nonreassuring. Although progression is more important than absolute parameters, persisting variable decelerations to less than 70 bpm lasting greater than 60 seconds are generally concerning. In addition to prolonged and deep variable decelerations, those with persistently slow return to baseline are also considered nonreassuring, as these reflect hypoxia persistent beyond the relaxation phase of the contraction (26). The response of the baseline FHR to the variable decelerations and the presence or absence of accelerations are important in formulating a management plan for the patient with significant variable decelerations. When nonreassuring variable decelerations are associated with the development of tachycardia and loss of variability, one begins to see substantial correlation with fetal acidosis.

Late decelerations may be secondary to transient fetal hypoxia in response to the decreased placental perfusion associated with uterine contractions. Occasional or intermittent late decelerations are not uncommon during labor. When late decelerations become persistent (ie, present with most contractions), they are considered nonreassuring, regardless of the depth of the deceleration. Late decelerations caused by reflex—those mediated by the CNS—generally become deeper as the degree of hypoxia becomes more severe. However, as metabolic acidosis develops from tissue hypoxia, late decelerations are believed to be the result of direct myocardial depression, and at this point, the depth of the late deceleration will not indicate the degree of hypoxia (27).

A prolonged deceleration, often incorrectly referred to as bradycardia, is an isolated, abrupt decrease in the FHR to levels below the baseline that lasts at least 60–90 seconds. These changes are always of concern and may be caused by virtually any mechanism that can lead to fetal hypoxia. The severity of the event causing the deceleration is usually reflected in the depth and duration of the deceleration, as well as the degree to which variability is lost during the deceleration. When such a deceleration returns to the baseline, especially with more profound episodes, a transient fetal tachycardia and loss of variability may occur while the fetus is recovering from hypoxia. The degree to which such decelerations are nonreassuring depends on their depth and duration, loss of variability, response of the fetus during the recovery period, and, most importantly, the frequency and progression of recurrence.

A sinusoidal heart rate pattern consists of a regular oscillation of the baseline long-term variability resembling a sine wave. This smooth, undulating pattern, lasting at least 10 minutes, has a relatively fixed period of three to five cycles per minute and an amplitude of 5–15 bpm above and below the baseline. Short-term variability is usually absent. This pattern may be associated with severe chronic, as opposed to acute, fetal anemia. It has also been described following the use of alphaprodine or other medications and, in such circumstances, may not represent fetal compromise. Additionally, severe hypoxia and acidosis occasionally manifest as a sinusoidal FHR; the reason for this is as yet not understood. True sinusoidal patterns are quite rare. Unfortunately, small, frequent accelerations of low amplitude are easy to confuse with sinusoidal patterns. The former are benign and occur more frequently while the latter, if they meet the strict criteria of a sinusoidal FHR, are always nonreassuring (28).

Evaluation and Management of Nonreassuring Patterns

With a persistently nonreassuring FHR pattern in labor, the clinician should approach the evaluation and management in a four-step plan as follows:

1. When possible, determine the etiology of the pattern.
2. Attempt to correct the pattern by specifically correcting the primary problem or by instituting general measures aimed at improving fetal oxygenation and placental perfusion.

3. If attempts to correct the pattern are not successful, fetal scalp blood pH assessment may be considered.
4. Determine whether operative intervention is warranted and, if so, how urgently it is needed.

The search for the cause of the nonreassuring FHR pattern should be directed by the clinician's interpretation of the pattern. If there are late decelerations, then excessive uterine contractions, maternal hypotension, or maternal hypoxemia should be considered. For severe variable or prolonged decelerations, a pelvic examination should be performed immediately to rule out umbilical cord prolapse or rapid descent of the fetal head. If no causes of such decelerations are found, one can usually conclude that umbilical cord compression is responsible.

General measures that may improve fetal oxygenation and placental perfusion include administering maternal oxygen by a tight-fitting face mask, ensuring that the woman is in the lateral recumbent position, discontinuing oxytocin, and, if maternal intravascular volume status is in question, beginning intravenous hydration.

Oxygen Therapy

The arterial Po_2 in the fetus is normally about one fourth of the arterial Po_2 in the mother. Despite this low Po_2, the fetal blood can carry a large amount of oxygen from the placenta because of the high concentration of fetal hemoglobin and its high affinity for oxygen. Oxygen is constantly and rapidly consumed and cannot be stored by the fetus. The fetus is thus dependent upon a constant supply of oxygen; a reduction in this supply cannot be tolerated for more than brief intervals.

When there is evidence of a nonreassuring pattern, administration of supplemental oxygen to the mother is indicated. A significant increase in maternal oxygenation is accomplished with a tight-fitting face mask and an oxygen flow rate of 8–10 L/min. Although such administration results in only a small increase in fetal Po_2, animal studies have suggested that a significant increase in fetal oxygen content may occur. Assuming both adequate placental exchange and delivery of oxygen through unobstructed umbilical cord circulation, the resultant increase in total fetal blood oxygen content is 30–40% or greater in animal studies, depending upon the degree to which the fetal Po_2 has fallen (29). When given for the usual duration of labor, maternal oxygen therapy has no known harmful effects on the fetus.

Maternal Position

Maternal position during labor can affect uterine blood flow and placental perfusion. In the supine position, there is an exaggeration of the lumbar lordotic curvature of the maternal spine facilitating compression of the vena cava and aortoiliac vessels by the gravid uterus. This results in decreased return of blood to the maternal heart leading directly to a fall in cardiac output, blood pressure, and uterine blood flow. In the supine position, aortic compression by the uterus may result in an increase in the incidence of late decelerations and a decrease in fetal scalp pH (30). The lateral recumbent position (either side) is best for maximizing cardiac output and uterine blood flow and is often associated with improvement in the FHR pattern (31). Other maternal positions may accomplish similar uterine displacement.

Epidural Block

Some degree of maternal hypotension is a relatively common complication of epidural block, occurring in 5–25% of procedures (32). Prophylactic intravascular volume expansion with 500–1,000 ml of lactated Ringer's injection is recommended prior to administration of an epidural anesthetic in order to diminish the likelihood of this complication. Treatment with an increase in intravenous fluids, left uterine displacement, or 2.5–10 mg of ephedrine intravenously or intramuscularly is recommended for hypotension occurring with administration of an epidural block. During the period of hypotension, uteroplacental perfusion may be compromised. This may be manifested by fetal tachycardia, prolonged decelerations, decreased beat-to-beat variability, late decelerations, or some combination of these.

The frequency of prolonged decelerations after administration of epidural analgesia has been reported to be 7.9–12.5% (33, 34). Uterine hypertonia with resultant prolonged decelerations has been observed in patients receiving epidural block during labor even in the absence of systemic hypotension (35). Management of epidural-associated decelerations should focus on treatment of the specific cause—either the increased uterine tone or maternal hypotension.

Oxytocin

Careful use of oxytocin is necessary to minimize uterine hyperstimulation and potential maternal and fetal morbidity. If nonreassuring FHR changes occur in patients receiving oxytocin, the infusion should be decreased or discontinued. Restarting the infusion at a lower rate or increasing it in smaller increments may be better tolerated.

Amnioinfusion

Variable decelerations are frequently encountered in both the first and second stages of labor. Those occurring prior to fetal descent at 8–9 cm of dilatation are most frequently seen in patients with oligohydramnios.

In patients with decreased amniotic fluid volume in either preterm or term pregnancies, replacement of amniotic fluid with normal saline infused through a transcervical intrauterine pressure catheter has been reported to decrease both the frequency and severity of variable decelerations (22, 23, 36). Replacement of amniotic fluid may be elected therapeutically in patients with progressive variable decelerations. Although randomized, controlled trials are lacking, it is reasonable to replace amniotic fluid prophylactically at the onset of labor in patients with known oligohydramnios. Studies also have demonstrated that amnioinfusion results in reductions in rates of cesarean delivery for "fetal distress," primarily due to variable decelerations, and fewer low Apgar scores at birth. Acute saline amnioinfusion has been reported to be an effective therapy that relieves most repetitive variable or prolonged intrapartum decelerations and is without apparent maternal or fetal risk (21). Investigators have also reported a decrease in newborn respiratory complications from meconium in patients who receive amnioinfusion. This results presumably from the dilutional effect of amnioinfusion and possibly from prevention of in utero fetal gasping that may occur during episodes of hypoxia caused by umbilical cord compression (37–39).

Generally, two techniques of amnioinfusion have been described: bolus infusion and continuous infusion. Originally described for patients requiring therapeutic amnioinfusion, bolus infusion of up to 800 ml can be administered at a rate of 10–15 ml/min until the decelerations abate; then, an extra 250 ml can be added (21). The infusion can be repeated when there is sudden or large fluid loss due to maternal position change or performance of the Valsalva maneuver or when an abnormal FHR tracing recurs. Ultrasound assessment of amniotic fluid volume can also be used to determine the need for repeat infusion (39).

Alternatively, a continuous infusion may be performed. While this was originally described for prophylactic amnioinfusion (22), it may also be used therapeutically. Continuous amnioinfusion usually begins with a loading dose of 10 ml/min for 1 hour followed by a maintenance dose of 3 ml/min. Use of an infusion pump, although not essential, can more accurately control both the volume and rate of infusion.

Warmed saline has been used in prophylactic amnioinfusions of preterm patients, but warming of infusate has not been shown to be of any specific value in term or preterm patients. For the term patient, there do not appear to be any adverse effects on maternal or newborn temperature or electrolytes when room temperature saline amnioinfusion is administered (36).

Care should be taken to avoid overdistending the uterine cavity. Increased basal uterine tone and sudden deterioration of FHR has been reported with infusion volumes of as little as 250 ml; abnormal FHR secondary to polyhydramnios has been reported following prolonged continuous amnioinfusion (40). With continuous amnioinfusion, intermittent discontinuation to assess basal uterine tone or the use of double-lumen uterine pressure catheters is recommended.

The onset of beneficial effects of amnioinfusion requires at least 20–30 minutes, so care should be taken when performing saline amnioinfusion to avoid delaying surgical intervention if there is no improvement in a significantly abnormal FHR. Preparations for expeditious delivery should be made simultaneously with saline amnioinfusion when worsening variable or prolonged decelerations occur.

Tocolytic Agents

Tocolytic agents are a potentially valuable tool in the management of certain intrapartum events. Changes in the FHR suggesting possible nonreassuring FHR patterns may accompany excessive uterine contractions. If a nonreassuring FHR pattern results from such excessive contractions, specific measures can be taken to decrease uterine activity. If oxytocin is being administered, the dose should be decreased or discontinued. In addition, a tocolytic agent sometimes may be injected. Terbutaline, 0.25 mg subcutaneously or 0.125–0.25 mg intravenously, has been used for this purpose. Both beta agonists and magnesium sulfate have been reported to be of value in rapidly improving fetal condition secondary to uterine relaxation during active labor (41, 42).

Even in the absence of uterine hypertonus, abnormal FHR patterns occurring in response to uterine contractions may be improved and newborn condition benefitted by the administration of tocolytic agents (43). This is especially true when unavoidable delays in effecting operative delivery are encountered.

Certain potential maternal and fetal side effects need to be considered when tocolytic agents are administered for a nonreassuring FHR. Beta agonists elevate both serum glucose levels and maternal and fetal heart rate. However, the direct effect on FHR is minor, and any improvement in FHR from a nonreassuring pattern following acute beta agonist therapy is not due to a direct effect of therapy on the fetal heart, but rather the result of a decrease in the uterine activity. Maternal pulse pressure is widened, and peripheral vascular resistance decreases. Additionally, reinstituting or augmenting uterine activity with oxytocin following acute administration of tocolytic agents may be necessary to reestablish a normal labor pattern. The administration of tocolytic therapy for nonreassuring FHR patterns should not delay necessary interventions.

Management of Persistent Nonreassuring Fetal Heart Rate Patterns

If the FHR pattern remains uncorrected, the decision to intervene depends on the clinician's assessment of the likelihood of severe hypoxia and the possibility of metabolic acidosis, as well as the estimated time to spontaneous delivery. For the fetus with persistent nonreassuring decelerations, normal FHR variability and the absence of tachycardia generally indicate the lack of acidosis. However, variability is difficult to quantify except in the extremes.

Persistent late decelerations or severe variable decelerations associated with the absence of variability are always nonreassuring and generally require prompt intervention unless they spontaneously resolve or can be corrected rapidly with immediate conservative measures (ie, oxygen, hydration, or maternal repositioning). The absence of variability or markedly decreased variability demonstrated on an external monitor is generally reliable. The presence of FHR variability is not confirmatory, however, and, in the presence of nonreassuring decelerations, a fetal electrode should be placed when possible.

The presence of spontaneous accelerations of greater than 15 bpm lasting at least 15 seconds virtually always ensures the absence of fetal acidosis. Fetal scalp stimulation or vibroacoustic stimulation can be used to induce accelerations; these also indicate the absence of acidosis (44, 45). Conversely, there is about a 50% chance of acidosis in the fetus who fails to respond to stimulation in the presence of an otherwise nonreassuring pattern (44, 45). In these fetuses, assessment of scalp blood pH, if available, may be used to clarify the acid–base status. This technique, while occasionally helpful, is used uncommonly in current obstetric practice (46). If the FHR pattern remains worrisome, either induced accelerations or repeat assessment of scalp blood pH is required every 20–30 minutes for continued reassurance. In cases in which the FHR patterns are persistently nonreassuring and acidosis is present or cannot be ruled out, the fetus should be promptly delivered by the most expeditious route, whether abdominal or vaginal.

Summary

Because alterations in fetal oxygenation occur during labor and because many complications can occur during this critical period, some form of FHR evaluation should be provided for all patients. The choice of technique is based on various factors, including the resources available. Nonreassuring FHR patterns are common and quite nonspecific. By understanding the physiologic and pathophysiologic basis of FHR monitoring, as well as its capabilities and limitations, the clinician can reduce the need for interventions.

REFERENCES

1. American College of Obstetricians and Gynecologists. Fetal and neonatal neurologic injury. ACOG Technical Bulletin 163. Washington, DC: ACOG, 1992

2. Low JA, Boston RW, Pancham SR. Fetal asphyxia during the intrapartum period in intrauterine growth-retarded infants. Am J Obstet Gynecol 1972;113:351–357

3. Westgren LMR, Malcus P, Svenningsen NW. Intrauterine asphyxia and long-term outcome in preterm fetuses. Obstet Gynecol 1986;67:512–516

4. Myers RE, Mueller-Huebach E, Adamsons K. Predictability of the state of fetal oxygenation from quantitative analysis of the components of late deceleration. Am J Obstet Gynecol 1973;115:1083–1094

5. Wakatsuki A, Murata Y, Ninomiya Y, Masaoka N, Tyner JG, Kutty KK. Autonomic nervous system regulation of baseline heart rate in the fetal lamb. Am J Obstet Gynecol 1992;167:519–523

6. Ball RH, Parer JT. The physiologic mechanisms of variable decelerations. Am J Obstet Gynecol 1992; 166:1683–1689

7. Davidson SR, Rankin JHG, Martin CB Jr, Reid DL. Fetal heart rate variability and behavioral state: analysis by power spectrum. Am J Obstet Gynecol 1992;167:717–722

8. Clark SL, Gimovsky ML, Miller FC. Fetal heart rate response to scalp blood sampling. Am J Obstet Gynecol 1982;44:706–708

9. Haverkamp AD, Orleans M, Langendoerfer S, McFee J, Murphy J, Thompson HE. A controlled trial of the differential effects of intrapartum fetal monitoring. Am J Obstet Gynecol 1979;134:399–412

10. Haverkamp AD, Thompson HE, Mcfee JG, Cetrulo C. The evaluation of continuous fetal heart rate monitoring in high-risk pregnancy. Am J Obstet Gynecol 1976;125: 310–320

11. Renou P, Chang A, Anderson I, Wood C. Controlled trial of fetal intensive care. Am J Obstet Gynecol 1976;126: 470–476

12. Kelso IM, Parsons RJ, Lawrence GF, Arora SS, Edmonds DK, Cooke ID. An assessment of continuous fetal heart rate monitoring in labor: a randomized trial. Am J Obstet Gynecol 1978;131:526–532

13. Wood C, Renou P, Oats J, Farrell E, Beischer N, Anderson I. A controlled trial of fetal heart rate monitoring in a low-risk obstetric population. Am J Obstet Gynecol 1981;141:527–534

14. MacDonald D, Grant A, Sheridan-Pereira M, Boylan P, Chalmers I. The Dublin randomized controlled trial of intrapartum fetal heart rate monitoring. Am J Obstet Gynecol 1985;152:524–539

15. National Institutes of Health. Antenatal diagnosis. Report of a consensus development conference. NIH publication #79-1973. Bethesda, Maryland: NIH, 1979

16. Leveno KJ, Cunningham FG, Nelson S, Roark M, Williams ML, Guzick D, et al. A prospective comparison of selective and universal electronic fetal monitoring in 34,995 pregnancies. N Engl J Med 1986;315;615–619

17. Vintzileos AM, Antsaklis A, Varvarigos I, Papas C, Sofatzis I, Montgomery JT. A randomized trial of intrapartum electronic fetal heart rate monitoring versus intermittent auscultation. Obstet Gynecol 1993;81:899–907

18. Shy KK, Luthy DA, Bennett FC, Whitfield M, Larson EB, van Belle G, et al. Effects of electronic fetal-heart-rate monitoring, as compared with periodic auscultation, on the neurologic development of premature infants. N Engl J Med 1990;322:588–593

19. Melone PJ, Ernest JM, O'Shea MD Jr, Klinepeter KL. Appropriateness of intrapartum fetal heart rate management and risk of cerebral palsy. Am J Obstet Gynecol 1991;165:272–277

20. Colditz PB, Henderson-Smart DJ. Electronic fetal heart rate monitoring during labour: does it prevent perinatal asphyxia and cerebral palsey? Med J Austr 1990;153:88–90

21. Miyazaki FS, Nevarez F. Saline amnioinfusion for relief of repetitive variable decelerations: a prospective randomized study. Am J Obstet Gynecol 1985;153:301–306

22. Nageotte MP, Freeman RK, Garite TJ, Dorchester W. Prophylactic intrapartum amnioinfusion in patients with preterm premature rupture of membranes. Am J Obstet Gynecol 1985;153:557–562

23. Strong TH Jr, Hetzler G, Sarno AP, Paul RH. Prophylactic intrapartum amnioinfusion: a randomized clinical trial. Am J Obstet Gynecol 1990;162:1370–1375

24. Ingemarsson I, Arulkumaran S, Ingemarsson E, Tambyraja RL, Ratnam SS. Admission test: a screening test for fetal distress in labor. Obstet Gynecol 1986;68: 800–806

25. Bissonnette JM. Relationship between continuous fetal heart rate patterns and Apgar score in the newborn. Br J Obstet Gynaecol 1975;82:24–28

26. Freeman RK, Garite TJ, Nageotte MP. Fetal heart rate monitoring. 2nd ed. Baltimore, Maryland: Williams and Wilkins, 1991

27. Martin CB Jr, de Haan J, van der Wildt B, Jongsma HW, Dieleman A, Arts THM. Mechanisms of late decelerations in the fetal heart rate. A study with autonomic blocking agents in fetal lambs. Eur J Obstet Gynecol Reprod Biol 1979;9:361–373

28. Modanlou HD, Freeman RK. Sinusoidal fetal heart rate pattern: its definition and clinical significance. Am J Obstet Gynecol 1982;142:1033–1038

29. Meschia G. Placental respiratory gas exchange and fetal oxygenation. In: Creasy RK, Resnik R, eds. Maternal fetal medicine: principles and practice. Philadelphia, Pennsylvania: WB Saunders, 1989:303–313

30. Abitbol MM. Supine position in labor and associated fetal heart rate changes. Obstet Gynecol 1985;65:481–486

31. Clark SL, Cotton DB, Pivarnik JM, Lee W, Hankins GDV, Benedetti TJ, et al. Position change and central hemodynamic profile during normal third-trimester pregnancy and post partum. Am J Obstet Gynecol 1991;164:883–887

32. Hood DD. Obstetric anesthesia: complications and problems. In: Problems in anesthesia. Philadelphia, Pennsylvania: JB Lippincott Co, 1989:1–17

33. Vroman S, Sian AYL, Thiery M, de Hemptinne D, Vanderheyden K, Van Kets H, et al. Elective induction of labor conducted under lumbar epidural block. I. Labor induction by amniotomy and intravenous oxytocin. Eur J Obstet Gynecol Reprod Biol 1977;7:159–180

34. Abboud TK, Afrasiabi A, Sarkis F, Daftarian F, Nagappala S, Noueihed R, et al. Continuous infusion epidural analgesia in parturients receiving bupivacaine, chloroprocaine, or lidocaine—maternal, fetal, and neonatal effects. Anesth Analg 1984;63:421–428

35. Steiger RM, Nageotte MP. Effect of uterine contractility and maternal hypotension on prolonged decelerations after bupivacaine epidural anesthesia. Am J Obstet Gynecol 1990;163:808–812

36. Nageotte MP, Bertucci L, Towers CV, Lagrew DL, Modanlou H. Prophylactic amnioinfusion in pregnancies complicated by oligohydramnios: a prospective study. Obstet Gynecol 1991;77:677–680

37. Sadovsky Y, Amon E, Bade ME, Petrie RH. Prophylactic amnioinfusion during labor complicated by meconium: a preliminary report. Am J Obstet Gynecol 1989;161:613–617

38. Wenstrom KD, Parsons MT. The prevention of meconium aspiration in labor using amnioinfusion. Obstet Gynecol 1989;73:647–651

39. Macri CJ, Schrimmer DB, Leung A, Greenspoon JS, Paul RH. Prophylactic amnioinfusion improves outcome of pregnancy complicated by thick meconium and oligohydramnios. Am J Obstet Gynecol 1992;167:117–121

40. Tabor BL, Maier JA. Polyhydramnios and elevated intrauterine pressure during amnioinfusion. Am J Obstet Gynecol 1987;156:130–131

41. Arias F. Intrauterine resuscitation with terbutaline: a method for the management of acute intrapartum fetal distress. Am J Obstet Gynecol 1978;131:39–43

42. Reece EA, Chervenak FA, Romero R, Hobbins JC. Magnesium sulfate in the management of acute intrapartum fetal distress. Am J Obstet Gynecol 1984;148:104–107

43. Tejani NA, Verma UL, Chatterjee S, Mittelmann S. Terbutaline in the management of acute intrapartum acidosis. J Reprod Med 1983;28:857–861

44. Clark SL, Gimovsky ML, Miller FC. The scalp stimulation test: a clinical alternative to fetal scalp blood sampling. Am J Obstet Gynecol 1984;148:274–277

45. Smith CV, Nguyen HN, Phelan JP, Paul RH. Intrapartum assessment of fetal well-being: a comparison of fetal acoustic stimulation with acid–base determinations. Am J Obstet Gynecol 1986;155:726–728

46. Clark SL, Paul RH. Intrapartum fetal surveillance: the role of fetal scalp blood sampling. Am J Obstet Gynecol 1985;153:717–720

This Technical Bulletin was developed under the direction of the Committee on Technical Bulletins of the American College of Obstetricians and Gynecologists as an educational aid to obstetricians and gynecologists. The committee wishes to thank Thomas J. Garite, MD, and Michael P. Nageotte, MD, for their assistance in the development of this bulletin. This Technical Bulletin does not define a standard of care, nor is it intended to dictate an exclusive course of management. It presents recognized methods and techniques of clinical practice for consideration by obstetrician–gynecologists for incorporation into their practices. Variations of practice taking into account the needs of the individual patient, resources, and limitations unique to the institution or type of practice may be appropriate.
ISSN 1074-8628

THE AMERICAN COLLEGE OF OBSTETRICIANS AND GYNECOLOGISTS
409 12th Street, SW
Washington, DC 20024-2188

12345/98765

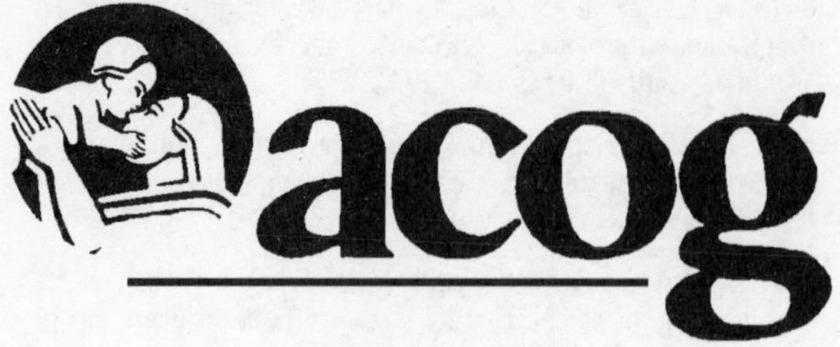

Number 208—July 1995

Technical Bulletin

An Educational Aid to Obstetrician–Gynecologists

Genetic Technologies

The elucidation of DNA structure by molecular techniques permits the study of human genes. Molecular biology is now applied to most branches of clinical medicine and therefore is relevant to practicing obstetrician–gynecologists. Awareness of the techniques integral to molecular biology is based on an understanding of DNA structure and genes.

This Technical Bulletin presents laboratory procedures based on molecular technologies that are currently being used in the diagnosis of genetic disorders. The role of restriction enzymes is addressed, as well as the principles and specifics of Southern blot analysis, restriction-fragment-length polymorphisms (RFLP), polymerase chain reaction (PCR), dot blot testing, and DNA sequencing. These procedures form the basis for the study of genetic disorders, and an understanding of them will help the clinician who sees patients with genetic concerns.

DNA Structure

DNA is a double-helical structure composed of two coils of nucleotide chains connected by nitrogenous bases. The precise complementary nature of nitrogenous bases provides the basis for the molecular analysis of DNA structure. The nitrogenous base adenine (A) specifically joins to thymine (T) by two hydrogen bonds, while guanine (G) joins to cytosine (C) by three hydrogen bonds. Therefore, GC bonds are more tightly held together than AT bonds and thus may be harder to separate. Uracil replaces T in RNA and is also complementary to A. These strands of DNA may be separated (denatured) or remain joined (annealed). Hybridization is the term commonly used to describe the joining of two different strands of DNA, such as DNA isolated from a patient with a genetic disorder and a DNA probe for the disease-producing gene.

Gene Structure

A gene is a strand of DNA that is transcribed into messenger RNA (mRNA) in the cell's nucleus, then translated into protein in the ribosomes. The amino acid sequence of the protein is determined by the RNA sequence (and ultimately DNA sequence), specifically by groups of 3 base pairs (bp) of nucleotides termed codons. This is referred to as the "genetic code." Individual genes make up only a small percentage of the 3×10^9 bp, or 3 million kilobases (kb), of nucleotides per haploid genome in humans. The function of the remainder of DNA is speculative, but it should be more fully understood with the completion of the human genome mapping project.

The human genome mapping initiative began in 1989 and should be completed around 2005. The purpose is to sequence the entire genomes of the human, mouse, nematode, and fruit fly. Characterization of the estimated 50,000–100,000 human genes should be beneficial for the understanding, diagnosis, and treatment of genetic diseases. Interspecies comparisons assume paramount importance for the understanding of gene structure, regulation, and function. New gene characterization continues at a rapid pace and will be markedly enhanced by the human genome mapping project.

A key point relating to the structure of DNA is the attachment of the phosphate to either of the two hydroxyl groups that are located on the deoxyribose sugar. These hydroxyl groups located at different sites on the deoxyribose molecule are numbered by convention as 3 prime (3′) and 5 prime (5′). Five prime and three prime refer to the carbon number of the deoxyribose sugar of DNA. The sugar phosphate backbone that is on the outside of the helix runs in 5′ to 3′ direction on one DNA strand and in 3′ to 5′ direction on the opposite strand. When nitrogenous bases are added to a growing DNA strand, they are added to the 3′ hydroxyl group of the phosphate (attached to the 3′ carbon).

The standard notation of gene structure is written as 5′ (upstream) on the left and 3′ (downstream) on the right (Fig. 1). The basic gene contains exons, which are DNA sequences that will be transcribed into mRNA, and introns (or intervening sequences), which are noncoding regions that lie between exons. The regions upstream and downstream to the exons are called the 5′ untranslated region and the 3′ untranslated region, respectively. These regions are also transcribed but not translated (as the name implies), and they are important in gene regulation.

When the gene is transcribed, the enzyme RNA polymerase II copies single-stranded DNA into mRNA. Once the mRNA is formed, the introns are removed, a chain of As (the poly-A tail) is added, and the mRNA leaves the nucleus and moves to the ribosomes for translation. The protein product is usually created in a precursor form, and the active protein is cleaved. The protein may be further modified in the Golgi apparatus of the cell by glycosylation.

Human genes usually contain consensus sequences, which are certain specific base pair arrangements present throughout most genes. These consensus sequences signal the location, initiation, and termination of transcription and translation, the locations of introns, and the location at which the poly-A tail will be added to the mRNA (Fig. 1). The DNA structure is the same in every cell of the body, but only certain tissues express certain mRNAs and produce certain proteins. The regulatory regions determine which tissues express the gene and quantitatively regulate its expression.

Restriction Enzymes

Since human genomic DNA is very large but specific genes are small (ranging from several kilobases to up to 1,000 kb in rare cases), cutting DNA into smaller pieces greatly facilitates its study. Enzymes in bacteria called restriction enzymes, or restriction endonucleases, enable digestion of DNA into smaller pieces. These restriction enzymes are native to the organism and protect against its destruction by foreign DNA, such as viruses. The restriction enzymes recognize specific sequences and cut every time this particular array of bases is encountered. They are named for the organism in which they were identified, as well as the strain. For example *Eco*RI was isolated from *Escherichia coli*, strain R, and was the first such enzyme obtained from this organism. This enzyme recognizes the sequence GAATTC and cuts between the G and A (Fig. 2). After this cleavage occurs, overhanging or

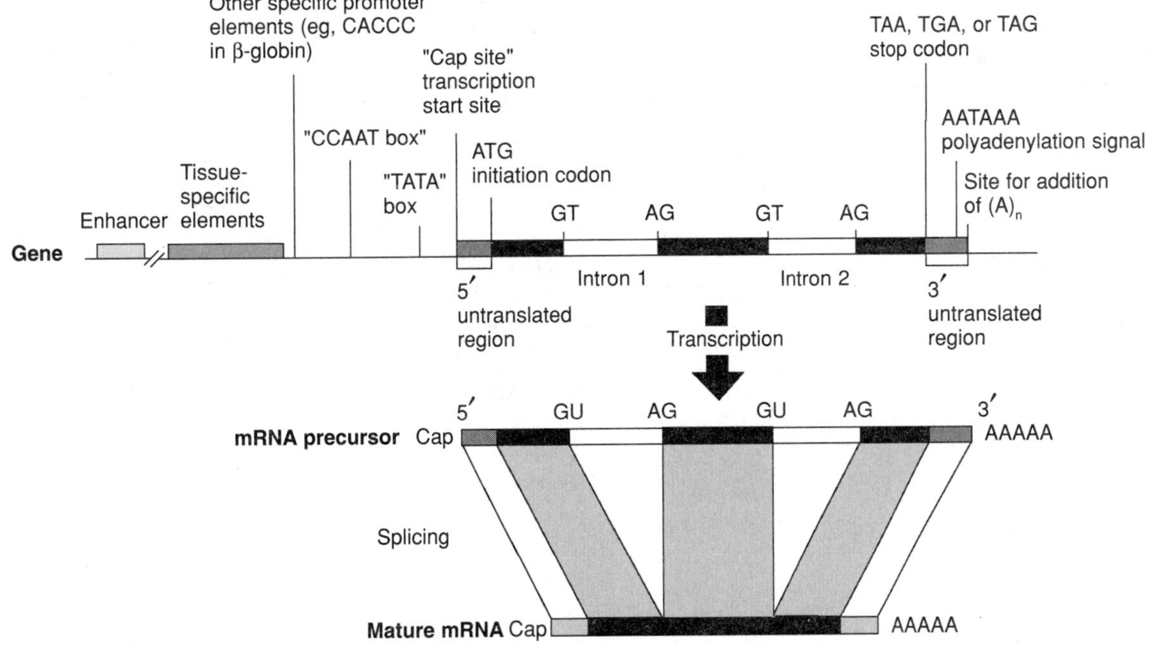

FIG. 1. The structure of a typical gene is demonstrated. The three exons are shown as solid dark regions, while the two introns are depicted as white regions bound by the consensus sequences GT and AG. The upstream region (5`) contains an enhancer, tissue-specific elements, and the promoter. Note the 5` untranslated region and the 3` untranslated region. Other consensus sequences are also shown, including the intron splice donor site (GT) and the splice acceptor site (AG). These sequences identify where introns are removed in mRNA production. Also depicted are the promoter elements, the CCAAT box and TATA box (which regulate expression), translation initiation site (ATG), and translation stop codons (TAA, TAG, TGA), and polyadenylation signal (AATAAA). (Gelehrter TD, Collins FS. Principles of medical genetics. Baltimore: Williams and Wilkins, 1990:91)

"sticky" single-stranded ends remain. These ends promote the religation or joining of two complementary pieces of DNA that have been cut with the same enzyme. Restriction enzymes allow cleavage of a specific fragment of DNA that then may be inserted into a vector such as a bacterial plasmid. This vector is capable of autonomous replication that allows milligram amounts of DNA to be produced (Fig. 3). The discovery of these important enzymes allowed investigators to join pieces of DNA cut with the same enzyme, a requirement to clone genes. Cloning genes is an essential step for the manipulation and study of disease-producing genes.

Southern Blot Analysis

Southern blot analysis provides a basis for studying genetic disorders at the DNA level. When a normal gene is identified, it can be used as a probe (ie, a DNA probe to study gene structure in an individual's DNA). If the subject's DNA and the DNA probe are each rendered single stranded and then hybridized, the complementary pairing should occur between the DNA probe and sample DNA. If the pairing does not occur, the subject's DNA does not contain the gene structures present in the probe. For convenience, subject DNA is commonly placed on some type of manageable substance, usually a nylon membrane. This is the Southern blot, named for E. M. Southern, not for a particular geographic region. A Northern blot, which identifies a specific sequence of RNA, consists of a membrane containing immobilized RNA, while a Western blot contains protein.

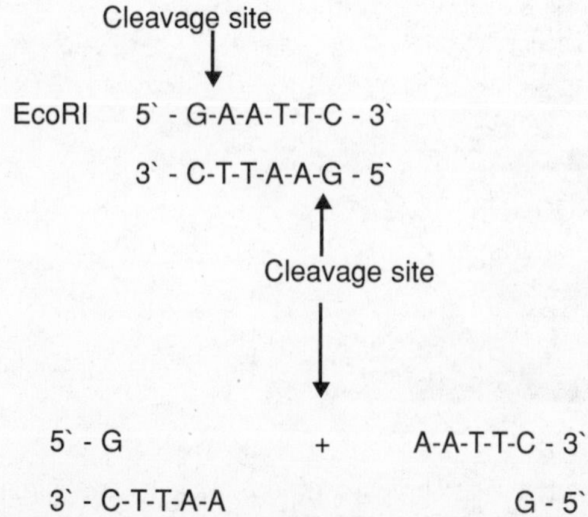

FIG. 2. Restriction enzymes (endonucleases) recognize specific sequences and cut every time this particular array is encountered. *Eco*RI recognizes the sequence GAATTC and cuts between the G and A.

Preparation of a Southern Blot

A series of steps is required to create a Southern blot (Fig. 4). DNA is first extracted from nucleated cells, such as leukocytes, trophoblasts, or amniocytes; mature erythrocytes do not contain DNA. The DNA is then digested with a restriction enzyme into innumerable small pieces. The gene of interest is among these many fragments, but its precise identification and size cannot be determined at this stage (although its presence can be ascertained by dot blots, which are described later). The DNA is loaded into an agarose gel, and electric current is applied. During this gel electrophoresis, the current causes smaller DNA fragments to migrate faster and farther than larger fragments (Fig. 4). The gel is then stained with ethidium bromide, which intercalates between the base pairs and allows visualization of the DNA when it is exposed to ultraviolet light. Because human genomic DNA is so large, the DNA in the lanes appears as a smear, but it is actually composed of many discrete fragments of varying size. Correct identification of the gene being studied is not yet possible at this point in the procedure.

The DNA contained within the agarose gel is still double stranded at this point. If the gel is exposed to alkali, the DNA will denature into single-stranded pieces. The gel now could be studied by hybridization to a single-stranded DNA probe, but, because of the fragility of the gel, the DNA is usually transferred to a nylon membrane (the Southern blot). The gel is placed on a platform (either glass or sponge) in a container with buffer. The nylon membrane is positioned directly above the gel followed by paper towels on top of the membrane (Fig. 4). The buffer passes up through the gel by capillary action, causing the single-stranded DNA to migrate to the nylon membrane. The membrane is then baked in a vacuum oven to permanently fix the DNA to the nylon blot. Transfer time may be shortened by using electroblotting or vacuum blotting.

The blot, containing a number of distinct specimens from both subjects and control(s), can now be hybridized to a DNA probe. For example, if congenital adrenal hyperplasia due to a deletion in the 21-hydroxylase gene is suspected, the blot could be hybridized to a DNA probe for 21-hydroxylase. For hybridization, a DNA probe is labeled with some type of marker, usually a radionuclide such as ^{32}P, although nonradioactive substances such as biotin–avidin may be used. Once the probe is labeled, if it is double stranded it is denatured by boiling or by using alkali and placed into a bag or tube with solution and the membrane for hybridization. DNA probes may be complementary DNAs (cDNAs), which are DNA sequences exactly complementary to the mRNA, lacking introns and regulatory regions, or they may be genomic clones containing parts of genes such as exons and introns or regulatory regions. Genomic probes and cDNA probes are

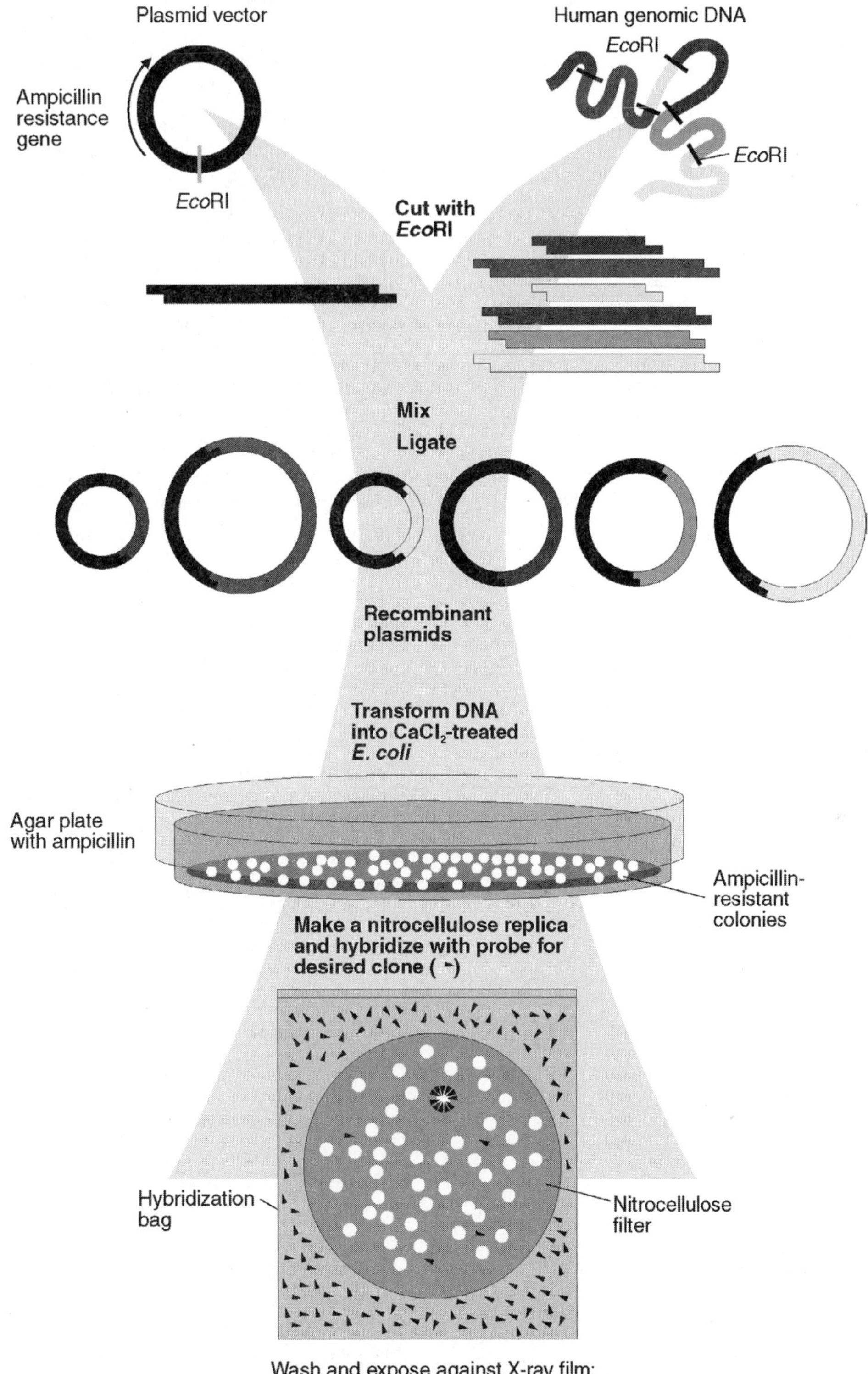

FIG. 3. Diagram of the process of generating a specific recombinant DNA molecule. Restriction enzymes allow the cleavage of a specific fragment of DNA. To produce a large quantity of the desired fragments, this fragment is inserted into a vector which is capable of autonomous replication. The overhanging or sticky ends can be ligated together using DNA ligase to generate a series of recombinant molecules in which different genomic fragments have been inserted into the vector. This mixture is then transfected into ampicillin-sensitive *Escherichia coli.* Only those bacteria that have taken the plasmid will form colonies when placed on ampicillin. To identify the specific recombinant carrying the desired genomic fragment, hybridization is carried out with a probe for the desired clone. (Gelehrter TD, Collins FS. Principles of medical genetics. Baltimore: Williams and Wilkins, 1990:74)

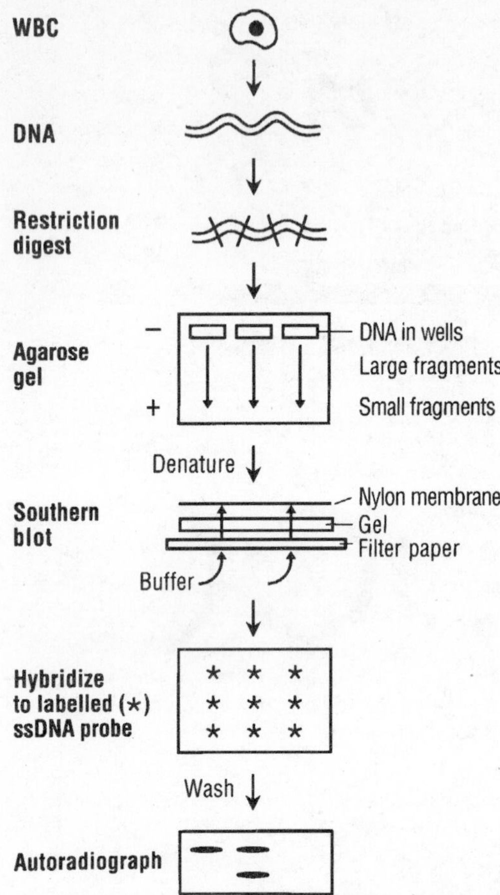

FIG. 4. The preparation of a Southern blot is shown. WBC indicates leukocytes; ssDNA, single-stranded DNA. The DNA is extracted from nucleated cells. The DNA is then digested with restriction enzyme into multiple small pieces. The DNA is loaded on an agarose gel and an electric current is applied. The smaller fragments migrate faster.

The gel is placed on a platform in a container with buffer. The nylon membrane (Southern blot) is placed directly above the gel. The single-stranded DNA migrates to the nylon membrane; the buffer passes up through the gel. The blot, containing a number of specimens from both subjects and control(s), can now be hybridized to a DNA probe.

Once hybridization is complete, the combined, labeled DNA probe is removed by washing. When washing is complete, the blot is placed in plastic wrap inside a cassette containing film at -70°C (autoradiography). The film is then developed, and the presence or absence of bands can be determined. (Layman LC. Basic concepts of molecular biology as applied to pediatric and adolescent gynecology. Obstet Gynecol Clin North Am 1992; 19:11)

both double stranded and require denaturation prior to hybridization. The DNA probes may also be short pieces of single-stranded DNA termed oligonucleotides, which usually range in size from 20 to 50 bp.

Once hybridization is complete, the unbound, labeled DNA probe is removed by washing. Washes are performed to remove as much of the nonspecific binding material as possible. By washing at high temperatures and low-salt concentrations (high stringency), only sequences that are exactly complementary remain hybridized. When washing is completed, the blot is placed in plastic wrap inside a cassette containing film at -70°C (a process called autoradiography). The film is then developed, and the presence or absence of bands can be determined (Fig. 4).

If the same number and size of bands are present in affected individuals and controls, the gene is present and no obvious large rearrangements of the gene are present. This does not preclude the possibility that smaller mutations, such as 2-bp deletions or point mutations, are present. In general, Southern blot analysis is not capable of detecting changes this small unless the mutation alters a restriction enzyme cut site (sickle mutation). If the band is absent, then a segment of the gene may be deleted. This can be confirmed by using blots of genomic DNA digested with several different restriction enzymes. The absence of a band on only one digest could be due to a polymorphism, not a deletion. Many diseases are characterized by deletions. Those particularly relevant to the practice of obstetrics and gynecology include deletions in the 21-hydroxylase gene in congenital adrenal hyperplasia (1), the α-globin gene in α-thalassemia (2), the dystrophin gene in Duchenne-type muscular dystrophy (3), and the transmembrane conductance regulator protein in cystic fibrosis (4). Unfortunately, not all individuals with a particular genetic disorder display the same deletion, so Southern analysis of deletions is not often clinically useful.

Restriction-Fragment-Length Polymorphisms

Frequently, a gene will be determined to be present by Southern blotting, but the number and fragment sizes may differ among subjects. If a difference exists in the pattern of bands on the Southern blot, the possibilities include the presence of true mutations altering the function of the normal gene and its product or the presence of benign base changes called polymorphisms, which do not produce deleterious phenotypic effects. Although these polymorphisms are not the cause of the genetic disorder, they may provide important diagnostic markers for the disease-producing gene, thus facilitating diagnosis.

For example, hybridization of a DNA probe to a Southern blot of DNA digested with the restriction enzyme *Hin*dIII yields fragments of 15 kb, 10 kb, and 5 kb for a certain genetic disorder (Fig. 5). On chromosome A, a 15-kb band is produced, but on chromosome B there is an additional *Hin*dIII site, so the 15-kb fragment is further cut into 10- and 5-kb fragments. Subjects may be homozygous or heterozygous for these alleles. This benign variation or dimorphism in DNA sequences may be useful for the diagnosis of a genetic disorder. If one of these fragments or alleles is found in individuals affected with the disorder and not found in unaffected individuals, then the DNA marker can be assumed to be segregating with the disease in such a family.

As shown in Fig. 5, both parents have one copy each of the 15-, 10-, and 5-kb fragments—they are heterozygous for these alleles. Each normal child is either homozygous for allele B (with two copies of the 10- and 5-kb fragments) or heterozygous like the parents. The individual with the genetic disorder has two copies of allele A (homozygous for the 15-kb fragment), but no unaffected individual has this pattern. In this family, the 15-kb fragment segregates with the disease, so it is a "marker" for this disorder. This marker is called an RFLP. Even though the 15-kb band may not contain the defect, it appears to segregate with the disease, and so it may be used for diagnosis.

The benign mutation or dimorphism may be identified as a restriction fragment (ie, the band on the radiograph) by using Southern blot analysis of family members. This restriction fragment usually results from a polymorphism causing a loss or gain of a restriction site. A polymorphism does not have a deleterious effect on the individual. The length refers to the size of the fragment or band. So an RFLP refers to a benign mutation in DNA sequences that alters an enzyme cut site, and the resulting fragment may segregate with a genetic disorder.

Several important aspects of RFLPs need to be considered further. The fragment or band on the radiograph is not the causative mutation; it is physically close (or linked) to the causative mutation. "Close" may mean several thousand kilobases away from the causative gene, which is why RFLPs may be identified long before the causative gene can be localized. Searching several thousand kilobases may take a tremendous amount of time, effort, and expense. These fragments follow Mendelian patterns of inheritance, as in the example shown. Since this fragment is not the cause of the disease, a study of family members is necessary. The RFLP is useful only if there is heterozygosity, as in this example. Here the 15-kb fragment segregates with the disease and is said to be "informative." Homozygosity for the 5- and 10-kb fragments or heterozygosity for the 15-, 10-, and 5-kb fragments do not occur in affected individuals. If affected and unaffected individuals in the same family were homozygous for the 15-kb fragment, it would be impossible to predict which individual has the disease with this RFLP (the RFLP would not be informative).

Restriction-fragment-length polymorphisms are perhaps the most useful tools in clinical genetic diagnosis. It is much easier to find a marker for a disorder than to find the exact causative gene. This is evidenced by the fact that diagnosis of Huntington disease by virtue of RFLP has been possible since the early 1980s, but the gene itself has only recently been identified. Since most genetic disorders are heterogenous, having different mutations among different families, RFLPs are generally more useful if family studies can be performed. There are many examples in the literature of diseases that can be diagnosed by RFLPs, such as Huntington disease, adult polycystic kidney disease, and congenital adrenal hyperplasia. Direct diagnosis of deletions is possible in most cases of cystic fibrosis and Duchenne-type muscular dystrophy; when deletions cannot be identified, RFLP analysis may be applicable.

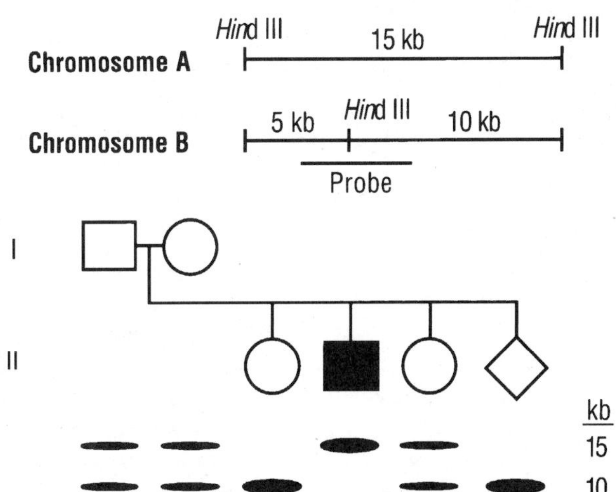

FIG. 5. The concept of restriction-fragment-length polymorphism is demonstrated. Above is the specific restriction map for HindIII with hybridization to a particular probe. The family is shown in the middle. A schematic radiograph from a Southern blot is shown at the bottom of the figure. Individual II-2 (solid block) is the affected family member and is homozygous for 15 kilobases (kb). Those family members heterozygous for 15, 10, and 5 kb (I-1, I-2, and II-3) and those homozygous for 10 and 5 kb (II-1 and II-4) are unaffected. (Layman LC. Basic concepts of molecular biology as applied to pediatric and adolescent gynecology. Obstet Gynecol Clin North Am 1992;19:13)

One specific example of a disorder detectable directly by Southern blot analysis is sickle cell anemia (5). Because the point mutation in the β-globin gene is identical in all patients with sickle cell anemia and because it results in the loss of a restriction site, diagnosis is possible by examining the restriction fragments. The difference here is that the point mutation causing the loss of a restriction site in sickle cell anemia is itself the causative mutation, not a benign polymorphism segregating with the disease. Genetic diagnosis would be much simpler if all genetic diseases had the same molecular basis of altering restriction cut sites, but this is not the case.

Polymerase Chain Reaction

Southern blot analysis is labor intensive and generally requires 5–10 μg of DNA for analysis. The development of the PCR has greatly simplified DNA analysis and shortened laboratory time. As mentioned previously, the target gene makes up a minority of the sequences in total chromosomal DNA. Rather than trying to identify a single gene among the many genes per haploid genome with a labeled probe as in Southern analysis, the PCR allows the exponential amplification of the targeted gene, so that its structure can be studied without the need for DNA probes. Only minute quantities of DNA, typically 0.1–1 μg, are necessary for PCR (although DNA can be amplified from a single cell) (6, 7). One important prerequisite of PCR not required for Southern blot analysis is that the sequence of the gene—or at least the borders of the region of DNA to be amplified—must be known.

The PCR procedure has three steps (Fig. 6). First, DNA is heated to 94–95°C to render it single stranded (or denatured). Second, the temperature is lowered to 37–55°C, which results in DNA annealing. The reaction solution contains primers, which are short pieces of DNA (oligonucleotides) usually about 20–30 bp in length. They are exactly complementary to the ends of each piece of the double-stranded DNA to be amplified. When the temperature is lowered, these primers will stick, or anneal, to their complementary regions of the DNA. This is the reason the sequence of part of the DNA template must be known. The primers are present in such excess that the DNA template is more likely to anneal to the primer rather than to itself. Third, the temperature is raised to about 72°C in the presence of an enzyme (a heat-stable DNA polymerase such as Taq polymerase) and the deoxynucleotide triphosphates (dNTPs) dATP, dCTP, dGTP, and dTTP so that the synthesis of the second complementary strand of DNA will be completed (6, 7). In practice, the primers, buffer, dNTPs, enzyme, and DNA are mixed together in a tube to a total volume of 25–100 μl and placed in a thermal cycler, an incubator that changes temperature rapidly. The exact cycling parameters and conditions for PCR must be determined empirically for each set of primers.

After one cycle of denaturation, annealing, and primer extension, the DNA content is doubled; one piece of double-stranded DNA becomes two double-stranded pieces of DNA. After two cycles there are four copies; after three cycles there are eight, and so on. The amount of DNA being amplified increases exponentially with each cycle so that the final amount of amplified DNA will be 2^n where n equals the number of cycles. After 30 cycles, which is the typical number of cycles used, the gene of interest may be amplified over 2^{30} or well over one million times. If agarose gel electrophoresis is performed on the amplified product of the PCR, the product will migrate to a specific point in the gel and appear as a distinct band (Fig. 7). Typically, fragments several kilobases in size can be amplified (6–8), but sequences up to 10 kb have been successfully amplified.

In the early stages of the PCR, some of the fragments will be longer than the desired product (Fig. 6). However, since the termini of the amplified regions are defined by the primers (they are physically incorporated into one strand as it is synthesized), as the number of cycles increases, successively more of the fragments become the desired length. For example, if a 1,230-bp fragment of DNA is to be amplified, some of the initial products may be 1,500 or 2,000 bp, but the final predominating product will be the 1,230-bp band (Figs. 6 and 7). The PCR process does not continue exponentially throughout all cycles. Eventually the primer substrate is so concentrated that the reaction does not progress as efficiently, and the product increases linearly rather than exponentially (9). This plateau effect is inevitable after many cycles, and most laboratories use 30–35 cycles of amplification for this reason.

A positive control (a sample known to be positive for the gene being amplified) and a negative control (a sample containing everything except DNA) should be run for every reaction (8). Because PCR is so sensitive, extreme care must be taken to avoid amplification of contaminant DNA from aerosolized secretions or sloughed skin cells. Therefore, PCR is often performed under a tissue culture hood by a technician wearing gloves and using sterile pipette tips, tubes, and reagents. These precautions are particularly important when DNA from a single cell is being amplified.

The PCR has greatly facilitated genetic diagnosis. If primers span a region of the gene known to be deleted in a certain disorder, deletions may be detected. The 3-bp deletion present in about 70% of American caucasians with cystic fibrosis may be detected by PCR analysis (4). If a variety of characterized deletions have been identified in patients with a certain disorder, they may be studied si-

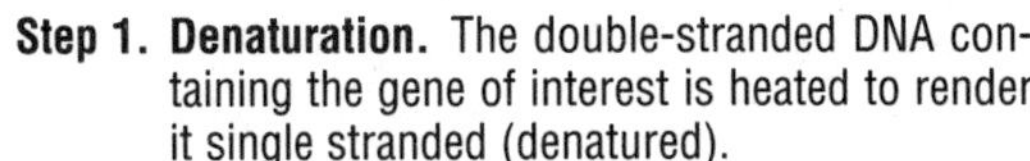

Step 1. Denaturation. The double-stranded DNA containing the gene of interest is heated to render it single stranded (denatured).

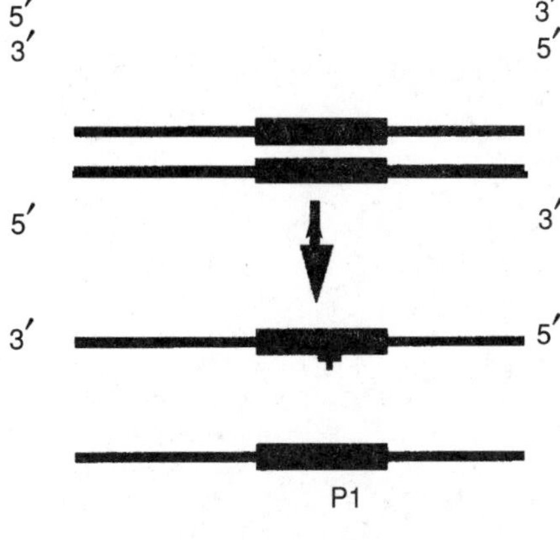

Step 2. Primer annealing. Short pieces of DNA that are complementary to the ends of the double-stranded DNA to be amplified (primers P1, 2) stick (anneal) to their complementary regions of DNA.

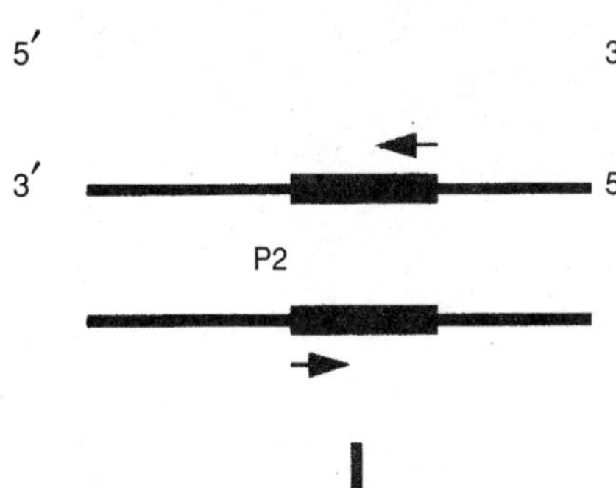

Step 3. Extension. In the presence of DNA polymerase and dNTPs, the synthesis of the second complementary strand of DNA is completed (extension). The DNA content has been doubled.

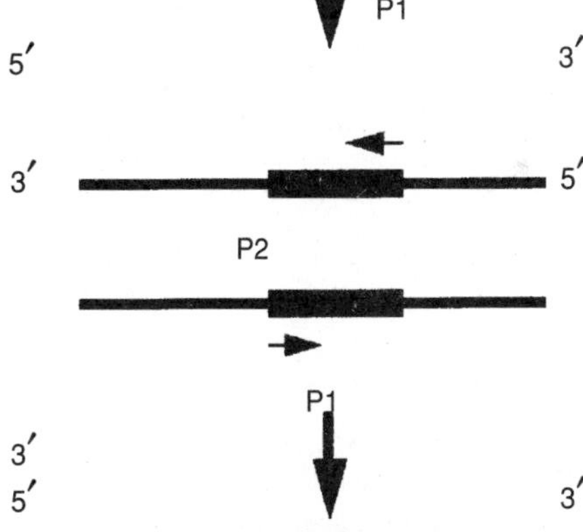

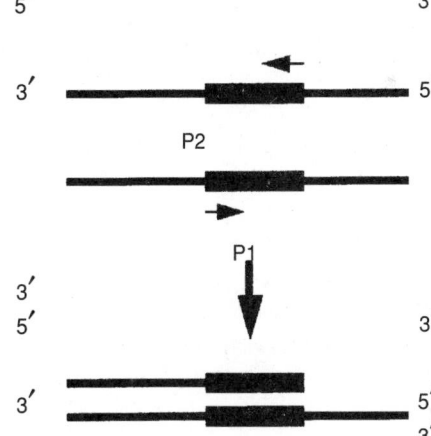

FIG. 6. Diagram of the polymerase chain reaction. One cycle is shown. The thickened region represents the sequence to be amplified.

multaneously in so-called multiplex PCR. The dystrophin gene is enormous, but since a large proportion of the deletions occurs in nine exons in patients with Duchenne type muscular dystrophy, these exons may be amplified in a single reaction (3). The resulting fragment sizes must be different so that they may be resolved by electrophoresis. Polyacrylamide gel electrophoresis allows resolution of smaller fragments than agarose gel electrophoresis. Analysis of RFLPs may also be performed by PCR if the primers are designed to amplify across the segment of DNA where the enzyme cut sites are located. In patients undergoing in vitro fertilization, analysis of PCR products is currently being investigated for its potential to permit the diagnosis of certain disorders such as cystic fibrosis, β-thalassemia, hemophilia A, Lesch–Nyhan syndrome, Duchenne type muscular dystrophy, and alpha-1-antitrypsin deficiency in single cells obtained from oocyte polar bodies and preembryo biopsy.

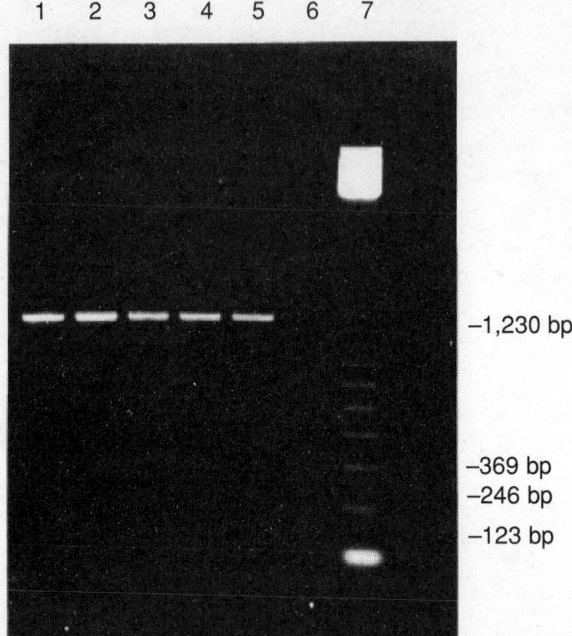

FIG. 7. Amplification of a 1,230-base pair (bp) region of the gonadotropin-releasing hormone gene. Lanes 1–4 are patients with idiopathic hypogonadotropic hypogonadism, lane 5 is a positive control, lane 6 is a negative control, and lane 7 contains a molecular weight marker. (Layman LC, Wilson JT, Huey LO, Lanclos KD, Plouffe L Jr, McDonough PG. Gonadotropin-releasing hormone, follicle-stimulating hormone beta, luteinizing hormone beta gene structure in idiopathic hypogonadotropic hypogonadism. Fertil Steril 1992;57:42–49. Reproduced with permission of the publisher, The American Fertility Society.)

Dot Blots and Other Methods

Southern blot analysis allows the detection of the size and basic structure of the gene as well as its presence. If the object is simply to determine whether the gene is present, dot blot analysis may be performed. In this method, undigested DNA is denatured, blotted onto nylon membranes, and hybridized to DNA probes. The use of both positive and negative controls is necessary because the lack of hybridization could indicate a procedural problem rather than a deletion. Because of this limitation, Southern blot analysis is usually preferred for clinical diagnosis. Dot blot analysis is usually reserved for probing by allele-specific probes.

When no mutations are obvious with Southern blot analysis or PCR, other techniques may be useful to search for point mutations or small deletions and insertions. Most genetic diseases are caused by point mutations in the coding regions. These single-base changes are detectable by DNA sequencing, which has been used extensively in basic research but generally has not been clinically applicable for genetic diagnosis (10). DNA sequencing is labor intensive and expensive, although it is amenable to automation (10). For this reason, one of the primary objectives of the human genome mapping project is to first identify markers scattered throughout the genome until the technique of sequencing is refined, automated, and less expensive (10).

If a point mutation for a particular genetic disorder is identified by DNA sequencing, dot blot analysis with allele-specific oligonucleotide probes can be performed. Two oligonucleotides, generally of 20–40 bases each, are synthesized and used for hybridization. One oligonucleotide is complementary to the normal (or wild-type) allele, and the other oligonucleotide is complementary to the mutant allele (Fig. 8). DNA (either uncut genomic DNA or a PCR product) may then be denatured, spotted onto a nylon membrane, and hybridized separately to each probe. A specimen from a homozygous normal individual hybridizes only to the normal oligonucleotide, while the homozygous mutant hybridizes only to the mutant probe. A specimen from a heterozygous individual hybridizes to both the mutant and wild-type oligonucleotides. This method of analysis is particularly suitable for sickle cell anemia, in which each affected individual has the same point mutation. Unfortunately, many genetic diseases, such as β-thalassemia and congenital adrenal hyperplasia, have different point mutations, so that the type of mutation would have to be known before this technique could be useful.

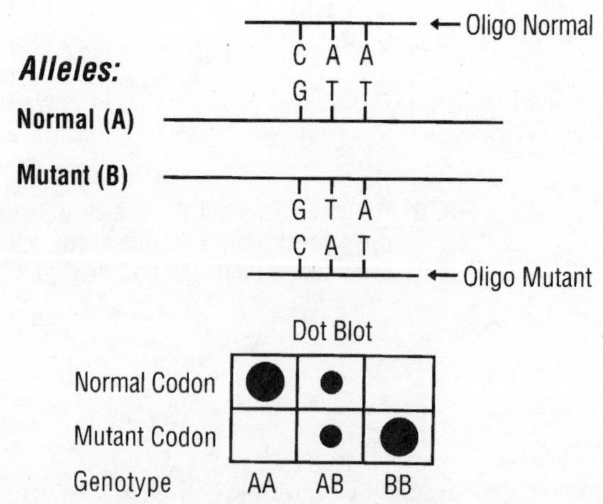

FIG. 8. Allele-specific oligonucleotide probing of a dot blot is shown. The normal and mutant alleles are shown at the top. Dot blot results are depicted at the bottom of the figure. (Layman LC. Basic concepts of molecular biology as applied to pediatric and adolescent gynecology. Obstet Gynecol Clin North Am 1992;19:21)

Recently, techniques such as denaturing gradient gel electrophoresis (11) and single-stranded conformation polymorphism (9) have been developed to detect single-base differences. Both procedures allow single-base changes to be identified as differentially migrating fragments on polyacrylamide gels, but they do not specify the mutation. Many more polymorphisms can be identified since detection is not limited to those polymorphisms altering restriction cut sites. DNA sequencing is required to identify which base is altered. Both denaturing gradient gel electrophoresis and single-stranded conformation polymorphism are excellent screening techniques, the results of which should be confirmed with DNA sequencing (9, 11).

Summary

Molecular techniques are now clinically useful for genetic diagnosis, and obstetrician–gynecologists should become familiar with their basic principles. Southern blot analysis and PCR are two of the most commonly used techniques to detect gene deletions and RFLPs. Analysis of RFLPs is perhaps the most widely applicable technique, but detailed family studies are required to determine whether an RFLP is informative.

REFERENCES

1. Reindollar RH, Gray MR. The molecular basis of 21-hydroxylase deficiency. Seminars in Reproductive Endocrinology 1991;9:34–45
2. Higgs DR, Vickers MA, Wilkie AOM, Pretorius I-M, Jarman AP, Weatherall DJ. A review of the molecular genetics of the human α–globin gene cluster. Blood 1989;73:1081–1104
3. Chamberlain JS, Gibbs RA, Ranier JE, Nguyen PN, Caskey CT. Deletion screening of the Duchenne muscular dystrophy locus via multiplex DNA amplification. Nucleic Acids Res 1988;16:11141–11156
4. Kerem B-S, Rommens JM, Buchanan JA, Markiewicz D, Cox TK, Chakravarti A, et al. Identification of the cystic fibrosis gene: genetic analysis. Science 1989;245:1073–1080
5. Wilson JT, Milner PF, Summer ME, Nallaseth FS, Fadel HE, Reindollar RH, et al. Use of restriction endonucleases for mapping the allele for β^S-globin. Proc Natl Acad Sci U S A 1982;79:3628–3631
6. Erlich A, Gelfand DH, Saiki RK. Specific DNA amplification. Nature 1988;331:461–462
7. Mullis KB, Faloona FA. Specific synthesis of DNA *in vitro* via a polymerase-catalyzed chain reaction. Methods Enzymol 1987;155:335–350
8. Layman LC. Basic concepts of molecular biology as applied to pediatric and adolescent gynecology. Obstet Gynecol Clin North Am 1992;19:1–26
9. Orita M, Iwahana H, Kanazawa H, Hayashi K, Sekiya T. Detection of polymorphisms of human DNA by gel electrophoresis as single-strand conformation polymorphisms. Proc Natl Acad Sci U S A 1989;86:2766–2770
10. Green ED, Waterston RH. The human genome project: prospects and implications for clinical medicine. JAMA 1991;266:1966–1975
11. Myers RM, Maniatis T, Lerman LS. Detection and localization of single base changes by denaturing gradient gel electrophoresis. Methods Enzymol 1987;155:501–527

SUGGESTED READING

McDonough PG. Molecular biology in reproductive endocrinology. In: Yen SSC, Jaffe RB, eds. Reproductive endocrinology: physiology, pathophysiology and clinical management. 3rd ed. Philadelphia: WB Saunders Co, 1990:25–64

Gelehrter TD, Collins FS. Structure and behavior of genes and chromosomes. In: Principles of medical genetics. Baltimore: Williams and Wilkins, 1990:9–25

This Technical Bulletin was developed under the direction of the Committee on Technical Bulletins of the American College of Obstetricians and Gynecologists as an educational aid to obstetricians and gynecologists. The committee wishes to thank Lawrence C. Layman, MD, and Paul G. McDonough, MD, for their assistance in the development of this bulletin. This Technical Bulletin does not define a standard of care, nor is it intended to dictate an exclusive course of management. It presents recognized methods and techniques of clinical practice for consideration by obstetrician–gynecologists for incorporation into their practices. Variations of practice taking into account the needs of the individual patient, resources, and limitations unique to the institution or type of practice may be appropriate. Requests for authorization to make photocopies should be directed to the Copyright Clearance Center, 222 Rosewood Drive, Danvers, MA 01923; telephone (508) 750-8400.

ISSN 1074-8628

THE AMERICAN COLLEGE OF OBSTETRICIANS AND GYNECOLOGISTS
409 12th Street, SW
Washington, DC 20024-2188

12345/87654

Number 193—June 1994
(Replaces #105, June 1987)

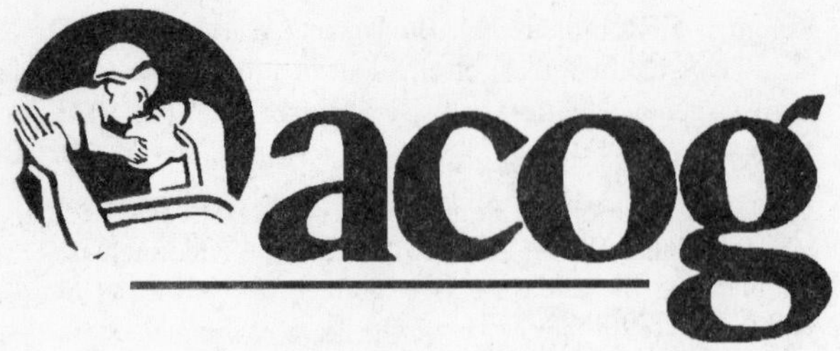

Technical Bulletin
An Educational Aid to Obstetrician–Gynecologists

Genital Human Papillomavirus Infections

Among women of reproductive age, the rate of detection of human papillomavirus (HPV) ranges from approximately 6% in those with apparently normal cervical cytology and examination to over 60% in those with cervical neoplasia (1). The frequency of HPV detection varies according to the detection method used and the population screened.

By international agreement, genital HPV infections are classified as latent (asymptomatic), subclinical, or clinical. Latent infections have no visible lesions and are detected only by DNA hybridization tests for HPV. Subclinical lesions are identified by application of 5% acetic acid and inspection under magnification. Clinical lesions can be identified without the aid of magnification and are typically called condylomata acuminata. The phenotypic expression of the virus is dependent on the type of epithelium, host interaction, and viral type. Infection in the genital tract may involve more than one site, including the vulva, vagina, cervix, urethra, perianal skin, and rectum.

Epidemiology

Although most HPV infections are related to sexual exposure, HPV DNA has been detected on underwear, biopsy instruments, and specula (2). In addition, HPV DNA has been detected on swabs of the cervix and vulva by sensitive polymerase chain reaction (PCR) probes in 20% of college-age women who had never had vaginal intercourse (3). Whether this DNA material can induce an infection has not been proven.

The natural history of subclinical and latent disease remains unknown. Transmissibility of these forms of HPV infection has been difficult to establish because there are no animal models and the virus cannot be grown in culture. Complicating the epidemiology of HPV are prospective longitudinal studies using DNA probes that demonstrate that latent infections come and go when asymptomatic women are repeatedly tested (4). It is unclear whether subclinical or latent disease can be transmitted.

Fifty percent of the male partners of women with condylomata acuminata have clinically visible lesions, and an additional 25% have subclinical lesions (5). While it is reasonable to identify and treat such partners, a retrospective study of treated versus untreated male partners did not demonstrate a decrease in the treatment failure rate for condylomata in the female partners (6). A similar study of male partners of women with cervical intraepithelial neoplasia (CIN) revealed no change in the recurrence rate for women whose male partners were treated (6.8%) versus those whose partners were not treated (7.5%) (7). Although the use of condoms has not been demonstrated to reduce the risk of reinfection, they are recommended to reduce the risk of other sexually transmitted diseases.

Virology

Human papillomaviruses are DNA viruses that are mucosotropic or cutaneotropic, most commonly involving the skin, lower genital tract, larynx, oral cavity, urethra, bladder, and anal and perianal epithelium. They belong to the family *Papovaviridae*, genus *Papillomavirus*. They have a capsid diameter of 45–55 nm, a molecular weight of 5×10^6, and a viral genome consisting of a double-stranded suprahelical DNA molecule of approximately 8,000 base pairs (8).

Over 60 HPV types have been identified, and more than 20 of these have been associated with lower genital tract infections (9). They have been subclassified according to their association with cervical neoplasia and carcinoma (see the box). The relationship of HPV 16 and 18 to cervical neoplasia appears to be a factor of the expression of E6 and E7 oncoproteins from the respective virus subtypes. E6 oncoprotein binds to P53 tumor suppressor protein, which results in loss of suppressor function (10). E7 oncoprotein links to the protein of the Rb retinoblastoma susceptibility gene (11). The E6 and E7 proteins of the low-risk viral types apparently have lower intrinsic biologic activity than do those of HPV 16 and 18, which may explain the usually benign character of HPV 6 and 11 (12). The E5 protein of HPV 16 can increase the number of keratinocyte cell surface epithelial growth factor receptors, contribute to the recycling of the surface receptor, increase the kinase activity of the receptor, as well as inhibit epithelial growth factor receptor degradation (13).

Human papillomavirus within the epithelial cell nucleus may exist either in an episomal (ie, extrachromosomal) location or integrated into the host DNA. Most cervical carcinomas associated with HPV 16 have viral DNA integrated into the host cell's DNA. In typical warts and intraepithelial neoplastic lesions (CIN, vaginal intraepithelial neoplasia, vulvar intraepithelial neoplasia [VIN]), HPV 16 usually exists in an episomal location (11).

Classification of HPV Types by Risk of Neoplasia and Cancer

High-risk types
- 16
- 18
- 45
- 56

Intermediate-risk types
- 30*
- 31
- 33
- 35
- 39
- 51
- 52
- 58
- 66

Low-risk types
- 6
- 11
- 42
- 43
- 44
- 53
- 54
- 55

*It is not clear whether HPV type 30 is of intermediate or high risk.

Lorincz AT, Reid R, Jenson AB, Greenberg MD, Lancaster W, Kurman RJ. Human papillomavirus infection of the cervix: relative risk associations of 15 common anogenital types. Adapted with permission from The American College of Obstetricians and Gynecologists (Obstetrics and Gynecology 1992, 79, 328–337)

Diagnosis of Vulvar, Vaginal, and Cervical Infection

Cytologic Screening

Detection of individuals with genital HPV infection often occurs through the process of cervical cytologic screening, in which koilocytosis and other cellular features of HPV infection may be identified. In the Bethesda System of cytologic classification, cytologic features of HPV infection are classified as low-grade squamous intraepithelial lesions. This category includes cellular features of mild dysplasia (CIN 1) and HPV infection. Koilocytosis is strictly defined as cellular changes demonstrating evidence of nuclear enlargement and atypia with a distinctive perinuclear halo (14). As an indication of HPV infection, the presence of koilocytes correlates better with results of DNA hybridization than any other single cytologic feature. It appears that subtle or nonclassic changes may not provide adequate sensitivity or specificity for detection of HPV and may result in overestimation of the frequency of infection when compared with molecular biologic methods of HPV detection (15).

Clinical Assessment

A broad spectrum of clinical findings may be associated with HPV that may be related to the HPV type and the host response to the infection. Individuals with evidence of HPV in one genital site have a significant risk of having HPV changes in another genital site. The anus and urethra should be evaluated. Typical genital warts of the vulva may be found anywhere on the vulva but are often multiple and involve the vulvar vestibule as well as medial aspects of the labia majora, perineal body, and periclitoral areas. Perianal involvement is common and does not necessarily imply anoreceptive sexual exposure.

Examination of the vulva with magnification and topical application of 3–5% acetic acid to identify acetowhite areas may assist in identification of sites of HPV infection that are not typically acuminate in nature. Such areas may represent associated VIN and are appropriate areas for biopsy.

Vulvar intraepithelial neoplasia (which includes bowenoid dysplasia, bowenoid papulosis, and carcinoma in situ) typically appears as multiple, variably sized and shaped lesions that are characteristically macular or papular and have irregular margins. They are acetowhite in approximately 70% of cases; however, the remainder may be red or pigmented. Approximately 70% of the cases are multicentric.

Within the vagina, the use of 3–5% acetic acid and colposcopy is of value in assessing vaginal epithelial changes when HPV infection is suspected. Colposcopic findings in the vagina are similar to those in the cervix. Acetowhite lesions should be biopsied to diagnose HPV changes or vaginal intraepithelial neoplasia. In some cases, the HPV changes may be extensive, essentially covering the entire vaginal mucosal surface.

On the cervix, papillomavirus-associated lesions may appear as typical condylomata or as squamous intraepithelial lesions of the cervix. The squamous intraepithelial lesions are typically acetowhite and occur either on the mature epithelium or in the transformation zone; they may be multiple and may have well-defined, sharp, discrete margins. The degree of acetowhite change and sharpness of margins correlates with the severity of the intraepithelial process. Biopsy of lesions within the transformation zone is indicated to establish the diagnosis. Latent HPV infection may be present in clinically and histologically normal epithelium surrounding the identifiable lesions (16).

Detection of Human Papillomavirus DNA

Human papillomavirus DNA may be detected by use of nucleic acid probes. In this technique, nucleic acid probes (labeled specific HPV RNA or DNA sequences) are hybridized to RNA or DNA within the cells in question. Hybridization by such specific probes is evidence of HPV infection. While Southern transfer hybridization was the primary research tool in the initial studies on genital HPV (11), dot filter hybridization correlates well with the Southern technique and is more cost-effective. In situ hybridization, in which either biotinylated or radioisotope-labeled probes may be used, correlates well with dot filter hybridization (9). If biotinylated probes are used, the sites of hybridization can be identified by light microscopy. Hybrid capture can be used to detect, type, and partially quantify genital HPV (17).

Polymerase chain reaction is the most sensitive of all the hybridization tests; it is significantly cheaper than Southern transfer (18). The sensitivity of PCR can be adjusted to approximate that of the Southern transfer, thereby reducing the risk of false-positive results.

All of these techniques can be performed on fresh tissue; however, in situ hybridization and PCR can also be used on fixed, paraffin-embedded tissue. In situ hybridization can identify the site of the virus within the tissue or cells under study. The pathologist can identify the areas of DNA hybridization by microscopic evaluation. With specific HPV primers, PCR is more sensitive than in situ hybridization and may eventually be partially automated to reduce cost. These techniques are the more prominent methods presently available for research and clinical studies.

The role of HPV testing in screening for cervical neoplasia is currently being studied. It cannot be routinely recommended at this time. Further studies are needed to prove the benefits of testing, but its value in certain circumstances is being explored:

- To determine whether atypical squamous cells of undetermined significance (ASCUS) are caused by HPV
- To determine which viral type(s) is present in women who have low-grade squamous intraepithelial lesions
- To determine whether HPV is present in histologic specimens in which the morphology is unclear
- To determine the origin of metastatic adenocarcinoma

Association with Gynecologic Disorders

Cervical Neoplasia

Epidemiologic studies have demonstrated that HPV detection is associated with a 10-fold or greater risk of cervical neoplasia when compared with controls (19). A prospective study of women who had negative cytology but tested positive for HPV demonstrated an 11-fold risk of developing CIN 2 or 3 within the 2-year follow-up period. Women with HPV 16 or 18 were more likely to develop CIN 2 or 3 than those with low- or intermediate-risk types. Each additional positive test was associated with a further increase in the risk of CIN 2 or 3 (20).

Over 75% of high-grade intraepithelial lesions are positive for high- or intermediate-risk HPV types. Among invasive cancers, 73% are positive for high-risk types only, and 10% are positive for intermediate-risk types (9). Patients with cervical carcinoma who are HPV negative have been found to have a significantly increased risk of dying from cervical carcinoma as compared with those who are HPV positive (21).

While HPV 16 is the most common type found in squamous carcinoma, HPV 18 is most common in adenocarcinoma (22) and neuroendocrine-positive, small-cell cervical carcinomas (23). The association of HPV 18 with these tumors suggests that women with HPV 18 may have a more significant risk of invasive neoplasm than those with other HPV types.

Vulvar Neoplasia

Vulvar condylomata acuminata are usually associated with HPV 6 or 11. Mosaic infections are possible. Both HPV 6 and its subtypes have also been associated with verrucous carcinoma and have been identified as a coinfection with HPV 16-containing vulvar squamous carcinomas (24).

Vulvar intraepithelial neoplasia is associated with HPV DNA in most patients (80–90%), with HPV 16 being the most common (25). Invasive vulvar carcinomas are positive for HPV in 20–50% of cases and are related to the cell type and morphology of the tumor, associated skin lesions, and the age of the patient (Table 1).

Several studies demonstrate that vulvar carcinoma may arise from at least two origins: one related to HPV and one not related to HPV (24, 26, 27). Younger women with VIN or vulvar squamous carcinoma are infected with HPV in approximately two thirds of cases, whereas in older women only slightly over one tenth of cases have evidence of HPV (24, 26–28). These studies demonstrate that vulvar squamous carcinoma in younger women with VIN may result from HPV 16 E6 inactivation of P53, while vulvar squamous cell carcinomas occurring in older women may result from spontaneous mutation or inactivation of P53 (25, 26).

Vulvar Vestibular Papillae

Although vulvar vestibular papillae may resemble small condylomata, they are rarely associated with HPV when analyzed by HPV DNA probes. An analysis of biopsy specimens from such patients revealed that 7% of 29 cases contained HPV which is the same as the background frequency of HPV in the normal vulva (29).

Vulvar Vestibulitis

Vulvar vestibulitis is a poorly understood clinical entity characterized by inflammation within the vulvar vestibule, exquisite point tenderness within the vestibule, and vulvar pain with severe external dyspareunia. Studies to identify HPV in the vulvar epithelium of patients with vulvar vestibulitis have had variable results. The evidence to date reveals no significant association with HPV 6, 11, 16, or 18 in this subset of patients. Some studies have suggested that there is a higher frequency of unidentified types of HPV. Histopathologic studies of vulvar vestibulitis, however, have reported that typical morphologic features of HPV infection are present in approximately 15% of cases (30). The glycogenated epithelium of the vestibule may be misinterpreted as koilocytosis, leading to a mistaken diagnosis of HPV infection. The limited success of the treatment of vulvar vestibulitis with interferon suggests that viral infection is not a primary etiology.

TABLE 1. CANCER OF THE VULVA CLINICAL PROFILES

	Associated with HPV DNA	
Characteristics	**Frequent (>60%)**	**Seldom (<15%)**
Age	35–65 years	55–85 years
Associated lesion	VIN*	Squamous cell hyperplasia, lichen sclerosus
Histology of tumor	Warty (condylomatous) or basaloid (poorly differentiated)	Keratinizing, well differentiated

*VIN indicates vulvar intraepithelial neoplasia.

Crum CP. Carcinoma of the vulva: epidemiology and pathogenesis. Adapted with permission from The American College of Obstetricians and Gynecologists (Obstetrics and Gynecology 1992, 79, 448–454)

Pregnancy and Genital Human Papillomavirus Infection

Genital warts may first appear or may grow markedly during pregnancy. The factors responsible may include up regulation and amplification of viral DNA secondary to the effects of progesterone and other hormones as well as suppression of immunity during pregnancy (11).

Podophyllin, 5-fluorouracil, and interferon are contraindicated in pregnancy. Small, asymptomatic lesions require no treatment. Larger, symptomatic lesions may be treated with trichloroacetic acid or bichloroacetic acid. Very large warts with secondary infection and maceration may be removed after the first trimester by simple excision or the use of laser or electrosurgery under appropriate anesthesia. If invasive carcinoma has been excluded by colposcopy and appropriate biopsies, intraepithelial lesions should be observed during pregnancy, with definitive treatment following delivery.

There is concern regarding the risk of maternal spread of HPV to the infant's larynx, resulting in laryngeal papillomatosis. This severely debilitating and potentially life-threatening HPV infection of the larynx usually appears within the first 5 years of life and is typically caused by HPV 6 or 11 and not by HPV types associated with warts in other cutaneous locations (31). The method of viral transmission to the infant's larynx is not known; however, possible routes are in utero exposure through the amniotic fluid or postnatal exposure of the larynx to the virus.

Approximately 60% of the mothers of infants with laryngeal papillomatosis have genital HPV infection. Based on the frequency of genital HPV infection in the U.S. population of pregnant women, it is estimated that 2–5% of all births are at risk for neonatal HPV exposure (31). The relatively low frequency of childhood laryngeal papillomatosis (approximately 1,550 cases per approximately 3.6 million births per year in the United States) suggests that vaginal delivery carries a risk of 0.04% of laryngeal infection in the neonate. This risk is not sufficient to recommend cesarean delivery for prevention of laryngeal papillomatosis; however, it may be indicated in situations in which genital warts are so large and severe as to obstruct or interfere with the course of labor or delivery or complicate the immediate postpartum course.

Therapy

A wide variety of chemical, mechanical, and ablative techniques are available to treat genital warts. Although visible lesions can be treated, removal of the virus from the genital tract cannot be guaranteed because no vaccine or specific antiviral therapy for HPV is currently available. Treatment strategies are aimed at destroying the visible lesions while waiting for the host immune response to control viral replication. Simple topical therapies are most cost-effective as initial treatment.

Topical concentrated trichloroacetic acid (50–85% solution) or bichloroacetic acid are dessicant acids which work best on moist mucosal warts. They are nontoxic and may be used in the vagina, on the cervix, and during pregnancy. They are best applied under colposcopic guidance to limit the area of skin damage.

Podophyllum resin in a 10–25% concentration in benzoin has been used for vulvar and perianal condylomata, but variable results and side effects have been reported due to the inconsistent concentration of the active chemical, podofilox. A purified preparation of podofilox is now available as a 0.5% solution (32). Podofilox treatment should not be used on the vagina or cervix or during pregnancy because of potential side effects of myelotoxicity and neurotoxicity.

Topical 5-fluorouracil is contraindicated for women who are or may become pregnant because it is reported to be teratogenic. It has been used to treat vaginal and vulvar condylomata and has been used in long-term management. A low concentration (1–2%) and careful weekly observation can be used to reduce side effects. Controlled long-term studies are needed to define its applicability.

Simple excision, electrosurgical excision, or laser vaporization are common therapeutic approaches used when simple topical treatment fails. These methods require anesthesia, and large lesions may require more than local anesthesia for treatment. Cryotherapy for vulvar condylomata is generally limited to small lesions that can be treated with small cryoprobes or topical liquid nitrogen. Thick, keratinized lesions that do not respond to topical treatment should be biopsied to rule out verrucous carcinoma. Verrucous carcinomas, which include giant condylomata (or Buschke-Löwenstein tumors) and some vulvar carcinomas with verrucous features, may have a warty appearance. These patients should be treated by radical local excision and not by destructive methods.

Condylomata acuminata that persist or recur after standard therapy may be treated with interferons. Interferons are proteins that have antiviral properties and have been used to treat HPV infections (33). Within the United States, various types of interferon are available which are interchangeable but differ in dose and length of treatment. Interferon may be given intramuscularly, subcutaneously, or intralesionally. The intralesional approach is commonly used for genital warts. Interferon is injected at the edge of and beneath the wart with a 26–32-gauge needle. Systemic symptoms, including fever, fatigue, myalgia, and headache, may occur; they diminish after the initial injection.

Human papillomavirus lesions of the cervix involving the transformation zone that are associated with low-grade squamous intraepithelial lesions have a 60–80% spontaneous regression rate and may not require treatment. They may be monitored by colposcopy and cytology until the course of the lesion has been determined. The cellular expression of an HPV infection may wax and wane so that only long-term follow-up will address the question of recurrence (34). The natural history of HPV lesions of the cervix remains under study.

High-grade CIN/HPV-associated lesions of the cervix are treated as CIN; these treatments include cryotherapy, electrosurgical excision (loop electrode excision procedure) of the cervical transformation zone, and laser ablation or excision of the transformation zone. Traditional cold-knife cone biopsy can also be therapeutic but is usually reserved for those cases in which invasive cancer cannot be ruled out by colposcopic evaluation and biopsy.

Summary

Knowledge of HPV infection is a rapidly changing area which presents a diagnostic and therapeutic dilemma. The clinical expression of HPV infection is highly variable and includes spontaneous regression and recurrence. A variety of molecular biologic methods are available for HPV detection and typing. The role of these diagnostic tools in clinical management is currently being defined. Several therapy options exist, and the choice of treatment depends on the physician and the circumstances and desires of the patient. The management of the patient with HPV includes recognition that the disease process cannot necessarily be cured, nor can the viral infection be totally or reliably eradicated from the genital tract with current methods.

REFERENCES

1. Becker TM, Wheeler CM, McGough NS, Jordan SW, Dorin M, Miller J. Cervical papillomavirus infection and cervical dysplasia in Hispanic, Native American, and non-Hispanic white women in New Mexico. Am J Public Health 1991;81:582–586

2. Ferenczy A, Bergeron C, Richart RM. Human papillomavirus DNA in fomites on objects used for the manage-

ment of patients with genital human papillomavirus infections. Obstet Gynecol 1989;74:950–954

3. Ley C, Bauer HM, Reingold A, Schiffman MH, Chambers JC, Tashiro CJ, et al. Determinants of genital human papillomavirus infection in young women. J Natl Cancer Inst 1991;83:997–1003

4. Schneider A, Kirchhoff T, Meinhardt G, Gissmann L. Repeated evaluation of human papillomavirus 16 status in cervical swabs of young women with a history of normal Papanicolaou smears. Obstet Gynecol 1992;79:683–688

5. Rosenberg SK, Greenberg MD, Reid R. Sexually transmitted papillomaviral infection in men. Obstet Gynecol Clin North Am 1987;14:495–512

6. Krebs H-B, Helmkamp BF. Treatment failure of genital condylomata acuminata in women: role of the male sexual partner. Am J Obstet Gynecol 1991;165:337–340

7. Krebs H-B, Helmkamp BF. Does the treatment of genital condylomata in men decrease the treatment failure rate of cervical dysplasia in the female sexual partner? Obstet Gynecol 1990;76:660–663

8. Koutsky LA, Galloway DA, Holmes KK. Epidemiology of genital human papillomavirus infection. Epidemiol Rev 1988;10:122–163

9. Lorincz AT, Reid R, Jenson AB, Greenberg MD, Lancaster W, Kurman RJ. Human papillomavirus infection of the cervix: relative risk associations of 15 common anogenital types. Obstet Gynecol 1992;79:328–337

10. Werness BA, Levine AJ, Howley PM. Association of human papillomavirus types 16 and 18 E6 proteins with P53. Science 1990;248:76–79

11. Zur Hausen H. Human papillomaviruses in the pathogenesis of anogenital cancer. Virology 1991;184:9–13

12. Barbosa MS, Vass WC, Lowy DR, Schiller JT. In vitro biological activities of the E6 and E7 genes vary among human papillomaviruses of different oncogenic potential. J Virol 1991;65:292–298

13. Straight SW, Hinkle PM, Jewers RJ, McCance DJ. The E5 oncoprotein of human papillomavirus type 16 transforms fibroblasts and effects the downregulation of the epidermal growth factor receptor in keratinocytes. J Virol 1993;67: 4521–4532

14. Tabbara S, Saleh ADM, Andersen WA, Barber SR, Taylor PT, Crum CP. The Bethesda classification for squamous intraepithelial lesions. Histologic, cytologic, and viral correlates. Obstet Gynecol 1992;79:338–346

15. Ward BE, Burkett B, Petersen C, Nuckols ML, Brennan C, Birch LM, et al. Cytologic correlates of cervical papillomavirus infection. Int J Gynecol Pathol 1990;9:297–305

16. Nuovo GJ, Nuovo MA, Cottral S, Gordon S, Silverstein SJ, Crum CP. Histological correlates of clinically occult human papillomavirus infection of the uterine cervix. Am J Surg Pathol 1988;12:198–204

17. Lorincz A. Diagnosis of human papillomavirus infection by the new generation of molecular DNA assays. Clin Immunol Newsletter 1992;12:123–128

18. Burmer GC, Parker JD, Bates J, East K, Kulander BG. Comparative analysis of human papillomavirus detection by polymerase chain reaction and Virapap/Viratype kits. Am J Clin Pathol 1990;94:554–560

19. Schiffman MH. Recent progress in defining the epidemiology of human papillomavirus infection and cervical neoplasia. J Natl Cancer Inst 1992;84:394–398

20. Koutsky LA, Holmes KK, Critchlow CW, Stevens CE, Paavonen J, Beckmann AM, et al. A cohort study of the risk of cervical intraepithelial neoplasia grade 2 or 3 in relation to papillomavirus infection. N Engl J Med 1992:327:1272–1278

21. DeBritton RC, Hildesheim A, De Lao SL, Brinton LA, Sathya P, Reeves WC. Human papillomaviruses and other influences on survival from cervical cancer in Panama. Obstet Gynecol 1993;81:19–24

22. Johnson TL, Kim W, Plieth DA, Sarker FH. Detection of HPV 16/18 DNA in cervical adenocarcinoma using polymerase chain reaction (PCR) methodology. Mod Pathol 1992;5:35–40

23. Stoler MH, Mills SE, Gersell DJ, Walker AN. Small-cell neuroendocrine carcinoma of the cervix. A human papillomavirus type 18-associated cancer. Am J Surg Pathol 1991;15:28–32

24. Bloss JD, Liao S-Y, Wilczynski SP, Macri C, Walker J, Peake M, et al. Clinical and histologic features of vulvar carcinomas analyzed for human papillomavirus status: evidence that squamous cell carcinoma of the vulva has more than one etiology. Hum Pathol 1991;22:711–718

25. Crum CP. Carcinoma of the vulva: epidemiology and pathogenesis. Obstet Gynecol 1992;79:448–454

26. Toki T, Kurman RJ, Park JS, Kessis T, Daniel RW, Shah KV. Probable nonpapillomavirus etiology of squamous cell carcinoma of the vulva in older women: a clinicopathologic study using in situ hybridization and polymerase chain reaction. Int J Gynecol Pathol 1991;10:107–125

27. Andersen WA, Franquemont DW, Williams J, Taylor PT, Crum CP. Vulvar squamous cell carcinoma and papillomaviruses: two separate entities? Am J Obstet Gynecol 1991;165:329–336

28. Park JS, Jones RW, McLean MR, Currie JL, Woodruff JD, Shah KV, et al. Possible etiologic heterogeneity of vulvar intraepithelial neoplasia. A correlation of pathologic characteristics with human papillomavirus detection by *in situ* hybridization and polymerase chain reaction. Cancer 1991;67:1599–1607

29. Moyal-Barracco M, Leibowitch M, Orth G. Vestibular papillae of the vulva. Lack of evidence for human papillomavirus etiology. Arch Dermatol 1990;126:1594–1598

30. Wilkinson EJ, Guerrero E, Daniel R, Shah K, Stone IK, Hardt NS, et al. Vulvar vestibulitis is rarely associated with human papillomavirus infection types 6, 11, 16, or 18. Int J Gynecol Pathol 1993;12:344–349

31. Shah K, Kashima H, Polk BF, Shah F, Abbey H, Abramson A. Rarity of cesarean delivery in cases of juvenile-onset respiratory papillomatosis. Obstet Gynecol 1986;68:795–798

32. Kirby P, Dunne A, King DH, Corey L. Double-blind randomized clinical trial of self-administered podofilox solution versus vehicle in the treatment of genital warts. Am J Med 1990;88:465–469

33. Friedman-Kien AE, Eron LJ, Conant M, Growdon W, Badiak H, Bradstreet PW, et al. Natural interferon alfa for treatment of condylomata acuminata. JAMA 1988;259: 533–538

34. Syrjänen K, Syrjänen S. Epidemiology of human papilloma virus infections and genital neoplasia. Scand J Infect Dis 1990;suppl 69:7–17

This Technical Bulletin was developed under the direction of the Committee on Technical Bulletins of the American College of Obstetricians and Gynecologists as an educational aid to obstetricians and gynecologists. The committee wishes to thank Edward J. Wilkinson, MD, for his assistance in the development of this bulletin. This Technical Bulletin does not define a standard of care, nor is it intended to dictate an exclusive course of management. It presents recognized methods and techniques of clinical practice for consideration by obstetrician–gynecologists for incorporation into their practices. Variations of practice taking into account the needs of the individual patient, resources, and limitations unique to the institution or type of practice may be appropriate.
ISSN 1074-8628

THE AMERICAN COLLEGE OF OBSTETRICIANS AND GYNECOLOGISTS
409 12th Street, SW
Washington, DC 20024-2188

12345/87654

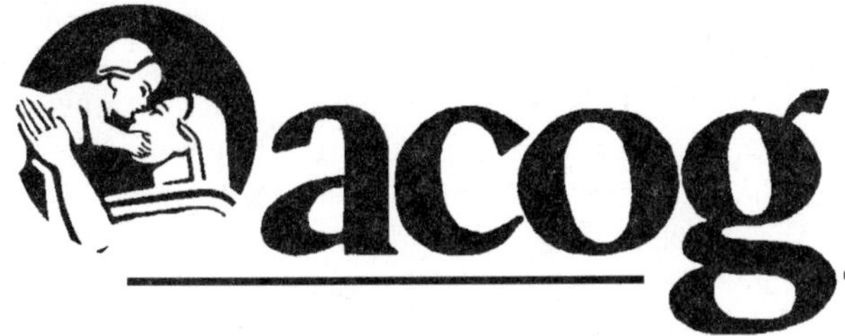

Number 215—November 1995

Technical Bulletin

An Educational Aid to Obstetrician–Gynecologists

Gynecologic Ultrasonography

Pelvic ultrasonography—both transvaginal and transabdominal—has proved to be beneficial in helping to establish an accurate diagnosis. It is an efficient technique for objective assessment of the size, location, and consistency (ie, cystic, solid, or mixed mass) of abnormal pelvic findings. This information, combined with that from the bimanual pelvic examination, allows for a more complete assessment of the patient. It should not be relied on as the sole diagnostic method but rather considered an adjunct to physical examination to confirm the presence or absence of a suspected problem (1). Ultrasound scans are considered part of the medical record. They should be documented and stored appropriately.

Indications for ultrasonography include, but are not restricted to, abnormal pregnancy (eg, bleeding, size–dates discrepancy, previous ectopic pregnancy, coexisting adnexal mass, pain), suspected or definite pelvic mass, evaluation of the endometrium, or the inability to perform an adequate pelvic examination to diagnose a clinical problem (eg, due to obesity) (2). Many of these indications are subjective and depend on the opinion of the individual clinician. However, whenever objective assessment of the size, location, and consistency of pelvic structures is required, vaginal ultrasonography is extremely helpful (3).

Types of Ultrasonography

Ultrasound is high-frequency sound waves that exceed 20,000 cycles per second. Frequency refers to the number of peaks or waves that traverse a given point per unit of time and is expressed as hertz (Hz). Instruments used in diagnostic ultrasonography operate at frequencies of 2 million–10 million Hz, or 2–10 megahertz (MHz). The higher the frequency of the sound, the shallower the depth of penetration, but the better the resolution of the image produced. Most abdominal ultrasound transducers operate at 3.5–5 MHz, while most vaginal transducers operate at 5–7.5 MHz.

Technologic advances in instrumentation have led to significant improvements in image production and resolution. Dynamic, or real-time, ultrasonography creates images faster than the flicker fusion rate of the eye so that the target appears to be moving in real time. Linear array real-time transducers use a longitudinal series of transducer crystals arranged in sequence to operate serially quite rapidly. Annular array scanners operate similarly but with the serial transducers arranged in concentric rings. Sector real-time ultrasonography uses a single transducer that moves through a prescribed arc. Curvilinear transducers have been introduced recently to incorporate principles of both linear array and sector transducers.

Real-time ultrasonography readily detects any kind of motion; for example, cardiac activity can be detected in an ectopic or early intrauterine pregnancy. This dynamic two-dimensional imaging also allows evaluation of the pelvic structures. Some transducers have been modified to allow insertion into the vagina. This has been one of the most significant advances for ultrasonography in the past decade.

Safety

During the 25 years that ultrasonography has been in clinical use in obstetrics and gynecology, it has not been known to cause harm to any patient (4). Many in vitro and animal studies have been carried out to study the bioeffects of ultrasonography (5–11). Thus far, there has been no independently reproduced study demonstrating a bioeffect on the patient when ultrasonography is delivered at diagnostic intensities.

Newer applications of ultrasound technology require higher energy output. Although no adverse fetal effects have been identified to date, increases in the power outputs of ultrasound instruments may increase the potential risks to the fetus. Because of these concerns, many machines are equipped with instruments that continuously display the power output as thermal and mechanical indices. These indices allow the operator to use exposure levels that are "as low as reasonably achievable" (12). The selection and maintenance of the equipment is the responsibility of the operator.

Transvaginal Versus Transabdominal Ultrasonography

The goal of pelvic ultrasonography is to obtain an image of the pelvic structures that has as much detail as possible. Each approach offers certain advantages and disadvantages toward that end.

Transabdominal ultrasonography provides a panoramic view with easily understood orientation of relative structures. However, it does not provide the anatomic detail that the vaginal probe affords. Furthermore, the transabdominal method requires that the bladder be full to act as an acoustic window and push loops of bowel cephalad. Waiting for the bladder to fill takes time, thus effectively lengthening the procedure. A full bladder can cause some patient discomfort.

The vaginal probe gives more detail because it is a highly focused approach. A disadvantage of transvaginal ultrasonography is that transducer movement is limited by the confines of the vagina at the introitus. Finally, due to limited penetration achieved with the vaginal probe, structures high in the pelvis (especially if adherent) may be out of the focal zone of the vaginal probe. Structures more than 6–8 cm beyond the vaginal apex may be beyond the range of the vaginal probe.

The decision of which modality to use first depends on the clinical entity suspected as a result of the physical examination. In many instances, transvaginal ultrasonography is performed and, if it is inconclusive, a transabdominal examination is required.

Transvaginal Imaging

There are two major kinds of vaginal probes: mechanical sector scanners and electronic solid-state phased array, or curvilinear, probes. Mechanical sector scanners are always end firing, and the field of view is symmetrically placed on both sides of the axis of the probe. Most solid-state electronic probes are not of the end-firing type. They usually cover a field of view that is off axis.

In mechanical sector probes, the handle is in axis with the shaft and the "firing window." However, in many solid-state probes (ie, phased array or curvilinear probes), the handle may be at an angle to the shaft; therefore, use of probes such as these requires the proper perception of the off-axis image produced.

Patient Preparation

The procedure should be fully explained to the patient in advance, and her involvement should be encouraged. Consideration should be given to the patient's privacy and sensitivity. Without proper preparation, the examination could be construed as offensive. Because of the sensitive nature of the examination, it may be advisable to have a chaperon present.

The initial ultrasound examination is best performed after taking a detailed history. The day of the cycle on which the examination is performed should be recorded.

The patient should have an empty bladder for the procedure. Ideally, a gynecologic examining table with leg supports should be used; however, if this is not available, the patient's hips should be elevated approximately 10 inches by a cushion. This will allow for full range of motion of the transducer.

Probe Preparation

A small amount of standard coupling gel is placed on the tip of the probe prior to insertion into a probe cover (eg, a latex condom, latex glove, or plastic bag). A special, clean lubricating gel should then be applied on top of the probe cover to allow for easy insertion of the probe. The probe should be disinfected between uses. The manufacturer's instructions should specify the compatibility of different cleansing agents with specific probes.

Many coupling gels and lubricants affect sperm motility and may act as a spermicide. Such lubricants should not be used in patients desiring pregnancy for examinations performed around mid-cycle or following intercourse.

Indications and Clinical Use

Evaluation of Pelvic Pathology

Ultrasonography is an adjunctive diagnostic aid; a definitive diagnosis cannot be established by ultrasonography. Management is based on an assessment of all the clinical factors.

The Uterus

When evaluating a suspected uterine mass, the practitioner should identify the appropriate anatomic structures. The initial step is to identify the bladder anteriorly and the rectosigmoid posteriorly. The position of the uterus depends on the distention of the bladder and rectosigmoid, masses that may be present extrinsic to the uterus, and intrinsic uterine masses. The normal uterus appears sonographically as a uniform structure.

By resting a hand on the abdomen and using the intermittent pressure of a transvaginal probe, the practitioner can determine the mobility of the uterus, the ovaries, or any pelvic structure. This sliding movement of the mentioned organs can be related to each other or the stationary pelvic floor ("sliding organs sign"). The origin of structures (eg, ovary versus a pedunculated fibroid) or adhesions can be diagnosed using this maneuver. Testing for pain is also possible with the vaginal probe identifying the touched structure in question on the screen.

Ultrasound examination is of benefit in determining the position of uterine masses—that is, whether they are pedunculated, serosal, intramural, submucosal, or endometrial. Serosal–pedunculated masses may be mistaken for structures originating extraneously from the uterus.

THE CERVIX. Scanning the uterine cervix is an integral part of the ultrasound examination. A wide variety of pathologies ranging from benign and prevalent Nabothian (inclusion) cysts to cervical fibroids or the rare cervical pregnancy can be identified. The importance of transvaginal ultrasound scanning of the cervix has increased in recent years.

THE MYOMETRIUM. The sonographic appearance of the myometrium and the arcuate vessels within the myometrium should be noted. Leiomyomata tend to be discrete, multiple, spherical masses of varying size. They can be found impinging on the endometrium (submucosal), within the myometrium (intramural), or on the surface of the uterus (subserosal).

Ultrasonographically, a leiomyoma often appears hypoechogenic. However, its appearance may vary depending on its location and whether it has undergone internal changes, such as hyaline degeneration, fatty degeneration, calcification, or hemorrhagic necrosis. These changes will alter the sonographic appearance of the leiomyoma; for example, the presence of calcium will result in an increase in echogenicity, whereas degeneration will produce a cystlike structure.

Submucosal leiomyomata give the appearance of a bulge in the endometrial lining. A more detailed investigation of this sign is warranted. This can be accomplished by instilling normal saline via a thin catheter placed in the uterine cavity. The saline will serve as a contrast medium and will outline the mass.

Serial ultrasonography can be used to determine whether the leiomyomata are growing or shrinking. This can be especially useful in patients entering menopause. When the uterus of a reproductive-age woman with leiomyomata is evaluated, the practitioner should be alert to the possibility of a small (4–6 weeks of gestation size) chorionic sac. These small gestations may be difficult to detect and may be found at odd locations.

Adenomyosis is diagnosed by noting the presence of endometrial tissue in the stroma of the myometrium. Although this condition may be suspected by the presence of small sonolucent areas within the myometrium, it cannot be confirmed on that basis. The diagnosis rests on clinical parameters and histologic confirmation.

THE ENDOMETRIUM. Sonographically, the interface of the two endometrial surfaces appears as a thin, echogenic line that can be evaluated throughout the menstrual cycle. The endometrium varies in thickness and appearance depending on the stage of the menstrual cycle or the use of exogenous hormones. Measurement of the endometrial thickness should be done on the long axis, with a combined anterior–posterior measurement. If fluid is found in the uterine cavity, the measurement should exclude that fluid interface.

In postmenopausal women with bleeding, studies indicate that, when there is a thin distinct endometrial echo less than 4–5 mm maximum anteroposterior thickness read from a long axis view, this finding is consistently associated with lack of significant tissue on sampling. Thus, such patients may be able to avoid invasive sampling and its risks, expense, and discomfort. Presence of an endometrial echo greater than 5 mm is not compatible with atrophy and thus, depending on hormonal status, may indicate the need for sampling. Saline infusion sonohysterography can be used to distinguish symmetrically thickened endometrium in which the process is global from endometrial changes that may be focal. In the former, blind sampling is appropriate, whereas the latter requires hysteroscopically directed evaluation. Finally, it is to be hoped that current research in three-dimensional techniques, particularly in volume rendering, may prove to be an added source of information distinguishing benign from malignant pathology.

It is also important to examine carefully the entire length of the myometrial–endometrial interface. If the endometrium is irregular or if there is an enlarged area of echogenicity, endometrial pathology should be suspected. An endometrial biopsy or dilation and curettage should be performed to determine the histologic status of the endometrium. The myometrial–endometrial interface should be evaluated by continuously shifting the transducer through its long axis and corresponding coronal planes.

Increasing attention is being given to the presence of heterogenous central uterine changes in women who receive tamoxifen for breast cancer. In some such cases, changes originally interpreted as endometrial are actually in the proximal myometrium (13). Sonohysterography may be used to determine the location (endometrial vs. proximal myometrial) of such heterogenous echoes.

During the follicular phase, the endometrium is thin, with a pencil-line echo of the cavity and hypoechoic functional endometrium on both sides of the cavity line (three-line sign). This phase is followed by gradual thickening, which reaches its peak immediately prior to ovulation. Following ovulation, coincidental with the rise in progesterone, the echogenicity of the endometrium on both sides of the cavity line increases and equals that of the cavity line, which gradually disappears within the hyperechoic endometrium. This hyperechoic endometrium is then "broken down" at the time of the menstrual flow. The endometrium can be measured throughout the first part of the cycle, therefore, to detect signs of endometrial maturity, which is relevant to the timing of ovulation. This changing echogenicity of the endometrium can serve as a natural contrast material in the uterus, leading to better definition of the endometrial–myometrial interface and detection of polyps or submucous leiomyomata or both.

Patients with irregular uterine bleeding may have an endometrial polyp, submucosal myoma, or adenomatous hyperplasia. Polyps can occur in patients of any age but tend to be more common in perimenopausal women. Polyps are usually seen as a prominent endometrial echo complex; rarely, discrete masses occupying the endometrial cavity are found. Sonohysterographic fluid enhancement through a thin intrauterine catheter may improve diagnostic capability (14).

Although neither transvaginal nor transabdominal ultrasound evaluation can confirm the presence or absence of cancer of the endometrium, ultrasonography can provide information to aid in diagnosis. In early stages, endometrial carcinoma can appear as a change in the thickness of the endometrial lining and changes in the endometrial echogenicity. Advanced endometrial or cervical carcinoma may appear as hydrometra, pyometra, or hematometra. These conditions will appear sonographically as cystic masses. The endometrial–myometrial interface should be defined and monitored to detect pathology at that level.

Other conditions that may be detected by ultrasound examination of the endometrium are Asherman syndrome and retained products of conception following spontaneous abortion, therapeutic abortion, or delivery. A diagnosis of Asherman syndrome can be strengthened by the presence of an irregular echogenic picture and, occasionally, by the finding of calcification. On ultrasonography, calcification is intensely echogenic and causes acoustic shadowing. The diagnosis can be firmly established by hysteroscopy. Retained products usually can be detected if an irregularly shaped, dilated endometrial cavity containing echogenic material is noted. Asherman syndrome can best be distinguished from retained products of conception by evaluating the patient's history. Uterine anomalies including septae, bicornuate uteri, and didelphis may be identified. Sonohysterography may be useful to measure a fundal septum prior to hysteroscopic resection when habitual abortion is present.

Adnexal Masses

Ultrasonographic examination of the adnexa encompasses evaluation of the ovaries, fallopian tubes, and parametrial areas. It is important that the examiner be familiar with other anatomic structures in this area, such as the external iliac artery and vein, internal iliac artery and vein, ureter, and bowel.

The ovaries usually lie in the ovarian fossa found along the lateral pelvic wall. The ovary can be located by identifying a pulsating linear echo; superior to this is the external iliac artery, and posterior and inferior to this is the ureter. The normal ovary of teenagers and young adults measures approximately 2 cm × 2 cm × 3 cm. The size of the ovary should be measured according to the largest diameter in the three planes. Some investigators have recommended determining ovarian volume, using the formula (length × width × height)/2. The ovarian volume in teenagers and young adults can reach 14 cm^3 (15). In postmenopausal women, the average ovarian volume is 2.5 cm^3 or less.

The following aspects of an adnexal mass should be evaluated:

- Mobility. The mass should be moved by the vaginal probe or by the hand of the operator that is resting on the abdomen.
- Pain. Location should be established.
- Wall structure. Features of an ovarian mass, such as thickness and outer and inner surface irregularities and papillae, should be described and measured.
- Septations. The thickness of the septations should be reported.
- Echogenicity of the mass. The mass can be completely sonolucent and may have low-level echogenic contents, may be with or without an echogenic core, may have mixed echogenicity containing all of these components, or may be completely echogenic.

The presence of the following conditions may make it more difficult to detect ovarian or adnexal masses with ultrasonography:

- Fluid-filled loop of bowel
- Feces in loop of bowel
- Closed-loop bowel obstruction
- Artifact of multipath reflection of sound waves (stratified echo pattern resulting from echoes bouncing back and forth) from fluid-filled structure (eg, bladder)
- Mesenteric cysts
- Peritoneal inclusion cysts
- Nabothian cysts
- Hydrosalpinges

The clinical findings of acute salpingitis may be strengthened by ultrasonographic findings of tuboovarian complexes of a fluid-containing structure with thickened walls sensitive to the touch of the probe, adnexa adherent to loop of bowels, or collection of fluid in the cul-de-sac. Chronic salpingitis can be diagnosed on the basis of a painless (to the touch of the probe), thin-walled, pear-shaped, fluid-filled adnexal structure. Abscesses can be detected by ultrasonography, which can also be used to characterize the abscess as unilocular or multilocular and determine the thickness of the abscess wall and anatomic location. This information should be integrated into clinical findings (eg, pain, fever) and is helpful in determining whether the abscess may be drained percutaneously or transvaginally or whether surgical intervention is required.

Peritoneal Fluid

Small amounts of fluid in the lower pelvis can be visualized with ultrasonography. The fluid should be examined for the presence or absence of floating debris, which will appear as low-level echoes. The tip of the probe can be used to rock the fluid slightly, thus aiding in the observation of floating particles. If the nature of the fluid must be determined, culdocentesis can be accomplished with the aid of transvaginal sonography, which offers the best guidance for needle placement through the needle guide mated to the shaft of the probe.

Attempts to assess the quantity of pelvic fluid have been reported in the literature. The smallest amount of fluid that can be detected is about 20–30 ml if a 5-MHz transvaginal probe is used. Although experienced sonographers can estimate the approximate amount, this should be done with extreme caution.

If a larger amount of abdominal or pelvic fluid is suspected, the space between the liver and the right kidney (the Morison pouch) should be examined. This can be achieved by placing an abdominal transducer parallel to the sagittal plane and overlying the right upper abdomen.

Urinary Bladder

Ultrasonography can be used to examine the bladder for the presence of extrinsic or intrinsic pathologic masses. The urethra and the bladder can be viewed on the sagittal end and on an extremely anteriorly directed coronal plane. A transverse scan through the superior portion of the bladder reveals the bladder to be rounded. If the bladder is scanned inferiorly, it will appear square, whereas a longitudinal scan will make it appear triangular. The thickness of the bladder and the presence of polyps or bladder stones will be outlined by the sonolucent urine. A scan performed at the base of the bladder, just proximal to the urethrovesical junction, will permit visualization of the urethral orifices. Ultrasonography may be used to estimate the volume of postvoid residual and, in incontinent women, the mobility of the urethrovesical junction.

Other Findings

Other pathologic processes that can affect organs in the lower pelvis can also be detected. The most prevalent bowel diseases that can be observed are diverticulosis and various degrees of dilatation of the small bowel. Dilatation of the bowel that can be mistaken for cystic structures can often be differentiated by the presence of peristalsis. Ectopic or low-lying horseshoe kidneys can also be detected by sonography. Transabdominal sonography can be used to identify appendicitis; however, considerable experience is required to do so.

Early Pregnancy Diagnosis

A gestational sac seen with ultrasonography at 4–5 weeks of gestation is the first definitive sign of pregnancy. It is characterized by a sonolucent center (the chorionic cavity) containing amnion, embryonic disc, and yolk sac (although these are still too small to be seen sonographically). The gestational sac is characterized by a symmetrical, thick, echogenic rind, which is formed by primary trophoblastic invasion symmetrically extending from the chorionic membrane into maternal decidua. When first seen, a normal gestational sac should be round, midposition to fundal in the uterus, and eccentric as it burrows into the endometrium. In any one "frozen" image, the sac may appear perfectly central in one two-dimensional plane yet it should be eccentrically located in three dimensions.

The point at which the sac can first be seen (ie, the threshold) is not as important as the point at which all normal sacs should be imaged (ie, the discriminatory level). The discriminatory level is 34.8 ± 2.2 days from the last menstrual period (16); however, menstrual dating can be inaccurate even when the menstrual history seems reliable. The discriminatory level in terms of levels of human chorionic gonadotropin (hCG) has been reported to range from 935 to 2,388 mIU/ml (by International Reference Preparation [IRP]; studies varied in use of first and second IRP) for transvaginal ultrasonography and is approximately 3,600 mIU/ml, IRP, for transabdominal ultrasonography (16–23). The presence of a leiomyoma, a coexisting intrauterine device, or a multiple gestation, however, may affect the discriminatory level (17, 21). Physicians should determine at what level of hCG they can determine pregnancy.

The mean diameter of the gestational sac increases approximately 1 mm/d during early pregnancy; when first seen, it may only be 2–3 mm in diameter. The yolk sac is a very round and regular structure. The discriminatory size of the gestational sac for transvaginal visualization of the yolk sac is reported to range from 8–10 mm in mean diameter (4, 18).

Embryonic heart activity is present prior to the ability to image the embryo as a structure distinct from the yolk sac. Cardiac motion may be seen occasionally along the edge of the yolk sac (24).

With further growth, the yolk sac should have a maximum mean diameter of 6 mm (25). As the amniotic cavity increases in size around the embryo, the yolk sac is seen as distinctly extraamniotic. The embryo begins as a straight structure until it reaches a length of 4 mm (at which point it has a caudal and rostral neuropore). It becomes a C-shaped, tadpolelike structure complete with tail. By 49 days of gestation, a measurement of its greatest length is 7 mm. Regression of the tail and extension of the head allow for identification of a true crown and rump and, thus, measurement of the sitting height of the embryo (crown–rump length) by 58 days of gestational age.

Assessment of Gestational Age

Gestational sac size expressed as a mean sac diameter has been used for correlation with menstrual age before visualization of an embryo. Measurement of the gestational sac is taken from the trophoblastic tissue–fluid interface and implies two perpendicular planes. Although numerous investigators have described formulas to relate gestational sac size to menstrual age (18, 26, 27), this is not the best method for assessing gestational age.

Embryonic Cardiac Activity

The S-shaped endothelial heart tube folds on itself and begins to beat by 21 days after conception. Thus, it is present and beating in a normal pregnancy before it can be seen with ultrasonography. Fetal cardiac activity should be seen any time a measurable fetal pole is detected. By others' criteria, however, cardiac motion can be detected by the time the embryo is 5 mm long or more (28, 29). Thus, embryos no more than 4 mm long that do not have discernable cardiac activity should demonstrate cardiac activity within 3–5 days because embryonic growth occurs at a rate of 1 mm/d. At 6 weeks and 1–2 days (by menstrual age), all normally developing embryos should have detectable heartbeats (30). The major concern regarding embryonic cardiac activity is at what point its absence can be considered a definitive sign of pregnancy failure. Some investigators have attempted to relate cardiac activity to hCG levels. These levels show a wide range from 6,636 to 26,356 mIU/ml, IRP (16, 19, 20, 31). This technique has much potential for error because of different standards of units for expressing hCG, the need to convert units, and the low reproducibility of quantitative levels from laboratory to laboratory.

It is preferable to relate the presence or absence of cardiac activity to embryonic size. The ability to show cardiac activity by ultrasonography depends on the type and frequency of equipment used, the degree of magnification available, the visual acuity of the operator, and any confounding anatomic variables (eg, maternal obesity, coexisting myomas).

Pathologic Pregnancy

Ectopic Pregnancy

The detection of an intrauterine pregnancy virtually excludes ectopic pregnancy. The exception is heterotopic pregnancy (simultaneous intrauterine and extrauterine pregnancies), which is said to occur in 1:30,000 spontaneous pregnancies (28). However, in women undergoing assisted reproductive procedures, the rate of heterotopic pregnancy increases to about 1:6,000 (32, 33).

The ability to diagnose an intrauterine pregnancy definitively depends on the milestones outlined. When no intrauterine gestation is seen on ultrasound examination, the quantitative hCG level should be determined. If the hCG level is less than the discriminatory level, then serial levels of hCG should be determined. In a normal early pregnancy, the hCG level will rise a minimum of 66% every 48 hours, or effectively double every 3 days. Once the hCG level surpasses a discriminatory level, an intrauterine gestation should be seen. The absence of an intrauterine gestation suggests that the pregnancy represents either a failing intrauterine gestation or an extrauterine pregnancy. Similarly, a subnormal rate of rise of hCG also indicates a failing intrauterine gestation or extrauterine pregnancy.

When an ongoing normal pregnancy has been excluded, curettage and examination of tissue for the presence or absence of chorionic villi may be useful. The presence of chorionic villi is proof of an intrauterine gestation. The presence of only decidual tissue raises the index of suspicion for ectopic pregnancy, although complete abortion (possibly tubal, as well) can account for such findings, especially when there has been previous bleeding. A follow-up measurement of quantitative hCG level (rising, plateauing, or falling) may help to distinguish ectopic pregnancy from a complete abortion.

Some intrauterine fluid collections may look like gestational sacs. The presence of the yolk sac and its location within the cavity of the uterus or along the cavity line preclude a diagnosis of such "pseudosacs." The pseudogestational sac of ectopic pregnancy occurs in 10–20% of cases. A true sac of an intrauterine pregnancy appears at 5 weeks of gestation and is identified by an intraendometrial fluid collection surrounded by an echogenic structure buried into the depth of the trophoblastic and decidual tissue on one or the other side of the cavity line. If any doubt exists about the legitimacy or normalcy of a gestational sac prior to the presence of a yolk sac or an embryo, a follow-up ultrasound examination and quantitative hCG measurement are warranted.

Among ectopic pregnancies, 15–28% will develop a yolk sac or cardiac activity or both (34, 35). Such pregnancies will often show normal doubling times of hCG. The familiar appearance of the gestational sac with its sonolucent center will be more easily seen on ultrasound examination, especially if there is cardiac activity.

Not all sonolucent or complex adnexal structures will be extrauterine gestations. The ovaries should be identified on the side in question to avoid identifying a corpus luteum or corpus luteum cyst as an extrauterine gestation.

Finally, the observation of free fluid in the cul-de-sac may be helpful but is not pathognomonic. It is present in 41–83% of extrauterine pregnancies (34, 36). The observation of free fluid in the cul-de-sac may be an indication of bleeding from an ectopic site. If it is still needed for diagnosis, ultrasound-directed culdocentesis can be performed easily. The aspiration of nonclotting blood suggests an ectopic pregnancy. However, it should be noted that the sensitivity, specificity, and positive and negative predictive values of culdocentesis are extremely low in comparison with those of transvaginal ultrasonography (37). If transvaginal ultrasonography is available, culdocentesis has no practical value in the diagnosis of ectopic pregnancy. Although rare, cornual or cervical pregnancies should be considered and evidence sought for such conditions.

Early Pregnancy Failure

Once ectopic pregnancy is excluded definitively, ultrasonography may assist the physician in determining the continued well-being of a pregnancy complicated by bleeding through a closed cervical os ("threatened abortion") or by a size–dates discrepancy. Follow-up measurements of quantitative hCG levels are of value only when ectopic pregnancy has not been ruled out. Prior to the documentation of an embryo, a failing pregnancy may be predicted by the presence of a distorted gestational sac. The observation of a collapsed or fragmented sac is highly suggestive of a pregnancy that has failed or is likely to fail. Once ectopic pregnancy is excluded, embryonic well-being is demonstrated by appropriate growth and achievements of the various landmarks outlined. A yolk sac should be seen on transabdominal ultrasonography when the gestational sac has achieved a mean diameter of 20 mm. If an embryo that is no more than 4 mm long is seen but no cardiac activity is discernable, a follow-up scan using a transvaginal probe should be conducted at an appropriate interval. Occasionally, embryonic demise with resorption will cause a sac to appear empty. The term *blighted ova* should be abandoned since there is gradual resorption of the demised embryo and extraembryonic structure.

Early pregnancy failure appears as either an embryo of sufficient size without cardiac activity or a gestational sac of sufficient size without yolk sacs or embryo present. In an incomplete abortion, the cavity may have variable sonographic appearances but should not have a true gestational sac and clinically should have an open os. A complete abortion may have a thin linear endometrial echo, since all tissue has been passed spontaneously. Therefore, in such cases, if an intrauterine gestation was not documented previously, the possibility of an ectopic pregnancy should be considered.

Gestational Trophoblastic Disease

Gestational trophoblastic disease is characterized by the proliferation of trophoblastic tissue that can be benign (hydatidiform mole) or malignant (choriocarcinoma). The incidence of hydatidiform mole is 1/1,000–1/1,200 pregnancies. The risk of recurrence for individuals who have had a previous hydatidiform mole is increased 10-fold. Hydatidiform mole has a grapelike appearance on ultrasound examination that corresponds to the hydropic vesicle changes of the trophoblast. Such a pattern often is not seen until after 10 weeks following the last menstrual cycle. Increasingly, however, with vaginal bleeding early in pregnancy, ultrasonography may simply show signs of a hyper-echoic uterine structure without sonographic signs of a pregnancy prior to the development of the classic molar appearance on ultrasound examination. Thus, microscopic pathologic study of curettage material should be performed routinely to confirm the diagnosis.

Ultrasonography may be an aid in the management of complications of gestational trophoblastic disease, which include bleeding and theca lutein cysts. Bleeding associated with gestational trophoblastic disease may appear on ultrasound examination as a crescent-shaped anechoic area surrounding the abnormal tissue. Theca lutein cysts occur in 20–50% of patients with gestational trophoblastic disease. The cysts tend to be multilocular. Following evacuation of the molar pregnancy, the cyst will resolve over the next 2–4 months.

Infertility Management

Ultrasonography in general, and transvaginal sonography in particular, may be helpful for the management of infertility. It can be used for the pretreatment, diagnostic, or baseline workup as well as for evaluation of follicular and endometrial development as a function of the menstrual cycle and evaluation of ovulation.

Pretreatment, Diagnostic, or Baseline Workup

The initial scan starts with the structural evaluation of the uterus in long axis and coronal planes. Uterine size, consistency, and the presence or absence of leiomyomata should be noted. The cervix should be evaluated by measuring its length from the internal to the external os; any pathologies, such as a Nabothian cyst or dilated external os, should be noted and measured as well. Measuring the cervix and the endometrium is accomplished on the sagittal long-axis view. The myometrium should then be evaluated by observing the myometrial–endometrial interface and describing its appearance.

Evaluation of Suspected Pelvic Abnormality

CONGENITAL UTERINE ANOMALIES. Ultrasonography is useful in detecting uterine malformations (lateral fusion defects) such as didelphic, bicornuate, or septate uteri. The sonographic hallmarks of the most common uterine malformation, bicornuate uterus, are the wide appearance of the uterine body with a fundal notch of the various signs and branching of the endometrial echoes into a right and left horn. In the case of a uterine malformation, however, laparoscopic or hysteroscopic confirmation should be considered. It is best to evaluate suspected uterine anomalies in the secretory phase of the cycle since the hyperechogenic endometrium tends to delineate the shape of the cavity or cavities. Alternatively, sonohysterography may be used in the early proliferative phase.

EVALUATION OF THE OVARIES. Transvaginal ultrasonography can be used to identify and describe the location, mobility, and appearance of the ovaries. In many cases, it may provide information about causes of infertility such as polycystic ovary syndrome or large bilateral masses. The size and number of follicles on each side should be reported. If detected, a corpus luteum or any other persistent structure should also be reported. The mobility of the ovaries, which can help assess pelvic adhesions, should be tested. This is best performed by using a combination of the transvaginal probe and the hand on the abdomen and observing the sliding of the ovary on the screen. Unusual locations of the ovary as well as possible fixation and possible masses should be noted.

Baseline transvaginal ultrasonography performed in the follicular phase can help to rule out conditions that may inhibit the development of the oocytes. These conditions can include a corpus luteum from a previous cycle, ovarian neoplasms, or endometriomas.

Sonographically, polycystic ovary syndrome may be characterized by a larger than usual ovary and the presence of multiple small subcapsular follicles, usually 4–6 mm in diameter. Although ultrasound findings alone are not specific enough to make the diagnosis of polycystic ovary syndrome, in combination with clinical signs and symptoms, ultrasonography may be of value.

Evaluation of Follicular and Endometrial Development and Ovulation

The ovaries should be evaluated for the presence of graafian follicles, and the size of the follicles should be noted. In a nonstimulated cycle, usually one dominant follicle is recruited by the ninth day, and it should be monitored throughout the follicular phase. If hormonal stimulation (eg, clomiphene citrate) is used, two or possibly three larger follicles may develop. In contrast, hormonal induction with menotropins usually results in a larger number of follicles in both ovaries. It is sufficient to measure the two largest diameters of the follicles. Each follicle should be measured on the plane showing its largest measurements. Once the follicles reach 2.0–2.5 cm, follicular maturity is presumed.

The sonographic signs of ovulation include:

- A sudden reduction in the size of a previously seen large follicle
- A concomitant change from the multilayered appearance of the endometrium to a more echo-filled texture on both sides of the cavity line
- The simultaneous appearance of small amounts of fluid in the cul-de-sac that were not previously seen

During cycles of ovulation induction with menotropins, the ultrasound findings may assist the clinician in deciding whether to trigger ovulation with hCG. If too many follicles have developed, withholding hCG may prevent hyperstimulation syndrome. If ovarian hyperstimulation does occur, ultrasonography can be used to document free peritoneal fluid and ovarian size. Sometimes the vaginal probe cannot encompass the entire size of the ovaries on one screen. The transabdominal scanning approach seems to yield a better and more comprehensive view of the ovaries, the uterus, and, at times, ascitic fluid.

Future Considerations

Color Doppler Studies

An increasing number of laboratories are now offering color-flow-directed flow measurements such as pulsatility and resistance indices as well as flow velocities (38–40). Color flow studies are considered investigational. The pulsatility index and resistance index express the relative resistance to blood flowing through the investigated vessel. The pulsatility index is calculated by the following formula:

$$\frac{\text{Systolic Velocity} - \text{Diastolic Velocity}}{\text{Mean Velocity}}$$

The resistance index is calculated by the following formula:

$$\frac{\text{Systolic Velocity} - \text{Diastolic Velocity}}{\text{Systolic Velocity}}$$

Preliminary results raise the possibility of detecting increased vascularity and new vessel formation in cases of malignant ovarian masses. In general, vessels in malignant tumors lack the muscle layer and have a lower impedance. However, increased flow may also be seen with pelvic inflammatory processes. The presence of a corpus luteum not only may be misleading in the structural evaluation of an adnexal finding but also may make the detection of an adnexal mass difficult since the flow–measurement values overlap with those found in ovarian cancer. The corpus luteum is known to have new vessel formation, which lowers the resistance to flow while present.

Recent studies have suggested a possible role for color Doppler in aiding the diagnosis of adnexal torsion. These studies suggest that, at the site of the torsion, the diameter of the vessels proximal to the occlusion is increased; the disruption of flow is identified on color Doppler. Within the torsed adnexa, there is significantly diminished flow or no flow at all. The cost–benefit ratio of color flow studies is still under investigation, and the value of such studies is as yet unproven. Moreover, the technique requires a great deal of training, and measurement remains a subjective process.

Screening for Ovarian Masses

Transvaginal sonography with or without color-flow-directed measurements of resistance to flow and flow velocities has been suggested as a means of screening for ovarian cancer. Although transvaginal sonography is probably the best means of determining the morphologic structure of adnexal masses, its efficacy in screening for ovarian cancer has not been established. Both modalities—transvaginal sonography and color-flow-directed measurements—are experimental for these uses.

Several studies are under way to determine whether transvaginal sonography and color Doppler can be used to screen a selected population at high risk for ovarian cancer (38, 40–42). Other studies are being done to examine the feasibility of using transvaginal sonography as a first-line modality for screening.

Summary

Advances in ultrasound imaging equipment have allowed increased applications of pelvic imaging by the practicing clinician. The myriad clinical uses presented here should provide the reader with a basic understanding of when ultrasonography may be helpful in different clinical conditions.

REFERENCES

1. Platt LD, Manning FA, Hill LM. Simultaneous real-time ultrasound scanning and pelvic examination in assessment of pelvic disease. Am J Obstet Gynecol 1980;136: 693–694
2. Timor-Tritsch IE, Rottem S, Thaler I. Review of transvaginal ultrasonography: a description with clinical application. Ultrasound Q 1988;6:1–3
3. Goldstein SR, ed. Endovaginal ultrasound. 2nd ed. New York: Wiley-Liss, 1991
4. American Institute of Ultrasound in Medicine. Bioeffects considerations for the safety of diagnostic ultrasound. J Ultrasound Med 1988;7(suppl 9):S1–S38
5. Sikov MR. Effect of ultrasound on development: I. Introduction and studies in inframammalian species. J Ultrasound Med 1986;5:577
6. Sikov MR. Effect of ultrasound on development: II. Studies in mammalian species and overview. J Ultrasound Med 1986;5:561
7. O'Brien WD. Determination of in situ exposure. Ultrasound Med Biol 1986;12:695
8. Abraham V, Ziskin MC, Heyner S. Temperature elevation in the rat fetus due to ultrasound exposure. Ultrasound Med Biol 1989;15:443
9. Tarantal AF, Chu F, O'Brien WD Jr, Hendricks AG. Measurement of sonographic heat generation in vivo in the gravid long-tailed macaque. J Ultrasound Med 1993; 12:285
10. Lele PP. Effects of ultrasound in "solid" mammalian tissues and tumors in vivo. In: Repacholi MH, Grandolofo M, Rindi A, eds. Ultrasound: medical applications, biological effects and hazard potential. New York: Plenum Press, 1987:275
11. Siddiqi TA, O'Brien WD Jr, Meyer RA, Sullivan JM, Miodovnik M. In situ exposimetry: the ovarian ultrasound examination. Ultrasound Med Biol 1991;17:257
12. American Institute of Ultrasound in Medicine. Bioeffects and safety of diagnostic ultrasound. Rockville, Maryland: AIUM, 1993
13. Goldstein SR. Unusual ultrasonographic appearance of the uterus in patients receiving tamoxifen. Am J Obstet Gynecol 1994;170:447–451
14. Goldstein SR. Use of ultrasonohysterography for triage of perimenopausal patients with unexplained uterine bleeding. Am J Obstet Gynecol 1994;170:565–570
15. Munn CS, Kiser LC, Wetzner SM, Baer JE. Ovary volume in young and premenopausal adults: US determination. Radiology 1986;159:731–732
16. Fossum GT, Davajan V, Kletzky OA. Early detection of pregnancy with transvaginal ultrasound. Fertil Steril 1988;49:788–791
17. Bateman BG, Nunley WC Jr, Kolp LA, Kitchin JD III, Felder R. Vaginal sonography findings and hCG dynamics of early intrauterine and tubal pregnancies. Obstet Gynecol 1990;75:421–427
18. Bernaschek G, Rudelstorfer R, Csaicsich P. Vaginal sonography versus serum human chorionic gonadotropin in early detection of pregnancy. Am J Obstet Gynecol 1988:158:608–612
19. Bree RL, Edwards M, Böhm-Vélez M, Beyler S, Roberts J, Mendelson EB. Transvaginal sonography in the evaluation of normal early pregnancy: correlation with hCG level. AJR 1989;153:75–79
20. Cacciatore B, Tiitinen A, Stenman U-H, Ylöstalo P. Normal early pregnancy: serum hCG levels and vaginal ultrasonography findings. Br J Obstet Gynaecol 1990;97: 889–903
21. Goldstein SR, Snyder JR, Watson C, Danon M. Very early pregnancy detection with endovaginal ultrasound. Obstet Gynecol 1988;72:200–204
22. Levi CS, Lyons EA, Lindsay DJ. Early diagnosis of nonviable pregnancy with endovaginal US. Radiology 1988;167:383–385

23. Nyberg DA, Mack LA, Laing FC, Jeffrey RB. Early pregnancy complications: endovaginal sonographic findings correlated with human chorionic gonadotropic levels. Radiology 1988;167:619–622
24. Fine C, Cartier M, Doubilet P. Fetal heart rates: values throughout gestation. J Ultrasound Med 1988;7(suppl): S105–S106
25. Lindsay DJ, Lovett IS, Lyons EA, Levi CS, Zheng X-H, Holt SC, et al. Yolk sac diameter and shape at endovaginal US: predictors of pregnancy outcome in the first trimester. Radiology 1992;183:115–118
26. Hellman LM, Kobayashi M, Fillisti L, Lavenhar M. Growth and development of the human fetus prior to the twentieth week of gestation. Am J Obstet Gynecol 1969;103:789–800
27. Daya S, Woods S, Ward S, Lappalainen R, Caco C. Early pregnancy assessment with transvaginal ultrasound scanning. Can Med Assoc J 1991;144:441–446
28. DeVoe RW, Pratt JH. Simultaneous intrauterine and extrauterine pregnancy. Am J Obstet Gynecol 1948;56:1119–1126
29. Goldstein SR. Significance of cardiac activity on endovaginal ultrasound in very early embryos. Obstet Gynecol 1992;80:670–672
30. Goldstein SR, Wolfson R. Endovaginal ultrasonographic measurement of early embryonic sizes—a means for assessing gestational age. J Ultrasound Med 1994;13:25–31
31. Nyberg DA, Filly RA, Mahony BS, Monroe S, Laing FC, Jeffrey RB Jr. Early gestation: correlation of hCG levels and sonographic identification. AJR 1985;144:951–954
32. Gamberdella FR, Marrs RP. Heterotopic pregnancy associated with assisted reproductive technology. Am J Obstet Gynecol 1989;160:1520–1524
33. Dimitry ES, Subak-Sharpe R, Mills M, Margara R, Winston R. Nine cases of heterotopic pregnancies in 4 years of in vitro fertilization. Fertil Steril 1990;53:107–110
34. Stiller RJ, De Regt RH, Blair E. Transvaginal ultrasonography in patients at risk for ectopic pregnancy. Am J Obstet Gynecol 1989;161:930–933
35. Fleischer AC, Pennell RG, Mckee MS, Worrell JA, Keefe B, Herbert CM, et al. Ectopic pregnancy: features at transvaginal sonography. Radiology 1990;174:375–378
36. DeCrespigny LC. Demonstration of ectopic pregnancy by transvaginal ultrasound. Br J Obstet Gynaecol 1988; 95:1253–1256
37. Vermesh M, Graczykowski JW, Sauer MV. Reevaluation of the role of culdocentesis in the management of ectopic pregnancy. Am J Obstet Gynecol 1990;162:411–413
38. Bourne T, Campbell S, Steer C, Whitehead MI, Collins WP. Transvaginal colour flow imaging: a possible new screening technique for ovarian cancer. BMJ 1989;299: 1367–1370
39. Kurjak A, Zalud I. Transvaginal colour flow imaging and ovarian cancer. BMJ 1990;300:330
40. Kurjak A, Zalud I, Schulman H. Adnexal masses. In: Kurjak A, ed. Transvaginal color Doppler: a comprehensive guide to transvaginal color Doppler sonography in obstetrics and gynecology. Park Ridge, New Jersey: Parthenon Group, 1990:103–123
41. Rodriguez MH, Platt LD, Medearis AL, Lacarra M, Lobo RA. The use of transvaginal sonography for evaluation of postmenopausal ovarian size and morphology. Am J Obstet Gynecol 1988;159:810–814
42. Karlan BY, Raffel LJ, Crvenkovic G, Smrt C, Chen MD, Lopez E, et al. A multidisciplinary approach to the early detection of ovarian carcinoma: rationale, protocol design, and early results. Am J Obstet Gynecol 1993;169:494–501

SUGGESTED READING

Goldstein SR, Timor-Tritsch IE. Ultrasound in gynecology. New York: Churchill Livingstone, 1995

This Technical Bulletin was developed under the direction of the Committee on Technical Bulletins of the American College of Obstetricians and Gynecologists as an educational aid to obstetricians and gynecologists. The committee wishes to thank Lawrence D. Platt, MD; Ilan E. Timor-Tritsch, MD; and Steven R. Goldstein, MD; for their assistance in the development of this bulletin. This Technical Bulletin does not define a standard of care, nor is it intended to dictate an exclusive course of management. It presents recognized methods and techniques of clinical practice for consideration by obstetrician–gynecologists for incorporation into their practices. Variations of practice taking into account the needs of the individual patient, resources, and limitations unique to the institution or type of practice may be appropriate.

ISSN 1074-8628

THE AMERICAN COLLEGE OF OBSTETRICIANS AND GYNECOLOGISTS
409 12th Street, SW, Washington, DC 20024-2188

12345/98765

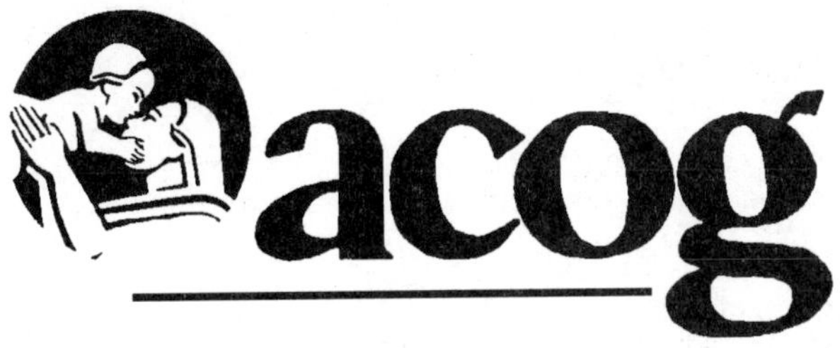

Number 210—August 1995

Technical Bulletin

An Educational Aid to Obstetrician–Gynecologists

Health Maintenance for Perimenopausal Women

Since 1960, the U.S. population has been increasing in age. As growing numbers of women of the post–World War II, baby-boom generation approach menopause, they will be faced with the transition from reproductive to postreproductive status. Attention to the special needs of these women can help prepare them for this transition and promote early interventions to improve health and well-being in the years to follow.

Transition

Menopause is the permanent cessation of menstruation following the decline of ovarian estrogen production. Perimenopause, or the climacteric, is the period extending from immediately before to after the menopause (generally around 45–55 years of age). For most women, this transition lasts approximately 4 years. This period is marked by altered ovarian function.

Prior to menopause when women are in their 40s, menstrual cycle length may begin to increase or decrease, and episodes of anovulation become more prevalent. Menstrual cycle changes during this time are associated with fluctuations in circulating follicle-stimulating hormone (FSH) levels which may be elevated or normal. Although measurement of circulating levels of FSH can be used to identify whether a woman is postmenopausal, it is not useful for monitoring the status of women taking postmenopausal hormone therapy because of failure of exogenous estrogen to suppress FSH.

Because ovarian function waxes and wanes during the perimenopausal years, contraception is necessary until the woman is amenorrheic for one year. Measurement of early follicular phase FSH may be clinically useful as a predictor of fecundity in perimenopausal women attempting to conceive. In women who have had a hysterectomy with their ovaries retained, serum FSH measurement can help to determine their menopausal status.

Screening and Counseling

The perimenopausal period offers an opportunity for counseling about factors that affect a woman's health. Physicians should develop preventive health programs based on each patient's needs and circumstances. The goal of a preventive health program is identification of an unhealthy life style that would benefit from intervention. Patients should undergo a complete medical history, physical examination, and selected laboratory studies and immunizations yearly or as appropriate based on risk factors (see the box).

Screening for Medical Disorders

Certain medical conditions are more prevalent in the perimenopausal woman. Routine assessments for these conditions improve the likelihood of early detection. Once identified, several of these conditions lend themselves to management by the obstetrician–gynecologist. Others may require referral.

Thyroid Disease

Thyroid disorders are common in women, and the incidence of hypothyroidism increases after age 65. Symptomatic women who have a strong family history of thyroid disorders or who have autoimmune dysfunction should be assessed by use of sensitive thyroid-stimulating hormone assays. Thyroid function tests can be misleading in women with systemic illness or those taking certain drugs. In healthy women, menopause and aging do not alter full thyroid hormone concentrations. Women being treated with thyroid replacement should also be moni-

Perimenopausal Health Maintenance

As a woman approaches age 45, her annual examination can be used as an opportunity for a perimenopausal assessment covering the following components, which relate to both menopause and routine health maintenance.

History

- Family history
  - Cardiovascular disease
  - Cancer
  - Diabetes
  - Osteoporosis
  - Other (Alzheimer disease, mental illness, obesity)
- Personal history
  - Health status (including symptoms of menopause)
  - Dietary/nutritional assessment
  - Physical activity
  - Substance use/abuse
  - Abuse or family violence
  - Sexual practices
  - Mental attitude (depression, anxiety, stress)
  - Psychosocial factors (marital status, work, family dynamics)

Physical Examination

- Height
- Weight
- Blood pressure
- Oral cavity
- Neck: adenopathy, thyroid gland
- Breasts, axillae
- Abdomen
- Pelvic and rectovaginal examination
- Skin

Laboratory Tests

- Pap test (physician discretion after three consecutive normal tests if patient is considered to be low risk)
- Mammography (every 1–2 years until age 50; yearly beginning at age 50)
- Cholesterol (every 5 years)
- Fecal occult blood test
- Sigmoidoscopy (every 3–5 years after age 50)
- Other tests (based on risk factors)

Immunizations

- Tetanus–diphtheria booster every 10 years
- Influenza vaccine (yearly beginning at age 55)
- Other (based on risk factors)

Education and Counseling

- Sexuality
  - High-risk behaviors
  - Contraceptive options
  - Sexually transmitted disease
  - Sexual function
- Fitness
  - Hygiene (including dental care)
  - Diet and weight control
  - Exercise
- Psychosocial
  - Family relationships
  - Domestic violence
  - Job/work satisfaction
  - Life style/stress
  - Sleep disorders
- Cardiovascular risk factors
  - Hypertension
  - Hyperlipidemia
  - Obesity/diabetes mellitus
- Health/Risk behaviors
  - Injury prevention
  - Breast self-examination
  - Exposure to ultraviolet rays
  - Suicide prevention
  - Substance abuse
- Hormone therapy
  - Risks versus benefits
  - Side effects
  - Therapeutic regimens

tored annually by thyroid-stimulating hormone assay; overtreatment is associated with osteoporosis.

Diabetes Mellitus

Fasting plasma glucose measurements are recommended every 3–5 years for women with one or more of the following risk factors:

- Family history of diabetes in parents or siblings
- Obesity (body weight greater than 120% of ideal)
- History of gestational diabetes

Diabetes can be diagnosed by assessment of fasting blood glucose levels or random blood glucose levels or use of a 2-hour oral glucose tolerance test. Screening should consist of fasting serum or plasma glucose measurement.

Concentrations of less than 115 mg/dl are normal. Concentrations of at least 140 mg/dl are consistent with diabetes and should be repeated to confirm the diagnosis. Concentrations of 115–139 mg/dl are abnormal, but they are not diagnostic for diabetes.

When diabetes has been diagnosed, it can be categorized as Type I (insulin dependent) or Type II (non-insulin dependent). If diabetes is overt and symptomatic, immediate drug therapy may be necessary. If it is not, dietary control, weight loss, and active exercise programs should be instituted and the patient educated about her disease. The patient's condition should be assessed to detect complications of the disease, such as organ damage from vascular changes. The goal of management is to ensure adequate glucose control.

Nutritional control for secondary and primary prevention (in the presence of insulin resistance with or without carbohydrate intolerance) is an integral component of care for women with overt or potential diabetes. Patients should be educated about the importance of fiber and limiting saturated fats and refined sugars. Women with overt diabetes need the services of a knowledgeable dietician with experience in diabetic diet education.

Insulin resistance can be a factor in diabetes and hypertension and is often linked to obesity. Regular physical exercise promotes weight loss and can improve insulin sensitivity and dyslipidemia in those people who are in high risk groups for cardiovascular and microvascular disease (1).

Breast Cancer

One of every nine American women who lives to 85 years of age will develop breast cancer. The incidence has increased over the past two decades but in 1987 reached a plateau at about 182,000 new cases per year. Mortality rates have remained constant at about 46,000 deaths per year. However, in view of an increasing incidence, a steady mortality rate may indicate an improvement in early diagnosis or therapy. The 5-year survival rate for women with localized breast cancer has risen from 78% in the 1940s to 93% in 1993. This is attributed to earlier diagnosis as a result of greater use of screening mammography. The breast is the leading site of cancer in women (32% of all cancers) and is the second leading cause of death from cancer in women, exceeded only by lung cancer.

Randomized, controlled trials have clearly demonstrated a decreased death rate from breast cancer in women who were offered mammography between the ages of 50 and 69 years old. After a review of the evidence showing the benefit of screening by mammography in women between 40 and 49 years old, the National Cancer Institute withdrew its recommendation for screening these women. It is ACOG's conclusion however, that the data are limited; thus ACOG guidelines continue to recommend offering screening by mammography every 1–2 years to women 40–49 years of age and annually to women over 50 years of age (2).

All women should have a thorough annual breast examination and perform monthly breast self-examination. Because of breast changes in response to the hormonal sequence of a normal menstrual cycle, self-breast examination is most effective during the follicular phase of the cycle.

Hypertension

Hypertension is the most common chronic disease in older women and a significant risk factor for stroke, congestive heart disease, and renal disease. Beginning at age 50, hypertension is more common in women than in men and more common in African Americans than in other racial groups.

The history and physical examination provide an opportunity to seek information regarding the following risk factors:

- Previous history of hypertension
- Previous history of antihypertensive treatment
- Family history of cardiovascular disease, especially with early age of onset
- Dietary history, especially excessive sodium or alcohol intake
- Relevant medications, such as glucocorticosteroids, sympathomimetic amines, or nasal decongestants
- Medical information of specific interest: headaches, coronary artery disease, chest pain, prior stroke, renal disease
- Other cardiovascular risk factors: smoking, high cholesterol or problematic lipid profile, obesity, diabetes mellitus, stress

The blood pressure classification for adults established in 1993 is shown in Table 1. A single elevated diastolic pressure less than 100 mm Hg should not be treated but should be rechecked within 2 months. When the diastolic pressure is 100 mm Hg or greater, the patient should be evaluated. A diastolic pressure greater than 120 mm Hg requires immediate attention. Malignant hypertension is a diastolic pressure greater than 140 mm Hg with papilledema. Evidence suggests that patients with a systolic blood pressure greater than 160 mm Hg will benefit from treatment (3).

The initial assessment of patients with hypertension should include at least the following laboratory evaluation: urinalysis; determination of levels of hemoglobin or hematocrit, creatinine, potassium, and fasting glucose; lipid profile; and electrocardiography. The first line of treatment for hypertension is dietary and life style changes. Weight loss, control of sodium and alcohol intake, exercise, stress management, and smoking cessation are all important treatment interventions for hypertension. If after 3 months these efforts have failed, pharmacologic

TABLE 1. CLASSIFICATION OF BLOOD PRESSURE FOR ADULTS AGED 18 YEARS AND OLDER

Category	Systolic (mm Hg)	Diastolic (mm Hg)
Normal	<130	<85
High normal	130–139	85–89
Hypertension		
Stage 1 (mild)	140–159	90–99
Stage 2 (moderate)	160–179	100–109
Stage 3 (severe)	180–209	110–119
Stage 4 (very severe)	210 or greater	120 or greater

Joint National Committee on the Detection, Evaluation, and Treatment of High Blood Pressure. The fifth report of the Joint National Committee on the Detection, Evaluation, and Treatment of High Blood Pressure (JNC V). Arch Intern Med 1993;153:161

therapy should be considered. Patients who respond to nonpharmacologic treatment require close monitoring, however, because a significant percentage will progress to higher levels of blood pressure and require pharmacologic therapy.

Women with diastolic blood pressures greater than 100 mm Hg should be treated with pharmacologic methods if nonpharmacologic methods fail to reduce blood pressures. Women with diastolic blood pressures of 90–100 mm Hg should be treated with medication if they are African American, have a systolic blood pressure greater than 160 mm Hg, or have other specific cardiovascular risk factors.

A Healthy Life Style

Maintaining a healthy life style is beneficial to women of all ages. For perimenopausal women, a healthy life style can also reduce the risk of several disorders prevalent in this age group. By making certain life style changes, these women can improve both their overall health and their quality of life.

Smoking

Certain health conditions that are more prevalent in perimenopausal women have been linked to smoking. The relationship of cigarette smoking to coronary heart disease, chronic obstructive pulmonary disease, lung cancer, and a number of other chronic diseases is well established. Smoking has a greater adverse effect on women when compared with men (4). Women who smoke only one to four cigarettes per day have a 2.5-fold increased risk of fatal coronary heart disease (5). In 1994, the incidence of lung cancer among women was estimated to be 72,000 cases, with an estimated 59,000 deaths (6).

Smokers should be repeatedly counseled to quit smoking, and follow-up visits just for this purpose are worthwhile. Approximately 65% of those who stop smoking relapse within 3 months, and another 10% resume smoking between 3 and 6 months, whereas only 3% relapse from 6 to 12 months (7). Nicotine replacement therapy, in the form of chewing gum or a transdermal patch, has been demonstrated to increase the effectiveness of smoking cessation programs when evaluated 6 months after the intervention. One study has demonstrated that smoking cessation at any age improves the health of the lungs, regardless of how long one has smoked (8).

Exercise

Although data in women are scarce, lack of physical activity is recognized as a risk factor for coronary artery disease in men. There is a significant positive relationship between levels of high-density lipoprotein (HDL) cholesterol and physical activity in postmenopausal women. Furthermore, in women with low levels of HDL cholesterol, aerobic exercise provides a greater increase in HDL cholesterol than it does in women with normal to high levels.

Vigorous exercise at least three times a week for 20 minutes should be strongly encouraged as part of an overall health plan for both cardiovascular health promotion and protection against osteoporosis. Cardiovascular training can be accomplished with aerobic exercise that elevates the heart rate into the patient's target heart rate. If this exercise is not weight bearing, strength training should be added two times per week. Weight-bearing physical activity, as little as 30 minutes a day for 3 days a week, may increase the mineral content of bone in older women. The exercise need not be extreme; walking 1.5 miles and performing ordinary calisthenics are sufficient to increase mineral content. More detailed information on exercise recommendations for women has been published elsewhere (9).

Alcohol Abuse

It is estimated that alcoholism occurs in up to 10% of older women, contributing significantly to functional disability (10). However, alcohol abuse is often overlooked and misdiagnosed. Women are at high risk for alcoholism if there is a family history of alcoholism or personal habitual alcohol use. The CAGE questionnaire may be helpful in detecting problem drinking (see the box).

Weight Control, Nutrition, and Diet

Weight control, exercise, and nutrition are keystones for good health, and there are some specific issues for perimenopausal women. Women in this age group commonly report weight gain, and this observation is validated by epidemiologic studies. Such studies indicate that 38% of women aged 40–49 and 52% of women aged 50–59 are overweight (11).

The traditionally recommended method for weight control is simple caloric reduction, although there is ample evidence that caloric reduction alone is ineffective for maintaining long-term weight reduction. Of particular

The CAGE Questions

- C Have you ever felt you ought to **C**ut down on your drinking?
- A Have people **A**nnoyed you by criticizing your drinking?
- G Have you ever felt bad or **G**uilty about your drinking?
- E Have you ever had a drink first thing in the morning to steady your nerves or get rid of a hangover (**E**ye opener)?

Ewing JA. Detecting alcoholism: the CAGE questionnaire. JAMA 1984;252:1907; Copyright 1984, American Medical Association

concern are regimens requiring marked caloric restriction. Efforts at weight reduction are optimized when dietary changes are combined with moderate cardiovascular exercise (30 minutes, three times per week) (12) and strength training (two sessions per week). Life style regimens that are most effective in reducing bone loss include weight-bearing cardiovascular exercise (13, 14), strength training, hormone therapy, and calcium supplementation. The best results occur in patients using more than one regimen (15–18). Use of hormone therapy, however, is the most important factor in reducing bone loss.

Strength training is assuming increasing importance in providing health benefits, particularly for perimenopausal women (19). In addition to conferring strength (20) and bone protection, strength training increases muscle mass, which in turn increases the metabolic rate and enhances weight control efforts (21, 22).

Good nutrition is an essential part of preventive health care. All evidence indicates that diet influences the risk of several major chronic diseases, especially atherosclerotic cardiovascular disease and hypertension. Diet may also play a positive role in preventing some cancers. Other health problems influenced by diet include dental caries, chronic liver disease, diabetes mellitus, and obesity.

While many clinicians do not routinely review dietary histories, it is important to assess calcium supplementation. In the absence of dietary calcium intake, 1,200–1,600 mg of elemental calcium should be ingested. Calcium carbonate has 40% elemental calcium; lactate, 13%; and gluconate, 9%. Although lactose intolerance increases with age, many patients consume some calcium in their diet. Dairy sources are calcium rich, but other foods, such as fortified orange juice, may also be excellent sources.

Even patients who appear well nourished may be malnourished. A 24-hour diet and fluid recall history is helpful to assess a patient's dietary habits.

Domestic Violence

Domestic violence includes both physical and mental abuse. It occurs in all segments of society. Obstetrician–gynecologists can play a vital role in identifying women who are the victims of abuse and offering them appropriate care.

Recognition of this problem requires a high index of suspicion; direct questioning is appropriate and recommended. Questions such as "Has anyone at home hit you or tried to injure you?" and "Have you ever been physically abused, either recently or in the past?" are appropriate ways in which to raise the subject. Physical examination may show evidence of injury, either recent or remote. Any such injuries should be noted in the medical record, and the patient should be asked how they occurred.

In addition to treating the patient's injuries, the physician should assess her emotional status. The physician should provide counseling and referral to legal and social resources and psychologic therapy.

Emotional Problems

Mood disorders, particularly depression, are among the most common psychiatric illnesses in women. Although depression can occur at any age, in 50% of patients the onset is between 20 and 50 years of age, with the mean being about 40 years. Depression can be overdiagnosed in women who have experienced grief reactions or who are undergoing situational stress (23).

Epidemiologic studies of the prevalence of depression in women have dispelled the notion of an increase in depression at the time of menopause or so-called *involutional melancholia*. The complex experience of menopause and midlife adjustment disorders must be considered within social, cultural, and psychologic contexts. Aging involves additional and unexpected losses of family and friends, physical changes, and concerns about premature aging or a loss of sexuality and femininity. The successful adjustment to living with chronic illness, uncertainties about developing cancer, or aging in general depends on the woman's past history of depression, her emotional resources, and the extended family and community support available to her. The obstetrician–gynecologist should be cognizant of the various factors that influence the presentation, diagnosis, and treatment of depression in women and refer patients for treatment as needed.

Reproductive Concerns

Perimenopausal women have reproductive concerns relating to fertility and infertility. Contraception may involve some adjustment in response to changing hormone levels. Those women who desire pregnancy may require special care.

Contraception

Prevention of unwanted pregnancy assumes increasing importance during the perimenopausal years. About 75% of pregnancies in women over age 40 are unintended (24). It may be difficult to know when it is safe to change from oral contraception to postmenopausal hormone treatment. Contraception can be discontinued when the FSH level is greater than 30 IU/L (measured at the end of the pill-free week in women on estrogen/progestin oral contraceptives).

Except for women who smoke, there is no limitation of contraceptive choice. The health risks and benefits of the contraceptive method should be discussed. Combination oral contraceptive pills are safe for women over 40 who don't smoke. Progestin-only methods, including the minipill, injectables (depot medroxyprogesterone acetate), or implants (Norplant), are excellent alternatives. The intrauterine device (IUD) is also an option, particularly the copper IUD, which is now approved for a 10-year duration of use. The progesterone IUD has an added benefit of reduced menstrual bleeding but requires replacement every year. Barrier methods that use nonoxynol-9 appear effective in reducing pregnancy and may reduce some sexually transmitted diseases as well.

Pregnancy

The proportion of births among women aged 35–49 is predicted to rise from 5% in 1982 to 8.6% in 2000, an increase of about 72% (25). Women considering pregnancy as they approach their perimenopausal years are faced with two concerns: the difficulty of achieving pregnancy later in life and the complications associated with being pregnant later in life.

There is a decline in fecundity with advancing age. A major contributor to the decline in delivery rates associated with increasing age is the risk of spontaneous abortion. The frequency of both euploid (normal) and aneuploid (abnormal) abortuses increases with maternal age. Clinically recognized abortion occurs in only 12% of women under age 20, but increases to at least 26% in women over age 40.

Traditionally, increased maternal age has been associated with an increased risk of obstetric complications. Statistics indicate that older women have a higher mortality rate with pregnancy. There is reason to believe, however, that the obstetric risks associated with advanced age can be minimized by attention to screening and modern obstetric care.

Hypoestrogenic Changes

Data from longitudinal studies uniformly indicate that approximately 80% of women experience menopause without significant difficulty as a normal physiologic event in their lives (26). Most women do experience some symptoms related to menopause, although the causal relation to estrogen deficiency is uncertain. The vasomotor flush is experienced to some degree by most menopausal women (26–28). Frequent problems include fatigue, nervousness, headaches, insomnia, depression, irritability, joint and muscle pain, dizziness, and palpitations. Emotional stability during the perimenopausal period can be disrupted by poor sleep patterns. The nature and severity of these symptoms vary considerably, so it can be difficult to differentiate among social, cultural, and biologic factors. Certain physiologic effects of estrogen deficiency can lead to long-term health problems such as osteoporosis and coronary heart disease.

Genitourinary Changes

Low levels of estrogen cause atrophy of mucosal surfaces accompanied by vaginitis, pruritus, dyspareunia, and stenosis. Genitourinary atrophy leads to a variety of symptoms that affect the ease and quality of living. Urethritis, urge incontinence, and urinary frequency are related to hypoestrogenism in the lower urinary tract. In discussing hypoestrogenic changes with patients, physicians should be sensitive to use of the term *atrophy* as patients may react negatively to its connotation of wasting away or decline.

Sexuality

Sexuality is an integral component of quality of life. Physicians should be prepared to bring up the subject of sexuality, because women may have questions but may be reluctant to ask them.

The major physical changes affecting sexuality that occur in perimenopausal women are a reduction in the rate of production and volume of vaginal fluid, some loss of vaginal elasticity, and thinning of vaginal tissues, which result in a decreased ability to tolerate deep thrusting or long-continuing thrusting. The dyspareunia associated with postmenopausal urogenital atrophy includes a feeling of dryness and tightness, vaginal irritation and burning with coitus, and postcoital spotting and soreness.

Coital activity correlates more closely with a woman's relationship with her partner than with hormone levels. Less vaginal atrophy is noted in sexually active women compared with inactive women; presumably, sexual activity maintains vaginal vasculature and circulation. However, objective measurements of the degree of lubrication have demonstrated that the vaginal factors that influence the enjoyment of sexual intercourse can be maintained by estrogen therapy (29).

Osteoporosis

Women who are thin, white, or of Asian descent; are hypoestrogenic with small frames; or have a family history of osteoporosis are considered to have an increased risk for the development of osteoporosis. Osteoporosis can also occur secondary to other disease processes. Other factors that have been implicated include alcohol, tobacco, and caffeine.

Measuring Bone Density

Screening bone density may be warranted in those women who are at high risk for osteoporosis and who cannot or will not take estrogen. If testing identifies rapid bone loss, referral to an appropriate specialist may be indicated. There is a 50–100% increase in the risk of fracture for each standard deviation decline in bone mass. Measurement of lower bone mass in the hip is even more predictive; one standard deviation is associated with a nearly threefold increase in risk of fracture (30). Despite the impressive correlation between fracture risk and bone density, it is not cost-effective to screen all postmenopausal women.

Preventing Osteoporosis

Preventive health efforts in this age group should be directed toward those factors that influence accumulation and loss of bone. Patients should be counseled about adequate calcium intake, weight-bearing exercise, and the elimination of risk factors to attain the best possible maximal bone density.

While exercise can have a beneficial effect on bone density, the impact of exercise on bone is significantly less than that achieved by hormone therapy (17). Women require a combination of hormone therapy, calcium supplementation, and exercise in order to fully minimize the risk of fractures. Women who do not take hormone therapy need higher levels of calcium supplementation.

Cardiovascular Disease

Cardiovascular disease is the leading cause of death for women in the United States; of the 550,000 people in the United States who die each year of heart disease, 250,000 are women (31). The risk factors are high blood pressure, smoking, high cholesterol levels, diabetes mellitus, and obesity. Men have a higher risk of developing coronary heart disease than women. With increasing age, however, the death rate of women approaches that of men.

Preventive measures—smoking cessation, blood pressure reduction, and lowered cholesterol levels—have helped improve mortality rates from coronary heart disease. It has also been shown that estrogen therapy protects against cardiovascular disease in women. Hormone therapy does not cause hypertension (except in very rare cases of idiosyncratic reaction) (32) and may provide cardiovascular protection to hypoestrogenic women with well-controlled hypertension.

In women, HDL cholesterol is an indicator of risk for coronary heart disease. For every increase in HDL cholesterol of 10 mg/dl there appears to be a 50% decrease in risk (33). After menopause, however, the ratio of low-density lipoprotein (LDL) cholesterol to HDL cholesterol rises. Estrogens increase HDL cholesterol and lower LDL cholesterol, and progestins are thought to have the opposite effect. It is unclear at present whether the addition of progestin to estrogen therapy diminishes the cardiovascular protection of estrogen.

Triglycerides are also an important risk factor for coronary heart disease in women. However, an increased rate of cardiovascular disease is observed only when increased triglyceride levels are present in association with low HDL cholesterol levels (34).

The correlation between total cholesterol and coronary heart disease rates is similar for men and women. Therefore, the National Cholesterol Education Program and the National Cholesterol Consensus Conference have concluded that the same levels of total cholesterol and HDL cholesterol should be used in assigning risk in both women and men (Table 2). If high levels of cholesterol are detected, the first steps in treatment are diet and exercise (35).

Abnormal Uterine Bleeding

Throughout the perimenopause, there is a significant incidence of abnormal uterine bleeding. Although the greatest concern provoked by this symptom is endometrial neoplasia, the usual finding is tissue that displays the effects of estrogen unopposed by progesterone. In premenopausal women, this results from anovulation, and in postmenopausal women, it results from extragonadal endogenous estrogen production or estrogen administration. Abnormal uterine bleeding should be evaluated and treated according to previously published guidelines (36).

Hormone Therapy

The issues of menopause and hormone therapy should be reviewed annually with perimenopausal patients. The variability in the symptoms and time course of the perimenopause, as well as the benefits, side effects, and risks of estrogen therapy, should be discussed.

If the patient has significant symptoms of hypoestrogenism, estrogen therapy can be offered even if the patient is menstruating. Measurement of FSH levels may be useful to document estrogen deficiency as the cause of symptoms when the clinical situation is not clear. In the asymptomatic patient who has been amenorrheic for 6 months, hormone therapy should be considered for its protective benefits. In the patient who has undergone hysterectomy with intact ovaries, the timing of initiation of therapy can be based on symptoms, signs, or the vaginal maturation index.

When considering the use of estrogen, the clinician should weigh benefits against side effects and risks for the

TABLE 2. INITIAL CLASSIFICATION BASED ON TOTAL CHOLESTEROL AND HDL CHOLESTEROL LEVELS*

Cholesterol Level	Initial Classification
Total Cholesterol	
<200 mg/dl (5.2 mmol/L)	Desirable blood cholesterol
200–239 mg/dl (5.2–6.2 mmol/L)	Borderline-high blood cholesterol
≥ 240 mg/dl (6.2 mmol/L)	High blood cholesterol
HDL Cholesterol	
<35 mg/dl (0.9 mmol/L)	Low HDL cholesterol

*HDL indicates high-density lipoprotein.

National Cholesterol Education Program. Expert panel on detection, evaluation, and treatment of high blood cholesterol in adults. Summary of the Second Report of the National Cholesterol Education Program (NCEP) Expert Panel on Detection, Evaluation, and Treatment of High Blood Cholesterol in Adults (Adult Treatment Panel II). JAMA 1993;269:3017

individual patient. A full discussion of these factors is presented elsewhere (37). Areas of controversy include assessing the level of altered risk (if any) of breast cancer with low-dose estrogen, the level of cardiovascular protection with the addition of progestin, and the use of estrogen in women who have had endometrial or breast cancer.

Summary

Perimenopausal women are assuming increasing importance in the practice of obstetrics and gynecology. While continuing to have reproductive concerns, such as attaining or preventing pregnancy, these women are confronted with a decline in estrogen levels and the inherent protection estrogen provides against osteoporosis and cardiovascular disease. Preventive care, life style modification, and early diagnosis and intervention can play a valuable role in maintaining patients' overall health and quality of life.

REFERENCES

1. Kitabchi AE, Ghawji M. Diabetes in the nonpregnant patient. Prim Care Update Ob/Gyns 1994;1:86–94
2. American College of Obstetricians and Gynecologists. Routine cancer screening. ACOG Committee Opinion 128. Washington, DC: ACOG, 1993
3. Joint National Committee on Detection, Evaluation, and Treatment of High Blood Pressure. The Fifth Report of the Joint National Committee on Detection, Evaluation, and Treatment of High Blood Pressure (JNC V). Arch Intern Med 1993;153:154–183
4. Davis DL, Dinse GE, Hoel DG. Decreasing cardiovascular disease and increasing cancer among whites in the United States from 1973 through 1987. JAMA 1994; 271:431–437
5. Willett WC, Green A, Stampfer MJ, Speizer FE, Colditz GA, Rosner B, et al. Relative and absolute excess risks of coronary heart disease among women who smoke cigarettes. N Engl J Med 1987;317:1303–1309
6. American Cancer Society. Cancer facts and figures—1994. Atlanta, Georgia: ACS, 1994
7. U.S. Department of Health and Human Services. The health benefits of smoking cessation: a report of the Surgeon General. Rockville, Maryland: U.S. Department of Health and Human Services, 1990; publication no. (CDC)90-8416:595
8. Anthonisen NR, Connett JE, Kiley JP, Altose MD, Bailey WC, Buist AS, et al. Effects of smoking intervention and the use of an inhaled anticholinergic bronchodilator on the rate of decline of FEV_1. The lung health study. JAMA 1994;272:1497–1505
9. American College of Obstetricians and Gynecologists. Women and exercise. ACOG Technical Bulletin 173. Washington, DC: ACOG, 1992
10. A federal response to a hidden epidemic: alcohol and other drug problems among women. Washington, DC: National Council on Alcoholism, 1987
11. Kuczmarski RJ, Flegal KM, Campbell SM, Johnson CL. Increasing prevalence of overweight among US adults. JAMA 1994;272:205–211
12. Johannessen S, Lui H. High-frequency, moderate-intensity training in sedentary middle-aged women. Physician Sportsmed 1986;14:99–102
13. Shimegi S, Yanagita M, Okano H, Yamada M, Fukui H, Fukumura Y, et al. Physical exercise increases bone mineral density in postmenopausal women. Endocrine Journal 1994;41:49–56
14. Michel BA, Lane NE, Block DA, Jones HH, Fries JF. Effect of changes in weight-bearing exercise on lumbar bone mass after age fifty. Ann Med 1991;23:397–401
15. Chestnut CH III. Bone mass and exercise. Am J Med 1993;95(5A):34S–36S
16. Gutin B, Kasper MJ. Can vigorous exercise play a role in osteoporosis prevention? A review. Osteoporos Int 1992;2(2):55–69
17. Prince RL, Smith M, Dick IM, Price RI, Webb PG, Henderson NK, et al. Prevention of postmenopausal osteoporosis. A comparative study of exercise, calcium supplementation, and hormone-replacement therapy. N Engl J Med 1991;325:1189–1195
18. Whatley JE, Gillespie WJ, Honig J, Walsh MJ, Blackburn AL, Blackburn GL. Does the amount of endurance exercise in combination with weight training and a very-low-energy diet affect resting metabolic rate and body composition? Am J Clin Nutr 1994;59:1088–1092
19. Mortell R, Tucker L. Effects of a 12-week resistive training program in the home using the body bar on dynamic and absolute strength of middle-age women. Percept Mot Skills 1993;76:1131–1138
20. Manning JM, Dooly Manning CF, White K, Kampa I, Silas S, Kesselhaut M, et al. Effects of a resistive training program on lipoprotein–lipid levels in obese women. Med Sci Sports Exerc 1991;23:1222–1226

21. Heislein DM, Harris BA, Jette AM. A strength training program for postmenopausal women: a pilot study. Arch Phys Med Rehabil 1994;75:198–204

22. Butts NK, Price S. Effects of a 12-week weight training program on the body composition of women over 30 years of age. J Strength Conditioning Res 1994;8:265–269

23. American College of Obstetricians and Gynecologists. Depression in women. ACOG Technical Bulletin 182. Washington, DC: ACOG, 1993

24. Brown SS, Eisenberg L, eds. The best intentions: unintended pregnancy and the well-being of children and families. Washington, DC: National Academy Press, 1995

25. Spencer G. Projections of the population of the United States, by age, sex, and race: 1983–2080. Current population reports—population estimates and projections; series P025, no. 952. Washington, DC: U.S. Department of Commerce, 1984

26. McKinlay SM, Brambilla DJ, Posner JG. The normal menopause transition. Maturitas 1992;14:103–115

27. Hunter M. The South-East England longitudinal study of the climacteric and postmenopause. Maturitas 1992;14: 117–126

28. Oldenhave A, Jaszmann LJB, Haspels AA, Everaerd WTAM. Impact of climacteric on well-being. A survey based on 5213 women 39 to 60 years old. Am J Obstet Gynecol 1993;168:772–780

29. Semmens JP, Tsai CC, Semmens EC, Loadholt CB. Effects of estrogen therapy on vaginal physiology during menopause. Obstet Gynecol 1985;66:15–23

30. Cummings SR, Black DM, Nevitt MC, Browner W, Cauley J, Ensrud K, et al. Bone density at various sites for prediction of hip fractures. Lancet 1993;341:72–75

31. Wenger NK, Speroff L, Packard B. Cardiovascular health and disease in women. N Engl J Med 1993;329:247–256

32. Lip GY, Beevers M, Churchill D, Beevers DG. Hormone replacement therapy and blood pressure in hypertensive women. J Hum Hypertens 1994;8:491–494

33. Kannel WB. Metabolic risk factors for coronary heart disease in women: perspective from the Framingham Study. Am Heart J 1987;114:413–419

34. Bass KM, Newschaffer CJ, Klag MJ, Bush TL. Plasma lipoprotein levels as predictors of cardiovascular deaths in women. Circulation 1993;153:2209

35. National Cholesterol Education Program. Expert panel on detection, evaluation, and treatment of high blood cholesterol in adults. Summary of the Second Report of the National Cholesterol Education Program (NCEP) Expert Panel on Detection, Evaluation, and Treatment of High Blood Cholesterol in Adults (Adult Treatment Panel II). JAMA 1993;269:3015–3023

36. American College of Obstetricians and Gynecologists. Dysfunctional uterine bleeding. ACOG Technical Bulletin 134. Washington, DC: ACOG, 1989

37. American College of Obstetricians and Gynecologists. Hormone replacement therapy. ACOG Technical Bulletin 166. Washington, DC: ACOG, 1992

SUGGESTED READING

American College of Obstetricians and Gynecologists. The battered woman. ACOG Technical Bulletin 124. Washington, DC: ACOG, 1989

American College of Obstetricians and Gynecologists. Carcinoma of the breast. ACOG Technical Bulletin 158. Washington, DC: ACOG, 1991

American College of Obstetricians and Gynecologists. Hormonal contraception. ACOG Technical Bulletin 198. Washington, DC: ACOG, 1994

American College of Obstetricians and Gynecologists. The intrauterine device. ACOG Technical Bulletin 164. Washington, DC: ACOG, 1992

American College of Obstetricians and Gynecologists. Management of medical disorders. In: Precis V. An update in obstetrics and gynecology. Washington, DC: ACOG, 1994:15–54

American College of Obstetricians and Gynecologists. Nonmalignant conditions of the breast. ACOG Technical Bulletin 156. Washington, DC: ACOG, 1991

American College of Obstetricians and Gynecologists. Osteoporosis. ACOG Technical Bulletin 167. Washington, DC: ACOG, 1992

American College of Obstetricians and Gynecologists. The role of the obstetrician–gynecologist in the diagnosis and treatment of breast disease. ACOG Committee Opinion 140. Washington, DC: ACOG, 1994

This Technical Bulletin was developed under the direction of the Committee on Technical Bulletins of the American College of Obstetricians and Gynecologists as an educational aid to obstetricians and gynecologists. The committee wishes to thank Leon Speroff, MD, for his assistance in the development of this bulletin. This Technical Bulletin does not define a standard of care, nor is it intended to dictate an exclusive course of management. It presents recognized methods and techniques of clinical practice for consideration by obstetrician–gynecologists for incorporation into their practices. Variations of practice taking into account the needs of the individual patient, resources, and limitations unique to the institution or type of practice may be appropriate.
ISSN 1074-8628

THE AMERICAN COLLEGE OF OBSTETRICIANS AND GYNECOLOGISTS
409 12th Street, SW
Washington, DC 20024-2188

12345/87654

ACOG EDUCATIONAL BULLETIN

Number 235, April 1997

Hemorrhagic Shock

The recognition of high-risk situations aids in the prevention and management of severe hemorrhage. Significant bleeding usually is of a limited nature and can be controlled, and blood can be replaced. The serious nature and frequent occurrences of life-threatening hemorrhage and hemorrhagic shock demand competence of the obstetrician–gynecologist in the management of these conditions.

This bulletin is intended to fulfill the following objectives:

- Identify gynecologic patients who are at risk for severe hemorrhage.
- Discuss the pathophysiology of hemorrhagic shock.
- Review current approaches to the management of severe, life-threatening hemorrhage and hemorrhagic shock.
- Describe the complications resulting from hemorrhagic shock and its treatment.

This Educational Bulletin was developed under the direction of the Committee on Educational Bulletins of the American College of Obstetricians and Gynecologists as an aid to obstetricians and gynecologists. The College wishes to thank Mitchel S. Hoffman, MD, and Marc A. Rozner, PhD, MD, for their assistance in the development of this bulletin. This document is not to be construed as establishing a standard of practice or dictating an exclusive course of treatment. Rather, it is intended as an educational tool that presents current information on obstetric–gynecologic issues.

Etiology

Shock is defined as hypoperfusion of the vascular bed with decreased cellular respiration. In shock, the circulating blood volume is less than the capacity of the vascular bed. The problem may arise from a decrease in effective circulating blood volume or an inability of the heart to pump. The result is a state of profound and widespread reduction in the effective delivery of oxygen and other nutrients to tissues, which leads to irreversible cellular injury if prolonged.

The most common cause of shock in obstetrics and gynecology is hemorrhage. However, other forms of shock occur and should be considered.

- Hypovolemic shock is caused by hemorrhage or loss of bodily fluids other than blood. Extensive fluid losses most often are related to problems of the gastrointestinal tract (vomiting, nasogastric tube output, diarrhea, proximal fistula output, sequestration during bowel obstruction), but occasionally can have other causes (postoperative reaccumulation of ascites, and inadequate replacement of fluid following extensive surgery).

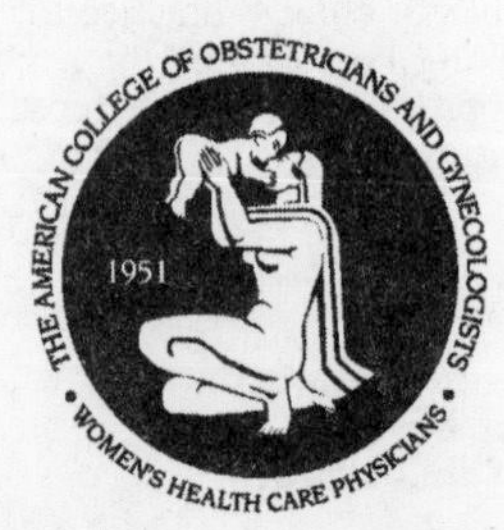

Replaces Number 82, December 1984

- Cardiogenic shock develops when the heart fails to pump an effective circulatory volume, resulting in hypoperfusion. In gynecologic patients, this is almost always due to myocardial injury.
- Systemic inflammatory response syndrome (formerly septic shock) results from the effects of endotoxin on the cardiovascular system. Endotoxin is a component of the gram-negative bacterial cell wall that is produced in sufficient quantities to cause profound effects on the vascular endothelium and cardiovascular function. The main initial finding of shock is a dramatic decrease in systemic vascular resistance.
- Neurogenic shock is caused by loss of sympathetic control of both resistance and capacitance vessels and loss of cardiac sympathetic tone. Acute vasodilation results in a significant decrease in effective circulatory volume.

Nonsurgical uterine bleeding from such conditions as leiomyomata and anovulation can be quite heavy and occasionally can cause profound anemia but will rarely result in shock. Bleeding from a gynecologic malignancy is seldom acute in nature. Sometimes, a ruptured corpus luteum cyst will cause intraperitoneal hemorrhage at a level sufficient to produce shock. Certain rare ovarian neoplasms, such as the granulosa cell tumor, are known for their occasional dramatic presentation of sudden rupture and hemorrhage. In gynecologic patients, however, shock most often is encountered intraoperatively or postoperatively. Potential for severe hemorrhage in pelvic surgery is greater with complicated or radical procedures.

Other sources of severe hemorrhage sometimes are encountered. Examples of disorders associated with bleeding include colon cancer, hemorrhagic radiation proctosigmoiditis, severe cystitis, and metastatic choriocarcinoma or severe preeclampsia with a subcapsular hematoma of the liver.

Clinical Manifestations

The initial clinical manifestations of hemorrhagic shock vary based on individual circumstances. A patient who is conscious and experiencing postoperative bleeding may manifest mental status changes, appear pale and diaphoretic, and have a fast, "thready" pulse and decreased urine output (Table 1).

The average adult woman has approximately 5 L (70 mL/kg) of blood. Depending upon a number of individual factors, hemodynamic decompensation and shock generally occur at an uncompensated loss of around 25–30% of the blood volume. A number of physiologic responses occur in the body's attempt to maintain tissue perfusion. The initial, predictable responses to hypotension are peripheral vasoconstriction and an increase in the rate and force of cardiac contraction. Vasoconstriction can reduce flow to "nonvital" organs, preferentially diverting cardiac output to the brain and the heart. Other compensatory effects include increased secretion of antidiuretic hormone, cortisol, aldosterone, and catecholamines. As a result of these increased hormones, blood flow to the kidneys will be reduced, producing a decrease in urine output. Also, blood sugar levels will increase and serum albumin levels will decrease.

During the early state of "primary" or "reversible" shock, control of hemorrhage and replacement of blood and fluid readily restore homeostasis. With continued hemorrhage, however, compensatory mechanisms become inadequate to preserve circulatory volume. A continued decrease in circulatory volume and hemoglobin

Table 1. The Clinical Picture in Hemorrhagic Shock and Expected Response to Volume Replacement

	Primary Shock		
Clinical Sign	**Early**	**Late**	**Secondary Shock**
Mental state	Alert and anxious	Confused	Coma
General appearance	Normal and warm	Pale and cold	Cyanotic and cold
Blood pressure	Slightly hypotensive	Moderately hypotensive	Markedly hypotensive
Respiratory system	Slight tachypnea	Tachypnea	Tachypnea and cyanosis
Urinary output	30–60 mL/h (0.5–1 mL/kg/h)	<30 mL/h (<0.5 mL/kg/h)	Anuria
Effect of volume challenge on			
Blood pressure	Increased	Slightly increased	No response
Urinary output	Increased	Slightly increased	No response

Modified from Marsden DE, Cavanagh D. Hemorrhagic Shock in the Gynecologic Patient. Clin Obstet Gynecol 1985;28:382.

results in reduced perfusion of tissues and tissue hypoxia. If peripheral vasoconstriction is not reversed, decompensation begins as damaged capillaries become dilated and leaky. Clinically, the patient's mental status deteriorates because perfusion of the brain becomes compromised. Blood pressure can no longer be maintained through the compensatory mechanisms described above, and the patient will become anuric. In this "late" or "decompensated" stage of primary shock, volume replacement is less likely to result in clinical improvement.

Without adequate treatment there is further tissue hypoxia and the patient develops other metabolic derangements. Peripheral vascular tone is lost and capillary leakage worsens. Organ perfusion becomes critically reduced and marked metabolic acidosis develops. Disseminated intravascular coagulation develops in some patients. Persistent metabolic acidosis in the face of volume replacement is an ominous sign. As decompensation progresses, failure of one or more organ systems occurs, and, if uncorrected, may lead to death.

Differential Diagnosis

When a patient develops clinical evidence of shock, the cause may not be immediately apparent. Depending on the clinical situation, even in patients with overt hemorrhage, other causes or factors may need to be considered.

In elderly patients, cardiac reserve may be low and significant hemorrhage may pose a risk for cardiac decompensation and possibly myocardial infarction. When managing hemorrhagic shock, especially in such patients at increased risk, the contribution of a cardiogenic component should be considered.

Massive pulmonary embolism occurring perioperatively or postoperatively may result in shock. Pulmonary embolism is unlikely to be confused with severe hemorrhage, but there are clinical situations where this possibility must be considered, such as the case of the cancer patient who rapidly develops shock seemingly out of proportion to blood loss.

Sepsis is another factor that should be considered with patients in shock. In many situations, conditions that pose a high index of suspicion, such as tuboovarian abscess or septic abortion, are present. The situation may be less clear, however, for the postoperative patient with unrecognized laceration of the bowel. Either sepsis or hemorrhage can lead to disseminated intravascular coagulation.

Prevention

Identification of the patient at risk for hemorrhage begins with a thorough knowledge of possible causes. A complete medical history is particularly helpful. A family history of conditions such as hemophilia will usually be well known to the patient. A tendency to bleed following a tooth extraction or to bruise easily should alert the practitioner to a potential problem. Patients taking anticoagulants are obviously at high risk for bleeding. However, many other drugs (particularly aspirin and nonsteroidal antiinflammatory drugs) can predispose a patient to excessive bleeding during gynecologic procedures. Physical examination may reveal ecchymoses or petechiae, which may indicate a coagulation problem. When there is a possibility of coagulation abnormality, the patient should undergo assessment of prothrombin time, partial thromboplastin time, platelet count, and bleeding time. In the presence of a particular coagulation disorder or strong clinical suspicion, a consultation with a hematologist should be sought.

Surgical techniques should be directed to the prevention of hemorrhage. During laparoscopy, trocars are introduced away from the large vessels. During hysterectomy, vascular pedicles are carefully ligated individually, traction is avoided, and the vaginal cuff is carefully sutured. In the presence of complex pelvic pathology, hemorrhage can be avoided by combining careful surgical technique with good exposure through a generous abdominal incision, use of a self-retaining retractor, and expert assistance.

Management

Preliminary Evaluation

When confronted with the patient who is hemorrhaging and is developing or has developed shock, evaluation and management must begin simultaneously. The source and rapidity of the bleeding and the extent of loss should be assessed. Based on these factors and the general condition of the patient, the physician can determine the urgency of the situation. The possibility of a cardiogenic component to the shock should be considered.

Initial evaluation begins with the assessment of vital signs. A trend in vital signs and urine output readings is much more meaningful than an individual reading. A pulse oximeter should be applied and if the Spo_2 is $<90\%$, supplemental O_2 should be administered.

Immediate hemoglobin and hematocrit levels do not predict the magnitude of acute blood loss, but baseline and serial determinations are needed. Baseline determinations of serum chemistry levels, coagulation studies, and arterial blood gas should also be obtained. The patient's blood should be typed and crossmatched and, depending on the severity or nature of the situation, platelets and fresh frozen plasma should be available.

Initiating Treatment

The goal of treatment is to restore adequate tissue perfusion in order to save the patient's life as well as to prevent irreparable damage to the vital organs. The essentials of treatment are to stop the bleeding and restore intravascular volume. In order to help establish a well-organized treatment plan for such an emergent and often chaotic situation, a couple of mnemonics have been described, one of which, called "ORDER," will be used here.

- Oxygenate
- Restore circulatory volume
- Drug therapy
- Evaluation
- Remedy the basic problem

Oxygenate

Reversal of a compromised respiratory system requires immediate supplementation to prevent tissue desaturation. Adequate pulmonary CO_2 and O_2 exchange must be assured. For the patient undergoing an operative procedure with general anesthesia, this aspect of care will be managed by the anesthesiologist. Supplemental oxygen by nasal cannula or mask will be satisfactory for most conscious patients. If there is any doubt about the patient's mental or ventilatory status, the anesthesiologist should be consulted about the need for endotracheal intubation.

Restore Circulatory Volume

At least two large-bore intravenous lines should be placed. A central line may be necessary for access or for monitoring, but the risk of pneumothorax with the subclavian approach must be considered. Initial therapy is directed toward restoration of the circulatory volume, which is accomplished effectively with isotonic crystalloid solutions (1). With critical hypotension, the intravascular volume will be more expediently reexpanded with the use of supplemental colloids. It may be necessary to use uncross-matched or type-specific blood in such patients (2, 3). Other immediate temporizing measures that can be useful include elevation of the legs and, in selected circumstances, placement of military antishock trousers.

Drug Therapy

Pharmacologic therapy generally is not needed to treat hemorrhagic shock and should be avoided in most cases. Occasionally, however, drugs may be used as necessary temporary adjuvants when the patient's condition is unstable when or complications are present. Because one of the predictable physiologic responses to severe blood loss is peripheral vasoconstriction, the addition of vasopressor agents might further compromise blood flow to vital organs. The use of these agents may be necessary, however, to temporize an unstable condition while hypovolemia is being corrected. Starting doses of ephedrine (10 mg) or epinephrine (5 μg) can provide a short-acting vasopressor effect with enhanced cardiac output. If more prolonged therapy is required, a titrated drip of dopamine is the best choice (Table 2). The dosage may start at a rate of 5–10 μg/kg/min increasing to 20 μg/kg/min to stimulate first β_1 receptors (to increase cardiac output) then α_1 receptors (to increase vascular tone). The half-life of dopamine is approximately 2 minutes, and the drip may be quickly titrated to achieve the desired effect.

Evaluation

In the initial management of a patient in hemorrhagic shock, many steps should be undertaken simultaneously to improve the situation. Careful attention should be directed to evaluation of the patient's condition before using invasive monitoring techniques. The vital signs are continually monitored to determine whether the patient's condition has improved and stabilized. In the conscious patient, the general appearance and neurologic status are important to assess. Urine output is a sensitive indicator of adequate tissue perfusion. An output of 30–60 mL/h

Table 2. Dose-Dependent Effects of Dopamine

Dose (μg/kg/min)	Effect
0.5–3	Primarily dopaminergic receptors resulting in: Increased RBF Increased splanchnic blood flow Marginal effect on CO, SVR
5–10	Mediated by dopaminergic and β_1 receptors, resulting in: Increased RBF Increased CO Possibly decreased SVR secondary to increased CO
10–20	Primarily an α_1 receptor effect with some β_1 stimulation. The α_1 receptor effects overcome the dopaminergic effects, resulting primarily in: Increased SVR Increased heart rate Increased inotropic response CO can be decreased secondary to increased SVR
>20	Substantial risk of dysrhythmias

Abbreviations: RBF, renal blood flow; CO, cardiac output; SVR, systemic vascular resistance

(0.5–1 mL/kg/h) indicates adequate volume replacement. If urine output is inadequate (<30 mL/h) despite presumed adequate volume replacement, or if shock is profound, the physician needs a better guide to prevent pulmonary edema. Patients without heart or lung disease may be assessed by serial measurements of central venous pressure (CVP). Normal mean CVP is 5 mm Hg, while the patient in hemorrhagic shock will have a very low CVP (<0 mm Hg). Once the venous system is refilled to normal capacity, additional fluid administration may not be handled readily and may substantially increase the CVP. While vigorous fluid therapy is being administered, the patient should be observed for signs of early pulmonary congestion, such as coughing, rales, or respiratory difficulty. If the CVP increases to the range of 15–20 mm Hg, either the intravascular space has been overloaded, introducing the danger of pulmonary edema, or the heart is failing.

Myocardial dysfunction may limit the usefulness of CVP measurements. In this situation, a pulmonary artery catheter is necessary to assess left ventricular function. A measure is needed of how well the left heart is pumping out the blood it is receiving from the pulmonary veins. A pressure-sensitive catheter is inserted through a central vein and the right heart into the pulmonary artery. Insertion through the central vein carries the same risk as insertion of other central lines. While the catheter passes through the heart, arrhythmias may occur, and there is a risk of rupture with insertion into the pulmonary artery (4). The inflated balloon tip of the catheter "floats" into the terminal arterial vasculature where it "wedges," allowing serial measurements. The pulmonary artery wedge pressure and cardiac output results (by thermodilution techniques) can be used to estimate left ventricular performance. Table 3 lists normal values for pulmonary artery catheterization.

In gynecologic patients with hemorrhagic shock, use of a pulmonary artery catheter usually is not necessary. When compared with a central venous line, it is more invasive and expensive and has more frequent and serious complications. In selected patients, however, serial measurements can guide fluid and drug administration. Expe-

Table 3. Normal Values for Pulmonary Artery Catheterization

Pressure	Typical (mm Hg)	Range (mm Hg)	Conditions Associated with Elevated Pressure	Conditions Associated with Decreased Pressure
Central venous or right atrium	5	0–8	Fluid overload Right ventricular failure Pulmonary embolus Severe tricuspid regurgitation Cardiac tamponade	Inadequate vascular volume Shock Anaphylaxis Sepsis
Right ventricle	20/0	15–30/0–10	Fluid overload Pulmonary embolus Left ventricular failure Pulmonic stenosis Pulmonary hypertension	Inadequate vascular volume Shock Anaphylaxis Sepsis
Pulmonary artery	12/7	10–30/5–15	Fluid overload Pulmonary embolus Left ventricular failure Pulmonary hypertension Mitral stenosis Severe mitral regurgitation	Inadequate vascular volume Shock Anaphylaxis Sepsis Right ventricular failure (without left ventricular failure)
Pulmonary artery occlusion	10	8–12	Fluid overload Mitral regurgitation Mitral stenosis Left ventricular failure Cardiac tamponade Pulmonary embolus	Inadequate vascular volume Shock Anaphylaxis Sepsis Right ventricular failure

rienced medical personnel should be consulted for placement and management of the catheter.

Further therapy is guided by the results of the initial laboratory tests as they become available. Oxygenation is monitored continually and adequate ventilation must be ensured. An arterial pressure catheter will allow continuous observation of the mean arterial pressure, blood gas analysis, and assessment of other blood values. Metabolic acidosis is corrected by adequate fluid resuscitation, but cautious administration of sodium bicarbonate is indicated when acidosis is severe. Assuming fluid replacement is adequate in the face of ongoing serious hemorrhage, effort should be made to keep the hemoglobin level sufficient to provide adequate tissue oxygenation (usually 6–10 g/dL depending upon the age and cardiac status of the patient). Tissue oxygenation can be assessed by following mixed venous oxygen saturation, arterial pH and bicarbonate levels, or blood lactate levels. Documented coagulopathy is corrected by appropriate blood component therapy (5). Clinically evident coagulopathy that interferes with hemostasis may need empiric treatment with fresh frozen plasma or platelets or both until further studies or laboratory results are available. The possibility of developing a coagulation defect must be considered when large volumes of blood are transfused.

If the patient remains in shock despite what would seem to be adequate resuscitative efforts, several possibilities should be considered. First, advanced irreversible shock is uncommon in the gynecologic patient and generally should not be considered as a reason for withholding vigorous therapy. Cardiac dysfunction because of intrinsic disease or myocardial hypoxia (and possible infarction) may be exacerbated secondary to the shock. A large pneumothorax following central venous line placement (usually from the subclavian approach rather than the jugular approach) can interfere significantly with resuscitative efforts and could lead to further deterioration of the patient's condition. In the gynecologic population, the likely cause of ongoing shock is continued extensive blood loss. If this is the case, the only remedy is to halt the bleeding. The type of intervention required to control the hemorrhage will depend on the primary cause.

Remedy the Basic Problem

Control of extensive bleeding in the gynecologic patient is usually a matter of obtaining operative hemostasis. This may require ligation or electrocoagulation of individual vessels or pressure combined with topical agents. When hemorrhage is massive, pressure on the aorta can control bleeding temporarily, allowing visualization of the bleeding site. In selected cases, ligation of the internal iliac arteries might be beneficial, usually in addition to other efforts. When massive bleeding continues despite these efforts, tight packing of the pelvis can be lifesaving. The pack may be brought out through the vagina within a plastic bag as an "umbrella pack," or brought out through a small opening in the abdominal wound along with a pressure-maintaining clamp tied to the fascia. There are several useful adjunctive agents such as "fibrin glue" (equal volumes of cryoprecipitate and bovine thrombin [1000 U/mL] in separate plastic syringes, sprayed into the field simultaneously) placed in the bleeding area just prior to packing. In selected cases of gynecologic hemorrhage, embolization is an alternative and may be preferable to surgery.

Massive Transfusion

Serious hemorrhage and shock may require transfusion of large quantities of blood. When one or more blood volumes has been given within a 24-hour period, the transfusion is considered to be "massive." Following rapid transfusion of more than half of a blood volume (10 U of packed cells or 35 mL/kg), crossmatching is no longer accurate. To prevent a graft versus host reaction, transfusion should be continued with the same blood type previously transfused until a stable crossmatch can be performed. Transfusion of such large volumes of blood is associated with some specific and significant problems (6). In general, the larger the volume of blood infused, the greater the risk of complications.

An experienced pelvic surgeon and an anesthesiologist should be part of the health care team of a seriously hemorrhaging patient who is receiving a massive transfusion. Close communication between this team and the blood bank must be maintained.

A number of electrolyte imbalances may develop during massive transfusion. During storage, potassium is released from the erythrocytes. Even large-volume transfusions actually result more often in hypokalemia, however, probably due to red cell redistribution, alkalosis, and the effects of a number of substances released in the physiologic response to shock (7). The large amount of citrate (preservative) infused with stored blood binds a significant amount of ionized calcium. Although the routine prophylactic administration of calcium is not recommended, calcium levels (as well as those of potassium and other electrolytes) should be checked frequently along with continuous cardiac monitoring.

Acid-base disturbances often occur during massive transfusion. Although stored blood does have a slightly lower pH, the presence of acidosis is more likely related to persistent shock. Transfusion of large volumes of blood is more likely to correct the acidotic state and typically results in alkalosis because of the metabolism of citrate to bicarbonate.

Erythrocytes are stored at a constant temperature of 4°C. When it is necessary to infuse large volumes of blood rapidly without warming, hypothermia may result. This effect is magnified by additional factors, including infusion of other unwarmed fluids, a relatively cold operating room, and loss of heat from the open peritoneal cavity. Hypothermia can lead to adverse effects that compound problems already resulting from massive blood loss, blood replacement, and shock. These effects include cardiac dysrhythmias, impaired citrate and lactate (anaerobic) metabolism, a shift to the left in the oxygen-hemoglobin dissociation curve (which decreases oxygen release), increased intracellular potassium release, delayed drug metabolism, increased blood viscosity, impaired erythrocyte deformability, and impaired coagulation (8, 9).

With massive transfusion, the patient's normal blood has been replaced with fluid and blood lacking platelets and coagulation factors. The platelet count drops during and after massive transfusion (a qualitative platelet deficit may also be present), and coagulation often becomes impaired (10, 11). However, there is no definite correlation with the volume transfused and abnormal coagulation studies. Studies have failed to demonstrate the benefit of routine prophylactic administration of platelets or fresh frozen plasma (12, 13). The cause of coagulopathy under these circumstances is unclear and is probably variable and multifactorial. Factors that have been implicated include the dilutional effect, consumptive coagulopathy, prolonged hypotension, the volume of crystalloid infused, and hypothermia (7, 13).

Coagulation studies (including platelet count, prothrombin time, partial thromboplastin time, fibrinogen level, and, perhaps, D-dimer assessments) should be performed after every 5–10 U of blood transfused. The care team should continually observe the patient for evidence of microvascular bleeding, including persistent oozing from suture sites and raw areas in the operative field, hematuria, and oozing from intravenous sites or from mucous membranes. In general, neither platelets nor coagulation factors should be administered without laboratory evidence of a specific deficiency. An exception is when there is evidence of microvascular bleeding or the situation is so extreme that there is ongoing hemorrhage and massive transfusion has taken place within the span of a few hours.

Ongoing hemorrhage in conjunction with an elevated prothrombin time or partial thromboplastin time should be treated with 10–15 mL/kg (or 2 U) of fresh frozen plasma repeated as needed, depending on the clinical course. Give platelets (6–8 platelet packs or 1 U/10 kg) if the platelet count is less than 20–50,000/mm^3 in the presence of continued hemorrhage. Platelet transfusions also provide factors V and VIII (one pooled pack gives the equivalent of about 1 U of fresh frozen plasma). Usually, administration of platelets and fresh frozen plasma will correct the coagulation abnormalities seen with massive transfusions. Cryoprecipitate is useful when there is evidence of consumptive coagulopathy with depleted fibrinogen and elevated D-dimer readings.

Other types of transfusion-related complications are described elsewhere (14). These problems include infection, alloimmunization, and transfusion reactions.

Complications of Shock

Following acute stabilization of the patient's condition, a number of problems or complications can persist or develop. Correction of electrolyte imbalances, acid-base disturbances, and coagulation abnormalities might take several days. Delayed transfusion reactions occasionally occur. Because the patient is at risk for stress-induced gastric ulceration, prophylaxis in the form of H_2 blockers should be given. The most serious complications developing subsequent to shock are related to ischemic organ injury (15).

Myocardial infarction is unlikely in an otherwise healthy person. Acute renal tubular necrosis is common and generally self-limited, requiring only careful fluid and electrolyte management. Occasionally, the patient incurs more severe kidney damage, necessitating temporary dialysis. The most common serious complication developing subsequently to shock is adult respiratory distress syndrome. Although research continues, much is unknown about this all-too-common entity, and the mortality rate remains high. Expert ventilatory and general intensive care is required for recovery.

Summary

Inevitably, the obstetrician–gynecologist will encounter severe hemorrhage and hemorrhagic shock. Although severe bleeding sometimes develops unexpectedly, quite often the physician can recognize a potentially high-risk situation and prevent or minimize hemorrhage.

Once faced with severe hemorrhage or shock, the physician must rapidly institute a plan of management such as that identified by the mnemonic "ORDER." The plan is based on an understanding of the pathophysiology of hemorrhagic shock and a thorough knowledge of the principles of fluid and blood replacement. A team approach is important.

Frequently, the obstetrician–gynecologist is confronted with massive ongoing hemorrhage and also must have an understanding of the problems associated with massive transfusion. Following stabilization of the patient's acute condition, the physician should be alert to the problems that can persist or develop.

References

1. Velanovich V. Crystalloid versus colloid fluid resuscitation: a meta-analysis of mortality. Surgery 1989;105: 65–71, 1989 (Meta-analysis)

2. Schwab CW, Shayne JP, Turner J. Immediate trauma resuscitation with type O uncrossmatched blood: a two-year prospective experience. J Trauma 1986;26:897–902 (Level III)

3. Lefebre J, McLellan BA, Coovadia AS. Seven years experience with group O unmatched packed red blood cells in a regional trauma unit. Ann Emerg Med 1987;16:1344–1349 (Level III)

4. American College of Obstetricians and Gynecologists. Invasive hemodynamic monitoring in obstetrics and gynecology. ACOG Technical Bulletin 175. Washington, DC: ACOG, 1992 (Level III)

5. Development Task Force of the College of American Pathologists. Practice parameter for the use of fresh-frozen plasma, cryoprecipitate, and platelets: fresh-frozen plasma, cryoprecipitate, and platelets administration practice guidelines. JAMA 1994;271:777–781 (Level III)

6. Nolan TE, Gallup DG. Massive transfusion: a current review. Obstet Gynecol Surv 1991;46:289–295 (Level III)

7. Carmichael D, Hosty T, Kastl D, Beckman D. Hypokalemia and massive transfusion. South Med J 1984;77:315–317 (Level III)

8. Valeri CR, Cassidy G, Khuri S, Feingold H, Ragno G, Altschule MD. Hypothermia-induced reversible platelet dysfunction. Ann Surg 1987;205:175–181 (Animal Study)

9. Luna GK, Maier RV, Pavlin EG, Anardi D, Copass MK, Oreskovich MR. Incidence and effect of hypothermia in seriously injured patients. J Trauma 1987;27:1014–1018 (Level III)

10. Counts RB, Haisch C, Simon TL, Maxwell NG, Heimbach DM, Carrico CJ. Hemostasis in massively transfused trauma patients. Ann Surg 1979;190:91–99 (Level II-3)

11. Reed RL, Heimbach DM, Counts RB, Ciavarella D, Baron L, Carrico CJ, et al. Prophylactic platelet administration during massive transfusion: a prospective, randomized, double-blind clinical study. Ann Surg 1986;203:40–48 (Level II-3)

12. Harrigan C, Lucas CE, Ledgerwood AM, Walz DA, Mammen EF. Serial changes in primary hemostasis after massive transfusion. Surgery 1985;98:836–844 (Level II-2)

13. Martin DJ, Lucas CE, Ledgerwood AM, Hoschner J, McGonigal MD, Grabow D. Fresh frozen plasma supplement to massive red blood cell transfusion. Ann Surg 1985; 202:505–511 (Animal Study)

14. American College of Obstetricians and Gynecologists. Blood component therapy. ACOG Technical Bulletin 199. Washington, DC: ACOG, 1994 (Level III)

15. Phillips TF, Soulier G, Wilson RF. Outcome of massive transfusion exceeding two blood volumes in trauma and emergency surgery. J Trauma 1987;27:903–910 (Level III)

The references in this bulletin are graded according to the method outlined by the U.S. Preventive Services Task Force:

- I Evidence obtained from at least one properly designed randomized controlled trial
- II-1 Evidence obtained from well-designed controlled trials without randomization
- II-2 Evidence obtained from well-designed cohort or case–control analytic studies, preferably from more than one center or research group
- II-3 Evidence obtained from multiple time series, with or without intervention, or dramatic results in uncontrolled experiments
- III Opinions of respected authorities, based on clinical experience, descriptive studies, or reports of expert committees

Other publications from ACOG:

- **Committee Opinions**, focused updates on emerging areas
- **Practice Patterns**, evidence-based guidelines
- **Criteria Sets**, baseline guidelines for review of diagnostic and management procedures

ISSN 1074-8628

The American College of Obstetricians and Gynecologists
409 12th Street, SW
PO Box 96920
Washington, DC 20090-6920

12345/10987

Number 198—October 1994
(Replaces #106, July 1987)

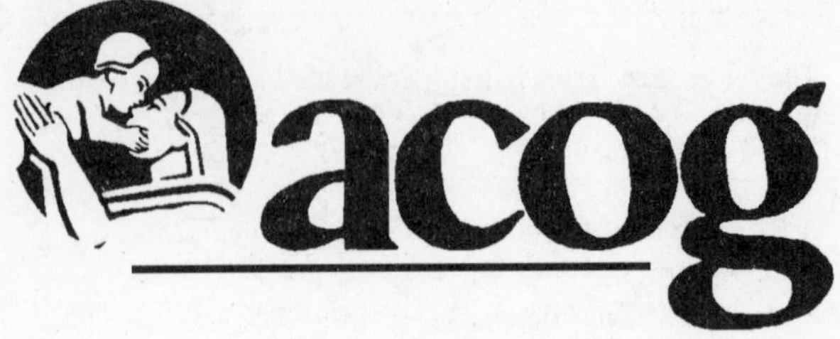

Technical Bulletin
An Educational Aid to Obstetrician–Gynecologists

Hormonal Contraception

Oral, injectable, and implantable hormonal contraceptives offer women safe, effective, and reversible fertility regulation. In some cases, their use also confers important noncontraceptive health benefits. This Technical Bulletin describes oral, injectable, and implantable contraceptives available in the United States, focusing on selection of the appropriate method, management, and counseling measures that maximize contraceptive efficacy and patient satisfaction.

Oral Contraceptives

Composition and Formulation

The dose of sex steroids in combination oral contraceptives (OCs) has declined dramatically since they first became available in the 1960s. This decline has resulted in the same contraceptive efficacy as that achieved with high-dose formulations but with fewer adverse metabolic effects. Oral contraceptives are considered high dose if they contain more than 50 μg of estrogen, moderate dose if they contain 50 μg, and low dose if they contain less than 50 μg. Today, the highest-dose formulations commercially available in the United States contain 50 μg.

Prior to 1992, OCs in the United States contained one of two estrogens (ethinyl estradiol or mestranol) and one of five progestins (norethindrone, levonorgestrel, norgestrel, norethindrone acetate, or ethynodiol diacetate). Since 1992, all preparations containing 35 μg of estrogen or less use ethinyl estradiol. Two new, less androgenic progestins—norgestimate and desogestrel—have been introduced recently (1). Another new progestin, gestodene, may become available soon.

Many different low-dose formulations exist. Although there are differences in the laboratory changes associated with various formulations, there is no convincing evidence that these differences adversely affect health outcome. Therefore, the choice of any particular formulation can be guided by such factors as physician or patient familiarity and cost.

Monophasic OCs have a constant dose of estrogen and progestin in each of the 21 tablets of active hormones in each cycle pack. Phasic OCs alter the dose of the progestin and (in some formulations) the estrogen component among the 21 active tablets in each pack. In formulating phasic OCs, manufacturers have lowered the total monthly steroid dose with the aim of reducing metabolic effects while maintaining contraceptive efficacy and cycle control.

Progestin-only oral contraceptives (mini-pills) are formulated with doses of progestins even lower than those in low-dose OCs (2). In contrast to OCs, each cycle of progestin-only pills consists of 28 tablets of active hormone. Progestin-only pills can be used by some women for whom estrogen is contraindicated.

Mechanism of Action, Efficacy, Administration, and Effect on Pregnancy

Combination OCs prevent ovulation by suppressing pituitary gonadotropin secretion (3). The progestin component of OCs causes changes in the cervical mucus and the endometrium that enhance the antifertility effect of OCs should ovulation occur. Because failure rates associated with combination OC use relate to individual compliance, they range from less than 1/100 woman-years in women who are highly compliant to greater than 15/100 woman-years in inner-city teens. Although some authorities estimate typical combination OC failure rates to be 3/100 woman-years (4), other methodologic approaches yield estimates as high as 8/100 woman-years (5). While many clinicians assume that progestin-only pills are less effective than combination OCs, existing data document progestin-only pill failure rates (1–7/100 woman-years) similar to those seen with combination pills (2, 4). Because progestin-only pills are often prescribed preferentially to lactating women and older women with cardiovascular risk factors—two groups of relatively less fertile women—higher failure rates might result if progestin-only pills were prescribed routinely to young women.

Oral contraceptives should be initiated on either the first day of menses or the first Sunday after menses begins. Oral contraceptives packaged with 28 pills, in which the last seven tablets are inactive, facilitate consistent daily pill-taking. Likewise, compliance may be enhanced by advising patients to associate pill-taking with a daily ritual (eg, toothbrushing). Compliance is critical to ensure efficacy. If a woman misses one or two combination OC tablets, she should take one tablet as soon as possible. She should then continue to take one tablet twice daily until each of the missed tablets has been taken. Women who have missed more than two consecutive tablets should be advised to use an additional form of contraception (eg, condoms and spermicide) while they complete taking the current pack of pills. Because of the increased risk of accidental pregnancy, women who persistently miss three or more combination OC tablets each cycle should be advised to consider other contraceptive choices that do not require daily compliance. Because progestin-only pills may be less effective than combination OCs, women should use back-up contraception for 48 hours if they are 3 hours or more late in taking a pill (6).

Reports have confirmed that OC use during early pregnancy does not increase the risk of fetal malformations (7). Upon discontinuation of the pill, fertility should be expected to return within 3 months in most patients.

Health Benefits

Although often overlooked, the health benefits associated with reliable contraception are substantial (8). Use of OCs is also associated with a variety of noncontraceptive health benefits, including quality-of-life benefits and protection from certain gynecologic malignancies (see the box).

Women taking OCs note that menses become regular and more predictable, the prevalence as well as severity of dysmenorrhea is reduced (9), and the number of days and amount of flow decline (10). In addition, iron stores increase in women with iron deficiency associated with menorrhagia (10). Use of OCs can restore regular menses in women with abnormal bleeding caused by chronic anovulation.

Women using OCs also enjoy relative protection from several benign but common conditions that cause morbidity. Benign breast disease, including fibroadenoma and cystic changes, occurs less frequently during OC use (11). Although older literature suggested that OC use prevented and suppressed functional ovarian cysts, it is not clear whether today's low-dose formulations have this effect (12, 13). The literature on rheumatoid arthritis is conflicting; however, a recent metaanalysis suggested that OC use modifies the natural history of rheumatoid arthritis, reducing the prevalence of severe disabling disease (14).

The incidences of pelvic inflammatory disease and ectopic pregnancy, two common and potentially life-threatening conditions, are reduced by use of OCs. In one study, the risk of being hospitalized for pelvic inflammatory disease was reduced by one half in OC users (15). Potential biologic explanations for this protection include the effects of OCs on cervical mucus and reduced menstrual blood and less retrograde menstruation associated with OCs. Because OCs prevent ovulation, ectopic pregnancies are rare, occurring 500-fold less often in OC users than in women using no contraceptive method (16).

Noncontraceptive Benefits of Oral Contraceptives

Menstrual Improvements
- More regular and predictable menses
- Reduced prevalence and severity of dysmenorrhea
- Reduction in days and amount of menstrual flow
- Increased iron stores in women with menorrhagia
- Restoration of regular menses in anovulatory women

Prevention of Benign Conditions
- Benign breast disease (fibroadenoma and cystic changes)
- Pelvic inflammatory disease
- Ectopic pregnancy

Prevention of Gynecologic Malignancies
- Epithelial ovarian cancer
- Endometrial adenocarcinoma

Possible Benefits
- Prevention of functional ovarian cysts
- Prevention of rheumatoid arthritis
- Increased bone mineral density

Prevention of epithelial ovarian and endometrial cancer is an important noncontraceptive benefit of use of combination OCs. In the United States, the most common cause of death from gynecologic malignancy is ovarian cancer. Worldwide, studies have consistently found that OC use is associated with an approximately 40% reduced risk of malignant as well as borderline epithelial ovarian cancer (17). The protection appears to last for at least 15 years following discontinuation of use and increases with duration of use, so that women who have used OCs for a decade or more experience an 80% risk reduction (18). In England and Wales, OC use has been estimated to have prevented nearly one quarter of deaths from ovarian cancer that would have otherwise occurred (19). The strong effect of OC use in preventing ovarian cancer is well established. The role of low-dose OCs is unclear; however, available data suggest that this protection against ovarian cancer may also be conveyed by use of low-dose OCs (18). Overall, women who use OCs can be confident that use will decrease the risk of ovarian cancer. This protective effect, however, has not been studied in women with genetic ovarian cancer syndromes (familial ovarian syndrome, Lynch II, ovary–breast syndrome). In contrast, life-table analyses suggest that a woman with only one relative with ovarian cancer may use OCs to reduce her risk of ovarian cancer (20).

Use of OCs is associated with a 50% reduced risk of endometrial adenocarcinoma (21), the most common gynecologic cancer in the United States. Protection occurs for each of the three principal histologic types of endometrial carcinoma and appears to persist for at least 15 years following discontinuation of OC use (22).

Whether estrogens and progestins have a positive impact on bone mineral density remains controversial. Three recent reports suggest that bone mineral density may be higher in long-term OC users (23–25), but other reports found no such increase.

Side Effects

Side effects of OCs are a major source of patient noncompliance and discontinuation. Clinicians can enhance their patients' contraceptive success by fully discussing side effects with them before OC initiation and managing these effects as they occur. Nausea and breast tenderness, caused by the estrogen component, commonly occur in OC users. Fortunately, the frequency and severity of these symptoms usually decline over the first several months of OC use. Although weight gain in some users may represent an anabolic response to the progestin component of OCs, it is not clear that, overall, OCs directly cause weight gain (26, 27). Because even low-dose OCs can cause an increase in blood pressure in some women, it is appropriate to monitor blood pressure annually in patients taking OCs.

Menstrual changes during OC use cause patient anxiety and are a common reason for discontinuation. Intermenstrual, or breakthrough, spotting and bleeding occur in approximately one quarter of women during the first 3 months of OC use but become much less common with ongoing use. Counseling patients to anticipate such early breakthrough bleeding and reassuring those who experience this side effect can maximize patients' desire to continue OC use. When intermenstrual bleeding occurs after 3 months of use, the patient should be examined for possible causes of bleeding unrelated to OC use, including cervical or endometrial infection and neoplasia. A short course of oral estrogen can be used to manage persistent or late-onset intermenstrual bleeding due to OCs (6).

Amenorrhea may occur with OC use, particularly in long-term users. Although such amenorrhea is not medically harmful, it may cause patient anxiety regarding pregnancy. Often pregnancy testing and reassurance will relieve patient anxiety. If patients continue to be disturbed by amenorrhea, oral estrogen taken with each of the 21 active OC tablets often will restore withdrawal bleeding (6). Alternatively, another low-dose combination OC can be prescribed.

Headaches are occasionally reported by women using combination OCs and require appropriate evaluation and management. Tension headaches are not related to OC use and can be treated with over-the-counter analgesics. Few published data regarding migraine headaches and the use of low-dose OCs are available. Clinical experience indicates that some women have improvement of migraine headaches with use of low-dose combination OCs, some have worsening, and some experience no effect. Some authorities suggest that only classic migraines, which are characterized by focal visual or other neurologic signs, require special attention. Women who experience classic migraines may be best served by using another form of contraception. Women who experience increased frequency or intensity of any type of migraine headaches should discontinue combination OC use. They may be candidates for use of progestin-only contraceptives. Some women using OCs experience migraine headaches only during menses. Elimination of the pill-free interval may be therapeutic in women with such menstrual migraines (28).

Health Risks

Extensive epidemiologic studies have evaluated the associations between OC use and the risk of cardiovascular disease and cancer. These studies indicate that OCs are a safe contraceptive choice for most women.

Cardiovascular Disease

During the 1960s and 1970s, studies suggested that women using high-dose OCs were at increased risk for thromboembolism, myocardial infarction, and stroke. The relevance of these observations to current clinical practice has been questioned for three reasons (29). First, current OC formulations have a three- to fourfold lower dose of estrogen and a 10-fold lower dose of progestin than older formulations. Second, early studies failed to take into account the effects of independent risk factors for vascular disease, including smoking and hypertension. Finally, physicians are now less likely to prescribe OCs to women at high risk for vascular disease, including older women who smoke.

Past use of OCs does not increase the risk of cardiovascular disease (30). Further, limited evidence suggests that OC use may even reduce the risk of atherosclerosis. An angiography-based German study of young women suffering myocardial infarctions observed that coronary atherosclerosis was less common in OC users than nonusers (31). Autopsy studies of female monkeys fed an atherogenic diet found less atherosclerosis in animals fed OCs than in those that were not fed OCs (32). These studies lead to two important insights regarding coronary artery disease and OC use. First, OC use does not cause coronary atherosclerosis, the leading cause of death of U.S. women. Second, in those rare cases in which myocardial infarctions occur in current OC users, they have a thrombotic rather than an atherosclerotic etiology.

Recent studies have clarified the dangers of smoking for OC users. In a large prospective British study, nonsmoking current OC users, regardless of age, were not at increased risk for myocardial infarction. Among current OC users who smoked, those who smoked fewer than 15 cigarettes daily experienced a more than threefold increased risk of infarction, while those who smoked more than 15 cigarettes daily were noted to have a dramatic 21-fold increased risk (33). While confirming that cigarette smoking is an important cause of myocardial infarction in women, this study also provides reassurance regarding OC use. Women over 35 years of age who smoke generally should not be prescribed combination OCs.

The increased risk of thromboembolism noted in women using OCs appears to be related to the estrogenic component. Use of low-estrogen OCs is associated with less risk of thromboembolism than is use of OCs with higher levels of estrogen (34). Whether the risk of thromboembolism is higher in women using low-dose OCs than in nonusers is not known. If women using low-dose OCs are at any increased risk, however, such risk is of low magnitude (35, 36). There is no documented evidence to support or reject the notion that combination OCs increase the risk of postoperative thrombosis in women without other risk factors. The risk of pregnancy must be weighed against any theoretical risk in women using low-dose preparations in deciding whether to discontinue OCs prior to surgery.

Cancer

Many women are concerned about the potential impact of OC use on breast cancer risk. Several studies have identified an increased risk of breast cancer associated with recent or current OC use. Detection bias, chance, or a late-stage promotion effect may explain these findings (37). Among studies conducted in women ages 20–54, nearly all studies of breast cancer and OC use have reached the conclusion that the overall risk of breast cancer is no different for women who have used OCs than for women who have not used them (37). The largest study assessed breast cancer risk in subgroups of OC users, including those with long duration of use, those with a history of benign breast disease, and those with a positive family history of breast cancer. Oral contraceptive use was not associated with an increased risk of breast cancer in any of these subgroups (38). These observations should reassure clinicians and patients regarding OC use in women with these characteristics.

The association of OC use and breast cancer in young women is an ongoing controversy. A reanalysis of one large study revealed the possibility that OC users experience an increased risk of breast cancer diagnosed at a young age and a reduced risk of breast cancer diagnosed later in life; this reduction in risk increases with increasing duration since last OC use (39). The age-specific risk of breast cancer is similar to the effect of parity on breast cancer risk (40). If this differential impact of OC use on breast cancer risk by age at diagnosis is real, its net effect would be to lower the overall incidence of breast cancer, because breast cancer is much more common in older women than in younger women.

The relationship between OC use and cervical cancer risk remains controversial (21). Conflicting findings of epidemiologic studies may be attributed to several potential biases, for which these studies have not been consistently controlled (41). If OC use is associated with any increased risk of cervical neoplasia, it is of small magnitude. A prudent approach is to perform annual cervical cytologic screening in OC users. A history of cervical intraepithelial neoplasia does not contraindicate the use of hormonal contraception.

In the 1980s, several British and U.S. reports raised concerns that OC use might increase the risk of liver cancer, a tumor that rarely occurs in developed countries. A large World Health Organization study of this association in developing countries, where liver cancer is more common, failed to confirm these concerns (42). Furthermore, in developed countries, no increase in mortality from liver cancer occurring in women has been noted since the introduction of OCs in the 1960s (29). Although benign hepatocellular adenomas can be produced by the estrogen component of OCs, these have become extremely rare since the advent of low-dose OCs (6).

Injectable Contraception

Several injectable preparations are used for contraception worldwide. The only formulation available in the United States, however, is depot medroxyprogesterone acetate (DMPA). Although DMPA has been marketed in the United States for several decades, concerns related to the occurrence of cancer in laboratory animals that received DMPA delayed its approval by the Food and Drug Administration for contraceptive use until October 1992 (43, 44).

Depot medroxyprogesterone acetate is injected as an aqueous suspension of microcrystals. The low solubility of the microcrystals at the injection site results in pharmacologically active levels persisting for 3–4 months following a 150-mg injection. Depot medroxy-progesterone acetate is marketed in the United States as a 150-mg/ml contraceptive solution and a 400-mg/ml solution for treating neoplasia. Because injection of the 400-mg/ml solution is associated with lower drug bioavailability and local pain, the high-strength DMPA solution should not be used for contraception.

Mechanism of Action, Efficacy, Administration, and Return to Fertility

As with OCs, DMPA acts primarily by inhibiting ovulation. When 150 mg of DMPA is injected every 3 months, its contraceptive efficacy is extremely high. Clinical trials have reported failure rates ranging from 0.0 to 0.7/100 woman-years. A typical failure rate associated with use of DMPA is 0.3/100 woman-years, comparable to the contraceptive efficacy of implants or surgical sterilization (4). The contraceptive efficacy of DMPA has not been reported to vary with patient weight or use of concurrent medications, apparently because of high circulating levels present.

The ideal time to initiate DMPA is within 5 days of the onset of menses. This approach ensures that the patient is not pregnant and prevents ovulation during the first month of use. After a 150-mg injection of DMPA, ovulation does not occur for at least 14 weeks. Therefore, a 2-week grace period exists for women receiving DMPA injections every 3 months. For women more than 2 weeks late for their DMPA injection, pregnancy should be excluded before administering DMPA. Use of DMPA in contraceptive doses does not increase the risk of congenital anomalies (7).

Although use of DMPA does not permanently suppress fertility, return of fertility may be delayed following discontinuation. The time between discontinuation and return to fertility is not related to the duration of DMPA use (45). Within 10 months of the last injection, 50% of women who discontinued use of DMPA to become pregnant will have conceived; in a small proportion of women, however, fertility is not reestablished until 18 months after the last injection (45). Before initiating DMPA contraception, candidates should be counseled about the possible prolonged duration of action. Women who may want to become pregnant within the next 1 or 2 years should choose an alternative contraceptive.

Side Effects

Menstrual changes occur in almost all women using DMPA. Episodes of unpredictable irregular bleeding and spotting lasting 7 days or more are common during the first months of use. With increasing duration of use, the frequency and duration of these episodes decrease, and amenorrhea becomes common. Approximately one half of women using DMPA for 1 year report amenorrhea (46). With further use, amenorrhea occurs in three quarters of DMPA users.

Menstrual changes are the most frequent cause for dissatisfaction with and discontinuation of DMPA. Appropriate patient education before initiation, as well as supportive follow-up measures, can markedly reduce patient discontent. Women clearly uncomfortable with the menstrual changes that inevitably accompany use of DMPA should be counseled to choose an alternative contraceptive. In many cases, patient anxiety over menstrual changes relates more to concerns that pregnancy or gynecologic disease may be present. Hence, well-informed and supportive clinicians who provide easy access to follow-up counseling and evaluation can do much to promote patient satisfaction and contraceptive continuation. Indeed, many women using DMPA view amenorrhea as a favorable aspect of their contraceptive choice.

As with OCs, persistent irregular bleeding can be treated with estrogen supplementation. Bleeding, however, frequently recurs after discontinuing estrogen. Endometrial sampling, hysteroscopy, and dilation and curettage have little role, if any, in managing menstrual changes in women using DMPA. Women persistently dissatisfied with the menstrual changes caused by DMPA may be better served by choosing an alternative method.

A variety of other side effects are reported by women using DMPA, including headaches, bloating of the abdomen or breasts, and mood changes. Few controlled studies conducted in developed countries have evaluated weight changes associated with use of DMPA. One Swedish study sponsored by the manufacturer noted that, overall, a cohort of DMPA users, most of whom had used injectable contraception for at least several years, experienced 1.3 kg (2.9 lb) more weight gain than a comparison group of women (47).

Benefits and Risks

Use of DMPA is associated with several noncontraceptive benefits. The tendency of DMPA to cause amenorrhea can make it a particularly appropriate contraceptive choice for women with menorrhagia, dysmenorrhea, iron deficiency anemia, or menstrual hygiene problems that are associated with severe mental retardation. Use of DMPA may, like use of OCs, reduce the risk of pelvic inflammatory disease (43). The use of DMPA has also been associated with hematologic improvement in women with sickle cell disease (48) and reduced seizure frequency in women with seizure disorders (49). Finally, some women choose DMPA because of the privacy associated with its use—no persons other than health care providers need know that DMPA is being used.

The World Health Organization examined the risks of breast, endometrial, ovarian, and cervical carcinoma associated with use of DMPA (43, 50). Results from these large case–control studies reveal that DMPA does not increase the risk of these tumors. The effect of DMPA on the risk of breast cancer appears to be similar to that for combination OC users. Use of DMPA was found to be associated with even greater prevention of endometrial cancer than is found with OC use.

A cross-sectional (nonprospective) study by New Zealand investigators reported that bone density in long-term DMPA users was lower than that in nonusers (51). No clinical evidence of osteoporosis, such as fractures, was noted. This bone density reduction reversed following DMPA discontinuation and may reflect relative lowering of ovarian estrogen production by DMPA. The Food and Drug Administration has asked the manufacturer to conduct a prospective study of bone density in DMPA users.

Contraceptive Implants

Composition and Formulation

As currently formulated, levonorgestrel implants (Norplant) consist of six 34 × 2.4-mm soft plastic implants, each filled with 36 mg of crystalline levonorgestrel. The initial overall daily rate of release by the six implants is 85 μg, gradually declining to approximately 30 μg by the fifth year of use (52). Plasma levonorgestrel levels in women using implants are considerably lower than those associated with use of levonorgestrel combination OCs. A new delivery system that uses fewer implants is in development.

Mechanism of Action, Efficacy, Administration, and Return to Fertility

Circulating progestin levels are sufficient to prevent ovulation in most women using implants. Cyclic luteal activity, however, manifested by progesterone levels lower than those associated with normal ovulation, occurs in about one third of users in the first year (53), becoming more common in later years. This luteal activity is associated with menstrual flow often perceived by users as normal menstrual cycles. Luteal insufficiency and impaired oocyte maturation appear to prevent fertilization in implant users in whom ovulatory activity occurs. Progestin-induced hostile cervical mucus also contributes to the high efficacy of implants (54).

Annual pregnancy rates among implant users average 0.8/100 users during 5 years of use. Pregnancy rates, however, gradually increase over time. Because these failure rates rise above 2/100 users in the sixth year of use, implants should be replaced after 5 years of use.

The 5-year cumulative pregnancy rates listed in the package insert for implants indicate initially higher failure rates for women who weigh more than 70 kg (154 lb). Clinical trials used to estimate these failure rates, however, combined experience involving two different implant systems: those using less dense and others using more dense tubing. Weight-specific failure rates associated with implant systems based on less dense tubing are substantially lower than those listed in the package labeling (55). For this reason, even women weighing greater than 90 kg (198 lb) should achieve high contraceptive efficacy with the implants currently marketed in the United States, which use less dense tubing.

Women using implants who experience cyclical menses consistent with ovulation have a higher risk of pregnancy than those with irregular bleeding or amenorrhea (56) and should be counseled regarding the need for pregnancy testing should menses cease. Studies of infants born to women who conceived while using implants have not suggested that implants are teratogenic (57).

Insertion of implants within 7 days of the onset of menses ensures that the patient is not pregnant and results in immediate contraception. Insertion and removal of implants are minor office procedures performed using local anesthesia. Instructions are included in package labeling and illustrate appropriate technique. However, as with any procedure, appropriate technique is best learned under direct supervision by an experienced clinician. Use of a template to mark the six insertion sites facilitates correct placement. Insertion of the implants in a superficial plane makes removal less difficult.

Because fibrous tissue forms around each implant, removal takes longer and is associated with more patient discomfort than insertion. An experienced clinician will require 10–30 minutes for removal. If removal is proceeding slowly or is associated with excessive patient discomfort, the removal procedure should be terminated and resumed in 4–6 weeks, at which time resolution of operative site tenderness and bruising should facilitate removal. If one or more implants were removed, back-up contraception should be used until the patient returns for the subsequent removal procedure. Because serum progestin levels fall to undetectable levels within 1 week following removal (58), return of fertility is rapid.

Side Effects

Menstrual changes are the most common side effect of implants. Most women experience an irregular bleeding pattern during the first year following implant insertion; this proportion declines to one third by the fifth year. Likewise, approximately one third of women experience regular cycles during their first year, with this proportion increasing to two thirds by the fifth year of implant use. During 5 years of implant use, 5–10% of women experience amenorrhea (56). Although these menstrual changes in implant users are distinct from those that occur in women using DMPA, counseling, method selection, and follow-up issues for DMPA also apply to implant users. As with DMPA, estrogen supplementation can be considered for implant users troubled by irregular bleeding, although the impact of estrogen supplementation on the contraceptive effectiveness of implants remains uncertain.

Headache is the nonmenstrual side effect that most frequently leads to implant removal (55). Cases of idiopathic intracranial hypertension have been reported in women using implants. A small number of women report increased hair loss.

Benefits and Risks

No epidemiologic data assessing risk of reproductive tract cancer in women using implants are available. Some women using implants develop ovarian cysts. Although such cysts may cause lower abdominal discomfort, more often they are asymptomatic and noted incidentally during pelvic examination. Functional ovarian cysts as large as 10 cm in diameter in implant users appear to be associated with persistent dominant follicles that gradually resolve spontaneously (53). Such ovarian cysts should be managed expectantly with follow-up clinical and sonographic examination. Surgical intervention is rarely necessary and should be reserved for cases in which a cyst fails to resolve or when torsion or rupture is suspected.

Selection of Methods

With the availability of oral, injectable, and implantable hormonal contraceptives, U.S. women have more safe, effective, and reversible birth control options than ever before. By individualizing their counseling and recommendations based on relevant behavioral and medical considerations, physicians can maximize their patients' success with hormonal contraception.

Compliance Issues

For healthy women, regardless of age, who are willing and able to take daily tablets, combination OCs often represent an appropriate contraceptive choice. Among married women initiating OCs to prevent pregnancy, approximately 72% will still be using them at 1 year of use (59). Because of their ease of compliance, however, DMPA or implants may be more suitable for some women. Teenagers, women with psychiatric problems, and those with mental retardation may experience particular problems with OC compliance and continuation. Injectable and implantable contraceptives are suitable for those with compliance problems.

Use After Abortion, After Birth, or During Lactation

Any method of hormonal contraception may be initiated immediately following induced or spontaneous termination of a first- or second-trimester pregnancy. Women remain at increased risk for thromboembolism for several weeks after childbirth. Women who do not breast-feed do not appear to ovulate before 3 weeks postpartum (60). Based on these observations, some physicians initiate combination OCs in non-breast-feeding women 2 weeks after childbirth (6), even though package labeling suggests that OCs not be initiated prior to 4 weeks postpartum. Because progestin-only OCs, DMPA, and implants do not contain estrogen, these latter methods may be initiated immediately postpartum.

It is reasonable to initiate hormonal contraception in lactating women once milk flow is established. Use of combination OCs can reduce the quantity and duration of lactation (61), although such use by well-nourished breast-feeding women does not appear to result in infant development problems (62). Progestin-only contraceptives may be an alternative to combination OCs. Progestin-only contraceptives do not impair lactation and in fact may increase the quality and duration of lactation (63, 64). When initiated within 1 week postpartum, progestin-only OCs have not been shown to adversely affect lactation or infant development (65). When initiated immediately or at 6 weeks postpartum, DMPA has not been demonstrated to decrease duration of lactation (66) or infant weight gain (67). In studies of women with implants inserted 6 weeks postpartum, no adverse impact on lactation or infant weight gain was noted (68). Because the manufacturers of DMPA and implants did not submit data regarding immediate postpartum use in lactating women, however, package labeling for these long-acting methods advises initiation 6 weeks postpartum in lactating women.

Use When Estrogen Is Contraindicated

Use of progestin-only OCs, DMPA, and implants may be appropriate when contraceptive doses of estrogen are contraindicated. Both pregnancy and combination OC use confer an increased risk of morbidity and mortality in women greater than 35 years of age who smoke or have hypertension, women with coronary artery disease, women at increased risk for thromboembolism, and women with systemic lupus erythematosus (69). Notwithstanding contraindications listed in package labeling, progestin-only methods should be considered safe and effective contraceptive choices for such women.

Active liver disease contraindicates combination OC use. A small clinical trial of oral medroxyprogesterone acetate in adults with chronic liver disease suggests that DMPA may be a safe contraceptive choice for women with liver ailments (70).

A personal history of breast cancer is listed in package labeling as a contraindication to use of all hormonal methods of contraception. The presence of uterine leiomyomata does not contraindicate use of hormonal contraception. There is no evidence that uterine leiomyomata increase in size in women using these methods.

Postcoital Contraception

Increased use of postcoital contraception could substantially reduce the number of unintended pregnancies and induced abortions performed each year. Used as an emergency method of contraception within 72 hours of unprotected coitus, it can be safe and effective. Women should be advised of the availability of postcoital contraception so they can request it promptly should the need arise.

Strategies used for postcoital contraception have included short courses of estrogen, estrogen plus progestin, danazol, or insertion of an intrauterine device (71). Published data suggest that the use of 100 μg of ethinyl estradiol and 1 mg of dl-norgestrel (eg, two pills containing 50 μg of estradiol and 0.5 mg of norgestrel each) taken by mouth within 72 hours of unprotected sexual intercourse and repeated 12 hours later significantly reduces the pregnancy rate. Regimens using contemporary low-dose pills may also be effective, although these have not been evaluated (72). Side effects such as nausea and vomiting occur in 15–30% of patients, and antiemetic medication may be appropriate in some circumstances. If menstruation does not begin when expected, a sensitive pregnancy test may be appropriate.

The antiprogestin mifepristone (RU 486) has also been successfully used for postcoital contraception and has been found to be more effective than OCs, with a lower evidence of side effects (73). This drug is not currently available in the United States.

Use of Concomitant Medications

Anticonvulsants and antibiotics that induce hepatic enzymes (eg, phenytoin, phenobarbital, carbamazepine, primidone, and rifampin) can reduce the contraceptive efficacy of OCs (74) and implants (75). The contraceptive efficacy of DMPA in women taking hepatic enzyme inducers has not been explicitly studied. However, physicians with substantial experience prescribing DMPA (150 mg every 3 months) for women taking anticonvulsants have not reported contraceptive failures in such patients (76). Pharmacokinetic studies suggest that the anticonvulsant valproic acid (77) and the antibiotics doxycycline (78) and tetracycline (79) do not appear to reduce OC efficacy and presumably do not impair implant efficacy.

Summary

Oral, injectable, and implantable contraceptives offer women safe, effective, and reversible fertility regulation. In some cases, their use also confers important noncontraceptive benefits. By individualizing counseling and recommendations based on relevant behavioral and medical considerations, clinicians can maximize their patients' success with hormonal contraceptives. Even in women with relative contraindications to the use of hormonal contraceptives, the risks associated with pregnancy may be sufficiently great so as to warrant their use.

REFERENCES

1. Klitsch M. The new pills: awaiting the next generation of oral contraceptives. Fam Plann Perspect 1992;24:226–228
2. Vessey MP, Lawless M, Yeates D, McPherson K. Progestogen-only oral contraception. Findings in a large prospective study with special reference to effectiveness. Br J Fam Plann 1985;10:117–121
3. Letterie GS, Chow GE. Effect of "missed" pills on oral contraceptive effectiveness. Obstet Gynecol 1992;79:979–982
4. Trussell J, Kost K. Contraceptive failure in the United States: a critical review of the literature. Stud Fam Plann 1987;18:237–283
5. Jones EF, Forrest JD. Contraceptive failure rates based on the 1988 NSFG. Fam Plann Perspect 1992;24:12–19
6. Speroff L, Darney P. A clinical guide for contraception. Baltimore: Williams and Wilkins, 1992
7. American College of Obstetricians and Gynecologists. Contraceptives and congenital anomalies. ACOG Committee Opinion 124. Washington, DC: ACOG, 1993
8. Kost K, Forrest JD, Harlap S. Comparing the health risks and benefits of contraceptive choices. Fam Plann Perspect 1991;23:54–61
9. Milsom I, Sundell G, Andersch B. The influence of different combined oral contraceptives on the prevalence and severity of dysmenorrhea. Contraception 1990;42:497–506
10. Larsson G, Milsom I, Lindstedt G, Rybo G. The influence of a low-dose combined oral contraceptive on menstrual blood loss and iron status. Contraception 1992;46:327–334
11. Brinton LA, Vessey MP, Flavel R, Yeates D. Risk factors for benign breast disease. Am J Epidemiol 1981; 113:203–214
12. Holt VL, Daling JR, McKnight B, Moore D, Stergachis A, Weiss NS. Functional ovarian cysts in relation to the use of monophasic and triphasic oral contraceptives. Obstet Gynecol 1992;79: 529–533
13. Lanes SF, Birmann B, Walker AM, Singer S. Oral con-traceptive type and functional ovarian cysts. Am J Obstet Gynecol 1992; 166:956–961
14. Spector TD, Hochberg MC. The protective effect of the oral contraceptive pill on rheumatoid arthritis: an overview of the analytic epidemiological studies using meta-analysis. J Clin Epidemiol 1990;43:1221–1230
15. Rubin GL, Ory HW, Layde PM. Oral contraceptives and pelvic inflammatory disease. Am J Obstet Gynecol 1982;144:630–635
16. Franks AL, Beral V, Cates W Jr, Hogue CJR. Contraception and ectopic pregnancy risk. Am J Obstet Gynecol 1990;163: 1120–1123
17. Hankinson SE, Colditz GA, Hunter DJ, Spencer TL, Rosner B, Stampfer MJ. A quantitative assessment of oral contraceptive use and risk of ovarian cancer. Obstet Gynecol 1992;80:708–714
18. The Cancer and Steroid Hormone Study of the Centers for Disease Control and the National Institute of Child Health and Human Development. The reduction in risk of ovarian cancer associated with oral-contraceptive use. N Engl J Med 1987;316:650–655
19. Villard-Mackintosh L, Vessey MP, Jones L. The effects of oral contraceptives and parity on ovarian cancer trends in women under 55 years of age. Br J Obstet Gynaecol 1989;96:783–788
20. Kerlikowske K, Brown JS, Grady DG. Should women with familial ovarian cancer undergo prophylactic oophorectomy? Obstet Gynecol 1992;80:700–707

21. Schlesselman JJ. Cancer of the breast and reproductive tract in relation to use of oral contraceptives. Contraception 1989;40: 1–38

22. The Centers for Disease Control Cancer and Steroid Hormone Study. Oral contraceptive use and the risk of endometrial cancer. JAMA 1983;249:1600–1604

23. Recker RR, Davies KM, Hinders SM, Heaney RP, Stegman MR, Kimmel DB. Bone gain in young adult women. JAMA 1992; 268:2403–2408

24. Kleerekoper M, Brienza RS, Schultz LR, Johnson CC. Oral contraceptive use may protect against low bone mass. Arch Intern Med 1991;151:1971–1976

25. Kritz-Silverstein D, Barrett-Connor E. Bone mineral density in postmenopausal women as determined by prior oral contraceptive use. Am J Public Health 1993; 83:100–102

26. Wiseman A, Bowie J, Cogswell D, Dewsbury J, Hamilton M, Hutchinson F, et al. Marvelon; clinical experience in the UK. Br J Fam Plann 1984;10(9):38–42

27. Goldzieher JW, Moses LE, Averkin E, Scheel C, Taber BZ. A placebo-controlled double-blind crossover investigation of the side effects attributed to oral contraceptives. Fertil Steril 1971;22:609–623

28. Mattson RH, Rebar RW. Contraceptive methods for women with neurologic disorders. Am J Obstet Gynecol 1993;168: 2027–2032

29. Grimes DA. The safety of oral contraceptives: epide-miologic insights from the first 30 years. Am J Obstet Gynecol 1992;166:1950–1954

30. Stampfer MJ, Willett WC, Colditz GA, Speizer FE, Hennekens CH. Past use of oral contraceptives and cardiovascular disease: a meta-analysis in the context of the Nurses' Health Study. Am J Obstet Gynecol 1990; 163:285–291

31. Engel H-J, Engel E, Lichtlen PR. Coronary atherosclerosis and myocardial infarction in young women—role of oral contraceptives. Eur Heart J 1983;4:1–8

32. Clarkson TB, Shively CA, Morgan TM, Koritnik DR, Adams MR, Kaplan JR. Oral contraceptives and coronary artery atherosclerosis of cynomolgus monkeys. Obstet Gynecol 1990;75:217–222

33. Croft P, Hannaford PC. Risk factors for acute myocardial infarction in women: evidence from the Royal College of General Practitioners' oral contraception study. BMJ 1989;298:165–168

34. Gerstman BB, Piper JM, Tomita DK, Ferguson WJ, Stadel BV, Lundin FE. Oral contraceptive estrogen dose and the risk of deep venous thromboembolic disease. Am J Epidemiol 1991; 133:32–37

35. Hirvonen E, Idänpään-Heikkilä J. Cardiovascular death among women under 40 years of age using low-estrogen oral contraceptives and intrauterine devices in Finland from 1975 to 1984. Am J Obstet Gynecol 1990;163:281–284

36. Thorogood M, Vessey MP. An epidemiologic survey of cardiovascular disease in women taking oral contraceptives. Am J Obstet Gynecol 1990;163:274–281

37. Harlap S. Oral contraceptives and breast cancer. Cause and effect? J Reprod Med 1991;36:374–395

38. The Cancer and Steroid Hormone Study of the Centers for Disease Control and the National Institute of Child Health and Human Development. Oral-contraceptive use and the risk of breast cancer. N Engl J Med 1986; 315:405–411

39. Wingo PA, Lee NC, Ory HW, Beral V, Peterson HB, Rhodes P. Age-specific differences in the relationship between oral contraceptive use and breast cancer. Obstet Gynecol 1991;78:161–170

40. Bruzzi P, Negri E, La Vecchia C, Decarli A, Palli D, Parazzini F, et al. Short term increase in risk of breast cancer after full term pregnancy. BMJ 1988;297:1096–1098

41. Kaunitz AM. Oral contraceptives and gynecologic cancer: an update for the 1990s. Am J Obstet Gynecol 1992;167:1171– 1176

42. The WHO Collaborative Study of Neoplasia and Steroid Contraceptives. Combined oral contraceptives and liver cancer. Int J Cancer 1989;43:254–259

43. Kaunitz AM. Long-acting injectable contraception with depot medroxyprogesterone acetate. Am J Obstet Gynecol 1994; 170:1543–1549

44. Klitsch M. Injectable hormones and regulatory controversy: an end to the long-running story? Fam Plann Perspect 1993; 25:37–40

45. Schwallie PC, Assenzo JR. The effect of depot-medroxy-progesterone acetate on pituitary and ovarian function, and the return of fertility following its discontinuation: a review. Contraception 1974;10:181–202

46. Belsey EM. Vaginal bleeding patterns among women using one natural and eight hormonal methods of contraception. Contraception 1988;38:181–206

47. Solheim F. An assessment of quality of life in women treated with Depo-Provera in Sweden. In: Zambrano D, ed. Depo-Provera® (medroxyprogesterone acetate) for contraception. A current perspective of scientific, clinical and social issues. Proceedings of an international symposium held on 19–20 November 1992. Oxford: Oxford Clinical Communcations, 1992:61–72

48. DeCeulaer K, Hayes R, Gruber C, Serjeant GR. Medroxy-progesterone acetate and homozygous sickle-cell disease. Lancet 1982;2:229–231

49. Mattson RH, Cramer JA, Caldwell BV, Siconolfi BC. Treatment of seizures with medroxyprogesterone acetate: preliminary report. Neurology 1984;34:1255–1258

50. The WHO Collaborative Study of Neoplasia and Steroid Contraceptives. Breast cancer and depot-medroxy-progesterone acetate: a multinational study. Lancet 1991;338:833– 838

51. Cundy T, Evans M, Roberts H, Wattie D, Ames R, Reid IR. Bone density in women receiving depot medroxy-progesterone acetate for contraception. BMJ 1991; 303:13–16

52. Robertson DN, Sivin I, Nash HA, Braun J, Dinh J. Release rates of levonorgestrel from Silastic® capsules, homogeneous rods and covered rods in humans. Contraception 1983;27:483–495

53. Shoupe D, Horenstein J, Mishell DR Jr, Lacarra M, Medearis A. Characteristics of ovarian follicular development in Norplant users. Fertil Steril 1991;55:766–770

54. Croxatto HB, Díaz S, Salvatierra AM, Morales P, Ebensperger C, Brandeis A. Treatment with Norplant® subdermal implants inhibits sperm penetration through cervical mucus in vitro. Contraception 1987;36:193–201

55. Sivin I. International experience with Norplant® and Norplant®-2 contraceptives. Stud Fam Plann 1988;19:81–94

56. Shoupe D, Mishell DR Jr, Bopp BL, Fielding M. The significance of bleeding patterns in Norplant implant users. Obstet Gynecol 1991;77:256–260

57. Díaz S, Pavez M, Herreros C, Johansson EDB, Croxatto HB. Bleeding pattern, outcome of accidental pregnancies and levonorgestrel plasma levels associated with method failure in Norplant® implants users. Contraception 1986;33:347–356

58. Croxatto HB, Díaz S, Pavez M, Cárdenas H, Larsson M, Johansson EDB. Clearance of levonorgestrel from the circulation

following removal of Norplant® subdermal implants. Contraception 1988;38:509–523

59. Hatcher RA, Trussell J, Stewart F, Stewart GK, Kowal D, Guest F, et al, eds. Contraceptive failure rates. In: Contraceptive technology. 16th rev ed. New York: Irvington Publishers, Inc, 1994: 637–653

60. Gray RH, Campbell OM, Zacur HA, Labbok MH, MacRae SL. Postpartum return of ovarian activity in nonbreastfeeding women monitored by urinary assays. J Clin Endocrinol Metab 1987; 64:645–651

61. Croxatto HB, Díaz S, Peralta O, Juez G, Herreros C, Casado ME, et al. Fertility regulation in nursing women: IV. Long-term influence of a low-dose combined oral contraceptive initiated at day 30 postpartum upon lactation and infant growth. Contraception 1983;27:13–25

62. WHO Special Programme of Research, Development and Research Training in Human Reproduction, Task Force on Oral Contraceptives. Effects of hormonal contraceptives on milk volume and infant growth. Contraception 1984;30:505–522

63. Koetsawang S. The effects of contraceptive methods on the quality and quantity of breast milk. Int J Gynaecol Obstet 1987; 25(suppl):115–127

64. McCann MF, Liskin LS, Piotrow PT, Rinehart W, Fox G. Breastfeeding, fertility, and family planning. Popul Rep [J] 1981;9:J525–J575

65. McCann MF, Moggia AV, Higgins JE, Potts M, Becker C. The effects of a progestin-only oral contraceptive (Levonorgestrel 0.03 mg) on breast-feeding. Contraception 1989;40:635–649

66. Guiloff E, Ibarra-Polo A, Zañartu J, Toscanini C, Mischler TW, Gómez-Rogers C. Effect of contraception on lactation. Am J Obstet Gynecol 1974;118:42–45

67. Karim M, Ammar R, El Mahgoub S, El Ganzoury B, Fikri F, Abdou I. Injected progestogen and lactation. BMJ 1971; 1:200–203

68. Díaz S, Herreros C, Juez G, Casado ME, Salvatierra AM, Miranda P, et al. Fertility regulation in nursing women: VII. Influence of Norplant® levonorgestrel implants upon lactation and infant growth. Contraception 1985;32:53–73

69. Jungers P, Dougados M, Pélissier C, Kuttenn F, Tron F, Lesavre P, et al. Influence of oral contraceptive therapy on the activity of systemic lupus erythematosus. Arthritis Rheum 1982;25:618–623

70. Sotaniemi EA, Hynnynen T, Ahlqvist J, Ahokas JT, Puoskari U, Pelkonen I. Effects of medroxyprogesterone on the liver function and drug metabolism of patients with primary biliary cirrhosis and chronic active hepatitis. J Med 1978;9:117–127

71. Fasoli M, Parazzini F, Cecchetti G, La Vecchia C. Post-coital contraception: an overview of published studies. Contraception 1989;39:459–468

72. Trussell J, Stewart F, Guest F, Hatcher RA. Emergency contraceptive pills: a simple proposal to reduce unintended pregnancies. Fam Plann Perspect 1992;24:269–273

73. Glasier A, Thong KJ, Dewar M, Mackie M, Baird DT. Mifepristone (RU 486) compared with high-dose estrogen and progestogen for emergency postcoital contraception. N Engl J Med 1992;327:1041–1044

74. Back DJ, Orme ML'E. Pharmacokinetic drug interactions with oral contraceptives. Clin Pharmacokinet 1990;18:472–484

75. Haukkamaa M. Contraception by Norplant® subdermal capsules is not reliable in epileptic patients on anti-convulsant treatment. Contraception 1986;33:559–565

76. Sapire KE. Depo-provera and carbamazapine. Br J Fam Plann 1990;15(4):130

77. Crawford P, Chadwick D, Cleland P, Tjia J, Cowie A, Back DJ, et al. The lack of effect of sodium valproate on the pharmacokinetics of oral contraceptive steroids. Contraception 1986;33:23–29

78. Neely JL, Abate M, Swinker M, D'Angio R. The effect of doxycycline on serum levels of ethinyl estradiol, norethindrone, and endogenous progesterone. Obstet Gynecol 1991;77:416–420

79. Murphy AA, Zacur HA, Charache P, Burkman RT. The effect of tetracycline on levels of oral contraceptives. Am J Obstet Gynecol 1991;164:28–33

This Technical Bulletin was developed under the direction of the Committee on Technical Bulletins of the American College of Obstetricians and Gynecologists as an educational aid to obstetricians and gynecologists. The committee wishes to thank Andrew M. Kaunitz, MD, and Elizabeth B. Connell, MD, for their assistance in the development of this bulletin. This Technical Bulletin does not define a standard of care, nor is it intended to dictate an exclusive course of management. It presents recognized methods and techniques of clinical practice for consideration by obstetrician–gynecologists for incorporation into their practices. Variations of practice taking into account the needs of the individual patient, resources, and limitations unique to the institution or type of practice may be appropriate.

ISSN 1074-8628

THE AMERICAN COLLEGE OF OBSTETRICIANS AND GYNECOLOGISTS
409 12th Street, SW
Washington, DC 20024-2188

12345/87654

ACOG EDUCATIONAL BULLETIN

Number 247, May 1998

Hormone Replacement Therapy

It has been estimated that more than 36 million women in the United States will become menopausal during the next decade. With the onset of menopause, ovarian production of estrogen is significantly reduced, leading to dramatic physiologic changes including:

- Hot flushes
- Mood disturbances
- Thinning of genitourinary tissues and a decrease in tissue elasticity
- Loss of calcium from the skeleton
- Metabolic shift to a more atherogenic lipoprotein profile

Previous studies have demonstrated unequivocally that estrogen replacement therapy can reduce significantly the incidence of osteoporotic fractures and vasomotor symptoms and improve genital atrophy (1, 2). Because estrogen receptors have been identified in almost all tissues in the body, it has been proposed that estrogen replacement can delay many of the undesired effects of aging. The results of a number of observational studies have suggested that estrogen replacement therapy is associated with reduced cardiovascular morbidity (3). Nevertheless, currently there is only one large-scale, long-term randomized trial under way to examine the effects of estrogen replacement therapy on cardiovascular disease. In this trial, the Women's Health Initiative, 25,000 menopausal women are being randomly selected to receive either estrogen replacement therapy or placebo. If the results of this 10-year trial support current observational data, hormone replacement therapy will be considered a major preventive public health strategy for all postmenopausal women.

Despite the many documented benefits of estrogen replacement therapy, compliance remains a significant problem. A substantial number of women who are prescribed estrogen either do not fill the prescription or discontinue therapy within less than 5 years because of perceived cancer risks (primarily breast cancer) or adverse side effects. In a study of 685 women who were screened, designated "at risk" for osteoporosis, and given estrogen therapy,

This Educational Bulletin was developed under the direction of the Committee on Educational Bulletins of the American College of Obstetricians and Gynecologists as an aid to obstetricians and gynecologists. The College wishes to thank James H. Liu, MD, for his assistance in the development of this bulletin. This document is not to be construed as establishing a standard of practice or dictating an exclusive course of treatment. Rather, it is intended as an educational tool that presents current information on obstetric–gynecologic issues.

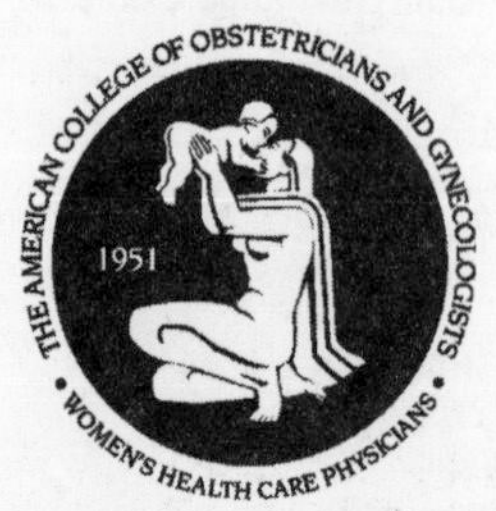

Replaces Number 166, April 1992

only 49% were still taking estrogen at the end of 1 year (4). The compliance rate was only marginally better in women who had undergone hysterectomy (59%). Even in prospective clinical trials where women were closely monitored, compliance rates were only in the 80% range (5). Widespread and long-term use will require coordinated strategies to educate physicians and women regarding the benefits and adverse effects of estrogen replacement therapy.

The use of antiestrogens, such as tamoxifen as adjuvant chemotherapy for breast cancer in menopausal women and as prophylactic treatment for women at high risk for breast cancer, is associated with improved lipid profiles and increased bone density (6). These unexpected beneficial effects suggest that certain estrogen analogs such as tamoxifen may function as weak estrogen agonists in specific tissues such as bone, liver, and endometrium. These differences in estrogen activity may be explained in part by the recent discovery of a second type of estrogen receptor, the estrogen beta receptor. Clinical trials are being conducted with other estrogen analogs (now called selective estrogen receptor modulators or SERMs) such as raloxifene to assess their use as an alternative to traditional estrogen replacement therapy. Raloxifene has been approved by the Food and Drug Administration for the prevention of postmenopausal osteoporosis. The effect of these agents on cognitive function has not been determined.

Substantial decreases in other circulating hormones besides estrogen occur during the transition into menopause or with aging. These hormones include progesterone, growth hormone (GH), and dehydroepiandrosterone sulfate (DHEAS) (7–10). Physiologic replacement therapies of these hormones are being evaluated in older men and postmenopausal women; however, a detailed discussion is beyond the scope of this bulletin. In contrast to estrogen, the postmenopausal ovary continues to secrete testosterone in significant amounts. The mean concentrations of circulating testosterone levels in postmenopausal women is approximately 250 pg/mL, which is only slightly less than in reproductive-age women (11).

Indications

Central Nervous System Symptoms

Changes in neurologic function such as increased irritability, mood disorders, mild depression, hot flushes, and sleep disturbances may arise during the perimenopausal transition even before the onset of menopause. Decreases in memory and other cognitive changes also have been reported in some menopausal women and younger women in whom menopause has been surgically induced (12–14). Estrogen replacement therapy is the most effective treatment for the relief of hot flushes. In a short-term crossover placebo study, treatment with 1.25 mg per day of conjugated estrogens was found to be significantly more effective than placebo in reducing central nervous system symptoms (ie, hot flushes, insomnia, irritability, poor memory, anxiety, and headaches) (15). Hormone replacement with adequate doses of estrogen can in many cases effectively reverse cognitive changes and improve function (16, 17).

In elderly menopausal women, recent observational and cross-sectional data suggest that estrogens may retard the progression of senile-associated dementia, especially Alzheimer's disease (18–21). The mechanism of estrogen action on brain function is unclear. However, estrogen can increase cerebral perfusion (22), and estrogen and other steroid receptors have been localized to multiple neuronal tissues (23). The impact of estrogen replacement therapy on senile-onset dementias will be evaluated in a prospective estrogen replacement randomized trial within the Women's Health Initiative study.

Progestins such as megestrol acetate, norethindrone, and medroxyprogesterone acetate can be effective in reducing vasomotor symptoms in women who are unable to take estrogens. However, these medications are less effective than estrogen in relieving hot flushes, must be administered in large doses to be effective, and have side effects. Other nonhormonal medications used to treat vasomotor symptoms include clonidine hydrochloride (0.1–0.3 mg patch) and a combination preparation containing phenobarbital, ergotamine, and belladonna alkaloids (24).

Sexual Function

There is no clear-cut evidence that sex drive is reduced significantly at the time of the menopause. For an interval of a few years, postmenopausally, the ovary remains a significant source of circulating androgens (11). Sexual function may be affected by other factors that may occur at the time of menopause, such as changes in body image, stress, or loss of a spouse. The use of combination estrogen and androgen therapy to increase libido is controversial because libido is affected by many variables and is difficult to quantitate objectively. Nevertheless, available literature suggests that the use of androgen alone or androgen with estrogen may induce a positive effect on mood and overall sense of well-being, particularly in women who have had their ovaries removed (14, 16, 17). The long-term use of estrogen and androgen in combination is not without risks.

Cardiovascular Symptoms

Coronary heart disease is the leading cause of death in women. Between the ages of 50 and 79 years, the incidence of coronary heart disease increases significantly. It accounts for approximately 400,000 deaths annually in the United States, with almost all deaths occurring in postmenopausal women. Many observational studies suggest that one mechanism by which estrogens protect against coronary heart disease is by lowering LDL cholesterol and increasing HDL cholesterol concentrations (25, 26). Currently, only one large randomized trial, the Postmenopausal Estrogen/Progestin Interventions (PEPI) study, has examined the effects of estrogen replacement therapy on risk factors for heart disease. This 3-year trial of 875 women demonstrated that conjugated estrogen (0.625 mg) given either alone or with progestin (medroxyprogesterone acetate [10 mg for 12 days per month], medroxyprogesterone acetate [2.5 mg per day], or oral micronized progesterone [200 mg for 12 days per month]) improves the lipoprotein profile by lowering LDL cholesterol and increasing HDL cholesterol levels (5). Although medroxyprogesterone acetate tended to reduce the magnitude of the increased HDL cholesterol levels, results of the PEPI trial indicate that this beneficial increase in HDL cholesterol remained significant when compared with placebo use. In contrast with medroxyprogesterone acetate, the administration of micronized progesterone did not reduce the beneficial lipid effects of estrogens. Fibrinogen levels, another marker for cardiovascular risk, also were decreased significantly in estrogen-treated groups relative to placebo.

It is estimated that the alteration in lipoprotein metabolism induced by estrogen therapy probably accounts for less than 50% of the cardioprotective effect of estrogens. It is postulated that estrogen may provide additional protection through other mechanisms such as its direct effect on arterial vasodilation and increased perfusion (19, 27), its intrinsic antioxidant properties (28), or its action on reducing the circulating levels of oxidized LDL (29).

Osteoporosis

A gradual loss of bone mineral density is associated with aging in both men and women. In contrast to bone loss in men, bone loss in women accelerates at the onset of menopause on average at a rate of approximately 3% per year for the first 5 years and 1% per year thereafter. However, in some women bone loss at this time may exceed 5% per year. Hip fractures frequently occur 15–25 years after menopause and result from the combination of severely reduced bone mass and falls. It is estimated that women hospitalized for hip fractures will have an overall mortality rate of 30% within 1 year of hip fracture. The projected health care costs for hip fractures alone is more than 7 billion dollars annually. Other fractures associated with osteoporosis include fractures of the vertebrae, distal forearm, and proximal humerus.

The loss of bone mineral density is the result of an alteration in the bone remodeling process. The rate of bone resorption increases, exceeding the rate of bone formation. Osteoporosis is diagnosed when bone mineral density decreases to less than 2.5 standard deviations below the young adult peak mean.

Estrogen therapy has been shown to be effective in preventing further bone loss by inhibiting osteoclastic activity in the bone remodeling process, thereby reducing bone resorption. Effective doses of estrogen for the prevention of osteoporosis are: 0.625 mg of conjugated estrogen, 0.5 mg of micronized estradiol, and 0.3 mg of esterified estrogen. Other therapies that are effective in preventing bone loss include alendronate, sodium fluoride (30), and intranasal use of calcitonin (31).

Genitourinary Symptoms

The tissues of the urethra and vagina are derived embryologically from the urogenital sinus and are classic examples of estrogen-responsive tissues. Withdrawal of estradiol during menopause results in a reduction in overall mitotic activity of vaginal and urethral mucosal epithelium, a decrease in exfoliation of surface cells, a decrease in tissue vascularity, and thinning of the mucosal layer. The vaginal and urethral mucosa appear pale, dry, and flattened. These hypoestrogenic changes in the vaginal mucosa are associated with vaginal dryness, dyspareunia, and a greater incidence of atrophic vaginitis. Atrophy of the urethral mucosa is associated with a greater incidence of urethritis, decreased urethral pressure, and a possible increased incidence of urinary incontinence.

Use of systemic estrogen replacement or local estrogen creams and urethral suppositories can reverse many if not all of these changes. Hormone replacement therapy can decrease the risk of urinary tract infection and microscopic hematuria (32). Even small amounts of estrogen preparations introduced onto the vaginal mucosa are more readily absorbed than oral preparations and can lead to significant increases in circulating levels of estrogen. For women who are unable to take estrogen but experience urogenital atrophy, there are estrogen creams or a polysiloxane estradiol-impregnated vaginal ring. The ring delivery system has been shown to relieve vaginal and urinary tract symptoms without increasing systemic estradiol levels; the device needs to be changed every three months.

Hypogonadal Conditions

Individuals who do not undergo pubertal maturation (ovarian failure secondary to cancer treatment, gonadal dysgenesis, isolated gonadotropin deficiency) require estrogen replacement therapy to induce the normal adult female phenotype. Treatment of these individuals generally requires gradually increasing estrogen doses to mimic the same pattern of changes that occurs during puberty. At reproductive age, these women may require twice as much estrogen as women of postmenopausal age. For women with a diagnosis of premature ovarian failure, hypothalamic amenorrhea, exercise-associated amenorrhea, anorexia nervosa, or hyperprolactinemia, estrogen replacement therapy should be considered for the same indications as for postmenopausal women.

Risk Factors

Thromboembolic Disease

Recent studies have shown a twofold to fourfold increase in the risk of venous thromboembolism in users of estrogen-only and combined estrogen–progestin hormone replacement therapy (33–35). Because the absolute risk of venous thromboembolism in both users and nonusers of estrogen is low, there is only a modest increase in the morbidity associated with hormone replacement therapy, and this increased risk must be weighed against documented benefits. At the least, however, the risk factors for venous thromboembolism—such as family history of venous thrombosis, gross obesity, an earlier episode of thromboembolism and intercurrent illness associated with immobilization—should be considered in weighing the benefits and risks of hormone replacement therapy for any individual.

Endometrial Hyperplasia and Endometrial Cancer

Long-term use of estrogen alone has been associated with the development of endometrial hyperplasia and endometrial cancer. The PEPI trial was the first large, prospective randomized study to examine the effects of unopposed estrogen over a 3-year follow-up period (36). During the trial, women who took conjugated estrogen (0.625 mg) only were more likely to develop simple cystic hyperplasia (27.7%), adenomatous hyperplasia (22.7%), or atypical adenomatous hyperplasia (11.8%) than the placebo group (<0.8%). Women who took conjugated estrogen (0.625 mg) in combination with either cyclic (10 mg of medroxyprogesterone acetate per day for 12 days or 200 mg of micronized oral progesterone per day for 12 days) (ie, 200 mg given as a single dose once daily for 12 days) or continuous progestin therapy (2.5 mg of medroxyprogesterone acetate per day) had the same rate of hyperplasia as the placebo group. In those developing adenomatous or atypical adenomatous hyperplasia, the endometrium reverted to normal in 94% of women after treatment with progestin therapy (10 mg of medroxyprogesterone acetate per day for 3 months). Thus, in women with a uterus, cyclic or continuous progestin therapy is required to protect the endometrium from hyperplastic transformation during estrogen replacement therapy (36).

For women with previously diagnosed endometrial cancer, hormone replacement therapy remains an option that should be viewed cautiously. In a survey of members of the Society of Gynecologic Oncologists, 83% of respondents approved the use of estrogen replacement therapy in patients with stage I, grade I, endometrial cancer; 56% favored using estrogen in cases of stage I, grade 2 cancer; and 39% would use estrogen in cases of stage I, grade 3 cancer. In women with a history of endometrial carcinoma, estrogens can be used for the same indications as for other women, except the selection of appropriate candidates should be based on prognostic indicators and the risk the patient is willing to assume. If the patient is free of tumor, the use of estrogen replacement therapy cannot result in recurrence. If an estrogen-dependent neoplasm is harbored somewhere in her body, it will eventually recur; however, the use of estrogen replacement therapy may result in an earlier recurrence (37).

Endometriosis

For women with a history of endometriosis, treatment with estrogen-only regimens is not contraindicated. However, because these women often are younger than most menopausal women and may have undergone bilateral oophorectomy, higher doses of estrogen may induce the recurrence of endometriosis (38). If this occurs, discontinuing the estrogen therapy and beginning a progestin-only regimen can be an option (see Table 1).

Breast Cancer

An increased risk of breast cancer has been associated with the extended duration of endogenous estrogen exposure such as that which occurs with early menarche, late menopause, and obesity. Although some studies have suggested that hormone replacement therapy is linked to an increased risk of breast cancer in postmenopausal wo-

TABLE 1. Commonly Used Progestin Preparations, Their Estimated Relative Potencies for Ability to Induce Endometrial Secretory Changes, and Recommended Progestin-Only Therapeutic Doses

Progestin	Relative Potency	Progestin-Only Dose
Medroxyprogesterone acetate (10 mg)	1.0	10–30 mg
Norethindrone (5 mg) (0.35 mg)	>6.0 ~0.5	1–5.0 mg
Micronized progesterone (200 mg)	1.0	Not reported
Progesterone vaginal suspension (90 mg)	1.0	Not reported
Megestrol acetate		40–80 mg

men (39, 40), other studies have shown little or no relationship between estrogen use and breast cancer (41, 42). Despite the more than 50 epidemiologic studies published on this topic, no consistent link between hormone replacement therapy and breast cancer has been found. One possible interpretation of the data is that either there is no increased risk or the risk is too small to be shown clearly by epidemiologic studies. As for all women, those taking hormone replacement therapy should be encouraged to perform monthly breast self-examinations, have regular physical examinations, and have mammography every 1–2 years after age 40 and annually after age 50.

Because progestins potentially may stimulate the growth of breast tumors, the effects of the combination of estrogen and progestin on breast cancer risk also should be considered. The results of studies that have examined this issue have been inconsistent (43). Various studies have shown estrogen–progestin therapy to increase, have no effect, or actually protect against breast cancer. The results of the Women's Health Initiative trial may help to reveal whether there is truly an increased breast cancer risk associated with long-term use of estrogen and estrogen–progestin therapy.

There are concerns that in women with previously diagnosed breast cancer, estrogen use may stimulate residual cancer cells to proliferate. However, there are no studies that support the concept that estrogen use leads to an increased risk of breast cancer recurrence or a change in the survival rate of these patients. Because women with prior breast cancer have an increased risk for a second primary breast cancer (44), close surveillance is warranted. Despite the well-recognized short-term and potential long-term benefits of hormone replacement therapy, it should be considered cautiously in women who have had breast cancer. Before starting this therapy, the patient should receive extensive counseling with input from her oncologist (45).

Hypertension and Weight Gain

In a large, randomized, prospective trial of women taking hormone replacement therapy, there were no significant differences in the mean systolic or diastolic blood pressures during the 3-year period of monitoring (5). Mean waist-to-hip ratios increased slightly over time for both the placebo and estrogen-treated groups. During the 3-year trial, the greatest weight gain (2.1 kg) occurred in the placebo group while the unopposed estrogen group had the lowest weight gain (0.7 kg).

Therapeutic Options

Hormone replacement therapy should be considered to relieve vasomotor symptoms, genital urinary tract atrophy, and mood and cognitive disturbances, as well as to prevent osteoporosis and cardiovascular disease. It also may be considered to help prevent colon cancer, Alzheimer's disease, and adult tooth loss. Before therapy is instituted, a thorough medical evaluation is appropriate. The medical history should focus on contraindications to estrogen and precautions against risk factors and side effects.

Estrogen Component

Although many estrogen preparations are available, the lowest effective estrogen dose that will relieve the patient's symptoms and provide cardiovascular and bone protection should be used. Table 2 outlines several of the more commonly used estrogen preparations and their relative potencies. Because oral estrogen preparations are initially transported to the liver via portal circulation, liver conversion and degradation will alter the expected ratio of estradiol to estrone. In contrast, transdermal, buccal, or vaginally administered estrogens are not subject to the hepatic "first pass" effect, and circulating estrogen levels will mimic a steady state. Because the impact on liver metabolism is greater with oral than with transdermal administration of estrogen, at equivalent doses, oral therapy results in greater increases in HDL cholesterol, decreases in LDL cholesterol, and increases in trigly-cerides. Measurement of circulating estradiol levels may be useful as an estimate of estrogen effects on symptoms for those taking transdermal or vaginal estradiol preparations. For those taking oral preparations, particularly conjugated estrogens, measurement of estradiol levels does not accurately reflect estrogen activity (see Table 2). Follicle-stimulating hormone (FSH) levels remain in the postmenopausal range (>40 mIU/mL) for women taking hormone replacement therapy.

Dietary sources of estrogen such as phytoestrogens are available from legumes (primarily soy-based products). Because phytoestrogens are weak estrogen agonists, relatively high doses must be taken to achieve the therapeutic effects derived from hormone replacement therapy. Preliminary studies suggest that a soy protein extract can reduce hot flushes by 45%, compared with a placebo response of 30% (46). Therefore, the estimated amounts of soy products that would need to be consumed to achieve therapeutic concentrations of phytoestrogens would be enormous.

Progestin Component

There are several types of progestins that can be used in hormone replacement therapy (see Table 1). The most commonly used progestin, medroxyprogesterone acetate, is a 21-carbon derivative of progesterone. A dose of 5–10 mg of medroxyprogesterone acetate during the last 12–14 days of estrogen administration is recommended to reduce

Table 2. Commonly Used Estrogen Preparations with Estimated Relative Potencies and Approximate Circulating Levels of Estradiol and Estrone

Estrogen	Relative Potency	Estradiol (pg/mL)	Estrone (pg/mL)
Oral conjugated estrogen			
0.625 mg*	1.0	40	150
0.3 mg	0.5	<40	<150
Oral micronized estradiol			
1 mg	1.0	30	260
0.5 mg*		<30	<260
Oral piperazine estrone sulfate			
0.75 mg estropipate*	1.0	~30–40	~120
Transdermal estradiol			
0.05 mg/day*	1.0	60	50
Oral esterified estrogen			
0.3 mg	0.5	<30	~60
Estradiol vaginal ring	<0.5	No detectable change	No detectable change

*Minimal effective dose for prevention of bone loss.

Modified from Lobo R, Mishell DR, Budoff PW, et al: Estrogen Replacement Therapy, Symposium Proceedings, San Francisco, May 9–10, 1984. Abbott Pharmaceuticals, Inc, p 9.

the incidence of hyperplasia and endometrial cancer. Lower doses (2.5 mg) will provide similar protection when given continuously with estrogen.

Oral micronized progesterone preparations are not standardized but are available from individual pharmacies. Absorption is affected by progesterone particle size, food intake, the use of oil vehicles, and the type of capsules (47–49). It appears that oral micronized progesterone in the dose range of 200–300 mg per day for 12 days per month (given in divided doses) is sufficient to protect against endometrial hyperplasia (50–52).

Norethindrone, a 19-carbon compound, is the most potent oral progestin compound available for hormone replacement therapy. Doses of 1 mg are sufficient to induce endometrial secretory changes. Higher doses of norethindrone have been associated with elevations in LDL cholesterol.

Therapeutic Regimens

In women who elect to begin hormone replacement therapy, annual physical examinations, including breast and pelvic examinations, should be performed. Routine assessments such as blood pressure evaluation, Pap tests, lipid profile assessment, and mammography should be performed. In those women with a uterus, a progestin should be given either in a sequential fashion (5–10 mg of medroxyprogesterone acetate for 12–14 days each month) or continuously (2.5 mg of medroxyprogesterone acetate per day). A baseline endometrial biopsy is not necessary unless there is irregular bleeding, but a biopsy should be considered for women with unexpected or excessive bleeding.

Estrogen–Progestin Combinations

For perimenopausal women (around ages 45–50) who use low-dose oral contraceptives, it is difficult to determine whether menopause has actually occurred. Two practical approaches can be considered. In women 50 years of age or older, evaluating FSH levels at the end of the placebo week will provide an assessment of residual ovarian function. Women with FSH levels >40 mIU/mL can be started on hormone replacement therapy. Alternatively, switching from oral contraceptives to hormone replacement therapy can be tried empirically between the ages of 50 and 51 years. Because hormone replacement therapy will not effectively suppress ovarian function, those women with ovarian activity will experience episodes of intermenstrual bleeding and increased breast tenderness.

In women who have an intact uterus, the addition of a progestin to the estrogen is necessary to prevent endometrial hyperplasia or endometrial cancer. In general, administration of progestins in sequential regimen is associated with cyclic, uterine withdrawal bleeding in a fairly predictable pattern. More recently, continuous administration of progestins has been studied in large multicenter trials. This approach results in a thin, atrophic endometrium, which can be associated with amenorrhea in up to 75% of individuals after 1 year. However, this amenorrheal response is not uniform, and many women will experience unpredictable vaginal spotting. Figure 1 shows several of the more common estrogen–progestin regimens.

Progestin-Only Regimens

For women who cannot take estrogens for various reasons but who are symptomatic with hot flushes or are con-

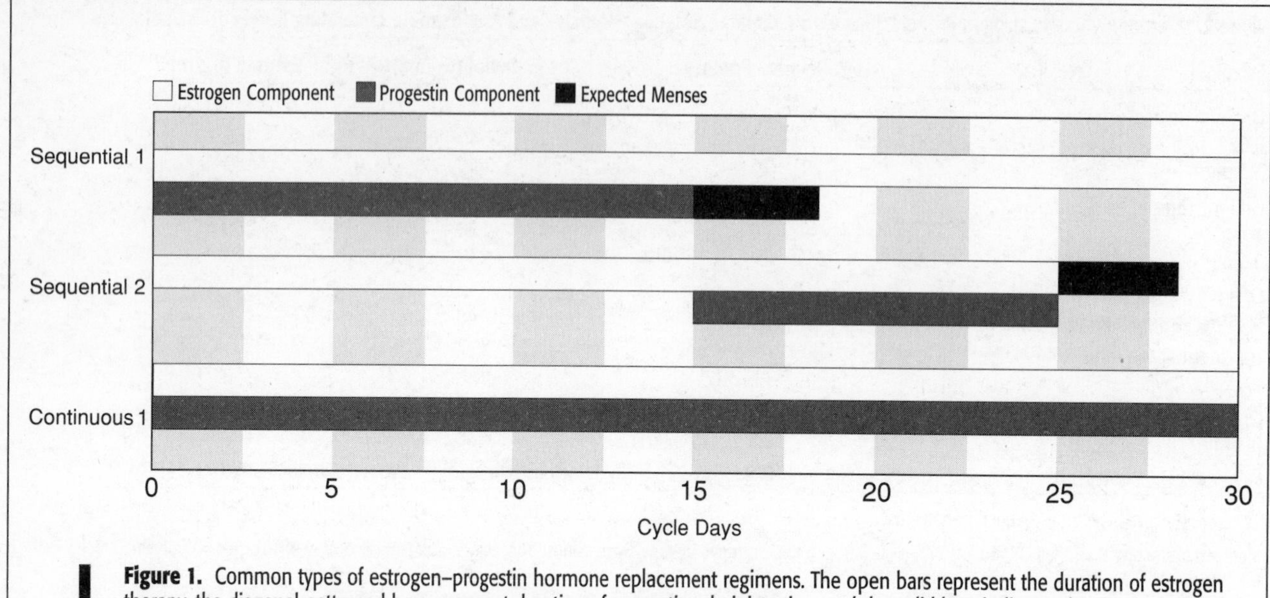

Figure 1. Common types of estrogen–progestin hormone replacement regimens. The open bars represent the duration of estrogen therapy, the diagonal-patterned bars represent duration of progestin administration, and the solid bars indicate when vaginal bleeding is expected.

cerned about osteoporosis, a progestin-only regimen is an option. The lowest doses of progestin that are effective for the treatment of vasomotor flushes are provided in Table 1.

Estrogen-Only Regimens

In women who do not have a uterus, there is no evidence that the addition of a progestin to estrogen replacement therapy provides any additional advantages or has any effect on the risk of breast cancer. For women who do not tolerate estrogen–progestin or progestin-only regimens, estrogen-only therapy can be considered if the patient can be monitored by endometrial biopsy to detect endometrial proliferation. In these circumstances, the risk of endometrial hyperplasia can approach 20% per year and require the addition of progestin therapy to reverse endometrial changes.

Estrogen–Androgen Regimens

Two estrogen–androgen dose preparations that contain 2.5 mg and 1.25 mg of methyltestosterone, respectively, are available. Absorption of methyltestosterone is excellent, allowing supraphysiologic levels of testosterone to be achieved. The use of androgens has been shown to increase total cholesterol (increase LDL cholesterol and decrease HDL cholesterol). Other side effects can include hirsutism, acne, and weight gain.

Selective Estrogen Modulators

A daily dose of 60 mg of raloxifene is currently recommended for osteoporosis prevention. In a prospective randomized multicenter trial of over 600 menopausal women, raloxifene was shown to effectively protect against bone loss and reduce LDL cholesterol levels without inducing endometrial proliferation (53). In contrast to oral estrogens, levels of HDL cholesterol and triglycerides were unchanged during treatment. The risk of venous thromboembolic phenomena associated with raloxifene use appears to be similar to that of estrogen. In this study, there were no significant differences in the proportions of women reporting hot flashes between the group receiving 60 mg of raloxifene daily and those taking placebo (26.3% and 22.7%). Thus, raloxifene would probably not be used in early menopausal women who are more likely to have hot flashes and other hypoestrogenic symptomatology.

Growth Hormone and Dehydroepiandrosterone Sulfate Replacement

Although GH and DHEAS decrease with aging, it has not been demonstrated that long-term empiric exogenous replacement of these compounds is effective in ameliorating the physiologic changes of aging. Several small studies have examined the short-term effects of GH replacement in older men and women (54). In general, short-term GH treatment will decrease body fat, increase muscle mass, and increase exercise capacity. However, the side effects of this treatment include decreased glucose tolerance, peripheral edema, and carpal tunnel syndrome. Preliminary studies suggest that short-term DHEAS therapy can increase circulating DHEAS levels in older women and by metabolic interconversion lead to increased testosterone levels (55). Both of these therapies should be considered investigational.

Strategies to Improve Compliance

Once a woman begins hormone replacement therapy, long-term compliance will become the major challenge if long-term benefits are to be realized. In a study of menopausal women between 46 and 63 years of age enrolled in a prescription plan, the stopping rate for estrogen replacement therapy was reported to be 20% at 6 months, 38% at 1 year, 51% at 18 months, and 59% at 2 years (56).

Several strategies proposed by the Women's Health Initiative may improve compliance significantly. A follow-up phone call at 6 weeks from a nurse inquiring about patient concerns seems to increase adherence. Women should be counseled regarding the development of breast tenderness, breast engorgement, and the timing of vaginal bleeding. The use of pill packs may reduce confusion of when to take estrogen–progestin regimens. For women who experience persistent or unpredictable vaginal spotting while on a continuous estrogen–progestin regimen, a switch to a cyclic regimen may increase compliance. A follow-up visit at 6 months after beginning hormone replacement therapy may help to identify any side effects. As with many compliance issues, establishing good rapport with ongoing communication between the patient and medical provider is key.

Summary

Traditionally, hormone replacement therapy has been started in menopausal women for treatment of vasomotor symptoms, mood disturbances, vaginal dryness, and osteoporosis prevention. However, because an increasing number of menopausal women are now better informed regarding menopausal changes and are beginning to embrace the concept of preventive health care, other additional benefits of hormone replacement therapy such as protection against cardiovascular disease and possible protection or delay in the onset of senile dementias make this option even more appealing. Alternatively, these perceived benefits must be assessed against the potential increased risk of breast cancer. Once the decision is made to begin hormone replacement therapy, it is important that patients continue treatment so that these long-term benefits are realized.

References

1. Cummings SR, Kelsey JL, Nevitt MC, O'Dowd KJ. Epidemiology of osteoporosis and osteoporotic fractures. Epidemiol Rev 1985;7:178–208
2. Steingold KA, Laufer L, Chetkowski RJ, DeFazio JD, Matt DW, Meldrum DR, et al. Treatment of hot flashes with transdermal estradiol administration. J Clin Endocrinol Metab 1985;61:627–632
3. Barrett-Connor E, Bush T. Estrogen and coronary heart disease in women. JAMA 1991;265:1861–1867
4. Torgerson DJ, Donaldson C, Russell IT, Reid DM. Hormone replacement therapy: compliance and cost after screening for osteoporosis. Eur J Obstet Gynecol Reprod Biol 1995;59:57–60
5. The Writing Group for the PEPI Trial. Effects of estrogen or estrogen/progestin regimens on heart disease risk factors in postmenopausal women. JAMA 1995;273:199–208
6. Love RR, Mazess RB, Barden HS, Epstein S, Newcomb PA, Jordan VC, et al. Effects of tamoxifen on bone mineral density in postmenopausal women with breast cancer. N Engl J Med 1992;326:852–856
7. Barrett-Connor E, Khaw KT. Absence of an inverse relation of dehydroepiandrosterone sulfate with cardiovascular mortality in postmenopausal women. N Engl J Med 1987;317:711
8. Musey VC, Collins DC, Musey PI, Martino-Saltzman D, Preedy JRK. Age-related changes in the female hormonal environment during reproductive life. Am J Obstet Gynecol 1987;157:312–317
9. Prior JC. Progesterone as a bone-trophic hormone. Endocr Rev 1990;11:386–398
10. Thompson JL, Butterfield GE, Marcus R, Hintz RL, Loan MV, Ghiron L, et al. The effects of recombinant human insulin-like growth factor-I and growth hormone on body composition in elderly women. J Clin Endocrinol Metab 1995;80:1845–1852
11. Judd HL, Judd GE, Lucas WE, Yen SS. Endocrine function of the postmenopausal ovary: concentration of androgens and estrogens in ovarian and peripheral vein blood. J Clin Endocrinol Metab 1974;39:1020–1024
12. Kampen DL, Sherwin BB. Estrogen use and verbal memory in healthy postmenopausal women. Obstet Gynecol 1994;83:979–983
13. Sherwin BB. The impact of different doses of estrogen and progestin on mood and sexual behavior in postmenopausal women. J Clin Endocrinol Metab 1991;72:336–343
14. Sherwin BB. Affective changes with estrogen and androgen replacement therapy in surgically menopausal women. J Affect Disord 1988;14:177–187
15. Campbell S, Whitehead M. Oestrogen therapy and the menopausal syndrome. Clin Obstet Gynaecol 1977; 4:31–47
16. Sherwin BB, Gelfand MM. Differential symptom response to parenteral estrogen and/or androgen administration in the surgical menopause. Am J Obstet Gynecol 1989;151: 153–160
17. Sherwin BB. Estrogen and/or androgen replacement therapy and cognitive functioning in surgically menopausal women. Psychoneuroendocrinology 1988;13:345–357
18. Fillit H, Weinreb H, Cholst I, Luine V, McEwen B, Amador R, et al. Observations in a preliminary open trial of estradiol therapy for senile dementia-Alzheimer's type. Psychoneuroendocrinology 1986;11:337–345

19. Funk JL, Mortel KF, Meyer JS. Effects of estrogen replacement therapy on cerebral perfusion and cognition among postmenopausal women. Dementia 1991;2:268–272

20. Henderson VW, Paganini-Hill A, Emanuel CK, Dunn ME, Buckwalter JG. Estrogen replacement therapy in older women. Arch Neurol 1994;51:896–900

21. Honjo H, Tanaka K, Kashiwagi T, Urabe M, Okada H, Hayashi M, et al. Senile dementia-Alzheimer's type and estrogen. Horm Metab Res 1995;27:204–207

22. Gangar KF, Vyas S, Whitehead M, Crook D, Meire H, Campbell S. Pulsatility index in internal carotid artery in relation to transdermal oestradiol and time since menopause. Lancet 1991;338:839–842

23. Sheridan PJ. Autoradiographic localization of steroid receptors in the brain. Clin Neuropharmacol 1984;7:281–295

24. Lebherz TB, French L. Nonhormonal treatment of the menopausal syndrome: a double-blind evaluation of an autonomic system stabilizer. Obstet Gynecol 1969; 33:795–799

25. Bush TL, Cowan LD, Barrett-Connor E, Criqui MH, Karon JM, Wallace RB, et al. Estrogen use and all-cause mortality. JAMA 1983;249:903–906

26. Stampfer MJ, Colditz GA. Estrogen replacement therapy and coronary heart disease: a quantitative assessment of the epidemiologic evidence. Prev Med 1991;20:47–63

27. Mikkola T, Turunen P, Avela K, Orpana A, Viinikka L, Ylikorkala O. 17 β-estradiol stimulates prostacyclin, but not endothelin-1, production in human vascular endothelial cells. J Clin Endocrinol Metab 1995;80:1832–1836

28. Tang M, Subbiah R. Estrogens protect against hydrogen peroxide and arachidonic acid induced DNA damage. Biochim Biophys Acta 1996;1299:155–159

29. Subbiah MT, Kessel B, Agrawal M, Rajan R, Abplanalp W, Rymaszewski Z. Antioxidant potential of specific estrogens on lipid peroxidation. J Clin Endocrinol Metab 1993;77: 1095–1097

30. Kleerekoper M, Mendlovic B. Sodium fluoride therapy of postmenopausal osteoporosis. Endocr Rev 1993;14: 312–323

31. Reginster JY, Deroisy R, Lecart MP, Sarlet N, Zegels B, Jupsin I, et al. A double-blind, placebo-controlled, dose-finding trial of intermittent nasal salmon calcitonin for prevention of postmenopausal lumbar spine bone loss. Am J Med 1995;98:452–458

32. Bergman A, Brenner PF. Beneficial effects of pharmacologic agents—genitourinary. In: Mishell DR, Jr, ed. Menopause: physiology and pharmacology. Chicago: Year Book Medical Publishers, Inc, 1987:151–164

33. Daly E, Vessey MP, Hawkins MM, Carson JL, Gough P, Marsh S. Risk of venous thromboembolism in users of hormone replacement therapy. Lancet 1996;348:977–980

34. Grodstein F, Stampfer MJ, Goldhaber SZ, Manson JE, Colditz GA, Speizer FE, et al. Prospective study of exogenous hormones and risk of pulmonary embolism in women. Lancet 1996; 348:983–987

35. Jick H, Derby LE, Myers MW, Vasilakis C, Newtom KM. Risk of hospital admission for idiopathic venous thromboembolism among users of postmenopausal oestrogens. Lancet 1996;348:981–983

36. The Writing Group for the PEPI Trial. Effects of hormone replacement therapy on endometrial histology in postmenopausal women. JAMA 1996;275:370–375

37. American College of Obstetricians and Gynecologists. Estrogen replacement therapy and endometrial cancer. ACOG Committee Opinion 126. Washington, DC: ACOG, 1993

38. Barbieri RL. Hormone treatment of endometriosis: the estrogen threshold hypothesis. Am J Obstet Gynecol 1992; 166:740–745

39. Colditz GA, Hankinson SE, Hunter DJ, Willett WC, Manson JE, Stampfer MJ, et al. The use of estrogens and progestins and the risk of breast cancer in postmenopausal women. N Engl J Med 1995;332:1589–1593

40. Steinberg KK, Thacker SB, Smith SJ, Stroup DF, Zack MM, Flanders WD, et al. A meta-analysis of the effect of estrogen replacement therapy on the risk of breast cancer. JAMA 1991;265:1985–1990

41. Dupont WD, Page DL. Menopausal estrogen replacement therapy and breast cancer. Arch Intern Med 1991;151: 67–72

42. Henrich JB. The postmenopausal estrogen/breast cancer controversy. JAMA 1992;268:1900–1902

43. Bergkvist L, Adami H, Persson I, Hoover R, Schairer C. The risk of breast cancer after estrogen and estrogen-progestin replacement. N Engl J Med 1989;321:293–297

44. Fornander T, Rutquist LE, Cedermark B, Glas U, Mattsson A, Silfversward C, et al. Adjuvant tamoxifen in early breast cancer: occurrence of new primary cancers. Lancet 1989;1: 117–120

45. American College of Obstetricians and Gynecologists. Estrogen replacement therapy in women with previously treated breast cancer. ACOG Committee Opinion 135. Washington, DC: ACOG, 1994

46. Albertazzi P, Pansini F, Bonaccorsi G, Zanotti L, Forini E, de Aloysio D. The effect of dietary soy supplementation on hot flushes. Obstet Gynecol 1998;91:6–11

47. Hargrove JT, Maxson WS, Wentz AC. Absorption of oral progesterone is influenced by vehicle and particle size. Am J Obstet Gynecol 1989;161:948–951

48. Nakajima ST, Gibson M. The effect of a meal on circulating steady-state progesterone levels. J Clin Endocrinol Metab 1989;69:917–919

49. Simon JA, Robinson DE, Andrews MC, Hildebrand JR, Rocci ML Jr, Blake RE, et al. The absorption of oral micronized progesterone: the effect of food, dose proportionality, and comparison with intramuscular progesterone. Fertil Steril 1993;60:26–33

50. Gillet JY, Andre G, Faguer B, Erny R, Buvat-Herbaut M, Domin MA, et al. Induction of amenorrhea during hormone replacement therapy: optimal micronized progesterone dose. A multicenter study. Maturitas 1994;19:103–115

51. Hargrove JT, Maxon WS, Wentz AC, Burnett LS. Menopausal hormone replacement therapy with continuous daily oral micronized estradiol and progesterone. Obstet Gynecol 1989;73:606–612

52. Lane G, Siddle NC, Ryder TA, Pryse-Davies J, King RJB, Whitehead MI. Dose dependent effects of oral progesterone on oestrogenised postmenopausal endometrium. BMJ 1983;287:1241–1245

53. Delmas PD, Bjarnason NH, Mitlak BH, Ravoux A-C, Shah AS, Huster WJ, et al. Effects of raloxifene on bone mineral density, serum cholesterol concentrations, and uterine endometrium in postmenopausal women. N Engl J Med 1997;337:1641–1647

54. Corpas E, Harman SM, Blackman MR. Human growth hormone and human aging. Endocr Rev 1993;14:20–39

55. Morales AJ, Nolan JJ, Nelson JC, Yen SSC. Effects of replacement dose of dehydroepiandrosterone in men and women of advancing age. J Clin Endocrinol Metab 1994;78:1360–1367

56. Berman RS, Epstein RS, Lydick EG. Compliance of women in taking estrogen replacement therapy. J Womens Health 1996;5:213–220

ISSN 1074-8628

The American College of Obstetricians and Gynecologists
409 12th Street, SW
PO Box 96920
Washington, DC 20090-6920

12345/21098

Number 202—February 1995

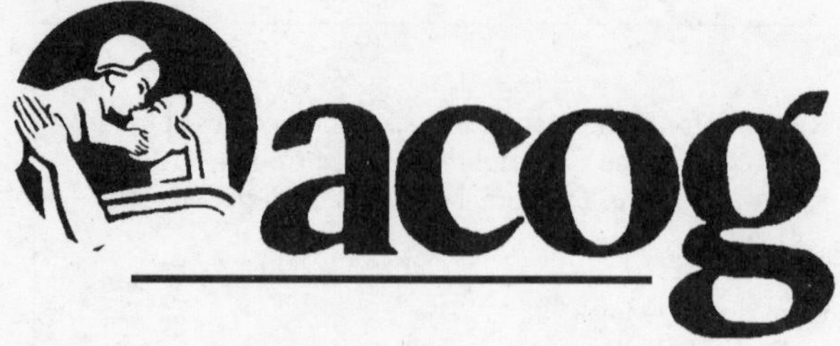

Technical Bulletin

An Educational Aid to Obstetrician–Gynecologists

Hyperandrogenic Chronic Anovulation

The process of ovulation requires the precise integration of hypothalamic, pituitary, and ovarian events. Dysfunction in these organs can result in oligoovulation or anovulation. In the presence of a normally functioning uterus, patients with anovulation can have a number of menstrual irregularities ranging from amenorrhea to abnormal uterine bleeding. In one Swedish population-based study, the prevalence of amenorrhea of 3 months' duration was 1.8%, and the prevalence of amenorrhea of 12 months' duration was 1.2% (1). This suggests that in the study population, the prevalence of chronic oligo-ovulation or anovulation was at least 1–2%.

In the absence of ovarian failure, there are many discrete disease processes that can cause anovulation; they can be divided into central and peripheral causes as shown in the box. In one population-based study of patients diagnosed with adult-onset amenorrhea in association with chronic anovulation, excluding anatomic causes and ovarian failure, 32% had hypothalamic chronic anovulation, 17% had hyperprolactinemic chronic anovulation, and 35% had hyperandrogenic chronic anovulation (2). Thus, hyperandrogenic chronic anovulation is one of the most common causes of anovulation and amenorrhea in women and is the focus of this bulletin. A detailed discussion of all three processes is beyond the scope of this bulletin. Further information is presented elsewhere (3–6), but general comments and principles follow.

Classification

The two most common causes of chronic anovulation are hypothalamic chronic anovulation and hyperandrogenic chronic anovulation (eg, polycystic ovary syndrome [PCO]).

Premature ovarian failure is a relatively common cause of anovulation. A repetitively elevated level of follicle-stimulating hormone (FSH) in serum suggests the diagnosis. The etiology of premature ovarian failure is diverse and includes causes of genetic (galactosemia, X chromosome abnormalities), immune, chemical (alkylating agents), radiation, and idiopathic origin.

There is no specific finding on physical examination or laboratory testing that has a high sensitivity or specificity for diagnosing "hypothalamic" anovulation. Consequently, hypothalamic anovulation is a diagnosis of exclusion. Withdrawal bleeding following a progestin challenge test is evidence of sufficient endogenous estrogen to stimulate growth of the endometrium and a patent

Causes of Chronic Anovulation

Central causes

- Hypothalamic chronic anovulation (dysfunctional pulsatile gonadotropin-releasing hormone secretion)
  - Anorexia nervosa and bulimia
  - Simple weight loss, diet, or malnutrition
  - Exercise-associated amenorrhea
  - Psychogenic amenorrhea
  - Pseudocyesis
  - Systemic debilitating illnesses
- Forms of isolated gonadotropin deficiency (female Kallmann syndrome)
- Pituitary chronic anovulation
  - Hypothalamic–pituitary damage from any of several causes
  - Idiopathic
- Hyperprolactinemic chronic anovulation (galactorrhea) of multiple etiologies (see box: "Conditions Associated with Inappropriate Prolactin Secretion")

Peripheral causes (due to inappropriate feedback)

- Neoplasms producing androgens or estrogens
- Neoplasms producing chorionic gonadotropin
- Liver and renal disease
- Obesity
- Congenital adrenal hyperplasia, classical and nonclassical

Combined central and peripheral causes (due to inappropriate feedback secondary to combined central–peripheral dysfunction)

- Polycystic ovary syndrome (functional androgen excess of adrenal or ovarian origin or both, hyperandrogenic chronic anovulation)
- Thyroid dysfunction
- Cushing syndrome
- Acromegaly

lower genital tract. It is nonspecific, however, and is not diagnostic of a particular disorder.

Anovulation caused by hypothalamic dysfunction (decreased gonadotropin-releasing hormone [GnRH] pulse frequency or amplitude or both) is not typically associated with a structural abnormality. Rather, abnormalities in neuroendocrine factors regulating GnRH secretion are the apparent cause of most cases of anovulation related to hypothalamic dysfunction. Preliminary evidence suggests that excessive hypothalamic levels of endogenous opioids, dopamine, melatonin, or a combination of these contribute to low GnRH secretion in some anovulatory women with hypothalamic dysfunction (7–9). Environmental "stress" may be an important factor causing hypothalamic alterations resulting in anovulation.

Hyperprolactinemia is noted in 15% of patients with amenorrhea. Consideration should be given to physiologic, pharmacologic, and pathologic causes of prolactin elevation in the patient with chronic anovulation. The box outlines the causes of hyperprolactinemia. Most patients with chronic anovulation are also hypoestrogenic. As a consequence, rapid bone loss is a concern in this subset of patients.

Chronic anovulation syndrome associated with signs of hyperandrogenism is a distinct subgroup of anovulatory women. This condition has been described by various names, such as Stein-Leventhal syndrome, PCO, functional ovarian hyperandrogenism, and hyperandrogenic chronic anovulation. Clinical features often associated with this syndrome include the following:

- Menstrual irregularity caused by oligoovulation or anovulation
- Signs of hyperandrogenism, such as hirsutism
- Obesity
- Perimenarchal onset
- Infertility due to anovulation
- Excess number of small antral follicles noted on ultrasonographic visualization of the ovaries
- Elevated levels of circulating androgen concentrations, such as elevated levels of free testosterone, total testosterone, androstenedione, dehydroepiandrosterone (DHEA), and DHEA sulfate (DHEAS)
- Elevated levels of circulating luteinizing hormone (LH)
- Insulin resistance and hyperinsulinemia

Conditions Associated with Inappropriate Prolactin Secretion

Physiologic
- Exercise
- Pregnancy
- Breast examination (physical examination of the breasts may elevate prolactin)

Pharmacologic
- Estrogen therapy
- Anesthesia
- Dopamine-depleting agents (reserpine, α-methyldopa)
- Dopamine receptor blocking agents (phenothiazine, metoclopramide)
- Histamine H_2-receptor antagonist (cimetidine)
- Serotoninergic stimulation (amphetamines)

Pathologic
- Hypothalamic lesions
- Pituitary tumors
- Empty sella syndrome
- Reflex causes (chest wall lesions)
- Hypothyroidism
- Renal failure
- Ectopic production
  - Bronchogenic carcinoma
  - Hypernephroma

Adapted from Yen SSC. Prolactin in human reproduction. In: Yen SSC, Jaffe RB, eds. Reproductive endocrinology: physiology, pathophysiology and clinical management. 3rd ed. Philadelphia: WB Saunders Co, 1991:364

Congenital Adrenal Hyperplasia

One example of a unique group of genetic disorders which can appear identical to hyperandrogenic chronic anovulation is congenital adrenal hyperplasia caused by mutations in enzymes of adrenal steroidogenesis. The function of the adrenal cortex is to synthesize glucocorticoids (cortisol), mineralocorticoids (aldosterone), and adrenal androgens. Five enzymes are required to convert cholesterol to cortisol (Fig. 1). Genetic disorders in three of these enzymes (21-hydroxylase, 11β-hydroxylase, and 3β-hydroxy-Δ^5-steroid dehydrogenase-isomerase) can be associated with overproduction of adrenal androgens and hyperandrogenic chronic anovulation. Disorders of the 21-hydroxylase genes are well characterized and occur in 2–4% of hyperandrogenic women (10). Disorders of the 11β-hydroxylase gene occur infrequently (less than 1% of hyperandrogenic women) (11). The genetics of human 3β-hydroxy-Δ^5-steroid dehydrogenase-isomerase are not fully understood, but there are probably multiple genes for this enzyme.

Mutations in the 21-hydroxylase gene that result in failure to synthesize a fully functional enzyme cause a decrease in the conversion of 17α-hydroxyprogesterone to 11-deoxycorticosterone. This causes a relative decrease in cortisol production, an increase in corticotropin (ACTH) secretion, and an increase in the production of 17α-hydroxyprogesterone, androstenedione, DHEA, DHEAS, and testosterone. If the mutation(s) causes near-complete loss of 21-hydroxylase activity, adrenal androgen production will be increased in utero, and a female infant may be born with the stigmata of classical congenital adrenal hyperplasia: clitoromegaly, labioscrotal fusion, and abnormal course of the urethra. If the mutation(s) causes a modest decrease in 21-hydroxylase activity, the phenotype may be nonclassical, or late-onset, adrenal hyperplasia, the signs of which include chronic anovulation, hirsutism, and menstrual irregularities.

For most genetic disorders, many different mutations can produce a similar phenotype. Dozens of different mutations in the 21-hydroxylase gene can cause adrenal hyperplasia; some common molecular changes include: nonsense, missense, and frame shift mutations; deletions; gene conversions between the active 21-hydroxylase gene (CYP21) and a pseudogene (CYP21P); and internal mutations within intron 2 that cause abnormal RNA splicing (12, 13). Many of the most severe cases of 21-hydroxylase adrenal hyperplasia, such as the salt-wasting form, are associated with gene deletion at the 5' end of the gene.

An unknown proportion of women believed to have PCO will in fact, if evaluated, demonstrate nonclassical (late-onset) adrenal hyperplasia. Although elevated levels of 17α-hydroxyprogesterone are diagnostic, the routine use of this test in PCO patients is controversial. Because of increased genetic susceptibility, women of Ashkenazic Jewish or Eskimo ancestry should be considered for testing.

Etiology

For most women with hyperandrogenic chronic anovulation, a specific etiology cannot be identified. These women appear to have multiple endocrine abnormalities that act in concert to cause chronic anovulation.

A critically important abnormality is increased LH secretion from the anterior pituitary gland. Detailed studies suggest that the increased circulating LH concentrations are caused by marked increases in LH pulse amplitude and modest increases in LH pulse frequency (14). The increase in LH pulse frequency is most likely caused by an increase in hypothalamic GnRH pulse frequency. The neuroendocrine events that produce an increase in GnRH pulse frequency are not well characterized but may involve hypothalamic opioid and catecholamine systems. The increase in LH pulse amplitude may be due to excess GnRH secretion or an excessively sensitive pituitary LH response to GnRH or both. Estradiol may play an important role in sensitizing the pituitary to GnRH. It is not clear whether the initial abnormality in most of these individuals is peripheral or central.

The chronic increase in LH secretion causes the ovarian stroma and theca of women with hyperandrogenism to secrete more androstenedione and testosterone per milligram of tissue than does ovarian tissue from ovulatory

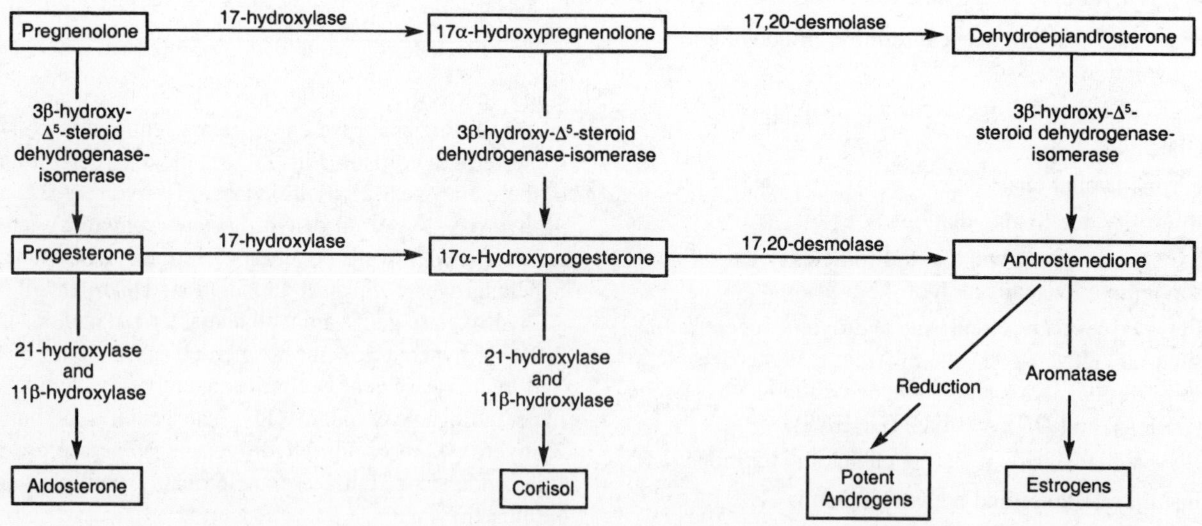

FIG. 1. The ovary, the testis, and the adrenal gland produce six common core steroids. The core Δ^5 steroids are pregnenolone, 17α-hydroxypregnenolone, and dehydroepiandrosterone. The core Δ^4 steroids are progesterone, 17α-hydroxyprogesterone, and androstenedione. The core steroids are the important precursors for the production of all gonadal steroids, glucocorticoids, and mineralocorticoids. Progesterone is an important gonadal steroid and is the precursor for all mineralocorticoids. 17α-Hydroxyprogesterone is the precursor for all glucocorticoids. Androstenedione is the precursor for the androgens and estrogens.

women (15). This ovarian androgen overproduction may be the result of chronic exposure of the ovary to excessive LH, increased sensitivity of the ovary to LH, or the effects of other growth factors (insulinlike growth factor-I, or somatomedin C) that act in concert with LH to stimulate ovarian androgen production.

Recent studies suggest that many hyperandrogenic women are insulin resistant and have compensatory hyperinsulinemia. These findings suggest a link between central metabolism and ovarian hyperandrogenism and may help explain the association between obesity and chronic anovulation.

Women with PCO have an increased frequency of glucose intolerance and lipid abnormalities. Consequently, these parameters should be evaluated in these patients. Chronic hyperinsulinemia may cause the ovary to secrete excess quantities of androgens. Mutations in the insulin receptor gene have been found in a small number of women with the HAIR-AN syndrome (a combination of hyperandrogenism, insulin resistance, and acanthosis nigricans). These women are typically obese and hirsute and are examples of the extreme effects of hyperandrogenic chronic anovulation.

Clinical Evaluation

In adult women with chronic anovulation and no evidence of hyperandrogenism, the clinical evaluation should focus on potential hypothalamic disorders (weight loss, anorexia, stress, strenuous exercise, infiltrative lesions), pituitary disorders (prolactinoma, empty sella, Sheehan syndrome, Cushing disease), and premature ovarian failure as potential etiologies. Measurements of FSH (to rule out ovarian failure), thyroid-stimulating hormone (to exclude the presence of hypothyroidism), and prolactin (to search for the presence of a prolactinoma or other hypothalamic–pituitary dysfunction) in serum are warranted. In addition, a progestin withdrawal test (medroxyprogesterone acetate, 10 mg/d for 10 days or progesterone in oil, 100–200 mg intramuscularly) is useful to evaluate the structural integrity of the uterus and to assess endogenous estrogen status.

In women with hyperandrogenic chronic anovulation, specific causes, such as ovarian or adrenal tumors or 21-hydroxylase deficiency, are unusual; most have a complex disorder caused by multiple endocrine abnormalities. These women should be evaluated as follows.

History

Key aspects of the history include the following:

- Time of onset of the syndrome. Many women with hyperandrogenic chronic anovulation note onset during the teenage years.
- Rate of progression. Clinically aggressive androgen-secreting tumors of the ovary and adrenal gland typically appear with a rapid onset of hirsutism and signs of virilization.
- State of menstrual cycles. In general, the level of androgen overproduction correlates with menstrual abnormalities. Marked androgen overproduction is most often associated with amenorrhea, while women with hirsutism and normal androgen levels often have regular menses. In addition, women with very high androgen levels may not respond to progestin withdrawal.

Physical Examination

Physical examination should include evaluation for signs of virilization, including deepening of the voice, balding, clitoromegaly, or increased body mass. Signs of Cushing disease, which include weakness, central obesity, spontaneous ecchymoses, purple striae of greater than 1 cm, hypokalemia, and osteoporosis, should be noted. Some women with hyperprolactinemia will initially have signs of hyperandrogenic chronic anovulation; therefore, patients should be evaluated for galactorrhea. Acanthosis nigricans may be present; it is a velvety, verrucous, hyperpigmented skin change that usually develops in intertriginous areas such as the nape of the neck, in the axillae, beneath the breasts, or on the medial aspects of the thighs. Its presence in a young, anovulatory woman strongly suggests insulin resistance and hyperinsulinemia. Patients should also be evaluated for adnexal masses.

There are various methods for the objective assessment of the severity of the hirsutism. Two of the most common are the Ferriman–Gallwey system (16) and the Bardin–Lipsett method (17). An effort should be made to document objectively the extent of the findings by a detailed description or photographs.

Laboratory Evaluation

The laboratory evaluation of hyperandrogenic chronic anovulation is controversial, and what is considered a standard evaluation varies substantially among physicians. It may include measurement of levels of: free or total testosterone or both, 8-AM 17α-hydroxyprogesterone during the follicular phase, DHEAS, and prolactin if amenorrhea is present.

Some authorities suggest that no laboratory studies are necessary for anovulatory women with mild hirsutism and uterine bleeding after a progestin challenge. However, this strategy will not identify women with 21-hydroxylase, late-onset adrenal hyperplasia (which requires measurement of 17α-hydroxyprogesterone). In addition, women with hyperandrogenic anovulation who are considering clomiphene citrate for ovulation induction will benefit from measurement of DHEAS to identify those who would be candidates for glucocorticoid therapy.

The purpose of the total testosterone assay is to aid in evaluating the severity of the hyperandrogenic process. In normal women, circulating levels of total testosterone average approximately 30 ng/dl, with an upper limit of normal near 75 ng/dl. Women with mild hyperandrogenism often have total testosterone levels of near 75 ng/dl. Severe hyperandrogenism is typically associated with total testosterone levels of greater than 200 ng/dl. If the level of total testosterone is greater than 200 ng/dl, the patient probably has ovarian stromal hyperthecosis or an adrenal or ovarian tumor; an adrenal or ovarian tumor is unlikely with lower levels. Clinicians must be aware that some commercial testosterone assays are not specific and assay for both testosterone and dihydrotestosterone (as well as other androgens). These assays typically yield testosterone results 50–100% higher than specific testosterone assays. Some medications, such as danazol, cross-react in the testosterone assay and are associated with falsely elevated testosterone measurements.

Testosterone circulates in three forms: free, weakly bound to albumin, and tightly bound to sex hormone-binding globulin (SHBG). Free and albumin-bound testosterone are the biologically active forms of circulating testosterone. In the hyperandrogenic state, SHBG levels are often decreased, resulting in a relative decrease in total testosterone and an increase in free testosterone. Measurement of free testosterone is a more sensitive test than total testosterone for identifying hyperandrogenic states. If free-testosterone and total-testosterone measurements are available at a similar cost, measurement of free testosterone may be preferable.

The purpose of measuring 17α-hydroxyprogesterone is to screen for nonclassical, late-onset adrenal hyperplasia resulting from a heterozygous state—21-hydroxylase deficiency. The practicality of screening all hyperandrogenic women for 21-hydroxylase deficiency is questionable because only 4% have this condition. However, therapy for this disorder is specific (glucocorticoids), and identification of a woman with late-onset adrenal hyperplasia may have implications for preconceptional counseling.

If the 8-AM measurement of 17α-hydroxyprogesterone in the follicular phase of the menstrual cycle is greater than 4 ng/ml, it is likely that the patient has nonclassical or late onset 21-hydroxylase adrenal hyperplasia (10). This can be confirmed by a 60-minute ACTH stimulation test: administering 0.25 mg of cosyntropin ($ACTH_{1-24}$) intravenously and measuring levels of 17α-hydroxyprogesterone 60 minutes later. Levels of greater than 10 ng/ml after ACTH stimulation strongly suggest the presence of 21-hydroxylase deficiency (18). If the 8-AM measurement is less than 2 ng/ml, then 21-hydroxylase adrenal hyperplasia is highly unlikely (10). If the same measurement yields concentrations of 2–4 ng/ml, an ACTH stimulation test may be needed to determine whether 21-hydroxylase deficiency is present.

A serum DHEAS measurement that is more than twice the upper limit of normal (typically 700 μg/dl) may signify the presence of an adrenal tumor. Although DHEAS is largely of adrenal origin, most women with late-onset adrenal hyperplasia do not have markedly elevated levels of DHEAS (19). In contrast, many women with an ovarian cause of hyperandrogenism do have somewhat elevated levels of DHEAS in the range of 300–700 μg/dl (19). This paradox limits the utility of the DHEAS measurement in identifying the source of hyperandrogenism. Measurement of DHEAS may have value in the evaluation of women with hyperandrogenism and infertility. In these women, if the level of DHEAS is greater than 200 μg/dl, treatment with dexamethasone may improve the ovarian response to clomiphene (20).

In a patient with a prior offspring with ambiguous genitalia secondary to congenital adrenal hyperplasia who conceives again, the possibility of an affected fetus must be considered. Once a positive pregnancy test is established, the patient should be counseled about the administration of glucocorticoid therapy (dexamethasone) to prevent virilization of a female fetus (21). Therapy is continued until either chorionic villus sampling or amniocentesis is performed. If the karyotype is 46,XX, treatment is continued.

Clinical Considerations and Management

Women with hyperandrogenic chronic anovulation often seek medical care for treatment of hirsutism, infertility due to anovulation, irregular uterine bleeding, or some combination of these.

Hirsutism

Hirsutism and acne caused by hyperandrogenism are best treated by simultaneously suppressing androgen production and action. Strategies and pharmacologic agents that may be effective include weight loss, estrogen–progestin oral contraceptives, antiandrogens such as spironolactone, and GnRH analogues (3).

In obese women with hyperandrogenic chronic anovulation, weight loss can often result in a decrease in levels of circulating testosterone and androstenedione. In one study of obese women, significant weight loss resulted in significant decreases in plasma androstenedione concentrations and plasma testosterone concentrations (22). Another study evaluated the effects of weight loss on 20 obese women with hyperandrogenic chronic anovulation (23). The mean body mass index of the subjects was 32.1 kg/m^2. Body mass index is calculated by dividing the subject's weight (in kilograms) by height (in meters) squared. A person with a body mass index greater than 26 kg/m^2 is considered overweight; a person with an index greater than 29 kg/m^2 is considered obese. After weight loss, levels of insulin, testosterone, progesterone, and LH were significantly reduced. Taken together, these studies clearly suggest that weight loss is associated with decreased circulating androgens in obese women with hyperandrogenic chronic anovulation.

Combined estrogen–progestin therapy is the cornerstone of pharmacologic treatment of hirsutism in women with hyperandrogenic chronic anovulation. Estrogen–progestin agents decrease LH and FSH secretion and ovarian production of androstenedione and testosterone, increase hepatic production of SHBG, and decrease levels of circulating DHEAS. The combination of estrogen–progestin agents with an antiandrogen such as spironolactone, 100–200 mg/d, may be especially useful in the treatment of hirsutism; however, spironolactone has not been approved by the U.S. Food and Drug Administration for treatment of hirsutism. Although some controversy exists with respect to cyproterone acetate versus spironolactone, current evidence suggests they are equally effective (24).

Recently, some investigators have used GnRH agonists in combination with estrogen–progestin in treatment of chronic anovulation with hyperandrogenism (25). However, this is considered investigational at present. Another investigational approach is the use of topical antiandrogens which inhibit hair follicle growth.

Ovulation Induction

Based on the clinical and laboratory evaluations, diagnosed disorders should be treated, which will likely result in ovulation. Primary treatment in the obese woman with hyperandrogenic chronic anovulation is weight loss. These patients may spontaneously ovulate if they lose as little as 10% of their body weight (22, 23). For the remainder of the patients, clomiphene citrate is the preferred therapy. Women with elevated DHEAS may benefit from pretreatment with glucocorticoids (20).

Unopposed Estrogen

Women with unopposed estrogen are at an increased risk for developing endometrial hyperplasia and carcinoma and possibly breast carcinoma (26). In one population-based study, the increased risk of carcinoma was threefold. Progestin replacement decreases the risk of developing endometrial carcinoma. In women with chronic anovulation and irregular uterine bleeding who have unopposed estrogen, sampling of the endometrium may be warranted.

Summary

The evaluation and treatment of chronic anovulation requires knowledge of the many disorders which may present as menstrual abnormalities. The evaluation should document physical findings suggestive of androgen excess. Initial evaluation includes an orderly approach to laboratory testing. Underlying disorders may include life-threatening diagnoses. The goals of therapy include correction of life-threatening disorders, protection of endometrial health, preservation or restoration of fertility, and reversal of cosmetically disturbing hirsutism.

REFERENCES

1. Pettersson F, Fries H, Nillius SJ. Epidemiology of secondary amenorrhea. I. Incidence and prevalence rates. Am J Obstet Gynecol 1973;117:80–86
2. Reindollar RH, Novak M, Tho SPT, McDonough PG. Adult-onset amenorrhea: a study of 262 patients. Am J Obstet Gynecol 1986;155:531–543
3. American College of Obstetricians and Gynecologists. Evaluation and treatment of hirsute women. ACOG Technical Bulletin 103. Washington, DC: ACOG, 1987
4. American College of Obstetricians and Gynecologists. Managing the anovulatory state: medical induction of ovulation. ACOG Technical Bulletin 197. Washington, DC: ACOG, 1994
5. American College of Obstetricians and Gynecologists. Amenorrhea. ACOG Technical Bulletin 128. Washington, DC: ACOG, 1989
6. American College of Obstetricians and Gynecologists. Women and exercise. ACOG Technical Bulletin 173. Washington, DC: ACOG, 1992
7. Berga SL, Loucks AB, Rossmanith WG, Kettel LM, Laughlin GA, Yen SSC. Acceleration of luteinizing hormone pulse frequency in functional hypothalamic amenorrhea by dopaminergic blockade. J Clin Endocrinol Metab 1991;72:151–156
8. Khoury SA, Reame NE, Kelch RP, Marshall JC. Diurnal patterns of pulsatile luteinizing hormone secretion in hypothalamic amenorrhea: reproducibility and responses to opiate blockade and an α_2-adrenergic agonist. J Clin Endocrinol Metab 1987;64:755–762
9. Laughlin GA, Loucks AB, Yen SSC. Marked augmentation of nocturnal melatonin secretion in amenorrheic athletes, but not in cycling athletes: unaltered opioidergic or dopaminergic blockade. J Clin Endocrinol Metab 1991;73:1321–1326
10. Azziz R, Zacur HA. 21-hydroxylase deficiency in female hyperandrogenism: screening and diagnosis. J Clin Endocrinol Metab 1989;69:577–584

11. Azziz R, Boots LR, Parker CR Jr, Bradley E Jr, Zacur HA. 11β-hydroxylase deficiency in hyperandrogenism. Fertil Steril 1991;55:733–741

12. Haglund-Stengler B, Ritzén EM, Luthman H. 21-hydroxylase deficiency: disease-causing mutations characterized by densitometry of 21-hydroxylase-specific deoxyribonucleic acid fragments. J Clin Endocrinol Metab 1990; 70:43–48

13. Owerbach D, Crawford YM, Draznin MB. Direct analysis of CYP21B genes in 21-hydroxylase deficiency using polymerase chain reaction amplification. Mol Endocrinol 1990;4:125–131

14. Waldstreicher J, Santoro NF, Hall JE, Filicori M, Crowley WF Jr. Hyperfunction of the hypothalamic–pituitary axis in women with polycystic ovarian disease: indirect evidence for partial gonadotroph desensitization. J Clin Endocrinol Metab 1988;66:165–172

15. Barbieri RL, Makris A, Randall RW, Daniels G, Kistner RW, Ryan KJ. Insulin stimulates androgen accumulation in incubations of ovarian stroma obtained from women with hyperandrogenism. J Clin Endrocrinol Metab 1986; 62:904–910

16. Ferriman D, Gallwey JD. Clinical assessment of body hair growth in women. J Clin Endocrinol Metab 1961; 21:1440–1447

17. Bardin CW, Lipsett MB. Testosterone and androstenedione blood production rates in normal women and women with idiopathic hirsutism or polycystic ovaries. J Clin Invest 1967;46:891–902

18. New MI, Lorenzen F, Lerner AJ, Kohn B, Oberfield SE, Pollack MS, et al. Genotyping steroid 21-hydroxylase deficiency: hormonal reference data. J Clin Endocrinol Metab 1983;57:320–326

19. Siegel SF, Finegold DN, Lanes R, Lee PA. ACTH stimulation tests and plasma dehydroepiandrosterone sulfate levels in women with hirsutism. N Engl J Med 1990;323:849–854

20. Daly DC, Walters CA, Soto-Albors CE, Tohan N, Riddick DH. A randomized study of dexamethasone in ovulation induction with clomiphene citrate. Fertil Steril 1984; 41:844–848

21. New MI. Prenatal diagnosis and treatment of adrenogenital syndrome (steroid 21-hydroxylase deficiency). Dev Pharmacol Ther 1990;15:200–210

22. Bates GW, Whitworth NS. Effect of body weight reduction on plasma androgens in obese, infertile women. Fertil Steril 1982;38:406–409

23. Pasquali R, Antenucci D, Casimirri F, Venturoli S, Paradisi R, Fabbri R, et al. Clinical and hormonal characteristics of obese and amenorrheic hyperandrogenic women before and after weight loss. J Clin Endocrinol Metab 1989;68: 173–179

24. O'Brien RC, Cooper ME, Murray RML, Seeman E, Thomas AK, Jerums G. Comparison of sequential cyproterone acetate/estrogen *versus* spironolactone/oral contraceptive in the treatment of hirsutism. J Clin Endocrinol Metab 1991;72:1008–1013

25. Andreyko JL, Monroe SE, Jaffe RB. Treatment of hirsutism with a gonadotropin-releasing hormone agonist (nafarelin). J Clin Endocrinol Metab 1986;63:854–859

26. Coulam CB, Annegers JF, Kranz JS. Chronic anovulation syndrome and associated neoplasia. Obstet Gynecol 1983;61:403–407

This Technical Bulletin was developed under the direction of the Committee on Technical Bulletins of the American College of Obstetricians and Gynecologists as an educational aid to obstetricians and gynecologists. The committee wishes to thank Robert L. Barbieri, MD, for his assistance in the development of this bulletin. This Technical Bulletin does not define a standard of care, nor is it intended to dictate an exclusive course of management. It presents recognized methods and techniques of clinical practice for consideration by obstetrician–gynecologists for incorporation into their practices. Variations of practice taking into account the needs of the individual patient, resources, and limitations unique to the institution or type of practice may be appropriate.

ISSN 1074-8628

THE AMERICAN COLLEGE OF OBSTETRICIANS AND GYNECOLOGISTS
409 12th Street, SW
Washington, DC 20024-2188

12345/98765

Number 219—January 1996
(Replaces #91, February 1986)

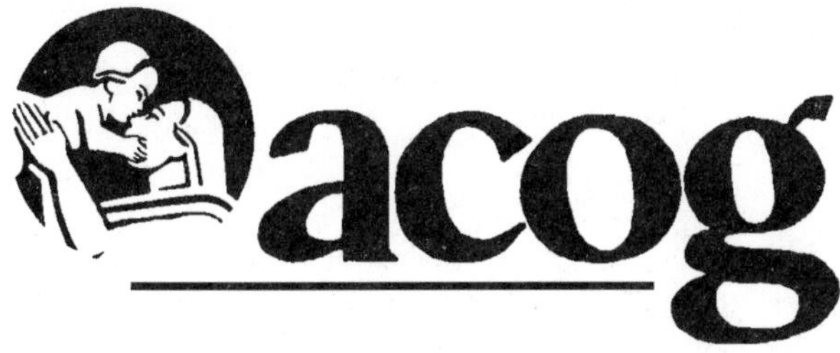

Technical Bulletin
An Educational Aid to Obstetrician–Gynecologists

Hypertension in Pregnancy

Hypertensive disease complicates roughly 6–8% of pregnancies in the United States and ranks second only to embolism as a cause of maternal mortality; it is directly responsible for 15% of maternal deaths in the United States (1). Maternal hypertension is also an important cause of perinatal morbidity and mortality, secondary to both direct fetal effects and iatrogenic preterm delivery performed for maternal indications. Despite the importance of this condition, its origin remains obscure, and the disease process is ultimately reversed only by delivery.

Terminology

Terminology used to describe hypertension in pregnancy is nonuniform, confusing, and steeped in tradition. Several overlapping terms are commonly applied to varying clinical manifestations of the same disease process. A variety of classifications have been proposed and used in the past. However, in clinical practice two distinct entities are commonly encountered in pregnant women: chronic hypertension and pregnancy-induced hypertension (PIH). These two conditions may also coexist; in fact, the risk of developing PIH is significantly increased in women with underlying chronic hypertension. Pregnancy-induced hypertension is a multiorgan disease process that may involve much more than elevated blood pressure. Several clinical subsets are recognized, depending on end-organ effects. Some such subsets have traditionally been given distinct labels, for example *preeclampsia* when renal involvement leads to proteinuria, *eclampsia* when central nervous system involvement leads to seizures, and, more recently, *HELLP syndrome* when the clinical picture is dominated by hematologic and hepatic manifestations. Although PIH may represent a final common pathway for a number of pathologic processes, given the limitations in our current understanding, such terminology should not be taken to connote intrinsically different disease entities. This bulletin will use the terms chronic hypertension and PIH with additional modifiers as necessary to describe clinically significant end-organ involvement.

Epidemiology

Several well-defined risk factors have been described for the development of PIH (Table 1). However, it is uncertain to what extent such observations actually reflect independent populations. For example, the observed relationship of racial and genetic factors to risk of PIH may be influenced by the underlying prevalence of chronic hypertension in certain demographic groups.

Clinical Manifestations

Blood Pressure

Hypertension is defined as a sustained blood pressure increase to levels of 140 mm Hg systolic or 90 mm Hg diastolic. Blood pressure may depend greatly on position, and ideally, measurements should be taken in a uniform manner at each prenatal visit with the proper cuff size while the patient is sitting. Although results of earlier reports suggested that an increase in blood pressure of 30 mm Hg systolic or 15 mm Hg diastolic from second-trimester values was also of diagnostic value, this concept is no longer considered valid. In one study, 73% of primigravid patients with normotensive pregnancies demonstrated an increase in diastolic blood pressure of more than 15 mm Hg at some stage during pregnancy, while 57% of these patients demonstrated an increase in diastolic pressure of more than 20 mm Hg during pregnancy (2). These observations were later confirmed by another study (3).

Ordinarily, PIH has its onset after 20 weeks of gestation, and chronic hypertension is defined as hypertension developing prior to 20 weeks of gestation. Patients with gestational trophoblastic disease are an exception; they

TABLE 1. RISK FACTORS FOR THE DEVELOPMENT OF PREGNANCY-INDUCED HYPERTENSION*

Factor	Risk Ratio
Nulliparity[1]	3:1
Age > 40 y[2]	3:1
African-American race [1]	1.5:1
Family history of pregnancy-induced hypertension [3]	5:1
Chronic hypertension [4]	10:1
Chronic renal disease [5]	20:1
Antiphospholipid [6] syndrome	10:1
Diabetes mellitus [7]	2:1
Twin gestation [8]	4:1
Angiotensinogen gene T235	
Homozygous [9]	20:1
Heterozygous [9]	4:1

*Low socioeconomic status and young maternal age are traditional risk factors; the actual independent contribution of these factors to the risk of pregnancy-induced hypertension is questionable.

[1] Cunningham FG, Leveno KJ. Management of pregnancy-induced hypertension. In: Rubin PC, ed. Handbook of hypertension, Vol X, hypertension in pregnancy. Amsterdam: Elsevier Science, 1988:290

[2] Spellacy WN, Miller SJ, Winegar A. Pregnancy after 40 years of age. Obstet Gynecol 1986;68:452–454

[3] Chesley LC, Cooper DW. Genetics of hypertension in pregnancy: possible single gene control of pre-eclampsia and eclampsia in the descendants of eclamptic women. Br J Obstet Gynaecol 1986;93:898–908

[4] Mabie WC, Pernoll ML, Biswas MK. Chronic hypertension in pregnancy. Obstet Gynecol 1986;67:197–205

[5] Cunningham FG, Cox SM, Harstad TW, Mason RA, Pritchard JA. Chronic renal disease and pregnancy outcome. Am J Obstet Gynecol 1990;163:453–459

[6] Branch DW, Silver RM, Blackwell JL, Reading JC, Scott JR. Outcome of treated pregnancies in women with antiphospolipid syndrome: an update of the Utah experience. Obstet Gynecol 1992;80:614–620

[7] Siddiqi T, Rosen B, Mimouni F, Khoury J, Miodovnik M. Hypertension during pregnancy in insulin-dependent diabetic women. Obstet Gynecol 1991;77:514–519

[8] Thompson SA, Lyons TL, Makowski EL. Outcomes of twin gestations at the University of Colorado Health Sciences Center, 1973–1983. J Reprod Med 1987;32:328–339

[9] Ward K, Hata A, Jeunemaitre X, Helin C, Nelson L, Namikawa C, et al. A molecular variant of angiotensinogen associated with preeclampsia. Nature Genetics 1993;4:59

can develop classic features of PIH during the first or second trimester.

Patients who develop PIH and, in addition, manifest end-organ involvement or fetal growth restriction are regarded as having severe disease. Early delivery should be considered for such women, often despite fetal immaturity. End-organ manifestations that can indicate severe disease are listed in the box.

Cardiovascular Effects

Blood pressure is a product of systemic vascular resistance and cardiac output. In patients with PIH, elevations of both factors may contribute to hypertension. A propensity to vasospasm is a well-established component of this disease process and likely is a major cause of many or most serious end-organ effects. Although the exact origin of such vasospasm is unknown, several intriguing observations have contributed significantly to the understanding of this process. Normal pregnancy is characterized by a blunted pressor response to infused angiotensin II; this blunted pressor response is not present in women with PIH (4). A classic study observed that women destined to develop PIH became progressively more sensitive to the pressor effects of infused angiotensin II after 18 weeks of gestation (5). Additional factors that may predispose a pregnant woman to PIH include a reduction in synthesis of prostacyclin relative to thromboxane (6) and alterations in the synthesis of endothelium-derived relaxing factor, endothelin-1, and nitric oxide (7, 8, 9).

Elevated cardiac output may also contribute to hypertension in women with PIH. One investigator showed a progressive increase in cardiac output from late first trimester in women destined to become hypertensive in late pregnancy (10). Similarly, a series of 45 patients with severe preeclampsia demonstrated systemic vascular resistances that, while higher than those seen in normal pregnancy, were similar to those observed in nonpregnant, normotensive women (11). However, cardiac output in these patients was increased above that seen during normotensive, third-trimester pregnancy, and the left ven-

Clinical Manifestations of Severe Disease in Patients with Pregnancy-Induced Hypertension

- Blood pressure > 160–180 mm Hg systolic or > 110 mm Hg diastolic
- Proteinuria > 5 g/24 h (normal < 300 mg/24 h)
- Elevated serum creatinine
- Grand mal seizures (eclampsia)
- Pulmonary edema
- Oliguria < 500 ml/24 h
- Microangiopathic hemolysis
- Thrombocytopenia
- Hepatocellular dysfunction (elevated alanine aminotransferase, aspartase aminotransferase)
- Intrauterine growth retardation or oligohydramnios
- Symptoms suggesting significant end-organ involvement: headache, visual disturbances, or epigastric or right-upper quadrant pain

tricular stroke work index was almost twice that reported in normotensive, third-trimester patients (12). Thus, both elevations in cardiac output and local or systemic vasospasm can contribute to clinical hypertension in patients with PIH.

Hematologic Effects

The most frequent hematologic consequence of PIH is plasma volume contraction, which can result in decreased regional perfusion and increase the risk of hypovolemic shock if hemorrhage occurs. This contraction is clinically reflected by a rise in hematocrit as the severity and duration of PIH increases. Such reductions in intravascular volume occur despite an actual increase in total body water.

Thrombocytopenia is the most frequent hematologic abnormality that occurs in women with PIH (13). The frequency and severity of this condition is increased when there is early onset of PIH or in the presence of chronic hypertension and superimposed PIH. Thrombocytopenia has traditionally been considered a manifestation of a more generalized microangiopathic hemolysis due to arteriolar spasm. However, vascular changes at the site of placental implantation may also play a role. Although extremely sensitive assays of intravascular coagulation activation are positive in many patients with PIH, clinical evidence of a consumptive coagulopathy is rare in the absence of coexistent placental abruption and is virtually never seen in the absence of moderate to severe thrombocytopenia (13). Levels of antithrombin III are reduced in patients with PIH (14), and a reduction in the ratio of factor VIII bioactivity to factor VIII antigen may also be seen (15). Although a qualitative defect in platelet function can be encountered in patients with PIH, this is only rarely of clinical significance (16).

A variant of severe PIH has been described in which hematologic abnormalities exist with severe preeclampsia/eclampsia (17). The syndrome of hemolysis, thrombocytopenia, and elevated hepatic transaminase levels has since become known as the HELLP syndrome (18). While HELLP syndrome was originally defined as including all of these factors, any one of these conditions can represent severe disease. Normal blood pressures are initially found in approximately 10–20% of patients with these manifestations, suggesting the need to be aware of the possibility of this condition in any woman in the third trimester with right-upper quadrant or epigastric pain (19, 20).

Renal Function

Both decreased glomerular filtration rate and proteinuria (urine protein exceeding 300 mg/24 h) are common in PIH, and sodium retention is virtually universal. Although the glomerular filtration rate is affected by decreased renal plasma flow, the filtration fraction (glomerular filtration rate/renal plasma flow) is decreased as well. Decreased clearance of uric acid is also seen and precedes changes in glomerular filtration rate (21). The results of a random dipstick assessment of proteinuria may not correlate with those of a 24-hour urine collection (22). Proteinuria occurs on the basis of glomerular damage (23) and subsequent leakage. Because of these renal function abnormalities, standard determinations of urine osmolality and electrolytes are not a reliable reflection of actual intravascular volume in severe PIH (24).

Neurologic Function

Hyperreflexia is commonly seen in patients with PIH. However, the degree of hyperreflexia has not been shown to correlate with the severity of the disease process. The presence or absence of hyperreflexia should not be a factor in making or excluding the diagnosis of PIH.

In severe cases, PIH can be complicated by grand mal seizures. Many cases of maternal mortality involve such events. Although seizures can occur during the postpartum period, other underlying neurologic processes should be considered when seizures occur more than 24 hours following delivery (25). The origin of seizures in patients with PIH is poorly understood. In one series, no differences were seen in central hemodynamic parameters among patients with severe PIH who suffered seizures and those who did not, although eclamptic patients had significantly lower colloid oncotic pressures than severely preeclamptic patients without seizures (26).

Other Organ Involvement

Pulmonary edema can occur in patients with PIH and can be related to decreased colloid oncotic pressure, pulmonary capillary leak, left heart failure, iatrogenic fluid overload, or a combination of these factors (27). Elevated hepatic transaminase levels reflect hepatocellular damage, probably secondary to vasospasm and ischemia. Pathologically, such changes can have varying manifestations ranging from focal periportal hemorrhage to infarction or rupture. Additional changes in the reninaldosterone axis, maternal immune system, and placenta have also been described and may play a role in the pathogenesis of PIH.

Effects on the Fetus

The decrease in placental perfusion that accompanies maternal vascular spasm in PIH is believed to account for the increased perinatal morbidity and mortality associated with this disease. Uteroplacental perfusion has been shown to be decreased with the use of several experimental approaches (28). Perinatal morbidity and mortality are increased, both secondary to intrauterine growth retardation (IUGR) and an increased incidence of placental abruption seen in women with PIH. Poor perinatal outcome, such as IUGR, is especially common in women with preexisting chronic hypertension complicated by PIH (29, 30).

Clinical Management

Prevention

Several studies have addressed the use of low doses of aspirin for the prevention of PIH. A metaanalysis of six controlled trials demonstrated a significant reduction in IUGR and cesarean delivery in women judged to be at high risk for PIH based on various criteria (31). No reduction in perinatal death was seen, and there were no adverse maternal or neonatal effects of the aspirin therapy.

In a subsequent study, 1,106 women deemed to be at moderate risk for PIH were randomized to receive aspirin therapy either prophylactically based on various risk factors or therapeutically following the development of hypertension or IUGR (32). No difference in maternal or perinatal outcome was seen, although the heterogenous nature of the study group may have influenced the results.

Another study randomized 3,135 normotensive nulliparous patients to receive 60 mg of aspirin or placebo (33). These investigators documented a lower incidence of preeclampsia in the treated group, principally among women whose initial systolic blood pressure was 120–134 mm Hg, but they did not demonstrate any improvement in perinatal morbidity. In this series, the treatment group exhibited a higher incidence of placental abruption, a finding not demonstrated in any other study.

In a study of 9,364 women at increased risk for either preeclampsia or IUGR, a small but potentially important effect of aspirin was demonstrated on delay of delivery in women with early onset preeclampsia (34). No effects were seen on stillbirths, neonatal deaths, or maternal outcome. These reports suggest that while administration of low-dose aspirin (60–80 mg) may be an appropriate option in women at high risk for developing PIH, use of this agent is, at the present time, not recommended for PIH prophylaxis in unselected, normotensive multiparous or nulliparous patients.

Calcium supplementation has also been reported to reduce the risk of PIH although confirmatory studies are needed (35). In a randomized, prospective study, a threefold reduction in preeclampsia was reported in angiotensin-sensitive patients who received 2 g of oral calcium gluconate per day (36).

Treatment of Pregnancy-Induced Hypertension

Delivery remains the only definitive treatment for PIH. For this reason, delivery is generally indicated in women at term with PIH of any severity and in preterm women with severe disease. However, there are several exceptions to these general rules.

Delivery is always an appropriate option in the term patient with hypertension. However, in the patient with an unfavorable cervix who exhibits only mild blood pressure elevations, minimal proteinuria, and no evidence of either maternal end-organ involvement or fetal compromise, delivery may be appropriately delayed in an effort to obtain a more favorable cervix prior to induction. In most cases, it is inappropriate to allow pregnancy in such patients to extend beyond 40 weeks of gestation.

Delivery should be considered in women who have signs and symptoms of severe PIH at 32–34 weeks of gestation. In some cases, the condition of women who initially manifest signs and symptoms of severe PIH will improve after observation and treatment with magnesium sulfate and various antihypertensive agents such as apresoline or labetolol. In such women, continued observation is reasonable and appropriate at less than 32 weeks of gestation. If severe PIH persists (ie, does not respond to initial observation and therapy) or recurs, delivery should be instituted. Some of the manifestations of severe PIH, such as maternal oliguria, renal failure, and HELLP syndrome (hemolysis, elevated liver enzymes, and low platelet count), mandate expedient delivery regardless of gestational age. Although the use of corticosteroids is appropriate at less than 34 weeks of gestation in many women who have PIH (including severe disease), the health of the mother or the fetus should not be jeopardized by delaying delivery solely for this reason.

An initial observation period and attempt at conservative management for women with severe preeclampsia who are remote from term have been supported in two randomized studies (37, 38). In both studies, however, the number of patients was small and only those at 28–34 weeks of gestation were included. Indications for delivery were persistent signs and symptoms of severe disease such as headache, scotomata, HELLP syndrome, or blood pressure persistently elevated to greater than or equal to 160/110. Moreover, patients were treated in a level III hospital with intensive observation of maternal and fetal status. Because most babies born at 32–34 weeks of gestation have normal long-term outcome, the conservative management of women with severe PIH at this gestational age has marginal benefit.

Management of severe PIH at less than 28 weeks of gestation poses a difficult clinical dilemma because it is often unsuccessful and may be hazardous. Attempts at conservative management in women with severe pre-eclampsia at 18–27 weeks of gestation have been associated with significant morbidity, including abruptio placentae (22%), eclampsia (17%), coagulopathy (8%), and renal failure (5%) (39). In addition, one woman had hypertensive encephalopathy and one had an intracerebral hemorrhage. The perinatal mortality rate was 87%.

In women who develop PIH prior to 34 weeks of gestation, consideration should be given to screening for the presence of antiphospholipid antibodies (40). If present, such antibodies portend an increased risk of adverse pregnancy outcome and an increased likelihood of recurrent severe hypertensive disease in future pregnancies (41).

For the preterm patient with mild PIH, conservative management is generally indicated. For any patient with PIH not undergoing delivery, it is essential to closely monitor blood pressure and proteinuria and evaluate renal and hepatic function and platelet count. Serial sonography for fetal growth and antepartum assessment of fetal well-being is also important. The optimal frequency with which any of these parameters should be evaluated has not been established but should depend on gestational age and the condition of the patient and fetus. For the stable patient with mild PIH who has had a thorough initial evaluation, either inpatient or outpatient management may be appropriate.

When delivery is indicated, parenteral magnesium sulfate is generally administered to prevent seizures. This is most commonly given as an intravenous loading bolus (4 g over 20 minutes) followed by a continuous infusion (2–3 g/h) administered via a controlled infusion device. Infusion of magnesium sulfate should be discontinued and a serum magnesium level obtained in any patient with loss of deep tendon reflexes, respiratory rate less than 12 per minute, and a decrease in urinary output to below 25 ml/h. The therapeutic range for magnesium is generally considered to be 4–8 mg/dl. When symptomatic magnesium overdose is suspected (eg, the presence of apnea, obtundation), it can be reversed by the intravenous administration of 1 g (10 ml of 10%) calcium gluconate intravenously over 2 minutes. Magnesium sulfate can also be given intramuscularly. When respiration has been depressed, it may be necessary to support ventilation mechanically until plasma levels have been reduced. Magnesium, while an effective anticonvulsant agent, does not substantially affect blood pressure; therefore, if blood pressure control is necessary, additional agents are mandatory (42).

Phenytoin sodium has been proposed as an alternative to magnesium sulfate for intrapartum seizure prophylaxis in patients with PIH (43). Recent evidence suggests that magnesium sulfate is superior to phenytoin in preventing seizures (44, 45).

During labor, several different antihypertensive agents have been used to control maternal blood pressure. Loss of autoregulation may predispose the patient to cerebral accident; therefore, when blood pressure exceeds 110 mm Hg diastolic or 180 mm Hg systolic, consideration should be given to lowering the blood pressure. One widely used agent is hydralazine hydrochloride given intravenously as a 5–10-mg bolus as often as every 20 minutes as necessary. Labetalol, 20 mg, given intravenously as often as every 10 minutes to a maximum dose of 300 mg, is an acceptable substitute. The maximum effect of a single dose occurs within 5 minutes. Both hydralazine and labetalol may be given as an intermittent bolus or a continuous infusion with continuous blood pressure monitoring. Other agents that can be used include verapamil and nifedipine. Occasionally, unresponsive blood pressure can require the administration of a more potent agent, such as sodium nitroprusside, usually with central hemodynamic monitoring (46). The use of calcium channel blockers may be especially efficacious in the postpartum period.

Delivery is indicated for any patient with persistent severe oliguria. If treatment is required before or after delivery, a fluid challenge of 500 ml may be given. If severe oliguria is unresponsive to a fluid challenge, additional volume may be withheld pending delivery or more precise hemodynamic definition of the origin of the oliguric state, generally necessitating central hemodynamic monitoring (47, 24, 48). In practice, such invasive techniques are only rarely necessary in patients with severe PIH. Acute renal failure is uncommon even in oliguric patients with severe PIH and generally does not result in residual renal dysfunction (49).

Vaginal delivery is generally preferable to cesarean delivery, even in patients with manifestations of severe disease (50). Under appropriate circumstances, cervical ripening with prostaglandin E_2 gel may be considered (51). In some cases, however, a seriously ill patient with an unfavorable cervix may be better served by cesarean delivery rather than a long induction of labor. Clearly, the decision must be based on the clinical circumstances.

Anesthesia

The relative merits of various types of anesthesia for patients with PIH have been debated. Every method of analgesia and anesthesia (with the possible exception of psychoprophylaxis) carries risks that can be minimized, but not eliminated.

For patients in labor with PIH, either parenteral analgesia or continuous conduction anesthesia is generally acceptable. Patients undergoing cesarean delivery may receive either general or conduction anesthesia, depending on the circumstances.

Continuous conduction anesthesia requires knowledge, skill, experience, and a clear understanding that most patients with PIH have a constricted intravascular volume, predisposing them to hypotension. Thus, the administration of an adequate preload is essential in these patients, and spinal anesthesia should be given only with great caution. Significant thrombocytopenia is a relative contraindication to conduction anesthesia. However, several series have demonstrated that patients with PIH receiving epidural anesthesia do not have an increased risk of hypotension compared with normotensive women (52). Improvement in intervillous blood flow has also been reported with epidural anesthesia in patients with PIH (53).

General anesthesia has been associated with marked elevations of blood pressure during induction and awakening, fluctuations which may prove hazardous to a hypertensive patient (54). Such fluctuations may be minimized with careful blood pressure monitoring and appropriate pharmacologic intervention with agents such as nitroglycerin, apresoline, or labetolol.

Chronic Hypertension

Mild to moderate chronic hypertension is unlikely to have significant deleterious maternal effects during a 40-week gestation. Elevations of blood pressure, however, may have significant detrimental effects on the fetus, including IUGR and fetal death. Severe elevations of blood pressure may require antihypertensive therapy to prevent maternal morbidity and mortality. Current evidence argues against starting pharmacologic treatment in patients with chronic hypertension and diastolic pressures below 100 mm Hg because it does not improve either maternal or fetal outcome (55).

Patients with chronic hypertension who conceive while taking antihypertensive medications may, with exceptions noted below, continue these medications during pregnancy. If antihypertensive therapy is to be initiated during gestation, alpha-methyldopa should be considered as a first-line agent because of extensive experience and documented fetal safety. Labetalol and atenolol are also acceptable alternatives. In pregnant patients taking beta-blocking agents, fetuses should be monitored carefully for IUGR, a condition that can be increased with the use of these drugs (56).

Two antihypertensive agents merit special consideration during pregnancy. Angiotensin-converting enzyme inhibitors may be associated with fetal hypocalvaria, renal failure, oligohydramnios, and fetal and neonatal death (57, 58). Women who conceive while using such agents should be advised to discontinue them immediately. In general, diuretics should not be initiated during pregnancy, as the associated plasma volume reduction theoretically may have adverse fetal effects (59). The use of diuretics is acceptable if blood pressure cannot be controlled with alternative agents. Patients who conceive while on chronic diuretic therapy may safely continue these agents. Other commonly used antihypertensive agents have not been studied extensively during pregnancy.

Women with chronic hypertension are at increased risk for having a fetus with growth retardation. Serial sonography and antepartum fetal heart rate assessment may be helpful in monitoring fetal well-being. Such women are also at significant risk for developing superimposed PIH. Serial assessment of blood pressure and urine protein will assist in the early identification of superimposed PIH. Because of the increased maternal and perinatal morbidity associated with this condition, induction of labor at term is an appropriate consideration for the woman with chronic hypertension and a favorable cervix.

REFERENCES

1. Rochat RW, Koonin LM, Atrash HK, Jewett JF, the Maternal Mortality Collaberative. Maternal mortality in the United States: report from the Maternal Mortality Collaborative. Obstet Gynecol 1988;72:91–97
2. MacGillivray I, Rose GA, Rowe D. Blood pressure survey in pregnancy. Clin Sci 1969;37:395
3. Villar MA, Sibai BM. Clinical significance of elevated mean arterial blood pressure in second trimester and threshold increase in systolic and diastolic blood pressure during third trimester. Am J Obstet Gynecol 1989; 160:419–423
4. Talledo OE, Chesley LC, Zuspan FP. Renin-angiotensin system in normal and toxemic pregnancies. III. Differential sensitivity to angiotension II and norepinephrine in toxemia of pregnancy Am J Obstet Gynecol 1968;100: 218–222
5. Gant NF, Daley GL, Chand S, Whalley PJ, MacDonald PC. A study of angiotensin II pressor response throughout primigravid pregnancy. J Clin Invest 1973;52:2682–2689
6. Mitchell MD, Koenig JM. Increased production of 15-hydroxyeiconsatetraenoic acid by placentae from pregnancies complicated by pregnancy-induced hypertension. Prostaglandins Leukot Essent Fatty Acids 1991; 43:61
7. Clark BA, Halvorson L, Sachs B, Epstein FH. Plasma endothelin levels in preeclampsia: elevation and correlation with uric acid levels and renal impairment. Am J Obstet Gynecol 1992;166:962–968
8. Chang J-K, Roman C, Heymann MA. Effect of endothelium-derived relaxing factor inhibition on the umbilical–placental circulation in fetal lambs in utero. Am J Obstet Gynecol 1992;166;727–734
9. Wang Y, Walsh SW, Guo J, Zhang J. The imbalance between thromboxane and prostacyclin in preeclampsia is associated with an imbalance between lipid peroxides and vitamin E in maternal blood. Am J Obstet Gynecol 1991;165:1695–1700
10. Easterling TR, Benedetti TJ, Schmucker BC, Millard SP. Maternal hemodynamics in normal and preeclamptic pregnancies: a longitudinal study. Obstet Gynecol 1990; 76:1061–1069

11. Cotton DB, Lee W, Huhta JC, Dorman KF. Hemodynamic profile of severe pregnancy-induced hypertension. Am J Obstet Gynecol 1988;158:523–529

12. Clark SL, Cotton DB, Lee W, Bishop C, Hill T, Southwick, et al. Central hemodynamic assessment of normal term pregnancy. Am J Obstet Gynecol 1989;161:1439–1442

13. Leduc L, Wheeler JM, Kirshon B, Mitchell P, Cotton DB. Coagulation profile in severe preeclampsia. Obstet Gynecol 1992;79:14–18

14. Weiner CP, Brandt J. Plasma antithrombin III activity: an aid in the diagnosis of preeclampsia–eclampsia. Am J Obstet Gynecol 1982;142:275–281

15. Redman CWG, Denson KWE, Beilin LJ, et al. Factor-VIII consumption in preeclampsia. Lancet 1977;2:1249

16. Socol ML, Weiner CP, Louis G, Rennberg K, Rossi EC. Platelet activation in preeclampsia. Am J Obstet Gynecol 1985;151:494–497

17. Pritchard JA, Weisman R Jr, Ratnoff OD, Vosburgh GJ. Intravascular hemolysis, thrombocytopenia and other hematologic abnormalities associated with severe toxemia of pregnancy. N Engl J Med 1954;250:87–98

18. Weinstein L. Syndrome of hemolysis, elevated liver enzymes, and low platelet count: a severe consequence of hypertension in pregnancy. Am J Obstet Gynecol 1982;142:159–167

19. Martin JN Jr, Blake PG, Pery KG Jr, McCaul JF, Hess LW, Martin RW. The natural history of HELLP syndrome: patterns of disease progression and regression. Am J Obstet Gynecol 1991;164:1500–1513

20. Sibai BM, Ramadan MK, Usta I, Salama M, Mercer BM, Friedman SA. Maternal morbidity and mortality in 442 pregnancies with hemolysis, elevated liver enzymes, and low platelets (HELLP syndrome). Am J Obstet Gynecol 1993;169:1000–1006

21. Gallery EDM, Gyory AZ. Glomerular and proximal renal tubuar function in pregnancy-associated hypertension: a prospective study. Eur J Obstet Gynecol Reprod Biol 1979;9:3

22. Meyer NL, Mercer BM, Friedman SA, Sibai BM. Urinary dipstick protein: a poor predictor of absent or severe proteinuria. Am J Obstet Gynecol 1994;170:137–141

23. Katz M, Berlyne GM. Differential renal protein clearance in toxemia of pregnancy. Nephron 1974;13:212

24. Kirshon B, Lee W, Mauer MB, Cotton DB. Effects of low-dose dopamine therapy in the oliguric patient with preeclampsia Am J Obstet Gynecol 1988;159:604–607

25. Sibai BM, Schneider JM, Morrison JC, Lipshitz, Anderson GD, Shier RW, et al. The late postpartum eclampsia controversy. Obstet Gynecol 1980;55:74–78

26. Clark SL, Divon MY, Phelan JP. Preeclampsia/eclampsia: hemodynamic and neurologic correlations. Obstet Gynecol 1985;66:337–340

27. Benedetti TJ, Kates R, Williams V. Hemodynamic observations in severe preeclampsia complicated by pulmonary edema. Am J Obstet Gynecol 1985;152:330–334

28. Gant NF, Worley RJ, eds. Hypertension in pregnancy: concepts and management. New York: Appleton-Century-Crofts, 1980:61–106

29. López-Llera M, Hernández-Horta JL, Huttich FC. Retarded fetal growth in eclampsia. J Reprod Med 1972; 9:229–232

30. Lin C-C, Lindheimer MD, River P, Moawad AH. Fetal outcome in hypertensive disorders of pregnancy. Am J Obstet Gynecol 1982;142:255–260

31. Imperiale TF, Petrulis AS. A meta-analysis of low-dose aspirin for the prevention of pregnancy-induced hypertensive disease. JAMA 1991;266:261–265

32. Italian Study of Aspirin in Pregnancy. Low-dose aspirin in prevention and treatment of intrauterine growth retardation and pregnancy-induced hypertension. Lancet 1993;341: 396–400

33. Sibai BM, Caritis SN, Thom E, Klebanoff M, McNellis D, Rocco L, et al. Prevention of preeclampsia with low-dose aspirin in healthy, nulliparous pregnant women. N Engl J Med 1993;329:1213–1218

34. Collaborative Low-Dose Aspirin Study in Pregnancy Collaborative Group. CLASP: a randomized trial of low-dose aspirin for the prevention and treatment of preeclampsia among 9364 pregnant women. Lancet 1994;343:619–629

35. Belizán JM, Villar J, Gonzalez L, Campodonico L, Bergel E. Calcium supplementation to prevent hypertensive disorders of pregnancy. N Engl J Med 1991;325:1399–1405

36. Sanchez-Ramos L, Del Valle GO, Briones D, Walker C, Delke I, Gaudier F. Prevention of preeclampsia by calcium supplementation in angiotensin-sensitive patients. Am J Obstet Gynecol 1994;170:408

37. Odendaal HJ, Pattinson RC, Bam R, Grove D, Kotze TJvW. Aggressive or expectant management for patients with severe preeclampsia between 28–34 weeks' gestation: a randomized controlled trial. Obstet Gynecol 1990;76:1070–1074

38. Sibai BM, Mercer BM, Schiff E, Friedman SA. Aggressive versus expectant management of severe preeclampsia at 28 to 32 weeks' gestation: a randomized controlled trial. Am J Obstet Gynecol 1994;171:818–822

39. Sibai BM, Taslimi M, Abdella TN, Brooks TF, Spinnato JA, Anderson GD. Maternal and perinatal outcome of conservative management of severe preeclampsia in midtrimester. Am J Obstet Gynecol 1985;152:32–37

40. Branch DW, Andres R, Digre KB, Rote NS, Scott JR. The association of antiphospholipid antibodies with severe preeclampsia. Obstet Gynecol 1989;73:541–545

41. Branch DW, Silver RM, Blackwell JL, Reading JC, Scott JR. Outcome of treated pregnancies in women with antiphospolipid syndrome: an update of the Utah experience. Obstet Gynecol 1992;80:614–620

42. Cotton DB, Gonik B, Dorman KF. Cardiovascular alterations in severe pregnancy-induced hypertension: acute effects of intravenous magnesium sulfate. Am J Obstet Gynecol 1984;148:162–165

43. Appleton MP, Kuehl TJ, Raebel MA, Adams HR, Knight AB, Gold WR. Magnesium sulfate versus phenytoin for seizure prophylaxis in pregnancy-induced hypertension. Am J Obstet Gynecol 1991;165:907–913

44. The Eclampsia Trial Collaborative Group. Which anticonvulsant for women with eclampsia? Evidence from the Collaborative Eclampsia Trial. Lancet 1995;345:1455–1463

45. Lucas MJ, Leveno KJ, Cunningham FG. A comparison of magnesium sulfate with phenytoin for the prevention of eclampsia. N Engl J Med 1995;333:201–205

46. Clark SL, Cotton DB. Clinical indications for pulmonary artery catheterization in the patient with severe preeclampsia. Am J Obstet Gynecol 1988;158:453–458

47. American College of Obstetricians and Gynecologists. Invasive hemodynamic monitoring in obstetrics and gynecology. ACOG Technical Bulletin 175. Washington, DC: ACOG, 1992

48. Clark SL, Greenspoon JS, Aldahl D, Phelan JP. Severe preeclamsia with persistent oliguria: management of hemodynamic subsets. Am J Obstet Gynecol 1986; 154:490–494

49. Sibai BM, Villar MA, Mabie BC. Acute renal failure in hypertensive disorders of pregnancy. Pregnancy outcome and remote prognosis in thirty-one consecutive cases. Am J Obstet Gynecol 1990;162:777–783

50. Pritchard JA, Cunningham FG, Pritchard SA. The Parkland Memorial Hospital protocol for treatment of eclampsia: evaluation of 245 cases. Am J Obstet Gynecol 1984; 148:951–963

51. American College of Obstetricians and Gynecologists. Induction of labor. ACOG Technical Bulletin 217. Washington, DC: ACOG, 1995

52. Gutsche B. The experts opine: is epidural block for labor and delivery and for cesarean section a safe form of analgesia in severe preeclampsia or eclampsia? Surv Anesth 1986;30:304

53. Jouppila P, Jouppila R, Hollmén A, Koivula A. Lumbar epidural analgesia to improve intervillous blood flow during labor in severe preeclampsia. Obstet Gynecol 1982;59:158–161

54. Hodgkinson R, Husain FJ, Hayashi RH. Systemic and pulmonary blood pressure during cesarean section in parturients with gestational hypertension. Can Anaesth Soc J 1980;27:389

55. Sibai BM, Mabie WC, Shamsa F, Villar MA, Anderson GD. A comparison of no medication versus methyldopa or labetalol in chronic hypertension during pregnancy. Am J Obstet Gynecol 1990;162:960–967

56. Butters L, Kennedy S, Rubin PC. Atenolol in essential hypertension during pregnancy. BMJ 1990;301:587–589

57. Barr M, Cohen MM. ACE inhibitor fetopathy and hypocalvaria: the kidney-skull connection. Teratology 1991; 44:485–495

58. Hanssens M, Keirse MJNC, Vankelecom F, Van Assche FA. Fetal and neonatal effects of treatment with angiotensin-converting enzyme inhibitors in pregnancy. Obstet Gynecol 1991;78:128–135

59. Gant NF, Madden JD, Siiteri PK, MacDonald PC. The metabolic clearance rate of dehyroisoandrosterone sulfate. IV. Acute effects of induced hypertension, hypotension, and naturesis in normal and hypertensive prenancies. Am J Obstet Gynecol 1976;124:143–148

This Technical Bulletin was developed under the direction of the Committee on Technical Bulletins of the American College of Obstetricians and Gynecologists as an educational aid to obstetricians and gynecologists. The committee wishes to thank Norman F. Gant, Jr., MD, and Larry C. Gilstrap III, MD for their assistance in the development of this bulletin. This Technical Bulletin does not define a standard of care, nor is it intended to dictate an exclusive course of management. It presents recognized methods and techniques of clinical practice for consideration by obstetrician–gynecologists for incorporation into their practices. Variations of practice taking into account the needs of the individual patient, resources, and limitations unique to the institution or type of practice may be appropriate.

ISSN 1074-8628

THE AMERICAN COLLEGE OF OBSTETRICIANS AND GYNECOLOGISTS
409 12th Street, SW, Washington, DC 20024-2188
12345/09876

Number 191—April 1994

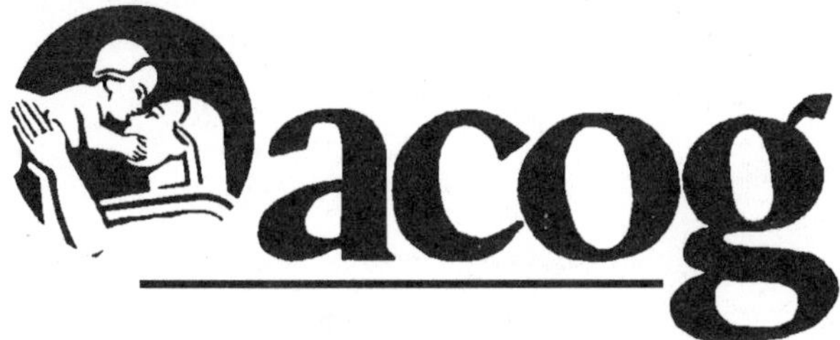

Technical Bulletin

An Educational Aid to Obstetrician–Gynecologists

Hysteroscopy

Hysteroscopy allows direct visualization of the endometrial cavity and the tubal ostia. It is performed to make or corroborate a diagnosis. Operative hysteroscopy allows the physician to obtain specimens, apply therapies, and perform a wide variety of surgical procedures under direct visualization. Specially designed mechanical, elec-trosurgical, and laser instruments can be used through the hysteroscope.

Instrumentation

Types of Hysteroscopes

There are several different types of hysteroscopes. The optics of the hysteroscope are designed to vary the focal length of the instrument so that the illuminated uterine cavity can be adequately and accurately visualized. The hysteroscope tip is generally angled to allow different perspectives of the endometrium. Several different fixed-angle scopes (0°, 12°, 30°, and 70°) are available.

Rigid hysteroscopes are constructed in a range of widths. Narrow hysteroscopes of 3–5 mm in diameter are being used increasingly in office settings. These diagnostic instruments often can be passed through the cervix with little or no cervical dilation required and produce minimal discomfort. The endometrial cavity can be directly inspected or a magnified image can be projected on a video screen in clear detail. Hysteroscopes greater than 5 mm in outer diameter can accommodate specially designed operative instruments. Large-caliber hysteroscopes of 8–10 mm have the advantage of maintaining optical integrity while introducing operative instruments. In addition, some larger instruments are capable of providing continuous laminar flow of distention medium in order to sustain the clarity of the operative field. A clear operative field is especially im-portant in cases in which bleeding is likely to occur.

Contact hysteroscopes are simple rigid instruments in which a single glass column serves the dual function of conducting light to the surface being examined and carrying the image back to the observer. The focal length is set so that the tissue is in focus when it is touching the surface of the hysteroscope. The main advantage of this instrument is that no distention medium is required; however, a disadvantage is the inability to obtain a panoramic view.

Flexible hysteroscopes are modelled after instruments used for gastrointestinal endoscopy. A tip deflection of 120–160° may be useful when an irregularly shaped uterus is encountered or when the practitioner wishes to hold the instrument in a fixed position while evaluating the uterine cavity. Flexion of the hysteroscope to the natural curve of a patient's uterus during insertion may also reduce discomfort during office evaluation. Flexible instruments also have an operating channel which can aid in taking a directed biopsy of the endometrium.

Operative Instrumentation

Operative instruments include rigid and flexible instruments such as scissors, biopsy forceps, and grasping instruments. When the goal is ablation of the endometrium, a roller bar or ball can be used. These instruments deliver a uniform coagulating current that desiccates the tissue as the bar or ball rolls over the endometrial surface. The loop electrode is a versatile tool that can be used in numerous procedures. When used for endometrial ablation, the loop can shave the endometrium off the supporting myometrium, providing a specimen for pathologic analysis. In addition, the loop can be used to excise or resect a uterine septum or leiomyomata. Knife electrodes concentrate cutting or coagulating current into a high-energy tip. Because the surface area of the knife electrode is small, its power density is higher at the tip at a given voltage than that of other instruments (eg, the roller ball).

Fiberoptic lasers constitute another class of hysteroscopic instruments. The Nd:YAG (neodymium–yttrium–aluminum–garnet), KTP (potassium–titanyl–phosphate), and argon lasers are all well suited for hysteroscopic use. Unlike the CO_2 laser, which cannot pass through fluids and is readily absorbed by water (therefore vaporizing tissue in its path), the Nd:YAG, argon, and KTP lasers are able to pass through flexible fibers and fluid media. The wavelengths of the argon and KTP lasers, 0.458–0.515 µm and 0.532 µm, respectively, make them most amenable to absorption by darkly pigmented tissue. These lasers will penetrate tissue to a depth of 1–2 mm with minimal scatter and can be used for their cutting action. The Nd:YAG laser wavelength of 1.064 µm allows it to pass deeply into tissue before it is absorbed (1). The Nd:YAG wave scatters upon contact with tissue, making this laser a poor cutting instrument but an excellent coagulator. The use of a sculpted sapphire tip can focus the beam and allow it to function as a laser scalpel.

Distention Media

Panoramic hysteroscopy requires distention of the uterine cavity. This goal can be accomplished by introducing either a gas or a fluid into the uterus. The refractive index of the distention medium will affect the magnification and visualization of the uterine cavity. Each medium has its own unique set of benefits and risks which must be weighed.

Among available gases, CO_2 is regarded as the agent of choice for diagnostic procedures. It is rapidly absorbed and easily cleared from the body. CO_2 affords a wider field of view and lower magnification than does a liquid medium (2). A hysteroscopic insufflator is required both to regulate flow and limit the maximum desired intrauterine pressure. Ordinarily, the flow is limited to 40–60 ml/min at a pressure of 100 mm Hg. However, CO_2 has significant disadvantages in an operative setting, including the loss of a clear field when bleeding occurs and the risk of embolism with exposed blood vessels.

Electrolyte solutions, such as normal saline and lactated Ringer's injection, are useful for diagnostic hysteroscopy. They are readily available, physiologic solutions that can be administered without complex equipment. Two major disadvantages limit the application of these solutions for operative hysteroscopy: the mixing of blood, which limits visualization, and the inability to use electrosurgery because electrolyte solutions are electrical conductors.

Nonelectrolyte solutions, such as 1.5% glycine, 3% sorbitol, mannitol, and high-molecular-weight dextran, are useful for both diagnostic and operative procedures. In contrast to electrolyte-containing distention media, these solutions do not conduct electrical current and can be used safely with electrosurgery. In addition, bleeding is less likely to interfere with visualization. A disadvantage of these products is that intravenous absorption may result in fluid overload, particularly during lengthy operative procedures.The rate and dosage of medium administered must be monitored.

Indications

Abnormal Uterine Bleeding

Evaluation of abnormal uterine bleeding is best accomplished in the context of the patient's history, symptoms, and physical examination. Abnormal bleeding is frequently due to an underlying endocrinopathy (3). Hormonal imbalance can be treated medically, generally using progestins, estrogens, or both. Depending on the age of the patient, endometrial biopsy can be used prior to the initiation of medical therapy to exclude the possibility of premalignant or malignant processes. Determining the efficacy of hormonal therapy may require 3–4 months. However, if medical therapy is not successful and an underlying anatomic cause is suspected, hysteroscopy may be performed. It is not cost-effective for every patient with abnormal uterine bleeding to undergo hysteroscopy; however, hysteroscopic technology augments the current diagnostic capabilities.

Endometrial ablation has been used to treat excessive uterine bleeding caused by benign disorders. Contrary to some patients' expectations, however, endometrial ablation does not routinely produce amenorrhea. In a study of 64 patients undergoing this procedure, 30% became amenorrheic, 26% reported spotting, and 34% reported decreased menstrual flow; 10% reported either no change or an increase in menstrual flow (4).

Uterine Leiomyomata

Hysteroscopy may be used to treat symptomatic submucous uterine leiomyomata. In contrast to myomectomy via laparotomy, hysteroscopic myomectomy generally decreases the direct and indirect morbidity associated with the procedure. It is most commonly performed on an outpatient basis. Enucleation of the entire leiomyoma can be achieved if the mass is predominantly submucous. When a large portion of the leiomyoma is intramural, a practical surgical compromise is to resect the accessible portion of the leiomyoma until it is flush with the remaining surfaces of the uterine cavity. This procedure is highly effective; of 94 patients who were monitored for 9 years after undergoing hysteroscopic myomectomy, only 16% underwent further surgery (5).

Intrauterine Adhesions

Intrauterine adhesions typically appear after operative trauma to the uterine cavity (such as dilation and curettage after pregnancy) or infection. Patients with intrauterine adhesions may be seeking treatment for amenorrhea or infertility. Hysteroscopy enables an accurate diagnosis and affords the opportunity for immediate treatment. Filmy adhesions frequently can be lysed under the pressure of the distention medium, while more dense adhesions can be cut or excised. The advantage of treatment under direct visualization is that surgical trauma to surrounding areas of normal endometrium can be avoided.

In a study of 187 patients with amenorrhea, hypomenorrhea, or dysmenorrhea, hysteroscopic lysis or removal of adhesions was followed by restoration of normal menstruation in 88.2% of patients and achievement of a term pregnancy in 79.7%. However, the outcome was directly related to the extent of uterine cavity occlusion. Term pregnancies were achieved in 81.3% of those with mild disease but in only 31.9% of those with severe disease (6).

Successful lysis of intrauterine adhesions, however, may not reduce the risk of abnormal placentation. The focal destruction of endometrium at the site of adhesion formation may prevent normal formation of the decidua basalis at that locus in pregnancy. This may alter normal placental implantation and increase the risk of placenta accreta, percreta, increta, and previa.

Proximal Tubal Obstruction

Hysteroscopic procedures have been performed for relief of proximal fallopian tube occlusion. There are no controlled data, however, to support the efficacy of these procedures. One reason for this may be the difficulty in making an accurate diagnosis of proximal obstruction. The confounding entity in some cases may be cornual spasm, which mimics pathologic obstruction.

Removal of Intrauterine Devices

The hysteroscope can be useful for removing a foreign body, such as an intrauterine device. If the string of the device is no longer visible in the vagina, one can conclude that the string has broken off, the string has been drawn up into the uterine cavity, the device has been expelled, or the device has penetrated or perforated the endometrium. Ultrasound visualization followed by unguided retrieval may succeed in recovering the device; if that fails, however, hysteroscopy allows removal under direct vision. String retraction can also be caused by an intrauterine pregnancy; therefore, this must be ruled out prior to performing hysteroscopy.

Müllerian Anomalies

Müllerian fusion defects (lateral fusion defects) are an important cause of second-trimester pregnancy loss. In the past, when a müllerian fusion defect was thought to be the cause of recurrent pregnancy losses, a Jones, Strassman, or Tompkins metroplasty was performed via laparotomy. Patients treated in this manner are subject to the risks of prolonged anesthesia time, significant blood loss, postoperative infection, and intraperitoneal adhesions. Because the uterine cavity is entered during the procedure, these patients also traditionally undergo cesarean delivery. Hysteroscopic management of the uterine septum significantly reduces surgical complications and has a comparable success rate. Approximately 80% of patients who undergo a transabdominal metroplasty are able to achieve a term pregnancy. In a study of 103 patients who underwent hysteroscopic metroplasty, 81% reported a term pregnancy (7).

Hysteroscopic visualization of a uterine septum alone, however, is not adequate for diagnosis, nor is evaluation of the cavity by hysterosalpingography. The apparent septum may be in fact a bicornuate uterus. Performing laparoscopy at the time of hysteroscopy can provide direct confirmation of a müllerian defect.

If the septum runs nearly the length of the uterine cavity and the hysteroscope is placed into one side of the cavity, a normal uterus can be diagnosed by mistake. In such a case, however, only one tubal ostium can be seen. Simultaneously performing laparoscopy may be of significant benefit as well; temporarily removing the laparoscopic light source allows transillumination of only the side of the uterus with the hysteroscopic light source.

Infertility Evaluation

Hysteroscopy is not routinely indicated for the evaluation of a woman with infertility; however, laparoscopy for unexplained infertility is often accompanied by hysteroscopic intrauterine evaluation. If hysterosalpingography shows an abnormality of the uterine cavity, hysteroscopic evaluation and treatment is warranted.

Procedure

Preoperative Consultation

The patient should be fully informed about the risks and benefits of the procedure, the cost, what the procedure involves, and alternative approaches. The choice of setting is dependent on whether the procedure is to be diagnostic or operative, the medical status of the patient, and the expected level of patient discomfort.

Support Staff

The importance of trained support staff cannot be overemphasized. They are needed to ensure that equipment is properly handled, set up, and stored.

Contraindications

Hysteroscopy generally should not be performed in patients who are pregnant, who have a genital tract infection, or who have medical contraindications such as cardiac disease. Active upper genital tract infection increases the risk of uterine perforation as well as widespread dissemination of pathogens. Lower genital tract infection should be treated before hysteroscopy to avoid possible spread to the upper genital tract (8).

Anesthesia and Analgesia

Sufficient anesthesia and analgesia should be provided to allay patient anxiety and discomfort. This allows the physician to complete a comprehensive examination or procedure in a timely fashion. Nonsteroidal anti-inflammatory medication or light sedation may suffice in many diagnostic situations; however, major surgical procedures usually require either regional or general anesthesia.

Complications: Prevention and Management

Fluid Overload

Fluid overload from direct uterine instillation of electrolyte solutions during diagnostic hysteroscopy is rare. Absorption of dextran 70, however, can result in significant fluid overload, especially during lengthy operative procedures. The entry of dextran into the circulation can produce pulmonary edema and disseminated intravascular coagulation. Although no more than 500 ml of dextran should be used during operative hysteroscopy, it has been demonstrated that even smaller volumes can still induce complications (9). If operative procedures using nonelectrolyte solutions other than dextran are lengthy and require large volumes of distention medium, close intraoperative and postoperative monitoring of serum electrolytes and fluid management is advisable. A lack of recovery of distention medium in excess of 1,000 ml is associated with significant risk of fluid overload. One potentially lethal consequence of fluid overload is hyponatremia. A rapid decrease in serum sodium concentration can result in generalized cerebral edema, seizures, and even death.

Infection

Infection following diagnostic and operative hysteroscopy is uncommon. Preoperative determination of upper or lower genital tract infection (and treatment of lower genital tract infection) can frequently prevent significant complications. Despite the fact that dextran is a compound of polymerized sucrose, infection following the use of this distention medium is rare in a previously uninfected patient. Routine use of prophylactic antibiotics is not advised. Antibiotics should be prescribed for patients who have been advised by their physicians to receive prophylaxis for endocarditis.

Perforation

Physical examination and determination of uterine position prior to placement of the hysteroscope are essential. Gentle assessment of the depth and direction of the uterine cavity can further aid in the procedure and prevent perforation. Forcing the hysteroscope through an inadequately dilated cervix further increases the risk of perforation. Laparoscopy can also be a useful adjunct in selected cases to reduce the likelihood of perforation.

A midline uterine perforation generally does not have significant sequelae. A lateral perforation, however, may lacerate major uterine vessels. Laparoscopy and direct visualization of the perforation site may be quite useful when lateral perforation has occurred to determine whether bleeding is present. Laparoscopic assessment is also useful for the uterus that has been perforated with an operative instrument, particularly an electrosurgical or laser device, which may injure the bowel and bladder.

If perforation occurs, it is advisable to discontinue the operative procedure. If a bowel injury occurs, laparotomy may be required.

Bleeding

Electrocautery frequently can diminish intraoperative bleeding. Postoperative bleeding often can be treated by the placement of a Foley catheter balloon in the uterine cavity. Uterine contraction around a 30-ml Foley balloon filled with 15–30 ml of saline will often tamponade bleeding surfaces.

Embolism

CO_2 and air embolization are rare but can cause circulatory collapse. An oxygen saturation monitor and a high index of suspicion can aid in detection of this problem. Management includes prompt placement of the patient on her left side, administration of oxygen, and percutaneous aspiration of the embolus.

Summary

The hysteroscope is a versatile instrument which can have significant benefit in both diagnostic and therapeutic situations. Appropriate patient selection, recognition of limitations in experience and skills, and adequate instrumentation and support staff can minimize complications.

As experience with the instrument and its applications grow, indications for its usage may change. It is unlikely, however, that the hysteroscope will replace other procedures completely.

In the future, some investigational procedures may find applications in practice. Passage of imaging systems through the tubal ostia may become a common adjunct to laparoscopy and hysteroscopy. Injection of polymers into the proximal fallopian tube for temporary or permanent sterilization may become a routine office practice.

Transfer or retrieval of gametes and embryos may find an application. Finally, continued improvement in optics technology may allow direct histologic examination in situ without need for tissue sampling.

REFERENCES

1. American College of Obstetricians and Gynecologists. Laser technology. ACOG Technical Bulletin 146. Washington, DC: ACOG, 1990
2. Siegler AM, Kemmann E. Hysteroscopy. Obstet Gynecol Surv 1975;30:567–588
3. American College of Obstetricians and Gynecologists. Dysfunctional uterine bleeding. ACOG Technical Bulletin 134. Washington, DC: ACOG, 1989
4. Daniell JF, Kurtz BR, Ke RW. Hysteroscopic endometrial ablation using the rollerball electrode. Obstet Gynecol 1992;80:329–332
5. Derman SG, Rehnstrom J, Neuwirth RS. The long-term effectiveness of hysteroscopic treatment of menorrhagia and leiomyomas. Obstet Gynecol 1991;77:591–594
6. Valle RF, Sciarra JJ. Intrauterine adhesions: hysteroscopic diagnosis, classification, treatment, and reproductive outcome. Am J Obstet Gynecol 1988;158:1459–1470
7. DeCherney AH, Russell JB, Graebe RA, Polan ML. Resectoscopic management of müllerian fusion defects. Fertil Steril 1986;45:726–728
8. Siegler AM, Valle RF. Therapeutic hysteroscopic procedures. Fertil Steril 1988;50:685–701
9. McLucas B. Hyskon complications in hysteroscopic surgery. Obstet Gynecol Surv 1991;46:196–200

This Technical Bulletin was developed under the direction of the Committee on Technical Bulletins of the American College of Obstetricians and Gynecologists as an educational aid to obstetricians and gynecologists. The committee wishes to thank Alan H. DeCherney, MD, and Alan S. Penzias, MD, for their assistance in the development of this bulletin. This Technical Bulletin does not define a standard of care, nor is it intended to dictate an exclusive course of management. It presents recognized methods and techniques of clinical practice for consideration by obstetrician–gynecologists for incorporation into their practices. Variations of practice taking into account the needs of the individual patient, resources, and limitations unique to the institution or type of practice may be appropriate.

THE AMERICAN COLLEGE OF OBSTETRICIANS AND GYNECOLOGISTS
409 12th Street, SW
Washington, DC 20024-2188

12345/87654

Number 160—October 1991
(Replaces #64, May 1982)

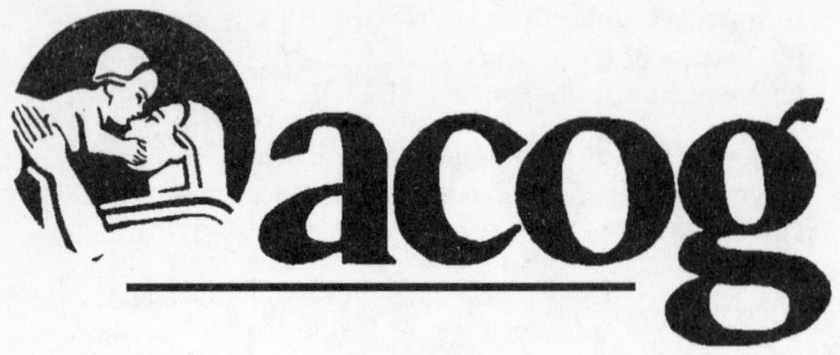

Technical Bulletin
An Educational Aid to Obstetrician–Gynecologists

Immunization During Pregnancy

In general, medications and procedures that may pose a risk to the fetus should be avoided during pregnancy. Risks from vaccination are largely theoretical, however, and the benefits of immunization usually outweigh potential risks in women with clear indications. Immunization may be indicated when the risk for exposure is high, infection poses a special risk to the mother or fetus, and the vaccine is not likely to cause harm.

The number of available vaccines has increased substantially since the early 1960s, and health care providers must continually update their knowledge about indications for vaccine use. This Technical Bulletin presents current recommendations of the Immunization Practices Advisory Committee (ACIP) for immunization of pregnant women (Table 1). Although new information continues to confirm the safety of vaccines inadvertently given during pregnancy, current information is subject to change because the effects of many diseases and vaccines on the pregnant woman or her fetus may be rare and infrequently reported.

Immunobiologic Agents

There are four types of immunobiologic agents commonly used in the United States (1). 1) *Toxoids* are preparations of chemically altered bacterial exotoxins. 2) *Inactivated vaccines* contain a suspension of heat-inactivated or chemically inactivated microorganisms or portions of microorganisms. 3) *Live viral and bacterial vaccines* are suspensions of viral or bacterial strains selected for their reduced virulence. Diminished virulence usually is produced by serial passages of the wild-type microorganism in tissue culture (attenuation). In all cases, although no significant illness is produced, the live viral or bacterial vaccine has sufficient antigenic properties in common with the infectious wild-type agent to stimulate protective immunity. 4) *Immune globulin preparations* are protein fractions of pooled human plasma containing antibodies that can produce transient, passive protection in the recipient. Specific immune globulins, which are produced from plasma of donors with very high antibody titers to a particular agent, are useful for protection against hepatitis B, rabies, tetanus, and varicella infections. Standard immune globulin is useful in providing protection against hepatitis A and measles. Bacterial polysaccharide immune globulin has been used for protection against *Haemophilus influenzae* type b, *Neisseria meningitidis*, and *Streptococcus pneumoniae*.

Criteria for Vaccination During Pregnancy

A systematic approach to vaccinating women of childbearing age is needed in order to ensure that every pregnant woman and her fetus are protected from preventable, serious diseases as well as from the possible risks that may accompany vaccination. Several factors should be weighed by the health care provider who is considering immunization for any adult female. Whenever possible, pregnant women should be immune to the diseases that pose the greatest and most common risks during pregnancy and for which there are effective vaccines. Accepted criteria for defining immunity vary by disease, and careful attention should be paid to prior illnesses, previous vaccination, and the results of past serologic tests.

Recommended Immunity for Women

Ideally, all women of childbearing age in the United States should be immune to measles, mumps, rubella, tetanus, diphtheria, and poliomyelitis, by virtue of either vaccination or natural infection. Most persons born prior to 1957 were infected naturally with measles and mumps and can be considered immune. For persons born since 1957, a history of physician-diagnosed disease, documentation of vaccination with live vaccine on or after the first birthday, or a positive antibody test with a reliable assay are considered indicators of immunity to measles or mumps. For some women—those entering institutions of higher education, newly hired medical personnel, and international travelers (2)—adequate measles vaccination consists of two doses of vaccine.

A documented history of vaccination on or after the first birthday or serologic evidence of any detectable antibody specific for rubella is considered evidence of immunity to rubella, but history of rubella disease is not (3). A clinical diagnosis of rubella is not reliable, since many other illnesses may mimic the signs and symptoms of this disease.

A person is considered immune to tetanus and diphtheria after receiving at least three doses of each toxoid, with the last dose administered at least 6–12 months after the preceding dose (4). A booster dose is required every 10 years.

Immunity to other diseases is important for women of childbearing age who have special risk factors. Hepatitis B vaccine is recommended for women at risk for hepatitis B (5, 6) (see "Current Vaccination Indications for Pregnant Women" in this Technical Bulletin). Influenza and pneumococcal vaccines are recommended for women with special conditions that put them at high risk for influenza or pneumococcal infection (7, 8) and complications; for example, women with certain chronic medical conditions should be given influenza vaccine, and patients who have undergone splenectomy should be given pneumococcal vaccine. In both pregnant and nonpregnant women, immune globulin or a specific immune globulin may be indicated following exposure to measles, hepatitis A or B, tetanus, chickenpox, or rabies (2, 4, 6, 9, 10). Likewise, immune globulin or vaccination against poliomyelitis, yellow fever, typhoid, or hepatitis B may be indicated for travelers to areas where these diseases are endemic or epidemic (6, 11–14).

Women should be immune to poliomyelitis prior to pregnancy. Because the risk for paralytic poliomyelitis in the United States is very small and most adults are already immune, routine poliomyelitis vaccination of adults without documentation of a primary series is not necessary. Adults who are not immune to poliomyelitis have only a very small risk for developing vaccine-associated poliomyelitis when children in the household are given oral polio vaccine. Therefore, administration of oral polio vaccine to children has been recommended regardless of the poliomyelitis vaccination status of adult household contacts, including the mother (11, 12). Alternatively, at least two doses of enhanced-potency inactivated poliomyelitis virus vaccine may be given to susceptible nonpregnant mothers before oral polio vaccine is given to their children, as long as complete immunization of the children is not delayed or jeopardized. Definitions of immunity as determined by the ACIP and recommendations for schedules of initial and booster immunization for all licensed vaccines are available from the Centers for Disease Control (1–4, 6–22).

Risk for Exposure

A second factor to be weighed is the woman's risk for exposure to disease. The ideal strategy is to induce immunity to a disease before pregnancy. When this has not been done, it is preferable to reduce exposure during pregnancy rather than to vaccinate, especially if a live viral or bacterial vaccine is required for immunization (15, 23). The pregnant woman should be advised against travel to areas where she is likely to be exposed to plague or yellow fever unless she was vaccinated against these diseases before pregnancy (13, 21). Appropriate hygienic precautions decrease the risk of cholera, hepatitis A, and typhoid in travelers to developing countries. It is not feasible to prevent exposure to diseases that are endemic to some parts of the United States, such as measles, mumps, and rubella. It is also difficult to prevent exposure to those diseases that periodically become epidemic, such as influenza. Some pregnant women will have risk factors for exposure to a specific disease. For example, women who are parenteral drug users, have multiple sexual partners, or who are sexual partners of persons infected with hepatitis B have a high risk for developing hepatitis B (6).

Risk from Disease

If the pregnant woman is susceptible and at risk for exposure, the morbidity and mortality from both maternal and fetal infection must be assessed. In the case of tetanus, the high rates of maternal morbidity and mortality are not altered because of pregnancy, and the newborn is at risk for neonatal tetanus. In the case of natural infection with poliomyelitis, paralysis may be more frequent when infection develops during pregnancy. Acute hepatitis B is always serious. Infants born to mothers who are infected with hepatitis B virus are at high risk for viral carriage and also have a risk for developing fulminant neonatal hepatitis. The pregnant woman herself is also at risk for serious illness. For these reasons, all pregnant women should be screened for hepatitis B virus infection (5, 24–27). A full description of risks of disease to both the pregnant woman and her fetus or infant is included in Table 1 for each immunobiologic agent.

Risk from Immunobiologic Agents

A vaccine must be assessed in terms of its effectiveness in conferring immunity and its potential for complicating pregnancy. Data on effectiveness are available for most of the agents listed in Table 1. Cholera vaccine is notable for the poor or transient immunity that it confers; live oral or inactivated parenteral typhoid vaccines induce immunity in less than 80% of recipients. Influenza vaccine provides protection for about 1 year after its administration. Tetanus immunization requires booster doses every 10 years. In contrast, many other vaccines have been shown to produce long-lasting and probably permanent immunity in over 90% of recipients.

Although limited information is available concerning the deleterious effects of most vaccines on a developing fetus, inactivated vaccines generally are considered safe to administer to pregnant women (15). There is no evidence that inactivated vaccines harm the fetus or increase the risk for abortion. Although there is no scientific evidence to support concerns about potential teratogenicity, when any vaccine is to be given during pregnancy, some physicians wait until after the first trimester to minimize concerns. Immune globulin and specific immune globulins, when indicated, are safe to administer during pregnancy.

There is concern that live viral or bacterial vaccine strains could potentially infect the fetus and cause congenital birth defects (15, 23). Therefore, live viral or bacterial vaccines should be avoided during pregnancy unless specifically indicated. Rubella vaccine is probably the best-studied immunobiologic agent with respect to risks for fetal infection (22, 28, 29). A total of 272 women who were known to be susceptible and who received the current RA 27/3 rubella vaccine shortly before becoming pregnant or early in pregnancy have been followed to term by the Immunization Division of the Centers for Disease Control. No infant had defects that suggested congenital rubella syndrome, although three had serologic findings consistent with subclinical rubella infection. These data indicate that the risk of rubella vaccine to the fetus is negligible (an observed risk of 0, with 95% confidence limits of 0–1.7%). Although the final decision rests with the woman and her physician, the ACIP believes that rubella vaccination during pregnancy should not be a reason to routinely recommend pregnancy termination. Nevertheless, pregnancy is a contraindication to rubella vaccination, as well as to measles and mumps vaccination, because of theoretical risks for fetal damage. Immune globulin usually will prevent or modify measles in the susceptible individual if given within 6 days after exposure and can be given to pregnant women exposed to measles. However, immune globulin has not been shown to prevent infection in a patient exposed to rubella or mumps. Moreover, immune globulin is probably of little benefit for pregnant women exposed to rubella infection because subclinical infection, with attendant fetal risks, still may develop. The ACIP believes that immune globulin has potential use only for the pregnant woman exposed to rubella who would not consider termination.

Even though yellow fever vaccine is an attenuated live vaccine, it can be administered to pregnant women who are at substantial risk for exposure to natural infection (13). The same is true for live attenuated oral polio vaccine when immediate protection is required during an outbreak (11, 12). Neither the live attenuated Ty 21a oral typhoid vaccine nor the inactivated parenteral typhoid vaccine has been studied and demonstrated to be safe in pregnancy. According to the ACIP, however, their use is not contraindicated during pregnancy (14).

Confirmation of Pregnancy

Before a woman is vaccinated, it should be determined whether she is pregnant. Because of the theoretical risk to the fetus of infection with live virus vaccines, women of childbearing age should receive measles, rubella, and mumps vaccines only if they are not pregnant. Testing for pregnancy, however, is not essential. Reasonable precautions before giving these vaccines include asking women if they are pregnant, explaining the theoretical risks, and advising them not to become pregnant for 3 months after vaccination (3). Pregnant women should not be vaccinated against mumps, measles, or rubella.

Current Vaccination Indications for Pregnant Women

The use of immunobiologic agents during pregnancy should be limited to a few well-defined situations. Preferably, women should be protected from preventable diseases by vaccination before they become pregnant. Live viral or bacterial vaccines, in particular, should not be given during pregnancy except when susceptibility and exposure are highly probable and the disease to be prevented poses a greater threat to the woman or fetus than does vaccination. An example would be yellow fever vaccine for a pregnant woman who moves to an area in which yellow fever is present.

In the United States, the only immunobiologic agents that are recommended for routine administration during pregnancy are tetanus and diphtheria toxoids. The hepatitis B vaccine series can be administered to pregnant women who are at high risk and who test negative for hepatitis B virus infection to protect them and their infants from infection during and after pregnancy (5). Women who are at high risk for hepatitis B virus infection and are thus candidates for vaccination during pregnancy include, but are not limited to, those with histories of the following (5, 6):

- Percutaneous use of illicit drugs
- Acute episode of any sexually transmitted disease
- Multiple sexual partners
- Work in a health care or public safety field
- Household contact with a hepatitis B carrier
- Work or residence in an institution for the developmentally disabled
- Work or treatment in a hemodialysis unit
- Receipt of clotting factor concentrates for bleeding disorders

Women already infected with hepatitis B may carry the virus unknowingly and pose a risk to their fetus or newborn. Because of the serious risk that hepatitis B poses for the fetus and newborn, all pregnant women should be screened for hepatitis B surface antigen. Screening pregnant women when they are admitted to the hospital in labor would be ideal if the results could be available within 12–24 hours. Because this is not always possible, the test for hepatitis B surface antigen should be added to the battery of routine prenatal tests (5, 26). The pregnant woman's need for influenza or pneumococcal immunization is determined on the basis of underlying high-risk conditions.

Measles, mumps, and rubella vaccine should be given to women at least 3 months prior to pregnancy or in the immediate postpartum period. Although virus shedding does occur, children given measles, mumps, or rubella vaccines do not transmit vaccine virus; thus, these vaccines can be administered safely to children of pregnant women. Pregnant women should be given yellow fever vaccine or primary vaccination against poliomyelitis when traveling to areas where the risk for exposure is high. As with all adults, the primary series for poliomyelitis vaccination usually comprises three doses of enhanced-potency inactivated poliomyelitis vaccine. During an outbreak, in which immediate protection is needed, however, one dose of oral polio vaccine can be used to begin the primary series.

The recommendations of the ACIP should be followed for the administration of immune globulin or specific immune globulins after exposure to measles, hepatitis A, hepatitis B, tetanus, chickenpox, or rabies (2, 4, 6, 9, 10). Varicella-zoster immune globulin, which is obtained from the American Red Cross, should be administered to the newborn if the mother developed chickenpox within 5 days prior to or 2 days following delivery (9). There is no evidence that maternal administration of varicella-zoster immune globulin reduces the rare occurrence of congenital varicella syndrome. Varicella-zoster immune globulin can be considered to treat the pregnant woman herself to prevent the complications of chickenpox.

Summary

Women of childbearing age in the United States should be immune to measles, rubella, mumps, tetanus, diphtheria, and, through childhood immunization, poliomyelitis. Of particular importance are rubella, because of the devastating effects of congenital infection; measles, because of its high risk for causing spontaneous abortion, preterm birth, and maternal morbidity; and tetanus, because transplacental transfer of antitoxin prevents neonatal tetanus. Protection against hepatitis B is critical for the pregnant woman and newborn who are at high risk for infection. Combined tetanus and diphtheria toxoids are the only immunobiologic agents routinely indicated for susceptible pregnant women. Other vaccines may be indicated for pregnant women under special circumstances. Measles, mumps, and rubella single-antigen vaccines, as well as the combined vaccine, are contraindicated in pregnancy but should ideally be given preconceptionally or postpartum.

In the decision of whether to immunize a pregnant woman with other vaccines, the risk for exposure to disease and its deleterious effects on the pregnant woman and her fetus must be balanced against the efficacy of the vaccine and any possible deleterious effects resulting from it. Preconception immunization of women to prevent disease in the offspring, when practical, is preferred to vaccination of pregnant women.

REFERENCES

1. Immunization Practices Advisory Committee/Centers for Disease Control. General recommendations on immunization. MMWR 1989;38:205–228

2. Immunization Practices Advisory Committee/Centers for Disease Control. Measles prevention: Recommendations of the Immunization Practices Advisory Committee (ACIP). MMWR 1989;38:S-9:1–18

3. Immunization Practices Advisory Committee/Centers for Disease Control. Rubella prevention. MMWR 1984;33: 301–318

4. Immunization Practices Advisory Committee/Centers for Disease Control. Diphtheria, tetanus, and pertussis: guidelines for vaccine prophylaxis and other preventive measures. MMWR 1985;34:405–414, 419–426

5. American College of Obstetricians and Gynecologists. Guidelines for hepatitis B virus screening and vaccination during pregnancy. ACOG Committee Opinion 78. Washington, DC: ACOG, 1990

6. Immunization Practices Advisory Committee/Centers for Disease Control. Protection against viral hepatitis. MMWR 1990;39:RR-2:1–26

7. Immunization Practices Advisory Committee/Centers for Disease Control. Pneumococcal polysaccharide vaccine. MMWR 1989;38:64–76

8. Immunization Practices Advisory Committee/Centers for Disease Control. Prevention and control of influenza. Part I, Vaccines. MMWR 1989;38:297–311

9. Immunization Practices Advisory Committee/Centers for Disease Control. Varicella-zoster immune globulin for the prevention of chickenpox. MMWR 1984;33:84–100

10. Immunization Practices Advisory Committee/Centers for Disease Control. Rabies prevention—United States, 1984. MMWR 1984;33:393–408

11. Immunization Practices Advisory Committee/Centers for Disease Control. Poliomyelitis prevention. MMWR 1982; 31:22–34

12. Immunization Practices Advisory Committee/Centers for Disease Control. Poliomyelitis prevention: enhanced-potency inactivated poliomyelitis vaccine-supplemental statement. MMWR 1987;36:795–798

13. Immunization Practices Advisory Committee/Centers for Disease Control. Yellow fever vaccine. MMWR 1990;39: RR-6:1–6

14. Immunization Practices Advisory Committee/Centers for Disease Control. Typhoid immunization. MMWR 1990;39: RR-10:1–5

15. Immunization Practices Advisory Committee/Centers for Disease Control. Adult immunization. MMWR 1984;33 (Suppl 1):1S–68S

16. Immunization Practices Advisory Committee/Centers for Disease Control. BCG vaccines. MMWR 1988;37

17. Immunization Practices Advisory Committee/Centers for Disease Control. Cholera vaccine. MMWR 1988;37:617–624

18. Immunization Practices Advisory Committee/Centers for Disease Control. Health information for international travel, 1989

19. Immunization Practices Advisory Committee/Centers for Disease Control. Meningococcal vaccines. MMWR 1985;34:255–259

20. Immunization Practices Advisory Committee/Centers for Disease Control. Mumps prevention. MMWR 1988; 38: 388–400

21. Immunization Practices Advisory Committee/Centers for Disease Control. Plague vaccine. MMWR 1982;31: 301–304

22. Immunization Practices Advisory Committee/Centers for Disease Control. Rubella vaccination during pregnancy—United States, 1971–1988. MMWR 1989;38; 289–293

23. Levine MM. Live-virus vaccines in pregnancy. Risks and recommendations. Lancet 1974;2(871):34–38

24. Amstey MS, Insel RA, Pichichero ME. Neonatal passive immunization by maternal vaccination. Obstet Gynecol 1984;63:105–109

25. Insel RA. Maternal immunization to prevent neonatal infections. N Engl J Med 1988;319:1219–1220

26. Kane MA, Hadler SC, Margolis HS, Maynard JE. Routine prenatal screening for hepatitis B surface antigen. JAMA 1988;259:408–409

27. Tong MJ, Thursby M, Rakela J, McPeak C, Edwards VM, Mosley JW. Studies on the maternal-infant transmission of the viruses which cause acute hepatitis. Gastroenterology 1981;80:999–1004

28. Preblud SR, Stetler HC, Frank JA Jr, Greaves WL, Hinman AR, Herrmann KL. Fetal risk associated with rubella vaccine. JAMA 1981;246:1413–1417

29. Preblud, SR. Some current issues relating to rubella vaccine. JAMA 1985;254:253–256

SUGGESTED READING

American College of Physicians. General recommendations for adult immunization, 1989

Amstey MS, Insel R, Munoz J, Pichichero M. Fetal-neonatal passive immunization against Hemophilus influenzae, type b. Am J Obstet Gynecol 1985;153:607-611

Baker CJ, Rench MA, Edwards MS, Carpenter RJ, Hays BM, Kasper DL. Immunization of pregnant women with a polysaccharide vaccine of group B streptococcus. N Engl J Med 1988;319:1180-1185

Cochi SL, Edmonds LE, Dyer K, Greaves WL, Marks JS, Rovira EZ, et al. Congenital rubella syndrome in the United States, 1970-1985. On the verge of elimination. Am J Epidemiol 1989;129:349-361

Gershon AA, Steinberg S, Brunell PA. Zoster immune globulin. A further assessment. N Engl J Med 1974;290:243-245

Hirschhorn N, Chowdhury AK, Lindenbaum J. Cholera in pregnant women. Lancet 1969;1(608):1230-1232

Jespersen CS, Littauer J, Sagild U. Measles as a cause of fetal defects. A retrospective cause of ten measles epidemics in Greenland. Acta Paediatr Scand 1977;66:367-372

Kaplan KM, Cochi SL, Edmonds LD, Zell ER, Preblud SR. A profile of mothers giving birth to infants with congenital rubella syndrome. An assessment of risk factors. Am J Dis Child 1990;144:118-123

Miller E, Cradock-Watson JE, Pollock TM. Consequences of confirmed maternal rubella at successive stages of pregnancy. Lancet 1982;2(8302):781-784

Newell KW, Duenas-Lehmann A, Leblanc DR, Garces-Osario N. The use of toxoid for the prevention of tetanus neonatorum. Final report of a double-blind controlled field trial. Bull World Health Organ 1966;35:863-871

Rubin DH, Palmer LS, Menasse L, Erenberg FG. Does breastfeeding protect infants from Haemophilus influenzae infection? J Pediatr 1987;110:162-163

Siegel M. Congenital malformations following chickenpox, measles, mumps, and hepatitis. Results of a cohort study. JAMA 1973;226:1521-1524

Siegel M, Fuerst HT. Low birth weight and maternal virus disease. A prospective study of rubella, measles, mumps, chickenpox, and hepatitis. JAMA 1966;197:680-684

Siegel M, Fuerst HT, Peress NS. Comparative fetal mortality in maternal virus diseases. A prospective study on rubella, measles, mumps, chickenpox, and hepatitis. N Engl J Med 1966;274:768

Yamauchi T, Wilson C, St Geme JW Jr. Transmission of live, attenuated mumps virus to the human placenta. N Engl J Med 1974;290:710-712

TABLE 1. IMMUNIZATION DURING PREGNANCY

Immunobiologic agent	Risk from disease to pregnant woman	Risk from disease to fetus or neonate	Type of immunizing agent	Risk from immunizing agent to fetus	Indications for immunization during pregnancy	Dose schedule*	Comments
			LIVE VIRUS VACCINES				
Measles	Significant morbidity, low mortality; not altered by pregnancy	Significant increase in abortion rate; may cause malformations	Live attenuated virus vaccine	None confirmed	Contraindicated (see immune globulins)	Single dose SC, preferably as measles–mumps–rubella[†]	Vaccination of susceptible women should be part of postpartum care
Mumps	Low morbidity and mortality; not altered by pregnancy	Probable increased rate of abortion in first trimester	Live attenuated virus vaccine	None confirmed	Contraindicated	Single dose SC, preferably as measles–mumps–rubella	Vaccination of susceptible women should be part of postpartum care
Poliomyelitis	No increased incidence in pregnancy, but may be more severe if it does occur	Anoxic fetal damage reported; 50% mortality in neonatal disease	Live attenuated virus (oral polio vaccine [OPV]) and enhanced-potency inactivated virus (e-IPV) vaccine[‡]	None confirmed	Not routinely recommended for women in U.S., except persons at increased risk of exposure	Primary: 2 doses of e-IPV SC at 4–8-week intervals and a 3rd dose 6–12 months after the 2nd dose. Immediate protection: 1 dose OPV orally (in outbreak setting)	Vaccine indicated for susceptible pregnant women traveling in endemic areas or in other high-risk situations
Rubella	Low morbidity and mortality; not altered by pregnancy	High rate of abortion and congenital rubella syndrome	Live attenuated virus vaccine	None confirmed	Contraindicated	Single dose SC, preferably as measles–mumps–rubella	Teratogenicity of vaccine is theoretic, not confirmed to date; vaccination of susceptible women should be part of postpartum care
Yellow fever	Significant morbidity and mortality; not altered by	Unknown	Live attenuated virus vaccine	Unknown	Contraindicated except if exposure is unavoidable	Single dose SC	Postponement of travel preferable to vaccination, if pregnancy possible

			INACTIVATED VIRUS VACCINES				
Influenza	Possible increase in morbidity and mortality during epidemic of new antigenic strain	Possible increased abortion rate; no malformations confirmed	Inactivated virus vaccine	None confirmed	Women with serious underlying diseases; public health authorities to be consulted for current recommendation	One dose IM every year	
Rabies	Near 100% fatality; not altered by pregnancy	Determined by maternal disease	Killed virus vaccine	Unknown	Indications for prophylaxis not altered by pregnancy; each case considered individually	Public health authorities to be consulted for indications, dosage, and route of administration	
Hepatitis B	Possible increased severity during third trimester	Possible increase in abortion rate and prematurity; neonatal hepatitis can occur; high risk of newborn carrier state	Recombinant vaccine	None reported	Pre- and post-exposure for women at risk of infection	Three- or four-dose series IM	Used with hepatitis B immune globulin for some exposures; exposed newborn needs vaccination as soon as possible
			INACTIVATED BACTERIAL VACCINES				
Cholera	Significant morbidity and mortality; more severe during third trimester	Increased risk of fetal death during third-trimester maternal illness	Killed bacterial vaccine	None confirmed	Indications not altered by pregnancy; vaccination recommended only in unusual outbreak situations	Single dose SC or IM, depending on manufacturer's recommendations when indicated	
Plague	Significant morbidity and mortality; not altered by pregnancy	Determined by maternal disease	Killed bacterial vaccine	None reported	Selective vaccination of exposed persons	Public health authorities to be consulted for indications, dosage, and route of administration	

(Continued, next page)

TABLE 1. IMMUNIZATION DURING PREGNANCY

Immunobiologic agent	Risk from disease to pregnant woman	Risk from disease to fetus or neonate	Type of immunizing agent	Risk from immunizing agent to fetus	Indications for immunization during pregnancy	Dose schedule*	Comments
Pneumococcus	No increased risk during pregnancy; no increase in severity of disease	Unknown	Polyvalent polysaccharide vaccine	No data available on use during pregnancy	Indications not altered by pregnancy; vaccine used only for high-risk individuals	In adults, 1 SC or IM dose only; consider repeat dose in 6 years for high-risk individuals	
Typhoid	Significant morbidity and mortality; not altered by pregnancy	Unknown	Killed or live attenuated oral bacterial vaccine	None confirmed	Not recommended routinely except for close, continued exposure or travel to endemic areas	Killed: Primary: 2 injections SC at least 4 weeks apart. Booster: Single dose SC or ID (depending on type of product used) every 3 years. Oral: Primary: 4 doses on alternate days Booster: Schedule not yet determined	
			TOXOIDS				
Tetanus–diphtheria	Severe morbidity; tetanus mortality 30%, diphtheria mortality 10%; unaltered by pregnancy	Neonatal tetanus mortality 60%	Combined tetanus–diphtheria toxoids preferred: adult tetanus–diphtheria formulation	None confirmed	Lack of primary series, or no booster within past 10 years	Primary: 2 doses IM at 1–2-month interval with a 3rd dose 6–12 months after the 2nd. Booster: Single dose IM every 10 years, after completion of primary series	Updating of immune status should be part of antepartum care

(Continued, next page)

			SPECIFIC IMMUNE GLOBULINS				
Hepatitis B	Possible increased severity during third trimester	Possible increase in abortion rate and prematurity; neonatal hepatitis can occur; high risk of carriage in newborn	Hepatitis B immune globulin	None reported	Postexposure prophylaxis	Depends on exposure; consult Immunization Practices Advisory Committee recommendations (IM)	Usually given with HBV vaccine; exposed newborn needs immediate postexposure prophylaxis
Rabies	Near 100% fatality; not altered by pregnancy	Determined by maternal disease	Rabies immune globulin	None reported	Postexposure prophylaxis	Half dose at injury site, half dose in deltoid	Used in conjunction with rabies killed virus vaccine
Tetanus	Severe morbidity; mortality 21%	Neonatal tetanus mortality 60%	Tetanus immune globulin	None reported	Postexposure prophylaxis	One dose IM	Used in conjunction with tetanus toxoid
Varicella	Possible increase in severe varicella pneumonia	Can cause congenital varicella with increased mortality in neonatal period; very rarely causes congenital defects	Varicella-zoster immune globulin (obtained from the American Red Cross)	None reported	Can be considered for healthy pregnant women exposed to varicella to protect against maternal, not congenital, infection	One dose IM within 96 hours of exposure	Indicated also for newborns of mothers who developed varicella within 4 days prior to delivery or 2 days following delivery; approx. 90–95% of adults are immune to varicella; not indicated for prevention of congenital varicella
			STANDARD IMMUNE GLOBULINS				
Hepatitis A	Possible increased severity during third trimester	Probable increase in abortion rate and prematurity; possible transmission to neonate at delivery if mother is incubating the virus or is acutely ill at that time	Standard immune globulin	None reported	Postexposure prophylaxis	0.02 ml/kg IM in one dose of immune globulin	Immune globulin should be given as soon as possible and within 2 weeks of exposure; infants born to mothers who are incubating the virus or are acutely ill at delivery should receive one dose of 0.5 ml as soon as possible after birth

(Continued, next page)

TABLE 1. IMMUNIZATION DURING PREGNANCY

Immunobiologic agent	Risk from disease to pregnant woman	Risk from disease to fetus or neonate	Type of immunizing agent	Risk from immunizing agent to fetus	Indications for immunization during pregnancy	Dose schedule*	Comments
Measles	Significant morbidity, low mortality; not altered by pregnancy	Significant increase in abortion rate; may cause malformations	Standard immune globulin	None reported	Postexposure prophylaxis	0.25 ml/kg IM in one dose of immune globulin, up to 15 ml	Unclear if it prevents abortion; must be given within 6 days of exposure

*Abbreviations: SC = subcutaneously; PO = orally; IM = intramuscularly; ID = intradermally.

† Two doses necessary for adequate vaccination of students entering institutions of higher education, newly hired medical personnel, and international travelers.

‡ Inactivated polio vaccine recommended for nonimmunized adults at increased risk.

This Technical Bulletin was developed under the direction of the Committee on Technical Bulletins of the American College of Obstetricians and Gynecologists as an educational aid to obstetricians and gynecologists. The committee wishes to thank Laura Fehrs, MD, Walter W. Williams, MD, Stephen L. Cochi, MD, Walter A. Orenstein, MD, and Carl W. Tyler, MD, for their assistance in the development of this bulletin. This Technical Bulletin does not define a standard of care, nor is it intended to dictate an exclusive course of management. It presents recognized methods and techniques of clinical practice for consideration by obstetrician–gynecologists for incorporation into their practices. Variations of practice taking into account the needs of the individual patient, resources, and limitations unique to the institution or type of practice may be appropriate.

THE AMERICAN COLLEGE OF OBSTETRICIANS AND GYNECOLOGISTS
409 12th Street, SW
Washington, DC 20024-2188

45/6

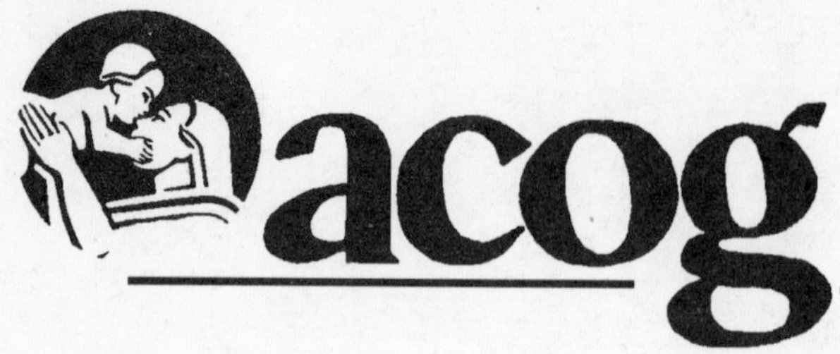

Number 125—February 1989

Technical Bulletin

An Educational Aid to Obstetrician–Gynecologists

Infertility

It is estimated that at least 14% of American couples of reproductive age who desire pregnancy are unable to conceive within a year (1). The 1980s have seen a geometric rise in annual numbers of physician visits for the diagnosis and treatment of infertility, with over 3 million affected couples (2). Although the sequelae of sexually transmitted infections have played a role, especially in younger women, the "infertility epidemic" is predominantly a cultural phenomenon of the "baby boom" generation. The postponement of pregnancy, combined with the attempt to condense childbearing into a shorter time interval, have resulted in an increasing proportion of infertile couples seeking medical care (3). At the same time, the demand by patients for sophisticated diagnosis and treatment has been met by an increasing number of physicians providing infertility services (4).

Infertility is a condition with unique and profound psychologic and emotional impacts. Infertility is experienced by most couples as a life crisis in which they feel isolated and powerless. Feelings of frustration, anger, depression, grief, guilt, and anxiety are common and should be anticipated and dealt with appropriately.

The commitment to provide infertility care is therefore not a trivial one. It is important for health care providers to understand and accept the emotional and educational needs and demands of infertility patients. Physicians must honestly appraise their interests, personalities, training, and experience and be prepared to refer patients to others when appropriate. In addition, a team approach may be helpful in ensuring that patients receive an adequate workup and counseling as the need arises.

This bulletin is intended to provide an overview of the evaluation of the infertile couple, with an emphasis on the investigation of frequently seen disorders associated with infertility. The evaluation of specific problem areas and therapeutic modalities will be covered elsewhere (5, 6).

Evaluation

The goals of an infertility evaluation are to provide a rational, organized approach to diagnosis, to present an accurate assessment of progress and prognosis during the evaluation, and to offer emotional and psychologic support.

The organization of an infertility evaluation requires consideration of each of the factors of reproduction (male, ovulatory, pelvic, and cervical), taking into account the expense, invasiveness, and risks of each procedure and the likelihood of a significant finding. The initial assessment is followed by the basic diagnostic workup, which determines treatment and further testing options.

Initial Assessment

The initial assessment begins with an extended fertility history and physical examination. Ideally, both partners should be present at the initial interview. The couple's ages, previous pregnancies, and length of time attempting conception are important factors to be noted. A sexual history includes the frequency of intercourse, use of lubricants (which can be spermicidal), anorgasmia, impotence, and dyspareunia.

A male factor is responsible for approximately 35% of cases of infertility. History of testicular surgery or injury, genitourinary infection (including sexually transmitted infections), postpubertal mumps, genital radiation, chemotherapy, hypospadias, or retrograde ejaculation should be noted. Physical examination of the male should include careful evaluation of genitalia, assessing testicular descent, size and consistency of testes, and possible presence of varicocele or penile anomalies. Excessive exposure to heat (hot tubs, saunas), toxic chemicals, or pesticides or use of marijuana or nicotine (7) should be eliminated. Alcohol consumption should be minimized.

A pelvic factor is responsible for approximately 25% of cases of infertility and includes abnormalities of the uterus, fallopian tubes, ovaries, and adjacent pelvic structures. It is suggested by a history of pelvic infection, including salpingitis (pelvic inflammatory disease), septic abortion, ruptured appendix, use of intrauterine devices, or pelvic tuberculosis. Secondary dysmenorrhea, dyspareunia, or cyclic abdominal or pelvic pain should prompt consideration of endometriosis. A history of ectopic pregnancy, adnexal surgery, leiomyomas, or exposure to diethylstilbestrol (DES) in utero are important considerations. Physical examination may reveal pelvic tenderness, pelvic mass, uterosacral nodularity, decreased uterine mobility, or irregular uterine contour.

An ovulatory factor is responsible for approximately 20% of cases of infertility and may present as secondary amenorrhea, irregular menses (ie, chronic anovulation or oligoovulation), or luteal phase defect. Irregular cycle lengths of less than 25 days or more than 36 days or a variation of more than 7 days in consecutive cycles are suggestive of ovulation defects, especially if premenstrual molimina, amount and duration of menstrual bleeding, and dysmenorrhea are variable. Signs and symptoms of hyperthyroidism or hypothyroidism, as well as hirsutism, galactorrhea, hot flushes, weight loss (particularly if associated with endurance exercise or a history of an eating disorder), obesity, and severe psychologic stress, should be taken into consideration.

A cervical factor is responsible for approximately 10% of cases of infertility and may be suggested by a history of cone biopsy, cautery, cervicitis, obstetric trauma, or DES exposure in utero.

Following the fertility history and physical examination, the initial assessment concludes with an overview of reproductive physiology and a formulation and explanation of the basic diagnostic steps in the infertility workup. Enough time should be allowed to assess and discuss the couple's emotional response in a supportive and unhurried manner. The initiation of the basic workup need not be postponed by prolonged temperature charting or nonspecific reassurance. Most couples feel that the admonition to "relax" implies that their anxiety is responsible for their infertility—an unsupported and hurtful suggestion.

Basic Workup

The more common infertility factors can be evaluated by a minimal number of tests. These include 1) semen analysis, 2) documentation of ovulation, 3) postcoital test, and 4) evaluation of tubal patency.

A semen sample should be collected for analysis after a 48-hour abstinence period (to reflect optimal coital frequency) and evaluated within 1 hour of ejaculation. Normal values for semen parameters are shown in Table 1. If any parameters are abnormal, two additional semen

TABLE 1. NORMAL SEMEN PARAMETERS

Determination	Normal value
Ejaculate volume	>1 ml
Concentration	>20 x 10^6/ml
Initial progressive motility	>50%
Normal morphology	>60%

analyses should be performed 2 weeks apart. If abnormalities persist, urologic consultation should be considered.

Ovulation may be assessed by three methods: basal body temperature, serum progesterone, or endometrial biopsy. Many clinicians prefer to use basal body temperature initially, rather than serum progesterone. Since progesterone is released into the circulation in a pulsatile fashion, a random progesterone level is valuable only if elevated. A low progesterone level may or may not be consistent with normal ovulation. If serum progesterone is used, levels should be measured 7 days after estimated ovulation. Laboratory values should be interpreted in light of an individual laboratory's standards. In general, values of greater than 15 ng/ml are consistent with normal ovulatory function, while levels of less than 5 ng/ml may indicate anovulation. Intermediate values may indicate a luteal phase defect and should be repeated in the following cycle for confirmation after ovulation has been detected by determination of luteinizing hormone (LH) surge in serum or urine (8). Endometrial biopsy, in addition to detecting ovulation, provides a more thorough evaluation of a luteal phase defect.

The postcoital test is an in vivo evaluation of sperm–cervical mucus interaction. The couple is asked to have intercourse after 48 hours of sexual abstinence, and the mucus is examined within 2–8 hours. The test is scheduled 24–48 hours prior to presumed ovulation in order to assess optimal mucus production. This can be most easily accomplished by the use of home test kits for detection of any increase in urinary LH or by identification of the ovulatory period by review of basal body temperature records from previous cycles as well as during the cycle in which the postcoital test is to be performed. For the postcoital test, mucus is removed from the endocervical canal and its quantity, clarity, pH, and spinnbarkeit are assessed. Although the evaluation of the postcoital test is subjective, the finding of 5–10 progressively motile sperm per high-power field in clear, acellular mucus with a spinnbarkeit of greater than 8 cm generally excludes a cervical factor.

Hysterosalpingography should be performed in the early proliferative phase of the cycle after the cessation of menstrual flow. Abnormal findings include congenital malformations of the uterus, submucous leiomyomas, intrauterine synechiae (Asherman syndrome), intrauterine polyps, salpingitis isthmica nodosa, tubal tuberculosis, and proximal or distal tubal block. Persistent dye collections suggestive of pelvic adhesions or hydrosalpinx may be seen on a delayed flat plate after dye instillation, the timing depending on the medium used. The procedure is contraindicated by the presence of a pelvic mass or tenderness or laboratory findings suggestive of pelvic inflammatory disease, as well as by an allergy to iodine or radiocontrast dye. Women with a history of pelvic infection are better evaluated directly by laparoscopy. The risks of hysterosalpingography include dye embolization (rare) and salpingitis (1–2%).

The results of the basic workup should be reviewed with the couple to confirm or eliminate any provisional diagnosis that may have been formulated at the initial assessment, to interpret new findings, and to discuss the options for treatment or further investigation. Frequent review sessions are essential to keep the couple informed as well as to provide emotional support and encouragement. Although couples often begin the fertility workup with hope and optimism, many find the diagnostic process itself to be stressful. Often there is ambivalence about test outcome—frustration may be felt if the results are normal, even while it is feared that poor results will mean sterility. Many couples find that participation in support groups during this time helps to alleviate feelings of isolation and provides an environment in which they can share their concerns with other infertile couples. RESOLVE, the national nonprofit infertility organization, has chapters in most areas of the country and is an excellent source of referrals for support groups and counseling.

Additional Evaluation and Management

The Male Factor

Repeated abnormality of any semen parameter may indicate the need for urologic consultation. Physical abnormalities such as hypospadias, cryptorchidism, or varicocele can be detected and genitourinary infection diagnosed and treated.

Serum testosterone, follicle-stimulating hormone (FSH), and prolactin abnormalities will identify men with germ cell aplasia, chromosomal abnormalities (such as Klinefelter syndrome), or pituitary adenomas. In cases of azoospermia or severe oligospermia, the combination of testicular biopsy and semen fructose measurement will distinguish ductal obstruction from spermatogenic failure. Hypogonadotropic men may respond to treatment with human menopausal gonadotropin (hMG) or gonadotropin-releasing hormone (GnRH), whereas treatment with clomiphene, human chorionic gonadotropin (hCG), or testosterone has generally been disappointing.

Although statistics from controlled trials are lacking, surgical ligation of a varicocele, when found in association with decreased motility and increased tapering sperm forms, will result in improvement in semen parameters in most men. When the semen volume is high or a varicocele is present, the first part of the ejaculate may contain a higher motility and concentration of sperm and be used for "split-ejaculate" artificial insemination. A history of diabetes or prostatectomy may be associated with retrograde ejaculation, which may respond to ephedrine or imipramine or to artificial insemination with sperm recovered via bladder catheterization.

The sperm penetration assay, or zona-free hamster egg assay, is an attempt to test the biologic fertilizing capacity of sperm. After a 48-hour abstinence, sperm is collected, washed, preincubated, and placed in contact with 20–30 hamster eggs from which the zona pellucidae have been enzymatically removed. The incubation medium and ambient gas composition are carefully controlled to allow sperm to capacitate, undergo the acrosome reaction, and penetrate eggs. Sperm from men of proven fertility almost consistently penetrate over 10% of the eggs, while failure to penetrate at least 10% of the eggs suggests a significant male factor. The sperm penetration assay may be useful in deciding whether to perform varicocele surgery, monitoring hormonal or antibiotic treatment, screening candidates for in vitro fertilization, and evaluating unexplained infertility. Both false-positive and false-negative results may be found, and care should be taken that the results of a single assay are not overinterpreted. All 0% penetration scores should be repeated for confirmation after all possible extenuating circumstances (inadequate abstinence, improper sample collection or handling, concurrent illness or medication, or a high semen white cell count) have been eliminated (9).

The most common male factor by far is idiopathic oligospermia, for which, unfortunately, there is no effective treatment. Artificial insemination with the husband's sperm has not been shown to yield pregnancy rates greater than in untreated couples. In the presence of abnormal male factors, in vitro fertilization remains an option. The discussion of donor insemination requires sensitivity and an individualized approach but should not be delayed unnecessarily in the face of long-standing male infertility. Risk of infection, legal ramifications, adjustments of pregnancy, and effects on offspring should be thoroughly discussed with the couple and counseling offered as appropriate. The American Fertility Society has recommended the use of frozen semen since 1988.

The Pelvic Factor

Laparoscopy with chromotubation is indicated if hysterosalpingography is contraindicated or yields abnormal results or if the history or physical findings strongly suggest a pelvic factor. Laparoscopy is also indicated if other infertility factors have not been found. Management depends on the specific diagnosis.

Tubal Disorders

Tubal disorders may result from prior salpingitis (pelvic inflammatory disease), endometriosis, adhesions from previous pelvic surgery, complications of intrauterine devices, previous ectopic pregnancy, tuberculous salpingitis, and salpingitis isthmica nodosa. Although lysis of mild peritubal adhesions may be accomplished under direct vision at the time of laparoscopy, many patients with tubal disease will require tuboplasty or in vitro fertilization and embryo transfer.

Tuboplasty success rates are dependent upon the degree of original inflammatory damage to the fimbriae and ciliated and secretory cells of the tube, the site of tubal closure (distal occlusion with hydrosalpinx has a poorer prognosis than does isthmic block), the causative pathogen (tuberculous salpingitis is a contraindication to tuboplasty), the postoperative length of viable tube, and the skill and experience of the surgeon. Most tubal surgery should be performed by those with specialized skills in microsurgical techniques, including use of magnification and fine suture material, atraumatic tissue handling and hemostasis, reperitonealization of raw surfaces, and adjuvant treatment to minimize adhesion formation. Pregnancy rates following tuboplasty may range from 15% or less for large hydrosalpinges to 70% or more for reversal of sterilization in which tissue trauma has been minimal. All tuboplasty patients have an increased risk of ectopic gestation.

In vitro fertilization has been successful in achieving human pregnancies since 1978. Pregnancy rates from successful in vitro fertilization programs range from 10–25% per cycle, with a 25–35% pregnancy loss rate. In vitro fertilization may be repeated several times, although it is a psychologically stressful procedure.

Uterine Disorders

DES syndrome results from in utero exposure to DES, which was given to pregnant women in the 1950s and 1960s. It is marked by characteristic changes in the vagina (adenosis), cervix (ectropion, "hood," "coxcomb"), and uterus (T shaped, hypoplastic cavity). An increased incidence of infertility, spontaneous abortion, and premature labor has been associated with DES syndrome (10). There is no specific treatment.

Intrauterine synechiae (Asherman syndrome) are adhesions formed as a result of surgical instrumentation of the uterus complicated by endometritis. They are most often associated with curettage following term pregnancy, spontaneous or therapeutic abortion, or myomectomy and may present as amenorrhea, hypomenorrhea, infertility, or habitual abortion. The true incidence of Asherman syndrome is not known, but this condition probably accounts for only a small percentage of patients with secondary amenorrhea (11). The appearance of filling defects on hysterosalpingography is diagnostic. Treatment is by hysteroscopically guided lysis of adhesions. Broad-spectrum antibiotics are given orally for 14 days, and a high-dose estrogen is given orally for 2 months to stimulate endometrial proliferation. Treated patients have an increased risk of spontaneous abortion, placenta previa or accreta, and abruptio placentae, although pregnancy rates as high as 70% may be achieved.

Submucous or large intramural myomas may cause infertility or repeated abortion. Congenital anomalies and leiomyomas are associated with habitual abortion but are less commonly a cause of infertility. They should be surgically treated only if the remainder of the evaluation is negative.

Endometriosis

Women with endometriosis are twice as likely to be infertile as women without this condition, an increase that is without complete explanation. Endometriosis is confirmed and classified by diagnostic laparoscopy. A uniform system of classification that takes into account the presence, location, and quality of adhesions, endometriomas, and tubal distortion has been formulated by the American Fertility Society and classifies the disease as minimal, mild, moderate, and severe (stages I–IV) (12).

Treatment of endometriosis may be surgical or hormonal and is based on a confirmed laparoscopic diagnosis, the patient's age, and the extent, location, and severity of the disease. Initial treatment can often be accomplished at the time of diagnostic laparoscopy with appropriate planning and expertise. The use of conventional electrocoagulation and laser technology aids in the aggressive laparoscopic treatment of minimal, mild, and moderate stages of endometriosis. Conservative surgery has the objective of restoring normal anatomic relationships while excising or fulgurating as much damaged tissue as possible. It should be reserved for more advanced stages of endometriosis (moderate to severe). Pregnancy rates vary inversely with the severity of the endometriosis, with rates of 60% following surgery for mild to moderate disease and 35% for severe disease. Most pregnancies occur in the first year after surgery.

Medical treatment for endometriosis may involve the use of danazol, which has a direct androgenic effect. This effect leads to the atrophy of endometrial implants and produces an anovulatory, hypoestrogenic state. Side effects are common and are related to both its androgenic properties and the hypoestrogenic environment it creates. Treatment is usually for 6 months, and pregnancy rates after treatment are approximately 45%. Oral contraceptives and progestogens alone may also be used as an alternative to danazol when the latter is not well tolerated.

GnRH analogs are long-acting agonists of GnRH that, when administered daily, impede pituitary gonadotropin release, causing ovarian estrogen secretion to fall to castrate levels. Although clinically available, GnRH analogs have not been approved for this usage. The risk and significance of associated osteopenia is currently under investigation.

The Ovulatory Factor

Adrenal and thyroid disorders should be excluded by history and physical examination. Determinations of serum concentrations of FSH, or LH and FSH, are needed to exclude ovarian failure. The appropriate treatment of the anovulatory patient can then be decided on the basis of serum prolactin levels and the results of a progesterone challenge. Hyperprolactinemia causes approximately 15% of ovulation disturbances and is associated with a clinical spectrum ranging from amenorrhea with galactorrhea to subtle luteal phase defects. An elevated prolactin measurement requires consideration and exclusion of primary hypothyroidism by measurement of thyroid-stimulating hormone (TSH) levels, drug-induced dopamine depletion (antihypertensives, psychoactive medication), and pituitary tumor. Diagnostic imaging should be performed to exclude a macroadenoma. Treatment may then proceed with bromocriptine mesylate (Parlodel), with the dose titrated to return serum prolactin levels to normal. Bromocriptine has side effects (nausea, headaches, orthostatic hypotension, nasal stuffiness) that are most prominent at the institution of therapy and that can be minimized by gradual increases in dosage (13).

Women with normal prolactin levels who bleed in response to a progesterone challenge (progesterone-in-oil, 100 mg intramuscularly; or medroxyprogesterone acetate, 10 mg daily for 7–10 days) are candidates for clomiphene treatment, as are women with irregular menses or confirmed midluteal serum progesterone levels of less than 15 ng/ml (14). Clomiphene citrate is administered at 50 mg for 5 days starting on day 3–5 after menstrual or withdrawal bleeding. The response of the patient may be monitored by basal body temperature recording or midluteal phase progesterone levels or both. If ovulation does not occur or the serum progesterone level in the midluteal phase remains less than 15 ng/ml, the dose is increased to 100 mg and the treatment repeated. If dysfunction persists after the daily dose has been increased to 150 mg, dehydroepiandrosterone sulfate levels should be measured and, if elevated, treated with a glucocorticoid (eg, dexamethasone, 0.5 mg per day; or prednisone, 5 mg per day) while clomiphene is restarted at 100 mg. Some patients who fail to ovulate may respond to clomiphene at higher doses (up to 250 mg per day) or a combination of clomiphene citrate followed by hMG. Moreover, some patients who develop follicle growth on clomiphene but do not ovulate may do so after intramuscular administration of hCG, 10,000 IU, when follicle diameter as determined by ultrasound is 20 mm or greater. If clomiphene is successful in inducing ovulation, intercourse can be timed by follicle measurements with ultrasound, urinary LH kits, or every other day beginning 5–7 days after the course of clomiphene is completed. If treatment is unsuccessful, a postcoital test is useful in evaluating mucus quality.

Clomiphene successfully induces ovulation in 70% of patients, although the pregnancy rate is only 40%. The incidence of twins is increased to 5–10%. Side effects of clomiphene include hot flushes, visual disturbances, headaches, abdominal bloating, nausea, and mood alterations. Ovarian enlargement may result from multiple follicle stimulation. Patients should be monitored with pelvic examinations in order to avoid administration of clomiphene to a patient with an enlarged ovary. There is no increased incidence of spontaneous abortion or congenital malformations with clomiphene therapy.

hMG is available as an equal combination of LH and FSH (Pergonal) or as FSH alone (Metrodin). These products are used to treat women who either do not bleed when challenged with progesterone or do not ovulate in response to clomiphene. Safe and effective treatment requires rapid serum estradiol measurements in conjunction with ultrasonic monitoring of the number and diameter of ovarian follicles. Pregnancy rates of 60–80% may be achieved in patients with hypogonadotropic hypogonadism, but success rates are significantly lower in patients with polycystic ovarian syndrome. Pregnancy rates are also affected by age and the number of ovulatory cycles completed; most pregnancies are achieved within six cycles. Because of its risks (elevated rates of multiple gestation, approximately 10–15%; hyperstimulation syndrome, 1%) and expense, hMG therapy should be selectively administered.

GnRH may be administered in a pulsatile manner by a portable infusion pump to successfully treat women with hypogonadotropic hypogonadism. Most women will respond to pulses of GnRH, 50–75 ng/kg given every 60–90 minutes for 10–20 days. The intravenous route of administration has been more successful than the more convenient subcutaneous route. Treatment costs are high, but lower than those of hMG therapy.

"Luteal phase defect" is a term applied to a poorly understood group of subtle hormonal alterations clinically linked with infertility and habitual abortion. The diagnosis is suggested by an elevation in basal body temperature lasting 10 days or less (short luteal phase) or an endometrial biopsy that is histologically more than 2 days out of phase. Luteal phase defects are known to occur sporadically in many women and should be documented in two successive cycles for diagnostic validity. Once hyperprolactinemia has been excluded, treatment options include clomiphene, clomiphene plus hCG, or progesterone suppositories (25 mg twice daily during the luteal phase).

The Cervical Factor

Few or absent sperm in the presence of good-quality mucus requires a reevaluation of the male factor. If a prior semen analysis was normal, faulty coital technique (including the use of spermicidal lubricants), low or high semen volume, semen liquefaction defects, or unexpected variations in sperm count should be suspected.

Poor-quality mucus is usually thick and tenacious with poor spinnbarkeit. Inaccurate timing relative to ovulation must be excluded. A scoring system has been devised and may be used to assess the quality of cervical mucus at the time of postcoital testing (15). If many leukocytes are present, cervicitis should be suspected; cultures for bacteria, *Ureaplasma urealyticum,* and chlamydia are useful in ensuring appropriate treatment.

Absent or low quantity of mucus may reflect inaccurate timing or cervical trauma, surgery, or DES syndrome. Treatment includes low-dose oral estrogen for 1 week prior to ovulation or intrauterine insemination with washed and incubated sperm.

The presence of nonmotile or nonprogressively motile sperm with a "shaking" pattern suggests the presence of sperm antibodies in either partner. Treatment options have not been extensively evaluated but include steroid suppression and intrauterine insemination.

Unexplained Infertility

In 5–10% of couples, completion of the basic workup will not reveal any abnormalities. The evaluation should be reviewed with the couple, and measurement of serum prolactin and androgens, cervical cultures for *U. urealyticum* and chlamydia, sperm antibody testing, and a sperm penetration assay should be considered. If laparoscopy has not been done, it should be performed. Since subtle anomalies of ovulation are occasionally associated with unexplained infertility, careful scrutiny of the ovulatory process is important to correct any abnormality. There is no rational therapy for unexplained infertility, yet the couple will often request empirical treatment. Referral to a specialist may be appropriate, with ultimate consideration of the use of new reproductive technologies, such as in vitro fertilization, gamete intrafallopian transfer, or ovum transfer (6). Discussion of adoption and other alternatives may be explored with the couple and emotional support continued.

Summary

Once a couple seeks medical help for infertility, their anxiety can be allayed only by prompt and accurate diagnosis, treatment, and education given in a setting of care and understanding. The initial assessment and basic workup can be completed in a single cycle if desired and will be diagnostic in the majority of couples. There are few couples in whom diagnosis and treatment, no matter how exhaustive, cannot be completed within 12–18 months if the physician is both organized and committed and the couple is kept well informed. Physicians must recognize and carefully weigh the expense and yield of each procedure individually if limited resources are to be optimally utilized.

REFERENCES

1. Mosher WD: Reproductive impairments in the United States, 1965–1982. Demography 22(3):415–430, 1985
2. Pratt WF, Mosher WD, Bachrach MC, et al: Infertility—United States, 1982. MMWR 34(14):197–199, 1985
3. Aral SO, Cates W: The increasing concern with infertility: Why now? JAMA 250(17):2327–2331, 1983
4. Speroff L, Wallach EE: The changing face of infertility. Contemp Obstet Gynecol 30(special issue):8–10+, 1987
5. American College of Obstetricians and Gynecologists: Medical Induction of Ovulation (ACOG Technical Bulletin 120). Washington DC, ACOG, 1988
6. American College of Obstetricians and Gynecologists: New Reproductive Technologies (ACOG Technical Bulletin). Washington DC, ACOG, 1990
7. Smith CG, Asch RH: Drug abuse and reproduction. Fertil Steril 48(3):355–373, 1987
8. Hull MGR, Savage PE, Bromham DR, et al: The value of a single serum progesterone measurement in the midluteal phase as a criterion of a potentially fertile cycle ("ovulation") derived from treated and untreated conception cycles. Fertil Steril 37(3):355–360, 1982
9. Rogers BJ: The sperm penetration assay: Its usefulness reevaluated. Fertil Steril 43(6):821–840, 1985
10. DeCherney AH, Naftolin F: Diethylstilbestrol—Effect on fertility. In: Behrman SJ, Kistner RW, Patton GW Jr (eds): Progress in Infertility, 3 ed. Boston, Little Brown, 1988, p 234
11. Vorys N: Menstrual dysfunction. In: Behrman SJ, Kistner RW, Patton GW Jr (eds): Progress in Infertility, 3 ed. Boston, Little Brown, 1988, p 352

12. American College of Obstetricians and Gynecologists: Management of Endometriosis (ACOG Technical Bulletin 85). Washington DC, ACOG, 1985

13. Physicians' Desk Reference, 42 ed: Parlodel (bromocriptine mesylate). Oradell NJ, Medical Economics Company Inc, 1988, p 1877

14. Speroff L, Glass RH, Kase NG: Clinical Gynecologic Endocrinology and Infertility, 3 ed. Baltimore, William & Wilkins, 1983, p 528

15. World Health Organization: WHO Laboratory Manual for the Examination of Human Semen and Semen Cervical Mucus Interaction. New York, Cambridge University Press, 1987

This Technical Bulletin was developed under the direction of the Committee on Technical Bulletins of the American College of Obstetricians and Gynecologists as an educational aid to obstetricians and gynecologists. The committee wishes to thank Robert D. Nachtigall, MD, for his assistance in the development of this bulletin. This Technical Bulletin does not define a standard of care, nor is it intended to dictate an exclusive course of management. It presents recognized methods and techniques of clinical practice for consideration by obstetrician–gynecologists for incorporation into their practices. Variations of practice taking into account the needs of the individual patient, resources, and limitations unique to the institution or type of practice may be appropriate.

Reviewed September 1992

THE AMERICAN COLLEGE OF OBSTETRICIANS AND GYNECOLOGISTS
409 12th Street, SW
Washington, DC 20024-2188

6789/76

Number 164—February 1992
(Replaces #104, May 1987)

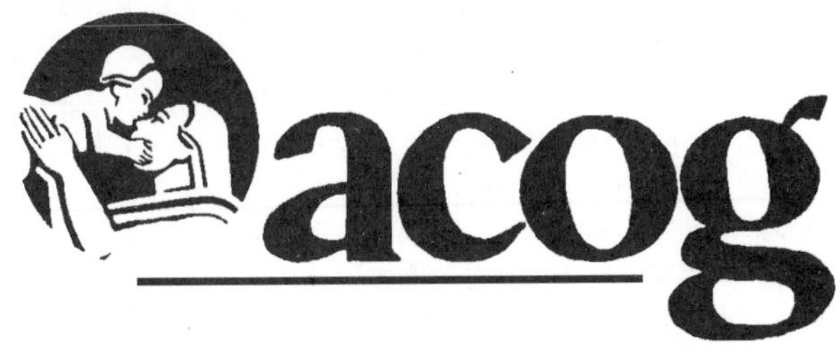

Technical Bulletin
An Educational Aid to Obstetrician–Gynecologists

The Intrauterine Device

Product liability and medical malpractice issues have had an impact on all contraceptive products, but none more so than the intrauterine device (IUD). In 1986, the sale of all IUDs except the steroid hormone-releasing IUD, Progestasert, was discontinued in the United States, although these devices were deemed safe and effective by the U.S. Food and Drug Administration (FDA). In 1988, a new copper IUD (Copper T380A; ParaGard) was approved for marketing by the FDA.

Both the ParaGard and the Progestasert IUDs are highly effective and safe methods of fertility regulation when used appropriately. Failure rates of IUDs are only slightly higher than those of oral contraceptives, and about 80% of women who have an IUD inserted will continue to use the device through the first year (1). The FDA has approved continuous use of the ParaGard for 96 months and of the Progestasert for 12 months. The progesterone hormone in the Progestasert is completely absorbed in about 14 months, requiring annual replacement of the device.

Although the incidence of side effects with IUD use is low, serious complications can occur. The physician must be cognizant of these potential adverse health effects.

Mechanisms of Action

Three independent mechanisms have been suggested for the contraceptive action of IUDs (2), although none has been conclusively established:

1. Interference with sperm transport from the cervix to the fallopian tube
2. Inhibition of sperm capacitation or survival
3. Endometrial changes that inhibit the process of implantation

Progesterone- and copper-releasing IUDs do not interfere with ovulation or with menstrual cyclicity. An IUD in the endometrial cavity alters the biochemical and cellular composition of cervical mucus, endometrial secretions, and tubal fluid. Significant increases in macrophages, lymphocytes, and plasma cells have been observed in both histologic sections of the endometrium and in endometrial fluid. Copper ions are detrimental to sperm capacitation and motility. Progesterone released in the endometrial cavity may alter tubal motility and sperm or egg viability in the tube. These changes are thought to impair fertilization (2). Studies detecting levels of human chorionic gonadotropin (hCG) reveal that this hormone is not present in IUD users during the luteal phase and implantation does not occur (3). As such, the IUD is not an abortifacient. There may be other mechanisms by which IUDs accomplish contraception.

Indications and Contraindications

The IUD is especially suited for older, parous women who wish to prevent further pregnancies but who are not ready to choose a permanent method of family planning; who are in stable relationships in which neither partner has any other sexual partners; and who have no history of pelvic inflammatory disease (PID) or ectopic pregnancy. Physicians should be aware of the absolute and relative contraindications to IUD insertion. Any relative contraindication can become an absolute contraindication when it poses a life-threatening complication, and in all cases the risk of IUD use must be weighed against the benefits. Women must be screened carefully with history and pelvic examination for any of the contraindications to IUD use (see box).

Absolute and Relative Contraindications to IUD Placement

Absolute

- Confirmed or suspected pregnancy
- Known or suspected pelvic malignancy
- Undiagnosed vaginal bleeding
- Known or suspected pelvic infection, acute or chronic, including sexually transmitted diseases and genital actinomycosis
- Reported behaviors placing an individual at high risk for sexually transmitted diseases
- Hyperbilirubinemia secondary to Wilson disease, which is relative only to devices containing copper

Relative

- Uterine size or shape incompatible with effective IUD use
- Medical conditions (eg, corticosteroid therapy, valvular heart disease, and any incidence of immune suppression) increasing the risk of infection
- Nulligravidity
- Abnormal Pap smear (until managed)
- History of ectopic pregnancy

Patient Counseling

Women should be informed about the availability, effectiveness, and potential risks of each method of contraception, particularly those that are appropriate for their age and parity. After considering these factors, if the patient indicates a preference for an IUD, the patient information brochure that is supplied by the manufacturer should be given to her. The patient should have the opportunity to review and discuss IUD use with the health care provider, who should fully explain the potential adverse health effects of the IUD.

Women who decide to have an IUD inserted should be informed that about 20% of women discontinue use of the IUD during the first year because of bleeding, cramping pain, or spontaneous expulsion. Other patients report increased menstrual flow. Patients should be advised that the failure rate of the IUD is about 1% per year and should be acquainted with the symptoms of pregnancy and complications of an IUD. If amenorrhea occurs, the patient must return promptly for evaluation. The patient should be made aware that when pregnancy occurs with IUD use, the relative likelihood of ectopic pregnancy and septic abortion is increased. The patient must be informed about the risks of pelvic infection and the factors (ie, having multiple sexual partners) that increase this risk. Patients with IUDs who develop flu-like symptoms within 1 month of insertion should be evaluated. Theoretically, patients with immune suppression may be at special risk of IUD-associated infection. Clinical judgment should be exercised accordingly.

Physician Liability

Liability issues, mostly product related, have had a significant impact on IUD use in the United States. Because of these issues, many physicians have discouraged patients from considering IUDs. A select group of patients, however, are excellent IUD candidates. By following certain steps, the physician can minimize the risk of liability:

- Inform the patient about the risks associated with IUD use.
- Obtain a thorough history and perform a thorough pelvic examination.
- Screen for gonococcus and chlamydia.
- Take immediate steps to locate and remove a displaced IUD, if it is still present.
- Inform the patient about the special risks associated with pregnancy when the IUD is in place.
- Provide appropriate counseling if pregnancy occurs.
- Instruct the patient to report any adverse effects associated with IUD use.
- Provide appropriate treatment if adverse effects occur.
- Document that counseling has occurred.

IUD Insertion and Removal

The manufacturer's physician information pamphlet should be read concerning the specifics of IUD insertion. The optimal time of insertion is during the latter part of the menstrual period, or 1 or 2 days after. Certain general recommendations can be made:

1. Administration of an analgesic or antiprostaglandin prior to insertion has been found useful in some women.
2. Antiseptic preparation of the cervix and vagina is imperative.
3. Paracervical block may be helpful to minimize insertional pain.
4. The cervical angle should be straightened with the use of a tenaculum. The uterus must be sounded; if the uterus is found to be less than 6 cm or greater than 9 cm, IUD insertion is contraindicated.

5. The patient should be taught how to find the IUD string and promptly report its absence.
6. The patient should return for a check-up after the next menses.
7. The use of an additional method of contraception during the first month of IUD use seems sensible. In addition, some patients use a second method each month at ovulation in order to gain even greater effectiveness.
8. The administration of prophylactic antibiotics may be considered, as IUD insertion almost always introduces cervical bacteria and other organisms into the endometrial cavity. Suggested regimens include doxycycline, 200 mg orally 1 hour before insertion, or erythromycin, 500 mg orally 1 hour before insertion and 500 mg 6 hours after insertion.

Removal of an IUD is accomplished by applying traction on the IUD tail string with forceps. When difficulty is encountered, removal may be facilitated by grasping the IUD itself after paracervical block. Should these measures prove unsuccessful, ultrasound or hysteroscopy should be performed. Occasionally, a device may have to be removed while the patient is under general anesthesia because of partial embedment in the uterine muscle.

Complications

Pelvic Infection

Unlike some other contraceptive methods, the IUD offers no protection against sexually transmitted infections. During the first several months of IUD use, there is an increased risk of pelvic infection, probably because of the introduction of organisms into the upper genital tract at the time of insertion. After this period, the increased risk of PID is probably related to sexually transmitted disease (4, 5). If signs and symptoms of upper-tract pelvic infection occur, the physician should perform appropriate bacteriologic culture studies and begin antibiotic treatment. In the presence of salpingitis, tuboovarian abscess, or severe pelvic infection, the IUD should be removed. The timing of removal in relation to the administration of antibiotics depends on clinical evaluation of the severity of the disease.

Displaced String

The physician should determine the reason for a displaced IUD string. Intrauterine pregnancy can cause upward displacement of an IUD and its string. When pregnancy has been ruled out, the location of the IUD can be determined by one or more of the following methods:

- Probing of the endocervical canal and intrauterine cavity for the retracted string or palpating the IUD with a uterine sound
- Ultrasonography
- Anteroposterior and lateral X-rays of the pelvis and abdomen with the position of the uterine cavity indicated by a radiopaque instrument or dye
- Hysteroscopic visualization of the intrauterine cavity

Perforation

Partial or complete perforation of the uterine wall by the IUD occurs in approximately 1/1,000–2,000 insertions (6). Probably, most perforations occur at the time of insertion; hence, the experience of the physician and the technique of insertion are important. Perforation is more likely to occur when insertions are done postpartum, ie, before complete involution of the uterus has occurred (7). Since all devices are capable of eliciting peritonitis, adhesions, and organ penetration, the IUD must be removed via laparoscopy, hysteroscopy, colpotomy, or laparotomy when IUD perforation is diagnosed.

Actinomyces Infections

Actinomyces, an anaerobic, gram-positive bacterium, is occasionally detected on cervical cytology in IUD users (8). If this occurs in an asymptomatic patient who wishes to continue using the IUD, treatment with an appropriate antibiotic (eg, ampicillin, 250 mg four times daily for 14 days) may be instituted and a repeat Pap test performed. If the results remain positive, or if the patient is symptomatic, she should have the IUD removed. When *Actinomyces* is found in a symptomatic patient, the IUD should be removed and antibiotic therapy initiated.

Pregnancy

If a woman using an IUD becomes pregnant, there is a 2–3% chance that the pregnancy will be ectopic (9). Therefore, careful evaluation for this possibility is essential (10, 11).

When intrauterine pregnancy is diagnosed in an IUD user and the patient elects to continue the pregnancy, the IUD should be removed as soon as possible if the string can be located. If the IUD is removed in the first trimester, the risk of a second- or third-trimester fetal loss is not increased. If the IUD remains in place, the woman should be advised of the increased risk of spontaneous abortion in the first trimester; of septic abortion, especially in the second trimester; and of premature birth in the third trimester (12). Because of these high risks of serious complications, she should be offered the option of pregnancy termination. If termination is elected, the IUD can be removed at the time of that procedure.

Should the woman elect to carry the pregnancy to term, the IUD can be removed under ultrasound guidance if it is located inferiorly to the gestational sac. However, abortion may still result. If located superiorly, the IUD usually cannot be removed without abortion. In either case, the pregnant woman with an IUD should be more closely monitored during the entire pregnancy. Available data indicate no increased risk of congenital anomalies in IUD-associated pregnancies.

Fertility After IUD Discontinuation

Pregnancy rates in women choosing to become pregnant after elective IUD removal are similar to those in women discontinuing the use of other methods of contraception (13–15). The relationship of past IUD use and tubal infertility secondary to salpingitis remains controversial. Pelvic infection due to sexually transmitted organisms occurs among IUD users and nonusers alike. Salpingitis may not be clinically apparent until the woman is trying to conceive. Limited data show little or no increased risk of infertility among IUD users who are in monogamous relationships (16). Following IUD discontinuation, the outcome of pregnancy appears to be no different than in women discontinuing use of other contraceptive methods.

Summary

The IUD is an excellent form of contraception for selected patients. As with all methods of contraception, the benefits and risks of the method and the needs of the patient must be considered. Counseling is an important part of the selection process and will identify those for whom the IUD is a suitable contraceptive choice.

REFERENCES

1. Sivin I, Tatum HJ. Four years of experience with the TCu 380A intrauterine contraceptive device. Fertil Steril 1981;36:159–163
2. Alvarez F, Brache V, Fernandez E, Guerrero B, Guiloff E, Hess R, et al. New insights on the mode of action of intrauterine contraceptive devices in women. Fertil Steril 1988;49:768–773
3. Segal SJ, Alvarez-Sanchez F, Adejuwon CA, Brache de Mejia V, Leon P, Faundes A. Absence of chorionic gonadotropin in sera of women who use intrauterine devices. Fertil Steril 1985;44:214–218
4. Lee NC, Rubin GL, Borucki R. The intrauterine device and pelvic inflammatory disease revisited: new results from the Women's Health Study. Obstet Gynecol 1988; 72:1–6
5. Kessel E. Pelvic inflammatory disease with intrauterine device use: a reassessment. Fertil Steril 1989;51:1–11
6. American College of Obstetricians and Gynecologists. Precis IV: an update in obstetrics and gynecology. Washington, DC: ACOG, 1990:10
7. Heartwell SF, Schlesselman S. Risk of uterine perforation among users of intrauterine devices. Obstet Gynecol 1983;61:31–36
8. Curtis EM, Pine L. Actinomyces in the vagina of women with and without intrauterine contraceptive devices. Am J Obstet Gynecol 1981;140:880–884
9. Tatum HJ, Schmidt FH, Jain AK. Management and outcome of pregnancies associated with the Copper T intrauterine contraceptive device. Am J Obstet Gynecol 1976;126:869–879
10. Sivin I. IUD-associated ectopic pregnancies, 1974-1984. In: Zatuchni GI, Goldsmith A, Sciarra JJ, eds. Intrauterine contraception: advances and future prospects. Philadelphia: Harper & Row, 1985:340–353
11. Ory HW. Ectopic pregnancy and intrauterine contraceptive devices: new perspective. The Women's Health Study. Obstet Gynecol 1981;57:137–144
12. Foreman H, Stadel BV, Schlesselman S. Intrauterine device usage and fetal loss. Obstet Gynecol 1981;58:669–677
13. Hasson HM. Clinical experience with intrauterine devices in a private practice. Adv Contracept 1985;1:51–61
14. Sandmire HF, Cavanaugh RA. Long-term use of intrauterine contraceptive devices in a private practice. Am J Obstet Gynecol 1985;152:169–175
15. Rioux JE, Cloutier D, Dupont P, Lamonde D. Pregnancy after IUD use. Adv Contracept 1986;2:185–192
16. Cramer DW, Schiff I, Schoenbaum SC, Gibson M, Belisle S, Albrecht B, et al. Tubal infertility and the intrauterine device. N Engl J Med 1985;312:941–947

This Technical Bulletin was developed under the direction of the Committee on Technical Bulletins of the American College of Obstetricians and Gynecologists as an educational aid to obstetricians and gynecologists. The committee wishes to thank Gerald I. Zatuchni, MD, for his assistance in the development of this bulletin. This Technical Bulletin does not define a standard of care, nor is it intended to dictate an exclusive course of management. It presents recognized methods and techniques of clinical practice for consideration by obstetrician–gynecologists for incorporation into their practices. Variations of practice taking into account the needs of the individual patient, resources, and limitations unique to the institution or type of practice may be appropriate.

THE AMERICAN COLLEGE OF OBSTETRICIANS AND GYNECOLOGISTS
409 12th Street, SW
Washington, DC 20024-2188

45678/21098

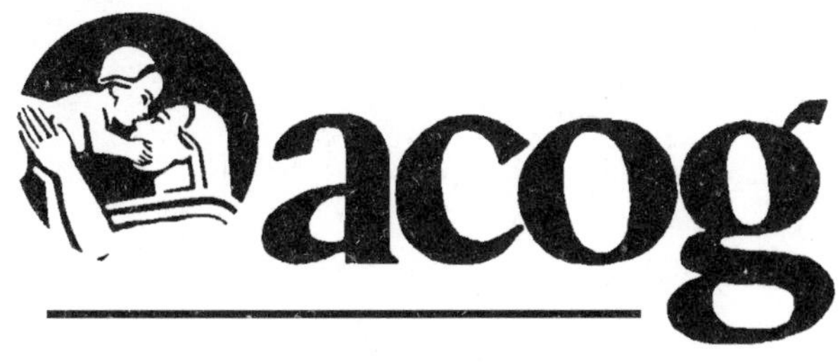

Number 175—December 1992
(Replaces #121, October 1988)

Technical Bulletin

An Educational Aid to Obstetrician–Gynecologists

Invasive Hemodynamic Monitoring in Obstetrics and Gynecology

Prior to the early 1970s, right heart catheterization was accomplished with semirigid catheters and fluoroscopy, thereby effectively limiting the procedure to cardiac catheterization laboratories (1). With the development of the flow-directed pulmonary artery catheter, however, the technology moved from the laboratory to intensive care units, operating rooms, and labor and delivery suites (2–7). Pulmonary artery catheterization provides information about left ventricular function that cannot be obtained with central venous pressure (CVP) monitoring. The combination of peripheral arterial and pulmonary arterial lines provides sufficient information to assess continuously both the cardiac and the pulmonary status of the patient. Use of pulse oximetry can provide continuous monitoring of arterial hemoglobin saturation (Sao_2). Clinical impressions can quickly be either reinforced or refuted with accurate hemodynamic measurements in critically ill patients, and therapeutic strategies can be calculated and their effects promptly evaluated.

Techniques

The decision to use invasive monitoring should include an assessment of the expertise of the physician to place the catheter and the expertise and availability of support staff to monitor the patient and maintain the equipment. Invasive monitoring should be carried out only in units with appropriate staffing ratios to allow continuous observation of the patient.

Cannulation of peripheral or central vessels for placement of intraarterial and pulmonary artery catheters should be accomplished by an individual skilled in these procedures and familiar with their associated complications. Detailed accounts of the technical aspects of line placement are available and will not be provided here. An increasing number of obstetrician–gynecologists are familiar not only with data collection and interpretation, but also with line placement (4). Additional assistance in line placement can usually be obtained from a trained intensive care specialist or anesthesiologist.

The standard flow-directed thermodilution pulmonary artery catheter (Fig. 1) includes a distal lumen at the catheter tip, a proximal lumen 30 cm from the catheter tip, a balloon lumen, and a thermistor. The distal lumen provides continuous measurement of the pulmonary artery pressure when the balloon is deflated and of the pulmonary capillary wedge pressure (PCWP) when the balloon is inflated. The proximal port can be used to monitor CVP or to administer fluids or drugs. Both the proximal and distal lumina of the catheter may be used to withdraw samples of venous blood for laboratory studies. Central core temperature can be measured and cardiac output calculated when the pulmonary artery catheter is used in conjunction with a thermodilution cardiac output computer. Additionally, fiberoptic pulmonary artery catheters are now being increasingly used, as they provide, in addition to all other parameters available from the standard pulmonary artery catheter, a continuous reading of the patient's mixed venous oxygen saturation.

Data Collection

Continuous measurements of CVP and pulmonary artery pressure and intermittent measurements of PCWP are afforded directly by use of the pulmonary artery catheter (Fig. 2). Cardiac output can be measured intermittently by thermodilution. Heart rate and rhythm are observed through the use of continuous electrocardiographic monitoring. Systemic arterial pressure can be measured by sphygmomanometer or percutaneous arterial cannulation;

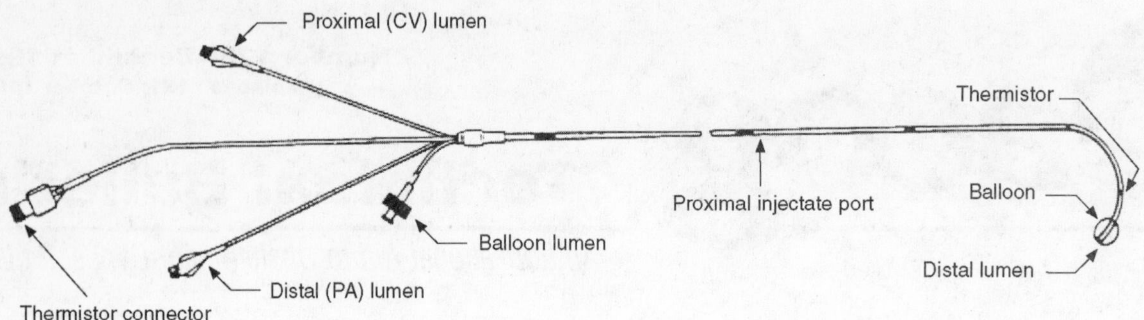

FIG. 1. Schematic diagram of a standard triple-lumen flow-directed pulmonary artery catheter.

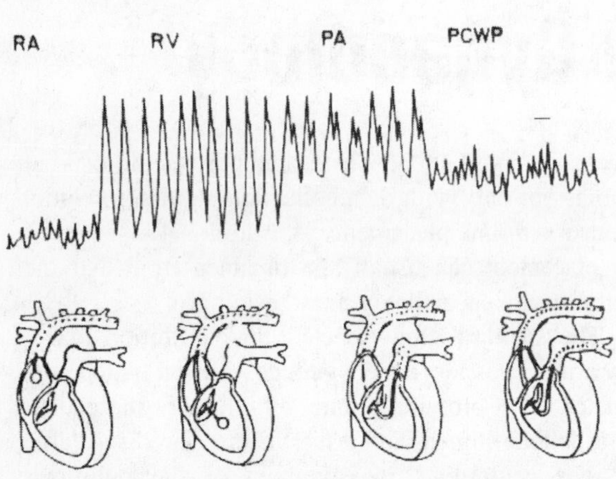

FIG. 2. Pressure waves in relation to catheter position from right atrium (RA) to right ventricle (RV) to pulmonary artery (PA) to pulmonary capillary wedge (PCW) position. (Dizon CT, Barash PG. The value of monitoring pulmonary artery pressure in clinical practice. Conn Med 1977;41:622)

the latter also provides easy access for arterial blood sampling. Mean pressure values can be determined for both the pulmonary arterial and the systemic circulation by electronic dampening of the respective tracing or by calculation with standard formulas. Additional hemodynamic values that reflect cardiopulmonary function and vascular resistance can be calculated as shown in the box. Stroke volume is a measure of the amount of blood pumped per contraction by the heart. Both cardiac output and stroke volume can be corrected for body size by dividing these values by body surface area to obtain the cardiac index and stroke index. Body surface area can be determined from standard nomograms (8); however, these data were collected in nonpregnant subjects, and comparable data are not available for pregnant women. Resistance to flow can be calculated from the right and left ventricles through determination of pulmonary and systemic vascular resistance, respectively. Pulmonary shunts and arterial–venous oxygen content differences are calculated by analysis of simultaneously obtained samples of mixed venous blood, drawn from the distal port of the pulmonary artery catheter, and arterial blood.

Hemodynamic values for healthy nonpregnant subjects (9) can be compared with those obtained in healthy primiparous women studied in the lateral recumbent position at 36–38 weeks of gestation and 11–13 weeks postpartum (10) (Table 1). Compared with a nonpregnant woman, a normal pregnant woman in the third trimester will have an increased cardiac output. The increased cardiac output is accounted for primarily by an increase in stroke volume, but also by increased heart rate. Mean arterial pressures were not different when measured in the late third trimester and at 3 months postpartum. In contrast, both the systemic and pulmonary vascular resis-

Formulas for Deriving Various Hemodynamic Parameters*

Mean arterial pressure
Mean pressure = [systolic pressure + 2 (diastolic pressure)]/3

Stroke volume (SV) (ml/beat)
SV = CO/HR

Stroke index (SI) (ml/beat/m^2)
SI = SV/BSA

Cardiac index (CI) (L/min/m^2)
CI = CO/BSA

Pulmonary vascular resistance (PVR) (dyne · cm · sec^{-5})
PVR = [(MPAP - PCWP)/CO] x 80†

Systemic vascular resistance (SVR) (dyne · cm · sec^{-5})
SVR = [(MAP - CVP)/CO] × 80†

*Abbreviations: BSA = body surface area (m$_2$); CO = cardiac output (L/min); CVP = central venous pressure (mm Hg); HR = heart rate (beats/min); MAP = mean systemic arterial pressure (mm Hg); MPAP = mean pulmonary artery pressure (mm Hg); PCWP = mean pulmonary capillary wedge pressure (mm Hg).

†Conversion factor: 1 mm Hg/1 L/min = 80 dynes · cm · sec^{-5}.

TABLE 1. HEMODYNAMIC VALUES IN HEALTHY NONPREGNANT, PREGNANT, AND POSTPARTUM SUBJECTS

	Hemodynamic Values in Subjects*		
Parameter (Units)	**Nonpregnant**	**36–38 Weeks of Gestation†**	**Postpartum**
Heart rate (beats/min)	60–100	83 ± 10	71 ± 10
Central venous pressure (mm Hg)	5–10	3.6 ± 2.5	3.7 ± 2.6
Mean pulmonary artery pressure (mm Hg)	15–20	—‡	—‡
Pulmonary capillary wedge pressure (mm Hg)	6–12	7.5 ± 1.8	6.3 ± 2.1
Mean arterial pressure (mm Hg)	90–110	90.3 ± 5.8	86.4 ± 7.5
Cardiac output (L/min)	4.3–6.0	6.2 ± 1.0	4.3 ± 0.9
Stroke volume (ml/beat)	57–71	74.7	60.6
Systemic vascular resistance (dyne · cm · sec^{-5})	900–1,400	1,210 ± 266	1,530 ± 520
Pulmonary vascular resistance (dyne · cm · sec^{-5})	<250	78 ± 22	119 ± 47

* Where available, data are given as mean ± standard deviation.

† Values in pregnant patients were determined with patient in left lateral decubitis position.

‡ — = Not reported.

Adapted from Rosenthal MH. Intrapartum intensive care management of the cardiac patient. Clin Obstet Gynecol 1981;24:789-807 and Clark SL, Cotton DB, Lee W, Bishop C, Hill T, Southwick J, et al. Central hemodynamic assessment of normal term pregnancy. Am J Obstet Gynecol 1989;161:1439-1442

tance, as determined by invasive monitoring, are significantly lower during the third trimester of pregnancy.

Data Interpretation

Assessment of cardiac function consists of evaluation of preload, afterload, heart rate, and myocardial contractility. If any of these four variables is abnormal, initial therapy should be targeted at correcting the specific dysfunction. Invasive monitoring allows for almost instantaneous assessment of therapeutic maneuvers. Additionally, significant pulmonary dysfunction in the face of normal cardiac function can quickly be determined to be due to a primary lung injury and therapy targeted for the specific pathophysiology involved. Assessment of cardiac function must include a systematic examination of each area that can lead to heart failure.

Preload

Preload is determined by end-diastolic intraventricular pressure and volume, thus setting the initial myocardial fiber length. Right and left ventricular end-diastolic filling pressures are clinically assessed by CVP and PCWP, respectively. Cardiac output plotted against PCWP gives a cardiac function curve for the left ventricle. The ventricular function curve shown in Fig. 3 demonstrates that a failing heart requires a higher preload (filling pressure) to achieve the same cardiac output as a normally functioning heart. Therapeutic manipulation of the ventricular filling pressures and simultaneous measurement of cardiac output allow calculation of the optimal preload (ie, the construction of a Starling ventricular function curve) at the patient's bedside. Preload can be increased by the administration of crystalloid solution, colloid solution, or blood and can be decreased by the use of a diuretic, a vasodilator, or by phlebotomy.

Afterload

Afterload is the tension of the ventricular wall during systole and is dependent on ventricular end-diastolic radius, aortic or pulmonary arterial diastolic pressure, and ventricular wall thickness (11). The magnitude of the increase in right or left intraventricular pressure during systole depends primarily on pulmonary or systemic vascular resistance, respectively (Fig. 4). In the presence of

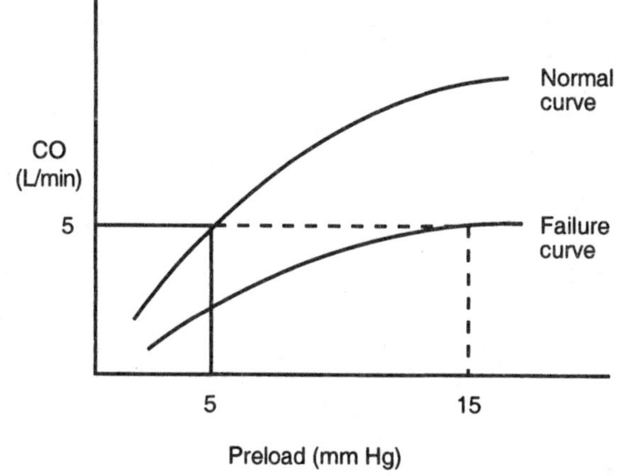

FIG. 3. Ventricular function (Starling) curve for a heart with both normal function and during failure. Pulmonary capillary wedge pressure or central venous pressure represents fiber length (preload), and cardiac output (CO) represents fiber shortening. Note that in order to maintain cardiac output, the failing heart is required to function at higher preloads.

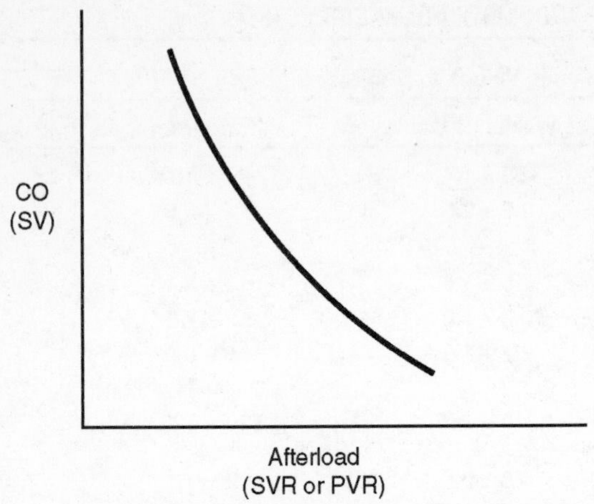

FIG. 4. Relationship of afterload (systemic or pulmonary vascular resistance—SVR or PVR) to cardiac output (CO) or stroke volume (SV) when preload is maintained constant. As afterload increases, cardiac output falls.

heart failure, increases in afterload worsen the degree of failure by decreasing both the stroke volume and the cardiac output. Afterload, like preload, can be increased or decreased as mandated by clinical circumstances. Increases can be mediated via alpha-adrenergic agonists such as phenylephrine, while decreases can be achieved with a number of vasodilating agents. Sodium nitroprusside infusions are used most commonly to decrease afterload in medical–surgical intensive care units, while hydralazine is the agent most commonly used in obstetrics.

Myocardial Contractility

The inotropic state of the heart is defined as the force and velocity of ventricular contractions when preload and afterload are held constant. Although cardiac output can be measured directly, its adequacy is best assessed by clinical parameters, including the patient's acid-base balance, mental status, urinary output, and, in pregnant patients, fetal heart rate tracing. In low-output cardiac failure, both preload and afterload should be optimized through therapeutic manipulation. If this fails to restore the cardiac output to an acceptable level, attention should be directed to improving myocardial contractility. Beta-sympathomimetic agents such as dopamine and isoproterenol are effective in improving cardiac output acutely. Depending on the cause of myocardial failure, either short- or long-term therapy with digitalis may be necessary.

Heart Rate

Although unusual in obstetric–gynecologic patients, heart block can compromise cardiac output. In this circumstance, treatment with either atropine or cardiac pacing is indicated. Similarly, sustained tachycardia can lead to heart failure due to shortened systolic ejection and diastolic filling times or myocardial ischemia, especially in the presence of stenotic cardiac valvular lesions. The pathophysiologic basis of tachycardia (eg, fever, hypovolemia, pain, hyperthyroidism) should be determined and corrected. Heart rate can also be controlled with propranolol or digoxin. Calcium channel blockers can also control heart rate, but the safety of these drugs for use in pregnant women is not known.

Indications for Invasive Monitoring

Clinical conditions for which invasive hemodynamic monitoring may assist in the management of obstetric–gynecologic patients are as follows:

- Sepsis with refractory hypotension or oliguria
- Unexplained or refractory pulmonary edema, heart failure, or oliguria
- Severe pregnancy-induced hypertension with pulmonary edema or persistent oliguria
- Intraoperative or intrapartum cardiovascular decompensation
- Massive blood and volume loss or replacement
- Adult respiratory distress syndrome
- Shock of undefined etiology
- Some chronic conditions, particularly when associated with labor or major surgery:
  - —New York Heart Association class III (symptoms with normal activity) or IV (symptoms at bed rest) cardiac disease (structural or physiologic) (12)
  - —Peripartum or perioperative coronary artery disease (ischemia, myocardial infarction)

Considerable controversy exists as to the need for routine use of a pulmonary artery catheter during the administration of either conduction or general anesthesia in women with severe pregnancy-induced hypertension. To date, no study has shown improved outcomes in such women.

Clearly, invasive monitoring will not be necessary in every patient with one of these conditions, nor is this an all-inclusive list of indications for monitoring. In most instances, the conditions and indications for invasive monitoring are identical to those found in other areas of medicine or surgery. Additionally, pregnancy is not a contraindication for invasive hemodynamic monitoring, and the same standards and criteria should be used in the selection of pregnant women for invasive monitoring as for nonpregnant patients.

Monitoring may be instituted prophylactically in the seriously ill or compromised obstetric–gynecologic patient preparatory to the stress of labor and delivery or a major surgical procedure. In the patient with acute and unexpected pulmonary edema, a primary lung injury (normal or low PCWP) can quickly be differentiated from heart failure (high PCWP) and specific targeted therapy administered. Volume status of the patient can be assessed by ventricular preload or filling pressures, which can be adjusted to optimize cardiac output. Assessment of volume status is often critical in patients with massive volume loss and replacement, sepsis, or oliguria that fails to respond to initial therapy. Although initial management of the majority of these acute events may not warrant invasive monitoring, failure to achieve the predicted clinical response to initial empirical therapy warrants consideration of invasive monitoring to collect additional information to guide and evaluate further therapeutic manipulations.

Central Venous Pressure

Right ventricular function and systemic vascular compliance can be assessed by CVP monitoring, which has been widely employed to establish the relationship of blood volume to vascular capacity. The primary disadvantages of this method relate to the fact that CVP levels may not necessarily be elevated in the presence of left ventricular failure and pulmonary congestion and, conversely, may be elevated in patients without evidence of pulmonary edema (13). Pulmonary capillary wedge pressure can be reliably assessed by CVP monitoring only in the absence of cardiopulmonary disease. It has been noted that in the presence of dissociated right and left heart function, absolute CVP values correlate poorly with left-sided filling pressures, and even changes in this modality may be misleading (13).

Complications

The complications of invasive hemodynamic monitoring can be subdivided into those occurring in conjunction with gaining vascular access and those related to the duration of monitoring. Peripheral arterial cannulation can be associated with hematoma formation, infection, and vessel thrombosis. Serious complications from insertion, such as gangrene and loss of a digit or extremity, occur in less than 1% of cases (Table 2) (14, 15). Gaining central venous access for either a pulmonary artery catheter or a CVP catheter can also be associated with vessel wall damage and hematoma formation, pneumothorax, inadvertent arterial puncture, and persistent bleeding. The pulmonary artery catheter, unlike CVP lines, frequently will cause transient arrhythmias as it is passed through the heart, but only 1% of patients will require pharmacologic treatment. A significant complication is hemorrhage as a result of disconnection of the catheter from the intravenous line. Rarer but reported complications include knotting of the catheter, rupture of the pulmonary artery, and thromboembolism. The risks of both sepsis and thromboembolism increase with duration of catheter placement, and all line complications are proportional to the experience of the operator. Given a broad range of medical and surgical patients with conditions necessitating invasive monitoring, 3% will sustain a major complication, including death (4, 14, 15). In assessing the need for monitoring, potential benefits must be weighed against the reported risks, taking into consideration that many complications, such as arrhythmias and pneumothoraces, are more likely to occur when dealing with a patient in extremis.

TABLE 2. COMPLICATIONS OF PULMONARY-ARTERY CATHETERIZATION

Complication	Incidence (%)
Premature ventricular contractions	15–27
Arterial puncture	8
Superficial cellulitis	3
Thromboembolism	?
Pneumothorax	1–2
Balloon rupture	<1
Pulmonary infarction/ischemia	1–7
Pulmonary artery rupture	<1
Catheter knotting	<1
Catheter-related sepsis	1

Hankins GDV, Cunningham FG. Severe preeclampsia and eclampsia: controversies in management. Williams obstetrics, supplement 1991; 18:11. Reprinted by permission of Appleton and Lange, Inc.

Summary

Indications for invasive hemodynamic monitoring in obstetrics and gynecology are much the same as in any other area of medicine and surgery. The clinical decision of whether to employ monitoring cannot be made according to absolute criteria but must be made on an individual basis. Obviously, not every patient will benefit from or need invasive hemodynamic monitoring; proper patient selection is important, as is the availability of skilled physicians, nurses, and ancillary support personnel. The information collected at the patient's bedside can be used to both guide and evaluate therapeutic maneuvers. Timely adjustment and titration of therapeutic maneuvers and treatments would logically have a significant impact on the outcome of a critical illness or on patients on the verge of cardiac or respiratory decompensation. Nonetheless, a randomized prospective study of the efficacy of the pulmonary artery catheter in obstetrics and gynecology does not currently exist, nor is such a study likely with the already widely accepted use of these technologies.

REFERENCES

1. Swan HJ, Ganz W, Forrester J, Marcus H, Diamond G, Chonette D. Catheterization of the heart in man with use of a flow-directed balloon-tipped catheter. N Engl J Med 1970;283:447-451

2. Berkowitz RL, Rafferty TD. Pulmonary artery flow-directed catheter use in the obstetric patient. Obstet Gynecol 1980;55:507-511

3. Cotton DB, Benedetti TJ. Use of the Swan-Ganz catheter in obstetrics and gynecology. Obstet Gynecol 1980; 56:641-645

4. Clark SL, Horenstein JM, Phelan JP, Montag TW, Paul RH. Experience with the pulmonary artery catheter in obstetrics and gynecology. Am J Obstet Gynecol 1985; 152:374-378

5. Benedetti TJ, Hargrove JC, Rosene KA. Maternal pulmonary edema during premature labor inhibition. Obstet Gynecol 1982;59(6 suppl):33s-37s

6. Hankins GD, Wendel GD Jr, Leveno KJ, Stoneham J. Myocardial infarction during pregnancy: a review. Obstet Gynecol 1985;65:139-146

7. Cunningham FG, Leveno KJ, Hankins GD, Whalley PS. Respiratory insufficency associated with pyelonephritis during pregnancy. Obstet Gynecol 1984;63:121-125

8. Boothby W, Sandiford RB. Nomographic charts for the calculation of the metabolic rate by the gasometer method. Boston Med Surg J 1921;185:337-354

9. Rosenthal MH. Intrapartum intensive care management of the cardiac patient. Clin Obstet Gynecol 1981;24:789-807

10. Clark SL, Cotton DB, Lee W, Bishop C, Hill T, Southwick J, et al. Central hemodynamic assessment of normal term pregnancy. Am J Obstet Gynecol 1989;161:1439-1442

11. Lappas DG, Powell WM Jr, Daggett WM. Cardiac dysfunction in the perioperative period: pathophysiology, diagnosis and treatment. Anesthesiology 1977;47:117-137

12. New York Heart Association. Nomenclature and criteria for diagnosis of diseases of the heart and great vessels. The Criteria Committee of the New York Heart Association. 8th ed. Boston: Little Brown, 1979

13. Cotton DB, Gonik B, Dorman K, Harrist R. Cardiovascular alterations in severe pregnancy-induced hypertension: relationship of central venous pressure to pulmonary capillary wedge pressure. Am J Obstet Gynecol 1985;151:762-764

14. Buchbinder N, Ganz W. Hemodynamic monitoring: invasive techniques. Anesthesiology 1976;45:146-155

15. Moser KM, Spragg RG. Use of the balloon-tipped pulmonary artery catheter in pulmonary disease. Ann Intern Med 1983;98:53-58

This Technical Bulletin was developed under the direction of the Committee on Technical Bulletins of the American College of Obstetricians and Gynecologists as an educational aid to obstetricians and gynecologists. This Technical Bulletin does not define a standard of care, nor is it intended to dictate an exclusive course of management. It presents recognized methods and techniques of clinical practice for consideration by obstetrician–gynecologists for incorporation into their practices. Variations of practice taking into account the needs of the individual patient, resources, and limitations unique to the institution or type of practice may be appropriate.

THE AMERICAN COLLEGE OF OBSTETRICIANS AND GYNECOLOGISTS
409 12th Street, SW
Washington, DC 20024-2188

12345/65432

ACOG EDUCATIONAL BULLETIN

Number 238, July 1997

Lower Urinary Tract Operative Injuries

Operative injuries to the urethra, bladder, and ureters can occur in general obstetric and gynecologic practice; these injuries can pose a major threat to a patient's well-being. Early detection and repair of intraoperative injuries to the lower urinary tract usually can restore normal function and prevent postoperative complications. Gynecologists should be skilled in the prevention and early detection of injuries and, when the need arises, be prepared to consult with surgeons with specialized skills in this area.

This Educational Bulletin was developed under the direction of the Committee on Educational Bulletins of the American College of Obstetricians and Gynecologists as an aid to obstetricians and gynecologists. The College wishes to thank William J. Mann, MD, for his assistance in the development of this bulletin. This document is not to be construed as establishing a standard of practice or dictating an exclusive course of treatment. Rather, it is intended as an educational tool that presents current information on obstetric–gynecologic issues.

Incidence

Injuries to the lower urinary tract are potentially devastating complications of gynecologic and obstetric surgery that can require corrective surgery and can lead to serious morbidity, kidney loss, and death. Injuries to the bladder or ureter occur in roughly 1.0% of major gynecologic procedures and cesarean deliveries, and 75% are associated with hysterectomy (1). The ratio of bladder injury to ureteral injury is approximately 5:1 (2). There are an estimated 500,000–600,000 hysterectomies performed each year. Based on this estimate, 5,000–6,000 women will experience an injury. The incidence of lower genital tract injuries is difficult to estimate because silent loss of an obstructed kidney or spontaneous resolution of partial ureteral obstruction may occur. Small vesicovaginal fistulae also may not be detected by the clinician.

In developing countries, most obstetric injuries to the bladder and urethra are the result of obstructed labor. In developed countries, most obstetric injuries to the bladder and ureters are the result of operative deliveries. Forceps deliveries complicated by periurethral, anterior vaginal, or lateral pelvic lacerations may result in injury to the genitourinary tract. Such injuries may be caused by the forceps or by repair of the laceration.

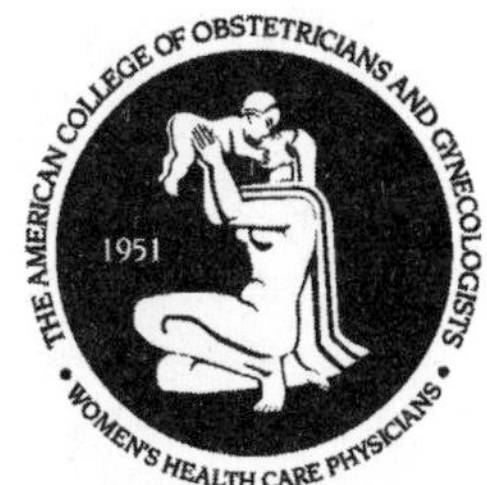

Predisposing Conditions

Most intraoperative lower urinary tract injuries occur in the absence of any recognized predisposing factors during otherwise uncomplicated surgical procedures. The occurrence of a bladder or a ureteral injury or a fistula is not in itself an indication of faulty technique. Some clinical conditions are associated with a higher risk of urinary tract injury because of loss of exposure or visibility, distorted normal anatomy, or both (see box).

Management of invasive and destructive conditions such as endometriosis, gynecologic and metastatic malignancies, suppurative infections, or radiation fibrosis may require dissection and even surgical resection of portions of the ureter, bladder, or urethra. As these disease processes infiltrate the pelvic tissues, they distort the normal pelvic anatomy, obliterate tissue planes, and may actually invade the lower urinary tract. In removing all involved tissues, the surgeon may injure the urinary tract, either directly by dissection or indirectly by interfering with its blood and nerve supply. When there is damage to the tissue blood supply, a period may elapse before there is evidence of injury. This delay can occur with fistulae as well as with operative procedures following extensive pelvic surgery, pelvic irradiation therapy, or chronic pelvic infection.

Conditions That May Contribute to Loss of Reduced Exposure or Visibility

- Large pelvic masses of any origin
- Pregnant uterus
- Obesity
- Pelvic hemorrhage
- Malignant disease
- Inadequate incision
- Inadequate retraction and lighting

Conditions That May Distort Anatomy

- Cervical and broad ligament myomas
- Cancer
- Endometriosis
- Chronic inflammatory disease (pelvic inflammatory diseases, diverticulitis)
- Prior pelvic surgery
- Radiation therapy
- Congenital anomalies
- Pelvic organ prolapse
- Pelvic adhesions

Prevention

Preoperative

Routinely performing preoperative intravenous pyelography in all hysterectomy patients does not prevent surgical injury to the urinary tract (3). However, preoperative imaging may be helpful in determining urinary tract function, defining anatomy, and detecting large pelvic tumors, endometriosis, advanced pelvic malignancies, or changes attributable to prior surgery.

Controversy exists over the value of placing preoperative ureteral stents to prevent ureteral injury. They may cause hematuria, edema, fibrosis, and ureteral perforation. The use of lighted ureteral stents has been promoted as a means of identifying the course of the pelvic ureter during laparoscopy or in the presence of abnormal pelvic anatomy. There are no data to support their effectiveness or routine use, however.

Operative

The risk of injury to the urinary tract can be reduced by proper exposure of the operative site, restoration of anatomic relationships before beginning the planned procedure, careful sharp dissection, and adequate hemostasis. During abdominal procedures, the ureters should be identified visually. Palpation alone for identification of the ureter may be insufficient because the characteristic "click" that occurs when pressure is applied also can be produced by vascular structures, dense connective tissue, and fibrosis. Once the ureters are identified, they should be retracted gently from the operative field. When dissecting the ureter, care should be taken to ensure its blood supply, which runs longitudinally in its adventitial sheath. It is best to leave the ureters attached to their overlying peritoneum. Prior surgery, radiation, and infection may damage the blood supply to the ureters, making subsequent dissection more likely to cause injury.

Ureteral injuries most commonly occur at the level of the infundibulopelvic ligament when ligation of the ovarian blood supply is performed. Another common site of injury is in the cardinal ligament where the ureter passes just lateral to and beneath the uterine vessels. The ureters also may be injured as they course medially and enter the base of the bladder. Elevating the infundibulopelvic ligament and identifying the ureter may help prevent injury at the pelvic brim. Reflecting the bladder inferiorly to allow displacement of the ureter laterally may prevent injury at the levels of the uterine artery and trigone. During hysterectomy, anterior intrafascial removal of the cervix displaces the ureters laterally and offers additional protection against ureteral injury.

Ureteral injuries also may occur during operative laparoscopic procedures when cautery, lasers, or stapling devices are used (4, 5). Prevention of these injuries again requires ureteral identification and sufficient mobilization to remove the ureters from the area.

Prevention of bladder injury begins with careful entry into the peritoneal cavity, particularly when the bladder is adherent to the anterior abdominal wall. The bladder can be drained prior to incision to help prevent cystotomy and to facilitate pelvic exposure. The bulb of the catheter can be elevated to help identify the bladder fundus.

When disease or prior surgery causes dense adhesions of the bladder to the anterior uterus, unsuccessful attempts at dissection may cause partial-thickness injury and subsequent fistulae. Sharp dissection may pose less risk. Preferably, the bladder can be filled with sterile milk or other nonstaining fluid in a retrograde fashion through the catheter, followed by sharp dissection. Alternatively, an extraperitoneal cystotomy can be performed and the vesicouterine reflection incised over a finger placed into the bladder. When sewing the vaginal cuff, a retractor should be placed to protect the bladder. This procedure prevents unintentional entrapment of the bladder in the cuff closure, with resulting necrosis and vesicovaginal fistula formation.

At the conclusion of the procedure, when hemostasis has been ensured, both ureters and the bladder should be inspected to confirm their integrity. Hematuria or oliguria during the procedure should signal the need to inspect these areas.

Diagnosis

If injury is suspected, 5 mL of indigo carmine may be given intravenously with a fluid challenge, with the catheter clamped. This will allow the bladder to fill with blue-dyed urine, and leaks in the ureters or bladder will spill dye into the pelvis. When leakage occurs, the pelvic tissues are quickly stained and other injuries may not be visible. It is best to carefully inspect and possibly even dissect both ureters to be sure additional injuries have not been missed. Absence of dye in the bladder can indicate bilateral ureteral obstruction; however, unilateral or partial ureteral obstruction can be present even if blue dye is seen in a distended bladder. Visible dilation of the ureter above a given point suggests obstruction. Alternatively, instead of distending the bladder, cystotomy can be performed or a cystoscope introduced through the dome of the bladder or the urethra to view the ureteral orifices and to confirm dye excretion.

Some physicians prefer to inject indigo carmine directly into the ureter above the affected area. Others prefer inserting ureteral stents, either through the opened bladder or transurethrally with a cystoscope. Finally, while cumbersome, intraoperative intravenous pyelography can be performed, although small leaks may be missed. If bladder injury is suspected, distending the bladder with sterile milk or other fluid allows leaks to be identified. Routine postoperative studies are not cost-effective in identifying occult ureteral injuries (6).

Obstruction

Complete bilateral ureteral obstruction will present with anuria, unresponsive to fluid challenge, and rising blood urea nitrogen and creatinine levels. Ultrasound or computed tomography scans showing bilateral dilation of the collecting systems suggest the diagnosis, but cystoscopy with retrograde dye injection into the ureters will confirm the diagnosis. With lesser degrees of obstruction, decreased urine volumes may not be noted. Unilateral ureteral entrapment may be associated with a mean increase of serum creatinine of 0.8 mg/dL (7). Abdominal and flank pain may be present, as well as leukocytosis and fever. An intravenous pyelogram or cystoscopy with retrograde dye study will be diagnostic.

Transection

Partial or complete ureteral transection may present as a clear vaginal discharge or abdominal distention, often associated with fever and leukocytosis. Intraperitoneal urine accumulation can cause ileus with nausea and vomiting. Serum creatinine levels may be normal or only slightly increased unless both ureters also are obstructed. An intravenous pyelogram will show nonvisualization of part or all of the transected ureter(s). Percutaneous nephrostomy with dye injection under fluoroscopy will allow identification of the site of injury. Retrograde ureteral catheterization or uretoscopy also can be used.

Fistulae

Fistulae may be preceded by fever, leukocytosis, or abdominal or flank pain or may simply present as a clear vaginal discharge without associated symptoms. Samples of fluid from a suspected fistula can be sent for blood urea nitrogen measurement, which will be markedly elevated relative to serum values. Fistulae may involve the bladder, ureter(s), or both. Ureteral fistulae usually are determined by use of intravenous pyelography combined with retrograde ureteral dye injection at cystoscopy.

Unrecognized bladder injuries may present as a clear watery vaginal discharge immediately or several days after surgery. Fever is seldom present. A speculum can be placed in the vagina and, if the fistula is not immediately apparent, dye or milk can be instilled through the urethra to identify the leak. Alternatively, sponges can be placed into the vagina and dye instilled into the bladder through the urethra. If only the upper sponge is stained, a vesicovaginal fistula is probably present. If only the lower sponge is stained, there is probably loss of urine through the urethra. If neither is stained, but the upper sponge is wet, a ureterovaginal fistula may be present. Intravenous pyelography and cystoscopy with retrograde studies are indicated to confirm the diagnosis and to exclude the presence of a complex injury.

Urethral injuries usually result from urethral diverticulum repair, anterior colporrhaphy, or procedures undertaken to repair previous urethral surgery. Sutures may transfix or surround the urethra, or the urethra may be lacerated by scalpel or scissors. Urethral injury usually is diagnosed by placing a transurethral catheter or performing urethroscopy.

Management

Bladder injuries can occur with laparoscopy, usually as a result of trocar injury. In the presence of a laparoscopic bladder injury, consideration should be given to the possibility of another visceral injury. Bladder and ureteral injuries can be repaired laparoscopically by experienced laparoscopists.

Urethral lacerations and fistulae should be repaired in layers. When the proximal urethra is injured, the continence mechanism is impaired and a bladder neck suspension is needed. Bulbocavernosus fat pad transplant (Martius operation) may provide bulk and a new blood supply at the site of the urethral repair.

Ureteral Injuries

Ureteral injuries should be managed by physicians skilled in their correction. Although immediate reexploration and repair is an option, cystoscopic or percutaneous stenting of the damaged ureter is a less aggressive approach associated with decreased morbidity (8, 9). Ureteral stents can be passed through areas of partial obstruction or leakage to allow healing to occur or sutures to dissolve. Balloon stents can be used to dilate areas of stenosis. Urinary sepsis is not a contraindication to percutaneous stenting; in fact, placing a percutaneous stent may allow drainage of the infected renal unit and facilitate treatment of the infection.

If surgical exploration is necessary, areas of obstruction can be lysed and sutures removed if necessary. While simple stenting may suffice, ureters that appear nonviable can be resected and ureteroureterostomy or ureteroneocystostomy performed. Leakage can be repaired by oversewing or resecting and creating a reanastomosis of the ureter. When massive portions of the pelvic ureter are destroyed, transureteroureterostomy can be performed, bladder flaps utilized, or segments of bowel interposed to breach the defect.

Fistulae

Traditionally, management of vesicovaginal fistulae required prolonged catheter drainage of the bladder, antibiotic therapy, and hormone replacement, if indicated. This approach theoretically allowed resolution of inflammation and occasional spontaneous healing (10, 11). Recently, there has been emphasis on early surgical repair after resolution of infection (12).

Most vesicovaginal fistulae should be repaired vaginally. The Latzko procedure, which is well suited for repair of posthysterectomy apical vesicovaginal fistulae, involves removal of at least 2 cm of vaginal epithelium around the fistula tract, followed by closure of the denuded tissue with rows of absorbable sutures. Midvaginal fistulae are closed in layers.

The abdominal approach is reserved for patients who have large or complex fistulae or fistulae from irradiation therapy, as well as for patients who have undergone previous attempts at vaginal repairs. With this approach, the entire fistulous tract is excised and the bladder and vagina are separated from each other and closed in layers. When possible, the omentum is interposed between the bladder and the vagina. A combined vaginal and abdominal approach also may be used, interposing tissue grafts from the thighs, labia, omentum, or other sites. With experienced surgeons, the rate of successful fistula repair is 90% with the first attempt and even higher with the second attempt (13, 14). Complications of vesicovaginal fistula repair may include incontinence, sepsis, and vaginal shortening.

Complex Injuries

Ureterovesicovaginal fistulae usually are repaired abdominally, with closure of the vaginal defect, ureteral reimplantation, and use of an omental graft to separate layers and provide new blood supply (15). Vesicovaginal fistulae in which much or all of the urethra has been lost require a more extended repair. Tissue from the bladder or the vagina can be used for reconstruction (14, 16).

Enterovesicovaginal fistulae may occur with pelvic malignancies, radiation, colitis, or diverticulitis. A two-step approach may be best: 1) diverting the gastrointestinal tract and closing the urinary fistula, and 2) reestablishing gastrointestinal continuity. Alternatively, the entire procedure may be completed at one time (17). Enterovesicovaginal fistulae resulting from colitis or irradiation therapy often require permanent diversion.

Summary

Injuries to the lower urinary tract may occur during a variety of obstetric and gynecologic procedures. A thorough knowledge of pelvic anatomy and the disease or condition requiring surgery, adequate exposure of the operative site, careful sharp dissection, and meticulous hemostasis will reduce but not eliminate these problems.

Intraoperative recognition of urinary tract injuries allows prompt repair and minimal postoperative morbidity. When injury to the lower urinary tract is suspected postoperatively, the diagnosis is based on thorough physical examination and testing, which may include endoscopy and imaging studies in selected patients. Because lower urinary tract injuries are infrequent, consultation with a surgeon experienced in the repair of such injuries may be appropriate.

References

1. Eisenkop SM, Richman R, Platt LD, Paul RH. Urinary tract injury during cesarean section. Obstet Gynecol 1982;60:591–596 (Level III)
2. Lee RA, Symmonds RE, Williams TJ. Current status of genitourinary fistula. Obstet Gynecol 1988;72:313–319 (Level III)
3. Piscitelli JT, Simel DL, Addison WA. Who should have intravenous pyelograms before hysterectomy for benign disease? Obstet Gynecol 1987;69:541–545 (Level II-2)
4. Grainger DA, Soderstrom RM, Schiff SF, Glickman MG, DeCherney AH, Diamond MP. Ureteral injuries at laparoscopy: insights into diagnosis, management, and prevention. Obstet Gynecol 1990;75:839–843 (Level III)
5. Kadar N, Lemmerling L. Urinary tract injuries during laparoscopically assisted hysterectomy: causes and prevention. Am J Obstet Gynecol 1994;170:47–48 (Level III)
6. St Martin EC, Trichel BE, Campbell JH, Locke CM. Ureteral injuries in gynecologic surgery. J Urol 1953;70:51–57 (Level III)
7. Stanhope CR, Wilson TO, Utz WJ, Smith LH, O'Brien PC. Suture entrapment and secondary ureteral obstruction. Am J Obstet Gynecol 1991;164:1513–1519 (Level II-3)
8. Tarkington MA, Dejter SW Jr, Bresette JF. Early surgical management of extensive gynecologic ureteral injuries. Surg Gynecol Obstet 1991;173:17–21 (Level III)
9. Dowling RA, Corriere JN Jr, Sandler CM. Iatrogenic ureteral injury. J Urol 1986;135:912–915 (Level III)
10. Davits RJAM, Miranda SI. Conservative treatment of vesicovaginal fistulas by bladder drainage alone. Br J Urol 1991;68:155–156 (Level III)
11. Waaldijk K. The immediate surgical management of fresh obstetric fistulas with catheter and/or early closure. Int J Gynaecol Obstet 1994;45:11–16 (Level III)
12. Blandy JP, Badenoch DF, Fowler CG, Jenkins BJ, Thomas NWM. Early repair of iatrogenic injury to the ureter or bladder after gynecological surgery. J Urol 1991;146: 761–765 (Level III)
13. Tancer ML. Observations on prevention and management of vesicovaginal fistula after total hysterectomy. Surg Gynecol Obstet 1992;175:501–506 (Level III)
14. Elkins TE. Surgery for the obstetric vesicovaginal fistula: a review of 100 operations in 82 patients. Am J Obstet Gynecol 1994;170:1108–1120 (Level III)
15. Fichtner J, Voges G, Steinbach F, Hohenfellner R. Ureterovesicovaginal fistulas. Surg Gynecol Obstet 1993; 176:571–574 (Level III)
16. Elkins TE, Ghosh TS, Tagoe GA, Stocker R. Transvaginal mobilization and utilization of the anterior bladder wall to repair vesicovaginal fistulas involving the urethra. Obstet Gynecol 1992;79:455–460 (Level III)
17. Pontari MA, McMillen MA, Garvey RH, Ballentyne GH. Diagnosis and treatment of enterovesical fistulae. Am Surg 1992;58:258–263 (Level III)

Suggested Reading

Brubaker LT, Wilbanks GD. Urinary tract injuries in pelvic surgery. Surg Clin North Am 1991;71:963–976

Falk HC, Tancer ML. Vesicovaginal fistula: an historical survey. Obstet Gynecol 1954;3:337–341

Gerber GS, Schoenberg HW. Female urinary tract fistulas. J Urol 1993;149:229–236

The references in this bulletin are graded according to the method outlined by the U.S. Preventive Services Task Force:

- I Evidence obtained from at least one properly designed randomized controlled trial
- II-1 Evidence obtained from well-designed controlled trials without randomization
- II-2 Evidence obtained from well-designed cohort or case–control analytic studies, preferably from more than one center or research group
- II-3 Evidence obtained from multiple time series, with or without intervention, or dramatic results in uncontrolled experiments
- III Opinions of respected authorities, based on clinical experience, descriptive studies, or reports of expert committees

Other publications from ACOG:

- **Committee Opinions**, focused updates on emerging areas
- **Practice Patterns**, evidence-based guidelines
- **Criteria Sets**, baseline guidelines for review of diagnostic and management procedures

ISSN 1074-8628

The American College of Obstetricians and Gynecologists
409 12th Street, SW
PO Box 96920
Washington, DC 20090-6920

12345/10987

Number 178—March 1993
(Replaces #59, December 1980)

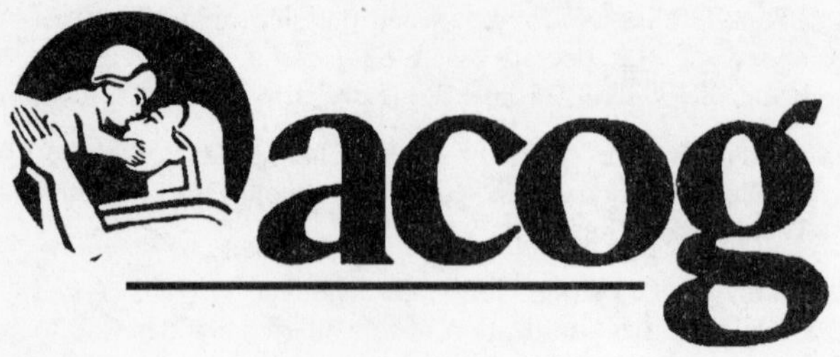

Technical Bulletin
An Educational Aid to Obstetrician–Gynecologists

Management of Gestational Trophoblastic Disease

Gestational trophoblastic disease (GTD) encompasses a spectrum of interrelated disease processes originating from the placenta. Several terms have been used to refer to these, including GTD, gestational trophoblastic neoplasia, and gestational trophoblastic tumors. The histologically distinct disease entities encompassed by this general terminology include complete and partial hydatidiform moles, invasive moles, placental site trophoblastic tumors (PSTT), and choriocarcinomas. Before the advent of sensitive assays for human chorionic gonadotropin (hCG) and efficacious chemotherapy, morbidity and mortality from all forms of GTD often occurred. However, with currently available quantitative assays for the beta subunit of hCG (β-hCG) for monitoring disease and current approaches to chemotherapy, most women with malignant GTD can be cured and their reproductive function can be preserved.

Estimates of the incidence of various forms of GTD vary. In the United States, hydatidiform moles are observed in approximately 1/600 therapeutic abortions and 1/1,000–1,200 pregnancies (1). Therefore, the practicing obstetrician–gynecologist may see approximately one or two molar pregnancies each year. Approximately 20% of patients with primary hydatidiform mole will develop malignant sequelae; the majority of these will be invasive moles and will not metastasize. Choriocarcinoma occurs in approximately 1/20,000–40,000 pregnancies; approximately 50% of gestational choriocarcinomas develop after term pregnancies, with 25% following molar gestations and 25% following other gestations (1). To allow optimal treatment, the obstetrician–gynecologist should be able to diagnose and manage women with primary molar gestations, diagnose malignant GTD, and assess risk in women with malignant GTD.

Hydatidiform Mole

Classification

Recent studies have defined two different forms of hydatidiform mole: partial and complete molar gestations. They are distinct cytogenetic disease processes with characteristic clinical and histopathologic findings and do not represent a "transition" from normal gestation to hydatidiform mole. The distinctive features of these two entities are outlined in Table 1. However, despite the clinical and pathologic differences, the management of patients with partial and complete moles should be similar.

Partial hydatidiform moles usually have 69 chromosomes derived from two paternal and one maternal haploid sets of chromosomes. Most have a 69,XXX or

TABLE 1. FEATURES OF PARTIAL AND COMPLETE HYDATIDIFORM MOLES

Feature	Partial Mole	Complete Mole
Karyotype	Most commonly 69,XXX or 69,XXY	46,XX or 46,XY
Pathology		
Fetus	Often present	Absent
Amnion, fetal red blood cells	Often present	Absent
Villose edema	Variable, focal	Diffuse
Trophoblastic proliferation	Variable, focal, slight to moderate	Variable, slight to severe
Clinical presentation		
Diagnosis	Missed abortion	Molar gestation
Uterine size	Small for dates	50% are large for dates
Theca lutein cysts	Rare	Occur in 25–30%
Medical complications	Rare	Frequent
Postmolar GTD	<5–10%	20%

69,XXY genotype derived from a haploid ovum with either reduplication of the paternal haploid set from a single sperm, or less frequently, from dispermic fertilization (2). Complete hydatidiform moles usually have a chromosomal complement totally derived from the paternal genome. The 46,XX genotype is most common, representing reduplication of the haploid genome of the sperm and exclusion of the chromosomal complement of the ovum (2). A smaller proportion of complete moles have a 46,XY karyotype consistent with dispermic fertilization.

Malignant sequelae occur in less than 5–10% of patients with partial hydatidiform moles and usually consist of nonmetastatic postmolar GTD (1). The volume and amount of trophoblastic proliferation in complete moles generally exceeds that observed in partial moles (2, 3). This proliferation is reflected by the clinical presentation. Initial β-hCG levels are higher than those seen in partial hydatidiform moles. The clinical and sonographic diagnosis is most frequently that of hydatidiform mole, with uterine enlargement beyond the expected gestational age observed in more than 50% of patients with complete moles (3). Patients often present with vaginal bleeding or expulsion of molar vesicles. Medical complications of molar pregnancy, including pregnancy-induced hypertension, hyperthyroidism, anemia, and hyperemesis, are more frequently seen in patients with complete moles (1). Approximately 15–25% of patients with complete moles will have theca lutein cysts of the ovaries with enlargement of greater than 6 cm (4, 5). Approximately 20% will develop malignant sequelae after evacuation of a complete hydatidiform mole (4, 6).

Diagnosis

Hydatidiform moles are usually diagnosed during the first trimester of pregnancy. The most common symptom of a mole is bleeding. Other symptoms include uterine enlargement greater than that expected for gestational dates, absence of fetal heart tones, cystic enlargement of the ovaries, hyperemesis, and an abnormally high serum level of β-hCG. The presence of these symptoms in the first trimester should alert the physician to the possibility of the presence of a mole. Pregnancy-induced hypertension in the first half of pregnancy is virtually diagnostic of hydatidiform mole. Ultrasound has replaced all other means of establishing the diagnosis preoperatively. It typically reveals the absence of a fetus and multiple echogenic areas of villi and clots.

Management

Occasionally, the diagnosis of a hydatidiform mole will be made on the basis of dilation and curettage for an incomplete abortion. In this instance, all patients should have serial determination of quantitative β-hCG levels. A baseline chest X-ray can be considered.

In patients in whom hydatidiform mole is suspected prior to evacuation, the following laboratory studies should be done: complete blood count with platelet determination, clotting function studies, renal and liver function studies, blood type and antibody screen, and determination of β-hCG level. A chest X-ray should also be obtained.

Common medical complications of hydatidiform mole include anemia, infection, hyperthyroidism, pregnancy-induced hypertension, and coagulopathy. As soon as patients with medical complications have been stabilized, the mole should be evacuated. The choice of location for the procedure should be based on the expertise of the physician, uterine size, and existing medical conditions and complications and the ability to manage them at the institution. In most patients, the preferred method of evacuation is suction curettage. Prostaglandins, oxytocin infusion, and hysterotomy are not usually recommended as the sole means of evacuation because they increase blood loss and may increase the risk for malignant sequelae after evacuation compared with suction curettage (4, 7). Furthermore, patients often require curettage after prostaglandins or oxytocin infusions are used to evacuate a mole (7). Evacuation is usually performed under general anesthesia, but local anesthesia may be used in a cooperative patient with a small uterus. After dilation of the cervix, uterine evacuation is accomplished with the largest cannula that can be introduced through the cervix. Intravenous oxytocin is begun after the cervix is dilated and continued postoperatively for several hours. After completion of suction curettage, gentle sharp curettage may be performed.

Pulmonary complications are frequently observed around the time of evacuation of hydatidiform mole in patients with marked uterine enlargement. Although the syndrome of trophoblastic embolization has been emphasized as an underlying cause for respiratory distress syndrome (8), there are many other potential causes of respiratory distress syndrome in these women. Respiratory distress syndrome can also be caused by high-output congestive heart failure caused by anemia or hyperthyroidism, preeclampsia, or iatrogenic fluid overload (9). In general, these complications should be treated aggressively with therapy directed by Swan–Ganz catheter monitoring and assisted ventilator support as required. Hyperthyroidism and pregnancy-induced hypertension usually abate promptly afterevacuation of the molar pregnancy and may not require specific therapy. Theca lutein cysts occur due to β-hCG stimulation and may take several months to resolve after molar evacuation (5).

Hysterectomy is an alternative to suction curettage in selected patients. Usually the adnexa may be preserved. Although hysterectomy reduces the risk of malignant sequelae, the chance of malignant GTD after hysterectomy for hydatidiform mole remains approximately 3–5% (4). Therefore, these patients should be monitored with serial β-hCG levels as follows.

After evacuation, it is important to monitor patients carefully in order to diagnose and treat malignant sequelae promptly. Serial quantitative β-hCG determinations should be performed utilizing radioimmunoassay or a comparable method. Qualitative pregnancy tests should not be used to monitor patients with hydatidiform mole. Human chorionic gonadotropin levels should be determined 48 hours after evacuation, every 1–2 weeks until levels are normal, and then at 1–2-month intervals for an additional 6–12 months (4, 6). Pelvic examinations are performed to monitor the involution of pelvic structures and to aid in the early detection of metastases. A chest X-ray is indicated if the β-hCG titer rises.

Contraception is recommended for at least 6 months to 1 year after remission. The rationale for an interval of monitoring during hCG remission is to allow identification of the rare patients who develop postmolar malignant sequelae after achieving normal hCG values. It should be noted, however, that virtually all episodes of malignant sequelae occurring after evacuation of a hydatidiform mole occur within approximately 6 months of molar evacuation (4, 6). Therefore, pregnancy after 6–12 months of documented remission of hCG levels minimizes the chance of obscuring a rise in hCG level caused by malignant GTD in this setting. Oral contraceptives do not increase the incidence of postmolar GTD or affect the pattern of regression of hCG levels (10). After completion of surveillance documenting remission, pregnancy can be permitted and hCG monitoring discontinued. Patients with a prior partial or complete molar gestation have a 10-fold increased risk (1–2% incidence) of a second mole in subsequent pregnancies (11). Therefore, all future pregnancies should be evaluated by ultrasound early in their course.

Although prophylactic chemotherapy has been shown to decrease the incidence of postmolar GTD in patients after evacuation of high-risk molar pregnancies, it is not routinely recommended (1). In compliant patients, the low morbidity and mortality achieved by monitoring patients with serial β-hCG determinations and instituting only indicated chemotherapy outweighs the potential risk and small benefit of routine prophylactic chemotherapy. As long as β-hCG values are declining, there does not appear to be any role for chemotherapy. However, if β-hCG values rise or plateau over more than 2 weeks, immediate workup and treatment for malignant postmolar GTD is indicated. Repeat curettage does not often induce remission and may result in uterine perforation (12). If malignant forms of GTD are diagnosed histologically or if patients develop clinical or radiographic evidence of malignant GTD, treatment is indicated (4, 6).

Malignant Gestational Trophoblastic Disease

Histologic Considerations

The clinical presentation of malignant GTD is more important in determining prognosis than the precise histologic diagnosis:

- *Invasive moles* are characterized by persistence of edematous chorionic villi with trophoblastic proliferation invading into the myometrium. They rarely metastasize but are usually treated with chemotherapy.
- *Gestational choriocarcinoma* is a pure epithelial neoplasm, comprising both neoplastic syncytiotrophoblast and cytotrophoblast elements without chorionic villi. Gestational choriocarcinoma tends to develop early systemic hematogenous metastases, and chemotherapy is indicated.
- *Placental site trophoblastic tumors* are very rare trophoblastic neoplasms characterized by absence of chorionic villi and proliferation of intermediate cytotrophoblast cells (13). The dimorphic population of syncytiotrophoblast and cytotrophoblast elements that are observed in choriocarcinoma are lacking in PSTT (13). They secrete amounts of β-hCG that are small in relation to the tumor volume. The PSTT generally are not sensitive to chemotherapy; therefore, it is important to distinguish them histologically from choriocarcinomas. Fortunately, they metastasize very rarely beyond the uterus; hysterectomy is the treatment of choice.

Clinical Diagnosis

Clinically, postmolar GTD is diagnosed on the basis of rising (increase of >10%) or plateauing (decline of <10% for at least three values over more than 14 days) β-hCG values. Women with GTD following nonmolar pregnancies may present with subtle signs and symptoms of disease, making a diagnosis difficult. Delayed diagnosis may lead to a worsened outcome. Abnormal bleeding following any pregnancy should be evaluated promptly with β-hCG testing and endometrial sampling to determine the presence of GTD. Metastases from gestational choriocarcinoma have been reported in virtually every body site; thus this diagnosis should be considered in any postpartum woman presenting with metastatic disease from an unknown primary site. Central nervous system metastases may produce neurologic abnormalities, intracranial hemorrhage, or mass lesions. A serum β-hCG determination and exclusion of normal pregnancy are all that are required to diagnose metastatic GTD in these circumstances.

Once the diagnosis of malignant GTD is suspected or established, immediate evaluation for metastases is mandatory. Along with history and physical examination, the following laboratory studies should be performed: complete blood count with platelet determination, clotting function studies, renal and liver function studies, blood type and antibody screen, and determination of baseline (pretherapy) β-hCG level. Modes of radiographic evaluation that may be used include chest X-ray or computed tomography (CT) scan, pelvic ultrasound, brain CT or magnetic resonance imaging scan, and abdominal–pelvic CT scan or magnetic resonance imaging scan of the liver. Systemic venous metastasis may result in pulmonary or vaginal lesions. Systemic arterial metastasis usually occurs after pulmonary metastases have been established. For a minimum evaluation, a chest X-ray should be performed. If it is positive, CT or magnetic resonance imaging of the brain and abdomen should be performed. However, if the chest radiograph is negative, a CT scan of the chest should be obtained because 40% of patients with negative chest X-rays have metastatic lesions seen on CT scan (14). If the chest CT is positive, the brain and abdomen should be evaluated as previously described.

Classification

Three systems have been proposed for categorization of patients with malignant GTD (1): those developed by the World Health Organization (WHO), the National Institutes of Health (NIH), and the International Federation of Gynecologists and Obstetricians (FIGO). The FIGO system is not clinically useful since it does not take into account other factors which may reflect disease outcome, such as volume of metastatic disease, antecedent pregnancy type, or duration of disease. Therefore, the WHO and NIH systems are used in the United States.

The WHO prognostic index score (Table 2) assigns a weighted value to several individual clinical variables. The total prognostic index score has been shown to correlate with prognosis and response to therapy (15).

The NIH's experience has led to a clinical classification system commonly used in the United States (1, 16, 17) (see the box: Classification of GTD). This system separates patients with nonmetastatic disease from those with metastatic disease, because virtually all patients with nonmetastatic disease can be cured using single-agent chemotherapy. Patients with metastatic GTD are further subdivided. Those with low-risk disease—who lack any clinical risk factors—are likely to respond to single-agent chemotherapy and are considered to have a good prognosis. In contrast, patients with high-risk disease—who have one or more clinical risk factors—are unlikely to respond to single-agent chemotherapy and are, therefore, considered to have a poor prognosis. Patients with a poor prognosis should be treated initially with multiagent chemotherapy.

Although the WHO prognostic index score may provide a more precise definition of prognosis in patients with high-risk disease (15), the NIH clinical classification system allows easy identification of patients with risk factors who are unlikely to respond to single-agent chemotherapy. Virtually all deaths from GTD occur among patients who fall into the poor prognosis, high-risk category (18). All patients identified as having high-risk malignant GTD should be treated in consultation with individuals who are experienced in the therapy of GTD.

TABLE 2. WORLD HEALTH ORGANIZATION PROGNOSTIC INDEX SCORE FOR GTD

	Score*			
Prognostic Factor	0	1	2	4
Age (y)	≤ 39	>39	—	—
Antecedent pregnancy	Hydatidiform mole	Abortion	Term	—
Interval (mo)†	<4	4–6	7–12	>12
β-hCG (IU/L)	$<10^3$	10^3–10	10^4–10^5	$>10^5$
ABO groups (female × male)	—	O×A, A×O	B, AB	—
Largest tumor, including uterine tumor	—	3–5 cm	>5 cm	—
Site of metastases	—	Spleen, kidney	Gastrointestinal tract, liver	Brain
Number of metastases identified	—	1–4	4–8	>8
Prior chemotherapy	—	—	Single drug	Two or more drugs

* The total score for a patient is obtained by adding the individual scores for each prognostic factor. Low risk = 0–4, intermediate risk = 5–7, high risk = ≥ 8.

† Interval is time between end of antecedent pregnancy and start of chemotherapy.

Classification of GTD

I. Benign GTD
   A. Complete hydatidiform mole
   B. Partial hydatidiform mole

II. Malignant GTD
   A. Nonmetastatic GTD
   B. Metastatic GTD
      1. Good prognosis, low risk—absence of any risk factor
      2. Poor prognosis, high risk—presence of any risk factor
         a. Duration >4 months
         b. Pretherapy level of β-hCG in serum >40,000 mIU/ml
         c. Brain or liver metastases
         d. GTD after term gestation
         e. Prior failed therapy

Management

Nonmetastatic

The primary remission rates of nonmetastatic GTD are similar, and essentially all patients with this condition ultimately can be cured with chemotherapy. Many chemotherapeutic regimens have been evaluated for the treatment of women with nonmetastatic GTD (see the box: Chemotherapy Regimens for Nonmetastatic GTD). Of the available regimens, the Gynecologic Oncology Group reports that weekly methotrexate is efficacious, minimally toxic, and most cost-effective (19). Chemotherapy is continued until β-hCG values have achieved normal levels, and then an additional course (two weekly doses) is administered after the first normal hCG value has been recorded. Since methotrexate is excreted entirely by the kidney, patients must have a normal creatinine level prior to each treatment.

In this group of women, it has been shown that early hysterectomy will shorten the duration and amount of chemotherapy needed to produce remission (20). Therefore, the patient's desire for further fertility should be evaluated at the onset of therapy. Hysterectomy may be performed during the first cycle of chemotherapy. However, continued chemotherapy remains mandatory until hCG values are normal.

Patients whose levels of β-hCG have leveled off or are rising during therapy should be switched to an alternative single-agent regimen. Dosages for dactinomycin and etoposide are shown in the box. The appearance of new metastasis or failure of alternative single-agent therapy mandates the use of multiagent chemotherapy. Hysterectomy should be considered for the treatment of patients with nonmetastatic disease that is refractory to single-agent chemotherapy (20).

Metastatic

Patients with metastatic GTD who lack any of the clinical factors that would suggest a poor prognosis have low-risk disease. They can be treated successfully with single-agent regimens (15, 18, 20). Traditionally, this has consisted of 5-day cycles of single-agent methotrexate or dactinomycin. Approximately 40% of patients will require alternative therapy to achieve remission; however, essentially all patients with low-risk disease can be cured with conventional chemotherapy. Hysterectomy as primary treatment in conjunction with chemotherapy may also decrease the amount of chemotherapy required to achieve remission in these patients (20).

Patients who have one or more high-risk clinical factors according to the NIH classification or who have a WHO prognostic index score greater than 7 have high-risk disease. These women may require some combination of chemotherapy, radiation, and surgery. Optimal survival in trophoblastic disease centers is 60–84% (15,

Chemotherapy Regimens for Nonmetastatic GTD*

First-line therapy: methotrexate†

- Weekly, 30 mg/m² IM‡, *or*
- Every 2 weeks, a 5-day regimen of 0.4 mg/kg IM (maximum 25 mg/d total), *or*
- Methotrexate, 1 mg/kg IM, on days 1, 3, 5, and 7 with folinic acid, 0.1 mg/kg IM, on days 2, 4, 6, and 8, *or*
- Methotrexate, 100 mg/m² IV bolus and 200 mg/m² IV infusion over 12 hours, followed by folinic acid, 15 mg PO every 6 hours for four doses (begun at the end of infusion)

Alternative therapy: dactinomycin†§ or etoposide†

Dactinomycin

- For 5 days, 9–13 μg/kg IV, every 2 weeks (maximum 500 μg/d), *or*
- Bolus, 1.25 mg/m² IV, every 2 weeks

Etoposide

- For 5 days, 200 mg/m² PO every 12–14 days¶

*Abbreviations: IM = intramuscularly, IV = intravenously, PO = orally.

†Gastrointestinal toxicity is common.

‡A weekly methotrexate regimen is described in Homesley HD, Blessing JA, Rettenmaier M, Capizzi RL, Major FJ, Twiggs LB. Weekly intramuscular methotrexate for nonmetastatic gestational trophoblastic disease. Obstet Gynecol 1988;72:413–418

§Caution: may produce extravasation injury.

¶Universal alopecia results.

18, 20, 21). In contrast to findings in patients with nonmetastatic or metastatic, low-risk disease, primary treatment with hysterectomy does not appear to improve the outcome in patients with metastatic, high-risk disease (20).

Initial multiagent chemotherapy is of primary importance. Triple therapy with methotrexate, dactinomycin, and either chlorambucil or cyclophosphamide (MAC) has been the standard regimen for many years in the United States. A multiagent regimen described by Bagshawe has also been used, but any superiority of this more complex regimen over MAC has not been demonstrated (22). With the identification of etoposide as an active agent in the treatment of GTD, a cyclic, non-cross-resistant chemotherapy regimen incorporating etoposide, methotrexate, and dactinomycin alternating with cyclophosphamide and vincristine (EMA/CO) has been used with a high rate of success in patients with high-risk disease (21).

Management of cerebral and hepatic metastases is controversial. Radiation therapy (2,000 cGy to the liver and 3,000 cGy to the brain) has been used with chemotherapy in an attempt to limit acute hemorrhagic complications from these sites of metastases (18). Although the use of brain irradiation with systemic chemotherapy is successful in controlling metastases (18), a high remission rate has been reported when a modification of the EMA/CO chemotherapeutic regimen was used without brain irradiation (23). Even with intense chemotherapy, additional surgery may be necessary to control bleeding, remove isolated metastases, or treat complications from metastatic disease (20).

Chemotherapy is continued until three consecutive normal β-hCG values have been obtained, and this is usually followed by three additional courses of chemotherapy in the hopes of eradicating all viable tumor. Despite using sensitive β-hCG assays and using maintenance chemotherapy, up to 13% of patients with high-risk disease will develop recurrence after achieving an initial remission (17).

Surveillance Following Chemotherapy

After hCG remission has been achieved, patients should be monitored with determinations of β-hCG values at 2-week intervals for the first 3 months of remission and then at 1-month intervals for the first year of remission. The risk of recurrence after one year of remission is less than 1%, but late recurrences have been observed (17). Therefore, it is recommended that patients undergo surveillance of hCG levels at approximately 6-month intervals.

Contraception, preferably with oral contraceptives, should be used during the first year of remission. Pregnancy may be considered after 1 year of remission. Because of the 1–2% risk of a second molar pregnancy in subsequent pregnancies, early ultrasound examination is recommended for all future pregnancies. There does not appear to be an increase in the risk of congenital malformations or complications of pregnancy with subsequent pregnancies.

Summary

Despite the potentially serious outcome of malignant GTD, most women with all forms of GTD can be successfully diagnosed and treated, with preservation of their normal reproductive function. It is important to manage hydatidiform mole properly in order to minimize acute complications, identify malignant sequelae promptly, and begin therapy. It is important to individualize therapy for women with malignant GTD based upon known risk factors, using less toxic therapy for patients with low-risk disease and aggressive multiagent therapy for patients with high-risk disease.

REFERENCES

1. Soper JT, Hammond CB. Gestational trophoblastic neoplasms. In: Scott JR, DiSaia PJ, Hammond CB, Spellacy WN, eds. Danforth's obstetrics and gynecology. 6th ed. Philadelphia: JB Lippincott Co, 1990:1141–1155
2. Szulman AE, Surti U. The syndromes of hydatidiform mole. I. Cytogenetic and morphologic correlations. Am J Obstet Gynecol 1978;131:665–671
3. Szulman AE, Surti U. The clinicopathologic profile of the partial hydatidiform mole. Obstet Gynecol 1982;59: 597–602
4. Curry SL, Hammond CB, Tyrey L, Creasman WT, Parker RT. Hydatidiform mole: diagnosis, management, and long-term followup of 347 patients. Obstet Gynecol 1975;45: 1–8
5. Montz FJ, Schlaerth JB, Morrow CP. The natural history of theca lutein cysts. Obstet Gynecol 1988;72:247–251
6. Lurain JR, Brewer JI, Torok EE, Halpern B. Natural history of hydatidiform mole after primary evacuation. Am J Obstet Gynecol 1983;145:591–595
7. Schlaerth JB, Morrow CP, Montz FJ, d'Ablaing G. Initial management of hydatidiform mole. Am J Obstet Gynecol 1988;158:1299–1306
8. Orr JW Jr, Austin JM, Hatch KD, Shingleton HM, Younger JB, Boots LR. Acute pulmonary edema associated with molar pregnancies: a high-risk factor for development of persistent trophoblastic disease. Am J Obstet Gynecol 1980;136:412–415
9. Twiggs LB, Morrow CP, Schlaerth JB. Acute pulmonary complications of molar pregnancy. Am J Obstet Gynecol 1979;135:189–194

10. Morrow P, Nakamura R, Schlaerth J, Gaddis O Jr, Eddy G. The influence of oral contraceptives on the postmolar human chorionic gonadotropin regression curve. Am J Obstet Gynecol 1985;151:906–914

11. Berkowitz RS, Goldstein DP, Bernstein MR, Sablinska B. Subsequent pregnancy outcome in patients with molar pregnancy and gestational trophoblastic tumors. J Reprod Med 1987;32:680–684

12. Schlaerth JB, Morrow CP, Rodriguez M. Diagnostic and therapeutic curettage in gestational trophoblastic disease. Am J Obstet Gynecol 1990;162:1465–1471

13. Driscoll SG. Placental-site chorioma. The neoplasm of the implantation-site trophoblast. J Reprod Med 1984; 29: 821–825

14. Mutch DG, Soper JT, Baker ME, Bandy LC, Cox EB, Clarke-Pearson DL, et al. Role of computed axial tomography of the chest in staging patients with non-metastatic gestational trophoblastic disease. Obstet Gynecol 1986;68: 348–352

15. DuBeshter B, Berkowitz RS, Goldstein DP, Cramer DW, Bernstein MR. Metastatic gestational trophoblastic disease: experience at the New England Trophoblastic Disease Center, 1965 to 1985. Obstet Gynecol 1987; 69: 390–395

16. Hammond CB, Borchert LG, Tyrey L, Creasman WT, Parker RT. Treatment of metastatic trophoblastic disease: good and poor prognosis. Am J Obstet Gynecol 1973;115:451–457

17. Mutch DG, Soper JT, Babcock CJ, Clarke-Pearson DL, Hammond CB. Recurrent gestational trophoblastic disease. Experience of the Southeastern Regional Trophoblastic Disease Center. Cancer 1990;66:978–982

18. Soper JT, Clarke-Pearson DL, Hammond CB. Metastatic gestational trophoblastic disease: prognostic factors in previously untreated patients. Obstet Gynecol 1988;71:338–343

19. Homesley HD, Blessing JA, Rettenmaier M, Capizzi RL, Major FJ, Twiggs LB. Weekly intramuscular methotrexate for nonmetastatic gestational trophoblastic disease. Obstet Gynecol 1988;72:413–418

20. Hammond CB, Weed JC Jr, Currie JL. The role of operation in the current therapy of gestational trophoblastic disease. Am J Obstet Gynecol 1980;136:844–858

21. Newlands ES, Bagshawe KD, Begent RHJ, Rustin GJS, Holden L, Dent J. Developments in chemotherapy for medium- and high-risk patients with gestational trophoblastic tumours (1979–1984). Br J Obstet Gynaecol 1986;93:63– 69

22. Curry SL, Blessing JA, DiSaia PJ, Soper JT, Twiggs LB. A prospective randomized comparison of methotrexate, dactinomycin, and chlorambucil versus methotrexate, dactinomycin, cyclophosphamide, doxorubicin, melphalan, hydroxyurea, and vincristine in "poor prognosis" metastatic gestational trophoblastic disease: a Gynecologic Oncology Group study. Obstet Gynecol 1989;73:357–362

23. Rustin GJS, Newlands ES, Begent RHJ, Dent J, Bagshawe KD. Weekly alternating etoposide, methotrexate, and actinomycin/vincristine and cyclophosphamide chemotherapy for the treatment of CNS metastases of choriocarcinoma. J Clin Oncol 1989;7:900–903

This Technical Bulletin was developed under the direction of the Committee on Technical Bulletins of the American College of Obstetricians and Gynecologists as an educational aid to obstetricians and gynecologists. The committee wishes to thank John T. Soper, MD, for his assistance in the development of this bulletin. This Technical Bulletin does not define a standard of care, nor is it intended to dictate an exclusive course of management. It presents recognized methods and techniques of clinical practice for consideration by obstetrician–gynecologists for incorporation into their practices. Variations of practice taking into account the needs of the individual patient, resources, and limitations unique to the institution or type of practice may be appropriate.

THE AMERICAN COLLEGE OF OBSTETRICIANS AND GYNECOLOGISTS
409 12th Street, SW
Washington, DC 20024-2188

345/76

ACOG EDUCATIONAL BULLETIN

Number 227, August 1996

Management of Isoimmunization in Pregnancy

When any fetal blood group factor inherited from the father is not possessed by the mother, antepartum or intrapartum fetal–maternal bleeding may stimulate an immune reaction by the mother. Maternal immune reactions can also occur from blood product transfusion. The formation of maternal antibodies to a foreign antigen may be followed by various degrees of transplacental passage of these antibodies into the fetal circulation. Depending on the degree of antigenicity and the amount and type of antibody involved, this transplacental passage may lead to hemolytic disease of the newborn.

The reproductive history of a woman with isoimmunization is of considerable importance in recognizing and determining the prognosis for a subsequent isoimmunized pregnancy. For example, if a D-negative, isoimmunized woman becomes pregnant with a D-positive fetus, the severity of the hemolytic disease will usually be equal to or greater than that of the previous pregnancy. Occasionally, the disease progression may be such that early-onset fetal hydrops may occur in a patient who experienced only mildly affected prior pregnancies. In rare cases, hemolytic disease in the current pregnancy may be less severe than in a prior pregnancy. Regardless of obstetric history, all pregnant women should undergo laboratory examinations at the first prenatal visit to determine the possibility of isoimmunization. Tests should include determination of ABO and D types as well as a screen for the presence of antibodies by an indirect Coombs test (antibody screen).

Factors that minimize the chance of isoimmunization to the D antigen are detailed elsewhere (1). There are no preventive strategies against sensitization to blood factors other than the D antigen. Although some of these antibodies are not clinically significant, most do gain access to the fetus across the placenta and can potentially cause fetal anemia and hydrops. Fortunately, ABO incompatibility, which is a common cause of subclinical and mild hemolytic disease of the newborn, does not cause clinical or severe erythroblastosis. Therefore, no antenatal testing, either by titer or by amniocentesis, is necessary when there is a history of ABO incompatibility.

This Educational Bulletin was developed under the direction of the Committee on Educational Bulletins of the American College of Obstetricians and Gynecologists as an aid to obstetricians and gynecologists. The College wishes to thank Michael L. Socol, MD, for his assistance in the development of this bulletin. This document is not to be construed as establishing a standard of practice or dictating an exclusive course of treatment. Rather, it is intended as an educational tool that presents current information on obstetric–gynecologic issues.

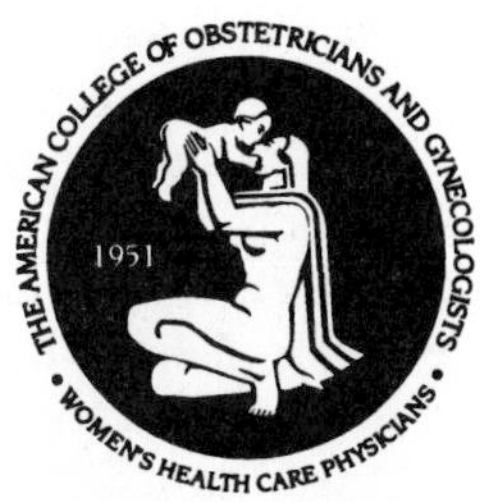

Replaces Number 148, October 1990

Clinically Significant Antibodies

CDE System

Anti-D isoimmunization remains the most common cause of erythroblastosis fetalis. Antibodies formed in response to the D antigen are of the immunoglobulin G (IgG) type. Consequently, they can cross the placenta and hemolyze fetal erythrocytes. Whereas most clinically significant blood group sensitizations noted during pregnancy are still secondary to anti-D incompatibility, sensitization to antigens other than D in the CDE system is not uncommon and can cause severe disease.

Other Antibodies

The most frequently encountered antibodies other than D are Lewis antibodies (Le^a and Le^b). Like most cold agglutinins, Lewis antigens do not cause erythroblastosis fetalis because they are predominantly of the IgM type and they are poorly expressed on fetal and newborn erythrocytes. In contrast, Kell antibodies (k, K, Kp^a, Kp^b, Js^a, Js^b) can produce erythroblastosis fetalis. Kell isoimmunization is often caused by prior transfusion, since Kell compatibility is usually not considered when blood is cross-matched. Fortunately, 90% of partners of Kell-immunized women are Kell negative themselves. Less common, but just as likely to cause erythroblastosis fetalis, are some of the Duffy antigens. Additional antibodies known to cause hemolytic disease are listed in Table 1. Care of patients with sensitization to antigens other than D that are known to cause hemolytic disease should be the same as that for patients with D isoimmunization. A possible exception is Kell sensitization, in which amniotic fluid analysis has been reported to correlate poorly with the severity of fetal anemia (2). These patients may benefit from more aggressive fetal assessment; however, optimal management of Kell-sensitized patients is controversial (3).

TABLE 1. ISOIMMUNIZATION RESULTING FROM IRREGULAR ANTIBODIES*

Blood Group System	Antigen
Rh	C, c, e, E
Kell	K, k, Ko, Kp^a, Kp^b, Js^a, Js^b
Duffy	Fy^a, Fy^b, Fy^3
Kidd	Jk^a, Jk^b, Jk^3
MNSs	M, N, S, s, U, Mi^a, Mt^a, Vw, Mur, Hil, Hut
Lutheran	Lu^a, Lu^b
Diego	Di^a, Di^b
Xg	Xg^a
P	$PP_1p^k(Tj^a)$
Public antigens	Yt^a, Yt^b, Lan, En^a, Ge, Jr^a, Co^a, $Co^{a\text{-}b\text{-}}$
Private antigens	Batty, Becker, Berrens, Biles, Evans, Gonzales, Good, Heibel, Hunt, Jobbins, Radin, Rm, Ven, $Wright^a$, $Wright^b$, Zd

* Lewis (Le^a, Le^b) and I antigens are not causes of hemolytic disease of the newborn.

Modified from Socol ML. Management of blood group isoimmunization. In: Gleicher N. Principles and practice of medical therapy in pregnancy. 2nd ed. Norwalk, Connecticut: Appleton and Lange, 1992:1051

Clinical Management

Once it has been established that a pregnant woman is sensitized to an antigen that may cause erythroblastosis, the genotype of the fetus's father should be determined. This is most useful for the atypical antigens because isoimmunization is often secondary to a transfusion. If the father of the fetus does not possess the antigen, the fetus is not at risk. If the father is a heterozygote there is only a 50% chance that the fetus has inherited the blood group antigen and the pregnancy is affected. The most likely zygosity for the D antigen can also be predicted as the alleles at the C, D, and E loci are inherited together, and some combinations are more frequent than others. Because it is not possible to test for the presence of D antigens, zygosity can be determined only by looking at the combination. Clinically, however, determining this genotype is of limited value for the couple receiving counseling after a severely affected pregnancy. Unless the D-positive partner has previously fathered a D-negative child, it is impossible to state with certainty that he is a heterozygote.

Antibody Titers

Maternal serum antibody titers can be measured by a variety of techniques (4). Agglutination of erythrocytes in saline measures maternal IgM antibody, and this is too large a molecule to cross the placenta. Albumin is a more viscous medium; therefore, the smaller IgG molecules are capable of agglutinating erythrocytes, but the contribution by IgM is not eliminated. The most sensitive and accurate barometer for clinical practice is the indirect Coombs test.

The usefulness of maternal serum antibody titers is determined by the patient's reproductive history. If a patient has never had a pregnancy complicated by Rh-related neonatal morbidity other than hyperbilirubinemia treated by phototherapy, antibody titers are the initial step of management. An antibody titer should be determined at the first prenatal visit, at 20 weeks of gestation, and approximately every 4 weeks thereafter. When the antibody titer is ≤ 1:8, whether directed to D or another paternal antigen capable of causing severe erythroblastosis, no intervention is necessary; when the titer is ≥ 1:16 in albumin or 1:32 by indirect antiglobulin (indirect Coombs test), amniocentesis or percutaneous umbilical cord blood sampling (cordocentesis) should be considered (5).

If a patient has had a prior affected pregnancy (neonatal exchange transfusion, early delivery, or intrauterine transfusion), antibody titers are not necessary because amniocentesis or percutaneous umbilical cord blood sampling will be required. The timing of the initial procedure is determined by past clinical history. It is usually performed at least 4–8 weeks earlier than the prior gestational age at which significant morbidity occurred, with some clinicians beginning at 20 weeks or even earlier.

Amniocentesis and Percutaneous Umbilical Cord Blood Sampling

Since the mid-1960s, amniocentesis with spectrophotometric examination of the amniotic fluid has been the accepted method for assessing the severity of erythroblastosis in utero. Amniotic fluid bilirubin is most likely derived from fetal tracheal and pulmonary secretions. It can be quantitated by spectrophotometrically measuring absorbance at the 450-nm wavelength in a specimen of amniotic fluid that has been shielded from light. The deviation from linearity (change in optical density at 450 nm [ΔOD_{450}]) is determined by measuring the difference between this absorbance and a straight line drawn from points 365 nm to 535 nm on the spectrophotometric curve. Contamination of amniotic fluid by meconium and by erythrocytes and their porphyrin breakdown products can significantly alter spectrophotometric analysis at 450 nm, but these problems can be largely overcome by chloroform extraction of the amniotic fluid (6). Heme pigment will also generate a peak at the 405-nm wavelength, and in the absence of blood contamination this may be indicative of severe hemolysis (4).

Fetal status is determined by plotting the ΔOD_{450} measurement on a Liley graph (Fig. 1) (7). Readings in zone III (uppermost zone) suggest severe hemolytic disease with a high probability of fetal death within 7–10 days. Readings in zone I (lowest zone) are reassuring although neonatal exchange transfusion may be necessary occasionally. There are no reliable data concerning the optimal frequency for repeated sampling. In general, amniocentesis is repeated every 1–4 weeks if the ΔOD_{450} measurement is in zone II (middle zone) and every 3–4 weeks if it has dropped into zone I. The frequency depends on where in zone II the value falls and the pattern established in previous procedures. Declining values are encouraging although they do not preclude mild hemolytic disease. Stable or rising ΔOD_{450} measurements are causes of concern.

Patients with results in zone I or low zone II can be allowed to proceed to term, at which point labor should be induced. In most cases, patients in the middle of zone II can progress to 36–38 weeks of gestation, at which time delivery should be accomplished, by induction of labor if possible. Depending on gestational age, patients in zone III should either be delivered or should receive intrauterine fetal transfusion. Similar considerations may apply to a rising titer in upper zone II. Delivery is often by cesarean birth because of an unfavorable cervix, but a trial of labor is not contraindicated.

Percutaneous umbilical cord blood sampling has improved the obstetric care of isoimmunized patients because of the ability to evaluate fetal status precisely. This is particularly true in the middle trimester, when amniotic fluid from unaffected fetuses will also contain bilirubin. Peak values of bilirubin are present between 20 and 24 weeks of gestation. The Liley curve was generated from pregnancies of at least 28 weeks of gestation. In the past, obstetricians have derived values for pregnancies of 20–27 weeks of gestation by extrapolating backwards from the Liley curve; however, such extrapolations may be inappropriate (8). In either the second or the third trimester, knowledge of the specific fetal hematocrit enables the physician to take a more rational approach to the need for, volume of, and timing of fetal transfusions. Hematologic values for normal fetuses from 15 to 30 weeks of gestation are shown in Table 2 (9, 10). In some instances, findings may even indicate that the fetus does not possess the blood group antigen in question and therefore requires no further evaluation. Perhaps most importantly, the use of amniocentesis in conjunction with percutaneous umbilical cord blood sampling allows a more aggressive approach at an earlier gestational age.

In spite of the enthusiasm that percutaneous umbilical cord blood sampling has generated for fetal diagnosis and therapy, some caution should be exercised. First, a chart of spectrophotometric measurements from sensitized pregnancies in the middle trimester has been constructed that may minimize the benefit of fetal blood sampling as the primary assessment of fetal status (11). Second, determination of fetal blood type, particularly for the D antigen, can be accomplished by polymerase chain reaction on fetal amniocytes and therefore does not always require a fetal blood sample (12). It should be emphasized, however, that these tests should be done in specialized laboratories with considerable experience in polymerase chain reaction testing. Third, liberal use of percutaneous umbilical cord blood sampling may induce an anamnestic immune response in the mother secondary to fetal–maternal hemorrhage, thereby accelerating the disease process (13, 14). Fourth, the loss rate with percutaneous umbilical cord blood sampling is generally agreed to be greater than that with amniocentesis. Consequently, whereas fetal blood sampling as the principal means of fetal assessment in isoimmunized pregnancies appears safe and effective in experienced hands (15, 16), most clinicians continue to rely primarily on amniocentesis.

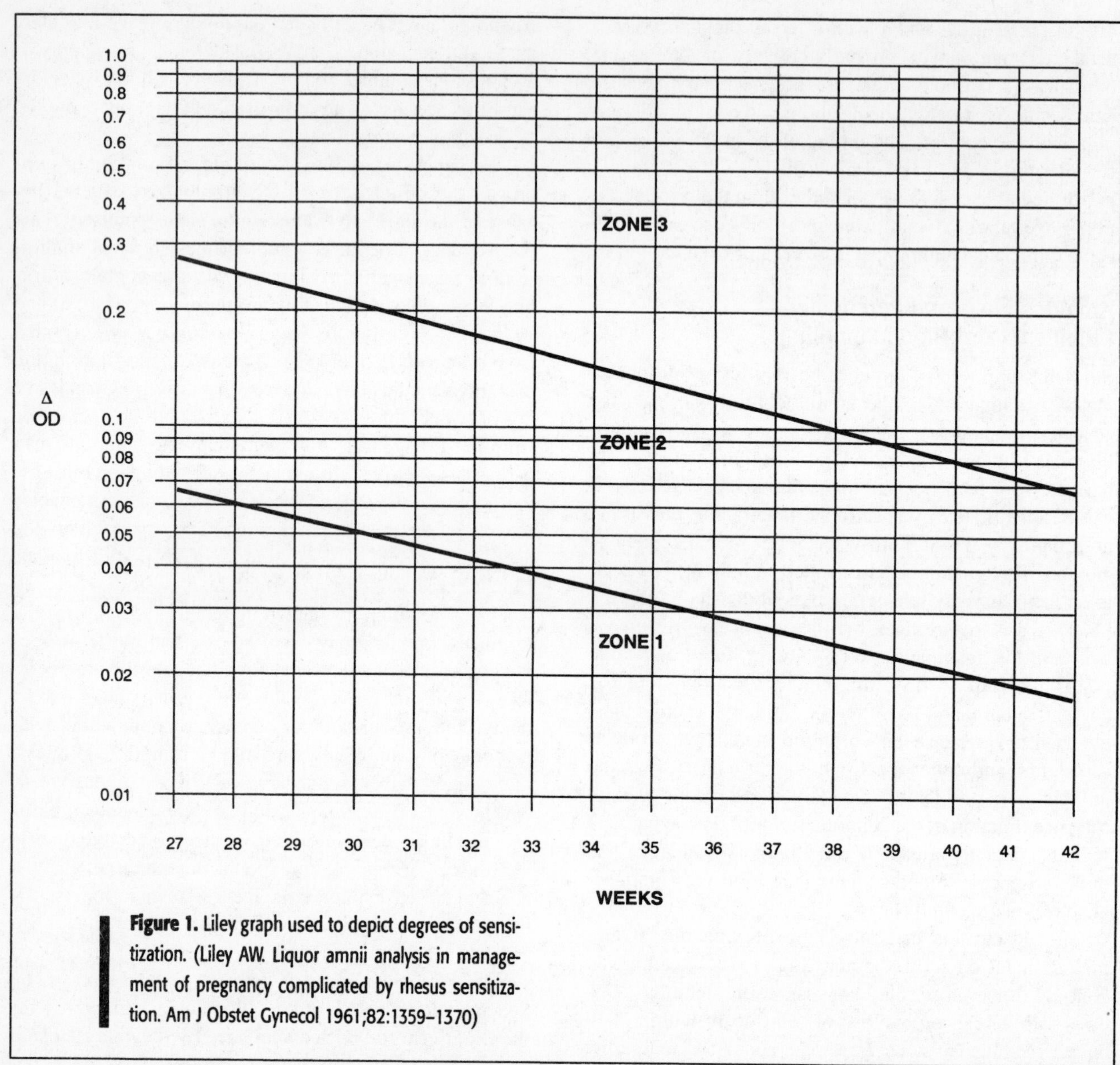

Figure 1. Liley graph used to depict degrees of sensitization. (Liley AW. Liquor amnii analysis in management of pregnancy complicated by rhesus sensitization. Am J Obstet Gynecol 1961;82:1359–1370)

TABLE 2. HEMATOLOGIC VALUES FOR NORMAL FETUSES*

Hematologic Value†	Gestational Age (Weeks)					
	15	16–17	18–20	21–22	23–25	26–30
Hgb (g/100 ml)	10.9 ± 0.7	12.5 ± 0.8	11.48 ± 0.78	12.29 ± 0.89	12.4 ± 0.77	13.36 ± 1.18
RBC (¥10^9/L)	2.43 ± 0.26	2.68 ± 0.21	2.66 ± 0.29	2.97 ± 0.27	3.06 ± 0.27	3.52 ± 0.32
MCV (±1)	143 ± 8	143 ± 12	133.9 ± 8.83	130 ± 6.17	126.2 ± 6.23	118.2 ± 5.7

*Values are for normal fetuses from 15 to 30 weeks of estimated gestational age.

†Hgb indicates hemoglobin; RBC, red blood cells; MCV, mean corpuscular volume.

Ancillary Testing

In the severely isoimmunized patient, signs of early hydrops appearing on ultrasonography may facilitate timely intervention. More problematic and controversial is the ability of ultrasonography to detect a deteriorating condition in the fetus before the onset of hydrops. Reported early signs of worsening fetal anemia include an increase in the size of the fetal liver, an increase in placental thickness, pericardial effusion, polyhydramnios, visualization of both sides of the fetal bowel, and abnormalities of pulsed Doppler flow-velocity waveforms. There is no evidence, however, that ultrasound markers can reliably distinguish mild from severe hemolytic disease in the absence of fetal hydrops (17). One study suggests that hydramnios is the earliest sign of significant fetal anemia (18), but it is not invariably present in severely affected cases.

Electronic fetal heart rate monitoring allows dynamic evaluation of fetal well-being and central nervous system reactivity. Some severely anemic fetuses exhibit a sinusoidal heart rate pattern, which has been attributed to the absence of autonomic nervous system control over the heart, high-output cardiac failure, or tissue hypoxia of the fetal heart and central nervous system. Nonreactive, suboptimal, or pathologic fetal heart rate patterns have also been reported more commonly in sensitized fetuses who were hypoxic and anemic than in those who had normal oxygen levels and were not anemic. Characteristics of the fetal heart rate pattern, however, did not accurately predict the degree of anemia or oxygenation (19).

Intrauterine Fetal Transfusion

Before physicians were able to gain direct access to the fetal circulation, intraperitoneal fetal transfusion was indicated if serial spectrophotometric measurements rose into upper zone II before 30 weeks of gestation or into zone III before 32–34 weeks of pregnancy. The infused blood was absorbed into the fetal circulation via the subdiaphragmatic lymphatic system. In the nonhydropic fetus, the rate of absorption was estimated to be 10–15% per 24 hours. Absorption was slower if hydrops was already evident (4).

Because of erratic absorption, especially in hydropic fetuses, intravascular fetal transfusion (20, 21) has largely replaced the intraperitoneal technique, although some investigators advocate a combined intravascular and intraperitoneal approach in select circumstances (22, 23). The fetal hematocrit level at which to initiate transfusion is somewhat arbitrary, but the value of 25% seems reasonable (24). Transfusions are performed using type O, Rh-negative, cytomegalovirus-negative, washed, irradiated packed cells cross-matched against maternal blood. After the fetal blood type is determined, it may occasionally be possible to use either maternal blood or a targeted donor whose blood is compatible with both mother and fetus (25). One method to estimate transfusion volume is by the formula described by Rodeck (26). Transfusion volumes usually range between 30 and 100 ml, and fetal blood is aspirated at the conclusion of the transfusion to determine the adequacy of therapy.

Repeat transfusions are planned for when the fetal hematocrit is predicted to be between 20% and 25%. This may be approximated by assuming a 1% decline per day or by using one of a number of published equations (27, 28). In fetuses with more severe hemolytic anemia, few fetal erythrocytes survive the initial transfusion interval. Therefore, the interval between first and second transfusions is usually 7–14 days, whereas the interval between subsequent transfusions or birth is 21–28 days.

Perinatal Outcome

Direct intravascular transfusion eliminates the erratic and incomplete absorption of erythrocytes inherent with the intraperitoneal approach. In addition, the intravascular technique allows more precise evaluation of the need for and adequacy of therapy by measurements of the initial and final fetal hematocrits. Consequently, it is not surprising that perinatal survival rates for severely isoimmunized fetuses following intravascular transfusion are now reported in excess of 80% (16, 21, 29–32). The improved survival rate is especially noteworthy when the early gestational ages at which therapy is being attempted are considered. Also encouraging is the improved outcome for hydropic fetuses. In one series, 16 of 20 pregnancies complicated by fetal hydrops had successful outcomes (33).

Although these results are promising, there are complications with any invasive procedure. Even in the most experienced hands, percutaneous umbilical cord blood sampling alone results in procedure-related pregnancy loss of approximately 1% (34). The procedure-related mortality for intravascular transfusion has been reported to be between 4% and 9% (29–31, 33). Additional significant morbidity has included nonremediable prolonged fetal heart rate decelerations that required emergent cesarean delivery (35) and increases in maternal antibody titer, presumably secondary to fetal–maternal hemorrhage (13, 14). When weighing the procedure-related risks against those for the neonate in the nursery, one should seriously consider delivery rather than performing an intravascular transfusion after 34 completed weeks of pregnancy.

Summary

Isoimmunization is diagnosed by a positive antibody screen and requires identification of the specific antigen responsible, classification of the antigen into either a clinically significant or a benign group, and titration of the level of antibody response. The paternal antigen status and zygosity should be determined whenever possible. Repetitive amniocentesis or fetal blood sampling may be required to monitor the fetal condition adequately. Early and continued consultation with experts in the management of this condition is key to developing an appropriate therapeutic plan that includes proper management at delivery and optimal neonatal support. New technologies and expertise now allow better outcome for severely affected fetuses.

References

1. American College of Obstetricians and Gynecologists. Prevention of D isoimmunization. ACOG Technical Bulletin 147. Washington, DC: ACOG, 1990 (Level III)
2. Caime ME, Mueller-Heubach E. Kell sensitization in pregnancy. Am J Obstet Gynecol 1986;154:85–90 (Level III)
3. Weiner CP, Widness JA. Decreased fetal erythropoiesis and hemolysis in Kell hemolytic anemia. Am J Obstet Gynecol 1996;174:547–551 (Level II-3)
4. Bowman JM. Maternal blood group isoimmunization. In: Creasy RK, Resnik R, eds. Maternal–fetal medicine: principles and practice. 3rd ed. Philadelphia: WB Saunders, 1994:711–743 (Level III)
5. Bowman JM, Pollock JM. Transplacental fetal hemorrhage after amniocentesis. Obstet Gynecol 1985;66:749–754 (Level II-3)
6. Brazie JV, Bowes WA Jr, Ibbott FA. An improved, rapid procedure for the determination of amniotic fluid bilirubin and its use in the prediction of the course of Rh-sensitized pregnancies. Am J Obstet Gynecol 1969;104:80–86 (Level III)
7. Liley AW. Liquor amnii analysis in the management of pregnancy complicated by rhesus sensitization. Am J Obstet Gynecol 1961;82:1359–1370 (Level III)
8. Nicolaides KH, Rodeck CH, Mibashan RS, Kemp JR. Have Liley charts outlived their usefulness? Am J Obstet Gynecol 1986;155:90–94 (Level III)
9. Forestier F, Daffos F, Galacteros F, Bardakjian J, Rainaut M, Beuzard Y. Hematological values of 163 normal fetuses between 18 and 30 weeks of gestation. Pediatr Res 1986; 20:342–346 (Level II-3)
10. Millar DS, Davis LR, Rodeck CH, Nicolaides KH, Mibashan RS. Normal blood cell values in the early midtrimester fetus. Prenat Diagn 1985;5:367–373 (Level III)
11. Queenan JT, Tomai TP, Ural SH, King JC. Deviation in amniotic fluid optical density at a wavelength of 450 nm in Rh-immunized pregnancies from 14 to 40 weeks' gestation: a proposal for clinical management. Am J Obstet Gynecol 1993;168:1370–1376 (Level III)
12. Fisk NM, Bennett P, Warwick RM, Letsky EA, Welch R, Vaughan JI, et al. Clinical utility of fetal RhD typing in alloimmunized pregnancies by means of polymerase chain reaction on amniocytes or chorionic villi. Am J Obstet Gynecol 1994;171:50–54 (Level III)
13. Nicolini U, Kochenour NK, Greco P, Letsky EA, Johnson RD, Contreras M, et al. Consequences of fetomaternal haemorrhage after intrauterine transfusion. BMJ 1988;297: 1379–1381 (Level III)
14. MacGregor SN, Silver RK, Sholl JS. Enhanced sensitization after cordocentesis in a rhesus-isoimmunized pregnancy. Am J Obstet Gynecol 1991;165:382–383 (Level III)
15. Weiner CP, Williamson RA, Wenstrom KD, Sipes SL, Grant SS, Widness JA. Management of fetal hemolytic disease by cordocentesis. I. Prediction of fetal anemia. Am J Obstet Gynecol 1991;165:546–553 (Level II-3)
16. Weiner CP, Williamson RA, Wenstrom KD, Sipes SL, Widness JA, Grant SS, et al. Management of fetal hemolytic disease by cordocentesis. II. Outcome of treatment. Am J Obstet Gynecol 1991;165:1302–1307 (Level II-3)
17. Nicolaides KH, Fontanarosa M, Gabbe SG, Rodeck CH. Failure of ultrasonographic parameters to predict the severity of fetal anemia in Rhesus isoimmunization. Am J Obstet Gynecol 1988;158:920–926 (Level II-2)
18. Chitkara U, Wilkins I, Lynch L, Mehalek K, Berkowitz RL. The role of sonography in assessing severity of fetal anemia in Rh- and Kell-isoimmunized pregnancies. Obstet Gynecol 1988;71:393–398 (Level III)
19. Nicolaides KH. Studies on fetal physiology and pathophysiology in Rhesus disease. Semin Perinatol 1989;13:328–337 (Level III)
20. Socol ML, MacGregor SN, Pielet BW, Tamura RK, Sabbagha RE. Percutaneous umbilical transfusion in severe rhesus isoimmunization: resolution of fetal hydrops. Am J Obstet Gynecol 1987;157:1369–1375 (Level III)
21. Harman CR, Bowman JM, Manning FA, Menticoglou SM. Intrauterine transfusion—intraperitoneal versus intravascular approach: a case–control comparison. Am J Obstet Gynecol 1990;162:1053–1059 (Level II-2)
22. Pattison N, Roberts A. The management of severe erythroblastosis fetalis by fetal transfusion: survival of transfused adult erythrocytes in the fetus. Obstet Gynecol 1989; 74:901–904 (Level II-3)
23. Moise KJ, Giancarlo M, Fisher DJ, Huhta JC, Cano LE, Carpenter RJ Jr. Acute fetal hemodynamic alterations after intrauterine transfusion for treatment of severe red blood cell alloimmunization. Am J Obstet Gynecol 1990;163: 776–784 (Level II-3)
24. Reece EA, Copel JA, Scioscia AL, Grannum PAT, DeGennaro N, Hobbins JC. Diagnostic fetal umbilical blood sampling in the management of isoimmunization. Am J Obstet Gynecol 1988;159:1057–1062 (Level III)

25. Gonsoulin WJ, Moise KJ Jr, Milam JD, Sala JD, Weber VW, Carpenter RJ Jr. Serial maternal blood donations for intrauterine transfusion. Obstet Gynecol 1990;75:158–162 (Level II-3)

26. Rodeck CH, Nicolaides KH, Warsof SL, Fysh WJ, Gamsu HR, Kemp JR. The management of severe rhesus isoimmunization by fetoscopic intravascular transfusions. Am J Obstet Gynecol 1984;150:769–774 (Level III)

27. Plecas DV, Chitkara U, Berkowitz GS, Lapinski RH, Alvarez M, Berkowitz RL. Intrauterine intravascular transfusion for severe erythroblastosis fetalis: how much to transfuse? Obstet Gynecol 1990;75:965–969 (Level II-3)

28. MacGregor SN, Socol ML, Pielet BW, Sholl JS, Silver RK. Prediction of hematocrit decline after intravascular fetal transfusion. Am J Obstet Gynecol 1989;161:1491–1493 (Level II-3)

29. Ney JA, Socol ML, Dooley SL, MacGregor SN, Silver RK, Millard DD. Perinatal outcome following intravascular transfusion in severely isoimmunized fetuses. Int J Gynaecol Obstet 1991;35:41–46 (Level II-3)

30. Berkowitz RL, Chitkara U, Wilkins IA, Lynch L, Plosker H, Bernstein HH. Intravascular monitoring and management of erythroblastosis fetalis. Am J Obstet Gynecol 1988;158: 783–795 (Level III)

31. Barss VA, Benacerraf BR, Frigoletto FD, Greene MF, Penso C, Saltzman DH, et al. Management of isoimmunized pregnancy by use of intravascular techniques. Am J Obstet Gynecol 1988;159:932–937 (Level III)

32. Parer JT. Severe Rh isoimmunization—current methods of in utero diagnosis and treatment. Am J Obstet Gynecol 1988;158:1323–1329 (Level III)

33. Grannum PAT, Copel JA, Moya FR, Scioscia AL, Robert JA, Winn HN, et al. The reversal of hydrops fetalis by intravascular intrauterine transfusion in severe isoimmune fetal anemia. Am J Obstet Gynecol 1988;158:914–919 (Level III)

34. Daffos F, Capella-Pavlovsky M, Forestier F. Fetal blood sampling during pregnancy with use of a needle guided by ultrasound: a study of 606 consecutive cases. Am J Obstet Gynecol 1985;153:655–660 (Level III)

35. Pielet BW, Socol ML, MacGregor SN, Ney JA, Dooley SL. Cordocentesis: an appraisal of risks. Am J Obstet Gynecol 1988;159:1497–1500 (Level III)

The references in this bulletin are graded according to the method outlined by the U.S. Preventive Services Task Force:

- I Evidence obtained from at least one properly designed randomized controlled trial
- II-1 Evidence obtained from well-designed controlled trials without randomization
- II-2 Evidence obtained from well-designed cohort or case–control analytic studies, preferably from more than one center or research group
- II-3 Evidence obtained from multiple time series, with or without intervention, or dramatic results in uncontrolled experiments
- III Opinions of respected authorities, based on clinical experience, descriptive studies, or reports of expert committees

Other publications from ACOG:

- **Committee Opinions**, focused updates on emerging areas
- **Practice Patterns**, evidence-based guidelines
- **Criteria Sets**, baseline guidelines for review of diagnostic and management procedures

ISSN 1074-8628

The American College of Obstetricians and Gynecologists
409 12th Street, SW
PO Box 96920
Washington, DC 20090-6920

12345/09876

Number 95—August 1986

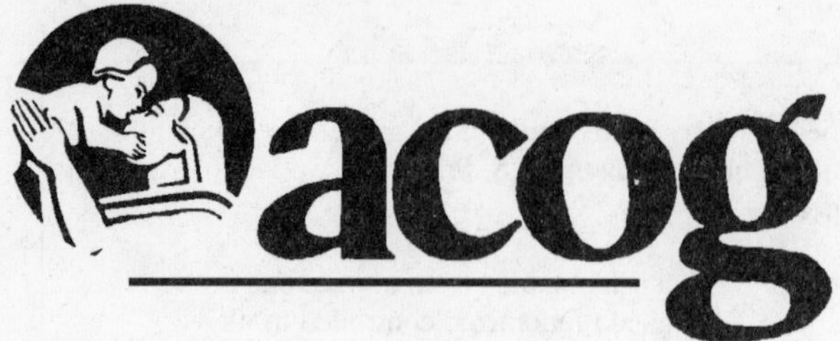

Technical Bulletin

An Educational Aid to Obstetrician–Gynecologists

Management of the Breech Presentation

During the past decade there has been an increasing trend to deliver the fetus in breech presentation by cesarean birth; thus the majority of mothers in labor with breech presentation are delivered abdominally (1). Despite this trend, there are many circumstances under which vaginal delivery of the breech presentation can proceed safely and with good outcome. Although there are general guidelines that may influence the mode of delivery, there is no consensus that will allow predetermination of the best route of delivery in all cases of breech presentation. This Technical Bulletin will discuss the confounding variables that affect the outcome of breech delivery and will describe some of the circumstances under which it is appropriate to consider vaginal delivery.

Confounding Variables Altering Outcome

The fetus in the breech presentation may already be at risk for untoward outcome, regardless of the route of delivery. Various reasons for untoward outcome in breech presentation include congenital anomalies, preterm labor, and maternal and fetal risk factors.

The incidence of congenital anomalies is higher in breech presentations; the overall incidence is 6.3%, compared with 2.4% in the total population (2). An increase in gross morphologic anomalies and other reasons for later diminished neurologic function associated with chromosomal anomalies have been documented in breech presentation infants (3).

Since at least 13% of fetuses are in the breech presentation at 30 weeks of gestation or less, the preterm infant, with its attendant complications, is often overrepresented in studies of breech deliveries. The preterm birth has a higher incidence of congenital anomalies, intracranial hemorrhage, growth retardation, neurologic disorders, and mortality. The susceptibility of the low-birth-weight fetus to intracerebral bleeding influences morbidity. Although bleeding may be precipitated by asphyxia and trauma, neonatal birth weight and gestational age account for 27% of neonatal mortality in frank breech presentations, whereas birth route accounts for less than 1% of the adverse outcomes. Findings are similar in vertex presentations.

Whether outcome can be improved by altering the birth route remains controversial (4–6). Two schools of thought exist. The first suggests that at some or all birth weights below 2.5 kg, breech presentation poses increased risk and assumes that trauma, cord prolapse, and head entrapment may be averted by cesarean delivery. The second holds that outcome data do not warrant the described risks. Results of some studies show that outcome is not improved by cesarean delivery, regardless of whether the presentation is breech or vertex, when equivalent weight groups are compared. Parity does not appear to be a factor (6).

Several maternal risk factors, such as placenta previa, abruptio placentae, and premature rupture of membranes, are associated with breech presentation. These risk factors are also associated with increased neonatal morbidity and mortality, as these complications are inevitably linked with higher risk of prematurity, chronic hypoxia, and infection (2).

This review of confounding variables that are important in considering outcome delineates the inherent and acquired risks present in breech presentations. In reviewing published data that may be helpful in making clinical decisions, the physician must be aware that in reports relating to choosing a method of delivery, outcome data may be influenced by these other factors rather than by presentation. In comparing reports, critical factors that influence the effect of delivery method on outcome include a live fetus at the onset of labor, gestational age, and the presence of major morphologic anomalies.

Management

Patient Information

Whether breech presentation is confirmed prior to or during labor, the exchange of information between obstetrician and family is an integral part of patient care. During these discussions, obstetricians should inform patients as to which method of delivery is considered to be best on the basis of the clinical situation and the circumstances of support facilities and personnel. It is important for the patient to be made aware of the clinical significance of other risk factors that may be present and that are not affected by the route of delivery.

Types of Breech Presentations

Since most reports review birth route with respect to the more common frank breech presentation, less information is available for the less common footling and complete breech presentations. It is generally believed that the risk of trauma to the fetus or the mother is increased with other than frank breech presentations. Unfortunately, there is not enough available information to make firm recommendations regarding the appropriate management of the nonfrank breech presentation.

Diagnosis

Leopold's four maneuvers are useful for determining presentation. Confirmation of suspected breech presentation is desirable. At earlier stages of gestation, however, 13% of fetal presentations may be breech, so immediate verification may not be indicated. Persistence of breech presentation in the third trimester warrants confirmation for proper delivery planning.

When available, ultrasonography can be used to confirm fetal presentation and head position. In addition, a large or hyperextended head, macrosomia, or major congenital anomalies can also be detected by ultrasonography. Ultrasonography may be repeated at the onset of labor if necessary to reconfirm fetal presentation and head position.

Assessment of the adequacy of the pelvis may influence management. Most reports recommend some form of pelvimetry for screening patients prior to undergoing a trial of labor (7). Documenting flexion or extension of the fetal head or excessive fetal size is generally performed at the onset of labor.

Antepartum Version

Conversion of breech to vertex presentation has been undertaken in late pregnancy to lower the incidence of breech presentations in labor. The option of version may be offered to the patient and the risks discussed (8). The procedure is usually performed after the 36th week, prior to the onset of labor (9). Version may be performed with the aid of tocolytic agents. The fetus is monitored during the procedure, and access to facilities for emergency cesarean delivery should be available if fetal distress is persistent. Reversion to the breech position may occur. Spontaneous conversion of breech to vertex presentation may occur at any time prior to birth (8).

The Delivery Environment

The availability of adequate support personnel, including anesthesiologists and neonatal staff, and operating room facilities will influence the method of delivery. Because breech presentation situations may require emergency cesarean delivery or neonatal intensive care, the choice of hospital and delivery mode warrant prospective planning. At lower fetal birth weights or in the presence of known fetal anomalies needing surgery, the mother should be transferred, if possible, to a suitably equipped and staffed perinatal care center. The need for assistance in the delivery room and the basic perinatal environment should be evaluated by each hospital and its obstetricians to establish guidelines for patient care in breech presentation.

Delivery of the Breech Presentation

In this section, breech delivery via both vaginal and cesarean routes is discussed, but the mechanics of breech presentation deliveries will not be described in detail. The final choice of birth route may depend upon the physician's delivery room experience and skills learned in performing breech deliveries.

The following are guidelines for consideration of vaginal delivery:

- **Facilities:** Capability of emergency cesarean delivery
- **Physician:** Experience in vaginal breech delivery
- **Anesthesia:** Personnel present for delivery
- **Type of breech:** Frank; other types need further evaluation
- **Fetal size:** Optimal estimated weight less than 4 kg
- **Head position and size:** Exclusion of hyperextension and macrocephaly
- **Pelvimetry:** Adequate pelvis
- **Labor:** Adequate progression in dilation, effacement, and descent

Management of Labor

The obstetrician should be readily available. Because emergencies may arise, intravenous lines should be in place, along with facilities for maternal surgery and blood transfusion. Fetal heart monitoring is required. If the tracings are of good quality, external monitoring is acceptable. If adequate information is not being obtained, internal heart rate and uterine pressure recordings should be obtained. Monitoring should continue in the delivery room in the event of vaginal birth.

As with all patients, timely vaginal examinations should document normal progress during the latent or active phases of labor. The use of oxytocin for protracted or arrested labor is controversial and cannot be resolved in this review. Local, pudendal, regional, and general anesthesia are all used in breech presentation deliveries.

Mechanics of Labor and Delivery

Many techniques and types of procedures are used, according to the experience and training of the obstetrician. The following points should be made.

Progress in labor, even if slow, should be left undisturbed while the presenting part is well engaged, on the perineum, or crowning and fetal heart rate patterns are normal. Slow, continuous dilation of the cervix assists delivery of the head. Rapid delivery can increase the likelihood of nuchal arms or extended head. Extraction of the fetus should not be performed unless clinically indicated.

Gentle suprapubic pressure over the aftercoming head may maintain flexion while the head engages in the pelvis. Continuing assistance from this abdominal pressure often leads to spontaneous delivery of the head.

Some obstetricians urge the routine use of Piper forceps for the aftercoming head, while others favor their use only in an emergency. The forceps should be available on the delivery table; their use requires an assistant.

The decision to perform an episiotomy is best made during delivery on the basis of the distensibility of the perineum and the size of the fetus. Performance of an episiotomy in a breech presentation is suggested in most reports in the literature.

After the rest of the body has been delivered, the Mauriceau–Smellie–Veit maneuver is most useful in rotating the aftercoming head to the anteroposterior diameter. It consists of pressure with the adjacent two fingers on the maxilla. This maneuver may also be used to maintain flexion, but some suprapubic pressure, as well as assistance in supporting the fetal body, also may be necessary.

It is generally necessary for the physician to be assisted by at least one person. To avoid trauma to the neck, the fetal body should not be elevated above the horizontal plane.

Physicians must be aware of the many complexities of breech extraction by cesarean birth. A well-developed lower uterine segment is often not present when there is a low-birth-weight fetus or ruptured membranes, and thus a vertical incision may be optimal. The decision for type of cesarean incision should be made by the obstetrician in the delivery room when all decision-making data are available. Cesarean extraction in breech presentation requires skills similar to those used in vaginal birth, including avoidance of hyperextension of the fetal head.

Summary

The controversies relating to breech birth cannot be answered by a consensus statement at this time. Many confounding variables affect risks to the fetus, independent of and dependent on the method of delivery. In light of the unresolved controversies and state of knowledge at this time, either cesarean section or vaginal delivery (in carefully selected cases) may be acceptable for the term frank breech presentation (10). Further information is needed before specific recommendations can be made regarding the nonfrank breech presentation.

REFERENCES

1. U.S. Department of Health and Human Services; Public Health Service; National Institutes of Health. Cesarean childbirth. NIH Publication No 82-2067. Washington, DC: U.S. Government Printing Office, 1981, p 379
2. Brenner WE. Breech presentation. Clin Obstet Gynecol 1978;21(2):511–513
3. Braun FH, Jones KL, Smith DW. Breech presentation as an indicator of fetal abnormality. J Pediatr 1975;86(3): 419–421
4. Premature breech: Vaginal delivery or caesarean section? Editorial. Br Med J 1979;1(6180):1747
5. Cruikshank DP, Pitkin RM. Delivery of the premature breech. Obstet Gynecol 1977;50(3):367–369
6. Rosen MG, Chik L. The effect of delivery route on outcome in breech presentation. Am J Obstet Gynecol 1984; 148(7):909–914
7. Ridley WJ, Jackson P, Stewart JH, et al. Role of antenatal radiography in the management of breech deliveries. Br J Obstet Gynaecol 1982;89(5):342–347
8. Wallace RL, VanDorsten JP, Eglinton GS, et al. External cephalic version with tocolysis. J Reprod Med 1984; 29(10):745–748
9. Hofmeyr GJ. Effect of external cephalic version in late pregnancy on breech presentation and caesarean section rate: A controlled trial. Br J Obstet Gynaecol 1983;90(5): 392–399
10. Collea JV, Chein C, Quilligan EJ. The randomized management of term frank breech presentation: A study of 208 cases. Am J Obstet Gynecol 1980;137(2):235–244

SUGGESTED READING

DeCrespigny LJ, Pepperell RJ. Perinatal mortality and morbidity in breech presentation. Obstet Gynecol 1979; 53(2): 141– 145

Goldenberg RL, Nelson KG, Hale CD, et al. Survival of infants with low birth weight and early gestational age, 1979 to 1981. Am J Obstet Gynecol 1984;149(5):508–511

Jenkins DM. Breech delivery. Clin Obstet Gynecol 1980; 7(3): 561– 580

Luterkort M, Persson PH, Weldner BM. Maternal and fetal factors in breech presentation. Obstet Gynecol 1984; 64(1): 55– 59

Rosen MG, Debanne S, Thompson K, et al. Long-term neurologic morbidity in breech and vertex births. Am J Obstet Gynecol 1985;151(6):718–720

Saling E, Mueller-Holve W. External cephalic version under tocolysis. J Perinat Med 1975;3(2):115–122

Stanley FJ, Alberman ED. Infants of very low birthweight. I: Perinatal factors affecting survival. Dev Med Child Neurol 1978;20(3):300–312

This Technical Bulletin was developed under the direction of the Committee on Technical Bulletins of the American College of Obstetricians and Gynecologists as an educational aid to obstetricians and gynecologists. The committee wishes to thank Mortimer Rosen, MD, for his assistance in the development of this bulletin. This Technical Bulletin does not define a standard of care, nor is it intended to dictate an exclusive course of management. It presents recognized methods and techniques of clinical practice for consideration by obstetrician–gynecologists for incorporation into their practices. Variations of practice taking into account the needs of the individual patient, resources, and limitations unique to the institution or type of practice may be appropriate.

Reviewed October 1991

THE AMERICAN COLLEGE OF OBSTETRICIANS AND GYNECOLOGISTS
409 12th Street, SW
Washington, DC 20024-2188

7/65

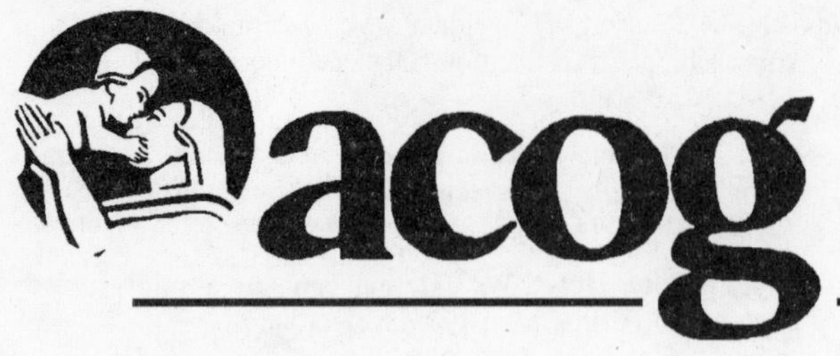

Number 197—September 1994
(Replaces #120, September 1988)

Technical Bulletin

An Educational Aid to Obstetrician–Gynecologists

Managing the Anovulatory State: Medical Induction of Ovulation

Advances in reproductive endocrinology have made ovulation induction one of the most successful means of treating infertility. Anovulation and ovulatory disorders are present in approximately 20% of infertile women. Ovulation and conception can be achieved in a significant number of these women.

General Pretreatment Considerations

It is important to establish the ovulatory status of the patient prior to beginning therapy. A brief history may be of the utmost importance. Uniformity of the menstrual interval, duration of flow, and amount of flow are strongly indicative of an ovulatory menstrual pattern. Of even greater importance is the presence of characteristic premenstrual molimina (bloating sensation, mood changes, uterine cramping, and breast tenderness). In contrast, an unpredictable menstrual pattern is highly suggestive of an anovulatory or oligoovulatory disorder.

Should the ovulatory status still be in doubt, several ancillary measures are available to resolve the issue. Measurement of serum progesterone concentrations in the luteal phase is a simple and accurate method for confirming presumptive ovulation. Although the pulsatile release of progesterone from the ovary may preclude the use of a single measurement to assess the adequacy of corpus luteum function, values in excess of 3–5 ng/ml may be viewed as compatible with presumptive ovulation. An endometrial biopsy performed during the luteal phase will not only confirm presumptive ovulation but will also permit dating of the endometrium. Serial vaginal sonographic examinations of the ovary provide an accurate, noninvasive means of monitoring follicular development and collapse.

There are also methods that the patient herself may use. Kits that measure the immunoreactive levels of luteinizing hormone (LH) in the urine can be used to document the onset of the midcycle LH surge. These kits allow prospective prediction of ovulation, thereby aiding in the timing of intercourse or artificial insemination. Basal body temperature charts continue to be an inexpensive (albeit, retrospective) means of ovulation detection. However, basal body temperature charts are sometimes inaccurate and often become a burden to the patient.

Given an accurate history, supported by the use of methods for ovulation detection, the ovulatory status of virtually any patient can be documented reliably. These same methods are also applicable to the monitoring of medically induced cycles.

Potentially reversible causes of anovulation (stress, weight gain or loss, drug use, medical illness, or strenuous physical activity) should be documented and addressed. Adrenal disorders (eg, Cushing syndrome or Addison disease), thyroid dysfunction (eg, hyperthyroidism or hypothyroidism), and liver disease should be ruled out prior to beginning therapy. The possibilities of occult hyperprolactinemia, incipient ovarian failure, or pregnancy should likewise be excluded.

Accordingly, it is strongly recommended that, at the minimum, the circulating concentrations of prolactin, thyroid-stimulating hormone, and follicle-stimulating hormone (FSH) be evaluated in all anovulatory patients. Endogenous estrogen production should be assessed. This can be accomplished through the measurement of the serum levels of estradiol but is rarely required because estrogen status can be assessed so simply clinically, for example, by evaluating the vaginal epithelium. Although frequently used, the use of exogenous progestin in an effort to induce withdrawal bleeding often leads to erroneous conclusions about the status of the patient, as approximately half of all women with ovarian failure will bleed in response to the progestin (1). Given such testing, accurate diagnosis of the nature of the anovulatory disorder should be possible, thereby allowing for the proper choice of a therapeutic regimen.

A semen analysis also should be obtained prior to ovulation induction; the sample tested should be adequate to allow fertilization. Routinely performing hysterosalpingography or diagnostic laparoscopy, however, is unnecessary prior to ovulation induction. These techniques should be used prior to induction of ovulation when there is strong historic evidence for tuboperitoneal pathology, the patient is of advanced age, or the expense, time commitment, or potential risk of gonadotropin-induced ovulation induction are not acceptable to the patient. Ovulation induction should not be undertaken indiscriminately in women with a known preexisting infertility factor other than anovulation. If pregnancy does not result after four to six cycles, a more intensive infertility evaluation is indicated in couples who have not been evaluated previously.

The process of ovulation induction should be explained to patients in sufficient detail to ensure realistic expectations. Information regarding the expense, time, and psychologic impact involved in completing a course of therapy should be provided. Potential complications and risks for both mother (eg, hyperstimulation) and fetus (eg, multiple gestation), as well as the chances of success, should be outlined (Table 1). Factors contributing to infertility, including age, must be taken into consideration when a prognosis is discussed. Full participation by the patient and her partner is helpful. Patients should be counseled that there are no data to indicate that any of the medications used for ovulation induction are associated with an increase in congenital anomalies (2).

Clomiphene Citrate

Clomiphene citrate, a nonsteroidal estrogen receptor antagonist, is a combination of active and inactive (racemic) isomers. Although its precise mechanism of action remains largely unknown (3), it is clear that the administration of clomiphene citrate is followed in short sequence by enhanced release of pituitary gonadotropins resulting in follicular recruitment, selection, assertion of dominance, and, ultimately, rupture. Clearly, then, an otherwise intact reproductive axis is required.

To date, clomiphene citrate is the medication of choice for ovulation induction in suitable patients because of its relative safety, efficacy, simple mode of administration (oral), and relatively low cost (4). The primary indication for the use of clomiphene citrate is ovulation induction in patients with adequate levels of estrogen and normal levels of FSH and prolactin. Patients with inappropriate gonadotropin release (with an increased ratio of LH to FSH), as occurs in polycystic ovary syndrome, are also candidates for therapy. In contrast, women with abnormally low levels of FSH and estrogen generally do not respond to clomiphene.

Although a wide range of figures has been reported, approximately 80% of well-selected patients can be expected to ovulate following treatment with clomiphene citrate. However, only about 40% of these patients ultimately become pregnant. If therapy is continued for six or more cycles, the pregnancy rate for ovulation initiated by clomiphene citrate in anovulatory women may approach that of spontaneously occurring cycles.

There are relatively few contraindications to the use of clomiphene citrate. A preexisting ovarian cyst or substantial (posttreatment) residual ovarian enlargement generally indicates that the use of clomiphene should be delayed. Pregnancy is an obvious contraindication. The inadvertent administration of clomiphene citrate during pregnancy can occur if appropriate evaluation to rule out pregnancy has not been performed. Along these lines, the old clinical dictum of "No period equals no clomiphene citrate," appears to be useful. Finally, the occurrence of otherwise poorly understood visual symptoms (night blindness and scotoma) in the course of clomiphene citrate therapy has generally been viewed as a contraindication to the continued use of the medication, although there are no data to support the practice.

TABLE 1. SUCCESS RATES AND SIDE EFFECTS OF VARIOUS AGENTS FOR INDUCTION OF OVULATION (IN APPROPRIATELY SELECTED PATIENTS)

Agent	Ovulation Rates	Pregnancy Rates	Multiple Pregnancy Rates	Common Side Effects
Clomiphene citrate	≤ 80%	≤ 40%	≤ 8%	Hot flashes, visual symptoms, nausea, breast tenderness
Bromocriptine	≤ 95%	≤ 85%	<1%	Gastrointestinal irritation, orthostatic hypotension, nasal congestion, headache
Gonadotropins	30–100%*	20–90%*	≤ 30%	Local (injection related), hyperstimulation syndrome
Gonadotropin-releasing hormone	30–100%*	20–90%*	≤ 12%	Local (injection related)

* Patients with low levels of estrogen and gonadotropins are likely to fare much better than those with normal levels.

Clomiphene citrate treatment is associated with hot flashes in up to 11% of patients. The incidence of multiple gestation ranges from 6.25–12.3%. The risk of spontaneous abortion does not increase with the use of clomiphene citrate. No interpretable data are available on the potential impact of clomiphene citrate on the incidence of breast or ovarian cancer.

Patients who are administered clomiphene citrate should be assessed for possible gestation and for ovarian enlargement as clinically indicated. The intense monitoring requirements characteristic of the use of gonadotropins are not generally necessary. Menses 3–4 weeks after completion of a course of clomiphene citrate is generally suggestive of ovulation, as are basal body temperature charts that reveal a biphasic pattern.

Hormonal monitoring is based on the premise that the successful initiation of ovulation with clomiphene citrate is associated with characteristic alterations in the serum levels of LH, estradiol, and progesterone. Increased circulating levels of progesterone (14 days after the last clomiphene citrate dose) are the hallmark of a presumptive luteal phase. An increased preovulatory level of estradiol occurring 7 days after the last dose of clomiphene citrate is taken to indicate at least some follicular development. Sonographic monitoring can document follicular development and collapse at ovulation. Although a growing body of information suggests a negative effect of clomiphene citrate on sonographically monitored endometrial thickness, the precise implication of these observations remains to be established.

Because of the safety record of clomiphene citrate, it is acceptable to administer it to anovulatory women for 4–6 months without completing an infertility evaluation. There are several approaches to the dosage of clomiphene citrate. The most commonly recommended initial dosage is 50 mg daily for 5 days, usually beginning on the fifth day of the cycle. Many clinicians recommend increasing the clomiphene citrate dosage in subsequent cycles as soon as it becomes apparent that the dosage is ineffective in inducing ovulation. Ideally, such a determination can and should be made at the conclusion of each treatment cycle. The simplest protocols call for therapy to be increased in increments of 50 mg at a time. More than 70% of conceptions related to clomiphene citrate will occur at dosages no higher than 100 mg daily for 5 days (5). Dosages of higher than 150 mg for 5 days are not usually effective. If patients do not respond to a 150-mg dosage, further evaluation and a change in therapy are warranted.

Several adjuncts to clomiphene citrate therapy have been proposed, including the use of glucocorticoids, human chorionic gonadotropin (hCG), or longer courses of clomiphene therapy. Patients with increased circulating levels of adrenal androgens (eg, dehydroepiandrosterone sulfate) may benefit from the addition of glucocorticoids (6). The addition of hCG to the clomiphene citrate regimen may be appropriate in cycles in which complete follicular development occurs in the absence of ovulation. High-dose therapy may be obviated by using lower doses of clomiphene for longer periods (7).

When ovulation occurs at a given dose, there is no advantage to increasing the dose in subsequent cycles of treatment. At that point, the patient should attempt to conceive for 4–6 months. Most conceptions initiated by clomiphene citrate occur within the first six ovulatory cycles (5). For optimal results, the patient should be advised to have intercourse every other day for 1 week beginning 5 days after the last day of clomiphene citrate administration. Use of ovulation predictor kits can provide one accurate approach to estimating the best time for intercourse, but false-positives do occur.

The significance of alterations in cervical mucus in response to clomiphene citrate remains a matter of controversy. Regardless, failure to conceive within six ovulatory clomiphene citrate cycles should prompt the physician to search for infertility factors other than anovulation.

Bromocriptine

Bromocriptine mesylate is a semisynthetic ergot alkaloid (8) with dopamine receptor agonist activity. It reduces the size of prolactin-producing pituitary tumors, lowers the level of serum prolactin, and restores reproductive cyclicity, thus enabling conception to occur in up to 80% of hyperprolactinemic anovulatory women (9). Several new longer-acting dopamine agonists are in various stages of clinical testing and development.

Both radiologically documented, prolactin-producing pituitary adenomas and idiopathic hyperprolactinemia are associated with anovulation. In patients with these conditions, bromocriptine is the treatment of choice for ovulation induction. It is not indicated in ovulatory patients with unexplained infertility (10).

Every effort should be made to use the minimal effective dose of bromocriptine as judged by the establishment of normal circulating levels of prolactin and by the resumption of normal menstrual cyclicity. The initial dose of 1.25 mg/d, orally, may be increased weekly in 1.25-mg increments. Dosages greater than 15 mg/d are seldom required. Vaginal administration of bromocriptine mesylate tablets has also proved successful (11).

Bromocriptine may induce nausea, vomiting, postural hypotension, headaches, and nasal congestion (8). However, these side effects are often transient and can be minimized by administering the medication at bedtime, avoiding large increases in dose (more than 2.5 mg), spacing increases in dosage a week apart, or providing the medication with meals. Vaginal administration may diminish side effects. No interpretable data are available on the potential impact of bromocriptine on the incidence of breast or ovarian cancer.

Less than 1% of women with microadenomas and less than 5% of women with macroadenomas will develop signs or symptoms of tumor growth during pregnancy. However, symptoms of headache and visual disturbances, as well as tumor growth in women with prolactinomas, are effectively treated with bromocriptine during pregnancy. Although the medication does cross the placenta, analysis of the outcome of more than 2,000 pregnancies did not reveal an increase in the incidence of congenital anomalies or spontaneous abortions (12). In addition, long-term follow-up of more than 350 children born to mothers receiving bromocriptine during pregnancy, some for more than 30 weeks, confirms the safety of the medication. Nevertheless, to avoid inadvertent use of bromocriptine during pregnancy, it is suggested that barrier contraception be used until normal menstrual cyclicity is established. Thereafter, bromocriptine should be continued until a positive pregnancy test is obtained at or around the time of the first missed menses. Earlier discontinuation (ie, following the midcycle gonadotropin surge) is feasible but somewhat impractical.

Gonadotropins

Human menopausal gonadotropins (hMG) consist of 75 or 150 IU each of LH and FSH per ampule. Urofollitropin consists of 75 IU of purified human FSH. More highly purified and genetically engineered products may be available in the near future.

Gonadotropins promote follicle growth and maturation as evidenced by increasing estradiol secretion and follicle size. They are the medications of choice for women with low levels of estrogen and gonadotropins. They may also be useful in patients who do not ovulate with clomiphene citrate therapy.

The success of gonadotropin therapy is related to the patient's diagnosis and age (13). Women with low levels of estrogen and gonadotropins fare better in nearly every series than those with normal levels of estrogen and gonadotropins. The cumulative pregnancy rate for the former group is up to 90% for women ages 35 and younger, with lower rates noted for older individuals. Pregnancy rates for women with normal levels of estrogen and gonadotropins are substantially lower (30–40% or less). The majority of pregnancies (95%) occur within the first 6 cycles of treatment. For unknown reasons, the rate of spontaneous abortion may be higher (30% or less) in gonadotropin-stimulated cycles than it is in unstimulated cycles (14, 15).

Gonadotropin therapy can be initiated regardless of uterine bleeding and administered on a daily (at times twice daily) basis. Careful hormonal and sonographic monitoring will aid the physician in determining when the state of the follicle(s) indicates that the patient is ready for an injection of hCG, intended to substitute for the endogenous LH surge. In some cases, a spontaneous LH surge will occur, thereby eliminating the need for exogenous hCG. However, this may be associated with premature luteinization of the leading, and thus immature, follicle.

The daily dosage of gonadotropins may vary broadly. It should be adjusted to individual needs, as patient sensitivity to the medication varies. Moreover, follicle development and the number of developing follicles may vary from cycle to cycle, even in patients given the same treatment regimen. Consequently, monitoring of the ovarian response with ultrasonography and serial estradiol measurements is imperative during each cycle of ovulation induction.

In general, gonadotropins are administered intramuscularly for 7–12 days, until a preovulatory follicle is developed. A suggested initial dose of hMG is 75–150 IU/d in most patients. If there is no ovarian response by the fourth day of therapy, the daily dose may be increased by 75–150 IU/d. Further increases may be required if there is no response.

Once the serum estradiol levels begin to increase (greater than 100 pg/ml in most laboratories), ultrasound examinations should be initiated to evaluate the number of follicles and their size. At that point, the daily gonadotropin dosage should remain constant unless further adjustment is indicated by daily monitoring. The subsequent rise in the serum levels of estradiol during the active phase of folliculogenesis is rapid and often exponential (16).

In order to trigger ovulation, the leading follicle should be 16–20 mm in diameter (as indicated by vaginal ultrasonography) at the time hCG is given. Follicles typically enlarge by about 2–3 mm/d, thus allowing anticipation of the day of ovulation. At that point, gonadotropin therapy should be discontinued, and a single dose of 5,000–10,000 IU of hCG is administered intramuscularly, usually 24 hours after the last dose of gonadotropin. Ovulation will usually occur within 36 hours after hCG administration. Therefore, intercourse should occur during the 2 days immediately following the hCG injection.

Subsequent doses of hCG to maintain corpus luteum function may not be required in chronically anovulating women with normal levels of estrogen and gonadotropins. In contrast, hCG supplementation may be required for chronic anovulation in women with low levels of estrogen and gonadotropins. In this case, smaller doses of hCG (eg, 2,500 IU) may be administered on at least two occasions (ie, 3 and 6 days after the ovulatory hCG dose).

The two major complications associated with the induction of ovulation with gonadotropins are ovarian hyperstimulation syndrome and multiple pregnancy. Close monitoring with measurements of serum estradiol and ultrasonography can help detect these complications and guide intervention. Although the use of a gonadotropin-releasing hormone (GnRH) agonist has been proposed as a means to reduce the incidence of ovarian hyperstimulation, no clear consensus has emerged in this regard.

Ideally, serum estradiol concentrations should fall within the range of 500–2,000 pg/ml when hCG is administered. However, this range is only a rough guideline; concentrations should correlate with the number of follicles seen by ultrasonography. To reduce ovarian hyperstimulation and multiple gestation, the cycle can be discontinued if serum estradiol levels exceed 2,000 pg/ml or if more than three preovulatory follicles are present. The presence of multiple secondary follicles (of 14–16 mm in diameter) may further increase the incidence of ovarian hyperstimulation. Ovarian hyperstimulation, however, can be avoided if the ovulating dose of hCG is withheld. The range of safety between normal ovulation and ovarian hyperstimulation is very narrow. Thus, hyperstimulation is sometimes an unavoidable complication of hMG therapy, despite extensive monitoring.

The symptoms of the ovarian hyperstimulation syndrome usually arise 5–7 days after hCG is administered (17). The ovarian hyperstimulation syndrome may be classified as mild, moderate, or severe:

- Mild cases result in ovarian enlargement not exceeding 5 cm, limited weight gain, and mild pelvic discomfort.
- Moderate cases result in ovarian enlargement of up to 10 cm in diameter and weight gain of 10 lb or more, often accompanied by nausea and vomiting.
- Severe cases result in ovarian enlargement of greater than 10 cm or ovarian enlargement to any size with ascites, hydrothorax, hemoconcentration, or oliguria.

Mild ovarian hyperstimulation occurs relatively commonly. Management is conservative (ie, observation). Pelvic or abdominal examinations should not be performed if hyperstimulation is suspected because the enlarged ovarian cysts are friable and prone to rupture; women with this condition should be evaluated only by gentle ultrasound examination.

Moderate ovarian hyperstimulation is less common. Women with this condition should be monitored closely by daily determination of weight, abdominal girth, and hematocrit.

Severe ovarian hyperstimulation is uncommon (less than 2%) but potentially life-threatening. It requires close monitoring, and hospitalization is generally required. The dominant complications are related to the migration of large amounts of fluid out of the intravascular space. Ascites and pleural effusion may occur. Weight gain, dyspnea, hypotension, oliguria, electrolyte imbalance, hemoconcentration, and increased coagulability are commonly noted. There is an increased risk of ovarian hemorrhage. In the event of frank intraabdominal bleeding, surgical therapy such as oophorectomy may be required.

When conception occurs, the symptoms of the ovarian hyperstimulation syndrome may persist for weeks (17). If no pregnancy occurs, the symptoms generally regress spontaneously within 7 days (ie, when menses ensues).

The overall risk of multiple gestation associated with gonadotropin therapy is estimated to be 10–30% (18). The majority of these multiple gestations are twin gestations.

Although recent studies have raised the possibility that gonadotropin-mediated ovulation induction may be associated with an enhancement of the risk of ovarian cancer (19), cause-and-effect relationships remain to be firmly established. Pending the conclusion of appropriate studies addressing this issue, no change in the prescription practices is deemed warranted.

Gonadotropin-Releasing Hormone

Gonadotropin-releasing hormone is an endogenous hypothalamic peptide capable of stimulating pituitary LH and FSH release. A synthetic peptide is now available.

The primary indication for pulsatile GnRH therapy is infertility associated with chronic anovulation in women with low levels of estrogen and gonadotropins. In appropriate individuals, pulsatile GnRH therapy can result in high rates of ovulation. Results in patients with chronic anovulation and normal levels of estrogen and gonadotropins, however, have been disappointing. Because both a functional pituitary and a functional ovary must be present for pulsatile GnRH therapy to be effective, patients with pituitary or ovarian failure should not be expected to respond to GnRH therapy.

The facts that the reproductive axis is largely intact and the mechanisms of feedback are preserved may account for the relatively low incidence of ovarian hyperstimulation and multiple births when pulsatile GnRH therapy is used, as compared with gonadotropin therapy. Both may still occur rarely in women who do not have a hypothalamic form of amenorrhea. No interpretable data are available on the potential impact of GnRH on the incidence of breast or ovarian cancer.

Additionally, the need for appropriate timing of the ovulating signal (hCG) is avoided because patients treated with pulsatile GnRH have an endogenous LH surge at the appropriate time in folliculogenesis. Most patients will ovulate after 10–20 days of pulsatile GnRH therapy.

Most series report the development of a single dominant follicle.

Gonadotropin-releasing hormone therapy may be administered either subcutaneously or intravenously (20). Considerable controversy exists as to the preferred route. Overall, intravenous therapy appears to be more predictable and less time consuming, require a lower dose per pulse, and result in higher rates of ovulation. On the other hand, intravenous therapy is clearly associated with a greater risk of phlebitis and needle displacement, thereby necessitating frequent infusion site inspection and relocation. Subcutaneous therapy is much easier to manage, more acceptable to patients, and virtually free of the risk of infection and needle displacement. It is generally agreed that intravenous delivery is often effective in cases refractory to subcutaneous therapy.

To be effective, GnRH must be administered in a pulsatile manner. The pump that delivers pulsatile GnRH can be thought of as an artificial hypothalamus. Pulse interval/volume-programmable infusion pumps are small enough to be concealed on the patient's body.

Intravenous therapy is usually effective at a dose of 5–10 μg per pulse. Subcutaneous therapy generally requires 10–20 μg per pulse, and few patients will ovulate at doses lower than 10 μg per pulse. Rarely are doses higher than 20 μg per pulse required. The lowest effective dose has obvious economic advantages and may also play a role in controlling the rate of multiple births.

Luteal phase maintenance in GnRH-induced cycles requires exogenous luteotropic support. If the pump is discontinued after ovulation, hCG or progesterone should be administered to support the luteal phase. Otherwise, support may be provided by continuing pulsatile GnRH delivery, which requires the patient to wear and maintain the pump for the entire luteal phase. When pregnancy is diagnosed, the pump is usually discontinued and the luteal phase supported with low doses of hCG or progesterone.

Summary

With proper diagnosis and selection of treatment, ovulation induction is an option for anovulatory women. Specialized skills, knowledge, and resources, as well as patient and physician commitment, are requisite to the appropriate application of these modalities. Patients should be provided with information, support, and access to the health care team to maximize success.

Current therapeutic options include the use of clomiphene citrate, bromocriptine, gonadotropins, and GnRH. Importantly, each and every one of these agents is best applied only in the appropriate clinical circumstances in keeping with the patient's individual needs. Whereas clomiphene citrate is particularly suited for the management of women with normal levels of FSH and prolactin and adequate levels of estrogen, gonadotropin therapy may be applied to both women with low levels of estrogen and gonadotropins as well as those with normal levels. Bromocriptine is only applicable for hyperprolactinemic women. Gonadotropin-releasing hormone therapy is best suited for circumstances characterized by low gonadotropin and estrogen levels as an alternative to gonadotropin therapy (assuming intact pituitary gonadotropin reserve).

REFERENCES

1. Rebar RW, Connolly HV. Clinical features of young women with hypergonadotropic amenorrhea. Fertil Steril 1990;53:804–810
2. Scialli AR. The reproductive toxicity of ovulation induction. Fertil Steril 1986;45:315–323
3. Adashi EY. Clomiphene citrate: mechanism(s) and site(s) of action—a hypothesis revisited. Fertil Steril 1984;42:331–344
4. Adashi EY. Clomiphene citrate-initiated ovulation: a clinical update. Semin Reprod Endocrinol 1986;4:255–276
5. Rust LA, Israel R, Mishell DR Jr. An individualized graduated therapeutic regimen for clomiphene citrate. Am J Obstet Gynecol 1974;120:785–790
6. Hoffman D, Lobo RA. Serum dehydroepiandrosterone sulfate and the use of clomiphene citrate in anovulatory women. Fertil Steril 1985;43:196–199
7. Lobo RA, Granger LR, Davajan V, Mishell DR Jr. An extended regimen of clomiphene citrate in women unresponsive to standard therapy. Fertil Steril 1982;37:762–766
8. Parkes D. Bromocriptine. N Engl J Med 1979;301:873–878
9. Cunnah D, Besser M. Management of prolactinomas. Clin Endocrinol 1991;34:231–235
10. Wright CS, Steele SJ, Jacobs HS. Value of bromocriptine in unexplained primary infertility: a double-blind controlled trial. BMJ 1979;1:1037–1039
11. Katz E, Weiss BE, Hassell A, Schran HF, Adashi EY. Increased circulating levels of bromocriptine after vaginal compared with oral administration. Fertil Steril 1991;55:882–884
12. Griffith RW, Turkalj I, Braun P. Outcome of pregnancy in mothers given bromocriptine. Br J Clin Pharmacol 1978;5:227–231
13. Ginsburg J, Hardiman P. Ovulation induction with human menopausal gonadotropins—a changing scene. Gynecol Endocrinol 1991;5:57–78
14. Schwartz M, Jewelewicz R. The use of gonadotropins for induction of ovulation. Fertil Steril 1981;35:3–12

15. Oelsner G, Serr DM, Mashiach S, Blankstein J, Snyder M, Lunenfeld B. The study of induction of ovulation with menotropins: analysis of results of 1897 treatment cycles. Fertil Steril 1978;30:538–544

16. Haning RV Jr, Austin CW, Kuzma DL, Shapiro SS, Zweibel WJ. Ultrasound evaluation of estrogen monitoring for induction of ovulation with menotropins. Fertil Steril 1982;37:627–632

17. Navot D, Relou A, Birkenfeld A, Rabinowitz R, Brzezinski A, Margalioth EJ. Risk factors and prognostic variables in the ovarian hyperstimulation syndrome. Am J Obstet Gynecol 1988;159:210–215

18. Navot D, Goldstein N, Mor-Josef S, Simon A, Relou A, Birkenfeld A. Multiple pregnancies: risk factors and prognostic variables during induction of ovulation with human menopausal gonadotrophins. Hum Reprod 1991;6:1152–1155

19. Whittemore AS, Harris R, Itnyre J, and the Collaborative Ovarian Cancer Group. Characteristics relating to ovarian cancer risk: collaborative analysis of 12 US case-control studies. Am J Epidemiol 1992;136:1184–1203

20. Filicori M, Flamigni C, Meriggiola MC, Cognigni G, Valdiserri A, Ferrari P, et al. Ovulation induction with pulsatile gonadotropin-releasing hormone: technical modalities and clinical perspectives. Fertil Steril 1991;56:1–13

This Technical Bulletin was developed under the direction of the Committee on Technical Bulletins of the American College of Obstetricians and Gynecologists as an educational aid to obstetricians and gynecologists. The committee wishes to thank Eli Y. Adashi, MD, and Howard D. McClamrock, MD, for their assistance in the development of this bulletin. This Technical Bulletin does not define a standard of care, nor is it intended to dictate an exclusive course of management. It presents recognized methods and techniques of clinical practice for consideration by obstetrician–gynecologists for incorporation into their practices. Variations of practice taking into account the needs of the individual patient, resources, and limitations unique to the institution or type of practice may be appropriate.

ISSN 1074-8628

THE AMERICAN COLLEGE OF OBSTETRICIANS AND GYNECOLOGISTS
409 12th Street, SW
Washington, DC 20024-2188

12345/87654

ACOG EDUCATIONAL BULLETIN

Number 228, September 1996

Maternal Serum Screening

Maternal serum screening is a noninvasive method of obtaining information about fetal development that can be used early in pregnancy. Maternal serum alpha-fetoprotein (MSAFP) was first used as a marker to identify patients at risk for having an infant with a fetal neural tube defect (NTD). Multiple serum markers have since been proved useful in identifying patients at risk for other fetal structural malformations and chromosomal anomalies.

The goal of a screening test is to identify from a large population a smaller group of patients that have an increased risk of a disorder and to offer that smaller group a more specific diagnostic examination. Screening should be voluntary, and the patient should be counseled about its limitations and benefits. A negative, or normal result of screening does not ensure that a child will not have a birth defect (including an NTD or fetal chromosomal anomaly). Conversely, a positive result is not a diagnosis of an abnormality but rather indicates that a patient has a level of risk sufficient to warrant further evaluation, such as ultrasonography or amniocentesis.

This Educational Bulletin was developed under the direction of the Committee on Educational Bulletins of the American College of Obstetricians and Gynecologists as an aid to obstetricians and gynecologists. The College wishes to thank Nancy C. Rose, MD, and Michael T. Mennuti, MD, for their assistance in the development of this bulletin. This document is not to be construed as establishing a standard of practice or dictating an exclusive course of treatment. Rather, it is intended as an educational tool that presents current information on obstetric–gynecologic issues.

Laboratory proficiency is paramount in ensuring that screening programs provide results for clinical interpretation of maternal serum markers. Proficiency testing, such as that supplied by the College of American Pathologists, is required for certified laboratories. Typically, alpha-fetoprotein (AFP) test results are reported as multiples of the median (MoM), a statistical convention introduced as a method by which different laboratories could compare their results (1). A laboratory should be able to verify medians and update them on a regular basis. It should track the MoM periodically and adjust medians accordingly. The appropriate controls should be run with each analyte for every assay, and data on the precision of each assay should be available.

When a patient's screen result is positive, the patient should be contacted without delay. The individual contacting the patient should be knowledgeable and be able to answer questions regarding the results of the test. It should be emphasized that a positive result does not mean that the fetus is affected with a disorder, but that further counseling and testing is available for the patient. Prenatal identification of fetal abnormalities enables families to make informed reproductive choices and allows the obstetrician to determine the most appropriate strategies for delivery and neonatal care. Alpha-fetoprotein, human chorionic gonadotropin (hCG), and unconjugated estriol (uE_3) are the markers currently used in maternal serum screening programs.

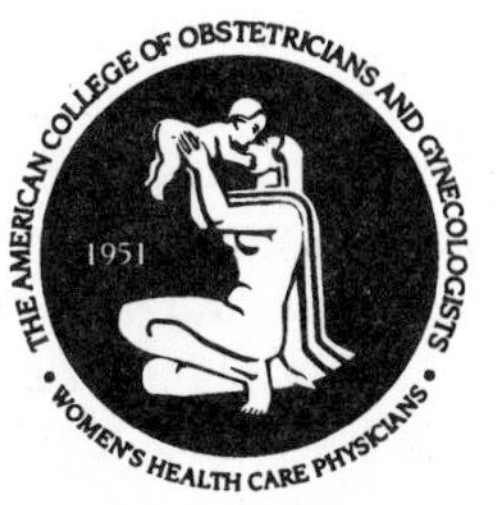

Replaces Number 154, April 1991

Alpha-Fetoprotein

Alpha-fetoprotein is produced by the fetus, making it an ideal marker of fetal development. Structurally and functionally, AFP is related to albumin. Genes that encode both proteins originate on chromosome 4, and each has a molecular weight of 69,000. Several functions have been postulated for AFP. Similar to albumin, it may be an intravascular transport protein or may play a role in maintaining oncotic pressure. An immunosuppressive role has also been suggested as a mechanism by which paternally derived fetal antigens are protected from provoking the development of maternal antibodies. Because there are reported cases of congenital AFP deficiency resulting in normal newborns (2), a critical role in fetal development is still speculative.

Fetal AFP is produced sequentially by the fetal yolk sac, the gastrointestinal tract, and the liver. It reaches a peak concentration in fetal serum at the end of the first trimester. Although the fetal liver continues to produce the same high levels of AFP, fetal serum levels decline in the second trimester as a result of the expanding fetal intravascular compartment. There is an abrupt decrease in AFP production at 30 weeks of gestation.

Filtration of blood through the fetal kidney results in high concentrations of AFP in the amniotic fluid. As the fetus swallows amniotic fluid, AFP is destroyed by gastrointestinal proteolytic enzymes. The decrease in amniotic fluid AFP during the second and third trimesters parallels that of fetal blood levels of AFP. The mechanism of transfer of AFP to the maternal circulation is both transplacental (two thirds) and transamniotic (one third) (3). In the maternal circulation, AFP levels gradually increase until 30 weeks of gestation and then decline until delivery. Therefore, during the second trimester, MSAFP levels continue to increase, while fetal levels decline (Fig. 1). Both high and low MSAFP levels may be predictive of a serious birth defect or adverse pregnancy outcome.

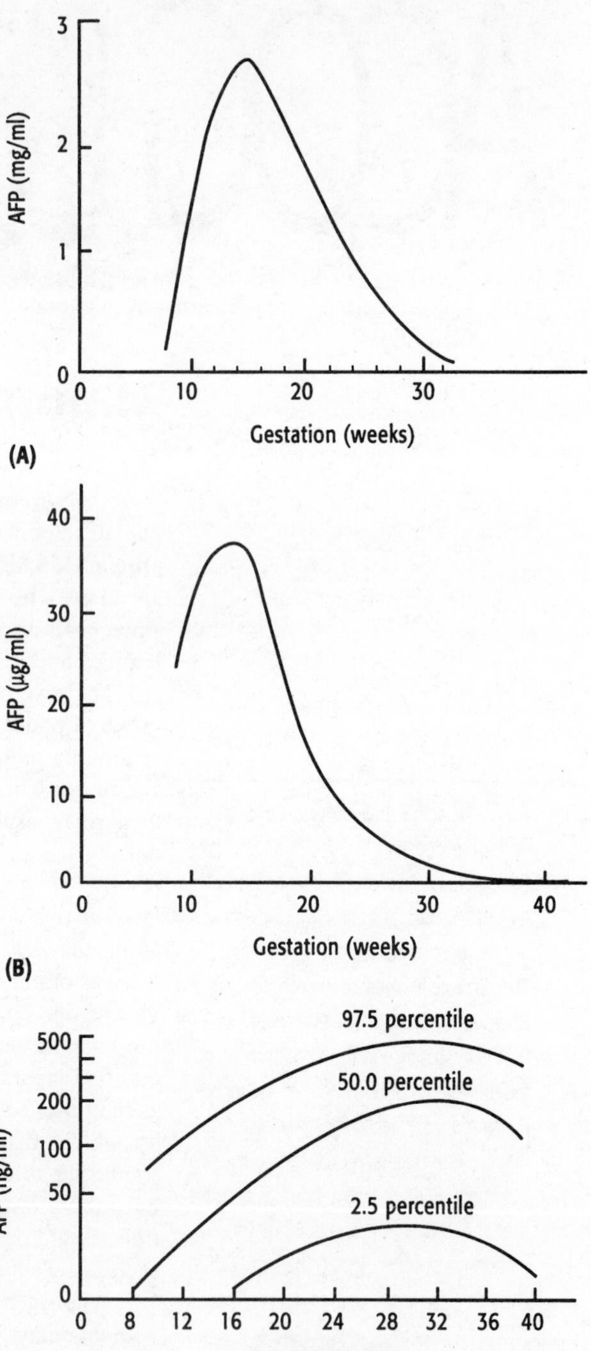

Figure 1. Approximate relationship between alpha-fetoprotein (AFP) values in fetal serum (A), amniotic fluid (B), and maternal serum (C). Note varying laboratory units for each graph. (Habib ZA. Maternal serum alpha-fetoprotein: its value in antenatal diagnosis of genetic disease and obstetrical–gynaecological care. Acta Obstet Gynecol Scand Suppl 1977;61:14; copyright 1977, Munksgaard International Publishers Ltd., Copenhagen, Denmark)

Neural Tube Defects

Neural tube defects are the second most frequent serious fetal malformation in the United States, surpassed only by congenital heart defects. They are a heterogeneous group of disorders that result from failure of the neural tube to close normally between the third and fourth week of embryologic development.

Evidence for multisite closure of the spinal cord has been demonstrated (4) and is reflected in humans by the relationship between the timing of specific teratogen exposure and sites of spinal cord disruption. During development, the cranial end of the neural tube becomes the forebrain, midbrain, and hindbrain; a failure of closure here results in anencephaly. A failure of closure distal to this region usually results in spina bifida. A third type of NTD, an encephalocele, is an extrusion of brain tissue through a skull defect, generally covered by overlying skin.

Clinical consequences of NTDs are variable. Anencephaly is incompatible with long-term survival. Among spina bifida survivors, disabilities correlate with the location and extent of the lesion as well as the presence or absence of hydrocephalus. Morbidity may include lack of specific motor function, often resulting in the inability to walk without assistance, incontinence, or developmental delay.

Incidence and Risk Factors

In the United States, the incidence of NTDs is approximately 1/1,000 births, with some temporal and geographic variation. More than 90% of NTDs occur in pregnancies in which there is no identifiable increased risk for these defects. Most NTDs (85%) are due to multifactorial inheritance—a genetic interplay between several genes and environmental factors. The most common factor that signals an increased risk for NTDs caused by multifactorial inheritance is a first- or second-degree family member with an isolated NTD.

Parents with an affected child have more than a 10-fold increased risk in a subsequent pregnancy as compared with the general population. The risk for these and other close relatives is shown in Table 1. About 12–15% of NTDs are caused by chromosomal anomalies, single gene defects, or teratogens (5). Neural tube defects have been associated with maternal diabetes mellitus as well as periconceptional ingestion of medications such as carbamazepine, valproic acid, and retinoic acid.

Folic acid has been shown to decrease the risk of development of NTDs except in diabetes. Several studies have shown that the use of folic acid decreased the rate of first occurrence of NTDs by about 50% in families not felt to have an increased risk for NTDs (6,7). Most NTDs occur in families without significant family history, and over 50% of pregnancies in the United States are unplanned (8). Thus, the U.S. Public Health Service has recommended that all reproductive-age women who are capable of becoming pregnant consume 0.4 mg of folic acid daily as a means of reducing their risk of having a pregnancy affected by an NTD. In those who have had a previous pregnancy with an isolated NTD, periconceptional folic acid supplementation of 4 mg/d, beginning at least 3 months before conception and continuing through the first trimester, has been shown to decrease the recurrence risk of NTDs by more than 70% (9). The mechanism of the effects of folic acid in the prevention of NTDs is not completely understood, and patients taking folic acid supplementation still have a residual risk for NTDs.

Table 1. Estimated Incidence of Neural Tube Defects Based on Specific Risk Factors in the United States

Population	Incidence/1,000 Live Births
Mother as reference	
General incidence	1.4–1.6
Women undergoing amniocentesis for advanced maternal age	1.5–3.0
Women with diabetes mellitus	20
Women on valproic acid in first trimester	10–20
Fetus as reference	
1 sibling with NTD*	15–30
2 siblings with NTD†	57
Parent with NTD	11
Half sibling with NTD	8
First cousin (mother's sister's child)	10
Other first cousins	3
Sibling with severe scoliosis secondary to 15–30 multiple vertebral defects	
Sibling with occult spinal dysraphism	15–30
Sibling with sacrococcygeal teratoma or hamartoma	≤15–30

*NTD indicates neural tube defect.

†Risk is higher in British studies. Risk increases further for three or more siblings or combinations of other close relatives.

Main DM, Mennuti MT. Neural tube defects: issues in prenatal diagnosis and counselling. Reprinted with permission from The American College of Obstetricians and Gynecologists (Obstetrics and Gynecology 1986, 67, 4)

Therefore, it is recommended that all patients, including those who are using folic acid supplementation, should be offered MSAFP screening or diagnostic testing based on risk factors.

Screening

Elevated levels of MSAFP have been associated with fetal NTDs. When appropriate laboratory cutoff levels are applied, MSAFP screening will detect about 85% of all open NTDs, which comprises about 80% of cases of open spina bifida and 90% of cases of anencephaly. Screening for MSAFP will not detect skin-covered defects, also known as closed defects (ie, most encephaloceles).

Because MSAFP levels increase in early gestation, individual laboratories should develop reference data with a median MSAFP level (1.0 MoM) for unaffected pregnancies for each week of gestation. Levels of MSAFP are influenced by several factors other than gestational age. These include an inverse relationship with maternal weight, a 10% higher level of MSAFP in African–American women, a decrease of about 15% in

MSAFP levels in women who have insulin-dependent diabetes mellitus, and doubling in twin gestation.

Most screening programs establish a cutoff of 2.0–2.5 times the median values (2.0–2.5 MoM) to be designated as a positive result. Most laboratories use 2.5 MoM, which produces about a 3–4% false-positive or at-risk rate. Selecting a cutoff requires striking a balance between the detection rate and the false-positive rate: the higher the screening cutoff, the lower the false-positive rate but the lower the detection rate.

Although MSAFP screening is most accurate when performed between 16 and 18 weeks of gestation, it can be performed between 15 and 22 weeks. Elevated MSAFP levels can detect defects other than NTDs such as those listed in the box. The log Gaussian distribution of MSAFP levels in unaffected pregnancies and abnormal pregnancies is shown in Fig. 2.

Other Abnormalities Identified by the Alpha-Fetoprotein Screening Process

- Ventral wall defects
  - Omphalocele
  - Gastroschisis
- Triploidy
- Trisomies 13, 18, and 21
- Unbalanced translocations
- Amniotic band sequence
- Pentalogy of Cantrell (omphalocele, lower sternal defect, deficiency of diaphragmatic pericardium, intracardiac abnormality, anterior diaphragm defect)
- Renal agenesis
- Fetal demise
- Multiple gestation
- Congenital nephrosis (Finnish type)
- Sacrococcygeal teratoma
- Dermatologic disorders
  - Epidermolysis bullosa
  - Congenital ichthyosiform erythroderma
- Chorioangioma
- Risk of poor perinatal outcome
- Maternal hepatoma
- Maternal ovarian teratoma

Diagnosis

When the patient's first MSAFP screening result is elevated, further evaluation should be undertaken. In some instances, a repeat MSAFP test may be performed when initial test results are elevated. The decision to repeat sampling in this circumstance may be based on a variety of factors such as gestational age, the level of the initial MSAFP result, and patient preference. Studies in which a repeat MSAFP screen was performed show that as many as 30% of repeat tests on moderately elevated MSAFP will be below the cutoff level, and this finding is not associated with an increased frequency of false-negative results of NTDs.

Ultrasonography

The most common reason for a false-positive MSAFP elevation is an underestimation of gestational age. Patients with one or two elevated MSAFP levels (depending

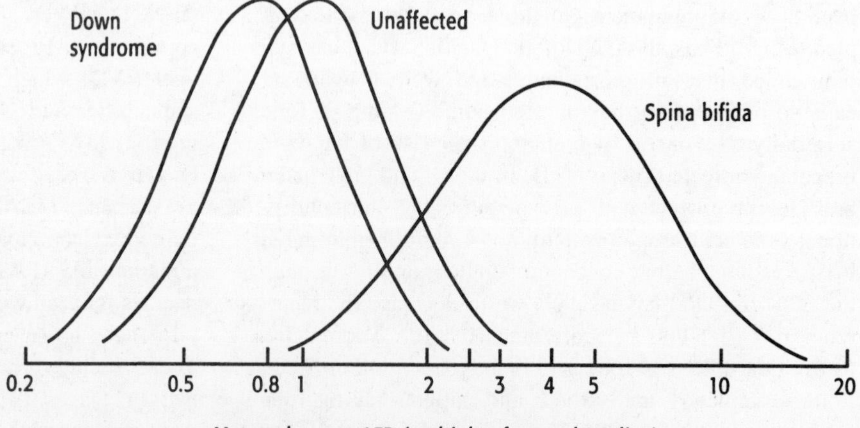

Figure 2. Log Gaussian distribution of alpha-fetoprotein (AFP) levels in maternal serum at 16–18 weeks of gestation in singleton pregnancies for open spina bifida, unaffected pregnancies, and Down syndrome. (Wald N, Cuckle HS. Recent advances in screening for neural tube defects and Down's syndrome. Baillieres Clin Obstet Gynaecol 1987;1:656; copyright 1987, WB Saunders Company Limited, London)

on the laboratory protocol) should undergo an ultrasound examination to determine gestational age. Clinicians should be aware that the biparietal diameter (BPD) in fetuses affected with spina bifida is often smaller than in normal fetuses (10). If the original gestational dating is inaccurate (eg, greater than a 7–14-day interval in the second trimester), depending on laboratory protocol, the MoM should be recalculated in light of the new gestational age.

If the initial ultrasound examination does not provide an explanation for the MSAFP elevation (such as inaccurate gestational dating, multiple gestation, or fetal demise), a comprehensive ultrasound examination should be performed to evaluate the fetus for malformations. Several second-trimester intracranial findings are observed with increased frequency in fetuses with NTDs. These include scalloping of the frontal bones (lemon sign) (11), downward displacement of the cerebellum (banana sign), and varying degrees of ventriculomegaly. Hydrocephalus is present at term or in the newborn period in about 80% of cases of NTDs. However, this finding may not appear at the time of second-trimester ultrasonography.

Some investigators have suggested that ultrasonography alone may be an acceptable alternative to amniocentesis for the diagnosis of an NTD (12). However, the prospective identification of NTDs may be limited by the location and extent of the lesion, fetal position, quality of the images, and experience of the ultrasonographer. The sensitivity of ultrasonography in detecting NTDs was about 90% in a large, prospective series (13). Other series (14, 15) have shown ultrasonography to have a higher degree of sensitivity in the detection of NTDs, but all these studies have been conducted in specialized centers and include patients referred for evaluation of elevated MSAFP levels (16). In such specialized centers, the patient may be counseled that the a priori risk of NTDs is decreased by 95%, assuming there is adequate visualization of fetal anatomy, including attention to the previously mentioned intracranial signs (14, 15). Based on such revised risk estimates, the patient may or may not choose to undergo invasive diagnostic procedures.

Amniocentesis

If further evaluation is desired, amniocentesis is performed. Many patients with an elevated MSAFP level will have normal amniotic fluid AFP levels. In contrast, an elevated amniotic fluid AFP level suggests an abnormality.

To differentiate an NTD from other types of open fetal defects, qualitative or quantitative assessment of acetylcholinesterase (AChE)—an enzyme contained in blood cells, muscle, and nerve tissue—may be performed. An elevation of both AFP and AChE levels suggests an open fetal NTD with a high degree of accuracy (>99%). An elevated amniotic fluid AFP level with a normal AChE level suggests a fetal defect other than an NTD. An elevated MSAFP, normal amniotic fluid AFP, normal AChE, and a normal ultrasound examination exclude almost all cases of open structural malformations. This last subgroup of patients, as well as those patients with an elevated MSAFP level and a normal ultrasound examination who decline amniocentesis, are considered to be at an increased risk for low birth weight, fetal death, and oligohydramnios (17). Increased fetal surveillance during the third trimester has been suggested for these patients; however, the benefits of these evaluations have not been established by prospective trials.

Chromosome analysis should be considered if an amniocentesis is performed to determine the cause of the MSAFP elevation whether or not a structural fetal defect is identified. Ultrasound examination should detect spina bifida in approximately 90% of patients tested (13). If a structural anomaly is identified, different outcome strategies may be used depending on whether the defect is due to a chromosomal aneuploidy or to an isolated defect. For example, with omphalocele there is a 20–30% incidence of chromosomal anomalies, and NTDs may be associated with trisomy 18 or trisomy 13. Further, a structural anomaly may be caused by a duplication or deficiency of a chromosomal segment. If an NTD is detected, additional ultrasound examinations, including a fetal cardiac evaluation, should be performed to detect other accompanying malformations and to monitor the development of hydrocephalus or hydramnios.

Management

Genetic counseling should include discussions of the cause, treatment, prognosis, recurrence risk, and future prevention of defects that are detected. The options available to the family, including termination, should be explained using a nondirective approach. As appropriate, the patient can be offered the opportunity to meet with a physician who cares for children with spina bifida, including pediatric neurosurgical specialists, and parental support groups.

The benefit of cesarean delivery of fetuses with an NTD has not been evaluated by prospective studies. In a retrospective analysis, however, the neonatal outcome for infants born before the onset of labor was compared with that for infants whose mothers underwent labor before cesarean or vaginal delivery (18). Infants who were delivered by cesarean birth without labor retained greater neurologic function at an average of 3.3 spinal segments above those born after labor, regardless of the ultimate mode of delivery. Hence, although the benefits of cesarean delivery have not been proved, this route of delivery should be considered for patients carrying a fetus affected with an isolated NTD.

Chromosomal Disorders

Fetal Down Syndrome

Down syndrome is the most common pattern of human malformation, with an incidence of about 1/800 live births. Affected individuals exhibit developmental delay and a characteristic facies and are at risk for congenital heart disease, gastrointestinal anomalies, and the development of childhood leukemias. Unlike NTDs, the incidence of fetuses with Down syndrome and several other types of chromosomal aneuploidies increases with advancing maternal age.

Although initially used to detect risk of open fetal defects, maternal serum screening is now used in part to screen for fetuses with Down syndrome. This screening is done with AFP plus several other serum markers. Therefore, the same serum sample can be used concurrently to screen for fetuses affected with either NTDs or Down syndrome.

Screening Techniques

The observation of an association between low MSAFP levels and fetal aneuploidy was first reported in 1984 (19) and subsequently verified by a prospective, multicenter collaborative study (20). Analysis of other serum markers, including hCG and uE_3, enhances the detection rate of fetuses with Down syndrome.

Maternal Serum Alpha-Fetoprotein. The median MSAFP level in pregnant women carrying fetuses with Down syndrome is about 0.8 MoM of that of control pregnancies. There is a more extensive overlap of MSAFP distributions between the unaffected fetuses and fetuses with Down syndrome than seen with NTDs (Fig. 2). With most laboratories, a patient's result is considered to be positive when the combination of her age and MSAFP level gives her a risk equivalent to the a priori risk of a 35-year-old woman. This is usually a 1:270 midtrimester risk for the occurrence of Down syndrome. In contrast to the absolute cutoff of 2.0 or 2.5 MoM used in NTD screening, Down syndrome screening uses a series of age-specific cutoff levels for each MSAFP level. That is, for the same MSAFP level, there is a direct relationship between the age of the patient and the chance of her result being designated as positive.

Human Chorionic Gonadotropin. Human chorionic gonadotropin is secreted by the syncytiotrophoblasts and is first detectable in maternal blood on about day 8 after ovulation. During the second trimester, hCG levels decline until about 20 weeks of gestation and remain at that level until term. Although it was previously suggested that serum levels of hCG might enhance the detection rate of a fetus with Down syndrome (21), supportive clinical data were first introduced in a study in which 11 of 17 pregnant women carrying fetuses with Down syndrome had an hCG elevation in maternal serum of at least 2.5 MoM (22). Because the median hCG level is so elevated in fetuses with Down syndrome in relation to control pregnancies, hCG is the most sensitive maternal screening marker for the detection of fetal Down syndrome (23). Additionally, the free beta subunit of hCG is equivalent to the measurement of the total hCG molecule in triple marker screening (24, 25).

Unconjugated Estriol. The synthesis of uE_3, a steroid hormone, is modulated by the placenta, fetal adrenal glands, and fetal liver. Lower second-trimester levels of maternal serum uE_3 have been reported in fetuses affected with Down syndrome (26). Like AFP, levels of uE_3 are about 25% lower in affected than unaffected pregnancies. The addition of uE_3 to maternal serum screening using AFP and hCG decreases the false-positive rate by about 25% (27), effectively decreasing the number of amniocenteses while achieving the same level of detection. The use of uE_3 also allows the ability to screen for trisomy 18.

Interpretation of Results

Given that all three analytes are independent of maternal age and are only weakly correlated with each other (28), they can be used in combination with maternal age to calculate a patient-specific risk for carrying a fetus with Down syndrome. The detection rate for fetuses with Down syndrome is 60%, with a false-positive rate of about 5%. Therefore, the detection rate using all three markers is superior to the 20–25% detection rate achieved using MSAFP alone (28). These results have since been prospectively verified by several groups (29, 30). The parameters should not be interpreted individually (ie, any one by itself), as this will significantly increase the false-positive rate without improving sensitivity substantially.

As with screening for NTDs, an accurate gestational age is essential. Unlike screening for NTDs, repeat MSAFP testing is not recommended because low values statistically tend to normalize toward the mean value; the effect of a repeat multiple marker result may be to erroneously reclassify a patient's result as negative. The BPD is a more sensitive estimation of gestational age in the second trimester because the long bones of fetuses with Down syndrome may be shorter when compared with other fetal measurements (31). If gestational age has been verified and the patient's result is found to be positive, she should be offered genetic counseling regarding the risks and benefits of amniocentesis.

Ultrasonography is the most accurate method of dating gestation. If an ultrasound examination places a patient at a gestational age at which maternal serum screening is inaccurate (that is, before 15 weeks of gestation in most laboratories), the maternal serum screening result should be disregarded, and repeat screening should be offered at an appropriate time in gestation (generally between 15 and 20 weeks of gestation). It should be emphasized that this is the only instance in which it is appropriate to repeat a multiple marker screening result. However, in patients with accurate dating of gestational age, caution must be exercised; a small-for-dates fetus may actually be growth restricted, secondary to aneuploidy. Ultrasonography may also help distinguish an affected fetus if findings such as hyperechoic bowel, increased nuchal skinfold measurements (≥ 6 mm), or complex heart disease are seen. However, it must be remembered that ultrasonography is also a screening test and that an affected fetus may have a normal sonographic evaluation.

Correction factors for maternal race, weight, and insulin-dependent diabetes mellitus are used for MSAFP in screening for fetuses with Down syndrome or an NTD. Currently, there are no data to interpret triple marker screening in multiple gestations.

Trisomy 18

In contrast to the biochemical profile of pregnancies with Down syndrome, in the screening pattern of some trisomy 18 pregnancies, all three markers are substantially lower than expected. In one study, 60% of fetuses with trisomy 18 were identified (32). Since fetuses affected with trisomy 18 may have NTDs or ventral wall defects, this method of screening is useful for affected fetuses without open defects. This pattern of screening markers is rare and cannot be due to poor gestational dating. The ability to screen for trisomy 18 pregnancies can be advantageous since it adds little to the positive rate and can help identify (through prenatal diagnosis) a serious, usually lethal disorder for which the family may have an earlier opportunity to make informed choices.

Screening in Women Age 35 and Older

Two prospective population studies with complete fetal chromosome ascertainment have demonstrated the effectiveness and limitations of serum screening for Down syndrome detection in older women. The first study evaluated 3,896 women who underwent only MSAFP screening before genetic amniocentesis for the indication of advanced maternal age (33). With a risk cutoff of at least 1:270, 85% of cases of fetal Down syndrome were detected, with an amniocentesis rate of 63%. A second report used a similar study protocol but performed multiple marker screening on 5,385 women of advanced maternal age before amniocentesis with a second-trimester cutoff of 1:200 (34). The detection rate of Down syndrome was 89%, with an amniocentesis rate of 25%. Both the amniocentesis rate and the detection rate increased with advancing maternal age. For example, in women age 40, the detection rate was 91% and the amniocentesis rate was 40%, but at age 35, the detection rate was only 65%.

The incidence of sex chromosome aneuploidies, which include 47,XXY and 47,XXX, increases with advancing maternal age. Serum MSAFP screening has been reported to detect 44–50% of such anomalies in women older than 35 (33, 34).

At this time, multiple marker testing in women over the age of 35 cannot be recommended for routine Down syndrome screening as an equivalent alternative to offering prenatal cytogenic diagnosis. However, it may be offered as an option for those women who do not accept the risk of amniocentesis or chorionic villus sampling or who wish to have this additional information prior to making a decision about having amniocentesis. If serum screening for Down syndrome is requested by a patient over the age of 35, the patient should be informed of the higher rate of a positive screening test in this age group. The patient should also be informed of the diminished ability of screening to detect Down syndrome and certain other chromosome abnormalities, such as 47,XXX and 47,XXY, when screening with this approach is compared with diagnostic testing by chorionic villus sampling or amniocentesis.

Other Screening Methods Currently Under Investigation

Although maternal serum screening with the use of double or triple markers is clearly superior to the use of MSAFP alone when screening for fetal Down syndrome, this method still fails to detect 40% of Down syndrome in women less than 35 years of age. Therefore, many other screening analytes, including PAPP-A, urinary beta-core, dimeric inhibin, and human placental lactogen, are currently being investigated for use in the first and second trimesters to determine whether they alone, or in combination, will increase detection to a rate greater than the current 60%. The extraction of fetal cells from the maternal circulation is a promising new technique that may eventually be used for screening or diagnosis, may improve diagnosis, and may decrease the need for serum markers or for invasive procedures.

Summary

Maternal serum screening offers women the ability to increase the detection of open fetal defects, Down syndrome, and trisomy 18. After being informed of the risks and advantages of serum screening, a patient may elect to be screened. Counseling must emphasize that serum screening for these disorders is voluntary, and patients must be aware that further evaluation, if their results are classified as positive, may include amniocentesis. Physicians should have access to genetic services and reliable laboratories to assist them in the management of maternal serum screening and genetic procedures. Special attention must be given to the older gravida to help her make an appropriate personal decision regarding screening and genetic testing. Patients receiving positive results from a definitive test (karyotype or, possibly, ultrasonography) should have access to adequate counseling, including the availability of support groups and pediatric surgeons.

References

1. Report of U.K. Collaborative Study on Alpha-fetoprotein in Relation to Neural-Tube Defects. Maternal serum alpha-fetoprotein measurement in antenatal screening for anencephaly and spina bifida in early pregnancy. Lancet 1977; 2:1323–1332 (Level II-3)
2. Faucett WA, Greenberg F, Rose E, Alpert E, Bancalari L, Kardon NB, et al. Congenital deficiency of alpha-fetoprotein. Am J Hum Genet 1989;45:1019A (Level III)
3. Los FJ, De Bruijn HWA, Van Beek Calkoen-Carpay T, Huisjes HJ. AFP transport across the fetal membranes in the human. Prenat Diagn 1985;5:277–281 (Level III)
4. Van Allen MI, Kalousek DK, Chernoff GF, Juriloff D, Harris M, McGillivray BC, et al. Evidence for multi-site closure of the neural tube in humans. Am J Med Genet 1993;47:723–743 (Level III)
5. Holmes LB, Driscoll SG, Atkins L. Etiologic heterogeneity of neural-tube defects. N Engl J Med 1976;294:365–369 (Level III)
6. Czeizel AE, Dudás I. Prevention of the first occurrence of neural-tube defects by periconceptional vitamin supplementation. N Engl J Med 1992;327:1832–1835 (Level II-2)
7. Vergel G, Sanchez LR, Heredero BL, Rodriguez PL, Martinez AJ. Primary prevention of neural tube defects with folic acid supplementation: Cuban experience. Prenat Diagn 1990;10:149–152 (Level II-2)
8. Grimes DA. Unplanned pregnancies in the United States. Obstet Gynecol 1986;67:438–442 (Level III)
9. MRC Vitamin Study Research Group. Prevention of neural tube defects: results of the Medical Research Council Vitamin Study. Lancet 1991;338:131–137 (Level I)
10. Wald N, Cuckle H, Boreham J, Turnbull AC. Effect of estimating gestational age by ultrasound cephalometry on the specificity of α-fetoprotein screening for open neural-tube defects. Br J Obstet Gynaecol 1982;89:1050–1053 (Level II-3)
11. Nicolaides KH, Campbell S, Gabbe SG, Guidetti R. Ultrasound screening for spina bifida: cranial and cerebellar signs. Lancet 1986;2:72–74 (Level III)
12. Nadel AS, Green JK, Holmes LB, Frigoletto FD Jr, Benacerraf BR. Absence of need for amniocentesis in patients with elevated levels of maternal serum alpha-fetoprotein and normal ultrasonographic examinations. N Engl J Med 1990;323:557–561 (Level III)
13. Platt LD, Feuchtbaum L, Filly R, Lustig L, Simon M, Cunningham GC. The California Maternal Serum α-Fetoprotein Screening Program: the role of ultrasonography in the detection of spina bifida. Am J Obstet Gynecol 1992; 166:1328–1329 (Level III)
14. Morrow RJ, McNay MB, Whittle MJ. Ultrasound detection of neural tube defects in patients with elevated maternal serum alpha-fetoprotein. Obstet Gynecol 1991;78:1055–1057 (Level III)
15. Hogge WA, Thiagarajah S, Ferguson JE, Schnatterly PT, Harbert GM Jr. The role of ultrasonography and amniocentesis in the evaluation of pregnancies at risk for neural tube defects. Am J Obstet Gynecol 1989;161:520–524 (Level III)
16. Wald NJ, Cuckle HS, Haddow JE, Doherty RA, Knight GJ, Palomaki GE. Sensitivity of ultrasound in detecting spina bifida. N Engl J Med 1991;324:769–770 (Level III)
17. Simpson JL, Elias S, Morgan CD, Andersen RN, Shulman LP, Sibai BM, et al. Does unexplained second-trimester (15 to 20 weeks' gestation) maternal serum α-fetoprotein elevation presage adverse perinatal outcome? Am J Obstet Gynecol 1991;164:829–836 (Level III)
18. Luthy DA, Wardinsky T, Shurtleff DB, Hollenbach KA, Hickok DE, Nyberg DA, et al. Cesarean section before the onset of labor and subsequent motor function in infants with meningomyelocele diagnosed antenatally. N Engl J Med 1991;324:662–666 (Level II-2)
19. Merkatz IR, Nitowsky HM, Macri JN, Johnson WE. An association between low maternal serum α-fetoprotein and fetal chromosomal abnormalities. Am J Obstet Gynecol 1984;148:886–891 (Level II-2)
20. New England Regional Genetics Group Prenatal Collaborative Study of Down Syndrome Screening. Combining maternal serum α-fetoprotein measurements and age to screen for Down syndrome in pregnant women under age 35. Am J Obstet Gynecol 1989;160:575–581 (Level III)
21. Chard T, Lowings C, Kitau MJ. Alphafetoprotein and chorionic gonadotropin levels in relation to Down's syndrome. Lancet 1984;2:750 (Level III)
22. Bogart MH, Pandian MR, Jones OW. Abnormal maternal serum chorionic gonadotropin levels in pregnancies with fetal chromosome abnormalities. Prenat Diagn 1987;7: 623–630 (Level II-2)
23. Bogart MH, Jones OW, Felder RA, Best RG, Bradley L, Butts W, et al. Prospective evaluation of maternal serum human chorionic gonadotropin levels in 3428 pregnancies. Am J Obstet Gynecol 1991;165:663–667 (Level II-3)
24. Spencer K, Coombes EJ, Mallard AS, Ward AM. Free beta human choriogonadotropin in Down's syndrome screen-

ing: a multicentre study of its role compared with other biochemical markers. Ann Clin Biochem 1992;29:506–518 (Level II-3)

25. Stone S, Henley R, Reynolds T, John R. A comparison of total and free β-HCG assays in Down syndrome screening. Prenat Diagn 1993;13:535–537 (Level III)

26. Canick JA, Knight GJ, Palomaki GE, Haddow JE, Cuckle HS, Wald NJ. Low second trimester maternal serum unconjugated oestriol in pregnancies with Down's syndrome. Br J Obstet Gynaecol 1988;95:330–333 (Level II-2)

27. MacDonald ML, Wagner RM, Slotnick RN. Sensitivity and specificity of screening for Down syndrome with alpha-fetoprotein, hCG, unconjugated estriol, and maternal age. Obstet Gynecol 1991;77:63–68 (Level II-2)

28. Wald NJ, Cuckle HS, Densem JW, Nanchahal K, Royston P, Chard T, et al. Maternal serum screening for Down's syndrome in early pregnancy. BMJ 1988;297:883–887 (Level II-2)

29. Phillips OP, Elias S, Shulman LP, Andersen RN, Morgan CD, Simpson JL. Maternal serum screening for fetal Down syndrome in women less than 35 years of age using alpha-fetoprotein, hCG, and unconjugated estriol: a prospective 2-year study. Obstet Gynecol 1992;80:353–358 (Level III)

30. Haddow JE, Palomaki GE, Knight GJ, Williams J, Pulkkinen A, Canick JA, et al. Prenatal screening for Down's syndrome with use of maternal serum markers. N Engl J Med 1992;327:588–593 (Level II-2)

31. Lockwood C, Benacerraf B, Krinsky A, Blakemore K, Belanger K, Mahoney M, et al. A sonographic screening method for Down syndrome. Am J Obstet Gynecol 1987; 157:803–808 (Level II-2)

32. Canick JA, Palomaki GE, Osathanondh R. Prenatal screening for trisomy 18 in the second trimester. Prenat Diagn 1990;10:546–548 (Level III)

33. Rose NC, Palomaki GE, Haddow JE, Goodman DBP, Mennuti MT. Maternal serum α-fetoprotein screening for chromosomal abnormalities: a prospective study in women aged 35 and older. Am J Obstet Gynecol 1994;170:1073–1080 (Level II-3)

34. Haddow JE, Palomaki GE, Knight GJ, Cunningham GC, Lustig LS, Boyd PA. Reducing the need for amniocentesis in women 35 years of age or older with serum markers for screening. N Engl J Med 1994;330:1114–1118 (Level II-2)

The references in this bulletin are graded according to the method outlined by the U.S. Preventive Services Task Force:

- I Evidence obtained from at least one properly designed randomized controlled trial
- II-1 Evidence obtained from well-designed controlled trials without randomization
- II-2 Evidence obtained from well-designed cohort or case–control analytic studies, preferably from more than one center or research group
- II-3 Evidence obtained from multiple time series, with or without intervention, or dramatic results in uncontrolled experiments
- III Opinions of respected authorities, based on clinical experience, descriptive studies, or reports of expert committees

Other publications from ACOG:

- **Committee Opinions,** focused updates on emerging areas
- **Practice Patterns**, evidence-based guidelines
- **Criteria Sets**, baseline guidelines for review of diagnostic and management procedures

ISSN 1074-8628

The American College of Obstetricians and Gynecologists
409 12th Street, SW
PO Box 96920
Washington, DC 20090-6920

12345/09876

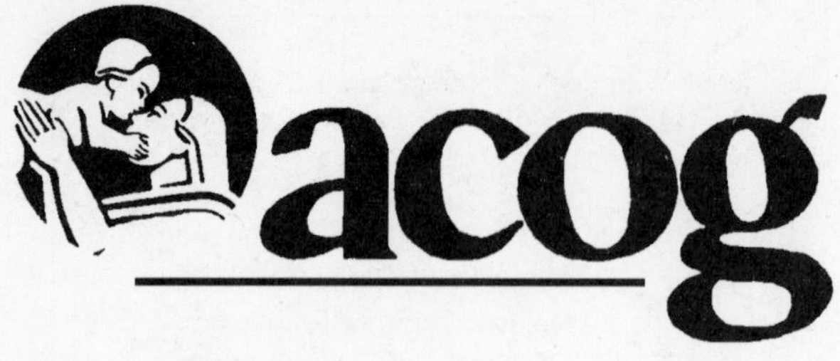

Number 109—October 1987
(Replaces #56, December 1979)

Technical Bulletin
An Educational Aid to Obstetrician–Gynecologists

Methods of Midtrimester Abortion

Despite reductions in the percentage of midtrimester abortions, each year in the United States over 100,000 women obtain legal abortions at 13 menstrual weeks of gestation or later. Regardless of personal moral beliefs, views, or practices in relation to abortion in the midtrimester, it is the physician's responsibility to remain aware of the current techniques and procedures in this area of the specialty to ensure the best possible care for patients faced with this eventuality.

In states where abortion methods and gestational ages were reported for 1981, dilation and evacuation (D&E) was the most commonly used method of abortion at 13 weeks of gestation or later, accounting for 67% of such abortions. Labor induction techniques in which hypertonic saline or urea or prostaglandin $F_{2\alpha}$ ($PGF_{2\alpha}$) were used accounted for 33% of midtrimester abortions. Hysterotomy and hysterectomy were responsible for less than 1% of second-trimester abortions (1).

Patients should be selected and counseled extensively for midtrimester termination of pregnancy because of the physical and emotional stress associated with these procedures. Health considerations include those which would change or prevent the procedure, such as sensitivity to medication and the presence of medical disorders. Performance of a second-trimester abortion should not be undertaken without special medical training and skills. Hemoglobin or hematocrit and blood type determinations are mandatory, and Rho(D) immunoglobulin should be administered to nonsensitized women according to the usual guidelines (2). The use of ultrasound has made estimation of fetal size more accurate and has contributed to the safety of second-trimester abortion (3).

Techniques

Dilation and Evacuation

Dilation and evacuation (D&E) is a generic term that encompasses cervical dilation followed by evacuation of the products of conception. Although midtrimester D&E is an extension of first-trimester suction and sharp curettage, special instruments are useful to evacuate the larger volumes of tissue encountered in the midtrimester pregnancy. Methods other than D&E may be preferred to obtain intact products of conception for autopsy.

As with curettage procedures performed early in pregnancy, paracervical or intracervical anesthesia may be used. Use of general anesthesia is associated with increased risk of hemorrhage and major visceral injury from the abortion procedure (3). Because the cervix must be dilated to a relatively large diameter in order to empty a large uterus, many physicians rely on placement of multiple intracervical osmotic dilators, either laminaria or synthetic types. Use of osmotic dilators is strongly recommended for abortions performed in the midtrimester. Others accomplish more rapid dilation with large-caliber dilators such as Pratt dilators. Thereafter, the uterus is emptied with a combination of forceps, suction curettage, and sharp curettage. Large-bore vacuum cannulas and large ovum forceps are available. In the event that retained products are suspected, ultrasound or contact hysteroscopy may be used to view the uterine contents and to guide the evacuation process. Total operating time is usually less than 30 minutes.

Intrauterine Instillation of Abortifacient Agents

Intrauterine infusion of hypertonic solutions, such as saline or urea and/or uterotonic agents such as $PGF_{2\alpha}$, induces uterine contractility, usually culminating in expulsion of the products of conception. These agents can be injected into either the intraamniotic space or the extraovular space (between the fetal membranes and the uterine wall). $PGF_{2\alpha}$ stimulates uterine contractions and produces faster abortions than do hypertonic agents, which act indirectly. The osmolar insult of hypertonic solutions generally causes fetal death; uterine contractility usually ensues, although the mechanism initiating uterine activity is unknown.

The technique for performing intraamniotic instillation of hypertonic saline is as follows (4–6). After the woman empties her bladder, the physician cleanses her lower abdomen with antiseptic and infiltrates her skin and subcutaneous tissue with local anesthetic. The physician then inserts a needle with an obturator (such as a no. 18 spinal needle) into the uterus, removes the obturator, and then adjusts the needle until a free flow of amniotic fluid is obtained. Testing the fluid for alkalinity with pH paper usually distinguishes amniotic fluid from urine (usually acidic).

Some physicians withdraw a volume of amniotic fluid before instillation of the abortifacient. Hoping to reduce the risk of displacing the needle as the uterus decreases in size, others avoid withdrawing amniotic fluid. Some clinicians pass a catheter into the amniotic cavity through the needle during intraamniotic infusion as an added safety measure to avoid intravascular injection of these agents. The most common dose of saline is 40 g (200 ml of 20% saline), which can be infused by gravity.

The technique of amniocentesis prior to instillation of $PGF_{2\alpha}$ is similar to that used for saline instillation (4–6). The usual initial dose is 20–40 mg (2.5–5-mg test dose followed by 17.5–35 mg of $PGF_{2\alpha}$). Some clinicians add 1 g of calcium gluconate to the intraamniotic injection (7). Approximately one-quarter of women who receive $PGF_{2\alpha}$ will require more than one injection.

The technique of instillation of hypertonic urea is analogous to that of hypertonic saline (4–6). One well-studied dosage is 80 g dissolved in 5% dextrose and water instilled into the amniotic cavity after drainage of most of the amniotic fluid. Because long induction-to-abortion times occur when urea is used as an abortifacient, augmentation (intravenous oxytocin or 5–10 mg of intraamniotic $PGF_{2\alpha}$) should be used after urea instillation.

Mechanical or pharmacologic techniques may be used to expedite instillation abortions (8). Placement of laminaria tents 12–16 hours prior to instillation of abortifacients appears to shorten induction-to-abortion times more than placement at the time of instillation. Intravenous oxytocin can be used to expedite abortions induced by hypertonic agents, although the decrease in induction-to-abortion times should be weighed against increased risks of coagulopathy, water intoxication, and uterine rupture when used in conjunction with saline abortions. The concurrent use of prostaglandins and oxytocin is potentially dangerous because excessive contractility may result, leading to uterine or cervical rupture. Small intraamniotic doses of $PGF_{2\alpha}$ (5–10 mg) have been used to accelerate midtrimester abortions with hypertonic solutions. If the placenta is not expelled within 1–2 hours, the use of forceps and curettage is recommended (5). Pitocin can be used to assist in placental expulsion after delivery of the fetus (6).

Instillation abortions are contraindicated in patients with active pelvic infection or in cases of intrauterine demise. Hypertonic solutions should not be used in patients who cannot tolerate the solute load, and use of $PGF_{2\alpha}$ in patients with preexisting asthma, epilepsy, glaucoma, pulmonary hypertension, or hypertensive cardiovascular disease may be inadvisable (5).

Extrauterine Administration of Abortifacient Agents

Only vaginal prostaglandin E_2 suppositories are currently approved as abortifacients by the U.S. Food and Drug Administration. The 20-mg prostaglandin E_2 suppositories may be used for abortions after 12 weeks of gestation, for missed abortions or cases of fetal death in utero up to 28 weeks of gestation, and management of hydatidiform mole. The suppositories are placed in the vagina every 3–5 hours until abortion occurs. Because nausea, vomiting, and diarrhea are frequent, this method is rarely the preferred primary technique of midtrimester abortion. Absorption through the vaginal vault, especially when membranes are ruptured or bleeding is present, may be incomplete and unpredictable. Similar problems may occur with other vaginally administered abortifacients now under development. In contrast, the prostaglandin E_2 suppository is often the preferred means of inducing abortion in cases of fetal death in utero at gestational ages when D&E is not satisfactory.

Intramuscular 15-methyl $PGF_{2\alpha}$ can be administered as an injection of 0.25 mg every 2–3 hours. Fever is reported to occur less frequently, and nausea and vomiting more frequently, than with prostaglandin E_2.

Hysterotomy and Hysterectomy

Because of their prohibitively high morbidity and mortality, hysterotomy and hysterectomy should be used as primary abortion methods only in unique circumstances. For hysterotomy, the abdominal approach is almost exclusively used, since it is technically simpler and allows access to the fallopian tubes for sterilization. Hysterectomy as an abortion method should be restricted to cases in which preexisting gynecologic pathology indicates removal of the uterus. Either the vaginal or abdominal approach may be used, depending on the size of the uterus. Although a hysterectomy provides surgical sterilization as well as abortion, it also entails the risks of major operation, a prolonged recuperation, and substantial expense.

Intrauterine Mechanical Devices

Insertion of a foreign body into the uterus is one of the oldest methods of abortion—and one of the least desirable. Devices used have included catheters, bougies (large, soft rubber catheters), plastic coils, balsa, laminaria tents, and metreurynters. A metreurynter is an intrauterine balloon (similar to a 30-ml Foley catheter) that is introduced through the cervix, inflated with a sterile solution, and then connected to traction at the foot of the woman's bed. All of these methods have the disadvantages of long abortion times and higher infection rates than alternative methods. Hence, none of these should be considered a primary method of abortion. Laminaria may be used to augment other methods when indicated.

Morbidity and Mortality

Satisfactory comparison of the complication rates associated with the principal methods of midtrimester abortion is difficult because of differences in patient populations, treatment protocols, physician experience, and definitions of complications in reported studies. The third phase of the Joint Program for the Study of Abortion (JPSA III) reported a death-to-case ratio of 4.9/100,000 abortions associated with D&E, 9.6/ 100,000 with instillation methods, and 60/100,000 with hysterotomy or hysterectomy (1).

At least six studies have documented the safety of D&E abortions after 12 menstrual weeks. Because D&E abortion does not require delay until 16 weeks of gestation or later, as does instillation abortion, most D&E abortions were performed at 13–16 weeks of gestation, while most instillation abortions were performed at 17 weeks of gestation or later. The later gestational ages necessitated by the choice of an instillation method contributed to the higher complication rates associated with instillation abortions than with D&E abortions. Fever, endometritis, retained products of conception, hemorrhage, and cervical injury requiring repair were each significantly more frequent among women undergoing instillation abortion, whereas uterine perforations were significantly more frequent among women undergoing D&E abortions (1).

Studies that have compared hypertonic saline and urea–$PGF_{2\alpha}$ as intraamniotic abortifacients have had various results. In the JPSA III report, urea–prostaglandin abortions were significantly safer than saline abortions. Most studies suggest that $PGF_{2\alpha}$ produces faster abortions than saline, with higher rates of vomiting, diarrhea, and incomplete abortion. Complications associated with intraamniotic urea augmented with intraamniotic $PGF_{2\alpha}$ or continuous intravenous oxytocin infusion include hemorrhage, infection, gastrointestinal side effects, and cervical lacerations. Use of hypertonic urea may be hypothetically safer than hypertonic saline, because the risk of hypernatremia and sodium load are not present and inadvertent intraperitoneal or intravascular administration may be less toxic. On the other hand, intramyometrial injection of either hypertonic saline or urea results in the same type of muscle necrosis.

Intrauterine mechanical devices are associated with high rates of infection and perforation as well as low rates of abortion. Existing data suggest that further trials of intrauterine mechanical devices are probably unwarranted. Although experience with prostaglandin E_2 suppositories is limited, the morbidity and mortality rates will likely be similar to those of $PGF_{2\alpha}$.

Nationwide abortion mortality surveillance data from 1972–1981 suggest that D&E may be safer than alternative methods of abortion after 12 weeks of gestation. Between 13–15 weeks of gestation, D&E had the lowest death-to-case rates and major operations had the highest rates, with instillation abortions intermediate. At 16–20 weeks, D&E had similar rates to instillation abortions, while major operations had higher rates than either. For all techniques combined, the risk of death increased with advancing gestational age.

Efficacy

Hysterotomy, hysterectomy, and D&E all have success rates approaching 100%. Of the instillation methods, $PGF_{2\alpha}$ may produce a higher proportion of abortions within given time intervals than do unaugmented hypertonic solutions. Although higher rates of abortion are seen at 24 and 48 hours with $PGF_{2\alpha}$ than with hypertonic saline, by 72 hours the rates are similar. For example, at 48 hours, about 86% of women receiving $PGF_{2\alpha}$ and 81% of those receiving saline will have aborted. About 97% of patients will have aborted by 72 hours with either agent. Additional prostaglandin therapy with vaginal prostaglandin E_2 or intramuscular 15-methyl $PGF_{2\alpha}$ may be administered 24 hours after the initial injection. The patient who fails to abort within a reasonable time period after this secondary method has begun may be treated by D&E if a skilled operator is available. Febrile morbidity increases with the length of the induction-to-abortion interval (6). Rarely, hysterotomy may be necessary as a backup method for failed abortion in the late midtrimester. Results will vary depending on the dose schedules and augmentation procedures used.

Acceptability

D&E appears to be more acceptable to women requesting midtrimester abortion than alternative techniques. Compared with instillation techniques, surgical evacuation spares women labor and abortion in bed. D&E usually costs less and takes less time than instillation abortions. Women who have had D&E abortions report less pain and fewer emotional symptoms than those who have undergone instillation abortions. On the other hand, D&E is more emotionally stressful and technically difficult for the physician and staff.

Among instillation techniques, $PGF_{2\alpha}$ alone and urea with $PGF_{2\alpha}$ result in a rapid abortion. At least half of these women, however, experience vomiting or diarrhea. $PGF_{2\alpha}$ is also associated with a higher rate of live-born fetuses than with hypertonic solutions; rates as high as 7% have been documented. The issue of the live-born fetus has become an important ethical, emotional, and medicolegal question.

Summary

D&E is the most common method of midtrimester abortion in the United States, with labor-inducing techniques accounting for most of the remainder. Data suggest that D&E may be faster, safer, and more acceptable to patients than induction of labor. Elucidation of the long-term sequelae of midtrimester abortion is a priority in abortion research.

Gestational age and abortion method are closely interrelated and are the two most important determinants of the safety and expense of the procedure. Early abortions by suction curettage are the safest and least expensive. Delays of any origin, whether administrative, social, or medical, increase the risk and cost. Specifically during the 13–16-week interval, prompt D&E by a skilled operator appears to be preferable to delaying the abortion until 17 weeks or later for an instillation technique.

Regardless of advances in abortion technology, midtrimester terminations are likely to remain more hazardous, expensive, and emotionally disturbing for women than early abortions. Providing prompt pregnancy confirmation, adequate counseling, and inexpensive, accessible first-trimester abortion services will minimize the need for midtrimester abortions.

REFERENCES

1. Centers for Disease Control: Abortion Surveillance 1981. Atlanta, CDC, 1985
2. American College of Obstetricians and Gynecologists: Management of Isoimmunization in Pregnancy (ACOG Technical Bulletin 90). Washington DC, ACOG, 1986
3. Grimes DA, Schulz KF: Morbidity and mortality from second-trimester abortions. J Reprod Med 30(7):505–514, 1985
4. Zatuchni GI, Sciarra JJ, Speidel JJ (eds): Pregnancy Termination: Procedures, safety, and new developments. Hagerstown, Harper & Row, 1979
5. Hern WM: Abortion Practice. Philadelphia, JB Lippincott Co, 1984
6. Berger GS, Brenner WE, Keith LG (eds): Second Trimester Abortion: Perspectives after a decade of experience. Boston, PSG Inc, 1981
7. Weinstein L, Droegemueller W, Greer B: The synergistic effect of calcium and prostaglandin $F_{2\alpha}$ in second trimester abortion: A pilot study. Obstet Gynecol 48(4):469–471, 1976
8. Brenner WE, Berger GS: Pharmacologic methods of producing midtrimester abortion: Risks and benefits. In: Sciarra JJ, Zatuchni GI, Speidel JJ (eds): Risks, Benefits and Controversies in Fertility Control. Hagerstown, Harper & Row, 1978, pp 292–321

This Technical Bulletin was developed under the direction of the Committee on Technical Bulletins of the American College of Obstetricians and Gynecologists as an educational aid to obstetricians and gynecologists. The committee wishes to thank John C. Morrison, MD, for his assistance in the development of this bulletin. This Technical Bulletin does not define a standard of care, nor is it intended to dictate an exclusive course of management. It presents recognized methods and techniques of clinical practice for consideration by obstetrician–gynecologists for incorporation into their practices. Variations of practice taking into account the needs of the individual patient, resources, and limitations unique to the institution or type of practice may be appropriate.

Reviewed February 1991

THE AMERICAN COLLEGE OF OBSTETRICIANS AND GYNECOLOGISTS
409 12th Street, SW
Washington, DC 20024-2188

2345/9012/2345

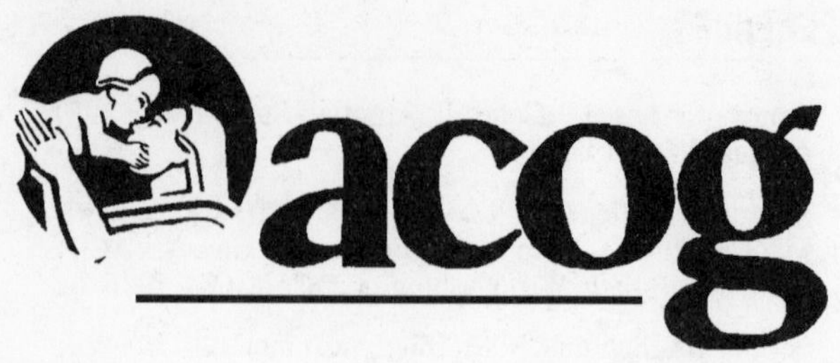

Number 156—June 1991
(Replaces #71, September 1983)

Technical Bulletin

An Educational Aid to Obstetrician–Gynecologists

Nonmalignant Conditions of the Breast

With increasing frequency women expect their obstetrician–gynecologists to assume responsibility for education, screening, counseling, and treatment concerning benign conditions of the breast. The obstetrician–gynecologist is in a favorable position to diagnose breast disease and should have a good understanding of the natural history as well as the diagnosis and treatment of these conditions. Established screening guidelines should be followed to allow early detection of breast cancer (1). The final diagnosis of a breast mass rests on histologic examination. Physical examination, imaging, and cytologic evaluations all contribute information but are not definitive.

This bulletin discusses the management of the signs and symptoms of breast disease and the basic postulates that are critical to the understanding of benign conditions of the breast. The need for patient education and counseling regarding self-examination should be stressed in any management protocol.

Diagnosis

The evaluation of breast disease is based on risk factors and age and is determined by history, physical examination, imaging studies, cytologic examination, and open biopsy.

History

In assessing benign conditions of the breast, attention should be focused on the following factors:

- Duration and onset of signs and symptoms
- Menstrual and reproductive history
- Hormone use
- Dietary habits

Factors that increase the risk of breast cancer should also be considered:

- Increased age
- Previous history of breast cancer
- Nulliparity
- Delayed childbearing (>30 years of age)
- Early menarche (before age 12)
- Late menopause (after age 53)
- Family history of breast cancer (first-degree relatives)
- Biopsy-proven ductal or lobular hyperplasia, particularly with atypia
- Higher socioeconomic status
- Obesity

Physical Examination

A visual examination should be performed while the patient is sitting or standing with her hands on her hips. The symmetry and contour of the breasts, position of the nipples, skin changes or scars, and appearance of a mass should be noted. The axillary and supraclavicular areas should be palpated to detect adenopathy. To assess any palpable dominant mass, the examiner should use the fingertips to palpate all of the breast tissue with the patient in both the upright and supine positions. To complete the examination, the examiner should check for nipple discharge; this may be difficult to elicit unless the patient is in an upright position. All positive findings should be documented in writing or with an appropriate drawing.

Imaging Techniques

Mammography can be used both as a screening technique and as a diagnostic method for symptomatic patients. Significant findings consist of alterations in density of breast tissue, calcifications, thickening of the skin, fibrous streaks, and nipple changes. Some of these mammography patterns may suggest early carcinoma and warrant further evaluation. Mammography can also aid in the identification of fibroadenomas, lymph nodes, or other benign masses such as a galactocele or areas of fat necrosis.

If a cystic mass is seen on mammography, ultrasound can characterize it with greater accuracy than mammography, particularly in the identification of a cystic structure. The technique, however, cannot identify microcalcifications, which can be hallmarks of early carcinoma.

Biopsy and Needle Aspiration

Excisional biopsy and needle aspiration are useful for both diagnosis and treatment of benign breast conditions. Needle aspiration of palpable macrocysts can be performed in an office setting, and local anesthesia is usually not necessary. Cytologic evaluation should be performed based on mammographic appearance and clinical features of the mass, the patient's age, history of breast disease, and risk factors. About 0.1–1% of cytologic specimens of breast fluid aspirations show evidence of malignancy. Most studies suggest a very low (0.2–0.5%) occurrence of intracystic carcinoma (2–4). It may be reasonable to perform repeat aspiration of a recurrent macrocyst, but if the lesion recurs twice, excision is warranted. Excisional biopsy is mandatory if a persistent mass eludes precise diagnosis with alternative means.

To aspirate a palpable mass, the lesion is immobilized with the fingers, and a 22–24-gauge needle is inserted. Occasionally a larger needle may be required because of the viscosity of the cyst fluid. If fluid is present, it should be aspirated and the needle withdrawn. If the mass is solid, several passes can be made through the mass while aspirating, until a small amount of fluid or tissue is seen in the syringe. The needle should be withdrawn and the specimen placed on a slide for cytologic evaluation. The method of slide preparation should be approved by the interpreting pathologist before preparation of slides for cytologic evaluation and handling of cyst fluid is started in an office setting.

Open biopsy is required if any of the following findings are present:

- Bloody cyst fluid on aspiration
- Failure of mass to disappear completely upon fluid aspiration
- Recurrence of cyst after one or two aspirations
- Solid dominant mass not diagnosed as fibroadenoma
- Bloody nipple discharge
- Nipple ulceration or persistent crusting
- Skin edema and erythema suspicious of inflammatory breast carcinoma

Open biopsy should be performed by specially trained personnel. Local anesthesia is preferred. The specimen should be sent for histologic analysis in order to determine the biologic characteristics of the tumor. The margins of the lesion should be carefully marked. If the biopsy is positive for carcinoma, estrogen and progesterone receptor studies and DNA evaluations should be completed.

Clinical Conditions

Fibrocystic Change

Fibrocystic change, the most common benign condition of the breast, occurs in approximately 10% of women under age 21 but becomes much more common in the premenopausal period. There is usually a regression of some of the signs of fibrocystic change during menopause, but it is common to find residual characteristics of the condition at the time of breast biopsy in postmenopausal women. The common symptoms are pain and tenderness and are usually bilateral and most often localized in the upper, outer quadrants of the breasts. They are noted most often during the 7–14 days of the premenstrual phase of the cycle. In 85–90% of women with significant fibrocystic change, discomfort is the leading symptom. Pain is due to breast stromal edema, ductal dilation, and some inflammatory response, with an increase in breast size noted in some women. The differential diagnosis of breast pain includes intercostal neuralgia, usually associated with respiratory infections; stretching of Cooper ligaments, noted with pendulous, large breasts; and chronic costochondritis.

The interactive etiologic factors contributing to fibrocystic change remain speculative. The ingestion of medications or foods containing methylxanthines is thought to inhibit cyclic adenosine 5'-monophosphate (cAMP) and cyclic guanosine 5'-monophosphate (cGMP) phosphodiesterase, leading to accumulation of increased amounts of cAMP and cGMP. High levels of cAMP and cGMP have been detected in patients with fibrocystic change and breast cancer (5, 6). Dietary ingestion of up to 500 mg of caffeine (the equivalent of four to five cups of coffee) has been associated with an increased risk of fibrocystic change (7). In some studies, reduction of dietary methylxanthines has been associated with a subjective reduction in pain, tenderness, and palpable nodularity, with exacerbation of symptoms upon resumption of methylxanthine ingestion (7). Other studies have failed to show a benefit from decreased methylxanthine ingestion.

The histologic characteristics of fibrocystic changes include cystic and epithelial proliferation within the ductal system plus stromal fibrosis. Proliferative changes of ductal or lobular structures, particularly those associated with atypia, are associated with an increased incidence of carcinoma.

Nonproliferative Changes

Cystic change refers to dilation of the ducts in the subareolar, lobular, or lobe areas. Most common is the development of microcysts 2 mm or less in size, which are often asymptomatic and do not produce clinical findings. Approximately 20–40% of microcysts progress to form macrocysts, probably as a result of aberrant endogenous hormonal stimulation.

Macrocysts often go unnoticed unless a patient performs breast self-examination on a regular basis or is aware of unique pain or tenderness associated with the development of menses. Although these cysts may regress after menses, they often return in the next cycle. Large macrocysts are more common in women in the later menstrual years and tend to undergo some degree of reduction in the postmenopausal period.

Fibrous change as a pure entity is very infrequent but generally occurs in the menstrual years. It is characterized by a firm, palpable mass that is usually located in the upper outer quadrant of the breast. The mass is generally 2–3 cm in size and develops following an inflammatory response to ductal irritation (8).

Proliferative Changes

Hyperplasia of ductal epithelium can be a simple proliferation with layering of the cells, occasionally three to five layers thick. On occasion, nuclear atypia may occur and is associated with a fivefold increase in the risk of breast cancer. Generally, these changes are noted when biopsy of a macrocyst formation is performed because of a persistent mass or abnormal calcifications detected at the time of screening mammography.

Adenosis is another proliferative pattern and is due to changes in the acini in the distal mammary lobule. These small ducts are often surrounded by a dense, fibrotic tissue that forms a firm, hard, plaque-like area, referred to as *sclerosing adenosis*. These areas are more common in women in their 30s and 40s and can easily be confused with a palpable early malignancy.

On occasion, ductal proliferation will result in an intraductal *papilloma*. These lesions are also more common in the later menstrual years but can continue up to age 65 or greater. Twenty to fifty percent of papillomas are accompanied by a serosanguineous nipple discharge, and up to 90% by a small, palpable mass adjacent to the areola, from which blood is seen effluxing on the nipple surface. Intraductal papillomas are rarely associated with a concurrent or subsequent papillary carcinoma but require excision to rule out the possibility of malignancy.

Management

Principles of management for fibrocystic changes include regular examinations, appropriate imaging, and medication, as well as excisional biopsy, when indicated. For minimal to moderate discomfort, a well-fitted brassiere with good support may be all that is necessary. This is particularly important for women who are physically active, such as runners.

Dietary modification may be useful. Specifically, restriction of methylxanthines may produce subjective improvement in as many as 65% of patients. The use of vitamins A and E has been touted as beneficial. A dose of 150,000 IU of vitamin A daily for 3 months has been suggested for patients with fibrocystic breast changes (9). In contrast, a study in which patients took 150, 300, and 600 IU of *dl*-α-tocopherol (vitamin E) per day for 2 months showed no improvement in symptoms of mammary dysplasia in patients with changes in the breast skin, pain, and subjective tenderness (10). Data regarding vitamins A and E are confusing, and it is difficult to state with certainty that either produces a significant, measurable benefit.

Diuretic therapy can be useful for moderate premenstrual mastalgia. This is of temporary benefit only and must be used on a regular, ongoing, monthly basis. Fluid retention is a result of cyclic hormonal stimulation. Analgesics such as ibuprofen (or other, similar agents), salicylates, or acetaminophen also may be helpful.

Oral contraceptives suppress symptoms of fibrocystic changes in 70–90% of patients with fibrocystic changes. Symptoms recur in up to 40% of patients when oral contraceptives are discontinued (11). Synthetic progestins may also be helpful. One study reported benefits in 80–85% of patients when medroxyprogesterone acetate, 5–10 mg, was used. When the medication was discontinued, however, 30–40% had a recurrence of symptoms. Undesirable side effects of hormonal therapy include weight gain, depression, abnormal bleeding, and alteration in lipid profile and may limit this therapy.

Other agents are of potential benefit but, because of their significant side effects, should be reserved for those patients in whom previous therapy has failed. Of these agents, bromocriptine is thought to be particularly useful, with an efficacy comparable to that of hormonal therapy.

Danazol (17α-norethisterone) in doses of 100–400 mg per day has also been reported to be effective. Unfortunately, the side effects are disturbing, compliance is poor, and symptoms recur after the medication is stopped (12, 13).

Fibroadenomas

Fibroadenomas are the most common lesions found in women under the age of 25 and are the second most common benign lesion of the breast. Fibroadenomas persist throughout the menstrual years, but there appears to be some regression in the postmenopausal period. Patients may palpate a mass, growth is generally gradual, and there may be occasional cyclic tenderness. Treatment by excisional biopsy is appropriate if the lesion is palpable, increasing in size, or psychologically disturbing. For women under age 25 with small palpable fibroadenomas, careful observation may be considered in selected situations. For very small masses that are identified as fibroadenomas by mammography or ultrasound and are not palpable, conservative management is appropriate. In either situation, the classical appearance of the lesion should be documented by imaging before a course of management is determined. Only 119 cases of carcinoma within a fibroadenoma have been reported in the world literature (14).

Phyllodes Tumor

Phyllodes tumor is an uncommon, generally slow-growing lesion representing both epithelial and stromal proliferation. It can occur in women of any age but is most common in premenopausal women. Although, like fibroadenomas, it is a fibroepithelial tumor, generally it is larger and contains a different type of connective tissue. In general, this connective tissue is hypercellular and has increased pleomorphism and mitotic activity. The cellularity of the connective tissue is the distinguishing characteristic of this tumor (15).

The clinical course of a phyllodes tumor is variable and often unpredictable. Attempts to determine the degree of potential malignancy by evaluating cellularity and pleomorphism have not met with uniform success. Approximately 10% of all phyllodes tumors contain some characteristics suggestive of a frankly malignant process. By far, however, most demonstrate equivocal histopathologic characteristics or appear benign. Rarely, a phyllodes tumor with a benign histologic appearance unexpectedly metastasizes and produces a lethal outcome. Phyllodes tumor should be treated by total excision with a wide margin of healthy tissue. Radical mastectomy or modified procedures are not indicated.

Superficial Thrombophlebitis

Superficial thrombophlebitis (Mondor disease) is an uncommon, benign process (16). Although it is usually associated with pregnancy, breast trauma, or operative procedures such as biopsy or mammary augmentation or reduction, it may also occur spontaneously. It presents as acute pain with erythema, usually in the upper lateral portion of the breast, and is most often associated with a superficial thrombophlebitis in the thoracoepigastric vein, which drains the upper outer quadrant of the breast. Occasionally, fibrosis occurs adjacent to the linear lesion, causing some skin retraction. The diagnosis is made on the basis of predisposing conditions and a characteristic linear, tender, erythematous mass.

Treatment is conservative, and biopsy is not necessary; analgesics and application of heat are effective in relieving discomfort. The condition resolves in 1–3 weeks. If perivenous fibrosis is not extensive, the breast returns to a normal appearance following resolution of inflammatory symptoms. Extensive perivenous fibrosis may cause some skin retraction superficial to the area of inflammation.

Mastitis

Mastitis is most common in lactating women, but it also may occur in nonpuerperal women, usually in association with galactorrhea. Common skin organisms such as *Staphylococcus aureus* and *Streptococcus* species may cause infection of the nipple and breast ducts. Nosocomial colonization of the infant is often associated with penicillin-resistant strains (17, 18) and may eventually lead to mastitis in the nursing mother. Patients typically present with tenderness, induration, and erythema of the breast, along with fever. If symptoms are acute or the patient demonstrates signs of severe sepsis, prompt implementation of appropriate intravenous antibiotic therapy is necessary, usually starting with a drug to treat resistant staphylococcal infection, such as dicloxacillin. During the puerperium, patients should be encouraged to breast-feed their infants from the unaffected breast and to express milk from the affected breast. If the infection does not resolve and an abscess forms, incision and drainage are mandatory. Appropriate aerobic and anaerobic cultures should be obtained at the time of drainage.

Galactocele

A galactocele is manifested as a cystic area with inspissated milk material. It usually occurs as a cystic, centrally located swelling developing shortly after the abrupt termination of lactation. Fluid accumulated within a galactocele and its fibrous capsule may appear clear or milky white. If present for an extended period, this material may become greenish yellow and appear purulent. When cultured, however, the material is generally sterile. In some patients, expression of the material in the galactocele, with temporary relief of the condition, may result when pressure is applied over the nodular area. Usually, however, the mass will recur. Initial treatment may include needle aspiration, but if the condition recurs, excision is necessary to avoid infection and abscess formation, as well as the development of calcifications that could be misinterpreted on mammography as early carcinoma.

Duct Ectasia

Duct ectasia is a condition usually occurring in perimenopausal or postmenopausal women. The patient may present with a tender, hard, erythematous mass adjacent to the areola in association with burning, itching, or a sensation of pulling in the nipple area. A thick, greenish-black discharge may be present. Histologic evaluation of the area shows dilated, distended terminal collecting ducts obstructed with inspissated, lipid-containing epithelial cells and phagocytic histiocytes. Occasionally, small abscesses form at the base of the nipple as a result of this infection. Treatment is excisional biopsy, although occasionally the symptoms dissipate when manual compression is applied to the nipple.

Subareolar Abscess

A subareolar abscess occurs most commonly in younger women. In this condition, the squamous epithelium of the terminal dilated portions of the collecting ducts (milk sinuses) located in the nipple structure undergo squamous metaplasia. Keratin is formed, plugging the duct and leading to accumulation of material in the duct, inflammation, and often, abscess formation at the base of the nipple. This condition is not associated with lactation. The small, abscessed area appears as a chronic inflammation and often recurs. Although antibiotics and incision and drainage may help, they will not permanently resolve the condition. Excision of the abscessed cavity and adjacent ductal structures is necessary.

Fat Necrosis

Fat necrosis is often associated with trauma to the breast and usually presents as a tender, firm mass that does not increase in size. The irregular mass is usually palpable, causes skin retraction, and may show multiple, small, stippled calcification on mammography. The clinical presentation and mammographic appearance may mimic those of carcinoma, requiring excisional biopsy.

Summary

The evaluation of benign conditions of the breast requires constant vigilance in relation to diagnosis, treatment, and, importantly, exclusion of carcinoma. Fortunately, the clinical presentation and epidemiologic considerations of the various benign lesions of the breast provide information permitting a fairly precise diagnosis. Fibrocystic changes, with its various subconditions, certainly is the most prominent benign condition, but other benign alterations occurring in the breast are also somewhat common.

The management of fibroadenomas requires precise judgment and depends partly on the patient's age and the characteristics of the growth. Acute infections such as mastitis require prompt intervention and treatment. Recurring infections such as a subareolar abscess should be treated specifically in an aggressive and definitive manner. Infrequently occurring problems such as superficial thrombophlebitis, galactocele, and fat necrosis can be very uncomfortable, and occasionally, their diagnosis will be more difficult to establish. They, however, demand accurate diagnosis and definitive treatment. The axiom of excisional biopsy and histologic evaluation of any lesion that does not respond to treatment is the most important guideline in the treatment of benign breast disease.

REFERENCES

1. American College of Obstetricians and Gynecologists. The role of the obstetrician–gynecologist in the diagnosis of breast disease. ACOG Committee Opinion 67. Washington, DC: ACOG, 1989

2. McSwain GR, Valicenti JF Jr, O'Brien PH. Cytologic evaluation of breast cysts. Surg Gynecol Obstet 1978;146: 921–925

3. Abramson DJ. A clinical evaluation of aspirations of cysts of the breast. Surg Gynecol Obstet 1974;139:531–537

4. Hindle WH, Navin J. Breast aspiration cytology: a neglected gynecologic procedure. Am J Obstet Gynecol 1983;146:482–487

5. Minton JP, Foeking MK, Webster DJ, Matthews RH. Response of fibrocystic disease to caffeine withdrawal and correlation of cyclic nucleotides with breast disease. Am J Obstet Gynecol 1979;135:157–158

6. Phelps HM, Phelps CE. Caffeine ingestion and breast cancer: a negative correlation. Cancer 1988;61:1051–1054

7. Boyle CA, Berkowitz GS, LiVolsi VA, Ort S, Merino MJ, White C, et al. Caffeine consumption and fibrocystic breast disease: a case-control epidemiologic study. J Natl Cancer Institute 1984;72(5):1015–1019

8. Drukker BH, DeMendonca W. Benign disease of the breast. In: Sciarra JW, ed. Gynecology and obstetrics. Philadelphia: Harper & Row, 1988

9. Band PR, Deschamps M, Falardeau M, Ladoucer J, Cote J. Treatment of benign breast disease with vitamin A. Preventive Medicine 1984:13:549–554

10. London RS, Sundaram GS, Murphy L, Manimekalai S, Reynolds M, Goldstein PJ. The effect of vitamin E on mammary dysplasia: a double blind study. Obstet Gynecol 1985;65:104–106

11. Vorherr H. Fibrocystic breast disease: pathophysiology, pathomorphology, clinical picture, and management. Am J Obstet Gynecol 1986;154(1):161–179

12. Nezhat C, Asch R, Greenblatt RB. Danazol for benign breast disease. Am J Obstet Gynecol 1980;137(5):604–607

13. Tobiassen T, Rasmussen T, Döberl A, Rannevik G. Danazol treatment of severely symptomatic fibrocystic breast disease and long-term follow-up—the Hjørring project. Acta Obstet Gynecol Scan Suppl 1984;123: 159–176

14. Yoshida Y, Takaoka M, Fukumoto M. Carcinoma arising in fibroadenoma: case report and review of the world literature. J Surg Oncol 1985;29132–140

15. Azzopardi JG. Sarcomas of the breast. In: Azzopardi JG, ed. Problems in breast pathology. London: W. B. Saunders, 1979:346

16. Haagensen CD. Thrombophlebitis of the superficial veins of the breast (Mondor's disease). In: Haagensen CD, ed. Diseases of the breast. Philadelphia: W. B. Saunders, 1986:379

17. Devereux WP. Acute puerperal mastitis: evaluation of its management. Am J Obstet Gynecol 1970;108:78–81

18. Brook L. Microbiology of non-puerperal breast abscesses. J Infect Dis 1988;157:377–379

This Technical Bulletin was developed under the direction of the Committee on Technical Bulletins of the American College of Obstetricians and Gynecologists as an educational aid to obstetricians and gynecologists. The committee wishes to thank Bruce H. Drukker, MD, for his assistance in the development of this bulletin. This Technical Bulletin does not define a standard of care, nor is it intended to dictate an exclusive course of management. It presents recognized methods and techniques of clinical practice for consideration by obstetrician–gynecologists for incorporation into their practices. Variations of practice taking into account the needs of the individual patient, resources, and limitations unique to the institution or type of practice may be appropriate.

Reviewed February 1994

THE AMERICAN COLLEGE OF OBSTETRICIANS AND GYNECOLOGISTS
409 12th Street, SW
Washington, DC 20024-2188

56789/87654

ACOG EDUCATIONAL BULLETIN

Number 229, October 1996

Nutrition and Women

The obstetrician–gynecologist is in an excellent position to improve women's health through attention to nutrition. This role involves nutritional assessment and education to promote reproductive and general health and to help prevent chronic disease. It also involves management of eating disorders and certain other health problems in which nutritional factors are involved.

This Educational Bulletin was developed under the direction of the Committee on Educational Bulletins of the American College of Obstetricians and Gynecologists as an aid to obstetricians and gynecologists. The College wishes to thank Ronald A. Chez, MD, and Carol W. Suitor, DSc, for their assistance in the development of this bulletin. This document is not to be construed as establishing a standard of practice or dictating an exclusive course of treatment. Rather, it is intended as an educational tool that presents current information on obstetric–gynecologic issues.

Nutrition-Related Health Problems

A woman's eating practices may influence her risk of cardiovascular disease, several types of cancer, diabetes mellitus, and osteoporosis, all of which are major causes of morbidity and mortality in the United States. Eating practices, along with physical activity, have a major effect on whether a woman is over-weight or obese. It has been found that even slight increases over the ideal weight pose health risks to women (1). Over the past 10–15 years, the prevalence of overweight among nonpregnant women aged 20–74 years increased from 26.5% to 34.9% (2). Data from 1988–1991 indicate that the prevalence of overweight increases gradually with age, from approximately 20% for women aged 20–29 years to 52% for women aged 50–59 years (2). Overweight is a particular problem among some minority groups. For example, non-Hispanic black women and Mexican–American women aged 20 years and older have a higher prevalence of overweight (48.5% and 47.2%, respectively) than do non-Hispanic white women (32.1%) (2).

On average, the U.S. population consumes higher-than-recommended amounts of fat (about 34% of their calories compared with the recommended level of 30%) and lower-than-recommended amounts of fiber (3). These eating habits are likely to increase their risk of cardiovascular disease and cancer. In general, women eat much less than the recommended amount of fruits and vegetables, especially if their income is low. Low fruit and vegetable consumption limits intake of many nutrients, such as folic acid and fiber, and is usually accompanied by excessive fat intake.

Undernutrition is relatively uncommon in the United States. It is more prevalent among low-income women in their childbearing years whose diet may be low in protein, vitamins A and C, folate, calcium, and iron (4). Data

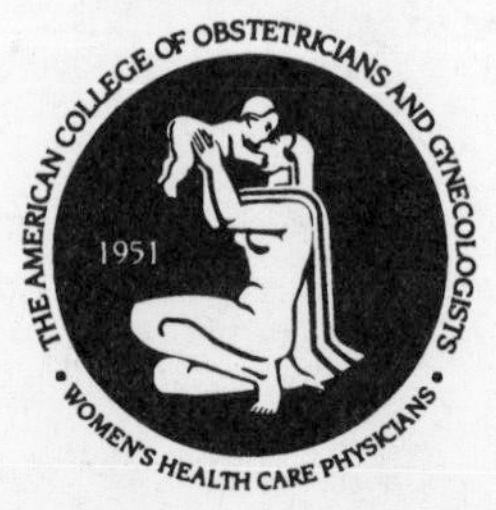

from the Second and Third National Health and Nutrition Examination Surveys indicated that approximately 6% of African–American adolescent and adult women and 5% of non-Hispanic whites had iron deficiency (5). A 12% prevalence of iron deficiency among Mexican-American women was also found.

At any one time, approximately 40% of women report that they are dieting—even though many of them are at normal weight (6). Severe eating disorders, such as anorexia nervosa, bulimia nervosa, and binge eating disorder, are seen most often in young women. Affected women may visit an obstetrician–gynecologist because of such associated reproductive abnormalities as amenorrhea, oligomenorrhea, and infertility.

Nutritional Recommendations and Guidelines

Nutrient and Food Intake

Since 1941, recommended dietary allowances (RDAs) have been used as nutrient reference values for populations and as goals for good nutrition (7). Some RDAs differ by age group, and most values are increased to meet the needs of pregnant or lactating women (Table 1). Because RDAs are judged to be adequate to meet the known nutrient needs of practically all healthy persons, the values are higher than the amounts required by some individuals.

Table 1. 1989 Recommended Dietary Allowances for Women

	Age in Years				Physiologic Status		
Nutrient	**15–18**	**19–24**	**25–50**	**51+**	**Pregnant**	**Lactating 1st 6 mo**	**Lactating 2nd 6 mo**
Protein, g	44	46	50	50	60	65	62
Vitamin A, μg RE*	800	800	800	800	800	1,300	1,200
Vitamin D, μg†	10	10	5	5	10	10	10
Vitamin E, mg α-TE‡	8	8	8	8	10	12	11
Vitamin K, μg	55	60	65	65	65	65	65
Vitamin C, mg	60	60	60	60	70	95	90
Thiamin, mg	1.1	1.1	1.1	1.0	1.5	1.6	1.6
Riboflavin, mg	1.3	1.3	1.3	1.2	1.6	1.8	1.7
Niacin, mg NE§	15	15	15	13	17	20	20
Vitamin B_6, mg	1.5	1.6	1.6	1.6	2.2	2.1	2.1
Folate, μg	180	180	180	180	400	280	260
Vitamin B_{12}, μg	2.0	2.0	2.0	2.0	2.2	2.6	2.6
Calcium, mg	1,200	1,200	800	800	1,200	1,200	1,200
Phosphorus, mg	1,200	1,200	800	800	1,200	1,200	1,200
Magnesium, mg	300	280	280	280	300	355	340
Iron, mg	15	15	15	10	30	15	15
Zinc, mg	12	12	12	12	15	19	16
Iodine, μg	150	150	150	150	175	200	200
Selenium, μg	50	55	55	55	65	75	75

*Retinol equivalents. 1 retinol equivalent = 1 μg retinol or 6 μg β-carotene.

†As cholecalciferol. 10 μg cholecalciferol = 400 IU of vitamin D.

‡α-Tocopherol equivalents. 1 mg D-α-tocopherol = 1 α-TE.

§1 NE (niacin equivalent) = 1 mg of niacin or 60 mg of dietary tryptophan.

Modified with permission from Recommended Dietary Allowances: 10th ed. Copyright 1989 by the National Academy of Sciences. Courtesy of the National Academy Press, Washington, D.C.

Dietary Guidelines for Americans

Eat a variety of foods.

Balance the food you eat with physical activity–maintain or improve your weight.

Choose a diet with plenty of grain products, vegetables, and fruits.

Choose a diet low in fat, saturated fat, and cholesterol.

Choose a diet moderate in sugars.

Choose a diet moderate in salt and sodium.

If you drink alcoholic beverages, do so in moderation.

U.S. Department of Agriculture, U.S. Department of Health and Human Services. Nutrition and your health: dietary guidelines for Americans. 4th ed. Home and Garden Bulletin no. 232. Washington, DC: U.S. Government Printing Office, 1995

The focus of *Dietary Guidelines for Americans*, a joint publication of the U.S. Department of Agriculture and the U.S. Department of Health and Human Services, is on foods rather than nutrients (8). These guidelines provide advice about eating to stay healthy (see the box). To achieve variety, the guidelines recommend eating foods from the following five major food groups daily: 1) vegetables, 2) fruits, 3) breads and cereals, 4) milk products, and 5) high-protein foods such as meats, poultry, fish, dry beans and peas, eggs, and nuts. A food pyramid has been developed to illustrate desirable quantities of these foods to consume each day (9) (Fig. 1).

Weight for Height

Increasingly, body mass index (BMI) is being used in establishing reference levels for body weight for women and men. Body mass index is computed as weight (in

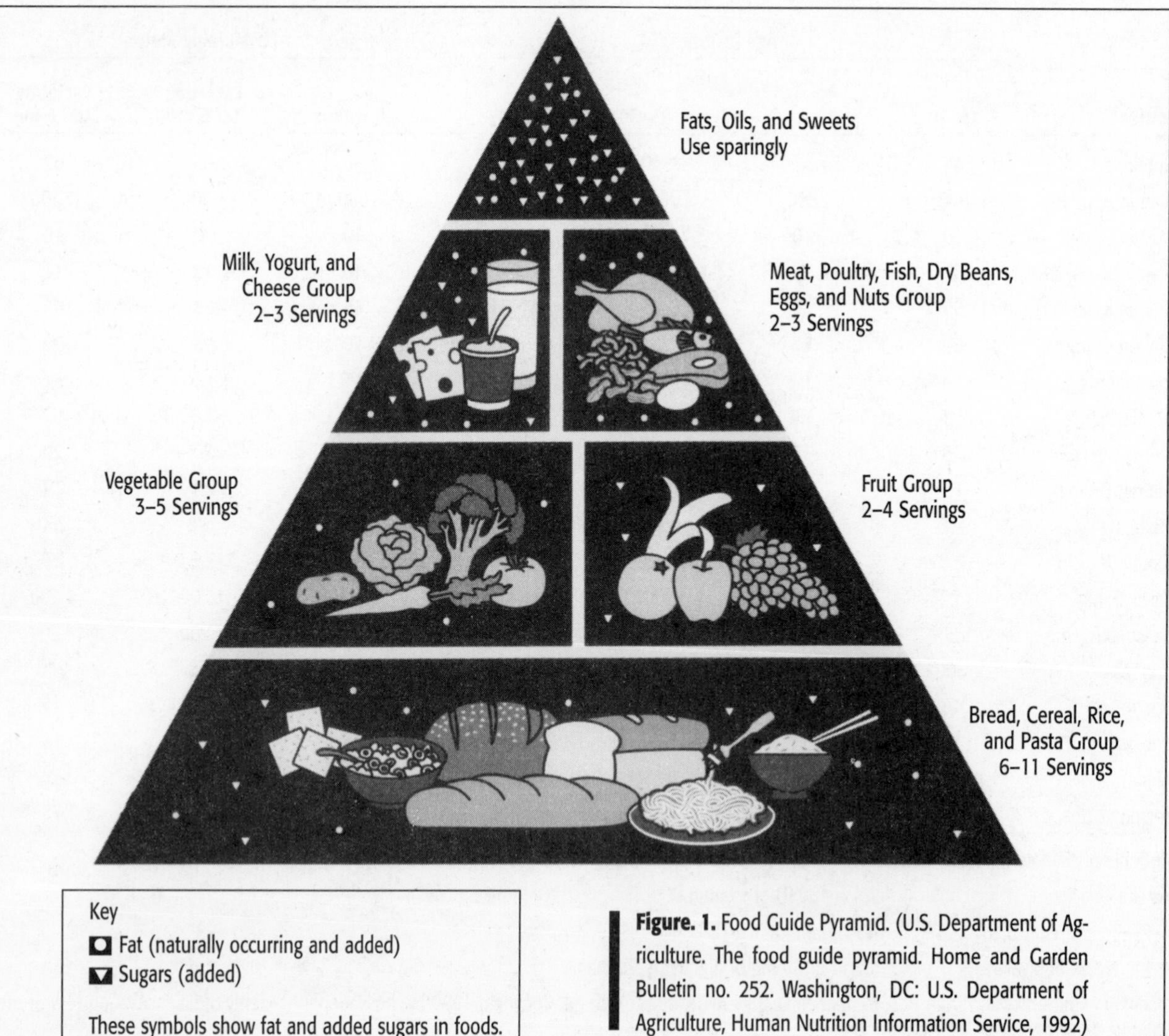

Figure. 1. Food Guide Pyramid. (U.S. Department of Agriculture. The food guide pyramid. Home and Garden Bulletin no. 252. Washington, DC: U.S. Department of Agriculture, Human Nutrition Information Service, 1992)

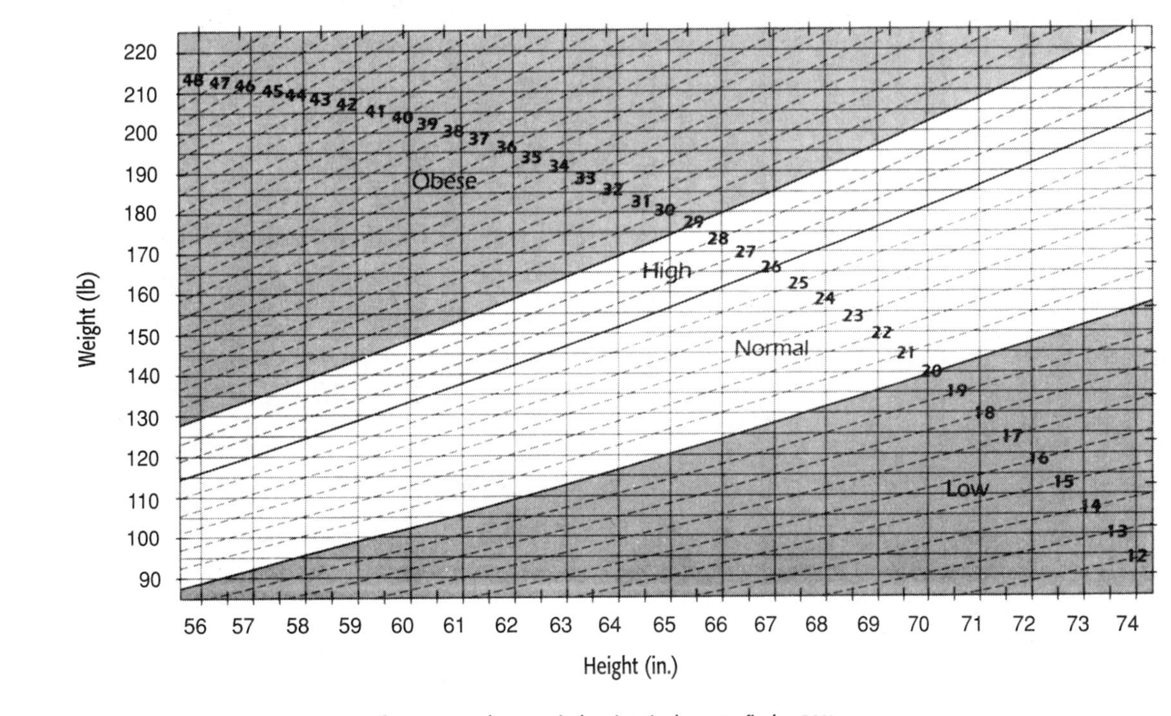

Figure 2. Body mass index (BMI) chart. To find a BMI category (eg, obese), find the point where the height and weight intersect. To estimate BMI, read the bold number on the dashed line that is closest to this point. (Institute of Medicine. Subcommittee for a Clinical Application Guide, Committee on Nutritional Status During Pregnancy and Lactation, Food and Nutrition Board, and the National Academy of Sciences. Nutrition during pregnancy and lactation. Washington, DC: National Academy Press, 1992)

kilograms) divided by height in meters squared. Using pounds and inches, multiply the division results by 700. Charts are available to eliminate the need to calculate BMI (Fig. 2). In a study by the Institute of Medicine, BMI cutoff values were used to determine prepregnancy weight-for-height status as follows (10):

- Underweight (<19.8)
- Normal weight (19.8–26.0)
- Overweight (26.0–29.0)
- Obese (>29.0)

The cutoff value for overweight used by the National Center for Health Statistics is equal to or greater than 27.3 (11). This value is approximately 120% of the midpoint of desirable weight for height from the 1983 Metropolitan Height and Weight tables for women (12).

The distribution of body fat appears to have a strong association with health. Women who have excess fat in the abdomen appear to be at greater risk for cardiovascular disease and diabetes mellitus than are those with excess fat in the hips and thighs (13).

Nutritional Assessment

Data that are useful in a nutritional assessment can be collected readily during the routine examination. This may involve asking a few extra questions, taking an extra measurement, and closely observing the patient for signs of nutritional problems.

History

When obtaining a medical history, the physician should take special note of nutrition-related illnesses (such as diabetes mellitus) that require diet modification. Food allergies, menorrhagia, use of prescription and nonpre-

Risk Factors for Nutritional Problems

Low income
Adolescence
Cigarette smoking
Substance abuse
Frequent dieting, fasting, or meal skipping
Vegan (complete vegetarian) diet
Pica
High parity
Menorrhagia
Physical or mental illness, including depression
Use of certain medications, such as phenytoin
Mental retardation
Problems with chewing, swallowing, or mobility
Decreased sense of smell or taste
Elderliness
Disability
Cancer and treatment
Chronic diseases

scription medications, parity, and recent pregnancy and lactation may influence diet and nutritional status (see box: "Risk Factors for Nutritional Problems").

A questionnaire may be a useful device in obtaining information about a patient's nutritional status (see box: "Sample Questions for Basic Nutrition and Lifestyle History"). Depending on the woman's responses, the physician can then ask related questions as needed.

Special attention should be directed to detecting the avoidance of all animal foods (vegan, or complete vegetarian, diet), frequent binging or crash dieting, or erratic eating patterns. The early manifestations of anorexia include an inappropriate and excessive concern about body image with a refusal to maintain body weight at a minimal normal level for the patient's age and height. Several questions in the box can provide clues to detect indications of an eating disorder.

Questions about physical activity and a planned program of exercise provide information that is valuable in assessing energy balance, likelihood of acquiring or losing fat, and risk of diseases such as osteoporosis and cardiovascular disease. Once the patient's needs have been identified, a management plan should be developed. Published resources exist that can be helpful in formulating the management plan (14, 15).

Sample Questions for Basic Nutrition and Lifestyle History

What did you eat and drink yesterday?

Do you avoid any foods for religious reasons? For health reasons? Which ones?

Do you drink alcoholic beverages? How often? How much?

Do you take any vitamin, mineral, or food supplements? What kind? How much?

Do you exercise? What kind? How often?

Do you smoke cigarettes?

Has your weight changed in the past 5 years? How?

Are you trying to lose (or gain) weight? How? Why?

How often do you skip meals?

Do you eat breakfast?

Does it bother you to know that you are going to be weighed?

Do you ever force yourself to vomit? Use laxatives or diuretics to lose weight?

Are you on a special diet? What kind? Why?

Do you have problems with planning and preparing meals for yourself or your family? If so, for what reasons:

- Too little time?
- Poor access to shopping?
- Financial constraints?
- Lack of equipment and space for storing food or preparing meals?
- Anything else?

The nutritional assessment addresses the use of harmful substances, including cigarettes, alcohol, and illicit drugs, because they have both direct and indirect effects on nutritional status. For example, smoking cigarettes increases the metabolic rate and changes lipoprotein lipase activity; thus, smoking cessation tends to lead to weight gain—a fact of great concern to many women. Smoking also increases the requirement for such nutrients as vitamin C and zinc, but nutrient intake tends to be lower for those who smoke than for nonsmokers. Alcohol provides 7 kcal/g and may interfere with the body's absorption, use, or excretion of such nutrients as vitamin A, thiamin, folic acid, and zinc (7). Stimulant drugs such as amphetamines and cocaine may contribute to low overall nutrient and energy intake while increasing energy requirements.

Physical Examination

Nutritional assessment includes accurate determination of height and weight, calculation of BMI, estimation of the distribution of body fat, and close observation for abnormalities of the teeth, gums, throat, or skin. The presence of physical illness or disability should be noted as well; physical illness may alter certain nutrient requirements, and disability may affect energy needs.

The physical examination may reveal findings that help direct the practitioner to the diagnosis of an eating disorder. Bulimic patients may have enlarged parotids, erosion of tooth enamel, lacerations of the hard palate, and signs of hypokalemia, including cardiac arrhythmias and hypotension. Physical findings in patients with anorexia nervosa may include dry skin with lanugo (hair), yellow palms, hypothermia, bradycardia, and hypotension. The obstetrician–gynecologist should assess whether a patient with an eating disorder is at risk of death. Indications for hospitalization may include 1) pulse less than 40 beats per minute, 2) temperature less than 36°C, and 3) systolic blood pressure less than 70 mm Hg. Patients with eating disorders should be treated on an inpatient or outpatient basis by an experienced multidisciplinary eating disorder team (16).

The estimate of a person's body fat usually is derived from subtracting lean body mass from total body weight. Lean body mass measurements through the use of total body water and total body potassium content are not clinically practical. The valid use of skinfold-thickness measurements with calipers requires extensive training, standardization tables, and purposeful monitoring for reproducibility. Therefore, most clinicians do not find this tool helpful. Newer methods to estimate body fat such as total body electric conductivity, bioelectric impedance analysis, and computerized axial tomography may become available in a form useful for office practice (17).

To quantify the body distribution of fat, the waist-to-hip ratio can be determined by the following method:

- Using a nonstretch tape, measure the waist in a horizontal plane at a point that is palpated and marked just above the right ilium on the midaxillary line (18). (This is below the point where the measurement is smallest.)
- Measure the hips at the maximum posterior extension between the iliac crest and buttocks.
- Divide the waist measurement by the hip measurement.

A value of one or more suggests an increased health risk compared with risk from the excess weight alone.

Routine laboratory tests are not helpful in screening for nutritional problems. Some tests (eg, hemoglobin, hematocrit, blood glucose, lipid profile) may be appropriate based on the history and physical examination. Radiographic assessment of bone density may be indicated for women who are at high risk for osteoporosis who do not take estrogen (19).

Patient Education, Counseling, and Referral

Patient education and counseling should focus on a healthy and complete diet. *Dietary Guidelines for Americans* (see the box) and the Food Guide Pyramid (Fig. 1) provide the basis for healthy eating and for the prevention of chronic disease, especially cardiovascular disease. The pyramid illustrates that grains, fruits, and vegetables should be the dietary foundation. Adults need only two to three servings daily of milk products and two to three small servings of meat, fish, or poultry daily. Low-fat, low-cholesterol choices and meat alternatives such as legumes are to be encouraged. Nutrition labels can be used to help distinguish low-fat from high-fat products. Some foods that have high levels of essential nutrients are listed in Table 2.

The National Cancer Institute's "5-a-Day" Campaign message is to eat at least five servings of fruits and vegetables daily for good health. The value of the fruits and vegetables in reducing risk of certain types of cancer appears to result from factors other than their content of antioxidant vitamins, such as β-carotene and vitamins C and E. For example, a randomized, controlled clinical trial to test the efficacy of supplemental β-carotene and vitamins C and E in preventing colorectal cancer showed no reduction in risk even though high fruit and vegetable intake is protective (20).

Table 2. Examples of Food Sources of Vitamins and Minerals

Nutrient	Food Source
Vitamin	
A	Green, leafy vegetables; dark yellow vegetables (eg, carrots and sweet potatoes); whole, fortified skim, and low-fat milks; liver
C	Citrus fruits (eg, oranges, lemons, grapefruit); strawberries; broccoli; tomatoes
D	Fortified milk; fish liver oils; exposure to sunshine
E	Vegetable oils; whole-grain cereals; wheat germ; green, leafy vegetables
Folic acid	Green, leafy vegetables; orange juice; strawberries; liver; legumes and nuts
Mineral	
Calcium	Milk and milk products; sardines and salmon with bones; collard, kale, mustard, and turnip greens
Iron	Meat; liver; dried beans and peas; iron-fortified cereals; prune juice

The "5-a-Day" approach can be a simple and very effective starting point for improving overall nutrition and controlling weight. Increasing fruit and vegetable intake leads to increased intake of fiber and many micronutrients (including folate) and can also lead to decreased fat intake. Nearly all fruits and vegetables are essentially fat free in their natural forms. If eaten with little or no added fats or oils, fruits and vegetables make a healthy replacement for higher-fat, higher-calorie, lower-fiber foods. Reduction of fat intake, especially saturated fat (21), may reduce the risk of certain kinds of cancer as well as of cardiovascular disease.

Regular physical activity including planned exercise programs helps achieve energy balance and prevent weight gain. It may also be helpful in preventing chronic diseases such as heart disease, non–insulin-dependent diabetes mellitus (22), and, if the exercise is weight bearing, osteoporosis (14, 23). Some emerging evidence suggests that exercise may help reduce the risk of breast cancer (24, 25).

Prevention of Neural Tube Defects

Consumption of folic acid before and during the first weeks of pregnancy may reduce the occurrence of neural tube defects. The U.S. Public Health Service recommends that all women of childbearing age capable of becoming pregnant consume 400 μg of folic acid daily to help prevent neural tube defects (26, 27). Except for women with unusually high intakes of fruits, vegetables, and legumes, achievement of an intake of 400 μg of folic acid daily is likely to require the use of fortified foods such as some breakfast cereals or a folic acid supplement.

The U.S. Food and Drug Administration has established new rules under which specified grain products will be required to be fortified with folic acid at levels ranging from 0.43–1.4 mg/lb of product. These amounts are designed to keep daily intake of folic acid below 1 mg. To ensure that women receive 400 μg of folic acid daily, however, the American College of Obstetricians and Gynecologists still recommends supplementation. The amount of fortified grain products consumed may provide less than the amount of folic acid recommended to prevent neural tube defects.

The Centers for Disease Control and Prevention recommend a very high intake of folic acid (4 mg daily—10 times the RDA for pregnant women) for women who have previously had a pregnancy affected by a neural tube defect and are planning a pregnancy (28). This level of folic acid should be ingested only as a single vitamin supplement and not as part of a multivitamin supplement to avoid ingestion of excessive amounts of other vitamins (27). In particular, amounts of vitamin A greater than 10,000 IU are associated with a risk of congenital anomalies.

Prevention of Iron Deficiency Anemia

Women in the childbearing years have higher iron requirements than do men. The physician can suggest two dietary strategies to help women decrease their risk of developing iron deficiency. One strategy is to include iron-rich foods in the diet. The other strategy is to consume vitamin C-rich foods, such as orange juice, with meals that do not contain meat. Vitamin C is a reducing agent that favors the conversion of ferric to ferrous iron in these foods and thereby increases bioavailability.

Routine iron supplementation has not been recommended for nonpregnant women. The Institute of Medicine recommends routine iron supplementation (30 mg/d) for pregnant women during the second and third trimesters (10, 29). This recommendation is based on the increased need for iron relative to usual dietary supply, the relatively common occurrence of iron deficiency among unsupplemented women, and the increase in hemoglobin concentration that occurs when pregnant women receive supplementation. In contrast, giving iron prophylactically is not standard practice in Great Britain or Europe (30). Low ferritin levels are indicative of iron deficiency anemia; thus, if this condition is suspected, ferritin studies can be confirmatory (31).

Adolescent Nutritional Needs

Teenage years are critically important with regard to developing healthy routines including life-long eating habits. For example, important accumulation of bone minerals occurs during this period. Therefore, a major nutritional concern for adolescents and adult women younger than age 25 years is adequate intake of calcium and vitamin D as can be obtained from eating sufficient amounts of milk products. As indicated in Table 1, the RDA for calcium is 1.5 times that for older women and the RDA for vitamin D is twice as high.

Prevention of Osteoporosis

A 1994 National Institutes of Health Consensus Conference (32) made recommendations regarding calcium intake to help women reduce their risk of developing osteoporosis (Table 3). Dairy products are the major sources of calcium because of their content and the frequency of their consumption. Food recommendations for women who believe they are lactose or milk intolerant include lactase-treated milk, lactase tablets (to be taken when eating foods containing lactose), hard cheeses, canned fish, seeds, nuts, and calcium-fortified foods such as breads, cereals, and fruit juices.

There are more than a dozen commonly prescribed calcium supplements. The bioavailability of calcium is affected by a number of factors:

Table 3. Recommended Calcium Intake by Age and Estrogen Use*

Age (y)	Estrogen Use	Recommended Calcium Intake (mg)†
25–50	Not applicable	1,000
50–65	Yes	1,000
50–65	No	1,500
>65	Yes or no	1,500

*The levels shown differ from recommended dietary allowances because they are directed specifically to prevention of osteoporosis.

†"Adequate" vitamin D is recommended to achieve optimal calcium absorption.

Adapted from National Institutes of Health. Consensus development conference statement. Optimal calcium intake. Bethesda, Maryland: NIH Office of Medical Applications of Research, 1994

- Solubility of the salt
- Interference from coingested medications
- Interference from coingested foodstuffs
- Amount of calcium per dose
- Number of doses per day
- Presence of vitamin D

The presence of certain medical conditions can affect the choice of supplement. Such conditions include lactase deficiency, impaired gastric acid secretion (as can occur in elderly patients), and a high-risk profile for kidney stone formation (33).

Vitamin D is essential to promote calcium absorption and metabolism. Exposure of the skin to sunshine is a major source of vitamin D for many U.S. women, even if only their faces and hands are exposed. Women who live at northern latitudes have limited exposure to the needed ultraviolet light during the winter months. Use of sunscreens decreases exposure to ultraviolet light and thus reduces vitamin D production by the skin. There is no clinically practical way to monitor vitamin D production from exposure to sunlight.

The principal dietary source of vitamin D is vitamin D–fortified milk. The amounts of vitamin D present in eggs, butter, and margarine are very small relative to the RDA (5 μg for women aged 25 years or older, 10 μg for younger women).

In postmenopausal women, nondietary methods to prevent or minimize the progression of osteoporosis include, in addition to estrogen replacement therapy, high-density strength training (23) and medication. The latter includes calcitonin, sodium fluoride, bisphosphonates such as etidronate and alendronate, and calcitriol. Each agent has its own mechanism of action, effect on bone, effect on fractures, recommendations, and risks (34).

Management of Nutrition-Related Problems

The identification and treatment of nutritional problems need to be addressed jointly by the patient, family (as applicable), physician, and other involved health team members. The process includes setting priorities and developing clear objectives for changed behavior. The health care team provides the patient and family members with information and opportunities to develop the skills needed for meeting the objectives. The patient may need help with planning menus, reading labels, obtaining food assistance, accepting the need for change, gaining family support, learning quick and easy food preparation methods, or learning other skills or attitudes that affect food habits.

For complex nutritional problems that require detailed diet management, referral to a registered dietitian is recommended. The dietitian will conduct an extensive nutritional assessment and will work closely with the patient and physician to develop and implement a nutritional care plan. For some nutrition-related problems, referral to social service, psychologic counseling, or substance abuse treatment may be indicated. Treatment by an eating disorders team is indicated for the woman with anorexia nervosa, bulimia, or other serious eating disorders.

Obesity is an especially difficult condition to treat successfully over the long term. Many women who lose substantial amounts of weight regain much of the weight within a year and all of it within 5 years. Because even small weight losses can reduce the risk of developing chronic diseases, the Institute of Medicine recommends focusing on weight management by dietary control and exercise rather than weight loss alone, "achieving the best weight possible in the context of overall health" (35).

The Institute of Medicine recommends consideration of the following three criteria in selecting a weight management program for an individual (35):

1. The match between the program and the consumer:
   - —Weight loss goals and the appropriateness of the goals
   - —The amount of attention and effort that the person can devote to the program
   - —Appropriate care by a health care provider for those with obesity-related comorbidities or other health problems
   - —Medical supervision for those with bulimia or significant medical problems.
2. The soundness and safety of the program:
   - —Assessment and monitoring of clients
   - —Qualifications and training of staff
3. The evidence of program benefits relative to the effort and cost involved:
   - —Evaluation of success in achieving small losses
   - —Ability to maintain long-term loss

Specific Nutritional Needs

Cardiovascular Disease

For the control of hypertension, dietary management may address weight loss and reduced sodium intake. Management depends on the findings of the nutritional assessment and any medication prescribed.

By lowering high serum cholesterol levels, mortality from coronary artery disease and the prevalence of cardiovascular disease may be decreased (36). Cholesterol levels can be lowered through a combination of exercise, limited intakes of saturated fat and cholesterol in the diet, and medication. Abnormal variations in a patient's lipid profile (dyslipidemia) can occur secondary to some disease states (37) or the use of certain drugs such as steroid hormones, retinoids, and phenothiazines (38). The relative importance of high-density lipoprotein cholesterol and the relation of hypertriglyceridemia to coronary artery disease (39) also should be taken into consideration.

Diabetes Mellitus

New guidelines for medical nutrition therapy of diabetes mellitus include substantial changes in recommended practice. The current emphasis is on individualized treatment plans that promote consistency in intake of fat, carbohydrate, and protein (40). The proportions of fat and carbohydrate in the diet plan are now based on individual assessment; they may vary with the woman's BMI, blood lipid levels, blood sugar levels, physical activity, and personal preferences. Recommended protein intake is 10–20% of calories. Sucrose is no longer contraindicated, but limits on sucrose consumption vary with individual circumstances.

The registered dietitian is an integral member of the health care team for the patient with diabetes mellitus. The dietitian can help the woman develop a workable diet plan that can be followed consistently and can provide concrete guidance for managing sick days and other stresses.

Perioperative Nutrition

When possible before elective surgery, women with poor nutritional status should be encouraged to improve their general dietary intake to promote optimal immunologic function and wound healing. Albumin, resorcinol, and ferritin levels should be measured if malnutrition is suspected. If a surgical procedure causes prolonged decreased bowel function that prevents enteral feeding for more than 5–7 days, total parenteral feeding may be indicated to avoid complications associated with malnutrition (5% dextrose in water or saline provides only 200 kcal/L). Whenever possible, enteral feeding is preferred over total parenteral nutrition because it is less expensive and has fewer complications.

Summary

Adoption by women of dietary practices that are based on *Dietary Guidelines for Americans* (8) can promote improved general and reproductive health and can help prevent chronic disease. Additional guidance is indicated for helping prevent neural tube defects, iron deficiency anemia, and osteoporosis. The obstetrician–gynecologist plays an important preventive role by providing basic nutritional assessment; nutrition education; counseling concerning diet, weight, and exercise; and referral for special nutritional care as needed. The physician needs to be especially alert for serious nutrition-related problems such as eating disorders that pose a serious health risk and to stress the importance of good nutrition particularly to adolescent and elderly patients.

References

1. Manson JE, Willett WC, Stampfer MJ, Colditz GA, Hunter DJ, Hankinson SE, et al. Body weight and mortality among women. N Engl J Med 1995;333:677–685 Level II-2)

2. Kuczmarski RJ, Flegal KM, Campbell SM, Johnson CL. Increasing prevalence of overweight among US adults: the National Health and Nutrition Examination Surveys, 1960–1991. JAMA 1994;272:205–211 (Level II-2)

3. McDowell MA, Briefel RR, Alaimo K, Bischof AM, Caughman CR, Carroll MD, et al. Energy and macronutrient intakes of persons ages 2 months and over in the United States: Third National Health and Nutrition Examination Survey, phase 1, 1988–91. Advance data from vital and health statistics; no. 255. Hyattsville, Maryland: National Center for Health Statistics, 1994 (Level II-2)

4. Block G, Abrams B. Vitamin and mineral status of women of childbearing potential. Ann N Y Acad Sci 1993;678: 244–254 (Level II-2)

5. Life Sciences Research Office, Federation of American Societies for Experimental Biology. Nutrition monitoring in the United States: an update report on nutrition monitoring. Prepared for the U.S. Department of Agriculture and the U.S. Department of Health and Human Services. Washington, DC: U.S. Government Printing Office, 1989; DHHS Publication No. (PHS) 89-1255 (Level III)

6. Horm J, Anderson K. Who in America is trying to lose weight? Ann Intern Med 1993;119:672–676 (Level II-2)

7. National Research Council. Subcommittee on the Tenth Edition of the RDAs, Food and Nutrition Board, Commission on Life Sciences. Recommended dietary allowances. 10th ed. Washington, DC: National Academy Press, 1989 (Level III)

8. U.S. Department of Agriculture, U.S. Department of Health and Human Services. Nutrition and your health: dietary guidelines for Americans. 4th ed. Home and Garden Bulletin no. 232. Washington, DC: U.S. Government Printing Office, 1995 (Level III)

9. U.S. Department of Agriculture. The food guide pyramid. Home and Garden Bulletin no. 252. Washington, DC: U.S. Department of Agriculture, Human Nutrition Information Service, 1992 (Level III)

10. Institute of Medicine. Subcommittee on Nutritional Status and Weight Gain During Pregnancy, Subcommittee on Dietary Intake and Nutrient Supplements During Pregnancy, Committee on Nutritional Status During Pregnancy and Lactation, Food and Nutrition Board. Nutrition during pregnancy: part I, weight gain: part II, nutrient supplements. Washington, DC: National Academy Press, 1990 (Level III)

11. National Institutes of Health Consensus Development Panel on the Health Implications of Obesity. Health implications of obesity: National Institutes of Health Consensus Development Conference Statement. Ann Intern Med 1985;103:1073–1077 (Level III)

12. Metropolitan Life Insurance Company. Metropolitan height and weight tables. Stat Bull Metrop Insur Co 1983;64:2–9 (Level III)

13. Wing RR, Matthews KA, Juller LH, Meilahn EN, Plantinga P. Waist to hip ratio in middle-aged women: associations with behavioral and psychosocial factors and with changes in cardiovascular risk factors. Arterioscler Thromb 1991; 11:1250–1257 (Level II-2)

14. American College of Obstetricians and Gynecologists. Women and exercise. ACOG Technical Bulletin 173. Washington, DC: ACOG, 1992 (Level III)

15. Patrick K, Sallis JF, Long B, Calfas KJ, Wooten W, Heath G, et al. A new tool for encouraging activity: project PACE. Physician Sportsmedicine 1994;22(11):45–46, 48–52, 55 (Level III)

16. Herzog DB, Copeland PM. Medical progress: eating disorders. N Engl J Med 1985;313:295–303 (Level III)

17. Roubenoff R, Dallal GE, Wilson PWF. Predicting body fatness: the body mass index vs estimation by bioelectrical impedance. Am J Public Health 1995;85:726–728 (Level II-3)

18. Chumlea WC, Kuczmarski RJ. Using a bony landmark to measure waist circumference. J Am Diet Assoc 1995;95:12 (Level III)

19. American College of Obstetricians and Gynecologists. Osteoporosis. ACOG Technical Bulletin 167. Washington, DC: ACOG, 1992 (Level III)

20. Greenberg ER, Baron JA, Tosteson TD, Freeman DH, Beck GJ, Bond JH, et al. A clinical trial of antioxidant vitamins to prevent colorectal adenoma. N Engl J Med 1994;331:141–147 (Level I)

21. Risch HA, Jain M, Marrett LD, Howe GR. Dietary fat intake and risk of epithelial ovarian cancer. J Natl Cancer Inst 1994;86:1409–1415 (Level II-2)

22. Manson JE, Rimm EB, Stampfer MJ, Colditz GA, Willett WC, Krolewski AS, et al. Physical activity and incidence of non-insulin-dependent diabetes mellitus in women. Lancet 1991;338:774–778 (Level II-2)

23. Nelson ME, Fiatarone MA, Morganti CM, Trice I, Greenberg RA, Evans WJ. Effects of high-intensity strength training on multiple risk factors for osteoporotic fractures: a randomized controlled trial. JAMA 1994; 272:1909–1914 (Level I)

24. Friedenreich CM, Rohan TE. A review of physical activity and breast cancer. Epidemiology 1995;6:311–317 (Level III)

25. Mittendorf R, Longnecker MP, Newcomb PA, Dietz AT, Greenberg ER, Bogdan GF, et al. Strenuous physical activity in young adulthood and risk of breast cancer (United States). Cancer Causes Control 1995;6:347–353 (Level II-2)

26. Centers for Disease Control. Recommendations for the use of folic acid to reduce the number of cases of spina bifida and other neural tube defects. MMWR 1992;41(RR-14):1–7 (Level III)

27. American College of Obstetricians and Gynecologists. Folic acid for the prevention of recurrent neural tube defects. ACOG Committee Opinion 120. Washington, DC: ACOG, 1993 (Level III)

28. Centers for Disease Control. Use of folic acid for prevention of spina bifida and other neural tube defects—1983–1991. MMWR 1991;40:513–516 (Level III)

29. American College of Obstetricians and Gynecologists. Nutrition during pregnancy. ACOG Technical Bulletin 179. Washington, DC: ACOG, 1993 (Level III)

30. Allen LH. Iron-deficiency anemia increases risk of preterm delivery. Nutr Rev 1993;51:49–52 (Level III)

31. Institute of Medicine. Committee on the Prevention, Detection, and Management of Iron Deficiency Anemia Among U.S. Children and Women of Childbearing Age. Iron deficiency anemia: recommended guidelines for the prevention, detection, and management among U.S. children and women of childbearing age. Washington, DC: National Academy Press, 1993 (Level III)

32. National Institutes of Health. Consensus development conference statement. Optimal calcium intake. Bethesda, Maryland: NIH Office of Medical Applications of Research, 1994 (Level III)

33. Levenson DI, Bockman RS. A review of calcium preparations. Nutr Rev 1994;7:221–232 (Level III)

34. Tilyard MW, Spears GF, Thomson J, Dovey S. Treatment of postmenopausal osteoporosis with calcitriol or calcium. N Engl J Med 1992;62:326–357 (Level II-3)

35. Institute of Medicine. Committee to Develop Criteria for Evaluating the Outcomes of Approaches to Prevent and Treat Obesity, Food and Nutrition Board, Institute of Medicine. Weighing the options: criteria for evaluating weight-management programs. Washington, DC: National Academy Press, 1995 (Level III)

36. Levine GN, Keaney JF Jr, Vita JA. Cholesterol reduction in cardiovascular disease: clinical benefits and possible mechanisms. New Engl J Med 1995;332:512–521 (Level III)

37. Cooper GR, Myers GL, Smith SJ, Schlant RC. Blood lipid measurements, variations and practical utility. JAMA 1992; 267:1652–1660 (Level III)

38. Henkin Y, Como JA, Oberman A. Secondary dyslipidemia, inadvertent effects of drugs in clinical practice. JAMA 1992;267:961–968 (Level III)

39. National Institutes of Health Consensus Development Panel on Triglyceride, High-Density Lipoprotein, and Coronary Artery Disease. Triglyceride, high-density lipoprotein, and coronary heart disease. JAMA 1993; 269:505–510 (Level III)

40. American Diabetes Association. Nutrition recommendations and principles for people with diabetes mellitus. Diabetes Care 1994;17:519–522 (Level III)

The references in this bulletin are graded according to the method outlined by the U.S. Preventive Services Task Force:

- I Evidence obtained from at least one properly designed randomized controlled trial
- II-1 Evidence obtained from well-designed controlled trials without randomization
- II-2 Evidence obtained from well-designed cohort or case–control analytic studies, preferably from more than one center or research group
- II-3 Evidence obtained from multiple time series, with or without intervention, or dramatic results in uncontrolled experiments
- III Opinions of respected authorities, based on clinical experience, descriptive studies, or reports of expert committees

Other publications from ACOG:

Other publications from ACOG:

- **Committee Opinions,** focused updates on emerging areas
- **Practice Patterns**, evidence-based guidelines
- **Criteria Sets**, baseline guidelines for review of diagnostic and management procedures

ISSN 1074-8628

The American College of Obstetricians and Gynecologists
409 12th Street, SW
PO Box 96920
Washington, DC 20090-6920

12345/09876

Number 225—July 1996
(Replaces #112, January 1988)

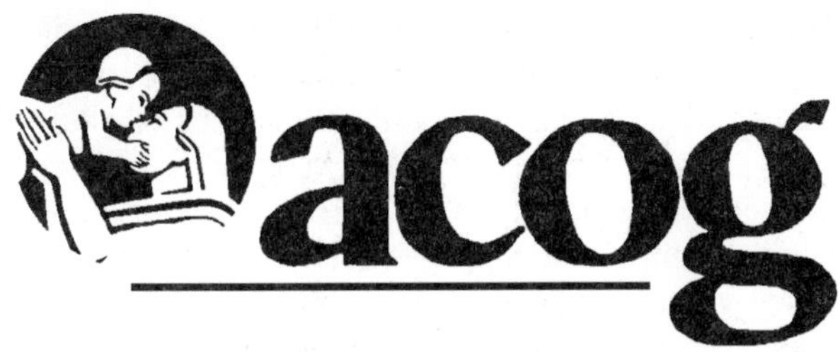

Technical Bulletin

An Educational Aid to Obstetrician–Gynecologists

Obstetric Analgesia and Anesthesia

Obstetric analgesia and anesthesia refer to the multiple techniques used to alleviate pain associated with labor and delivery. Analgesia is relief of pain without loss of consciousness. Regional analgesia implies partial sensory blockade, with or without partial motor blockade, over a specific region of the body. Regional anesthesia is the loss of sensation, motor function, and reflex activity over a specific region of the body. Regional blocks used for labor or vaginal delivery or both include lumbar epidural, caudal epidural, spinal, paracervical block, lumbar sympathetic block, pudendal block, and perineal infiltration. In the past, lumbar epidural analgesia often resulted in significant relaxation of skeletal muscle. In contemporary practice, many physicians administer dilute solutions of local anesthetic, with or without an opioid, which typically result in little or no motor blockade.

General anesthesia results in a loss of consciousness. Systemic agents capable of producing anesthesia may produce modest analgesia when administered in low concentrations. The term *balanced anesthesia* refers to a technique in which a combination of drugs is used to provide hypnosis, amnesia, analgesia, and skeletal muscle relaxation, while exposing the fetus to small amounts of anesthetic agents.

General Considerations

All physicians who provide care for obstetric patients should understand the physiologic changes that occur during normal pregnancy. For example, blood volume, heart rate, and cardiac output all increase, while systemic vascular resistance decreases. Tidal volume and minute ventilation increase, while functional residual capacity decreases.

Anesthesia remains a significant cause of maternal mortality. Anesthetic complications were the sixth leading cause of maternal death after a live birth in the United States and Puerto Rico between 1979 and 1986 (1). Anesthetic complications accounted for 3.3% of maternal deaths during this 8-year interval. Failed intubation and pulmonary aspiration of gastric contents remain the two leading causes of maternal mortality associated with anesthesia (2).

Pregnant women are at increased risk for failed tracheal intubation when compared with nonpregnant women (3). Factors that may predispose to difficult intubation in healthy pregnant women include full dentition, the normal weight gain of pregnancy, breast enlargement, and airway edema. Other factors that predispose to difficult intubation include obesity, a short neck or limited head and neck movement or both, limited jaw movement, a receding mandible, protruding maxillary incisors, severe facial and neck edema, arthritis of the neck, and anatomic abnormalities of the face or mouth (4, 5).

Pregnant women are also at increased risk for pulmonary aspiration of gastric contents. Pregnancy results in decreased competence of the lower esophageal sphincter. In addition, the pain of labor (as well as the presence of opioids used to provide analgesia) delays gastric emptying. Beyond midpregnancy, all pregnant women are considered to be at risk for a "full stomach," regardless of the interval since the last meal. Obstetric patients should not receive general anesthesia via mask, except perhaps in the rare circumstance of failed tracheal intubation in a patient whose fetus requires immediate delivery. An apparent decline in the incidence of maternal mortality secondary to pulmonary aspiration of gastric contents should not lessen the physician's concern for this complication. Many cases of maternal aspiration result in severe maternal morbidity, if not mortality.

All obstetricians should understand the general principles and techniques for obstetric analgesia and anesthesia and the necessary qualifications for those individuals who administer obstetric anesthesia (6). These qualifications include the need for persons administering or supervising obstetric anesthesia to be able to manage the infrequent but occasionally life-threatening complications of major regional anesthesia. Mastering and retaining the skills and knowledge necessary to manage these complications require adequate training and frequent application.

Labor

The pain of labor and delivery includes both a visceral and a somatic component. During the first stage of labor, pain results primarily from uterine contractions and cervical dilation. Painful impulses are transmitted via visceral afferent nerve fibers, which travel with sympathetic nerve fibers and enter the spinal cord at T-10, T-11, T-12, and L-1. During the second stage of labor, descent of the fetus results in distension of the pelvic floor, vagina, and perineum, which results in somatic pain. These painful impulses are transmitted primarily through the pudendal nerve and enter the spinal cord at S-2, S-3, and S-4. The pudendal nerve innervates the vagina, vulva, and perineum, and it also supplies motor fibers to some skeletal muscles of the pelvic floor and the perineum.

The pain of labor varies and can be severe for many women. In no other circumstance is it considered acceptable for a person to experience severe pain, amenable to safe intervention, while under a physician's care. Therefore, maternal request is sufficient justification for pain relief during labor (7). The full range of pain relief should be available and should not be denied because of an absence of other "medical indications."

Systemic Analgesia

Opioids

Systemic opioids can relieve the pain of labor. Large doses are often needed to provide effective analgesia during active labor, but such large doses may result in excessive maternal sedation and an increased risk of neonatal respiratory depression. Other maternal side effects include nausea, vomiting, pruritus, decreased gastrointestinal motility, hypotension, and obtunded protective airway reflexes. Other fetal and neonatal side effects include decreased fetal heart rate (FHR) variability, impaired early breast-feeding, and altered early neonatal neurobehavior. In general, all opioids have similar effects on the fetus and neonate when administered to the mother in equipotent doses.

Historically, meperidine has achieved the widest popularity for use as a systemic analgesic during labor. The usual dosage is 25–50 mg intravenously every 1–2 hours or 50–100 mg intramuscularly every 2–4 hours. Some physicians prescribe small intravenous bolus doses of meperidine by patient-controlled administration. The onset of analgesia is within 5 minutes after intravenous administration and within 30–45 minutes after intramuscular administration. A phenothiazine (eg, promethazine) is sometimes administered at the same time to diminish nausea and vomiting.

Meperidine rapidly crosses the placenta by passive diffusion. The half-life of meperidine is approximately 2 1/2 hours in the woman and approximately 13 hours in the neonate. Maximal fetal tissue uptake of meperidine occurs approximately 2–3 hours after maternal administration. The neonate is at greatest risk for respiratory depression when delivery occurs 2–3 hours after maternal meperidine administration.

Fentanyl is a highly lipid-soluble synthetic opioid with a potency approximately 100 times that of morphine and 800 times that of meperidine. It has a rapid onset of action and is highly protein bound. When given in small doses, fentanyl has a short duration of activity (20–30 minutes) as a result of its rapid redistribution from plasma. The usual dosage is 50–100 μg intravenously, administered as often as every hour at maternal request during active labor. Physicians sometimes prescribe small intravenous bolus doses of fentanyl by patient-controlled administration. Maternal side effects include sedation, nausea, vomiting, and decreased gastrointestinal motility. Administration of fentanyl may result in a period of decreased FHR variability, which may persist for up to 30 minutes, but no other nonreassuring FHR patterns have been reported (8). There is no evidence that fentanyl results in an increased risk of neonatal respiratory or neurobehavioral depression when compared with equipotent doses of other opioids.

The synthetic opioid agonist–antagonists butorphanol and nalbuphine, like morphine, result in maternal respiratory depression when given in modest equianalgesic doses. However, with increasing doses, both butorphanol and nalbuphine demonstrate a ceiling effect for maternal respiratory depression. For example, 2 mg of butorphanol produces similar respiratory depression to that which occurs with 10 mg of morphine. However, 4 mg of butorphanol results in less respiratory depression than 20 mg of morphine (9).

During labor, the usual dose of butorphanol is 1–2 mg intravenously or intramuscularly. The usual dose of nalbuphine is 10 mg. Administration of either drug results in a rapid onset of analgesia and sedation. The sedation often resembles that which occurs after administration of meperidine combined with phenothiazine. There is no evidence that butorphanol or nalbuphine results in either an increased or decreased risk of neonatal respiratory or neurobehavioral depression when compared with equipotent doses of other opioids.

Because all opioids may produce maternal or neonatal respiratory depression, the availability of an effective antagonist is essential. Naloxone is a pure opioid antagonist that is the drug of choice in the treatment of respiratory and neurobehavioral depression secondary to opioid agonist drugs. This agent works primarily by displacing the opioid from its receptor sites. Because it is a pure antagonist, it does not cause additional respiratory depression. In adults, the usual initial dose is 0.04–0.40 mg intravenously, with the total dose titrated to the desired effect. The recommended dose for neonates (including preterm neonates) is 0.1 mg/kg. If there is no response, the initial dose may be repeated in 3–5 minutes. Naloxone should be given intravenously when possible. Although naloxone may be given intramuscularly or subcutaneously, absorption may be delayed in the neonate who is stressed and vasoconstricted. Because naloxone has a relatively short duration of action, it may be necessary to repeat the dose to maintain reversal of the neonatal respiratory and neurobehavioral depression.

There is no fetal or neonatal benefit to the maternal administration of naloxone during labor or just before delivery. This results in antagonism of maternal analgesia, and it provides uncertain or incomplete reversal of the opioid's effects on the neonate.

In summary, general recommendations for the use of systemic opioids during labor include the use of the smallest dose possible and minimal use of repeated doses to reduce accumulation of the drug and its metabolites in the fetus. Unfortunately, small doses often do not result in substantial analgesia, especially during advanced labor.

Inhalation Analgesia

Intermittent inhalation of 40–50% nitrous oxide may provide modest analgesia, although it is administered infrequently in the first stage of labor. Appropriate equipment must be available to ensure safety. A device that limits the concentration of nitrous oxide is required, and it must be checked at regular intervals to prevent the unintentional administration of a high concentration of nitrous oxide and a hypoxic concentration of gas. Reports of the use of this technique during labor have noted variable analgesic efficacy and varied effects on maternal oxygen saturation.

Sometimes either nitrous oxide or one of the potent halogenated anesthetic agents (eg, halothane, enflurane, isoflurane) is administered during the second stage of labor. Inhalation analgesia is most safely accomplished when it is administered by a fully trained anesthesia care provider with appropriate monitoring in a fully equipped delivery room. The goal should be conscious analgesia, not anesthesia. Potential problems include maternal amnesia and, more importantly, the loss of protective airway reflexes, which may result in pulmonary aspiration of gastric contents. The latter problem has prompted some obstetric anesthesiologists to avoid giving inhalation analgesia.

Epidural Analgesia

Lumbar epidural analgesia has become the most widely used form of regional block for the relief of pain during labor. It typically provides analgesia without significant sedation. Lumbar epidural analgesia involves the insertion of a 16- or 18-gauge needle through the ligamentum flavum into the epidural space, usually at L2–3, L3–4, or L4–5. An 18- or 20-gauge catheter is passed through the epidural needle in a cephalad direction for a distance of 2–4 cm within the epidural space. The catheter is securely taped in place and serves as a route for either intermittent or continuous injection of local anesthetic or opioid or both. During early labor, some practitioners may prefer to provide a segmental block (ie, blockade of spinal segments T-10, T-11, T-12, and L-1) to eliminate the pain of uterine contractions and cervical dilation during the first stage of labor. In practice, partial blockade of lumbar and sacral sensory nerves often occurs. However, administration of a dilute solution of local anesthetic minimizes the extent of motor blockade and preserves the woman's perception of pelvic pressure during descent of the fetus.

Indications and Contraindications

In most patients, the primary indication for epidural analgesia is the patient's desire for pain relief. Medical indications for epidural analgesia during labor may include anticipated difficulty in intubation, a history of malignant hyperthermia, selected forms of cardiovascular and respiratory disease, or prevention or treatment of autonomic hyperreflexia in parturients with a high spinal cord lesion. Obstetric indications are more controversial and may include breech presentation, multiple gestation, or an increased risk for emergency cesarean delivery.

Epidural analgesia is the preferred analgesic/anesthetic technique for most preeclamptic women for the following reasons: 1) it provides analgesia superior to that provided by other techniques; 2) it decreases circulating concentrations of catecholamines, facilitates control of maternal blood pressure, and in some cases improves uteroplacental perfusion (10); and 3) it allows the anesthesiologist to avoid laryngoscopy and intubation, which may precipitate severe hypertension in preeclamptic women. Also, intubation may be difficult or impossible because some preeclamptic women have severe pharyngolaryngeal edema. In the absence of experience in administering epidural anesthesia to women with severe preeclampsia, general anesthesia may be an acceptable alternative for cesarean delivery (11).

Contraindications to epidural or spinal analgesia include the following:

- Patient refusal or inability to cooperate
- Increased intracranial pressure secondary to a mass lesion
- Infection at the site of needle placement
- Clinical coagulopathy
- Uncorrected maternal hypovolemia
- Unavailability of qualified medical personnel trained or experienced in the technique

It is controversial whether mild or isolated abnormalities discovered in the results of blood coagulation tests contraindicate the administration of epidural or spinal analgesia.

Selection of Agents

Bupivacaine is the epidural local anesthetic agent used most commonly during labor. In the past, administration of a concentrated solution (0.5%) provided profound anesthesia and a prolonged duration of action; however, this resulted in an excessive density of sensory and motor blockade and an unnecessary increase in maternal risk for systemic toxicity or high spinal anesthesia. Analgesia with incremental bolus doses of 0.125–0.250% bupivacaine, followed by a continuous epidural infusion of 0.0625–0.1250% bupivacaine, is commonly used today. The continuous epidural infusion of local anesthetic results in a more uniform, stable level of analgesia, and it decreases the need for repetitive bolus injections.

Physicians may prefer to administer either 1% lidocaine or 2% 2-chloroprocaine during the first stage of labor. These agents have a more rapid onset of action than bupivacaine. However, they also have a shorter duration of action and cause more intense motor blockade. Furthermore, epidural administration of 2-chloroprocaine interferes with the subsequent efficacy of bupivacaine and some opioids.

A local anesthetic and an opioid may be used in combination to provide epidural analgesia during labor. The opioid produces analgesia by binding to opioid receptors in the spinal cord. Systemic absorption of opioid also occurs, which may result in transient maternal euphoria, sedation, or both. Many physicians include a lipid-soluble opioid (eg, 50 μg of fentanyl or 10 μg of sufentanil) with the initial bolus of local anesthetic and then administer a continuous epidural infusion of local anesthetic with opioid (eg, 0.0625% bupivacaine with 1–2 μg of fentanyl per milliliter or 0.2–0.4 μg of sufentanil per milliliter) (12). The administration of both local anesthetic and opioid results in an additive (and perhaps synergistic) effect, which hastens the onset of analgesia and prolongs its duration. The addition of opioid allows administration of a smaller total dose of local anesthetic, which decreases the likelihood of local anesthetic complications and results in a decreased intensity of motor block.

Complications and Side Effects

One of the most common side effects of epidural analgesia is maternal hypotension. Before initiation of epidural analgesia, the patient should receive prophylactic intravascular volume expansion with an injection of 500–1,000 ml of non-glucose-containing, isotonic crystalloid solution (eg, lactated Ringer's injection) (13–15). Rapid infusion of dextrose-containing solutions should be minimized during labor because of the potential for fetal acidemia. If hypotension occurs, it should be corrected by giving additional intravenous fluids or by intravenous administration of 5–10 mg of ephedrine or both. In addition, aortocaval compression should be avoided at all times. The patient may lie supine with approximately 30° left uterine displacement, or she may lie in the full left or right lateral decubitus position. In general, it seems appropriate to alter the patient's position at 30- to 60-minute intervals.

The use of bupivacaine for epidural analgesia has been associated with transient FHR decelerations (16). One retrospective study observed an association between prolonged FHR decelerations (defined as a decrease of the FHR below 120 beats per minute of at least 2 minutes in duration) and uterine hypertonus in patients who had received epidural bupivacaine during labor (17). In contrast, a prospective study observed no abnormal FHR patterns after the administration of either epidural bupivacaine or lidocaine with epinephrine for elective cesarean delivery (18). When maternal hemodynamics are changing, such as with maternal hypotension from regional anesthesia or maternal hemorrhage, increased fetal surveillance may be indicated. Otherwise, patients who receive epidural analgesia should be monitored in a manner similar to that used for any patient in labor.

The most serious immediate complications of epidural analgesia include systemic local anesthetic toxicity and high/total spinal anesthesia. Signs and symptoms of local anesthetic drug toxicity include drowsiness, lightheadedness, tinnitus, circumoral paresthesias, a metallic taste in the mouth, slurred speech, blurred vision, unconsciousness, convulsions, and cardiac dysrhythmias and arrest. Signs and symptoms of high spinal anesthesia include numbness and weakness of the upper extremities, dyspnea, whispered speech, inability to speak, and finally, apnea and loss of consciousness.

Measures that may minimize the likelihood of these complications include aspiration of the catheter before each dose of local anesthetic and administration of a test dose of local anesthetic before administration of a therapeutic dose. The test dose should allow recognition of unintentional intravenous or subarachnoid injection of local anesthetic without causing systemic toxicity or total spinal anesthesia. The inclusion of 15 μg of epinephrine in the test dose may facilitate recognition of unintentional intravenous injection. Intravenous injection of 15 μg of epinephrine typically results in transient maternal tachycardia. If little or no block is produced after injection of an appropriate therapeutic dose of local anesthetic, one should consider the possibility that it was injected intravenously. Other precautions should include use of dilute solutions of local anesthetic, injection of no more than 5 ml of local anesthetic as a single bolus, and continual verbal communication with the patient.

Treatment of systemic local anesthetic toxicity includes administration of 100% oxygen, with use of positive-pressure ventilation if necessary. Endotracheal intubation will facilitate ventilation and help protect the airway. A small dose of thiopental (25–50 mg) or diazepam (2.5–5.0 mg) will stop convulsions. Alternatively, administration of succinylcholine (1 mg/kg) will stop skeletal muscle activity and facilitate endotracheal intubation. Aortocaval compression must be avoided at all times, and intravenous fluids and vasoactive drugs should be administered to support the maternal circulation. Bradycardia should be treated with atropine (0.6–1.0 mg), and ventricular tachycardia should be treated with bretylium (5 mg/kg). Ventricular fibrillation should be treated with bretylium, epinephrine, and defibrillation.

Treatment of total spinal anesthesia includes administration of 100% oxygen and use of positive-pressure ventilation, preferably via an endotracheal tube. Aortocaval compression must be avoided at all times. Intravenous fluids and vasoactive drugs (eg, ephedrine) should be administered to support maternal circulation. If profound hypotension exists and the patient does not respond to an appropriate dose of ephedrine, a resuscitation dose of epinephrine (0.5–1.0 mg) should be given. Likewise, epinephrine should be administered in cases of severe, refractory bradycardia (19).

In cases of maternal cardiac arrest followed by unsuccessful resuscitation, the physician should consider immediate delivery of the infant. Delivery of the infant within 4–5 minutes of the arrest will maximize the chances of infant survival (20). This approach has not been shown to be harmful to the mother. Because evacuation of the uterus may relieve aortocaval compression, such an approach may be beneficial, although this has not been proven.

Other complications of epidural analgesia include antepartum urinary retention and postpartum headache (as a result of unintentional dural puncture). Postpartum headache occurs in less than 2% of cases of attempted epidural analgesia. Conservative measures (eg, bed rest, oral or intravenous caffeine, oral theophylline) may ameliorate symptoms in a minority of patients. The definitive treatment of postdural puncture headache is autologous epidural blood patch.

Serious long-term sequelae (eg, paralysis secondary to epidural hematoma or abscess) are rare. However, an epidural hematoma or abscess should be suspected if recovery from the block is slow or absent or if neurologic function worsens after a period of initial recovery. The primary symptoms are pain and weakness (and fever in the patient with an epidural abscess), which may progress rapidly to paralysis. Early laminectomy and surgical drainage are the only recourse for preserving or restoring neurologic function.

There is controversy regarding the effects of epidural analgesia on the progress of labor in both the first and second stages and its effect on the operative delivery rate. Randomized controlled trials have shown conflicting results (21–24). Some physicians believe that there is a cause-and-effect relationship between epidural analgesia, prolonged labor, and operative delivery. Others contend that women at increased risk for operative delivery are more likely to experience severe pain and request epidural analgesia during labor.

Spinal Analgesia

Recently, some anesthesiologists have advocated the administration of spinal (ie, intrathecal) analgesia during the first stage of labor. This technique typically involves the intermittent or continuous spinal administration of an opioid without a local anesthetic. Intrathecal administration of morphine (0.25–0.50 mg) provides satisfactory analgesia for most of the first stage of labor. Unfortunately, it results in a high incidence of side effects (eg, nausea, pruritus), it does not provide effective relief of the somatic component of pain during advanced labor, and it entails some risk of postpartum respiratory depression.

Alternatively, a small dose of a lipid-soluble opioid (eg, fentanyl, sufentanil) results in a rapid onset of effective analgesia, but the duration of action is only 1–2 hours. The introduction of small-gauge spinal catheters allowed continuous administration of spinal opioid analgesia during labor with a low incidence of postdural puncture headache. However, anecdotal reports of neurologic deficits (eg, cauda equina syndrome, primarily in nonpregnant patients who had received hyperbaric lidocaine) prompted the U.S. Food and Drug Administration to remove these catheters from the market. There is a high incidence of postdural puncture headache when a larger epidural catheter is used to provide continuous spinal analgesia. Nonetheless, this remains a useful technique in cases of unintentional dural puncture during attempted epidural anesthesia in morbidly obese parturients.

In a combined spinal–epidural technique, a small-gauge spinal needle is used to give a small dose of a lipid-soluble opioid (eg, 10 μg of sufentanil) intrathecally. Subsequently, a catheter is placed in the epidural space. The intrathecal opioid will provide 1–2 hours of analgesia, and physicians sometimes allow patients to ambulate during this time. When pain recurs, analgesia is reestablished by injecting local anesthetic (with or without opioid) through the epidural catheter. Initial reports suggested that intrathecal opioid analgesia did not result in hypotension. Subsequently, others have noted the occurrence of modest hypotension in some patients treated by this technique (25). Therefore, intravenous access should be established, and blood pressure should be measured at regular intervals in patients who receive intrathecal opioid analgesia.

Paracervical Block

Paracervical block is occasionally used to provide analgesia during the first stage of labor. The goal is to block transmission of painful impulses through the paracervical ganglion (also known as the Frankenhauser ganglion), which lies immediately lateral and posterior to the uterocervical junction. Paracervical block does not adversely affect the progress of labor. Also, it may provide good analgesia without the sensory and motor blockade that may occur during administration of epidural analgesia. Disadvantages of paracervical block include its short duration of action (ie, 45–60 minutes) and the fact that it does not relieve the somatic component of pain during advanced labor.

The major complication of paracervical block is fetal bradycardia, the cause of which is unclear. If fetal bradycardia should occur, the patient should be placed in the lateral position and should receive 100% oxygen. In most cases, the bradycardia is self-limiting, with a duration of 6–10 minutes.

The technique should be avoided in patients with evidence of uteroplacental insufficiency or nonreassuring FHR tracings. Also, the block should not be administered if delivery is imminent.

The FHR should be monitored closely before, during, and after performance of paracervical block. The injection of local anesthetic should be superficial (ie, just beneath the vaginal mucosa, so as to raise a wheal) at the 4-o'clock and 8-o'clock positions, adjacent to the cervix. Aspiration for blood should be performed before each injection. The usual total volume of local anesthetic is 10–20 ml (ie, 5–10 ml on each side). Following the injection of local anesthetic on one side, the physician should wait 3–5 minutes to observe for fetal bradycardia before injecting local anesthetic on the other side. The local anesthetics most often used for paracervical block are 2% 2-chloroprocaine and 1% lidocaine. 2-Chloroprocaine undergoes rapid enzymatic hydrolysis and has the shortest intravascular half-life among the local anesthetics used clinically. This rapid metabolism seems advantageous in the event of unintentional intravascular or fetal injection. According to the *Physicians' Desk Reference*, the use of bupivacaine is contraindicated for paracervical block in obstetric patients.

Vaginal Delivery

Regional methods used for analgesia during labor can be used for anesthesia during delivery. The patient remains awake and alert, and in most cases she is able to actively participate in the delivery process.

Epidural Anesthesia

Epidural analgesia/anesthesia may be initiated de novo for vaginal delivery, or segmental epidural analgesia may be augmented by administering a larger dose (10–15 ml) of local anesthetic solution to achieve perineal analgesia/anesthesia. 2-Chloroprocaine is often administered for this purpose because of its rapid onset of action. Administration of 3% 2-chloroprocaine will result in profound motor block, which will facilitate instrumental vaginal delivery.

Spinal Anesthesia

Spinal anesthesia has a rapid onset of action, is relatively easy to administer, and provides more reliable sacral blockade than does epidural anesthesia. Only a small dose of local anesthetic is needed, which reduces the risk of systemic local anesthetic toxicity. Spinal anesthesia typically results in profound sensory and motor blockade. Thus, it is an ideal technique for operative vaginal delivery. However, unless one limits the block to the sacral segments (ie, the so-called "saddle block"), spinal anesthesia impairs maternal expulsive efforts. Thus, spinal anesthesia typically is not administered until delivery is imminent or the obstetrician has made a decision to perform operative vaginal delivery. If the obstetrician plans a trial of forceps and is uncertain as to whether vaginal delivery may be accomplished safely, the anesthesiologist should either administer a spinal dose of local anesthetic that will provide sufficient anesthesia for subsequent cesarean delivery or perform an epidural or combined spinal–epidural block.

Spinal anesthesia has become less popular for vaginal delivery because of the increased use of epidural analgesia during labor. However, it is an excellent choice for those patients who require operative vaginal delivery and who do not have preexisting epidural analgesia.

Pudendal Block

Obstetricians often perform pudendal nerve block in patients without epidural or spinal anesthesia. Pudendal nerve block may provide satisfactory anesthesia for spontaneous vaginal delivery and uncomplicated outlet or low forceps delivery. However, it may not provide adequate anesthesia for midforceps delivery and may not allow comfort during postpartum examination of the upper vagina and cervix and manual exploration of the uterus.

Pudendal block is usually performed by the transvaginal technique. A needle guide is used to prevent injury to the vagina and fetus. The needle and needle guide are introduced into the vagina with the left hand for the left side of the pelvis and with the right hand for the right side. The needle is introduced through the vaginal mucosa and sacrospinous ligament just medial and posterior to the ischial spine. The pudendal artery lies in proximity to the pudendal nerve. Thus, the physician must aspirate before and during the injection of local anesthetic. Typically, 7–10 ml of local anesthetic solution is injected on each side. The most commonly used local anesthetics are 1% lidocaine and 2% 2-chloroprocaine. There is no need to use a more concentrated solution of local anesthetic for performance of pudendal block.

The major disadvantage of pudendal block is its high rate of failure. Maternal complications are uncommon but may be serious (eg, laceration of the vaginal mucosa, systemic local anesthetic toxicity, vaginal and ischiorectal hematoma, retropsoal and subgluteal abscess). Fetal complications are rare but may result from needle trauma or direct fetal injection of local anesthetic.

Perineal Infiltration

Pudendal nerve block and perineal infiltration may be used in combination. Several milliliters of 0.5% or 1% lidocaine or 2% 2-chloroprocaine are injected into the posterior fourchette. The obstetrician must take precautions to avoid injection of the local anesthetic into the fetal scalp. The onset of anesthesia is rapid because there are no large nerve fibers to be blocked. Perineal infiltration provides anesthesia only for episiotomy and repair; it provides no muscle relaxation. The total dose of plain lidocaine (without epinephrine) should not exceed 4.5 mg/kg (ie, 30 ml of a 1% solution in a 70-kg patient).

Cesarean Delivery

Most cesarean deliveries are performed with spinal or epidural anesthesia. When cesarean delivery is performed for FHR abnormality, the severity of the abnormality should be considered in determining the urgency of the delivery and the type of anesthesia to be administered (26, 27). Cesarean deliveries performed for a nonreassuring FHR pattern do not necessarily preclude the use of regional anesthesia (26–28).

Before cesarean delivery, the fetus as well as the mother should be evaluated. Fetal heart rate monitoring should be continued until the abdominal preparation is begun.

Regardless of the choice of anesthesia, an oral nonparticulate antacid (eg, 0.3 M sodium citrate) should be administered to decrease the mother's risk of developing aspiration pneumonitis. In addition, some anesthesiologists give an H_2-receptor antagonist (eg, cimetidine, ranitidine), metoclopramide, or both to decrease gastric acidity and accelerate gastric emptying.

Pulse oximetry should be used in all patients who undergo major surgery (eg, cesarean delivery). In patients who undergo endotracheal intubation for general anesthesia, CO_2 in the expired gas should be positively identified. In addition, the continuous use of end-tidal CO_2 analysis in those patients who undergo endotracheal intubation is encouraged (29).

Epidural Anesthesia

Epidural anesthesia is an excellent choice for most patients who receive epidural analgesia during labor and who subsequently require cesarean delivery. The obstetric care team should be alert to the presence of risk factors that place the parturient at increased risk for complications from emergency general or regional anesthesia. For those patients at risk, consideration should be given to the planned placement in early labor of an intravenous line and an epidural or spinal catheter, with confirmation that the catheter is functional (26). The density of the preexisting epidural block and the choice of local anesthetic will affect the time required to establish satisfactory anesthesia for surgery.

When time permits, surgical anesthesia may be established by administering incremental bolus injections of 2% lidocaine with epinephrine, 3% 2-chloroprocaine, or 0.5% bupivacaine. Bupivacaine (0.75%) is no longer approved for epidural administration in obstetric patients because of the increased cardiotoxicity associated with unintentional systemic administration of large doses of bupivacaine. This should not be confused with the administration of a small dose of 0.75% hyperbaric bupivacaine for spinal anesthesia. Additional non-glucose-containing crystalloid solution should be administered to decrease the likelihood of hypotension secondary to the more extensive level of sympathetic blockade. A sensory level of at least T-4 is desirable to minimize visceral discomfort during surgery.

If the need for cesarean delivery is more urgent, the following protocol may be used. While the urethral catheter is inserted and the abdomen is prepared and draped, a bolus of lactated Ringer's injection is given intravenously and 15–20 ml of 3% 2-chloroprocaine or 2% lidocaine with epinephrine is injected in the epidural space in 5-ml increments. If anesthesia is not satisfactory when the physician is ready to make the skin incision, local infiltration or general anesthesia should be considered unless circumstances permit awaiting the onset of satisfactory regional anesthesia.

Epidural anesthesia results in a slower onset of sympathetic blockade than does spinal anesthesia and thus is appropriate for those patients who undergo elective cesarean delivery and who may benefit from the slow onset of sympathetic blockade (eg, those with severe preeclampsia or cardiovascular disease). Finally, epidural anesthesia may be preferred for those patients who prefer regional anesthesia but may require prolonged surgery (eg, patients with morbid obesity or a history of several previous cesarean deliveries).

Spinal Anesthesia

Spinal anesthesia is an excellent choice for most healthy patients scheduled for elective cesarean delivery. Also, it may be administered to some patients who require emergency cesarean delivery and who do not have preexisting epidural analgesia (28). Lidocaine (60–75 mg) will provide anesthesia for 45–75 minutes, bupivacaine (12 mg) will provide anesthesia for 1–2 hours, and tetracaine (8–10 mg, with or without epinephrine) will provide anesthesia for 2–4 hours. Local anesthetics used for spinal anesthesia are generally administered as hyperbaric solutions (ie, they include dextrose).

Advantages of spinal anesthesia for cesarean delivery include its simplicity, reliability, and rapid onset of action. Spinal anesthesia also provides more reliable sacral blockade than does epidural anesthesia. The most common complication of spinal anesthesia is maternal hypotension. When possible, the patient should receive approximately 1,000–1,500 ml of non-glucose-containing crystalloid solution before initiation of spinal anesthesia. To avoid aortocaval compression, uterine displacement should be maintained until the fetus is delivered. Ephedrine may be given prophylactically during administration of spinal anesthesia. Hypotension should be treated aggressively with ephedrine (intravenous bolus, 5–10 mg) and administration of additional non-glucose-containing crystalloid intravenously.

In the past, a major disadvantage of spinal anesthesia was the high incidence of postdural puncture headache. The introduction of noncutting "pencil-point" spinal needles (eg, Sprotte, Whitacre) has resulted in a significant decrease. Use of a 24-gauge Sprotte or a 25-gauge Whitacre needle may result in an incidence of 1% or less.

When time permits, the anesthesiologist should ensure the presence of satisfactory anesthesia before the abdomen is prepared and draped. Unfortunately, some patients experience inadequate epidural or spinal anesthesia. When this occurs, options include the following:

- Administration of a second epidural or spinal procedure
- Supplemental infiltration with local anesthetic
- Administration of supplemental systemic analgesia (eg, 40–50% nitrous oxide or a small intravenous dose of an opioid or ketamine)
- Rapid-sequence induction of general anesthesia (which includes placement of a cuffed endotracheal tube).

General Anesthesia

Some patients have conditions (eg, coagulopathy, hemorrhage) that contraindicate administration of regional anesthesia. In addition, there are some circumstances (eg, a prolapsed umbilical cord with severe fetal bradycardia) in which a rapid induction of general anesthesia may be preferable to administration of regional anesthesia (26).

To minimize the risks of maternal aspiration and neonatal depression, the following sequence of events is followed when general anesthesia is used:

1. Administration of a clear, nonparticulate antacid
2. Administration of 100% oxygen
3. Application of cricoid pressure to occlude the esophagus and decrease the likelihood of pulmonary aspiration of gastric contents
4. Intravenous administration of either sodium thiopental (4 mg/kg) or ketamine (1 mg/kg)
5. Intravenous administration of succinylcholine (1.0–1.5 mg/kg) to provide a rapid onset of muscle relaxation to facilitate endotracheal intubation
6. Insertion and confirmation of the proper placement of a cuffed endotracheal tube
7. Administration of a high concentration of inspired oxygen (eg, 50% oxygen and 50% nitrous oxide) until delivery
8. Administration of a low concentration of a potent halogenated agent (eg, halothane, enflurane, or isoflurane) to reduce the incidence of maternal awareness

In the past, some physicians emphasized the importance of a brief induction-to-delivery interval in those patients who received general anesthesia for cesarean delivery. A prolonged induction-to-delivery interval (ie, more than 10 minutes) may result in delivery of an infant who appears sleepy immediately after delivery. Such an infant may have a depressed 1-minute Apgar score, but the 5-minute Apgar score generally does not differ from those found in infants of mothers who receive regional anesthesia. In contrast, a prolonged uterine incision-to-delivery interval (ie, more than 3 minutes) is associated with an increased incidence of low umbilical cord blood pH measurements and low Apgar scores, regardless of the anesthetic technique used (30).

Regardless of the indication for cesarean delivery, the anesthesiologist should not perform a rapid-sequence induction of general anesthesia in patients with a suspected difficult airway. In these cases, alternatives to rapid-sequence induction of general anesthesia include either regional anesthesia or awake intubation (eg, oral fiberoptic laryngoscopy and intubation). Unfortunately, some cases of difficult intubation occur unexpectedly. Every obstetric unit should have the necessary equipment and supplies for use in patients with a difficult airway. Every anesthesiologist and obstetrician should have a predetermined plan for management of unexpected failed intubation and failed ventilation. An example of a simplified protocol for such circumstances is shown in the box (31). The laryngeal mask airway may be helpful in some cases of failed intubation and failed ventilation.

Local Infiltration Anesthesia

Cesarean delivery may be performed with local infiltration anesthesia in extreme emergencies when a skilled anesthesia care provider is not available. In most cases, local infiltration anesthesia should be used only as a last resort.

Sample Protocol for Management of Unexpected Failed Intubation and Failed Ventilation

The following protocol summarizes key points in managing unexpected failed intubation and failed ventilation. However, every case requires individualized management.

1. Call for help.
2. Avoid multiple attempts at intubation.
3. Maintain cricoid pressure.
4. Ventilate patient with 100% oxygen. Place an oral airway if necessary.
5. Make a decision regarding surgery:
   a. If the fetus does not require immediate delivery,
      (1) ventilate until spontaneous respiration returns.
      (2) awaken the patient.
      (3) perform regional anesthesia or awake, oral fiberoptic intubation.
   b. If either the fetal or maternal condition requires immediate delivery,
      (1) ventilate with oxygen and a potent halogenated agent.
      (2) if ventilation is satisfactory, deliver the fetus.
      (3) allow spontaneous respiration if possible.
      (4) after delivery, either maintain mask ventilation or perform oral fiberoptic intubation.
6. If unable to ventilate via mask, place a laryngeal mask airway*. Alternatively, place a large-gauge intravenous cannula through the cricothyroid membrane and proceed with transtracheal oxygenation/ventilation†.

*Procedure discussed in Pennant JH, White PF. The laryngeal mask airway. Anesthesiology 1993;79:144–163 and Gataure PS. The laryngeal mask airway in obstetrical anaesthesia. Can J Anaesth 1995;42:130–133.

†Procedure discussed in Benumof JL, Scheller MS. The importance of transtracheal jet ventilation in the management of the difficult airway. Anesthesiology 1989;71:769–778.

Modified from American Society of Anesthesiologists Task Force on Management of the Difficult Airway. Practice guidelines for management of the difficult airway. Anesthesiology 1993;78:597–602

Postoperative Analgesia

Use of epidural or spinal anesthesia for cesarean delivery allows the anesthesiologist to provide prolonged postoperative analgesia via administration of epidural or intrathecal opioids. Alternatives include opioids administered intravenously, intramuscularly, or by patient-controlled administration.

Summary

Many agents and techniques are available for analgesia and anesthesia in obstetric patients. The choice of technique, agent, and dosage is based on numerous factors, including patient preference, medical status, and contraindications. Decisions regarding anesthesia should be closely coordinated among the obstetrician, the anesthesiologist, the patient, and skilled support personnel.

REFERENCES

1. Atrash HK, Koonin LM, Lawson HW, Franks AL, Smith JC. Maternal mortality in the United States, 1979–1986. Obstet Gynecol 1990;76:1055–1060
2. Department of Health, Welsh Office; Scottish Home and Health Department; Department of Health and Social Security, Northern Ireland. Report on confidential enquiries into maternal deaths in the United Kingdom 1985–87. London: HMSO Publications, 1991:73–87
3. Samsoon GLT, Young JRB. Difficult tracheal intubation: a retrospective study. Anaesthesia 1987;42:487–490
4. Wilson ME, Spiegelhalter D, Robertson JA, Lesser P. Predicting difficult intubation. Br J Anaesth 1988;61:211–216
5. Rocke DA, Murray WB, Rout CC, Gouws E. Relative risk analysis of factors associated with difficult intubation in obstetric anesthesia. Anesthesiology 1992;77:67–73
6. American Academy of Pediatrics, American College of Obstetricians and Gynecologists. Guidelines for perinatal care. 3rd ed. Elk Grove Village, Illinois: AAP; Washington, DC: ACOG, 1992
7. American College of Obstetricians and Gynecologists. Pain relief during labor. ACOG Committee Opinion 118. Washington, DC: ACOG, 1993
8. Rayburn W, Rathke A, Leuschen MP, Chleborad J, Weidner W. Fentanyl citrate analgesia during labor. Am J Obstet Gynecol 1989;161:202–206
9. Nagashima H, Karamanian A, Malovany R, Radnay P, Ang M, Koerner S, et al. Respiratory and circulatory effects of intravenous butorphanol and morphine. Clin Pharmacol Ther 1976;19:738–745
10. Jouppila P, Jouppila R, Hollmen A, Koivula A. Lumbar epidural analgesia to improve intervillous blood flow during labor in severe preeclampsia. Obstet Gynecol 1982; 59:158–161

11. Gutsche B. The experts opine: is epidural block for labor and delivery and for cesarean section a safe form of analgesia in severe preeclampsia or eclampsia? Surv Anesth 1986;30:304–311

12. Chestnut DH, Owen CL, Bates JN, Ostman LG, Choi WW, Geiger MW. Continuous infusion epidural analgesia during labor: a randomized, double-blind comparison of 0.0625% bupivacaine/0.0002% fentanyl versus 0.125% bupivacaine. Anesthesiology 1988;68:754–759

13. Kenepp NB, Shelley WC, Gabbe SG, Kumar S, Stanley CA, Gutsche BB. Fetal and neonatal hazards of maternal hydration with 5% dextrose before caesarean section. Lancet 1982;1:1150–1152

14. Philipson EH, Kalhan SC, Riha MM, Pimentel R. Effects of maternal glucose infusion on fetal acid-base status in human pregnancy. Am J Obstet Gynecol 1987;157:866–873

15. Piquard F, Hsiung R, Schaefer A, Haberey P, Dellenbach P. Does fetal acidosis develop with maternal glucose infusion during normal labor? Obstet Gynecol 1989;74:909–914

16. Abboud TK, Afrasiabi A, Sarkis F, Daftarian F, Nagappala S, Noueihed R, et al. Continuous infusion epidural analgesia in parturients receiving bupivacaine, chloroprocaine, or lidocaine—maternal, fetal, and neonatal effects. Anesth Analg 1984;63:421–428

17. Steiger RM, Nageotte MP. Effect of uterine contractility and maternal hypotension on prolonged decelerations after bupivacaine epidural anesthesia. Am J Obstet Gynecol 1990;163:808–812

18. Loftus JR, Holbrook RH, Cohen SE. Fetal heart rate after epidural lidocaine and bupivacaine for elective cesarean section. Anesthesiology 1991;75:406–412

19. Caplan RA, Ward RJ, Posner K, Cheney FW. Unexpected cardiac arrest during spinal anesthesia: a closed claims analysis of predisposing factors. Anesthesiology 1988;68:5–11

20. American Heart Association. Special resuscitation situations. JAMA 1992;268:2242–2250

21. Thorp JA, Hu DH, Albin RM, McNitt J, Meyer BA, Cohen GR, et al. The effect of intrapartum epidural analgesia on nulliparous labor: a randomized, controlled, prospective trial. Am J Obstet Gynecol 1993;169:851–858

22. Chestnut DH, Vincent RD Jr, McGrath JM, Choi WW, Bates JN. Does early administration of epidural analgesia affect obstetric outcome in nulliparous women who are receiving intravenous oxytocin? Anesthesiology 1994;80:1193–1200

23. Chestnut DH, McGrath JM, Vincent RD Jr, Penning DH, Choi WW, Bates JN, et al. Does early administration of epidural analgesia affect obstetric outcome in nulliparous women who are in spontaneous labor? Anesthesiology 1994;80:1201–1208

24. Morton SC, Williams MS, Keeler EB, Kahn KL. Effect of epidural analgesia for labor on the cesarean delivery rate. Obstet Gynecol 1994;83:1045–1052

25. Cohen SE, Cherry CM, Holbrook RH Jr, El-Sayed YY, Gibson RN, Jaffe RA. Intrathecal sufentanil for labor analgesia—sensory changes, side effects, and fetal heart rate changes. Anesth Analg 1993;77:1155–1160

26. American College of Obstetricians and Gynecologists. Anesthesia for emergency deliveries. ACOG Committee Opinion 104. Washington, DC: ACOG, 1992

27. American College of Obstetricians and Gynecologists. Fetal distress and birth asphyxia. ACOG Committee Opinion 137. Washington, DC: ACOG, 1994

28. Marx GF, Luykx WM, Cohen S. Fetal-neonatal status following caesarean section for fetal distress. Br J Anaesth 1984;56:1009–1013

29. American Society of Anesthesiologists. Standards for basic anesthetic monitoring. Park Ridge, Illinois: ASA, 1993

30. Datta S, Ostheimer GW, Weiss JB, Brown WU Jr, Alper MH. Neonatal effect of prolonged anesthetic induction for cesarean section. Obstet Gynecol 1981;58:331–335

31. American Society of Anesthesiologists Task Force on Management of the Difficult Airway. Practice guidelines for management of the difficult airway. Anesthesiology 1993;78:597–602

This Technical Bulletin was developed under the direction of the Committee on Technical Bulletins of the American College of Obstetricians and Gynecologists as an educational aid to obstetricians and gynecologists. The committee wishes to thank David H. Chestnut, MD, for his assistance in the development of this bulletin. This Technical Bulletin does not define a standard of care, nor is it intended to dictate an exclusive course of management. It presents recognized methods and techniques of clinical practice for consideration by obstetrician–gynecologists for incorporation into their practices. Variations of practice taking into account the needs of the individual patient, resources, and limitations unique to the institution or type of practice may be appropriate. Requests for authorization to make photocopies should be directed to the Copyright Clearance Center, 222 Rosewood Drive, Danvers, MA 01923; telephone (508) 750-8400.

ISSN 1074-8628

THE AMERICAN COLLEGE OF OBSTETRICIANS AND GYNECOLOGISTS
409 12th Street, SW
PO Box 96920
Washington, DC 20090-6920

12345/09876

ACOG EDUCATIONAL BULLETIN

Number 251, September 1998

Obstetric Aspects of Trauma Management

Trauma has become one of the leading causes of morbidity and mortality of women in the world, resulting in nearly one million deaths each year. It also has become one of the leading causes of morbidity and mortality during pregnancy (1, 2). It is estimated that physical trauma complicates approximately 1 in every 12 pregnancies, with motor vehicle crashes being the most significant contributor to fetal death due to trauma (3). Nearly 50,000 of the estimated 250 million people in the United States die each year from motor vehicle crashes. This rate is equivalent to approximately 20 deaths due to motor vehicle crashes for every 100,000 persons in the United States.

The incidence and severity of injuries can be lessened by the appropriate use of automobile safety restraints. Physicians should counsel patients about such use and reassure them of the safety of these devices during pregnancy. Despite these precautions, injuries will occur during pregnancy and obstetrician–gynecologists should be equipped to handle them.

Optimum management of the seriously injured pregnant woman requires an integrated effort of multiple specialties, starting with emergency medical technicians, emergency medicine physicians, trauma surgeons, and other specialists, depending on the type of injury. Obstetricians play a central role in the management of injured pregnant women. Their knowledge and expertise are vital to management decisions regarding both the woman and the fetus. The effects of various drugs on uterine blood flow, potential teratogenic and mutagenic effects of diagnostic radiation and medications, the effect of surgery on pregnancy, and the assessment of gestational age are critical management issues. In addition, complications of pregnancy unrelated to the trauma may be superimposed in the injured gravida (eg, pregnancy-induced hypertension, placenta previa) and are best managed by the obstetrician. The obstetrician may be consulted regarding the condition of a pregnant trauma patient or, more commonly, may be the primary physician caring for the patient following trauma. In either case, the approach must be systematic, ensuring that the woman is medically stable prior to evaluation of the fetus.

Obstetricians who are involved with the care of pregnant trauma patients should seek consultation with experienced trauma surgeons. It also is helpful for all physicians to be knowledgeable about advanced trauma life-support measures.

This Educational Bulletin was developed under the direction of the Committee on Educational Bulletins of the American College of Obstetricians and Gynecologists as an aid to obstetricians and gynecologists. The College wishes to thank Mark Pearlman, MD, and Cosmas van de Ven, MD, for their assistance in the development of this bulletin. This document is not to be construed as establishing a standard of practice or dictating an exclusive course of treatment. Rather, it is intended as an educational tool that presents current information on obstetric–gynecologic issues.

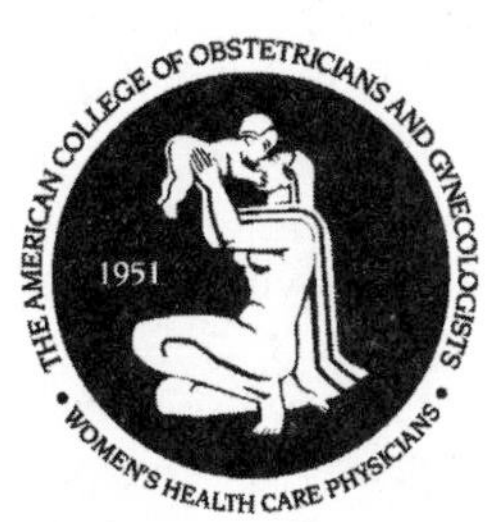

Replaces Number 151, January 1991, and Number 161, November 1991

Incidence

In industrialized nations, approximately two thirds of all trauma during pregnancy results from motor vehicle crashes. Other frequent causes of trauma during pregnancy are falls and direct assaults to the abdomen (3, 4). According to the National Safety Council, female drivers are more likely to be involved in automobile accidents than male drivers (84 female drivers versus 73 male drivers per 10 million miles driven) (5).

Domestic violence has reached epidemic proportion in the United States. It is estimated that approximately 2 million women per year are reported to have been assaulted by their male partners (6). Researchers have found a prevalence of violence against pregnant women ranging from 1% to 20% (7). Domestic violence and battery were found to occur in 1 of every 12 pregnant women in an inner-city setting (8). Among victims of physical abuse, moderate or severe violence during pregnancy was reported by 20% of women in the Baltimore area, 17% in Houston, 7% in Galveston, and 7% in Toronto (9, 10). Sixty percent of victims report two or more episodes of physical assault during pregnancy (11). This latter statistic emphasizes the importance of early identification of physical abuse during pregnancy and implementation of effective intervention methods, which are discussed elsewhere (6).

Maternal Mortality

Trauma, either accidental (as in traffic accidents) or intentional (as in homicide or domestic violence), is a leading cause of death in women of reproductive age (1). Trauma also is the leading cause of nonobstetric maternal death (12); for example, it accounted for an average of 22% of all maternal deaths in Iowa and caused nearly one half of 95 maternal deaths from 1986 to 1989 in Cook County, Illinois (2).

Fetal Mortality

Accurate statistics on the number of fetal losses due to trauma each year are not available. Estimates extrapolated from published case series suggest that between 1,300 and 3,900 pregnancies are lost each year in the United States as a result of trauma (13).

Life-threatening maternal trauma (eg, maternal shock, head injury resulting in coma, emergency laparotomy for maternal indications) is associated with a 40–50% fetal loss rate, whereas minor or non–life-threatening injuries resulted in a 1–5% pregnancy loss (14). Because minor injuries are more common, most fetal losses result from minor maternal injuries (4, 15, 16). It is estimated that abruptio placentae is a complication in 40–50% of pregnant women who sustain severe trauma, compared with the 1–5% incidence in pregnant women who experience non–life-threatening trauma (4, 16–19).

Several series of fetal losses resulting from trauma indicate that more than 50% of fetal losses occur in association with seemingly minor or insignificant maternal trauma (4, 15, 16, 18, 20).

Numerous retrospective studies have attempted to predict fetal or neonatal outcome based on an injury severity score. However, one study suggests that injury severity scoring is not a good predictor of adverse fetal outcome (21).

Types of Trauma

Blunt Abdominal Trauma

The evaluation and management of blunt abdominal trauma during pregnancy involves several key issues. Gestational age at the time of injury, extent and severity of maternal injury, and mechanism of injury should be considered.

The gestational age at the time of injury is valuable in determining the need for fetal assessment as well as in managing the mother's condition. The possibility of fetal viability in an extrauterine environment (ie, beyond 24–26 weeks of gestation) can significantly change management decisions if there is evidence of fetal compromise. Furthermore, enlargement of the uterus beyond 18–20 weeks of gestation compresses both the inferior vena cava and aorta in the supine position, increasing the likelihood of hypotension and decreased uterine perfusion. Finally, the type of maternal and fetal injury patterns may depend to a great extent on gestational age at the time of injury. For example, direct injury to the uterus and fetus prior to 13 weeks of gestation is extremely unlikely because they are protected by the bony pelvis. Generally, trauma in the first trimester does not cause pregnancy loss, with the exception of profound hypotension and associated hypoperfusion of the uterus and its contents. Although it is not the highest priority in managing the injured gravida, gestational age should be assessed as soon as feasible.

Fetal loss resulting from blunt abdominal trauma may result from abruptio placentae or other placental injury, direct fetal injury, uterine rupture, maternal shock, or death or some combination thereof. Several studies of trauma and fetal loss show that at least 50% of fetal losses with known etiology were the result of abruptio placenta (4, 15, 16, 18). In one report of severe car crashes involving pregnant women, maternal loss of life was the most frequent cause of fetal death (17).

There are several potential mechanisms of abruptio placentae due to trauma. Differences in tissue properties between the elastic myometrium and the relatively inelastic placenta can result in a shearing at the tissue interface.

Because fluid is noncompressible, intrusion of the elastic uterine wall will result in displacement of amniotic fluid and distention of the other parts of the uterus. Therefore, a shear force can occur regardless of placental location. The risk of abruptio placentae appears to be independent of the placental location (3).

Direct fetal injury (eg, skull fracture) complicates less than 1% of all pregnancies in which trauma occurs. Although case reports of fetal skull fractures have been described following relatively minor trauma, most cases result from significant maternal injury later in gestation (22, 23).

Uterine rupture is an infrequent but life-threatening complication of trauma. It occurs in only 0.6% of all injuries during pregnancy and tends to complicate trauma resulting from direct abdominal impact associated with substantial force (24, 25). The extent of uterine injury can be variable, and it may result in serosal hemorrhage or abrasions; avulsion of the uterine vasculature with hemorrhage; complete disruption of the myometrial wall with extrusion of the fetus, placenta, or umbilical cord into the abdominal cavity; or complete uterine avulsion. Approximately 75% of reported cases of uterine rupture involve the fundus. The presentation of uterine rupture can range from subtle findings (eg, uterine tenderness, nonreassuring fetal heart rate patterns) without changes in maternal vital signs, to rapid onset of maternal hypovolemic shock. Signs of peritoneal irritation, such as distention, rebound tenderness, guarding, and rigidity are frequently detected upon examination but may be less pronounced during pregnancy.

Pelvic Fractures

Pelvic fractures may result in significant retroperitoneal bleeding, which is associated with substantial morbidity and mortality. When combined with the possibility of intraperitoneal bleeding, pelvic fractures are frequently associated with hypovolemic shock. Associated injuries of the bladder or urethral disruption can result in hematuria and also may pose difficulty in placing a urinary catheter.

Pelvic fracture is not a definite contraindication for vaginal delivery. Even in the presence of a slightly displaced pelvic fracture, safe vaginal delivery can be accomplished. However, a severe, dislocated, or unstable fracture or a large healing callus may preclude an attempt at vaginal delivery.

Penetrating Trauma

Most penetrating abdominal trauma results from gunshot wounds or stab wounds. Penetrating abdominal trauma during pregnancy has a remarkably disparate prognosis for the fetus and the woman (26, 27). Fetal loss due to penetrating trauma usually occurs through direct injury or by injury to the cord or placenta. Maternal outcome generally is more favorable because the maternal viscera are shielded by the uterus and its contents, which absorbs much of the projectile energy.

The extent and severity of maternal and fetal injury due to gunshot wounds depends on a number of factors including the size and velocity of the bullet; the anatomic region penetrated; the angle of entry; deflection of the bullet's trajectory by muscle, bone, or viscera; the gestational age of the fetus; and the distance from which the bullet was fired. Frequently, more internal damage occurs than that suggested by the appearance of the entrance wound.

The enlarged uterus tends to protect the bowel from injury when stab wounds penetrate the lower abdomen because the bowel is displaced into the upper abdomen. However, as a result of cephalad displacement of the bowel by the enlarging uterus, stab wounds to the upper abdomen can frequently result in more complex bowel injury than in the nonpregnant woman.

Management

The primary goal and initial efforts in managing the injured pregnant woman should be evaluation and stabilization of maternal vital signs. If attention is drawn to the fetus before the woman is stabilized, serious or life-threatening maternal injuries may be overlooked, or circumstances that can compromise fetal oxygenation (eg, maternal hypoxemia, hypovolemia, or supine hypotension) may be ignored, lessening the likelihood of both maternal and fetal survival.

A systematic approach begins with a primary survey of the woman by securing and maintaining an airway, ensuring adequate breathing, and maintaining adequate circulatory volume. The placement of two large-bore (14–16 gauge) intravenous lines is necessary in most seriously injured trauma patients. Supplemental oxygen should be administered by nasal cannula, mask, or endotracheal intubation as required to maintain a hemoglobin saturation of 90% or greater. Crystalloid in the form of lactated Ringer's solution or normal saline should be given over the first 30–60 minutes of acute resuscitation as a 3:1 replacement based on blood loss. The use of vasopressors to restore maternal blood pressure should be avoided until appropriate volume replacement has been administered. Although these agents may reduce uterine blood flow in normovolemic patients, they should not be withheld if needed in the resuscitation of the mother. Displacement of the uterus off the inferior vena cava and abdominal aorta with the patient in a supine position is helpful in trauma patients beyond midpregnancy. This can be effected by having the patient lie in the lateral decubitus position. If the patient must remain supine (eg, if a spinal injury is suspected or if cardiopulmonary resuscitation is being administered), manual displacement of the uterus laterally with a hand or placement of a wedge under a backboard will accomplish this goal.

Following stabilization, a more detailed secondary survey of the patient, including fetal evaluation, should be performed. All body regions must be thoroughly examined. Pregnancy should not alter necessary treatment and evaluation of the trauma patient. The abdomen is of particular importance, because a substantial percentage of serious injuries involve the uterus, intraperitoneal structures, and retroperitoneum. The uterus should be examined for evidence of gross deformity, tenderness, or contractions.

Computed tomography can be used to evaluate patients who have suffered significant trauma. Computed tomographic scanning of the abdomen exposes the fetus to approximately 3.5 rad, depending on the number and thickness of the images and the equipment used. As with any procedure involving ionizing radiation, scanning closer to the uterus increases fetal exposure. Fetal exposure exceeding 20 rad may be sufficient to induce adverse effects in early pregnancy (28).

Open peritoneal lavage can be effective in the diagnosis of intraperitoneal hemorrhage during pregnancy (29). Open lavage with sharp dissection and opening of the anterior abdominal peritoneum under direct vision, usually periumbilically, is advocated over a blind needle insertion to lessen the likelihood of injury to the uterus or to other displaced intraabdominal organs. Peritoneal lavage is unnecessary if clinically obvious intraperitoneal bleeding is present. Following are some indications for peritoneal lavage after trauma during pregnancy:

- Abdominal signs or symptoms suggestive of intraperitoneal bleeding
- Altered sensorium
- Unexplained shock
- Major thoracic injuries
- Multiple major orthopedic injuries

Penetrating trauma requires the complete undressing of the patient for careful inspection of all entrance and exit wounds because occasionally victims are shot or stabbed multiple times, and entrance and exit wounds of high-velocity projectiles are unpredictable. Radiographs of the area in multiple projections often are helpful to localize a bullet if an exit wound is not seen. The uterus and its contents can often stop the progression of a projectile, limiting the extent of maternal injury to the abdominal wall and the uterus. Signs of peritoneal irritation are less reliable during pregnancy, however, and changes in vital signs due to blood loss may occur relatively late because of the increase in blood volume related to pregnancy. The general approach to management of abdominal gunshot wounds involves exploratory laparotomy, although laparotomy can be used selectively (26). Although stab wounds that do not appear to penetrate beyond the abdominal wall have been managed nonoperatively, evidence of peritoneal penetration usually requires exploratory laparotomy, particularly if there are signs of intraperitoneal hemorrhage or bowel perforation (30). The indications for tetanus prophylaxis do not change in pregnancy, and appropriate candidates should be vaccinated.

If adequate oxygenation and uterine perfusion are maintained, the fetus usually tolerates surgery and anesthesia well. Intraoperative fetal heart rate monitoring should be considered if the fetus is viable. A Doppler device or ultrasound transducer wrapped in a sterile plastic bag may be used for this purpose. When the uterus has been penetrated by an object or projectile, the fetus probably has been injured. If the fetus is alive, the decision to perform cesarean delivery should be weighed against the likelihood of fetal survival. Factors involved in this decision include gestational age, the condition of the fetus based on any antenatal testing that may have been performed, the extent of injury to the uterus (ie, a cesarean hysterectomy may be necessary with extensive injuries), and whether the gravid uterus allows adequate exploration of the peritoneal cavity. These decisions often are made jointly with the trauma surgeon. The need to perform a laparotomy, by itself, is not an indication to proceed with cesarean delivery. If the uterus has been penetrated and delivery must proceed, a pediatric surgeon and a neonatologist should be available if possible.

Fetal Assessment

The use of electronic fetal cardiac and uterine activity monitoring in pregnant trauma victims beyond 20 weeks of gestation may be predictive of abruptio placentae. Placental abruption did not occur in trauma patients in whom uterine contractions occurred at a frequency of less than one every 10 minutes during 4 hours of monitoring (16, 18). Of those women who had uterine contractions of greater frequency, however, almost 20% had placental abruption (16). Abnormal fetal heart tracings, including tachycardia and late deceleration, were seen frequently in cases of abruptio placentae.

Because abruption usually becomes apparent shortly after injury, monitoring should be initiated as soon as the woman is stabilized. Recommended minimum time of posttrauma monitoring includes 4 hours (3, 18) and 2–6 hours (31). However, none of these times have been validated by large, prospective studies. Monitoring should be continued and further evaluation carried out if uterine contractions, a nonreassuring fetal heart rate pattern, vaginal bleeding, significant uterine tenderness or irritability, serious maternal injury, or rupture of the amniotic membranes is present. If these findings are not present, the patient may be discharged or transferred (20). Upon discharge, the patient should be instructed to return if she develops vaginal bleeding, leakage of fluid, decreased fetal movement, or severe abdominal pain.

The use of ultrasonography following trauma during pregnancy does not appear to be as sensitive as cardiotocographic monitoring for diagnosing abruptio placentae (4, 16, 18, 20). However, ultrasonography is useful in the setting of trauma during pregnancy for establishing gestational age, locating the placenta, determining fetal well-being and extent of fetal injury or demise, and estimating amniotic fluid volume. In the woman, ultrasonography also may reveal the presence of intraabdominal fluid and increase the index of suspicion for intraperitoneal hemorrhage.

Fetal–Maternal Hemorrhage

Complications of fetal–maternal hemorrhage in trauma patients include fetal and neonatal anemia, fetal cardiac arrhythmias, and fetal death. There is no evidence that laboratory testing for fetal–maternal hemorrhage (eg, Kleihauer–Betke test) can predict adverse immediate sequelae due to hemorrhage (32). Among women who exhibit signs of fetal–maternal hemorrhage due to trauma, the mean estimated blood volume of injected fetal blood usually is less than 15 mL, and more than 90% of the hemorrhages are less than 30 mL (4, 16). Therefore, administration of 300 μg (one ampule) of D immune globulin would protect nearly all D-negative trauma victims from D alloimmunization. The routine use of the Kleihauer–Betke assay or other similar quantitative assays of fetal–maternal hemorrhage may be useful in identifying those few unsensitized, D-negative trauma patients who are found to have more than 30 mL transfusion. Additional D immune globulin (300 μg for every 30 mL of whole blood transfused) may be administered to these patients. Administration of D immune globulin at any time within the first 72 hours following fetal–maternal hemorrhage appears to provide protection from alloimmunization. Consideration should be given to administering D immune globulin to all unsensitized D-negative pregnant patients who have experienced abdominal trauma.

Special Considerations

Perimortem Cesarean Delivery

Although there are no clear guidelines regarding perimortem cesarean delivery, fetal survival is unlikely if more than 15–20 minutes have transpired since the loss of maternal vital signs. There are insufficient data on which to base conclusions regarding the appropriateness of abdominal delivery when efforts at resuscitation have failed. Based on isolated case reports, cesarean delivery should be considered for both maternal and fetal benefit 4 minutes after a woman has experienced cardiopulmonary arrest in the third trimester (33).

Safety Restraint Use During Pregnancy

There is substantial evidence that seat belt use during pregnancy protects both the mother and the fetus (17, 34, 35). Nonetheless, many pregnant women do not wear seat belts properly (13). Prenatal education on the use of seat belts improves compliance of seat belt use as well as improves knowledge of proper use (13). Current recommendations indicate that throughout pregnancy, safety belts should be used with both the lap belt and shoulder harness in place. The lap belt portion should be placed under the pregnant woman's abdomen, over both anterior superior iliac spines and the pubic symphysis. The shoulder harness should be positioned between the breasts. There should not be excessive slack in either belt, and both the lap and shoulder restraints should be applied as snugly as comfort will allow. Placement of the lap belt over the dome of the uterus significantly increases pressure transmission to the uterus and has been associated with significant uterine and fetal injury (36, 37). Based on preliminary data using a crash dummy that simulates a pregnant woman, there does not appear to be extraordinary force transmission to the pregnant uterus when seat belts are properly placed (37).

Airbag deployment during pregnancy does not appear to be associated with an increased risk for either maternal or fetal injury. Based on limited existing information, it does not appear reasonable to recommend disabling airbags during pregnancy.

Summary

Trauma is one of the leading causes of death of young people in this country; in many cases, it is preventable. The appropriate use of safety restraint systems in automobiles, compliance with traffic laws, and early identification and intervention in suspected cases of domestic violence are all preventive measures that may reduce the likelihood of both maternal and fetal morbidity and mortality. The obstetrician–gynecologist plays a central role both in the education of pregnant women and in the early identification of suspected abuse.

When trauma has occurred, an organized approach to management is critically important to optimize outcome. The first priority is treatment and stabilization of the woman; only then should attention be directed to the fetus. Electronic fetal and uterine monitoring is an important component of management beyond midtrimester trauma.

References

1. Dannenberg AL, Carter DM, Lawson HW, Ashton DM, Dorfman SF, Graham EH. Homicide and other injuries as causes of maternal death in New York City, 1987 through 1991. Am J Obstet Gynecol 1995;172:1557–1564

2. Fildes J, Reed L, Jones N, Martin M, Barrett J. Trauma: the leading cause of maternal death. J Trauma 1992;32:643–645

3. Pearlman MD, Tintinalli JE, Lorenz RP. A prospective controlled study of outcome after trauma during pregnancy. Am J Obstet Gynecol 1990;162:1502–1510

4. Goodwin TM, Breen MT. Pregnancy outcome and fetomaternal hemorrhage after noncatastrophic trauma. Am J Obstet Gynecol 1990;162:665–671

5. National Safety Council. Accident facts. Chicago: National Safety Council, 1997

6. American College of Obstetricians and Gynecologists. Domestic violence. ACOG Technical Bulletin 209. Washington, DC: ACOG, 1995

7. Gazamararian JA, Lazorick S, Spitz AM, Ballard TJ, Saltzman LE, Marks JS. Prevalence of violence against pregnant women. JAMA 1996;275:1915–1920

8. Helton AS, McFarlane J, Anderson ET. Battered and pregnant: a prevalence study. Am J Public Health 1987;77: 1337–1339

9. Berenson AB, Stiglich NJ, Wilkinson GS, Anderson GD. Drug abuse and other risk factors for physical abuse in pregnancy among white non-Hispanic, black, and Hispanic women. Am J Obstet Gynecol 1991;164:1491–1499

10. McFarlane J, Parker B, Soeken K, Bullock L. Assessing for abuse during pregnancy. Severity and frequency of injuries and associated entry into prenatal care. JAMA 1992;267: 3176–3178

11. Stewart DE, Cecutti A. Physical abuse in pregnancy. Can Med Assoc J 1993;149:1257–1263

12. Varner MW. Maternal mortality in Iowa from 1952 to 1986. Surg Gynecol Obstet 1989;168:555–562

13. Pearlman MD, Phillips ME. Safety belt use during pregnancy. Obstet Gynecol 1996;88:1026–1029

14. Pearlman MD, Tintinalli JE. Evaluation and treatment of the gravida and fetus following trauma during pregnancy. Obstet Gynecol Clin North Am 1991;18:371–381

15. Fries MH, Hankins GDV. Motor vehicle accident associated with minimal maternal trauma but subsequent fetal demise. Ann Emerg Med 1989;18:301–304

16. Pearlman MD, Tintinalli JE, Lorenz RP. Blunt trauma during pregnancy. N Engl J Med 1990;323:1609–1613

17. Crosby WM, Costiloe JP. Safety of lap-belt restraint for pregnant victims of automobile collisions. N Engl J Med 1971;284:632–636

18. Dahmus MA, Sibai BM. Blunt abdominal trauma: are there predictive factors for abruptio placentae or maternal–fetal distress? Am J Obstet Gynecol 1993;169:1054–1059

19. Rothenberger D, Quattlebaum FW, Perry JF Jr, Zabel J, Fischer RP. Blunt maternal trauma: a review of 103 cases. J Trauma 1978;18:173–179

20. Williams JK, McClain L, Rosemurgy AS, Colorado NM. Evaluation of blunt abdominal trauma in the third trimester of pregnancy: maternal and fetal considerations. Obstet Gynecol 1990;75:33–37

21. Biester EM, Tomich PG, Esposito TJ, Weber L. Trauma in pregnancy: normal revised trauma score in relation to other markers of maternofetal status—a preliminary study. Am J Obstet Gynecol 1997;176:1206–1212

22. Evrard JR, Sturner WQ, Murray EJ. Fetal skull fracture from an automobile accident. Am J Forensic Med Pathol 1989;10:232–234

23. Hartl R, Ko K. In utero skull fracture: case report. J Trauma 1996;41:549–552

24. Astarita DC, Feldman B. Seat belt placement resulting in uterine rupture. J Trauma 1997;42:738–740

25. Buchsbaum HJ. Accidental injury complicating pregnancy. Am J Obstet Gynecol 1968;102:752–769

26. Awwad JT, Azar GB, Seoud MA, Mroueh AM, Karam KS. High-velocity penetrating wounds of the gravid uterus: review of 16 years of civil war. Obstet Gynecol 1994;83: 259–264

27. Kissinger DP, Rozycki GS, Morris JA Jr, Knudson M, Copes WS, Bass SM, et al. Trauma in pregnancy: predicting pregnancy outcome. Arch Surg 1991;126:1079–1086

28. American College of Obstetricians and Gynecologists. Guidelines for diagnostic imaging during pregnancy. ACOG Committee Opinion 158. Washington, DC: ACOG, 1995

29. Esposito TJ, Gens DR, Smith LG, Scorpio R. Evaluation of blunt abdominal trauma occurring during pregnancy. J Trauma 1989;29:1628–1632

30. Grubb DK. Nonsurgical management of penetrating uterine trauma in pregnancy: a case report. Am J Obstet Gynecol 1992;166:583–584

31. American Academy of Pediatrics, American College of Obstetricians and Gynecologists. Guidelines for perinatal care. 4th ed. Elk Grove Village, Illinois: AAP; Washington, DC: ACOG, 1997

32. Boyle J, Kim J, Walerius H, Samuels P. The clinical use of the Kleihauer–Betke test in Rh positive patients. Am J Obstet Gynecol 1996;174:343

33. Katz VL, Dotters DJ, Droegemueller W. Perimortem cesarean delivery. Obstet Gynecol 1986;68:571–576

34. Crosby WM, King AI, Stout LC. Fetal survival following impact: improvement with shoulder harness restraint. Am J Obstet Gynecol 1972;112:1101–1106

35. Wolf ME, Alexander BH, Rivara FP, Hickok DE, Maier RV, Starzyk PM. A retrospective cohort study of seatbelt use and pregnancy outcome after a motor vehicle crash. J Trauma 1993;34:116–119

36. McCormick RD. Seat belt injury: case of complete transection of pregnant uterus. J Am Osteopath Assoc 1968;67:1139–1141

37. Pearlman MD, Viano D. Automobile crash simulation with the first pregnant crash test dummy. Am J Obstet Gynecol 1996;175:977–981

ISSN 1074-8628

The American College of
Obstetricians and Gynecologists
409 12th Street, SW
PO Box 96920
Washington, DC 20090-6920

12345/21098

ACOG EDUCATIONAL BULLETIN

Number 239, August 1997

Operative Laparoscopy

The laparoscope has evolved into an important tool used in operative gynecology. Nearly all gynecologic surgical procedures can be performed using laparoscopic techniques, but there are little data documenting the advantage of laparoscopy over laparotomy. Theoretical advantages include shorter operative time, faster recovery, decreased adhesion formation, and decreased cost, depending on the skill of the operator and the disease being treated (1, 2).

This bulletin is designed to present the principles of management of operative laparoscopy. It is not intended to describe techniques but rather to provide direction on general approaches for all operative laparoscopic procedures regardless of their complexity. As with all surgical procedures, referral to an experienced laparoscopist may be appropriate for complicated cases.

This Educational Bulletin was developed under the direction of the Committee on Educational Bulletins of the American College of Obstetricians and Gynecologists as an aid to obstetricians and gynecologists. The College wishes to thank Thomas G. Stovall, MD, and Ana Alvarez-Murphy, MD, for their assistance in the development of this bulletin. This document is not to be construed as establishing a standard of practice or dictating an exclusive course of treatment. Rather, it is intended as an educational tool that presents current information on obstetric–gynecologic issues.

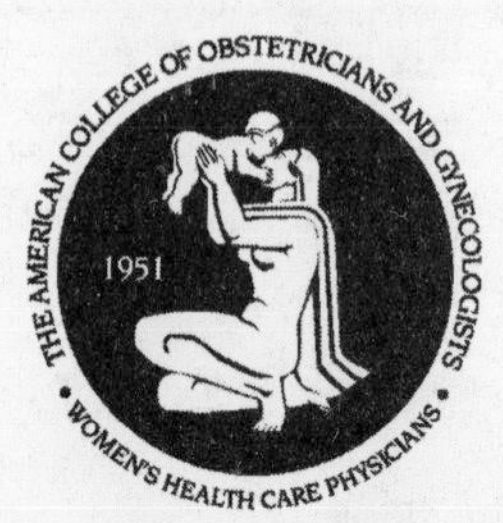

Principles of Laparoscopic Safety

Patient Positioning

The patient should be placed in the supine position and kept flat (0° angle) until after general anesthesia has been administered. She then can be placed in a dorsal lithotomy position using padded stirrups. Care must be taken to ensure that the legs or arms are not overextended and that there are no points of excessive pressure on the extremities.

Trocar Placement and Closure

Trocars are available in several sizes, in disposable and nondisposable forms. The type of trocars chosen can be based on the surgeon's preference, the type of procedure to be performed, and equipment costs.

The primary trocar is most commonly placed infraumbilically or supraumbilically and can be placed with (indirect) or without (direct) prior abdominal insufflation. Direct and indirect methods have similar risk of injury to the bowel and major blood vessels. Injuries can be caused by placement of the pneumoperitoneum needle and the primary trocar. The use of the direct entry method has been shown to decrease the amount of intraabdominal gas required and reduce operative time for laparoscopic sterilization (3). The method chosen is dependent on the desire of the surgeon.

Trocar site closure is advocated by some gynecologic surgeons in an effort to prevent incisional bowel herniation. Closure may be accomplished by using the traditional surgical techniques of fascial edge identification and re-approximation. A number of specialized surgical instruments and needles have been developed for fascial closure with laparoscopic guidance. The true incidence of incisional herniation is unknown, although it seems to be more common when multiple ancillary ports and larger-diameter cannulas are required (4–6).

Electrosurgery and Laser Surgery

Instruments used to deliver electrical energy include needle tip electrodes, scissors, and spatulas. These instruments also are available in combined forms, allowing a needle electrode to provide suction and irrigation. Instrumentation also is available to detect breaks in the electrical ground or any breaks in the electrical circuits to enhance patient safety.

It is unclear whether lasers offer any real advantage over electrosurgery. As with any type of surgical tool, special requirements and precautions are required (7).

The Team Concept

Laparoscopy requires special instrumentation, connections, skill, and special care in handling equipment. In most institutions, special teams have been assembled in the various surgical disciplines to maintain this equipment. As with any team approach, it is imperative that backup personnel be trained and used regularly and that backup equipment be available in the event of malfunctions. This issue is less of a problem now that virtually all surgical disciplines are using endoscopic equipment on a regular basis.

Credentialing and Surgeon Experience

Credentialing a surgeon to perform a particular procedure has received more attention with the introduction of operative laparoscopy because it represents a "new" approach to a given surgical procedure (8). Surgeons should have formal training and didactic and guided experience in laboratory and operative settings.

Limitations of Laparoscopy

The surgeon should understand the limitations of the proposed procedure. One such limitation with laparoscopy is that at times the intended surgical procedure cannot be completed because of poor visualization or lack of hemostasis, instrumentation, or surgical expertise. At other times, the risks of proceeding with operative laparoscopy are greater than the risks of converting the procedure to a laparotomy. The decision to convert to laparotomy incision should be made when laparoscopy no longer allows safe or effective management. Laparoscopic procedures should be undertaken only by surgeons experienced in performing surgery by means of laparotomy.

Choice of Procedure

The choice of the surgical approach (laparotomy, vaginal, or laparoscopic) should be based on the surgical indication, patient condition, surgeon's expertise and training, informed patient preference, and the data supporting the chosen approach. Cost should not be an overriding consideration unless all approaches have been shown to produce similar outcomes. Laparoscopy may be used whenever there is a need to evaluate the pelvic or other intraabdominal tissues. There are no absolute contraindications to laparoscopy.

Principles of Complication Prevention and Management

As laparoscopic surgical procedures become more complex, the number of complications has increased. The most common site of vascular injury is the inferior epigastric vessels, which can be punctured easily at the time of secondary trocar placement. These vessels usually can be avoided by placing the secondary trocar lateral to the rectus muscles or by transilluminating the lower abdominal wall or by both. Placing the lateral trocar approximately 8 cm from the midline and at least 5 cm above the symphysis has been suggested to minimize the risk of vessel injury (9). When injury to the inferior epigastric vessels occurs, the proximal and distal ends should be sutured using a variety of techniques. Attempts to cauterize these vessels usually are not successful.

Perforation of the aorta or vena cava is a rare, life-threatening event. Most of these injuries result from Verres needle placement (10). Immediate laparotomy is required to manage this complication.

Injury to the bowel can result from electrosurgical injury, placement of the needle to produce the pneumoperitoneum, or trocar placement. When the injury is caused by puncture with the pneumoperitoneum needle, usually no further management is required. In contrast, most trocar punctures require surgical repair. Burn injuries require resection of "viable" tissue around the injury site to ensure that only undamaged tissue remains (11–13). Bowel injury often is very difficult to diagnose due to the subtle nature of its presentation. Bowel injury should be considered when patients present postoperatively with pain and fever, which may be 5–10 days postoperatively in the case of thermal injury.

Urinary tract injury most commonly occurs during secondary trocar insertion. Injury to the bladder can be minimized by placing the secondary trocar under direct visualization and by making certain that the bladder is emptied prior to trocar placement. As with bowel injury, if the bladder is punctured with a Verres needle, no treatment generally is required. With a trocar injury, however, the perforation should be sutured if recognized at the time of the initial surgery. If the injury is unrecognized, the patient most often presents later with urinary ascites and accompanying abdominal pain, distention, and fever. These patients will have an elevated blood urea nitrogen and creatinine concentration and should be treated with bladder drainage and aggressive hydration. The injury may heal with catheter drainage, but surgical repair may be necessary.

Ureteral injury is becoming more common as a result of the increasing numbers of laparoscopic hysterectomies and retroperitoneal laparoscopic procedures that are being performed. When diagnosed at the time of surgery, the injury should be repaired immediately. When the injury is not diagnosed until after the surgery is completed, management is similar to ureteral injury repair after open surgery (14–18).

Evaluation of New Technology

In evaluating the feasibility of laparoscopy, as with any new therapy, physicians should consider its impact on patient care, the advantages and disadvantages of the technology, its safety, and the costs involved with its use. Laparoscopic surgical procedures usually are performed in an effort to replicate procedures successfully performed with laparotomy. Generally, a new procedure is described first in a case report or small case series, and rapid proliferation and quick adoption follow. In contrast, when a new medical treatment is described or drug therapy discovered, multiple, randomized double-blind controlled trials are required before the drug is given approval for use.

There are disadvantages to using case reports for introducing a surgical technique. Reported studies derived from experienced individuals do not always reflect the long learning curve involved in mastering the procedure, and outcome data do not exist. Although many reports suggest that the complication rates are similar to or less than those achieved with traditional surgical approaches, these reports are limited by their lack of a control group and specific inclusion and exclusion criteria. Additionally, the question exists as to whether a less complex procedure or medical treatment would have been sufficient to treat the patient appropriately.

Cost and charge data are very complex and can be used and reported in a variety of ways. This variation explains why reports comparing laparoscopic and laparotomy approaches have conflicting findings. For some procedures, a laparoscopic approach seems to be less costly, whereas for others, the costs appear to be greater. In general, the costs are less with reusable equipment and minimal use of lasers. These data must be interpreted with some caution, however, because they are generated from nonrandomized studies.

Summary

Despite the limitations of the technology and of current scientific evidence, laparoscopic surgery has made a substantial impact on gynecologic surgery. Its future impact can only be imagined as surgical techniques and instrumentation continue to evolve. Surgeons must be careful not to embrace a technique just because it is new. As with any surgical technique, adequate training and education are necessary to obtain the best long-term results.

References

1. Azziz R, Steinkampf MP, Murphy A. Postoperative recuperation: relation to the extent of endoscopic surgery. Fertil Steril 1989;51:1061–1064 (Level II-3)

2. Lundorff P, Hahlin M, Kallfelt B, Thorburn J, Lindblom B. Adhesion formation after laparoscopic surgery in tubal pregnancy: a randomized trial versus laparotomy. Fertil Steril 1991;55:911–915 (Level II-2)

3. Borgatta L, Gruss L, Barad D, Kaali SG. Direct trocar insertion vs. Verres needle use for laparoscopic sterilization. J Reprod Med 1990;35:891–894 (Level II-2)

4. Montz FJ, Holschneider CH, Munro MG. Incisional hernia following laparoscopy: a survey of the American Association of Gynecologic Laparoscopists. Obstet Gynecol 1994; 84:881–884 (Level III)

5. Boike GM, Miller CE, Spirtos NM, Mercer LJ, Fowler JM, Summitt R, et al. Incisional bowel herniations after operative laparoscopy: a series of nineteen cases and review of the literature. Am J Obstet Gynecol 1995;172:1726–1733 (Level III)

6. Kadar N, Reich H, Liu CY, Manko GF, Gimpelson R. Incisional hernias after major laparoscopic gynecologic procedures. Am J Obstet Gynecol 1993;168:1493–1495 (Level III)

7. American College of Obstetricians and Gynecologists. Laser technology. ACOG Technical Bulletin 146. Washington, DC: ACOG, 1990 (Level III)

8. American College of Obstetricians and Gynecologists. Credentialing guidelines for new operative procedures. ACOG Committee Opinion 142. Washington, DC: ACOG, 1994 (Level III)

9. Hurd WW, Bude RO, DeLancey JOL, Pearl ML. The relationship of the umbilicus to the aortic bifurcation: impli-

cations for laparoscopic technique. Obstet Gynecol 1992; 80:48–51 (Level III)

10. Baadsgaard SE, Bille S, Egeblad K. Major vascular injury during gynecologic laparoscopy. Acta Obstet Gynecol Scand 1989;68:283–285 (Level III)
11. Birns MT. Inadvertent instrumental perforation of the colon during laparoscopy: nonsurgical repair. Gastrointest Endosc 1989;35:54–56 (Level III)
12. Thompson BH, Wheeless CR Jr. Gastrointestinal complications of laparoscopy sterilization. Obstet Gynecol 1973; 41:669–676 (Level III)
13. Shell JH Jr, Myers RC Jr. Small bowel injury after laparoscopic sterilization. Am J Obstet Gynecol 1973;115:285 (Level III)
14. American College of Obstetricians and Gynecologists. Lower urinary tract operative injuries. ACOG Educational Bulletin 238. Washington, DC: ACOG, 1997 (Level III)
15. Grainger DA, Soderstrom RM, Schiff SF, Glickman MG, DeCherney AH, Diamond MP. Ureteral injuries at laparoscopy: insights into diagnosis, management, and prevention. Obstet Gynecol 1990;75:839–843 (Level III)
16. Gomel V, James C. Intraoperative management of ureteral injury during operative laparoscopy. Fertil Steril 1991;55: 416–419 (Level III)
17. Woodland MB. Ureter injury during laparoscopic-assisted vaginal hysterectomy. Am J Obstet Gynecol 1992;167: 756–757 (Level III)
18. Kadar N, Lemmerling L. Urinary tract injuries during laparoscopically assisted hysterectomy: causes and prevention. Am J Obstet Gynecol 1994;170:47–48 (Level III)

The references in this bulletin are graded according to the method outlined by the U.S. Preventive Services Task Force:

- I Evidence obtained from at least one properly designed randomized controlled trial
- II-1 Evidence obtained from well-designed controlled trials without randomization
- II-2 Evidence obtained from well-designed cohort or case–control analytic studies, preferably from more than one center or research group
- II-3 Evidence obtained from multiple time series, with or without intervention, or dramatic results in uncontrolled experiments
- III Opinions of respected authorities, based on clinical experience, descriptive studies, or reports of expert committees

Other publications from ACOG:

- **Committee Opinions,** focused updates on emerging areas
- **Practice Patterns**, evidence-based guidelines
- **Criteria Sets**, baseline guidelines for review of diagnostic and management procedures

ISSN 1074-8628

The American College of Obstetricians and Gynecologists
409 12th Street, SW
PO Box 96920
Washington, DC 20090-6920

12345/10987

ACOG EDUCATIONAL BULLETIN

Number 256, December 1999

Oral Contraceptives for Adolescents: Benefits and Safety

Correct and consistent use of all forms of contraception is an integral part of the prevention of adolescent pregnancy. The percentage of women using any method of birth control at first intercourse increased from 50% among those beginning coitus before 1980 to 76% for those beginning coitus in the 1990s (1). Oral contraceptive pills are the most popular method of contraception among female adolescents. In a 1995 survey, 44% of adolescents at risk for pregnancy chose oral contraceptives (OCs) compared with 37% who chose condoms, 10% who chose injectable contraceptives, and 3% who chose contraceptive implants (2). However, only 40% of adolescents seek medical contraceptive services within the first year of sexual activity (3).

Oral contraceptives are highly effective at preventing pregnancy when used consistently and correctly, with a reported failure rate of 0.1% (4). The failure rate of OCs for all women in the first year of use varies by age, income, and whether they are married, unmarried, or cohabiting. Low-income adolescents who cohabit have the highest OC failure rates (5). Adolescents are more likely to miss pills and may take OCs in an on-again, off-again fashion, depending on their patterns of sexual activity, which often includes serial monogamy (3, 6, 7). Only 40% of adolescents who use OCs took the pill every day and only 19% took it at the same time every day (3). The failure rate of OCs among adolescents is as high as 32% compared with 5% among all typical users (4, 5).

Special attention must be given to the adolescent during every visit for contraceptive services. Components of the initial visit should include comprehensive counseling and provision of information about human sexuality and the prevention of sexually transmitted diseases (STDs). The initial visit does not have to include a pelvic examination if the patient requests that it be deferred (8). Health care providers also should educate adolescents about the value of emergency oral contraception, explain how it is used, and consider providing an advance prescription (9). The information provided should be reinforced at subsequent visits.

Confidentiality concerns are a deterrent to the use of contraceptive services by adolescents and should be allayed during the heath care visit. As of

This Educational Bulletin was developed under the direction of the Committee on Adolescent Health Care of the American College of Obstetricians and Gynecologists as an aid to obstetricians and gynecologists. The College wishes to thank Paula Hillard, MD, and Andrew Kaunitz, MD, for their assistance in the development of this bulletin. This document is not to be construed as establishing a standard of practice or dictating an exclusive course of treatment. Rather, it is intended as an educational tool that presents current information on obstetric–gynecologic issues.

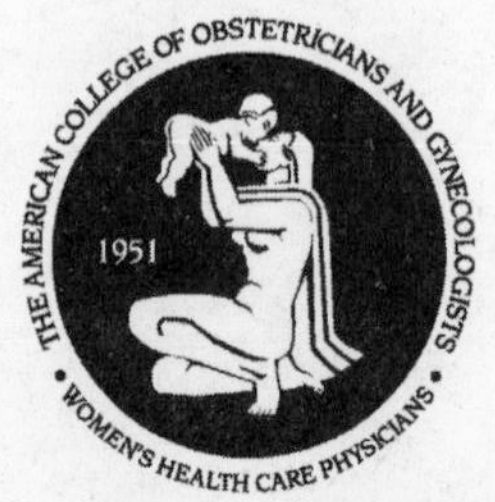

Replaces Committee Opinion Number 90, February 1991

1997, 23 states and the District of Columbia have laws that explicitly give minors the authority to consent to contraceptive services (10). Clinicians should be familiar with current state and local statutes on the rights of minors to consent to health care services, as well as those laws that affect confidentiality. Providers should encourage and, when appropriate, facilitate communication between a minor and her parent(s) (11).

The costs associated with OCs also are a deterrent to adolescent use. To ensure confidentiality, adolescents who have insurance coverage through their parents may not want to use the benefit to obtain OCs. Others may be uninsured or have insurance that excludes coverage of OCs. In all of these cases, referral to a publicly funded clinic may be appropriate.

Benefits of Oral Contraceptives

In addition to preventing pregnancy, the health benefits of combination OCs for almost all healthy adolescents outweigh the minimal risks. There are a small number of individuals with specific medical conditions, such as a history of venous thromboembolism, for whom OCs containing estrogen are contraindicated. However, even for adolescents with medical conditions, such as diabetes mellitus, pregnancy may pose a much greater risk than OC use.

Combination OCs have a beneficial effect on a number of conditions that can affect an adolescent's quality of life, including dysmenorrhea, benign breast disease, functional ovarian cysts, iron deficiency anemia, acne, and menstrual irregularity. In the United States, adult women and adolescents remain misinformed about the health effects of OCs. In a 1998 survey, half of the respondents were not aware of any OC benefits beyond preventing pregnancy (12).

Dysmenorrhea is one of the most frequent and debilitating conditions experienced by adolescents. Most women have moderate to complete relief within a few months after starting OC use (13). Adolescents who experience relief of dysmenorrhea are more likely to use OCs consistently and correctly(14). Studies have documented a significant reduction in the risk of benign breast disease among OC users (15). Similarly, numerous studies have documented a significant reduction in the frequency of functional ovarian cysts requiring surgery among users of high-dose monophasic OC pills with more than 35 μg of estrogen. These findings may be extended to users of newer OC pills with lower levels of hormones (16). Many adolescents have marginal iron stores and iron deficiency anemia is a common problem. Because menstrual flow and its duration are decreased by nearly 50% with the use of OCs, iron stores can increase significantly (13).

Acne improves significantly with most OC pill formulations. This is contrary to the common belief among adolescents that most OCs worsen acne. In particular, OCs containing third generation progestins may have an additional benefit for adolescents with acne. Based on the results of placebo-controlled randomized clinical trials of the triphasic norgestimate OC, the U.S. Food and Drug Administration recently added treatment of acne to the labeling for this formulation (17).

Chronic anovulation, which may have its onset in the adolescent years, can be treated with OCs. Oral contraceptives not only induce regular cyclic menses, but also suppress the hormone imbalance that occurs with chronic anovulation. This has a positive effect on the lipoprotein profile, thereby theoretically decreasing the long-term risk of cardiovascular disease. Oral contraceptive use also interrupts the steady state effect of estrogen associated with anovulation on the endometrium preventing dysfunctional uterine bleeding and endometrial hyperplasia (18).

Oral contraceptive use helps reduce the risk of life-threatening conditions, such as ovarian and endometrial cancers, pelvic inflammatory disease (PID), ectopic pregnancy, and toxic shock syndrome. Endometrial and ovarian cancers are rare among adolescents, but, if OCs are taken for more than 1 year, the protective effects last for at least 19 years after discontinuation of use (19). Adolescents have the highest rate of hospitalization for PID in the United States. Oral contraceptives reduce the risk of developing PID by altering the cervical mucus (4, 20). Other mechanisms for this risk reduction may include altering the endometrial lining and decreasing the ascent of bacteria into the upper genital tract (20). Epidemiologic studies (though not specific to adolescents) also indicate that the risk of toxic shock syndrome is reduced by about 50% in OC users (21). Use of OCs also may improve bone mineral density in women who are hypoestrogenic because of eating disorders or extreme exercise, although concurrent psychological management is essential (22).

Potential Deterrents to the Use of Oral Contraceptives

Fear of complications or side effects is a major deterrent to the use of OCs by adolescents, and many may not start taking OCs once they have been prescribed. Common fears may include blood clots, cancer, impaired fertility, absence of withdrawal bleeding, and stunted growth (23). Most of these fears are unfounded and must be addressed by proper counseling (see the box).

Common Concerns of Adolescents

Following are some of the common concerns of adolescents and an appropriate response to be given by the physician.

I'm going to get fat if I go on the pill. Some women gain weight, some women lose weight. With the pills we can prescribe now, weight gain isn't as much of a problem as it used to be. If it becomes a problem for you, we can try a different pill. Don't stop taking the pill, though. Call me and we can talk about our options, and remember you'll gain a lot more weight if you get pregnant.

Pills are dangerous. For most teenagers, it is very safe to take the pill. This is true even if you smoke, which I hope you don't. In fact, taking the pill lowers your risk of some cancers and many other health problems. Plus, it is less dangerous for you to take the pill than it is for you to be pregnant and have a child.

My friend who is on the pill says she bleeds when she isn't suppose to. The pill can cause what is called "breakthrough bleeding." Most breakthrough bleeding is due to missed pills, but sometimes it happens in the first few months after you start taking the pill. It is not harmful to your health and usually stops after a few months if you are taking the pill correctly. If you are taking the pills every day at the same time and have this problem for more than a few months, come in and see me. Just don't stop taking the pill. We can always try another pill until we get one that is right for you.

My friend who is on the pill doesn't get her period any more. Missing a period may happen, but it is even more likely that you will have a lighter flow, shorter periods, and less cramps. If you miss one period and have taken the pill correctly, you should keep taking the pill. If you have forgotten some pills and miss one period, call me, but keep taking the pill.

The pill causes acne. Actually, many pills help get rid of acne. If acne is a problem for you and the pills prescribed don't help it, call me and we'll try a different pill.

You have to tell my parents I'm on the pill. I understand that confidentiality is a big concern for you. We will keep this just between you and me, if that is what you want. I do want to encourage you, though, to talk with your parents about your decision to go on the pill.

Thromboembolism

Epidemiologic studies have shown an association between combination OC use by women of all ages and an approximate fourfold increased relative risk of venous thrombosis and embolism compared with nonusers (24). The increased risk of thromboembolism noted in women currently using OCs appears to be related to the estrogenic component. Although low-dose OCs carry less risk of thromboembolism than the higher dose preparations used in the past, increased risk remains. However, venous thromboembolism occurs considerably less frequently with use of modern combination OCs than during pregnancy. The overall risk of death from thromboembolic phenomena in adolescents is very low. There were too few cases in 1992 for the number to meet the standards of reliability (25). Thus, even with a small increase in relative risk, the absolute risk of death from thromboembolism among adolescents using the low-dose OC pills available today approaches zero (26). There also has been concern over the risk of thromboembolism associated with the use of third-generation progestagens. Although the differences in the rates of nonfatal venous thromboembolism are small and the use of these pills may be beneficial to some patients, the decision regarding their use should be left to the physician and the patient. It should be noted that the risk of thromboembolism in adolescents with factor V Leiden and other familial thrombophilic conditions is increased when they use OCs. However, routine screening of adolescents prior to initiating combination OCs is not currently recommended (27).

Cardiovascular Disease

Use of OCs in healthy nonsmoking adult women does not increase the risk of cerebrovascular disease (28) or myocardial infarction (29). These observations are reassuring regarding the safety of OC use in adolescent patients. Although adolescents, as well as all women, should be encouraged not to smoke, cigarette smoking does not contraindicate use of combination OCs by adolescents as it does for women older than age 35 who smoke. This is due to the low risk of cardiovascular disease among adolescents.

Preexisting hypertension is considered to be a relative contraindication to OC use (30). The prevalence of hypertension in the United States is strongly related to age and to smoking, with the lowest rates in young people (31). The risk that OCs would precipitate hypertension is remote for adolescents (32).

Cancer

Women remain concerned about the risk of cancer associated with OC use despite compelling epidemiologic evidence that use of OCs provides significant protection against endometrial and ovarian cancer (33). In a 1998 survey, 27% of the women surveyed indicated that use of OCs causes cancer (12). Many women, including adolescents, are concerned that OC use will increase their risk of breast cancer. A recent pooled analysis of data on breast cancer and OC use has clarified this relationship. This analysis combined data from 54 studies, including over 53,000 breast cancer patients and over 100,000 controls, with reassuring overall findings. No increased risk of breast cancer was associated with past (10 or more years since OC discontinuation) OC use, regardless of duration of use. The presence or absence of a family history of breast cancer did not affect these observations, nor did the use of OCs formulated with various types or doses of hormones (34).

The association of OC use and breast cancer in young women remains an ongoing controversy, however. A reanalysis of one large study revealed that women aged 20–34 years who had ever used OCs had a slightly increased risk of being diagnosed with breast cancer at a young age (35). In addition, a slightly elevated breast cancer risk has been noted with current or recent (within 10 years of stopping) OC use, but the background risk of breast cancer among adolescents and young women is extremely small (34, 36). This excess risk involves tumors less advanced clinically than those diagnosed in OC nonusers. Overall, these observations indicate that OC use does not cause breast cancer. The elevated risk associated with current or recent use is unexplained. Some speculate that this reflects surveillance bias; because OC users are more likely to have contact with the health care system, tumors are detected earlier.

Cervical Neoplasia

Cervical neoplasia's unique epidemiology, similar to that of an STD, makes assessing any association with OC use challenging. However, recent publication of studies that control for potential confounding factors, including STD risk factors and cytology screening, have clarified our understanding of this subject. Several recent case-control studies found that the risk of invasive cervical cancer with OC use was not significantly different than in nonusers (37, 38, 39). Likewise, recent well-controlled studies have found no association between OC use and cervical intraepithelial neoplasia (CIN) (39, 40). Most studies have found no association between OC use and genital human papillomavirus infection (41, 42, 43, 44). Adenocarcinoma, which accounts for approximately 10% of cervical cancers, may have an epidemiology distinct from that of the more common squamous tumor. Two large and well-controlled studies found that OC use was associated with a significantly increased relative risk of cervical adenocarcinoma (38, 45); the absolute risk is extremely small. From 1992 to 1996, the age-specific rate was 1 in 350,000 females aged 15–19 years (36).

All adolescents at risk for cervical neoplasia (those who have had intercourse), including those who use OCs, should receive regular cytology screening. Adolescents with a history of CIN (including those who have had conization, cryotherapy, or laser or loop excision) as well as those being evaluated for CIN remain appropriate candidates for OCs.

Amenorrhea and Delayed Fertility

Rather than causing oligomenorrhea or amenorrhea, OCs merely mask it by inducing cyclic withdrawal bleeding (30). The risk of amenorrhea after OC pill discontinuation is less than 1%,and appears to be more common in women who had irregular menses prior to using OCs. Misunderstanding about the rapid resumption of ovulation has led to many unplanned pregnancies among adolescents, who mistakenly believe that protection against pregnancy lasts several months after discontinuation (46).

Effect on Height

Medical providers and parents may fear that OC use by adolescents will stunt physical growth. Oral contraceptives do not cause premature closure of the epiphyses or inhibit skeletal growth. By the time menarche occurs, endogenous estrogen production has already initiated epiphyseal closure, and this process cannot be altered by exogenous steroids (47). Therefore, use of OCs after menarche is appropriate.

Contraindications

Conditions contraindicating use of combination OCs are rarely encountered in adolescents. Clinicians should be aware of contraindications listed in package labeling for OCs. In addition, progestin-only methods (including injections, implants, and progestin-only pills or mini-pills) may be more appropriate than combination OCs in adolescents with the rare conditions of refractory hypertension, severe hypertriglyceridemia, systemic lupus erythematosus associated with renal disease or antiphospholipid antibodies, and those with migraine headaches. Although progestin-only pills may be helpful in specific medical circumstances, they are prescribed infrequently, particularly for adolescents, because their efficacy is even more dependent on consistent and correct use than are combination OCs.

Causes of Discontinuation

Weight

Adolescents are extremely sensitive about their appearance, and weight gain related to OCs was a major worry for 85% of suburban adolescents in one study (48). Even the perception of weight gain as a side effect may result in discontinuation of OCs. Weight gain is infrequent with the low-dose OCs. Placebo-controlled studies with high-dose OC pills show similar rates of weight gain in the two groups (49). In addition, a randomized, blinded clinical trial of a triphasic norgestimate–ethinyl estradiol OC found that the occurrence of weight gain was similar in the OC and placebo groups (50).

Menstrual Irregularities

The side effects of breakthrough bleeding and failure to experience withdrawal bleeding can cause anxiety and are common reasons for pill discontinuation (48). Adolescents should be counseled that breakthrough bleeding is most common in the first months of use, is not medically harmful, frequently is due to missed pills, and tends to resolve within a few cycles. Physicians should be aware that OCs formulated with 20 μg of estrogen are associated with substantially more breakthrough bleeding than OCs formulated with 30–35 μg of estrogen (51). Although lack of withdrawal bleeding can occur with consistent pill use, it should be investigated in adolescents to rule out pregnancy, given their high rates of missed pills. There is no substantive evidence that the use of any contraception during early pregnancy is associated with fetal anomalies. If a pregnancy occurs while OCs are being used, the method should be discontinued (9).

Irregular bleeding in adolescents using OCs can be due to missed pills, incorrect use of the pill, cervicitis, endometritis, and neoplasia (52). Adolescents who experience irregular bleeding should be screened for pregnancy, STDs, and counseled about consistent pill use.

Other Side Effects

Other side effects of OC use, such as nausea, breast tenderness, and headaches may prompt an individual to discontinue usage. These side effects are rare with lower dose OCs. Often these symptoms resolve spontaneously and can be managed with reassurance. Should these side effects persist after 2–3 cycles, an alternative OC pill can be chosen.

Sexually Transmitted Diseases

Oral contraceptives are not intended to provide protection against STDs. Nearly 87% of girls and 80% of boys aged 15–17 years report considerable knowledge about STDs. However, these adolescents radically underestimate the incidence of STDs and possibly their risk of becoming infected (53). Sexually transmitted diseases affect 4 million adolescents annually (54). The common adolescent behavior of serial monogamy exposes each partner indirectly to infections of previous partners and emphasizes the need for education about STDs, including information about HIV infection and its prevention. There are also data suggesting that adolescent girls who use hormonal contraception, such as OCs, are less likely to use condoms (55). Dispensing condoms and demonstrating their correct use is important whenever OCs are prescribed (56).

Encouraging Correct and Consistent Use of Oral Contraceptives

Oral contraceptives can be initiated on either the first day of menses or the first Sunday after menses begins. Oral contraceptives packaged with 28 pills facilitate consistent daily pill taking. Likewise, advising patients to associate pill taking with a daily ritual (eg, toothbrushing) may enhance compliance. Compliance is critical to ensure efficacy of OCs and is a particular problem for adolescents.

Patients should be told what to do when a pill is missed. If a woman misses one or two combination OC tablets, she should take one tablet as soon as possible. She should then continue to take one tablet twice daily until each of the missed tablets has been taken. If more than two consecutive tablets are missed, an additional form of contraception (eg, condoms and spermicide) is advised while they complete taking the current pack of pills (57). Because of the increased risk of accidental pregnancy, adolescents who consistently miss three or more combination OC tablets each cycle should be advised to consider other contraceptive choices that do not require daily compliance, such as injectable or implantable methods.

Postpartum Use

Pregnant adolescents should be counseled prior to delivery about the need for contraception postpartum. All options, including OCs, should be discussed. Progesterone-only pills or mini-pills do not appear to have adverse effects on lactation and may be useful in the postpartum months during lactation (58). Package labeling for norethindrone mini-pills has been updated. Patient instructions now state that this formulation can be started within 3 weeks postpartum in women who are partially nursing and at 6 weeks in those who are nursing exclusively (59). Mini-pills must be taken according to a rigorous daily schedule (18) and should be prescribed for adolescents with caution and counseling.

Summary

In the United States, adolescent pregnancy rates are higher than in nearly all other industrialized nations of the world despite comparable levels of sexual activity (3). Approximately 50% of female high school students have had sexual intercourse (60). In the United States, approximately 880,000 pregnancies occurred in females aged 15–19 years in 1996. Of these pregnancies, approximately 56% resulted in births, 35% in induced abortions, and 9% in spontaneous abortion or stillbirths (61).

Pregnancy rates among those adolescents who are sexually active have declined while the use of contraceptives has increased (62). Oral contraceptive pills remain the most popular method of contraception among adolescents. Sexually active adolescents should be advised to use condoms consistently with OCs to decrease the risk of STDs, including HIV infection. Adolescents who are not sexually active should be encouraged to remain abstinent.

For almost all adolescents, the benefits associated with the use of OCs for pregnancy prevention outweigh the medical risks. Adolescent compliance with OCs remains a substantial problem. Health care providers have the capacity to reduce this problem and help adolescents avoid the potentially disastrous outcome of an unintended pregnancy by educating them about the need for consistent use of OCs, explaining the appropriate way to take pills and respond to a missed pill, and allaying fears about side effects.

References

1. Abma JC, Chandra A, Mosher WD, Peterson LS, Piccinino LJ. Fertility, family planning, and women's health: new data from the 1995 National Survey of Family Growth. Vital Health Stat 1997;19:6
2. Piccinino LJ, Mosher WD. Trends in contraceptive use in the United States: 1982–1995. Fam Plann Perspect 1998; 30:4–10, 46
3. Alan Guttmacher Institute. Sex and America's teenagers. New York: AGI, 1994
4. Hatcher RA, Trussell J, Stewart F, Cates W, Stewart GK, Guest F, et al. Contraceptive technology. 17th ed. New York: Ardent Media Inc, 1998
5. Fu H, Darroch JE, Haas T, Ranjit N. Contraceptive failure rates: new estimates from the 1995 National Survey of Family Growth. Fam Plann Perspect 1999;31:56–63
6. Oakley D, Sereika S, Bogue EL. Oral contraceptive pill use after an initial visit to a family planning clinic. Fam Plann Perspect 1991;23:150–154
7. Hillard PJ. The patient's reaction to side effects of oral contraceptives. Am J Obstet Gynecol 1989;161:1412–1415
8. American College of Obstetricians and Gynecologists. Guidelines for women's health care. Washington, DC: ACOG, 1996
9. American College of Obstetricians and Gynecologists. Emergency oral contraception. ACOG Practice Pattern 3. Washington, DC: ACOG, 1996
10. Alan Guttmacher Institute. Teenagers' right to consent to reproductive health care. Issues Brief. New York: AGI, 1997
11. American College of Obstetricians and Gynecologists. Confidentiality in Adolescent Health Care. ACOG Educational Bulletin 249. Washington, DC: ACOG, 1998
12. Association of Professors of Gynecology and Obstetrics. Gallup survey finds health benefits are the best kept secret of the pill (press release). Washington, DC: APGO, October 6, 1998
13. Larsson G, Milsom I, Lindstedt G, Rybo G. The influence of a low-dose combined oral contraceptive on menstrual blood loss and iron status. Contraception 1992;46:327–334
14. Robinson JC, Plichta S, Weisman CS, Nathanson CA, Ensminger M. Dysmenorrhea and use of oral contraceptives in adolescent women attending a family planning clinic. Am J Obstet Gynecol 1992;166:578–583
15. Charreau I, Plu-Bureau G, Bachelot A, Contesso G, Guinebretiere JM, Le MG. Oral contraceptive use and risk of benign breast disease in a French case-control study of young women. Eur J Cancer Prev 1993;2:147–154
16. Lanes SF, Birmann B, Walker AM, Singer S. Oral contraceptive type and functional ovarian cysts. Am J Obstet Gynecol 1992;166:956–961
17. Redmond GP, Olson WH, Lippman JS, Kafrissen ME, Jones TM, Jorizzo JL. Norgestimate and ethinyl estradiol in the treatment of acne vulgaris: a randomized, placebo-controlled trial. Obstet Gynecol 1997;89:615–622
18. Speroff L, Darney PD. A clinical guide for contraception. 2nd ed. Baltimore: Williams and Wilkins, 1996
19. Rosenberg L, Palmer JR, Zauber AG, Warshauer ME, Lewis JL Jr, Strom BL. A case-control study of oral contraceptive use and invasive epithelial ovarian cancer. Am J Epidemiol 1994;139:654–661
20. Pasner LA, Phipps WR. Type of oral contraceptive in relation to acute, initial episodes of pelvic inflammatory disease. Contraception 1991;43:91–99
21. Gray RH. Toxic shock syndrome and oral contraception. Am J Obstet Gynecol 1987;156:1038
22. Hergenroeder AC, Smith EO, Shypailo R, Jones LA, Klish WJ, Ellis K. Bone mineral changes in young women with hypothalamic amenorrhea treated with oral contraceptives,

medroxyprogesterone, or placebo over 12 months. Am J Obstet Gynecol 1997;176:1017–1025

23. Rosenberg M, Waugh MS. Causes and consequences of oral contraceptive noncompliance. Am J Obstet Gynecol 1999;180:276–279

24. Carr BR, Ory H. Estrogen and progestin components of oral contraceptives: relationship to vascular disease. Contraception 1997;55:267–272

25. National Center for Health Statistics. Vital Statistics of the United States, 1987. Vol II, Mortality, part A. Washington DC: Public Health Service 1990:276; DHHS Publication No. (PHS) 90-1101

26. Porter JB, Jick H. Walker AM. Mortality among oral contraceptive users. Obstet Gynecol 1987;70:29–32

27. Kaunitz AM. Oral contraceptive use and venous thromboembolism: translating epidemiologic data into clinical practice. ACOG Clinical Review 1999;4(4):1–2, 11–12

28. Petitti DB, Sidney S, Bernstein A, Wolf S, Quesenberry C, Ziel HK. Stroke in users of low-dose oral contraceptives. N Engl J Med 1996;335:8–15

29. Sidney S, Siscovick DS, Petitti DB, Schwartz SM, Quesenberry CP, Psaty BM, et al. Myocardial infarction and use of low-dose oral contraceptives: a pooled analysis of 2 US studies. Circulation 1998;98:1058–1063

30. Andrews WC. Principles of oral contraception. In: Corson SL, Derman RJ, Tyrer LB, eds. Fertility control. Boston: Little, Brown, 1985:157–169

31. Benson V, Marano MA. Current estimates from the National Health Interview Survey, 1995. National Center for Health Statistics. Vital Health Stat 1998;199:78

32. Petitti DB, Klatsky AL. Malignant hypertension in women aged 15 to 44 years and its relation to cigarette smoking and oral contraceptives. Am J Cardiol 1983;52:297–298

33. Grimes DA, Economy KE. Primary prevention of gynecologic cancers. Am J Obstet Gynecol 1995;172:227–235

34. Breast cancer and hormonal contraceptives: collaborative breast cancer reanalysis of individual data on 53,297 women with breast cancer and 100,239 women without breast cancer from 54 epidemiological studies. Collaborative Group on Hormonal Factors in Breast Cancer. Lancet 1996;347: 1713–1727

35. Wingo PA, Lee NC, Ory HW, Beral V, Peterson HB, Rhodes P. Age-specific differences in the relationship between oral contraceptive use and breast cancer. Obstet Gynecol 1991;78:161

36. National Cancer Institute. SEER Cancer Statistics Review, 1973-1996 "Initial Content." Available at: (http://www-seer.ims.nci.nih.gov/Publications/CSR1973_1996/): Retrieved September 24, 1999

37. Parazzini F, la Vecchia C, Negri E, Maggi R. Oral contraceptive use and invasive cervical cancer. Int J Epidemiol 1990;19:259–263

38. Brinton LA, Reeves WC, Brenes MM, Herrero R, de Britton RC, Gaitan E, et al. Oral contraceptive use and risk of invasive cervical cancer. Int J Epidemiol 1990;19:4–11

39. Kjaer SK, Engholm G, Dahl C, Bock JE, Lynge E, Jensen OM. Case-control study of risk factors for cervical squamous-cell neoplasia in Denmark. III. Role of oral contraceptive use. Cancer Causes Control 1993;4:513–519

40. Coker AL, McCann MF, Hulka BS, Walton LA. Oral contraceptive use and cervical intraepithelial neoplasia. J Clin Epidemiol 1992;45:1111–1118

41. Ley C, Bauer HM, Reingold A, Schiffman MH, Chambers JC, Tashiro CJ, et al. Determinants of genital human papillomavirus infection in young women. J Natl Cancer Inst 1991;83:997–1003

42. Bauer HM, Hildesheim A, Schiffman MH, Glass AG, Rush BB, Scott DR, et al. Determinants of genital human papillomavirus infection in low-risk women in Portland, Oregon. Sex Transm Dis 1993;20:274–278

43. Wheeler CM, Parmenter CA, Hunt WC, Greer CE, Hildesheim A, Manos MM. Determinants of genital human papillomavirus infection among cytologically normal women attending the University of New Mexico student health center. Sex Transm Dis 1993;20:286–289

44. Fairley CK, Chen S, Ugoni A, Tabrizi SN, Forbes A, Garland SM. Human papillomavirus infection and its relationship to recent and distant sexual partners. Obstet Gynecol 1994;84:755–759

45. Ursin G, Peters RK, Henderson BE, d'Ablaing G, Monroe KR, Pike MC. Oral contraceptive use and adenocarcinoma of cervix. Lancet 1994;344:1390–1394

46. Kisker EE. Teenagers talk about sex, pregnancy, and contraception. Fam Plann Perspect 1985;17:83–90

47. Bolton GC. Adolescent contraception. Clin Obstet Gynecol 1981;24:977–986

48. Emans SJ, Grace E, Woods ER, Smith DE, Klein K, Merola J. Adolescents' compliance with the use of oral contraceptives. JAMA 1987;257:3377–3381

49. Goldzieher JW, Moses LE, Averkin E, Scheel C, Taber BZ. A placebo-controlled double-blind crossover investigation of the side effects attributed to oral contraceptives. Fertil Steril 1971;22:609–623

50. Lippman JS, Godwin A, Olson W. The tolerability of a triphasic norgestimate/EE containing OC: results from a double-blind, placebo-controlled trial. Prim Care Update Ob/Gyn 1998;5:173–174

51. Sulak P, Lippman J, Siu C, Massaro J, Godwin A. Clinical comparison of triphasic norgestimate/35 micrograms ethinyl estradiol and monophasic norethindrone acetate/20 micrograms ethinyl estradiol. Cycle control, lipid effects, and user satisfaction. Contraception 1999; 59: 161–166

52. Krettek JE, Arkin SI, Chaisilwattana P, Monif GR. Chlamydia trachomatis in patients who used oral contraceptives and had intermenstrual spotting. Obstet Gynecol 1993;81:728–731

53. The Henry J. Kaiser Family Foundation. What teens know and don't (but should) about sexually transmitted diseases: A national survey of 15 to 17 year-olds. Menlo Park, California: Kaiser Family Foundation, 1999

54. American Social Health Association. Sexually transmitted diseases in America: how many cases and at what cost? Menlo Park, California: Kaiser Family Foundation, 1998

55. Roye CF. Condom use by Hispanic and African-American adolescent girls who use hormonal contraception. J Adolesc Health 1998;23:205–211

56. Rosenfeld WD, Bassoon Swedler J. Role of hormonal contraceptives in prevention of pregnancy and sexually transmitted diseases. Adolesc Med 1992;3:207–222

57. American College of Obstetricians and Gynecologists. Hormonal contraception. ACOG Technical Bulletin 198. Washington, DC: ACOG, 1994

58. American Academy of Pediatrics, American College of Obstetricians and Gynecologists. Guidelines for perinatal care. 4th ed. Elk Grove Village, Illinois: AAP; Washington, DC: ACOG, 1997

59. Kaunitz AM. Revisiting progestin-only OCs. Contemporary Ob/Gyn 1997;42(12):91–92, 97–98, 101, 104

60. Trends in sexual risk behaviors among high school students—United States, 1991–1997. MMWR Morb Mortal Wkly Rep 1998;47:749–752

61. Alan Guttmacher Institute. Teenage pregnancy: overall trends and state-by-state information. Available at: (http://www.agi-usa.org/pubs/teen_preg_stats.html): Retrieved September 24, 1999

62. Saul R. Teen pregnancy: progress meets politics. Guttmacher Rep 1999;2(3):6–9

ISSN 1074-8628

The American College of
Obstetricians and Gynecologists
409 12th Street, SW
PO Box 96920
Washington, DC 20090-6920

12345/32109

ACOG EDUCATIONAL BULLETIN

Number 246, April 1998

Osteoporosis

Osteoporosis is an important health problem affecting mature women. The health care costs of osteoporosis are staggering and estimated to be in the range of $14 billion annually. Of the 28 million Americans with osteoporosis or with low bone mass, approximately 80% are women. Osteoporosis-related fractures will occur in more than 40% of women over the age of 50 (1). An estimated 1.3 to 1.5 million fractures occurring annually are attributed to osteoporosis and disproportionately affect women. Hip fracture, a serious manifestation of osteoporosis, accounts for about 15% of the total. Within 1 year after a hip fracture, up to 20% of the victims will die, 25% of the survivors will be confined to long-term care facilities, and 50% will experience long-term loss of mobility. Hip fractures are associated with more death, greater disability, and higher costs than all other types of osteoporotic fractures combined. Spinal fractures can be associated with pain, loss of height, and deformities (Dowager hump). Osteoporosis also is associated with tooth loss and the resorption of the alveolar ridge. Numerous studies suggest that osteoporosis increases the risk of edentia. Obstetrician–gynecologists play a major role in the prevention, diagnosis, and treatment of osteoporosis as outlined in this bulletin.

This Educational Bulletin was developed under the direction of the Committee on Educational Bulletins of the American College of Obstetricians and Gynecologists as an aid to obstetricians and gynecologists. The College wishes to thank Robert L. Barbieri, MD, for his assistance in the development of this bulletin. This document is not to be construed as establishing a standard of practice or dictating an exclusive course of treatment. Rather, it is intended as an educational tool that presents current information on obstetric–gynecologic issues.

Definition

Osteoporosis is a systemic skeletal disease characterized by low bone mass and microarchitectural deterioration of bone tissue, with a consequent increase in bone fragility and susceptibility to fracture (2). Until recently, the diagnosis of osteoporosis usually was made after a woman had suffered a clinically significant fracture. Advances in the measurement of bone mass now make the diagnosis of osteoporosis possible prior to the occurrence of clinically significant fractures. The World Health Organization suggests that low bone density, or osteopenia, be defined as a bone mineral density between 1 and 2.5 standard deviations below the young adult mean and that osteoporosis be defined as a bone mineral density 2.5 standard deviations or more below the young adult peak mean (3). Other authorities define osteoporosis as a bone mineral density more than 2 standard deviations below the young adult peak mean (4). At the spine and hip, a 1 standard deviation decrease in bone mass is associated with approximately a twofold increase in fracture risk.

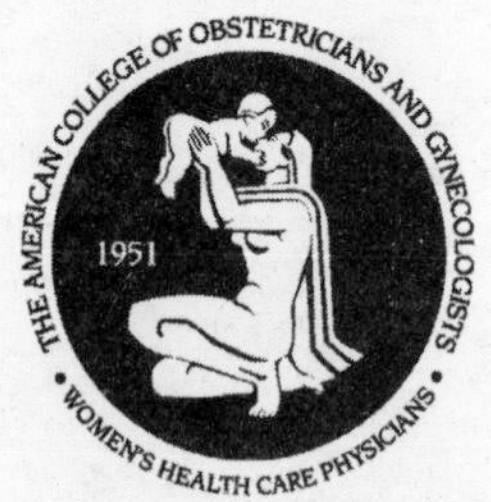

Replaces Number 167, May 1992

Pathophysiology

The functional part of bone is the remodeling unit. The bone-remodeling unit is the site on the surface of the bone where osteoblasts and osteoclasts work to make and resorb bone. Bone is constantly being remodeled in order to provide optimal support and to repair damage occurring from daily activities. The remodeling cycle can be conveniently divided into four phases: resting, resorption, reversal, and formation. Each remodeling cycle may take several months to complete.

During the resting phase, stem cells from the bone marrow are attracted to the bone surface and differentiate into osteoclasts. During the resorption phase, the osteoclasts remove bone using an acid pH to dissolve the minerals and proteolytic enzymes to digest the bone proteins. During the reversal phase, the osteoclasts cease removing the bone and mesenchymal stem cells are attracted to the bone surface and differentiate into osteoblasts. During the formation phase, osteoblasts make new bone by first laying down a protein matrix (osteoid), which is then mineralized. Type I collagen constitutes 90% of the osteoid. The protein matrix accounts for much of the tensile strength, and the minerals provide compressional strength. Cytokines (interleukin-1, -3, -6, and -11) and growth factors (transforming growth factor-beta, platelet derived growth factor, and insulinlike growth factors I and II) may modulate osteoclast and osteoblast function and mediate the coordination of these two cell types.

Bone conveniently can be divided into two major types: cortical and trabecular. Cortical bone forms the outer shell of all bones and accounts for 75% of total bone mass. Trabecular bone is the spongy, interlacing network of struts that forms the internal support within the cortical bone. Trabecular bone is concentrated in the vertebral bodies and pelvis and at the ends of the long bones. Trabecular bone accounts for 25% of total bone mass, but because of its spongy, open architectural structure it accounts for most of the surface area of the bone. Bone remodeling units are limited to the bone surface. Because trabecular bone has a large surface area, it has a higher turnover rate than cortical bone.

Bone formation and resorption is an ongoing process that usually is balanced in young adults who have adequate nutrition and exercise and normal puberty (5). Bone mass peaks at approximately 30 years in both men and women. After reaching peak bone mass, about 0.4% of bone is lost per year in both sexes. In addition to this loss, women also lose approximately 2% of cortical bone and 5% of trabecular bone per year for the first 5 to 8 years following menopause. With aging, the coordinated balance between osteoclasts and osteoblasts may be disturbed, resulting in excessive bone loss. In women who are recently menopausal, excess bone loss is commonly due to excessive osteoclast resorption. In later postmenopausal years, suppressed osteoblast activity and inadequate formation of bone may play a major role in the progression of osteoporosis. The excessive number of women as compared to men with osteoporosis is due in part to the accelerated loss of bone that occurs following menopause.

Factors Affecting Bone Mass

Bone mass is influenced by numerous factors. These factors include: family history, hormone levels, lifestyle and habits, nutrition, medications, and diseases that affect bone metabolism.

Many studies have shown that the risk of osteoporosis is greater for white and Asian women than for African American women. Mexican American women have an intermediate risk. These racial differences are probably due, in part, to genetic determinants of body size, body composition, and bone metabolism. Family studies also suggest that genetic factors play a role in determining bone mass. Female children and relatives of women with osteoporosis have lower bone mass than children and relatives of women without osteoporosis.

Estradiol, testosterone, progesterone, cortisol, parathyroid hormone, thyroxine, growth hormone, and insulin all can influence bone mass. The effect of estradiol on bone mass is probably both dose and time dependent. Marked deficiency in circulating estradiol (<20 pg/mL) appears to produce greater bone loss than modest deficiencies in estradiol (in the range of 40 pg/mL). Short periods of estrogen deficiency appear to be associated with less total bone loss than long periods of estradiol deficiency. Estrogen deficiency also is associated with many physiologic conditions and disease states (breastfeeding; menopause; surgical oophorectomy; and hypothalamic and pituitary causes of hypogonadotropic hypogonadism, such as nutritional and weight loss-associated amenorrhea, stress-associated amenorrhea, and amenorrhea associated with prolactin-secreting pituitary tumors). The mechanisms by which estradiol regulates bone mass are not completely defined.

Many lifestyle factors and habits influence bone mass. Cigarette smoking, excessive use of alcohol, and high caffeine intake may be associated with decreased bone mass and an increased risk of hip fracture (6). Most studies show that women who smoke cigarettes have lower bone mass than nonsmokers and a twofold increased risk of hip fracture. Alcohol consumption of 7 ounces or more per week has been associated with low bone mass and increased fracture rate (7).

Dietary calcium intake is an important modulator of bone mass, especially during childhood, adolescence, and advanced age (8). Childhood calcium intake appears to influence adult hipbone mass (9). In elderly hypoestrogenic women, the efficiency of gastrointestinal absorption of calcium may be reduced, requiring greater calcium intake to maintain calcium balance.

Vitamin D and its metabolites are essential to calcium metabolism and maintenance of mineral balance. In the United States, vitamin D deficiency rarely occurs except in select populations, such as those who are institutionalized with inadequate dietary intake and insufficient exposure to the sun. High protein diets acutely increase calcium excretion, but long-term, high-protein diets are not associated with excess bone loss. Diets high in phosphorus can result in excess calcium loss, but daily phosphorus intake less than 2,000 mg is not harmful to bone (recommended daily allowance in menopausal women is 700 mg [10]).

Systemic medications such as glucocorticoids, thyroxine, and heparin can cause decreased bone mass. Glucocorticoids are commonly used to treat rheumatic, allergic, and pulmonary diseases and to reduce rejection in patients with organ transplants. They have a direct effect on bone, causing inhibition of bone formation and enhancing bone resorption, and also decrease calcium absorption from the intestine and increase renal excretion of calcium. A dose of less than 10 mg daily of prednisone or equivalent is associated with minimal bone loss. At high doses, glucocorticoids are associated with bone loss in the range of 10% in the first year of treatment. Hyperthyroidism is associated with decreased bone mass. The effect may persist for many years after the hyperthyroidism is successfully treated. Thyrox-ine replacement at doses of 200 µg or more daily also is associated with osteoporosis. Thyroxine replacement that normalizes thyroid-stimulating hormone but does not completely suppress it appears to be associated with normal bone density (11). Chronic heparin therapy (12,000–50,000 U/d) is associated with bone loss in approximately one third of women.

Many metabolic bone diseases are associated with bone loss. These diseases often can be differentiated based on the measurement of serum calcium, phosphorus, and alkaline phosphatase (Table 1). The clinician should be aware that serum calcium rises slightly in hypoestrogenic states. Menopausal women may have a different normal range, with a higher upper normal limit, than women who are premenopausal or than men. Many laboratories do not account for this observation in their published normal ranges for serum calcium.

Osteoporosis can be caused by systemic diseases of the endocrine, hematopoietic, gastrointestinal, and connective tissue systems. When osteoporosis is caused by a systemic disease it often is referred to as secondary osteoporosis. The endocrine diseases most commonly associated with secondary osteoporosis are Cushing's disease, hyperthyroidism, hyperparathyroidism, and diabetes mellitus. The diseases of the hematopoietic system most commonly associated with secondary osteoporosis are lymphoma and multiple myeloma. Gastrointestinal diseases can cause osteoporosis by impairing the action of vitamin D and reducing calcium absorption. Gastrointestinal diseases that can cause osteoporosis include malabsorption syndromes due to systemic diseases (celiac disease) or surgical resection of stomach or bowel. Connective tissue disease such as Marfan syndrome and Ehlers–Danlos syndrome also can be associated with osteoporosis.

Table 1. Summary of Clinical Laboratory Data in Common Metabolic Diseases of the Bone

Bone Disorder	Serum Calcium	Serum Phosphorus	Alkaline Phosphatase
Osteoporosis	Normal	Normal	Normal
Osteomalacia	Low	Low	Elevated
Hyperparathyroid	Elevated	Low	Elevated
Renal failure, renal Elevated osteodystrophy	Low	Elevated	
Paget's disease	Normal	Normal	Very elevated

Screening

Development of screening guidelines for osteoporosis raises many complex issues. There is no single guideline for testing bone density. Figure 1 illustrates one possible screening algorithm for osteoporosis. In this algorithm, menopausal women taking hormone replacement therapy are not routinely offered bone mass measurements. Women who decline hormone replacement therapy are offered bone mass measurements if clinical risk factors for osteoporosis are present. In contrast, one consensus development conference concluded that: "assessment of clinical risk factors does not accurately predict the likelihood of fracture. Hence, bone mass measurement is recommended as the best approach to screen individuals for their risk of developing osteoporosis" (2). However, not all authorities support population-wide screening for osteoporosis.

Diagnosis

Imaging technology is now available to determine bone mass with minimal radiation exposure, high accuracy, and high precision. For measurement of the axial, proximal appendicular, and total body bone mass, dual X-ray absorptiometry (DXA) is preferred by most authorities. The precision of the measurement is approximately 1%. The radiation dose is less than 5 mrem (12). Almost all

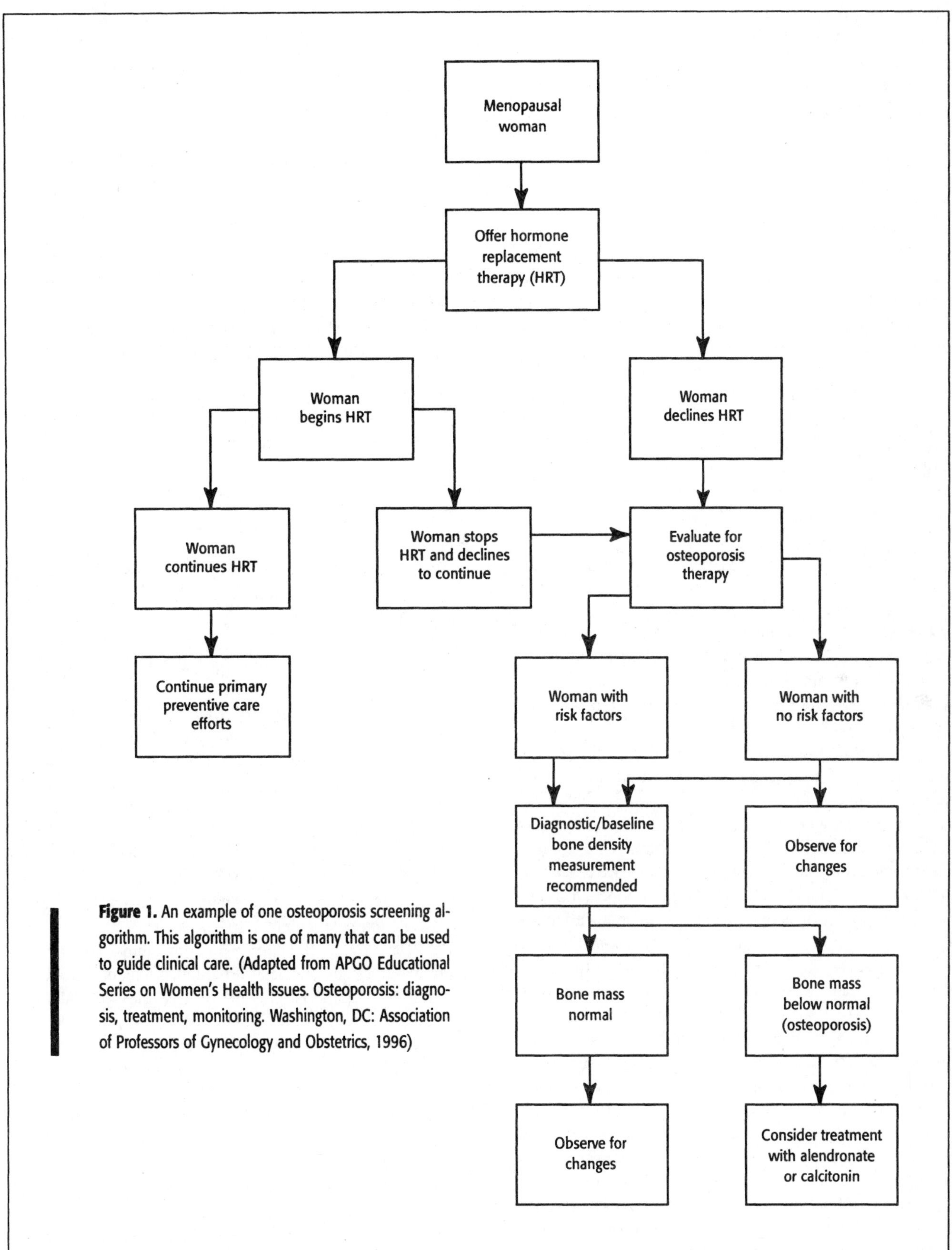

Figure 1. An example of one osteoporosis screening algorithm. This algorithm is one of many that can be used to guide clinical care. (Adapted from APGO Educational Series on Women's Health Issues. Osteoporosis: diagnosis, treatment, monitoring. Washington, DC: Association of Professors of Gynecology and Obstetrics, 1996)

modern DXA devices have an examination time in the range of 5 minutes. The fastest devices use high-power X-ray generators or fan beams and can complete an examination in 2 minutes. For clinical purposes in identifying a population at high risk for fracture, the reproducibility of DXA measurement of bone mass is excellent. Dual X-ray absorptiometry instruments are available, which measure bone mass at peripheral sites such as in the forearm. Measurement of forearm, wrist, or hand bone density may not predict hip fractures as accurately as the direct measurement of hipbone mass. However, some authorities state that "measurement at any site is a competent predictor of fracture at all sites" (2). One disadvantage of DXA is that bone spurs, aortic calcium, and arthritis may falsely elevate the reported bone density.

Dual-photon absorptiometry utilizes a gadolinium 135 source, which emits gamma photons at two different energy levels. Dual X-ray absorptiometry has largely replaced dual-photon absorptiometry instruments because of higher resolution and the avoidance of the cost and maintenance required for the radionuclide source. Quantitative computed tomography has been adapted for bone mass measurements, but radiation dosage, cost issues, and accessibility have limited its widespread use. Single-photon absorptiometry at peripheral sites such as the wrist or heel has less precision than DXA and, as noted previously, measurements at the wrist may not predict hip fracture as well as direct measurement of hipbone density. Ultrasound bone mass measurement is a new technique that offers the potential advantage of avoiding exposure to ionizing radiation.

Bone mass tests typically report three values: 1) an absolute value for the bone mass expressed as grams per square centimeter, 2) a value for bone mass relative to a sex- and age-matched reference population, usually called a Z-score, and 3) a value for bone mass relative to the mean peak bone mass, usually called a T-score or a young adult Z-score (13). The T-score describes bone mass compared with the mean peak bone mass of a young adult reference population using standard deviations as the measure. A T-score of -2 indicates that the bone mass is 2 standard deviations below the mean peak bone mass. A T-score of –2 is associated with an approximate fourfold increased fracture risk. Some authorities contend that measurement of bone mass is a better predictor of fracture than blood pressure measurement is of stroke, or blood cholesterol is of heart disease (4).

In addition to bone density instruments, bone mass can be estimated through serial height measurements. Measurement of current height and comparison to reported maximal adult height can help establish the presumptive diagnosis of osteoporosis. Osteoporosis is likely to be present if the patient has lost more than 1 inch in height from her maximal adult height and the clinical setting is consistent with a diagnosis of osteoporosis.

Biochemical markers can be useful to help identify women with high bone turnover. Biochemical markers of bone turnover also may prove to be useful to monitor the effects of osteoporosis treatment. Markers that measure the rate of bone formation include serum bone alkaline phosphatase, serum osteocalcin, and serum procollagen I extension peptides. Markers that show the rate of bone resorption include urinary N-telopeptide collagen cross-links, urinary deoxypyridinoline, and urinary hydroxyproline. The technology for measurement of bone biochemical markers is evolving rapidly.

For premenopausal and postmenopausal women who have osteoporosis documented by bone mass measurement or who have lost significant height or who have had a fracture, the presence of metabolic bone disease should be considered. Common secondary causes of metabolic bone disease are shown in Table 1.

Prevention

The most effective approach to osteoporosis prevention is to ensure each woman reaches her genetically endowed peak bone mass and to minimize the amount of bone loss during menopause. Interventions to prevent osteoporosis span the continuum of life and extend into menopause with the addition of estrogen. Several options are outlined in Table 2.

Prevention of osteoporosis begins in childhood and adequate calcium intake is important. Recommendations for daily calcium intake are listed in Table 3. Many children and adolescents do not achieve the recommended daily intake of calcium. For children and adolescents, calcium supplementation is not widely practiced. Calcium supplementation is indicated to ensure that genetically determined peak bone mass is achieved (9). Insufficient calcium intake also can accelerate age-associated bone loss. Calcium supplementation may provide a convenient means for reaching the daily dietary calcium goal without adding significant calories to the diet. Elemental calcium is present in various preparations (Table 4). Calcium citrate is more soluble and better absorbed than calcium carbonate in both fasting normal and achlorhydric individuals.

Sedentary lifestyle is associated with reduced bone mass. Weight-bearing exercise stimulates osteoblasts to form new bone (14). Observational studies suggest that exercise stimulates an increase in muscle mass and that exercise and increased muscle mass both contribute to the development of an increased bone mass. The benefits of exercise can be demonstrated into the ninth decade of life, but persist only when the exercise is continued (15). In

Table 2. Options for Osteoporosis Prevention and Treatment

Agent	Mechanism of Action	Effect on Bone	Effect on Fractures	Recommended for	Risks	Comment
Calcium	Increased availability	Deficiency causes loss; supplements reduce loss	Reduction in fracture risk by use of calcium with vitamin D	Adolescents, lactating women, hypoestrogenic women, osteoporosis risk factors including age	Should not exceed 2,000 mg/d; hypercalciuria, hypercalcemia	Revised daily requirement
Vitamin D	Increased intestinal absorption of CA + +	Direct effect unknown; increases mass when combined with calcium	Reduction in fracture risk by use of calcium with vitamin D	Institutionalized elderly and women over 70	Hypercalcuria and hypercalcemia with increased doses	Overdosage in elderly can lead to renal failure
Estrogen	Reduces bone resorption by inhibiting osteoclasts	Slows bone loss; increases mass slightly; affects all types of bones	Documented reduction of all fractures; as high as 50% reduction of hip fractures	First-line choice for prevention in absence of contraindication; indicated for proven osteoporosis or abnormal bone density	Uterine bleeding, endometrial hyperplasia, endometrial carcinoma	Additional cardiovascular and other benefits have been described
Alendronate	Reduces bone resorption by inhibiting osteoclasts	Slows bone loss; increases bone mass	Significant reduction (48%) in new vertebral fractures	Treatment of osteoporosis (10 mg dose); prevention of repeat vertebral fractures	Not recommended for patients with renal insufficiency or upper gastrointestinal problems	Use as a preventive in normal population (5 mg dose)
Calcitonin	Reduces bone resorption by inhibiting osteoclasts	Increases vertebral bone mass	Significant reduction in new vertebral fractures	Alternative to estrogen therapy	Development of neutralizing antibodies—effect unknown	Objection to injections now avoided by intranasal spray; absorption is variable
Raloxifene	Reduces bone resorption by inhibiting osteoclasts	Slight increase in bone mass over 2–3 years of use	—	Prevention of osteoporosis	—	Low rate of uterine bleeding
Progestogens	Reduces bone resorption by inhibiting osteoclasts	Slows bone loss	Long-term study of progestins alone unavailable	Women on estrogen replacement therapy unless hysterectomized; not recommended as sole agent	Doses required to positively affect bone; causes reduction in high-density lipoprotein and elevation of low-density lipoprotein	—
Fluoride	Deposited and concentrated in bone; slowly reabsorbed	Increases bone mass in continuous manner; new bone is structurally abnormal	No demonstrated reduction in vertebral fracture; may increase nonvertebral fractures	Not recommended in the United States	New bone may be weaker and increase fracture risk	Slow-release formulations may improve effectiveness of fluoride
Etidronate	Inhibits bone resorption by reducing ability of osteoclasts to reabsorb bone	Increases bone mass; reduces bone remodeling	Reduction not clearly demonstrated	Not FDA approved for this purpose	Inhibits mineralization at slightly higher doses; long-term effects unknown	Approved for osteoporosis treatment in Canada
Tamoxifen	Assumed to be an antiabsorptive agent with an effect of a weak estrogen	Laboratory evidence of reduced bone loss in rats	No long-term data	Not recommended as an agent specific for osteoporosis prevention	Endometrial carcinoma incidence is reportedly increased	Level of protection against osteoporosis unknown; other agents should be added

Table 3. Optimal Calcium Requirements

Age or Clinical State	Recommended Elemental Calcium Intake (mg)
Children	
Age 1–5 years	800
Age 6–10 years	800–1,200
Adolescents	1,200–1,500
Adult women (premenopausal)	1,000
Adult women (menopausal or hypoestrogenic on estrogen replacement therapy)	1,000
Adult women (menopausal or hypoestrogenic not on estrogen replacement therapy)	1,500

Adapted from Optimal Calcium Intake. NIH Consensus Statement 1994;12(4):7

menopausal women, weight-bearing exercise for 22 months was shown to result in a 6.1% increase in bone density of the lumbar spine (16). The benefits of physical exercise include maintenance of bone mass and an increase in muscle strength and coordination.

The risk of falling increases substantially with aging. Diseases and sensory impairments that can promote falling should be treated. Medications that reduce strength and balance should be avoided, if possible. Most falls that result in hip fractures occur indoors. The living environment should be monitored to reduce the risk of falling. Cessation of smoking and reducing alcohol and caffeine intake may all contribute to a decreased risk of developing a fracture.

Raloxifene, a nonsteroidal benzothiophene, has been approved by the Food and Drug Administration for the prevention of osteoporosis at a dose of 60 mg daily. Raloxifene is a selective estrogen receptor modulator, which displays estrogen agonist properties in the bone (inhibits osteoclast function) and the liver (decreases low-density lipoprotein cholesterol). Because raloxifene has no estrogen agonist activity in the endometrium, raloxifene treatment is associated with minimal uterine bleeding. At doses of 60 mg daily for 24 months, raloxifene is associated with a 1–2% increase in lumbar spine and hip bone density (17).

Treatment

In women with established osteoporosis, calcium, vitamin D supplementation, and an exercise program should be considered. As outlined in Figure 1, estrogen replacement therapy is the primary preventive and therapeutic modality for hypoestrogenic women with osteoporosis.

Many women who start estrogen replacement therapy discontinue the treatment. For menopausal women with established osteoporosis who decline estrogen replacement, alendronate and calcitonin are effective treatment options. All women with osteoporosis should be offered estrogen replacement as the first line of therapy, which decreases bone loss, reduces the incidence of fracture, and prevents height loss (18–20). Estrogen replacement initiated during perimenopause or soon after the onset of menopause prevents the early phase of menopausal bone loss and decreases the subsequent risk of fracture by approximately 50%. Estrogen also is effective if initiated many years after the onset of menopause (19, 21, 22). For menopausal women taking estrogen replacement therapy, the addition of a progestin does not significantly increase bone mass; the optimum duration of this therapy is not well established. When estrogen replacement therapy is discontinued, bone loss can increase to a rate similar to that seen following oophorectomy (23).

Alendronate is a bisphosphonate that has been demonstrated to increase bone mineral density and reduce the fracture rate in menopausal women with osteoporosis. Biphosphonates are analogues of inorganic pyrophosphate, and a number of other biphosphonates are currently under development. Alendronate binds tightly to the bone's hydroxyapatite crystal surface and inhibits the function of nearby osteoclasts, reducing bone resorption. At the doses used to treat osteoporosis, alendronate does not significantly inhibit osteoblast function. Menopausal women treated with alendronate for 3 years gained significant bone mass at the hip trochanter (6–8%) and the spine (6–9%) (24). Vertebral fractures were reduced by 48% in the women treated with alendronate. Loss of height was greater in the women who were treated with

Table 4. Amount of Elemental Calcium Present in Various Preparations

Generic Name	Amount of Elemental Calcium (%)	Dose	Elemental Calcium Present in Preparation (mg)
Calcium carbonate	40	600–1,500 mg tablet	600
		500–1,250 mg tablet	500
		500 mg tablet	200
Calcium citrate	21.2	950 mg tablet	200
Calcium lactate	13	325 mg tablet	42.2
		650 mg tablet	84.5

placebo plus 500 mg of calcium than in the women treated with alendronate.

Alendronate is approved by the Food and Drug Administration for the prevention of osteoporosis (5 mg daily) and for the treatment of established osteoporosis (10 mg daily). Alendronate is poorly absorbed from the gastrointestinal tract (1% absorption). It is recommended that alendronate be taken in the morning with 8 ounces of water, prior to any food or beverage. No food or beverage should be taken for the next 30 minutes to allow the alendronate to be absorbed. After taking alendronate, the woman should remain in an upright position, either sitting or standing, to minimize the possibility of abdominal discomfort. The major side effects associated with alendronate treatment are abdominal pain and musculoskeletal pain. Alendronate use can be associated with upper gastrointestinal bleeding. One potential advantage of alendronate is that it remains tightly bound to the surface of the bone for many years. Because of the long half-life of alendronate, estimated to be greater than 10 years, there may not be rapid bone loss during the period just after discontinuation of the drug that occurs after the discontinuation of estrogen.

Calcitonin is produced endogenously by the parafollicular C cells of the thyroid gland. Calcitonin inhibits bone resorption. Currently, the most convenient route of administration of calcitonin is as a nasal spray. One spray in one nostril delivers the recommended dose of 200 IU of salmon calcitonin. Intranasal calcitonin has been demonstrated to increase bone mass and reduce the risk of vertebral fractures (25, 26). The most frequent side effect of nasal salmon calcitonin is rhinitis.

Progestins, fluoride, androgens, and parathyroid hormone have been demonstrated to be effective in the treatment of osteoporosis. In a hypoestrogenic state, progestins can decrease biochemical markers of bone resorption and preserve bone density. Progestins, used as monotherapy for osteoporosis may be more effective at preserving bone in the wrist than the spine.

Fluoride is a mineral that stimulates osteoblasts to produce new bone. When fluoride is administered at doses of 75 mg daily or more, the new bone formed is dense but may be structurally weak and susceptible to fracture (27). Lower doses of fluoride, administered in a slow-release formulation for 28 months, have been demonstrated to both improve bone density and simultaneously decrease fracture risk (28). The most common side effects of treatment with fluoride are gastric irritation and lower extremity pain. Currently, there is insufficient evidence to support the safety and efficacy of sodium fluoride therapy for the treatment of osteoporosis (29).

Parathyroid hormone is not approved by the Food and Drug Administration for the treatment of osteoporosis. On an experimental basis, exogenously administered parathyroid hormone and biologically active fragments of parathyroid hormone appear to stimulate bone growth if given intermittently or at low doses (30).

Summary

Advances in imaging technology allow clinicians to diagnose osteoporosis before a clinically significant fracture occurs. In addition, advances in pharmacology give clinicians a broad range of estrogens and nonestrogen treatments for osteoporosis. These advances in imaging technology and treatment are timely. As the population ages, a large increase in osteoporotic fractures is expected. It is key that women at increased risk are identified. Premenopausal and menopausal women should be encouraged to exercise and maintain adequate calcium intake. Menopausal women should be encouraged to consider estrogen replacement therapy, and those with risk factors who decline estrogen replacement therapy should be recommended for bone density measurements. Women with low bone density or established osteoporosis should be offered estrogen replacement, alendronate, or calcitonin therapy. Application of these new tools and treatments by obstetrician–gynecologists may reduce the number of osteoporotic fractures experienced by our aging population.

References

1. Genant HK, Jergas M, Palermo L, Nevitt M, Valentin RS, Black D, et al. Comparison of semiquantitative visual and quantitative morphometric assessment of prevalent and incident vertebral fractures in osteoporosis. The Study of Osteoporotic Fractures Research Group. J Bone Miner Res 1996;11:984–996

2. Consensus Development Conference: Diagnosis, prophylaxis, and treatment of osteoporosis. Am J Med 1993; 94:646–650

3. World Health Organization. Assessment of fracture risks and its application to screening for postmenopausal osteoporosis. WHO Technical Report Series. Geneva: WHO, 1994

4. Nordin BEC. Guidelines for bone densitometry. Med J Aust 1994;160:517–520

5. Boot AM, DeRidder MAJ, Pols HAP, Krenning EP, DeMuinck Keizer-Schrama SMPF. Bone mineral density in children and adolescents: relation to puberty, calcium intake, and physical activity. J Clin Endocrinol Metab 1997;82:57–62

6. Hernandez-Avila M, Colditz GA, Stampfer MJ, Rosner B, Speizer FE, Willett WC. Caffeine, moderate alcohol intake, and risk of fractures of the hip and forearm in middle-aged women. Am J Clin Nutr 1991;54:157–163

7. Felson DT, Kiel DP, Anderson JJ, Kannel WB. Alcohol consumption and hip fractures: the Framingham study. Am J Epidemiol 1988;128:1102–1110

8. Matkovic V, Illich J. Calcium requirements for growth: are current recommendations adequate? Nutr Rev 1993;51: 171–180

9. Nieves JW, Golden AL, Siris E, Kelsey JL, Lindsay R. Teenage and current calcium intake are related to bone mineral density of the hip and forearm in women aged 30–39 years. Am J Epidemiol 1995;141:342–351

10. Institute of Medicine. Standing Committee on the Scientific Evaluation of Dietary Reference Intakes. Dietary reference intakes for calcium, phosphorus, magnesium, vitamin D, and fluoride. Washington, DC: National Academy Press, 1997 (prepublication copy)

11. Marcocci C, Golia F, Bruno-Bossio G, Vignali E, Pinchera A. Carefully monitored levothyroxine suppressive therapy is not associated with bone loss in premenopausal women. J Clin Endocrinol Metab 1994;78:818–823

12. Jergas M, Genant HK. Current methods and recent advances in the diagnosis of osteoporosis. Arthritis Rheum 1993;36:1649–1662

13. Compston JE, Cooper C, Kanis JA. Bone densitometry in clinical practice. BMJ 1995;310:1507–1510

14. Gutin B, Kasper MJ. Can vigorous exercise play a role in osteoporosis prevention? A review. Osteoporos Int 1992;2: 55–69

15. Fiatarone MA, Marks EC, Ryan ND, Meredith CN, Lipsitz LA, Evans WJ. High-intensity strength training in nonagenarians: effects on skeletal muscle. JAMA 1990;263: 3029–3034

16. Dalsky GP, Stocke KS, Ehsani AA, Slatopolsky E, Lee WC, Birge SJ Jr. Weight-bearing exercise training and lumbar bone mineral content in postmenopausal women. Ann Intern Med 1988;108:824–828

17. Delmas PD, Bjarnason NH, Mitlak BH, Ravoux A-C, Shah AS, Huster WJ, et al. Effects of raloxifene on bone mineral density, serum cholesterol concentrations, and uterine endometrium in postmenopausal women. N Engl J Med 1997;337:1641–1647

18. Ettinger B, Genant HK, Cann CE. Long-term estrogen replacement therapy prevents bone loss and fractures. Ann Intern Med 1985;102:319–324

19. Lindsay R, Tohme JF. Estrogen treatment of patients with established postmenopausal osteoporosis. Obstet Gynecol 1990;76:290–295

20. Nachtigall LE, Nachtigall RH, Nachtigall RD, Beckman EM. Estrogen replacement therapy; I: a 10-year prospective study in the relationship to osteoporosis. Obstet Gynecol 1979;53:277–281

21. Lufkin EG, Wahner HW, O'Fallon WM, Hodgson SF, Kotowitcz MA, Lane AW, et al. Treatment of postmenopausal osteoporosis with transdermal estrogen. Ann Intern Med 1992;117:1–9

22. Schneider DL, Barrett-Connor EL, Morton DJ. Timing of postmenopausal estrogen for optimal bone mineral density: the Rancho Bernardo study. JAMA 1997;277:543–547

23. Christiansen C, Christensen MS, Transbol I. Bone mass in postmenopausal women after withdrawal of oestrogen/gestagen replacement therapy. Lancet 1981;1:459–461

24. Liberman UA, Weiss SR, Broll J, Minne HW, Quan H, Bell NH, et al. Effect of oral alendronate on bone mineral density and the incidence of fractures in postmenopausal osteoporosis. The Aldendronate Phase III Osteoporosis Treatment Study Group. N Engl J Med 1995;333: 1437–1443

25. Overgaard K, Hansen MA, Jensen SB, Christiansen C. Effect of salcatonin given intranasally on bone mass and fracture rates in established osteoporosis: a dose-response study. BMJ 1992;305:556–561

26. Rico H, Hernandez ER, Revilla M, Gomez-Castresana F. Salmon calcitonin reduces vertebral fracture rate in postmenopausal crush fracture syndrome. Bone Miner 1992;16:131–138

27. Riggs BL, Hodgson SF, O'Fallon WM, Chao EYS, Wahner HW, Muhs JM, et al. Effect of fluoride treatment on the fracture rate in postmenopausal women with osteoporosis. N Engl J Med 1990;322:802–809

28. Pak CYC, Sakhaee K, Piziak V, Peterson RD, Breslau NA, Boyd P, et al. Slow-release sodium fluoride in the management of postmenopausal osteoporosis: a randomized controlled trial. Ann Intern Med 1994;120:625–632

29. American Medical Association. Drug evaluations annual. Chicago: AMA, 1995.

30. Finkelstein JS, Klibanski A, Schaefer EH, Hornstein MD, Schiff I, Neer RM. Parathyroid hormone for the prevention of bone loss induced by estrogen deficiency. N Engl J Med 1994;331:1618–1623

ISSN 1074-8628

The American College of Obstetricians and Gynecologists
409 12th Street, SW
PO Box 96920
Washington, DC 20090-6920

12345/21098

ACOG EDUCATIONAL BULLETIN

Number 250, August 1998

Ovarian Cancer

Ovarian cancer is the leading cause of death from gynecologic malignancy and the fourth leading cause of cancer death in American women. An estimated 25,400 new cases are reported in the United States yearly, and approximately 14,500 women die annually from the disease (1). Unfortunately, ovarian cancer often is detected only when it has spread throughout the peritoneal cavity. Despite aggressive surgical resection and adjunctive therapy, most patients die in a period of months from malnutrition and small bowel obstruction caused by intraperitoneal tumor.

Nearly 80% of all ovarian cancers are epithelial ovarian carcinomas arising from the germinal epithelium of the ovary. Epithelial ovarian carcinomas may be subclassified by cell type to include serous, mucinous, endometrioid, clear cell, and undifferentiated carcinomas. However, because there appears to be little difference in the prognosis based on cell type, epithelial carcinomas will be considered together in discussing therapy, prognosis, and survival. The tumors of low malignant potential (borderline tumors) are considered separately because they are less aggressive than invasive carcinomas. Also discussed are other malignancies of the ovary, which include those of germ cell origin (dysgerminoma, endodermal sinus tumor, immature teratoma, choriocarcinoma, and embryonal cell carcinoma), stromal and sex cord tumors (granulosa–theca, Sertoli–Leydig, hilar, lipoma, and thecoma), mesenchymal tumors, and cancer metastatic to the ovary, in particular from the gastrointestinal tract (Krukenberg tumor) and breast.

This Educational Bulletin was developed under the direction of the Committee on Educational Bulletins of the American College of Obstetricians and Gynecologists as an aid to obstetricians and gynecologists. The College wishes to thank Daniel L. Clarke-Pearson, MD, and Anthony C. Evans, MD, PhD, for their assistance in the development of this bulletin. This document is not to be construed as establishing a standard of practice or dictating an exclusive course of treatment. Rather, it is intended as an educational tool that presents current information on obstetric–gynecologic issues.

Epidemiology and Risk Factors

A woman has a 1-in-70 risk of developing ovarian cancer in her lifetime. The incidence is 1.4 per 100,000 women under age 40, increasing to approximately 45 per 100,000 for women over age 60 (2). The median age at diagnosis is 61. A higher incidence of ovarian cancer is seen in women who have never been pregnant or are of low parity. Women who have had either breast or colon cancer or have a family history of these cancers also are at higher risk of developing ovarian cancer.

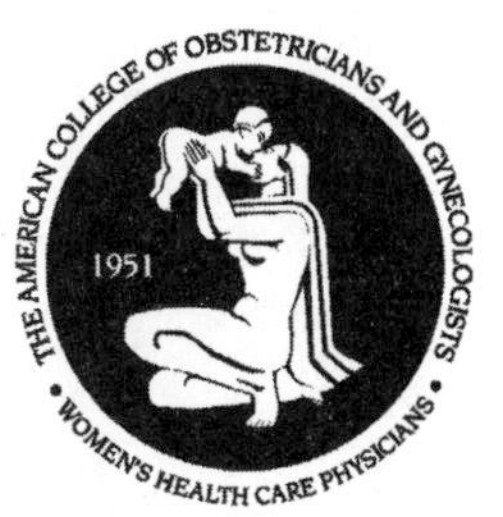

Replaces Number 141, May 1990

The cause of ovarian cancer is not clear but may be associated with environmental factors because its incidence is higher in industrialized countries. Factors that have been suspected of increasing the risk of ovarian cancer include high dietary fat intake, use of talc compounds in the perineal area, and mumps infection before menarche. Protective factors include multiparity, oral contraceptive use, a history of breastfeeding, and anovulatory disorders. Although an association between ovarian cancer and ovulation induction in infertile patients has been suggested, these data have been questioned (3).

Only about 5–10% of ovarian cancer patients have a significant family history of cancer. Three familial syndromes have been identified. Typically, women affected by these syndromes tend to develop ovarian cancer at a younger age than those who develop sporadic ovarian cancer. The cancer family syndrome (Lynch type II) is characterized by development of nonpolyposis colon cancer and either breast, ovarian, or endometrial adenocarcinoma. Site-specific ovarian cancer is a less common familial pattern. Familial breast–ovarian cancer syndrome is associated with early-onset breast and ovarian cancers. All of these syndromes are transmitted in an autosomal dominant fashion with varying degrees of penetrance.

The site-specific ovarian cancer and familial breast–ovarian cancer syndromes have been demonstrated to be associated with allelic deletion at the *BRCA1* locus on chromosome 17q21. This pattern is characteristic of loss of activity of a tumor suppressor gene. Although involved in the development of many familial cases of ovarian cancer, the *BRCA1* tumor suppressor gene rarely is mutated in sporadic ovarian cancers. Women with *BRCA1* mutation have a 90% lifetime risk of developing either ovarian or breast cancer (4).

Screening

Because most cases of ovarian cancer are advanced at the time of diagnosis and current treatment rarely is curative, significant effort has been expended to identify a cost-effective screening strategy that would allow earlier diagnosis and, therefore, higher cure rates. Currently, there is no proven method of screening for ovarian cancer. Suggested methods include pelvic examination, abdominal and transvaginal ultrasound, and analysis of CA 125 levels in serum. Unfortunately, pelvic examination alone has not been found to be effective in reducing the mortality rate from ovarian cancer. Measurements of CA 125 in serum appear to have a high false-negative rate for early-stage disease. Additionally, this method appears to have a high false-positive rate in premenopausal women, a group in whom most ovarian enlargements are benign. Abdominal and transvaginal ultrasound also have high false-positive rates, particularly in premenopausal women.

Until a prospective study has established the effectiveness of screening in a large population, routine screening by abdominal or vaginal ultrasound or measurement of CA 125 levels in serum cannot be recommended for women with no known risk factors. For women with a documented, familial ovarian cancer syndrome who wish to maintain their reproductive capacity, some authorities have suggested the use of transvaginal ultrasonography, analysis of levels of CA 125 in serum, or both, in combination with frequent pelvic examinations. The efficacy of this approach has not been established.

In women with proven Lynch II syndrome, periodic endometrial biopsy, mammography, and colonoscopy also may be considered. The use of oral contraceptives has been shown to result in a decreased incidence of ovarian cancer in the general population. The protective effect of these medications is not related to the type or dose of estrogen and progesterone. However, the effect of oral contraceptive use on the risk of ovarian cancer in women with familial cancer syndromes has not been evaluated.

Women who have demonstrated familial ovarian or hereditary breast–ovarian cancer syndromes and who do not wish to maintain their reproductive capacity may be offered prophylactic bilateral salpingo-oophorectomy. Preferably, a familial syndrome should be established by a full pedigree analysis by a geneticist. Further, genetic testing for the *BRCA1* gene would lead to identification of women at highest risk while avoiding surgery in those who do not have the gene mutation. The ethical implications of genetic testing must be fully understood by the patient and her physician. These women should be informed that removal of the tubes and ovaries does not provide 100% protection; primary peritoneal carcinoma has been reported after bilateral salpingo-oophorectomy (5).

Diagnosis

History

There are no early symptoms of cancer of the ovary. Most presenting symptoms are those associated with increasing tumor mass, spread of tumor along the serosal surfaces of the bowel, and ascites. Abdominal discomfort, upper abdominal fullness, and early satiety are associated with cancer of the ovary. Other frequently encountered signs and symptoms are fatigue, increasing abdominal girth, urinary frequency, and shortness of breath caused by pleural effusion or massive ascites.

Physical Findings

The most frequently noted physical finding of ovarian cancer is a pelvic mass. Although the character of an adnexal mass (either cystic or solid) is not necessarily diagnostic, an adnexal mass that is bilateral, irregular, solid, or fixed suggests malignancy. Other findings suggestive of malignancy are ascites or a nodular cul-de-sac. The risk of ovarian cancer is significantly higher in premenarcheal and postmenopausal women with an adnexal mass than in women of reproductive age.

Diagnostic Workup

The initial workup should be aimed at evaluating whether an adnexal mass requires surgical intervention. Further, preoperative recognition of masses likely to represent ovarian cancer facilitates patient preparation, surgical staging, and cytoreduction. Finally, the workup should exclude other causes of an adnexal mass.

Initial evaluation with a thorough history, physical examination, and vaginal probe ultrasonography will distinguish most benign masses from malignant masses. Ultrasound characteristics suggesting a higher probability of ovarian cancer include evidence of bilaterality, solid and cystic components, excrescences, thick septations, and the presence of free peritoneal fluid. Chest X-ray is performed to rule out parenchymal or pleural involvement with effusion. Screening mammography, if it has not been done within 6–12 months, should be performed preoperatively to rule out another primary source.

Other studies that may be helpful in the diagnostic workup of selected patients include barium enema, upper gastrointestinal series, colonoscopy, upper gastrointestinal endoscopy, intravenous pyelography, and computed tomography (CT) scan or magnetic resonance imaging. The use of one or more of these studies should be based on patient symptoms and physical findings. These studies also may be helpful in identifying other primary tumor sites (bowel, pancreas), which may present with metastases to the ovary, or in evaluating symptoms of obstruction, bleeding, or pain. None of these tests is absolutely diagnostic for ovarian cancer.

The tumor marker CA 125 may assist in evaluation, although its limitations must be understood. Sustained elevation of CA 125 levels occurs in more than 80% of patients with nonmucinous epithelial ovarian carcinomas but in only 1% of the general population (6, 7). Levels of CA 125 in serum also may be elevated in patients with conditions such as endometriosis, leiomyomata, pelvic inflammatory disease, hepatitis, congestive heart failure, cirrhosis, and malignancies other than ovarian carcinomas. In postmenopausal patients with pelvic masses, CA 125 levels in serum greater than 65 U/mL are predictive of a malignancy in 75% of cases. Elevated levels of CA 125 in serum in these patients should therefore alert the physician to suspect ovarian, endometrial, or other gynecologic malignancies. Although increased specificity can be achieved using other tumor-associated antigens (see the box), this is accompanied by a decrease in sensitivity and is not generally helpful for diagnosis. Other serum tumor markers such as alpha-fetoprotein, human chorionic gonadotropin, and lactate dehydrogenase may be useful in the management of ovarian germ cell malignancies although they are not sufficiently specific or sensitive to be diagnostic.

In general, diagnostic paracentesis should not be performed when ascites is accompanied by a pelvic mass. Ascites due to other conditions such as congestive heart failure, liver failure, or pancreatitis usually may be excluded after careful medical evaluation. In addition, because cytologic examination of ascites may be negative in patients with advanced ovarian cancer, negative cytology does not preclude the need for exploratory laparotomy. Occasionally, a patient who is thought to have a large amount of ascites actually has a large ovarian cyst filling the abdomen. In such cases, paracentesis may result in rupture of the cyst capsule and the release of malignant cells into the peritoneal cavity. Paracentesis may be useful in the rare patient with respiratory compromise due to extreme elevation of the diaphragm by fluid. In these cases, several liters of ascites may be removed before surgery in order to improve respiratory function.

Serum Tumor Markers Useful in the Management of Ovarian Neoplasms

Epithelial ovarian cancer
- CA 125
- CA 15-3
- CA 19-9
- Carcinoembryonic antigen
- Lipid-associated sialic acid
- NB/70K

Germ cell tumors
- Alpha-fetoprotein
- Human chorionic gonadotropin
- Lactic dehydrogenase
- CA 125

Stromal tumors
- Inhibin
- Estrogens
- Androgens
- Alpha-fetoprotein

Preoperative Preparation

If a high probability of ovarian malignancy exists, the physician should consider consultation with a gynecologic oncologist. The oncologist should ensure that the patient is fully informed about the surgery and obtain consent for the variety of surgical procedures often necessary in treating ovarian cancer, including mechanical or antibiotic preparation of the bowel in the event that colon resection is necessary. Prophylaxis to prevent infection and venous thromboembolism usually is beneficial. Nutrition-al support also may be indicated.

Primary Treatment

Epithelial Ovarian Cancer

Primary therapy for ovarian cancer is complete staging and optimal reduction of tumor volume. Subsequent therapy depends on the operative findings. Many patients thought to have early-stage ovarian carcinoma have occult metastases beyond the pelvis that are not detected by an incomplete surgical staging procedure. The prognosis for advanced disease is influenced by the amount of tumor remaining after surgery. Accurate documentation of residual tumor mass is necessary to determine response to treatment. Some patients may need second procedures to accomplish the goals of therapy. Timely referral for surgery is critical.

Staging

Ovarian cancer staging is based on surgical evaluation. Therefore, it is imperative for the operating surgeon to be familiar with the staging criteria and have the surgical skills necessary to perform all steps of the staging procedure. Accurate staging is of utmost importance for the patient's further therapy and in discussing prognosis. The staging classification is shown in Table 1. Staging is determined by clinical, surgical, histologic, and pathologic findings, including results of cytologic testing of effusions or peritoneal washings. Therefore, pleural effusion should be sampled in all cases.

Operative Techniques

The incision used should provide maximum exposure of the pelvis and allow thorough evaluation of the upper abdomen. When the abdomen is entered, the surgeon should note the presence or absence of ascites. If present, ascites should be aspirated and sent for cytopathologic evaluation. A small amount of heparin should be added to prevent clotting of bloody or mucoid specimens. If ascites is not present, abdominal washings with saline should be obtained from the pericolic gutters, the suprahepatic space, and the pelvis. A Pap test of the diaphragm should be taken. The abdominal cavity should then be explored systematically. The lower surface of the diaphragm, the upper abdominal recesses, the liver, and retroperitoneal nodes should be carefully noted for tumor involvement. In addition, the intestines, mesentery, and omentum should be examined. The presence or absence of metastases in the pelvis and abdomen should be noted, and the exact location and size of tumor nodules should be described in detail. The presence and location of adhesions between the tumor and bowel also should be noted.

In cases in which disease is grossly confined to the pelvis, efforts should be made to detect occult metastasis with peritoneal cytologies, biopsies of peritoneum from the pelvis and pericolic gutters, and resection of the greater omentum. In addition, selective pelvic and para-aortic lymphadenectomy also should be carried out at this operation to evaluate potential retroperitoneal spread.

Inadequate surgical staging is common in presumed early-stage disease and usually results from the surgeon not performing a lymphadenectomy (8). In a study of 100 patients initially thought to have stage I and II disease, occult metastases resided in the retroperitoneal nodes in approximately 10% of patients. Fifteen percent of patients had disease in the omentum, and 10% of patients had microscopic disease on the diaphragm (9). Any of these findings would advance the disease to stage III.

Cytoreductive Surgery

Although never tested in a randomized trial, maximal tumor cytoreduction appears to improve response to chemotherapy and survival of women with advanced ovarian cancer. Accordingly, operative management is designed to remove as much tumor as is safely possible. When a malignant tumor is present, a thorough abdominal exploration, total abdominal hysterectomy, bilateral salpingo-oophorectomy, lymphadenectomy, omentectomy, and removal of all gross cancer consistent with good surgical judgment are standard therapy.

Maximal cytoreductive surgery must be tempered by surgical judgment and the avoidance of significant operative morbidity. In addition to using the retroperitoneal approach to bilateral salpingo-oophorectomy, other pelvic techniques that are useful to achieve pelvic debulking include en bloc rectosigmoid resection, pelvic peritoneotomy, and "reverse" hysterectomy (10). The development of surgical intestinal staplers has facilitated the use of rectosigmoid resection with low end-to-end rectosigmoid anastomosis, thus avoiding colostomy. Removal of a large omental mass may be expedited by dividing the omentocolic ligament to separate the infracolic omentum from the transverse colon. This gives access to the lesser sac and allows resection of disease involving the lesser omentum. At times, splenectomy is required to allow debulking of an omental mass.

Table 1. Definitions of the Stages in Primary Carcinoma of the Ovary

Stage	Definition
I	Growth is limited to the ovaries
IA	Growth is limited to one ovary; no ascites present containing malignant cells; no tumor on the external surface; capsule is intact
IB	Growth is limited to both ovaries; no ascites present containing malignant cells; no tumor on the external surfaces; capsules are intact
IC*	Tumor is classified as either stage IA or IB but with tumor on the surface of one or both ovaries; or with ruptured capsule(s); or with ascites containing malignant cells present or with positive peritoneal washings
II	Growth involves one or both ovaries with pelvic extension
IIA	Extension and/or metastases to the uterus and/or tubes
IIB	Extension to other pelvic tissues
IIC*	Tumor is either stage IIA or IIB but with tumor on the surface of one or both ovaries; or with capsule(s) ruptured; or with ascites containing malignant cells present or with positive peritoneal washings
III	Tumor involves one or both ovaries with peritoneal implants outside the pelvis and/or positive retroperitoneal or inguinal nodes; superficial liver metastasis equals stage III; tumor is limited to the true pelvis but with histologically proven malignant extension to small bowel or omentum
IIIA	Tumor is grossly limited to the true pelvis with negative nodes but with histologically confirmed microscopic seeding of abdominal peritoneal surfaces
IIIB	Tumor involves one or both ovaries with histologically confirmed implants of abdominal peritoneal surfaces, none exceeding 2 cm in diameter; nodes are negative
IIIC	Abdominal implants greater than 2 cm in diameter and/or positive retroperitoneal or inguinal nodes
IV	Growth involves one or both ovaries with distant metastases; if pleural effusion is present, there must be positive cytology findings to assign a case to stage IV; parenchymal liver metastasis equals stage IV

*To evaluate the impact on prognosis of the different criteria for assigning cases to stage IC or IIC, it would be of value to know whether the rupture of the capsule was spontaneous or caused by the surgeon and if the source of malignant cells detected was peritoneal washings or ascites.

Modified from International Federation of Gynecology and Obstetrics. Annual report on the results of treatment in gynecological cancer. 22nd edition. Stockholm: FIGO, 1994

Because ovarian carcinoma typically involves the peritoneal surfaces, individual metastases involving the mesentery of the intestine, pericolic gutters, and diaphragm often can be resected. Enlarged lymph nodes can be removed to effect debulking. Resection of the bowel with reanastomosis in patients with ovarian carcinoma does not greatly increase the morbidity rate of the primary procedure and may allow resection of a significant amount of gross tumor. There is no advantage to resecting intestine with nonobstructive involvement if a large tumor mass is to be left elsewhere.

Surgery for Preservation of Fertility

Conservative surgical therapy should be considered in patients who desire preservation of fertility. To be a candidate for conservative surgery, the patient must have surgically documented stage IA disease with a well-to-moderately differentiated or borderline lesion. It is important that unilateral salpingo-oophorectomy rather than cystectomy or oophorectomy be performed and that a careful pathologic analysis of the original tumor, consisting of at least one histologic section per 0.5–1 cm of maximal tumor diameter, be used to assess the degree of differentiation and to exclude occult metastasis to the ipsilateral tube. Cytology from the pelvis, pericolic gutters, and diaphragm should be obtained along with multiple random biopsies of the pelvis, uterine serosa, and pericolic gutters. An infracolic omentectomy should be performed as well as selective para-aortic lymphadenectomy and ipsilateral pelvic lymphadenectomy. The contralateral ovary should be inspected carefully and biopsy of suspicious areas performed. Removal of the remaining ovary should be considered following childbearing to exclude an occult contralateral lesion.

Low Malignant Potential Tumors

Conservative surgery may be recommended for epithelial ovarian tumors of low malignant potential. These tumors account for approximately 15% of all epithelial ovarian cancers and occur predominantly in premenopausal women. Serous tumors appear to be the most common borderline tumors, of which 70–85% are stage I. Treatment of patients with stage I tumors should take into consideration the high cure rate of these tumors, age of the patient, and bilateral rate of 20–40%. Those patients who desire preservation of fertility may be managed conservatively with a unilateral salpingo-oophorectomy. However, careful surgical staging as described previously must be done to evaluate accurately the extent of disease. Patients with stage I borderline tumors have a 10-year survival rate of approximately 95%, and it is generally agreed that they do not require adjuvant therapy (11).

Adjuvant Therapy

Patients with stage IA or IB disease (who have been completely surgically staged) and who have borderline, well- or moderately-differentiated tumors do not benefit from additional chemotherapy because their prognosis is excellent with surgery alone. It should be stressed that these results should not be extrapolated to patients who have undergone less than adequate surgical staging procedures.

Chemotherapy

The use of chemotherapy improves survival and is an effective means of palliation of ovarian cancer. In patients who are at increased risk of recurrence (stage I G3 and all IC–IV), chemotherapy is recommended. Sequential clinical trials of chemotherapy agents demonstrate that cisplatin (or carboplatin) given in combination with paclitaxel is the most active combination identified (12). This drug combination generally is given intravenously every 3 weeks for a total of six courses unless disease progression is recognized.

Cisplatin and paclitaxel also may be administered directly into the peritoneal cavity. In patients who have minimal residual intraperitoneal disease, intraperitoneal administration of cisplatin appears to be more effective when compared with intravenous administration (13). Other chemotherapy agents also have activity against ovarian cancer and might be considered for second-line therapy or in initial treatment of patients who for special reasons cannot tolerate cisplatin or paclitaxel. These drugs include: cyclophosphamide, topotecan, docetaxel, hexamethylmelamine, ifosfamide, etoposide, and doxorubicin. High-dose chemotherapy combined with autologous bone marrow transplant or stem cell support is still experimental.

Patients should be monitored for side effects of therapy including neutropenia, sepsis, thrombocytopenia, anemia, neuropathy, nephropathy, and nausea and vomiting. Effective methods to reduce toxicity include the use of colony-stimulating factors, erythropoietin, antibiotics, transfusion of specific blood products, chemoprotective agents, and antiemetics.

Radiation Therapy

Because the majority of ovarian cancer spreads beyond the pelvis, pelvic radiation therapy is not considered useful as primary treatment of ovarian cancer. Whole abdominal radiation with a pelvic boost can be effective treatment when all macroscopic disease has been surgically resected. Inclusion of large portions of bone marrow may limit subsequent tolerance of salvage chemotherapy (14).

Follow-up

Evaluation of disease status during therapy is important in order to identify both patients who are receiving benefit from treatment and patients who are failing treatment and should have it changed.

In women with elevated levels of CA 125 in serum, serial determinations are useful in monitoring disease status. Depending on the distribution and size of tumor nodules following primary surgical therapy, CA 125 in serum often is a more sensitive determinant of tumor burden than physical examination or radiologic studies. About 90% of patients will have a direct correlation between serial CA 125 levels in serum and disease progression, regression, or stability (6). A favorable chemotherapeutic response is predicted in cases where CA 125 levels in serum decrease dramatically. A reduction of CA 125 in serum to the normal range within 3 months of surgery predicts a negative second-look assessment and improved survival (15). Conversely, patients who have elevated levels of CA 125 in serum at 3 months after primary debulking rarely achieve a complete chemotherapeutic response. Increasing levels of CA 125 in serum during therapy almost always suggest treatment failure.

Computed Tomography

Computed tomography scans may be useful for monitoring tumor burden during therapy. Computed tomography imaging allows bidimensional measurements of tumor nodules. These masses can be monitored periodically to assess the effectiveness of therapy. Alternatively, at completion of therapy, a CT scan that fails to show any evidence of cancer can provide reassurance. However, the false-negative rate for CT scans in this setting is approximately 45% (16). If there remains any question of persistent or recurrent disease following therapy, CT imaging may allow needle-directed biopsy of suspicious areas.

Second-look Laparotomy

No prospective clinical trials have demonstrated a survival benefit for patients undergoing second-look laparotomy. Therefore, this procedure usually is performed in conjunction with research protocols to monitor the effectiveness of new therapies. There may be a benefit to the surgery in some patients who can be further cytoreduced (17) or rapidly placed on second-line therapy if persistent cancer is found. Second-look procedures are not considered standard of care for treatment of ovarian cancer. The risks, costs, benefits, and morbidity of the operation must be considered for each individual.

Follow-up after a negative second-look laparotomy or in patients who are clinically free of disease should include a general physical and pelvic examination every 3 months for the first 2 years and every 6 months thereafter. In addition, CA 125 in serum, if elevated before treatment, may be a useful marker of early (subclinical) recurrence. The value of serial CT scans is limited and the study is not recommended routinely.

Recurrent or Progressive Ovarian Cancer

Most patients with ovarian cancer ultimately will develop progressive or recurrent disease after initial surgery and adjuvant therapy. There is no single "best" treatment, and individualized treatment options should be developed in conjunction with a gynecologic oncologist who has a comprehensive understanding of treatment choices.

Patients with progressive disease during primary chemotherapy, residual cancer at second-look laparotomy, or clinical recurrence within 6 months of initial therapy usually are treated with second-line chemotherapy. Typical response rates are in the range of 10–30%, depending upon the clinical situation and the type of chemotherapy employed.

Treatment choices might include investigational clinical trials or treatment with a readily available drug that the patient has not yet received. Because of the limited response rate of most second-line therapies, patients should be considered seriously for clinical trials evaluating new therapy. Hormonal agents such as tamoxifen or megestrol are attractive alternatives given their limited toxicity.

Patients who have demonstrated a good response to treatment with cisplatin or carboplatin and who have a recurrence after at least 12 months of clinical remission commonly will have a second response when retreated with cisplatin or carboplatin (18). Patients with minimal or no gross intraperitoneal disease might be considered for treatment with intraperitoneal chemotherapy or whole abdomen radiation therapy.

Palliation

At present, most patients with advanced ovarian cancer ultimately succumb to their disease, and it is imperative that the physician be skilled in managing the preterminal events in order to make the remaining weeks and days as comfortable and useful as possible. Ovarian cancer progresses as an intraperitoneal process with tumor implants growing on peritoneal and mesenteric surfaces. The usual course is that of intermittent small bowel obstruction with diminished bowel peristalsis due to mesenteric involvement, as well as mechanical obstruction. Progressive ascites also may contribute to decreased intestinal function. The patient's general nutritional status diminishes to a picture of cachexia with muscle wasting and a distended abdomen full of ascites, tumor, and small bowel gas. Less frequently, a malignant pleural effusion may lead to respiratory compromise.

After an adequate trial of chemotherapy or radiation therapy, operative intervention in patients with progressive disease is tempered by good surgical judgment and a perspective of the disease process. Patients with a pelvic mass leading to complete rectosigmoid colonic obstruction benefit from a colostomy. A patient with small bowel obstruction secondary to adhesions or radiation therapy also may benefit from surgery. The survival of patients after surgery for small bowel obstruction is on the order of 2–3 months, and many times bowel function never adequately returns postoperatively. Therefore, every attempt should be made to manage medically the patient with partial small bowel obstruction. Passage of a nasogastric tube for decompression and management of fluids and electrolytes may resolve the patient's symptoms at least temporarily. The role of total parenteral nutrition is controversial. Although it may increase the success of surgical repair, it also may only unduly prolong the patient's terminal course. Ultimately, the patient with ovarian cancer–induced small bowel obstruction that does not resolve by medical management must be seriously considered for some sort of small bowel bypass surgery. Consideration also should be made to placement of a gastrostomy, which may be used to relieve the patient's obstructive symptoms without the need for an indwelling nasogastric tube. Although the patient's life may be short, relief of the obstruction may allow the patient to spend the remaining weeks at home in comfort with her family.

Malignant ascites may at times become so severe as to lead to significant patient discomfort, intermittent small bowel obstruction, or respiratory compromise. This problem can be managed by performing paracentesis with a large trocar to remove all ascites. Some patients have had this procedure performed many times over several months with good symptomatic relief. Patients with symptomatic malignant pleural effusion may benefit from placement of a chest tube for drainage and then intrapleural instillation of a sclerosing agent.

Germ Cell Tumors

Germ cell tumors are the most common type of ovarian cancer in women under the age of 30. These tumors comprise less than 5% of ovarian cancers.

Dysgerminoma

Approximately 50% of germ cell malignancies are pure dysgerminomas. With a median age of occurrence of 17 years, dysgerminoma is one of the most common ovarian neoplasms diagnosed during pregnancy. Approximately 70% of dysgerminomas are confined to the ovary at diagnosis. They are bilateral 5–10% of the time and spread most commonly to lymph nodes. Unilateral oophorectomy is adequate therapy for most of these patients, but full surgical staging should be performed. Routine biopsy of a normal-appearing contralateral ovary is not recommended because scarring and adhesions may compromise fertility. Occasionally, dysgerminoma is found in association with gonadoblastoma in patients with dysgenetic gonads and at least a portion of a Y chromosome. Under these circumstances, both ovaries should be removed because these patients are infertile and are likely to develop a gonadoblastoma in the contralateral ovary.

With metastatic disease, intraperitoneal tumor masses that are easily resectable should be removed. Although dysgerminoma is exquisitely radiosensitive, it also is chemosensitive. Several effective regimens include vincristine, dactinomycin, and chlorambucil; methotrexate, dactinomycin, and chlorambucil; and vinblastine, bleomycin, and cisplatin (19). In stage I disease, 15–23% will develop recurrences; 90% of recurrences appear within 2 years of initial therapy. Seventy-five percent of patients with recurrent dysgerminoma have been salvaged with radiation therapy. Overall survival for all patients is approximately 85%. Lactate dehydrogenase can be a tumor marker for dysgerminoma. If elevated initially, it may be helpful in follow-up.

Other Germ Cell Malignancies

Endodermal sinus tumor is the second most common germ cell malignancy occurring at a median age of 19 years. Most are associated with elevation of serum alpha-fetoprotein levels, and often these rapidly growing tumors are found to have spread outside the ovary at diagnosis.

Immature teratomas have anaplastic germ cell elements and are graded histologically on the basis of the amount and degree of cellular immaturity. The prognosis is closely related to the histologic grade. Immature teratomas rarely are bilateral, but frequently spread throughout the peritoneal cavity.

Embryonal carcinomas, choriocarcinomas, and polyembryomas are exceedingly rare and are all highly malignant. Embryonal carcinoma and choriocarcinomas frequently secrete human chorionic gonadotropin and may produce symptoms of precocious puberty, hirsutism, or abnormal uterine bleeding. Embryonal carcinoma frequently secretes alpha-fetoprotein, which can be a useful tumor marker in follow-up.

As for dysgerminomas, therapy consists of unilateral salpingo-oophorectomy, debulking of peritoneal implants, and thorough surgical staging. Most patients, including those with widely disseminated metastases, can be treated successfully with vincristine, dactinomycin, and chlorambucil or bleomycin, etoposide, and cisplatin chemotherapy (20). Following chemotherapy, some may have persistent peritoneal implants, which are microscopically free of immature elements and lack the potential to become immature again.

There is no indication for second-look laparotomy in germ cell tumors. Close surveillance, including use of serum tumor markers and periodic CT scans of the abdomen and pelvis, is adequate follow-up. Many patients who subsequently develop recurrent disease can now be cured with cisplatin-containing chemotherapy regimens.

Sex Cord–Stromal Tumors

Sex cord–stromal tumors account for 5–8% of all ovarian malignancies. The most common are pure stromal cell tumors (granulosa cell tumor, thecomas, and fibromas), but mixed tumors also are seen (eg, granulosa–theca cell tumor). The granulosa cell tumor is considered a low-grade malignancy. It may occur at any point in a woman's life. In the prepubertal girl, secretion of estrogen often leads to sexual pseudoprecocity. In the reproductive age group, menstrual irregularity or secondary amenorrhea are common. Postmenopausal bleeding may signal a granulosa cell tumor in the older woman.

The unopposed secretion of estrogen by many of these tumors may result in endometrial hyperplasia (25–50% of cases) or endometrial adenocarcinoma (5% of cases). Other presenting signs and symptoms may be nonspecific and are associated with the presence of a pelvic mass or intraperitoneal spread. Ascites is present in only 10% of cases, and the tumor is confined to one ovary (stage IA) in more than 90% of patients. Surgical resection (unilateral oophorectomy) with thorough staging is appropriate management in early cases where the patient desires preservation of fertility. The endometrium should also be evaluated for coexistent adenocarcinoma or hyperplasia. There is no evidence that adjuvant chemotherapy or radiation therapy improves survival. Recurrences are rare and typically occur 5–30 years after initial diagnosis. In cases that present with metastases or that recur later, surgical resection followed by chemotherapy or local radiation therapy generally is suggested. Because of the rarity of these tumors, there is no established chemotherapy regimen. Combination therapy with vincristine, doxorubicin and cyclophosphamide or bleomycin, etoposide, and cisplatin are commonly used, however, and complete responses have been reported.

Sertoli–Leydig tumors occur most commonly in the third and fourth decades of life. They account for less than 0.2% of ovarian cancers and are most frequently considered low-grade malignancies. Production of androgens leads to clinical virilization (oligomenorrhea, amenorrhea, breast atrophy, acne, clitoromegaly, hirsutism, receding hairline or deepening of the voice) in 70–85% of cases. Rarely, these tumors are associated with symptoms of estrogenization. Serum androgens (testosterone and androstenedione) may be elevated. Because less than 1% are bilateral and most are low-grade, conservation of the contralateral ovary is reasonable in reproductive-aged women. In older women, hysterectomy and bilateral salpingo-oophorectomy is appropriate. Adjuvant therapy has not been demonstrated to offer any survival advantage, but chemotherapy usually is given to patients with advanced stage or recurrent disease.

References

1. American Cancer Society. Cancer facts and figures. Altanta: ACS, 1998:5008
2. Harlap S. The epidemiology of ovarian cancer. In Markman M, Hoskins WJ, eds. Cancer of the ovary. New York: Raven Press Ltd, 1993:79–93
3. Bristow RE, Karlan BY. Ovulation induction, infertility, and ovarian cancer risk. Fertil Steril 1996;66:499–507
4. Easton DF, Ford D, Bishop DT, Breast Cancer Linkage Consortium. Breast and ovarian cancer incidence in BRCA1-mutation carriers. Am J Hum Genet 1995;56:265–271
5. Piver MS, Jishi MF, Tsukada Y, Nava G. Primary peritoneal carcinoma after prophylactic oophorectomy in women with a family history of ovarian cancer: a report of the Gilda Radner Familial Ovarian Cancer Registry. Cancer 1993;71:2751–2755
6. Bast RC Jr, Klug TL, St John E, Jenison E, Niloff JM, Lazarus H, et al. A radioimmunoassay using a monoclonal antibody to monitor the course of epithelial ovarian cancer. N Engl J Med 1983;309:883–887
7. Olt GJ, Berchuck A, Bast RC Jr. Gynecologic tumor markers. Semin Surg Oncol 1990;6:305–313
8. Munoz KA, Harlan LC, Trimble EL. Patterns of care for women with ovarian cancer in the United States. J Clin Oncol 1996;15:279
9. Young RC, Decker DG, Wharton JT, Piver S, Sindelar WF, Edwards BK, et al. Staging laparotomy in early ovarian cancer. JAMA 1983;250:3072–3076
10. Barnes W, Johnson J, Waggoner S, Barter J, Potkul R, Delgado G. Reverse hysterocolposigmoidectomy (RHCS) for resection of panpelvic tumors. Gynecol Oncol 1991;42:151–155
11. Massad LS Jr, Hunter VJ, Szpak CA, Clarke-Pearson DL, Creasman WT. Epithelial ovarian tumors of low malignant potential. Obstet Gynecol 1991;78:1027–1032
12. McGuire WP, Hoskins WJ, Brady MF, Kucera PR, Partridge EE, Look KY, et al. Cyclophosphamide and cisplatin compared with paclitaxel and cisplatin in patients with stage III and stage IV ovarian cancer. N Engl J Med 1996;334:1–6
13. Alberts DS, Liu PY, Hannigan EV, O'Toole R, Williams SD, Young JA, et al. Intraperitoneal cisplatin plus intravenous cyclophosphamide versus intravenous cisplatin plus intravenous cyclophosphamide for Stage III ovarian cancer. N Engl J Med 1996;335:1950–1955
14. Dembo AJ. Abdominopelvic radiotherapy in ovarian carcinoma: a 10-year experience. Cancer 1985;55:2285–2290
15. Sevelda P, Schemper M, Spona J. CA 125 as an independent prognostic factor for survival in patients with epithelial ovarian cancer. Am J Obstet Gynecol 1989;161:1213–1216
16. Stehman FB, Calkins AR, Wass JL, Smirz LR, Sutton GP, Ehrlich CE. A comparison of findings at second-look laparotomy with preoperative computed tomography in patients with ovarian cancer. Gynecol Oncol 1988;29:37–42
17. Podczaski E, Manetta A, Kaminski P, Ricelli A, Larson J, DeGeest K, et al. Survival of patients with ovarian epithelial carcinomas after second-look laparotomy. Gynecol Oncol 1990;36:43–47
18. Gore ME, Frayatt I, Wiltshaw E, Dawson T. Treatment of relapsed carcinoma of the ovary with cisplatin or carboplatin following initial treatment with these compounds. Gynecol Oncol 1990;36:207–211
19. Williams SD, Blessing JA, Hatch KD, Homesley HD. Chemotherapy of advanced dysgerminoma: trials of the Gynecologic Oncology Group. J Clin Oncol 1991;9:1950–1955
20. Gershenson DM, Morris M, Cangir A, Kavanagh JJ, Stringer CA, Edwards CL, et al. Treatment of malignant germ cell tumors of the ovary with bleomycin, etoposide, and cisplatin. J Clin Oncol 1990;8:715–720

ISSN 1074-8628

The American College of Obstetricians and Gynecologists
409 12th Street, SW
PO Box 96920
Washington, DC 20090-6920

12345/21098

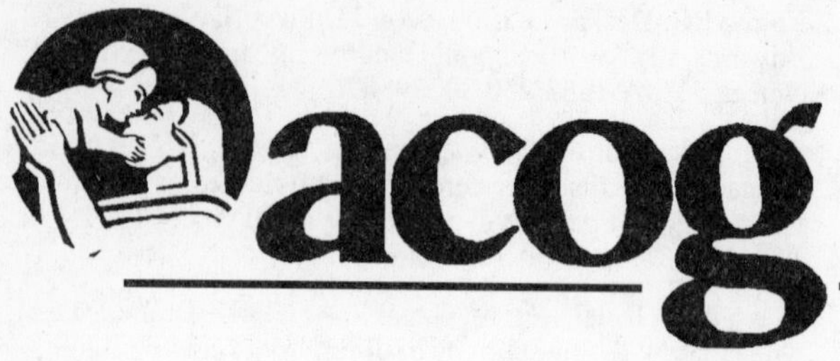

Number 201—January 1995

Technical Bulletin

An Educational Aid to Obstetrician–Gynecologists

Pediatric Gynecologic Disorders

Increased awareness of sexual abuse of children and of sexually transmitted diseases (STDs) has brought to light the need for gynecologists to be aware of gynecologic conditions that should be detected and treated in prepubertal and peripubertal girls. The evaluation and management of such challenging problems in young girls is age dependent and necessitates clinician expertise in assessing physiologic maturity and in special examination techniques specific to pediatric patients. Care of pediatric patients begins in the delivery room, with examination of the neonate, and extends to management of pediatric disorders in children and young women.

Evaluation

Neonates should be examined immediately upon delivery. Rare, life-threatening conditions should be suspected if the external genitalia are ambiguous. Physical examination should include the breasts and genitalia. Often breast tissue will be palpable and nipple discharge will be present, which are reflections of the presence of estrogen derived secondarily from the mother. The labia should be separated to inspect the clitoris, introitus, and hymen. A rectal examination should be performed to determine patency and the presence of a pelvic midline structure—the uterus. No masses should be palpable in the adnexal areas or abdominal cavity. During the first few weeks of life, there may be a white mucoid vaginal discharge as a result of maternal estrogen. The neonate may exhibit a small amount of vaginal bleeding as a result of withdrawal from maternal estrogen.

The examination of prepubertal and peripubertal patients should focus on the main symptoms to identify in this population: pruritus, dysuria, skin color changes, and discharge. Children do not typically develop symptomatic discharge. Therefore, the color and amount of any discharge should be noted; bloody discharge is a serious problem that may have a number of causes. Specifically, questions focusing on the possibility of trauma to the genital organs caused by accident or sexual abuse should be raised.

The presence or absence of estrogen influences the child's vaginal microflora and the clinician's ability to evaluate the child's lower genital tract without causing trauma. Therefore, clinicians should recognize these hormonal patterns:

- Infants to toddlers (up to 2–3 years of age): Vulvovaginal epithelium reflects waning effects of residual maternal estrogen.
- Toddlers to prepubertal girls (2–3 years to 8–10 years of age): Epithelium becomes atrophic.
- Prepubertal to peripubertal girls (8–10 years to 12–14 years of age): Epithelium demonstrates effects of rising estrogen levels.

When performing a genital evaluation of a child, the physician should obtain adequate information to determine that appropriate growth is proceeding, as well as to respond properly to any complaint. Before a genital examination is performed, the gynecologist should explain to the patient what is to take place during the examination and assure her that she has control over what takes place during the examination. Explaining the purpose of the examination, describing what the patient may experience, and allowing the child to see any instruments that may be used will help reduce anxiety, promote trust, and result in a much more productive examination. The gynecologist can also use this opportunity to educate patients about their genital region.

Most pediatric gynecologic problems can be diagnosed by inspection of the external genitalia. Compliance may be achieved by stressing to the child that the examiner is only going to look and involving her in the examination by using a handheld mirror or requesting her assistance in labial retraction. The genitals of a small, anxious child can often best be evaluated by allowing the child to remain on the parent's lap with the child's legs spread open and draped over the parent's thighs. Positioning the child and demonstrating the use of the handheld mirror while she is fully clothed will greatly decrease her anxiety as well as that of her parent or guardian. The larger child can be positioned supine with feet in the examination table stirrups. The lateral Sims position may also be a useful alternative. In either case, having the patient's buttocks at the end of the examination table and having a focused, intense light source aids the examination. Children have small genitalia, and they do not hold still for very long. Therefore, the use of low-power magnification or a colposcope will aid the examiner in evaluating the genitalia.

Once the child is properly positioned, the examiner should note any abnormalities of the labia majora, mons pubis, intracrural folds, labia minora, and the clitoral glans and hood. The urethra, the periurethral area, the hymen, the vestibule, and the posterior fourchette should be examined. In order to examine the entire vestibule adequately, gentle simultaneous bilateral labial retraction is usually necessary. The physician should also be able to identify characteristics of variant hymens—such as the microperforate, septate, or imperforate hymen—which may be present in up to 3–4% of all patients. Surgical intervention is usually not justified until puberty for the imperforate hymen and after puberty for the others. Many cases of suspected imperforate hymen actually turn out to be instances of microperforate hymen, which may or may not resolve at puberty.

If the child is cooperative, she should also be examined in the knee–chest position and instructed to relax her abdominal muscles and take deep breaths. This position causes the vagina to open. When the labia majora are then simultaneously spread laterally and superiorly by the examiner or an assistant, the upper vagina and cervix can be visualized (1).

The physician examining the prepubertal child should be able to distinguish the erythema of normal vulvar epithelium from that of inflammation. In the former, the capillary network is easily visualized; in the latter, the accompanying tissue edema and engorgement obscure the capillaries. The diameter of the vaginal orifice will vary considerably based on the degree of muscle relaxation of the perineal musculature, the technique used to spread the labia to visualize the vestibule, and the normal variations in hymenal configurations.

The unestrogenized prepubertal lower genital tract is easily traumatized and does not readily tolerate speculum examinations or bimanual examinations. Material for a wet mount, Gram stain, forensic studies, or cultures, if needed, can be obtained through vaginal irrigation. One method of vaginal irrigation involves creating a catheter-in-a-catheter by passing a 4-inch segment of the plastic tubing from a butterfly intravenous set into the distal 4 inches of a soft number-12 bladder catheter and inserting this into the vagina. The distal end of the intravenous tubing is attached to a 1-ml tuberculin syringe. This instrument can also be used for irrigating the vagina to obtain specimens for culture and microscopic examination. Irrigation should be performed with sterile physiologic saline; the solution should not contain any bacteriostatic agent (2).

In cases in which visual assessment of the vagina is inadequate, vaginoscopy can be helpful to minimize the trauma. This is sometimes possible in the office if the child is cooperative and if the vulva is initially anesthetized with 2% viscous lidocaine. The ideal instrument for vaginal examinations in the premenarchal female is a small-diameter endoscope with an irrigating capacity that does not traumatize the hymen. After the endoscope is inserted into the vagina, gently closing the labia majora around the scope causes the retained irrigating fluid to expand the vagina, thus permitting a good view of the entire vaginal canal and cervix. If office examination is unsuccessful or if pathology that requires further definition or treatment is found, an examination with anesthesia is indicated. In the selected, well-estrogenized peripubertal girl who is premenarchal, a narrow, 8-cm long speculum can be used with extreme caution to visualize the cervix and vagina without causing trauma to the hymen.

Diagnosis and Management

Vulvovaginitis

Vulvitis in the prepubertal child is diagnosed primarily by visualizing inflammatory erythema on the medial aspects of the labia majora or excoriations associated with the symptoms of vulvar pain, dysuria, and pruritus; discharge is not a primary symptom. The gynecologist should attempt to determine whether the pruritus is clitoral or anal, whether the child is masturbating or seeking relief of symptoms, or whether it is related to overzealous hygienic practices. Common symptoms of vulvovaginitis and related causes, which are indications for further evaluation, are shown in the box.

Commonly, diaper rash is a chemical dermatitis. Candidal vulvovaginitis can occur in the early months after birth because maternal estrogen has made the vulvovaginal epithelium receptive to adherence by yeast cells. By 3–4 years of age, the vulvovaginal epithelium becomes atrophic, and therefore, candidal vulvovaginitis is not as common. However, the atrophic epithelium of the older child is very easily irritated by fecal contamination, irritating soaps, and trauma.

Vulvar–labial agglutination is a common sequela of prepubertal vulvitis. The parent or patient may report that

Common Symptoms and Causes of Vulvovaginopathies

Bleeding
- Prolapsed urethra
- Infection, especially with condylomata acuminata
- Trauma, including foreign object in the vagina
- Endocrine disorders
- Benign and malignant neoplasms
- Sexual abuse

Discharge
- Infection
  - Fecal flora
  - Sexually transmitted diseases
  - Enterobiasis
- Hygienic practices (overzealous or inadequate)
- Labial adhesions
- Foreign body

Dermatitis
- Lichen sclerosis
- Lichen planus
- Seborrheic dermatitis
- Atopic dermatitis
- Contact dermatitis
- Vulvar psoriasis

the external genital anatomy is grossly distorted. Spontaneous resolution occurs but can be expedited by applying topical estrogen cream daily for 7–10 days; prolonged use may result in precocious development. Physical separation by labial traction is traumatic to the child and should be avoided. Recurrence is common if the cause of the vulvitis is not eliminated. Vulvar–labial agglutination that does not respond to estrogen therapy may require mechanical separation with the patient anesthetized. Once the labia are separated, estrogen cream should be applied until reepithelialization of the surface has occurred.

Vaginitis is usually associated with copious asymptomatic discharge; it may be helpful to examine soiled undergarments to quantify the amount of discharge. The child may ultimately develop symptoms of vulvitis secondary to the chafing caused by the discharge. Vaginal discharge in the prepubertal female is associated with significant vaginal inflammation and is suggestive of a single-organism vaginitis, foreign object, neoplasm, or, rarely, an anatomic abnormality such as an ectopic ureter.

Foreign bodies, often toilet paper, in the vagina are the most common cause of vaginitis. Foreign objects can cause a bloody vaginal discharge that is otherwise asymptomatic. X-ray and ultrasound studies are not recommended routinely, since they fail to detect most vaginal foreign objects. Removal of the foreign body can be accomplished by lavaging the vagina with normal saline passed through a small catheter. If this is unsuccessful, the child should receive a general anesthetic and the object should be removed. Objects that have remained in the vagina for prolonged periods may become embedded in the vaginal wall or even penetrate the wall. Therefore, they should be removed with great care and examined thoroughly. The vulva and vaginal mucosa are usually inflamed and should be treated with topical estrogen cream for 1–2 weeks.

Vaginal discharge may appear as estrogen levels rise when a girl approaches menarche. A wet-mount suspension of the discharge confirms the effect of estrogen by identifying mature squamous cells. If the wet mount suggests inflammation (eg, if white blood cells, clue cells, or numerous bacteria are present), information regarding possible sexual activity or abuse should be elicited, and other causes of vaginitis should be considered. Cultures for *Neisseria gonorrhoeae* and *Chlamydia trachomatis* should be obtained.

Most studies of the microflora of the prepubertal vagina are flawed by a lack of control subjects and failure to consider the estrogen status of the subjects. Enteric organisms are frequently and transiently present in the prepubertal child's vagina. Only when a large inoculum occurs (for example, after a bout of diarrhea) will the child develop a symptomatic copious and frequently bloody discharge. When a culture is obtained to identify the predominant organism, it is important to inform the laboratory that identification of a specific organism(s) is desired. Otherwise, the results will be described as "normal vaginal flora" and thus will be inconclusive. Hemorrhagic discharge is particularly common with *Shigella* and certain strains of streptococcus, but an overgrowth of any enteric organism can have the same effect (3).

Abnormalities of Sexual Differentiation

Ambiguous Genitalia

When an infant is born with ambiguous genitalia, the immediate concerns of the obstetrician are to prevent dehydration of the newborn and to counsel the parents. Congenital adrenal hyperplasia is the most common cause of ambiguous genitalia (accounting for more than 90% of cases), and salt-wasting forms may lead to rapid dehydration and fluid and electrolyte imbalance. Therefore, fluid intake and output, serum electrolytes, and glucose concentration should be monitored carefully.

The parents should be counseled that the infant's genitalia are "incompletely formed" and further evaluation is warranted. As a general rule, the presence of a midline frenulum on the phallus may suggest the infant is a genetic male, whereas paired attachments of the "labia" to the phallus suggest a genetic female. Usually, the more severe the ambiguity, the simpler it is to raise the child as a female regardless of genetic sex. Intensive investigation and a multidisciplinary approach are helpful in making this decision. Rectal examination, selected imaging studies, measurement of 17α-hydroxy-progesterone (which is elevated in 21-hydroxylase deficiency) and karyotype analysis are all warranted.

Precocious Puberty

Puberty, the transition period between childhood and maturity, is characterized by marked changes in growth and sexual development. In females, these changes are triggered by the action of an intact hypothalamic–pituitary–ovarian axis. Environmental factors, such as high altitude, strenuous exercise, poor nutrition, chronic disease, and severe obesity, may delay the onset of puberty. Moderate obesity may be associated with earlier onset of puberty.

The first sign of puberty is thelarche (breast development), which occurs between the ages of 9–11 years. Breast development is usually complete—Tanner stage 5 (adult contour)—within 3–3 1/2 years after the onset of thelarche. Associated with the initiation of breast development is the production of estrogen, which creates a vaginal environment suitable for the growth of *Lactobacillus* species.

Adrenarche, the development of pubic hair, is the second stage in maturation and typically occurs between ages 11–12 years. This is an important event that is associated with increased levels of dehydroepian-drosterone sulfate, which indicates that the hypothalamic–pituitary–adrenal axis is intact. Axillary hair usually does not appear until after the growth of pubic hair is complete.

Menarche usually occurs 2 1/2 years after thelarche at approximately 12.8 years of age. The initial cycles are usually anovulatory. After about 12–18 months, cycles become regular, and this indicates that ovulation is occurring. Premature menarche (menses before the age of 10) is rare and usually occurs with other secondary sexual changes seen in precocious puberty, not as an isolated symptom. Thus, other causes of lower genital tract bleeding, such as trauma resulting from sexual abuse, should be ruled out by physical examination. Laboratory evaluation should include screening for hematologic disorders and coagulopathies.

When females less than 8 years of age have premature onset of a single secondary sexual characteristic, such as premature adrenarche or thelarche, it often can be attributed to end-organ sensitivity to low circulating levels of sex steroids. Close observation, including the use of growth charts, is required. In the presence of accelerated growth and evidence of multisite organ stimulation (eg, thelarche and vestibular epithelial changes or advancing pubarche and clitorimegaly or acne), a thorough evaluation is warranted.

The goal of the evaluation is to determine the source of the hormonal stimulation. Magnetic resonance imaging, computed tomography, and ultrasonography may be helpful in ruling out adrenal or ovarian neoplastic or functional enlargement. Even when the results of these studies are normal, the site of sex steroid overproduction is not necessarily within the central nervous system. Over the course of a few weeks, the prepubertal ovary can rapidly and autonomously enlarge due to simple follicular cyst formation, produce estradiol, and then regress in size spontaneously. Surgical intervention is not necessary unless the cyst persists for several months or there is progression of signs and symptoms. When the hypothalamic–pituitary axis is suspected of premature activity, the gonadotropin-releasing hormone stimulation test is helpful in establishing the diagnosis of true (central) precocious puberty.

Therapy specific to the cause should be initiated with the goal of preventing the excessively short stature and the psychologic sequelae that result from premature sexual development. Centrally driven precocious puberty is treated with gonadotropin-releasing hormone analogues that will inhibit rapid bone growth and prevent premature epiphyseal closure. In addition, further development of secondary sexual characteristics will also be arrested. The effect of simultaneous treatment with growth hormone is being investigated. McCune–Albright syndrome (polyostotic fibrous dysplasia, patchy dermal pigmentation, and endocrine dysfunction) is difficult to treat; however, there have been some promising results with the aromatase inhibitor testolactone (4).

Developmental Breast Disorders

Premature thelarche is relatively common in prepubertal girls. This usually consists of bilateral breast buds (Tanner stage 2) appearing in girls younger than 8 years old, but it can be as advanced as Tanner stage 3. It is likely that premature thelarche is due to increased sensitivity of breast tissue to low levels of circulating estrogens. Reassurance is all that is required for patients prior to the age of 8 years. In the absence of other signs of pubertal development (such as a growth spurt or the development of pubic and axillary hair), examination at 3-month intervals is warranted to rule out precocious puberty. Breast buds should not be mistaken for neoplasia. Biopsy can lead to marked distortion in the mature breast and thus should not be done without an absolute indication (5).

Abnormal Vaginal Bleeding

Vaginal bleeding in a prepubertal child is abnormal and should be evaluated. Rarely does menstrual bleeding occur without premature thelarche and other evidence of estrogen stimulation, such as thickening of the hymen or development of vaginal rugae. Data exist that have demonstrated a rise in gonadotropins associated with developmental breast change from Tanner stage 1 to Tanner stage 2 (6).

Trauma

Contusions and abrasions can be treated conservatively as long as there is no evidence of uncontrolled bleeding and they do not interfere with bodily functions. The following questions should be considered in the evaluation of trauma resulting in lacerations:

- Is the report of how the injury occurred compatible with the wound?
- How will the extent of the wound be determined without causing the patient further trauma?
- Will the wound close by secondary intention or is surgical debridement and closure warranted?

Lacerations extending beyond the levator ani that may result in retroperitoneal or intraabdominal extension require thorough evaluation by vaginoscopy, and most of these examinations should be performed under anesthesia. When the injury transects the hymen, sexual assault should be suspected. Therefore, if the alleged abuse has occurred within the past 72 hours, specimens should be obtained for forensic studies before the perineum is prepared for surgical repair. Small wounds that do not require suturing may be controlled with pressure and perineal care. A small hematoma can be managed by keeping the child supine and quiet for several hours. The child should be examined frequently to determine whether the hematoma is expanding and requires intervention. If there is no evidence that the hematoma is enlarging and the patient is hemodynamically stable and can void, hospital admission is not required.

Benign and Malignant Neoplasms

URETHRAL PROLAPSE. Prolapse can sometimes be difficult to distinguish from a neoplasm. It can be precipitated by straining or increased intraabdominal pressure such as that from constipation. Use of stool softeners or dietary advice may be helpful. The most common symptom of urethral prolapse in the prepubertal, unestrogenized girl is painless genital bleeding. Symptoms of urethral irritation, such as dysuria and frequency, sometimes occur; urinary retention is rarely present. A distinguishing characteristic is the proximal location of the external urethral meatus in the center of the prolapsed tissue. Initial treatment consists of local application of estrogen cream for a few weeks and frequent sitz baths. Surgical excision of the redundant tissue should be performed in those patients who do not respond to topical estrogen therapy. Surgery is also indicated when the accompanying symptoms are extreme or if there is any question as to the diagnosis.

CONDYLOMATA ACUMINATA. Condylomata acuminata are a cause of painless genital bleeding in the prepubertal child. On the unestrogenized vulva, the lesions are commonly flesh colored, and small red punctations cover their surface. The latter are the capillaries, which course to the tips of each papule and are visible due to the thinness of the atrophic epithelium; these same capillaries cause the extreme friability of these exophytic epithelial lesions.

Therapeutic placement of caustic agents and ablative office procedures are usually not feasible methods of treatment for most children due to poor compliance. Treatment, therefore, consists of observation, biopsy, or ablative procedures performed under general anesthesia. Because condylomata acuminata are frequently sexually transmitted, the possibility of sexual abuse should be addressed.

SARCOMA BOTRYOIDES (EMBRYONAL RHABDOMYOSARCOMA). Although rare, hymenal and cervical polyps may exist. These must be distinguished from sarcoma botryoides. Sarcoma botryoides, although exceedingly rare, is the most common malignancy of the lower genital tract in the very young female. In children younger than 5 years of age, it frequently appears as a bloody vaginal discharge. The friable polypoid neoplasm typically arises from the anterior vaginal wall near the cervix and can appear benign; a careful histologic search must be made for immature rhabdomyoblasts in these lesions. The use of chemotherapy prior to surgery has resulted in a great improvement in the long-term prognosis for these once almost uniformly fatal tumors (7).

Sexual Abuse

For a number of reasons, young children who have been sexually abused usually do not have physical signs of genital injury when first examined: the alleged abuse may have occurred some time ago, the abusive activity may not have involved attempts to penetrate the vagina in the unestrogenized child, or the penetration may have occurred when the vulvar tissues were primed by estrogen. Estrogen induces rapid healing and elastic properties in the vulvovaginal tissues which allow distension, frequently without laceration. Nevertheless, the physician should be able to differentiate a normal and an altered hymen. Statutes vary from state to state as to the need for a parent's or legal guardian's consent to perform genital examination of a child in cases of suspected sexual abuse or molestation.

The hymen is normally smooth and contiguous. The lacerated hymen is usually discontinuous at some point from the 3-o'clock position clockwise to the 9-o'clock position (8). When there has been severe stretch trauma to the hymen, it will retract into hymenal caruncles or remnants; this is an important sign because some children who have been sexually penetrated may never undergo surgical repair of the acute injury.

Identification of an STD in a young girl is another means of substantiating allegations of sexual abuse. Cultures for *N. gonorrhoeae* and *C. trachomatis*, wet mounts for trichomonads, and a thorough examination of the external genitalia for condylomata are indicated. Current data indicate that a prepubertal child with gonorrhea most likely has had genital-to-genital exposure. The exact mode of transmission of other STDs is controversial, although many such cases have been found to involve sexual abuse. The dose of antibiotic used to treat any infection depends on the child's weight (9).

If an STD or other signs of abuse are found, all state laws require the findings to be reported to protective service agencies for investigation of sexual abuse. Physicians should be aware of their state's laws. When the issue of sexual abuse arises, physicians should consider their role as the patient's advocate. They should also remain medically objective and work closely with other professionals in the legal, law enforcement, and protective service areas to help these children. In addition, physicians should be sensitive to the fact that when a child is involved in allegations of sexual abuse, the situation may be traumatic for a parent (presumably not the perpetrator), and a parent(s) may require emotional support.

Summary

There is a broad spectrum of pathophysiologic genital conditions affecting young patients. With patience and sensitivity, physicians can modify their gynecologic practices to incorporate even very young girls. These modifications include awareness of various childhood hormonal patterns. Issues of parental consent and involvement are an important aspect of such a practice. Modifications may allow for primary prevention of a broad array of problems and may be one of the most rewarding efforts the physician will put forth.

REFERENCES

1. Blake J. Gynecologic examination of the teenager and young child. Obstet Gynecol Clin North Am 1992;19:27–38
2. Pokorny SF, Stormer J. Atraumatic removal of secretions from the prepubertal vagina. Am J Obstet Gynecol 1987;156:581–582
3. Altchek A. Pediatric vulvovaginitis. J Reprod Med 1984;29:359–375
4. Layman LC, Plouffe L Jr, McDonough PG. Case report: McCune–Albright syndrome: evidence for periodic estrogen secretion. Adolesc Pediatr Gynecol 1988;1:131–136
5. Simmons PS. Diagnostic considerations in breast disorders of children and adolescents. Obstet Gynecol Clin North Am 1992;19:91–102
6. Cacciatore B, Apter D, Alfthan H, Stenman U-H. Ultrasonic characteristics of the uterus and ovaries in relation to pubertal development and serum LH, FSH, and estradiol concentrations. Adolesc Pediatr Gynecol 1991;4:15–20
7. Gordon AN, Montag TW. Sarcoma botryoides of the cervix: excision followed by adjuvant chemotherapy for preservation of reproductive function. Gynecol Oncol 1990;36:119–124
8. Emans SJ, Woods ER, Flagg NT, Freeman A. Genital findings in sexually abused, symptomatic and asymptomatic, girls. Pediatrics 1987;79:778–785
9. Paradise JE. The medical evaluation of the sexually abused child. Pediatr Clin North Am 1990;37:839–862

SUGGESTED READING

Dewhurst J. Practical pediatric and adolescent gynecology. New York: Marcel Dekker, 1980

Emans SJH, Goldstein DP, eds. Pediatric and adolescent gynecology. 3rd ed. Boston: Little, Brown and Co, 1990

Pokorny SF. Configuration of the prepubertal hymen. Am J Obstet Gynecol 1987;157:950–956

This Technical Bulletin was developed under the direction of the Committee on Technical Bulletins of the American College of Obstetricians and Gynecologists as an educational aid to obstetricians and gynecologists. The committee wishes to thank Susan F. Pokorny, MD, for her assistance in the development of this bulletin. This Technical Bulletin does not define a standard of care, nor is it intended to dictate an exclusive course of management. It presents recognized methods and techniques of clinical practice for consideration by obstetrician–gynecologists for incorporation into their practices. Variations of practice taking into account the needs of the individual patient, resources, and limitations unique to the institution or type of practice may be appropriate. Requests for authorization to make photocopies should be directed to the Copyright Clearance Center, 222 Rosewood Drive, Danvers, MA 01923; telephone (508) 750-8400.

ISSN 1074-8628

THE AMERICAN COLLEGE OF OBSTETRICIANS AND GYNECOLOGISTS
409 12th Street, SW
Washington, DC 20024-2188

12345/98765

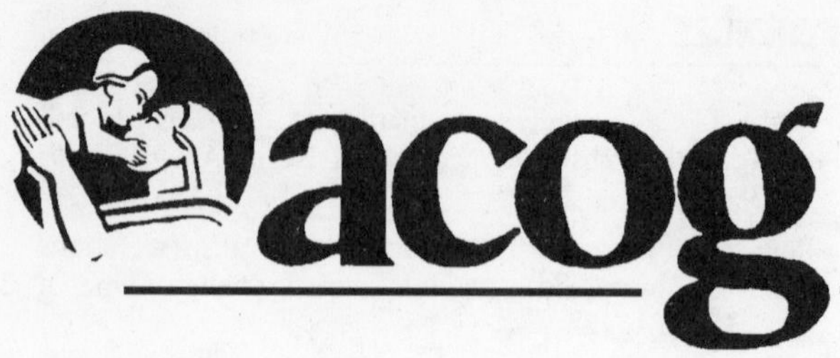

Number 214—October 1995

Technical Bulletin

An Educational Aid to Obstetrician–Gynecologists

Pelvic Organ Prolapse

Pelvic organ prolapse refers to protrusions of the pelvic organs into or out of the vaginal canal. It is a condition limited almost entirely to adult women. Teleologically, it is the result of a woman having attained an erect, bipedal posture. Etiologically, most cases appear to be the result of vaginal childbirth and chronic increases in intraabdominal pressure. Anatomically, pelvic organ prolapse is primarily a vaginal problem (1) that is the result of damage, both direct and indirect, to the vagina and its pelvic support system. Direct injuries include detachments and lacerations of the vaginal support system or stretching and lacerations of the vaginal wall. Indirect injuries include hypoestrogenic atrophy and denervation injuries (2–5). Secondarily, prolapse may involve the urethra, bladder, uterus, intestine, and rectum. The symptoms caused by pelvic organ prolapse are highly variable. They depend to a great extent on which organs are involved, their degree of displacement, and their physiologic compromise.

There are prophylactic measures that, over a lifetime, may help prevent the onset and progression of pelvic organ prolapse. Once symptoms and clinical findings indicate the need for intervention, a variety of nonsurgical and surgical methods may be used singly or in combination to treat the condition. It is important that each patient's management be individualized.

Contributing Factors

Because pelvic organ prolapse is rarely a problem in neurologically normal nulliparous women, pregnancy, labor, and vaginal childbirth are thought to be primary contributing factors. There are insufficient data to determine the relationship between episiotomy and pelvic prolapse. Chronic and repetitive increases in intraabdominal pressure increase the risk of developing pelvic organ prolapse. Therefore, obesity, chronic coughing, constipation, pelvic tumors, ascites, and strenuous physical exertion that increases intraabdominal pressure contribute to the progression of the disorder.

In some patients, pelvic organ prolapse is thought to develop as a result of congenital or inherited weaknesses within the pelvic support system. The increased incidence of prolapse in women with spina bifida occulta and the observation that some women appear to be "hernia-prone" are evidence of the effects that neurologic problems and tissue factors might have on the development of prolapse. Conversely, it has been reported that Asian women are less likely than Caucasian women to develop prolapse (6). The reason for the differences in incidence among races is unknown but may be due to differences in pelvic architecture, the quality of musculature and supporting tissues, the ability to heal neuromuscular injury, or women's life styles.

Estrogen replacement therapy at the time of the menopause helps preserve the integrity of the vaginal support system and prevents atrophy of the vagina itself. Although little is known about the natural history of prolapse, it is the impression of many clinicians that estrogen therapy may slow the onset or impede progression of pelvic organ prolapse. It also improves the tolerance of pessary usage, diminishes the sensitivity and vulnerability of prolapsed tissues, and may contribute to the durability of surgical repairs.

There are a number of iatrogenic factors that may contribute to pelvic organ prolapse. These include failure to adequately correct all pelvic support defects at the time of surgery. Additionally, procedures that alter the direction of pelvic forces may cause areas that had been adequately supported to prolapse. Examples include ventral suspensions of the urethra, uterus, or vagina that increase the exposure of the cul-de-sac to increases in intraabdominal pressure; posterior fixation of the vaginal apex (1); failure to detect and correct an occult enterocele; and excessive shortening of the vagina. Every pelvic surgeon should be aware of the role these factors play in initiating or contributing to the progression of pelvic organ prolapse.

Pelvic Support Systems

Anatomically, the pelvic organs are maintained within the pelvis by the bilaterally paired and posteriorly fused levator ani muscles. Collectively, they are referred to as the pelvic floor. The levator ani muscles are attached to the bony pelvis anteriorly and posteriorly; laterally, they are attached to the arcus tendineus musculi levatoris ani, which overlie the obturator internus muscles of the pelvic side walls. The anterior separation between the levator ani is called the levator hiatus. Inferiorly, the levator hiatus is covered by the urogenital diaphragm. The urethra, vagina, and rectum pass through the levator hiatus and urogenital diaphragm as they exit the pelvis. The posterior joining of the levator ani in the midline by the anococcygeal ligament forms the levator plate.

The endopelvic fascia is a visceral fascia that invests the pelvic organs and forms bilateral condensations referred to as ligaments (ie, pubourethral, cardinal, and uterosacral ligaments). These ligaments attach the organs to the fascia of the pelvic sidewalls and bony pelvis. The ligaments should be preserved at the time of surgery and used in reconstructive procedures. The bony pelvis is the ultimate point of attachment of all pelvic support systems.

The vagina and its ligamentous attachments are responsible for much of the support of those organs that lie outside it, especially those just outside its anterior wall (7). Damage to the vagina and its support system allows the urethra, bladder, rectum, and small bowel to protrude into the vaginal canal.

The perineal body is a central point for the attachment of the perineal musculature. It lies beneath and supports the pelvic diaphragm. The distal posterior wall of the vagina is fused to the ventral surface of the perineal body. The perineal body is also important to the support of the rectum.

It is important that the pelvic organs, their interrelationships, and their support systems be thought of conceptually and functionally in three dimensions. Although the contents of the abdominal cavity bear down on the pelvic organs, they remain suspended in their relation to each other and to the underlying levator sling and perineal body. Each organ is capable of independent function as a result of its separation by connective tissue spaces within the endopelvic connective tissue support system. The normal tonic contraction of the levator ani muscles supports the pelvic organs from below and contributes to urinary and fecal continence. Relaxation of the levator ani muscles allows descent of the pelvic organs and aids urination and defecation.

Signs and Symptoms

Signs and symptoms commonly attributed to pelvic organ prolapse are listed in the box. The different presentations of this condition often make it difficult to correlate symptoms and clinical findings. It appears that some patients become accustomed to marked degrees of prolapse and feel very little discomfort or inconvenience as a result of it. The rate of progression of the prolapse is better correlated with the individual patient's expression of concern regarding symptoms and anatomic findings.

A frequent sign is that of a protrusion of the vagina. There may be a feeling of pelvic pressure, a "bearing-down" sensation, or a perception that something is "falling out." Some patients may feel "pulling" in the inguinal areas or low backache. Symptoms are often accentuated by standing and lifting; they are usually relieved by lying down.

Anterior vaginal wall prolapse has a strong association with urinary urgency and frequency, urinary incontinence, incomplete emptying, and voiding dysfunction. If incontinence is a prominent symptom accompanying prolapse, evaluation and management are required. Urinary incontinence may be absent or masked by the prolapse until the prolapse is reduced or surgically corrected and may then become a predominant symptom (8). Posterior vaginal wall prolapse may be associated with difficult defecation. Although constipation is frequently associated with pelvic organ prolapse, this symptom is amenable to medical therapy. Constipation (as opposed to difficulty with defecation) is not an indication for rectocele repair. Straining with untreated constipation, however, may contribute to the progression of rectocele and pelvic organ prolapse (3, 5). The cardinal symptoms of a rectocele are stool trapped in the rectocele pocket and the need to support the rectocele or perineum to complete defecation.

Signs and Symptoms Associated with Pelvic Organ Prolapse

Pelvic pressure
Bearing-down sensation
Bilateral groin pain
Sacral backache
Coital difficulty
Protrusion from vagina
Spotting, ulceration, bleeding
Urinary frequency or urgency, nocturia
Urinary incontinence or retention
Difficult defecation

Evaluation

One limitation of the physical examination is that only the vaginal side of the protrusion can be seen. In patients who have had prior surgery for prolapse, the pelvic viscera may protrude into the vagina in an unusual and sometimes unpredictable manner. Also, there may be detachment of the vaginal wall, which is separate from the organs that lie outside it. Site-specific vaginal examination can differentiate midline from lateral support weakness or defects (9).

Prolapses are traditionally subclassified according to which pelvic organs are secondarily involved. One such classification is given in the box below.

Pelvic organ prolapse is accentuated in the standing position and by having the patient perform Valsalva maneuvers. The patient should strain until the prolapse becomes fully distended and all elements are evident. Unfortunately, it is inconvenient and somewhat difficult to determine and grade all weaknesses within the vagina and pelvic support system by examining patients in the standing position. The lithotomy position, on the other hand, even during a maximum Valsalva effort, tends to obscure some pelvic support defects. Therefore, it is recommended that women with symptoms that may be caused by pelvic organ prolapse be examined in the lithotomy, sitting, and standing positions. They should be examined before, during, and after a maximum Valsalva effort. Their protruding organs should be replaced and observed as they descend during subsequent Valsalva maneuvers.

Some physicians have recommended that traction be applied to the uterine cervix and other protruding organs to determine their maximum degree of descent (10); however, this is often uncomfortable for the patient and is unphysiologic. It is important, however, that each area of weakness within the pelvic support system be determined and graded individually according to its maximum degree of descent within the vaginal canal or outside the introitus. Although there is no universally agreed upon system for grading these disorders, the box above suggests one such system (9).

Clinical Classification of Pelvic Organ Prolapse

Anterior vaginal prolapse
- Cystourethrocele
- Cystocele

Apical vaginal prolapse
- Uterovaginal
- Vaginal vault (posthysterectomy)

Posterior vaginal prolapse
- Enterocele*
- Rectocele

* Enteroceles usually involve the posterior vaginal fornix and posterior vaginal wall; they also may involve the anterior and lateral vaginal walls.

Clinical Grading of Descent in Pelvic Organ Prolapse*

Grade 0: No descent

Grade 1: Descent between normal position and ischial spines

Grade 2: Descent between ischial spines and hymen

Grade 3: Descent within hymen

Grade 4: Descent through hymen

* Each organ that descends within the vaginal canal should be given a grade that corresponds to its maximum degree of descent, whether the patient is in the lithotomy, sitting, or standing position. Those grading descent should state the patient's position and whether or not a maximum Valsalva effort was performed. If traction is used to determine the maxi-mum descent of an organ, this should also be stated.

Management

Prophylactic measures for preventing pelvic organ prolapse include diagnosis and treatment of chronic respiratory and metabolic disorders; correction of constipation (2, 3) and intraabdominal disorders that may cause chronic increases in intraabdominal pressure; and administration of estrogen to menopausal women who have no contraindication to its use. Patients should be counseled about the preventive effects of weight control and proper nutrition, smoking cessation, and the avoidance of strenuous occupational and recreational stresses that could damage the pelvic support system. Women should be taught and encouraged to perform pelvic muscle exercises as a method of strengthening their pelvic diaphragm and as prophylaxis against the development of pelvic organ prolapse (11).

Failure to recognize and treat significant support defects at the time of concomitant gynecologic surgery may lead to progression of prolapse. Disabilities that may occur include urinary incontinence or retention; urinary tract infections; an inability to void or defecate without manual replacement of the uterus, bladder, or rectum; sexual dysfunction; and vaginal ulceration.

There are nonsurgical and surgical methods of managing symptomatic pelvic organ prolapse. Treatment is determined by the age of the patient, the desire for future fertility, the desire for coital function, the severity of symptoms and degree of disability, and the presence of medical complications. It is the physician's responsibility to inform women of their management options and the potential benefits and risks of each.

Nonsurgical Management

In addition to strengthening pelvic muscles and administering estrogen to menopausal women, nonsurgical management of pelvic organ prolapse mainly involves fitting the patient with a vaginal pessary. There are numerous vaginal pessaries designed to support specific types of pelvic organ prolapse (12). Pessaries press against the walls of the vagina and are retained within the vagina by the tissues of the vaginal outlet. On occasion, the vagina and its outlet will be so dilated that it will not hold a pessary. If there is no other reasonable therapeutic option for such a patient, a perineorrhaphy may be performed with the patient under local anesthesia, constricting the vaginal outlet to enable it to retain a pessary.

Pessaries may cause vaginal irritation and ulceration. They are better tolerated when the vaginal epithelium is well estrogenized; exogenous estrogen may be required in the hypoestrogenic patient. Periodically, vaginal pessaries should be removed, cleaned, and reinserted (12). Failure to do so may result in serious consequences, including fistula formation.

Patients may be managed successfully with a pessary for years. Indications for surgery include the desire for definitive surgical correction, recurrent vaginal ulcerations with a pessary, and genuine stress incontinence that the patient finds unacceptable.

Surgical Management

Many surgical procedures, both vaginal and abdominal, have been described for the correction of pelvic organ prolapse. The goals of pelvic reconstructive surgery for support defects are to relieve symptoms, restore normal anatomic relationships, restore normal visceral function, allow satisfactory coital function, and obtain a durable result. Pelvic reconstruction is a challenge for even the most skilled pelvic surgeon. To accomplish all of the goals of surgery, the surgeon will have to select the combination of surgical procedures that will most likely meet the needs of the patient. In addition, it is of utmost importance that the surgeon be adaptable in performing each operation because intraoperative findings may dictate the need to alter the planned surgical procedure or approach.

Vaginal Procedures

VAGINAL HYSTERECTOMY. Patients who have completed childbearing and who have significant uterovaginal prolapse or uterine pathology may benefit by having a vaginal hysterectomy as a part of their surgical procedure. The performance of a hysterectomy, in and of itself, is insufficient for the cure of uterovaginal prolapse. The vaginal apex should be resuspended either by using pelvic ligaments preserved at the time of hysterectomy or by using an alternative procedure if these ligaments are found to be attenuated.

After removal of the uterus, it is important to look for an occult enterocele. If an occult enterocele is present, the redundant cul-de-sac peritoneum, and possibly the posterior vagina apex (13, 14), should be excised and McCall sutures (15) should be placed within the uterosacral ligaments to obliterate the posterior cul-de-sac. Care should be taken to prevent any of the culdoplasty sutures from kinking or otherwise injuring either ureter. The culdoplasty sutures may be brought through the posterior vaginal cuff to resuspend the vaginal apex posteriorly over the levator ani muscles and within the hollow of the sacrum. The horizontal axis of the upper vagina and the obliteration of the posterior cul-de-sac prevent subsequent enterocele formation and vaginal vault prolapse.

The vaginal apex is further suspended by its fixation to the uterosacral and cardinal ligaments. If these ligaments have become elongated and attenuated as a result of uterovaginal prolapse, they should be shortened before they are reattached to the vaginal apex. When the uterosacral and cardinal ligaments are shortened, it is important to locate the ureters to prevent injuring them. When the uterosacral and cardinal ligaments are too attenuated for use in resuspending the vaginal apex, the vaginal apex may be suspended from one or both sacrospinous ligaments (16, 17) or the iliococcygeus fascia (18).

ANTERIOR COLPORRHAPHY. Anterior colporrhaphy is indicated when there is a cystocele resulting from an anterior midline vaginal wall defect. It should provide differential support to the urethrovesical junction, while also supporting the trigone and base of the bladder. The basic surgical procedure has undergone many modifications to improve results. Anterior colporrhaphy may have variable effects on the delicate tissues of the urethra and the urinary continence mechanism. Therefore, a clear understanding of the patient's lower urinary tract function prior to surgery, including the potential for developing incontinence, is important (19).

The procedure is initiated by a midline anterior vaginal wall incision that extends from the vaginal apex to within 1 cm of the external urethral meatus. The anterior vaginal wall flaps are carefully dissected to leave endopelvic fascia attached to the urethra and the trigone and base of the bladder. The dissection is continued bilaterally to the descending pubic rami. Interrupted horizontal mattress sutures are used to elevate and provide differential support to the urethrovesical junction. Additional interrupted horizontal mattress sutures are placed, as needed, to repair any fascial defect beneath the urethra and bladder. Care must be taken not to "overcorrect" any cystocele, thereby diminishing the effect of the prior attempt to elevate the bladder neck. Any redundancy of the anterior vaginal wall flaps is trimmed to preserve the vaginal caliber. The cut edges of the anterior vaginal wall are approximated in the midline.

Disadvantages of this operation include the possibility of damage to the urethra, damage to the urinary continence mechanism, and scarring of the vesicovaginal space. The operation may be a technical challenge in patients with recurrent prolapse following prior anterior colporrhaphy and those who have a markedly narrowed, stenotic vaginal canal.

TRANSVAGINAL ENTEROCELE REPAIR. It is best to anticipate the need for treatment of the cul-de-sac when planning an operative procedure for pelvic organ prolapse. The enterocele component of prolapse is often underdiagnosed and, therefore, undertreated. Diagnosing enteroceles requires a high index of suspicion and evaluation of the patient's maximum Valsalva maneuvers in the standing position. As prophylaxis against the development of an enterocele, the surgeon should obliterate the cul-de-sac when the operative procedure predisposes the patient to future enterocele formation (20).

Most enteroceles involve the posterior vaginal fornix and posterior wall of the vagina. The overlying vaginal wall is longitudinally incised. The peritoneal sac of the enterocele is identified, dissected free of the surrounding tissues, and opened at its distal end. The small bowel within the sac is reduced into the abdominal cavity. The neck of the enterocele sac is closed in a purse string fashion, and the distal sac is excised. The peritoneal closure is reinforced by the approximation of the underlying endopelvic fascia (21). This should be done in a way that pulls the upper vagina over the levator plate so that increases in abdominal pressure force the vagina against the rectum and close any potential enterocele space.

POSTERIOR COLPORRHAPHY. A posterior colporrhaphy should be performed when there is a symptomatic rectocele that is caused by a rectovaginal fascial defect. This is in contrast to the outdated dictum that posterior colporrhaphy should always accompany anterior colporrhaphy. These rectoceles may be diagnosed by physical examination as well as imaging studies. It is wise to consider preoperative radiologic evaluations of unusual rectoceles or those associated with rectal prolapse. Detachment of the posterior vaginal wall does not necessarily confirm the presence of a rectocele. Posterior colporrhaphy should be considered as a distinct and separate procedure when pelvic organ prolapse is repaired (22). It should be performed in a deliberate and precise manner, as it may be a cause of dyspareunia.

Depending on the need for reconstruction of the perineum, the skin may be incised in a V fashion over the perineum or transversely along the external margin of the posterior fourchette. The vaginal wall of the posterior fourchette is sharply dissected from the underlying tissues of the perineal body. The rectovaginal space is entered and widely dissected all the way to the vaginal apex. The pararectal fascia is plicated over the rectum with interrupted delayed absorbable or permanent sutures from the vaginal apex to the introitus (21). As each suture is placed, the diameter of the vagina is assessed to be sure there is no transverse constriction that may result in dyspareunia. Linear, lateral relaxing incisions will relieve any constrictions that occur. If necessary, redundancy of the posterior vaginal wall flaps is trimmed and care is taken to preserve the vaginal caliber. The cut edges of the upper posterior vaginal wall are approximated in the midline. If there is a defective perineal body, its connective tissue is plicated in the midline. It is not necessary to plicate muscle per se but rather the capsule of the muscle. This is most commonly the pubis rectalis muscle. The remaining cut edges of the posterior vaginal wall and perineum are approximated.

PERINEORRHAPHY. After vaginal repair, when there is a deficient perineal body, consideration should be given to performing a perineorrhaphy. The perineal deficit may be due to attenuation, laceration, or hypermobility of the perineal body. Controversy is ongoing as to whether levator ani plication adds to the success of the operation. If any muscles are approximated in the midline, they should not be strangulated or destroyed. Care should be taken not to constrict the posterior fourchette, as this may be a cause of dyspareunia.

VAGINAL VAULT SUSPENSION. Vaginal vault suspension should be considered when there is symptomatic prolapse of the vaginal apex. The vaginal vault usually can be suspended by attaching it to the uterosacral and cardinal ligaments and to the pararectal fascia. When these tissues are so attenuated that they do not adequately support the vaginal apex, it may be suspended either unilaterally or bilaterally from the sacrospinous ligaments (16, 17) or the iliococcygeus fascia (18).

VAGINAL OBLITERATION. A few older patients with marked degrees of pelvic organ prolapse are not and never will be sexually active. In these cases, with informed consent, it may be reasonable to stenose or even close the vagina to obtain a satisfactory and more durable repair. Particular attention must be given to the evaluation of lower urinary tract function before obliterating the vagina. Otherwise, it may be difficult to restore urinary continence should incontinence result from the procedure.

If a uterus is present, a dilation and curettage may be performed to detect significant endometrial pathology, and, if none is found, a LeFort procedure may be performed to replace the uterus and partially close the vagina. When the LeFort procedure is performed, a wide sheet of anterior vaginal epithelium is removed, leaving the underlying fascia attached to the bladder (23). A similar sheet of posterior vaginal epithelium is removed. The cut vaginal wall is approximated horizontally in front of the cervix. The denuded areas of the anterior and posterior vaginal walls are approximated with horizontal layers of interrupted absorbable suture. Plicating mattress sutures are placed beneath the bladder neck to prevent postoperative urinary incontinence and across the anterior rectal wall. At the completion of these procedures a mucosal tunnel remains across the cervix and on either side of the vagina. This tunnel serves as a route for any subsequent uterine discharge.

Some patients with a uterus may be treated with a vaginal hysterectomy and colpectomy–colpocleisis, whereas those without a uterus may be treated with a colpectomy–colpocleisis alone. Colpectomy is performed by incising the vaginal epithelium in the midline, anteriorly and posteriorly (24). The vaginal epithelium is widely dissected from the underlying fibromuscular wall of the vagina to its 3-o'clock and 9-o'clock positions. The lateral flaps of the vaginal epithelium are then excised to within 2 cm of the introitus. Any enterocele sac is dissected, closed, excised, and supported. Plicating mattress sutures are placed beneath the bladder neck to prevent postoperative urinary incontinence and across the anterior rectal wall. The medial margins of the levator ani are approximated in the midline, closing the lower three quarters of the levator hiatus. The cut edges of the vagina are reapproximated in the midline.

Abdominal Procedures

HYSTERECTOMY. Removal of the uterus may benefit patients who have completed childbearing and who have significant uterovaginal prolapse or uterine pathology. Removal of the uterus, without correction of other support defects, is likely to result in early evidence of postoperative pelvic organ prolapse. It is unusual for hysterectomy alone to be sufficient treatment of prolapse. Postoperative pelvic organ prolapse usually can be avoided by the careful planning and execution of a procedure that will correct all pelvic support defects.

After removal of the uterus, it is important to examine the posterior cul-de-sac for size and potential for developing an enterocele. In an effort to resuspend the vaginal apex and prevent subsequent vaginal vault prolapse and enterocele development, the surgeon should reattach the cut ends of the cardinal and uterosacral ligaments to the vaginal apex. If uterine prolapse has caused elongation and attenuation of these ligaments, they should be shortened or plicated to suspend the vaginal apex over the posterior cul-de-sac and create a flap–valve mechanism to protect the cul-de-sac from subsequent enterocele formation. On occasion, it may be best to obliterate the cul-de-sac with permanent suture placed in a Moschcowitz or Halban fashion (25, 26). If this is done, care should be taken to avoid any ureteral injury or compromise of the lumen of the sigmoid colon.

PARAVAGINAL REPAIR. Abdominal or vaginal paravaginal repairs are performed primarily for the correction of a cystourethrocele associated with stress urinary incontinence. The abdominal approach is more easily accomplished and is the more durable of the two (9). The retropubic space (of Retzius) is widely dissected. Interrupted permanent sutures are used to reattach bilaterally the anterior superior vaginal sulci to the arcus tendineus fasciae pelvis ("white line") from the ischial spine to the lower edge of the pubic ramus (27).

VAGINAL VAULT SUSPENSION. When a hysterectomy has been performed, it is important that the vaginal apex be resuspended by the uterosacral and cardinal ligaments. If these ligaments are inadequate for the suspension, a sacral colpopexy may be performed (28–30). In performing a sacral colpopexy, the deepest portion of the cul-de-sac is obliterated with permanent sutures placed in a Moschcowitz or Halban fashion (25, 26). The peritoneum is incised over the vaginal apex. The bladder is dissected from the upper anterior vaginal wall, and the peritoneum is dissected from the upper posterior vaginal wall. A fascial or synthetic graft is securely sewn with permanent sutures to a broad portion of the fibromuscular wall of the vaginal apex. The posterior parietal peritoneum is incised in the midline from the promontory of the sacrum to the obliterated cul-de-sac. The cephalad end of the suspending strap is subsequently sewn, without tension, to the anterior longitudinal ligament of the sacrum, and the cut edges of the parietal peritoneum are approximated to leave the suspending strap outside the peritoneal cavity. A paravaginal repair or retropubic urethropexy is recommended to prevent postoperative stress urinary incontinence.

Special Considerations

REDUNDANT ANTERIOR VAGINAL WALL. The apex of the anterior vaginal wall may be so dilated that it requires narrowing. This has been referred to as abdominal cystocele repair. It is performed by removing a full-thickness wedge of the vaginal wall from the anterior vaginal apex (31). The cut edges of the vaginal wall are then reapproximated in the midline. The anterior lateral sulci of the vagina may then require reattachment to the white line (arcus tendineus fascia pelvis).

GENUINE STRESS INCONTINENCE. Patients with documented genuine stress incontinence should have a continence procedure performed at the time of their prolapse surgery. Vaginal procedures lend themselves to concomitant needle urethropexies or colposuspensions; abdominal procedures are appropriately followed by retropubic urethropexies or colposuspensions. In some cases, the correction of a cystourethrocele by a paravaginal repair or an anterior repair will be sufficient to correct genuine stress incontinence.

FERTILITY-SPARING APPROACHES. Since pelvic organ prolapse is thought to be initiated by childbearing, it is best to defer the surgical treatment of the condition until childbearing is complete. Pelvic muscle exercises (11) and vaginal pessaries help in managing patients with symptomatic pelvic organ prolapse who wish to preserve their childbearing potential. If it becomes necessary to consider surgery for uterovaginal prolapse, a number of procedures may be performed to resuspend the uterus. Vaginal procedures include the Manchester–Fothergill procedure and sacrospinous ligament fixation of the cervix (32). Abdominal procedures include sacral cervicopexy–hysteropexy (33) or the Shirodkar sling cervicopexy (34).

VENTRAL SUSPENSIONS. Historically, ventral suspensions of the anterior vaginal wall, the uterus, and the vaginal apex have been performed to correct anterior vaginal and uterine prolapse. If performed, they should not be allowed to interfere with urethral and bladder function or expose the posterior cul-de-sac, thus leading to the development of an enterocele.

Follow-Up

In addition to complications associated with anesthesia, immediate complications of surgery for pelvic organ prolapse include hemorrhage, infection of the operative site or lower urinary tract, and injury of contiguous organs, blood vessels, or nerves. Possible long-term complications include postoperative urinary incontinence and recurrent pelvic organ prolapse (35). Postoperative urinary incontinence or retention and recurrent prolapse are less likely to occur when the surgical procedure is designed to correct abnormalities that are discovered during preoperative assessment of lower urinary tract function and the determination of all pelvic support defects.

Patients and their physicians share responsibility for improving the likelihood that surgical repair of pelvic organ prolapse will succeed. Patients should be aware of those factors that are thought to contribute to the progression of the disorder. Practitioners should continue to give special attention to the detection and treatment of chronic respiratory and metabolic disorders. If they have not already done so, patients should stop smoking, control their weight, avoid constipation, and avoid engaging in repetitive occupational and recreational activities that cause marked increases in intraabdominal pressure. Hypoestrogenic women should receive estrogen replacement therapy unless its use is contraindicated.

Summary

Management of pelvic organ prolapse must be individualized. Patients who are candidates for surgical correction should undergo a careful preoperative assessment that includes treatment of contributing medical problems, identification of all support defects, and evaluation of the lower urinary tract function. Surgeons who perform reconstructive procedures for pelvic organ prolapse should be familiar with multiple surgical procedures because intraoperative modification of the preoperative plan may be required. A thorough knowledge of the disorder and its impact on physiologic functions allows the selection of a surgical approach that usually is successful in relieving symptoms and restoring and preserving anatomic relationships, visceral function, urinary function, and coital function on a lasting basis.

REFERENCES

1. Bonney V. The principles that should underlie all operations for prolapse. J Obstet Gynaecol Br Empire 1934; 41:669–683
2. Gilpin SA, Gosling JA, Smith ARB, Warrell DW. The pathogenesis of genitourinary prolapse and stress incontinence of urine. A histological and histochemical study. Br J Obstet Gynaecol 1989;96:15–23
3. Kiff ES, Barnes PRH, Swash M. Evidence of pudendal neuropathy in patients with perineal descent and chronic straining at stool. Gut 1984;25:1279–1282
4. Snooks SJ, Swash M, Henry MM, Setchell M. Risk factors in childbirth causing damage to the pelvic floor innervation. Int J Colorectal Dis 1986;1:20–24
5. Smith ARB, Hosker GL, Warrell DW. The role of partial denervation of the pelvic floor in the aetiology of genitourinary prolapse and stress incontinence of urine. A neurophysiological study. Br J Obstet Gynaecol 1989; 96:24–28
6. Zacharin RF. "A Chinese anatomy"—the pelvic supporting tissues of the Chinese and Occidental female compared and contrasted. Aust N Z J Obstet Gynaecol 1977;17:1–11
7. DeLancey JOL. Anatomic aspects of vaginal eversion after hysterectomy. Am J Obstet Gynecol 1992;166:1717–1728
8. Richardson DA, Bent AE, Ostergard DR. The effect of uterovaginal prolapse on urethrovesical pressure dynamics. Am J Obstet Gynecol 1983;146:901–905
9. Baden WF, Walker T. Surgical repair of vaginal defects. Philadelphia: JB Lippincott, 1992
10. Beecham CT. Classification of vaginal relaxation. Am J Obstet Gynecol 1980;136:957–958
11. Kegel AH. Progressive resistance exercise in the functional restoration of the perineal muscles. Am J Obstet Gynecol 1948;56:238–248
12. Miller DS. Contemporary use of the pessary. In: Sciarra JJ, ed. Gynecology and obstetrics. Vol 1. Philadelphia: JB Lippincott, 1992:1–12

13. Torpin R. Excision of the cul-de-sac of Douglas for the surgical cure of hernias, through the female caudal wall, including prolapse of the uterus. J Int Coll Surg 1955; 24:322–330
14. Waters EG. Vaginal prolapse: technic for correction and prevention at hysterectomy. Obstet Gynecol 1956;8:432–436
15. McCall ML. Posterior culdeplasty. Surgical correction of enterocele during vaginal hysterectomy: a preliminary report. Obstet Gynecol 1957;10:595–602
16. Randall CL, Nichols DH. Surgical treatment of vaginal inversion. Obstet Gynecol 1971;38:327–332
17. Morley GW, DeLancey JOL. Sacrospinous ligament fixation for eversion of the vagina. Am J Obstet Gynecol 1988;158:872–881
18. Shull BL, Capen CF, Riggs MW, Kuehl TJ. Bilateral attachment of the vaginal cuff to iliococcygeus fascia: an effective method of cuff suspension. Am J Obstet Gynecol 1993;168:1669–1677
19. American College of Obstetricians and Gynecologists. Urinary incontinence. ACOG Technical Bulletin 213. Washington, DC: ACOG, 1995
20. Given FT Jr. "Posterior culdoplasty": revisited. Am J Obstet Gynecol 1985;153:135–139
21. Thornton NW Jr, Peters WA III. Repair of vaginal prolapse after hysterectomy. Am J Obstet Gynecol 1983;147:140–148
22. Nichols DH. Posterior colporrhaphy and perineorrhaphy: separate and distinct operations. Am J Obstet Gynecol 1991;164:714–721
23. Hanson GE, Keettel WC. The Neugebauer–LeFort operation. A review of 288 colpocleises. Obstet Gynecol 1969;34:352–357
24. Percy NM, Perl JI. Total colpectomy. Surg Gynecol Obstet 1961;113:174–184
25. Moschcowitz AV. The pathogenesis, anatomy, and cure of prolapse of the rectum. Surg Gynecol Obstet 1912;15:7–21
26. Halban J. Gynakologische Operationslehre. Berlin: Urban and Schwarzenberg, 1932
27. Richardson AC, Lyon JB, Williams NL. A new look at pelvic relaxation. Am J Obstet Gynecol 1976;126:568–573
28. Addison WA, Timmons MC, Wall LL, Livengood CH III. Failed abdominal sacral colpopexy: observations and recommendations. Obstet Gynecol 1989;74:480–483
29. Hendee AE, Berry CM. Abdominal sacropexy for vaginal vault prolapse. Clin Obstet Gynecol 1981;24:1217–1226
30. Timmons MC, Addison WA, Addison SB, Cavenar MG. Abdominal sacral colpopexy in 163 women with posthysterectomy vaginal vault prolapse and enterocele. Evolution of operative techniques. J Reprod Med 1992; 37:323–327
31. Macer GA. Transabdominal repair of cystocele, a 20 year experience, compared with the traditional vaginal approach. Am J Obstet Gynecol 1978;131:203–206
32. Kovac SR, Cruikshank SH. Successful pregnancies and vaginal deliveries after sacrospinous uterosacral fixation in five of nineteen patients. Am J Obstet Gynecol 1993; 168:1778–1786
33. Nichols DH. Fertility retention in the patient with genital prolapse. Am J Obstet Gynecol 1991;164:1155–1158
34. Shirodkar VN. The problem of prolapse. In: Contributions to obstetrics and gynecology. Edinburgh: E & S Livingstone 1960:46–64
35. Shull BL, Capen CV, Riggs MW, Kuehl TJ. Preoperative and postoperative analysis of site-specific pelvic support defects in 81 women treated with sacrospinous ligament suspension and pelvic reconstruction. Am J Obstet Gynecol 1992;166:1764–1771

RECOMMENDED READING

Nichols DH, Randall CV. Vaginal surgery. 3rd ed. Baltimore: Williams and Wilkins, 1989

This Technical Bulletin was developed under the direction of the Committee on Technical Bulletins of the American College of Obstetricians and Gynecologists as an educational aid to obstetricians and gynecologists. The committee wishes to thank Raymond A. Lee, MD, for his assistance in the development of this bulletin. This Technical Bulletin does not define a standard of care, nor is it intended to dictate an exclusive course of management. It presents recognized methods and techniques of clinical practice for consideration by obstetrician–gynecologists for incorporation into their practices. Variations of practice taking into account the needs of the individual patient, resources, and limitations unique to the institution or type of practice may be appropriate.

ISSN 1074-8628

THE AMERICAN COLLEGE OF OBSTETRICIANS AND GYNECOLOGISTS
409 12th Street, SW
Washington, DC 20024-2188

12345/98765

ACOG EDUCATIONAL BULLETIN

Number 243, January 1998

Postpartum Hemorrhage

To define postpartum hemorrhage, one must first define normal blood loss at delivery. In a classic study by Pritchard and colleagues, average blood losses at vaginal delivery, cesarean delivery, and repeat cesarean delivery plus hysterectomy were approximately 500 mL, 1,000 mL, and 1,500 mL, respectively (1).

Excessive blood loss, or hemorrhage, may be difficult to define clinically, because the diagnosis usually is based on subjective observations. Postpartum hemorrhage has been defined as either a 10% change in hematocrit between admission and the postpartum period or a need for erythrocyte transfusion (2). Based on these definitions, vaginal delivery has been associated with a 3.9% incidence (2) and cesarean delivery has been associated with a 6.4% incidence of postpartum hemorrhage (3).

Early postpartum hemorrhage occurs during the first 24 hours after delivery, whereas late postpartum hemorrhage occurs after 24 hours but before 6 weeks after delivery. Early postpartum hemorrhage is far more common than late postpartum hemorrhage, and it is associated with a greater degree of blood loss and morbidity.

Several additional factors regarding postpartum hemorrhage should be considered by the obstetrician. First, blood loss is often clinically underestimated by as much as 30–50%, sometimes resulting in a delay in addressing an important problem. Second, the blood volume expansion that occurs during pregnancy compensates for normal blood loss at delivery. This expansion occurs to a lesser degree in preeclamptic women, who also experience greater blood loss at delivery than do normotensive women. Third, postpartum hemorrhage is likely to recur in subsequent pregnancies.

This Educational Bulletin was developed under the direction of the Committee on Educational Bulletins of the American College of Obstetricians and Gynecologists as an aid to obstetricians and gynecologists. The College wishes to thank Gary A. Dildy III, MD, for his assistance in the development of this bulletin. This document is not to be construed as establishing a standard of practice or dictating an exclusive course of treatment. Rather, it is intended as an educational tool that presents current information on obstetric–gynecologic issues.

Role in Maternal Mortality

The maternal mortality rate was 7.1 per 100,000 live births in the United States during 1995 (4). Embolism and hypertensive disease are the two most common causes of direct maternal mortality in advanced gestations, with hemorrhage usually ranking third (5–7). In a study of maternal mortality in Massachusetts from 1954 to 1985, a decline was observed in hemorrhage-related maternal deaths. This decline was thought to be secondary to a reduction in the incidence of uterine atony and more timely blood trans-

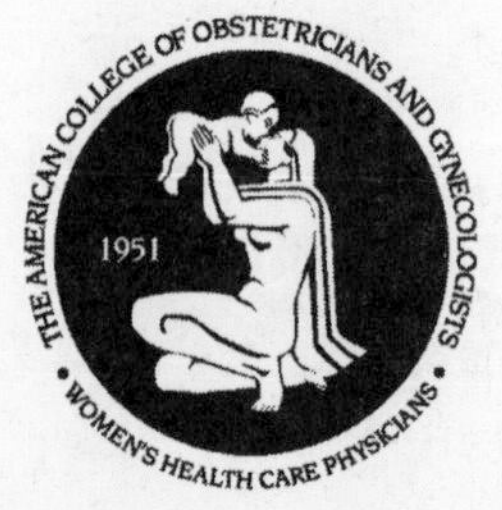

Replaces Number 143, July 1990

fusions (8). Of the 500,000 pregnancy-related deaths that occur each year worldwide, postpartum hemorrhage remains a significant problem, contributing to 30% of these deaths in the developing world (9).

Predictors and Causes of Postpartum Hemorrhage

Uterine atony and lacerations of the vagina and cervix are the most common causes of postpartum hemorrhage (10). Other causes are listed in the box. Risk factors for uterine atony include uterine overdistention secondary to hydramnios, multiple gestation, oxytocin use, and fetal macrosomia. High parity, rapid or prolonged labor, intraamniotic infection, and use of uterine-relaxing agents (terbutaline, magnesium sulfate, halogenated anesthetic agents, and nitroglycerin) are other associated risk factors.

Lower genital tract lacerations secondary to obstetric trauma occur more commonly with forceps delivery or vacuum extraction than with spontaneous vaginal delivery. Other risk factors associated with lower genital tract trauma include fetal macrosomia, precipitous labor and delivery, and use of episiotomy. The possibility of a laceration should be considered when bleeding persists in the presence of adequate uterine tone. Deep lacerations may result in hematoma formation, which may not be palpable if located above the pelvic diaphragm. Pelvic pain and shock may be the only presenting signs and symptoms.

Retained placental tissue may result in incomplete uterine involution and persistent bleeding. Occasionally, retention of a complete or partial cotyledon may occur in a placenta that appears otherwise normal. In some cases, this may be due to a succenturiate lobe; in other cases placenta accreta, increta, or percreta may be the cause of hemorrhage. The incidence of placenta accreta is 1 in 2,500 deliveries, and predisposing conditions are previous puerperal curettage, cesarean delivery, hysterotomy, placenta previa, and high parity. Especially prominent as a factor predisposing to placenta accreta is one or more prior cesarean delivery scars in the presence of a placenta previa, in which case the risk of accreta may be 25% or higher.

Acquired coagulopathies are rare complications of pregnancy that are life threatening. Anticoagulant administration (eg, heparin for deep venous thrombosis) occasionally may lead to significant postpartum hemorrhage if the anticoagulant is not discontinued before delivery or if it is not pharmacologically reversed with protamine sulfate. However, moderate prolongation of activated partial thromboplastin time is unlikely to lead to significant hemorrhage if the platelet count is adequate and uterine atony is not present. Severe infections such as gram-negative enteric bacteria (*Escherichia coli*, *Klebsiella*, *Enterobacter*, *Pseudomonas*, *Serratia*), gram-negative anaerobes (*Bacteroides*), gram-positive bacteria (*Streptococcus pyogenes*), viruses (varicella), and fungal infections may result in disseminated intravascular coagulopathy. Several conditions unique to obstetric patients (abruptio placentae, amniotic fluid embolism, and retained dead fetus syndrome) also may be associated with the development of disseminated intravascular coagulopathy. Severe preeclampsia may be associated with thrombocytopenia and cause bleeding. Inherited disorders of coagulation occasionally are encountered in women of reproductive age. In general, women with these disorders have a history of heavy menstrual bleeding.

Uterine rupture is a potentially catastrophic event for both mother and fetus. The incidence is approximately 1 in 2,000 deliveries. Uterine rupture may occur spontaneously in obstructed labor, with multiple gestations, with abnormal fetal lie, and especially in women of high parity (11). Previous uterine surgery, particularly deep myomectomy or transfundal cesarean delivery, is a significant risk factor for uterine rupture and postpartum hemorrhage. Obstetric interventions such as midforceps delivery and internal podalic version with breech extraction may precipitate uterine rupture.

Uterine inversion may be associated with uterine atony and excessive cord traction during the third stage of labor; however, some cases occur spontaneously. The incidence is estimated to be 1 in 2,500 deliveries. Risk factors for uterine inversion include fetal macrosomia, fundal placentation, use of oxytocin, and primiparity (12). Placenta accreta and uterine anomalies also have been associated with uterine inversion.

Reported risk factors for hemorrhage at the time of cesarean delivery are preeclampsia, disorders of active

Etiologies of Postpartum Hemorrhage

Early postpartum hemorrhage (≤24 hours postdelivery)
- Uterine atony
- Retained placental fragments
- Lower genital tract lacerations
- Uterine rupture
- Uterine inversion
- Placenta accreta
- Hereditary coagulopathy

Late postpartum hemorrhage (>24 hours to 6 weeks postdelivery)
- Infection
- Placental site subinvolution
- Retained placental fragments
- Hereditary coagulopathy

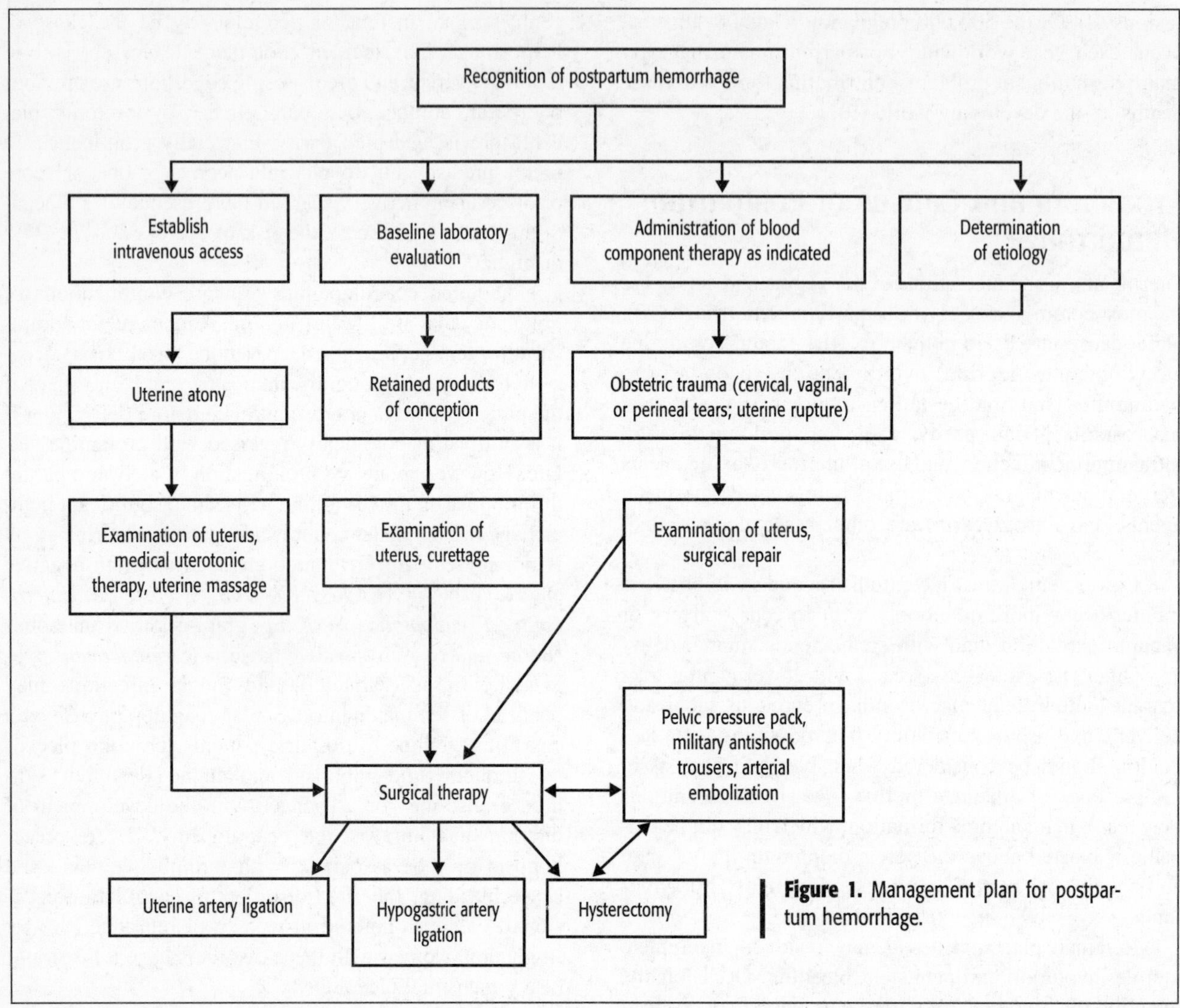

Figure 1. Management plan for postpartum hemorrhage.

labor, history of previous hemorrhage, obesity, use of general anesthesia, and intraamniotic infection (3, 13, 14). Late postpartum hemorrhage is less common than early postpartum hemorrhage. Etiologies include subinvolution, retained products of conception, and endometritis (15). Ultrasonography may be useful for detecting retained placental tissue (16). Treatment may require uterotonic agents, antibiotics, and uterine curettage.

Management of Postpartum Hemorrhage

The management of postpartum hemorrhage is summarized in Figure 1. The antepartum or early intrapartum assessment of risk factors for postpartum hemorrhage may allow advanced preparation and avoidance of more severe sequelae. ABO and D (RhoD) blood type determination and antibody screen should be performed in anticipation of the need for blood component therapy. Adequate intravascular access should be obtained via one or two 16–18-gauge intravenous catheters in women in whom significant risk factors have been identified.

Concurrent steps should be undertaken to evaluate and treat the patient. The etiology of the abnormal bleeding is determined by physical examination consisting of uterine palpation, visual inspection of the lower genital tract, and careful inspection of the placenta. Uterine atony will be evident by bimanual examination. Placenta accreta usually is recognized by difficult or incomplete separation at the time of placental delivery.

Supplemental oxygen administration will enhance cellular oxygen delivery, and placement of an indwelling urinary catheter will facilitate assessment of intravascular volume resuscitation. Careful documentation of vital signs, pharmacologic agents, transfused blood products, and laboratory data in a flow sheet facilitates care.

Table 1. Uterotonic Agents for Postpartum Hemorrhage*

Medication	Dose	Primary Route (Alternate)	Frequency of Dose	Side Effects	Comments and Contraindications
Oxytocin	10–40 U in 1,000 mL of normal saline or lactated Ringer solution	IV (IM, IMM)	Continuous infusion	Usually none, but nausea, vomiting, and water intoxication have been reported	No contraindications
Methylergonovine	0.2 mg	IM (IMM)	Every 2–4 h	Hypertension, hypotension, nausea vomiting	Contraindications include hypertension/toxemia
15-m $PGF_{2\alpha}$	0.25 mg	IM (IMM)	Every 15–90 min, not to exceed 8 doses	Vomiting, diarrhea, nausea, flushing or hot flashes, chills or shivering	Contraindications include active cardiac, pulmonary renal, or hepatic disease
Dinoprostone (PGE_2)	20 mg	PR	Every 2 h	Vomiting, diarrhea, nausea, fever, headache, chills or shivering	Should be avoided in hypotensive patient because of vasodilatation; if available, 15-m $PGF_{2\alpha}$ is preferable

*Abbreviations: IV, intravenous; IM, intramuscular; IMM, intramyometrial; 15-m $PGF_{2\alpha}$, 15-methyl prostaglandin $F_{2\alpha}$; PR, per rectum. Adapted from Dildy GA, Clark SL. Postpartum hemorrhage. Contemp Obstet Gynecol 1993;38:21–29

Initial laboratory evaluation includes a complete blood count with platelet concentration and blood type with antibody screen if not previously performed. The clotting mechanism is assessed by measurement of fibrinogen, fibrin split products, prothrombin time, and partial thromboplastin time.

Treatment of Underlying Problems

Uterine atony initially is managed by bimanual uterine massage and compression. Bimanual compression is performed by massaging the uterus between a hand on the abdomen and a hand or fist in the vagina or within the uterus. Emptying of an overdistended bladder may assist in obtaining adequate uterine contractility. Medical therapy should begin with intravenous oxytocin administration (Table 1). Oxytocin also may be given by the intramuscular or intramyometrial route. Methylergonovine is a powerful contractile agent but is contraindicated in the presence of hypertensive disease states, when severe hypertension may ensue secondary to intense vasoconstriction.

Prostaglandin derivatives (15-methyl prostaglandin $F_{2\alpha}$ [15-methyl $PGF_{2\alpha}$]) have been reported to have success rates that are quite high when used alone (88%) or in combination with other oxytocic agents (95%) for treatment of postpartum hemorrhage (17). 15-Methyl $PGF_{2\alpha}$ usually is administered by deltoid intramuscular injection, but it may be given by intramyometrial injection at cesarean delivery (18) or transabdominally after vaginal delivery (19). Prostaglandin treatment failures may be secondary to delay in administration (18). Potential side effects of prostaglandin administration include diarrhea, hypertension, hypotension, vomiting, and fever (17). Arterial oxygen desaturation has been reported after 15-methyl $PGF_{2\alpha}$ administration (20). 15-Methyl $PGF_{2\alpha}$ is preferable to prostaglandin E_2, which may cause vasodilatation and exacerbation of hypotension, although the prostaglandin E_2 may be helpful in patients with heart or lung disease in whom 15-methyl $PGF_{2\alpha}$ is contraindicated. When medical therapy for uterine atony fails, reevaluation for genital tract lacerations and retained placental tissue should be considered.

Uterine packing was once commonly used for persistent postpartum bleeding, but its use has become less common because of concern for concealed hemorrhage and further cardiovascular compromise (10). Uterine packing occasionally may be useful for control of hemorrhage secondary to uterine atony, placenta previa, and placenta accreta (21).

Surgical therapy is used for direct indications (eg, uterine curettage for suspected retained placental tissue) or if medical therapy is unsuccessful. Obstetric lacerations are repaired by placing the initial suture above the apex of the laceration to control retracted arteries.

Uterine artery ligation may easily be performed at laparotomy (22–24). The ascending branches of the uterine arteries are ligated, usually at the level of the vesicouterine peritoneal reflection. To reduce uterine perfusion further, ligation of uteroovarian and infundibulopelvic vessels also may be performed.

Hypogastric artery ligation reduces arterial pulse pressure to the pelvic organs (25). The procedure may be technically difficult and is successful in less than half of the patients (26); therefore, it is increasingly being replaced by other forms of management. The anterior trunk of the hypogastric artery distal to the posterior division is singly ligated but is not divided. Care must be exercised to avoid injury to the hypogastric vein, which lies posterior to the artery. Indications for hypogastric artery ligation include hemorrhage secondary to atony, hysterotomy extension, and placenta accreta. In general, use of the procedure should be reserved for hemodynamically stable patients of low parity in whom future childbearing is of paramount concern (26).

Hysterectomy may be a lifesaving maneuver in cases of postpartum hemorrhage when other therapies are unsuccessful (27). The most common indications for emergency hysterectomy include uterine atony, placenta accreta, uterine rupture, extension of a low transverse uterine incision, and leiomyomata, which prevent uterine closure and hemostasis (28).

Conservative as well as radical surgical attempts to control hemorrhage may fail in some cases. Other maneuvers to control persistent obstetric hemorrhage have been reported in relatively small series. Selective arterial embolization may be a therapeutic option in centers with interventional radiologists when bleeding is not immediately life threatening (29). Fever, contrast media nephrotoxicity, and buttock claudication are reported complications of this procedure. Failure of arterial embolization does not preclude later attempts at surgical maneuvers; however, hypogastric artery ligation reduces access for subsequent selective arterial embolism. A pelvic pressure pack may work to tamponade persistent posthysterectomy hemorrhage (30), especially when the bleeding is exacerbated by coagulopathy. Military antishock trousers also have been used in cases of postpartum hemorrhage (31).

With uterine inversion, the uterus is replaced and the placenta is removed, either before or after the uterus is replaced (32). Uterine-relaxing agents (magnesium sulfate, terbutaline, halogenated anesthetic agents, nitroglycerin) may be administered if manual replacement is unsuccessful because of uterine contraction. The intravenous infusion of oxytocic agents is initiated after successful uterine repositioning. Surgical maneuvers to reposition the uterus (Spinelli, Haultain, and Huntington procedures) usually are not required in acute cases of inversion.

Further Considerations

Blood component therapy is an integral part of the proper management of postpartum hemorrhage. Specific details regarding the use of erythrocytes, platelets, fresh-frozen plasma, and cryoprecipitate are available (33). Whole blood transfusion is indicated infrequently. The use of blood component therapy is a better treatment option because the specific required component is provided and various components from a single unit of donated blood can be used to treat several patients.

Resuscitation of a depleted intravascular blood volume by infusion of crystalloid solutions or blood products may be monitored indirectly by assessing urine output with an indwelling urinary catheter. Attempts should be made to maintain the urine output above 0.5 mL/kg/h. As a general rule, 3 mL of crystalloid solution is infused for each 1 mL of estimated blood loss. A second large-bore intravenous line is useful to allow simultaneous intravascular volume replacement and drug administration.

Pulmonary artery catheterization usually is not indicated unless hemorrhage is accompanied by additional complications. Examples of complications include sepsis, cardiac or pulmonary disease, or severe hypertension secondary to preeclampsia.

Complications of Postpartum Hemorrhage

The complications of postpartum hemorrhage are varied, and the range of degree of severity is quite broad. Hypovolemia may lead to maternal hypotension, shock, acute tubular necrosis, dilutional coagulopathy, cardiac arrest, and death. Further detail regarding the pathophysiology and complications of hemorrhagic shock is provided elsewhere (34). Blood transfusion complications include hemolysis due to ABO incompatibility, viral diseases, acute lung injury, transmission of bacteria or endotoxins, transmission of parasitic agents, graft-versus-host disease, alloimmunization to blood products, and transfusion-related immunosuppression (35).

Summary

Multiple improvements in obstetric care, including technical advances in blood banking, antibiotic therapy, obstetric anesthesia, and oxytocic agents have led to improved maternal outcome and survival. Yet, postpartum hemorrhage is still a significant contributor to maternal morbidity and mortality in modern obstetrics. Uterine atony remains the most common contributor to this potentially lethal clinical problem. Patients experiencing postpartum hemorrhage usually respond to medical and conservative surgical therapies, but may ultimately require hysterectomy for hemostasis. Early recognition of risk factors and preparation for medical and surgical intervention may reduce the degree of initial blood loss and thus result in less severe complications.

References

1. Pritchard JA, Baldwin RM, Dickey JC, Wiggins KM. Blood volume changes in pregnancy and the puerperium. II. Red blood cell loss and changes in apparent blood volume during and following vaginal delivery, cesarean section, and cesarean section plus total hysterectomy. Am J Obstet Gynecol 1962;84:1271–1282
2. Combs CA, Murphy EL, Laros RK Jr. Factors associated with postpartum hemorrhage with vaginal birth. Obstet Gynecol 1991;77:69–76
3. Combs CA, Murphy EL, Laros RK Jr. Factors associated with hemorrhage in cesarean deliveries. Obstet Gynecol 1991;77:77–82
4. Anderson RN, Kochanek KD, Murphy SL. Report of final mortality statistics, 1995. Monthly vital statistics report; vol 45, no. 11. Hyattsville, Maryland: National Center for Health Statistics, 1997
5. Kaunitz AM, Hughs JM, Grimes DA, Smith JC, Rochat RW, Kafrissen ME. Causes of maternal mortality in the United States. Obstet Gynecol 1985;65:605–612
6. Kochanek KD, Hudson BL. Advance report of final mortality statistics, 1992. Monthly vital statistics report; vol 43, no. 6, suppl. Hyattsville, Maryland: National Center for Health Statistics, 1995
7. Rochat RW, Koonin LM, Atrash HK, Jewett JF. Maternal mortality in the United States: report from the maternal mortality collaborative. Obstet Gynecol 1988;72:91–97
8. Sachs BP, Brown DAJ, Driscoll SG, Schulman E, Acker D, Ransil BJ, et al. Hemorrhage, infection, toxemia, and cardiac diseases, 1954–1985: causes for their declining role in maternal mortality. Am J Public Health 1988;78:671–675
9. AbouZahr C, Royston E, eds. The global picture: the causes of maternal death. In: Maternal mortality: a global factbook. Geneva: World Health Organization, 1991:7–11
10. Cunningham FG, MacDonald PC, Gant NF, Leveno KJ, Gilstrap LC III. Williams obstetrics. 19th ed. Norwalk, Connecticut: Appleton & Lange, 1993
11. Fuchs K, Peretz B-A, Marcovici R, Paldi E, Timor-Tritsh I. The "grand multipara"—is it a problem? A review of 5785 cases. Int J Gynaecol Obstet 1985;23:321–325
12. Brar HS, Greenspoon JS, Platt LD, Paul RH. Acute puerperal uterine inversion: new approaches to management. J Reprod Med 1989;34:173–177
13. Gilstrap LC III, Hauth JC, Hankins GDV, Patterson AR. Effect of type of anesthesia on blood loss at cesarean section. Obstet Gynecol 1987;69:328–332
14. Naef RW III, Chauhan SP, Chevalier SP, Roberts WE, Meydrech EF, Morrison JC. Prediction of hemorrhage at cesarean delivery. Obstet Gynecol 1994;83:923–926
15. Khong TY, Khong TK. Delayed postpartum hemorrhage: a morphologic study of causes and their relation to other pregnancy disorders. Obstet Gynecol 1993;82:17–22
16. Lee CY, Madrazo B, Drukker BH. Ultrasonic evaluation of the postpartum uterus in the management of postpartum bleeding. Obstet Gynecol 1981;58:227–232
17. Oleen MA, Mariano JP. Controlling refractory atonic postpartum hemorrhage with Hemabate sterile solution. Am J Obstet Gynecol 1990;162:205–208
18. Bruce SL, Paul RH, van Dorsten JP. Control of postpartum uterine atony by intramyometrial prostaglandin. Obstet Gynecol 1982;59:47S–50S
19. Bigrigg A, Chui D, Chissell S, Read MD. Use of intra myometrial 15-methyl prostaglandin $F_2\alpha$ to control atonic postpartum haemorrhage following vaginal delivery and failure of conventional therapy. Br J Obstet Gynaecol 1991;98:734–736
20. Hankins GDV, Berryman GK, Scott RT Jr, Hood D. Maternal arterial desaturation with 15-methyl prostaglandin F_2 alpha for uterine atony. Obstet Gynecol 1988;72: 367–370
21. Maier RC. Control of postpartum hemorrhage with uterine packing. Am J Obstet Gynecol 1993;169:317–323
22. O'Leary JL, O'Leary JA. Uterine artery ligation in the control of intractable postpartum hemorrhage. Am J Obstet Gynecol 1966;94:920–924
23. O'Leary JL, O'Leary JA. Uterine artery ligation for control of postcesarean section hemorrhage. Obstet Gynecol 1974; 43:849–853
24. Waters EG. Surgical management of postpartum hemorrhage with particular reference to ligation of uterine arteries. Am J Obstet Gynecol 1952;64:1143–1148
25. Burchell RC. Internal iliac artery ligation: hemodynamics. Obstet Gynecol 1964;24:737–739
26. Clark SL, Phelan JP, Yeh S-Y, Bruce SR, Paul RH. Hypogastric artery ligation for obstetric hemorrhage. Obstet Gynecol 1985;66:353–356
27. Plauché WC. Cesarean hysterectomy: indications, technique, and complications. Clin Obstet Gynecol 1986;29: 318–328
28. Clark SL, Yeh S-Y, Phelan JP, Bruce S, Paul RH. Emergency hysterectomy for obstetric hemorrhage. Obstet Gynecol 1984;64:376–380
29. Vendantham S, Goodwin SC, McLucas B, Mohr G. Uterine artery embolization: an underused method of controlling pelvic hemorrhage. Am J Obstet Gynecol 1997;176:938–948
30. Hallak M, Dildy GA III, Hurley TJ, Moise KJ Jr. Transvaginal pressure pack for life-threatening pelvic hemorrhage secondary to placenta accreta. Obstet Gynecol 1991;78: 938–940
31. Pearse CS, Magrina JF, Finley BE. Use of MAST suit in obstetrics and gynecology. Obstet Gynecol Surv 1984;39: 416–422
32. Dildy GA, Clark SL. Acute puerperal uterine inversion. Contemp Obstet Gynecol 1993;38:13–21
33. American College of Obstetricians and Gynecologists. Blood component therapy. ACOG Technical Bulletin Number 199. Washington, DC: ACOG, 1994
34. American College of Obstetricians and Gynecologists. Hemorrhagic shock. ACOG Educational Bulletin Number 235. Washington, DC: ACOG, 1997
35. Fresh-Frozen Plasma, Cryoprecipitate, and Platelets Administration Practice Guidelines Development Task Force of the College of American Pathologists. Practice parameter for the use of fresh-frozen plasma, cryoprecipitate, and platelets. JAMA 1994;271:777–781

ISSN 1074-8628

The American College of Obstetricians and Gynecologists
409 12th Street, SW
PO Box 96920
Washington, DC 20090-6920

12345/21098

Number 205—May 1995

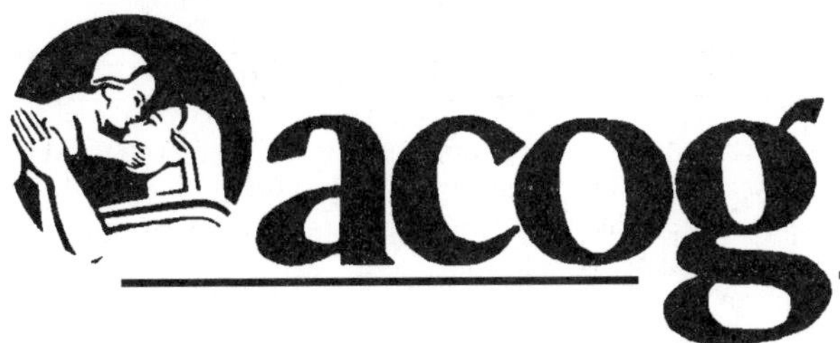

Technical Bulletin

An Educational Aid to Obstetrician–Gynecologists

Preconceptional Care

Many obstetric practitioners have encountered a patient at the first prenatal visit with a maternal complication or fetal malformation that might have been prevented by appropriate counseling and intervention prior to pregnancy. Some patients are unaware that their medical conditions, medications, occupational exposures, or social practices may have consequences in the earliest weeks of pregnancy. Because organogenesis begins around 17 days after fertilization, steps to provide the ideal environment for the developing conceptus are most likely to be effective if they precede the traditional initiation of prenatal care. Awareness of this fact has resulted in recent emphasis on preconceptional counseling.

A number of situations demonstrate the benefit of preconceptional intervention. These include patients with diabetes, phenylketonuria, or infectious diseases (such as congenital rubella syndrome). In addition, the use of folic acid to prevent neural tube defects (NTDs), the avoidance of certain prescription medications, and the institution of dietary changes before conception also have been shown to affect the pregnancy outcome positively.

Along with the potential opportunity for primary prevention of some congenital anomalies and other complications of pregnancy, preconceptional counseling offers an ideal time to educate women about the advantages of planning their pregnancies. Even among married women in the United States, the unintended pregnancy rate is nearly 40% (1). Preconceptional counseling also allows for the timely sharing of information about the importance of prenatal care, its content, and its frequency. Such counseling can help the patient establish realistic expectations about pregnancy outcome.

Targeting only self-referred women who are planning their next conception or women referred with risk factors will result in a significant number of missed opportunities for primary prevention. Women who experience unintended pregnancies are at least as likely to have risk factors for poor pregnancy outcome as are women who deliberately choose to become pregnant.

Therefore, a routine visit by any woman who may, at some time, become pregnant presents an opportunity to emphasize the importance of preconceptional health and habits. Focusing on all women of childbearing age allows for the timely identification of risks; the initiation of appropriate interventions, if desired; and the opportunity to stress the advantages of planned pregnancies. This approach also makes it possible to convey the importance of the earliest weeks of pregnancy and of adhering to good health habits even before the start of prenatal care.

During each routine visit to the practitioner's office, the patient should be questioned about her use of family planning techniques and her plans for having children. Her response and her history can determine whether preconceptional care should be initiated. It may be necessary to schedule an additional visit for a systematic preconceptional assessment. Physical examination related to preconceptional care should be directed by the patient's specific risk profile.

A coordinated multispecialty effort directed by the obstetrician–gynecologist can provide a comprehensive framework for preconceptional health care for all women of childbearing potential. Patients and practitioners alike must understand the limitations of medical knowledge. While most babies are born healthy, there are spontaneous abortions, congenital anomalies, and fetal, neonatal, and maternal complications even under ideal circumstances. Preconceptional care does not guarantee good pregnancy outcomes.

Components of Preconceptional Health Care

Preconceptional counseling should include the thorough and systematic identification of risks, the provision of education individualized to the patient's needs, and the initiation of any desired interventions (see the box). Risk identification encompasses queries about the patient's medical, reproductive, and family histories; nutritional habits; drug and environmental exposures; and social issues.

The clinician may be familiar with all of the issues raised; however, in some patients, issues identified by the history, such as the fetal effects of specific maternal diseases, drug use, or chemical exposures, may require further research by the clinician. Once information is available, the patient can be informed about the certainty or limitations of available information, what the risks of pregnancy may be, and precautions that may be beneficial. After women have been informed of the increased risks pregnancy may pose to their health or to the health of a fetus or both, they can accept the increased risks, choose to modify their risks, or opt to avoid childbearing.

Components of Preconceptional Care

Systematic identification of preconceptional risks through assessment of reproductive, family, and medical histories; nutritional status; drug exposures; and social concerns of all fertile women

Provision of education based on risks

Discussion of possible effects of pregnancy on existing medical conditions for both the prospective mother and the fetus and introduction of interventions, if appropriate and desired

Discussion of genetic concerns and referral, if appropriate and desired

Determination of immunity to rubella and immunization, if indicated

Determination of hepatitis status and immunization, if indicated

Laboratory tests, as indicated

Nutritional counseling on appropriate weight for height, sources of folic acid, and avoidance of vitamin oversupplementation; referral for in-depth counseling, if appropriate and desired

Discussion of social, financial, and psychologic issues in preparation for pregnancy

Discussion regarding desired birth spacing and real and perceived barriers to achieving desires, including problems with contraceptive use

Emphasis on importance of early and continuous prenatal care and discussion of how care may be structured based on the woman's risks and concerns

Recommendation to patient to keep menstrual calendar

Modified from Jack B, Culpepper L. Preconception care. In: Merkatz IR, Thompson JE, eds. New perspectives on prenatal care. New York: Elsevier, 1990:84

Reproductive History

The preconceptional reproductive history is an important tool for identifying factors that contributed to earlier poor pregnancy outcomes and that may be amenable to intervention (2). Diagnosis and treatment of factors such as uterine malformations, maternal autoimmune disease, endocrine abnormalities, and genital infection may lessen the risk of recurrent pregnancy losses. Review of the obstetric history when a woman is not pregnant may allow prospective parents to explore their fears, concerns, and questions in a less emotionally charged environment.

Family History

Preconceptional assessment of the family history for genetic risks offers a number of advantages over making inquiries at the first prenatal visit. Carrier screening is of special significance because it allows for relevant counseling before the first affected pregnancy. Such screening can be offered based on family history or the ethnic or racial background of the couple. Examples include testing for Tay-Sachs disease for people of Eastern European Jewish or French Canadian ancestry; β-thalassemia for those of Mediterranean, Southeast Asian, Indian, Pakistani, or African ancestry; α-thalassemia for people of Southeast Asian or African ancestry; and sickle cell anemia for people of African, Mediterranean, Middle Eastern, Caribbean, Latin American, or Indian descent. Screening for cystic fibrosis may be offered to patients with a family history of the disease. Preconceptional recognition of carrier status allows women and their partners to understand autosomal recessive risks outside of the emotional context of pregnancy. This understanding allows both informed decision making about conception and planning for further desired testing should pregnancy occur.

The family history may reveal other risks for genetic diseases such as fragile X or Down syndromes. The latter risk may become apparent either because of parental age or familial occurrence. Genetic counseling should be offered to couples with identifiable risks so that they may understand the risks and, if desired, prepare for appropriate diagnostic tests in pregnancy such as chorionic villus sampling or amniocentesis (3). Patients should be informed of the risks of these tests, including the small risk of miscarriage. In some instances, genetic counseling may result in couples deciding to forgo pregnancy or to use assisted reproductive technologies that may obviate the risk.

Medical Assessment

Preconceptional care for women with significant medical problems should include an assessment of potential risk not only to the fetus but also to the woman, should she become pregnant. For women with conditions that pose little or no risk, the preconceptional visit should provide realistic reassurance and discussion of the advantages of carefully timed conception. Care must be taken to identify and counsel all women whose life expectancy could be markedly reduced by pregnancy or whose fetus would have a high likelihood of complications. For instance, primary pulmonary hypertension has a maternal mortality rate that approaches 50% and a fetal mortality rate that exceeds 40% (4).

The increased rate of congenital malformations in infants born to mothers with insulin-dependent diabetes mellitus is significantly reduced when these women maintain excellent blood glucose control during organogenesis (5, 6). Practitioners should emphasize to insulin-dependent women of reproductive age the importance of preventing unplanned pregnancies and preparing for pregnancy (6).

The medical assessment should also investigate the risks of infectious diseases. Congenital rubella syndrome can be prevented by preconceptional screening and vaccination. Women with social or occupational risks for exposure to hepatitis B virus (HBV) should be identified and offered vaccination. Each year in the United States, approximately 16,500 births occur in HBV-infected women (7); their infants, through prenatal exposure, have a high likelihood of becoming chronic HBV carriers, with 25% of them eventually dying of liver-related disease (8). Those patients at risk for exposure to tuberculosis or cytomegalovirus (people who work in neonatal intensive care units, child care facilities, or dialysis units) or toxoplasmosis (cat owners and people who eat or handle raw meat) can be offered preconceptional testing for these diseases. Voluntary and confidential human immunodeficiency virus (HIV) antibody testing, with appropriate counseling and consent, should be offered to all women. Because some jurisdictions have laws or regulations regarding HIV testing, clinicians should be familiar with their state's requirements. In addition, risk factors may suggest other laboratory testing, such as that for *Neisseria gonorrhoeae*, *Chlamydia trachomatis*, or *Treponema pallidum*.

To assess and minimize the risk of exposure to medications, the practitioner should ask about use of prescription and nonprescription drugs and provide information on the safest choices and how to avoid drugs associated with fetal risk (9). For instance, isotretinoin (Accutane), an oral treatment approved by the U.S. Food and Drug Administration for severe, recalcitrant cystic acne, is highly teratogenic, causing craniofacial defects, malformations of the cardiovascular and central nervous systems, and defects of the thymus. Among fetuses who survive until 20 weeks of gestation, the malformation rate is 23% (10). An estimated 4,000 women ages 15–44 have an approved indication for this drug per year, but 65,000 women of reproductive age receive a prescription (11).

Occasionally, a drug profile will identify medications for which alternative therapies exist that are safer to a developing fetus. For instance, the anticoagulant coumarin and its derivatives have been associated with warfarin embryopathy. Because heparin is not teratogenic, women requiring anticoagulation should be encouraged to switch to heparin therapy before conception. Similarly, the offspring of women treated for epilepsy are at increased risk for congenital malformations. Debate exists as to whether the disease process, the medication, or a combination of both causes the malformations; however, an attempt at withdrawal of anticonvulsants from women who have not had a seizure in at least 2 years may eliminate at least one of the proposed contributors (12). For women who are not candidates for withdrawal, a drug regimen that poses the least threat should be recommended.

The risk to the fetus of new drugs may not have been fully explored. For example, angiotensin-converting enzyme inhibitors, a relatively recent addition to the options for treating hypertension, originally were used in a substantial number of pregnant women; they have subsequently been reported to have a 30% incidence of fetal morbidity, including renal disease ranging from dysfunction to complete failure following second- and third-trimester exposure (13). To decrease fetal risk and parental anxiety, drug regimens should be altered when possible in the preconceptional period to include those drugs that have been most thoroughly assessed in human pregnancy and that have been determined to pose the least risk.

Although there is no evidence that oral contraceptives or contraceptive implants are teratogens, it appears prudent for a patient to avoid systemic hormones as she prepares for pregnancy, allowing the body to regain its normal menstrual rhythm. Longer-acting hormonal contraceptives, such as injectable methods, require longer periods for menstrual rhythm to resume. Vaginal spermicides are not teratogenic in the offspring of women who conceive while using this form of contraception or immediately after discontinuing its use (14, 15).

Nutritional Assessment

Dietary evaluation and recommendation of alterations that may benefit the fetus's development are important components of preconceptional care. Access to a registered dietician is useful for patient consultations.

Evaluation of nutritional status should include assessment of the appropriateness of weight for height and discussion of eating habits such as vegetarianism, fasting, pica, eating disorders, and use of megavitamin supplementation. Appropriate dietary modifications should be suggested. Some nutritional problems may require referral and counseling. On the other hand, a vegetarian diet may require only minor alterations to ensure adequate intake of all the nutrients necessary for normal embryonic development (2).

Infants born to women with classic phenylketonuria and a maternal blood phenylalanine level greater than 20 mg/dl are likely to have microcephaly and mental retardation and are at increased risk of congenital heart disease and intrauterine growth retardation. Dietary restrictions that result in lowered levels of maternal phenylalanine during the earliest weeks of gestation appear to reduce the risk of fetal malformation (16–18).

Periconceptional intake of folic acid appears to reduce the risk of NTDs. A large cohort study not confined to high-risk patients found a 73% reduction in NTDs in well-nourished women using folate-containing multiple vitamins during the first 6 weeks of gestation and no reduction in those initiating use after 6 weeks (19). One prospective, randomized, controlled study has demonstrated that the use of 0.8 mg of folic acid was associated with significant reduction of first occurrence of NTDs (20). The U.S. Public Health Service recommends daily supplementation with 0.4 mg of folic acid for all U.S. women capable of becoming pregnant (21). Further studies are needed to determine the most effective dose, particularly for undernourished women. Unless contraindicated by pernicious anemia, women who have previously had a fetus affected with an NTD should be offered preventive treatment with 4.0 mg of folic acid daily, preferably starting 1 month before the time they plan to conceive and continuing through the first 3 months of pregnancy (22).

Social Assessment

Queries regarding a patient's social and life style history should seek to identify behaviors and exposures that may compromise reproductive outcome and should elicit information about social, financial, and psychologic issues that could affect the optimal timing of conception. Routine assessment of hobbies, habits, and home and employment environments may identify exposures that have been associated with adverse reproductive consequences and that can be minimized in the periconceptional period. Examples include exposures to organic solvents, vinyl monomers used in the manufacturing of plastics, pesticides, and heavy metals such as lead and mercury (2). Although data are limited, once specific concerns have been identified, information about the known reproductive effects may be obtained from a variety of sources.

While environmental exposures are a frequent concern of couples considering pregnancy, women should be informed that, in general, maternal use of alcohol, tobacco, and other mood-altering drugs is more hazardous for a fetus than most other life style choices (23). Alcohol is a known teratogen. Evidence is accumulating about the teratogenic properties of cocaine (24, 25); however, its ability to cause prematurity, abruption, and other complications has been well documented (26). In addition, tobacco use has been identified as the leading preventable cause of low birth weight (27).

While self-reporting of substance use is often inaccurate, the prevalence of substance exposures in American women of childbearing age is significant, varying by geographic area. Approximately 25–38% of pregnant women smoke cigarettes (28, 29). Results from the 1990 National Institute of Drug Abuse Household Survey indicate that as many as 73% of 12–34-year-old women expose their fetuses to alcohol at some time during pregnancy (28). Of women of childbearing age, 2.6–28% report use of cocaine, 3–27% report use of marijuana, and 0.3–3.9% report use of opiates (24, 30, 31).

Although many women understand the risks of substance exposures following confirmation of pregnancy, they are generally unaware of the importance of the earliest weeks of conception and the fact that no amount of ingestion has been proven safe. If substance exposure is complicated by addiction, structured recovery programs are usually needed to effect behavioral change.

For these reasons, all patients should be asked about use and abuse of alcohol, tobacco, and illicit drugs. These queries are critical for identifying patterns that pose immediate or long-term health or reproductive risks for the patient. The preconceptional interview allows for timely education about drug use and abuse in pregnancy, informed decision making about the risks of conception, and the introduction of interventions for those who abuse substances.

Victims of domestic violence should be identified preconceptionally, as they are likely to be abused during pregnancy. Approximately 37% of obstetric patients are physically abused while pregnant (32). Such assaults can result in placental separation; antepartum hemorrhage; fetal fractures; rupture of the uterus, liver, or spleen; and preterm labor (32). Information about available community, social, and legal resources and a plan for dealing with the abusive partner should be made available to women who are abused.

The cost of childbearing in the United States is considerably higher than many women and couples realize. In addition, many women and couples do not know the eligibility requirements or amount of maternity coverage provided by their insurance. Some have no medical coverage. The preconceptional interview is an appropriate time to raise these issues for all women. Some women may choose to delay conception until coverage is available.

Similarly, many women are unaware of their employers' policies regarding leave benefits for complicated and uncomplicated pregnancies and the postpartum period.

Investigation of these issues before conception can only result in better preparation for pregnancy.

Summary

Preconceptional health care offers an important opportunity for practitioners involved in women's health to expand their primary care and prevention roles. Preconceptional counseling has been shown to benefit the fetus in various ways. Efforts to provide information may also lead to improvements in the patient's health.

REFERENCES

1. Westoff CF. Contraceptive paths toward the reduction of unintended pregnancy and abortion. Fam Plann Perspec 1988;20:4–13
2. Cefalo RC, Moos MK. Preconceptional health care: a practical guide. 2nd ed. St Louis: Mosby, 1995
3. Jack B, Culpepper L. Preconception care. In: Merkatz IR, Thompson JE, eds. New perspectives on prenatal care. New York: Elsevier, 1990:69–88
4. Dawkins KD, Burke CM, Billingham ME, Jamieson SW. Primary pulmonary hypertension and pregnancy. Chest 1986;89:383–388
5. Fuhrmann K, Reiher H, Semmler K, Glöckner E. The effect of intensified conventional insulin therapy before and during pregnancy on the malformation rate in offspring of diabetic mothers. Exp Clin Endocrinol 1984;83:173–177
6. Kitzmiller JL, Gavin LA, Gin GD, Jovanovic-Peterson L, Mann EK, Zigrang WD. Preconception care of diabetes. Glycemic control prevents congenital anomalies. JAMA 1991;265:731–736
7. Centers for Disease Control. Recommendations of the Immunization Practices Advisory Committee. Prevention of perinatal transmission of hepatitis B virus: prenatal screening of all pregnant women for hepatitis B surface antigen. MMWR 1988;37:341–346
8. Beasley RP, Hwang L-Y, Chin-Yun Lee G, Lan C-C, Roan C-H, Huang F-Y, et al. Prevention of perinatally transmitted hepatitis B virus infections with hepatitis B immune globulin and hepatitis B vaccine. Lancet 1983;2:1099–1102
9. American College of Obstetricians and Gynecologists. Teratology. ACOG Technical Bulletin 84. Washington, DC: ACOG: 1985
10. Lammer EJ, Hayes AM, Schunior A, Holmes LB. Unusually high risk for adverse outcomes of pregnancy following fetal isotretinoin exposure. Am J Hum Genet 1988;43:A58
11. Teratology Society. Recommendations for isotretinoin use in women of childbearing potential. Teratology 1991; 44:1–6
12. Callaghan N, Garrett A, Goggin T. Withdrawal of anticonvulsant drugs in patients free of seizures for two years: a prospective study. N Engl J Med 1988;315:942–946
13. Barr M Jr, Cohen M Jr. ACE inhibitor fetopathy and hypocalvaria: the kidney–skull connection. Teratology 1991;44:485–495
14. Simpson JL, Phillips OP. Spermicides, hormonal contraception and congenital malformations. Adv Contracept 1990;6:141–167
15. American College of Obstetricians and Gynecologists. Contraceptives and congenital anomalies. ACOG Committee Opinion 124. Washington, DC: ACOG, 1993
16. Lenke RR, Levy HL. Maternal phenylketonuria—results of dietary therapy. Am J Obstet Gynecol 1982;142:548–553
17. Drogari E, Smith I, Beasly M, Lloyd JK. Timing of strict diet in relation to fetal damage in maternal phenylketonuria. Lancet 1987;2:927–930
18. Platt LD, Koch R, Azen C, Hanley WB, Levy HL, Matalon R, et al. Maternal phenylketonuria collaborative study, obstetric aspects and outcome: the first 6 years. Am J Obstet Gynecol 1992;166:1150–1162
19. Milunsky A, Jick H, Jick S, Bruell CL, MacLaughlin DS, Rothman KJ, et al. Multivitamin/folic acid supplementation in early pregnancy reduces the prevalence of neural tube defects. JAMA 1989;262:2847–2852
20. Czeizel AE, Dudás I. Prevention of the first occurrence of neural-tube defects by periconceptional vitamin supplementation. N Engl J Med 1992;327:1832–1835
21. Centers for Disease Control and Prevention. Recommendations for the use of folic acid to reduce the number of cases of spina bifida and other neural tube defects. MMWR 1992;41(RR-14):1–7
22. Centers for Disease Control. Use of folic acid for prevention of spina bifida and other neural tube defects. 1983–1991. MMWR 1991;40:513–516
23. Shepard TH. Counseling pregnant women exposed to potentially harmful agents during pregnancy. Clin Obstet Gynecol 1983;26:478–483
24. Zuckerman B, Frank DA, Hingson R, Amaro H, Levenson SM, Kayne H, et al. Effects of maternal marijuana and cocaine use on fetal growth. N Engl J Med 1989;320:762–768
25. Chávez GF, Mulinare J, Cordero JF. Maternal cocaine use during early pregnancy as a risk factor for congenital urogenital anomalies. JAMA 1983;262:795–798
26. American College of Obstetricians and Gynecologists. Substance abuse in pregnancy. ACOG Technical Bulletin 195. Washington, DC: ACOG, 1994
27. U.S. Department of Health and Human Services. The health consequences of smoking for women: a report of the Surgeon General. Washington, DC: Government Printing Office, 1980; publication no. HHS396
28. Gomby DS, Shiono PH. Estimating the number of substance-exposed infants. The Future of Children 1991;1:17-25
29. Floyd RL, Zahniser C, Gunter E, Kendrick JS. Smoking during pregnancy: prevalence, effects, and intervention strategies. Birth 1991;18:48–53
30. Centers for Disease Control. Statewide prevalence of illicit drug use by pregnant women—Rhode Island. MMWR 1990;39:225–227

31. Chasnoff IJ, Landress HJ, Barret ME. The prevalence of illicit-drug or alcohol use during pregnancy and discrepancies in mandatory reporting in Pinellas County, Florida. N Engl J Med 1990;322:1202–1206

32. American Medical Association, Council on Scientific Affairs. Violence against women. Relevance for medical practitioners. JAMA 1992;267:3184–3189

SUGGESTED RESOURCES

Professional

Briggs GG, Freeman RK, Yaffe SJ. Drugs in pregnancy and lactation. 3rd ed. Baltimore: Williams and Wilkins, 1990

Cefalo RC, Moos MK. Preconceptional health care: a practical guide. 2nd ed. St Louis: Mosby, 1995

Chamberlain G, Lumley J, eds. Prepregnancy care: a manual for practice. New York: John Wiley and Sons, 1986

Garver KL, Marchese SG. Genetic counseling for clinicians. Chicago: Year Book Medical Publishers, 1986

Paul M. Occupational and environmental reproductive hazards: a guide for clinicians. Baltimore: Williams and Wilkins, 1993

Schardein JL. Chemically induced birth defects. 2nd ed. New York: Marcel Dekker, 1993

Sever JL, Larsen SW, Grossman JH. Handbook of perinatal infections. 2nd ed. Boston: Little, Brown and Co, 1989

Reproductive Toxicology Center. This center markets, at a reasonable fee, an on-line information database called Reprotox. The database includes information on the reproductive effects of industrial and environmental chemicals; prescription, over-the-counter, and illicit drugs; and nutritional agents. Telephone: (202) 293-5137.

Patient

American College of Obstetricians and Gynecologists. ACOG guide to preconception care. Washington, DC: ACOG, 1990

Barnes B, Bradley SG. Planning for a healthy baby: essential readings for all future parents. London: Eubury Press, 1990

Cherry SH. Planning ahead for pregnancy. New York: Penguin Press, 1987

Queenan JT, Leslie KK, eds. Preconceptions: preparation for pregnancy. Boston: Little Brown Co, 1989

Reuben C. The healthy baby book. Los Angeles: Jeremy P. Tarcher, Inc, 1992

Before pregnancy. A comprehensive pregnancy planning guide which, based on the responses to a unique preconceptional assessment, is individualized to the health issues of a woman and her partner. Comprehensive Information for Perinatal Health, Inc (CIPHI). Citrus Heights, California

This Technical Bulletin was developed under the direction of the Committee on Technical Bulletins of the American College of Obstetricians and Gynecologists as an educational aid to obstetricians and gynecologists. The committee wishes to thank Merry K. Moos, BSN, FNP, MPH, and Robert C. Cefalo, MD, PhD, for their assistance in the development of this bulletin. This Technical Bulletin does not define a standard of care, nor is it intended to dictate an exclusive course of management. It presents recognized methods and techniques of clinical practice for consideration by obstetrician–gynecologists for incorporation into their practices. Variations of practice taking into account the needs of the individual patient, resources, and limitations unique to the institution or type of practice may be appropriate.
ISSN 1074-8628

THE AMERICAN COLLEGE OF OBSTETRICIANS AND GYNECOLOGISTS
409 12th Street, SW
Washington, DC 20024-2188

12345/98765

Number 206—June 1995
(Replaces #133, October 1989)

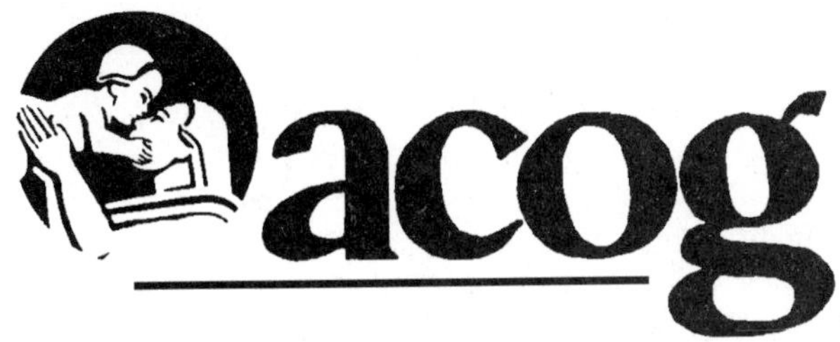

Technical Bulletin
An Educational Aid to Obstetrician–Gynecologists

Preterm Labor

Preterm labor is defined as labor occurring prior to the completion of 37 weeks of gestation (less than 259 days from the last menstrual period). It is a major cause of preterm delivery, a complication that affects approximately one in 10 births in the United States.

Preterm birth is the cause of at least 75% of neonatal deaths that are not due to congenital malformations. An infant born weighing less than 1,500 g is approximately 200 times more likely to die in the first year of life than a baby born weighing more than 2,500 g; those low-birth-weight infants who survive are 10 times more likely to be neurologically impaired. Preterm birth disproportionately contributes to developmental delay, visual and hearing impairment, chronic lung disease, and cerebral palsy. Even in seemingly healthy preterm infants, school failure and family disruption are more common than in term infants (1). Given the high rates of these complications and their close relationship with birth weight, it is apparent that significant improvements in infant, child, and family health rely on preventing preterm birth.

Although preterm birth has long been one of the most pressing and important problems in obstetrics, the rate of preterm births has not changed over the past 40 years. Despite a great deal of research and the introduction of new diagnostic and therapeutic technologies, there has been little or no improvement in outcome. Although there are many different therapies available, there is great controversy over their effectiveness in the prevention of prematurity and the management of patients in preterm labor. Lack of consensus over criteria for diagnosis of preterm labor, variations in administration and dosage of tocolytic agents, and differences in interpretation of success with therapy add to this dilemma. In addition, a clinician's personal experience with successful inhibition of preterm labor in individual patients may differ from the findings of published controlled studies. The purpose of this Technical Bulletin is to identify the issues involved in managing this condition and discuss different management options.

Etiology and Epidemiology

Predisposing Factors

In most cases of preterm labor, the cause is unknown. Epidemiologic studies have consistently reported as risk factors low socioeconomic status, nonwhite race, maternal age of 18 years or less or of 40 years or more, and low prepregnancy weight.

Although multiple gestations account for only 1.1% of all pregnancies, they result in 10% of all preterm births. A history of one previous preterm birth is associated with a recurrence risk of 17–37% (2, 3); the risk increases with the number of prior preterm births and decreases with the number of term deliveries.

There is also a clear increase in subsequent preterm deliveries in women who have experienced one or more spontaneous second-trimester abortions. One spontaneous or induced first-trimester abortion does not increase the risk of preterm birth. There is still debate, however, over whether multiple first-trimester induced abortions are associated with a higher preterm delivery rate.

Certain maternal behaviors have been linked to higher rates of preterm deliveries. Maternal smoking and cocaine use correlate significantly with preterm delivery. Women who do not seek prenatal care, regardless of socioeconomic background, are significantly more likely to deliver before term (4). It is unclear which specific aspects of prenatal care help minimize prematurity. In general, women who work outside the home do not have a higher risk of preterm birth than women who do not. However, one epidemiologic study did demonstrate an increased risk of preterm delivery in women who maintained long working hours with intensive occupational fatigue, especially if there were additional factors that predisposed the patient to preterm birth (5). Coitus and orgasm have been linked to prematurity in some studies but not in others; there are no prospective studies, however, that support sexual abstinence for the prevention of preterm labor.

In addition to idiopathic preterm labor, other conditions that could lead to preterm delivery include preterm premature rupture of membranes, maternal medical or obstetric complications, and antepartum fetal compromise or death. The relative contribution of each of these immediate obstetric causes of preterm birth appears to vary depending on the population studied (6). Preterm deliveries in predominantly white, middle-class populations are more likely to result from preterm labor. Conversely, in a racially mixed group of patients receiving public assistance, preterm premature rupture of membranes is a more common cause of preterm birth (6).

Uterine Causes of Prematurity

Women with uterine malformations such as unicornuate or bicornuate uterus are at increased risk for preterm delivery. The risk varies with the abnormality. Uterine myomata, particularly those that are submucosal or subplacental, are associated with antepartum bleeding and preterm labor (7).

Cervical incompetence, whether secondary to trauma from a prior obstetric or gynecologic procedure, associated with diethylstilbestrol exposure in utero, or of unknown etiology, may lead to painless cervical dilation and premature loss. Once dilation has occurred, uterine contractions or rupture of membranes often follows, making it difficult to establish the cause of the preterm birth. Although the prevalence of cervical incompetence is unknown, it is estimated to affect from 0.1% to 2% of all pregnancies (8). Between the late 1940s and 1971, it is estimated that 1 million to 1.5 million women were exposed in utero to diethylstilbestrol (9). These women are at increased risk for preterm delivery (15–28% of pregnancies affected) and spontaneous abortions (20–40% affected) (10).

Infectious Causes

Maternal genital tract colonization and infection may be important causes of preterm births. Sexually transmitted diseases and preterm labor have common risk factors. The association between chorioamnionitis and preterm birth is well established. Although an increased rate of preterm delivery has been described in women with cervical colonization with group B streptococci, *Neisseria gonorrhoeae, Chlamydia trachomatis, Ureaplasma urealyticum, Treponema pallidum, Trichomonas vaginalis,* or *Gardnerella vaginalis* (11), the actual contribution of these organisms to preterm labor remains ill defined. The practice of obtaining antenatal cultures (including for group B streptococci, *C. trachomatis,* and *N. gonorrhoeae*) in select patients is based primarily on the need to prevent perinatal transmission, and neither culture nor treatment has been established as beneficial for the prevention of preterm birth.

Risk Assessment

Several risk-scoring systems have been developed to identify women likely to deliver preterm or low-birth-weight infants. Of these, the system devised by Papiernik and modified by Creasy has been applied most extensively (12). It was validated prospectively in New Zealand, although only 30% of women classified as high risk actually delivered prior to term. When applied in the United States, however, similar screening systems have shown varying degrees of success. The best results have been found in upper socioeconomic populations (12); these systems have been poorly predictive of preterm labor and delivery in inner-city populations (13). Overall, the sensitivity (the likelihood that a patient will be correctly identified) of such systems is less than 50%, and the positive predictive value (the likelihood of a high-risk patient delivering prematurely) has been less than 20%. These scoring systems are more accurate for multigravid women because of the importance of prior pregnancy complications as a predictor.

There is controversy as to whether routine cervical examinations in the late second and early third trimesters are a useful screening technique for women with uncomplicated pregnancies. Cervical dilatation of at least 2 cm at 28 weeks of gestation was associated with an increased risk of prematurity in one study of unselected women (14), and another study demonstrated increased risk with internal os dilatation of 1 cm or more in the early third trimester (15). In two earlier series, however, cervical dilatation was present in at least 7% of patients at 28 weeks of gestation, increasing to 32% or more at 32 weeks of gestation, and was not associated with a greater likelihood of preterm delivery (16, 17). A 1995 multinational, randomized trial compared policies of either attempting to perform a cervical examination at each prenatal visit (2,803 women, mean six exams) or avoiding a cervical examination if possible (2,797 women, mean one exam). There were no significant differences between the experimental and control groups with respect to preterm delivery (6.7% versus 6.4%), low birth weight (6.6% versus 7.7%), or premature rupture of membranes (27.1% versus 26.5%). This large study suggests that there is no predictive advantage to routine cervical examinations in pregnant women at average risk (18).

Better indicators are needed to identify women who will develop preterm labor. Approaches that have not yet been validated include weekly monitoring for baseline uterine activity (19) and periodic evaluation of vaginal pH (20). Identification of fetal fibronectin from cervico-vaginal secretions is a marker of decidual disruption (21). Although not yet available commercially, serial use of this marker in high-risk patients or single use in patients in whom the diagnosis of premature labor may be in question holds promise if further studies confirm the initial results.

Prevention

A number of approaches to prevention have been promoted, although none has emerged as clearly effective. These approaches include intensive patient education programs, cervical examination, home uterine activity monitoring, prophylactic tocolysis, modification of daily activities, and the liberal use of cerclage.

In one nonrandomized study, the incidence of preterm delivery in a group of high-risk patients was 50% lower when compared with retrospective data following the institution of a program of educating patients and physicians about preterm labor and examining the woman's cervix weekly (22). However, two randomized controlled trials using this approach have failed to demonstrate a benefit (13, 23). Both of these studies were performed with indigent populations, who are more likely to have preterm rupture of membranes as the cause of preterm delivery. In contrast, one large, regional evaluation of this approach has suggested benefit for nonindigent patients who received care from private providers (24). Use of this method must be considered investigational.

Home uterine activity monitoring has been used as a method of early detection of uterine contractions in patients at high risk for preterm labor. The technique is based on the fact that women who subsequently go into labor before term exhibit higher uterine contraction rates earlier in gestation than women who first experience labor at term (25). Even women carefully educated to be aware of the signs and symptoms of preterm contractions may be unaware of most contractions identified by monitoring (26). However, the contributions of such contractions to preterm labor and birth are uncertain.

Several randomized controlled trials have been performed to evaluate the efficacy of home uterine activity monitoring and daily nurse contact in preventing preterm delivery. A review of these studies suggested methodologic deficiencies (27). Two studies demonstrated reductions in preterm delivery compared with traditional care for patients at risk (28, 29). Three randomized controlled trials established some benefit of daily nurse contact but showed no additional benefit of the monitor (30–32). Multiple gestation is the only subgroup in which benefit of the monitor in addition to nurse contact has been shown (30). The U.S. Food and Drug Administration approved a single home uterine activity monitoring system for use as an early warning device of preterm labor for women with a history of preterm birth. This approval was based on a randomized controlled trial that demonstrated that patients who used home uterine activity monitoring were identified in preterm labor earlier (ie, they exhibited less cervical dilatation) (33).

Substantial controversy exists over whether there is sufficient evidence of benefit to warrant recommendation in high-risk groups of routine or even selective use of home uterine activity monitoring. While it is clear that women who subsequently deliver prematurely are more likely to exhibit increased uterine contractions 24 hours or more prior to the onset of symptoms and that the monitor can demonstrate these contractions, it is not clearly demonstrated that this expensive and burdensome system can be used to actually affect the rate of preterm delivery. However, this may be a limitation of the relatively ineffective therapy available to prevent preterm delivery. In addition, considering the overdiagnosis of preterm labor, the use of home uterine activity monitoring and subsequent treatment has the potential for substantially increasing costs. Further studies are needed to address these issues.

Another approach that has been suggested to prevent preterm labor is initiating oral tocolytic therapy prior to the onset of regular uterine contractions associated with cervical change. Despite the widespread use of tocolytic agents for prophylaxis against preterm labor, however, this approach has not been evaluated extensively, particularly in singleton gestations. At least six placebo-controlled studies have used prophylactic beta-mimetic agents in women with multifetal gestations. Two studies demonstrated minor benefit, though an aggregate analysis demonstrated no overall benefit (34). Pregnancy was not prolonged significantly in any of the studies limited to high-risk singleton gestations (34). Because of the lack of clearly demonstrated benefit and the potential for tachyphylaxis and side effects with beta-mimetic drugs, these agents should be avoided prior to the onset of true preterm labor.

Reduced activity or bed rest in the late second and early third trimesters is commonly recommended to prevent preterm births. This therapy is often prescribed for women with multiple gestations, although randomized studies do not demonstrate that it results in a prolongation of gestation. There are no studies of the efficacy of bed rest for preventing preterm labor in high-risk singleton pregnancies. Furthermore, there is very little agreement as to what actually constitutes "reduced activity." Although sexual abstinence or stress reduction programs are often recommended, no clear consensus exists regarding the efficacy of these measures.

Prophylactic cervical cerclage is typically recommended for women with clear-cut histories of cervical incompetence (ie, recurrent painless dilation of the cervix associated with midtrimester or early third-trimester loss); there have been no randomized trials to support or refute the efficacy of this approach. A randomized trial of prophylactic cerclage in twin pregnancies revealed no benefit (35). Two randomized trials of cerclage studied more than 700 patients at high risk for preterm birth but excluded those with a classic history for incompetent cervix; neither showed a benefit from cerclage (36, 37). In the Medical Research Council/Royal College of Obstetricians and Gynaecologists cervical cerclage trial (38), 1,292 patients whose obstetricians were not sure whether cerclage was indicated were randomized to either receive a cerclage if possible (92% obtained a cerclage) or to avoid a cerclage unless clearly indicated (8% obtained cerclage). A statistically significant decrease in deliveries prior to 33 weeks of gestation from 17% to 13% was noted for the group randomized to routine cerclage (P = 0.03). There was a corresponding difference in very low birth weight deliveries (13% versus 10%, P = 0.05). The difference in the overall rate of miscarriage, stillbirth, and neonatal death (11% versus 9%) was less marked and not statistically significant. The use of cervical cerclage was associated with increased medical intervention and a doubling of the risk for puerperal pyrexia. The relatively small potential benefit of prophylactic cerclage in patients with marginal histories should be weighed against the risks and expense of the procedure.

One common approach to such patients is frequent cervical examinations—perhaps weekly or biweekly—combined with education designed to raise the patient's awareness of symptoms such as lower abdominal or vaginal pressure or discomfort or increased discharge. In some centers, serial ultrasound monitoring of cervical width and length is used instead of, or as an adjunct to, digital examinations. Significant cervical dilation is considered an indication for emergency cerclage. Such approaches have not been evaluated in controlled trials.

The use of cerclage is associated with more intensive management, including more frequent hospital admissions, increased use of oral tocolytics, induction of labor, and cesarean delivery. Potential adverse effects include cervical trauma, increased likelihood of infection if membranes rupture prematurely, and difficulty in removing the stitch, as well as anesthetic and surgical risks.

Management

During the initial phase of management, the patient should be evaluated carefully and the frequency of uterine contractions should be assessed. Contributing causes such as infection or preterm rupture of membranes should be noted. A history and physical examination should help identify those patients for whom tocolysis or specific tocolytic agents would be likely to have adverse effects. At this time, the physician can estimate the gestational age and observe the patient for cervical change.

Intravenous hydration with 500 ml of isotonic crystalloid solution is a commonly used initial approach to treatment although it is not of established benefit for the patient who appears to be normally hydrated (39). Excessive hydration is best avoided because of the association of pulmonary edema with tocolytic therapy. If intravenous fluid is given, administration of a hypo-tonic solution (5% dextrose in water or 0.25% normal saline) will help minimize the risk of pulmonary edema (40). In patients with advanced cervical change or very early gestational age, hydration may delay prompt initiation of intravenous tocolysis. Thus, the use of initial hydration based on the status of the individual patient is appropriate.

In assessing whether a patient is a candidate for tocolysis, gestational age should be confirmed, uterine contractions should be documented, and cervical dilatation and effacement should be assessed. Certain maternal or fetal conditions may contraindicate tocolytic treatment of preterm labor (see the box). Each case must be judged individually by weighing the risks of continuing the pregnancy versus those of delivery.

Tocolysis

There are no established criteria for when to initiate tocolytic therapy, but the presence of regular uterine contractions with documentation of cervical change (effacement or dilatation) appears to be the most widely used. Awaiting changes in cervical effacement or dilatation prior to initiation of tocolytic therapy may not compromise treatment outcome if the patient is dilated less than 3 cm (41). Cervical dilatation of at least 3 cm is associated with less effective treatment. Nonetheless, patients with more advanced cervical dilatation may benefit from tocolytic therapy if it results in gaining time to allow safe transport of the woman to a tertiary medical center or, if indicated, treatment with corticosteroids to reduce the incidence and severity of neonatal respiratory distress syndrome (RDS). Although tocolytic agents are commonly used, there are no data to suggest that tocolysis improves any index of long-term perinatal morbidity or mortality.

When tocolytic agents are selected for the treatment of preterm labor, most clinicians begin treatment prior to 34 weeks of gestation but approach the management of preterm labor at 34–37 weeks on an individualized basis. When statistics from many neonatal centers across the country are compared, it appears that the survival rate for babies born at 34 weeks of gestation (mean weight of 2,000–2,400 g) is within 1% of the survival rate beyond 37 weeks.

Furthermore, while there is certainly additional neonatal morbidity at 34–36 weeks, it is usually of a less severe variety—mild RDS, hyperbilirubinemia, or poor feeding—and rarely a cause of long-term sequelae.

Contraindications to Tocolysis for Preterm Labor*

General Contraindications

Acute fetal distress (except intrauterine resuscitation)
Chorioamnionitis
Eclampsia or severe preeclampsia
Fetal demise (singleton)
Fetal maturity
Maternal hemodynamic instability

Contraindications for Specific Tocolytic Agents

Beta-mimetic agents
— Maternal cardiac rhythm disturbance or other cardiac disease
— Poorly controlled diabetes, thyrotoxicosis, or hypertension

Magnesium sulfate
— Hypocalcemia
— Myasthenia gravis
— Renal failure

Indomethacin
— Asthma
— Coronary artery disease
— Gastrointestinal bleeding (active or past history)
— Oligohydramnios
— Renal failure
— Suspected fetal cardiac or renal anomaly

Nifedipine—Maternal liver disease

* Relative and absolute contraindications to tocolysis based on clinical circumstances should take into account the risks of continuing the pregnancy versus those of delivery.

However, there is a small group of patients in this age range who have severe RDS and the potential for sequelae.

Cost–benefit studies (in which maternal and neonatal charges assessed for patients beyond 33 weeks of gestation treated with tocolytic agents were compared with those assessed for untreated patients) have not documented either an improvement in neonatal survival rate or a decrease in cost (42). Assessment of fetal lung maturity, certainty of clinical dating, estimated fetal weight, and extenuating maternal (eg, diabetes) or family history (late-onset, severe RDS) can sometimes help the clinician select appropriate treatment between 34 and 37 weeks of gestation.

It is very important to involve the patient and her family in the decision to start or stop tocolytic therapy. Discussion of the potential risks and benefits of tocolytic agents will help the patient to better understand the goals and limitations of therapy.

Efficacy

Evaluation of the efficacy of tocolytic agents is complicated by several factors: the difficulty in establishing an accurate diagnosis of labor; the fact that preterm labor has a multitude of etiologies, some of which may be more responsive to tocolytic therapy; and the lack of consensus as to what constitutes success or failure. Some suggested definitions of "success" include extending gestation until 37 weeks; until 34–35 weeks, when nearly all neonates do well; or for 48 hours, to allow administration of cortico-steroids. Another criterion of "success" may be improved perinatal morbidity and mortality data. A review of outcome data from 16 randomized placebo-controlled trials of beta-mimetic tocolytic agents demonstrated that these tocolytic agents are relatively more successful in delaying delivery for a few days than until term (43). No cumulative reduction in neonatal morbidity or mortality has been shown, although this may be the result of relatively small sample sizes.

A recent randomized, placebo-controlled multicenter study evaluating ritodrine for tocolysis demonstrated a significant reduction in the proportion of women delivering within 48 hours of randomization in the ritodrine group (44). In addition, ritodrine was more successful in delaying delivery for 7 days than the placebo. This study found no significant beneficial effect, however, on perinatal mortality, frequency of prolongation to term, or birth weight.

Many of the published studies demonstrating the efficacy of different tocolytic therapies have been trials comparing one tocolytic agent with another. Several randomized, controlled comparisons of ritodrine and magnesium sulfate have demonstrated statistically comparable efficacy and incidence of side effects. In one randomized study with sequential design, magnesium sulfate was discontinued more frequently because of continued uterine contractions while the beta-mimetic agents were discontinued because of maternal side effects (45). Substitution of the alternative first-line agent resulted in effective tocolysis in 90% of the cases in which the initial agent failed. A randomized trial comparing indomethacin and ritodrine showed these forms of therapy had similar efficacy (46).

Few placebo-controlled studies evaluating magnesium sulfate or indomethacin have been published. A randomized study comparing magnesium sulfate with no therapy showed no significant differences in duration of gestation, birth weight, neonatal morbidity, or perinatal mortality (47). This study used a "clinically safe" maximum infusion of 3 g/h with mean maximum levels of magnesium in serum of 5.5 meq/L. Whether higher infusion rates would be more efficacious remains to be determined.

More than 20 uncontrolled studies and at least two placebo-controlled studies suggest that tocolytic therapy with indomethacin, a prostaglandin inhibitor, is efficacious (48). In one study, indomethacin was found to effectively delay delivery for at least 48 hours when compared with placebo (49).

No placebo-controlled trials of the calcium channel blocker nifedipine have been published. However, three small, randomized trials suggest that nifedipine may have efficacy comparable to that of ritodrine as a tocolytic agent.

To date, no studies have convincingly demonstrated an improvement in survival or any index of long-term neonatal outcome with the use of tocolytic therapy. On the other hand, the potential damages of tocolytic therapy to the mother and the neonate are well documented (50–52). Because of the clear benefit of corticosteroid administration before 34 weeks of gestation, the use of tocolytic agents for short-term prolongation of pregnancy is justified. Otherwise, the question of whether to use tocolytic agents at any gestational age cannot be answered at this time, especially beyond 34 weeks of gestation.

Treatment Protocols

Once the decision to treat preterm labor is made, pharmacologic tocolysis is begun. Ritodrine and magnesium sulfate are usually administered intravenously, while terbutaline (a beta-mimetic) may be given intravenously or subcutaneously. Protocols for tocolysis are similar in that they use the minimum amount of agent necessary to stop contractions, advocate reduction or cessation of the drug when significant side effects are noted, and switch to an oral agent after intravenous or subcutaneous therapy is successful for 12–48 hours. The goal of treatment is to reduce the frequency of uterine contractions and arrest cervical change. Following successful cessation of uterine contractions with use of an intravenous agent, a maintenance oral dosage of either terbutaline or ritodrine is commonly used. A benefit to oral maintenance has not been demonstrated consistently. In fact, a metaanalysis of four controlled randomized trials has demonstrated no benefit to oral maintenance therapy over observation alone (53).

One concern with oral long-term terbutaline therapy is its common adverse effect on glucose tolerance. Therefore, the 50-g oral glucose screening test for gestational diabetes mellitus should be repeated in most patients who receive terbutaline therapy for over a week (54). Oral ritodrine therapy does not significantly alter glucose tolerance. Oral magnesium has been used for maintenance tocolysis in patients in whom beta-mimetic agents are contraindicated, but data demonstrating efficacy are lacking.

Once oral maintenance therapy with either terbutaline or ritodrine is started, it is commonly continued until 35–37 weeks of gestation. The dosage is adjusted on the basis of perceived uterine contractility and maternal side effects. Some practitioners have found an elevated maternal pulse rate of 90–105 beats per minute to be a useful index of tocolytic effect.

Based on the results of in vitro and animal data, intermittent pulsatile administration of subcutaneous terbutaline has been promoted as an alternative to oral maintenance therapy for select, very-high-risk patients (55). At present, there is no evidence to support the efficacy of this costly and complicated approach.

Side Effects

Individual tocolytic agents have been shown to have a variety of side effects. The potentially serious effects are listed in the box. Both beta-mimetic medications and magnesium sulfate carry some risk for maternal pulmonary edema, although this risk appears greater with the beta-mimetic agents. The etiology of pulmonary edema associated with tocolytic therapy is not completely clear. Associated risk factors include excessive intravenous hydration, multiple gestation, occult sepsis, and underlying cardiac disease. Although adjunctive corticosteroids were initially implicated, both physiologic and statistical

Potential Complications of Tocolytic Agents

Beta-Adrenergic Agents
- Hyperglycemia
- Hypokalemia
- Hypotension
- Pulmonary edema
- Cardiac insufficiency
- Arrhythmias
- Myocardial ischemia
- Maternal death

Magnesium Sulfate
- Pulmonary edema
- Respiratory depression*
- Cardiac arrest*
- Maternal tetany*
- Profound muscular paralysis*
- Profound hypotension*

Indomethacin
- Hepatitis†
- Renal failure†
- Gastrointestinal bleeding†

Nifedipine—Transient hypotension

*Effect is rare; seen with toxic levels.

†Effect is rare; associated with chronic use.

data reveal that it is unlikely that such medications are involved. Total fluid restriction to less than 2,500–3,000 ml/d, limitation of the salt content in intravenous solutions, and maintenance of maternal pulse below 130 beats per minute can reduce the frequency of this serious complication. Development of pulmonary edema in the first 24 hours of therapy is uncommon. When used appropriately, magnesium sulfate appears to result in fewer side effects. Since toxic effects of magnesium are rarely seen below concentrations of 8 mg/dl, it may be helpful to monitor serum magnesium concentrations. Most women with preterm labor can be treated safely and effectively with either magnesium sulfate or a beta-mimetic agent. Dual therapy has been associated with a significantly increased risk of maternal side effects (51).

Indomethacin has been shown to have significant fetal effects. A number of studies have suggested decreased amniotic fluid volume and constriction of the ductus arteriosus after exposure to indomethacin (52, 56–58). Additionally, a recent retrospective analysis found that very preterm infants (less than 30 weeks) delivered after recent exposure to indomethacin experienced significantly more intracranial hemorrhage, patent ductus arteriosus, and necrotizing enterocolitis when compared with gestational age-matched controls (50).

Few data are available on nifedipine, but few adverse maternal or fetal effects have been noted. More studies are needed to clarify the role of nifedipine in tocolytic therapy. Both indomethacin and nifedipine presently are considered second-line agents for use when the primary therapy has failed. Case reports have suggested that concurrent use of magnesium sulfate and calcium channel blockers may precipitate severe hypotension.

Adjunctive Therapy

Corticosteroids should be considered for the induction of fetal lung maturity. All women between 24 and 34 weeks of pregnancy at risk for preterm delivery are candidates for antenatal corticosteroid therapy (59). Fetal race, gender, and availability of surfactant therapy should not influence the decision to use antenatal corticosteroid therapy. Optimal benefits begin 24 hours after initiation of therapy and last 7 days. Because evidence suggests that mortality, RDS, and intraventricular hemorrhage are reduced even when treatment lasts for less than 24 hours, antenatal corticosteroids should be given unless immediate delivery is anticipated. In addition, a consensus conference of the National Institutes of Health concluded that antenatal corticosteroid use is beneficial in women with preterm premature rupture of membranes at less than 30–32 weeks of gestation in the absence of clinical chorioamnionitis because of the high risk of intraventricular hemorrhage at these early gestational ages. However, further research is needed to evaluate the risks and benefits of using corticosteroids in women who have preterm premature rupture of membranes (60).

Antibiotics have been used successfully in addition to tocolytic therapy in several randomized, placebo-controlled studies of women in preterm labor. In some, but not all, studies, women treated with erythromycin, ampicillin, or clindamycin had significantly longer intervals to delivery than did controls, although there was no difference in neonatal morbidity (61, 62). More studies are needed to confirm the value of adjunctive antibiotic therapy and to define the population of women who will benefit from it.

Considerations for Delivery

When preterm delivery is imminent, decisions regarding intrapartum management of the low-birth-weight fetus may also critically affect the ultimate outcome. Over the past few decades, as neonatal and perinatal care has improved, the lower limit of viability has decreased progressively. A few recent reports describe infants born at 22 weeks of gestation who survive to hospital discharge, although these are rare cases (and often involve larger-than-expected babies). Survival at 23 weeks is also unusual, with rates ranging from 0–8%. By 24 weeks of gestation, approximately 15–20% of all live-born neonates of this age will survive to hospital discharge. Recent studies from tertiary centers often reveal that 50–60% of neonates born at 25 weeks of gestation survive, as do up to 85% of those born at 26–28 weeks of gestation. By 29 weeks, survival rates are often in excess of 90%. Although survival beyond 24 weeks of gestation is possible, long-term neurologic effects are common in the very-low-birth-weight infant and should be considered during patient counseling and management.

Aggressive obstetric and neonatal interventions have had a minimal effect on the survival of infants born at 22 or 23 weeks of gestation. This suggests a current viability threshold of approximately 24 weeks of gestation or an estimated birth weight of 600 g (63). However, recommendations for this threshold should be considered in light of the perinatal outcome statistics of the hospital's or region's own tertiary center, which should be reviewed periodically.

Survival rates of preterm infants born in a facility with an intensive care nursery are higher than those of infants of similar birth weight born in a smaller facility (64, 65). Thus, if time is available for safe maternal transport, any woman likely to deliver an infant too small or too sick to be well cared for in her intended hospital may be considered a candidate for transport to a facility better able to care for the infant. Transfer procedures must be consistent with applicable federal and state legal requirements. It is usually best if the obstetrician and the pediatrician can agree in advance on the approximate gestational age at which deliveries can safely take place in their hospital. The value of maternal transport should be weighed against the risks. Transports should not interfere with prompt initiation of therapy. Ideally, all preterm deliveries occurring after 24 weeks of gestation should be performed in the labor and delivery suite, with an individual qualified to perform resuscitation present. Difficult decisions such as these must be made in cooperation with the prospective parent(s).

Summary

Premature delivery is the leading cause of perinatal mortality and long-term neurologic morbidity. Despite intensive efforts, prematurity rates remain unchanged. Although different forms of therapy, such as tocolytic therapy and home uterine activity monitoring, are being used to prevent prematurity, their true benefit and the proper place for their application remain to be established. Continued efforts at risk identification, accurate and early diagnosis, and prompt intervention hold the most promise for prevention of premature delivery. In addition, when preterm birth is imminent, intensive intrapartum care and delivery in a location where access to the appropriate level of neonatal intensive care is available will optimize perinatal outcome.

REFERENCES

1. McCormick MC. The contribution of low birth weight to infant mortality and childhood morbidity. N Engl J Med 1985;312:82–90
2. Hoffman HJ, Bakketeig LS. Risk factors associated with the occurrence of preterm birth. Clin Obstet Gynecol 1984; 27:539–552
3. Keirse MJNC, Rush RW, Anderson AB, Turnbull AC. Risk of pre-term delivery in patients with a previous pre-term delivery and/or abortion. Br J Obstet Gynaecol 1978;85: 81–85
4. Greenberg RS. The impact of prenatal care in different social groups. Am J Obstet Gynecol 1983;145:797–801
5. Mamelle N, Laumon B, Lazar P. Prematurity and occupational activity during pregnancy. Am J Epidemiol 1984; 119:309–322
6. Meis PJ, Ernest JM, Moore ML. Causes of low birth weight births in public and private patients. Am J Obstet Gynecol 1987;156:1165–1168
7. Davis JL, Ray-Mazumder S, Hobel CJ, Baley K, Sassoon D. Uterine leiomyomas in pregnancy: a prospective study. Obstet Gynecol 1990;75:41–44
8. Harger JH. Cervical cerclage: patient selection, morbidity, and success rates. Clin Perinatol 1983;10:321–341
9. U.S. Department of Health, Education, and Welfare. DES Task Force summary report. DHEW publication no. (NIH) 79-1688. Washington, DC: DHEW, 1978
10. Stillman RJ. In utero exposure to diethylstilbestrol: adverse effects on the reproductive tract and reproductive performance in male and female offspring. Am J Obstet Gynecol 1982;142:905–921
11. Romero R, Mazor M. Infection and preterm labor. Clin Obstet Gynecol 1988;31:553–583
12. Creasy RK, Gummer BA, Liggins GC. System for predicting spontaneous preterm birth. Obstet Gynecol 1980; 55: 692–695
13. Main DM, Richardson DK, Hadley CB, Gabbe SG. Controlled trial of a preterm labor detection program: efficacy and costs. Obstet Gynecol 1989;74:873–877
14. Leveno KJ, Cox K, Roark ML. Cervical dilatation and prematurity revisited. Obstet Gynecol 1986;68:434–435
15. Bouyer J, Papiernik E, Dreyfus J, Collin D, Winisdoerffer B, Gueguen S. Maturation signs of the cervix and prediction of preterm birth. Obstet Gynecol 1986;68:209–214
16. Schaffner F, Schanzer SN. Cervical dilatation in the early third trimester. Obstet Gynecol 1966;27:130–133
17. Parikh MN, Mehta AC. Internal cervical os during the second half of pregnancy. J Obstet Gynaecol Br Commw 1961;68:818–821
18. Buekens P, Alexander S, Boutsen M, Blondel B, Kaminski M, Reid M, et al. Randomised controlled trial of routine cervical examinations in pregnancy. Lancet 1994;344: 841–844
19. Main DM, Katz M, Chiu G, Campion S, Gabbe SG. Intermittent weekly contraction monitoring to predict preterm labor in low-risk women: a blinded study. Obstet Gynecol 1988;72:757–761
20. Ernest JM, Meis PJ, Moore ML, Swain M. Vaginal pH: a marker of preterm premature rupture of the membranes. Obstet Gynecol 1989;74:734–738
21. Lockwood CJ, Senyei AE, Dische MR, Casal D, Shah KD, Thung SN, et al. Fetal fibronectin in cervical and vaginal secretions as a predictor of preterm delivery. N Engl J Med 1991;325:669–674
22. Herron MA, Katz M, Creasy RK. Evaluation of a preterm birth prevention program: preliminary report. Obstet Gynecol 1982;59:452–456
23. Goldenberg RL, Davis RO, Copper RL, Corliss DK, Andrews JB, Carpenter AH. The Alabama Preterm Birth Prevention Project. Obstet Gynecol 1990;75:933–939
24. Buescher PA, Meis PJ, Ernest JM, Moore ML, Michielutte R, Sharp P. A comparison of women in and out of a prematurity prevention project in a North Carolina perinatal care region. Am J Public Health 1988;78:264–267
25. Nageotte MP, Dorchester W, Porto M, Keegan KA Jr, Freeman RK. Quantitation of uterine activity preceding preterm, term, and postterm labor. Am J Obstet Gynecol 1988;158:1254–1259
26. Newman RB, Gill PJ, Wittreich P, Katz M. Maternal perception of prelabor uterine activity. Obstet Gynecol 1986;68:765–769
27. Grimes DA, Schulz KF. Randomized controlled trials of home uterine activity monitoring: a review and critique. Obstet Gynecol 1992;79:137–142

28. Hill WC, Fleming AD, Martin RW, Hamer C, Knuppel RA, Lake MF. Home uterine activity monitoring is associated with a reduction in preterm birth. Obstet Gynecol 1990;76(1 suppl):13S–18S

29. Morrison JC, Martin JN Jr, Martin RW, Gookin KS, Wiser WL. Prevention of preterm birth by ambulatory assessment of uterine activity: a randomized study. Am J Obstet Gynecol 1987;156:536–543

30. Dyson DC, Crites YM, Ray DA, Armstrong MA. Prevention of preterm birth in high-risk patients: the role of education and provider contact versus home uterine monitoring. Am J Obstet Gynecol 1991;164:756–762

31. Iams JD, Johnson FF, O'Shaughnessy RW. A prospective random trial of home uterine activity monitoring in pregnancies at increased risk of preterm labor. Am J Obstet Gynecol 1988;159:595–603

32. Porto M. Home uterine activity monitoring: essential tool or expensive accessory? Contemp Ob/Gyn 1990;35: 114–123 (special issue)

33. Mou SM, Sunderji SG, Gall S, How H, Patel V, Gray M, et al. Multicenter randomized clinical trial of home uterine activity monitoring for detection of preterm labor. Am J Obstet Gynecol 1991;165:858–866

34. Keirse MJNC, Grant A, King JF. Preterm labour. In: Chalmers I, Enkin M, Keirse MJNC, eds. Effective care in pregnancy and childbirth. Oxford: Oxford University Press, 1989:694–745

35. Dor J, Shalev J, Mashiach S, Blankstein J, Serr DM. Elective cervical suture of twin pregnancies diagnosed ultrasonically in the first trimester following induced ovulation. Gynecol Obstet Invest 1982;13:55–60

36. Lazar P, Gueguen S, Dreyfus J, Renaud R, Pontonnier G, Papiernik E. Multicentred controlled trial of cervical cerclage in women at moderate risk of preterm delivery. Br J Obstet Gynaecol 1984;91:731–735

37. Rush RW, Isaacs S, McPherson K, Jones L, Chalmers I, Grant A. A randomized controlled trial of cervical cerclage in women at high risk of spontaneous preterm delivery. Br J Obstet Gynaecol 1984;91:724–730

38. MRC/RCOG Working Party on Cervical Cerclage. Final report of the Medical Research Council/Royal College of Obstetricians and Gynaecologists multicentre randomized trial of cervical cerclage. Br J Obstet Gynaecol 1993; 100:516–523

39. Pircon RA, Strassner HT, Kirz DS, Towers CV. Controlled trial of hydration and bed rest versus bed rest alone in the evaluation of preterm uterine contractions. Am J Obstet Gynecol 1989;161:775–779

40. Hankins GDV. Complications of beta-sympathomimetic tocolytic agents. In: Clark SL, Cotton DB, Hankins GDV, Phelan JP, eds. Critical care obstetrics. 2nd ed. Oxford: Blackwell Scientific Publications, 1991:223–250

41. Utter GO, Dooley SL, Tamura RK, Socol ML. Awaiting cervical change for the diagnosis of preterm labor does not compromise the efficacy of ritodrine tocolysis. Am J Obstet Gynecol 1990;163:882–886

42. Korenbrot CC, Aalto LH, Laros RK Jr. The cost effectiveness of stopping preterm labor with beta-adrenergic treatment. N Engl J Med 1984;310:691–696

43. King JF, Grant A, Keirse MJNC, Chalmers I. Beta-mimetics in preterm labour: an overview of the randomized controlled trials. Br J Obstet Gynaecol 1988;95:211–222

44. Canadian Preterm Labor Investigators Group. Treatment of preterm labor with the beta-adrenergic agonist ritodrine. N Engl J Med 1992;327:308–312

45. Beall MH, Edgar BW, Paul RH, Smith-Wallace T. A comparison of ritodrine, terbutaline, and magnesium sulfate for the suppression of preterm labor. Am J Obstet Gynecol 1985;153:854–859

46. Besinger RE, Niebyl JR, Keyes WG, Johnson TRB. Randomized comparative trial of indomethacin and ritodrine for the long-term treatment of preterm labor. Am J Obstet Gynecol 1991;164:981–988

47. Cox SM, Sherman ML, Leveno KJ. Randomized investigation of magnesium sulfate for prevention of preterm birth. Am J Obstet Gynecol 1990;163:767–772

48. Higby K, Xenakis EM-J, Pauerstein CJ. Do tocolytic agents stop preterm labor? A critical comprehensive review of efficacy and safety. Am J Obstet Gynecol 1993;168: 1247–1259

49. Niebyl JR, Blake DA, White RD, Kumor KM, Dubin NH, Robinson JC, et al. The inhibition of preterm labor with indomethacin. Am J Obstet Gynecol 1980;136:1014–1019

50. Norton ME, Merrill J, Cooper BAB, Kuller JA, Clyman RI. Neonatal complications after the administration of indomethacin for preterm labor. N Engl J Med 1993;329: 1602–1607

51. Wilkins IA, Lynch L, Mehalek KE, Berkowitz GS, Berkowitz RL. Efficacy and side effects of magnesium sulfate and ritodrine as tocolytic agents. Am J Obstet Gynecol 1988;159:685–689

52. Moise KJ, Huhta JC, Sharif DS, Ou CN, Kirshon B, Wasserstrum N, et al. Indomethacin in the treatment of premature labor: effects on the fetal ductus arteriosus. N Engl J Med 1988;319:327–331

53. Macones GA, Berlin M, Berlin J. Efficacy of oral beta-agonist maintenance therapy in preterm labor: a meta-analysis. Obstet Gynecol 1995;85:313–317

54. Main EK, Main DM, Gabbe SG. Chronic oral terbutaline tocolytic therapy is associated with maternal glucose intolerance. Am J Obstet Gynecol 1987;157:644–647

55. Lam F, Gill P, Smith M, Kitzmiller JL, Katz M. Use of the subcutaneous terbutaline pump for long-term tocolysis. Obstet Gynecol 1988;72:810–813

56. Goldenberg RL, Davis RO, Baker RC. Indomethacin-induced oligohydramnios. Am J Obstet Gynecol 1989; 160:1196–1197

57. Hickok DE, Hollenbach KA, Reilley SF, Nyberg DA. The association between decreased amniotic fluid volume and treatment with nonsteroidal anti-inflammatory agents for preterm labor. Am J Obstet Gynecol 1989;160:1525–1531

58. Kirshon B, Moise KJ, Wasserstrum N, Ou CN, Huhta JC. Influence of short-term indomethacin therapy on fetal urine output. Obstet Gynecol 1988;72:51–53

59. National Institutes of Health Consensus Development Conference. Effect of corticosteroids for fetal maturation on perinatal outcomes. National Institutes of Health

Consensus Development Conference Statement, May 27, 1994:1–18

60. American College of Obstetricians and Gynecologists. Antenatal corticosteroid therapy for fetal maturation. Committee Opinion 147. Washington, DC: ACOG, 1994

61. McGregor JA, French JI, Reller LB, Todd JK, Makowski EL. Adjunctive erythromycin treatment for idiopathic preterm labor: results of a randomized, double-blinded, placebo-controlled trial. Am J Obstet Gynecol 1986; 154: 98–103

62. Morales WJ, Angel JL, O'Brien WF, Knuppel RA, Finazzo M. A randomized study of antibiotic therapy in idiopathic preterm labor. Obstet Gynecol 1988;72:829–833

63. Hack M, Fanaroff AA. Outcomes of extremely-low-birth-weight infants between 1982 and 1988. N Engl J Med 1989;321:1642–1647

64. Harris TR, Isaman J, Giles HR. Improved neonatal survival through maternal transport. Obstet Gynecol 1978;52: 294–300

65. Paneth N, Kiely JL, Wallenstein S, Susser M. The choice of place of delivery: effect of hospital level on mortality in all singleton births in New York City. Am J Dis Child 1987;141;60–64

This Technical Bulletin was developed under the direction of the Committee on Technical Bulletins of the American College of Obstetricians and Gynecologists as an educational aid to obstetricians and gynecologists. The committee wishes to thank Denise M. Main, MD, for her assistance in the development of this bulletin. This Technical Bulletin does not define a standard of care, nor is it intended to dictate an exclusive course of management. It presents recognized methods and techniques of clinical practice for consideration by obstetrician–gynecologists for incorporation into their practices. Variations of practice taking into account the needs of the individual patient, resources, and limitations unique to the institution or type of practice may be appropriate.

ISSN 1074-8628

THE AMERICAN COLLEGE OF OBSTETRICIANS AND GYNECOLOGISTS
409 12th Street, SW
Washington, DC 20024-2188

12345/98765

ACOG EDUCATIONAL BULLETIN

Number 254, November 1999

Primary and Preventive Health Care for Female Adolescents

Adolescence is a time of transition from childhood to adulthood, marked by a number of developmental milestones. For many, this passage is relatively smooth; for others, however, it may be a time of difficulty. Adolescent girls, in particular, are confronted with numerous challenges, and the decisions they make can have both short- and long-term consequences for their health and well being. The primary health risks to adolescents are no longer the traditional medical causes of illness; rather, they are behavioral. These risks include a sedentary lifestyle, poor nutritional habits, cigarette smoking, alcohol and illicit drug use, driving under the influence of alcohol, early initiation of sexual activity, and poor use of contraception. Most adolescents will engage in one of these unhealthy and risky behaviors, and data from the 1997 Youth Risk Behavior Surveillance Report indicate that nearly 1 in 12 adolescents engage in two or more of these risky behaviors, posing an even greater threat to their health and lives (1). Furthermore, 75% of all deaths among youth and young adults (10–24 years of age) in 1996 resulted from four preventable causes: motor vehicle crashes (32%); homicide (20%); suicide (13%); and other unintentional injuries (10%) (2). Guidance from a physician can greatly facilitate a young girl's healthy transition to adulthood. Physicians can provide preventive guidance to both parents and adolescents. They can screen for health-risk behaviors and early disease and can either provide or refer patients for the necessary immunizations against infectious diseases. This Educational Bulletin will address female adolescent development and primary and preventive health care intervention, including timing of health care visits, health guidance for parents and adolescents, screening, and immunization.

This Educational Bulletin was developed under the direction of the Committee on Adolescent Health Care of the American College of Obstetricians and Gynecologists as an aid to obstetricians and gynecologists. This document is not to be construed as establishing a standard of practice or dictating an exclusive course of treatment. Rather, it is intended as an educational tool that presents current information on obstetric–gynecologic issues.

Female Adolescent Development

The delivery of preventive services to adolescents differs from the delivery of preventive services to adults. Although diseases and behaviors among

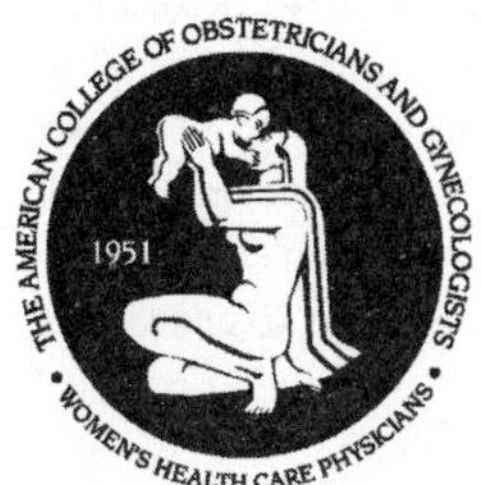

adolescents and adults may or may not be similar, an adolescent's unique developmental stage dictates the framing of preventive services. Furthermore, not all adolescents of the same age are at the same stage of development, thus necessitating further examination of the adolescent's physical, sexual, psychosocial, and cognitive development. Understanding the milestones and developmental stages of adolescence is beneficial to the obstetrician–gynecologist treating adolescents.

Sexual Development

Thelarche, or breast-budding, the first sign of secondary sexual development in most adolescent females, occurs for most young girls in North America at 8–10 years of age. Production of low amounts of estrogen stimulates long bone growth, with a peak height velocity of 9 cm per year. When higher levels of estrogen are produced, breast development progresses, long bone growth decelerates, and the epiphyses close. Menarche occurs during this deceleration phase. On average, the first menses occurs between 12–13 years of age, with regular ovulation established by approximately 20 cycles later. The average duration of puberty is 4 years, with a range of 1.5–8 years. Data from a large-scale cross-sectional study indicate that at every age and for the development of each pubertal characteristic, African-American girls are more advanced than white girls (3). Absence of thelarche by age 13 years or menarche by age 15 years represents a 2.5 standard deviation from the mean and warrants evaluation. Likewise, breast development at younger than age 8 years in the white population, or 7 years in the African-American population, is outside the range for normal development. In addition, tempo and sequence aberrancies during an otherwise established pubertal process should be included for evaluation of delayed or precocious sexual development.

Psychosocial and Cognitive Development

Adolescence is a prolonged period of transition during which a young person's expanding horizons, self-discovery, and quest for independence lead to the formation of a separate and distinct identity (4). It is particularly challenging because the processes of physical, psychologic, and cognitive development occur on separate tracks, with different timetables, which rarely are synchronous. Thus, the obstetrician–gynecologist often will encounter a young girl who has matured physically but not accomplished important psychologic and cognitive developmental tasks that will allow her to: 1) understand the consequences of present behaviors on future health outcomes and make crucial decisions about the future, 2) understand the saliency of risks and internalize those risks, and 3) form and maintain stable and healthy relationships while evolving and learning to communicate a value system of her own.

The adolescent often believes that she is different from others and, therefore, not liable to the risks that threaten her peers. Although on an intellectual level these risks may be well understood, adolescent behaviors tend to reflect an assumption of invulnerability. Such egocentrism generally is outgrown with continuing cognitive development and a young person's perception of "self" relative to "others." As the girl progresses through adolescence, she becomes increasingly capable, both cognitively and emotionally, of comprehending abstract ideas, relating present actions to future outcomes, and understanding the consequences of her own behaviors. Thus, the clinical approach to counseling a younger adolescent will differ from the approach taken with an older adolescent or an adult.

Timing of Health Care Visits

Initial Visit

The obstetrician–gynecologist frequently is asked by adult patients at what age should their adolescent daughter visit an ob-gyn. The first visit to the obstetrician–gynecologist for health guidance, screening, and the provision of preventive health care services should take place between the ages of 13 and 15 years (5). Because the obstetrician–gynecologist can function as either a primary care physician or a consultant specialist, it is important to determine whether or not the adolescent patient has a primary care provider. If so, a collaborative relationship between physicians should be established.

The exact timing and scope of the initial visit to the obstetrician–gynecologist will depend on the individual girl and her physical and emotional development. Parents and adolescent females should be reassured that the initial visit at this age serves primarily to establish rapport between the obstetrician–gynecologist and the young woman, and generally does not include a pelvic examination. This visit is an ideal opportunity to discuss with both parents and adolescents normal adolescent development and other concerns related to adolescence.

In order to provide optimum health care, physicians should discuss issues of confidentiality with both the adolescent and her parent(s) (6). Confidentiality frequently is identified as a major obstacle to the delivery of health care services to adolescents. To overcome this barrier, physicians should initiate discussion of this topic, advise the adolescent patient and her parent(s) of relevant state and local statutes, and stress the importance of open communication between all parties. Physicians are encouraged to consult other sources for an in-depth examination of the issues surrounding confidentiality (6).

The provision of additional services beyond guidance and screening should be based on the information obtained at this initial visit. If the patient has had sexual intercourse, or if other gynecologic concerns exist, a pelvic examination, Pap test, and cervical screening for sexually transmitted diseases (STDs) are appropriate (5).

Annual Visits

Because the potential for unhealthy behaviors and poor health outcomes is significant during adolescence, the initial consultation visit should be followed by annual preventive health care visits.

Annual visits contribute to the formation of a trusting relationship between the adolescent patient and her physician. This, in turn, eases the disclosure of high-risk behaviors and facilitates the early diagnosis of physical and emotional disorders. Such visits also enhance the physician's credibility as a caring adult and, therefore, lend weight to recommendations that promote good health. Finally, annual visits enable the adolescent to assume increasingly greater responsibility for her health and well-being.

The proactive, annual preventive health care visit should focus on health guidance for both patient and parent(s), including a discussion of normal adolescent development; screening for physical, emotional, and behavioral conditions; and immunizations. Primary and preventive health care for adolescents should be based on the guidelines summarized in this bulletin. Physicians should tailor the content of their health guidance, screening, and level of parental involvement to the unique requirements of each patient. A physical examination is not required at every visit, but should be included at least once during early adolescence (12–14 years), middle adolescence (15–17 years), and late adolescence (18–21 years). A pelvic examination should be performed on all adolescents who are either sexually active or older than 18 years and when indicated by the medical history (eg, pubertal aberrancy, abnormal bleeding, or abdominal or pelvic pain). If the patient has had sexual intercourse, a Pap test and screening for STDs also are appropriate.

To help adolescents navigate the transition from childhood to adulthood, a number of organizations have formulated guidelines for adolescent preventive health care services. *Guidelines for Adolescent Preventive Services (GAPS)*, developed for the American Medical Association by a national group of experts, including representatives from ACOG, forms the basis of the following recommendations (7). These recommendations are grouped into three categories: health guidance for both parents and adolescents, screening, and immunization.

Health Guidance

Periodic health guidance for parents and adolescents is a critical component of primary and preventive health care. This is different from obtaining the past medical history because it involves the counseling and discussion component of the health care visit. Health guidance provides an opportunity for physicians, adolescent patients, and their parents to address current and potential health care needs.

For the Parents

Parents and other adult caregivers should receive health guidance at least once during their child's early adolescence, once during middle adolescence, and preferably once during late adolescence. Such guidance can be provided either concurrent to the adolescent's visit or as a separate visit. Health guidance for parents includes information about the following areas:

- Normal adolescent development, including information about physical, sexual, and emotional development
- Signs and symptoms of common diseases and morbidities in adolescents, including depression and emotional distress, to alert parents to the potential health risks facing their children
- Physical and psychosocial benefits gained from participation in sports and other supervised extracurricular activities
- Parenting behaviors that promote healthy adolescent adjustments:
  - Allowing increased autonomy and responsibility
  - Anticipating challenges to parental authority
  - Establishing jointly family rules and the consequences for breaking them, and enforcing those rules and consequences
  - Enhancing self-esteem with praise and recognition of positive behaviors and achievements
  - Minimizing criticism
  - Respecting privacy
  - Spending time with the adolescent
- Ways to minimize potentially harmful behaviors by:
  - Monitoring and managing the adolescent's use of motor vehicles

— Avoiding weapons in the home or ensuring that adolescents follow weapon safety procedures
— Removing weapons and potentially lethal medications from the home of a suicidal adolescent
— Monitoring the adolescent's social and recreational activities, including the use of tobacco, alcohol, drugs, and sexual behavior, particularly in early and middle adolescence
— Remaining involved in the adolescent's use of her free time, including television and internet usage, particularly in early and middle adolescence
— Monitoring peer relationships
— Recognizing their daughter's vulnerability in unequal relationships, such as those with older partners or when the partner is in a position of relative authority over the adolescent (8)
— Encouraging the regular use of sunscreen

Additionally, it is important for parents to recognize the influential role of the media, particularly as a source of sexual information for adolescents. At an age when many girls experience a decline in self-esteem (9), youth-oriented magazines reinforce sexual stereotypes, emphasize physical appearances, and advise girls on attracting adolescent males. In these popular publications, sexually explicit materials and abstinence-only messages are included together, and little or no information is provided to help readers make healthy, safe, and responsible decisions. Such materials further contribute to the difficult choices that increasingly younger girls are forced to consider. Recognition of these sources of information can help both parents and physicians in their efforts to ensure the health of adolescent girls.

For the Adolescent

Adolescents should receive annual health guidance to promote a better understanding of their physical, psychosocial, and psychosexual development. Such guidance should emphasize health promotion and risk reduction strategies. The importance of becoming actively involved in decisions regarding their own health care also should be emphasized.

Screening provides an excellent opportunity to counsel adolescents about healthy lifestyles. Because of concerns regarding mutual trust, issues of confidentiality, and individual comfort levels when discussing sensitive topics, eliciting an accurate response can be difficult. Often, repeated questioning over time is necessary to obtain accurate and complete information.

Health guidance for the adolescent is important. This discussion should address diet and physical activity, healthy sexual lifestyle, and injury prevention as follows:

- Dietary habits, including ways to achieve a healthy diet and safe weight management
- The benefits of physical activity and encouragement to engage regularly in safe physical activities
- Responsible, consensual sexual behavior, including counseling on:
  — Abstinence from sexual intercourse and information that this method is the most effective way to prevent pregnancy and STDs, including HIV infection
  — HIV transmission and the dangers of the disease
  — The effectiveness of latex condoms in reducing the risk of pregnancy and STDs, including HIV infection
  — Responsible sexual behavior for adolescents who are not currently sexually active and for those who are using birth control and condoms appropriately
  — Reducing the risk of sexual victimization and acquaintance rape, including the role of alcohol and other drugs (8)
  — Information on emergency contraception, including the 24-hour, national toll-free hotline number 1-888-NOT-2-LATE
- Prevention of injuries, including:
  — Avoiding the use of alcohol or other substances
  — Avoiding driving a motor vehicle or other recreational vehicle if the teen has consumed alcohol or other substances
  — Avoiding riding in a car or other recreational vehicle if the driver has consumed alcohol or other substances
  — Encouraging adolescents and their parents to develop agreements for picking-up adolescents who have consumed alcohol or other substances
  — Using safety devices, including seat belts, motorcycle and bicycle helmets, and appropriate athletic protective devices
  — Nonviolent conflict resolution
  — Avoiding the use of weapons or promoting weapon safety
  — Promoting appropriate physical conditioning before exercise

Screening

Blood Pressure

All adolescents should be screened annually for hypertension according to the protocol developed by the National Heart, Lung, and Blood Institute Task Force on High Blood Pressure in Children and Adolescents (10). Although the incidence of hypertension in adolescence is low, early detection of elevated blood pressure and evaluation for hypertension risk factors may prevent later cardiovascular diseases.

Body size is the single most important determinant of blood pressure in children and adolescents (10). By accounting for different levels of growth when evaluating blood pressure, a more precise classification can be made thus avoiding misclassification of those adolescents at the extremes for normal growth (Fig. 1). Listed in the box are steps for assessing classification of blood pressure.

The National Heart, Lung, and Blood Institute's task force has defined normal blood pressure as systolic blood pressure (SBP) and diastolic blood pressure (DBP) below the 90th percentile for age and sex. High-normal blood pressure is average SBP or DBP greater than or equal to the 90th percentile, but below the 95th percentile. Hypertension in adolescence is defined as average systolic or diastolic blood pressure greater than or equal to the 95th percentile for age and sex measured on at least three separate occasions.

Adolescents with either SBP or DBP at or above the 90th percentile for age (Fig. 2. A) should have blood pressure measurements repeated at three different times within 1 month, under similar physical conditions, to confirm baseline value. After a baseline value has been confirmed, adolescents with baseline blood pressure values greater than the 95th percentile for age (Fig. 2. B) should have a complete biomedical evaluation to establish treatment options. Adolescents with blood pressure values between the 90th and 95th percentiles should be assessed for predisposing factors such as obesity, and their blood pressure should be monitored every 6 months.

Steps for Assessing Classification of Blood Pressure

1. Use the standard height chart to determine the height percentile.
2. Measure the adolescent's blood pressure. Record SBP and DBP.
3. Find the adolescent's age on the right side of the 90th percentile chart. Follow the age line horizontally across the chart to the intersection of the line for the height percentile (vertical line).
4. Move up or down the height percentile line to the intersection of measured blood pressure.

Result on 90th Percentile Chart

- If you move down on the height percentile line, blood pressure is normal. Repeat steps 3 and 4 on the chart for 90th percentile SBP.
- If you move up on the height percentile line, you must repeat steps 3 and 4 on the chart for 95th percentile DBP.

Result on 95th Percentile Chart

- If you move down on the height percentile line, blood pressure is high-normal. Repeat steps 3 and 4 on the chart for 95th percentile SBP.
- If you move up on the height percentile line, hypertension* is indicated. Repeat steps 3 and 4 on the chart for 95th percentile SBP.

*Note that hypertension is diagnosed after three consecutive blood pressure readings above the 95th percentile on three separate occasions.

Modified from National High Blood Pressure Education Program. Update on the Task Force Report (1987) on High Blood Pressure in Children and Adolescents: a working group report from the National High Blood Pressure Education Program. National Institutes of Health, National Heart, Lung, and Blood Institute. Bethesda, MD: National High Blood Pressure Education Program, 1996; NIH publication no. 96-3790

Cholesterol

Adolescents should be screened by history using the following guidelines to determine their risk of developing hyperlipidemia and adult coronary heart disease. Selected adolescents should have lipid testing according to the protocol developed by the Expert Panel on Blood Cholesterol in Children and Adolescents (11):

- Adolescents whose parents have a serum cholesterol level greater than 240 mg/dL should be screened for total blood cholesterol (nonfasting) at least once.
- Adolescents with either an unknown family history or multiple risk factors for future cardiovascular disease (eg, smoking, hypertension, obesity, diabetes mellitus, excessive consumption of dietary saturated fats and cholesterol) may be screened for total serum cholesterol level (nonfasting) at least once at the discretion of the physician.
- Adolescents with blood cholesterol values less than 170 mg/dL should have the test repeated in 5 years. Those with values between 170 and 199 mg/dL should have a repeat test. If the average value of the two tests is below 170 mg/dL, total blood cholesterol level should be reassessed within 5 years. A lipoprotein analysis should be done if the average choles-

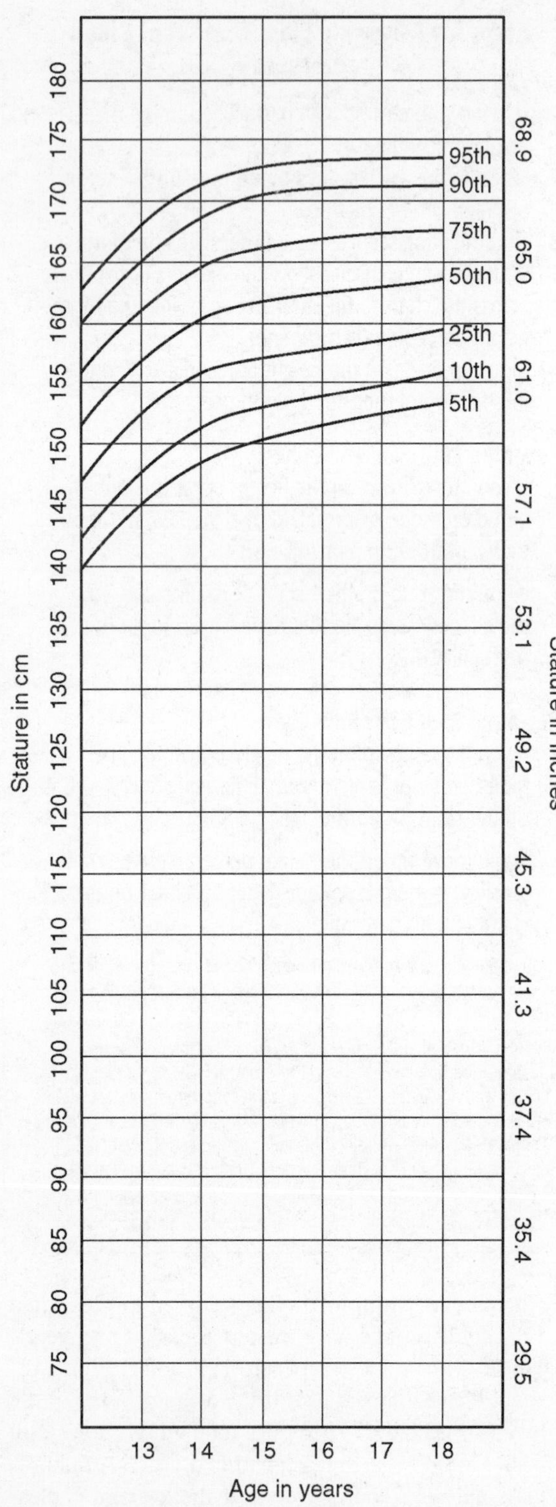

Figure 1. Girls stature by age percentiles. (Modified from National Center for Health Statistics, NCHS growth charts, 1976. Monthly vital statistics report; Vol 25, no. 3 [suppl]. Rockville, Maryland: National Center for Health Statistics, 1976)

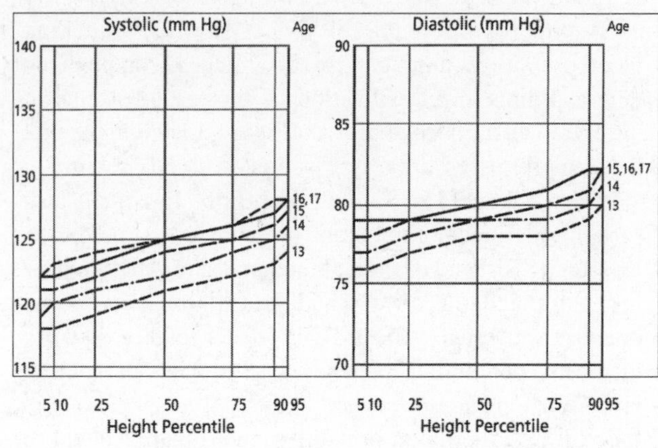

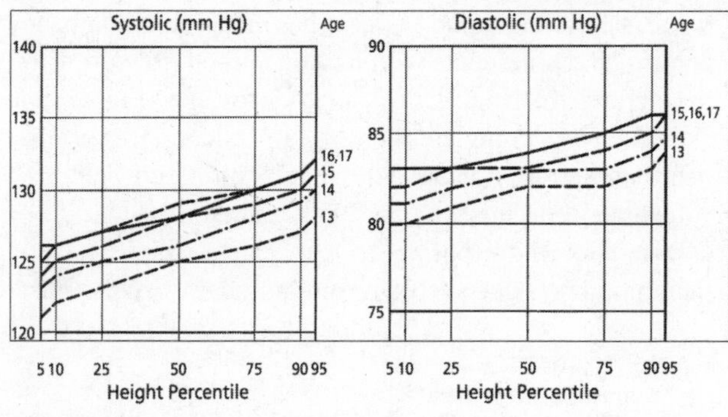

Figure 2. Systolic and diastolic blood pressure by height and age for girls in the 90th percentile **(A)** and girls in the 95th percentile **(B).** (Modified from National High Blood Pressure Education Program. Update on the Task Force Report [1987] on High Blood Pressure in Children and Adolescents: a working group report from the National High Blood Pressure Education Program. National Institutes of Health, National Heart, Lung, and Blood Institute. Bethesda, MD: National High Blood Pressure Education Program, 1996; NIH publication no. 96-3790)

terol value from the two tests is 170 mg/dL or higher, or if the result of the initial test was 200 mg/dL or greater.

- Adolescents who have a parent or grandparent with coronary artery disease, peripheral vascular disease, cerebrovascular disease, or sudden cardiac death at age 55 or younger should be screened with a fasting lipoprotein profile.
- Treatment options are based on the average of two assessents of low-density lipoprotein cholesterol. Values below 110 mg/dL are acceptable; values between 110 and 120 mg/dL are borderline, and the lipoprotein status should be re-evaluated in 1 year. Adolescents with values of 130 mg/dL or greater will need further evaluation.

Eating Disorders

All adolescents should be screened annually for eating disorders and obesity by determining weight and stature, calculating a body mass index (BMI) (Fig. 3), and asking about body image and eating patterns. For many young women, significant weight loss or preoccupation with dieting should alert the obstetrician–gynecologist to the possibility of an eating disorder. Additionally, test results of vital signs may help to confirm the suspicion of eating disorders and identify patients needing emergency hospitalization. The following general guidelines should be used:

- Adolescents should be assessed for organic disease, anorexia nervosa, or bulimia if any of the following are found:
  - Amenorrhea or abnormal menses
  - Refusal to maintain body weight at or above a normal weight for age and height (12)
  - Recurrent dieting when not overweight
  - Use of self-induced emesis, laxatives, starvation, or diuretics to lose weight
  - Distorted body image
  - BMI below the 5th percentile
  - Hypotension, bradycardia, cardiac arrhythmia, or hypothermia
- Adolescents with a BMI greater than or equal to 95th percentile for age (Fig. 4) are overweight and should have an in-depth dietary and health assessment to determine psychosocial morbidity and risk for future cardiovascular disease.
- Adolescents with a BMI between the 85th and 94th percentile for age are at risk for becoming overweight. A dietary and health assessment to determine psychosocial morbidity and risk for future cardiovascular disease should be performed on these youth if:
  - Their BMI has increased by two or more units during the previous 12 months
  - There is a family history of premature heart disease, obesity, hypertension, or diabetes mellitus
  - They express concern about their weight
  - They have elevated blood pressure or cholesterol levels in serum

Tobacco

All adolescents should be asked annually about their use of tobacco products. Approximately 1 in 4 high school seniors currently uses tobacco, and females are as likely as males to be smokers. Screening for tobacco use should include the following:

- Adolescents who smoke or use any tobacco products should be assessed further to determine their pattern of use.
- A cessation plan should be provided for adolescents who smoke or use any tobacco products. Appropriate nicotine replacement therapy should be considered when there is strong evidence of nicotine dependence and a clear desire to quit tobacco use (13).
- Because of an adolescent's preoccupation with body image, all teens should be counseled on the effects of smoking and use of other tobacco products on hair, skin, and breath.
- Counseling also should include long-term health consequences, including the possible impact on a female's reproductive potential.

Alcohol and Other Drugs

All adolescents should be asked annually about their use of alcohol and other drugs, including street drugs, over-the-counter and prescription drugs for nonmedical purposes, and inhalants. Substance abuse occurs frequently in adolescence, is a major factor in injuries and deaths among adolescents, and contributes to motor vehicle accidents, homicide, and suicide. Screening for alcohol and drug use should include the following recommendations:

- Adolescents who report any use of alcohol or other drugs, or inappropriate use of medications during the past year should be assessed further regarding family history, circumstances surrounding use, amount and frequency of use, attitudes and motivation to use, use of other drugs, and the adequacy of physical, psychosocial, and school functioning.
- Adolescents whose substance use endangers their health should receive counseling and mental health treatment.

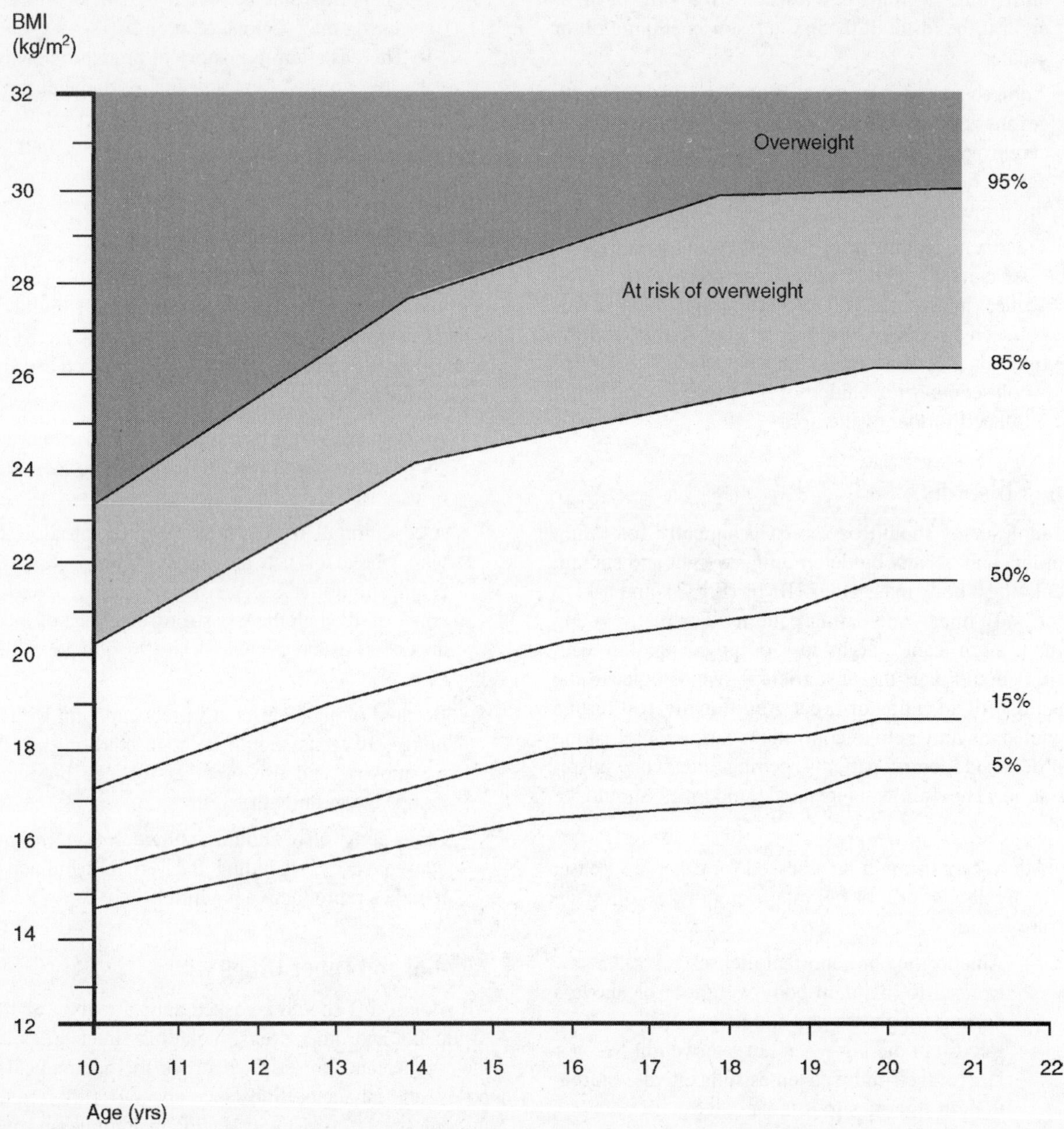

Figure 3. Height, weight, and body mass index (BMI) by age: female. (Guidelines for Adolescent Preventive Services [GAPS] Implementation Training Workbook. 2nd ed. Chicago, Illinois: American Medical Association, Copyright 1996)

	Stature m (in)																											
Weight kg (lb)	**1.24 (49)**	**1.27 (50)**	**1.30 (51)**	**1.32 (52)**	**1.35 (53)**	**1.37 (54)**	**1.40 (55)**	**1.42 (56)**	**1.45 (57)**	**1.47 (58)**	**1.50 (59)**	**1.52 (60)**	**1.55 (61)**	**1.57 (62)**	**1.60 (63)**	**1.63 (64)**	**1.65 (65)**	**1.68 (66)**	**1.70 (67)**	**1.73 (68)**	**1.75 (69)**	**1.78 (70)**	**1.80 (71)**	**1.83 (72)**	**1.85 (73)**	**1.88 (74)**	**1.90 (75)**	**1.93 (76)**
20 (45)	13	13	12	12	11	11	10	10	10	9	9	9	8															
23 (50)	15	14	13	13	12	12	12	11	11	10	10	10	9	9	9	9	8											
25 (55)	16	15	15	14	14	13	13	12	12	12	11	11	10	10	10	9	9	9										
27 (60)	18	17	16	16	15	15	14	13	13	13	12	12	11	11	11	10	10	10	9	9								
29 (65)	19	18	17	17	16	16	15	15	14	14	13	13	12	12	12	11	11	10	10	10	10							
32 (70)	21	20	19	18	17	17	16	16	15	15	14	14	13	13	12	12	12	11	11	11	10	10						
34 (75)	22	21	20	20	19	18	17	17	16	16	15	15	14	14	13	13	12	12	12	11	11	11	10					
36 (80)	24	22	21	21	20	19	19	18	17	17	16	16	15	15	14	14	13	13	13	12	12	11	11	11				
39 (85)	25	24	23	22	21	21	20	19	18	18	17	17	16	16	15	15	14	14	13	13	13	12	12	12	11			
41 (90)	27	25	24	23	22	22	21	20	19	19	18	18	17	17	16	15	15	14	14	14	13	13	13	12	12	12		
43 (95)	28	27	25	25	24	23	22	21	20	20	19	19	18	17	17	16	16	15	15	14	14	13	13	13	12	12		
45 (100)	29	28	27	26	25	24	23	22	22	21	20	20	19	18	18	17	17	16	16	15	15	14	14	14	13	13	13	12
48 (105)	31	30	28	27	26	25	24	24	23	22	21	21	20	19	19	18	17	17	16	16	16	15	15	14	14	13	13	13
50 (110)	32	31	30	29	27	27	25	25	24	23	22	22	21	20	19	19	18	18	17	17	16	16	15	15	15	14	14	13
52 (115)	34	32	31	30	29	28	27	26	25	24	23	23	22	21	20	20	19	18	18	17	17	16	16	16	15	15	14	14
54 (120)	35	34	32	31	30	29	28	27	26	25	24	24	23	22	21	20	20	19	19	18	18	17	17	16	16	15	15	15
57 (125)	37	35	34	33	31	30	29	28	27	26	25	25	24	23	22	21	21	20	20	19	19	18	17	17	17	16	16	15
59 (130)	38	37	35	34	32	31	30	29	28	27	26	26	25	24	23	22	22	21	20	20	19	19	18	18	17	17	16	16
61 (135)	40	38	36	35	34	33	31	30	29	28	27	27	25	25	24	23	22	22	21	20	20	19	19	18	18	17	17	16
64 (140)	41	39	38	36	35	34	32	31	30	29	28	27	26	26	25	24	23	22	22	21	21	20	20	19	19	18	18	17
66 (145)	43	41	39	38	36	35	34	33	31	30	29	28	27	27	26	25	24	23	23	22	21	21	20	20	19	19	18	18
68 (150)	44	42	40	39	37	36	35	34	32	31	30	29	28	28	27	26	25	24	24	23	22	21	21	20	20	19	19	18
70 (155)	46	44	42	40	39	37	36	35	33	33	31	30	29	29	27	26	26	25	24	23	23	22	22	21	21	20	19	19
73 (160)	47	45	43	42	40	39	37	36	35	34	32	31	30	29	28	27	27	26	25	24	24	23	22	22	21	21	20	19
77 (170)	50	48	46	44	42	41	39	38	37	36	34	33	32	31	30	29	28	27	27	26	25	24	24	23	23	22	21	21
79 (175)		49	47	46	44	42	40	39	38	37	35	34	33	32	31	30	29	28	27	27	26	25	24	24	23	22	22	21
82 (180)		51	48	47	45	44	42	40	39	38	36	35	34	33	32	31	30	29	28	27	27	26	25	24	24	23	23	22
84 (185)			50	48	46	45	43	42	40	39	37	36	35	34	33	32	31	30	29	28	27	26	26	25	25	24	23	23
86 (190)				49	47	46	44	43	41	40	39	37	36	35	34	32	32	31	30	29	28	27	27	26	25	24	24	23
88 (195)				51	49	47	45	44	42	41	39	38	37	36	35	33	32	31	31	30	29	28	27	26	26	25	25	24
91 (200)					50	48	46	45	43	42	40	39	38	37	35	34	33	32	31	30	30	29	28	27	27	26	25	24
93 (205)						50	47	46	44	43	41	40	39	38	36	35	34	33	32	31	30	29	29	28	27	26	26	25
95 (210)							49	47	45	44	42	41	40	39	37	36	35	34	33	32	31	30	29	28	28	27	26	26
98 (215)							50	48	46	45	43	42	41	40	38	37	36	35	34	33	32	31	30	29	28	28	27	26
100 (220)								49	47	46	44	43	42	40	39	38	37	35	35	33	33	31	31	30	29	28	28	27
102 (225)								51	49	47	45	44	42	41	40	38	37	36	35	34	33	32	31	30	30	29	28	27
104 (230)									50	48	46	45	43	42	41	39	38	37	36	35	34	33	32	31	30	30	29	28
107 (235)										49	47	46	44	43	42	40	39	38	37	36	35	34	33	32	31	30	30	29
109 (240)										50	48	47	45	44	43	41	40	39	38	36	36	34	34	33	32	31	30	29
111 (245)											49	48	46	45	43	42	41	39	38	37	36	35	34	33	32	31	31	30
113 (250)											50	49	47	46	44	43	42	40	39	38	37	36	35	34	33	32	31	30
116 (255)												50	48	47	45	44	42	41	40	39	38	37	36	35	34	33	32	31
118 (260)													49	48	46	44	43	42	41	39	39	37	36	35	34	33	33	32
120 (265)													50	49	47	45	44	43	42	40	39	38	37	36	35	34	33	32
122 (270)														50	48	46	45	43	42	41	40	39	38	37	36	35	34	33
125 (275)															49	47	46	44	43	42	41	39	38	37	36	35	35	33
127 (280)															50	48	47	45	44	42	41	40	39	38	37	36	35	34
129 (285)															50	49	47	46	45	43	42	41	40	39	38	37	36	35
132 (290)																50	48	47	46	44	43	42	41	39	38	37	36	35
134 (295)																50	49	47	46	45	44	42	41	40	39	38	37	36
136 (300)																	50	48	47	45	44	43	42	41	40	39	38	37

Figure 4. Body mass index for selected weight and stature. (Guidelines for Adolescent Preventive Services [GAPS] Implementation Training Workbook. 2nd ed. Chicago, Illinois: American Medical Association, Copyright 1996)

- Urine screening for drug use in adolescents without prior informed consent is not recommended and is illegal in many states.

Sexual Activity

All adolescents should be asked annually about involvement in sexual behaviors that may result in unintended pregnancy and STDs, including HIV infection. High rates of sexual activity, coupled with inconsistent use of contraception, contribute to the United States having one of the highest adolescent pregnancy rates in the developed world. Currently, 1 out of every 10 adolescent females aged 15–19 years becomes pregnant annually (14).

Adolescents should be counseled that abstinence is the only health choice that assures protection from STDs and pregnancy. Sexually active patients must be educated about the safety and efficacy of current contraceptive options. The most effective protection against unintended pregnancy and STDs, other than abstinence, includes a combination of latex condoms and hormonal methods of birth control. Adolescents also should be counseled about emergency contraception pills. Although emergency contraception pills can prevent unintended pregnancies after episodes of unprotected sexual intercourse or method failure, they afford no protection against STDs. Pregnant adolescents whose pregnancies are unintended (either mistimed or unwanted) should be counseled about pregnancy options, including adoption, raising the baby, and termination. The practitioner must be knowledgeable about local support services and state laws regarding parental notification and consent for elective termination of pregnancy. If the adolescent continues with the pregnancy, the importance of prenatal care should be emphasized, and appropriate follow-up care should be arranged. For pregnant school-aged adolescents, the importance of completing high school should be stressed. Screening for sexual activity should include the following points:

- Sexually active adolescents should be asked about their sexual orientation, partner use of condoms, contraceptive methods, number of current and previous sexual partners, exchange of sex for money or drugs, and history of prior pregnancy or STDs.
- Adolescents should be questioned about the age and the relationship with their partners to screen for possible sexual abuse.
- Adolescents at risk for pregnancy, STDs (including HIV), or sexual exploitation should be counseled on how to reduce their risk.

Sexually Transmitted Diseases

Because most adolescent patients become sexually active prior to high school graduation, STDs are a major health issue for this population. Sexually transmitted diseases are the most common infectious diseases among adolescents, and as a group they are at greatest risk. Each year, nearly 4 million adolescents are infected with STDs, accounting for 25% of the 15 million new cases of sexually transmitted diseases in the United States annually (15). As such, sexually active adolescents should be screened annually for STDs, including:

- Screening for gonorrhea and chlamydia
- Serologic testing for syphilis if they have:
  - — History of prior STDs
  - — Multiple sexual partners
  - — Exchanged sex for drugs or money
  - — Used illicit drugs
  - — Been admitted to jail or other detention facility
  - — Lived in an endemic area
- Evaluation for human papillomavirus by visual inspection and Pap test

Human Immunodeficiency Virus

All adolescents should be evaluated for HIV risk status. Those found to be at risk should be offered HIV testing according to the following recommendations:

- Adolescents are at high risk if they have any of the following characteristics:
  - — Multiple sexual partners
  - — High-risk partner, eg, HIV positive, injectable drug user, bisexual, or has had more than one sexual partner
  - — Prior STDs
  - — Exchanges sex for drugs or money
  - — Long-term residence or birth in an area with high prevalence of HIV infection
  - — History of blood transfusion prior to 1985
  - — Use of intravenous drugs
- Testing of nonpregnant adolescents should be performed only after informed consent is obtained, consistent with state legal requirements.
- Testing should be performed only in conjunction with both pretest and posttest counseling.
- The frequency of screening for HIV infection should be determined by risk factors.
- Universal HIV testing, with patient notification, should be a routine component of prenatal care for

all pregnant adolescents. If the adolescent declines testing, this should be noted in the medical record (16).

Human Papillomavirus

All sexually active adolescents and all patients 18 years of age or older should be screened annually for human papillomavirus with a Pap test. Abnormal cervical cytology should be evaluated in accordance with ACOG guidelines (5, 17).

Depression

All adolescents should be asked annually about behaviors or emotions that indicate recurrent or severe depression and risk of suicide. Feelings of sadness should not be dismissed as mere moodiness in this patient population. Situational losses, relationship and school problems, parental loss, and parental conflicts may lead to depression. Recognition of depression and subsequent intervention can reduce suicidal behaviors in adolescent women. Recommendations for screening for depression are as follows:

- Screening for depression or suicidal risk should be performed on adolescents who exhibit cumulative risk as determined by declining school grades, chronic sadness, family dysfunction, problems with sexual orientation, physical or sexual abuse, alcohol or other drug use, family history of suicide, previous suicide attempt, and suicidal plans (18).
- If suicidal risk is suspected, adolescents should be evaluated immediately and, based on degree of risk, referred to a mental health professional or hospitalized.
- Nonsuicidal adolescents with symptoms of severe or recurrent depression should be assessed and, if necessary, referred to a mental health professional for treatment.

Abuse

According to the Commonwealth Fund's Commission on Women's Health, 26% of adolescent girls in grades 9–12 report experiencing physical or sexual abuse, including date-rape (9). Given this high incidence, all adolescents should be asked annually about a history of abuse, including emotional, physical, and sexual abuse.

Following are screening recommendations:

- If abuse is suspected, adolescents should be questioned regarding the circumstances surrounding the abuse; assessed for physical, emotional, and psychosocial consequences; and screened for involvement in risky health behaviors.
- Health providers should be aware of local laws requiring breach of confidentiality and reporting of abuse to appropriate state officials.
- Adolescents who report emotional or psychosocial sequelae from abuse should be referred to a mental health professional for evaluation and treatment.

School Performance

All adolescents should be assessed annually for learning or school-related problems. Adolescents with a history of truancy, repeated absences, or poor or declining performance should be assessed or referred to other professionals to screen for the presence of conditions that could interfere with school success. These include learning disabilities, attention deficit hyperactivity disorder, medical problems, abuse, family dysfunction, mental disorder, and alcohol or other drug use. This assessment and the subsequent management should be coordinated with school personnel, the primary medical care provider (if different from the obstetrician–gynecologist), and the adolescent's parents or caregivers.

Tuberculosis

Adolescents should be evaluated for tuberculosis risk status. Adolescents should receive a tuberculin skin test if they:

- Have been exposed to active tuberculosis
- Have lived in a homeless shelter, been incarcerated, or lived in another long-term care facility
- Have lived in or come from an area with high prevalence of tuberculosis, or lived with persons known or suspected to have tuberculosis
- Are currently working in a health care setting
- Are HIV positive
- Are medically underserved or low-income status
- Have a history of alcoholism
- Have medical risk factors known to increase the risk of disease if infected

The frequency of testing depends upon the individual adolescent's risk factors. Adolescents with a positive tuberculin test should be treated according the treatment guidelines put forth jointly by the Centers for Disease Control and Prevention and the American Thoracic Society (19).

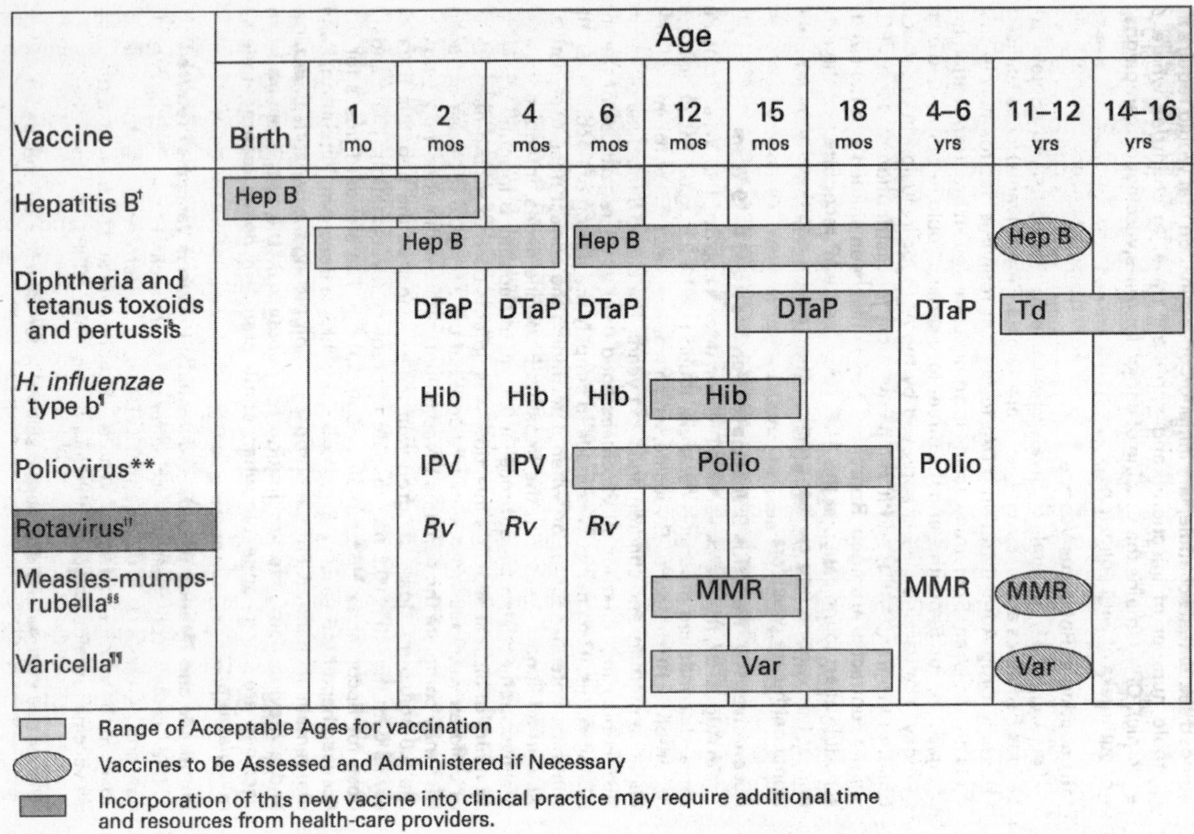

Vaccine	Age: Birth	1 mo	2 mos	4 mos	6 mos	12 mos	15 mos	18 mos	4–6 yrs	11–12 yrs	14–16 yrs
Hepatitis B†	Hep B										
		Hep B			Hep B					Hep B	
Diphtheria and tetanus toxoids and pertussis§			DTaP	DTaP	DTaP		DTaP		DTaP	Td	
H. influenzae type b¶			Hib	Hib	Hib	Hib					
Poliovirus**			IPV	IPV		Polio			Polio		
Rotavirus††			*Rv*	*Rv*	*Rv*						
Measles-mumps-rubella§§						MMR			MMR	MMR	
Varicella¶¶						Var				Var	

*This schedule indicates the recommended ages for routine administration of currently licensed childhood vaccines. Any dose not given at the recommended age should be given as a "catch-up" vaccination at any subsequent visit when indicated and feasible. Combination vaccines may be used whenever any components of the combination are indicated and its other components are not contraindicated. Providers should consult the manufacturers' package inserts for detailed recommendations.

†Infants born to hepatitis B surface antigen (HBsAg)-negative mothers should receive the second dose of hepatitis B (Hep B) vaccine at least 1 month after the first does. The third dose should be administered at least 4 months after the first dose and at least 2 months after the second dose, but not before age 6 months. Infants born to HBsAg-positive mothers should receive Hep B vaccine and 0.5 mL hepatitis B immune globulin (HBIG) within 12 hours of birth at separate injection sites. The second dose is recommended at age 1–2 months and the third dose at age 6 months. Infants born to mothers whose HBsAg status is unknown should receive Hep B vaccine within 12 hours of birth. Maternal blood should be drawn at the time of delivery to determine the mother's HBsAg status; if the HBsAg test is positive, the infant should receive HBIG as soon as possible (no later that age 1 week). All children and adolescents (through age 18 years) who have not been vaccinated against hepatitis B may begin the series during any visit. Special efforts should be made to vaccinate children who were born in or whose parents were born in areas of the world where hepatitis B virus infection is moderately or highly endemic.

§Diptheria and tetanus toxoids and acellular pertussis vaccine (DTaP) is the preferred vaccine for all doses in the vaccination series, including completion of the series in children who have received one or more doses of whole-cell diphtheria and tetanus toxoids and pertusis vaccine (DTP). Whole-cell DTP is an acceptable alternative to DTaP. The fourth dose (DTP or DTaP) may be administered as early as age 12 months, provided 6 months have elapsed since the third dose and if the child is unlikely to return at age 15–18 months. Tetanus and diphtheria toxoids (Td) is recommended at age 11–12 years if at least 5 years have elapsed since the last does of DTP, DTaP, or DT. Subsequent routine Td boosters are recommended every 10 years.

¶Three Haemophilus influenzae type b (Hib) conjugate vaccines are licensed for infant use. If Hib conjugate vaccine (PRP-OMP) is administered at ages 2 and 4 months, a dose at age 6 months is not required. Because clinical studies in infants have demonstrated that using some combination products may induce a lower immune response to the Hib vaccine component, DTaP/Hib combination products should not be used for primary vaccination in infants at ages 2, 4, or 6 months unless approved by the Food and Drug Administration for these ages.

**Two poliovirus vaccines are licensed in the United States: inactivated poliovirus vaccine (IPV) and oral poliovirus vaccine (OPV). The ACIP, AAFP, and IPV administered at ages 2 and 4 months followed by two doses of OPV at age 12–18 months and age 4–6 years. Use of IPV for all doses also is acceptable and is recommended for immunocompromised persons and their household contacts. OPV is no longer recommended for the first two doses of the schedule and is acceptable only for special circumstances (eg, children of parents who do not accept the recommended number of injections, late initiation of vaccination that would require an unacceptable number of injections, and imminent travel to areas where poliomyelitis is endemic. OPV remains the vaccine of choice for mass vaccination campaigns to control outbreaks of wild poliovirus.

††The first dose of Rv vaccine should not be administered before age 6 weeks, and the minimum interval between doses is 3 weeks. The Rv vaccine series should not be initiated at age 7 months, and all doses should be completed by the first birthday. The AAFP opinion is that the decision to use rotavirus (Rv) vaccine should be made by the parent or guardian in consultation with the physician or other health care provider.

§§The second dose of measles, mumps, and rubella vaccine (MMR) is recommended routinely at age 4–6 years but may be administered during any visit provided at least 4 weeks have elapsed since receipt of the first does and that both doses are administered beginning at or after age 12 months. Those who have not previously received the second dose should complete the schedule no later than the routine visit to a health care provider at age 11–12 years.

¶¶Varicella (Var) vaccine is recommended at any visit on or after the first birthday for susceptible children (ie, those who lack a reliable history of chickenpox [as judged by a health care provider] and who have not been vaccinated). Susceptible persons aged ≥13 years should receive two doses given at least 4 weeks apart.

Figure 5. Recommended childhood immunization schedule*–United States, January–December 1999. (Centers for Disease Control and Prevention. Recommended Childhood Immunization Schedule–United States, 1999. MMWR Morb Mortal Wkly Rep 1999;48:14–15)

Immunization

National immunization policies have changed in response to the development of a vaccination against Hepatitis B virus and the resurgence of measles and rubella among adolescent and adult populations. All adolescents should receive prophylactic immunizations according to the guidelines established by the federally convened Advisory Committee on Immunization Practices (20) (Fig. 5). Physicians should determine the number and type of previous vaccinations to assess the immunization needs of the adolescent.

Ideally, all vaccinations should be administered at the scheduled 11–12-year visit. In many instances, however, it will be necessary for physicians to administer vaccines to those who have fallen behind the recommended schedule, or who were older than 11–12 years when the recommendations were formulated. Prior to administering immunizations, physicians should ensure that, if required, the necessary parental consent has been obtained. Following are recommendations for determining what immunizations are needed:

- Adolescents should receive a bivalent tetanus–diptheria vaccine booster at the 11–12-year visit if not previously vaccinated within 5 years. With the exception of the tetanus–diptheria booster at 11–12 years, routine boosters should be administered every 10 years.
- Adolescents should receive a second dose of measles, mumps, and rubella vaccine at age 11–12 years, unless there is documentation of two vaccinations earlier during childhood. Measles, mumps, and rubella vaccine should not be administered to pregnant adolescents.
- Hepatitis B immunization is administered in three parts and generally is provided to infants. Older children should be assessed and if unvaccinated, should receive immunization at 11–12 years of age. The immunization status of older adolescents should also be assessed and the vaccine administered, if necessary (21).
- Hepatitis A vaccination should be given to adolescents who are traveling to or living in countries with high or intermediate endemicity of hepatitis A virus, live in communities with high endemic rates of hepatitis A virus, have chronic liver disease, or are injecting drug users.
- Varicella should be administered at the 11–12 year-visit to all unvaccinated persons or those lacking a reliable history of chickenpox. Susceptible persons 13 years of age or older should receive two doses, at least 1 month apart.

Summary

Although most adolescents enjoy good health, many of their behaviors put them at risk for negative health outcomes. Consequently, a fundamental change in the provision of health care services is required. Increasingly, services must be directed at primary and secondary prevention. As such, physicians should respond by making preventive services a greater component of their clinical practice. The approach outlined previously can help in this transition and can ensure that adolescents receive the services their health status demands.

References

1. Centers for Disease Control and Prevention. CDC Surveillance Summaries, 1998. MMWR Morb Mortal Wkly Rep 1998;47(No. SS-3)
2. National Center for Health Statistics. Deaths: Final data for 1997. National vital statistics report; vol 47, no. 19. Hyattsville, Maryland: National Center for Health Statistics, 1999
3. Herman-Giddens ME, Slora EJ, Wasserman RC, Bourdony CJ, Bhapkar MV, Koch GG. Secondary sexual characteristics and menses in young girls seen in office practice: a study from the Pediatric Research in Office Settings Network. Pediatrics 1997;99:505–512
4. Carnegie Council on Adolescent Development. Great transitions: preparing adolescents for a new century. Abridged version. New York: Carnegie Corporation of New York, 1996
5. American College of Obstetricians and Gynecologists. Guidelines for women's health care. Washington, DC: ACOG, 1996
6. American College of Obstetricians and Gynecologists. Confidentiality in adolescent health care. ACOG Educational Bulletin 249. Washington, DC: ACOG, 1998
7. American Medical Association. AMA Guidelines for adolescent preventative services (GAPS) recommendations and rationale. Baltimore: Williams & Wilkins, 1994
8. American College of Obstetricians and Gynecologists. Adolescent victims of sexual assault. ACOG Educational Bulletin 252. Washington, DC: ACOG, 1998
9. The Commission on Women's Health. The Commonwealth Fund survey of the health of adolescent girls. New York: The Commonwealth Fund, 1997
10. National High Blood Pressure Education Program. Update on the task force report (1987) on high blood pressure in children and adolescents: a working group report from the National High Blood Pressure Education Program. National Institutes of Health, National Heart, Lung, and Blood Institute. Bethesda, MD: National High Blood Pressure Education Program, 1996; NIH publication no. 96-3790
11. National Cholesterol Education Program. Report of the Expert Panel on Blood Cholesterol in Children and Adolescents. National Institutes of Health, National Heart,

Lung, and Blood Institute. Bethesda, MD: National Cholesterol Education Program, 1991; NIH publication no. 91-2732

12. American Psychiatric Association. Diagnostic and statistical manual of mental disorders. 4th ed. Washington, DC: American Psychiatric Association, 1994
13. Fiore MC, Bailey WC, Cohen SJ, Dorfman SF, Goldstein MG, Gritz ER, et al. Smoking cessation. Clinical Practice Guideline No 18. Rockville, MD: U.S. Department of Health and Human Services, Public Health Service, 1996; AHCPR publication no. 96-0692
14. Ventura SJ, Mathews TJ, Curtin SC. Declines in teenage birth rates, 1991–97: national and state patterns. National Vital Statistics Report; vol 47, no. 12. Hyattsville, Maryland: National Center for Health Statistics, 1998
15. Cates W Jr. Estimates of the incidence and prevalence of sexually transmitted diseases in the United States. American Social Health Association Panel. Sex Transm Dis 1999;26(suppl 4):S2–7
16. American Academy of Pediatrics, American College of Obstetricians and Gynecologists. Joint statement on human immunodeficiency virus screening. Elk Grove Village, Illinois: AAP; Washington, DC: ACOG, 1999
17. American College of Obstetricians and Gynecologists. Cervical cytology: evaluation and management of abnormalities. ACOG Educational Bulletin 183. Washington, DC: ACOG, 1993
18. American College of Obstetricians and Gynecologists. Prevention of adolescent suicide. ACOG Committee Opinion 190. Washington, DC: ACOG, 1997
19. Bass JB Jr, Farer LS, Hopewell PC, O'Brien R, Jacobs RF, Ruben F, et al. Treatment of tuberculosis and tuberculosis infection in adults and children. American Thoracic Society and the Centers for Disease Control and Prevention. Am J Respir Crit Care Med 1994;149:1359–1374
20. Centers for Disease Control and Prevention. Recommended childhood immunization schedule—United States, 1999. MMWR Morb Mortal Wkly Rep 1999; 48:12–16
21. American College of Obstetricians and Gynecologists. Hepatitis B immunization for adolescents. ACOG Committee Opinion 184. Washington, DC: ACOG, 1997

ISSN 1074-8628

The American College of Obstetricians and Gynecologists
409 12th Street, SW
PO Box 96920
Washington, DC 20090-6920

12345/32109

ACOG EDUCATIONAL BULLETIN

Number 255, November 1999

Psychosocial Risk Factors: Perinatal Screening and Intervention

The American College of Obstetricians and Gynecologists has long been concerned about the psychosocial issues faced by women and their families during the childbearing years that affect their mental and physical well being. Many of these issues are more prevalent in the adolescent population. Screening for psychosocial risk factors may help predict a woman's attentiveness to personal health matters, her use of prenatal services, and the health status of her offspring (1).

Many physicians who care for women have had little training in managing the psychosocial issues that women encounter (2). An emerging body of evidence indicates that patients place high value on attention to these issues and report greater satisfaction with physician visits when there is more "psychosocial talk" and less "biomedical talk" (3). Health care providers, therefore, need to be encouraged to screen for psychosocial risk factors and to provide or refer patients for essential services to manage psychosocial problems. This can be accomplished through training to increase provider awareness of and interest in these issues as well as ways to respond to them. Adequate reimbursement by third-party payers for the necessary services also is essential.

Background

Although it is acknowledged that addressing psychosocial issues during pregnancy is important and has the potential to reduce costs to the individual and society (4), there are no screening tools widely available that have been shown to have high degrees of sensitivity and specificity. The Healthy Start Program of the Florida Department of Health, however, has designed one particularly well-regarded screening system, which has been used and refined by this program since 1992. Other tools exist, but none have been identified that have been evaluated as extensively as the Healthy Start tool. In addition, the Healthy Start tool provides a more concise and simple

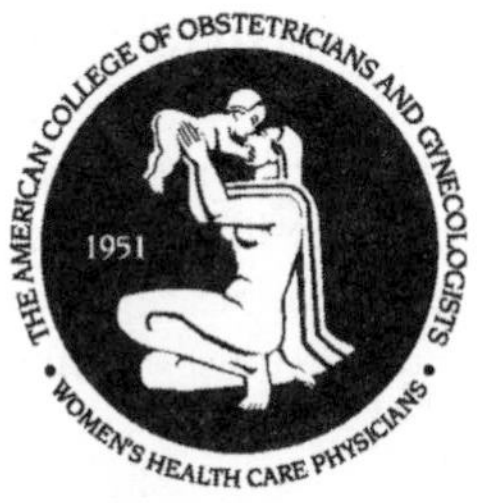

Psychosocial Screening Tool

1. Do you have any problems that prevent you from keeping your health care appointments?
2. How many times have you moved in the past 12 months? 0 1 2 3 >3
3. Do you feel unsafe where you live?
4. Do you or any members of your household go to bed hungry?
5. In the past 2 months, have you used any form of tobacco?
6. In the past 2 months, have you used drugs or alcohol (including beer, wine, or mixed drinks)?
7. In the past year, has anyone hit you or tried to hurt you?
8. How do you rate your current stress level—low or high?
9. If you could change the timing of this pregnancy, would you want it earlier, later, not at all, or no change?

Modified and reprinted with permission from Florida's Healthy Start Prenatal Risk Screening Instrument. Florida Department of Health. DH 3134. September 1997

means of collecting psychosocial data that can be used for self-reporting or interview style information retrieval (see the box for a modified version of this screening tool). Each topic identified in this tool will be discussed in this Educational Bulletin. Many of the topics are discussed more fully in various ACOG documents (see ACOG Resources).

Even though at first glance some of the questions appear to be relevant only for low-income populations, psychosocial screening of all patients presenting for pregnancy evaluation or prenatal care is an important step toward improving women's health and birth outcomes. When screening is done, every effort should be made to provide the brief interventions that are described in the following discussion. Through a brief intervention, the provider can identify areas of concern, validate major issues with the patient, provide information and, if indicated, make suggestions for possible changes. If necessary, the provider can refer the patient for further evaluation or intervention. For screening to be effective, a well-developed process for referrals is necessary. If assistance is needed with locating appropriate referral sites, local or state health officials can be contacted.

Given the sensitive nature of psychosocial assessment, every effort should be made to screen in private, especially when inquiring about domestic or intimate partner violence. Even then, patients may not be comfortable discussing problems with physicians until a trusting relationship has been formed. Because problems may arise during the pregnancy that were not present at the initial visit, it is best to perform psychosocial screening once each trimester to increase the likelihood of identifying important issues and reducing poor birth outcomes. A recent study indicates that women who were screened for psychosocial issues once each trimester were half as likely as women who were not screened to have a low-birth-weight or preterm baby (5). Documentation should include the nature of any problems identified, the chosen intervention(s), and plans for follow-up. A suggested format for this documentation, suitable for copying and inserting into the patient's chart, can be found at the end of this document.

Psychosocial risk factors also should be considered in discharge planning after delivery. Many of the psychosocial issues that increase the risk for poor pregnancy outcome also can affect the health and welfare of the newborn. It is essential that women with significant psychosocial problems stay in the hospital after delivery as long as necessary to assess adequately the health of the mother and the newborn; education of the woman about postpartum and infant care also occurs during this time. In the absence of complications, a 48-hour hospital stay after a normal vaginal delivery and a 96-hour stay after a cesarean delivery is recommended (6).

Barriers to Care

Inadequate insurance coverage, inability to pay for health care services, and not knowing where to go to receive care are a few of the most common barriers to health care. Others include lack of transportation and day care and language difficulties (7). These barriers are especially problematic for adolescents. For individuals faced with these barriers, referral to an appropriate social service agency may be useful. These agencies can sometimes help women navigate the health care system. In particular, they can help her enroll in Medicaid, which covers the costs of medical care and transportation to and from medical and social service appointments and also subsidizes or provides free day care. Through flexible scheduling of appointments, inquiring about difficulties a patient may have with keeping appointments, and assisting with solutions, the provider increases the likelihood of compliance with prenatal care recommendations. Following are brief interventions for several of the most common barriers to care.

Transportation

Transportation difficulties are commonly cited as a barrier to prenatal visits (8), particularly for women residing in rural areas (9). Many women lack transportation to and from health care appointments and rely on either public transportation or the willingness of friends and family to transport them. If a patient is not certain how she will get to appointments, the health care provider should discuss options available to her.

Day Care

For a patient who already has children, finding and paying for appropriate child care while attending appointments can be another barrier to care (10). Caring for elderly or disabled family members may pose a similar challenge. For patients who cannot arrange day care, establishing an office setting that can accommodate children and relatives is helpful.

Interference by Others

Sometimes a patient's spouse, partner, or parent may not want her to keep medical appointments. Although patients often are not directly forthcoming with this information, providers can obtain important details about the patient by asking about interference from family members, domestic or family violence, and safety issues when patients miss appointments. Flexible scheduling, assistance with transportation, or social service assistance may improve compliance with ongoing perinatal care.

Language

Because barriers to care are magnified when the patient does not speak English, it is important to use translators when possible. If this is not possible, providers can ask the patient to identify a family member or friend who can act as a translator. This may be a less desirable choice, however, because information may be intentionally or unintentionally translated incorrectly. For example, in cases of domestic violence, if the abusive spouse is translating, he might omit a question about safety in the home, misrepresent the patient's response, or retaliate. Another partial solution is to provide written materials in appropriate languages for patients who do not speak English. If communication is not adequate, it must be decided whether the patient should remain in the practice or be referred to a facility with better access to translators.

Frequent Moves

Frequent moves can indicate a variety of problems. For example, the patient may be having difficulty finding acceptable housing that is affordable. If this is the case, the patient can be referred to the appropriate social service agency for assistance. These local agencies also can provide information about other resources in the area, including health services, social support groups, and child care resources. Inquiring about the patient's feelings of isolation also is important. If this is a problem, referral to any available neighborhood support groups or a counselor can be helpful. In addition, frequent moves may reflect violence in the home or may indicate problems with the law that can cause stress.

Safety

Safety concerns can pertain to either safety in the house or safety in the neighborhood. In either case, if there is immediate danger to the patient, alternative housing should be discussed. If there are children who are not safe in the household, a referral to the state's child protection agency may be required. The state agency can be contacted for specific reporting requirements. If the safety concern relates specifically to the house, such as structural defects, rat or insect infestation, or sanitation issues, further inquiry can determine the necessary referral or intervention.

If the danger is a result of intimate partner violence, referrals, including one to a battered women's shelter, should be made. If there are no shelters or safe houses available, hospital beds may be provided on an emergency basis in some cases. It is important to assess the potential for life-threatening situations and develop safety plans with the patient, understanding that the likelihood of serious injury often is highest when the woman attempts to leave her abuser. Physicians need to be aware that the patient is the best judge of her own safety. She, therefore, may choose to return home despite receiving advice to the contrary, and the physician must honor her decision.

Nutrition

Nutritional problems can be found in women of every socioeconomic status and range from an inability to acquire and prepare food to eating disorders. If the woman cannot afford a sufficient supply of food, she should be referred to food pantries and soup kitchens in her area. All low-income women should receive information about the Special Supplemental Food Program for Women, Infants and Children (WIC) and food stamp programs. Referrals to the appropriate social service agency to apply for these or other available benefits can be helpful.

Women of low socioeconomic status often live in environments that do not allow for the storage, refrigeration, or preparation of food. Many nutritionists are trained in alternative methods of food storage and preparation and would, therefore, be able to assist the patient upon referral. The nutritionist also could assess the patient's diet and suggest healthy foods that are inexpensive.

Additional questions should be asked, especially of adolescents and young women, about eating habits such as fasting or meal skipping, which are indicative of anorexia and bulimia. If it is determined that the patient has an eating disorder, referral to a psychiatrist who specializes in this issue and a nutritionist for counseling about food management is essential. All WIC programs have nutritionists who are required to counsel patients on these matters. Hospitalization also may be required for patients with eating disorders. Poor weight gain also may reflect substance abuse, domestic violence, or depression.

Tobacco Use

Smoking tobacco is associated with increased perinatal mortality; bleeding complications of pregnancy; and a higher incidence of small-for-gestational age babies, low-birth-weight babies, and preterm delivery (11). It is estimated that a 10% reduction in fetal and infant deaths would be achieved if all pregnant women stopped smoking (12). There also is increasing evidence that Attention Deficit Hyperactivity Disorder (ADHD) and other behavioral or learning problems that affect school-aged children may be linked to maternal smoking during pregnancy (13). Therefore, it is essential that patients be screened for tobacco use and provided information on smoking cessation and why it is necessary to stop smoking during pregnancy. Interventions by clinicians that are as brief as 5–15 minutes have been shown to be effective at increasing smoking cessation rates (14).

Substance Use

Women who use substances have increased risks of preterm delivery, fetal growth restriction, fetal alcohol syndrome, fetal death, and possible long-term neurobehavioral effects (15). They also are at increased risk for sexually transmitted diseases, including human immunodeficiency virus (HIV). Women who use substances often obtain prenatal care late in the pregnancy, achieve poor weight gain, and frequently miss appointments, all of which can have negative effects on the health of the woman and the fetus. Substance abuse, by either the woman or her partner, also is associated with domestic violence. Asking patients about substance abuse at the time of the first prenatal visit is essential; questions about her partner's use of substances also may be helpful. If either inquiry indicates an area of concern, additional assessment is required (15).

Intimate Partner Violence

The incidence of abuse during pregnancy is high, with reports ranging from 1% to 20% of all pregnant women (16). Many studies report that violence often begins in pregnancy; if already present, it may escalate (17). Research also suggests that violence may increase during the postpartum period (18). Given these findings, it would be useful to screen every woman for intimate partner violence at least once in each trimester; whenever bruising, improbable injury, or depressed mood is noted; and at the postpartum visit. It also is important to know the various characteristics that may serve as markers for abuse. Women who are abused are more likely to receive inadequate prenatal care. In particular, abused pregnant women seek prenatal care later in pregnancy (19), miss more appointments, and are more likely to cancel appointments on short notice than nonabused pregnant women (20).

Stress

Stress is defined as any real or perceived trauma—whether it is physical or psychologic—that results in the release of stress hormones. Folklore has always taken it for granted that stress, such as acute anxiety, sorrow, or worry disturbs the fetus and causes physical harm (21). The observation that maternal stress is measurably related to neonatal activity and irritability in both lower animals and in humans has been documented by research during the past 30 years (22). Recent studies support that women who are anxious during pregnancy tend to have smaller babies and that women with high levels of stress hormones are more likely to deliver preterm (23, 24).

Practitioners should identify patients under stress. The stress associated with pregnancy itself, concerns about labor and delivery, and projected fears about parenting can sometimes be reduced by providing counseling and information during the course of prenatal care. Other patients may require evaluation and treatment by mental health practitioners to help identify and resolve distress.

Unintended Pregnancy

Approximately 49% of all pregnancies are unintended at the time of conception (25). This percentage is considerably higher among adolescents. An unintended pregnancy generally is defined as a pregnancy that was mistimed or unwanted at the time of conception. Research has shown that having an unintended pregnancy is a predictor of insufficient prenatal care, which results in an increased risk of a poor birth outcome. Women with unintended pregnancies are more likely to smoke and drink and have a greater likelihood of delivering a low-birth-weight infant. Their infants are more likely to die within the first year of life (26). In addition, the incidence of unintended pregnancy is higher among women who have been battered (27) and battering is more common during an unplanned pregnancy (28).

Unintended pregnancies often become accepted pregnancies that produce much-loved and wanted children. However, women with pregnancies that remain unwanted should be counseled about the full range of reproductive options, which include abortion and adoption. Women must be allowed to make independent decisions about their own pregnancies. This choice remains a woman's right and must be respected.

Summary

Addressing the broad range of psychosocial issues with which pregnant women are confronted is an essential step toward improving women's health and birth outcomes. This may be difficult to do completely in a private physician's office setting, therefore, an effective system of referrals is helpful. To increase the likelihood of successful interventions, psychosocial screening should be performed on a regular basis and documented in the patient's prenatal record.

ACOG Resources

American College of Obstetricians and Gynecologists. Depression in women. ACOG Technical Bulletin 182. Washington, DC: ACOG, 1993

American College of Obstetricians and Gynecologists. Domestic violence: the role of the physician in identification, intervention, and prevention. Slide lecture kit. Washington, DC: ACOG, 1995

American College of Obstetricians and Gynecologists. Domestic violence. ACOG Educational Bulletin 209. Washington, DC: ACOG, 1995

American College of Obstetricians and Gynecologists. Mandatory reporting of domestic violence. ACOG Committee Opinion 200. Washington, DC: ACOG, 1998

American College of Obstetricians and Gynecologists. Nutrition and women. ACOG Educational Bulletin 229. Washington, DC: ACOG, 1996

American College of Obstetricians and Gynecologists. Smoking and women's health. ACOG Educational Bulletin 240. Washington, DC: ACOG, 1997

American College of Obstetricians and Gynecologists. Substance abuse. ACOG Technical Bulletin 194. Washington, DC: ACOG, 1994

American College of Obstetricians and Gynecologists. Substance abuse in pregnancy. ACOG Technical Bulletin 195. Washington, DC: ACOG, 1994

Bibliography

American Academy of Pediatrics Committee on Drugs. The transfer of drugs and other chemicals into human milk. Pediatrics 1994;93:137–150

Briggs GG, Freeman RK, Yaffe SJ. Drugs in pregnancy and lactation. 5th ed. Baltimore: Williams & Wilkins, 1998

Dolan-Mullen P, Ramirez G, Groff JY. A meta-analysis of randomized trials of prenatal smoking cessation interventions. Am J Obstet Gynecol 1994;171:1328–1334

Haller E. Eating disorders. A review and update. West J Med 1992;157:658–662

Henningfield JE. Nicotine medications for smoking cessation. N Engl J Med 1995;333:1196–1203

Hutchins E, DiPietro J. Psychosocial risk factors associated with cocaine use during pregnancy: a case-control study. Obstet Gynecol 1997;90:142–147

Laken MP, Hutchins E. Building and sustaining systems of care for substance-using pregnant women and their infants: Lessons learned. Arlington, Virginia: National Center for Education in Maternal and Child Health, 1995

MacGregor SN, Keith LG, Bachicha JA, Chasnoff IJ. Cocaine abuse during pregnancy: correlation between prenatal care and perinatal outcome. Obstet Gynecol 1989;74:882–885

Morse B, Gehshan S, Hutchins E. Screening for substance abuse during pregnancy: improving care, improving health. Arlington, Virginia: National Center for Education in Maternal and Child Health, 1997

Tofler IR, Stryer BK, Micheli LJ, Herman LR. Physical and emotional problems of elite female gymnasts. N Engl J Med 1996;335:281–283

Working Group on Nicotine Dependence. Practice guideline for the treatment of patients with nicotine dependence. American Psychiatric Association. Am J Psychiatry 1996;153:1–31

References

1. Goldenberg RL, Patterson ET, Freese MP. Maternal demographic, situational and psychosocial factors and their relationship to enrollment in prenatal care: a review of the literature. Women Health 1992;19:133–151
2. Goldberg D. A classification of psychological distress for use in primary care setting. Soc Sci Med 1992;35:189–193
3. Bertakis KD, Roter D, Putnam SM. The relationship of physician medical interview style to patient satisfaction. J Fam Pract 1991;32:175–181
4. Curry MA. Nonfinancial barriers to prenatal care. Women Health 1989;15:85–99

5. Wilkinson DS, Korenbrot CC, Greene J. A performance indicator of psychosocial services in enhanced prenatal care of Medicaid-eligible women. Matern Child Health J 1998;2:131–143
6. American Academy of Pediatrics, American College of Obstetricians and Gynecologists. Guidelines for perinatal care. 4th ed. Elk Grove Village, Illinois: AAP; Washington, DC: ACOG, 1997
7. Brown SS. Drawing women into prenatal care. Fam Plann Perspect 1989;21:73–80
8. Aved BM, Irwin MM, Cummings LS, Findeisen N. Barriers to prenatal care for low-income women. West J Med 1993;158:493–498
9. McDonald TP, Coburn AF. Predictors of prenatal care utilization. Soc Sci Med 1988;27:167–172
10. Kugler JP, Yeash J, Rumbaugh PC. The impact of sociodemographic, health care system, and family function variables on prenatal care utilization in a military setting. J Fam Pract 1993;37:143–147
11. American College of Obstetricians and Gynecologists. Smoking and women's health. ACOG Educational Bulletin 240. Washington, DC: ACOG, 1997
12. Kleinman JC, Pierre MB Jr, Madans JH, Land GH, Schramm WF. The effects of maternal smoking on fetal and infant mortality. Am J Epidemiol 1988;127:274–282
13. Milberger S, Biederman J, Faraone SV, Chen L, Jones J. Is maternal smoking during pregnancy a risk factor for attention deficit hyperactivity disorder in children? Am J Psychiatry 1996;153:1138–1142
14. Dolan Mullen P, Melvin CL, Windsor RA. A Review of the Evidence to Recommend Cessation Counseling for Pregnant Women Who Smoke. Smoke-Free Families Program, Department of Obstetrics and Gynecology, School of Medicine, University of Alabama at Birmingham, Birmingham, Alabama, 1999
15. American College of Obstetricians and Gynecologists. Substance abuse in pregnancy. ACOG Technical Bulletin 195. Washington, DC: ACOG, 1994
16. Gazmararian JA, Lazorick S, Spitz AM, Ballard TJ, Saltzman LE, Marks JS. Prevalence of violence against pregnant women. JAMA 1996:1915–1920
17. Hillard PJ. Physical abuse in pregnancy. Obstet Gynecol 1985;66:185–190
18. Stewart DE. Incidence of postpartum abuse in women with a history of abuse during pregnancy. CMAJ 1994;151: 1601–1604
19. McFarlane J, Parker B, Soeken K, Bullock L. Assessing for abuse during pregnancy. Severity and frequency of injuries and associated entry into prenatal care. JAMA 1992; 267:3176–3178
20. American Medical Association. Diagnostic and treatment guidelines on domestic violence. Chicago: AMA, 1994
21. Benedek T. The psychobiology of pregnancy. In: Anthony EJ, Benedek T, eds. Parenthood: Its psychology and psychopathology. London: J & A Churchill Ltd., 1970: 137–151
22. Herrenkohl LR. The impact of prenatal stress on the developing fetus and child. In: Cohen RL, ed. Psychiatric consultation in childbirth settings. New York: Plenum, 1988:21–35
23. Teixeira JM, Fisk NM, Glover V. Association between maternal anxiety in pregnancy and increased uterine artery resistance index: cohort based study. BMJ 1999;318: 153–157
24. Wadhwa PD, Porto M, Garite TJ, Chicz-DeMet A, Sandman CA. Maternal corticotropin-releasing hormone levels in the early trimester predict length of gestation in human pregnancy. Am J Obstet Gynecol 1998;179: 1079– 1085
25. National Center for Health Statistics. Healthy People 2000 review, 1998-99. Hyattsville, Maryland: Public Health Service, 1999
26. The best intentions: unintended pregnancy and the well-being of children and families. Committee on Unintended Pregnancy, Institute of Medicine, National Academy of Sciences. Washington, DC: National Academy Press, 1995
27. Stewart DE, Cecutti A. Physical abuse in pregnancy. CMAJ 1993;149:1257–1263
28. Fergusson DM, Horwood LJ, Kershaw KL, Shannon FT. Factors associated with reports of wife assault in New Zealand. J Marriage Fam 1986;48:407–412

ISSN 1074-8628

The American College of Obstetricians and Gynecologists
409 12th Street, SW
PO Box 96920
Washington, DC 20090-6920

12345/32109

Psychosocial Risk Assessment

YES	NO	
☐	☐	1. Do you have any problems that prevent you from keeping your health care appointments?
0 1 2 3	>3	2. How many times have you moved in the past 12 months?
☐	☐	3. Do you feel unsafe where you live?
☐	☐	4. Do you or any members of your household go to bed hungry?
☐	☐	5. In the past 2 months, have you used any form of tobacco?
☐	☐	6. In the past 2 months, have you used drugs or alcohol (including beer, wine, and mixed drinks)?
☐	☐	7. In the past year, has anyone hit you or tried to hurt you?
low	high	8. How do you rate your current stress level–low or high?
a b c	d	9. If you could change the timing of this pregnancy, would you want it (a) earlier, (b) later, (c) not at all, (d) no change?

Patient Name: ____________________

Patient No.: ____________________

Date	Area of Concern	Intervention	Recommendation/Referral	Follow-up	Initials

Modified and reprinted with permission from Florida's Healthy Start Prenatal Risk Screening Instrument. Florida Department of Health. DH 3134. October 1996

Number 224—June 1996

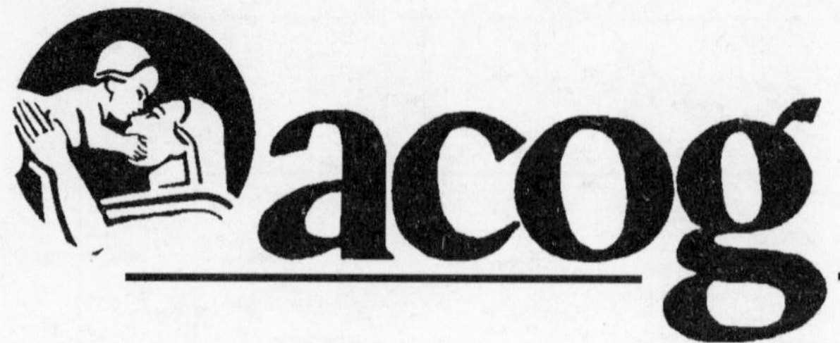

Technical Bulletin

An Educational Aid to Obstetrician–Gynecologists

Pulmonary Disease in Pregnancy

Pulmonary diseases have become more prevalent in general and in pregnancy. The incidence of asthma has increased by over 30%, and mortality from asthma increased by 46% during the 1980s (1). The rising incidence of tuberculosis has caused the Centers for Disease Control and Prevention to draft new guidelines to prevent transmission of the disease. Drug-resistant strains of *Mycobacterium tuberculosis* have also dramatically increased in some areas of the country. Women with cystic fibrosis who become pregnant, face a "new" complication of pregnancy. Additionally, bronchitis and pneumonia still occur during pregnancy, and bacterial resistance may become a problem with these conditions.

This bulletin will address changes that occur in respiratory physiology during pregnancy. In addition, it will review the diagnosis and management of asthma, bronchitis, pneumonia, tuberculosis, and cystic fibrosis in pregnant women.

Physiologic Changes in Pregnancy

When a woman is pregnant, anatomic changes occur in her chest. Her lower ribs flare out, and the subcostal angle increases as the transverse diameter of her chest increases by about 2 cm. Her diaphragm also rises by about 4 cm, although its excursions are not hampered by her enlarged uterus. Despite anatomic changes, a pregnant woman's ability to move air in and out of the lungs is not impeded.

Progesterone derived from the placenta appears to stimulate the respiratory centers in the brain to produce hyperventilation and a sensation of dyspnea. Hyperventilation decreases the alveolar CO_2 tension and the arterial P_{CO_2}, producing respiratory alkalosis. This hypocarbia results in a decreased plasma bicarbonate level, resulting in minimal change in pH. Normal pregnancy is thus a state of compensated respiratory alkalosis. Normal blood gas measurements during pregnancy are shown in Table 1.

TABLE 1. BLOOD GAS VALUES IN PREGNANT AND NON-PREGNANT WOMEN

Status	pH	P_{O_2} (mm Hg)	P_{CO_2} mm Hg)
Nonpregnant	7.4	93	35–40
Pregnant	7.4	100–105	30

Tests of pulmonary function that are important during pregnancy include the forced vital capacity (FVC), the forced expiratory volume in 1 second (FEV_1), and the peak expiratory flow rate (PEFR). By comparing the FEV_1 to the FVC, one can determine the degree of obstruction to airflow present in the lungs. This is often used clinically to monitor efficacy of treatment. Normal pulmonary function test values are shown in Table 2. Spirometry is necessary to assess the FVC and FEV_1. Assessing the PEFR, however, requires only an inexpensive, portable flow meter. The PEFR is effort dependent, and the patient must be cooperative and able to exhale as vigorously as possible each time the PEFR is measured. Measurement of PEFR is clinically useful in various settings as well as in the patient's home to measure airflow obstruction and response to therapy (2). Figure 1 shows the pulmonary changes in pregnancy.

Asthma

Asthma is a chronic disease with acute exacerbations; it is characterized by recurrent bouts of wheezing and dyspnea resulting from airway obstruction. Airway obstruction is more marked in expiration than in inspiration, resulting in a prolonged expiratory phase. The airways of a person with asthma are hyperresponsive to stimuli such as allergens, viral infections, air pollutants, exercise, and cold air. The hyperactivity is manifested by bronchospasm, mucosal edema, and mucus plugging that results in air trapping and hyperinflation of the lungs. Inflammatory changes are present in the submucosa of

TABLE 2. NORMAL PULMONARY VALUES IN PREGNANT AND NONPREGNANT WOMEN

Term	Definition	Values: Nonpregnant	Values: Pregnant	Clinical significance in pregnancy
Tidal volume (V_T)	The amount of air moved in one normal respiratory cycle	450 ml	600 ml (increases up to 40%)	
Respiratory rate (RR)	Number of respirations per minute	16/min	Changes very little	
Minute ventilation	The volume of air moved per minute; product of RR and V_T	7.2 L	9.6 L (increases up to 40% because of the increase in V_T)	Increases oxygen available for the fetus
Forced expiratory volume in one second (FEV_1)		Approximately 80–85% of the vital capacity	Unchanged	Valuable to measure because there is no change due to pregnancy
Peak expiratory flow rate (PEFR)			Unchanged	Valuable to measure because there is no change due to pregnancy
Forced vital capacity (FVC)	The maximum amount of air that can be moved from maximum inspiration to maximum expiration	3.5 L	Unchanged	If over 1 L, pregnancy is usually well tolerated.
Residual volume (RV)	The amount of air that remains in the lung at the end of a maximal expiration	1,000 ml	Decreases by around 200 ml to around 800 ml	Improves gas transfer from alveoli to blood

airways in all cases of asthma, and this fact has led to new thinking about the optimal treatment of asthma (3). Measurement of the FEV_1 or PEFR can quantify objectively the degree of obstruction present and is often used to monitor treatment. Hypoxia occurs during acute exacerbation, and with severe attacks, there is alveolar hypoventilation with retention of CO_2 and respiratory insufficiency.

Acute Exacerbations

Typically, pregnant women with asthma have had previous episodes and know when they are experiencing an exacerbation. Occasionally, the first asthmatic attack may occur during pregnancy, and this situation can present more of a diagnostic challenge. The differential diagnosis of asthma includes conditions such as pulmonary edema, pulmonary embolism, bronchitis, pneumonia, mechanical obstruction of the upper airway, and cystic fibrosis.

For patients having an acute attack, historical data should be obtained, including history of similar attacks and their management. The onset and duration of the current attack as well as events leading up to the episode should be recorded. Current medications and the presence of fever or productive cough should be noted. The patient should be questioned about other pulmonary or cardiac diseases.

On physical examination the general appearance of the patient should be noted: Is she cyanotic? Can she speak in complete sentences without pausing for air? Can she walk across the room? Does she use accessory respiratory muscles? The respiratory rate and temperature should be recorded.

Laboratory evaluation includes FEV_1 or PEFR for all patients and should be repeated after each bronchodilator treatment. Arterial blood gas determinations should be performed in all but the mildest cases. If there is a productive cough or fever or if neutrophils are noted in the sputum, a chest X-ray should be obtained to look for bronchopneumonia.

During an asthma attack, the severity is best judged by clinical appearance, as reflected by FEV_1 or PEFR. Oxygenation should be monitored to ensure sufficiency for mother and fetus. Initially, the Pco_2 decreases, but as the patient hyperventilates, the Po_2 increases. A rising Pco_2 (> 35 mm Hg) in the presence of hypoxia suggests imminent respiratory collapse and the need for intubation. Pulse oximetry provides no information on the patient's

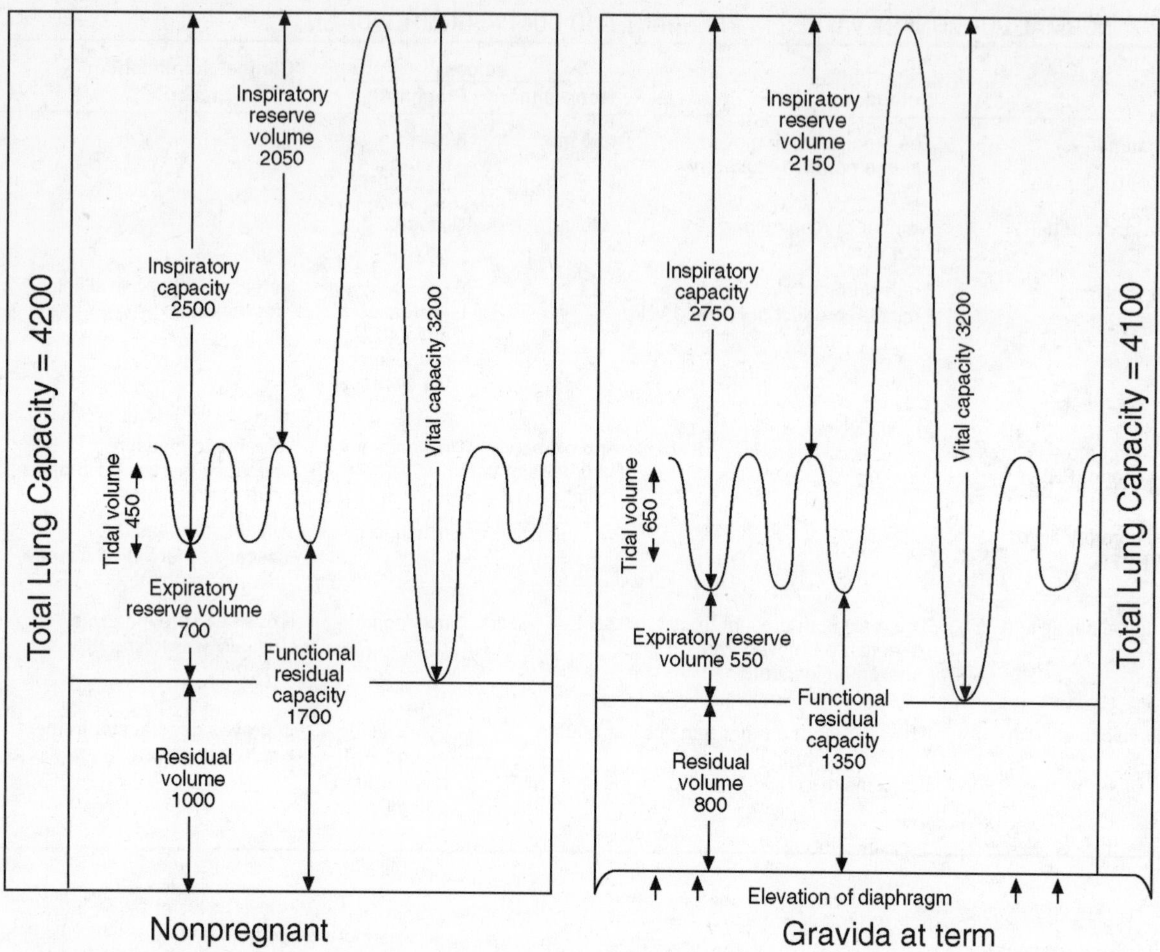

FIG. 1. Respiratory changes during pregnancy. All values shown are in milliliters. (Bonica JJ. Maternal anatomic and physiologic alterations during pregnancy and parturition. In: Bonica JJ, McDonald JS. Principles and practice of obstetric analgesia and anesthesia. Baltimore: Williams & Wilkins, 1995:49; copyright Lea & Febiger.)

ability to clear carbon dioxide, and its use is not a substitute for arterial blood gas evaluation.

Medication dosages for treatment of acute exacerbations of asthma in pregnancy are listed in Table 3. Inhaled beta$_2$-agonists have become the primary agents to treat acute exacerbations of asthma. Bronchodilation begins within 5 minutes of therapy. Treatments can be repeated every 20–30 minutes unless there are adverse side effects. Inhalation of epinephrine or isoproterenol should be avoided because of the higher incidence of cardiovascular side effects due to beta$_1$ stimulation. Subcutaneous terbutaline can be used in place of the inhaled agents at a dosage of 0.25 mg every 20–30 minutes for three doses, but current practice favors inhalation therapy. Oxygen should be given to all pregnant women with acute asthma to maintain the Po_2 over 70 mm Hg or O_2 saturation over 95%.

For women who respond rapidly (an FEV_1 or PEFR greater than 70% of predicted value) to bronchodilator therapy, follow-up may be continued on an outpatient basis. Patients with an incomplete response to beta$_2$-agonist bronchodilator therapy may be treated for up to 4 hours to determine whether admission to the hospital is warranted. Most patients with an FEV_1 or PEFR of less than 40% after 1 hour of bronchodilator therapy or less than 70% after 4 hours require hospitalization.

The use of methylxanthines such as theophylline or aminophylline is discouraged in acute cases. They have not been shown to be more effective than beta$_2$-agonists, and they require close monitoring to achieve therapeutic, nontoxic levels.

Corticosteroids should be given intravenously if the exacerbation is severe, if the exacerbation occurs while the patient is taking oral steroids, or if the response to bronchodilator therapy is incomplete or poor after 1 hour of bronchodilator treatment. An incomplete response would be an FEV_1 or PEFR of 40–70% of the predicted value; a poor response would be an FEV_1 or PEFR less than 40% of predicted value.

TABLE 3. DOSAGES OF MEDICATIONS FOR ASTHMA DURING PREGNANCY*

Drug Class	Medication	Dosage
	Acute Exacerbation	
Beta-Agonists Inhaled	Albuterol	2.5 mg (0.5 ml of a 0.5% solution, diluted with 2–3 ml of normal saline)
	or	
	Metaproterenol	15 mg (0.3 ml of a 5% solution, diluted with 2–3 ml of normal saline)
Subcutaneous	Terbutaline	0.25 mg
Corticosteroids Intravenous	Methylprednisolone	60–80 mg IV bolus every 6–8 hours
	or	
	Hydrocortisone	2.0 mg/kg IV bolus every 4 hours
	or	
	Hydrocortisone	2.0 mg/kg IV bolus, then 0.5 mg/kg/h continuous intravenous infusion
Oral	A typical oral regimen that may be used as a substitute for IV corticosteroids might be prednisone or methylprednisolone	60 mg given immediately, then 60–120 mg/d in divided doses, tapered over several days at the discretion of the physician With improvement in the patient's condition (eg, stabilized PEFR), corticosteroids are usually tapered to a single daily dose of oral prednisone or methylprednisolone (eg, 60 mg/d) or divided doses (eg, 20 mg three times daily), then gradually further reduced over 7–14 days. If the patient requires a prolonged course of oral corticosteroids, side effects may be minimized by a single morning dose given on alternate days.
	Ambulatory Management of Chronic Asthma	
Antiinflammatory	Cromolyn sodium	2 puffs qid (inhalation)
		2 sprays in each nostril bid–qid (intranasally for nasal symptoms)
	Beclomethasone	2–5 puffs bid–qid (inhalation)
		2 sprays in each nostril bid (intranasally for allergic rhinitis)
	Prednisone	Burst for active symptoms: 40 mg/d, single or divided dose for 1 week, then taper for 1 week.
		If prolonged course is required, single morning dose on alternate days may minimize adverse effects.
Bronchodilator	Inhaled beta$_2$-agonist	2 puffs every 4 hours as needed
	Theophylline	Oral: Dose needed to reach serum concentration level of 8–12 μg/ml

*Abbreviations: IV, intravenous; PEFR, peak expiratory flow rate; qid, four times daily; bid, two times daily.

National Asthma Education Program. Report of the Working Group on Asthma in Pregnancy. Management of asthma during pregnancy. Bethesda, Maryland: Department of Health and Human Services, 1993:29, 41; NIH publication no. 93-3279

Antibiotics are not used routinely in the management of acute asthma. In the presence of fever, elevated leukocyte count or purulent sputum, their use is appropriate. Dehydration may be evidenced by the state of mucous membranes, urine output, urine specific gravity, or electrolytes, indicating the need for hydration. Sedatives, mucolytics, anticholinergics, and chest physical therapy have not been shown to be beneficial in acute attacks, and they may be harmful (2).

Fortunately, acute exacerbations of asthma are rare during labor and delivery; they should be managed in the manner outlined here. Fetal status should be monitored closely in all cases of acute exacerbations of asthma.

Chronic Asthma

The National Asthma Educational Program clearly states that the amount of data present on the treatment of asthma in pregnancy is limited and that "animal data, therapeutic principles and expert judgment and experience . . . were used to form the recommendations" (2). Medications used for the ambulatory management of asthma are listed in Table 3.

Chronic mild asthma results in brief, intermittent symptoms occurring up to twice a week. The PEFR is generally over 80% of expected or even 80% of the patient's personal best value established through repeated self-measurement. Therapy for these patients consists of an inhaled beta$_2$-agonist, two puffs every 3–4 hours for the duration of symptoms.

Patients with moderate asthma have symptoms more often than twice a week; symptoms may last several days, affect sleep, or require emergency care. The PEFR is usually 60–80% of baseline. Therapy consists of inhaled corticosteroid or inhaled cromolyn to reduce inflammation and an inhaled beta$_2$-agonist for bronchodilation. Sustained-release theophylline may be of value for patients who have symptoms at night.

Patients with severe chronic asthma have continuous symptoms, limited activity, and frequent nocturnal symptoms and exacerbations that may require emergency treatment and hospitalization. Their PEFR may be below 60% of baseline, established by standardized norms or by percentage of the patient's best PEFR. Vigorous use of inhaled corticosteroids, inhaled cromolyn, and inhaled beta$_2$-agonist is warranted. Administering oral corticosteroids in a short burst (40 mg daily for 7 days and then tapering for a week) may be necessary to relieve symptoms.

A number of side effects of inhaled corticosteroids have been described, including cataract formation, purpura, and dermal thinning. Hypothalmic–pituitary–adrenal axis suppression has also been noted. Inhaled corticosteroids can also lead to development of oral candidiasis, so the mouth and throat should be rinsed thoroughly after each treatment to decrease the risk (4, 5). Correct use of metered dose inhalers is a technique some patients find difficult to master. For these people, the use of a spacer between the inhaler and the mouth may prove beneficial.

The National Asthma Education Program identified four components for the successful management of asthma in pregnancy. The first component is objective assessment of pulmonary function. Women are encouraged to perform PEFR recordings at home to assess symptoms, predict exacerbations, and adjust asthma therapy. Tests of fetal status, such as ultrasound measurements, and antepartum fetal assessment should be used as needed to evaluate the fetus. The second component of asthma management is to identify and then avoid or control the substances or situations that trigger asthmatic attacks. Pharmacologic therapy is the third component of asthma management (Table 3). The fourth component is patient education. Pregnant women should be informed about the importance of taking medication to control asthma and be reassured that the medication is not harmful.

During labor and delivery, women whose asthma is well controlled may continue taking their usual medications. Intravenous hydrocortisone (100 mg every 8 hours for 24 hours) should be given to women who have received systemic corticosteroids during the pregnancy. The choice of analgesic and anesthetic may be adjusted because of asthma. Narcotics such as morphine and meperidine are best avoided, whereas fentanyl may be used. Lumbar epidural is probably the anesthetic of choice for women with asthma.

Induction of labor with oxytocin or prostaglandin E_2 gel is not contraindicated by asthma. Oxytocin or intrarectal prostaglandin E_2 suppositories may be used in the treatment of uterine atony with postpartum hemorrhage. The use of 15-methyl prostaglandin $F_{2\alpha}$ may worsen asthma and should be avoided.

Patients whose asthma is well controlled during pregnancy generally have a normal pregnancy outcome. The incidence of preeclampsia is slightly higher in women with asthma (6). Low FEV_1 measurements during pregnancy have been associated with fetal growth restriction (7). This implies that the clinician should not only aim to control the symptoms of pregnant women with asthma but also try to optimize pulmonary function.

Approximately 33–40% of women with asthma experience no change in their asthma during pregnancy. Worsening of symptoms is noted by 35–42%, and improvement occurs in 18–28% of women. There is a tendency for the course of asthma to be concordant in subsequent pregnancies (8).

Bronchitis

Bronchitis is an inflammation/infection of the tracheobronchial tree that spares the alveoli. Acute bronchitis is often viral but may be caused by species of *Mycoplasma*, *Streptococcus*, *Haemophilus*, or *Chlamydia*. Bronchitis is diagnosed on the basis of productive cough and fever in the absence of alveolar involvement.

In the absence of chronic bronchitis, there is no proven benefit to antibiotic therapy for acute bronchitis in healthy adults. If therapy is needed, erythromycin or amoxicillin–clavulanate may be prescribed. Acute exacerbations of chronic bronchitis are more likely to be bacterial and should be treated with amoxicillin–clavulanate, trimethoprim–sulfamethoxazole, or cefuroxime (9). Doxycycline is a recommended therapy for nonpregnant patients but is contraindicated in pregnancy because of the potential damage to fetal bone and teeth. Trimethoprim–sulfamethoxazole is recommended for nonpregnant patients but may be used after the first trimester. Although trimethoprim–sulfamethoxazole traditionally has been avoided at term as it was thought to increase neonatal hyperbilirubinemia, data are inadequate to confirm such an association.

Pneumonia

Pneumonia is an inflammation or infection of the lower respiratory tract, including the alveoli and respiratory bronchioles. Pneumonia complicates 0.1–1% of all pregnancies, and it can have devastating results. Mortality rates have decreased dramatically with the advent of antibiotics (10). Despite this, the disease continues to be a cause of death in pregnant women. Co-infections with human immunodeficiency virus (HIV) may further worsen the prognosis.

Pneumonia in pregnancy may be bacterial, viral, or chemical, the last as the result of aspiration of gastric contents. Pneumonia from fungal or parasitic infection is exceedingly rare and generally limited to immunocompromised women. Viral and aspiration pneumonias are commonly complicated by the secondary growth of bacteria. In all cases of suspected pneumonia, an adequate sputum sample containing few epithelial cells and many leukocytes should be obtained for Gram stain and culture. A chest X-ray is an essential part of the evaluation. Obtaining blood cultures and serology such as cold agglutinins for diagnosing *Mycoplasma* or paired titers (acute and convalescent) may also assist in identifying causative organisms.

Bacterial Pneumonia

The classic presentation of bacterial pneumonia is an acute illness accompanied by fever, chills, productive cough, and a lobar pattern on chest X-ray. A classic presentation resulting from infection by *Streptococcus pneumoniae* is the most common type of pneumonia seen in pregnancy (30–50%). However, *Haemophilus influenzae*, *Klebsiella pneumoniae*, and *Staphylococcus aureus* are also common causes. Streptococcal pneumonia produces a "rusty" sputum with gram-positive diplococci and asymmetric consolidation with air bronchograms on chest X-ray. *H. influenzae* is a gram-negative coccobacillus that produces consolidation with air bronchograms, often in the upper lobes. *K. pneumoniae*, a gram-negative rod, causes extensive tissue destruction with air bronchograms, pleural effusion, and cavitation. *S. aureus* pneumonia produces pleuritic chest pain, purulent sputum with gram-positive cocci, and a chest X-ray picture of consolidation without air bronchograms because the bronchi themselves are involved and atelectasis is present.

Atypical pneumonia is slowly progressive and accompanied by headache, low-grade fever, muscle aches, and a nonproductive cough. The chest X-ray shows a diffuse bronchopneumonia pattern, the severity of which is out of proportion to the mild clinical symptoms. *Mycoplasma pneumoniae* is the most common organism responsible for an atypical pneumonia, but other organisms occasionally may be involved. *M. pneumoniae* is best detected by the presence of cold agglutinins, which are present in 70% of cases.

Frequently, therapy is begun with broad-spectrum antibiotics. Once the causative organism and its sensitivity are known, antibiotic therapy may be directed more specifically. Nosocomial infection requires a third-generation cephalosporin combined with an aminoglycoside to ensure adequate coverage for gram-negative organisms and *S. aureus* (10, 11). Erythromycin, 500 mg every 6 hours, is the recommended therapy for atypical pneumonia. It may be given orally or intravenously, depending on the clinical status of the patient (10).

Influenza Pneumonia

Pneumonia due to influenza A infection and the secondary bacterial pneumonia that may result are severe, acute illnesses with high fever, malaise, headache, and cough. The chest X-ray may be clear and the cough nonproductive with uncomplicated influenza pneumonia. When bacterial superimposition occurs (commonly *S. aureus*), the cough produces purulent sputum and radiographic findings include peribronchial infiltrates with cavitation and a pleural effusion.

Uncomplicated influenza pneumonia should spontaneously resolve in 3–4 days and does not usually require therapy. Persistent or worsening symptoms point to superimposed bacterial infection, and broad-spectrum antibiotic coverage with an agent such as a cephalosporin is required. Amantadine and ribavirin have been used in nonpregnant patients to decrease the severity of influenza A infections. Both agents, however, are embryotoxic and teratogenic in animal studies and thus are reserved for life-threatening disease in pregnancy such as fulminant respiratory failure (11). The use of acyclovir is currently recommended for varicella infections in pregnancy only if pneumonia or encephalitis develops. Prophylactic acyclovir use to prevent varicella pneumonia in pregnant women has not been recommended.

Varicella Pneumonia

Pneumonia may occur in up to 20% of adults with varicella infection (chicken pox), and its severity is increased in pregnancy. The mortality rate for varicella pneumonia in pregnancy may exceed 35%. The pneumonia generally begins 2–6 days after onset of the rash, with pleuritic chest pain, dyspnea, cough, and hemoptysis. The chest X-ray shows a diffuse miliary or nodular pattern. Aggressive therapy with acyclovir, 8–10 mg/kg every 8 hours intravenously, and rigorous supportive therapy must be initiated immediately to avoid mortality. Acyclovir has been used extensively in pregnancy with no reported increase in birth defects or fetal loss; however, the life-threatening nature of this illness mandates its use regardless of any potential fetal effect (11).

Aspiration Pneumonia

Aspiration of gastric contents at the time of labor and delivery was a major cause of maternal mortality in the past. Aspiration of particulate matter and gastric acid causes an immediate chemical pneumonitis followed, in 24–48 hours, by a secondary bacterial pneumonia. Pregnant women, especially at term, are at increased risk for aspiration, due to relaxation of the gastroesophageal sphincter, elevated intraabdominal pressure, and delayed gastric emptying. The cornerstone of therapy for aspiration in pregnancy is prevention. Use of nonparticulate antacids (sodium citrate), regional anesthesia, and rapid sequence induction of general anesthesia with cricoid pressure have dramatically decreased the incidence of aspiration-related maternal mortality.

Aspiration must be suspected in any case of postpartum respiratory distress, particularly following general anesthesia. Broad-spectrum coverage for gram-negative enteric organisms, many of which are anaerobic, is required and may include imipenem, ticarcillin–clavulanate, ceftazidime and clindamycin, or clindamycin/gentamicin. Supportive therapy is of paramount importance. Previous recommendations for the use of corticosteroids in aspiration pneumonia have been withdrawn (11).

Tuberculosis

Once considered rare in the United States, tuberculosis is increasing dramatically in women of childbearing age. In endemic areas, the incidence of tuberculosis may approach 0.1% of pregnancies (12). All pregnant women at high risk for tuberculosis should be screened with a purified protein derivative (PPD) skin test when they begin prenatal care. High-risk factors for tuberculosis include:

- HIV infection
- Close contact with persons known or suspected to have tuberculosis
- Medical risk factors known to increase risk of disease if infected
- Birth in a country with high tuberculosis prevalence
- Medically underserved status
- Low income
- Alcohol addiction
- Intravenous drug use
- Residency in a long-term care facility (eg, correctional institutions, mental institutions, nursing homes and facilities)
- Health professionals working in high-risk health care facilities

In endemic urban areas, universal screening may be warranted, as essentially all patients meet risk criteria.

Women with a positive PPD skin test must be evaluated for active tuberculosis with a thorough physical examination for extrapulmonary disease and a chest x-ray once they are beyond the first trimester (abdominal shielding may be used) (13). Symptoms of active disease include cough, fever, malaise, weight loss, night sweats, and hemoptysis. Symptomatology and the progression of the disease are unaltered by pregnancy. In most cases of tuberculosis diagnosed by screening in pregnancy, patients are asymptomatic with no evidence of active disease.

Treatment regimens for tuberculosis are based on the presence or absence of active disease and, in the absence of active disease, the duration of PPD positivity (13, 14). The risk of progression to active disease is highest in the 2 years after conversion. Therefore, in women with a known recent conversion (2 years) to a positive PPD and no evidence of active disease, recommended medication is isoniazid, 300 mg/d, starting after the first trimester and continuing for 6–9 months. Women less than 35 years of age with an unknown or prolonged duration of PPD positivity (more than 2 years) should receive isoniazid, 300 mg/d, for 6–9 months following delivery. For women older than 35 years of age, isoniazid prophylaxis is not recommended for unknown or prolonged PPD positivity in the absence of active disease because of concerns about hepatotoxicity.

Treatment of active tuberculosis in pregnancy should commence immediately with dual-agent therapy for a full 9 months. Isoniazid, 300 mg/d, combined with rifampin, 600 mg/d, is the standard therapeutic regimen. If resistance to isoniazid is identified, ethambutol, 2.5 g/d, is substituted for the rifampin dose (isoniazid plus ethambutol regimen). Pyridoxine (vitamin B_6) supplementation, 50 mg/d, is essential for all patients receiving isoniazid therapy.

Isoniazid, rifampin, and ethambutol have been used extensively in pregnancy with no adverse effects. Antituberculous agents not recommended for use in pregnancy include ethionamide, streptomycin, capreomycin, kanamycin, cycloserine, and pyrazinamide.

Breast-feeding is considered safe during maternal antituberculous therapy as long as the infant is not concurrently taking oral antituberculous therapy. (If both mother and infant are on antituberculosis therapy, excessive drug levels may be reached in the neonate.) Breast-fed infants of women taking isoniazid therapy should receive a multivitamin supplement, including pyridoxine.

All newborn infants of women taking antituberculous therapy should receive a PPD skin test at birth and again at 3 months of age. Infants born to women with active tuberculosis at the time of delivery should receive isoniazid prophylaxis (10 mg/kg/d) until maternal disease has been inactive for 3 months (negative maternal sputum cultures). Failure to diagnose and treat congenital or neonatal tuberculosis results in significantly elevated morbidity and mortality (10, 14). Active tuberculosis in a neonate should be treated with isoniazid and rifampin immediately upon diagnosis. Multiagent therapy with isoniazid, rifampin, streptomycin, and pyrazinamide is recommended for drug-resistant organisms. If appropriate therapy is given, most long-term morbidity can be avoided.

Cystic Fibrosis

Cystic fibrosis is an autosomal recessive genetic disorder resulting from a mutation on chromosome 7. It is a complex disorder affecting a membrane-bound Cl^- ion transport protein. The effects are seen mainly in the pulmonary and gastrointestinal tracts, where secretions are abnormally thick (15). With current methods of treatment, the median survival is about 29 years of age.

As patients with cystic fibrosis live longer, issues related to reproduction arise. Women with cystic fibrosis are thought to have lower fertility; they also have abnormally dense cervical mucus, which has been thought to be a cause of decreased fertility. Approximately 95% of men with cystic fibrosis are sterile due to abnormalities of the derivatives of the Wolffian duct. Spermatogenesis does occur, and techniques have been devised to obtain epididymal sperm from these men to be used to overcome their azoospermia (15).

The first reports of pregnancy and cystic fibrosis painted a gloomy picture, with a high rate of prematurity, stillbirth, and neonatal death, as well as a high death rate of mothers within 6 months of delivery (16). More recent studies, however, have shown that women with milder disease are more likely to have a successful pregnancy. Characteristics of these women include a later age at diagnosis, more normal weight, absence of pancreatic insufficiency, and stable pulmonary function (15, 17, 18). Formerly, it was thought that if the FVC was less than 50% of the predicted value, there was an absolute contraindication to pregnancy in a patient with cystic fibrosis. Among such women with stable pulmonary function prior to pregnancy, however, there have since been several pregnancies with successful outcomes. Pulmonary hypertension, a rare complication of cystic fibrosis, is considered a contraindication to pregnancy.

Studies of cystic fibrosis and pregnancy have small numbers of patients, and most are retrospective, but some generalizations can be made: the spontaneous abortion rate is not increased, the prematurity rate is around 25%, and the death rate among pregnant and postpartum women with cystic fibrosis is not higher than in nonpregnant women of a similar age with cystic fibrosis. Congenital anomalies are not increased, and breast-feeding is possible (18).

Ideally, women with cystic fibrosis should have preconceptional counseling and should be in optimal health prior to pregnancy. Consultation with a specialist may be advisable. The services of a dietitian are important for the total care of the woman. Genetic counseling about the risk of cystic fibrosis in the offspring should be provided, and carrier testing for the father, as well as prenatal diagnosis, should be discussed (19).

During pregnancy, the woman should be monitored closely for pulmonary infection, which should be treated promptly and vigorously, if present. Maternal nutrition and weight gain should be monitored and fetal growth evaluated. Because diabetes occurs more often in this population, women should be screened early in pregnancy for gestational diabetes.

Summary

As pulmonary disorders become more prevalent overall, obstetricians will see an increasing number of these conditions in their pregnant patients. Management of respiratory disorders during pregnancy is not markedly different from management in the nonpregnant state, but the physician must be aware of the respiratory changes in pregnancy and how these affect the fetus in order to optimize treatment.

REFERENCES

1. Centers for Disease Control. Asthma—United States, 1980–1990. MMWR 1992;41:733–735
2. National Asthma Education Program. Report of the Working Group on Asthma in Pregnancy. Management of asthma during pregnancy. Bethesda, Maryland: Department of Health and Human Services, 1993; NIH publication no. 93-3279
3. Barnes PJ. A new approach to the treatment of asthma. N Engl J Med 1989;321:1517–1527
4. Cotton P. Asthma consensus is unconvincing to many. JAMA 1993;270:297
5. Medical Letter, Inc. Drugs for asthma. Med Lett Drugs Ther 1995;37(939):1–4
6. Stenius-Aarniala B, Piirilä P, Teramo K. Asthma and pregnancy: a prospective study of 198 pregnancies. Thorax 1988;43:12–18
7. Schatz M, Zeiger RS, Hoffman CP. Intrauterine growth is related to gestational pulmonary function in pregnant asthmatic women. Chest 1990;98:389–392
8. Schatz M, Harden K, Forsythe A, Chilingar L, Hoffman C, Sperling W, et al. The course of asthma during pregnancy, post partum, and with successive pregnancies: a prospective analysis. J Allergy Clin Immunol 1988;81:509–517
9. Mandell GL, Douglas RG, Bennett JE, Dolin R, eds. Principles and practice of infectious diseases: antimicrobial therapy 1993/1994. New York: Churchill Livingstone, 1993:48–49
10. Maccato ML. Pneumonia and pulmonary tuberculosis in pregnancy. Obstet Gynecol Clin North Am 1989;16: 417–430
11. Rodrigues J, Niederman MS. Pneumonia complicating pregnancy. Clin Chest Med 1992;13:679–691
12. Margono F, Mroueh J, Garely A, White D, Duerr A, Minkoff HL. Resurgence of active tuberculosis among pregnant women. Obstet Gynecol 1994;83:911–914
13. American Thoracic Society. Treatment of tuberculosis and tuberculosis infection in adults and children. Am J Respir Crit Care Med 1994;149:1359–1374
14. Sanders CV, Hill MK. Tuberculosis in pregnancy. In: Mead PB, Hager WD, eds. Infection protocols for obstetrics and gynecology. Montvale, New Jersey: Medical Economics Publishing, 1992:66–71
15. Kotloff RM, FitzSimmons SC, Fiel SB. Fertility and pregnancy in patients with cystic fibrosis. Clin Chest Med 1992;13:623–635
16. Cohen LF, di Saent'Agnese PA, Friedlander J. Cystic fibrosis and pregnancy. A national survey. Lancet 1980;2: 842–844
17. Canny GJ, Corey M, Livingstone RA, Carpenter S, Green L, Levison H. Pregnancy and cystic fibrosis. Obstet Gynecol 1991;77:850–853
18. Kent NE, Farquharson DF. Cystic fibrosis in pregnancy. Can Med Assoc J 1993;149:809–813
19. Canny GJ. Pregnancy in patients with cystic fibrosis. Can Med Assoc J 1993;149:805–806

SUGGESTED READING

Clark SL. Asthma in pregnancy. Obstet Gynecol 1993; 82: 1036–1040

National Asthma Education Program. Expert panel report. Guidelines for the diagnosis and management of asthma. Bethesda, Maryland: Department of Health and Human Services, 1991; NIH publication no. 91-3042

National Asthma Education Program. Report of the Working Group on Asthma in Pregnancy. Management of asthma during pregnancy. Bethesda, Maryland: Department of Health and Human Services, 1993; NIH publication no. 93-3279

This Technical Bulletin was developed under the direction of the Committee on Technical Bulletins of the American College of Obstetricians and Gynecologists as an educational aid to obstetricians and gynecologists. The committee wishes to thank Robert W. Huff, MD, and Jeanna M. Piper, MD, for their assistance in the development of this bulletin. This Technical Bulletin does not define a standard of care, nor is it intended to dictate an exclusive course of management. It presents recognized methods and techniques of clinical practice for consideration by obstetrician–gynecologists for incorporation into their practices. Variations of practice taking into account the needs of the individual patient, resources, and limitations unique to the institution or type of practice may be appropriate.

ISSN 1074-8628

THE AMERICAN COLLEGE OF OBSTETRICIANS AND GYNECOLOGISTS
409 12th Street, SW
PO Box 96920
Washington, DC 20090-6920

12345/09876

Number 171—August 1992
(Replaces #62, July 1981)

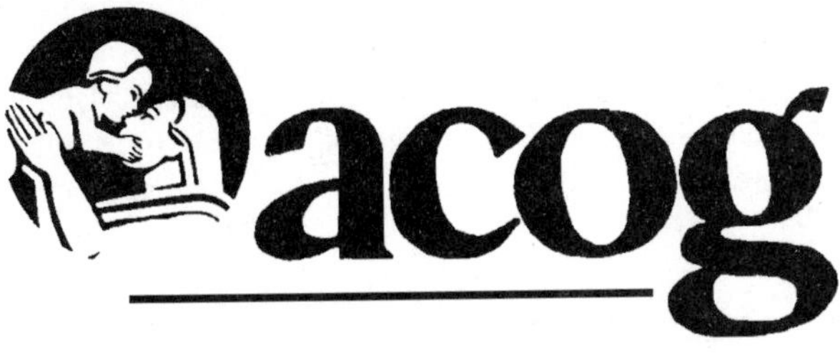

Technical Bulletin

An Educational Aid to Obstetrician–Gynecologists

Rubella and Pregnancy

Preventing maternal rubella infection and its subsequent teratogenic effects (1) on the fetus is the major objective of rubella immunization programs. The initial strategy for rubella control was to vaccinate all preschool and elementary school children. Pregnant women would be protected from rubella by reducing their risk of being exposed to infected children at home or in the community. By the mid-1970s, the incidence of rubella had been reduced considerably, but it had become evident that many pregnant women were still at risk for rubella infection. Persons 15 years of age or older, who had not been targeted in the childhood vaccination strategy, made up a greater proportion of reported cases. Outbreaks continued to occur in settings where young adults congregated. In 1977, the rubella control strategy was augmented to include recommendations that all susceptible adults, particularly postpubertal women, be vaccinated. After the implementation of this strategy, the number of reported cases of postnatal rubella and congenital rubella syndrome (CRS) steadily dropped (2, 3).

In 1988, an all-time low of 225 cases of rubella were reported to the National Notifiable Disease Surveillance System at the Centers for Disease Control (CDC). However, from 6–11% of postpubertal women may remain seronegative, according to data from premarital screening programs in selected states, and even higher rates of seronegativity were reported in special populations. These data suggested that cases of CRS might continue to occur.

A moderate resurgence of rubella and a dramatic increase in CRS occurred between 1988 and 1991 (4, 5). The reported incidence of rubella increased nearly fivefold during 1988–1990 to a provisional annual total of 1,093 cases, the highest total reported since 1982. In 1990, there were 17 confirmed or compatible cases and 5 provisional cases of CRS (6). While the reason for the resurgence of rubella is unclear, it appears to be associated with a failure to vaccinate susceptible persons rather than a failure of rubella vaccine. Cases of CRS occurred primarily in infants of unvaccinated mothers.

Rubella Vaccines

In 1969, three live attenuated rubella vaccines were licensed for use in the United States: the HPV-77 (DE-5 and DK-12) vaccines and the Cendehill vaccine. RA 27/3 vaccine, a live attenuated vaccine produced in human diploid cells, is more immunogenic than previous vaccines and has been used exclusively in the United States since 1979. Experience with the HPV/77 strains of rubella virus vaccine showed that a single dose of vaccine given at 12 months of age or older induced antibodies in over 95% of susceptible individuals.

A number of studies have been conducted to evaluate the persistence of rubella antibody following rubella vaccination, as measured by hemagglutination inhibition or enzyme-linked immunosorbent assay (ELISA). Long-term follow-up studies conducted 16 years after immunization with the HPV/77 vaccines or the Cendehill vaccine indicated a loss of antibody detectable by ELISA in 8% of persons receiving vaccine. Other studies of long-term persistence of immunity have shown that vaccinees lacking hemagglutination inhibition antibody are often found to have antibody by other laboratory tests, such as neutralizing antibody, passive hemagglutination, or ELISA, or cell-mediated immune responses, suggesting that most, if not all, such persons are immune. RA 27/3-induced antibody levels, which are present in at least 95% of vaccinees, have been shown to persist for at least 18 years in 92% of vaccinees who had originally seroconverted (6). Further evidence for persisting immunity comes from revaccination studies of persons with low levels of antibody, who typically have an anamnestic response; viremia, when studied, has been rare.

The rubella vaccine virus can be recovered from the respiratory secretions of recipients up to 28 days after subcutaneous or intranasal administration. However, studies have documented the lack of communicability of the vaccine virus in usual circumstances. Even though the vaccine virus may be excreted in the mother's milk and seroconversion in the feeding infant may occur, there appears to be no contraindication to vaccinating a susceptible mother if she plans to breast-feed her infant. Thus, the susceptible mother should be vaccinated whether or not she plans to breast-feed.

Side Effects

Some recipients may develop mild and brief rubella-like signs and symptoms, such as fever, rash, and lymphadenopathy, usually 5–21 days after vaccination. Joint symptoms following vaccination are more common in women than in men or children. Joint complaints occur in approximately 25% of susceptible adult women vaccinated with the RA 27/3 vaccine, and frank arthritis in about 10%. Joint reactions attributable to vaccine appear to occur only in susceptible persons. Chronic or recurrent arthralgia or arthritis has been rarely reported to follow rubella vaccination of susceptible adult women, and a comparative study documented that such illnesses were substantially less frequent after vaccination than after natural rubella.

Rubella Vaccine in Pregnancy

Rubella vaccine virus is known to cross the placenta and may infect the fetus during the early stages of development; however, there is no evidence that it causes birth defects or illness (7). Between 1971 and 1988, the Centers for Disease Control collected data on 307 infants born to susceptible women who had received rubella vaccine up to 3 months before conception or during the first trimester of pregnancy. Ninety-four infants were born to mothers who had received the previously used Cendehill or HPV/77 vaccines, and 212 were born to mothers who had received the RA 27/3 vaccine. None of the infants had defects indicative of CRS. Three of the infants born to mothers receiving the Cendehill or the HPV-77 vaccine and three born to mothers receiving the RA 27/3 vaccine had laboratory evidence of subclinical fetal infection but no illness or defects. The observed risk of congenital malformations following rubella vaccination with the RA 27/3 vaccine therefore is 0; the theoretic risk may be as high as 1.7%.

Although the observed risk of congenital malformations following rubella vaccination is no greater than the risk of malformations occurring by chance, pregnancy remains a contraindication to rubella vaccination on theoretic grounds. Reasonable precautions should be taken to preclude vaccination of pregnant women, including asking women if they are pregnant, excluding those who say they are, and explaining the theoretic risks to the others. Because of the theoretic risk to the fetus, women who have been vaccinated should be advised to avoid conception for 3 months. If a woman who is vaccinated is discovered to be pregnant, the Immunization Practices Advisory Committee, which plays a major role in recommendations for U.S. immunization policy, has stated that "the risk of vaccine-associated defects is so small as to be negligible and should not ordinarily be a reason in itself to consider interruption of pregnancy." The pregnant patient and her physician should make the final decision.

Rubella Exposure or Suspected Infection

The risk of CRS abnormalities in infants varies according to the gestational age at which the infection occurs; therefore, counseling regarding the risk and management of pregnant women who have evidence of primary rubella infection must be individualized. Prospective studies of infection during pregnancy have demonstrated that when maternal infection occurred in the first trimester, the average incidence of abnormalities was 25%, compared with an incidence of less than 1% following infection during the second trimester. The risk was estimated to be at least 50%, 25%, and 10% during the first, second, and third month, respectively. In 1982, even higher rates overall of anomalies were reported (8). This latter study may provide a more accurate determination of risk, since all maternal cases were serologically confirmed and sensitive antibody assays were used to detect congenital infection. The risk for congenital defects in this study was 90% when maternal infection occurred before 11 weeks of gestation, 33% for infection during 11–12 weeks, 11% for 13–14 weeks, 24% for 15–16 weeks, and 0% after 16 weeks (8). Termination of pregnancy is usually considered when there is clear evidence of primary infection during the first trimester of pregnancy. Instances of rubella between 16–20 weeks of pregnancy are rare and are manifested by bilateral sensorineural deafness (often severe) in the newborn. No studies have documented congenital defects following maternal infection after 20 weeks of gestation. Routine postexposure rubella prophylaxis with immunoglobulin is not recommended because it has not been shown to be effective.

Diagnosis of Recent Rubella Infection

An accurate diagnosis of acute primary rubella infection in the pregnant woman is imperative if appropriate management is to be undertaken. Since a large proportion of cases are subclinical and clinical diagnosis is unreliable, the diagnosis of acute rubella infection requires serologic testing. Pregnant women who present with a rubella-like illness or recent exposure to rubella but have tested positive for rubella-specific antibody during prenatal or preconception screening can be presumed to be immune.

The definition of a significant rise in rubella immunoglobulin G (IgG) antibody level or a minimal IgG antibody level indicative of immunity varies by the type of assay and by the laboratory performing the testing and must be elucidated by the laboratory. A relatively sensitive assay (ie, one that is able to detect ≥ 10 IU) should be used. The serologic diagnosis of recent rubella infection requires either of the following:

1. Detection in acute and convalescent sera of a significant rise in rubella antibody levels, either total or IgG
2. Presence of rubella IgM antibody

In the United States, the most commonly used assays for the diagnosis of acute rubella infection are hemagglutination inhibition, ELISA, and indirect fluorescent immunoassay (9). Complement fixation tests are now used infrequently; they are less sensitive, and complement fixation antibodies appear later in the course of disease than do antibodies measured by other assays. Passive hemagglutination and passive latex agglutination tests are fast and convenient tests that are useful for detecting evidence of immunity but are not recommended for quantitating antibody or for confirming rubella illness. Neutralization tests are very sensitive but not usually available in clinical laboratories.

Hemagglutination inhibition, ELISA, and indirect fluorescent immunoassays have been developed for detection of the serum rubella IgM fraction as well as for measurement of IgG antibody levels. Total rubella antibodies are rarely measured now by commercial laboratories, since most ELISA and indirect fluorescent immunoassays use conjugates specific for IgG. Therefore, in this bulletin, reference will generally be made only to rubella IgG or rubella IgM antibodies. In the case that an assay for total rubella antibodies is used for immunity screening in the absence of exposure to virus, it can be assumed that the majority of the antibody is IgG class antibody.

Rubella IgM antibody can be detected from early after onset of illness, reaching a peak at 7–10 days, and persisting up to 4 weeks after the appearance of rash. Some sensitive assays may detect IgM antibody longer than 4 weeks. False-positive tests for IgM antibody can occur with any indirect assay, such as ELISA or indirect fluorescent immunoassay, if the laboratory technique used does not avoid nonspecific reactions due to complexes with rheumatoid antibody. A negative IgM test, unless supported by additional laboratory or other data, cannot definitively prove lack of infection because of the potential for a false-negative result due to early waning of IgM antibody.

Low levels of rubella total or IgG antibodies, while not excluding the possibility of recent rubella infection, are not characteristic of the antibody response that is seen within the first 6 months following acute rubella infection. On the other hand, high total or IgG antibody levels may be present in up to 15% of the normal population and, by themselves, do not indicate a recent infection. Thus, a single measurement of rubella total or IgG antibody is generally not helpful in making a definitive diagnosis of acute rubella infection; rubella IgM antibody testing and/or collection of a second serum specimen for evidence of seroconversion to rubella are needed. Most commercial laboratories do not routinely save serum specimens; when recent rubella infection is suspected, the clinician should specifically order that acute specimens be saved to be tested in parallel with convalescent specimens.

It can be difficult to establish a diagnosis of rubella infection in a pregnant woman who is vaccinated but who has a significant rise in total or IgG antibody level after recent exposure to rubella. If IgM is present, then acute infection or reinfection has occurred. If no IgM antibody is detected, the rise in IgG level probably represents a boosting of antibody due to reinfection, rather than a primary response to infection. Boosting of IgG antibody has been seen in persons whose immunity was documented prior to exposure. Maternal reinfections usually pose no risk to the fetus.

Figure 1 shows a guide to assessing the risk of CRS in a fetus of a woman who is exposed to rubella or who has a rubella-like illness during pregnancy. Figure 2 shows a schematic representation of the rubella antibody responses following exposure and infection. The following guidelines amplify the evaluation suggested in the figures:

1. All women not known to be immune to rubella who have exposure to rubella or a rubella-like illness during pregnancy should be evaluated serologically for evidence of recent infection. If testing indicates that recent infection is likely to have occurred, then the woman should receive appropriate counseling, including the information that there is a high risk of CRS for the fetus if the primary infection occurred during the first trimester of pregnancy.
2. Women who have documented positive tests for rubella-specific antibody at some point prior to pregnancy can be presumed to be immune. Should these women have a significant rise in rubella IgG antibody titer without detection of IgM antibody, they should be counseled that asymptomatic reinfection is most likely to have occurred.
3. Serologic testing for diagnosis of recent rubella infection should include testing of acute sera for both IgG and IgM antibody. The presence of rubella-specific IgM antibody indicates acute infection. If tests for IgM are negative or unavailable, testing of paired acute and convalescent sera for IgG antibody should be carried out. In the setting of rubella-like illness during pregnancy, the acute specimen should be drawn as soon after rash onset as possible, followed by a convalescent specimen 2–3 weeks later if the ini-

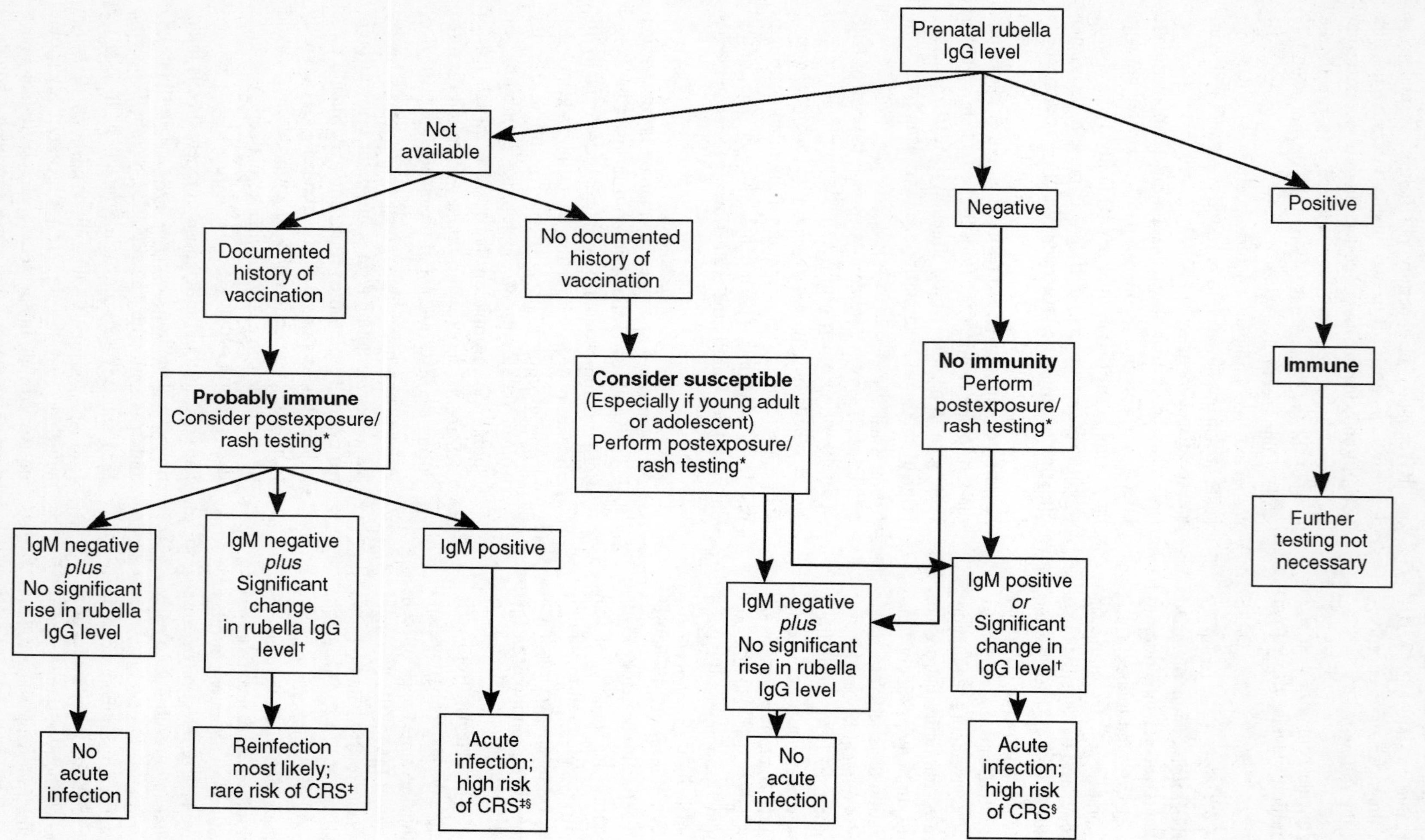

FIG. 1. Diagnosis of acute rubella in pregnancy.

* Should include IgM and IgG testing of acute specimen and paired acute and convalescent sera for IgG levels. Acute specimens should be drawn as soon as possible after rash onset, followed by a convalescent specimen 2–3 weeks later. For exposure to rubella, acute specimens should be drawn immediately, followed by convalescent specimen 4–5 weeks later.

† Since what constitutes a significant change in IgG level or low IgG level varies by type of assay and laboratory, interpretation of levels by laboratory is needed.

‡ Consultation with clinical virologist or other expert in diagnosis of rubella is warranted.

§ If infection occurred in first trimester of pregnancy.

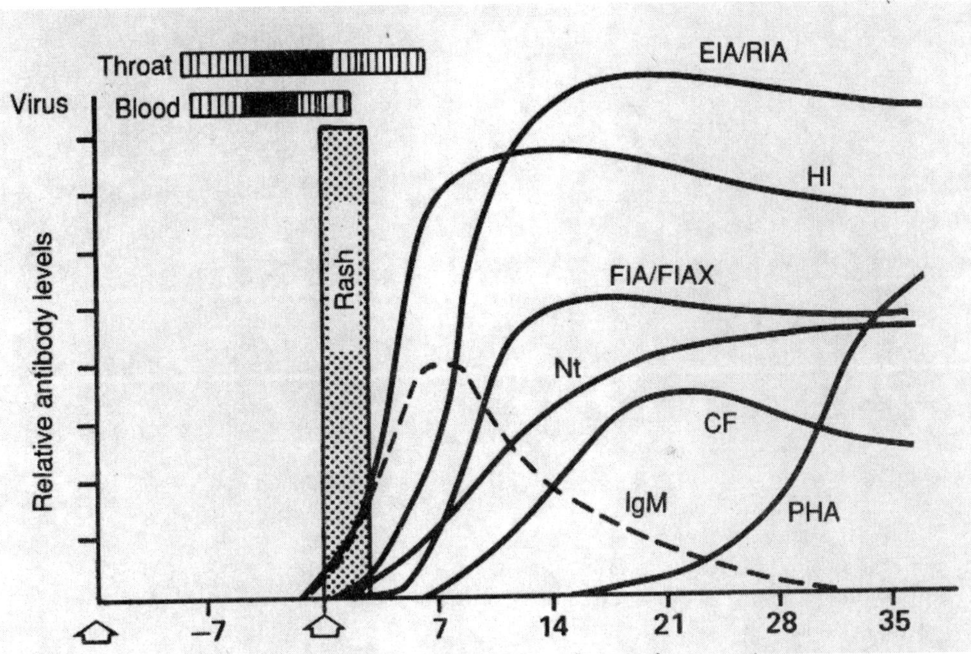

FIG. 2. Schema of immune response in acute rubella infection. EIA/RIA, enzyme immunoassay/radioimmunoassay; HI, hemagglutination inhibition; FIA/FIAX, indirect flourescence immunoassay; Nt, neutralization test; CF, complement fixation; IgM, immunoglobulin M; PHA, passive hemagglutination. Adapted with permission from: Herrmann KL. Available rubella serologic tests. Rev Infect Dis 1985; 7 Suppl 1:S108-S112.

tial test for IgM is negative. When suspected exposure to rubella has occurred, the acute specimen should be drawn immediately, followed by a convalescent specimen 4–5 weeks later. A relatively sensitive assay, such as ELISA, hemagglutination inhibition, or indirect fluorescent immunoassay, should be used.

4. Another difficult diagnostic dilemma is posed by the patient whose immune status is not known through prior prenatal or earlier rubella testing and who presents 5 weeks or more after exposure to a rash illness or 4 weeks or more after onset of a rash. If no rubella IgG antibody is detected, the patient is clearly susceptible to rubella and has no evidence of a recent infection. If IgG antibody is detected, there is evidence of a previous rubella infection. The date of infection and the risk to the fetus are difficult to determine, although a low level of antibody suggests more remote infection. Testing for rubella IgM antibody or repeating the test for IgG antibody levels to determine whether there is a significant rise or decline may be considered.
5. When the risk of CRS for the fetus is unclear because maternal serologic tests are not diagnostic, other information may be useful. This includes historical and epidemiologic information, such as recent maternal exposure to rubella, rash illness, vaccination history, stage of pregnancy in which infection is thought to have occurred, and timing of laboratory specimens (10). These patients need to be counseled about the uncertainties involved in assessing their degree of risk.

Recommendations to Prevent Rubella Exposure

In order to decrease both the number of pregnant women who are susceptible to rubella and the incidence of CRS, the following practices are encouraged:

1. Rubella vaccination of all children 12–15 months of age or older should be routine. All prepubertal school children without a record of previous rubella immunization should be vaccinated. Mothers should be given a copy of the vaccination records. Since there is conclusive evidence that the vaccine virus is not transmitted from person to person, children may be vaccinated even when there is a pregnant woman in the household.
2. All adolescents and adults not known to be immune to rubella, especially women of childbearing age, should be vaccinated unless they are pregnant or have other contraindications to vaccination. Only persons with detectable antibodies or a physician-signed record of rubella immunization should be considered immune. A history of rubella disease is not sufficient evidence of prior immunity. Any woman with no history of vaccination and no contraindications for vaccination can be vaccinated without prior serologic testing. Immunization of adult women of childbear-

ing age is particularly important, as is immunization of health care personnel who may transmit rubella to pregnant women or who might themselves contract rubella while pregnant. Because of the theoretic risk to the fetus, women of childbearing age should not receive rubella vaccine if they are pregnant, and they should understand that they should not become pregnant for 3 months after vaccination.

3. All prenatal patients should be screened for susceptibility to rubella as early in pregnancy as practical. Seronegative women, including those who are breastfeeding, should be vaccinated in the postpartum period, prior to discharge from the hospital. Since the vaccine is usually effective in immunizing the seronegative woman, postvaccination antibody testing is not necessary until a subsequent pregnancy. Although antenatal or postpartum administration of D immune globulin (human) or other blood products is not a contraindication for postpartum vaccination, in this situation, antibody testing should be done 6–8 weeks following vaccination to ensure seroconversion. If seroconversion does not occur, a second vaccination is necessary.
4. All suspected cases of rubella should be reported immediately to the local or state health department. While the clinical evaluation is being completed, the health department can determine what exposures may have occurred and initiate appropriate rubella control measures. Suspected cases of CRS should also be reported.

REFERENCES

1. Dudgeon JA. Congenital rubella: Pathogenesis and immunology. Am J Dis Child 1969;118:35–44
2. Centers for Disease Control. Rubella and congenital rubella syndrome—United States, 1985–1988. MMWR 1989; 38:173–182
3. Cochi SL, Edmonds LE, Dyer K, Greaves WL, Marks JS, Rovira EZ, et al. Congenital rubella syndrome in the United States, 1970–1985. On the verge of elimination. Am J Epidemiol 1989;129:349–361
4. Centers for Disease Control, Immunization Practices Advisory Committee. Increase in rubella and congenital rubella syndrome—United States, 1988–1990. MMWR 1991;40: 93–99
5. Centers for Disease Control, Immunization Practices Advisory Committee. Outbreaks of rubella among the Amish—United States, 1991. MMWR 1991; 40:264–265
6. O'Shea S, Best JM, Banatvala JE, Marshall WC, Dudgeon JA. Persistence of rubella antibody 8–18 years after vaccination. BMJ 1984;288:1043
7. Centers for Disease Control. Rubella vaccination during pregnancy—United States, 1971–1988. MMWR 1989;38: 289–293
8. Miller E, Cradock-Watson JE, Pollock TM. Consequences of confirmed maternal rubella at successive stages of pregnancy. Lancet 1982;2:781–784
9. Herrmann KL. Available rubella serologic tests. Rev Infect Dis 1985;7 Suppl 1:S108–S112
10. Mann JM, Preblud SR, Hoffman RE, Brandling-Bennett AD, Hinman AR, Herrmann KL. Assessing risks of rubella infection during pregnancy. A standardized approach. JAMA 1981;245:1647–1652

RECOMMENDED READING

Centers for Disease Control, Immunization Practices Advisory Committee. Rubella prevention. MMWR 1990;39 (RR-15):1–18

Enders G, Knotek F. Rubella IgG total antibody avidity and IgG subclass-specific antibody avidity assay and their role in the differentiation between primary rubella and rubella reinfection. Infection 1989;17:218–226

Hedman K, Hietala J, Tiilikainen A, Hartikainen-Sorri AL, Raiha K, Suni J, et al. Maturation of immunoglobulin G avidity after rubella vaccination studied by an enzyme linked immunosorbent assay (avidity-ELISA) and by haemolysis typing. J Med Virol 1989;27:293–298

Herrmann KL. Rubella virus. In: Lennette EH, Schmidt NJ. eds. Diagnostic procedures for viral, rickettsial and chlamydial infections. 5th ed. Washington: American Public Health Association, 1979

Orenstein WA, Bart KJ, Hinman AR, Preblud SR, Greaves WL, Doster SW, et al. The opportunity and obligation to eliminate rubella from the United States. JAMA 1984;251: 1988–1994

Preblud SR, Serdula MK, Frank JA Jr, Brandling-Bennett AD, Hinman AR. Rubella vaccination in the United States: a ten-year review. Epidemiol Rev 1980;2:171–194

Schum TR, Nelson DB, Duma MA, Sedmak GV. Increasing rubella seronegativity despite a compulsory school law. Am J Public Health 1990;80:66–69

Stehr-Green PA, Cochi SL, Preblud SR, Orenstein WA. Evidence against increasing rubella seronegativity among adolescent girls. Am J Public Health 1990;80:88

This Technical Bulletin was developed under the direction of the Committee on Technical Bulletins of the American College of Obstetricians and Gynecologists as an educational aid to obstetricians and gynecologists. The committee wishes to thank Laura J. Fehrs, MD; Walter W. Williams, MD; Stephen L. Cochi, MD; Walter A. Orenstein, MD; and Carl W. Tyler, MD; for their assistance in the development of this bulletin. This Technical Bulletin does not define a standard of care, nor is it intended to dictate an exclusive course of management. It presents recognized methods and techniques of clinical practice for consideration by obstetrician–gynecologists for incorporation into their practices. Variations of practice taking into account the needs of the individual patient, resources, and limitations unique to the institution or type of practice may be appropriate.

THE AMERICAN COLLEGE OF OBSTETRICIANS AND GYNECOLOGISTS
409 12th Street, SW
Washington, DC 20024-2188

3456/76

ACOG EDUCATIONAL BULLETIN

Number 231, December 1996

Seizure Disorders in Pregnancy

Seizure disorders are the most frequent major neurologic complication encountered in pregnancy, affecting approximately 1% of the general population. Seizure disorders may be categorized as acquired or idiopathic. Acquired seizure disorders, which account for less than 15% of all seizures, may result from trauma, infection, space-occupying lesions, or metabolic disorders. The remaining seizure disorders are classified as idiopathic and are known as epilepsy; they are the focus of this Educational Bulletin. Idiopathic seizures can be divided into different types, such as tonic–clonic, partial complex with or without generalization, myoclonic, focal, or absence seizures.

The treatment of pregnant patients with seizure disorders can be for both the obstetrician and neurologist due to the interrelationship of the effects of epilepsy and pregnancy, the variable effects of anticonvulsant medications on mother and fetus, and the changes in the pharmacokinetics of these medications during pregnancy. In addition, the current neurologic status of a patient with epilepsy may be unknown for a variety of reasons. Often the patient has been doing well and has not seen her neurologist in several years. The obstetrician and neurologist should work together prior to conception and throughout the patient's pregnancy to determine the safest and most effective medical therapy. Furthermore, the pediatrician selected by the patient to care for her baby should be included in prepregnancy discussions to address the potential increase in congenital malformations, the potential for neonatal sedation with certain medications, and questions concerning breast-feeding.

This Educational Bulletin was developed under the direction of the Committee on Educational Bulletins of the American College of Obstetricians and Gynecologists as an aid to obstetricians and gynecologists. The College wishes to thank Philip Samuels, MD, for his assistance in the development of this bulletin. This document is not to be construed as establishing a standard of practice or dictating an exclusive course of treatment. Rather, it is intended as an educational tool that presents current information on obstetric–gynecologic issues.

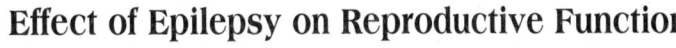

Effect of Epilepsy on Reproductive Function

Women with seizure disorders should seek care from an obstetrician–gynecologist as soon as they become sexually active. The use of certain antiepileptic medications may interfere with the action of oral contraceptive agents. Carbamazepine, phenobarbital, and phenytoin enhance the activity of hepatic microsomal oxidative enzymes (1). These medications, as well as the steroid hormones, share the cytochrome *P*-450 system. The resulting increased enzymatic activity may lead to rapid clearance of steroid hormones, which may allow ovulation. Therefore, patients taking low-dose oral

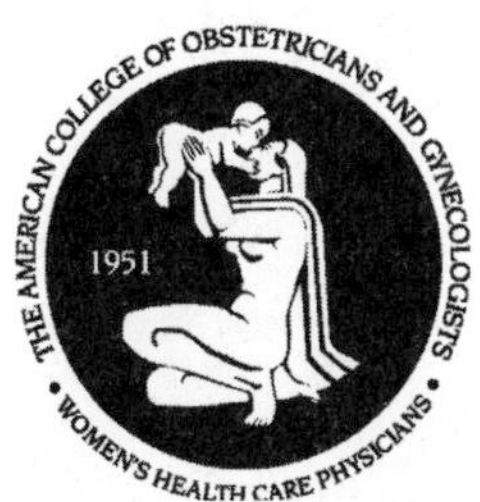

contraceptives and certain antiepileptic medications may have more breakthrough bleeding (2) and may be at increased risk for unplanned pregnancy (3, 4). This rapid clearance does not appear to be induced by use of valproate or benzodiazepines (1).

Although fertility rates may be lower in patients with epilepsy, most patients with epilepsy are able to conceive without difficulty (1, 5, 6). Based upon the patient's age, gravidity, and health status, an infertility evaluation should be undertaken when the obstetrician determines it is appropriate.

Effects of Pregnancy on Epilepsy

Patients with seizure disorders may be treated with single medications or a combination of medications, based on the type of seizure and side effects (Table 1). Serum levels of the most frequently used anticonvulsant medications (phenytoin, carbamazepine, and phenobarbital) can change dramatically during pregnancy, generally decreasing in total concentration as pregnancy progresses. Many factors contribute to this decrease, including altered protein binding, accelerated hepatic metabolism, nausea and vomiting, delayed gastric emptying, changes in plasma volume, and frequent antacid use. Although total levels fall, the free (active) levels tend to increase because of a decline in serum albumin and other proteins throughout pregnancy. This increase is most significant with phenytoin (90% protein bound) but is also noted with carbamazepine (76% protein bound) and phenobarbital (variable protein binding).

The drug dosage should be adjusted according to the total serum level and the patient's condition. If drug levels are carefully monitored, pregnancy should have little effect on seizure frequency. Drug toxicity varies with the drug being taken; therefore, patients should be monitored for symptoms of toxicity even if the drug level is within the normal therapeutic range (Table 1). This can be best accomplished by close cooperation between the neurologist and obstetrician. Such teamwork will help ensure that the woman receives the most efficacious and safest anticonvulsant regimen.

Effects of Epilepsy on Pregnancy

Most women with seizure disorders who become pregnant will have an uneventful pregnancy with an excellent outcome. However, several complications have been reported to occur more commonly in pregnant women with epilepsy. These include an increased incidence of depressed Apgar scores, low birth weight, diminished head circumference, preeclampsia, and stillbirth (7–11). Whether these complications are related to the seizure disorder or to anticonvulsant therapy is unclear. Other studies, however, are reassuring in that no increase in the rates of perinatal mortality, preeclampsia, preterm labor, or cesarean delivery could be demonstrated in women with epilepsy (10, 12).

Fetal and Neonatal Effects

Vitamin Deficiencies

All anticonvulsants interfere with folic acid metabolism. Thus, patients taking anticonvulsants may develop folic acid deficiency. Folic acid deficiency during embryogenesis has been associated with neural tube defects and other congenital malformations (13, 14). Because organogenesis occurs during the first weeks after conception, folic acid supplementation (0.4 mg/d) has been recommended for all patients before conception and in the first trimester (15). A dosage of 4 mg/d is recommended for all patients who have had a prior pregnancy affected by a neural tube defect. A similar preconceptional dose (4 mg/d) would seem appropriate for the patient taking anticonvulsant medication, as carbamazepine and valproate have been associated with an increased risk of neural tube defects, which occur early in the first trimester (16, 17).

Table 1. Potential Toxic Effects of Commonly Used Anticonvulsants

Medication	Maternal Effects	Characteristic Potential Fetal/Neonatal Effects
Carbamazepine	Drowsiness, leukopenia, ataxia, mild hepatotoxicity	Facial dysmorphisms, neural tube defects, hypoplasia of distal phalanges
Phenobarbital	Drowsiness, ataxia	Neonatal withdrawal, neonatal coagulopathy
Phenytoin	Nystagmus, ataxia, hirsutism, gingival hyperplasia, megaloblastic anemia	Facial clefting, hypoplasia of distal phalanges, hypertelorism, neonatal coagulopathy
Primidone	Drowsiness, ataxia, nausea	Neonatal withdrawal, neonatal coagulopathy
Valproic acid	Ataxia, drowsiness, alopecia, hepatotoxicity, thrombocytopenia	Facial dysmorphisms, neural tube defects

The optimal dose of folic acid needed to prevent neural tube defects in women with seizure disorders has not been established. In an investigation of the relationship between folate deficiency and malformations in infants born to mothers with epilepsy, no difference was found in major malformations between infants of patients and infants of controls with normal folate levels (18). In addition, increasing folic acid ingestion may increase the activity of hepatic microsomal enzymes and thus the clearance of anticonvulsant medications. Serum levels of medications should be checked frequently after folic acid therapy is implemented.

Neonatal hemorrhage due to decreased vitamin K–dependent clotting factors (II, VII, IX, X) has occurred in infants born to mothers taking phenobarbital, phenytoin, or primidone. In one series, 8 of 16 infants exposed to these medications had an umbilical cord blood coagulation pattern similar to that occurring with vitamin K deficiency (19). These infants responded to vitamin K infusion. Similar conclusions were reached in a review of the literature, and it was recommended that such infants be given 1 mg of vitamin K intramuscularly at birth (20). Some authors recommend prophylactic oral vitamin K during the last month of pregnancy (21), although the utility of this oral medication in preventing hemorrhage has not been proved definitively (22).

Therapy with phenobarbital, phenytoin, or primidone may also result in increased metabolism of vitamin D, leading to decreased vitamin D levels. Accordingly, patients should be encouraged to take prenatal vitamins that include an adequate amount of vitamin D (23).

Congenital Malformations

Seizure disorders are associated with an increase in congenital malformations, but the magnitude of the risk and whether drug therapy or specific drugs affect the incidence of certain anomalies remain uncertain. Although there are variations within the published literature, there appears to be a 6–8% chance of birth defects in infants born to women taking anticonvulsant medication. This represents a risk two to three times that of the general population. Each of the commonly used anticonvulsant medications (phenytoin, phenobarbital, carbamazepine, valproate, and primidone) has been implicated in some studies as teratogenic, but there is no clear consensus concerning which anticonvulsant has the most teratogenic potential. It is of paramount importance to treat the patient with the medication that best controls her seizures.

In a major, multiinstitutional study of the teratogenicity of antiepileptic medications, 902 pregnancies in mothers with idiopathic epilepsy were examined (24). The incidence of malformations in infants of mothers receiving anticonvulsant therapy was about five times that of those in the nonmedicated group (24). The predominant malformations were cleft lip/palate and cardiovascular malformations. At least two investigators (24, 25) noted that as the number of anticonvulsant medications used in combination during pregnancy increased, so did the incidence of fetal malformations. In one of these studies, there was no dose-dependent increase in the incidence of malformations associated with any single medication (25). In contrast, no difference between the rate of malformations in mothers receiving polytherapy and mothers receiving a single medication was found in another study (26).

A specific fetal hydantoin syndrome has been identified consisting of growth and performance delays, cranial facial abnormalities (including clefting), and limb anomalies (including hypoplasia of nails and distal phalanges) (27). Approximately 10–30% of infants born to women taking these drugs have been reported to have some aspects of the syndrome (28, 29). The proportion of exposed infants having the complete syndrome is much smaller.

Facial clefting has a multifactorial inheritance pattern, which reflects a combination of genetic and environmental factors (30). In one study, epilepsy alone showed a slight increase in the risk of cleft lip, with anticonvulsant medications increasing the risk even further (31). In another epidemiologic study, however, no evidence of a familial association between epilepsy and clefting disorders was found (32).

Teenagers with seizure disorders are often treated with valproate because it has few side effects in this age group. It has, however, been associated with specific anomalies. In 1984, investigators reported a specific fetal valproate syndrome of cranial–facial defects (33) that was confirmed by others (34, 35). A 1.5% risk of a neural tube defect was noted if the mother took valproate in the first trimester (17). In almost all cases of neural tube defects among infants exposed to anticonvulsant medications, the mothers were exposed to either valproate or carbamazepine. In most of the cases, the neural tube defects were lumbosacral. In the general population, however, spina bifida and anencephaly are equally distributed (ie, lumbosacral and higher defects are equally common). This suggests that valproate and carbamazepine have a predisposition to cause lumbosacral defects. The development of neural tube defects in infants of mothers taking valproate appears to be dose dependent. Other investigators have shown that valproate alters folic acid metabolism in mouse embryos, which could account for the increased risk of neural tube defects in infants born to mothers who have taken valproate (36).

Until recently, carbamazepine was considered safer than other anticonvulsant medications for use in pregnancy. Carbamazepine, however, has been linked to spina bifida, as noted previously. A 1% risk of spina bifida has been demonstrated in infants of mothers taking carbamazepine (16). A pattern of minor cranial–facial defects, fingernail hypoplasia, and developmental delay also has been reported in infants exposed to carbamazepine in utero (37). Because this spectrum of defects is similar to that seen in the fetal hydantoin syndrome, investigators hypothesized that, as both drugs are metabolized through an arene oxide pathway, perhaps an epoxide intermediary is the teratogenic agent (37). Those fetuses with low levels of epoxide hydrolase are exposed to higher levels of epoxide intermediaries, which may lead to an increase in malformations. Phenytoin, phenobarbital, and, to a lesser extent, carbamazepine are metabolized through this pathway (38).

Infants born to mothers who have been taking barbiturates during pregnancy may exhibit some withdrawal symptoms that begin about 1 week after birth and usually last 1–2 weeks (39). These symptoms usually involve minor irritability but occasionally may be more serious.

There has been much debate over whether epilepsy, the use of antiepileptic medications, or both are associated with psychomotor delays or mental retardation. The difficulties and controversy in determining the effects of anticonvulsants on cognitive and intellectual development have been presented elsewhere (40). A recent study indicated that individuals exposed to phenobarbital in utero might have slightly decreased verbal IQ scores (41).

Researchers have found a statistically significant difference in IQ among children of mothers with seizure disorders compared with controls (9). However, other factors associated with maternal epilepsy such as seizures during pregnancy, inherited brain disorders, and a nonoptimal psychosocial environment can also affect a child's psychomotor development (42). There appears to be a small, undefined risk of a slightly decreased IQ in children born to mothers with epilepsy; however, it does not appear that the use of any particular anticonvulsant medication increases this risk.

Management

Preconceptional Counseling

It is preferable to discuss the relationship of seizure disorders and pregnancy with an epileptic woman before she becomes pregnant. She generally can be counseled that most women with seizure disorders can have a successful pregnancy although there is a small increased risk of congenital malformation. The types and frequencies of malformations should be discussed. A detailed history should be obtained to determine any family history of seizure disorders or congenital malformations, as well as the patient's medication use and seizure frequency. Adequate rest and sleep should be recommended during pregnancy because sleep deprivation can increase the frequency of seizures.

The patient should be informed that if she has frequent seizures before conception, this pattern will probably continue. Women with frequent seizures should delay conception until seizures can be better controlled, even if this delay entails a change of medication. In patients who have tonic–clonic seizures, controlling seizures is of primary importance.

If the patient has had no seizures during the past 2–5 years, the obstetrician may ask the neurologist to consider withdrawing anticonvulsant medications. This is usually achieved by slowly reducing the amount of medication over a 1–3-month period. However, up to 50% of patients will experience a relapse and need to resume taking medication. Patients should not drive during this period.

If medications are necessary to control seizures, a single medication is preferred over multiple medications. Some patients receiving multiple medications can be switched to monotherapy over a period of several months. As medications are gradually withdrawn, the level of the remaining medication should be monitored frequently to make certain that it remains therapeutic. Ideally, the patient should refrain from conceiving until seizures are well controlled for several months on the minimum dose of medication.

Pregnant women with idiopathic epilepsy frequently want to know whether their child is at risk for developing epilepsy. Children of women who do not have a seizure disorder have a 0.5–1% risk of developing epilepsy, whereas infants born to mothers with a seizure disorder of unknown cause are four times more likely to develop idiopathic epilepsy (43). Epilepsy in the father does not increase a child's risk of developing a seizure disorder.

During Pregnancy

The patient's anticonvulsant level should be monitored periodically and dosages adjusted accordingly. For patients without seizures, it is reasonable for the obstetrician to monitor medication levels each trimester. Physicians should avoid monitoring levels and adjusting dosages too frequently, however, because it takes four to five half-lives for a medication to reach a steady state (Table 2). Drug levels should be determined immediately before the next dose (trough levels) in order to assess whether the dose is adequate. If the patient is showing signs of toxicity, the dosage should be decreased or the medication discontinued and serum levels assessed.

Patients taking anticonvulsants should be evaluated for possible fetal neural tube defects with a combination of maternal serum alpha-fetoprotein determination and ultrasonography. Amniocentesis should be offered if the preceding tests are equivocal. At 18–22 weeks of gestation, the patient should undergo a comprehensive ultrasound examination to look for congenital malformations, including cardiac malformations, which occur more often in women taking antiepileptic medications. If the

Table 2. Commonly Used Anticonvulsants During Pregnancy

Medication	Therapeutic Level (mg/L)	Nonpregnant Dosage*	Usual Half-Life
Carbamazepine	4–10	600–1,200 mg/d in 3 or 4 divided doses	36 h (initially) 16 h (with chronic therapy)
Phenobarbital	15–40	90–180 mg/d in 2 or 3 divided doses	100 h
Phenytoin	10–20 (total) 1–2 (free)	300–500 mg/d in single or divided doses[†]	Average 24 h
Primidone	5–15	750–1,500 mg/d in 3 divided doses	8 h
Valproic acid	50–100	550–2,000 mg/d in 3 or 4 divided doses	Average 13 h

*Due to changes in volume of distribution and metabolism, dosages in pregnancy are often higher. The dosages must be individualized and may be dramatically higher than those listed.

[†]If a total dose greater than 300 mg is needed, dividing the dose will result in a more stable serum concentration.

patient's weight gain and fundal growth appear appropriate, regular ultrasound examinations for fetal growth assessment may be unnecessary. If there is any question concerning fetal growth, serial sonography should be performed to determine the estimated fetal weight and the amniotic fluid index. The benefit of routine antepartum fetal heart rate assessment in the management of patients with epilepsy remains unclear; it should be undertaken for the usual obstetric indications.

Labor and Delivery

With appropriate fetal monitoring, the availability of good obstetric anesthesia, and the ability to measure maternal anticonvulsant levels, vaginal delivery can be accomplished safely in the patient with a seizure disorder. Administration of anticonvulsant medications during a prolonged labor does, however, present a challenge. During labor, oral absorption of medications is erratic; if the patient vomits, it is almost negligible. When administration of anticonvulsants is necessary during labor, levels should be determined to help ascertain the appropriate dosage. If the patient's phenytoin level is normal, the usual daily dose may be administered intravenously. In patients with therapeutic serum levels of phenobarbital, a single 60–90-mg intramuscular dose will usually be sufficient for maintenance throughout labor and delivery.

Management is more complex in a patient taking carbamazepine, which is not manufactured in a parenteral form. Oral administration may be attempted, but if the patient has seizures or a preseizure aura, she is often best treated with a therapeutic dose of phenytoin to last through labor. The usual loading dosage is 10–15 mg/kg administered intravenously at a rate no faster than 50 mg/min. The patient's cardiac activity should be monitored because life-threatening dysrhythmias, although rare, may occur if the medication is administered too rapidly. Benzodiazepines also may be used for acute seizures, but they can cause early neonatal depression as well as maternal apnea (44). The delivery plan should include the availability of personnel to perform neonatal resuscitation if necessary.

Occasionally, seizures will be diagnosed for the first time during pregnancy. If the seizures occur in the third trimester, they may be confused with eclampsia. It is often difficult to distinguish eclampsia from an epileptic seizure. The patient may be hypertensive initially after an epileptic seizure and may exhibit some myoglobinuria secondary to muscle breakdown. The diagnosis often becomes clearer over time, but in either case action must be undertaken to prevent additional seizures. In these cases, it is best to assume the patient has eclampsia.

If a patient has recurrent generalized seizures (status epilepticus), immediate treatment is essential. Consultation with an anesthesiologist and a neurologist may be helpful. The drug of choice is intravenous phenytoin, which is highly effective, has a long duration of action, and has a low incidence of serious side effects. Alternatively, phenobarbital or diazepam may be used. These drugs cause respiratory depression, however, and the physician must have the ability to intubate the patient, if necessary, when they are used. Status epilepticus may lead to maternal and fetal hypoxemia. The patient should be placed on her left side if possible as this will increase uterine blood flow as well as decrease the risk of maternal aspiration. Oxygen should also be administered if possible. A theoretic risk of placental abruption also exists with prolonged seizures.

Postpartum Period

The levels of anticonvulsant medications may rise rapidly during the first few weeks postpartum and should be monitored frequently. One approach is to measure the serum level approximately 1 week postpartum to guide dosage adjustments. If the patient's medication dosages were increased during pregnancy, they will often need to be decreased rather rapidly after delivery to prepregnancy doses.

All of the major anticonvulsant medications cross into breast milk (44, 45). The use of these medications, however, is not a contraindication to breast-feeding unless the infant shows signs of excessive sedation. Primidone, phenobarbital, and benzodiazepines may have a sedative effect on the infant. If breast-feeding is suddenly stopped, some infants who had been exposed to these medications may experience withdrawal symptoms. These usually occur in the first few days after breast-feeding is stopped (46). Infants may need to be started on low-dose phenobarbital and undergo gradual withdrawal (46).

Women should be counseled about contraception postpartum. No method is contraindicated for patients with epilepsy, although if oral contraceptives are selected higher doses may be required. The patient should be encouraged to continue to receive care to control her condition and receive preconceptional care for a future anticipated pregnancy.

Summary

With close cooperation and communication among the obstetrician, neurologist, pediatrician, and patient, most women with idiopathic epilepsy who become pregnant will have an uneventful pregnancy with an excellent outcome. To optimize the neonatal outcome in a patient requiring medication, using a single drug at the lowest possible dose that keeps her free of seizures is preferable. The prevention of tonic–clonic seizures, however, is of utmost importance. Simple interventions such as avoiding sleep deprivation, having the patient take folic acid before conception, and giving the infant a vitamin K injection at birth will help optimize the outcome. There is an increase of congenital malformations in infants born to women with epilepsy; however, the incidence is low. Most women with epilepsy will experience normal pregnancy and labor and will have spontaneous vaginal deliveries of healthy babies.

References

1. Cramer JA, Jones EE. Reproductive function in epilepsy. Epilepsia 1991;32(Suppl 6):S19–S26 (Level III)
2. Back DJ, Bates M, Bowden A, Breckenridge AM, Hall MJ, Jones H, et al. The interaction of phenobarbital and other anticonvulsants with oral contraceptive steroid therapy. Contraception 1980;22:495–503 (Level III)
3. Coulam CB, Annegers JF. Do anticonvulsants reduce the efficacy of oral contraceptives? Epilepsia 1979;20: 519–526 (Level II-3)
4. Janz D, Schmidt D. Anti-epileptic drugs and failure of oral contraceptives. Lancet 1974;1:1113 Level (III)
5. Webber MP, Hauser WA, Ottman R, Annegers JF. Fertility in persons with epilepsy: 1935–1974. Epilepsia 1986; 27:746–752 (Level II-3)
6. Dansky LV, Andermann E, Andermann F. Marriage and fertility in epileptic patients. Epilepsia 1980;21:261–271 (Level II-3)
7. Yerby M, Koepsell T, Daling J. Pregnancy complications and outcomes in a cohort of women with epilepsy. Epilepsia 1985;26:631–635 (Level II–2)
8. Knight AH, Rhind EG. Epilepsy and pregnancy: a study of 153 pregnancies in 59 patients. Epilepsia 1975;16:99–110 (Level II–3)
9. Nelson KB, Ellenberg JH. Maternal seizure disorder, outcome of pregnancy, and neurologic abnormalities in the children. Neurology 1982;32:1247–1254 (Level II–2)
10. Källén B. A register study of maternal epilepsy and delivery outcome with special reference to drug use. Acta Neurol Scand 1986;73:253–259 (Level II–2)
11. Mastroiacovo P, Bertollini R, Licata D. Fetal growth in the offspring of epileptic women: results of an Italian multicentric cohort study. Acta Neurol Scand 1988;78:110–114 (Level II-2)
12. Hiilesmaa VK, Bardy A, Teramo K. Obstetric outcome in women with epilepsy. Am J Obstet Gynecol 1985;152: 499–504 (Level II–2)
13. Ogawa Y, Kaneko S, Otani K, Fukushima Y. Serum folic acid in epileptic mothers and their relationship to congenital malformations. Epilepsy Res 1991;8:75–78 (Level II–2)
14. Milunsky A, Jick H, Jick SS, Bruell CL, MacLaughlin DS, Rothman KJ, et al. Multivitamin/folic acid supplementation in early pregnancy reduces the prevalence of neural tube defects. JAMA 1989;262:2847–2852 (Level II–2)
15. Centers for Disease Control and Prevention. Recommendations for the use of folic acid to reduce the number of cases of spina bifida and other neural tube defects. MMWR 1992;41(RR14):1–7 (Level III)
16. Rosa FW. Spina bifida in infants of women treated with carbamazepine during pregnancy. N Engl J Med 1991;324: 674–677 (Level II–2)
17. Lindhout D, Schmidt D. In-utero exposure to valproate and neural tube defects. Lancet 1986;2:1392–1393 (Level II–2)
18. Yerby MS, Leavitt A, Erickson DM, McCormick KB, Loewenson RB, Sells CJ, et al. Antiepileptics and the development of congenital anomalies. Neurology 1992;42(Suppl 5):132–140 (Level II–2)
19. Mountain KR, Hirsh J, Gallus AS. Neonatal coagulation defect due to anticonvulsant drug treatment in pregnancy. Lancet 1970;1:265–268 (Level II–2)
20. Bleyer WA, Skinner AL. Fatal neonatal hemorrhage after maternal anticonvulsant therapy. JAMA 1976;235:626–627 (Level II–3)
21. Delgado-Escueta AV, Janz D. Consensus guidelines: preconception counseling, management, and care of the pregnant woman with epilepsy. Neurology 1992; 42(Suppl 5):149–160 (Level III)
22. Cornelissen M, Steegers-Theunissen R, Kollée L, Eskes T, Motohara K, Monnens L. Supplementation of vitamin K in pregnant women receiving anticonvulsant therapy prevents neonatal vitamin K deficiency. Am J Obstet Gynecol 1993;168:884–888 (Level II-2)

23. Friis B, Sardemann H. Neonatal hypocalcaemia after intrauterine exposure to anticonvulsant drugs. Arch Dis Child 1977;52:239–247 (Level II–3)

24. Nakane Y, Okuma T, Takahashi R, Sato Y, Wada T, Sato T, et al. Multi-institutional study on the teratogenicity and fetal toxicity of antiepileptic drugs: a report of a collaborative study group in Japan. Epilepsia 1980;21:663–680 (Level II–2)

25. Kaneko S, Otani K, Fukushima Y, Ogawa Y, Nomura Y, Ono T, et al. Teratogenicity of antiepileptic drugs: analysis of possible risk factors. Epilepsia 1988;29:459–467 (Level II–2)

26. Koch S, Lösche G, Jager-Romän E, Jakob S, Rating D, Deichl A, et al. Major and minor birth malformations and antiepileptic drugs. Neurology 1992;42(Suppl 5):83–88 (Level II–2)

27. Hanson JW, Smith DW. The fetal hydantoin syndrome. J Pediatr 1975;87:285–290 (Level II–3)

28. Hanson JW, Myrianthopoulos NC, Harvey MAS, Smith DW. Risks to the offspring of women treated with hydantoin anticonvulsants, with emphasis on the fetal hydantoin syndrome. J Pediatr 1976;89:662–668 (Level II–3 and Level II–2)

29. Gaily E, Granström M-L, Hiilesmaa V, Bardy A. Minor anomalies in offspring of epileptic mothers. J Pediatr 1988; 112:520–529 (Level II–2)

30. Kelly TE, Rein M, Edwards P. Teratogenicity of anticonvulsant drugs. IV. The association of clefting and epilepsy. Am J Med Genet 1984;19:451–458 (Level II–2)

31. Friis ML, Holm NV, Sindrup EH, Fogh-Andersen P, Hauge M. Facial clefts in sibs and children of epileptic patients. Neurology 1986;36:346–350 (Level II–2)

32. Hecht JT, Annegers JF, Kurland LT. Epilepsy and clefting disorders: lack of evidence of a familial association. Am J Med Genet 1989;33:244–247 (Level II–2)

33. DiLiberti JH, Farndon PA, Dennis NR, Curry CJR. The fetal valproate syndrome. Am J Med Genet 1984;19:473–481 (Level II–3)

34. Ardinger HH, Atkin JF, Blackston RD, Elsas LJ, Clarren SK, Livingstone S, et al. Verification of the fetal valproate syndrome phenotype. Am J Med Genet 1988;29:171–185 (Level II–3)

35. Jäger-Roman E, Deichl A, Jakob S, Hartmann A-M, Koch S, Rating D, et al. Fetal growth, major malformations, and minor anomalies in infants born to women receiving valproic acid. J Pediatr 1986;108:997–1004 (Level II–2)

36. Wegner C, Nau H. Alteration of embryonic folate metabolism by valproic acid during organogenesis: implications for mechanism of teratogenesis. Neurology 1992;42(Suppl 5):17–24 (Level I)

37. Jones KL, Lacro RV, Johnson KA, Adams J. Pattern of malformations in the children of women treated with carbamazepine during pregnancy. N Engl J Med 1989;320: 1661–1666 (Level II–2)

38. Finnell RH, Buehler BA, Kerr BM, Ager PL, Levy RH. Clinical and experimental studies linking oxidative metabolism to phenytoin-induced teratogenesis. Neurology 1992;42(Suppl 5):25–31 (Level I–2)

39. Desmond MM, Schwanecke RP, Wilson GS, Yasunaga S, Burgdorff I. Maternal barbiturate utilization and neonatal withdrawal symptomatology. J Pediatr 1972;80:190–197 (Level II–3)

40. Dessens AB, Boer K, Koppe JG, van de Poll NE, Cohen-Kettenis PT. Studies on long-lasting consequences of prenatal exposure to anticonvulsant drugs. Acta Paediatr Suppl 1994;404:54–64 (Level III)

41. Reinisch JM, Sanders, SA, Mortensen EL, Rubin DB. In utero exposure to phenobarbital and intelligence deficits in adult men. JAMA 1995;274:1518–1525 (Level II-2)

42. Granström M-L, Gaily E. Psychomotor development in children of mothers with epilepsy. Neurology 1992; 42(Suppl 5):144–148 (Level III)

43. Annegers JF, Hauser WA, Elveback LR, Anderson VE, Kurland LT. Seizure disorders in offspring of parents with a history of seizures—a maternal–paternal difference? Epilepsia 1976;17:1–9 (Level II–2)

44. Yerby MS. Problems and management of the pregnant woman with epilepsy. Epilepsia 1987;28(Suppl 3):S29–S36 (Level III)

45. Kaneko S, Sato T, Suzuki K. The levels of anticonvulsants in breast milk. Br J Clin Pharmacol 1979;7:624–627 (Level II–3)

46. Knott C, Reynolds F, Clayden G. Infantile spasms on weaning from breast milk containing anticonvulsants. Lancet 1987;2:272–273 (Level III)

The references in this bulletin are graded according to the method outlined by the U.S. Preventive Services Task Force:

I	Evidence obtained from at least one properly designed randomized controlled trial
II-1	Evidence obtained from well-designed controlled trials without randomization
II-2	Evidence obtained from well-designed cohort or case–control analytic studies, preferably from more than one center or research group
II-3	Evidence obtained from multiple time series, with or without intervention, or dramatic results in uncontrolled experiments
III	Opinions of respected authorities, based on clinical experience, descriptive studies, or reports of expert committees

Other publications from ACOG:

- **Committee Opinions**, focused updates on emerging areas
- **Practice Patterns**, evidence-based guidelines
- **Criteria Sets**, baseline guidelines for review of diagnostic and management procedures

ISSN 1074-8628

The American College of Obstetricians and Gynecologists
409 12th Street, SW
PO Box 96920
Washington, DC 20090-6920

12345/09876

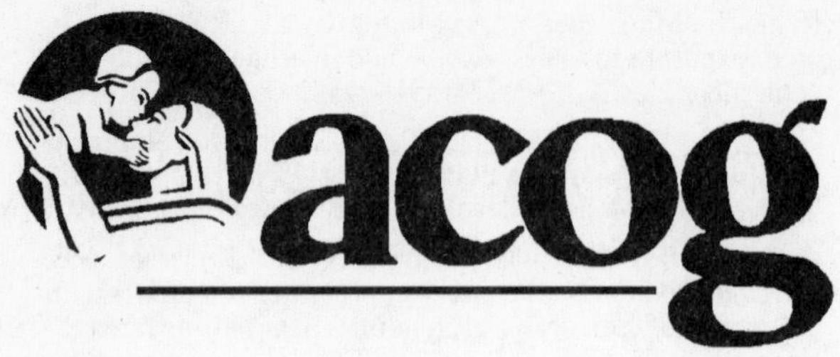

Number 204—April 1995
(Replaces #75, March 1984)

Technical Bulletin
An Educational Aid to Obstetrician–Gynecologists

Septic Shock

Septic shock is a response to infection resulting in peripheral circulatory failure and inadequate tissue perfusion. This condition ultimately leads to cell dysfunction or death. While this definition is accurate, its clinical utility is not readily apparent. There have been various terms recommended to describe serious infections and their inflammatory response; however, they tend to be inconsistent and confusing. Consistent terminology is crucial to determine both appropriate treatment and prognosis in individual cases of serious infections and also to establish reproducible groups of infected patients to compare efficacy of new treatments. Recently, a consensus conference agreed on a set of definitions that could be applied to patients with serious infections (Table 1) (1). These definitions constitute a continuum in severity of infection, from simple sepsis to septic shock with multiple organ dysfunction.

Septicemia is defined by the Centers for Disease Control and Prevention as systemic disease associated with the presence and persistence of pathogenic microorganisms or their toxins in the blood. It is the 13th leading cause of death in the United States, resulting in 200,000 deaths per year and $5 billion to $10 billion in direct annual expenditures. The Centers for Disease Control and Prevention's National Hospital Discharge Summary indicates that the septicemia rate increased from 73.6/100,000 persons to 175.9/100,000 from 1979 to 1987, a 139% increase (2). This trend was seen in all geographic areas in the United States and in all age groups, particularly among persons over 65 years of age. Even when adjusted for the upward trend in population age, there was a 111% increase from 1979 to 1987 in this age range. Factors that account for this increased rate include an increased number of immunocompromised persons (eg, those infected with human immunodeficiency virus [HIV], organ transplant recipients, and those undergoing chemotherapy); increased use of invasive medical devices, both inside and outside of the hospital; and improved ability to diagnose septicemia.

The incidence of bacteremia in obstetric–gynecologic patients has been documented infrequently. One study reported a 0.7% incidence of bacteremia among all patients admitted to an obstetrics–gynecology ward in a large county hospital (3). Of the 144 documented instances of bacteremia, there were four deaths, all of which occurred in patients who had clinical evidence of septic

TABLE 1. CLINICAL DEFINITIONS OF SERIOUS INFECTIONS

State	Definition
Infection	Microbial phenomenon characterized by an inflammatory response to the presence of microorganisms or the invasion of normally sterile host tissue by those organisms
Bacteremia	The presence of viable bacteria in the blood
Sepsis (simple)	The systemic response to infection, manifested by two or more of the following conditions as a result of the infection: (1) temperature >38°C or <36°C; (2) heart rate > 90 beats per minute; (3) respiratory rate >20/min or $Paco_2$ <32 mm Hg; and (4) leukocyte count >12,000/mm^3, <4,000 mm^3, or >10% immature (band) forms.
Severe sepsis	Sepsis associated with organ dysfunction, hypoperfusion, or hypotension. Hypoperfusion and perfusion abnormalities may include, but are not limited to, lactic acidosis, oliguria, or an acute alteration in mental status.
Septic shock	Sepsis with hypotension despite adequate fluid resuscitation along with the presence of perfusion abnormalities that may include, but are not limited to, lactic acidosis, oliguria, or an acute alteration in mental status. Patients who are receiving inotropic or vasopressor agents may not be hypotensive at the time that perfusion abnormalities are measured
Multiple organ dysfunction	Presence of altered organ function in an acutely ill patient such that homeostasis cannot be maintained without intervention

Modified from Bone RC, Balk RA, Cerra FR, Dellinger RP, Fein AM, Knaus WA, et al. ACCP/SCCM consensus conference: definitions for sepsis and organ failure and guidelines for the use of innovative therapies in sepsis. Chest 1992;101:1646

shock with multiorgan system dysfunction prior to death. In a separate report of bacteremia in an indigent obstetric population, the incidence of documented bacteremia was 0.75%, with no deaths reported (4). When septic shock does develop, permanent disability may result. Mortality occurs in 20–50% of cases (3).

Pathogenesis of Septic Shock

Septic shock usually results from infection with gram-negative organisms, although it also may result from gram-positive bacteria, fungi, and probably viruses. Gram-negative organisms are responsible for 30–80% of all cases of septic shock, while 6–24% of cases result from gram-positive organisms.

The development of gram-negative septic shock is initiated by a lipopolysaccharide component of the gram-negative cell wall, termed *endotoxin*. Endotoxin is composed of a series of antigenically variable oligosaccharides often termed *O antigen*. Internal to these variable oligosaccharides are core oligosaccharides, which are antigenically similar across different species of gram-negative bacteria. The core oligosaccharides are bound to a highly conserved lipid component, lipid A. It is the lipid A component that is responsible for much of the toxicity of endotoxin. Recent study has determined that endotoxin can stimulate macrophages to produce cytokines, particularly tumor necrosis factor (TNF, formerly called cachectin) and interleukins (IL), which are in large part responsible for the myriad of subsequent events that appear clinically as septic shock. It is this indirect activation of the host's own inflammatory systems that is responsible for most of the serious clinical manifestations seen in septic shock.

Endotoxin (as well as certain exotoxins and the cell wall of many gram-positive bacteria) can activate at least three separate pathways in the host: 1) the complement pathway, 2) the coagulation cascade, and 3) cytokine production by macrophages. The mechanisms by which activation of these pathways may cause the pathophysiologic changes seen in septic shock are important in understanding many of the concepts involved in the management of septic shock.

Cytokines are a group of soluble intercellular signaling molecules that have a wide spectrum of effects. It appears that TNF plays an important role in the development of septic shock. Monocytes/macrophages incubated with endotoxin will produce TNF within 40 minutes (5). Injection of lipopolysaccharide into mice causes release of TNF. In addition, direct injection of TNF results in changes typical of septic shock (eg, adult respiratory distress syndrome [ARDS], acute tubular necrosis, adrenal hemorrhage, and bowel changes typical of endotoxic shock) (6, 7). The importance of the role of TNF in septic shock is further supported by data demonstrating that the lethal effects of bacteremia can be reversed by administering monoclonal antibody against TNF in baboons (8). Other cytokines, including IL-1, IL-6, and IL-8; interferon-gamma; and granulocyte-stimulating factor, have been isolated in elevated concentrations in the serum of humans with septic shock. Their role in the pathogenesis of septic shock appears to be important, as antagonists to these cytokines have been associated with improved survival. Certain cytokines directly cause toxic effects, while others may potentiate the effects of TNF.

Microbiology and Clinical Settings of Septic Shock

Most clinical series of septic shock (including obstetric septic shock) demonstrate that gram-negative facultative anaerobic organisms, particularly the Enterobacteriaceae, are the most frequently isolated. Of these, *Escherichia coli* is found in approximately 50% of all cases, with *Klebsiella* species, *Serratia* species, and *Enterobacter* species accounting for 30%. The remaining 20% of cases result from gram-positive infections (eg, *Streptococci* and *Staphylococci*) and obligate anaerobic infections (eg, *Prevotella* species [formerly *Bacteroides* species], *Bacteroides fragilis*, *Peptostreptococci* species, *Clostridium perfringens*, and *Fusobacterium* species).

The clinical circumstances surrounding obstetric septic shock vary. Endometritis after cesarean delivery is the most common predisposing infection leading to obstetric septic shock and is responsible for up to 85% of cases in some studies. Other infections that can lead to septic shock include endometritis following vaginal delivery (1–4%), urinary tract infection (1–4%), septic abortion (1–2%), chorioamnionitis (0.5–1%), toxic shock syndrome (less than 1%), and necrotizing fasciitis (less than 1%) (9). Prolonged rupture of membranes (over 48 hours), retained products of conception, and insertion of instruments into the genitourinary tract have all been associated with septic shock (10).

Clinical Manifestations of Septic Shock

Septic shock may affect a number of organ systems, including the cardiovascular system, the pulmonary system, and the renal system; hematologic and neurologic effects may also occur (Table 2). In pregnancy, the fetus may be affected.

Cardiovascular Effects

There is a continuum of change in the hemodynamic pattern of patients with septic shock, beginning with a hyperdynamic vasodilated state ("warm shock") and progressing to a vasoconstricted state with diminished cardiac output ("cold shock") and eventually to an irreversible state of shock. Septic shock progresses through three clinical stages (preshock, early shock, and late shock), each accompanied by specific changes in the cardiopulmonary systems (11). Preshock is characterized by tachypnea and respiratory alkalosis (Pco_2 less than 30 mm Hg), often the first sign of impending sepsis. This tachypnea is associated with a moderate hyperdynamic state (increased cardiac output and a diminished systemic vascular resistance [SVR]) with little change in blood pressure. This is the stage at which intervention is most successful and cardiovascular changes improve with volume expansion.

Early shock state displays a more marked hyperdynamic state, characterized by hypotension (systolic pressure less than 60 mm Hg) which results from a dramatic decrease in SVR which may overwhelm the increase in cardiac output. Systemic vascular resistance as low as 400 dynes/s/cm^{-5} may be seen. Patients who have a prolonged early shock state (over 24 hours) are apparently less likely to survive, presumably because the inciting bacteria have not been adequately controlled (12).

The late shock state is characterized by a decreasing cardiac index as a result of dysfunctional left ventricular performance and an increase in SVR. Blood pressure remains low and is refractory to attempts at volume expansion. Tissue perfusion is inadequate, and inotropic and vasoactive agents are necessary to maintain blood pressure. Reduced oxygen delivery and tissue extraction result in anaerobic metabolism, lactate accumulation, and metabolic acidosis, pulmonary shunting with hypoxemia, decreased uterine perfusion and fetal acidosis in pregnant women, and other end-organ hypoperfusion. This composite is demonstrated by the advanced clinical picture of hypotension: cold and clammy skin, hypoxemia, oliguria, and altered mentation.

There is strong experimental and clinical evidence that the major cause of diminished myocardial function is a result of a circulating myocardial depressant factor pro-

TABLE 2. COMMON CLINICAL MANIFESTATIONS OF SEPTIC SHOCK

Organ System	Clinical Findings	Mechanism
Cardiovascular		
Hypotension	Systolic BP <60 mm Hg	Vasodilation Decreased circulating volume due to increased vascular permeability
Cardiac dysfunction	Increase in cardiac index (early) Decrease in cardiac index (late) Decrease in ejection fraction	Myocardial depressant factor Decreased myocardial blood flow
Pulmonary (ARDS)	Bilateral diffuse infiltrates on CXR Hypoxemia Normal PCWP (<18 mm Hg)	Increased vascular permeability Direct endothelial damage
Renal		
Oliguria	<30 ml/h	Hypotension and renal vasoconstriction
ATN		Prolonged cortical hypoxia secondary to decreased renal blood flow
Interstitial nephritis		Immune mechanism
Hematologic		
DIC	Elevated FDP, PT, PTT Decreased platelets and fibrinogen Spontaneous bleeding (uncommon)	Endotoxin activation of Hageman factor
Leukocytosis	>20,000 cells/mm^3	Demargination Neutrophil-releasing substance
Neurologic (mental status changes)	Somnolence, coma, combativeness (uncommon, usually due to hypoxia)	Decreased cerebral blood flow Hypoxia
Fever	Temperature >38°C	Direct endotoxin/TNF effect on hypothalamus

BP indicates blood pressure; ARDS, adult respiratory distress syndrome; CXR, chest X-ray; PCWP, pulmonary capillary wedge pressure; ATN, acute tubular necrosis; DIC, disseminated intravascular coagulopathy; FDP, fibrin degradation products; PT, prothrombin time; PTT, partial thromboplastin time; TNF, tumor necrosis factor.

Pearlman MD, Faro S. Obstetric septic shock: a pathophysiologic basis for management. Clin Obstet Gynecol 1990;33:485

duced by the pancreas (13). There is also speculation that endotoxin contributes to myocardial dysfunction, either directly or by release of other mediators that depress myocardial function activities. Also, investigators have demonstrated diminished oxygen extraction by the myocardium in septic patients, which may reflect an anatomic shunting of myocardial blood flow away from the capillary beds, resulting in further myocardial depression (13).

Adult Respiratory Distress Syndrome and Oxygen Use

Sepsis is the most frequent predisposing factor of ARDS, and these two disease states in combination result in a mortality rate exceeding 80% (14). Various definitions have been used to describe ARDS; one that incorporates both the pathophysiology and the clinical sequelae is most useful. Adult respiratory distress syndrome is characterized pathophysiologically by increased pulmonary capillary permeability resulting in increased extravascular lung water, a widening of the alveolar–arterial O_2 tension gradient (A-a gradient), and decreased pulmonary compliance. This leads to the clinical syndrome of hypoxemia (Po_2 less than 65 mm Hg) despite efforts at increased oxygenation (40–50% O_2 by mask). Diffuse bilateral infiltrates are present on chest X-ray consistent with pulmonary edema without evidence of volume overload or cardiac failure (pulmonary capillary wedge pressure [PCWP] less than 18 mm Hg).

Both macrophage-produced IL-1 and TNF have been implicated in causing the altered vascular permeability seen in ARDS. In addition, macrophages may produce other substances (lysosomes, prostaglandins, and oxyradicals) that cause further damage to endothelial cells and contribute to the altered respiratory mechanics and increased vascular permeability seen in ARDS. The increased A-a gradient is generally not a result of increased intraalveolar fluid, as might be intuitively expected. An anatomic redistribution of blood flow (shunting) away from affected areas of low oxygen tension has been demonstrated to be the predominant mechanism causing arterial hypoxemia. Indeed, shunting away from areas of low alveolar Po_2 tension is seen more frequently in survivors of ARDS, suggesting that this is a protective mechanism and that nonsurvivors do not appropriately regulate pulmonary blood flow (14).

Pregnancy-Specific Complications

Most of the available data regarding the relationship of septic shock and pregnancy come from animal models. One study compared the effect of injecting *E. coli* endotoxin in pregnant and nonpregnant animals (15). The pregnant animals died significantly more quickly (3.5 hours versus 14 hours), had a more pronounced metabolic acidosis, and exhibited a significant diminution in uterine tissue oxygenation compared with the nonpregnant animals.

Another study evaluated the effect of "sublethal" endotoxin administration in pregnant baboons, which resulted in increased uterine activity followed by profound maternal hypotension and metabolic acidosis (16). The fetal heart rate declined steadily after injection even prior to the onset of maternal hypotension. All fetuses had profound metabolic acidosis at 2 hours, and all died within 6 hours without concomitant maternal death. Abruptio placentae and cerebral hemorrhage were also seen in two fetuses. These profoundly adverse fetal effects appear to result from altered uteroplacental blood flow (ie, selective shunting away from the uterine vasculature). This shunting and diminished gas exchange appear to be the major effectors of fetal acidosis.

An additional study showed that the fetus is particularly resistant to the direct effects of endotoxin (17). In a model using pregnant ewes, the median lethal dose of endotoxin in the fetus was 10 times that of the mother. This resistance of the fetus and neonate to direct endotoxin effect likely relates to an immature ability of the fetal immune system to mount a vasoactive response.

Renal Effects

The effect of sepsis on altered renal function ranges over a wide spectrum from minimal proteinuria with no changes in renal function to acute tubular necrosis, renal failure, and death. Diminished effective circulating volume and hypotension both contribute to renal hypoperfusion with ischemia resulting in destruction of the more sensitive cortical portion of the kidney and acute tubular necrosis (18). Another potential mechanism of renal damage associated with sepsis involves immune complex deposition (ie, glomerular deposits of immunoglobulin G, immunoglobulin M, complement 3, and bacterial antigen) resulting in a diffuse proliferative glomerulonephritis. Antigen–antibody complexes may also accumulate in the interstitium, resulting in an interstitial nephritis.

It is critically important to remember that the improper use or monitoring of nephrotoxic antibiotics in septic patients, particularly aminoglycosides, may potentiate the adverse effects of sepsis, hypotension, and immune reactions on renal function. For example, critically ill patients taking aminoglycosides should have levels of the medication in serum determined following the third or fourth dose. Peak levels in serum (drawn 30–60 minutes after administration of the medication) should be between 5 and 10 μg/ml for gentamicin or tobramycin and between 15 and 30 μg/ml for amikacin to ensure adequate antimicrobial levels while reducing the likelihood of renal toxicity and ototoxicity. Many experts believe that monitoring trough levels in serum (drawn just prior to administration of the medication) is also helpful in reducing the likelihood of toxicity; optimal trough levels for gentamicin and tobramycin are less than 1–2 μg/ml and for amikacin, less than 10 μg/ml. Determining levels of medication in serum is often helpful to guide changes in dosing, frequency of administration, or both.

Hematologic Effects

Disseminated intravascular coagulopathy (DIC) occurs with regularity in patients with sepsis, and at the same time, serious infections are the most frequent cause of DIC. Activation of the coagulation cascade results in intravascular thrombin generation, consumption of platelets and coagulation factors, fibrin deposition within small vessels, and fibrinolysis. In severe DIC, death can result from organ necrosis secondary to extensive fibrin deposition in the microvasculature, the so-called generalized Schwartzman reaction (19).

The most likely mechanism of initiation of DIC is direct endotoxin activation of Hageman factor (factor XII) with subsequent initiation of the intrinsic coagulation cascade (20). Also, direct endothelial damage with exposure of the basement membrane can activate the intrinsic pathway. Recently, attention has been drawn to production of procoagulants by the monocyte/macrophage system (11). Monocyte-produced TNF may intermediate and induce endothelial expression of tissue procoagulant activity and activation of the extrinsic pathway. With an endotoxin-initiated mechanism of intrinsic pathway activation, it is recognized that DIC is a much more frequent sequela of gram-negative than gram-positive sepsis.

Clinically, this syndrome can appear with hemorrhage, thrombosis, or microangiopathic hemolysis. Some patients will have no clinical evidence of DIC and only altered coagulation values (biochemical DIC). Laboratory findings include decreased platelets and fibrinogen with elevated prothrombin time, partial thromboplastin time, and fibrin degradation products. Red blood cell schistocytes can also be seen, as they are damaged passing through the narrowed thrombus-laden microvasculature. Treatment with platelets, coagulation factors, and fibrinogen replacement is generally reserved for those patients with clinically significant bleeding.

The most common hematologic change seen in sepsis is neutrophilic leukocytosis with many band forms (left shift). This is due to demargination of leukocytes from vessel walls and release of immature leukocytes from marrow storage pools. Endotoxin can stimulate the release of neutrophil-releasing substance (presumably activated complement, C3a), which is the substance responsible for the leukocyte release (21). Pronounced neutrophilia (more than 50,000/mm^3), sometimes referred to as the leukemoid reaction, is caused by an exaggerated release of leukocytes due to the release of several sialated glycoproteins called colony-stimulating factors. These substances increase granulocyte production by activating committed stem cells. Neutropenia, in contrast, is much less common and tends to occur in infants, the elderly, alcoholics, and others with poor marrow reserves. Leukopenia in the face of sepsis is a poor prognostic sign.

Management

The initial steps taken to resuscitate the septic patient are likely to be the most important steps in preventing mortality both for the patient and, during pregnancy, for the fetus. The management of septic shock can be divided into seven steps (see the box). The initial components of primary concern are ensuring adequate oxygenation and effective cardiac output and administering broad-spectrum antibiotics. Consultation with specialists in infections or critical care medicine is frequently helpful in assisting in the management of these often complex cases.

Pulse oximetry measures oxyhemoglobin saturation by means of a photosensor applied noninvasively to the fingertip, nose, toes, or earlobe. Pulse oximetry saturation (Spo_2) correlates predictably with arterial oxygen saturation (Sao_2) over a wide range of oxygen saturations (pulse oximetry has a ±2% accuracy), but it is limited in circumstances of low hemoglobin or impaired local perfusion. This technology can be quite useful in measuring oxygen saturation when hypoxemia is suspected or continuously monitoring oxygen saturation in the patient who has begun oxygen therapy. In the patient with sepsis and no underlying disease, oxygen therapy should be started if there is documented arterial hypoxemia: Sao_2 less than 90%, Spo_2 less than 92%, or Pao_2 less than 60 mm Hg. In some patients, such as those with underlying cardiac disease, oxygen therapy might be started sooner. The Spo_2 can be titrated to keep pulse oximetry in a target range of 95–97% for cardiac patients with a myocardial infarction or angina, 90–92% for patients with chronic obstructive

Management of Septic Shock

1. Maintain adequate oxygenation.
2. Maintain adequate circulating volume.
3. Transfer to intensive care unit.
4. Obtain appropriate laboratory data.
5. Institute inotropic or vasopressor therapy to maximize cardiac performance.
6. Administer appropriate antimicrobial agents.
7. Surgically remove infected abscess or drain abscess or both, if necessary.

pulmonary disease and CO_2 retention, and 92–94% for all other patients.

Fluid resuscitation can begin with the rapid infusion of crystalloid solution (1–2 L of lactated Ringer's injection or normal saline over 15–20 minutes) and may begin without invasive hemodynamic monitoring. However, because of the frequent need for large volumes of crystalloid solution and the risk of pulmonary edema, ARDS, and myocardial dysfunction, most subsequent hemodynamic therapy should be performed with the aid of a flow-directed pulmonary artery catheter (Swan-Ganz catheter). An understanding of the use of flow-directed pulmonary artery catheters is critical to the management of septic shock; this has been described elsewhere (22). One useful guide to further fluid resuscitation is the "7–3 rule." Crystalloid solution is administered at 10 ml/min for 15 minutes. If the PCWP does not increase by 3 mm Hg, the fluid bolus is repeated. However, if the PCWP increases by 7 mm Hg or more, the fluid bolus is held. If the PCWP increases by 3–7 mm Hg, continued fluid management is based on several factors, including PCWP, blood pressure, cardiac output, oxygenation, and pulmonary status. Optimal PCWP is in the range of 12–16 mm Hg and can often be achieved with fluid therapy alone. Appropriate laboratory tests should be performed (see the box).

If after appropriate fluid administration cardiovascular function remains suboptimal, vasoactive or inotropic agents or both are necessary. Dopamine is the initial drug of choice for improving cardiac function and blood pressure in patients with septic shock (23). The effects of dopamine are numerous and dose dependent. At low doses (1–3 μg/kg/min), dopamine reacts with dopaminergic receptors, causing vasodilation and increased blood flow in the renal, mesenteric, coronary, and cerebral vasculature. At intermediate doses (5–10 μg/kg/min), beta-adrenergic effects are predominant, which increase myocardial contractility and improve cardiac function. At high doses (more than 20 μg/kg/min), the principal effect is alpha-adrenergic, and vasoconstriction is seen in all vascular beds (including the uterine vasculature). At these high doses, fetal hypoxia is seen with regularity (24).

If dopamine does not adequately support blood pressure, an attempt should be made to differentiate whether this is due to persistent vasodilation (blood pressure less than 80 mm Hg with SVR less than 1,400 dynes/s/cm^{-5}) or a depressed left ventricular function curve (low left ventricular stroke work index despite adequate PCWP) (10). If a depressed myocardium is the major cause, inotropic therapy (eg, dobutamine or epinephrine) should be started; if persistent vasodilation is the problem, a peripheral vasoconstrictor (phenylephrine or norepinephrine) should be started. Table 3 lists common medications and dosages used for managing septic shock.

Frequently Ordered Laboratory Tests for Serious Infections

- Complete blood count, including leukocyte differential and platelet count
- Electrolytes
- Arterial blood gases
- Blood urea nitrogen and creatinine
- Urinalysis
- Prothrombin time, partial thromboplastin time, fibrinogen
- Serum lactate
- Cultures with antibiotic sensitivities
  - Blood
  - Urine
  - Endometrium (if endometritis suspected)
  - Amniotic fluid (if chorioamnionitis suspected)
  - Wound or episiotomy site (if suspected)
  - Other sites (eg, sputum, drains) if appropriate
- Chest X-ray
- Adjunctive imaging studies as necessary (eg, computed tomography, magnetic resonance imaging, abdominal X-ray)

Modified from Pearlman MD, Faro S. Obstetric septic shock: a pathophysiologic basis for management. Clin Obstet Gynecol 1990;33:488

Oxygenation problems are frequent in septic shock, with the development of ARDS in 30–40% of patients. The progression to respiratory failure requiring mechanical ventilation is common in these patients, although respiratory failure can also be seen in septic shock without ARDS. This latter situation is most likely due to respiratory muscle fatigue, when energy supply fails to meet the enormous energy demands seen in septic shock. The decision to initiate mechanical ventilation in sepsis depends on the presence of respiratory failure. A PO_2 less than 50 mm Hg on room air, or a PCO_2 over 50 mm Hg with a decreasing pH are general indicators of respiratory failure. In patients on mechanical ventilation with ARDS, positive end-expiratory pressure is frequently necessary to maintain adequate oxygenation (O_2 saturation greater than 90%). This produces positive pressure across the alveoli and airway walls at end expiration, which allows otherwise collapsed alveoli to be recruited for oxygen exchange, increasing the functional respiratory capacity.

Eradication of the infecting organisms(s) is of primary importance in the management of septic shock. Prompt administration of appropriate antibiotics and, when necessary, extirpation of infected tissue are critical in improving patient survival rates. Because of the polymicrobial nature of pelvic infections, broad-spectrum coverage is necessary in such critically ill patients. There

TABLE 3. COMMONLY USED VASOACTIVE AND INOTROPI DRUGS

Agent	Usual Dose
Dopamine	1–3 µg/kg/min (dopaminergic range, "renal dose")
	5–10 µg/kg/min (beta-adrenergic)
	>20 µg/kg/min (alpha-adrenergic)
Isoproterenol	1–4 µg/min
Dobutamine	2–20 µg/kg/min
Norepinephrine	2–8 µg/min
Phenylephrine	20–200 µg/min
Epinephrine	1–8 µg/min

Modified from Pearlman MD, Faro S. Obstetric septic shock: a pathophysiologic basis for management. Clin Obstet Gynecol 1990;33:488

are numerous effective antibiotics that can be used to treat septic shock. A combination of ampicillin, clindamycin, and gentamicin has long been the initial treatment for pelvic infections. Imipenam and cilastatin combined with vancomycin has been successfully used in many centers for the treatment of polymicrobial septic shock. The extended-spectrum penicillins in combination with aminoglycosides (eg, ticarcillin and tobramycin) have also been used with comparable success rates. As there is real potential for nephrotoxicity and ototoxicity with the use of aminoglycosides, peak and trough levels should be obtained when this class of drugs is used. With the vast array of antimicrobial agents available, there are many other regimens that are equally appropriate in the treatment of septic shock, and the choice of antibiotic for these critically ill patients should be made with an understanding of the usual pattern and sensitivity pattern of the organisms involved in pelvic infection in the physician's institution.

There are clinical circumstances in which the treatment of septic shock requires surgical intervention. Investigators have demonstrated that 40% of septic obstetric patients required surgical removal of infected products of conception, and all of these patients survived (10). If chorioamnionitis is present in the septic patient, prompt delivery is a critical part of overall treatment. The route of delivery depends on the overall clinical picture (eg, stability of the patient, fetal well-being, and inducibility of the cervix). Delivery usually is not indicated in the septic pregnant patient in whom the pregnancy is not the source of the infection (eg, pyelonephritis).

In the postpartum septic patient whose condition is worsening despite appropriate antibiotic therapy, a thorough search for an infected nidus should be performed. Possible infected sites include retained products of conception, uterine microabscesses, pelvic abscess, wound infection, and septic pelvic vein thrombosis. Similarly, in the postoperative gynecologic patient, the possibility of cuff abscess, tuboovarian abscess, or, rarely, ovarian abscess should be considered. Operative intervention with the removal of infected tissue or drainage of abscesses should be performed.

Summary

Septic shock remains an important cause of death and permanent disability in obstetric and gynecologic patients. Prompt recognition and diagnosis are critical to optimizing outcome. A thorough understanding of the pathophysiologic mechanisms operative in septic shock is important in treating these critically ill women. Immediate attention to oxygenation and hemodynamic stability is of paramount importance in effecting the best possible outcome. The use of sophisticated technology, including pulmonary artery monitoring and mechanical ventilation is frequently necessary, requiring intensive monitoring. Consultation with practitioners experienced in the management of septic shock is often helpful.

REFERENCES

1. Bone RC, Balk RA, Cerra FR, Dellinger RP, Fein AM, Knaus WA, et al. ACCP/SCCM consensus conference: definitions for sepsis and organ failure and guidelines for the use of innovative therapies in sepsis. Chest 1992; 101:1644–1655
2. Centers for Disease Control. Increase in national hospital discharge survey rates for septicemia—United States, 1979–1987. MMWR 1990;39:31–34
3. Ledger WJ, Norman M, Gee C, Lewis W. Bacteremia on an obstetric–gynecologic service. Am J Obstet Gynecol 1975;121:205–212
4. Blanco JD, Gibbs RS, Castandeda YS. Bacteremia in obstetrics: clinical course. Obstet Gynecol 1981;58:621–625
5. Hofsli E, Bakke O, Nonstad U, Espevik T. A flow cytometric and immunofluorescence microscopic study of tumor necrosis factor production and localization in human monocytes. Cell Immunol 1989;122:405–415
6. Remick DG, Kunkel RG, Larrick JW, Kunkel SL. Acute *in vivo* effects of human recombinant tumor necrosis factor. Lab Invest 1987;56:583–590
7. Tracey KJ, Beutler B, Lowrey SF, Merryweather J, Wolpe S, Milsark IW, et al. Shock and tissue injury induced by recombinant human cachectin. Science 1986;234:470–474
8. Tracey KJ, Fong Y, Hesse DG, Manogue KR, Lee AT, Kuo GC, et al. Anti-cachectin/TNF monoclonal antibodies prevent septic shock during lethal bacteremia. Nature 1987; 330:662–664
9. Gonik B. Septic shock in obstetrics. Clin Perinatol 1986; 13:741–754
10. Lee W, Clark SL, Cotton DB, Gonik B, Phelan J, Faro S, et al. Septic shock during pregnancy. Am J Obstet Gynecol 1988;159:410–416

11. Harris RL, Musher DM, Bloom K, Gathe J, Rice L, Sugarman B, et al. Manifestations of sepsis. Arch Intern Med 1987;147:1895–1906

12. Parker MM, Shelhamer JH, Natanson C, Alling DW, Parrillo JE. Serial cardiovascular variables in survivors and nonsurvivors of human septic shock: heart rate as an early predictor of prognosis. Crit Care Med 1987;15:923–929

13. Cunnion RE, Parillo JE. Myocardial dysfunction in sepsis. Crit Care Clin 1989;5:99–118

14. Bersten A, Sibbald WJ. Acute lung injury in septic shock. Crit Care Clin 1989;5:49–79

15. Beller FK, Schmidt EH, Holzgreve W, Hauss J. Septicemia during pregnancy: a study in different species of experimental animals. Am J Obstet Gynecol 1985;151:967–975

16. Morishima HO, Niemann WH, James LS. Effects of endotoxin on the pregnant baboon and fetus. Am J Obstet Gynecol 1978;131:899–902

17. Bech-Jansen P, Brinkman CR III, Johnson GH, Assali NS. Circulatory shock in pregnant sheep. I. Effects of endotoxin on uteroplacental and fetal umbilical circulation. Am J Obstet Gynecol 1972;112:1084–1094

18. Lucas CE. The renal response to acute injury and sepsis. Surg Clin North Am 1976;56:953–975

19. McKay DG, Jewett JF, Reid DE. Endotoxin shock and the generalized Schwartzman reaction in pregnancy. Am J Obstet Gynecol 1959;78:546–566

20. Beller FK. Sepsis and coagulation. Clin Obstet Gynecol 1985;28:46–52

21. Edwards RL, Rickles FR. Macrophage procoagulants. Prog Hemost Thromb 1984;7:183–209

22. American College of Obstetricians and Gynecologists. Invasive hemodynamic monitoring in obstetrics and gynecology. ACOG Technical Bulletin 175. Washington, DC: ACOG, 1992

23. Boyd JL III, Stanford GG, Chernow B. The pharmacotherapy of septic shock. Crit Care Clin 1989;5:133–150

24. Rolbin SH, Levinson G, Shnider SM, Biehl DR, Wright RG. Dopamine treatment of spinal hypotension decreases uterine blood flow in the pregnant ewe. Anesthesiology 1979;51:36–40

This Technical Bulletin was developed under the direction of the Committee on Technical Bulletins of the American College of Obstetricians and Gynecologists as an educational aid to obstetricians and gynecologists. The committee wishes to thank Mark D. Pearlman, MD, for his assistance in the development of this bulletin. This Technical Bulletin does not define a standard of care, nor is it intended to dictate an exclusive course of management. It presents recognized methods and techniques of clinical practice for consideration by obstetrician–gynecologists for incorporation into their practices. Variations of practice taking into account the needs of the individual patient, resources, and limitations unique to the institution or type of practice may be appropriate. Portions of this text are modified from Pearlman MD, Faro S. Obstetric septic shock: a pathophysiologic basis for management. Clin Obstet Gynecol 1990;33:482–492. Used with permission.

ISSN 1074-8628

THE AMERICAN COLLEGE OF OBSTETRICIANS AND GYNECOLOGISTS
409 12th Street, SW
Washington, DC 20024-2188

12345/98765

ACOG EDUCATIONAL BULLETIN

Number 242, November 1997

Sexual Assault

Sexual assault may be defined as any sexual act performed by one person on another without the person's consent, although legal definitions vary from state to state. Sexual assault includes genital, anal, or oral penetration by a part of the accused's body or by an object. It may result from force, the threat of force either on the victim or another person, or the victim's inability to give appropriate consent. While the actual incidence of sexual assault in the United States is not known, it appears to be rising. Although most definitions center on forced carnal knowledge without consent of a woman by a man, newer definitions are often gender neutral.

This Educational Bulletin was developed under the direction of the Committee on Educational Bulletins of the American College of Obstetricians and Gynecologists as an aid to obstetricians and gynecologists. The College wishes to thank Morton A. Stenchever, MD, and Diane H. Stenchever, MSW, for their assistance in the development of this bulletin. This document is not to be construed as establishing a standard of practice or dictating an exclusive course of treatment. Rather, it is intended as an educational tool that presents current information on obstetric–gynecologic issues.

Incidence

In 1994, the U.S. Department of Justice indicated that the annual incidence of sexual assault was 200 per 100,000 persons (1), up from 73 per 100,000 persons in 1987, which accounted for 6% of all violent crimes at that time (2). An American Medical Association report on sexual assault suggests that one in five women is sexually assaulted by the time she is 21 years of age (3). According to the National Crime Victimization Survey, approximately 700,000 women are sexually assaulted every year (1). Victims are often reluctant to report sexual assault because of embarrassment, fear of retribution, feelings of guilt, or simply a lack of knowledge of their rights. It has been reported that as many as 44% of women have been victims of actual or attempted sexual assault at some time in their life, and as many as 50% of these women have been victims on more than one occasion (4). Researchers have noted that of 188 women agreeing to complete a questionnaire at a family medicine residency clinic, 54 (28.7%) reported being a victim of some sort of sexual assault in the past. In this sample, 15% reported being the victim of rape, 8% the victim of attempted rape, and 5.3% the victim of forced sexual contact; 41.4% of the rape victims reported that they had been red more than once, but only 18.2% sought medical attention and 21% sought counseling (5).

Society has many misconceptions about the victims of sexual assault, particularly those who are female. These misconceptions include the beliefs that women who have been assaulted encouraged the assault by their behavior or dress, that they did not offer sufficient resistance to the assault, and that they were promiscuous. In addition, female victims of sexual assault are often

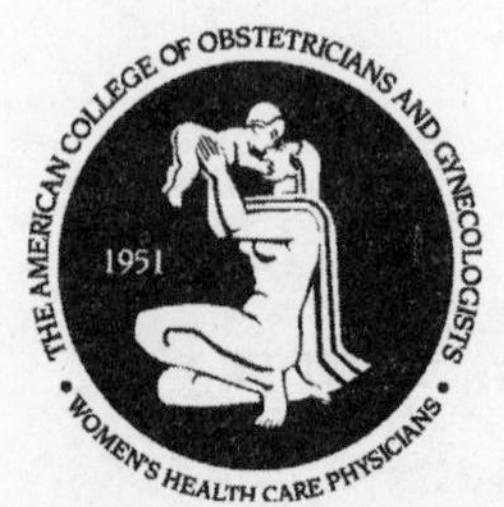

Replaces Number 172, September 1992

believed to have ulterior motives for pressing charges. Blame is often placed on the woman, despite the fact that she is a victim of a criminal act.

Sexual assault occurs in all age, racial, and socioeconomic groups. The very young, the mentally and physically handicapped, and the very old are particularly susceptible. Although the act may be committed by a stranger, it frequently is committed by someone who is known to the victim (6).

Some situations have been defined as variants of sexual assault. One example is "marital rape," which is defined as forced coitus or related sexual acts within a marital relationship without the consent of a partner; it often occurs in conjunction with physical abuse. A second is "date or acquaintance rape." In this situation, the woman may voluntarily participate in sexual play but coitus occurs, often forcibly, without her consent (7). Date rape is frequently not reported because the victim may think that she contributed to the act by participating up to a point or that she will not be believed. In one study, 942 female college students were surveyed with an 85% return rate; 25% of those responding indicated that they had been victims of sexual aggression by an acquaintance at some time beyond the age of 16. Fifty-five percent of these victims indicated that they had been at least somewhat drunk at the time of the sexual aggression, which in some instances led to a higher level of sexual assault (8). Rohypnol, known as the "date rape" drug, has been used to diminish a woman's ability to consent or to remember much of the assault.

All states have statutes criminalizing sexual intercourse with a female younger than a specific age. This is often referred to as statutory rape. Consent of the female is irrelevant in this situation because she is defined, by statute, as being incapable of consenting. Many states also have laws addressing aggravated criminal sexual assault, which have the following attributes: weapons are used; victims' or others' lives are endangered; bodily harm or physical violence is inflicted; the act is committed in relation to another felony; or the victim is older than age 60, physically handicapped, or mentally retarded (9). Physicians should be aware of the laws in their states.

Psychologic Impact

A woman who is sexually assaulted loses control over her life during the period of the assault. Her integrity and sometimes her life are threatened. She may experience intense anxiety, anger, or fear. After the assault, a "rape-trauma" syndrome often occurs (10, 11). The immediate response (acute phase) may last for hours or days and is characterized by a distortion or paralysis of the individual's coping mechanisms. The outward responses vary from complete loss of emotional control to an apparently well-controlled behavior pattern. The signs may include generalized pain throughout the body; headache; chronic pelvic pain; eating and sleep disturbances; physical symptoms such as vaginal discharge, itching, and rectal pain; and emotional complaints such as depression, anxiety, and mood swings.

The next phase—the delayed (or organization) phase—is characterized by flashbacks, nightmares, and phobias, in addition to gynecologic and menstrual complaints. This phase often occurs months or years after the event and may involve major life adjustments (10, 11).

This rape-trauma syndrome is similar to a grief reaction in many respects. As such, it can only be resolved when the victim has emotionally worked through the trauma and loss of the event and replaced it with other life experiences. The counseling offered to the victim is specific for her current phase.

Assault Assessment Kits

The physician evaluating the victim of sexual assault has a number of responsibilities, both medical and legal, and should be aware of state statutory requirements that may involve the use of kits for gathering evidence. Specific responsibilities are determined by the patient's needs and by state law (see box).

Many jurisdictions and several clinics have developed a sexual assault assessment kit, which lists the steps necessary and the items to be obtained so that as much in-

Physicians' Role

Medical
- Obtain informed consent from patient
- Obtain accurate gynecologic history
- Assess and treat physical injuries
- Obtain appropriate cultures and treat any existing infections
- Provide prophylactic antibiotic therapy and offer immunizations
- Provide therapy to prevent unwanted conception
- Offer baseline serologic tests for hepatitis B virus, human immunodeficiency virus (HIV), and syphilis
- Provide counseling
- Arrange for follow-up medical care and counseling

Legal
- Provide accurate recording of events
- Document injuries
- Collect samples (pubic hair, fingernail scrapings, vaginal secretions, saliva, blood-stained clothing)
- Report to authorities as required
- Assure chain of evidence (orderly and unbroken progress of specimens to legal authorities)

formation as possible can be prepared for forensic purposes. Many clinics have nurses who are trained to collect needed samples and information. If these individuals are available, it is appropriate to request their assistance. Rape crisis counselors also can provide valuable support.

Medical Evaluation

Informed consent must be obtained before the examination of a sexual assault victim is begun and specimens are collected. In addition to fulfilling legal requirements, this informed consent process also helps the victim participate in regaining control of her body and her life. Physicians should treat the injuries of a sexual assault victim and perform appropriate tests to detect, prevent, and treat infections and to detect and, if desired, prevent pregnancy. Up to 40% of victims who are sexually assaulted sustain injuries (12), depending upon the violence of the attack and whether the victim attempted to protect herself. Most injuries are minor and require simple therapy. About 1% of the injuries require hospitalization and major operative repair, and 0.1% are fatal (12).

After acute injuries have been determined and stabilized, a careful history and physical examination should be performed (13). A chaperon or victim advocate should be present during the history taking and physical examination to reassure the victim and provide support. The patient should be asked to state in her own words what happened. The physician may also ask her to identify her attacker if possible. If the attacker is not known to her, it is helpful to obtain a detailed description. Obtaining this description is the responsibility of the police, but it may be facilitated by what the patient tells the doctor. The patient should also be asked to provide details of the act(s) performed.

A history of previous obstetric and gynecologic conditions should be recorded, particularly infections, pregnancy, use of contraception, and date of the last menstrual period. It is necessary to determine whether the patient may have a preexisting pregnancy, be at risk for pregnancy, or have a preexisting infection.

A careful physical examination of the entire body should be performed and photographs or drawings made of the injured areas. These pictures should be labeled with the patient's name and incorporated into her record. The physician should search for bruises, abrasions, or lacerations about the neck, back, buttocks, and extremities. Injuries may be present around the vulva and rectum because of manipulation of these areas with the hand or penis. Such lesions are more common in children who have not had sexual intercourse before and in older women. Superficial or extensive lacerations of the hymen and vagina, injury to the urethra, and occasionally rupture of the vaginal vault into the abdominal cavity may be noted. Bite marks are common and should be looked for in all regions of the body, particularly about the genitalia and breasts. Occasionally, foreign objects may be found in the vagina, urethra, or rectum. If oral penetration has occurred, injuries to the mouth and pharynx may be noted.

A pelvic examination should be performed to assess the status of the reproductive organs, collect samples from the cervix and vagina, and to test for *Neisseria gonorrhoeae* and *Chlamydia trachomatis* (see box). The Centers for Disease Control and Prevention recommends obtaining a serum sample for later testing if test results are positive; however, it may be more practical to perform these tests initially. Such tests can provide information that aids management and should be offered with the proper informed consent. Lesions may be noted that suggest human papillomavirus infection and trichomoniasis, and candidal infections may be determined with the appropriate slide preparations.

If a Wood light is available, it can be used to find semen on the patient's body, because dried semen will fluoresce under such a lamp. Such fluorescence can be documented in the record, although the accuracy of materials collected from such areas is controversial and false-positive results are known to occur (3). Sperm and other Y-chromosome–bearing cells may be identified from materials collected from victims by using fluorescence in situ hybridization with a DNA probe specific for the Y chromosome. Where available, this test may be applied to materials collected from the victim (14, 15).

Few studies are available to predict the actual risk of acquiring a sexually transmissible infection during a sexual assault, but *Trichomonas* infections may be the most likely to be acquired (16). The current risk of acquiring human immunodeficiency virus (HIV) is thought to be low during a single act of heterosexual intercourse (<1%), but the risk depends on the population involved and the sexual acts performed. Results of a study from the Centers for Disease Control and Prevention show that the risk for adult rape victims of acquiring gonorrhea ranges from 6% to 12%, and that of acquiring syphilis is up to 3% (16). In children who are sexually abused, the most frequently documented sexually transmissible infections are gonorrhea and chlamydial infections (16).

Hepatitis B virus is 20 times more infectious than HIV during sexual intercourse. It is recommended that hepatitis B immune globulin (0.06 mL of hepatitis B immune globulin per kilogram) be administered intramuscularly as soon as possible (during the acute care visit) but certainly within 14 days of exposure. It is followed by the standard three-dose immunization series with hepatitis B vaccine (0, 1, and 6 months) beginning at the time of hepatitis B immune globulin administration.

Screening and Treatment of Sexually Transmissible Infections Following Sexual Assault

Initial Examination

Infection

Testing for and N gonorrhoeae and C trachomatis from specimens from any sites of penetration or attempted penetration

Wet mount and culture, if available, or a vaginal swab specimen for Trichomonas vaginalis infection (and bacterial vaginosis and yeast if malodor of discharge is present)

Collection of serum sample for subsequent serologic analysis if test results are positive

Pregnancy Prevention (see Table 1)

Prophylaxis

Hepatitis B virus vaccination

Empiric recommended antimicrobial therapy for chlamydial, gonococcal, and trichomonal infections and for bacterial vaginosis:

- Ceftriaxone, 125 mg intramuscularly in a single dose, plus
- Metronidazole, 2 g orally in a single dose, plus
- Doxycycline 100 mg orally two times a day for 7 days

Alternative treatments may be given as recommended by the Centers for Disease Control and Prevention

Follow-Up Examination (2 weeks)

Cultures for N gonorrhoeae and C trachomatis (not needed if prophylactic treatment has been provided)

Wet mount and culture, if available, for T vaginalis

Collection of serum sample for subsequent serologic analysis if test results are positive

Follow-Up Examination (12 weeks)

Examination for infectious agents

Serologic tests to be considered:

- T pallidum
- HIV (repeat test at 6 months)
- Hepatitis B virus (not needed if hepatitis B virus vaccine was given)

If the patient is found to be at risk for pregnancy as a result of the assault, "emergency contraception" can be offered. The risk of pregnancy after sexual assault has been estimated to be 2–4% in victims who were not protected by some form of contraception at the time of the attack. An appropriate regimen is one dose of combination oral contraceptive tablets at the time the victim is seen and an additional dose in 12 hours (17) (Table 1). Although it was originally suggested that oral contraceptives be given within 72 hours after exposure, some researchers suggest that emergency contraception can be effective up to 120 hours after unprotected coitus. There are insufficient data to evaluate the effectiveness of the treatment when initiated more than 72 and up to 120 hours after a single act of unprotected sexual intercourse (18, 19). A pregnancy test should be performed at the time of the 2-week return visit if conception is suspected. If pregnancy is diagnosed, the patient should be counseled concerning all of her available options, including abortion.

Legal Concerns

Rape and *sexual assault* are legal terms that should not be used in medical records. Rather, the physician should report findings as "consistent with the use of force." The physician should attempt to obtain a careful history describing the event. In addition to performing a physical examination to determine the condition of the patient, the physician should collect physical evidence that a sexual assault has taken place. It is best for this evidence to be collected as soon as possible after the attack. Victims should be encouraged to come immediately to a medical facility where they can be evaluated before they bathe, urinate, defecate, wash out their mouths, or clean their fingernails. In general, evidence of coitus will be present in the vagina for as long as 48 hours after the attack but other orifices may retain evidence only up to 6 hours. In caring for the patient, however, the physician must always place her well-being before legal considerations and tend to her most immediate needs first.

The physician should document the physical and emotional condition of the patient as judged by direct observations, her history, and the physical examination. Data should be included to document the evidence of force and the evidence of sexual contact. Materials (such as hair, fingernail scrapings, blood-stained clothing) that may help identify the offender also should be obtained. Each injury should be described carefully in detail from the standpoint of documenting whether force was used.

If the victim is a minor, the physician should report the incident to the appropriate authorities. Physicians should contact their state or local child protective service agency about child abuse.

Table 1. Prescriptive Equivalents for the Yuzpe Method of Emergency Contraception*

Trade Name	Formulation	Number of Pills Taken with Each Dose
Ovral	0.05 mg of ethinyl estradiol 0.50 mg of norgestrel	2
Lo-Ovral	0.03 mg of ethinyl estradiol 0.30 mg of norgestrel	4
Nordette	0.03 mg of ethinyl estradiol 0.15 mg of levonorgestrel	4
Levlen	0.03 mg of ethinyl estradiol 0.15 mg of levonorgestrel	4
Triphasil	(Yellow pills only) 0.03 mg of ethinyl estradiol 0.125 mg of levonorgestrel	4
Trilevlen	(Yellow pills only) 0.03 mg of ethinyl estradiol 0.125 mg of levonorgestrel	4

*Treatment consists of two doses taken 12 hours apart. Use of an antiemetic agent before taking the medication will lessen the risk of nausea, a common side effect.

Reprinted from American College of Obstetricians and Gynecologists. Emergency oral contraception. ACOG Practice Pattern 3. Washington, DC: ACOG, 1996

In addition to the description of the assault and documentation of sexual contact, the physician should include a history of when the patient last had consensual intercourse before the attack. Secretions from the vagina should be obtained to detect motile sperm, and samples should be collected to detect the presence of acid phosphatase, an enzyme found in high concentrations of seminal fluid. Several authorities do not consider the Pap test to be a forensic test, but if the appropriate chain of evidence is maintained, many consider it useful for this purpose. Vaginal secretions should be collected for acid phosphatase reaction and DNA evaluation by wet and dry swab and refrigerated until a pathologist can evaluate them. Although DNA evaluation may not be readily available in all areas, it is rapidly becoming so and is admissible in many jurisdictions.

Motile sperm may be present in the vagina for up to 8 hours after intercourse but may be present in the cervical mucus for as long as 2–3 days. Nonmotile sperm may be noted in the vagina for up to 24 hours and in the cervix for up to 17 days (20). If no sperm are noted, evidence for acid phosphatase should still be sought because the attacker may have had a vasectomy.

Because seminal fluid is rapidly destroyed by bacteria in salivary enzymes, identification of seminal fluid in the mouth after a few hours is difficult. Seminal fluid may be found staining the skin or clothing for several hours after an attack, and these areas should be evaluated. Skin washings and clothing should be investigated for the presence of acid phosphatase. Motile sperm may be present in the rectum for an undetermined amount of time. In general, nonmotile sperm can be found for up to 24 hours. Acid phosphatase may also be detected in the rectum (20).

Secretion of a major blood group antigen is found in the saliva of 80% of people. Saliva should be collected from the victim to ascertain whether she is a secretor and therefore to help differentiate her secretions from those of the attacker. If the patient is not a secretor and blood group antigens are found in the vaginal washings, they are probably from the semen of the attacker (20). Fingernail scrapings should be obtained and evaluated for skin or blood of the attacker. Specific blood or DNA from the materials may help identify the attacker.

All clothing closely associated with the area of assault should be collected and labeled. Pubic hair combings should be collected in an attempt to obtain pubic hair from the attacker. All labeled materials should be turned over to the authorities and a receipt retained for the patient's chart. For evidence to be of use, it should be given directly to the proper authorities by a physician along with the appropriate paper work.

Counseling

When the physical and medical–legal needs of the patient have been addressed and the circumstances of the attack carefully documented, the physician should discuss with the patient the degree of injury and the probability of infection or pregnancy. The physician should describe the general course that the patient may be expected to follow and how follow-up will be carried out. The victim should be invited to express her anxieties and should state her understanding of what has happened and what will happen. Misconceptions should be corrected. She should be reassured about her concerns whenever possible.

Other health personnel, particularly those trained to handle rape-trauma victims, should be consulted to facilitate counseling and follow-up. The patient should not be released from the facility until specific follow-up plans are made and explained to her. The follow-up plan should be agreed to by the patient, the physician, and the counselors who have become involved. The plan should reflect the patient's needs and may involve her desire to see her regular physician for follow-up. An emergency resource should be provided in the event that psychologic symptoms arise prior to the scheduled visit. Because patients often do not remember what is said to them at the time of the visit, all plans should be described in writing.

Regardless of the extent of her injuries, the victim may perceive the experience as life threatening. Many patients appear to be in control emotionally when seen immediately after a sexual assault. This response should not be misinterpreted to indicate that the patient is coping with the circumstances. Regardless of the patient's apparent emotional state, it is important to follow the recommendations made here and to anticipate that the patient will probably experience aspects of rape-trauma syndrome at some time in the future. She should be made aware of the symptoms she may experience, such as difficulty in making decisions, depression, anxiety, and flashbacks. The patient should be advised to seek help if and when these symptoms occur. At that time, appropriate therapy and counseling can be arranged.

Follow-Up

The patient should be seen subsequently to reevaluate her medical and psychologic status. The scheduling of examinations should depend on the history of assault or abuse. If initial exposure is recent, infectious agents acquired through the exposure may not have produced sufficient concentrations of organisms to result in positive tests. A follow-up visit approximately 2 weeks after the last sexual exposure should include a repeat physical examination and collection of additional specimens. Another follow-up visit approximately 12 weeks after the last sexual exposure also is necessary to collect sera and to allow sufficient time for antibodies to develop.

The patient should be reevaluated psychologically approximately 2 weeks after the initial medical evaluation. Follow-up counseling should be discussed at this visit. Future visits should be determined on the basis of the patient's individual needs. It is important during each visit to emphasize to the patient that she is not to blame for the attack and allow her to discuss her feelings and current perceptions of her problem. Patients should be encouraged to seek help as the need arises.

Special Circumstances

A physician may be confronted with special circumstances with respect to sexual assault. They may include the assault of babies and infants, incestuous assaults on children, and assaults on the handicapped or elderly (21–25). In each circumstance, the proper diagnosis that such an assault has taken place may require the physician's awareness and suspicion of the possibility that an assault has occurred. Once the diagnosis is made, the physician should apply the recommendations in this bulletin. In addition to reporting the assault to the authorities, the physician may be able to work with them to place the individual in a protective environment away from potential assaulters and to arrange for specific care and counseling for the victim of sexual assault and those intimately involved with her.

References

1. U.S. Department of Justice. Criminal Victimization 1994. Bureau of Justice statistics bulletin. National crime victimization survey. Washington, DC: U.S. Government Printing Office, 1996
2. U.S. Federal Bureau of Investigation. Uniform crime reports for the United States 1987. Washington, DC: U.S. Government Printing Office, 1988
3. American Medical Association. Strategies for treatment and prevention of sexual assault. Chicago: AMA, 1995
4. Russell D. The prevalence and incidence of forcible rape and attempted rape offenders. Victimology 1982;7:81–93
5. Beebe DK, Gulledge KM, Lee CM, Replogle W. Prevalence of sexual assault among women patients seen in family practice clinics. Fam Pract Res J 1994;14:23–28
6. Bowie SI, Silverman DC, Kalick SM, Edbril SD. Blitz rape and confidence rape: implications for clinical intervention. Am J Psychother 1990;44:180–188
7. American College of Obstetricians and Gynecologists. Adolescent acquaintance rape. ACOG Committee Opinion 122. Washington, DC: ACOG, 1993
8. Harrington NT, Leitenberg H. Relationship between alcohol consumption and victim behaviors immediately preceeding sexual aggression by an acquaintance. Violence Vict 1994;9:315–324
9. Tuit EP. Ignorance of the law is no excuse. Chicago: Kendall Hall Publishing, 1992
10. Burgess AW, Holmstrom LL. Rape trauma syndrome. In: Burgess AW, Holmstrom LL, eds. Rape: victims of crisis. Bowie, Maryland: Robert J. Brady Co, 1974:37–50
11. van der Kolk BA. The body keeps the score: memory and the evolving psychobiology of posttraumatic stress. Harvard Rev Psychiatry 1994;1:253–265
12. Marchbanks PA, Lui K-J, Mercy JA. Risk of injury from resisting rape. Am J Epidemiol 1990;132:540–549
13. Renshaw DC. Treatment of sexual exploitation. Rape and incest. Psychiatr Clin North Am 1989;12:257–277
14. Collins KA, Rao PN, Hayworth R, Schnell S, Tap MP, Lantz PE, et al. Identification of sperm and non-sperm male cells in cervicovaginal smears using fluorescence in situ hybridization: applications in alleged sexual assault cases. J Forensic Sci 1994;39:1347–1355
15. Roa PN, Collins KA, Geisinger KR, Parsons LH, Schnell S, Hayworth-Hodge R, et al. Identification of male epithelial cells in routine postcoital cervicovaginal smears in fluorescence in situ hybridization. Application in sexual assault and molestation. Am J Clin Pathol 1995;104:32–35

16. Schwarcz SK, Whittington WL. Sexual assault and sexually transmitted diseases: detection and management in adults and children. Rev Infect Dis 1990;12:S682–S690

17. Yuzpe AA, Smith RP, Rademaker AW. A multicenter clinical investigation employing ethinyl estradiol combined with dl-norgesterol as a postcoital contraceptive agent. Fertil Steril 1982;37:508–513

18. Grou F, Rodrigues I. The morning after pill—how long after? Am J Obstet Gynecol 1994;171:1529–1534

19. American College of Obstetricians and Gynecologists. Emergency oral contraception. ACOG Practice Pattern 3. Washington, DC: ACOG, 1996

20. Braen GR. Physical assessment and emergency medical management for adult victims of sexual assault. In: Warner CG, ed. Rape and sexual assault: management and intervention. Germantown, Maryland: Aspen Publishers, 1980:47–66

21. American College of Obstetricians and Gynecologists. Pediatric gynecologic disorders. ACOG Technical Bulletin 201. Washington, DC: ACOG, 1995

22. Cartwright PS, Moore RA. The elderly victim of rape. South Med J 1989;82:988–989

23. Gentry CE. Incestuous abuse of children: the need for an objective view. Child Welfare 1978;57:355–364

24. Jones JG. Sexual abuse of children. Current concepts. Am J Dis Child 1982;136:142–146

25. Rimsza ME, Niggemann EH. Medical evaluation of sexually abused children: a review of 311 cases. Pediatrics 1982;69: 8–14

ISSN 1074-8628

The American College of Obstetricians and Gynecologists
409 12th Street, SW
PO Box 96920
Washington, DC 20090-6920

12345/10987

Number 211—September 1995

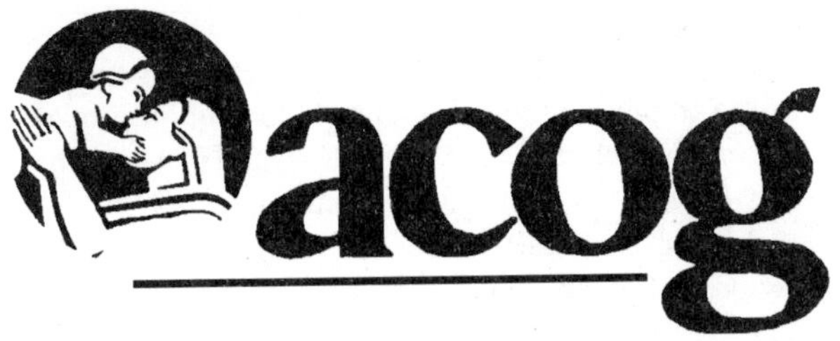

Technical Bulletin

An Educational Aid to Obstetrician–Gynecologists

Sexual Dysfunction

According to a survey of sexual practices in the United States, a minority of Americans experience sexual problems, but women are much more affected by sexual problems than are men (1). Because many women consider their obstetrician–gynecologist to be their primary care physician, and this relationship includes concerns related to their sexual health, obstetrician–gynecologists should be prepared to discuss their patients' concerns about sexuality.

Physicians should respond appropriately to these concerns so patients will be encouraged to discuss their sexuality. A physician–patient relationship based on mutual trust and respect offers a nurturing environment that limits the potential for discomfort in discussing these issues. It is generally preferable for the physician to introduce the subject rather than assume the patient will do so if she chooses. The physician's time limitations, experience, and the nature of the problem may warrant referral for counseling.

Through evaluation, the physician can determine whether a patient's sexual concerns are organic or psychologic in nature. Sexual dysfunction may be the result of physiologic changes or of disease or treatment. In such cases, candid discussion about effects on sexual well-being may be helpful, and treatment may be possible. When helping a woman deal with problems arising from psychologic issues, the physician may offer education, counseling, and techniques that are appropriate for brief evaluation and treatment within the context of regular medical practice. At times, basic information about the variety of relationship, family, and sexual patterns is helpful. By developing a clinical awareness of the interplay between relationship and family stresses and illness and having resources for referrals when they are indicated, the physician can be very helpful.

This bulletin provides an overview of sexual practices and describes the components of an assessment of sexual health. The various manifestations of dysfunction and their sources are considered within the context of basic sexual response, and several treatment approaches are outlined. Some treatments may be within the scope of the obstetrician–gynecologist's office practice, or referral may be appropriate depending on the nature and extent of the problem. Referrals for various problems of sexual dysfunction are typically made to psychologists, marriage or relationship counselors, or sex therapists.

Assessment

A woman may have concerns about her sexual health at any time and for many reasons, but certain specific events may produce changes sufficient to cause concern:

- Pubertal development
- Sexual activity and intercourse
- Contraception
- Surgical procedures that affect future childbearing, menstruation, or sexual function
- Menopause
- Change in status of marriage or intimate relationship
- Infection with a sexually transmitted disease

In an assessment of sexual health, a nonjudgmental approach on the part of the physician creates security for both patient and physician. It allows the patient to speak without fear of disapproval and permits the physician to ask as many questions as needed to obtain the necessary information (2). Counselors should be aware of their own biases and, in a therapeutic setting, should learn to listen to and discuss ideas and behaviors that conflict with these biases without displaying discomfort.

Sexuality involves a broad range of expressions of intimacy, and the physician should not make assumptions about the woman's behavior. Sexual practices may be influenced by race and education. The physician should keep in mind the possibility of cultural and personal variation in sexual practices when counseling patients.

For example, it may be inappropriate to assume that the woman's partner is a man. In one survey, 1.2% of women reported having sex exclusively with other women over the past year (1), but the actual number of women who participate in homosexual activity is widely disputed. For lesbians, the traditional health history questions about marital status, intercourse, and birth control should be replaced by the use of gender-inclusive terms without heterosexual assumptions. Phrases such as "partner" instead of "husband" and "sexual activity" instead of "intercourse" are clearly preferred. Increased sensitivity and knowledge about lesbian sexuality will help promote communication and facilitate assessment of any problems.

During the initial interview, questions should be as open and as general as possible. Some basic questions are: 1) Are you sexually active? 2) Is it satisfying for you? 3) Do you think it is satisfying for your partner? 4) Do you have any concerns about your sexual life or functioning? The physician should be aware of non-verbal communication. Discrepancy between verbal content and nonverbal communication may indicate a problem. In these instances it may be helpful for the physician to ask the patient to explain the discrepancy.

The physician should ask the patient about the sexual behaviors involved in her relationship(s). For each of the behaviors described by the patient, the physician should ask whether the behavior is acceptable to the woman; whether she has any concerns about it; the level of arousal or, if applicable, pain produced; and whether the woman achieves an orgasm. If the woman appears uncomfortable and unable to describe her sexual behaviors, the physician may assist her by describing some of the most common behaviors.

Vaginal intercourse is by far the most common sexual practice among Americans (1). Oral sex is a distant second but not uncommon practice. Regarding frequency of sexual activity, there is a wide range of normal responses. Overall, the average frequency of sex is seven times per month for men and six times per month for women (1). By talking with patients, explaining normal feelings and activities as well as specific suggestions, the physician essentially gives the patient "permission" to use this knowledge.

If time is limited, it may be helpful to schedule additional visits to discuss sexuality topics further. For the physician to only half listen and be distracted by other concerns may leave the woman feeling that her sexual concerns are not important or not worthy of discussion.

If initial questioning about the patient's sexual history reveals that she is sexually active but that it is not satisfying for her or that she has concerns that merit attention, taking a more detailed sexual history may be helpful. When a woman states that she is not sexually satisfied, the difficulty can often be identified as a lack of communication, insufficient or ineffective stimulation, a lack of understanding about what constitutes adequate sexual response, lack of a nurturing environment, physical discomfort, or fear of pregnancy or infection such as with human immunodeficiency virus (HIV).

With regard to assessment of sexual function, it is important to evaluate the effectiveness of sexual stimulation. For example, if clitoral touching is the initial form of sexual contact between a woman and her partner, the behavior may be more irritating than stimulating. If the same behavior occurs after what the woman deems to be an appropriate amount of kissing, general body caressing, and possibly breast stimulation, effective stimulation may be achieved. Personal preferences and effective communication play an important role in determining the appropriate sequence of behaviors.

Stimulation must last long enough and be intense enough to allow adequate opportunity for arousal. Many women are unaware that psychologic stimulation is an important component of arousal. When combined with physical stimulation, the use of sexual fantasy may result in a higher level of sexual arousal than physical stimulation alone. One study evaluated the relationship between guilt regarding sexual fantasies and sexual satisfaction. It found that those who felt guilty reported having fewer sexual fantasies during intercourse than those who did not feel guilty, and this led to higher levels of sexual dissatisfaction and sexual dysfunction (3).

Many women believe that intercourse should be the source of most of their own arousal. As a consequence, a woman may automatically cut short other stimulating behaviors with the hope and expectation that intercourse will provide both arousal and orgasm. Many of these women repeatedly find that intercourse does not produce the amount of stimulation expected but have very little idea of what is needed to enhance stimulation.

Similarly, many women assume that it is natural to achieve an orgasm as a part of normal sexual response. Because of this belief, they may develop a sense of inadequacy if they are unable to fulfill these expectations during every encounter. In fact, sexual response may not culminate in orgasm (Table 1). Survey results do not show a strong relationship between having orgasms and sexual satisfaction.

A nurturing environment allows a woman to be responsive sexually. For many women, sexual interest and response are affected by the emotional tone of the relationship. If the emotional tone is positive, then sexual interest and responsiveness may be maximized. In this area, female sexuality differs somewhat from male sexuality. Although men can and do desire a nurturing environment and find that their sexual responsiveness is enhanced by it, a relative lack of nurturing typically does not have as much of a negative impact on men as it does on women.

Cohabitation, with or without marriage, also positively affects satisfaction. Survey results indicate that sexual satisfaction is reported to be highest among married people and those cohabiting and lowest among those who were not married and not living with someone (1).

TABLE 1. FREQUENCY OF ORGASM DURING SEX WITH PRIMARY PARTNER BY GENDER, AGE, AND MARITAL STATUS (%)

Social Characteristics	Frequency of Orgasm (%)				
	Always	**Usually**	**Sometimes**	**Rarely**	**Never**
Gender					
Men	75	20	3	1	1
Women	29	42	21	4	4
Age (y)					
Men					
18–24	70	22	6	0	2
25–29	73	21	3	2	2
30–39	77	20	2	0	1
40–49	79	18	2	0	0
50–59	72	19	3	2	4
Women					
18–24	22	39	26	5	8
25–29	31	40	21	3	5
30–39	29	41	22	5	4
40–49	34	44	16	4	2
50–59	26	47	20	5	2
Marital/Residential Status					
Men					
Non-cohabiting	74	20	3	1	1
Cohabiting	74	21	1	2	1
Married	75	20	3	0	1
Women					
Non-cohabiting	30	32	24	6	8
Cohabiting	24	44	28	2	2
Married	29	46	18	4	2

The major obstacles to a nurturing environment are either personal or interpersonal. The common personal obstacles are unrealistic expectations, feelings of fear (of pregnancy or disease) or guilt, physical pain, and mental distraction. Interpersonal obstacles include difficulties with the partner, either in regard to the relationship in general or sexuality in particular. Because the partner plays such an important role in sexual satisfaction, it is often helpful for the partner to be involved in treatment and counseling.

Contraceptive techniques, particularly those that are dependent on coitus, can affect sexual activity. If the couple is not comfortable or satisfied with a particular method, contraception may not be used or may interfere with sexual expression. During the assessment, the physician should inquire about whether the couple uses birth control, the method used, and their level of satisfaction with the method.

Sexual Response

Adequate sexual function is a complex interaction of hormonal events and psychosocial relationships. There is a recognized pattern of sexual response, but individual variation clearly exists.

The first stage of sexual response is desire. This is comparable to the energy that allows an individual to initiate or respond to sexual stimulation (4).

The second stage of sexual response is arousal. Both physical and emotional stimulation may lead to breast and genital vasodilation and clitoral engorgement. In the female, dilation and engorgement of the blood vessels in the labia and tissue surrounding the vagina produce the "orgasmic platform," an area at the distal third of the vagina where blood becomes sequestered. Localized perivaginal swelling and vaginal lubrication make up the very early changes in this stage of sexual response. Subsequently, ballooning of the proximal portion of the vagina and elevation of the uterus occurs. In the male, vasodilation of the cavernosal arteries and closure of the venous channels that drain the penis produce an erection.

The third stage in the sexual response cycle is orgasm. The physical and emotional excitement that has been generated is maximized. This requires the individuals to relinquish their sense of control. Physiologically, women experience a series of involuntary 0.8-second contractions of the bulbocavernosus and ischiocavernosus muscles (4). In one study, 42% of women reported experiencing multiple orgasms, primarily with masturbation (5).

The fourth stage of the cycle is resolution. Most congestion and tension resolves within seconds, although complete resolution may take up to 60 minutes.

Interruption or absence of any of the stages of the sexual response cycle can result in sexual dysfunction. Daily stresses, such as the demands of one's children or insufficient time alone with one's partner, or inability to relax may contribute to decreased desire. Performance anxiety, misconceptions about human sexual response, a generally discordant relationship, a reaction to illness, and specific medical or surgical treatments may create barriers that may lead to sexual difficulties.

Sexual Dysfunction

Treatment of patients with sexual dysfunction involves a series of steps in behavior modification aimed at reducing the demand for performance, identifying and modifying the emotions that inhibit appropriate responses, and teaching the woman and her partner what types of physical and psychologic behaviors are needed to augment their responsiveness. The physician's immediate task is to help reduce the patient's anxiety and gather enough information to diagnose and treat the condition or to provide a referral. Before treatment starts, the physician needs to assess his or her capability for and interest in providing this type of treatment. The most common sexual difficulties in men and women are shown in Fig. 1.

Lack of Desire

There is much that is not known about sexual desire, and more research is needed to help increase physicians' understanding of this important aspect of sexual function. What is known is that some disturbances of sexual desire are interpersonal in origin.

Conditioning may also inhibit the sexual response cycle at this level. In the psychology of sexual response, an individual may review and evaluate what has happened and may also interpret a sexual encounter in terms of success or failure. This interpretation contributes to greater or lesser desire for future sexual experiences. If experiences are pleasant and enjoyable, desire will be enhanced; experiences that are painful, uncomfortable, or psychologically threatening will contribute to decreased desire. For example, a woman who has had difficulty experiencing orgasm for a number of years may develop a defeatist attitude about her ability to be orgasmic. Over time, she may find that her ability to be aroused is also decreased. As sexual interaction continues, the process may further erode, so that by the time she sees a gynecologist, her chief complaint will be the lack of desire. Most women with low sexual desire have some difficulty with arousal or orgasm (6–8).

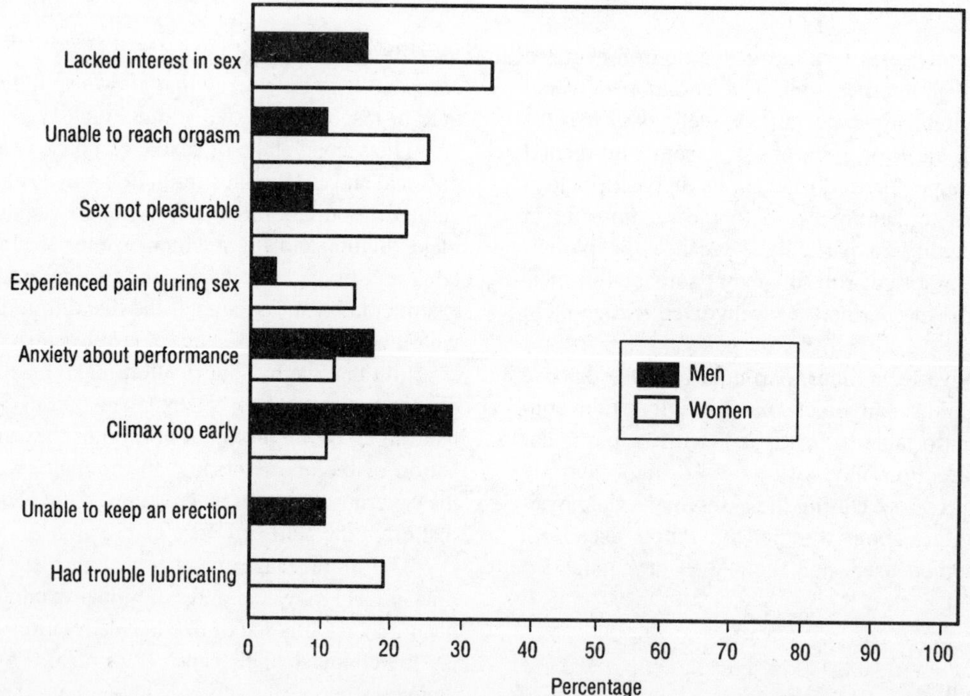

FIG. 1. Percentage of men and women who had sexual difficulties for at least one of the past 12 months. (From SEX IN AMERICA by Michael et al. Copyright © 1994 by CSG Enterprises, Inc., Edward O. Laumann, Robert T. Michael, and Gina Kolata. By permission of Little, Brown and Company)

Some women with low levels of desire are capable of arousal and orgasm with relative ease, but they simply have relatively little interest in starting the process or in having the process initiated by their partner. Occasionally, a woman's desire is inhibited by repressed sexual fantasies or homosexual impulses which she worries may be acted out if she were to become sexually interested.

Lack of Arousal

Difficulty becoming sexually aroused may occur if there is insufficient foreplay (holding, touching, kissing, or caressing) or if either partner is emotionally distracted. Arousal phase dysfunction may be manifested either physiologically by insufficient vasocongestion or psychologically.

If a woman is unable to become aroused with appropriate stimulation, other psychologic causes of arousal phase dysfunction should be explored. Possible causes include failure to acknowledge sexual arousal as part of her self-image, difficulty communicating to her partner her specific likes or dislikes, or her partner's inability or refusal to please her. Neurosensory physical problems should be ruled out.

Sensate focus exercises, as originally described by Masters and Johnson, can be very helpful in this regard (9). One purpose of these exercises is to help the couple successfully relate to each other physically without experiencing performance pressure or anxiety. In these exercises, the woman and her partner take turns caressing each other's body except for the genital area. When caressing becomes pleasurable for both partners, they move on to manual genital stimulation and, if desired, further sexual activity. Through these exercises, the couple develops nonverbal means to communicate to each other their desired types of stimulation.

Lack of Orgasm

At one time, women who were unable to have an orgasm during intercourse were considered to be dysfunctional or frigid. This is no longer the case. Lack of orgasm is now seen as a problem only if the patient or her partner perceives it as one. Over 90% of women are able to experience orgasm. For some of these women, orgasms occur by self-stimulation or by partner stimulation manually, orally, or with a vibrator.

One study demonstrated that, when compared with women who were orgasmic, women who were anorgasmic experienced greater difficulty discussing with their partner sexual activities that included direct clitoral stimulation. They also had more negative attitudes about masturbation, subscribed to more myths about sex, and had more guilt about sex (10).

Orgasmic dysfunction is categorized as either primary (existing from the beginning of sexual activity) or secondary (existing either with one partner and not another or under one set of circumstances and not another; also called situational). In some cases, the woman may have difficulty experiencing orgasm, and specific questioning may reveal that she also has an arousal phase dysfunction. Orgasms can only occur with high levels of arousal; a woman who has never experienced an orgasm may have trouble differentiating high from low levels of arousal.

For a woman with primary dysfunction who has never had any experience with self-stimulation, a very effective behaviorally oriented, time-limited treatment program has been described. The recommended steps the patient can perform are summarized in the following nine steps (11):

1. Increase self-awareness by examining the body and genitals.
2. Explore the genitals with her fingertips.
3. Identify sensitive areas of the genitals that produce pleasurable feelings.
4. Manually stimulate the pleasure-producing areas.
5. Increase the intensity and duration of stimulation and increase psychologic stimulation by means of sexual fantasy.
6. If after completing step 5 an orgasm has not been reached, use a vibrator on or around the clitoris to increase stimulation.
7. Once masturbation has resulted in orgasm, masturbate with the partner present in order to demonstrate effective and pleasurable techniques of stimulation.
8. Guide the partner in manual stimulation through nonverbal communication (eg, place a hand on top of the partner's hand).
9. Once high levels of arousal and, possibly, orgasm have occurred in step 8, engage in intercourse. The so-called bridge technique, in which the clitoris or clitoral area is manually stimulated during intercourse, can be helpful.

Various support groups have become quite popular for women who want and need the support of other women dealing with a similar problem.

Dyspareunia and Vaginismus

Dyspareunia is a general term for pain during intercourse. This may include pain during entry, pain with deep thrusting, or pain following intercourse. Organic disorders that may contribute to dyspareunia include hypoestrogenism, endometriosis, ovaries in the cul-de-sac, fibroids, and pelvic infection, among others. Therefore, evaluation for dyspareunia should include careful assessment of the genital tract with an effort to reproduce symptoms during bimanual examination prior to treatment. The sensitive nature of this examination requires that the physician thoroughly discuss the procedure with the patient before it is begun; it is also advisable to have a chaperon present.

Vaginismus is a spasm of the levator ani muscle that makes penetration into the vagina painful, difficult, or impossible. The diagnosis covers a spectrum: some women may be unable to undergo gynecologic examination; others may be quite comfortable in the gynecologist's office but fearful of sexual vaginal penetration. In some cases of vaginismus, the onset may be related to a previous painful episode, either psychologic or physiologic.

Most cases of vaginismus are primary in nature (ie, the problem is present at the first coital attempt). The appropriate treatment consists of a combination of vaginal dilation exercises, muscle awareness exercises, and counseling.

Vaginal dilation exercises enable a woman to recognize that something inserted into her vagina under her control does not cause pain. Although plastic syringe covers can be used, vaginal dilators are preferred by a number of women. Dilators are available in sets of four graduated sizes and can be obtained from medical supply stores. The smallest dilator is approximately the size of the fifth finger and is the first placed in the vagina by the woman. As each dilator is replaced by the next larger size without pain, a change from muscle spasm to muscle relaxation occurs. It should be emphasized that, in the absence of scars or stenosis, dilators do not cause mechanical dilation or stretching of the introitus. Symptom resolution is highest when the woman inserts the dilators into her vagina herself.

For muscle awareness exercises, the examiner places one finger inside the vaginal introitus, and the woman is instructed to contract the same muscle that she uses to stop the flow of urine. Once this muscle has been identified, the woman inserts her own finger into the vagina. The next step is for the woman to transfer her conscious attention from her finger being squeezed to the contracting vaginal muscles. Most women are able to identify the sensation of their finger being squeezed before they can identify the sensation of the contracting vaginal muscles. With a relatively normal pubococcygeal muscle, the primary objective of these exercises is to help the woman develop a cognitive awareness of the sensations of the lower vagina. This includes recognition of the distinction between a contracted and a relaxed pubococcygeal muscle. The process is continued at home. Once a woman can identify clearly the appropriate muscles, isometric vaginal contractions can be done without placing a finger in the vagina.

Relationship and Psychologic Factors

In some instances of sexual difficulty, the cause may be traced to problems in the relationship with the partner. If relationship problems are chronic or progressive, it is probably only a matter of time before this leads to a sexual problem. In other cases, the difficulty is sexually based; for example the partner may not know what is appropriate or the woman may be unable or unwilling to respond. Communication between partners is a first step toward sexual health.

Psychologic problems that may affect sexual function sometimes stem from inappropriate learning or conditioning in childhood or adolescence. Inhibitions may be the result of specific traumatic events and their emotional sequelae, such as sexual abuse. Some women who have been abused as children feel that their sense of trust has been violated and may have extraordinary difficulties relating in an intimate and sensual way to their partners. Other women may respond by losing their sexual desire or their ability to experience orgasm. When a psychologic factor is the cause of sexual problems, there usually will be other manifestations of the psychologic damage.

When a woman is reacting to angry feelings toward her partner and this is secondary to repeated negative sexual experiences in the past, a qualified sex therapist can intervene effectively. If the problem is primarily due to difficulties in the relationship, referral to an appropriate marriage or relationship counselor is indicated.

Factors Affecting Sexual Function

Some conditions and diseases may have a significant impact on sexuality. The physiologic changes that accompany pregnancy and menopause, for example, as well as medical conditions and their treatment, may affect sexual expression. Conditions or diseases may be acute, single occurrences or long-term processes that require adjustment and treatment.

Pregnancy

One study of sexual changes during pregnancy found that the frequency of sexual relations decreased in the first trimester (mostly because of psychologic factors), increased in the second trimester (allegedly because of increased pelvic congestion), and decreased in the third trimester (because of physical discomfort) (4). Most investigators have not been able to confirm an increase in sexual activity in the second trimester, but the decrease in both the first and third trimesters has been confirmed. A misconception exists that intercourse during the first trimester might interrupt the pregnancy, and this may contribute to decreased frequency of sexual activity during this time.

Another study found a linear decrease not only in intercourse but also in orgasmic ability and sexual interest during pregnancy (12). This study also provided the first normative data on masturbation, genital stimulation, and oral–genital stimulation during pregnancy. Retrospective measurement of sexual activity 2 years before, 1 year before, and during pregnancy identified a consecutive decrease in nearly all types of sexual behaviors. Another study focused on women's desire to be held during pregnancy (13). More than one half of the women noted a change in their wish to be held, and of those who did, approximately three fourths reported increased desire. Future research should include longitudinal studies on the same subjects before, during, and after pregnancy, as well as information from the women's partners.

Postpartum, the combination of a new baby, fatigue, hormonal changes, and perhaps a healing episiotomy scar may contribute to decreased coitus. As the woman readjusts over time, sexual frequency should resume.

Menopause

Most women experience some change in sexual function during the years before and after menopause. Common sexual complaints include loss of desire, decreased frequency of sexual activity, painful intercourse, diminished sexual response, and dysfunction of the male partner (14).

If the male develops erectile dysfunction, the couple has the following choices—either to stop having sex (intercourse) or to have sex without intercourse. Couples who engage in sexual stimulation to orgasm without intercourse are much more likely to maintain sexual frequency. Such behaviors may include manual stimulation of the partner's genitals, oral–genital stimulation, or rubbing the partially erect penis against the vaginal opening or clitoris. For other couples who are not comfortable with sexual stimulation other than intercourse, sexual frequency may decrease dramatically. For some couples, infrequent or no sexual activity may be well tolerated and accepted, but for others, it may have significantly detrimental effects on the relationship.

Ovarian hormone levels are among the factors that can affect sexual arousal, desire, and frequency of sexual activity (14). Postmenopausal women who do not receive hormone replacement therapy typically have more difficulty with vaginal lubrication and may experience dyspareunia at times. Use of a vaginal lubricant may be helpful. Because the vaginal epithelium is thinner and more atrophic, it is more susceptible to trauma and abrasions (4). Unless contraindicated, hormone replacement therapy and, in some circumstances, the use of a vaginal dilator for a short time may help alleviate these sexual difficulties. However, interest and desire may increase in some women who do not undergo hormone replacement therapy because of the higher proportion of androgen to estrogen that exists after menopause.

Cancer

When a woman has been diagnosed as having cancer, early communication with the patient about the effects of the disease and its treatment on her sexuality is beneficial. After patients have dealt with the initial shock of diagnosis and have begun treatment, they frequently experience anxiety about future sexual capacity but are reluctant to ask questions about sex.

Pelvic Cancer

Treatment for gynecologic cancer has significant physiologic and psychologic effects. The physiologic effects are a result of surgery, radiation, and chemotherapy. The primary psychologic issues faced are fear of death, disfigurement, or a partner's rejection.

Surgery for cancer of the vulva may require extensive resection of the labia, mons pubis, or clitoris. In addition to altering physical appearance, this surgery may narrow the vaginal introitus. Conservative surgical resection with preservation of normal anatomy or reconstruction has replaced the standard "en bloc" radical vulvectomy. It provides similar cure rates and improved appearance and function. Occasional reports have demonstrated that some women continue to be capable of having orgasms after clitoridectomy, but there are insufficient data to predict which women will continue to be capable of having orgasms.

Cervical and endometrial cancer are treated by radical hysterectomy. This may shorten the vagina and affect a woman's sexual response. Counseling about the effects can help prepare patients for changes and minimize their impact (see "Hysterectomy").

Colorectal cancer is the third leading cause of death from cancer in women in the United States (15). If the rectum and distal colon are surgically removed, damage to the pelvic autonomic nerves can adversely affect sexual response. Also, after surgical removal of the rectum, the posterior vaginal wall may lack both cushioning and support.

Radiation therapy is often used in treatment of cervical, vaginal, and endometrial cancer. It produces significant physiologic changes. The vagina becomes atrophic, loses its elasticity, and decreases in caliber and length, and this may lead to complete agglutination. To help minimize the adverse effects, the woman should be given vaginal dilators and instructed in their use. As soon as the risk of hemorrhage is past, dilation should be performed daily. Coating the dilator with estrogen cream will provide lubrication, and the cream will maintain some estrogenic effect. If estrogen is contraindicated, a vaginal lubricant should be used. Dilation should be performed for several months after radiation therapy since the stenosis continues to develop. Sexual activity should be encouraged after the risk of hemorrhage has passed.

Chemotherapy often causes complete hair loss, decrease in energy, disruption of bowel function, and atrophic changes of the vagina. All of these may decrease sexual desire and function. Vaginal estrogen therapy, adequate antinausea therapy, and maintenance of physical appearance with wigs or head coverings may improve the patient's self-image and sexual function.

Return to sexual activity may be hampered by the sexual partner's fear that sex may injure the patient. Less often, the partner may fear contracting cancer or being burned by residual radiation. These concerns should be dealt with by counseling the couple before, during, and after treatment. One study showed that women who had undergone pelvic radiation therapy were not prepared for the subsequent side effects, including the effects on sexuality, leading some to choose to avoid sexual contact altogether (16). Sexual rehabilitation counseling significantly increases the number of women who resume sexual activity after cancer treatment (17). Resumption of sexual activity also correlates with other quality-of-life measurements.

Breast Cancer

In one study of 60 women who had had a mastectomy, only 4 reported having had discussions with their physician on how mastectomy might affect their sexuality (18). In contrast, almost 50% of the women indicated a desire for such a discussion but thought it was an inappropriate topic because no health care professional had mentioned it.

Mastectomy for breast cancer has been shown to have the following effects on sexual function (18):

- Forty-nine percent of women resume intercourse within 1 month of discharge from the hospital, but one third do not resume intercourse by 6 months after discharge.
- The number of women who never use the female superior position for intercourse increases threefold after mastectomy, suggesting that directly viewing the mastectomy site is discomforting for the woman, her partner, or both.
- The frequency of breast stimulation decreases substantially, indicating both avoidance of the remaining breast by the partner and a definite avoidance of single-breast stimulation by some women.
- Thirty-eight percent of partners do not view the mastectomy scar in the first 3 months after the operation.

The sexual implications of breast cancer, and mastectomy in particular, relate to the psychologic and physiologic effects of the disease on the patient and the psychologic effect on her partner. In some cases, the woman may feel deformed or mutilated, resulting in low self-esteem and an inability to function sexually (19). In other cases, sexual function may be inhibited by the woman's fear of rejection by her partner (20). In situations in which sexual function is affected, therapeutic counseling may be helpful. However, counseling the patient and her partner in advance on what to anticipate after treatment for breast cancer may serve as a preventive measure.

Numerous reports have documented that a significant proportion of emotional problems associated with mastectomy is due to the fact that the loss of the breast may have a negative impact on body image (21). One investigator concluded that women who sought reconstruction of the breast were exhibiting evidence of positive coping and asserting effective problem-solving behavior (22). Other authors further supported the value of seeking breast reconstruction (23). Women who sought reconstruction were seen as well adjusted and able to maintain a high level of psychosocial functioning. In one study, women who had undergone breast reconstruction after mastectomy were more comfortable with their sexuality than before the reconstruction (24). Also, although the frequency of sexual activity did not increase, satisfaction did and more closely approximated levels of satisfaction reported for the patient's best time prior to mastectomy.

Interestingly, most women who sought reconstruction did so on their own initiative: 60% of the women said their husband or significant other was neutral or opposed to the surgery. The antiquated notion that only discontented women who cannot accept their defect or adjust to it undergo breast reconstruction has been laid to rest (21).

The American Cancer Society's Reach to Recovery program offers support to breast cancer patients as they adjust to their disease and treatment. The Young Women's Christian Association (YWCA) has developed a national program for postoperative cancer patients, ENCORE (encouragement, normalcy, counseling, opportunity, reaching out, energies revived).

Pelvic Surgery

Any surgical procedure involving the female genital area may have sexual implications. While discomfort, pain, or bleeding may be expected by the physician and thus are not a cause for alarm, these symptoms may cause considerable anxiety for the woman and her partner. Which sexual activities are "permitted" after the procedure, what is prohibited, for what reason, and for how long should be discussed with the patient clearly and explicitly. If long-term sexual or emotional adjustment is required, it is best to include the partner in relevant discussions and, if appropriate, consider referral.

Hysterectomy

Preoperative discussion of the sexual implications of hysterectomy may help alleviate many fears and anxieties. Hysterectomy may result in a shortened vagina, and this may be a more significant problem for women who are postmenopausal than for those who are not. If a woman experiences dyspareunia on deep thrusting after hysterectomy, she may find it helpful to control the depth of penetration either by assuming the female superior position during intercourse or by bringing her legs closer together while in the female supine position. Sufficient lubrication will help alleviate some of this difficulty. After hysterectomy, a woman will no longer have uterine contractions at the time of orgasm. Some women will experience this change in sensation as both a qualitative and quantitative decrease in enjoyment.

Some women may experience adverse psychologic sequelae to hysterectomy, but most do not experience psychosexual problems postoperatively (25). Those women who do develop problems appear more apt to have decreased estrogen secretion postoperatively (because of concomitant bilateral oophorectomy), to have preoperative sexual conflicts, or to believe that hysterectomy diminishes one's femininity. Women with postoperative problems also are often poorly educated and have little understanding of the proposed surgery or what to expect afterward. Women who are asymptomatic before hysterectomy or who undergo removal of a normal uterus from a normal pelvis to alleviate pelvic symptoms may also develop psychosexual problems.

To minimize postoperative problems, the patient's psychologic profile as well as her physical problems and fantasies should be considered preoperatively. Preoperative preparation that includes a detailed discussion of anatomy, physiology, sexual response, and psychologic concerns and fears is very helpful. Women at risk for adverse psychosexual sequelae may benefit from extensive education and counseling before therapy.

Pelvic Exenteration

When pelvic exenteration is required, the patient is often referred to a new physician or a new location or both, and there is usually insufficient time to develop a relationship with a new physician. Exenteration may be required when cancer is either extensive or recurrent. In addition to these negative factors, the treatment will remove the vagina and may leave the patient with one or two stomas on her abdominal wall; these may occasionally smell of urine or pass flatus. Postexenteration, there may be a hole in the woman's pelvis, and this may contribute to a feeling of asexuality. Each of these may damage the woman's self-esteem.

No sexual option after pelvic exenteration is perfect. Without vaginal reconstruction, the options include no sexual activity, intercrural sex, direct penile–clitoral contact, masturbation, use of a vibrator, manual stimulation of the partner's genitals, and oral stimulation of the partner's genitals. There is no one decision that is right for all couples. The most acceptable options for a given couple depend on their ages, the status of the relationship, previous sexual frequency, sexual attitudes, and each partner's level of enjoyment of past sexual activity. The role of the physician is to help the couple reach agreement.

Chronic Medical Illness

Chronic disease may have a significant negative impact on a woman's ability to feel and be sexual. Some illnesses have a strong negative influence on a woman's self-image, others affect her physiologic response, and still others may affect her partner. In some instances, the illness may adversely affect all of these. As obstetrician–gynecologists and primary care providers, physicians should appreciate how such conditions as cardiovascular disease, arthritis, chronic lung disease, urinary stress incontinence, and long-standing pain may affect women's sexual function.

Commonly used medications that interfere with sexual function in women do so by decreasing desire or libido, delaying or preventing orgasm, or causing painful clitoral tumescence (Table 2). The most common of such medications are antihypertensive agents, antipsychotics, and antidepressants. Medications can also cause erectile dysfunction in men and contribute to the sexual dysfunction of a couple.

Male Factors

Sometimes a patient's concerns may be related to the sexual health of her male partner. It is helpful for the physician to be familiar with some of the common causes of male sexual dysfunction and their treatments. While it is unlikely that the physician would be involved in treating the male partner, such knowledge may provide reassurance to the patient, who may in turn encourage her male partner to seek counseling or treatment.

Erectile Dysfunction

Erectile dysfunction, or impotence, is difficulty either obtaining a penile erection of sufficient rigidity to allow for vaginal penetration or maintaining the erection until ejaculation, assuming there is no ejaculatory disorder. The term *erectile dysfunction* is a more accurate and acceptable term than *impotence*. While it is commonly believed that erectile dysfunction is mostly of psychogenic etiology, for many men over age 40, erection problems are caused by pathophysiologic changes. Significant factors are arteriosclerosis or atherosclerosis, diabetes mellitus, neurologic disorders, and medical treatments—pharmacologic, radiotherapeutic, or surgical. Hormonal abnormalities are rare causes of erection difficulties.

When taking a sexual history, the clinician may find the following questions to be helpful in establishing a diagnosis:

TABLE 2. MEDICATIONS THAT CAUSE SEXUAL DYSFUNCTION IN WOMEN

	Effect		
Medication	**Decreased Libido**	**Delayed or No Orgasm**	**Painful Clitoral Tumescence**
Amphetamines and related anorexic drugs		•	
Bromocriptine			•
Cimetidine	•		
Clomipramine	•	•	
Diazepam		•	
Fenfluramine	•		
Fluoxetine		•	
Imipramine		•	
Isocarboxazid		•	
Methadone		•	
Methazolamide	•		
Methyldopa	•		
Phenelzine		•	
Propranolol	•		
Reserpine	•		
Spironolactone	•		
Timolol	•		
Trazodone			•

Modified from The Medical Letter, Inc. Drugs that cause sexual dysfunction: an update. Med Lett Drugs Ther 1992;34:74–77

- Does your male partner wake up in the morning with an erection? If so, is it rigid enough for vaginal penetration?
- During the time your partner has had an erection problem, has he masturbated to ejaculation? If so, were those erections rigid enough for vaginal penetration?
- When you and your partner are sexually involved, do you manually or orally stimulate his penis? If so, how rigid does the penis get?
- When was the last time you and your partner were able to have intercourse with a reasonably normal erection?
- Was the onset of the erectile dysfunction sudden or gradual?
- Since the onset of the problem, has it occurred intermittently or has it been progressive?

The answers to these questions provide insight into the nature of the problem and the need for intervention. Most investigators have found that a sudden onset of erectile dysfunction that occurs intermittently is mostly associated with psychologic causes. Erectile dysfunction that has a gradual onset and is persistent or progressive is mostly associated with organic causes. While dysfunctions have traditionally been defined as either organic or psychogenic in nature, it is becoming increasingly clear that this is an oversimplification.

Diagnostic techniques are nocturnal penile tumescence monitoring or vascular assessment or both. The treatment of erectile dysfunction depends in part on the diagnosis. For erectile dysfunction secondary to a well-defined organic etiology, the treatment options include abstention from sex, stimulation to orgasm without intercourse, vacuum devices, pharmacologic treatment to induce erections (including direct injection of vasoactive medications into the shaft of the penis by the patient at home), penile implant, or, in selected cases, penile vascular surgery.

Psychologic Effects

A man's sexual dysfunction—whether resulting from low sexual desire, difficulty obtaining or maintaining an erection for intercourse, or some other problem—may be deleterious to a woman's sexual arousal. If the woman equates an erection with love, lack of an erection may be equated with lack of love, and this interpretation may mentally distract her from potential arousal. In a similar fashion, early ejaculation, either before penetration or immediately at vaginal penetration, or difficulty ejaculating may result in both partners focusing more on male function than on their mutual enjoyment. Relationship difficulties commonly interfere with sexual function. Overt hostility, withdrawal, or communication patterns that lead to repetitive misunderstanding are perceived by many women as variables that either cause or contribute to sexual difficulty.

Summary

Sexual dysfunction may adversely affect a woman's self-esteem and her overall sense of well-being. The obstetrician–gynecologist can play an important role by asking the patient about any problems with sexual function.

Physiologic changes, disease, surgery, or medical therapy may result in sexual dysfunction. The physician should recognize the potential effects of these conditions on a patient's sexuality and provide the patient with appropriate education and counseling. Patients should also be advised about alternatives for sexual expression, particularly after pelvic surgery. Specific support groups of others facing similar conditions may also be helpful.

If, after taking a history of the patient's psychologic status, relationship, and a sexual history, the physician does not see an obvious cause and course of treatment, the best choice may be referral to a marriage or relationship counselor or a sexual therapist, particularly if the problem is of a psychologic nature or of long duration. Counseling or referral can be helpful and rewarding for the patient, her partner, and the physician.

REFERENCES

1. Michael RT, Gagnon JH, Laumann EO, Kolata G. Sex in America: a definitive survey. Boston: Little, Brown and Co, 1994
2. Burchell RC. Counseling in gynecologic practice: an overview. In: Clinical obstetrics and gynecology. Hagerstown, Maryland: Harper and Row, 1978:165–172
3. Cado S, Leitenberg H. Guilt reactions to sexual fantasies during intercourse. Arch Sex Behav 1990;19:49–63
4. Masters WH, Johnson VE. Human sexual response. Boston: Little, Brown and Co, 1966:141–168
5. Darling CA, Davidson JK Sr, Jennings DA. The female sexual response revisited: understanding the multiorgasmic experience in women. Arch Sex Behav 1991;20: 527–540
6. Kaplan HS. The new sex therapy: active treatment of sexual dysfunction. New York: Brunner/Mazel, 1974
7. Cutler WB. Sexual life after hysterectomy. In: Hysterectomy: before and after. New York: Harper and Row, 1988:225–250
8. Morgan S. Sexuality! In: Coping with a hysterectomy. New York: Dial Press, 1982:131–170
9. Masters WH, Johnson VE. Human sexual inadequacy. Boston: Little, Brown and Co, 1970
10. Kelly MP, Strassberg DS, Kircher JR. Attitudinal and experiential correlates of anorgasmia. Arch Sex Behav 1990;19:165–177
11. LoPiccolo J, Lobitz WC. The role of masturbation in the treatment of orgasmic dysfunction. In: LoPiccolo J, LoPiccolo L, eds. Handbook of sex therapy. New York: Plenum Press, 1978:187–195
12. Solberg DA, Butler J, Wagner NN. Sexual behavior in pregnancy. New Engl J Med 1973;288:1098–1103
13. Hollender MH, McGehee JB. The wish to be held during pregnancy. J Psychosom Res 1974;18:193–197
14. Sarrel PM. Sexuality and menopause. Obstet Gynecol 1990;74 (4 suppl)26S–30S
15. American Cancer Society. Cancer facts and figures—1994. Atlanta: ACS, 1994
16. Lancaster J. Women's experience of gynaecological cancer treated with radiation. Curationis 1993;16:37–42
17. Capone MA, Good RS, Westie KS, Jacobson AF. Psychosocial rehabilitation of gynecologic oncology patients. Arch Phys Med Rehab 1980;61:128–132
18. Frank D, Dornbush RL, Webster SK, Kolodny RC. Mastectomy and sexual behavior: a pilot study. Sexuality and Disability 1978;1:16–26
19. Rollin B. First, you cry. New York: New York American Library, 1977
20. Witkin MH. Sex therapy and mastectomy. J Sex Marital Ther 1975;1:290–304
21. Schain WS. Psychosocial factors in mastectomy and reconstruction. In: Noone AB, Decker BC, eds. Plastic and reconstructive surgery of the breast. Philadelphia: Decker, 1991:327–343
22. Clifford E. The reconstructive experience. The search for restitution. In: Georgiade NG, ed. Breast construction following mastectomy. St Louis: CV Mosby, 1979:22–35
23. Holland JC, Rowland JH. Patient rehabilitation and support. Psychosocial reactions to breast cancer and its treatment. In: Harris JR, Hellman S, Henderson IC, Kinne DW, eds. Breast diseases. Philadelphia: JB Lippincott Co, 1987:632–647
24. Rowland JH, Holland JC, Chaglassian T, Kinne D. Psychological response to breast reconstruction: expectations for and impact on postmastectomy functioning. Psychosomatics 1993;34:241–250
25. Bachmann GA. Psychosexual aspects of hysterectomy. Women's Health Issues 1990;1:41–49

SUGGESTED READING

Barbach LG. The book for yourself: the fulfillment of female sexuality. New York: Doubleday, 1975

Schover LR, Jensen SB. Sexuality and chronic illness. New York: Guilford Press, 1988

Wabrek AJ. Sexual counseling in office practice. In: Glass RH, ed. Office gynecology. 4th ed. Baltimore, Maryland: Williams and Wilkins, 1993:189–210

This Technical Bulletin was developed under the direction of the Committee on Technical Bulletins of the American College of Obstetricians and Gynecologists as an educational aid to obstetricians and gynecologists. The committee wishes to thank Alan J. Wabrek, MD, MPH, for his assistance in the development of this bulletin. This Technical Bulletin does not define a standard of care, nor is it intended to dictate an exclusive course of management. It presents recognized methods and techniques of clinical practice for consideration by obstetrician–gynecologists for incorporation into their practices. Variations of practice taking into account the needs of the individual patient, resources, and limitations unique to the institution or type of practice may be appropriate.

ISSN 1074-8628

THE AMERICAN COLLEGE OF OBSTETRICIANS AND GYNECOLOGISTS
409 12th Street, SW
Washington, DC 20024-2188

12345/98765

ACOG EDUCATIONAL BULLETIN

Number 240, September 1997

Smoking and Women's Health

Cigarette smoking is the largest preventable cause of death and disability among women in the United States. More than 22 million American women smoke cigarettes despite the overwhelming medical evidence about the harmful effects of smoking (1). From 1965 to 1990, there was a 40% decline in the overall prevalence of smoking, but since 1990, the prevalence has plateaued.

Among high school students, the percentage of those smoking cigarettes increased from 27% in 1991 to 35% in 1995. In the 1995 Youth Risk Behavior Survey, 34.3% of high school girls reported that they smoked cigarettes during the past 30 days (2). Adolescence is the critical period during which most women begin to smoke. Of adult smokers, 91% had their first cigarette before age 20 and 77% became daily smokers by age 20. Very few women begin smoking after age 20 (3).

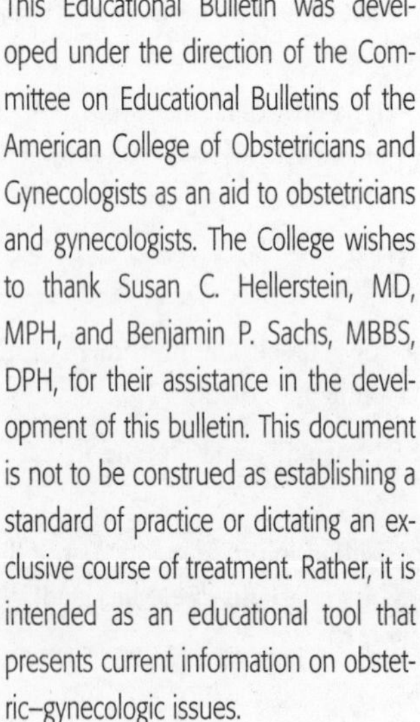

This Educational Bulletin was developed under the direction of the Committee on Educational Bulletins of the American College of Obstetricians and Gynecologists as an aid to obstetricians and gynecologists. The College wishes to thank Susan C. Hellerstein, MD, MPH, and Benjamin P. Sachs, MBBS, DPH, for their assistance in the development of this bulletin. This document is not to be construed as establishing a standard of practice or dictating an exclusive course of treatment. Rather, it is intended as an educational tool that presents current information on obstetric–gynecologic issues.

Among women of reproductive age, 29% smoke. Smoking is more prevalent among women living in poverty and those with less than a high school education (4). Between 19% and 30% of pregnant women continue to smoke, putting themselves and their fetuses at risk for a number of adverse reproductive events (2, 5). From 1992 to 1993, restrictive work site and public smoking policies helped transform a significant number of women from daily smokers into occasional smokers, but the overall number of smokers did not change.

Most American women who smoke want to quit. In the 1992–1993 National Health Interview Survey, 72.5% of female smokers reported that they wanted to quit; 34% attempt to quit each year, but only 2.5% successfully stop each year (1).

Physicians, nurses, and medical staff can be instrumental in preventing the initiation of smoking among adolescents. Obstetric and gynecologic prac-titioners can accurately inform women of the medical consequences of smok-ing and facilitate successful smoking cessation.

Effects of Smoking on Women

Composition of Tobacco Smoke

There are more than 2,500 chemicals identified in tobacco smoke. Many components have not been evaluated for their effects on health. Two of the major components that are thought to be responsible for the adverse effects

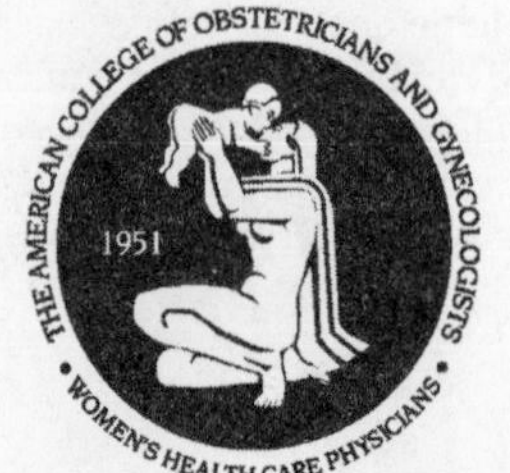

Replaces Number 180, May 1993

of cigarette smoke are nicotine and carbon monoxide (6). Both active and passive smoking involve the inhalation of smoke, with systemic absorption via the pulmonary vasculature.

Nonreproductive Effects

Cancer

Smoking is responsible for approximately 29% of all cancers. Since 1987, lung cancer has been the leading cause of cancer deaths among women. In 1997, an estimated 66,000 women will die of lung cancer. Women who smoke are 12 times more likely to die from lung cancer than those who never smoked. Smoking cessation for 10 years reduces the risk of lung cancer to that of a nonsmoker. In addition, smoking increases the risks of cancer of the pharynx, esophagus, kidney, bladder, pancreas, and cervix (7). Cotinine, a product of nicotine, has been found in the cervical mucus of smokers (8).

Coronary Artery Disease

Smoking is responsible for 55% of the cardiovascular deaths in women less than 65 years old. The Nurses Health Study prospectively followed 117,006 female nurses aged 30–55 years. In that study, the relative risk of total coronary heart disease among smokers was four times higher than that of the women who never smoked. The risk of coronary heart disease was highest among those who initiated smoking before 15 years of age (relative risk = 9.25). In women who stopped smoking, the relative risk of coronary heart disease immediately decreased to 1.5. Two years after smoking cessation, the risk of coronary heart disease decreased to the level of those who had never smoked (9). Smoking is also a risk factor for coronary artery disease in women younger than 30 years old (10). Women over the age of 35 who use oral contraceptives and smoke have higher risks of deep venous thrombosis, myocardial infarction, and cerebrovascular accidents. Therefore, oral contraceptives generally are not recommended for smokers older than age 35.

Menopause

At least 13 studies indicate that smokers cease menstruating 1–2 years earlier than nonsmokers. This effect is dose dependent, and the difference persists after controlling for subjects' weight (6, 11). Moreover, female smokers 60 years of age and older have significantly reduced bone mineral density of the hip compared with nonsmokers (12).

Other Effects

Women who smoke cigarettes are more likely to develop bronchitis and emphysema. Gastric ulcers and cerebrovascular disease also are associated with smoking (7).

Reproductive Effects

Overall, there is evidence that women who smoke have decreased fertility. Tobacco smoking has been implicated in disorders of ovulatory function, tubal function, implantation physiology, oocyte depletion, and early pregnancy loss (5). Smoking also alters the characteristics of sperm. In addition, treatment of invasive cancer, which is much more likely to occur in women who smoke, can result in infertility.

Ovulatory Dysfunction

Animal studies have shown that nicotine can alter gonadotropin release in a dose-dependent fashion, decrease the luteinizing hormone surge, and inhibit the release of prolactin. Changes in the midcycle luteinizing hormone surge may explain the effect of smoking on the menstrual cycle (13).

Few well-designed studies have addressed the issue of ovulatory dysfunction in women. In a classic study of 24,000 women, the frequency of abnormal vaginal bleeding was found to be 67% higher in heavy smokers (those who smoked more than 21 cigarettes per day) than in nonsmokers (14).

Tubal Function

Nicotine alters tubal motility in rhesus monkeys and rabbits (9). In humans, ectopic pregnancy may be a manifestation of altered tubal function. Several case–control studies have shown an approximately doubled risk of ectopic pregnancy when the mother smoked at the time of conception (15). In a multinational study of 1,108 women with confirmed ectopic pregnancies, the frequency of ectopic pregnancy was higher in smokers than in nonsmokers (odds ratio, 2.2–4.0, depending on the subgroup) (16). The analysis was adjusted for pelvic inflammatory disease and intrauterine device use.

Spontaneous Abortion

In a review of in vitro fertilization (IVF) studies that controlled for the number of eggs retrieved, fertilization rates, and implantation rates, the incidence of spontaneous abortion was 42.1% in smokers compared with 18.9% in non-smokers (17). Researchers evaluated 979 karyotyped spontaneous abortions (18). Spontaneous abortions of smokers were 39% more likely to be chromosomally normal than those of nonsmokers. This suggests a nongenetic mechanism.

In studies of patients who have undergone IVF, the nicotine metabolite cotinine is found in higher concentrations in follicular fluid of smokers than nonsmokers (19). Despite initial small studies showing lower IVF success rates for smokers, two larger studies have elucidated the issue. There is no difference in the number of eggs retrieved, fertilization rates, implantation rates, or the overall pregnancy rate per embryo transferred between smokers and nonsmokers (17, 20). However, in both studies there were significantly more spontaneous abortions in smokers than nonsmokers (42% versus 19% [17] and 73% versus 24% [20]). Thus, the overall result is fewer successful IVF pregnancies for women who smoke.

Effects on Pregnancy

Various effects of cigarette smoking on pregnancy have been studied. They include placental changes, pregnancy complications, and perinatal loss. Carbon monoxide and nicotine are thought to be the main ingredients in cigarette smoke responsible for adverse fetal effects linked to smoking. These products cause decreased availability of oxygen to maternal tissues and to the fetus.

Placental changes found in smokers include hypertrophy, thickening of the trophoblastic basement membrane (21), and calcification (22), changes typically seen in cases of chronic hypoxia and ischemia. The volume density of fetal vessels in terminal villi is decreased, signifying a loss in the exchange area of the placentas in women who smoke (23).

Pregnancy Complications

In the Collaborative Perinatal Project, abruptio placentae was 1.5 times more common in smokers than in nonsmokers and was more likely to result in perinatal mortality. When women stopped smoking before their first prenatal visit, there were 50% fewer fetal and neonatal deaths due to abruptio placentae (23). In several studies, women who smoked cigarettes during pregnancy had placenta previa twice as often as nonsmokers (24, 25).

Low Birth Weight

There is a consistent association in the medical literature between smoking and lower birth weight. This is from a combination of preterm deliveries of appropriate-weight babies and term deliveries of intrauterine growth-restricted babies. The mean birth weight of infants of women who smoke during pregnancy is 170–200 g less than that of infants of nonsmokers. This difference persists even after controlling for confounding variables such as maternal age, parity, maternal weight gain and energy intake, social class, level of education, and alcohol consumption (26).

Studies have shown a consistent relationship between preterm premature rupture of membranes and smoking (27, 28). Further studies controlling for differences in maternal sexual activity and in maternal genital tract pathogens are needed to assess the association between smoking and premature rupture of membranes. In a study attempting to characterize reasons for higher rates of preterm births in African–American women compared with white women, 10% of the excess risk in African–American women was attributed to cigarette smoking (29).

Smokers also have a 3.5–4.0-fold increase in small-for-gestational-age infants compared with nonsmokers (30). Newborns of smokers are smaller at every gestational age. Women who stop smoking before 16 weeks of gestation have infants with birth weights similar to those of babies of women who never smoked (31).

Perinatal Outcomes

Multiple studies have demonstrated a clear association between maternal smoking and perinatal loss. Placenta previa, abruptio placentae, and preterm premature rupture of membranes are a factor in most of the perinatal losses in smokers.

A study of sudden infant death syndrome (SIDS) showed that maternal smoking during pregnancy significantly increased the risk of death from SIDS twofold. When prenatal smoking was combined with postnatal exposure to tobacco smoke, the relative risk of SIDS increased to 2.93 (32). According to a population-based cohort study, after controlling for other factors, prenatal exposure to tobacco smoke accounts for up to 30% of SIDS deaths, which could be prevented with prenatal smoking cessation (33). Infants exposed to tobacco smoke have an increased risk of acute respiratory illnesses and an increase in chronic respiratory symptoms.

Smoking Cessation

Physician Training and Counseling

Physician advice can help women stop smoking, but often physicians do not inquire routinely about smoking and do not advise patients to quit. In the Stanford five-city project, only 50% of smokers reported that their physician had ever advised them to stop smoking. They were less likely to be counseled if they were adolescents or young adults, non–oral contraceptive users, or without cigarette-related disease. Only 3.6% of former smokers stated that their physician had helped them quit (34).

Although there are conflicting data on the magnitude of the effect, physician counseling motivates some patients to quit. The physician's effectiveness in increasing actual cessation rates depends on a systematic approach to identifying smokers and supporting smoking cessation. Results of five randomized controlled trials showed that brief physician training in smoking cessation (3 hours) and intervention protocols produced cessation rates of up to 15% at 1-year follow-up (35). The major conclusions of the randomized trials regarding physician training are as follows (35):

- Training physicians in the treatment of nicotine dependence will result in more consistent and effective patient care.

- When trained physicians are routinely prompted to intervene with patients who smoke, they can achieve a significant reduction in smoking prevalence.
- Patients of trained physicians who receive routine reminders were up to six times more likely to stop smoking than patients of control physicians.

Intervention Guidelines

Physician guidelines for patient smoking cessation have been published by the National Cancer Institute (Box 1). More recently, the Agency for Health Care Policy and Research of the Centers for Disease Control and Prevention has published recommendations for smoking cessation specialists (Box 2).

The physician and office staff can encourage smoking cessation by ensuring that all smokers are identified, monitored, and counseled appropriately at every office visit. The health team can discuss with patients nicotine addiction and treatment and address fears about weight gain, stress management, and support systems. Office staff can identify a smoking cessation coordinator and educator, make the office smoke free, put in place ways to

Box 1
Smoking Cessation Guidelines for Physicians

Ask

All patients about smoking and document the following in the chart: brand, quantity, age at initiation, prior attempts to quit

Advise

All smokers to stop—personalize the message to quit

Assist

Patient in quitting:

1. Establish a quit date within 4 weeks
2. Consider signing a stop smoking contract with the patient
3. Provide self-help materials
4. Consider nicotine replacement for those who smoke more than one pack a day or who smoke their first cigarette within 30 minutes of waking

Arrange

Patient follow-up care:

1. Office staff member to call or write patient within 7 days of the initial visit to reinforce the decision
2. Follow-up visit within 1–2 weeks after the quit date
3. At follow-up visit, provide support and help prevent relapse; if relapse happens, encourage patient to try again immediately
4. Second follow-up visit in 1–2 months; for patients who have relapsed, discuss circumstances and special concerns

National Cancer Institute. How to help your patients stop smoking. Bethesda, Maryland: NCI, 1995; NIH Publication No. 95-3064

Box 2
Recommendations for Smoking Cessation Specialists

Assess the smoker who has entered a program—Assess whether participants in smoking cessation programs are motivated to quit.

Use a variety of clinical specialists—Medical/health care clinicians can deliver messages about health risks and benefits, and nonmedical clinicians can deliver psychosocial or behavioral interventions.

Ensure the program is intensive enough—Program should include four to seven sessions 20–30 minutes in length for at least 2 weeks.

Use a variety of program formats—Individual or group counseling may be used in addition to supplementary self-help materials.

Include effective counseling techniques—Interventions should include problem-solving/skill training content as well as clinican-delivered social support for quitting.

Target the smoker's motivation to quit—Make the motivation relevant to the person's disease status, family or social situation, health concerns, age, gender, and other characteristics, such as prior quitting. Review with the individual the potential risks associated with smoking and have him or her highlight those that seem most relevant. Repeat the motivational intervention as needed.

Provide relapse prevention intervention—Specialists should work to prevent long-term risks of relapse and make dietary, exercise, or lifestyle recommendations, or include the person in a program that focuses on these issues. These interventions can occur during treatment sessions or during follow-up contacts.

Include nicotine replacement therapy—Except in special circumstances, every smoker should be offered nicotine replacement therapy. The nicotine patch and nicotine gum are particularly useful in helping smokers quit.

Adapted from Fiore MC, Bailey WC, Cohen SJ, et al. Smoking Cessation: Information for Specialists. Clinical Practice Guideline. Quick Reference Guide for Smoking Cessation Specialists, No. 18. Rockville, MD: U.S. Department of Health and Human Services, Public Health Service, Agency for Health Care Policy and Research and Centers for Disease Control and Prevention, 1996 April; AHCPR Publication No. 96-0694.

identify and monitor smokers, remind the health providers to intervene, and assist in follow-up phone calls and arranging visits. Many smokers benefit from self-help smoking cessation materials. A list of some available smoking cessation materials is provided in Table 1.

Nicotine Medications

The use of nicotine-containing medications can double or triple success rates in smoking cessation if prescribed in a setting with ancillary support programs (36). The short-term cessation rates with nicotine medications are between 20% and 40%, compared with 10–20% with placebo; however, the long-term efficacy depends on the context of the treatment (37). Most smokers who quit relapse within a week, when the symptoms of nicotine withdrawal peak. Nicotine is highly addictive, and withdrawal symptoms begin within a few hours, peak in several days, and often last up to a month. Typically the symptoms include dysphoria, insomnia, irritability, anxiety, difficulty in concentrating, restlessness, decreased heart rate, and increased appetite.

Nicotine-containing medications can provide relief of withdrawal symptoms while smokers adapt to life without cigarettes. In cigarette smoke, nicotine is rapidly absorbed and with large variability in plasma concentrations. By contrast, the medications result in slower, lower,

Table 1. Self-Help Smoking Cessation Materials

Organization	Address/Phone	Available Materials
American Cancer Society	1599 Clifton Rd, NE Atlanta, GA 30329 (800)-ACS-2345 (404) 320-3333	Don't Bite Off More Than You Should Chew How to Stay Quit Over the Holidays Why Start Life Under a Cloud? (for pregnant women) Smart Move
American College of Obstetricians and Gynecologists	ACOG Resource Center 409 12th St, SW PO Box 96920 Washington, DC 20090-6920 (202) 863-2518	It's Time to Quit Smoking
American Dental Association	211 East Chicago Ave Chicago, IL 60611 (312) 440-2500	Smokeless Tobacco: Think Before You Chew
American Heart Association	7272 Greenville Ave Dallas, TX 75231-4596 (214) 373-6300	Calling It Quits Guidelines for a Weight Control Component in a Smoking Cessation Program
American Lung Association	1740 Broadway New York, NY 10019 (800) 586-4872 (212) 315-8700	A Healthy Beginning: The Smoke-Free Family Guide for New Parents (kit) A Lifetime of Freedom from Smoking: A Maintenance Program for Ex-Smokers Freedom from Smoking Program Freedom from Smoking for You and Your Baby (kit) In Control: A Home Video Smoking and Pregnancy Program Reducing the Health Risks of Secondhand Smoke Quit Smoking Forever
Health Promotion Resource Center	Stanford Center for Research in Disease Prevention 1000 Welch Rd Palo Alto, CA 94304-1885 (415) 723-0003	Calling It Quits (videotape) Cool Turkey Quitting Guide: A Day-by-Day Program to Help You Quit Smoking Como dejar de fumar en tres pasos Quit Smoking Kit
National Cancer Institute	Office of Cancer Communications 31 Center Dr, MSC 2580 Building 31, Room 10A-29 Bethesda, MD 20892-2580 (800)-4-CANCER	Chew or Snuff Is Real Bad Stuff Clearing the Air–How to Quit Smoking and Quit for Keeps Guia para dejar de fumar Why Do You Smoke?
Princeton Health Systems	9 Mercer St Princeton, NJ 08540 (800) 437-6668	Free and Clear

and less variable plasma concentrations. The available forms include nicotine gum, patch, and the recently approved nasal spray. The effectiveness of oral inhalers are being investigated (36).

Nicotine medications should be recommended for smokers who are likely to be nicotine dependent (36). Most often, nicotine dependence is found in those who smoke greater than one pack of cigarettes per day, smoke within 30 minutes of getting up in the morning, or have experienced nicotine withdrawal symptoms with prior attempts at cessation. Nicotine medications are contraindicated for patients with hypersensitivity or allergies to nicotine, with a recent myocardial infarction, worsening angina, or life-threatening arrhythmia. Patients who smoke while using these medications should be cautioned that there is a much higher risk of myocardial infarction and stroke. Recommendations from the Agency for Health Care Policy and Research for the use of nicotine replacement are listed in Box 3.

Nicotine Gum

Generally, nicotine polacrilex gum is recommended according to the number of cigarettes smoked each day (see Box 4):

- Fewer than 20 cigarettes per day, one dose of 2 mg for every two cigarettes
- More than 20 cigarettes per day, 4 mg for every 3–4 cigarettes per day

After 1–2 months, weaning can begin with the total daily intake decreased by one unit dose per week. Use for more than 6 months is not recommended. Side effects of nico-

Box 3
Clinical Guidelines for Recommending Nicotine Replacement Products

Who should receive nicotine replacement?

Available research shows that nicotine replacement generally increases rates of smoking cessation. Therefore, except in the presence of serious medical precautions, the clinician should encourage the use of nicotine replacement with patients who smoke. Little research is available on the use of nicotine replacement with light smokers (eg, those smoking 10–15 cigarettes/day or less). If nicotine replacement is to be used with light smokers, a lower starting dose of the nicotine patch or nicotine gum should be considered.

Should nicotine replacement therapy be tailored to the individual smoker?

Research does not support the tailoring of nicotine patch therapy (except with light smokers as noted above). Patients should be prescribed the patch dosages outlined in Box 5.

Research supports tailoring nicotine gum treatment. Specifically, 4-mg gum, as opposed to 2-mg gum, can be used with patients who are highly dependent on nicotine (eg, those smoking more than 20 cigarettes/day, those who smoke within 30 minutes of awakening, and those who report that it is difficult to refrain from smoking where it is forbidden[1]). Clinicians may also recommend the higher gum dosage if patients request it or have failed to quit using the 2-mg gum.

Should patients be encouraged to use the nicotine patch or nicotine gum?

Although both pharmacotherapies are efficacious, nicotine patch therapy is preferable for routine clinical use. This preference is based on the following comparisons with nicotine gum therapy:

- Nicotine patch therapy is associated with fewer compliance problems that interfere with effective use
- Nicotine patch therapy requires less clinician time and effort to train patients in its effective use

The following factors support the use of nicotine gum:

- Patient preference
- Previous failure with the nicotine patch
- Contraindications specific to nicotine patch use (eg, severe skin reactions)

[1]Heatherton TF, Kozlowski LT, Frecker RC, Fagerstrom K-O. The Fagerstrom Test for Nicotine Dependence: a revision of the Fagerstrom Tolerance Questionnaire. Br J Addiction 1991;86:1119–1127

Adapted from Fiore MC, Bailey WC, Cohen SJ, et al. Smoking Cessation. Clinical Practice Guideline No. 18. Rockville, MD: U.S. Department of Health and Human Services, Public Health Service, Agency for Health Care Policy and Research, 1996 April; AHCPR Publication No. 96-0692.

tine polacrilex gum include jaw fatigue and gastrointestinal symptoms.

Transdermal Nicotine

Transdermal nicotine patches are available in a variety of doses and can be recommended as follows: For women who smoke more than 20 cigarettes a day, 20–22 mg per 24 hours should be the initial dose depending on the brand. After 4 weeks, wean to successively lower dosages, each for 2–4 weeks (see Box 5). The patient should be seen and counseled at each dose reduction. Patients who smoke less than 20 cigarettes per day should start with midrange transdermal doses. Those who smoke five cigarettes or less are not likely to have withdrawal symptoms or to benefit from transdermal nicotine medication. Side effects of transdermal nicotine may include skin reaction and sleep disturbance, which can be alleviated by removing the patch at night.

Weight Gain

Many women smokers are concerned about weight gain associated with smoking cessation. Although not all women who stop smoking will gain weight, in a recent study of smoking cessation and weight gain, women who stopped smoking gained significantly more weight than those who had never smoked or those who continued to smoke (38). Over a 10-year period, the average weight

Box 4
Suggestions for the Clinical Use of Nicotine Gum

Patient selection

Appropriate as a primary pharmacotherapy for smoking cessation. For suggestions regarding use in special populations, see Box 3.

Precautions

Pregnancy—Pregnant smokers should first be encouraged to attempt cessation without pharmacologic treatment. Nicotine gum should be used during pregnancy only if the increased likelihood of smoking cessation, with its potential benefits, outweighs the risk of nicotine replacement and potential concomitant smoking.

Cardiovascular disease—Although not an independent risk factor for acute myocardial events, nicotine gum should be used only after consideration of risks and benefits among particular cardiovascular patient groups: those in the immediate (within 4 weeks) postmyocardial infarction period, those with serious arrhythmias, and those with severe or worsening angina pectoris.

Side effects—Common side effects of nicotine chewing gum include mouth soreness, hiccups, dyspepsia, and jaw ache. These effects are generally mild and transient, and can often be alleviated by correcting the patients' chewing technique (see prescribing instructions below).

Dosage

Nicotine gum is available in 2-mg and 4-mg (per piece) doses. Patients should be prescribed the 2-mg gum except in special circumstances outlined in Box 3. The gum is most commonly prescribed for the first few months of a quit attempt. Clinicians should tailor the duration of therapy to fit the needs of each patient. Patients using the 2-mg strength should use not more than 30 pieces/day, whereas those using the 4-mg strength should not exceed 20 pieces/day. (Information on tailoring the dose of nicotine gum is presented in Box 3.)

Prescribing instructions

No smoking while using the gum.

Chewing technique—Gum should be chewed slowly until a "peppery" taste emerges, then "parked" between the cheek and gum to facilitate nicotine absorption through the oral mucosa. Gum should be slowly and intermittently "chewed and parked" for about 30 minutes.

Absorption—Acidic beverages (eg, coffee, juices, soft drinks) interfere with the buccal absorption of nicotine, so eating and drinking anything except water should be avoided for 15 minutes before and during chewing.

Scheduling of dose—Patients often do not use enough gum to get the maximum benefit; they chew too few pieces per day and they do not use the gum for a sufficient number of weeks. Instructions to chew the gum on a fixed schedule (at least one piece every 1–2 hours) for at least 1–3 months may be more beneficial than ad lib use.

Adapted from Fiore MC, Bailey WC, Cohen SJ, et al. Smoking Cessation. Clinical Practice Guideline No. 18. Rockville, MD: U.S. Department of Health and Human Services, Public Health Service, Agency for Health Care Policy and Research, 1996 April; AHCPR Publication No. 96-0692.

Box 5
Suggestions on the Clinical Use of the Nicotine Patch

Patient selection

Appropriate as a primary pharmacotherapy for smoking cessation. For suggestions regarding use in special populations, see Box 3.

Precautions

Pregnancy—Pregnant smokers should first be encouraged to attempt cessation without pharmacologic treatment. The nicotine patch should be used during pregnancy only if the increased likelihood of smoking cessation, with its potential benefits, outweighs the risk of nicotine replacement and potential concomitant smoking. Similar factors should be considered in lactating women.

Cardiovascular diseases—Although not an independent risk factor for acute myocardial events, the nicotine patch should be used only after consideration of risks and benefits among particular cardiovascular patient groups: those in the immediate (within 4 weeks) postmyocardial infarction period, those with serious arrhythmias, and those with severe or worsening angina pectoris.

Skin reactions—Up to 50% of patients using the nicotine patch will have a local skin reaction. Skin reactions are usually mild and self-limiting, but may worsen over the course of therapy. Local treatment with hydrocortisone cream (5%) or triamcinolone cream (0.5%) and rotating patch sites may ameliorate such local reactions. In less than 5% of patients do such reactions require the discontinuation of nicotine patch treatment.

Dosage

Treatment of 8 weeks or less has been shown to be as efficacious as longer treatment periods.[1] Based on this finding, the following treatment schedules are suggested as reasonable for most smokers. Clinicians should consult the package insert for other treatment suggestions. Finally, clinicians should consider individualizing treatment based on specific patient characteristics, such as previous experience with the patch, amount smoked, degree of addictiveness, etc.*

Brand	Duration	Dosage
Nicoderm and Habitrol	4 weeks	21 mg/24 hours
	then 2 weeks	14 mg/24 hours
	then 2 weeks	7 mg/24 hours
Prostep	4 weeks	22 mg/24 hours
	then 4 weeks	11 mg/24 hours
Nicotrol	4 weeks	15 mg/16 hours
	then 2 weeks	10 mg/16 hours
	then 2 weeks	5 mg/16 hours

Prescribing instructions

No smoking while using the patch.

Location—At the start of each day, the patient should place a new patch on a relatively hairless location between the neck and waist.

Activities—No restrictions while using the patch.

Time—Patches should be applied as soon as patients waken on their quit day.

[1]Fiore MC, Smith SS, Jorenby DE, Baker TB. The effectiveness of the nicotine patch for smoking cessation: a meta-analysis. JAMA 1994;271:1940–1947

*These dosage recommendations are based on a review of the published research literature and do not necessarily conform to packet insert information.

Adapted from Fiore MC, Bailey WC, Cohen SJ, et al. Smoking Cessation. Clinical Practice Guideline No. 18. Rockville, MD: U.S. Department of Health and Human Services, Public Health Service, Agency for Health Care Policy and Research, 1996 April; AHCPR Publication No. 96-0692.

gain for women associated with smoking cessation was 5.0 kg; however, only about one sixth of the increase in prevalence of overweight in the United States can be attributed to smoking cessation.

Weight gain is not caused by a change in chronic resting metabolic rates after smoking cessation; tobacco smoke is not an anorectic or a thermogenic agent (39). Weight gain with smoking cessation seems to be caused by a transient increase in oral intake without any change in physical activity. In the Nurses Health Study, middle-aged women who quit smoking and simultaneously increased their exercise level minimized weight gain associated with smoking cessation (40). A nutritious diet of low-fat foods and regular exercise can help smokers cope with withdrawal symptoms and minimize weight gain.

Stress Management

Many smokers are concerned about how to manage stress when they have stopped smoking. Restlessness and the inability to concentrate are symptoms of nicotine withdrawal, which will become less acute after 3 days and may disappear within a few weeks. After a few weeks of not smoking, most women actually feel less nervous. By knowing what to expect, women can mobilize their personal resources, willpower, family, and friends to get through the particularly difficult first few weeks of smoking cessation. Patients should be encouraged to exercise and use other techniques for stress management.

Smoking Cessation During Pregnancy

Approximately one third of women who become pregnant are smokers at the time of conception. Approximately 20% of smokers quit by the time of their first prenatal visit (5). It has been estimated that if all pregnant women stopped smoking, a 10% reduction of infant and fetal deaths would be seen (37).

The most successful efforts in smoking cessation during pregnancy involve interventions that do not just provide antismoking advice but also emphasize how to stop smoking. Experience teaches that smoking cessation materials should be targeted toward pregnant women rather than the general smoking population (41). A prospective, randomized, controlled clinical trial of an intensive smoking reduction program with substantial patient contact and supervision (initial visit plus telephone contact at least monthly) has been shown to aid in smoking cessation during pregnancy and to increase birth weights (5). Use of a smoking cessation chart may help health care providers to monitor patient contacts with the goal of achieving smoking cessation as well as reinforcing that behavior throughout and after pregnancy.

A recent meta-analysis of 10 randomized controlled trials showed a 50% increase in smoking cessation between the sixth and ninth months of pregnancy with organized prenatal smoking interventions (41). In the third trimester, smoking cessation rates of up to 32% were achieved with the prenatal program. Two important points stood out about the successful programs: 1) All used smoking cessation materials geared toward pregnant women rather than the general population; and 2) more intensive intervention with multiple contacts and in multiple formats was most effective.

In the general population, approximately 65% of those who stop smoking relapse within 3 months of quitting and another 10% relapse between 3 to 6 months, whereas only 3% relapse from 6 to 12 months (42). This suggests that women who quit smoking for the 9 months of pregnancy may have a low relapse rate. The high motivation of pregnant women to protect their health and that of their babies may provide an excellent window of opportunity for achieving smoking cessation and should be encouraged because even short-term cessation has benefit. Physician support is warranted not only during the pregnancy but immediately following because as many as two thirds of pregnant women who quit smoking have been shown to relapse within 3 months of delivery (43).

Nicotine gum was initially deemed contraindicated in pregnancy because of uncertainties regarding the risks associated with its use. In 1992, the Food and Drug Administration downgraded it to pregnancy category C (risk cannot be ruled out). Transdermal systems are graded at pregnancy category D (positive evidence of risk). Generally, in pregnancy, it is reasonable to use the nicotine medications if prior attempts to quit smoking without medications have failed and if the smoker is still smoking more than 10–15 cigarettes per day (36). If the patient smokes at this level, the use of a nicotine replacement system may pose fewer risks than smoking.

Circulating nicotine levels attained with this method usually are less than those observed in smokers of 20 or more cigarettes per day (44). In the absence of direct data concerning use of the patch and gum during pregnancy, it is appropriate to inform the patient about the presumed risks and benefits of this approach and to make therapeutic decisions on an individual basis.

Summary

Smoking tobacco increases the risk of cancer, cardiovascular conditions, and other health problems for all women. It also is associated with numerous reproductive health problems including increased perinatal mortality, bleeding complications of pregnancy, decreased mean birth weight, and higher incidences of small-for-gestational-age babies, low-birth-weight babies, and preterm deliveries.

The ultimate goal of the provider is to identify all women who smoke and counsel them to stop. A concrete smoking cessation plan, coupled with the use of nicotine replacement when indicated, and proper follow-up care can help women quit smoking and avoid relapse.

References

1. Centers for Disease Control and Prevention. Cigarette smoking among adults—United States, 1993. MMWR 1994;43:925–929
2. Centers for Disease Control and Prevention. Tobacco use and usual source of cigarettes among high school students—United States, 1995. MMWR 1996;45:413–418
3. Nelson DE, Giovino GA, Shopland DR, Mowery PD, Mills SL, Eriksen MP. Trends in cigarette smoking among US adolescents 1974 through 1991. Am J Public Health 1995; 85:34–40
4. Centers for Disease Control and Prevention. Cigarette smoking among women of reproductive age—United States, 1987–1992. MMWR 1994;43:789–791
5. Sexton M, Hebel JR. A clinical trial of change in maternal smoking and its effect on birth weight. JAMA 1984;251: 911–915
6. U.S. Department of Health and Human Services. The health benefits of smoking cessation: a report of the Surgeon General. Washington, DC: U.S. Government Printing Office, 1990; U.S. Department of Health and Human Services publication no. (CDC)90-8416
7. American Cancer Society. Cancer facts and figures. Atlanta: ACS, 1997:5008
8. McCann MF, Irwin DE, Walton LA, Hulka BS, Morton JL, Axelrad CM. Nicotine and cotinine in the cervical mucus of smokers, passive smokers, and nonsmokers. Cancer Epidemiol Prev 1992;1:125–129
9. Kawachi I, Colditz GA, Stampfer MJ, Willett WC, Manson JE, Rosner B, et al. Smoking cessation and time course of decreased risks of coronary heart disease in middle-aged women. Arch Intern Med 1994;154:169–175
10. Arnold AZ, Moodie DS. Coronary artery disease in young women: risk factor analysis and long-term follow-up. Cleve Clin J Med 1993;60:393–398
11. McKinlay SM, Bifano NL, McKinlay JB. Smoking and age at menopause in women. Ann Intern Med 1985;103: 350–356
12. Hollenbach KA, Barrett-Connor E, Edelstein SL, Holbrook T. Cigarette smoking and bone mineral density in older men and women. Am J Public Health 1993;83:1265–1270
13. Mattison DR, Plowchalk DR, Meadows MJ, Miller MM, Malek A, London S. The effect of smoking on oogenesis, fertilization, and implantation. Semin Reprod Endocrinol 1989;7:291–304
14. Hammond EC. Smoking in relation to physical complaints. Arch Environ Health 1961;3:28–46
15. Chow W-H, Daling JR, Weiss NS, Voigt LF. Maternal cigarette smoking and tubal pregnancy. Obstet Gynecol 1988; 71:167–170
16. Campbell OM, Gray RH. Smoking and ectopic pregnancy: a multinational case-control study. In: Rosenberg MJ, ed. Smoking and reproductive health. Littleton, Massachusetts: PSG Publishing, 1987:70–75
17. Pattinson HA, Taylor PJ, Pattinson MH. The effect of cigarette smoking on ovarian function and early pregnancy outcome of in vitro fertilization treatment. Fertil Steril 1991;55:780–783
18. Kline J, Levin B, Shrout P, Stein Z, Susser M, Warburton D. Maternal smoking and trisomy among spontaneously aborted conceptions. Am J Hum Genet 1983;35:421–431
19. Rosevear SK, Holt DW, Lee TD, Ford WCL, Wardle PG, Hull MG. Smoking and decreased fertilisation rates in vitro. Lancet 1992;340:1195–1196
20. Maximovich A, Beyler SA. Clinical assisted reproduction: cigarette smoking at time of in vitro fertilization cycle initiation has negative effect on in vitro fertilization–embryo transfer success rate. J Assist Reprod Genet 1995;12:75–77
21. Van Der Veen F, Fox H. The effects of cigarette smoking on the human placenta: a light and electron microscopic study. Placenta 1982;3:243–256
22. Brown HL, Miller JM Jr, Khawli O, Gabert HA. Premature placental calcification in maternal cigarette smokers. Obstet Gynecol 1988;71:914–917
23. Naeye RL. Abruptio placentae and placenta previa: frequency, perinatal mortality, and cigarette smoking. Obstet Gynecol 1980;55:701–704
24. Williams MA, Mittendorf R, Lieberman E, Monson RR, Schoenbaum SC, Genest DR. Cigarette smoking during pregnancy in relation to placenta previa. Am J Obstet Gynecol 1991;165:28–32
25. Handler AS, Mason ED, Rosenberg DL, Davis FG. The relationship between exposure during pregnancy to cigarette smoking and cocaine use and placenta previa. Am J Obstet Gynecol 1994;170:884–889
26. Haworth JC, Ellestad-Sayed JJ, King J, Dilling LA. Fetal growth retardation in cigarette-smoking mothers is not due to decreased maternal food intake. Am J Obstet Gynecol 1980;137:719–723
27. Hadley CB, Main DM, Gabbe SG. Risk factors for preterm premature rupture of the fetal membranes. Am J Perinatol 1990;7:374–379
28. Harger JH, Hsing AW, Tuomala RE, Gibbs RS, Mead PB, Eschenbach DA, et al. Risk factors for preterm premature rupture of fetal membranes: a multicenter case-control study. Am J Obstet Gynecol 1990;163:130–137
29. Lieberman E, Ryan KJ, Monson RR, Schoenbaum SC. Risk factors accounting for racial differences in the rate of premature birth. N Engl J Med 1987;317:743–748
30. Ounsted M, Moar VA, Scott A. Risk factors associated with small-for-dates and large-for-dates infants. Br J Obstet Gynaecol 1985;92:226–232
31. MacArthur C, Knox EG. Smoking in pregnancy: effects of stopping at different stages. Br J Obstet Gynaecol 1988;95: 551–555
32. Blair PS, Fleming PJ, Bensley D, Smith I, Bacon C, Taylor E, et al. Smoking and sudden infant death syndrome:

results from 1993–5 case-control study for confidential inquiry into stillbirths and deaths in infancy. BMJ 1996;313:195–198

33. Taylor JA, Sanderson M. A reexamination of the risk factors for sudden infant death syndrome. J Pediatr 1995;126:887–891
34. Frank E, Winkleby MA, Altman DG, Rockhill B, Fortmann SP. Predictors of physicians' smoking cessation advice. JAMA 1991;266:3139–3144
35. Manley M, Epps RP, Husten C, Glynn T, Shopland D. Clinical interventions in tobacco control: a National Cancer Institute training program for physicians. JAMA 1991;266:3172–3173
36. Henningfield JE. Nicotine medications for smoking cessation. N Engl J Med 1995;333:1196–1203
37. Kleinman JC, Pierre MB Jr, Madans JH, Land GH, Schramm WF. The effects of maternal smoking on fetal and infant mortality. Am J Epidemiol 1988;127:274–282
38. Flegal KM, Troiano RP, Pamuk RE, Kuczmarski RJ, Campbell SM. The influence of smoking cessation on the prevalence of overweight in the United States. N Engl J Med 1995;333:1165–1170
39. Perkins KA. Metabolic effects of cigarette smoking. J Appl Physiol 1992;72:401–409
40. Kawachi I, Troisi RJ, Rotnitzky AG, Coakley EH, Colditz GA. Can physical activity minimize weight gain in women after smoking cessation? Am J Public Health 1996;86:999–1004
41. Dolan-Mullen P, Ramirez G, Groff JY. A meta-analysis of randomized trials of prenatal smoking cessation interventions. Am J Obstet Gynecol 1994;171:1328–1334
42. Lumley J, Astbury J. Advice for pregnancy. In: Chalmers I, Enkin M, Keirse MJNC, eds. Effective care in pregnancy and childbirth. Oxford: Oxford University Press, 1989:237–254
43. Fingerhut LA, Kleinman JC, Kendrick JS. Smoking before, during, and after pregnancy. Am J Public Health 1990;80:541–544
44. Benowitz NL. Nicotine replacement therapy during pregnancy. JAMA 1991;266:3174–3177

ISSN 1074-8628

The American College of
Obstetricians and Gynecologists
409 12th Street, SW
PO Box 96920
Washington, DC 20090-6920

12345/10987

ACOG EDUCATIONAL BULLETIN

Number 260, September 2000

Smoking Cessation During Pregnancy

Smoking during pregnancy is associated with maternal, fetal, and infant morbidity and mortality (1). An office-based protocol that systematically identifies pregnant women who smoke and offers treatment has been proven to increase quit rates (2). For pregnant women who smoke less than 20 cigarettes per day, the provision of a 5–15 minute, five-step counseling session and pregnancy-specific educational materials increases cessation by 30–70% (3). This bulletin outlines this office-based intervention and addresses treatment issues pertaining to pregnant women who smoke heavily, smoking reduction, pharmacotherapy, health care support systems, and coding.

Epidemiology

Between 15% and 29% of pregnant women smoke during pregnancy (4). Health risks associated with smoking during pregnancy include ectopic pregnancy, intrauterine growth restriction, placenta previa, and abruptio placentae (1). Adverse pregnancy outcomes include preterm birth, low birth weight, and perinatal mortality (1). It is estimated that there would be a 10% reduction in perinatal mortality (5) and an 11% reduction in the incidence of low birth weight (6) if smoking during pregnancy were eliminated. Infant health risks include sudden infant death syndrome (SIDS), hospitalization, and neurodevelopmental abnormalities (1).

Intervention

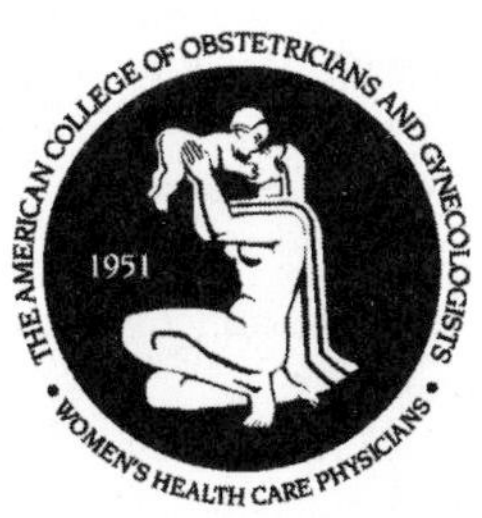

The 5–15 minute intervention is most effective with pregnant women who smoke less than 20 cigarettes per day (3). The intervention is appropriate for use during routine prenatal office visits and includes the following five steps: **Ask, Advise, Assess, Assist,** and **Arrange** (2). It is adapted from the U.S. Public Health Service clinical practice guideline, Treating Tobacco Use and Dependence (2) and is based, in part, on earlier work by the

National Cancer Institute (7). The obstetrician–gynecologist or auxiliary health care provider, after appropriate training, can perform the five steps with pregnant women who smoke. The steps are outlined as follows and on the chart (see the box). The chart guides the provider through the interaction and documents the treatment (3).

1. **Ask** about smoking status. Providers should ask the patient at the first prenatal visit to choose a statement that best describes her smoking status from a list of statements on smoking behavior (see the box). Using this multiple-choice method is more likely to elicit an accurate response than asking a simple "Yes or No" question. The smoking cessation chart, a tobacco use sticker, or a vital signs stamp that includes smoking status should be used in the medical record to remind providers to ask patients about smoking status at follow-up visits.

2. **Advise** patients who smoke to stop by providing clear, strong advice to quit with personalized messages about the benefits of quitting and the impact of continued smoking on the woman, fetus, and newborn. Congratulate patients who report having stopped smoking and affirm their efforts with a statement about the benefits of quitting.

3. **Assess** patients' willingness to attempt to quit smoking within the next 30 days. One approach to this assessment is to say, "Quitting smoking is one of the most important things you can do for your health and your baby's health. If we can give you some help, are you willing to try?" If the patient is willing, then the provider can move to the next step. If the patient is unwilling to try, providers may consider having a brief discussion with the patient to educate and reassure her about quitting (2). Quitting advice, assessment, and assistance should be offered at subsequent prenatal care visits.

4. **Assist** patients who are interested in quitting by providing pregnancy-specific, self-help smoking cessation materials. Enhance the patient's problem-solving skills by asking when and where she typically smokes and suggesting how she might avoid these "trigger situations." Offer support around the importance of having smoke-free space at home; seeking out a "quitting buddy" such as a former smoker or nonsmoker both at work and at home; and what to expect in terms of nicotine withdrawal, such as irritability and cravings. Communicate caring and concern and encourage the patient to talk about the process of quitting.

5. **Arrange** during regular follow-up visits to track the progress of the patient's attempt to quit smoking. Smoking status should be monitored throughout pregnancy, providing opportunities to congratulate and support success, reinforce steps taken towards quitting, and advise those still considering a cessation attempt.

Although counseling and pregnancy-specific materials are effective cessation aids for many pregnant women, some women continue to smoke. These women often are heavily addicted and should be encouraged at follow-up visits to stop smoking. Clinicians also may consider offering or referring patients for additional psychosocial treatment (2). Although quitting smoking early in pregnancy yields the greatest benefits for the pregnant woman and fetus, quitting at any point can be beneficial (2). For instance, pregnant women who stop smoking at any time up to the 30th week of gestation have infants with higher birth weights than women who smoke throughout pregnancy (8). The benefits of "cutting down" are difficult to measure or verify. So, the effort of women who cut down should be reinforced, but they also should be reminded that quitting entirely brings the best results for their health and that of their babies (3).

Pharmacotherapy

The use of nicotine replacement products or other pharmaceuticals as smoking cessation aids during pregnancy has not been sufficiently evaluated to determine its efficacy or safety. Nicotine gum and patches should be considered for use during pregnancy only when nonpharmacologic treatments (eg, counseling) have failed, and if the increased likelihood of smoking cessation, with its potential benefits, outweighs the unknown risk of nicotine replacement and potential concomitant smoking. Research to determine the safety and efficacy of pharmacotherapy is strongly recommended because potential benefits seem to outweigh potential risks. Optimally, smokers can be treated with these pharmacotherapies before conception.

Support Systems

The Agency for Healthcare Research and Quality has recommended systems changes to help health care providers identify and treat tobacco users (2). These changes require the partnership of health care administrators, insurers, and purchasers and include the following strategies: 1) provide education, resources, and feedback to promote provider involvement in smoking cessation; 2) promote hospital policies that support and provide smoking cessation services; 3) include effective smoking cessation treatments as paid or covered services in all health benefits packages; and 4) reimburse clinicians and specialists for delivery of effective tobacco dependence treatments and include these interventions among the defined duties of the clinicians (2).

Smoking Cessation Intervention for Pregnant Patients

ASK–1 minute

- Ask the patient to choose the statement that best describes her smoking status:

  A. I have NEVER smoked or have smoked LESS THAN 100 cigarettes in my lifetime. ❑

  B. I stopped smoking BEFORE I found out I was pregnant, and I am not smoking now. ❑

  C. I stopped smoking AFTER I found out I was pregnant, and I am not smoking now. ❑

  D. I smoke some now, but I have cut down on the number of cigarettes I smoke SINCE I found out I was pregnant. ❑

  E. I smoke regularly now, about the same as BEFORE I found out I was pregnant. ❑

  If the patient stopped smoking before or after she found out she was pregnant (B or C), reinforce her decision to quit, congratulate her on success in quitting, and encourage her to stay smoke free throughout pregnancy and postpartum.

  If the patient is still smoking (D or E), document smoking status in her medical record, and proceed to Advise, Assess, Assist, and Arrange.

ADVISE–1 minute

- Provide clear, strong advice to quit with personalized messages about the benefits of quitting and the impact of smoking and quitting on the woman and fetus. ❑

ASSESS–1 minute

- Assess the willingness of the patient to attempt to quit within 30 days. ❑

  If the patient is ready to quit, proceed to Assist.

  If the patient is not ready, provide information to motivate the patient to quit and proceed to Arrange.

ASSIST–3 minutes +

- Suggest and encourage the use of problem-solving methods and skills for smoking cessation (eg, identify "trigger" situations). ❑
- Provide social support as part of the treatment (eg, "we can help you quit"). ❑
- Arrange social support in the smoker's environment (eg, identify "quit buddy" and smoke-free space). ❑
- Provide pregnancy-specific, self-help smoking cessation materials. ❑

ARRANGE–1 minute +

- Assess smoking status at subsequent prenatal visits and, if patient continues to smoke, encourage cessation.

Data from Melvin C, Dolan Mullen P, Windsor RA, Whiteside HP, Goldenberg RL. Recommended cessation counselling for pregnant women who smoke: a review of the evidence. Tobacco Control 2000;9:1–5

Coding

Office visits specifically addressing smoking cessation may be coded as follows (note that not all payers reimburse for counseling outside of the global package and some do not cover preventive services at all):

- International Classification of Diseases, Ninth Revision, Clinical Modification (ICD-9-CM) code 305.1 (tobacco use disorder, tobacco dependence from the Mental Health section) *with* Current Procedural Terminology* (CPT) code 99401 *or* 99211
  - — CPT code 99401 (preventive medicine counseling lasting approximately 15 minutes): If counseling is done by the physician at the time of a regular antepartum visit, use modifier 25 on code 99401. If counseling is done by the physician at another encounter, separate from the antepartum visit, no modifier is needed with code 99401.
  - — CPT code 99211: If a nurse counsels the patient, and if nurses are recognized by the insurance company as "qualified" providers of the service, then code 99211 would be used instead of code 99401. If the nurse is not recognized as a caregiver, the services will not be covered unless provided by the physician.

References

1. American College of Obstetricians and Gynecologists. Smoking and women's health. ACOG Educational Bulletin 240. Washington, DC: ACOG, 1997
2. Fiore MC, Bailey WC, Cohen SJ, et al. Treating tobacco use and dependence. Clinical practice guideline. Rockville, MD: U.S. Department of Health and Human Services. Public Health Service, June 2000
3. Melvin C, Dolan Mullen P, Windsor RA, Whiteside HP, Goldenberg RL. Recommended cessation counselling for pregnant women who smoke: a review of the evidence. Tobacco Control 2000;9:1–5
4. Ventura SJ, Martin JA. Report of final natality statistics, 1996. Monthly vital statistics report; vol 46, no. 11 (suppl). Hyattsville, Maryland: National Center for Health Statistics, June 30, 1998
5. Kleinman JC, Pierre MB, Madans JH, Land GH, Schramm WF. Effects of maternal smoking on fetal and infant mortality. Am J Epidemiol 1998;127:274–282
6. DiFranza JR, Lew RA. Effect of maternal cigarette smoking on pregnancy complications and sudden infant death syndrome. J Fam Pract 1995;40:385–394
7. Glynn TJ, Manley MW. How to help your patients stop smoking: a National Cancer Institute manual for physicians. Smoking and Tobacco Control Program, Division of Cancer Prevention, NCI, U.S. Department of Health and Human Services, Washington, DC, November 1990; NIH publication no. 90-3064
8. U.S. Department of Health and Human Services. The health benefits of smoking cessation. U.S. Department of Health and Human Services, Public Health Service, Centers for Disease Control, Center for Chronic Disease Prevention and Health Promotion, Office on Smoking and Health, 1990; DHHS publication no. (CDC) 90-8416

ISSN 1074-8628

The American College of Obstetricians and Gynecologists
409 12th Street, SW
PO Box 96920
Washington, DC 20090-6920

12345/43210

ACOG EDUCATIONAL BULLETIN

Number 253, November 1998

Special Problems of Multiple Gestation

The incidence of twin and higher-order multiple gestations has increased significantly over the past 15 years primarily because of the availability and increased use of ovulation-inducing drugs and newly developed assisted reproductive technologies such as in vitro fertilization. Multiple pregnancies and their various complications have, therefore, become more common (1). The incidence of twins, triplets, and higher-order multiple gestations now has reached approximately 3% of all pregnancies (2). When considering only those pregnancies resulting from assisted reproductive techniques, the rate of twin deliveries is from 25% to 30%; triplets account for 5% of deliveries, whereas the rate of higher-order multiple gestations is 0.5–1% of deliveries (3). Significant maternal and neonatal consequences are affected by this increase in multiple births.

Multifetal gestation is associated with an increased risk of perinatal morbidity and mortality (see Tables 1–3). Women who are undergoing treatment for infertility should be aware of the risks and potential fetal and maternal complications of multiple gestation. Such women can benefit from preconceptional counseling.

Obstetrician–gynecologists should be prepared to manage, with consultation when necessary, the special problems and complications of twin and higher-order multiple gestations. Because of the many variables associated with higher-order gestations and the need for specialized care based on individual circumstances, this Educational Bulletin will focus on twin gestations.

This Educational Bulletin was developed under the direction of the Committee on Educational Bulletins of the American College of Obstetricians and Gynecologists as an aid to obstetricians and gynecologists. This document is not to be construed as establishing a standard of practice or dictating an exclusive course of treatment. Rather, it is intended as an educational tool that presents current information on obstetric–gynecologic issues.

Antepartum Management

Nutritional Considerations

It is recommended that maternal dietary intake in a multiple gestation be increased daily by approximately 300 kcal above that for a singleton pregnancy (4). Supplementation should include iron and folic acid. Although optimal weight gain for women with multiple gestations has not been deter-

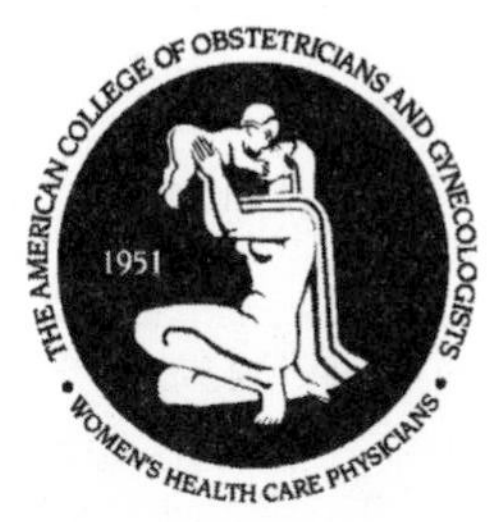

Replaces Number 131, August 1989

Table 1. Singleton Fetal Death Rates (per 1,000 conceptions)

	Weeks of Gestation										
Birth Weight (g)	**24–25**	**26–27**	**28–29**	**30–31**	**32–33**	**34–35**	**36–37**	**38–39**	**40–41**	**≥ 42**	**Birth Weight Alone**
≥ 4,900	—	—	—	—	—	—	—	—	—	—	—
4,600 < 4,900	—	—	—	—	—	—	—	3.6	1.9	2.1	2.3
4,300 < 4,600	—	—	—	—	—	—	—	1.7	1.2	1.6	1.4
4,000 < 4,300	—	—	—	—	—	—	3.0	1.1	1.0	1.3	1.1
3,700 < 4,000	—	—	—	—	—	—	2.2	0.9*	0.9	1.4	1.0†
3,400 < 3,700	—	—	—	—	—	—	2.2	1.0	1.1	1.5	1.2
3,100 < 3,400	—	—	—	—	—	2.9	2.6	1.3	1.4	1.8	1.5
2,800 < 3,100	—	—	—	—	6.4	5.0	3.5	2.0	2.2	2.6	2.5
2,500 < 2,800	—	—	—	—	12.1	8.8	6.5	4.1	4.5	4.8	5.3
2,200 < 2,500	—	—	—	21.4	19.4	14.2	13.9	10.3	11.2	12.0	12.9
1,900 < 2,200	—	—	49.2	37.1	29.6	27.8	31.1	26.2	24.4	—	29.1
1,600 < 1,900	—	68.9	72.1	43.7	49.8	61.8	72.3	—	—	—	57.0
1,300 < 1,600	150.2	99.2	66.2	68.4	103.2	127.3	—	—	—	—	89.4
1,000 < 1,300	193.2	93.5	95.1	142.9	212.5	—	—	—	—	—	128.6
700 < 1,000	173.7	151.5	221.7	287.9	353.4	—	—	—	—	—	200.7
500 < 700	318.1	355.2	447.0	509.7	—	—	—	—	—	—	361.2
Gestational Age Alone	231.3	157.3	126.7	86.8	45.2	15.1	5.9	1.9	1.6‡	1.9	4.3§

*Lowest fetal death rate by birth weight and gestational age: 0.9.

†Lowest fetal death rate by birth weight alone: 1.0.

‡Lowest fetal death rate by gestational age alone: 1.6.

§Overall fetal death rate: 4.3.

Modified from Luke B. Reducing fetal deaths in multiple births: optimal birthweights and gestational ages for infants of twin and triplet births. Acta Genet Med Gemellol 1996;45:333–348.

mined, it has been suggested that women with twins gain 35–45 pounds (5).

Prenatal Diagnosis

The usual indications for prenatal diagnosis and counseling in a singleton pregnancy apply to twin and higher-order gestations. Because the incidence of twin gestation increases with maternal age, women with multiple gestations often are candidates for prenatal genetic diagnosis. Genetic counseling should make clear to the patient the need to obtain a sample from each fetus, the risk of a chromosomal abnormality, potential complications of the procedure, the possibility of discordant results, and the ethical and technical concerns when one fetus is found to be abnormal. Some research has shown that the combined risk of fetal chromosome abnormality is higher in dizygotic twin gestations than in a singleton gestation (6, 7). Structural anomalies are more common in monozygotic twins.

Maternal Serum Screening

Maternal serum alpha-fetoprotein (MSAFP) screening programs contribute to the detection of multiple gestations. Multiple gestation is the second most common reason after incorrect dating for the reported increase in the MSAFP level during the second trimester. Maternal serum alpha-fetoprotein screening will identify approximately 60% of unsuspected twin gestations and virtually all higher-order gestations. About 10% of pregnancies with an elevated MSAFP level will be explained by the presence of more than one fetus. The median value of MSAFP levels in twins from 14 to 20 weeks of gestation is 2.5 times that for singleton pregnancies (8). The levels in triplets and quadruplets are three and four times as high, respectively (9). Genetic screening programs, there-

Table 2. Twin Fetal Death Rates (per 1,000 conceptions)

	Weeks of Gestation										
Birth Weight (g)	**24–25**	**26–27**	**28–29**	**30–31**	**32–33**	**34–35**	**36–37**	**38–39**	**40–41**	**≥ 42**	**Birth Weight Alone**
≥ 4,900	—	—	—	—	—	—	—	—	—	—	—
4,600 < 4,900	—	—	—	—	—	—	—	—	—	—	—
4,300 < 4,600	—	—	—	—	—	—	—	—	—	—	—
4,000 < 4,300	—	—	—	—	—	—	—	—	—	—	—
3,700 < 4,000	—	—	—	—	—	—	—	—	—	—	—
3,400 < 3,700	—	—	—	—	—	—	7.7	6.2	7.6	13.6	7.3
3,100 < 3,400	—	—	—	—	—	8.9	4.5	5.8	5.7	11.6	5.9
2,800 < 3,100	—	—	—	—	11.1	6.2	3.6	4.8	4.8	9.7	4.8
2,500 < 2,800	—	—	—	—	9.5	4.3	3.3*	4.1	7.7	11.4	4.7†
2,200 < 2,500	—	—	—	22.0	9.4	5.2	5.9	9.1	12.2	17.5	7.8
1,900 < 2,200	—	—	29.9	19.8	9.3	9.1	12.4	19.4	22.2	30.1	13.4
1,600 < 1,900	—	—	22.5	17.5	14.2	17.3	33.1	42.4	58.3	76.2	23.8
1,300 < 1,600	—	55.8	24.0	26.0	35.7	60.0	90.7	105.5	73.8	—	44.6
1,000 < 1,300	142.9	57.4	41.5	58.0	97.2	126.2	—	—	—	—	65.1
700 < 1,000	86.4	68.5	106.7	180.8	185.4	—	—	—	—	—	99.6
500 < 700	157.1	187.6	214.7	191.7	—	—	—	—	—	—	176.2
Gestational Age Alone	123.4	85.5	57.0	41.0	21.5	11.7	8.1‡	8.2	10.1	16.7	15.5§

*Lowest fetal death rate by birth weight and gestational age: 3.3.
†Lowest fetal death rate by birth weight alone: 4.7.
‡Lowest fetal death rate by gestational age alone: 8.1.
§Overall fetal death rate: 15.5.
Modified from Luke B. Reducing fetal deaths in multiple births: optimal birthweights and gestational ages for infants of twin and triplet births. Acta Genet Med Gemellol 1996;45:333–348.

fore, redefine an elevated MSAFP level for a twin gestation because there are two fetuses and a larger volume of placenta. Depending on the laboratory, a value greater than 4.5 multiples of the median in an uncomplicated twin gestation is abnormal, requiring further comprehensive ultrasound evaluation by an experienced ultrasonographer and possible amniocentesis for the detection of amniotic fluid alpha-fetoprotein and acetylcholinesterase.

Although maternal serum screening for neural tube defects can be useful in the twin pregnancy, its effectiveness in screening for trisomy 21 is not well defined (10). Further investigation is necessary to determine the clinical usefulness of multiple marker screening for Down syndrome in twin and higher-order pregnancies.

Amniocentesis

Although the risks may be increased, amniocentesis, using continuous ultrasound guidance, of both sacs can be performed successfully in most patients with a twin gestation (11). One technique is ultrasound-guided amniocentesis of each sac with approximately 1–2 mL of a dilute (approximately 0.08%) indigo carmine dye instilled into the first amniotic sac (12). A second amniocentesis of clear fluid confirms specimens from each sac. Methylene blue dye, which is associated with fetal bowel atresia and other complications, should not be used (13). If the twins are without question monozygotic, there is no reason to tap more than one sac.

Chorionic Villus Sampling

Chorionic villus sampling (CVS) is an appropriate method of first-trimester prenatal diagnosis in multiple gestations (14). The procedure is best performed by or under the supervision of an experienced operator who samples both placentas under ultrasound guidance between 10.0 and 12.9 weeks of gestation. Difficulties that can arise with CVS in twin gestations include the inability to obtain an adequate sample and contamination of one sample with tissue from the second. In approximately 1% of patients, tissue can be obtained only from

Table 3. Triplet Fetal Death Rates (per 1,000 conceptions)

	Weeks of Gestation										
Birth Weight (g)	**24–25**	**26–27**	**28–29**	**30–31**	**32–33**	**34–35**	**36–37**	**38–39**	**40–41**	**≥ 42**	**Birth Weight Alone**
≥ 4,900	—	—	—	—	—	—	—	—	—	—	—
4,600 < 4,900	—	—	—	—	—	—	—	—	—	—	—
4,300 < 4,600	—	—	—	—	—	—	—	—	—	—	—
4,000 < 4,300	—	—	—	—	—	—	—	—	—	—	—
3,700 < 4,000	—	—	—	—	—	—	—	—	—	—	—
3,400 < 3,700	—	—	—	—	—	—	—	—	—	—	—
3,100 < 3,400	—	—	—	—	—	—	—	—	—	—	—
2,800 < 3,100	—	—	—	—	—	27.8	22.2	39.0	117.6	—	34.0
2,500 < 2,800	—	—	—	—	41.7	14.3	9.5	32.0	78.9	200.0	23.0
2,200 < 2,500	—	—	—	—	15.2	6.8	9.0	18.8	59.7	130.4	13.8
1,900 < 2,200	—	—	—	16.7	7.0	5.2*	8.1	15.5	40.8	100.0	9.3†
1,600 < 1,900	—	—	22.7	11.0	7.0	7.2	21.8	46.2	76.9	125.0	13.4
1,300 < 1,600	—	29.4	15.7	11.4	12.0	24.6	54.3	60.6	93.8	272.7	21.5
1,000 < 1,300	—	37.4	15.9	24.2	34.7	54.8	80.0	133.3	—	—	29.1
700 < 1,000	31.3	30.4	32.6	25.0	153.8	214.3	—	—	—	—	41.0
500 < 700	73.8	105.3	172.4	—	—	—	—	—	—	—	94.5
Gestational Age Alone	54.2	43.8	25.5	15.5	14.2	11.4‡	15.0	31.5	69.9	147.7	21.0§

*Lowest fetal death rate by birth weight and gestational age: 5.2.
†Lowest fetal death rate by birth weight alone: 9.3.
‡Lowest fetal death rate by gestational age alone: 11.4.
§Overall fetal death rate: 21.0.
Modified from Luke B. Reducing fetal deaths in multiple births: optimal birthweights and gestational ages for infants of twin and triplet births. Acta Genet Med Gemellol 1996;45:333–348.

one placenta. When CVS is performed at centers with experienced operators, twin–twin contamination occurs in approximately 4–6% of samples, causing prenatal diagnostic errors. When CVS or amniocentesis is performed in the twin gestation, documentation of the location of the fetuses and the membrane separating the sacs is important because discordant results can occur, and the location of the abnormal fetus may need to be known for future management.

Multifetal Reduction

The greater the number of fetuses within the uterus, the greater the risk for preterm delivery and adverse perinatal outcome. Multifetal pregnancy reduction may be performed to decrease the risk of serious perinatal morbidity and mortality associated with preterm delivery by reducing the number of fetuses (15, 16). Preferably, this problem can be avoided by carefully monitoring patients receiving ovulation-inducing drugs and by minimizing the number of embryos transferred during in vitro fertilization or embryo transfer programs. The ethical dilemmas can be considerable (17). Patients with higher-order multiple gestations may be faced with the possibility of terminating the entire pregnancy, continuing the pregnancy and taking the risk of delivering severely preterm infants, or reducing the pregnancy in an effort to decrease the risk of perinatal morbidity and mortality.

Pregnancy loss is the main risk of multifetal pregnancy reduction and ranges from 10% to 26%. The benefit of this procedure is most clear in quadruplet and higher-order gestations because it increases the length of gestation of the surviving fetuses (18). It is unclear and remains to be determined whether multifetal pregnancy reduction improves long-term neonatal outcome of a triplet gestation reduced to twins. Elevations in MSAFP levels occur after selective reduction to twins (19); nonetheless, these patients should undergo a detailed ultrasound examination of the surviving fetuses in the middle of the second trimester.

Dizygotic twins can be discordant for congenital anomalies. Selective fetal termination allows a pregnancy to continue with a normal twin after the termination of an abnormal twin. In one study, selective fetal termination was performed successfully in 183 multifetal pregnancies, most of which were twin gestations (20). Indications for selective fetal termination were twins discordant for chromosomal abnormalities, fetal structural anomalies, or one twin affected by a Mendelian disorder. The preferred method for selective fetal termination was intracardiac injection of potassium chloride. The procedure caused loss of the entire pregnancy if there was a monochorionic placentation. The pregnancy loss rate before 24 weeks of gestation was 12.6%; an additional 3.8% of patients gave birth between 24 and 28 weeks of gestation. The authors of this study concluded that selective fetal termination for an abnormal pregnancy is a safe procedure when performed by experienced physicians provided there is a dichorionic placentation. Ligation of the umbilical cord under endoscopic visualization has been performed for selective termination in a monochorionic pregnancy, but the safety and efficacy of this procedure requires further study (21).

Ultrasonography

Ultrasonography can be useful in both prenatal diagnosis and antepartum surveillance. With its use, less than 10% of twin gestations are undiagnosed before labor and delivery. Although the value of routine screening to promote early diagnosis is subject to debate, ultrasonography has a role in evaluating the progress of pregnancy once the diagnosis is established.

Screening

In the randomized clinical Routine Antenatal Diagnostic Imaging With Ultrasound (RADIUS) trial, special attention was given to multiple gestation. In the study, 129 multiple gestations were included. The RADIUS study concluded that multiple pregnancies were consistently diagnosed at an earlier gestational age in the screened group; however, this finding did not result in any overall alteration in management improving adverse perinatal outcome. This conclusion is not consistent with findings of other studies. In a 10-year study of 22,400 women having 43,000 routine ultrasound examinations involving 249 multiple gestations, earlier detection improved perinatal outcome (22). When multiple gestation is suspected on the basis of clinical examination, family history, a history of assisted reproduction, or an elevated MSAFP value, an ultrasound examination should be performed. Often, ultrasound examinations are performed early in gestation in twins to document viability; this examination also can be helpful in defining chorionicity.

Evaluation

A detailed ultrasound evaluation of a multiple gestation should be performed during the second trimester. This examination should include determination of placentation, amnionicity, and chorionicity; the number of fetuses; evaluation for fetal amniotic fluid or placental abnormalities; and an assessment of the growth of each fetus. If two separate placentas are identified or if the fetuses are of different sex, the placentation is dichorionic. A thick membrane also suggests dichorionicity. When a thin, wispy membrane is seen between two sacs with a single placenta, and the fetuses are of the same sex, monochorionicity is suggested. "Stuck twin syndrome," where there is polyhydramnios for one twin and extreme oligohydramnios for the other, can be very difficult to differentiate from a monochorionic pregnancy because the membrane may be so near the stuck twin that it is difficult to detect. Determination of chorionicity is most accurate in the first trimester; as the pregnancy progresses, it becomes less accurate (23, 24).

Visualization of a membrane confirms the diagnosis of a diamniotic gestation. When dichorionicity is diagnosed, the pregnancy must also be diamniotic. The number of fetuses should be identified; this number, however, may decrease as the pregnancy progresses. Until the third trimester, twins follow the same growth curves that apply to singleton pregnancies. There is no clear clinical advantage to the use of twin- or triplet-specific ultrasound growth tables. Evaluation of serial fetal growth should include estimated fetal weight of each fetus and appropriate and concordant interval growth.

Routine Cervical Evaluation

Routine cervical evaluation by either clinical or ultrasonographic assessment has been investigated as an approach to predict preterm birth in the multiple gestation. A cervical scoring system, calculated as cervical length (in centimeters) minus cervical dilatation at the internal os (in centimeters) has been used (25). This system has been associated with a positive predictive value of 75%, which is associated with a fourfold increased relative risk of preterm delivery (26). Weekly digital cervical examination for clinical assessment of the cervix has not been associated with adverse maternal or fetal outcome (27).

Vaginal ultrasonography has been used to measure cervical width, length, and funneling and to examine the relationship of these measurements to the risk of preterm birth (28). In this study, the risk of spontaneous preterm delivery was increased in women who were found to have a short cervix. Although this is a promising technique, further evaluation of transvaginal ultrasonography by a prospective randomized study is necessary to determine its role in the prevention of preterm birth.

Several investigators have studied the use of cervical cerclage in multiple gestations to prevent preterm birth (29). Because there is no clear-cut benefit to this approach, and its use is associated with both maternal and fetal risks, this procedure is not recommended for multiple gestations.

Bed Rest

The role and value of bed rest at home or in the hospital in the prevention of preterm delivery of a multiple gestation remains controversial. Not only is hospital bed rest costly, stressful, and disruptive, there is no clear consensus that it is of any benefit. Numerous studies have failed to show that bed rest decreases the incidence of preterm delivery, lengthens gestation, or improves neonatal morbidity in multiple gestation (30). Also, there are little data to support activity reduction in multiple or singleton gestations. Antepartum hospitalization may be necessary in the multiple gestation for managing complications such as preterm labor and abnormal fetal growth.

Antepartum Surveillance

The routine use and benefit of antepartum fetal surveillance in the uncomplicated multifetal gestation has not been shown to be of benefit. When intrauterine growth restriction, abnormal fluid volumes, growth discordance, pregnancy-induced hypertension, fetal anomalies, monoamnionicity, or other pregnancy complications occur, fetal surveillance, including nonstress testing or the modified or standard biophysical profile, is indicated (31). The biophysical profile is as reliable in multiple gestations as in singleton gestations (32).

Although some patients may find it difficult to distinguish between fetal movement of each twin, fetal movement counting can be an adjunct to these antepartum surveillance techniques. Umbilical cord velocimetry may be helpful in evaluating the severely growth-restricted fetus, but its role in antepartum fetal surveillance of the singleton or multiple gestation is yet to be determined (33).

Home Uterine Activity Monitoring

The use of the home uterine activity monitor has been advocated by some to prevent or manage preterm labor in singleton or multiple gestations. There are, however, no data to support its use (34–36).

Management of Complications

Preterm Labor

The most significant and common complication of multiple pregnancy is preterm labor resulting in preterm delivery. Perinatal morbidity and mortality are affected by gestational age and weight at delivery as well as by the number of fetuses. The presence of a single anomalous fetus in a twin gestation increases the risk of preterm delivery compared with nonanomalous twin gestations (37). Patient education, risk assessment, serial cervical evaluation by manual or transvaginal ultrasound examinations, specialized antepartum clinics, and home uterine activity monitoring have been used with mixed results to detect preterm labor early and prevent preterm birth in multiple gestations.

Preterm labor in twins is preceded by an increase in uterine contraction frequency; however, this does not hold true with triplets (38). Women with triplet gestations have more uterine irritability than do those with twin or singleton pregnancies. The management of preterm labor is discussed elsewhere (39).

A number of medications are available for inhibition of preterm labor. These agents include magnesium sulfate, beta-adrenergic agents, indomethacin, and the calcium channel blockers. Whenever tocolysis is used, recognition of contraindications and close maternal and fetal monitoring are necessary to detect complications. Women pregnant with multiple gestations are at a higher risk for the development of pulmonary edema because of higher blood volume, lower colloid osmotic pressure, and anemia. Older women with multiple gestations also are at increased risk for myocardial ischemia and cardiac arrhythmias as a result of tocolytic therapy. No benefit has been shown from the use of oral tocolysis in multiple gestations to prevent the onset of preterm labor or preterm birth (40, 41).

Corticosteroids should be administered for induction of fetal lung maturation to women with multiple pregnancies who are experiencing preterm labor (less than 34 weeks of gestation) (42). The National Institutes of Health also recommends corticosteroid therapy for women with preterm premature rupture of membranes at less than 30–32 weeks of gestation. Because steroid administration in triplet and higher-order multiple gestation may actually increase contractions, close surveillance of uterine activity following administration of corticosteroids is recommended (43).

Preterm Rupture of Membranes

Preterm premature rupture of membranes occurs more frequently in twin gestations than in singleton gestations (44). A matched-control study of preterm premature rupture of membranes in twins concluded that the nonpresenting twin more frequently had hyaline membrane disease, respiratory complications, and required more oxygen therapy than the presenting infant. There were no significant differences between twin and singleton gestations in infectious morbidity, cord prolapse, abruptio placentae, or latency to delivery. Infant morbidity and mortality were high for the nonpresenting infant at significantly increased risk of respiratory complications (44).

Preterm rupture of the presenting sac occurs most frequently. Although the incidence is unknown, membrane rupture of the nonpresenting sac also can occur. When preterm rupture of membranes occurs in the multiple gestation, it most frequently occurs prior to fetal lung maturation. Preterm premature rupture of membranes occurs more frequently in the triplet gestation than in the twin gestation, resulting in a higher incidence of preterm labor, delivery, and perinatal mortality (45). The management of the multifetal gestation complicated by preterm premature rupture of membranes depends on the gestational age, fetal lung maturation, number of fetuses, and the presence of maternal or fetal complications. The use of tocolysis, antibiotics, and glucocorticoids when preterm premature rupture of membranes occurs remains controversial. When there is evidence of fetal lung maturation, delivery may be indicated. In rare cases, prolongation of pregnancy after preterm premature rupture of membranes after delivery of the first twin may be considered.

Fetal Disorders

Intrauterine Growth Restriction

Intrauterine growth restriction occurs more frequently in twins and higher-order multiple gestations than in a singleton pregnancy and is a significant cause of increased neonatal morbidity and mortality. Antepartum management of the multiple gestation should include early identification of intrauterine growth restriction by ultrasonography and increased fetal surveillance to improve perinatal outcome. There is no single definition for the diagnosis of intrauterine growth restriction or discordant growth in twins. Estimated fetal weight is helpful in making the diagnosis of intrauterine growth restriction and discordance between fetuses.

Intrauterine growth restriction usually is diagnosed either when the estimated fetal weight decreases below the 10th percentile for a singleton gestation or when there is discordance (ie, a difference in estimated fetal weight of greater than 20% between twin A and twin B expressed as a percentage of the larger twin's weight). Once intrauterine growth restriction has been diagnosed, the multiple gestation should be monitored more closely with serial ultrasonography every 2–3 weeks to assess fetal growth and amniotic fluid volume. Frequent fetal antenatal surveillance by the nonstress test or biophysical profile is necessary. Early delivery should be considered. When amniocentesis is necessary to assess fetal lung maturity, results obtained from amniotic fluid of either twin usually will represent lung maturity of both twins (46).

Other Complications

Twin–twin transfusion syndrome, monoamniotic twinning, conjoined twins, and acardia (or twin reversed arterial perfusion sequence) are fetal complications of monochorionic gestations that are rarely encountered by the obstetrician–gynecologist. Patients with these complications should be cared for by or in collaboration with specialists familiar with their management.

Death of One Twin

Death of one fetus of a multiple gestation can occur at any time during pregnancy although it is more common in the first trimester. These patients can benefit from perinatal grief counseling. Only 50% of twin gestations diagnosed in the first trimester result in delivery of two live infants. Early fetal demise of one twin may not be recognized clinically but may be diagnosed by first-trimester ultrasonography. A documented multiple gestation that spontaneously loses one or more fetuses during the first trimester is called the vanishing twin phenomenon. This occurs most commonly in the twin gestation, but also has been reported in the higher-order multiple pregnancy (47). The true incidence of this phenomenon is unknown, but one study reported a vanishing twin rate of 21.2% (48). Another study reported a 25% loss rate of a single twin in multiple gestations arising from assisted reproductive procedures (49). No adverse maternal outcome occurs as the result of a vanishing embryo, and the prognosis for the surviving twin is excellent (48).

Single fetal demise after the first trimester is more common with monochorionic placentation, ranging in incidence from 0.5% to 6.8% (50). When death of one fetus occurs, the probability of harm to the surviving twin or to the mother is low. Death or damage in the remaining twin was previously thought to be caused by intravascular coagulation. Recent evidence, however, suggests that acute hypotension in the surviving twin with partial exsanguination into the dying twin through anastomoses within the placenta is more likely responsible. The surviving twin can develop fetal morbidity consisting more often of renal cortical necrosis and multicystic encephalomalacia. The incidence of morbidity and mortality in the surviving co-twin is highest with monochorionic twins compared with dichorionic twins, in whom the risk is negligible (51). Preterm birth is one of the greatest risks to the surviving co-twin (52, 53).

Once a single fetal demise is diagnosed, the gestational age of the pregnancy and the condition of the surviving fetus will dictate clinical management. When death of one fetus occurs prior to 34 weeks of gestation, fetal movement counting and increased antepartum fetal surveillance of the surviving twin should be undertaken. Fetal compromise or the presence of fetal lung maturation suggest a need for delivery. Maternal consumptive coagulopathy with hypofibrinogenemia occasionally may develop under these circumstances (54, 55). Delivery may be appropriate if the death of one twin occurs after 34 weeks of gestation.

Intrapartum Management

Timing

Ideally, women with multiple pregnancies should undergo delivery by 40 weeks of gestation; however, the clinician must frequently weigh the risks to the fetuses if intrauterine life is continued versus the risk to the mother if the pregnancy is continued. For example, preterm labor, discordance, abnormal fetal surveillance, or pregnancy-induced hypertension may mandate earlier intervention. The ideal time of delivery for uncomplicated pregnancies is uncertain; however, if elective delivery is considered before 38 weeks of gestation, fetal lung maturity should be assessed. Although there are few data pertaining to multiple gestations beyond 40 weeks of gestation, delivery should probably be effected by this time.

Labor and Delivery

When a woman with a known or suspected multiple gestation presents in labor, confirmation as soon as possible by ultrasound examination of fetal number and presentations is indicated. Both twins should be monitored continuously during labor. Ultrasonography should be available to determine the heart rate of the second twin as well as its orientation following delivery of the first twin. Appropriate, experienced pediatric and anesthesia personnel should be notified and available at delivery. Capability for emergency cesarean delivery is necessary and blood should be available because the likelihood of operative intervention, as well as postpartum hemorrhage, is increased.

Route of Delivery

Controversy surrounds the preferred route of delivery for some multiple gestations, especially twins. Delivery should be based on individual needs and may depend on the clinician's practice and experience. The various twin presentations should be taken into account. All combinations of twin presentations and their frequency essentially can be classified into the following groups (56):

Twin A–Vertex with Twin B–Vertex. Vaginal delivery is anticipated for vertex–vertex twins. Cesarean delivery should only be performed for the same indications applied to singleton gestations. In one series, 81.2% of the vertex–vertex twin gestations were successfully delivered vaginally (57).

Twin A–Vertex with Twin B–Nonvertex. There are conflicting data on the management of twins in vertex–breech or vertex–transverse presentation. Because depressed Apgar scores and an increased perinatal mortality rate have been associated with vaginal delivery of the second twin, cesarean delivery has been advocated by some whenever the second twin is in a nonvertex presentation (58). Cesarean delivery, however, is not always necessary. Vaginal delivery of twin B in the nonvertex presentation is a reasonable option for a neonate with an estimated weight greater than 1,500 g. Under these circumstances, it has been reported that perinatal mortality and low 5-minute Apgar scores are not increased when a second breech twin is delivered vaginally after the criteria for vaginal delivery of a singleton breech are met (57, 59–61). There are insufficient data to advocate a specific route of delivery (vaginal or abdominal) of twin B whose birth weight is less than 1,500 g, although cesarean delivery is performed frequently (57, 62).

Twin A–Nonvertex. In general, cesarean delivery is the method of choice when the first twin is nonvertex, such as a breech or transverse presentation. The safety of vaginal delivery for this group has not been documented. When the first twin is breech and the second is in a vertex presentation, the possibility of locked twins exists, in which case vaginal delivery would be contraindicated, if not impossible. Locked twins, however, appear to be exceedingly rare.

Interval Between Deliveries

The interval between delivery of each twin is not critical in determining the outcome of twin B (57, 63). Surveillance of twin B with real-time ultrasonography and continuous monitoring of the fetal heart rate, however, are advised after the delivery of twin A. Rapid delivery may be required because of complications, such as abruptio placentae, cord prolapse, or a decrease in the fetal heart rate. If labor has not resumed within a reasonable time after the delivery of twin A, oxytocin augmentation with careful fetal heart rate surveillance can be initiated. Once the vertex is in the pelvic inlet, amniotomy can be performed. When fetal condition dictates the need to expedite delivery, internal podalic version and breech extraction may be an acceptable alternative.

There are insufficient data to assess the safety of vaginal delivery of twins after previous cesarean delivery. The modes of delivery used for twins and higher-order multiple gestations in the presence of a prior cesarean delivery are areas under study (64, 65). Obstetricians should select the delivery technique with which they are most comfortable.

Summary

The incidence of twins, triplets, and higher-order multiple gestations has increased dramatically because of widespread use of ovulation-inducing drugs and advanced assisted reproductive techniques. There is considerable perinatal/maternal morbidity and mortality associated with multifetal gestations. The practicing obstetrician managing these high-risk patients should be familiar with their special antepartum and intrapartum problems. The obstetrician–gynecologist unaccustomed to caring for patients with a multifetal gestation should consult with maternal–fetal medicine specialists who have expertise in managing these pregnancies. Better use of infertility modalities, early diagnosis of the multiple pregnancy, prevention of preterm birth, close fetal surveillance, and atraumatic labor and delivery can improve perinatal outcome in the multifetal gestation.

References

1. Luke B. The changing pattern of multiple births in the United States: maternal and infant characteristics, 1973 and 1990. Obstet Gynecol 1994;84:101–106
2. Ventura SJ, Martin JA, Curtin SC, Mathews TJ. Report of final natality statistics, 1996. Monthly vital statistics report; vol 46, no. 11 (suppl). Hyattsville, Maryland: National Center for Health Statistics, 1998
3. American Fertility Society, Society for Assisted Reproductive Technology. Assisted reproductive technology in the United States and Canada: 1992 results generated from the American Fertility Society/Society for Assisted Reproductive Technology registry. Fertil Steril 1994;62:1121–1128
4. National Research Council. Subcommittee on the Tenth Edition of the RDAs, Food and Nutrition Board, Commission on Life Sciences. Recommended dietary allowances. 10th ed. Washington, DC: National Academy Press, 1989
5. Abrams B. Maternal nutrition. In: Creasy RK, Resnick R, eds. Maternal-fetal medicine, principles and practice. 3rd ed. Philadelphia: WB Saunders, 1994:162–170
6. Rodis JF, Egan JFX, Craffey A, Ciarleglio L, Greenstein RM, Scorza WE, et al. Calculated risk of chromosomal abnormalities in twin gestations. Obstet Gynecol 1990; 76:1037–1041
7. Meyers C, Adam R, Dungan J, Prenger V. Aneuploidy in twin gestations: when is maternal age advanced? Obstet Gynecol 1997;89:248–251
8. Johnson JM, Harman CR, Evans JA, MacDonald K, Manning FA. Maternal serum alpha-fetoprotein in twin pregnancy. Am J Obstet Gynecol 1990;162:1020–1025
9. Wald N, Cuckle H. Maternal serum alpha-fetoprotein levels in triplet and quadruplet pregnancy. Br J Obstet Gynaecol 1978;85:124–126
10. Wald N, Cuckle H, Wu T, George L. Maternal serum unconjugated oestriol and human chorionic gonadotrophin levels in twin pregnancies: implications for screening for Down's syndrome. Br J Obstet Gynaecol 1991;98:905–908
11. Tabsh KM, Crandall B, Lebherz TB, Howard J. Genetic amniocentesis in twin pregnancy. Obstet Gynecol 1985; 65:843–845
12. Elias S, Gerbie AB, Simpson JL, Nader HL, Sabbagha RE, Shkolnik A. Genetic amniocentesis in term gestation. Am J Obstet Gynecol 1980;138:169–174
13. Van der Pol JG, Wolf H, Boer K, Treffers PE, Leschot NJ, Hey HA, et al. Jejunal atresia related to the use of methylene blue in genetic amniocentesis in twins. Br J Obstet Gynaecol 1992;99:141–143
14. Wapner RJ, Johnson A, Davis G, Urban A, Morgan P, Jackson L. Prenatal diagnosis in twin gestations: a comparison between second-trimester amniocentesis and first-trimester chorionic villus sampling. Obstet Gynecol 1993; 82:49–56
15. Berkowitz RL, Lynch L, Chitkara U, Wilkins IA, Mehalek KE, Alvarez E. Selective reduction of multifetal pregnancies in the first trimester. N Engl J Med 1988;318:1043–1047
16. American College of Obstetricians and Gynecologists. Multifetal pregnancy reduction and selective termination. Committee Opinion 94. Washington, DC: ACOG, 1991
17. Evans MI, May M, Drugan A, Fletcher JC, Johnson MP, Sokol RJ. Selective termination: clinical experience and residual risks. Am J Obstet Gynecol 1990;162:1568–1575
18. Evans MI, Dommergues M, Wapner RJ, Lynch L, Dumez Y, Goldberg JD, et al. Efficacy of transabdominal multifetal pregnancy reduction: collaborative experience among the world's largest centers. Obstet Gynecol 1993;82:61–66
19. Lynch L, Berkowitz RL. Maternal serum alpha-fetoprotein and coagulation profiles after multifetal pregnancy reduction. Am J Obstet Gynecol 1993;169:987–990
20. Evans MI, Goldberg JD, Dommergues M, Wapner RJ, Lynch L, Dock BS, et al. Efficacy of second-trimester selective termination for fetal abnormalities: international collaborative experience among the world's largest centers. Am J Obstet Gynecol 1994;171:90–94
21. Quintero RA, Reich H, Puder KS, Bardicef M, Evans MI, Cotton DB, et al. Brief report: umbilical-cord ligation of an acardiac twin by fetoscopy at 19 weeks of gestation. N Engl J Med 1994;330:469–471
22. Persson PH, Kullander S. Long-term experience of general ultrasound screening in pregnancy. Am J Obstet Gynecol 1983;146:942–947
23. D'Alton ME, Dudley DK. The ultrasonographic prediction of chorionicity in twin gestation. Am J Obstet Gynecol 1989;160:557–561

24. Kurtz AB, Wapner RJ, Mata J, Johnson A, Morgan P. Twin pregnancies: accuracy of first-trimester abdominal US in predicting chorionicity and amnionicity. Radiology 1992; 185:759–762

25. Houlton MCC, Marivate M, Philpott RH. Factors associated with preterm labour and changes in the cervix before labour in twin pregnancy. Br J Obstet Gynaecol 1982; 89:190–194

26. Newman RB, Godsey RK, Ellings JM, Campbell BA, Eller DP, Miller MC. Quantification of cervical change: relationship to preterm delivery in the multifetal gestation. Am J Obstet Gynecol 1991;165:264–269

27. Bivins HA Jr, Newman RB, Ellings JM, Hulsey TC, Keenan A. Risks of antepartum cervical examination in multifetal gestations. Am J Obstet Gynecol 1993;169:22– 25

28. Iams JD, Goldenberg RL, Meis PJ, Mercer BM, Moawad A, Das A, et al. The length of the cervix and the risk of spon-taneous premature delivery. N Engl J Med 1996;334: 567–572

29. Mordel N, Zajicek G, Benshushan A, Schenker JG, Laufer N, Sadovsky E. Elective suture of uterine cervix in triplets. Am J Perinatol 1993;10:14–16

30. Andrews WW, Leveno KJ, Sherman ML, Mutz J, Gilstrap LC, Whalley PJ. Elective hospitalization in the management of twin pregnancies. Obstet Gynecol 1991;77:826– 831

31. American College of Obstetricians and Gynecologists. Antepartum fetal surveillance. ACOG Technical Bulletin 188. Washington, DC: ACOG, 1994

32. Newman RB, Ellings JM. Antepartum management of the multiple gestation: the case for specialized care. Semin Perinatol 1995;19:387–403

33. American College of Obstetricians and Gynecologists. Utility of antepartum umbilical artery Doppler velocimetry in intrauterine growth restriction. Committee Opinion 188. Washington, DC: ACOG, 1997

34. Dyson DC, Crites YM, Ray DA, Armstrong MA. Prevention of preterm birth in high-risk patients: the role of education and provider contact versus home uterine monitoring. Am J Obstet Gynecol 1991;164:756–762

35. Dyson DC, Danbe KH, Bamber JA, Crites YM, Field DR, Maier JA, et al. Monitoring women at risk for preterm labor. N Engl J Med 1998;338:15–19

36. American College of Obstetricians and Gynecologists. Home uterine activity monitoring. Committee Opinion 172. Washington, DC: ACOG, 1996

37. Malone FD, Craigo SD, Chelmow D, D'Alton ME. Outcome of twin gestations complicated by a single anomalous fetus. Obstet Gynecol 1996;88:1–5

38. Newman RB, Gill PJ, Campion S, Katz M. The influence of fetal number on antepartum uterine activity. Obstet Gynecol 1989;73:695–699

39. American College of Obstetricians and Gynecologists. Preterm labor. ACOG Technical Bulletin 206. Washington, DC: ACOG, 1995

40. Newton ER. Antepartum care in multiple gestation. Semin Perinatol 1986;10:19–29

41. Ashworth MF, Spooner SF, Verkuyl DAA, Waterman R, Ashurst HM. Failure to prevent preterm labour and delivery in twin pregnancy using prophylactic oral salbutamol. Br J Obstet Gynaecol 1990;97:878–882

42. National Institutes of Health. Consensus development conference statement. Effect of corticosteroids for fetal maturation on perinatal outcomes. Bethesda, Maryland: NIH Office of Medical Applications of Research, 1994

43. Elliott JP, Radin TG. The effect of corticosteroid administration on uterine activity and preterm labor in high-order multiple gestations. Obstet Gynecol 1995;85:250–254

44. Mercer BM, Crocker LG, Pierce WF, Sibai BM. Clinical characteristics and outcome of twin gestation complicated by preterm premature rupture of the membranes. Am J Obstet Gynecol 1993;168:1467–1473

45. Sassoon DA, Castro LC, Davis JL, Hobel CJ. Perinatal outcome in triplet versus twin gestations. Obstet Gynecol 1990;75:817–820

46. Leveno KJ, Quirk JG, Whalley PJ, Herbert WNP, Trubey R. Fetal lung maturation in twin gestation. Am J Obstet Gynecol 1984;148:405–411

47. Seoud MA-F, Toner JP, Kruithoff C, Muasher SJ. Outcome of twin, triplet, and quadruplet in vitro fertilization pregnancies: the Norfolk experience. Fertil Steril 1992;57: 825–834

48. Landy HJ, Weiner S, Corson SL, Batzer FR, Bolognese RJ. The "vanishing twin": ultrasonographic assessment of fetal disappearance in the first trimester. Am J Obstet Gynecol 1986;155:14–19

49. Corson SL, Dickey RP, Gocial B, Batzer FR, Eisenberg E, Huppert L, et al. Outcome in 242 in vitro fertilization-embryo replacement or gamete intrafallopian transfer-induced pregnancies. Fertil Steril 1989;51:644–650

50. Dudley DKL, D'Alton ME. Single fetal death in twin gestation. Semin Perinatol 1986;10:65–72

51. Burke MS. Single fetal demise in twin gestation. Clin Obstet Gynecol 1990;33:69–78

52. Fusi L, Gordon H. Twin pregnancy complicated by single intrauterine death. Problems and outcome with conservative management. Br J Obstet Gynaecol 1990;97:511–516

53. Eglowstein MS, D'Alton ME. Single intrauterine demise in twin gestation. J Matern Fetal Med 1993;2:272–275

54. Romero R, Duffy TP, Berkowitz RL, Chang E, Hobbins JC. Prolongation of a preterm pregnancy complicated by death of a single twin in utero and disseminated intravascular coagulation. Effects of treatment with heparin. N Engl J Med 1984;310:772–774

55. Landy HJ, Weingold AB. Management of a multiple gestation complicated by an antepartum fetal demise. Obstet Gynecol Surv 1989;44:171–176

56. Hays PM, Smeltzer JS. Multiple gestation. Clin Obstet Gynecol 1986;29:264–285

57. Chervenak FA, Johnson RE, Youcha S, Hobbins JC, Berkowitz RL. Intrapartum management of twin gestation. Obstet Gynecol 1985;65:119–124

58. Cetrulo CL. The controversy of mode of delivery in twins: the intrapartum management of twin gestation. Part I. Semin Perinatol 1986;10:39–43

59. Acker D, Lieberman M, Holbrook RH, James O, Phillipe M, Edelin KC. Delivery of the second twin. Obstet Gynecol 1982;59:710–711

60. Chervenak FA, Johnson RE, Berkowitz RL, Grannum P, Hobbins JC. Is routine cesarean section necessary for vertex-breech and vertex-transverse gestations? Am J Obstet Gynecol 1984;148:1–5

61. Gocke SE, Nageotte MP, Garite T, Towers CV, Dorcester W. Management of the nonvertex second twin: primary cesarean section, external version, or primary breech extraction. Am J Obstet Gynecol 1989;161:111–114

62. Barrett JM, Staggs SM, Van Hooydonk JE, Growdon JH, Killam AP, Boehm FH. The effect of type of delivery upon neonatal outcome in premature twins. Am J Obstet Gynecol 1982;143:360–367

63. Rayburn WF, Lavin JP Jr, Miodovnik M, Varner MW. Multiple gestation: time interval between delivery of the first and second twins. Obstet Gynecol 1984;63:502–506

64. Miller DA, Mullin P, Hou D, Paul RH. Vaginal birth after cesarean section in twin gestation. Am J Obstet Gynecol 1996;175:194–198

65. Essel JK, Opai-Tetteh ET. Twin delivery after a cesarean section—always a section? S Afr Med J 1996;86:279–280

Suggested Reading

American College of Obstetricians and Gynecologists. Antepartum fetal surveillance. ACOG Technical Bulletin 188. Washington, DC: ACOG, 1994

American College of Obstetricians and Gynecologists. Hypertension in pregnancy. ACOG Technical Bulletin 219. Washington, DC: ACOG, 1996

American College of Obstetricians and Gynecologists. Maternal serum screening. ACOG Educational Bulletin 228. Washington, DC: ACOG, 1996

American College of Obstetricians and Gynecologists. Preconceptional care. ACOG Technical Bulletin 205. Washington, DC: ACOG, 1995

Berkowitz RL, Lynch L, Stone J, Alvarez M. The current status of multifetal pregnancy reduction. Am J Obstet Gynecol 1996; 174:1265–1272

Chervenak FA, D'Alton ME, eds. Multiple gestation. Semin Perinatol 1995;19:341–434

Gall SA. Multiple pregnancy and delivery. St. Louis, Missouri: Mosby-Year Book, 1996

Keith LG, Papiernik E, Keith DM, Luke B. Multiple pregnancy: epidemiology, gestation and perinatal outcome. New York: The Parthenon Publishing Group, 1995

The American College of Obstetricians and Gynecologists
409 12th Street, SW
PO Box 96920
Washington, DC 20090-6920

12345/21098

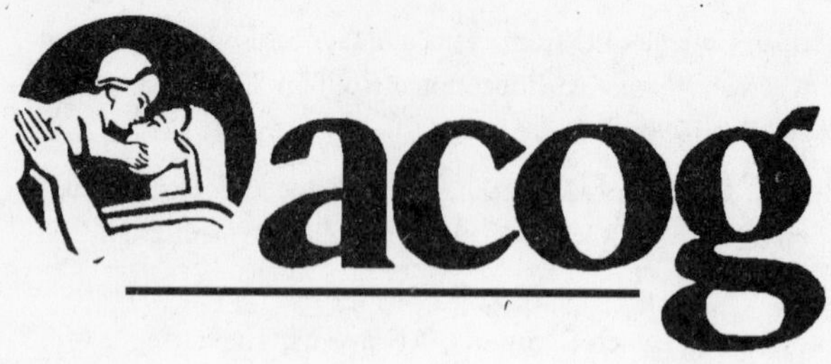

Number 222—April 1996
(Replaces #113, February 1988)

Technical Bulletin

An Educational Aid to Obstetrician–Gynecologists

Sterilization

Over 170 million couples worldwide use surgical sterilization as a safe and reliable method of contraception. In the United States, sterilization is the most commonly used method among married or formerly married women. An estimated 640,000 female sterilization procedures and 500,000 male sterilization procedures are performed each year (1, 2). In 1988, sterilizations accounted for 39% of contraceptive method use by all women 15–44 years old; 27.5% of women using contraception had undergone tubal sterilization, and 11.7% reported that their partners had undergone vasectomy (3).

Patient Counseling and Selection

Patients should be informed about both male and female sterilization as well as the risks and benefits of alternative long-acting, temporary contraceptive methods (see the box). When appropriate, the male partner can be included in such initial counseling. Many men and women have the impression that sterilization operations are easily reversible. The clinician should make clear to the patient that all operative sterilizations are intended to be permanent. Counseling should take into account risk factors that affect regret of sterilization. In the United States, the strongest indicator of future regret is young age at the time of sterilization, regardless of parity or marital status. Women between the ages of 20 and 24 years at sterilization are twice as likely to experience poststerilization regret as women sterilized between the ages of 30 and 34 years (4). Marital instability increases the probability of regret. Approximately 6% of sterilized women report regret or request information about sterilization reversal within 5 years of the procedure; urologists estimate that close to 1–2% of the total number of men they sterilize seek information on vasectomy reversal (4, 5). Although success rates in vas and tubal reanastomosis have improved dramatically in recent years, successful reversal and subsequent pregnancy depend on many factors, including the type of sterilization, interval between sterilization and reversal, age, and length of the remaining tube.

Preoperative counseling should include an explanation of the causes and probability of sterilization failure. When the patient has considered and accepted the risks of regret or failure, the physician can provide information about operative approaches, including a review of the possible complications from both the operation and the anesthesia. The patient should be informed about the advantages and disadvantages of local and general anesthesia, pain likely to be associated with the operation, and possible complications, including damage to organs or major vessels, infection, and subsequent ectopic pregnan-

Components of Presterilization Counseling

- Alternative methods available, including male sterilization
- Reasons for choosing sterilization
- Screening for risk indicators for regret
- Details of the procedure, including anesthesia with attendant risks and benefits
- The permanent nature of the procedure and information on reversal
- The possibility of failure, including ectopic pregnancy
- Post tubal ligation physiology, including the possibility of unrelated change in menstruation
- The need to use condoms for protection against sexually transmitted diseases and human immunodeficiency virus infection if at risk of exposure
- Answers to all questions to the satisfaction of the patient
- Completion of informed consent document

Modified from Pollack AE, Soderstrom RM. Female tubal sterilization. In: Corson SL, Derman RJ, Tyrer LB, eds. Fertility control. 2nd ed. London, Ontario: Goldin Publishers, 1994:295–296

cy. The patient should be informed of her need for adequate postoperative care and support, and she should plan accordingly.

The patient should be given an opportunity to ask questions about the procedure. Both this discussion and the fact that the patient was given the opportunity to ask questions should be noted in the patient's record by the physician. All this is best accomplished at a preoperative visit scheduled far enough in advance of the operation to allow the patient ample time to weigh the factors involved in the decision. Physicians should be aware of state laws or insurance regulations that may require a specific interval between obtaining consent and performance of sterilization procedures. State law may mandate the use of special consent forms. Written informed consent should be obtained following counseling in a relaxed and unpressured environment. It is best not to obtain consent concurrent with labor or an abortion procedure because these events are associated with stress and a high incidence of regret of sterilization.

Patients should be advised that female and male sterilization offer no protection against sexually transmitted diseases (STDs) such as human immunodeficiency virus (HIV) infection. Patients should be encouraged to use condoms or have their partners use condoms when they are at risk of exposure. In the United States, studies indicate that sterilized women with risk factors for STDs have low rates of condom use and infrequently attend clinics for preventive reproductive health services (6, 7).

Tubal Sterilization

Timing

Tubal sterilization can be performed postpartum, postabortion, or as an interval procedure (unrelated in time to a pregnancy). The timing of the procedure will influence both the surgical approach and the method of tubal occlusion used.

Postpartum sterilizations are performed at the time of cesarean delivery while the abdomen is open or following a vaginal delivery using a 2–5-cm subumbilical minilaparotomy incision. The subumbilical minilaparotomy approach allows for easy entry into the abdomen and access to the tubes because the anterior abdominal wall is thin just below the umbilicus over the fundus. It is best to perform postpartum minilaparotomy before the onset of significant uterine involution but following full assessment of maternal and neonatal well being. The likelihood of postpartum hemorrhage in multiparous women subsides after the first 12 hours postpartum. Postpartum minilaparotomy may be performed safely and comfortably using local anesthesia with sedation or regional or general anesthesia.

Postabortion sterilizations can be performed safely following uncomplicated spontaneous or induced abortion. Following a first-trimester abortion, laparoscopic sterilization or minilaparotomy using a suprapubic approach are both acceptable. In either case, a single anesthetic for the abortion and the sterilization may be used to avoid additional risk. Following a second-trimester abortion, minilaparotomy via a small midline vertical incision at the level of the fundus can be used safely. Open laparoscopy or the Hasson cannula may be used, thereby avoiding the risk of perforation of the soft, enlarged uterus associated with introduction of the laparoscopic trocar. Alternatively, an interval procedure can be performed once complete uterine involution has occurred.

Tubal sterilization can be performed as an interval procedure at any time during the menstrual cycle. Although performance of the sterilization procedure during the patient's estimated follicular phase and confirmation of patient use of a highly effective method of contraception before sterilization will reduce the risk of luteal phase pregnancy (a pregnancy diagnosed after sterilization in which conception occurred before sterilization), highly sensitive pregnancy testing will further reduce the risk. A same-day presterilization urine test capable of detecting human chorionic gonadotropin levels as low as 20 mIU/ml or a qualitative serum assay for the beta subunit of human chorionic gonadotropin will suffice (8). Tests this sensitive will allow for pregnancy detection as early as 1 week after conception. Performance of dilation and curettage concurrent with all interval sterilizations as a routine practice is not recommended on the basis of effectiveness, cost, and morbidity (9). Interval sterilization is usually performed using laparoscopy or minilaparotomy with local, regional, or general anesthesia. Transvaginal approaches have been described, and transcervical hysteroscopic approaches are being investigated.

Surgical Approach

Laparoscopy

Modern laparoscopy was first developed in Europe in the 1960s and became a popular method for direct visualization of the abdominal and pelvic organs. In the 1970s, it was introduced in the United States for tubal sterilization. In 1987, approximately one third of all tubal sterilizations in the United States were laparoscopic procedures. Most of these were performed under short-acting, general anesthesia in an outpatient setting.

In the United States, closed laparoscopy is used more often than open laparoscopy. In laparoscopic sterilization, an endoscope is inserted through a small incision made just below the umbilicus. Closed laparoscopy is performed through a small subumbilical skin incision just large enough to admit a sharp trocar. The trocar is used to puncture the abdominal wall, gaining entry into the peritoneal cavity blindly. Open laparoscopy is performed through a 1.5-cm semilunar or vertical subumbilical incision made through the layers of the abdominal wall until the peritoneal cavity has been entered under direct visualization (10).

Advantages of laparoscopy over other surgical approaches for sterilization include the opportunity to inspect the abdominal and pelvic organs, barely visible incision scars, and a rapid return to full activity for the patient. The disadvantages of laparoscopic sterilization include the cost and the fragility of the equipment, the special training required, and the risk of bowel, bladder, or major vessel injury following insertion of the needle or trocar.

With special training and experience, both closed and open laparoscopy can be performed with local anesthesia while maintaining a high level of patient comfort. Small studies have indicated that many women prefer the use of local anesthesia for sterilization procedures (11).

Minilaparotomy

The minilaparotomy approach may be performed by using local anesthesia with sedation, regional anesthesia, or general anesthesia. In contrast to laparoscopy, minilaparotomy requires only basic surgical instruments and training. Minilaparotomy is performed by using a 2–3-cm incision placed in relation to the uterine fundus. For interval sterilization, a uterine manipulator may be used to bring the uterine fundus toward the incision. For women undergoing either laparoscopic or minilaparotomy procedures with local anesthesia, placement of a paracervical block before insertion of the uterine manipulator reduces discomfort (12). Although most surgeons prefer to perform tubal occlusion using suture ligation and excision techniques, clips or rings may be applied through the minilaparotomy incision. With minilaparotomy, a segment of the tube can be removed for pathologic confirmation that both tubes were sterilized.

Methods of Occlusion

Electrocoagulation

Electrocoagulation for tubal occlusion is used exclusively with laparoscopic sterilization. Unipolar electrocoagulation with or without tubal excision was the first laparoscopic method of tubal occlusion. However, because uncommon but serious complications, including thermal bowel injury, were reported, bipolar coagulation was introduced and is now the most commonly used laparoscopic method in the United States. Bipolar coagulation also results in a more localized injury to the fallopian tube than does the unipolar method. Therefore, to maximize its effectiveness, at least 3 cm of the isthmic portion of the fallopian tube must be completely coagulated. Adequate coagulation requires sufficient energy of 25 W delivered in a cutting waveform (13). Use of a current meter, rather than a visual endpoint or a defined period of time, more accurately indicates complete coagulation.

Mechanical Methods

Mechanical occlusion devices commonly used in the United States include the silicone rubber band (Falope ring) and the spring-loaded clip (Hulka-Clemens clip). A new titanium clip lined with silicone rubber (Filshie clip) has been widely used in Great Britain with low reported failure rates (14, 15).

Special applicators are necessary for each of the mechanical occlusive devices, and each requires skill for proper application. The band can only be applied to a fallopian tube that is sufficiently mobile to allow it to be drawn into the applicator. Both types of clips should be applied perpendicular to the long axis of the proximal isthmus of the fallopian tube. Both types of clips and the silicone rubber band are most likely to be effective when used to occlude a normal tube. Tubal adhesions or a thickened or dilated fallopian tube increase the risk of misapplication and subsequent failure (16).

All of the mechanical methods of tubal occlusion destroy much less oviduct (about 5 mm for clips and 2 cm for rings) than do electrocoagulation methods. Therefore, if reversal is attempted, there is a greater chance of success.

Ligation Methods

Tubal occlusion at the time of cesarean delivery, laparotomy for other indications, or minilaparotomy is usually performed by using ligation techniques. A variety of techniques have been well described (17). Care should be taken to excise a sufficient section of fallopian tube to ensure complete transection of the tubal lumen.

Efficacy

Failure

Precise failure rates for each method of tubal occlusion and long-term cumulative failure rates have been difficult to measure because of the methods' high effectiveness rates. A generally accepted failure rate of less than 1% is based on combined small studies in which different occlusion methods were used (18). Preliminary findings from the U.S. Collaborative Review of Sterilization indicate that cumulative failure rates are higher than expected, with significant differences between methods (19). The risk of failure persists for years after the procedure and varies by method of tubal occlusion and age. In a total of 143 sterilization failures, cumulative 10-year probabilities of pregnancy were highest after spring-loaded clip sterilization (36.5 per 1,000 procedures) and lowest after unipolar coagulation (7.5 per 1,000) and postpartum partial salpingectomy (7.5 per 1,000). The cumulative risk of pregnancy was highest among women sterilized at a young age with bipolar coagulation (54.3 per 1,000) and spring-loaded clip application (52.1 per 1,000). It is important to note, however, that in another study of sterilization failures, all spring-loaded clip failures were found to be due to misapplication (16).

Fecundity declines significantly after the age of 35 years. In one study, patients younger than 35 years were 1.7 times more likely to become pregnant following sterilization than women over the age of 35 years (20). In another study, among women 18–27 years of age who underwent bipolar coagulation, 2.8% became pregnant between 5 and 10 years after the procedure (19).

Pregnancies after sterilization may occur without any technical error. Technical error leading to failure occurs less frequently with minilaparotomy regardless of the occlusion method used (21). In one study, the location of the suture on the ligated tube affected estimated minilaparotomy failure rates, which were approximately 3% in 3 years for fimbriectomy with infundibular ligation, approximately 1.7% for ampullary ligation, and approximately 0.34% for isthmic ligation (20).

Ectopic Pregnancy

When sterilization failure occurs, the subsequent pregnancy is more likely to be ectopic than intrauterine. The degree of increased risk depends on the occlusion method used. The results of several reports suggest that over half of the pregnancies that occur after electrocoagulation sterilization procedures may be ectopic (22, 23). If an ectopic pregnancy occurs, the physician should evaluate both proximal tubes and manage any acute problems that are present.

Complications

In the United States, female sterilization has a mortality rate of 1–2 deaths per 100,000 procedures (24). Complications of general anesthesia are the leading cause of death from tubal sterilization. Other causes include sepsis and hemorrhage. Between 1977 and 1981, most of those deaths from sepsis resulted from thermal bowel injury following unipolar electrocoagulation, while most of those deaths from hemorrhage followed major vessel lacerations associated with abdominal entry for laparoscopic sterilization (25).

Studies in the United States indicate that women undergoing interval minilaparotomy are at approximately twice the risk of having any complication than are women undergoing interval laparoscopic sterilization. However, women who undergo minilaparotomy often have medical risk factors, including certain cardiac and pulmonary problems, that are contraindications to laparoscopy and therefore are intrinsically at greater surgical risk (26, 27).

Late Sequelae

The long-term health effects of tubal sterilization on menstrual pattern disturbance, pelvic pain, and the need for pelvic surgery are controversial. Early studies of menstrual disturbance following sterilization failed to account for confounding variables such as presterilization use of hormonal contraceptives that generally mask underlying menstrual dysfunction. Most recent prospective studies that account for these factors have found little or no difference in menstrual function between women before and after sterilization, or between sterilized women and nonsterilized control subjects in the first 2 years of follow up. Findings from reports that include follow up for more than 2 years have been less consistent, yet no single method of occlusion, regardless of the amount of tubal destruction, has been associated with an increase in risk for poststerilization menstrual disturbance (28).

Two studies have evaluated the likelihood of hospitalization for menstrual disorders in women who have undergone sterilization. A U.S. population-based cohort study showed an increased relative risk of 1.6 (95% confidence interval of 1.3–2.1) for hospitalization for menstrual disorders compared with a control group of wives of men who have had vasectomies (29). Follow up of a large British cohort for 6 years failed to identify a significant increase in risk (30).

Some sterilized women may be more likely to undergo subsequent hysterectomy. Women who have been sterilized before age 30 have a higher risk of a hysterectomy than women sterilized after age 30. This risk has not been related to an increase in menstrual disturbance or the extent of tissue damage based on the method of occlusion used (31).

Ovarian Cancer

In several older studies, an inverse relationship between tubal occlusion and subsequent ovarian cancer has been found, although the strength of this relationship has varied widely (32, 33, 34). A controlled, prospective study reported a reduced risk of ovarian cancer among women who had tubal occlusion or hysterectomy (35). The study monitored 77,544 women for 12 years. For those women who had a tubal ligation, the relative risk of ovarian cancer was 0.33. The reduced risk persisted after the investigators controlled for risk factors such as smoking and protective factors (eg, use of oral contraceptives). Cases of reported ovarian cancer, identified within the first 4 years after sterilization, were excluded to eliminate possible screening bias (32, 33).

Pelvic Inflammatory Disease

It has long been believed that tubal sterilization protects against pelvic inflammatory disease. This would seem to make intuitive sense, as this condition is thought to be caused by the ascent of bacteria through the cervix, uterus, and fallopian tubes and into the peritoneal cavity. This protection is, however, not absolute. Case reports of pelvic inflammatory disease and tuboovarian abscess in women who have undergone sterilization are rare but do exist in the literature (36, 37).

Sterilization in Men

Vasectomy performed as an outpatient procedure has been popular in the United States since 1965. More than 5 million men in the United States have had a vasectomy (38). When compared with tubal sterilization, vasectomy is safer, less expensive, and equally as effective. In the United States, urologists, general surgeons, and family physicians perform vasectomy procedures in their offices using local anesthesia.

Traditionally, vasectomy was performed through two incisions in the scrotum, one overlying each vas deferens. The incisions were then closed with a suture. In 1985, the no-scalpel vasectomy technique was introduced (39). This method makes use of two specially designed instruments: one allows the vas to be fixed externally, while the second is used to puncture the scrotal skin without using a scalpel (40). The technique was developed to increase acceptability of vasectomy by reducing the apprehension related to making an incision on the scrotum (41, 40). It reduces the already low rate of minor complications (less than 3%) seen with traditional vasectomy, such as wound hematoma and infection (42).

Both traditional and no-scalpel vasectomy use the same methods to occlude the vas. These include excising a segment of the vas and sealing the ends via ligation, electrocoagulation or thermocoagulation, or clips. To decrease the incidence of recanalization, some surgeons further separate the severed ends by folding them back on one another or burying one end in the scrotal fascia.

Pregnancy rates following vasectomy are less than 1% in most studies and usually result from failure to occlude the correct structure, unprotected intercourse too soon after the operation, or spontaneous recanalization. Unlike tubal occlusion in women, vasectomy is not immediately effective: about 3 months or 20 ejaculations are needed to flush the vasa of viable sperm. Postvasectomy semen analysis should be performed to determine the effectiveness of the procedure.

The possibility of long-term side effects from vasectomy has received considerable attention. Nine separate epidemiological studies in men have failed to show a relationship between atherosclerosis and vasectomy (43). An original study in monkeys that suggested such a relationship has not been confirmed (44, 45). Other consequences of vasectomy have been suggested, but none has been proven. In addition, several studies report that in the United States, men who have chosen vasectomies are often healthier than control counterparts (46, 47).

In Western countries, white, upper-middle-class men are more likely to choose vasectomy and are also the group more likely to have testicular cancer. A study of nearly 74,000 men who have had vasectomies showed the incidence of testicular cancer in this group to be no higher than that of the general population (48). It also showed that vasectomy does not accelerate the growth of preexisting testicular tumors.

In 1993, researchers published the first large cohort studies to show a weak but statistically significant increased risk for prostate cancer in a subgroup of men at least 20 years after vasectomy (49, 47). Two subsequent studies have failed to support these findings (50, 51).

The U.S. National Institutes of Health convened a group of experts in 1993 to review the published reports on prostate cancer. The committee found that although additional research into a possible causal relationship between vasectomy and prostate cancer should be conducted, a change in the current practice of vasectomy was not warranted. The National Institutes of Health made the following recommendations (52):

- Providers should continue to offer vasectomy and perform the procedure
- Vasectomy reversal is not warranted to prevent prostate cancer
- Screening for prostate cancer should not be any different for men who have had a vasectomy than for those who have not

Summary

Sterilization provides a safe and effective contraceptive method. Both female and male sterilization have few long-term sequelae. Several new methods of transcervical sterilization are under development, but laparoscopy and minilaparotomy are likely to remain the most popular methods of female sterilization.

REFERENCES

1. Schwartz DB, Wingo PA, Antarsh L, Smith JC. Female sterilizations in the United States, 1987. Fam Plann Perspect 1989;21:209–212
2. Marquette CM, Koonin LM, Antarsh L, Gargiullo PM, Smith JC. Vasectomy in the United States, 1991. Am J Public Health 1995;85:644–649
3. Mosher WD. Contraceptive practice in the United States, 1982–1988. Fam Plann Perspect 1990;22:198–205
4. Wilcox LS, Chu SY, Eaker ED, Zeger SL, Peterson HB. Risk factors for regret after tubal sterilization: 5 years of follow-up in a prospective study. Fertil Steril 1991; 55:927–933
5. Wilcox LS, Chu SY, Peterson HB. Characteristics of women who considered or obtained tubal reanastomosis: results from a prospective study of tubal sterilization. Obstet Gynecol 1990;75:661–665
6. Centers for Disease Control. HIV-risk behaviors of sterilized and nonsterilized women in drug-treatment programs—Philadelphia, 1989–1991. MMWR 1992;41: 149–152
7. Centers for Disease Control. Surgical sterilization among women and use of condoms-Baltimore, 1989–1990. MMWR 1992;41:568–575
8. Lipscomb GH, Spellman JR, Ling FW. The effect of same-day pregnancy testing on the incidence of luteal phase pregnancy. Obstet Gynecol 1993;82:411–413
9. Lichter ED, Laff SP, Friedman EA. Value of routine dilation and curettage at the time of interval sterilization. Obstet Gynecol 1986;67:763–765
10. Penfield AJ. Female sterilization by minilaparotomy or open laparoscopy. Baltimore, Maryland: Urban & Schwarzenberg, 1980
11. Handa VL, Berlin M, Washington AE. A comparison of local and general anesthesia for laparoscopic tubal sterilization. Journal of Women's Health 1994;3:135–141
12. Poindexter AN III, Abdul-Malak M, Fast JE. Laparoscopic tubal sterilization under local anesthesia. Obstet Gynecol 1990;75:5–8
13. Soderstrom RM, Levy BS, Engel T. Reducing bipolar sterilization failures. Obstet Gynecol 1989;74:60–63
14. Filshie GM, Casey D, Pogmore JR, Dutton AGB, Symonds EM, Peake ABL. The titanium/silicone rubber clip for female sterilization. Br J Obstet Gynaecol 1981;88:655–662
15. Green-Thompson RW, Popis M, Cairncross NWA. Outpatient laparoscopic tubal sterilization under local anaesthesia: a review of three years at King George V Hospital, Durban. Obstet Gynecol Forum August 1993:4–14,44
16. Stovall TG, Ling FW, O'Kelley KR, Coleman SA. Gross and histologic examination of tubal ligation failures in a residency training program. Obstet Gynecol 1990;76: 461–465
17. Wheeless CR Jr. Tubal sterilization. In: Thompson JD, Rock JA. Te Linde's operative gynecology. 7th ed. Philadelphia: JB Lippincott Co, 1992:343–359
18. The Johns Hopkins University. Population Information Program. Minilaparotomy and laparoscopy: safe, effective, and widely used. Popul Rep C 1985;9:C-125–C-167
19. Peterson HB, Xia Z, Hughes JM, Wilcox LS, Tylor LR, Trussel J. The risk of pregnancy after tubal sterilization: findings from the U.S. Collaborative Review of Sterilization. Am J Obstet Gynecol 1996;174:1161–1170
20. Cheng MCE, Wong YM, Rochat RW, Ratnam SS. Sterilization failures in Singapore: an examination of ligation techniques and failure rates. Stud Fam Plann 1977; 8:109–115
21. Chi I-C, Laufe LE, Gardner SD, Tolbert MA. An epidemiologic study of risk factors associated with pregnancy following female sterilization. Am J Obstet Gynecol 1980;136:768–773
22. McCausland A. High rate of ectopic pregnancy following laparoscopic tubal coagulation failures: incidence and etiology. Am J Obstet Gynecol 1980;136:97–101
23. Kjer JJ, Knudsen LB. Ectopic pregnancy subsequent to laparoscopic sterilization. Am J Obstet Gynecol 1989; 160:1202–1204
24. Escobedo LG, Peterson HB, Grubb GS, Franks AL. Case-fatality rates for tubal sterilization in U.S. hospitals, 1979 to 1980. Am J Obstet Gynecol 1989;160:147–150
25. Peterson HB, DeStefano F, Rubin GL, Greenspan JR, Lee NC, Ory HW. Deaths attributable to tubal sterilization in the United States, 1977 to 1981. Am J Obstet Gynecol 1983;146:131–136
26. DeStefano F, Greenspan JR, Dicker RC, Peterson HB, Strauss LT, Rubin GL. Complications of interval laparoscopic tubal sterilization. Obstet Gynecol 1983;61: 153–158
27. Layde PM, Peterson HB, Dicker RC, DeStefano F, Rubin GL, Ory HW. Risk factors for complications of interval tubal sterilization by laparotomy. Obstet Gynecol 1983;62:180–184
28. Wilcox LS, Martinez-Schnell B, Peterson HB, Ware JH, Hughes JM. Menstrual function after tubal sterilization. Am J Epidemiol 1992;135:1368–1381
29. Shy KK, Stergachis A, Grothaus LG, Wagner EH, Hecht J, Anderson G. Tubal sterilization and risk of subsequent hospital admission for menstrual disorders. Am J Obstet Gynecol 1992;166:1698–1706
30. Vessey M, Huggins G, Lawless M, McPherson K, Yeates D. Tubal sterilization: findings in a large prospective study. Br J Obstet Gynaecol 1983;90:203–209
31. Rulin MC, Davidson AR, Philliber SG, Graves WL, Cushman LF. Long-term effect of tubal sterilization on menstrual indices and pelvic pain. Obstet Gynecol 1993;82:118–121
32. Irwin KL, Weiss NS, Lee NC, Peterson HB. Tubal sterilization, hysterectomy, and the subsequent occurrence of epithelial ovarian cancer. Am J Epidemiol 1991;134:362–369
33. Whittemore AS, Wu ML, Paffenbarger RS Jr, Sarles DL, Kampert JB, Grosser S, et al. Personal and environmental characteristics related to epithelial ovarian cancer. II. Exposures to talcum powder, tobacco, alcohol, and coffee. Am J Epidemiol 1988;128:1228–1240
34. Mori M, Harabuchi I, Miyake H, Casagrande JT, Henderson BE, Ross RK. Reproductive, genetic, and dietary risk factors for ovarian cancer. Am J Epidemiol 1988;128:771–777

35. Hankinson SE, Hunter DJ, Colditz GA, Willett WC, Stampfer MJ, Rosner B, et al. Tubal ligation, hysterectomy, and risk of ovarian cancer: a prospective study. JAMA 1993;270:2813–2818

36. Vermesh M, Confino E, Boler LR, Friberg J, Gleicher N. Acute salpingitis in sterilized women. Obstet Gynecol 1987;69:265–267

37. Huggins GR, Sondheimer SJ. Complications of female sterilization: immediate and delayed. Fertil Steril 1984;41:337–355

38. Mosher WD, Pratt WF. Contraceptive use in the United States, 1973–88. Advance data from vital and health statistics; no. 182. Hyattsville, Maryland: National Center for Health Statistics, 1990

39. Huber D. No-scalpel vasectomy: the transfer of a refined surgical technique from China to other countries. Adv Contracept 1989;5:217–218

40. Schlegel PN, Goldstein M. No-scalpel vasectomy. Semin Urol 1992;10:252–256

41. Nirapathpongporn A, Huber DH, Krieger JN. No-scalpel vasectomy at the King's birthday vasectomy festival. Lancet 1990;335:894–895

42. Li S, Goldstein M, Zhu J, Huber D. The no-scalpel vasectomy. J Urol 1991;145:341–344

43. Peterson HB, Huber DH, Belker AM. Vasectomy: an appraisal for the obstetrician-gynecologist. Obstet Gynecol 1990;76:568–572

44. Alexander NJ, Clarkson TB. Vasectomy increases the severity of diet-induced atherosclerosis in *Macaca fascicularis*. Science 1978;201:538–541

45. Clarkson TB, Alexander NJ, Morgan TM. Atherosclerosis of cynomolgus monkeys hyper- and hyporesponsive to dietary cholesterol: lack of effect on vasectomy. Arteriosclerosis 1988;8:488–498

46. Massey FJ Jr, Bernstein GS, O'Fallon WM, Schuman LM, Coulson AH, Crozier R, et al. Vasectomy and health: results from a large cohort study. JAMA 1984; 252:1023–1029

47. Giovannucci E, Tosteson TD, Speizer FE, Ascherio A, Vessey MP, Colditz GA. A retrospective cohort study of vasectomy and prostate cancer in US men. JAMA 1993;269:878-882

48. Møller H, Knudsen LB, Lynge E. Risk of testicular cancer after vasectomy: cohort study of over 73 000 men. BMJ 1994;309:295–299

49. Giovannucci E, Ascherio A, Rimm EB, Colditz GA, Stampfer MJ, Willett WC. A prospective cohort study of vasectomy and prostate cancer in US men. JAMA 1993;269:873-877

50. Hayes RB, Pottern LM, Greenberg R, Schoenberg J, Swanson GM, Liff J, et al. Vasectomy and prostate cancer in US blacks and whites. Am J Epidemiol 1993;137: 263– 269

51. Coulson AH, Crozier R, Massey FJ Jr, O'Fallon WM, Schuman LM, Spivey GH. Health status of american men—a study of post-vasectomy sequelae: results. J Clin Epidemiol 1993;46:857–920

52. Healy B. Does vasectomy cause prostate cancer? JAMA 1993;269:2620

This Technical Bulletin was developed under the direction of the Committee on Technical Bulletins of the American College of Obstetricians and Gynecologists as an educational aid to obstetricians and gynecologists. The committee wishes to thank Amy E. Pollack, MD, MPH, for her assistance in the development of this bulletin. This Technical Bulletin does not define a standard of care, nor is it intended to dictate an exclusive course of management. It presents recognized methods and techniques of clinical practice for consideration by obstetrician–gynecologists for incorporation into their practices. Variations of practice taking into account the needs of the individual patient, resources, and limitations unique to the institution or type of practice may be appropriate.

ISSN 1074-8628

THE AMERICAN COLLEGE OF OBSTETRICIANS AND GYNECOLOGISTS
409 12th Street, SW
Washington, DC 20024-2188

12345/09876

Number 194—July 1994

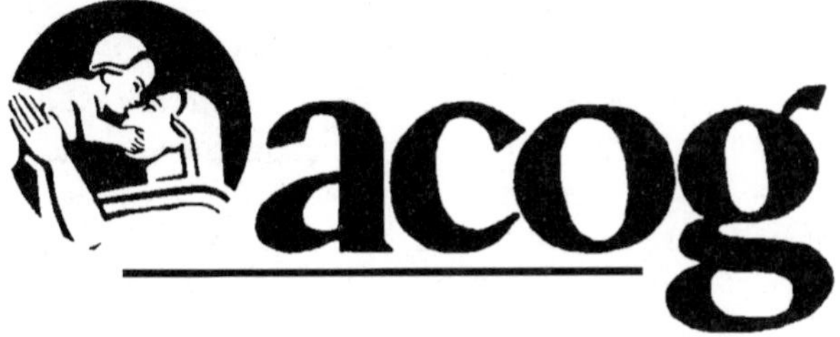

Technical Bulletin

An Educational Aid to Obstetrician–Gynecologists

Substance Abuse

The obstetrician–gynecologist can play a role in substance abuse prevention and treatment. This role may include screening patients by use of questionnaires; providing education, treatment, and referral; guiding and referring high-risk patients; advising patients of social and support groups; practicing safe prescription writing; and addressing the needs of adolescents.

Misuse of illegal and controlled drugs, alcohol, and tobacco constitutes a significant national health problem. Data from the most recent National Household Survey on Drug Abuse (1) indicate that 29% of Americans smoke cigarettes, up to 6.7% abuse beverage alcohol, 2% use psychotherapeutic drugs (eg, sedatives, tranquilizers, stimulants, and analgesics), and 7% use illicit drugs (eg, marijuana, cocaine, opioids). Of the nearly 60 million women of childbearing age (15–44 years), over 5 million (9%) have used marijuana or cocaine in the past month.

Substance abuse is typified by a wide variety of use patterns, chronic relapsing patterns of dependence, and variation in individual responses and prognosis. Many of those who abuse substances use more than one substance—either an illicit substance or alcohol or tobacco. Typically with alcohol, a woman begins drinking in her teens with problem drinking beginning after 25 years of age. She is often introduced to alcohol or other drug abuse by a codependent male partner.

Substances of Abuse and Their Side Effects

Substance abuse can have serious implications for the health of women. Among them are adverse effects on reproductive function and pregnancy (2).

In addition to the substance-specific effects described in this bulletin, there are also more generic risks of substance abuse. Abuse of substances is associated with unhealthy life styles. For example, the abuser may trade sex for drugs, exposing her to sexually transmitted diseases. Substance abusers are also at risk for malnutrition. Drug users who share needles are at risk of contracting blood-borne infections such as infection with human immunodeficiency virus or hepatitis B virus.

Tobacco

Chronic cigarette smoking has been well documented to have a major adverse impact on women's health (3). Nicotine is the most studied and most pharmacologically active substance found in cigarette smoke. It is readily inhaled into the lungs as particulate matter in smoke, and blood levels vary depending on the inhalation habits of the smoker, nicotine content of tobacco smoked, and presence or absence of filters. This water- and lipid-soluble substance is metabolized by the liver, kidneys, and lungs, with most eliminated from the body through urinary excretion within 2 hours of cigarette smoking. Coronary artery and peripheral vascular disease, respiratory illness (chronic obstructive lung disease), peptic ulcer disease, esophageal reflux, and cancer (lung, oropharynx, larynx, esophagus, bladder) are morbidities associated with chronic tobacco smoking.

Marijuana

Marijuana is derived from the plant *Cannabis sativa.* Its principal psychoactive ingredient is 1,9-tetrahydrocannabinol, which is present in large quantities in each marijuana cigarette. This lipophilic substance accumulates in fatty tissues for days before being metabolized by the liver and eliminated in the feces. Marijuana smoking has been associated with tachycardia, exercise intolerance, bronchitis, sinusitis, and pharyngitis. Chronic consumption leads to anovulation and decreased sperm count and motility.

Alcohol

Beverage alcohol is a water-soluble compound that is readily distilled from a variety of plants. It undergoes first-order metabolism in the liver, and metabolic products are excreted by the kidneys. In 1984, alcohol abuse or dependence was the fourth most frequent psychiatric diagnosis in 18–24-year-old women (4). Approximately 100,000 deaths per year can be attributed to the misuse of alcohol (5). Alcohol use is associated with 50% of fatal automobile accidents, 68% of drownings, 54% of fires, and 48% of serious falls.

Chronic alcohol consumption has multiple adverse health effects and is associated with a number of cancers. It is also linked to malnutrition, including deficiencies in thiamine, riboflavin, pyridoxine, niacin, and vitamin C.

Cocaine

Cocaine is a lipophilic alkaloid extracted from the leaves of *Erythroxylon coca*. It is generally consumed by snorting, "free-basing" (inhaling cocaine vapors combined with an organic solvent), or smoking the alkaloid itself as "crack." Cocaine's major site of action is at the nerve terminal, where it inhibits dopamine, norepinephrine, and serotonin uptake. This results in intense vasoconstriction, arrhythmia, and a concomitant rise in blood pressure (6). Other adverse consequences are seizures, cerebrovascular accidents, psychosis, nasal septal perforation, malnutrition, and hyperthermia. Some cocaine users may trade sex for drugs, resulting in a higher incidence of infectious disease complications, including but not limited to syphilis, hepatitis, and acquired immunodeficiency syndrome (AIDS).

Opioids

Opioids are a class of drugs derived from opium and synthetic compounds with similar actions. The prototypical opioid is morphine. Heroin (diacetylmorphine) is more potent on a gram-for-gram basis but is believed to exert its effects chiefly by being metabolized to morphine. Codeine is methylated morphine and is also metabolized to the parent compound. Other opioids, such as meperidine (Demerol), methadone (Dolophine), and oxycodone (Percodan), are structurally dissimilar to morphine but share its pharmacologic properties, probably by stimulating the same receptors. These agents produce euphoria, somnolence, and decreased sensitivity to pain. Adverse effects of opioid use include constipation, nephrotic syndrome, and overdose.

Inhalants

Use of inhalants ("glue sniffing," solvent abuse) tends to be limited to adolescents. These substances are lipophilic and readily pass through the respiratory tract. Their use may be accompanied by arrhythmias leading to sudden death. They may also cause bone marrow toxicity, liver damage, renal failure, peripheral neuropathy, atrophy, parethesias, cerebellar signs, and organic brain syndrome.

Hallucinogens

Phencyclidine (PCP, "angel dust") is an amphetamine-like compound. Lysergic acid diethylamide (LSD) shares many similar properties. Both of these agents are thought to aggravate latent schizophrenia. Their use may lead to chronic psychosis, flashbacks, and violent behavior.

Amphetamines and Barbiturates

Abuse of medications may occur alone or in combination with other substances to reduce the uncomfortable side effects of polydrug abuse. Use of amphetamines ("uppers") may be accompanied or followed by use of barbiturates ("downers"); benzodiazepines may be taken with cocaine ("moon-walking"). Repeated ingestion of these central nervous system stimulants and depressants may lead to cognitive impairment and psychologic depression.

Prevention

Obstetrician–gynecologists have important opportunities for prevention of substance abuse. Three of the key areas in which they can make an impact are prescribing appropriately, encouraging healthy behaviors through providing appropriate information and education, and identifying and referring patients already abusing drugs.

Several occasions for substance abuse screening and prevention exist in daily practice. Pregnancy and visits for medical problems which may be exacerbated by substance abuse are two examples. Awareness of populations that may be at higher risk for substance abuse can aid clinicians in their prevention efforts:

- Biological daughter of alcoholic or drug-abusing parent(s)
- Spouse of an alcoholic or drug abuser
- Women who have recently experienced a traumatic life event
  - —Divorce or separation
  - —Death of spouse or significant other
  - —Job loss
  - —Retirement
  - —Rape or sexual abuse
  - —Witness to a traumatic event
- Women with a physical handicap or disability
- Health care professionals
- Women who have a psychiatric disorder (eg, depression, psychosis, anxiety, hyperactivity)

When prescribing potentially addictive substances, the clinician should carefully assess the risks of drug treatment and should consider nonpharmacologic treatments or nonaddicting medications whenever possible (7). Potentially addictive drugs should be initially prescribed at a dose adequate to relieve symptoms and then be reduced gradually to the smallest effective dose. Use of the following guidelines may be helpful:

- Take a thorough history of current and past prescription drug use, over-the-counter and other nonprescription drug use, and alcohol use.

- Prescribe according to a fixed schedule to minimize the reinforcement of symptoms, medication-seeking behavior, and illness behavior that occurs with "as needed" dosing.
- Prescribe for short periods of time during treatment of acute syndromes. Avoid more than one refill and telephone refills. Reassess the patient at frequent intervals.
- Write prescription orders in such a way as to make them impossible to alter. As an example, write the prescription as "dispense 30 (thirty)."
- Document prescription rationale, including the exact quantity prescribed.

The clinician should remain alert for clues that a patient might be seeking psychoactive medication by exaggerating symptoms (8). These individuals may complain of losing prescriptions or medications and repeatedly report running out of medications before the time that would be expected if medications were taken as prescribed. They often seek narcotic or tranquilizer prescriptions from multiple physicians or claim that another doctor, who is now unavailable, prescribed a certain narcotic that now needs to be refilled. They may insist on a particular drug by brand name and claim that nothing else works or demand an immediate prescription of a strong narcotic for a chronic illness.

Educating all patients about the effects of drugs is important. Activities to be avoided while taking the medication and potential interactions with other medications need to be understood. The clinician should describe the potential for a drug to produce dependence if directions are not followed and make clear the dosage and effect when mixed with other substances. The clinician should also warn about the dangers of misuse of a drug and assess the patient's understanding.

History

Directing questions in the history to levels of use of alcohol, tobacco, and other drugs helps to indicate when further investigation is needed. Patients tend to minimize substance abuse problems and often give inaccurate information regarding quantity consumed. Alcoholics may underreport the actual amount of alcohol consumed but may be more accurate regarding frequency of use. When asked questions regarding quantity and frequency of substance use, patients may feel threatened or defensive or may be concerned about confidentiality. Self-report of use is more accurate when patients are sober and less accurate when they are intoxicated. The best quantitative data are obtained when asking about the specific use on a specific memorable day (eg, "Tell me what you drank yesterday").

Several instruments have been developed that can be very useful as brief screening tests in the office and can be integrated into a patient intake questionnaire. The most widely known of these is a four-question screening test known as the CAGE questionnaire (9). This questionnaire has a 91% sensitivity and 77% specificity for detecting problem drinking. One positive response indicates reason for concern; two positive responses indicate that a problem is likely. The CAGE questions are shown in the box.

At the time of the comprehensive initial office visit or annual checkup, patients should be asked whether they consume alcohol. If the patient states that she does not drink, usually no further screening is necessary. Patients who respond that they do drink should be asked the CAGE questions to help ascertain the level of their alcohol consumption. By combining the CAGE with the broader, standard office interview questions, the primary care clinician has a reasonably effective means of detecting current or developing alcohol dependence. Patients who reply affirmatively to only one of the first three CAGE questions may respond to brief office intervention, often combined with more frequent follow-up visits.

The need for an "eye opener" is generally considered a more serious indication of alcohol dependence. Whether treatment consists of office interventions or referral depends upon the individual physician's experience and judgment. Use of CAGE questions in patient interviews and brief office intervention techniques have been integrated into the curricula of many medical school and residency programs.

Other questionnaires that may assist the clinician in discovering problem drinking include the T-ACE (10), the MAST (Michigan Alcohol Screening Test) and Brief MAST (11), and a Trauma Scale (12).

Psychologic and Physical Findings

There are a variety of common presenting complaints that are associated with substance use problems. Psychologic

CAGE Questionnaire

C = Have you ever felt you ought to Cut down on your drinking?

A = Have people Annoyed you by criticizing your drinking?

G = Have you ever felt bad or Guilty about your drinking?

E = Have you ever had a drink first thing in the morning to steady your nerves or get rid of a hangover (Eye opener)?

Ewing JA. Detecting alcoholism: the CAGE questionnaire. JAMA 1984;252:1907

problems associated with substance abuse or dependence frequently are brought to the attention of the clinician by a relative. Vague physical symptoms such as fatigue, insomnia, headaches, sexual problems, and loss of appetite should prompt early suspicion of substance use. Definitive psychologic and physical evidence of substance abuse usually does not become apparent until late in the disease process. Findings considered to be "red flags" for substance abuse are summarized in the box.

Laboratory Tests for Screening and Diagnosis

Blood Alcohol Level

Screening for alcohol abuse by questionnaire has a higher probability of detecting problem alcohol use than laboratory tests. Tests are best used to aid the assessment of alcohol abuse. Determining the blood alcohol level has limited application since ethanol is eliminated relatively rapidly. It will not predict the patient's overall drinking behaviors. Important indicators of tolerance to alcohol are blood alcohol levels of greater than:

- 300 mg/dl at any time
- 100 mg/dl during a routine physical examination
- 150 mg/dl without evidence of gross neurologic impairment

Signs and Symptoms of Substance Abuse

Physical Findings

Track marks and other evidence of intravenous drug use
Alcohol on the breath
Scars, injuries
Hypertension
Tachycardia or bradycardia
Tremors
Slurred speech
Self-neglect or poor hygiene
Liver or renal disease
Runny nose
Chronic cough
Cheilosis
Nervous mannerisms (eg, frequently licking lips, jitters, foot tapping)
Pinpoint or dilated pupils
Reproductive dysfunction (hypogonadism, irregular menses, miscarriage, infertility, fetal alcohol syndrome)

Psychologic Problems

Memory loss
Depression
Anxiety
Panic
Paranoia
Unexplained mood swings
Personality changes
Intellectual changes
Sexual promiscuity
Dishonesty
Unreliability

Adapted from Cyr MG. Assessment and diagnosis. In: Dubé CE, Goldstein MD, Lewis DC, Myers ER, Zwick WR, eds. Project ADEPT curriculum for primary care physician training. Vol 1. Providence, Rhode Island: Brown University, 1989

Liver Function Tests

Liver function tests are of some use in assessing the severity of alcohol consumption. An assessment of γ-glutamyltransferase is the most sensitive liver function test for alcohol abuse but is only about 50% sensitive in detecting problem drinking. It is one of the best early indicators of alcoholism and is elevated in 75% of subjects who have been drinking for several weeks. After a patient stops drinking, several weeks must pass before this test returns to normal. Aspartate aminotransferase and alanine aminotransferase (formerly known as serum glutamic-oxaloacetic transaminase and serum glutamate pyruvate transaminase, respectively) have low sensitivity and specificity for alcohol consumption.

Hematologic Tests

An elevated mean corpuscular volume in the complete blood count may reflect the macrocytosis associated with chronic alcohol abuse. This may be due to direct toxic effects of ethanol upon the developing erythroblasts in bone marrow, associated folate or vitamin B_{12} deficiency, or liver disease. Anemia may be due to folate deficiency, gastrointestinal bleeding, or suppression of bone marrow. Blood panels show some promise for identification of alcohol abuse but have not been particularly useful in clinical practice.

Toxicology

Urine toxicology screens are widely used to detect common drugs of abuse. Immunoassay procedures are the most sensitive of these techniques, but confirmatory testing with gas chromatography/mass spectrometry is used by many laboratories to reduce false-positives. Certain foods (eg, poppy seeds) and medications (eg, decongestants) produce false-positives.

Urine drug screening is not foolproof, just as questionnaires will not always identify substance abuse problems because of patient denial. When used appropriately, a urine drug screen can identify a substance abuse problem when other detection methods have not. A total drug-screening program should consist of both questionnaires and drug testing.

Most laboratories perform a standard "drug panel" aimed at the most commonly used illicit drugs (eg, marijuana, cocaine, amphetamines, barbiturates, opioids). Less commonly used illicit drugs (eg, LSD) may not be detected. Population and regional trends in illicit drug use are often known by local emergency medicine departments. These may serve as a source for more specific information about local trends in drug abuse and prompt more specific testing.

When the physician suspects that drug use is associated with clinical behavior or outcome, directed questioning may be informative. Sometimes the patient may have consumed an adulterated substance or the phenomenon of denial may prohibit discovery of the substance in this way. In these circumstances, the physician must use any local knowledge of what drugs are "on the street" combined with information from emergency departments and, finally, observation of the patient's behavioral status (eg, hallucinations, agitation, drowsiness) and examination (eg, alcoholic fetor, white powder in nares) to assist in drug testing.

Individuals wishing to avoid detection of their substance use may attempt to adulterate the specimen or dilute or "washout" a substance by consuming large quantities of water prior to testing. The increased sensitivity of modern drug tests usually results in detection despite these attempts. Screening with prior approval can be random and is useful in helping persons in denial who are resistant to therapy.

Ethics of Drug Testing

Since positive results have implications for patients that transcend their health, they should give informed consent prior to testing. When there is no suspicion of substance abuse, random checks of a patient's urine for substances are unethical. A false-positive from such testing might have devastating consequences for the patient and clinician. The patient's medical records are confidential, and protection of her rights is of the utmost importance.

Medical circumstances occasionally arise in which this consent is considered unnecessary or unobtainable. Patients who are in a stupor, unconscious, or show obvious signs of intoxication need to be tested in order to direct further medical interventions.

Role of the Obstetrician–Gynecologist in Diagnosis and Treatment

Obstetrician–gynecologists generally are unaware of options and community resources available for substance abuse intervention and treatment. Hospital social workers are among the best resources for this information. There are several important roles the primary care provider fills in the diagnosis and treatment of substance abuse that benefit these patients.

Often, encouragement and support provided by the physician may lead the patient to reduce or eliminate substance use. This aids in preventing medical and psychosocial complications of substance use. Patient education and early diagnosis and referral for treatment are key parts of this total patient care. As the most significant health care practitioner for many women, the obstetrician–gynecologist may be influential in a patient's decision to accept treatment or referral.

The obstetrician–gynecologist may wish to offer or participate in treatment for low-level substance abuse. This may consist of follow-up office visits to monitor substance use, substance abuse, or treatment compliance. Providing additional information through directed readings and educational materials about substance abuse is beneficial. Self-help and other treatment programs like Narcotics Anonymous, Alcoholics Anonymous, and Al Anon are important resources. Family members may be involved to help address different aspects of the substance abuse problem.

Finally, the obstetrician–gynecologist should be willing to encourage the patient's participation in her treatment plan. Prescription of potentially addictive medications should be avoided. Treatment or referral for medical or psychiatric complications and comorbidities should be managed in accordance with the physician's expertise in this field and the patient's wishes.

Barriers to Diagnosis and Treatment

Not all patients will readily acknowledge a substance abuse problem and cooperate with a treatment plan. It is helpful, therefore, for the clinician to be aware of certain common impediments to diagnosis and treatment.

Denial is a psychologic defense against acknowledging the personal pain caused by a substance abuse problem. This contributes to underreporting of consumption and resistance to treatment. The denial may be subconscious, thus keeping patients from getting relevant information and treatment. If tolerance to a substance develops, it may contribute to denial. With continued use of an addicting drug, the patient experiences fewer and fewer effects of the drug over time. Higher doses are required to achieve the desired effect. Patients often do not feel or appear intoxicated, even after recent drug use.

Attempts by others to "help" the substance abuser by smoothing over problems which result from substance abuse are known as "enabling." This may consist of covering at work or school, hiding the substance use problem from superiors, supplying alcohol or drugs to avoid confrontation or other unpleasant effects, and minimizing or ignoring the substance abuse problem.

The physician may actually be an enabler through the provision of inappropriate prescription drugs, providing doctor's notes for work missed because of substance abuse, or by giving tacit approval for substance abuse by not addressing the problem. Physicians may have their own uncertainty about the appropriateness of personal substance use habits. They often misunderstand the chronic, relapsing nature of alcohol or psychoactive substance abuse and dependence. They may not appreciate the intensity of the urge to use and the preoccupation with the substance the patient experiences. Physicians should avoid contributing to addiction by prescribing nonaddictive medications whenever they are available.

If the patient has a significant other who has adapted to the substance use problem in order to maintain equilibrium in their relationship, this codependency is particularly important to consider when the patient is resistant to referral or seeking help. Treatment or counseling aimed at the issues of codependency is often required.

Pharmacologic Agents Used in Treatment

While clinicians already play a prominent role in promoting smoking cessation programs, it is anticipated that the introduction of new oral and transdermal nicotine substitutes will bring increasing numbers of patients for therapy. A recent review of these systems suggests that physician support and education must be used in conjunction with any prescription for these therapies (13).

Introduction of nicotine gum was the first attempt to provide a substitute for cigarettes. Early popularity of this approach has been dampened by recognition that cigarette craving is not reduced since peak and trough swings occur with gum consumption. The recently approved transdermal systems may overcome this limitation by achieving sustained trough levels over long periods of time. Short-term results suggest that the number of active nicotine patch users who quit smoking is about twice that of placebo patch users. There is little evidence to suggest that the patch should be used longer than 6–8 weeks.

Relapse prevention is just as important with cigarettes as with other substances, and long-term behavior modification and reinforcement are extremely important. Data on the use of nicotine gum and patches in special populations (eg, those with coronary artery disease, pregnant women) are limited.

Patients in treatment programs for other drugs may be taking supplemental pharmacologic agents. The three most commonly used agents are disulfiram (Antabuse), methadone, and naltrexone (Trexan). Disulfiram is used to ensure abstinence from alcohol in conjunction with supportive therapy. Ingestion of alcohol while taking this medication results in nausea and vomiting. Liver functions should be monitored regularly in these patients. Methadone is used to treat narcotic withdrawal. This long-acting narcotic is used in maintenance treatment of narcotic addiction. Naltrexone is used to block the "high" associated with opioid drug use. It is used in detoxified, formerly opioid-dependent patients to help prevent relapse. Patients with intact families and jobs benefit most from this treatment.

Summary

Obstetrician–gynecologists have a clear role in substance abuse prevention and treatment. Knowledge of key risk factors, familiarity with substance abuse screening techniques, and identification of the symptoms and signs of abuse are all components in this process.

REFERENCES

1. National Institute on Drug Abuse. National Household Survey on Drug Abuse: highlights, 1988. Rockville, Maryland: U.S. Department of Health and Human Services, 1990; DHHS publication no. (ADM)90-1681
2. American College of Obstetricians and Gynecologists. Substance abuse in pregnancy. ACOG Technical Bulletin 195. Washington, DC: ACOG, 1994
3. American College of Obstetricians and Gynecologists. Smoking and reproductive health. ACOG Technical Bulletin 180. Washington, DC: ACOG, 1993
4. Blume SB. Women and alcohol: a review. JAMA 1986; 256:1467–1469
5. U.S. Department of Health and Human Services. Prevention 89/90: federal programs and progress. Washington, DC: U.S. Government Printing Office, 1990
6. Ritchie JM, Greene NM. Local anesthetics. In: Gilman AG, Goodman LS, Rall TW, Murad F, eds. The pharmacological basis of therapeutics. 7th ed. New York: Macmillan, 1985:302–321
7. Schuckit MA, ed. Drug and alcohol abuse: a clinical guide to diagnosis and treatment. 3rd ed. New York: Plenum Medical Book Co, 1989:45–95
8. Dubovsky SL, Weissberg MP. Use of addictive drugs. In: Clinical psychiatry in primary care. 2nd ed. Baltimore, Maryland: Williams & Wilkins, 1982:130–133
9. Ewing JA. Detecting alcoholism. The CAGE questionnaire. JAMA 1984;252:1905–1907
10. Sokol RJ, Martier SS, Ager JW. The T-ACE questions: practical prenatal detection of risk-drinking. Am J Obstet Gynecol 1989;160:863–870
11. Pokorny AD, Miller BA, Kaplan HB. The brief MAST: a shortened version of the Michigan Alcoholism Screening Test. Am J Psychiatry 1972;129:342–345
12. Skinner HA, Holt S, Schuller R, Roy J, Israel Y. Identification of alcohol abuse using laboratory tests and a history of trauma. Ann Intern Med 1984;101:847–851
13. Fiore MC, Jorenby DE, Baker TB, Kenford SL. Tobacco dependence and the nicotine patch: clinical guidelines for effective use. JAMA 1992;268:2687–2694

This Technical Bulletin was developed under the direction of the Committee on Technical Bulletins of the American College of Obstetricians and Gynecologists as an educational aid to obstetricians and gynecologists. The committee wishes to thank Robert A. Welch, MD, and Robert J. Sokol, MD, for their assistance in the development of this bulletin. This Technical Bulletin does not define a standard of care, nor is it intended to dictate an exclusive course of management. It presents recognized methods and techniques of clinical practice for consideration by obstetrician–gynecologists for incorporation into their practices. Variations of practice taking into account the needs of the individual patient, resources, and limitations unique to the institution or type of practice may be appropriate.

ISSN 1074-8628

**THE AMERICAN COLLEGE OF OBSTETRICIANS AND GYNECOLOGISTS
409 12th Street, SW
Washington, DC 20024-2188**

12345/87654

Number 195—July 1994
(Replaces #96, September 1986)

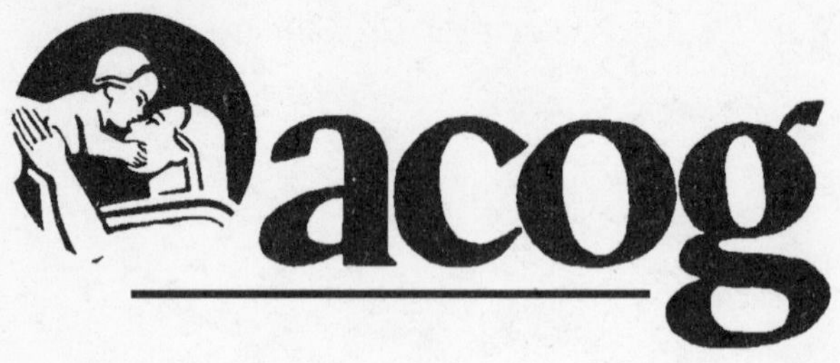

Technical Bulletin
An Educational Aid to Obstetrician–Gynecologists

Substance Abuse in Pregnancy

Substance abuse by pregnant women is considered by many to be one of the major problems in modern obstetrics. The potential deleterious effects of substance abuse on the developing fetus raise numerous medical, ethical, legal, and economic questions. Few subjects have generated more controversy and debate in both the medical and lay press. In some states, the legal requirements regarding reporting substance abuse threaten to interfere with patient confidentiality and the entire patient–physician relationship. Despite intensive research into the problem of substance abuse by pregnant women, many questions remain unanswered. The purpose of this Technical Bulletin is to review the known effects of specific substances on pregnancy outcome, treatment guidelines, and currently available methods of detecting substance abuse.

Substance abusers rarely abuse a single substance. Those who abuse illicit substances frequently also abuse tobacco or alcohol or both (1). The potential impact of multiple substance abuse must be taken into account when attempting to evaluate the effects of individual substances on the fetus or on pregnancy outcome. Another confounding factor is the unknown potential effect of the multiple diluents that are often added to drugs purchased on the street. For all of these reasons, it is probably more accurate to speak of problems associated with substance abuse by pregnant women than only those problems caused by illicit drug abuse.

The true prevalence of substance abuse by pregnant women is difficult, if not impossible, to establish. In urban populations receiving care at large medical centers, routine urine testing at the time of labor has demonstrated rates of illicit substance abuse of 20% or higher (2). Because of the high-risk populations surveyed, however, many feel that these studies overestimate the magnitude of the problem in the general population.

In 1990, Chasnoff and associates presented the results of a cross-sectional study of substance abuse by pregnant women in Pinellas County, Florida (3). In that study, all patients who presented for prenatal care to a public- or private-sector health provider had urine samples analyzed for evidence of recent alcohol or illicit substance abuse. Approximately 15% of unselected women had toxicologic evidence of recent use. Importantly, there was no difference in the prevalence of recent substance abuse when those with private insurance were compared with medically indigent patients. In a statewide prevalence study from Rhode Island, 7.5% of patients admitted to the hospital in labor had toxicologic evidence of recent substance abuse (4).

It would appear, then, that 10% is a reasonable minimal estimate of the prevalence of urine toxicologic evidence of substance abuse in the general population of pregnant women in the United States. Given the poor sensitivity of urine screening for the detection of anything but very recent use, however, the number of women who abuse substances during pregnancy is almost certainly higher.

Effects of Specific Substances

The pregnancies of substance abusers are often complicated by other problems such as sexually transmitted diseases, late access to prenatal care, and poor nutrition. Most studies of the effects of substance abuse on pregnancy have analyzed urban, primarily minority populations which are at high risk for poor pregnancy outcome even in the absence of substance abuse. Nonetheless, there are some complications that may be attributed to individual substances.

Alcohol

Fetal alcohol syndrome (FAS) was first described in 1973; however, the deleterious effect of alcohol has been suspected for centuries. A congenital syndrome, FAS is characterized by three findings: growth retardation (which may occur in the prenatal period, the postnatal period, or both), facial abnormalities, and central nervous system dysfunction (5). In addition to a history of maternal alcohol use during pregnancy, at least one finding from each of these three categories must be present to make the diagnosis of FAS (6). The facial abnormalities include shortened palpebral fissures, low-set ears, midfacial hypoplasia, a smooth philtrum, and a thin upper lip. Central nervous system abnormalities that are considered part of FAS include microcephaly, mental retardation, and behavioral disorders such as attention deficit disorder.

Skeletal abnormalities and structural cardiac defects are also seen with increased frequency in the children of women who use alcohol during pregnancy but are not required for the diagnosis of FAS. These skeletal anomalies include abnormalities of position or function or both and, occasionally, abnormal palmar crease patterns. The most common cardiac structural anomalies are ventricular septal defects, but a number of others occur.

Performance deficits in children with FAS are striking. Intelligence is profoundly affected in some; the average IQ of children with FAS is 63 (7). Affected children may display fine motor dysfunction. Irritability is common in infancy, and hyperactivity is a common finding in later childhood.

Ethanol freely crosses the placenta and the fetal blood–brain barrier. The deleterious effects of ethanol are presumed to be mediated by direct toxicity as well as through toxic metabolites such as acetaldehyde. In addition, the poor nutritional status of heavy alcohol users may play a role. There is substantial evidence that toxicity is dose related and that the exposure time of greatest risk is the first trimester (8). The most severe effects are on the brain, however, and this organ continues to develop throughout gestation.

The exact risk incurred by maternal alcohol use is difficult to establish. In the United States, FAS is noted once in every 500–1,000 deliveries. It is the most common identified cause of mental retardation (9). Even among chronic alcoholics, the incidence of FAS is highly variable, ranging from as low as 6% to as high as 30–50% (10, 11). Moreover, use of lesser amounts of alcohol have been associated with fully developed FAS. Of the offspring of moderate to heavy drinkers (who consume 1–2 oz of absolute alcohol per day), approximately 10% can be expected to develop some characteristics of FAS (12, 13). Although an occasional drink during pregnancy has not been shown to be of harm, patients should be counseled that there is no level of alcohol use during pregnancy that is known to be safe.

A neonatal abstinence syndrome characterized by jitteriness, irritability, and poor feeding may occur within the first 12 hours of life. This syndrome is less common and less severe than that seen following opiate withdrawal. Short-term treatment with barbiturates is sometimes necessary to ameliorate the symptoms.

Long-term effects of FAS include failure to thrive, dental malalignment and malocclusion, as well as eustachian tube dysfunction from midfacial hypoplasia. Recurrent otitis media is a frequent complication. Ocular development may be impaired, resulting in severe degrees of myopia.

Tobacco

No discussion of substance abuse by pregnant women is complete without addressing the potential problems of tobacco use. It has been estimated that 25–30% of women of reproductive age smoke (14, 15). Patients who use alcohol or illicit substances during pregnancy are more than twice as likely than those who do not use these substances to admit to concurrent tobacco use (52% versus 20%) (16).

The effects of cigarette smoking on pregnancy outcome have been studied extensively over the last 20 years. A number of pregnancy complications appear to occur more frequently among heavy smokers than nonsmokers. Spontaneous abortion, placental abruption, premature rupture of membranes, and preterm delivery have all been shown to be significantly associated with cigarette smoking (17–19). In addition, in a number of studies, the infants of heavy cigarette smokers have been shown to have lower birth weights than those of nonsmokers; the mean difference was 200 g (20). The exact causes of these adverse outcomes have not been fully elucidated, but it appears that quitting smoking before 16 weeks of gestation ameliorates many of these adverse effects (21).

Marijuana

Marijuana is derived from the plant *Cannabis sativa*; its active ingredient is tetrahydrocannabinol. There is no evidence that marijuana is a significant teratogen in humans. Initial reports suggested an increased frequency of meconium-stained amniotic fluid and precipitate labor in heavy marijuana users, but these results have not been reproducible (22).

Due to their high lipid solubility and large molecular weight, cannabinoid metabolites can be detected in the urine of users for days to weeks—much longer than for alcohol and most other illicit substances. Given that marijuana is commonly used by multiple substance abusers, the presence of cannabinoid metabolites in the urine may identify patients who are at high risk for being current users of other substances as well.

Cocaine

The development of "crack" cocaine, an inexpensive, easily manufactured form of cocaine, has resulted in its widespread use. By some estimates, at least 10 million Americans have used cocaine and at least five million are regular users. The practice of exchanging crack cocaine for sex has been associated with large numbers of pregnancies complicated by cocaine use. Indeed, in some inner-city municipal hospitals, 15% of parturients have evidence of recent cocaine use (23).

Cocaine is rapidly absorbed across all mucous membranes. Its effects are due to blockade of reuptake of norepinephrine and dopamine. Central inhibition of reuptake results in euphoria, while the peripheral effects result in vasoconstriction, tachycardia, and local anesthesia. Cocaine appears to be metabolized through a number of different pathways in humans. The action of both plasma and liver esterases on cocaine results in the formation of ecgonine methyl ester. This water-soluble compound accounts for 30–50% of the cocaine metabolites found in urine. In addition, there appears to be spontaneous nonenzymatic hydrolysis of cocaine to benzoyl ecgonine, which is also excreted primarily in the urine. This compound also accounts for 30–50% of the cocaine metabolites found in urine and is the compound that most commercially available enzyme assays are designed to detect in urine tested for evidence of recent cocaine use (24). The fate of cocaine in the fetus has not been well defined; however, the facts that cholinesterases are poorly developed in the fetus and that early neonatal urine is frequently positive for cocaine metabolites when maternal urine is negative suggest that there may be some concentration of cocaine metabolites in the fetus.

Crack cocaine is extremely addictive. This alkaloid form of cocaine is not destroyed by heating; smoking crack results in rapidly attained, extremely high blood levels of cocaine. The intense euphoria associated with these high levels increases the desire to use the drug and results in rapid escalation of use.

The maternal hazards of cocaine use are similar to the complications seen in adult users in general. High levels of cocaine can result in profound vasoconstriction leading to malignant hypertension, cardiac ischemia, and cerebral infarction. In addition, high levels of cocaine have been shown to have a direct cardiotoxic effect and have been associated with many well-publicized episodes of sudden death. Despite the fact that cholinesterase activity is somewhat decreased in pregnant women, there is no evidence that pregnancy increases one's susceptibility to cocaine's toxic effects.

A number of complications of pregnancy have been noted to occur with increased frequency among cocaine users. Cocaine use has been associated with an increased incidence of spontaneous abortion and fetal death in utero (25). In addition, pregnant cocaine users have been shown to be at high risk for premature rupture of membranes (20%), preterm labor and delivery (25%), intrauterine growth retardation (25–30%), meconium-stained amniotic fluid (29%), and placental abruption (6–8%) (1, 26, 27). There have been well-documented cases of in utero fetal cerebral infarction (28).

The teratogenic effects of cocaine, if any, have not been conclusively demonstrated. In addition to growth retardation, several studies have noted an increased frequency of microcephaly in association with cocaine use (29, 30). Limb reduction defects and genitourinary malformations have also been reported with first-trimester cocaine use (31–33). The malformations are hypothesized to be due to vascular interruption during development caused by cocaine's intense vasoconstrictive effects. The number of cases reported to date is small and the studies subject to design deficiencies thus precluding any valid conclusions regarding the teratogenicity of cocaine.

Infants born to cocaine-using women are also at risk for neurobehavioral abnormalities. Cocaine-exposed infants have significant impairments in orientation, motor, and state regulation neurobehaviors (29). Cocaine exposure has also been linked to sudden infant death syndrome (34).

Opiates

Narcotic addiction during pregnancy poses serious health threats to both the woman and the fetus. Studies analyzing the pregnancy outcomes of heroin addicts have demonstrated rates of stillbirth, fetal growth retardation, prematurity, and neonatal mortality three to seven times higher than those of the general population (35). Whether these problems are a direct effect of the narcotics or a result of the myriad health and social problems typical of narcotic addicts is difficult to establish. It is clear, however, that treatment with methadone is associated with improved pregnancy outcome, and, in one study, the perinatal outcome of patients enrolled in methadone maintenance programs was as good as that of the general population (36).

The newborn infant of a narcotic addict is at risk for a severe, potentially fatal, narcotic withdrawal syndrome. As many as two thirds of infants born to heroin addicts will develop signs and symptoms of narcotic withdrawal. Although the incidence of clinically significant withdrawal appears to be slightly lower among methadone-treated addicts, it can be just as severe (37). Neonatal withdrawal is characterized by a high-pitched cry, poor feeding, hypertonicity, tremors, irritability, sneezing, sweating, vomiting, diarrhea, and, occasionally, seizures. With heroin, the signs of withdrawal usually appear 24–72 hours after birth. Signs of withdrawal occur 1–2 days later in infants born to mothers taking methadone. Occasionally, withdrawal symptoms do not appear until 10 days of life—after the infant has been discharged.

Although all illicit substance abusers must be considered at increased risk for human immunodeficiency virus (HIV) infection, this is especially true for narcotic addicts. While the primary route of administration for cocaine is smoking, the primary route for narcotics is intravenous. The frequent sharing of needles has resulted in extremely high rates of HIV infection (greater than 50%) and hepatitis among this population.

Amphetamines

The illicit use of amphetamines by pregnant women has never been as prevalent as cocaine or narcotic use, and so there is relatively little information available. The use by pregnant women of crystal methamphetamine ("ice," "blue ice"), a potent stimulant administered intravenously, has been associated with decreased fetal head circumference and increased risk for placental abruption, intrauterine growth retardation, and fetal death in utero (38, 39). This pattern of abnormalities is similar to that seen in cocaine users and may be related to the vasoconstrictive properties of amphetamines. In addition, the well-known anorectic properties of amphetamines may severely impair nutrition during pregnancy.

Hallucinogens

There is no evidence that lysergic acid diethylamide (LSD) or other hallucinogens cause chromosomal damage, as was once reported (40). Although there are no known deleterious effects of this group of drugs on human pregnancy, there have been few controlled studies. There have been no studies on the potential long-term effects on neuro-development in the neonate.

Prenatal and Early Postpartum Care for the Pregnant Substance Abuser

Intensive prenatal care has been shown to ameliorate the maternal and neonatal complications associated with substance abuse. For example, among pregnant cocaine users, the obstetric outcome for those who receive multidisciplinary prenatal care is significantly improved compared with users who receive little or no prenatal care (41). However, matched controls had better outcomes than either cocaine-using group. The favorable pregnancy outcomes seen in opiate addicts enrolled in methadone maintenance programs throughout pregnancy attest to the beneficial effects of prenatal care.

The pregnant substance abuser often has a multitude of nonmedical problems. Some users have no job, are undereducated, live in substandard housing, or have psychiatric disorders. Where possible, it is helpful to have a multidisciplinary team of health care and social service providers to address the multiple problems of substance abusers. At each prenatal encounter, substance abuse treatment should be offered to those who have not quit.

A thorough substance abuse history should be taken from all patients as part of the medical and obstetric history. Those with significant alcohol use should be counseled regarding the risk and effects of FAS. All substance abusers should be counseled about the potential risks of preterm delivery, fetal growth retardation, fetal death, and possible long-term neurobehavioral effects of continued substance abuse.

In addition to routine laboratory testing, HIV testing should be encouraged. Periodic urine toxicology testing may be offered as a motivational tool to encourage abstinence. The reliability of urine toxicology, however, is limited by the rapid clearance of most substances. In addition, overaggressive urine testing could be perceived by the patient as threatening and thus decrease patient compliance.

Because growth retardation is a relatively frequent finding among fetuses of substance abusers, accurate assessment of gestational age is essential for optimal management. Early ultrasound confirmation of gestational age may obviate the need for more intensive testing or intervention later in pregnancy. Furthermore, because of the increased frequency of structural anomalies among substance abusers, a fetal anatomic survey may be indicated. Antepartum testing is appropriate when there is reason to expect fetal compromise (eg, size small for dates, decreased fetal movement, suspected growth retardation). When there is normal growth and an active fetus, there is no compelling evidence that regular antepartum testing is associated with improved perinatal outcome in this group of patients.

The labor and delivery of substance abusers should be managed like that of any high-risk pregnancy. Fetal well-being should be documented throughout labor, and the indications for anesthesia or operative delivery are the same as those for most obstetric patients. It is critical that the health care provider(s) caring for the baby be informed of the mother's substance abuse since the infant may need prolonged observation for signs of withdrawal and for potential future developmental abnormalities.

Encouraging substance abusers to receive treatment should continue through the postpartum period. Adequate contraception should be provided to prevent undesired pregnancies. The mother should be counseled that the infant may be exposed through breast-feeding to substances she is using. Mothers whose infants are at risk for neurobehavioral handicaps should be informed of the importance of early and frequent developmental examinations. Follow-up should be encouraged. In addition, a number of states mandate the reporting and follow-up of these mothers and infants. Physicians should be familiar with the requirements of their state.

Screening

Substance abuse is one of the most important risks encountered in contemporary obstetrics. Therefore, all patients should be questioned thoroughly about substance abuse (including alcohol and tobacco) at the time of their first prenatal visit (see the box).

Although denial is a major component of addictive behavior and limits the reliability of self-reporting, the patient should be given the opportunity to admit to substance abuse. In instances in which a constellation of signs and symptoms suggest substance abuse, she should be made aware of the potential association of these signs with substance abuse and the need to share information with her health care provider. Several screening questionnaires have been developed to detect problem drinking which also may prove helpful in detecting substance abuse. For example, the T-ACE questions (see the box), the CAGE questionnaire (42), the brief MAST questionnaire (43), and the Trauma Scale (44) all pose a brief series of nonthreatening questions about alcohol use.

Relatively inexpensive qualitative urine assays are available to aid in the detection of most illicit substances. The opiates and their metabolites are detectable in urine specimens of nonpregnant adults for only 48–72 hours after the most recent use (45). Cocaine undergoes rapid metabolism; its subsequent urinary excretion results in a short window (no more than 2–3 days) during which the drug can be detected in the urine of nonpregnant adults. The ability of urine toxicology to detect recent substance abuse may be further hampered in pregnant women by the increase in renal plasma flow (and therefore, clearance) of up to 50% associated with normal pregnancy. These factors limit the ability of urine testing to detect substance abuse in pregnant women.

Periodic urine testing may be desirable, however, in a pregnant woman who admits to substance abuse prior to or during pregnancy in order to encourage and reinforce continual abstinence. Since positive results have implications for patients that transcend their health, patients should give informed consent prior to testing. The requirements for consent vary from state to state. Physicians should be familiar with their own state laws regarding consent for drug screening of pregnant women and newborns. Universal toxicology screening is not recommended. Testing the mother or neonate or both may be useful in some clinical situations, such as the presence of unexplained fetal growth retardation, unexpected prematurity, or abruptio placentae in a woman not known to have hypertensive disease, even when substance abuse has not been suspected previously.

Both meconium and neonatal hair samples have been used to document substance abuse by pregnant women (46, 47). Both of these techniques, however, have limitations. Complete collection of meconium is difficult to ensure, and neither technique provides in-formation on substance abuse until after the completion of pregnancy. However, these samples may help identify neonates who may be at risk for developing long-term sequelae as a result of in utero exposure and who may benefit from early identification and intervention.

Recent legislation in some states considers in utero drug exposure to be a form of child abuse or neglect under the law and requires reporting of positive drug tests in

"T-ACE" Questions

T How many drinks does it take to make you feel high (TOLERANCE)?

A Have people ANNOYED you by criticizing your drinking?

C Have you felt you ought to CUT DOWN on your drinking?

E Have you ever had a drink first thing in the morning to steady your nerves or get rid of a hangover (EYE OPENER)?

For the Tolerance question, an answer of more than two drinks is considered a positive response. A score of 2 is assigned for a positive response to the Tolerance question, and a score of 1 is assigned to all others for a positive response. A T-ACE score of 2 or greater is considered positive for problem drinking.

Sokol RJ, Martier SS, Ager JW. The T-ACE questions: practical prenatal detection of risk-drinking. Am J Obstet Gynecol 1989;160:865

Signs and Symptoms of Substance Abuse

Because of the frequency of complications seen in substance abusers, it is important that the clinician be alert for clinical and historical clues that may indicate the possibility of substance abuse.

Behavior Patterns
- Sedation
- Inebriation
- Euphoria
- Agitation
- Disorientation

Physical Signs
- Dilated or constricted pupils
- Track marks or abscesses
- Inflamed nasal mucosa
- Increased pulse and blood pressure
- Hallucinations
- Nystagmus

Medical History
- Unusual infections (cellulitis, endocarditis, atypical pneumonias, HIV)
- Cirrhosis
- Hepatitis
- Pancreatitis

pregnant women or their newborns to the state's child protection agency. One must be familiar with state laws regarding testing and reporting.

Summary

Substance abuse by pregnant women continues to be one of the leading problems in modern obstetrics. The frequency of abuse of more than one substance, especially with alcohol and tobacco, makes interpretation of the literature difficult; however, there is little doubt that substance abuse is associated with poor pregnancy outcome. Furthermore, abstinence and prenatal care are associated with improved perinatal outcomes. Despite the positive impact of perinatal care, however, continued abuse of substances during pregnancy can result in infant impairment.

Clinicians who provide care to pregnant women should be alert to the possibility of substance abuse in all women so that treatment can be offered and complications can be anticipated, or better, avoided. At the time of the first prenatal visit, all pregnant women should be questioned thoroughly about past and present drug use. While toxicology screening may be helpful in some circumstances, universal screening is not recommended. Practitioners should be familiar with testing and reporting requirements in their state.

Substance abusers should be counseled about the risks posed by continued substance use. At each prenatal and postpartum visit, substance abuse treatment should be offered to those who have not quit. When possible, it is helpful to work with a multidisciplinary team to address the various problems associated with substance abuse.

REFERENCES

1. Little BB, Snell LM, Klein VR, Gilstrap LC III. Cocaine abuse during pregnancy: maternal and fetal implications. Obstet Gynecol 1989;73:157–160
2. Gillogley KM, Evans AT, Hansen RL, Samuels SJ, Batra KK. The perinatal impact of cocaine, amphetamine, and opiate use detected by universal intrapartum screening. Am J Obstet Gynecol 1990;163:1535–1542
3. Chasnoff IJ, Landress HJ, Barrett ME. The prevalence of illicit-drug or alcohol use during pregnancy and discrepancies in mandatory reporting in Pinellas County, Florida. N Engl J Med 1990;322:1202–1206
4. Centers for Disease Control. Statewide prevalence of illicit drug use by pregnant women—Rhode Island. MMWR 1990;14:225–227
5. Jones KL, Smith DW, Ulleland CN, Streissguth AP. Pattern of malformation in offspring of chronic alcoholic mothers. Lancet 1973;1:1267–1271
6. Rosett HL. A clinical perspective of the fetal alcohol syndrome. Alcohol Clin Exp Res 1980;4:119–122
7. Jones KL, ed. Smith's recognizable patterns of human malformation. 4th ed. Philadelphia: WB Saunders, 1988: 491–494
8. Ernhart CB, Sokol RJ, Martier S, Moron P, Nadler D, Ager JW, et al. Alcohol teratogenicity in the human: a detailed assessment of specificity, critical period, and threshold. Am J Obstet Gynecol 1987;156:33–39
9. Abel EL, Sokol RJ. Fetal alcohol syndrome is now leading cause of mental retardation. Lancet 1986;2:1222
10. Olegård R, Sabel KG, Aronsson M, Sandin B, Johansson PR, Carlsson C, et al. Effects on the child of alcohol abuse during pregnancy. Acta Paediatr Scand Suppl 1979;275: 112–121
11. Abel EL, Sokol RJ. Incidence of fetal alcohol syndrome and economic impact of FAS-related anomalies. Drug Alcohol Depend 1987;19:51–70
12. Hanson JW, Streissguth AP, Smith DW. The effects of moderate alcohol consumption during pregnancy on fetal growth and morphogenesis. J Pediatr 1978;92:457–460
13. Autti-Ramo I, Gaily E, Granstrom ML. Dysmorphic features in offspring of alcoholic mothers. Arch Dis Child 1992;67:712–716
14. Centers for Disease Control. Cigarette smoking among reproductive-aged women—Behavioral Risk Factor Surveillance System, 1989. MMWR 1991;40:719–723
15. Centers for Disease Control. Cigarette smoking among adults—United States, 1988. MMWR 1991;40:757–765
16. Christmas JT, Knisley JS, Dawson KS, Dinsmoor MJ, Weber SE, Schnoll SH. Comparison of questionnaire screening and urine toxicology for detection of pregnancy complicated by substance use. Obstet Gynecol 1992;80:750– 754
17. Harlap S, Shiono PH. Alcohol, smoking, and incidence of spontaneous abortions in the first and second trimester. Lancet 1980;2:173–176
18. Naeye RL. Abruptio placentae and placenta previa: frequency, perinatal mortality, and cigarette smoking. Obstet Gynecol 1980;55:701–704
19. Naeye RL. Factors that predispose to premature rupture of the fetal membranes. Obstet Gynecol 1982;60:93–98
20. American College of Obstetricians and Gynecologists. Smoking and reproductive health. ACOG Technical Bulletin 180. Washington, DC: ACOG, 1993
21. MacArthur C, Knox EG. Smoking in pregnancy: effects of stopping at different stages. Br J Obstet Gynaecol 1988;95:551–555
22. Fried PA, Buckingham M, Von Kulmiz P. Marijuana use during pregnancy and perinatal risk factors. Am J Obstet Gynecol 1983;146:992–994
23. Spence MR, Williams R, DiGregorio GJ, Kirby-McDonnell A, Polansky M. The relationship between recent cocaine use and pregnancy outcome. Obstet Gynecol 1991;78:326–329
24. Stewart DJ, Inaba T, Lucassen M, Kalow W. Cocaine metabolism: cocaine and norcocaine hydrolysis by liver and serum esterases. Clin Pharmacol Ther 1979;25:464–468

25. Chasnoff IJ, Burns WJ, Schnoll SH, Burns KA. Cocaine use in pregnancy. N Engl J Med 1985;313:666–669

26. MacGregor SN, Keith LG, Chasnoff IJ, Rosner MA, Chisum GM, Shaw P, et al. Cocaine use during pregnancy: adverse perinatal outcome. Am J Obstet Gynecol 1987;157:686–690

27. Neerhof MG, MacGregor SN, Retzky SS, Sullivan TP. Cocaine abuse during pregnancy: peripartum prevalence and perinatal outcome. Am J Obstet Gynecol 1989; 161:633–638

28. Heier LA, Carpanzano CR, Mast J, Brill PW, Winchester P, Deck MDF. Maternal cocaine abuse: the spectrum of radiologic abnormalities in the neonatal CNS. Am J Neuroradiol 1991;12:951–956

29. Chasnoff IJ, Griffith DR, MacGregor S, Dirkes K, Burns KA. Temporal patterns of cocaine use in pregnancy. Perinatal outcome. JAMA 1989;261:1741–1744

30. Cherukuri R, Minkoff H, Feldman J, Parekh A, Glass L. A cohort study of alkaloidal cocaine ("crack") in pregnancy. Obstet Gynecol 1988;72:147–151

31. Chasnoff IJ, Chisum GM, Kaplan WE. Maternal cocaine use and genitourinary tract malformations. Teratology 1988;37:201–204

32. Chávez GF, Mulinare J, Cordero JF. Maternal cocaine use during early pregnancy as a risk factor for congenital urogenital anomalies. JAMA 1989;262:795–798

33. Hoyme HE, Jones KL, Dixon SD, Jewett T, Hanson JW, Robinson LK, et al. Prenatal cocaine exposure and fetal vascular disruption. Pediatrics 1990;85:743–747

34. Durand DJ, Espinoza AM, Nickerson BG. Association between prenatal cocaine exposure and sudden infant death syndrome. J Pediatr 1990;117:909–911

35. Fricker HS, Segal S. Narcotic addiction, pregnancy, and the newborn. Am J Dis Child 1978;132:360–366

36. Newman RG, Bashkow S, Calko D. Results of 313 consecutive live births of infants delivered to patients in the New York City Methadone Maintenance Treatment Program. Am J Obstet Gynecol 1975;121:233–237

37. Blinick G, Wallach RC, Jerez E, Ackerman BD. Drug addiction in pregnancy and the neonate. Am J Obstet Gynecol 1976;125:135–142

38. Little BB, Snell LM, Gilstrap LC III. Methamphetamine abuse during pregnancy: outcome and fetal effects. Obstet Gynecol 1988;72:541–544

39. Oro AS, Dixon SD. Perinatal cocaine and methamphetamine exposure: maternal and neonatal correlates. J Pediatr 1987;111:571–578

40. Long SY. Does LSD induce chromosomal damage and malformations? A review of the literature. Teratology 1972;6:75–90

41. MacGregor SN, Keith LG, Bachicha JA, Chasnoff IJ. Cocaine abuse during pregnancy: correlation between prenatal care and perinatal outcome. Obstet Gynecol 1989;74:882–885

42. Ewing JA. Detecting alcoholism. The CAGE questionnaire. JAMA 1984;252:1905–1907

43. Pokorny AD, Miller BA, Kaplan HB. The brief MAST: a shortened version of the Michigan Alcoholism Screening Test. Am J Psychiatry 1972;129:342–345

44. Skinner HA, Holt S, Schuller R, Roy J, Israel Y. Identification of alcohol abuse using laboratory tests and a history of trauma. Ann Intern Med 1984;101:847–851

45. Way EL, Adler TK. The pharmacologic implications of the fate of morphine and its surrogates. Pharmacol Rev 1960;12:383–446

46. Graham K, Koren G, Klein J, Schneiderman J, Greenwald M. Determination of gestational cocaine exposure by hair analysis. JAMA 1989;262:3328–3330

47. Ostrea EM Jr, Brady M, Gause S, Raymundo AL, Stevens M. Drug screening of newborns by meconium analysis: a large-scale, prospective, epidemiologic study. Pediatrics 1992;89:107–113

This Technical Bulletin was developed under the direction of the Committee on Technical Bulletins of the American College of Obstetricians and Gynecologists as an educational aid to obstetricians and gynecologists. The committee wishes to thank James T. Christmas, MD, for his assistance in the development of this bulletin and Robert A. Welch, MD, and Robert J. Sokol, MD, for their contributions to this bulletin. This Technical Bulletin does not define a standard of care, nor is it intended to dictate an exclusive course of management. It presents recognized methods and techniques of clinical practice for consideration by obstetrician–gynecologists for incorporation into their practices. Variations of practice taking into account the needs of the individual patient, resources, and limitations unique to the institution or type of practice may be appropriate.
ISSN 1074-8628

THE AMERICAN COLLEGE OF OBSTETRICIANS AND GYNECOLOGISTS
409 12th Street, SW
Washington, DC 20024-2188

12345/87654

ACOG EDUCATIONAL BULLETIN

Number 236, April 1997

Teratology

Teratology is the study of abnormal fetal development. Major defects are apparent at birth in about 3% of the general population, and in about 4.5% by 5 years of age. An exact cause or mechanism for the defect can be determined in less than 50% of cases. Some substances, organisms, and physical agents are known to be teratogens, capable of causing abnormal fetal development.

Although obstetricians are often asked about potentially teratogenic agents, the present discussion is limited to those agents proved by cumulative information to be harmful to a fetus. Other agents are suspected but not documented teratogens. Expert consensus on the safety of such agents does not exist and may be impossible to achieve.

Practical information for determining the teratogenicity of common environmental, infectious, and pharmacologic agents is outlined in this bulletin. Important factors to consider in determining the risk of teratogenesis include the exact identity and dose of the apparent teratogen, the stage of embryogenesis during which the exposure occurred, and the genetic sensitivity of the mother and fetus.

This Educational Bulletin was developed under the direction of the Committee on Educational Bulletins of the American College of Obstetricians and Gynecologists as an aid to obstetricians and gynecologists. This document is not to be construed as establishing a standard of practice or dictating an exclusive course of treatment. Rather, it is intended as an educational tool that presents current information on obstetric–gynecologic issues.

Factors Influencing Teratogenic Effect

Some agents cause major defects if fetal exposure occurs during a specific critical period but cause no harmful effect at another time. For example, rubella can cause multiple anatomic defects when fetal infection occurs during the first trimester of pregnancy but causes only chronic infection in the newborn when exposure occurs during the third trimester. After organogenesis has been completed (13 weeks of gestation), the observable effect of an environmental agent may be limited to fetal growth restriction or a minimal reduction in organ size and to functional rather than gross structural defects.

Individual variation in susceptibility to a constant dose of a given agent also influences teratogenic effect. Each child of a chronic alcoholic may display different manifestations of fetal alcohol syndrome, possibly because of genotypic differences in sensitivity to alcohol. This may also explain why high doses of a known teratogen have no effect on some exposed fetuses. The occurrence of threshold phenomena can explain why low doses of some agents have no teratogenic effect. Furthermore, an effect of a low dose that

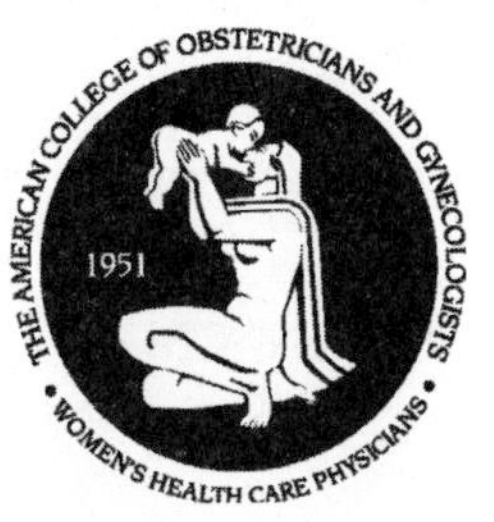

Replaces Number 233, February 1997

is statistically insignificant in a small sample might be shown to be biologically significant if a larger population were studied.

Study of Teratogenic Drugs

For most drugs, animal studies have been used extensively to determine possible teratogenic effects. Although such studies may be helpful, their results do not always reliably predict human response.

When studies of birth defects in humans are evaluated, the statistics presented should be reviewed with caution. Results of retrospective and uncontrolled studies, as well as individual case reports, may be misleading about the risk of exposure to specific drugs during pregnancy, especially those commonly used during gestation. Some offspring of any large population of women using a drug during pregnancy will be born with birth defects. These events may lead to spurious claims of a causal relationship. Differentiating the effects of a specific pharmacologic agent from the effects of the illness for which it was prescribed can also be difficult as it involves determining the natural prevalence rate—the rate at which the defect occurs in a population—and the increased risk known to be attributable to the drug used to treat that population. Often, studies of large populations are required to determine the risk from teratogenic agents. Large, carefully done, controlled prospective studies can help resolve questions raised by retrospective studies and case reports. Current data from well-designed prospective studies, when available, should be emphasized in counseling.

Counseling

Counseling regarding environmental or teratogenic exposure should be performed in a sympathetic, supportive, and informative manner so that the patient is not unduly alarmed or burdened by guilt. Most patient inquiries are related to low-level risks.

Certain patients, however, have been exposed to agents that are known to be associated with significant increased risk for fetal malformation or mental retardation. The physician may wish to consult with or refer such a patient to a health professional with special education or experience in teratology and birth defects. Prenatal testing also may be indicated. After patients are fully informed of the risks, some request pregnancy termination. Psychologic support of the patient's decision should be provided. In particular, follow-up counseling is advised for patient education and emotional support after abortion or after the birth of an affected baby. Technical multispecialty support for the abnormal infant is essential.

Specific techniques for prenatal diagnosis and management of teratogenic effects are beyond the scope of this bulletin. Amniocentesis for chromosome karyotyping is not appropriate for detecting birth defects caused by environmental teratogens. Detailed targeted ultrasonography may be used to diagnose some structural defects and effects produced by teratogenic agents (1). Serologic testing, ultrasonography, chorionic villus sampling, amniocentesis, and fetal blood sampling may be used in the prenatal diagnosis of congenital cytomegalovirus, rubella, toxoplasmosis, and varicella infections. Open neural tube defects and midline ventral fusion defects may often be detected by ultrasonography or maternal serum screening (2). However, patients should be counseled that ultrasonography can never exclude the presence of teratogenic effects.

Although general statements may be made about the teratogenetic potential of prescription drugs, maternal condition and treatment needs should also be considered, weighing the benefit to the mother with the risk to the fetus. The U.S. Food and Drug Administration has defined five risk categories (A, B, C, D, X) that are used by manufacturers to rate their products for use during pregnancy and are reported in the *Physicans' Desk Reference* (3):

- **Category A**: Controlled studies in women fail to demonstrate a risk to the fetus in the first trimester (and there is no evidence of a risk in later trimesters), and the possibility of fetal harm appears remote. Vitamin C is an example of a category A substance when its use does not exceed the recommended daily allowance.
- **Category B**: Either animal reproduction studies have not demonstrated fetal risk but no controlled studies in pregnant women have been reported, or animal reproduction studies have shown an adverse effect (other than a decrease in fertility) that was not confirmed in controlled studies in women in the first trimester (and there is no evidence of risk in later trimesters). Ampicillin is an example of a category B drug.
- **Category C**: Either studies in animals have revealed adverse effects on the fetus (teratogenic, embryocidal, or other) but no controlled studies in women have been reported, or studies in women and animals are not available. Drugs should be given only if the potential benefit justifies the potential risk to the fetus. Zidovudine used to decrease perinatal transmission of human immunodeficiency virus (HIV) is an example of a category C drug.
- **Category D**: Positive evidence of human fetal risk exists, but the benefits from use in pregnant women may be acceptable despite the risk (eg, if the drug is

needed for a life-threatening condition or for a serious disease for which safer drugs cannot be used or are ineffective). Phenytoin is an example of a category D drug.

- **Category X**: Studies in animals or human beings have demonstrated fetal abnormalities, or evidence exists of fetal risk based on human experience, or both, and the risk in pregnant women clearly outweighs any possible benefit. The drug is contraindicated in women who are or may become pregnant. Isotretinoin is an example of a category X drug.

Agents Not Documented Teratogens*

Following are examples of agents for which there is limited evidence of varying degrees to document teratogenicity:

Drugs and chemicals
- Acetaminophen
- Acyclovir
- Antiemetics (eg, phenothiazines, trimethobenzamide)
- Antihistamines (eg, doxylamine)
- Aspartame
- Aspirin
- Caffeine
- Hair spray
- Marijuana
- Metronidazole
- Minor tranquilizers (eg, meprobamate, chlordiazepoxide, fluoxetine)
- Occupational chemical agents
- Oral contraceptives
- Pesticides
- Trimethoprim–sulfamethoxazole
- Vaginal spermicides
- Zidovudine

Infections
- Herpes simplex type 2 virus
- Parvovirus B19

Electromagnetic fields from video display terminals

Heat

*Paternal exposure to any agent has not been shown to be teratogenic.

Examples of agents of common concern to pregnant patients but for which there is not adequate evidence to document teratogenicity or adverse effect are listed in the box. Paternal exposure to any agent is not thought to be teratogenic.

Table 1 lists some drugs, chemicals, and infectious agents for which the preponderance of evidence suggests a significant teratogenic risk, as well as the most commonly encountered effects. The organisms that cause cytomegalovirus infections, rubella, syphilis, toxoplasmosis, and varicella infections are classified as fetal pathogens because they damage fully or partially formed tissues by direct infection. However, they are not limited to inducing abnormal development during organogenesis. Causes of neonatal damage (eg, herpes infection passed from mother to child during labor) rather than fetal damage are excluded from the table. Also excluded are agents such as cigarette smoke, which causes fetal hypoxia, ischemia, and growth restriction, but does not cause structural defects. The omission of certain agents is not meant to imply that their safety has been proved.

The use of illicit substances is poorly reported so it is difficult to delineate the precise incidence of use in the general population and in the population of women who have infants with particular birth defects. Thus, it is difficult to know if such drugs are teratogenic.

Sources of Current Teratogen Information

Several sources of useful current information regarding potential teratogens are available. These include computerized databases both on-line and on diskette. Another source is the Organization of Teratogen Information Services, which consolidates teratology information nationwide and reports it by region. Numerous teratogen information services are available throughout the United States to serve specific geographic areas. For information on the teratogen service in a particular area, contact:

Eastern United States
Massachusetts Teratogen Information Service
Boston, Massachusetts
(617) 466-8474

or

Western United States
Pregnancy Riskline
Salt Lake City, Utah
(801) 328-2229

Computerized teratology and reproductive risk databases provide up-to-date summaries of electronic resource teratology information. Databases commonly available are listed in the box.

Computer Teratology and Reproductive Risk Information Databases

Micromedex, Inc.
REPRORISK (REPROTEXT, REPROTOX, Shepard's Catalog of Teratogenic Agents and TERIS)
Englewood, CO
(800) 525-9083

National Library of Medicine, MEDLARS Service Desk
GRATEFUL MED (TOXLINE, TOXNET and MEDLINE)
Bethesda, MD
(800) 638-8480

Reproductive Toxicology Center
REPROTOX
Columbia Hospital for Women Medical Center
Washington, DC
(202) 293-5137

Shepard's Catalog of Teratogenic Agents
University of Washington
Seattle, WA
(206) 543-3373

Teratogen Information System
TERIS and Shepard's Catalog of Teratogenic Agents
Seattle, WA
(206) 543-2465

References

1. American College of Obstetricians and Gynecologists. Ultrasonography in pregnancy. ACOG Technical Bulletin 187. Washington, DC: ACOG, 1993 (Level III)
2. American College of Obstetricians and Gynecologists. Maternal serum screening. ACOG Educational Bulletin 228. Washington, DC: ACOG, 1996 (Level III)
3. U.S. Food and Drug Administration. Pregnancy labeling. FDA Drug Bulletin 1979;9:23–24 (Level III)

Suggested Reading

American College of Obstetricians and Gynecologists. Diagnosis and management of fetal death. ACOG Technical Bulletin 176. Washington, DC: ACOG, 1993

American College of Obstetricians and Gynecologists. Early pregnancy loss. ACOG Technical Bulletin 212. Washington, DC: ACOG, 1995

American College of Obstetricians and Gynecologists. Maternal serum screening. ACOG Educational Bulletin 228. Washington, DC: ACOG, 1996

American College of Obstetricians and Gynecologists. Perinatal viral and parasitic infections. ACOG Technical Bulletin 177. Washington, DC: ACOG 1993

American College of Obstetricians and Gynecologists. Preconceptional care. ACOG Technical Bulletin 205. Washington, DC: ACOG, 1995

American College of Obstetricians and Gynecologists. Seizure disorders in pregnancy. ACOG Educational Bulletin 231. Washington, DC: ACOG, 1996

American College of Obstetricians and Gynecologists. Substance abuse in pregnancy. ACOG Technical Bulletin 195. Washington, DC: ACOG, 1994

American Medical Association Drug Evaluation Annual 1995. Chicago: AMA, 1995

Briggs GG, Freeman RK, Yaffe SJ. Drugs in pregnancy and lactation. 4th ed. Baltimore: Williams and Wilkins, 1994

Cefalo RC, Moos MK. Preconceptional health care: a practical guide. 2nd ed. St Louis: Mosby, 1995

Friedman JM, Polifka JE. Teratogenic effects of drugs: a resource for clinicians (TERIS). Baltimore: Johns Hopkins University Press, 1994

Gilstrap LC, Little BB. Drugs and pregnancy. New York: Elsevier, 1992

Heinonen OP, Slone D, Shapiro S. Birth defects and drugs in pregnancy. Boston: John Wright, PSG Inc, 1982

Paul M. Occupational and environmental reproductive hazards: a guide for clinicians. Baltimore: Williams and Wilkins, 1993

Rayburn WH, Zuspan FP. Drug therapy in obstetrics and gynecology. 3rd ed. St Louis: Mosby Year Book, Inc, 1992

Shepard TH. Catalog of teratogenic agents. 8th ed. Baltimore: Johns Hopkins University Press, 1995

Table 1. Teratogenic Agents

Agent	Effects	Comments
Drugs and chemicals		
Alcohol	Growth restriction before and after birth, mental retardation, microcephaly, midfacial hypoplasia producing atypical facial appearance, renal and cardiac defects, various other major and minor malformations	Nutritional deficiency, smoking, and multiple drug use confound data. Risk due to ingestion of one to two drinks per day is not well defined but may cause a small reduction in average birth weight. Fetuses of women who ingest six drinks per day are at a 40% risk of developing some features of the fetal alcohol syndrome.
Androgens and testosterone derivatives (eg, danazol)	Virilization of female, advanced genital development in males	Effects are dose dependent and related to the stage of embryonic development at the time of exposure. Given before 9 weeks of gestation, labioscrotal fusion can be produced; clitoromegaly can occur with exposure at any gestational age. Risk related to incidental brief androgenic exposure is minimal.
Angiotensin-converting enzyme (ACE) inhibitors (eg, enalapril, captopril)	Fetal renal tubular dysplasia, oligohydramnios, neonatal renal failure, lack of cranial ossification, intrauterine growth restriction	Incidence of fetal morbidity is 30%. The risk increases with second- and third-trimester use, leading to in utero fetal hypotension, decreased renal blood flow, and renal failure.
Coumarin derivatives (eg, warfarin)	Nasal hypoplasia and stippled bone epiphyses are most common; other effects include broad short hands with shortened phalanges, ophthalmologic abnormalities, intrauterine growth restriction, developmental delay, anomalies of neck and central nervous system	Risk for a seriously affected child is considered to be 15–25% when anticoagulants that inhibit vitamin K are used in the first trimester, especially during 6–9 weeks of gestation. Later drug exposure may be associated with spontaneous abortion, stillbirths, central nervous system abnormalities, abruptio placentae, and fetal or neonatal hemorrhage.
Carbamazepine	Neural tube defects, minor craniofacial defects, fingernail hypoplasia, microcephaly, developmental delay, intrauterine growth restriction	Risk of neural tube defect, mostly lumbosacral, is 1–2% when used alone during first trimester and increased when used with other antiepileptic agents.
Folic acid antagonists (methotrexate and aminopterin)	Increased risk for spontaneous abortions, various anomalies	These drugs are contraindicated for the treatment of psoriasis in pregnancy and must be used with extreme caution in the treatment of malignancy. Cytotoxic drugs are potentially teratogenic. Effects of aminopterin are well documented. Folic acid antagonists used during the first trimester produce a malformation rate of up to 30% in fetuses that survive.
Cocaine	Bowel atresias; congenital malformations of the heart, limbs, face and genitourinary tract; microcephaly; intrauterine growth restriction; cerebral infarctions	Risks may be affected by other factors and concurrent abuse of multiple substances. Maternal and pregnancy complications include sudden death and placental abruption.
Diethylstilbestrol	Clear-cell adenocarcinoma of the vagina or cervix, vaginal adenosis, abnormalities of cervix and uterus, abnormalities of the testes, possible infertility in males and females	Vaginal adenosis is detected in more than 50% of women whose mothers took these drugs before 9 weeks of gestation. Risk for vaginal adenocarcinoma is low. Males exposed in utero may have a 25% incidence of epididymal cysts, hypotrophic testes, abnormal spermatozoa, and induration of the testes.
Lead	Increased abortion rate, stillbirths	Fetal central nervous system development may be adversely affected. Determining preconceptional lead levels for those at risk may be useful.
Lithium	Congenital heart disease, in particular, Ebstein anomaly	Risk of heart malformations due to first-trimester exposure is low. The effect is not as significant as reported in earlier studies. Exposure in the last month of gestation may produce toxic effects on the thyroid, kidneys, and neuromuscular systems.

(Continued)

Table 1. Teratogenic Agents (continued)

Agent	Effects	Comments
Drugs and Chemicals (continued)		
Organic mercury	Cerebral atrophy, microcephaly, mental retardation, spasticity, seizures, blindness	Cerebral palsy can occur even when exposure is in the third trimester. Exposed individuals include consumers of fish and grain contaminated with methyl mercury.
Phenytoin	Intrauterine growth restriction, mental retardation, microcephaly, dysmorphic craniofacial features, cardiac defects, hypoplastic nails and distal phalanges	The full syndrome is seen in less than 10% of children exposed in utero, but up to 30% have some manifestations. Mild to moderate mental retardation is found in some children who have severe physical stigmata. The effect may depend on whether the fetus inherits a mutant gene that decreases production of epoxide hydrolase, an enzyme necessary to decrease the teratogen phenytoin epoxide.
Streptomycin and kanamycin	Hearing loss, eighth-nerve damage	No ototoxicity in the fetus has been reported from use of gentamicin or vancomycin.
Tetracycline	Hypoplasia of tooth enamel, incorporation of tetracycline into bone and teeth, permanent yellow–brown discoloration of deciduous teeth	Drug has no known effect unless exposure occurs in second or third trimester.
Thalidomide	Bilateral limb deficiencies, anotia and microtia, cardiac and gastrointestinal anomalies	Of children whose mothers used thalidomide between 35 and 50 days of gestation, 20% show the effect.
Trimethadione and paramethadione	Cleft lip or cleft palate; cardiac defects; growth deficiency; microcephaly; mental retardation; characteristic facial appearance; ophthalmologic, limb, and genitourinary tract abnormalities	Risk for defects or spontaneous abortion is 60–80% with first-trimester exposure. A syndrome including V-shaped eyebrows, low-set ears, high arched palate, and irregular dentition has been identified. These drugs are no longer used during pregnancy due to the availability of more effective, less toxic agents.
Valproic acid	Neural tube defects, especially spina bifida; minor facial defects	Exposure must occur prior to normal closure of neural tube during first trimester to produce open defect (incidence of approximately 1%).
Vitamin A and its derivatives (eg, isotretinoin, etretinate, and retinoids)	Increased abortion rate, microtia, central nervous system defects, thymic agenesis, cardiovascular effects, craniofacial dysmorphism, microphthalmia, cleft lip and palate, mental retardation	Isotretinoin exposure before pregnancy is not a risk because the drug is not stored in tissue. Etretinate has a long half-life and effects occur long after drug is discontinued. Topical application does not have a known risk.
Infections		
Cytomegalovirus	Hydrocephaly, microcephaly, chorioretinitis, cerebral calcifications, symmetric intrauterine growth restriction, microphthalmos, brain damage, mental retardation, hearing loss	Most common congenital infection. Congenital infection rate is 40% after primary infection and 14% after recurrent infection. Of infected infants, physical effects as listed are present in 20% after primary infection and 8% after secondary infection. No effective therapy exists.
Rubella	Microcephaly, mental retardation, cataracts, deafness, congenital heart disease; all organs may be affected	Malformation rate is 50% if the mother is infected during first trimester. Rate of severe permanent organ damage decreases to 6% by midpregnancy. Immunization of children and nonpregnant adults is necessary for prevention. Immunization is not recommended during pregnancy, but the live attenuated vaccine virus has not been shown to cause the malformations of congenital rubella syndrome.
Syphilis	If severe infection, fetal demise with hydrops; if mild, detectable abnormalities of skin, teeth, and bones	Penicillin treatment is effective for Treponema pallidum eradication to prevent progression of damage. Severity of fetal damage depends on duration of fetal infection; damage is worse if infection is greater than 20 weeks. Prevalence is increasing; need to rule out other sexually transmitted diseases.

(Continued)

Table 1. Teratogenic Agents (continued)

Agent	Effects	Comments
Infections (continued)		
Toxoplasmosis	Possible effects on all systems but particularly central nervous system: microcephaly, hydrocephaly, cerebral calcifications. Chorioretinitis is most common. Severity of manifestations depends on duration of disease.	Low prevalence during pregnancy (0.1–0.5%); initial maternal infection must occur during pregnancy to place fetus at risk. Toxoplasma gondii is transmitted to humans by raw meat or exposure to infected cat feces. In the first trimester, the incidence of fetal infection is as low as 9% and increases to approximately 59% in the third trimester. The severity of congenital infection is greater in the first trimester than at the end of gestation. Treat with pyrimethamine, sulfadiazine, or spiramycin.
Varicella	Possible effects on all organs, including skin scarring, chorioretinitis, cataracts, microcephaly, hypoplasia of the hands and feet, and muscle atrophy	Risk of congenital varicella is low, approximately 2–3% and occurs between 7 and 21 weeks of gestation. Varicella–zoster immune globulin is available regionally for newborns exposed in utero during last 4–7 days of gestation. No effect from herpes zoster.
Radiation	Microcephaly, mental retardation	Medical diagnostic radiation delivering less than 0.05 Gy* to the fetus has no teratogenic risk. Estimated fetal exposure of common radiologic procedures is 0.01 Gy or less (eg, intravenous pyelography, 0.0041 Gy).

*1 gray = 100 rad.

The references in this bulletin are graded according to the method outlined by the U.S. Preventive Services Task Force:

- I Evidence obtained from at least one properly designed randomized controlled trial
- II-1 Evidence obtained from well-designed controlled trials without randomization
- II-2 Evidence obtained from well-designed cohort or case–control analytic studies, preferably from more than one center or research group
- II-3 Evidence obtained from multiple time series, with or without intervention, or dramatic results in uncontrolled experiments
- III Opinions of respected authorities, based on clinical experience, descriptive studies, or reports of expert committees

Other publications from ACOG:

- **Committee Opinions**, focused updates on emerging areas
- **Practice Patterns**, evidence-based guidelines
- **Criteria Sets**, baseline guidelines for review of diagnostic and management procedures

ISSN 1074-8628

The American College of Obstetricians and Gynecologists
409 12th Street, SW
PO Box 96920
Washington, DC 20090-6920

12345/10987

Number 181—June 1993

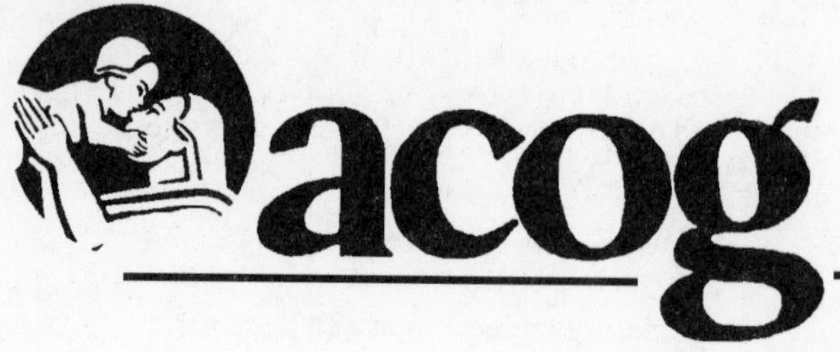

Technical Bulletin

An Educational Aid to Obstetrician–Gynecologists

Thyroid Disease in Pregnancy

Thyroid disease often occurs in women of reproductive age. Changes induced by pregnancy may stimulate either remission or exacerbation of certain thyroid disorders. In addition, certain obstetric abnormalities, such as gestational trophoblastic disease and hyperemesis gravidarum, may result in clinically significant changes in thyroid function. This bulletin will address the effects of thyroid disorders and their treatment during pregnancy and the postpartum period.

Physiology

Pregnancy has a significant impact on maternal thyroid physiology. Changes in the structure and function of the thyroid gland during pregnancy can mimic some of the effects of hyperthyroidism; consequently, proper evaluation of thyroid disorders and accurate interpretation of thyroid function tests require an understanding of these changes. The results of commonly used thyroid function tests may be altered in normal pregnant women and in women with hyperthyroidism (Table 1). Glandular hyperplasia and increased vascularity result in moderate thyroid enlargement but not thyromegaly. Any goiter or nodule recognized during pregnancy should be considered pathologic.

TABLE 1. EFFECTS OF PREGNANCY AND HYPERTHYROIDISM ON TESTS COMMONLY USED TO EVALUATE THYROID FUNCTION

Test	Normal Pregnancy	Hyperthyroidism
TSH	No change	Decreased*
TBG	Increased	No change
Total T_4	Increased	Increased
Free T_4	No change	Increased
Total T_3	Increased	Increased
Free T_3	No change	Increased
Thyroid radioiodine uptake	Increased	Increased
T_3RU	Decreased	Increased

*In rare cases of hyperthyroidism, TSH may be increased.

Most of the pregnancy-induced changes in thyroid physiology are stimulated by hyperestrogenemia. High estrogen levels cause production of altered thyroxine-binding globulin (TBG) (1), resulting in an increase in TBG and, as a direct consequence, a decrease in triiodothyronine resin uptake (T_3RU) and increases in the levels of thyroxine (T_4) and triiodothyronine (T_3) in the serum. The reported value of the T_3RU is inversely proportional to the amount of TBG. Therefore, values of T_3RU decrease in pregnancy as TBG levels increase. Total serum levels of T_4 begin to rise during the first trimester and ultimately increase to 9–16 μg/dl, compared with 5–12 μg/dl in nonpregnant, euthyroid women. In early pregnancy, when chorionic gonadotropin levels reach their peak, levels of free T_4 in serum also increase and those of thyroid-stimulating hormone (TSH) decrease (2). For most of the pregnancy, however, serum levels of free T_4, free T_3, and TSH are within the normal, nonpregnant range and overt hyperthyroidism does not occur.

It is not generally practical for the clinician to measure either TBG or T_4 in its metabolically active free state. Consequently, T_3RU is measured to provide an indirect assessment of TBG and to allow the calculation of the free T_4 index. The free T_4 index and similar values are not measured directly but are derived from various calculations using T_4 and T_3RU. They may be useful in compensating for the changes of pregnancy.

Hyperthyroidism

Thyrotoxicosis is seen in 1/2,000 pregnant women. It is most often caused by Graves disease, an organ-specific autoimmune process associated with thyroid-stimulating antibody (TSAb) activity. These autoantibodies mimic TSH in its ability to stimulate thyroid function and appear to be the pathogenic agents responsible for both thyroid hyperfunction and gland growth in Graves disease (3). However, there is no direct correlation between levels of antibody activity and clinical or laboratory indications of disease severity.

Although thyrotoxicosis in Graves disease generally results from stimulation of TSH receptors by TSAb (stimulation-induced thyrotoxicosis), clinical hyperthyroidism may also result from glandular disruption and release of stored thyroid hormone (destruction-induced thyrotoxicosis). In the latter group of women, antimicrosomal antibody titers may be elevated. Assessment of TSAb and antimicrosomal antibody titers may assist in the differentiation of these two groups; differentiation is potentially important for therapy.

Pregnancy may affect the natural history of Graves disease. Most women between the ages of 20 and 40 who have new-onset Graves disease have delivered within 12 months of initial diagnosis (4). In addition, women with inactive Graves disease may experience transient increases in free T_4 at 10–15 weeks of gestation without associated changes in TSAb activity (5, 6). This suggests a response of an abnormal thyroid gland to stimulation by placental human chorionic gonadotropin or chorionic thyrotropin during pregnancy (2). Postpartum exacerbation of thyrotoxicosis is seen in 78% of such women (5).

The outcome of pregnancy in women with thyrotoxicosis largely depends upon whether metabolic control is achieved. Women who remain hyperthyroid despite therapy and those whose disease remains untreated are at increased risk of preeclampsia, congestive heart failure, and adverse perinatal outcome (7). The adverse outcomes include an increased rate of preterm labor, preterm delivery, and stillbirths, with a resultant increase in the overall perinatal mortality.

Diagnosis

Mild thyrotoxicosis may be difficult to diagnose during pregnancy. Helpful diagnostic signs include resting tachycardia (>100 beats per minute), thyromegaly, exophthalmos, onycholysis, and failure of a nonobese woman to gain weight despite normal or increased food intake. Thyrotoxicosis usually results in markedly elevated serum T_4 levels even above the increase normally expected in pregnancy. In addition, the decrease in T_3RU characteristic of normal pregnancy does not occur; consequently, the free T_4 index is increased. Because of the potential for damage to the fetal thyroid gland, radioiodine uptake studies should not be performed during pregnancy.

Management

Thyrotoxicosis

Thyrotoxicosis during pregnancy usually can be controlled medically and generally does not pose a serious threat to the mother. Treatment may require medication directed at blocking either thyroid hormone production (eg, thiourea compounds) or the peripheral manifestations of thyroid hormone, such as tachycardia (eg, beta blockers). Since propylthiouracil (PTU) and methimazole both cross the placenta, medical treatment has the potential for causing fetal complications, including hypothyroidism and goiter. Accordingly, one of the first tenets of treatment is to use the least amount of medication required to achieve clinical euthyroidism. It has been reported by some investigators that newborns exposed in utero to methimazole are at increased risk for an unusual scalp defect called aplasia cutis (8); at present, however, there is no convincing evidence that either methimazole or PTU is teratogenic (9, 10). Fetal and neonatal thyroid dysfunction may also result from maternal thyroid-stimulating and blocking antibodies, which may cross the placenta and bind to the fetal thyroid gland, thus affecting its function.

Propylthiouracil is generally considered the drug of choice for treating thyrotoxicosis during pregnancy; its use has resulted in satisfactory pregnancy outcomes for women who become euthyroid on treatment (7). The dose of PTU is based on experience (11); depending on symptoms, the starting dose is 300–450 mg daily. If necessary, this dose is increased until the woman appears minimally thyrotoxic on clinical assessment and her total serum T_4 level is reduced to the upper normal range for pregnancy. Response to a given dose may take up to 3–4 weeks to be reflected in the laboratory values. Further adjustments should be based on clinical response and laboratory values.

Beta blocking agents may be of great utility in diminishing the symptoms of hyperthyroidism. The onset of action of the beta blockers, which act peripherally to blunt the effects of the thyroid hormone, is much faster than that of the thiourea compounds, whose mechanism of action is dependent upon blocking the synthesis of new thyroid hormones. The greatest experience is with propranolol, but other beta blockers should be equally effective. The dosage is titrated to effect, with a goal of reducing the resting maternal heart rate to less than 100 beats per minute. Depending upon the severity of symptoms, the beta blockers may be administered intravenously or orally. When signs or symptoms of pulmonary edema occur, it is important to evaluate the patient's myocardial function and determine the mechanism of the pulmonary edema prior to treatment with beta blockers. Depression of ventricular function is a known side effect of beta blockers.

Thyroidectomy may be carried out after thyrotoxicosis has been controlled medically. For women who cannot adhere to outpatient medical treatment or for those in whom medical treatment is ineffective, subtotal thyroidectomy may be the treatment of choice regardless of trimester after appropriate pharmacologic control is achieved.

Thyroid Storm

Thyroid storm is rarely encountered during pregnancy or the puerperium, even in untreated women (7). Much more common is heart failure, apparently caused by the long-term myocardial effects of T_4 and intensified by other pregnancy complications that include severe preeclampsia, infection, anemia, or combinations of these (12). If thyroid storm or heart failure is suspected, treatment consists of 1 g each of PTU and potassium iodide given orally or, if the woman is unable to swallow, through a nasogastric tube. Beta blockers may be given intravenously to blunt peripheral manifestations such as tachycardia, but these agents should be used with caution in the presence of heart failure. Other important tenets of treatment are adequate rehydration and thermoregulation. A thorough search for underlying infection should also be initiated. Aggressive treatment of hypertension, infection, and anemia is crucial to successfully reversing heart failure by reducing cardiac workload.

Hyperthyroidism Secondary to Gestational Trophoblastic Disease

Although serum T_4 levels in women with molar pregnancy usually are remarkably elevated, clinically apparent hyperthyroidism is identified in only 2% of cases (13). Serum T_4 elevation may be the effect primarily of estrogen, as in normal pregnancy, in which case free T_4 levels are not elevated and the T_3RU is decreased. It is possible that free T_4 is elevated as the direct consequence of the TSH-like effect of chorionic gonadotropin or a variant of this hormone, although this theory is controversial (13, 14).

Effects of Therapy on the Fetus and Infant

Estimates of the adverse fetal effects of thiourea drugs vary. In one study in which 52 women were treated, evidence for hypothyroidism was observed in only one infant (7). In another series, cord serum T_4 levels were lower in neonates born to thyrotoxic mothers taking PTU until delivery than in infants born to mothers who discontinued the drug earlier. However, no dose–response relationship was found, and none of the infants was hypothyroid (10). Generally, morbidity and mortality predominate in infants born to women who remain thyrotoxic despite therapy, or who do not receive adequate prenatal care and treatment. In one long-term study, intellectual and physical development and thyroid function were evaluated in children born to thyrotoxic mothers treated with PTU during pregnancy. No adverse effects on subsequent growth and development were identified (15).

Prolonged maternal administration of iodide significantly increases the likelihood of hypothyroidism and obvious goiter in the infant. Iodide readily crosses the placenta by 10–12 weeks of gestation and is avidly taken up by the fetal thyroid for the duration of pregnancy. Accordingly, iodide therapy has no role in the routine management of these women and should be given only preceding the time of thyroidectomy or acutely for severe disease such as heart failure or impending thyroid storm.

Breast-feeding has been considered by some investigators to be contraindicated when the mother is taking antithyroid drugs. Concentrations of these drugs in breast milk are low, however, and the amount of drug ingested by the infant is quite small. The American Academy of Pediatrics has therefore stated that neither PTU nor methimazole use is a contraindication to breast-feeding (16).

Even after successful treatment with surgery or radiation, euthyroid women with Graves disease may give birth to infants who manifest thyrotoxicosis, including goiter and exophthalmos. In this situation, neonatal thyrotoxicosis probably results from transplacental passage of maternal TSAbs (17). This condition is suggested by a maternal history of thyrotoxicosis, identification of appreciable TSAb activity in maternal serum, a history of a previously affected infant, or persistent fetal tachycardia. Fetal thyrotoxicosis secondary to transplacental passage of maternal TSAbs has been reported recently as a cause of fetal demise (18, 19).

Neonatal thyrotoxicosis occurs in about 1% of in-fants of mothers with Graves disease. These newborns may require antithyroid treatment for several weeks until the TSAbs are metabolized. The infant who has been exposed in utero to these antibodies and whose mother was treated until the time of delivery with PTU may be euthyroid at birth only to become hyperthyroid a few days later as the drug is cleared while the thyrotoxic effect of the immunoglobulins persists.

Hypothyroidism

Hypothyroidism is diagnosed if the rise in the level of circulating T_4 expected during pregnancy fails to take place and the level of TSH is elevated. Hypothyroidism includes women with either clinical symptoms or abnormally low (for pregnancy) serum T_4 levels or both. Overt hypothyroidism complicating pregnancy is uncommon, probably because it is often associated with infertility. Women with uncorrected hypothyroidism who do become pregnant have an inordinate number of low-birth-weight and stillborn infants. In addition, one study showed that uncorrected hypothyroidism results in a high incidence of preeclampsia and placental abruption (20). Heart failure is also encountered with increased frequency. Adequate replacement therapy is important in these women.

Some believe that hypothyroid women receiving maintenance levels of thyroid hormone before pregnancy rarely require an increased dose during pregnancy. Studies suggest, however, that pregnancy is associated with an increase in T_4 requirement (21, 22). One study evaluated hypothyroid women who, before pregnancy, had normal TSH and free T_4 index levels on a mean daily dose of 0.1 mg of T_4 (22). During pregnancy, serum TSH levels increased and free T_4 index levels decreased; as a result, the mean daily dose of T_4 was increased to 0.15 mg. These women were not thought to be clinically hypothyroid at any point in the study.

Subclinical hypothyroidism, which is characterized by a lack of symptoms in conjunction with elevated serum TSH levels and normal serum T_4 and T_3 levels, is more common than overt disease. The effects of subclinical hypothyroidism on pregnancy outcome are not clearly defined, and generally, the need for T_4 replacement will hinge on the patient's clinical history. A high incidence of subclinical hypothyroidism has been reported in pregnant women with type I diabetes and normal T_4 levels prior to conception (23).

Effects on the Fetus and Infant

In general, infants of hypothyroid mothers appear healthy and without evidence of thyroid dysfunction (24). In some situations, however, the infant of a hypothyroid mother may be similarly affected. For example, if maternal hypothyroidism was caused by use of iodine 131 during pregnancy, the fetal thyroid gland may also have been damaged or destroyed. Any infant whose mother was so treated during pregnancy should be evaluated carefully after delivery. If neonatal hypothyroidism is found, thyroid replacement therapy should be instituted promptly. Environmental factors, such as dietary iodine deficiency or excess, may also be important. Appropriate iodine supplements given prenatally to iodinedeficient women elevate T_4 and decrease TSH levels in both the mother and the neonate (25).

Because congenital hypothyroidism is difficult to diagnose clinically and early and aggressive T_4 replacement therapy is critical in these infants, biochemical screening of all newborns is recommended (26). Mass screening of newborns can detect congenital hypothyroidism, which occurs in 1/4,000–7,000 infants. Based on the results of 5- to 7-year follow-up, it appears that most, if not all, sequelae of congenital hypothyroidism, including intellectual impairment, can be prevented with prompt and adequate treatment (27).

Nodular Thyroid Disease

In nonpregnant patients, evaluation of a thyroid nodule commonly includes radioiodine scanning to demonstrate hyper- or hypofunction. Radioactive iodine should be avoided in pregnancy, although the likelihood of associated fetal injury seems remote, especially with first-trimester exposure. Ultrasound examination reliably detects nodules larger than 0.5 cm and can disclose whether they are solid or cystic. Although cystic lesions are associated with a lower incidence of malignancy than solid masses, definitive diagnosis requires fine-needle aspiration or tissue biopsy (28, 29). Aspiration has been reported to have a false-positive rate of 0–2% and a false-negative rate of 1–3% for distinguishing malignant from benign disease. Although most thyroid carcinomas are well differentiated and have an indolent course, surgical therapy should not be delayed simply on the basis of an ongoing pregnancy.

Postpartum Thyroid Dysfunction

Clinical or biochemical evidence of thyroid dysfunction, either hyperthyroidism or hypothyroidism, can be found in 5–10% of postpartum women (30–33). Because postpartum thyroid dysfunction usually develops 1–8 months postpartum and the symptoms are vague and nonspecific, it is diagnosed infrequently (34). Affected women may manifest symptoms such as fatigue, palpitations, depression, and memory and concentration impairment well after the routine postpartum visit. Patients and physicians should be aware of these symptoms and their need for evaluation.

Postpartum thyroid dysfunction, characterized histologically as a destructive, lymphocytic thyroiditis, is an autoimmune disorder in which thyroid microsomal autoantibodies play a central role (35, 36). Women who test positive for microsomal autoantibodies early in pregnancy or shortly after delivery are at risk for developing postpartum thyroid dysfunction (31, 32, 37). Women at the highest risk for postpartum thyroid dysfunction include those who have a history of this disorder and those who have a personal or family history of other thyroid or autoimmune disease.

Thyrotoxic Phase

Between 1 and 4 months postpartum, approximately 4% of women develop transient thyrotoxicosis (38). The onset is abrupt, and often a small, painless goiter is found on physical examination. Although there may be many symptoms, only fatigue and palpitations are more frequent in affected women than in normal postpartum women. Neither leukocytosis nor elevated erythrocyte sedimentation rate is usually present.

Thyrotoxicosis results from an excessive release of stored hormone secondary to glandular disruption (destruction-induced thyrotoxicosis), rather than from excessive hormone production. In contrast to Graves disease (stimulation-induced thyrotoxicosis), thyroid uptake of either radioiodine or technetium is low and TSAbs are not detectable. In this condition, PTU is ineffective and may even hasten development of a subsequent hypothyroid phase. Treatment usually is not given, but if peripheral manifestations of excessive thyroid hormone are severe, a beta blocker may be useful. Approximately two thirds of women who develop transient thyrotoxicosis return directly to a euthyroid state; the other third subsequently experience hypothyroidism.

Hypothyroid Phase

Between 4 and 8 months postpartum, 2–5% of women develop hypothyroidism (33). At least a third of these women will have experienced the thyrotoxic phase of postpartum thyroid dysfunction previously. Hypothyroidism can develop rapidly. Goiter, depression, and memory and concentration impairment are common and are more prominent in the hypothyroid phase than during the thyrotoxic phase. Clinical evaluation and thyroid function tests are valuable in making or confirming the diagnosis. T_4 replacement is initiated if hypothyroidism develops and the severity of symptoms warrant. Most patients can be given T_4 replacement therapy for 12–18 months after delivery; thereafter, it can be withdrawn gradually (33).

Approximately 10–30% of women with postpartum thyroid dysfunction will develop permanent hypothyroidism. Long-term follow-up is important in these women.

Summary

To accurately evaluate thyroid disorders in pregnancy, the physician must understand the physiologic changes that occur both in thyroid gland size and in thyroid function tests.

The effect of thyrotoxicosis on pregnancy outcome largely depends on whether metabolic control is achieved. Women who become euthyroid on treatment usually can expect satisfactory outcomes. Propylthiouracil is considered to be the drug of choice for treating thyrotoxicosis during pregnancy. Because of the significant risk of hypothyroidism and obvious goiter in the infant, the use of iodide should be reserved for severe disease, such as thyroid storm or heart failure. Thyrotoxic infants may need antithyroid treatment until TSAbs are metabolized.

Since overt hypothyroidism is often associated with infertility, it is uncommon in pregnancy. Hypothyroid women who do become pregnant, however, have an increased risk of low-birth-weight or stillborn infants. These women may require a greater dosage of thyroid hormone during pregnancy. The effects of subclinical hypothyroidism are not well defined. Accordingly, the need for treatment hinges on the woman's clinical history. Infants of hypothyroid mothers usually show no evidence of thyroid dysfunction, but those who are hypothyroid should receive prompt thyroid replacement therapy. To minimize the sequelae of congenital hypothyroidism, mass screening of infants and prompt treatment of those affected is recommended.

During pregnancy, thyroid nodules should be evaluated by ultrasound and fine-needle aspiration or tissue biopsy. Radioiodine scanning should be avoided during pregnancy. If thyroid cancer is diagnosed, pregnancy should not delay treatment.

Because postpartum thyroid dysfunction is fairly common yet difficult to detect, physicians and patients should be aware of the symptoms and risk factors. When a thyrotoxic phase develops, treatment is not usually required. If peripheral manifestations are severe, however, beta blockers may be helpful. Women who experience the hypothyroid phase later in the postpartum period face risks of goiter, impaired memory, depression, and lethargy. A significant proportion of these hypothyroid women will go on to develop permanent hypothyroidism and will require long-term follow-up.

REFERENCES

1. Ain KB, Mori Y, Refetoff S. Reduced clearance rate of thyroxine-binding globulin (TBG) with increased sialylation: a mechanism for estrogen-induced elevation of serum TBG concentration. J Clin Endocrinol Metab 1987;65:689–696
2. Kimura M, Amino N, Tamaki H, Mitsuda N, Miyai K, Tanizawa O. Physiologic thyroid activation in normal early pregnancy is induced by circulating hCG. Obstet Gynecol 1990;75:775–778
3. Mariotti S, Chiovato L, Vitti P, Marcocci C, Fenzi GF, Del Prete GF, et al. Recent advances in the understanding of humoral and cellular mechanisms implicated in thyroid autoimmune disorders. Clin Immunol Immunopathol 1989;50:S73–S84
4. Jansson R, Dahlberg PA, Winsa B, Meirik O, Säfwenberg J, Karlsson A. The postpartum period constitutes an important risk for the development of clinical Graves' disease in young women. Acta Endocrinol (Copenh) 1987;116: 321–325
5. Amino N, Tanizawa O, Mori H, Iwatani Y, Yamada T, Kurachi K, et al. Aggravation of thyrotoxicosis in early pregnancy and after delivery in Graves' disease. J Clin Endocrinol Metab 1982;55:108–112
6. Tamaki H, Amino N, Aozasa M, Mori M, Tanizawa O, Miyai K. Serial changes in thyroid-stimulating antibody and thyrotropin binding inhibitor immunoglobulin at the time of postpartum occurrence of thyrotoxicosis in Graves' disease. J Clin Endocrinol Metab 1987;65:324–330
7. Davis LE, Lucas MJ, Hankins GDV, Roark ML, Cunningham FG. Thyrotoxicosis complicating pregnancy. Am J Obstet Gynecol 1989;160:63–70
8. Milham S Jr. Scalp defects in infants of mothers treated for hyperthyroidism with methimazole or carbimazole during pregnancy. Teratology 1985;32:321
9. Van Dijke CP, Heydendael RJ, De Kleine MJ. Methimazole, carbimazole, and congenital skin defects. Ann Intern Med 1987;106:60–61

10. Momotani N, Noh J, Oyanagi H, Ishikawa N, Ito K. Antithyroid drug therapy for Graves' disease during pregnancy. Optimal regimen for fetal thyroid status. N Engl J Med 1986;315:24–28

11. Burrow GN. The management of thyrotoxicosis in pregnancy. N Engl J Med 1985;313:562–565

12. Hankins GDV, Lowe TW, Cunningham FG. Dilated cardiomyopathy and thyrotoxicosis complicated by septic abortion. Am J Obstet Gynecol 1984;149:85–86

13. Amir SM, Osathanondh R, Berkowitz RS, Goldstein DP. Human chorionic gonadotropin and thyroid function in patients with hydatidiform mole. Am J Obstet Gynecol 1984;150:723–728

14. Mann K, Schneider N, Hoermann R. Thyrotropic activity of acidic isoelectric variants of human chorionic gonadotropin from trophoblastic tumors. Endocrinology 1986;118: 1558–1566

15. Burrow GN, Klatskin EH, Genel M. Intellectual development in children whose mothers received propylthiouracil during pregnancy. Yale J Biol Med 1978;51:151–156

16. American Academy of Pediatrics. Committee on Drugs. Transfer of drugs and other chemicals into human milk. Pediatrics 1989;84:924–936

17. Matsuura N, Konishi J, Fujieda K, Kasagi K, Iida Y, Hagisawa M, et al. TSH-receptor antibodies in mothers with Graves' disease and outcome in their offspring. Lancet 1988;1:14–17

18. Houck JA, Davis RE, Sharma HM. Thyroid-stimulating immunoglobulin as a cause of recurrent intrauterine fetal death. Obstet Gynecol 1988;71:1018–1019

19. Page DV, Brady K, Mitchell J, Pehrson J, Wade G. The pathology of intrauterine thyrotoxicosis: two case reports. Obstet Gynecol 1988;72:479–481

20. Davis LE, Leveno KJ, Cunningham FG. Hypothyroidism complicating pregnancy. Obstet Gynecol 1988;72:108–112

21. Tamaki H, Amino N, Takeoka K, Mitsuda N, Miyai K, Tanizawa O. Thyroxine requirement during pregnancy for replacement therapy of hypothyroidism. Obstet Gynecol 1990;76:230–233

22. Mandel SJ, Larsen PR, Seely EW, Brent GA. Increased need for thyroxine during pregnancy in women with primary hypothryoidism. N Engl J Med 1990;323:91–96

23. Jovanovic-Peterson L, Peterson CM. De novo clinical hypothyroidism in pregnancies complicated by type I diabetes, subclinical hypothyroidism, and proteinuria: a new syndrome. Am J Obstet Gynecol 1988;159:442–446

24. Montoro M, Collea JV, Frasier SD, Mestman JH. Successful outcome of pregnancy in women with hypothyroidism. Ann Intern Med 1981;94:31–34

25. Thilly CH, Delange F, Lagasse R, Bourdoux P, Ramioul L, Berquist H, et al. Fetal hypothyroidism and maternal thyroid status in severe endemic goiter. J Clin Endocrinol Metab 1978;47:354–360

26. American Academy of Pediatrics, American Thyroid Association. Newborn screening for congenital hypothyroidism: recommended guidelines. Pediatrics 1987;80:745–749

27. Fisher DA, Foley BL. Early treatment of congenital hypothyroidism. Pediatrics 1989;83:785–789

28. Ashcraft MW, Van Herle AJ. Management of thyroid nodules. II: scanning techniques, thyroid suppressive therapy, and fine-needle aspiration. Head Neck Surg 1981;3: 297–322

29. Rosen IB, Walfish PG. Pregnancy as a predisposing factor in thyroid neoplasia. Arch Surg 1986;121:1287–1290

30. Amino N, Mori H, Iwatani Y, Tanizawa O, Kawashima M, Tsuge I, et al. High prevalence of transient postpartum thyrotoxicosis and hypothyroidism. N Engl J Med 1982;306:849–852

31. Fung HYM, Kologlu M, Collison K, John R, Richards CJ, Hall R, et al. Postpartum thyroid dysfunction in Mid Glamorgan. BMJ 1988;296:241–244

32. Hayslip CC, Fein HG, O'Donnell VM, Friedman DS, Klein TA, Smallridge RC. The value of serum antimicrosomal antibody testing in screening for symptomatic postpartum thyroid dysfunction. Am J Obstet Gynecol 1988;159:203–209

33. Jansson R, Dahlberg PA, Karlsson FA. Postpartum thyroiditis. Bailliere's Clin Endocrinol Metab 1988; 2:619–635

34. Ramsay I. Postpartum thyroiditis—an underdiagnosed disease. Br J Obstet Gynaecol 1986;93:1121–1123

35. Iwatani Y, Amino N, Tamaki H, Aozasa M, Kabutomori O, Mori M, et al. Increase in peripheral large granular lymphocytes in postpartum autoimmune thyroiditis. Endocrinol Jpn 1988;35:447–453

36. Vargas MT, Briones-Urbina R, Gladman D, Papsin FR, Walfish PG. Antithyroid microsomal autoantibodies and HLA-DR5 are associated with postpartum thyroid dysfunction: evidence supporting an autoimmune pathogenesis. J Clin Endocrinol Metab 1988;67:327–333

37. Jansson R, Bernander S, Karlsson A, Levin K, Nilsson G. Autoimmune thyroid dysfunction in the postpartum period. J Clin Endocrinol Metab 1984;58:681–687

38. Walfish PG, Chan JYC. Postpartum hyperthyroidism. Clin Endocrinol Metab 1985;14:417–447

This Technical Bulletin was developed under the direction of the Committee on Technical Bulletins of the American College of Obstetricians and Gynecologists as an educational aid to obstetricians and gynecologists. The committee wishes to thank Thomas W. Lowe, MD, for his assistance in the development of this bulletin. This Technical Bulletin does not define a standard of care, nor is it intended to dictate an exclusive course of management. It presents recognized methods and techniques of clinical practice for consideration by obstetrician–gynecologists for incorporation into their practices. Variations of practice taking into account the needs of the individual patient, resources, and limitations unique to the institution or type of practice may be appropriate.

THE AMERICAN COLLEGE OF OBSTETRICIANS AND GYNECOLOGISTS
409 12th Street, SW
Washington, DC 20024-2188

12345/76543

Number 187—December 1993
(Replaces #116, May 1988)

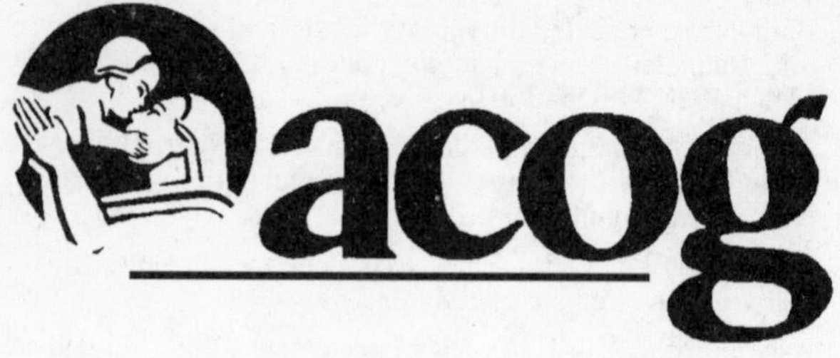

Technical Bulletin
An Educational Aid to Obstetrician–Gynecologists

Ultrasonography in Pregnancy

Diagnostic ultrasonography is widely used in the assessment of pregnancy and the fetus. Although clinical benefits of routine ultrasonography during pregnancy have not been established, approximately 70% of pregnancies in the United States undergo ultrasound evaluation (1).

Instrumentation

Ultrasound is defined as high-frequency sound waves, exceeding 20,000 cycles per second. Frequency refers to the number of peaks or waves that traverse a given point per unit of time and is expressed as hertz (Hz). Instruments used in diagnostic ultrasonography operate at frequencies of 2 million–10 million Hz or 2–10 megahertz (MHz). The higher the frequency of the sound, the shallower the depth of penetration, but the better the resolution of the image produced. Most abdominal ultrasound transducers operate at 3.5–5 MHz, while most vaginal transducers operate at 5–7.5 MHz.

Technologic advances in instrumentation have led to significant improvements in image production and resolution. Dynamic, or real-time, ultrasonography creates new images faster than the flicker fusion rate of the eye so that the fetus, or target, appears to be moving in real time. Linear array real-time transducers use a longitudinal series of transducer crystals arranged in sequence to operate serially quite rapidly. Annular array scanners operate similarly but with the serial transducers arranged in concentric rings. Sector real-time ultrasonography uses a single transducer which moves through a prescribed arc. Curvilinear transducers have been introduced recently to incorporate principles of both linear array and sector transducers.

Real-time ultrasonography readily detects fetal body motion, cardiac activity, and breathing movements. This dynamic two-dimensional imaging allows evaluation of both structural and functional characteristics of the fetus.

Safety

Ultrasound energy delivered to a target, such as the fetus, varies with the ultrasound frequency, intensity (power), duration of exposure, and distance from the transducer. A safe level of ultrasound exposure to tissue has been defined arbitrarily as less than 100 mW/cm^2 (2). Most instruments used in diagnostic ultrasonography produce energies no greater than 10–20 mW/cm^2 at the transducer face.

Ultrasound exposure at intensities usually produced by diagnostic ultrasound instruments has not been found to cause any harmful biologic effects on instrument operators, pregnant women, fetuses, or other patients. Infants exposed in utero have shown no significant differences in birth weight or length, childhood growth, cognitive function, acoustic or visual ability, or rates of neurologic deficits (3, 4).

Newer applications of ultrasound technology require higher output potentials. Although no adverse fetal effects have been identified to date, increases in the power outputs of ultrasound instruments may increase the potential risks to the fetus. Because of these concerns, many manufacturers include instrumentation on the machines which will continuously display the power output as thermal and mechanical indices. Two principles have been established as guidelines for the ultrasound practitioner. First, the "prudent use" of the equipment is the responsibility of the operator. Second, the operator is responsible for completing the examination using scan modes and power outputs which result in energy exposures which are "as low as reasonably achievable" (5).

Ultrasound Examinations

Indications for ultrasonography during pregnancy are multiple and diverse (see the box). The type of examination may vary according to the information sought.

Indications for Ultrasonography During Pregnancy

Estimation of gestational age for patients with uncertain clinical dates, or verification of dates for patients who are to undergo scheduled elective repeat cesarean delivery, indicated induction of labor, or other elective termination of pregnancy
Evaluation of fetal growth
Vaginal bleeding of undetermined etiology in pregnancy
Determination of fetal presentation
Suspected multiple gestation
Adjunct to amniocentesis
Significant uterine size/clinical dates discrepancy
Pelvic mass
Suspected hydatidiform mole
Adjunct to cervical cerclage placement
Suspected ectopic pregnancy
Adjunct to special procedures
Suspected fetal death
Suspected uterine abnormality
Intrauterine contraceptive device localization
Biophysical evaluation for fetal well-being
Observation of intrapartum events
Suspected polyhydramnios or oligohydramnios
Suspected abruptio placentae
Adjunct to external version from breech to vertex presentation
Estimation of fetal weight and/or presentation in premature rupture of membranes and/or premature labor
Abnormal serum alpha-fetoprotein value
Follow-up observation of identified fetal anomaly
Follow-up evaluation of placental location for identified "placenta previa"
History of previous congenital anomaly
Serial evaluation of fetal growth in multiple gestation
Evaluation of fetal condition in late registrants for prenatal care

(Adapted from U.S. Department of Health and Human Services. Diagnostic ultrasound in pregnancy. National Institutes of Health publication no. 84-667. Bethesda, Maryland: National Institutes of Health, 1984)

When indicated, a *basic* ultrasound examination suffices for most obstetric patients. When technically feasible and within the limits of the gestational age at which it is performed, a basic examination should provide the following information:

- Fetal number
- Fetal presentation
- Documentation of fetal life
- Placental location
- Assessment of amniotic fluid volume
- Assessment of gestational age
- Survey of fetal anatomy for gross malformations
- Evaluation for maternal pelvic masses

A basic ultrasound examination is primarily a metric examination. Nonetheless, a brief survey of fetal anatomy and maternal pelvic organs should be performed. Some major structural malformations of the fetus may be identified during basic examinations, and some basic examinations may suggest the need for a more comprehensive survey.

In certain circumstances, a *limited* ultrasound examination may be appropriate and desirable. Such circumstances commonly relate to the specific nature of the information required or the urgent nature of the clinical situation. A limited examination may be useful to collect information such as the following:

- Assessment of amniotic fluid volume
- Fetal biophysical profile testing
- Ultrasonography-guided amniocentesis
- External cephalic version
- Confirmation of fetal life or death
- Localization of placenta in antepartum hemorrhage
- Confirmation of fetal presentation

A *comprehensive* ultrasound examination may be indicated for a patient who is suspected of carrying a physiologically or anatomically defective fetus by history, clinical evaluation, or prior ultrasound examination. A limited examination, as defined above, may be performed by ultrasonographers or specially trained personnel. The basic examination, however, should be performed or reviewed by an appropriately trained operator. The comprehensive examination should be performed by an operator with experience and expertise in such scanning.

In some situations, it may not be possible to perform a full fetal survey. These include:

- Oligohydramnios
- Hyperflexed position of the fetus
- Engagement of the head
- Compression of some fetal parts
- Maternal obesity

First-Trimester Pregnancy

Ultrasound scanning in the first trimester may be performed either abdominally or vaginally. The following information should be obtained:

- Presence or absence of an intrauterine gestational sac
- Identification of embryo or fetus
- Fetal number
- Presence or absence of fetal cardiac activity

- Crown–rump length
- Evaluation of uterus and adnexal structures

Transvaginal scanning with higher-frequency transducers often allows better first-trimester assessment of pregnancy, with earlier detection of fetal echoes and activity. While abdominal scanning reliably detects the gestational sac at 6 weeks of gestation by menstrual dating (6), transvaginal scanning can identify the sac by 5 menstrual weeks of gestation (7, 8). Similarly, fetal echoes should be seen by 7 weeks of gestation via abdominal scanning but prior to 6 weeks of gestation when vaginal scanning is used (7). Generally, fetal heart activity can be detected with abdominal scanning at 7 weeks of gestation by menstrual dating and at 6 weeks of gestation with transvaginal scanning (9).

First-trimester bleeding is the most common indication for early ultrasonography. Blighted ovum, or an embryonic pregnancy, can be diagnosed by the failure to detect a fetus within a normal gestational sac after 6 weeks of gestation by menstrual dating. Missed abortion is diagnosed by the absence of cardiac activity in a fetus after 7 weeks of gestation. In patients with suspected ectopic pregnancy, the main contribution of ultrasonography is the demonstration of a gestational sac within the uterus, thereby confirming intrauterine pregnancy. Very rarely, intrauterine and extrauterine (heterotopic) pregnancies may coexist. Although ectopic pregnancy occasionally may be confirmed by demonstration of a gestational sac outside the uterus, both false-positive and false-negative findings hinder the success of ultrasonography alone in diagnosing ectopic gestation. Determining quantitative titers of the beta subunit of human chorionic gonadotropin (β-hCG) in serum may help to confirm the diagnosis. Appropriate correlation of ultrasound findings with β-hCG titers requires knowledge of whether the First or Second International Standard is being used (10). Transvaginal scanning may allow earlier detection of the gestational sac than transabdominal scanning.

Multiple pregnancy should be diagnosed on first-trimester ultrasonography only when multiple fetuses, preferably with documented cardiac activity, are demonstrated. Variability in fusion between amnion and chorion in early pregnancy may give the mistaken appearance of more than one gestational sac.

Measurement of fetal crown–rump length between 8 and 13 weeks can define gestational age to within 5 days in 95% of cases (11). When measuring the crown–rump length, care must be taken to avoid confusing the yolk sac with the fetal head.

Second-Trimester Pregnancy

Obstetric ultrasonography is most often performed to determine gestational age when clinical dating is equivocal or when there is a discrepancy between uterine size and menstrual history. The most commonly used fetal measurements are biparietal diameter, length of the femur or other long bones, and abdominal and head circumferences. Less frequently used parameters are outer orbital diameters, transcerebellar diameter, and length of the foot. It is preferable to use more than one parameter in determining gestational age. The average of the gestational age predictions of biparietal diameter, head circumference, abdominal circumference, and femur length is the best estimate of fetal age (12, 13). This averaging method, however, may be affected adversely by one measurement which is incompatible with other measurements, for example, a small biparietal diameter secondary to compression of the head in oligohydramnios or breech presentation. In such situations, the outlying value can be omitted from the calculation of the mean ultrasound age. Nonetheless, it must be recognized that such outlying values occasionally may indicate an abnormality characterized by an unusual growth pattern of a part, such as a small head or short limbs.

When the placental site is being localized in the second trimester, the term "placenta previa" should be used very cautiously because of the potential for relative change secondary to lengthening of the lower uterine segment later in pregnancy. When an abdominal ultrasound examination is performed at this stage, a distended bladder may give an erroneous impression of placenta previa. This can be resolved by completing the examination after the patient has emptied her bladder. Most placentas that appear to reach the internal os on second-trimester ultrasonography will not prove to be placenta previa in the third trimester. The appearance of placenta completely covering the internal os is an indication for a repeat ultrasound evaluation in the third trimester.

Third-Trimester Pregnancy

The uniformity of fetal growth that characterizes early pregnancy is lost later in gestation. Consequently, large variations (±3 weeks) in normal fetal measurements at any given age in the third trimester compromise the accuracy of late pregnancy ultrasonography in establishing gestational age. Nonetheless, measurements in late pregnancy do allow estimation of fetal weight and assessment of fetal growth rate. Estimates of fetal weight are based on regression models which use measurements of two or more gestational age parameters, including head, abdomen, and femur (14). These formulas allow estimation of fetal weight with a 95% confidence interval of 15–20%; that is, one standard deviation is generally 7.5–10% of the estimated weight. Unfortunately, fetal weight estimates are much less accurate in predicting the very-low-birth-weight or macrosomic fetus.

Fetal growth can be evaluated by measuring growth parameters on serial ultrasound studies. Serial measurements done after 28 weeks of gestation must be spaced at least 2 weeks apart to allow for the inherent error of ultrasound measurements and the decreasing fetal growth rate which occurs normally as gestational age progresses (12, 15).

Ultrasound measurements in early pregnancy should be more accurate in determining fetal age and estimating the delivery date than studies done in late pregnancy. When comparing the results of a later study with one done earlier, one must consider the increasing variability (±2 standard deviations) among later gestational age assessments (Table 1). Difficulties encountered particularly in late-third-trimester ultrasonography include a relative paucity of amniotic fluid, the hyperflexed position of the fetus, engagement of the fetal head, and compression of some fetal parts.

Methods of evaluating possible intrauterine growth retardation (IUGR) have progressed from biparietal diameter measurement through measurement of abdominal circumference (AC), calculation of the ratios of head circumference (HC) and femur length (FL) to AC, and estimation of fetal weight. When compared with a fetus with normal growth, the AC measurement is relatively small in the fetus with asymmetric IUGR, most likely because of decreased liver glycogen storage. In the normal fetus, the HC/AC ratio falls steadily throughout pregnancy, from a mean of 1.2 at 18 weeks of gestation to 1.0 at 36 weeks. In asymmetric IUGR, the HC remains significantly larger than the AC, and HC/AC ratios are more than two standard deviations above the expected mean value (16). While the FL/AC ratio in a fetus with normal growth remains approximately 0.22, a ratio greater than 0.24 suggests asymmetric IUGR (17). Assessment of amniotic fluid volume may provide useful information when IUGR is suspected. The value of placental grading is unproven.

Fetuses with symmetric IUGR typically have normal HC/AC and FL/AC ratios. Such fetuses comprise approximately 20–25% of cases of IUGR. These cases usually are detected by ultrasonography when all growth parameters lag significantly behind a gestational age confirmed by accurate menstrual history or early ultrasound dating.

Vaginal bleeding in the third trimester is an indication for assessing the location of the placenta. Placenta previa may be diagnosed by either transabdominal or transvaginal ultrasonography. With transabdominal scanning, a false-positive diagnosis may occur when the bladder is overdistended, as mentioned previously, or when a contraction occurs in the lower segment of the uterus (18). A contraction in the region of the internal os may bear an ultrasound textural similarity to placental tissue (19). A false-negative diagnosis of placenta previa is very uncommon but may occur when visualization of a posterior placenta previa is prevented by the overlying fetal head or when one fails to scan laterally over the lower uterine segment to identify a lateral placenta previa.

TABLE 1. ASSESSMENT OF GESTATIONAL AGE

Parameter	Gestational Age (wk)	Range (2SD*) (d)
Crown–rump length	5–12	±5
Biparietal diameter	12–20	±8
	20–30	±14
	>30	±21
Femur length	12–20	±7
	20–36	±11
	>36	±16

* SD = standard deviation.

(Adapted from Iams JD, Gabbe SG. Intrauterine growth retardation. In: Iams JD, Zuspan FP, Quilligan EJ, eds. Manual of obstetrics and gynecology, 2nd ed. St Louis: Mosby, 1990:165–172)

In cases of suspected placenta previa, transvaginal scanning may be used to obtain optimal visualization of the placenta and its relationship to the internal os (20). This procedure is performed when the maternal bladder is empty. The ultrasound transducer should be gently inserted into the vagina, avoiding pressure on the cervix and lower uterine segment.

Survey of Fetal Anatomy

Ultrasound evaluation of fetal anatomy may detect some major structural anomalies. It must be emphasized that it is unrealistic to expect to detect fetal anomalies with 100% accuracy even with the most expert and thorough scanning. A 1989 survey of selected ACOG Fellows revealed that 67% had detected one or more fetal anomalies by ultrasonography, and 51% had missed one or more anomalies (1). Gross malformations such as anencephaly and hydrocephaly were detected most commonly and were seldom overlooked. Anomalies which were more difficult to detect and overlooked more frequently included heart defects, facial clefts, diaphragmatic hernias, skeletal abnormalities, and neural tube defects.

Recent studies have shown that transvaginal scanning can detect some anomalies in the first trimester (21, 22). Nonetheless, most of these anomalies will be more readily apparent when ultrasound examination is performed later in pregnancy. The basic ultrasound examination should include a survey of fetal anatomy. During the second or third trimester, this examination should include a survey of the following: cerebral ventricles, four-chamber view of the heart (including its position within the thorax), spine, stomach, urinary bladder, umbilical cord insertion site on the anterior abdominal wall, and renal region (9). Where the initial scan shows possible evidence of fetal abnormality, or in cases referred because of a specific risk of a fetal abnormality, a more detailed examination will be required. The following guidelines for fetal anatomical survey are designed to aid the practitioner in performing a comprehensive ultrasound examination of the fetus.

Head

The fetal head is normally elliptical. In some fetal abnormalities, the cranial configuration may provide valuable diagnostic information. For example, a cloverleaf-shaped cranium may accompany thanatophoric dysplasia or aneuploidy and a lemon-shaped skull may indicate spina bifida. Although the diagnosis of microcephaly can be quite challenging, it must be suspected when fetal head measurements are inappropriately small in relation to other biometric parameters.

During a basic ultrasound examination, the appearance of the ventricles should be noted. If they appear to be abnormal, a comprehensive ultrasound examination should be recommended. Hydrocephaly is characterized by enlargement of the ventricular system of the brain, most commonly resulting from obstruction of cerebrospinal fluid circulation. The diagnosis of hydrocephaly may be suspected when any of the following conditions is observed: abnormally increased ratio of lateral ventricular width to hemispheric width, a lateral ventricular atrial (posterior horn of the lateral ventricle) width greater than 1 cm, a free-floating appearance of the choroid plexus, or asymmetric appearance of the choroid plexus. The ratio of the lateral ventricular width to hemispheric width is normally high during early pregnancy, exceeding 50% from 15–20 weeks of gestation. This ratio decreases with advancing age, falling to 33% by 24 weeks and remaining at this level through delivery. A ratio above 50% after 24 weeks of gestation is considered abnormal (23). The width of the ventricular atrium varies up to 10 mm between 15 and 35 weeks of gestation. Atrial width greater than 10 mm strongly suggests hydrocephaly (24, 25). There is frequent association of hydrocephaly with other anomalies, especially spina bifida, and assessment for other anomalies must be completed in making management decisions regarding hydrocephaly.

Holoprosencephaly and hydranencephaly also show significant increases of cerebrospinal fluid within the brain. These anomalies generally can be differentiated from hydrocephaly by the absence of midline echoes.

Transcerebellar measurements can be studied. Recent evidence indicates that in over 90% of cases of open spina bifida, the cerebellar structures are distorted, presumably by downward traction, resulting in an inability to identify the cerebellar bulbs ("banana sign") or to obtain a transcerebellar measurement that is appropriate for the gestational age (26).

The reported incidence of choroid plexus cysts varies from 0.18–3.6% in second-trimester fetuses (27–29). Usually located in the posterior aspect of the lateral ventricle, these cysts may be unilateral or bilateral and may vary in size from 2–20 mm. The majority are benign and will resolve by approximately 24 weeks of gestation. Several reports, however, have associated choroid plexus cysts with chromosomal abnormalities (28, 30, 31). The most commonly noted abnormality is trisomy 18, which occurs in approximately 1% or less of second-trimester fetuses with identified cysts. When choroid plexus cysts are visualized, more extensive scanning should be performed to look for additional abnormalities. Although fetuses with trisomy 18 commonly have multiple anomalies, there are cases in which choroid plexus cysts are the only abnormalities seen (28, 30, 31).

Fetal cystic hygromas are congenital malformations of the lymphatic system which occur most frequently in the nuchal region. On ultrasound examination, a membranelike elevation is seen that is distinct and separate from the skin line of the posterior fetal neck. The area within appears sonolucent and may be septated. Cystic hygromas are commonly associated with hydrops fetalis and chromosomal abnormalities, and additional anomalies have been reported (32). Although monosomy XO is the most common chromosomal abnormality identified in second- or third-trimester fetuses with cystic hygromas, recent studies in first-trimester fetuses demonstrate a predominance of fetal aneuploidy (33, 34). Although spontaneous resolution of the hygroma may occur, these fetuses are still at risk for aneuploidy. Fetuses with normal karyotypes and spontaneous resolution of the hygroma have a relatively good prognosis.

Spine

Ultrasound study of the fetal spine is easier in the second trimester than in the third. A sagittal view of the spine should reveal two parallel sets of echoes emanating from the vertebral body and a spinal pedicle. In a coronal view, the pedicles produce a set of parallel echogenic tracts. With these views and a series of transverse scanning ultrasonograms, a spinal defect may be identified if splaying of the lamina or the presence of a sac is detected. Disruption of overlying skin may support the diagnosis. Approximately 10% of neural tube defects are covered by intact skin.

Thorax

The fetal lungs are routinely visualized by the middle of the second trimester and normally produce midrange echoes on ultrasound examination. The lungs grow at a rate similar to that of the heart and thorax such that the ratio between cardiac diameter and thoracic circumference remains relatively constant throughout the second and third trimesters (35). A variety of abnormalities may appear as sonolucent, echogenic, or complex areas within the chest, including diaphragmatic hernias, cystic adenomatoid malformations, bronchopulmonary sequestrations, pericardial teratomas, and pleural effusions.

A four-chambered view of the fetal heart should be studied. This view is generally obtained by placing the transducer perpendicular to the long axis of the fetal spine. In this view, the heart normally lies in the left anterior quadrant of the chest. The axis of the heart is approximately 45° with a range of 22–75° (36). Deviation of the fetal heart from its normal position is suggestive of an intrathoracic mass or fluid collection. Good visualization of the atria and ventricles, cardiac septa, and outflow tracts should allow detection of 83–92% of structural cardiac anomalies (37, 38).

Developmental abnormalities of the fetal diaphragm occur in approximately 1/2,000–1/3,000 births. Identification of an apparently intact diaphragmatic outline does not rule out diaphragmatic hernia, especially when a mass or cystic lesion is identified within the fetal chest (39). Prenatal diagnosis of an abnormally small or deformed fetal thoracic cage is most often associated with skeletal dysplasia or prolonged oligohydramnios. An extremely small, bell-shaped chest secondary to either condition correlates highly with lung hypoplasia (40).

Abdomen

The fetal stomach and urinary bladder usually can be visualized by 14 weeks of gestation. Gastrointestinal obstruction is suspected when one notes an enlarged stomach or dilated loops of bowel or both. Hyperechogenic bowel is a nonspecific finding in a small number of normal fetuses. However, it has been observed with increased frequency in fetuses with Down syndrome (41) or cystic fibrosis (42). Although the cause of this hyperechogenicity is uncertain, in fetuses with cystic fibrosis it most likely represents inspissated meconium.

Urinary tract obstruction is suspected when an enlarged fetal bladder or dilated renal pelves are noted. Slight dilatation of the renal pelves is probably physiologic, usually transient, and rarely progressive. The anteroposterior (AP) diameter of the renal pelvis rarely exceeds 10 mm, and the ratio between this pelvic diameter and the AP diameter of the kidney is usually less than 50%. A pelvic diameter greater than 15 mm and a pelvis:kidney ratio of greater than 50% usually indicates significant hydronephrosis, especially when the renal calyces appear rounded and blunted (43). Fetal kidneys usually can be demonstrated after 16 weeks of gestation. In bilateral renal agenesis, the accompanying oligohydramnios may cause great difficulty in visualizing the fetal abdominal organs and in diagnosing the absence of kidneys. When the kidneys are absent, the adrenal glands enlarge to fill the void and may be mistaken for the kidneys.

Extremities

Length of the femur should be measured in the basic examination. If the length of the femur is abnormal, a comprehensive examination should be used to determine the lengths of the other long bones. Various skeletal dysplasias may be suggested by abnormalities in the measurements of the long bones, the shape of these bones, their density, the presence of fractures, or the absence of specific bones.

Umbilical Cord and Abdominal Wall

When a transverse view of the umbilical cord fails to reveal three vessels, the possibilities of other fetal malformations or karyotypic abnormalities should be considered (44). If only two vessels are seen, a comprehensive ultrasound examination is indicated. Most abdominal wall defects can be excluded by the demonstration of an intact abdomen in the area of umbilical cord insertion.

Fetal Assessment

Amniotic Fluid Index

Abnormalities of amniotic fluid volume are associated with adverse perinatal outcomes. The increased frequencies of congenital anomalies, growth retardation, and perinatal death require careful evaluation of the fetal status when polyhydramnios or oligohydramnios is present (45–47). Although subjective assessment of amniotic fluid volume offers an appropriate screening method, measurement of the amniotic fluid index is a more reproducible and quantitative technique for assessing volume abnormalities (48). The amniotic fluid index represents the sum of the largest vertical pocket of fluid measured in centimeters in each of the four quadrants of the uterus (Fig. 1). These measurements are made with the patient lying supine and the uterus divided into quadrants longitudinally by the midline and transversely midway up the fundus. The scanning transducer is aligned parallel to the midline and perpendicular to the plane of the floor in each quadrant (49). Brief movement of the umbilical cord or a fetal extremity into a fluid pocket does not prevent measurement of the full depth of the pocket.

Biophysical Profile

Biophysical profile testing consists of a nonstress test with the addition of four observations made by real-time ultrasound. The five components are as follows:

- Reactive nonstress test

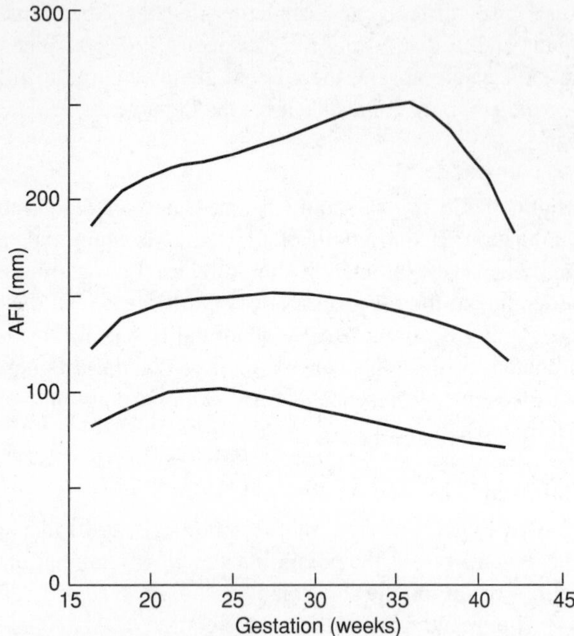

FIG. 1. Amniotic fluid index (AFI) data from normal patients plotted against gestational week. Upper, middle, and lower lines represent 95th, 50th, and 5th percentile, respectively. (Adapted from Moore TR. Superiority of the four-quadrant sum over the single-deepest-pocket technique in ultrasonographic identification of abnormal amniotic fluid volumes. Am J Obstet Gynecol 1990;163:762–767)

- Fetal breathing movements (one or more episodes of rhythmic fetal breathing movements of 30 seconds or more within 30 minutes)
- Fetal movement (three or more discrete body or limb movements within 30 minutes)
- Fetal tone (one or more episodes of extension of a fetal extremity with return to flexion)
- Quantitation of amniotic fluid volume. There is no universal agreement as to the optimal method of assessing amniotic fluid volume. Some investigators consider the detection of a single pocket of amniotic fluid exceeding 2 cm in two perpendicular planes to be adequate. A semi-quantitative, four-quadrant assessment of amniotic fluid depth (amniotic fluid index) is widely used, and cross-sectional nomograms have been developed (48, 49). Ideal cutoff levels for intervention using the amniotic fluid index have yet to be established.

With this method, a score of 2 (normal) or 0 (abnormal) is assigned to each of the five observations. A score of 8 or 10 is normal; a score of 6 is considered equivocal (a fetus should be retested in 12–24 hours); and a score of 4 or less is abnormal. In the presence of oligohydramnios, further evaluation may be warranted (50).

Should All Patients Be Screened?

Controversy continues regarding whether ultrasound screening of all obstetric patients improves pregnancy outcome. A consensus development conference convened by the National Institute of Child Health and Human Development in 1984 concluded that no clinical benefit is derived from routine obstetric ultrasonography. However, this workshop did propose 27 indications for ultrasonography during pregnancy (see the box).

Commonly advanced arguments in favor of routine scanning include early detection of unsuspected fetal anomalies, early detection of multiple gestation, accurate determination of gestational age leading to improved diagnosis and management of postdatism and fetal growth retardation, and decreased perinatal mortality rate (51–54).

Routine ultrasonography in early pregnancy can help to reduce the incidence of labor induction for suspected postdatism and decrease the frequency of undiagnosed major fetal anomalies and undiagnosed twins. However, significant effects on infant outcome are not confirmed by randomized, controlled trials (51, 52, 55–60). Although obstetric ultrasound studies are performed routinely in many European countries, in the United States the routine use of ultrasonography cannot be supported from a cost–benefit standpoint.

REFERENCES

1. Horger EO III, Tsai CC. Ultrasound and the prenatal diagnosis of congenital anomalies: a medicolegal perspective. Obstet Gynecol 1989;74:617–619
2. American Institute of Ultrasound in Medicine. Bioeffects considerations for the safety of diagnostic ultrasound. J Ultrasound Med 1988;7(9 Suppl):S1–S38
3. Stark CR, Orleans M, Haverkamp AD, Murphy J. Short- and long-term risks after exposure to diagnostic ultrasound in utero. Obstet Gynecol 1984;63:194–200
4. Lyons EA, Dyke C, Toms M, Cheang M. In utero exposure to diagnostic ultrasound: a 6-year follow-up. Radiology 1988;166:687–690
5. American Institute of Ultrasound in Medicine. Bioeffects and safety of diagnostic ultrasound. Rockville, Maryland: AIUM, 1993
6. Batzer FR, Weiner S, Corson SL, Schlaff S, Otis C. Landmarks during the first forty-two days of gestation by the β-subunit of human chorionic gonadotropin and ultrasound. Am J Obstet Gynecol 1983:146:973–979
7. Fossum GT, Davajan V, Kletzky OA. Early detection of pregnancy with transvaginal ultrasound. Fertil Steril 1988;49:788–791

8. Shapiro BS, Escobar M, Makuch R, Lavy G, DeCherney AH. A model-based prediction for transvaginal ultrasonographic identification of early intrauterine pregnancy. Am J Obstet Gynecol 1992;166:1495–1500

9. American Institute of Ultrasound in Medicine. Guidelines for the performance of the antepartum obstetrical ultrasound examination. Rockville, Maryland: AIUM, 1991

10. American College of Obstetricians and Gynecologists. Ectopic pregnancy. ACOG Technical Bulletin 150. Washington, DC: ACOG, 1990

11. Robinson HP, Fleming JEE. A critical evaluation of sonar "crown-rump length" measurements. Br J Obstet Gynaecol 1975;82:702–710

12. Hadlock FP, Deter RL, Harrist RB, Park SK. Estimating fetal age: computer-assisted analysis of multiple fetal growth parameters. Radiology 1984;152:497–501

13. Ott WJ. Accurate gestational dating. Obstet Gynecol 1985;66:311–315

14. Hadlock FP, Harrist RB, Carpenter RJ, Deter RL, Park SK. Sonographic estimation of fetal weight. The value of femur length in addition to head and abdomen measurements. Radiology 1984;150:535–540

15. Kurtz AB, Wapner RJ, Kurtz RJ, Dershaw DD, Rubin CS, Cole-Beuglet C, et al. Analysis of biparietal diameter as an accurate indicator of gestational age. J Clin Ultrasound 1980;8:319–326

16. Campbell S, Thoms A. Ultrasound measurement of the fetal head to abdomen circumference ratio in the assessment of growth retardation. Br J Obstet Gynaecol 1977;84:165–174

17. Hadlock FP, Deter RL, Harrist RB, Roecker E, Park SK. A date-independent predictor of intrauterine growth retardation: femur length/abdominal circumference ratio. Am J Roentgenol 1983;141:979–984

18. Townsend RR, Laing FC, Nyberg DA, Jeffrey RB, Wing VW. Technical factors responsible for "placental migration": sonographic assessment. Radiology 1986;160: 105–108

19. Artis AA III, Bowie JD, Rosenberg ER, Rauch RF. The fallacy of placental migration: effect of sonographic techniques. Am J Roentgenol 1985;144:79–81

20. Brown JE, Thieme GA, Shah DM, Fleischer AC, Boehm FH. Transabdominal and transvaginal endosonography: evaluation of the cervix and lower uterine segment in pregnancy. Am J Obstet Gynecol 1986;155:721–726

21. Timor-Tritsch IE, Farine D, Rosen MG. A close look at early embryonic development with the high-frequency transvaginal transducer. Am J Obstet Gynecol 1988; 159:676-681

22. Cullen MT, Green J, Whetham J, Salafia C, Gabrielli S, Hobbins JC. Transvaginal ultrasonographic detection of congenital anomalies in the first trimester. Am J Obstet Gynecol 1990;163:466–476

23. Johnson ML, Dunne MG, Mack LA, Rashbaum CL. Evaluation of fetal intracranial anatomy by static and real-time ultrasound. J Clin Ultrasound 1980;8:311–318

24. Pretorius DH, Davis K, Manco-Johnson ML, Manchester D, Meier PR, Clewell WH. Clinical course of fetal hydrocephalus: 40 cases. Am J Neuroradiol 1985;6:23–27

25. Siedler DE, Filly RA. Relative growth of the higher fetal brain structures. J Ultrasound Med 1987;6:573–576

26. Pilu G, Romero R, Reece EA, Goldstein I, Hobbins JC, Bovicelli L. Subnormal cerebellum in fetuses with spina bifida. Am J Obstet Gynecol 1988;158:1052–1056

27. Clark SL, DeVore GR, Sabey PL. Prenatal diagnosis of cysts of the fetal choroid plexus. Obstet Gynecol 1988;72:585–587

28. Platt LD, Carlson DE, Medearis AL, Walla CA. Fetal choroid plexus cysts in the second trimester of pregnancy: a cause for concern. Am J Obstet Gynecol 1991; 164:1652–1656

29. Chinn DH, Miller EI, Worthy LM, Towers CV. Sonographically detected fetal choroid plexus cysts: frequency and association with aneuploidy. J Ultrasound Med 1991;10:255–258

30. Achiron R, Barkai G, Katznelson MB-M, Mashiach S. Fetal lateral ventricle choroid plexus cysts: the dilemma of amniocentesis. Obstet Gynecol 1991;78:815–818

31. Perpignano MC, Cohen HL, Klein VR, Mandel FS, Streltzoff J, Chervenak FA, Goldman MA. Fetal choroid plexus cysts: beware the smaller cyst. Radiology 1992;182:715–717

32. Chervenak FA, Isaacson G, Blakemore KJ, Breg WR, Hobbins JC, Berkowitz RL, et al. Fetal cystic hygroma: cause and natural history. N Engl J Med 1983;309:822–825

33. Johnson MP, Johnson A, Holzgreve W, Isada NB, Wapner RJ, Treadwell MC, et al. First-trimester simple hygroma: cause and outcome. Am J Obstet Gynecol 1993;168:156–161

34. Shulman LP, Emerson DS, Felker RE, Phillips OP, Simpson JL, Elias S. High frequency of cytogenetic abnormalities in fetuses with cystic hygroma diagnosed in the first trimester. Obstet Gynecol 1992;80:80–82

35. Chitkara U, Rosenberg J, Chervenak FA, Berkowitz GS, Levine R, Fagerstrom RM, et al. Prenatal sonographic assessment of the fetal thorax: normal values. Am J Obstet Gynecol 1987;156:1069–1074

36. Comstock CH. Normal fetal heart axis and position. Obstet Gynecol 1987;70:255–259

37. Copel JA, Pilu G, Green J, Hobbins JC, Kleinman CS. Fetal echocardiographic screening for congenital heart disease: the importance of the four-chamber view. Am J Obstet Gynecol 1987;157:648–655

38. Bromley B, Estroff JA, Sanders SP, Parad R, Roberts D, Frigoletto FD Jr, et al. Fetal echocardiography: accuracy and limitations in a population at high and low risk for heart defects. Am J Obstet Gynecol 1992;166:1473—1481

39. Benacerraf BR, Adzick NS. Fetal diaphragmatic hernia: ultrasound diagnosis and clinical outcome in 19 cases. Obstet Gynecol 1987;156:573–576

40. Songster GS, Gray DL, Crane JP. Prenatal prediction of lethal pulmonary hypoplasia using ultrasonic fetal chest circumference. Obstet Gynecol 1989;73:261–266

41. Nyberg DA, Resta RG, Luthy DA, Hickok DE, Mahony BS, Hirsch JH. Prenatal sonographic findings of Down syndrome: review of 94 cases. Obstet Gynecol 1990;76: 370–377

42. Caspi B, Elchalal U, Lancet M, Chemke J. Prenatal diagnosis of cystic fibrosis: ultrasonographic appearance of meconium ileus in the fetus. Prenat Diagn 1988;8:379–382

43. Grignon A, Filion R, Filiatrault D, Robitaille P, Homsy Y, Boutin H, et al. Urinary tract dilatation in utero: classification and clinical applications. Radiology 1986;160:645–647

44. Saller DN Jr, Keene CL, Sun C-CJ, Schwartz S. The association of single umbilical artery with cytogenetically abnormal pregnancies. Am J Obstet Gynecol 1990;163: 922–925

45. Chamberlain PF, Manning FA, Morrison I, Harman CR, Lange IR. Ultrasound evaluation of amniotic fluid volume. I. The relationship of marginal and decreased amniotic fluid volumes to perinatal outcome. Am J Obstet Gynecol 1984;150:245–249

46. Chamberlain PF, Manning FA, Morrison I, Harman CR, Lange IR. Ultrasound evaluation of amniotic fluid volume. II. The relationship of increased amniotic fluid volume to perinatal outcome. Am J Obstet Gynecol 1984;150:250–254

47. Carlson DE, Platt LD, Medearis AL, Horenstein J. Quantifiable polyhydramnios: diagnosis and management. Obstet Gynecol 1990;75:989–993

48. Moore TR. Superiority of the four-quadrant sum over the single-deepest-pocket technique in ultrasonographic identification of abnormal amniotic fluid volumes. Am J Obstet Gynecol 1990;163:762–767

49. Rutherford SE, Phelan JP, Smith CV, Jacobs N. The four-quadrant assessment of amniotic fluid volume: an adjunct to antepartum fetal heart rate testing. Obstet Gynecol 1987;70:353–356

50. Manning FA, Harman CR, Morrison I, Menticoglou SM, Lange IR, Johnson JM. Fetal assessment based on fetal biophysical profile scoring. IV. An analysis of perinatal morbidity and mortality. Am J Obstet Gynecol 1990; 162:703–709

51. Bennett MJ, Little G, Dewhurst J, Chamberlain G. Predictive value of ultrasound measurement in early pregnancy: a randomized controlled trial. Br J Obstet Gynaecol 1982;89:338–341

52. Saari-Kemppainen A, Karjalainen O, Ylöstalo P, Heinonen OP. Ultrasound screening and perinatal mortality: controlled trial of systematic one-stage screening in pregnancy. Lancet 1990;336:387–391

53. Waldenström U, Nilsson S, Fall O, Axelsson O, Eklund G, Lindeberg S, et al. Effects of routine one-stage ultrasound screening in pregnancy: a randomised controlled trial. Lancet 1988;2:585–588

54. Warsof SL, Cooper DJ, Little D, Campbell S. Routine ultrasound screening for antenatal detection of intrauterine growth retardation. Obstet Gynecol 1986;67:33–39

55. Eik-Nes SH, Økland O, Aure JC, Ulstein M. Ultrasound screening in pregnancy: a randomised controlled trial. Lancet 1984;1:1347

56. Neilson JP, Munjanja SP, Whitfield CR. Screening for small for dates fetuses: a controlled trial. BMJ 1984; 289:1179–1182

57. Secher NJ, Kern Hansen P, Lenstrup C, Sindberg Eriksen P, Morsing G. A randomized study of fetal abdominal diameter and fetal weight estimation for detection of light-for-gestation infants in low-risk pregnancies. Br J Obstet Gynaecol 1987;94:105–109

58. Ewigman B, LeFevre M, Hesser J. A randomized trial of routine prenatal ultrasound. Obstet Gynecol 1990;76: 189–194

59. Ewigman BG, Crane JP, Frigoletto FD, LeFevre ML, Bain RP, McNellis D, et al. Effect of prenatal ultrasound screening on perinatal outcome. N Engl J Med 1993; 329: 821–827

60. LeFevre ML, Bain RP, Ewigman BG, Frigoletto FD, Crane JP, McNellis D, et al. A randomized trial of prenatal ultrasonographic screening: impact on maternal management and outcome. Am J Obstet Gynecol 1993;169:483–489

This Technical Bulletin was developed under the direction of the Committee on Technical Bulletins of the American College of Obstetricians and Gynecologists as an educational aid to obstetricians and gynecologists. The committee wishes to thank Edgar O. Horger III, MD, for his assistance in the development of this bulletin. This Technical Bulletin does not define a standard of care, nor is it intended to dictate an exclusive course of management. It presents recognized methods and techniques of clinical practice for consideration by obstetrician–gynecologists for incorporation into their practices. Variations of practice taking into account the needs of the individual patient, resources, and limitations unique to the institution or type of practice may be appropriate.

THE AMERICAN COLLEGE OF OBSTETRICIANS AND GYNECOLOGISTS
409 12th Street, SW
Washington, DC 20024-2188

12345/76543

Number 216—November 1995
(Replaces #127, April 1989)

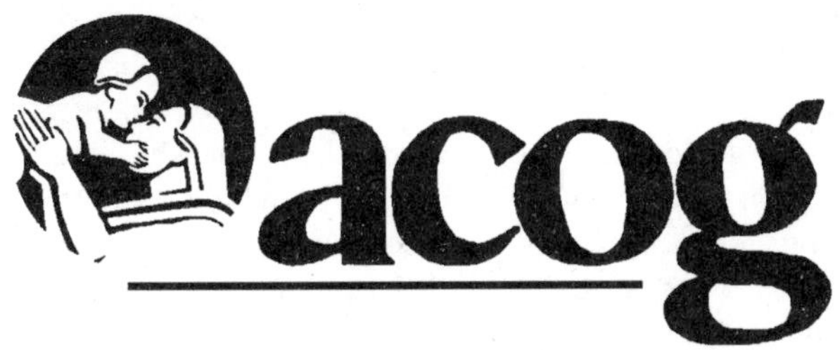

Technical Bulletin

An Educational Aid to Obstetrician–Gynecologists

Umbilical Artery Blood Acid–Base Analysis

Umbilical cord blood acid–base analysis provides an objective method of assessing a newborn's condition. Classically, the Apgar scoring system, first published in1953, has been used to assess newborn condition. Over time, however, the Apgar score has come to be used inappropriately to define asphyxia, a misapplication since many other conditions (eg, congenital anomalies, prematurity, maternal drug administration) can result in low scores that are not reflective of asphyxia. Asphyxia implies hypoxia to a degree leading to metabolic acidosis. Thus, the Apgar score alone cannot be used to define or classify asphyxia. A more appropriate tool for defining this condition is assessment of fetal and newborn acid–base status. A review of fetal and neonatal acid–base regulation and response to acute or chronic hypoxic stress can assist the practitioner in properly interpreting fetal capillary or umbilical cord blood pH and other measurements.

Fetal Acid–Base Physiology

For the purposes of this bulletin, the following definitions will be used:

Hypoxemia:	Decreased oxygen content in blood
Hypoxia:	Decreased level of oxygen in tissue
Acidemia:	Increased concentration of hydrogenions in the blood
Acidosis:	Increased concentration of hydrogenions in tissue
Asphyxia:	Hypoxia with metabolic acidosis

The fetus produces two major types of acids during metabolism—carbonic and noncarbonic. Carbonic acid (H_2CO_3) is formed by the hydration of carbon dioxide (CO_2) during oxidative metabolism. This volatile acid is found in very low concentrations in plasma. Carbon dioxide diffuses across the placenta very rapidly, and the rate of elimination is directly related to blood flow rates on both sides of the placenta. Several noncarbonic acids, including lactic and β-hydroxybutyric acids, are products of anaerobic metabolism. The fetus disposes of these acids across the placenta, but diffusion is much slower than for CO_2. This is of clinical importance because fetal metabolic acidosis takes longer to develop and to correct than does respiratory acidosis.

The pH of blood or tissue is directly related to the concentration of base (bicarbonate) and inversely related to the concentration of acid (H_2CO_3). The fetus has a system of buffers in blood and other tissues that permits the maintenance of the pH at a relatively constant level despite the continuous production of acid by cellular metabolism. Plasma bicarbonate and hemoglobin are the two most important buffers and account for approximately 70% of the total buffers in blood (1). Other buffers include erythrocyte bicarbonate (18%), plasma protein (7%), and inorganic phosphate (5%). The buffer base can be depleted from buffering a fixed acid. The terms *base deficit* and *base excess* refer to the amounts of buffer below and above normal levels, respectively. When depletion of the buffer base occurs, a base deficit exists. Base deficit or excess is not measured directly but can be calculated from a nomogram (2) when two of the three following components are known: pH, HCO_3^-, and CO_2.

Types of Acidemia

Generally, fetal or newborn acidemia is classified as respiratory, metabolic, or mixed, based on the PCO_2 and bicarbonate concentrations (Table 1). Classically, a high PCO_2 has been defined as greater than two standard deviations above the mean, and a low HCO_3^- has been defined as two standard deviations below the mean (3–5).

However, these definitions do not take into consideration that with marked elevations of the PCO_2 there can be a compensatory increase of 1 meq of HCO_3^- per liter

TABLE 1. CLASSIFICATION OF FETAL OR NEWBORN ACIDEMIA

Acidemia Type	Pco_2 (mm Hg)	HCO_3^- (meq/L)
Respiratory	High	Normal
Metabolic	Normal	Low
Mixed	High	Low

for each increase in Pco_2 of 10 mm Hg (6). If the HCO_3^- concentration is not corrected, a mixed acidemia could be classified erroneously as purely respiratory in nature.

It should be noted that maternal acid–base status can influence fetal acid–base status. Because the difference in maternal–fetal pH is usually between 0.05 and 0.10 units, differences within this range may reflect maternal contribution to the acidosis. However, unless the mother is suspected to be severely acidemic or alkalotic, it is not necessary to routinely measure maternal blood pH and blood gas values to assess newborn acid–base status accurately.

Umbilical Cord Blood Acid–Base Determinations

Umbilical cord blood pH and blood gas values are a useful adjunct to the Apgar score in assessing the immediate condition of the newborn. The technique is simple and relatively inexpensive, and the results are readily available.

Technique

A segment of umbilical cord approximately 10–20 cm in length is doubly clamped. This should be accomplished immediately after delivery, as delays of as short as 20–30 seconds can alter the arterial blood Pco_2 and pH (7). Because the umbilical artery contains blood that is returning from the fetus to the placenta, values from the umbilical artery provide the most accurate information regarding fetal and newborn acid–base status. In fact, the pH and blood gas values obtained from the umbilical vein could be in the normal range in the presence of an extremely low umbilical artery blood pH. Such findings have been documented with umbilical cord prolapse (3). If the practitioner encounters difficulty in obtaining arterial blood from the umbilical cord (ie, in the very premature infant), a sample obtained from an artery on the chorionic surface of the placenta will provide accurate results (3). These arteries are relatively easy to identify, as they cross over the veins.

Once the umbilical cord has been clamped, blood is drawn into a 1–2-ml plastic or glass syringe which has been flushed with heparin solution (1,000 U/ml) or into syringes with lyophilized heparin. Any residual air or heparin should be ejected and the needle capped. Umbilical cord segments can be left at room temperature for up to 1 hour without clotting or significant changes in pH, Po_2, or Pco_2 (8). Thus, it is not necessary to sample the umbilical artery immediately once the umbilical cord has been clamped. After the blood sample has been aspirated into a syringe, the specimens are relatively stable for 30–60 minutes at room temperature (9). Consequently, transport of the specimens in ice to a laboratory is not necessary if the analysis is to be performed within 30 minutes of collection. Recently, a mathematic model has been proposed that allows one to perform umbilical artery blood pH determinations up to 60 hours after delivery (10). This model allows the clinician without 24-hour laboratory facilities to transport specimens in ice to other laboratories for analysis. The technique permits the true acid–base status of the fetus at birth to be assessed.

Normal Values

The mean "normal" values for umbilical cord blood pH and blood gas values for term infants from three studies are summarized in Table 2. In two of the studies, the values were obtained from the infants of selected patients with uncomplicated labors who had spontaneous vaginal deliveries (4, 11). In the third study, values were obtained from the infants of unselected patients who delivered vaginally (3). The three mean values reported for normal umbilical arterial blood pH in the term newborn range from 7.27 to 7.28, with a lower limit of 7.15 (ie, two standard deviations below the mean).

The normal values for premature infants from three studies are summarized in Table 3 (3, 11, 12). Although the Apgar scores for premature infants may be significantly lower than those for term infants, the pH and acid–base status are similar. The three mean values reported for normal umbilical arterial blood pH in the preterm newborn range from 7.26 to 7.29, with a lower limit of 7.13–7.14.

Pathologic Fetal Acidemia

Traditionally, fetal or newborn acidemia has been defined as an umbilical artery blood pH of less than 7.20. However, most newborns with acidemia so defined will be vigorous at birth with normal Apgar scores and manifest no obvious neurologic sequelae (6, 13). Therefore, some investigators have recommended that a pH concentration of two standard deviations below the mean pH (7.10–7.18) be used to define significant fetal acidemia (4, 5, 14). Even with this lower threshold, most newborns will have normal Apgar scores. For example, in a prospective study of 1,210 consecutive deliveries comparing Apgar scores and acid–base status, 73% and 86% of newborns with an umbilical artery pH of 7.10 or less had normal Apgar scores at 1 and 5 minutes, respectively (15).

TABLE 2. NORMAL UMBILICAL CORD BLOOD PH AND BLOOD GAS VALUES IN TERM NEWBORNS (MEAN ± ONE STANDARD DEVIATION)

Value	Yeomans* (n = 146)	Ramin* (n = 1,292)	Riley† (n = 3,522)
Arterial blood			
pH	7.28 (0.05)	7.28 (0.07)	7.27 (0.069)
Pco_2 (mm Hg)	49.2 (8.4)	49.9 (14.2)	50.3 (11.1)
HCO_3^- (meq/L)	22.3 (2.5)	23.1 (2.8)	22.0 (3.6)
Base excess (meq/L)	—‡	-3.6 (2.8)	-2.7 (2.8)
Venous blood			
pH	7.35 (0.05)	—	7.34 (0.063)
Pco_2 (mm Hg)	38.2 (5.6)	—	40.7 (7.9)
HCO_3^- (meq/L)	20.4 (4.1)	—	21.4 (2.5)
Base excess (meq/L)	—	—	-2.4 (2)

* Data are from infants of selected patients with uncomplicated vaginal deliveries.

† Data are from infants of unselected patients with vaginal deliveries.

‡ Data were not obtained.

Ramin SM, Gilstrap LC III, Leveno KJ, Burris J, Little BB. Umbilical artery acid–base status in the preterm infant. Obstet Gynecol 1989;74:256–258

Riley RJ, Johnson JWC. Collecting and analyzing cord blood gases. Clin Obstet Gynecol 1993;36:13–23

Yeomans ER, Hauth JC, Gilstrap LC III, Strickland DM. Umbilical cord pH, Pco_2 and bicarbonate following uncomplicated term vaginal deliveries. Am J Obstet Gynecol 1985;151:798–800

TABLE 3. NORMAL UMBILICAL ARTERY BLOOD PH AND BLOOD GAS VALUES IN PREMATURE INFANTS (MEAN ± ONE STANDARD DEVIATION)

Value for Arterial Blood	Ramin* (n = 77)	Dickinson† (n = 949)	Riley† (n = 1,015)
pH	7.29 (0.07)	7.27 (0.07)	7.28 (0.089)
Pco_2 (mm Hg)	49.2 (9.0)	51.6 (9.4)	50.2 (12.3)
HCO_3^- (meq/L)	23.0 (3.5)	23.9 (2.1)	22.4 (3.5)
Base excess (meq/L)	-3.3 (2.4)	-3.0 (2.5)	-2.5 (3)

* Data are from infants of selected patients with uncomplicated vaginal deliveries.

† Data are from infants of unselected patients with vaginal deliveries.

Dickinson JE, Eriksen NL, Meyer BA, Parisi VM. The effect of preterm birth on umbilical cord blood gases. Obstet Gynecol 1992;79:575–578

Ramin SM, Gilstrap LC III, Leveno KJ, Burris J, Little BB. Umbilical artery acid–base status in the preterm infant. Obstet Gynecol 1989;74:256–258

Riley RJ, Johnson JWC. Collecting and analyzing cord blood gases. Clin Obstet Gynecol 1993;36:13–23

It has been demonstrated that a more realistic pH threshold for significant or pathologic fetal acidemia (ie, that pH associated with adverse neonatal sequelae, including death) is 7.00 (6, 13, 16). An umbilical artery blood pH of less than 7.00 with a metabolic pattern appears to be an important component of a definition of birth asphyxia or hypoxia to a degree of severity that might be associated with subsequent neurologic dysfunction. Even when this low pH threshold is used to define significant acidemia, most newborns in this category will be neurologically normal, with no apparent morbidity (17, 18).

Recommendations

Should umbilical cord blood pH and blood gas analysis be performed on all newborns? According to a survey of 128 university departments of obstetrics and gynecology in the United States, approximately 27% used umbilical cord blood pH and acid–base determinations in all deliveries (19). Three fourths of the programs used umbilical cord blood sampling specifically for newborns with low Apgar scores and abnormal fetal heart rate patterns, and 50% used it routinely with delivery of a premature infant.

Because only newborns who are severely depressed (ie, those with persistent Apgar scores of 0–3 for 5 minutes or longer and an umbilical artery blood pH of less than 7.00) are at risk of manifesting hypoxic ischemic encephalopathy and subsequent neurologic dysfunction, it seems logical that umbilical cord blood acid–base determination offers little in the evaluation of a vigorous term newborn with normal Apgar scores. Moreover, the routine use of umbilical cord blood gas analysis in all deliveries has not been shown to be cost-effective.

Umbilical cord blood pH and acid–base analysis is most useful in association with the delivery of an infant with a low Apgar score. There is little doubt that the most significant role of umbilical cord blood acid–base analysis is in the evaluation of the very premature infant with low Apgar scores. Apgar scores of otherwise uncomplicated preterm infants are typically lower than those of term infants (11, 20, 21). Many such infants could be classified incorrectly as asphyxiated based solely on the Apgar score. Moreover, premature infants are at higher risk for intracranial hemorrhage and subsequent neurologic dysfunction, such as cerebral palsy. Without umbilical cord blood gas analysis, these neurologic complications could be incorrectly attributed to intrapartum or birth asphyxia, especially if the latter is based solely on Apgar scores. Normal umbilical cord blood gas values in the premature infant virtually eliminate the diagnosis of significant intrapartum hypoxia or birth asphyxia.

Umbilical cord blood pH and acid–base analysis to assess newborn acid–base status can be useful also in pregnancies complicated by meconium staining of the amniotic fluid. Tracheal visualization, intubation, or suctioning could lead to low Apgar scores that might be incorrectly attributed to newborn asphyxia. In situations such as postterm birth or delivery complications (eg, breech birth or twins), identification and documentation of a normal pH value excludes birth asphyxia as a cause of any subsequently detected neonatal abnormality.

One reasonable protocol for umbilical cord blood pH and blood gas analysis is as follows (22):

- Double clamp a segment of the umbilical cord immediately after birth in all deliveries.
- If a serious abnormality that arose in the delivery process or a problem with the neonate's condition or both persist at or beyond the first 5 minutes, obtain an umbilical artery blood specimen for pH and acid–base determinations in a syringe flushed with heparin and have it analyzed.
- If a specimen cannot be obtained from the umbilical artery, obtain a specimen from an artery on the chorionic surface of the placenta.
- If the 5-minute Apgar score is satisfactory and the newborn appears stable and vigorous, the segment of umbilical cord can be discarded.

REFERENCES

1. Towell ME. Fetal acid–base physiology and intrauterine asphyxia. In: Goodwin JW, Godden JO, Chance GW, eds. Perinatal medicine: the basic science underlying clinical practice. Baltimore: Williams and Wilkins, 1976:187–208
2. Siggaard Andersen O. The pH-log P_{CO_2} blood acid–base nomogram revised. Scand J Clin Lab Invest 1962;14: 598–604
3. Riley RJ, Johnson JWC. Collecting and analyzing cord blood gases. Clin Obstet Gynecol 1993;36:13–23
4. Yeomans ER, Hauth JC, Gilstrap LC III, Strickland DM. Umbilical cord pH, P_{CO_2} and bicarbonate following uncomplicated term vaginal deliveries. Am J Obstet Gynecol 1985;151:798–800
5. Thorp JA, Sampson JE, Parisi VM, Creasy RK. Routine umbilical cord blood gas determinations? Am J Obstet Gynecol 1989;161:600–605
6. Goldaber KG, Gilstrap LC III, Leveno KJ, Dax JS, McIntire DD. Pathologic fetal acidemia. Obstet Gynecol 1991;78:1103–1107
7. Lievaart M, de Jong PA. Acid–base equilibrium in umbilical cord blood and time of cord clamping. Obstet Gynecol 1984;63:44–47
8. Duerbeck NB, Chaffin DG, Seeds JW. A practical approach to umbilical artery pH and blood gas determinations. Obstet Gynecol 1992;79:959–962
9. Strickland DM, Gilstrap LC III, Hauth JC, Widmer K. Umbilical cord pH and P_{CO_2}: effect of interval from delivery to determination. Am J Obstet Gynecol 1984;148:191–193
10. Chauhan SP, Cowan BD, Meydrech EF, Magann EF, Morrison JC, Martin JN Jr. Determination of fetal acidemia at birth from a remote umbilical arterial blood gas analysis. Am J Obstet Gynecol 1994;170:1705–1712
11. Ramin SM, Gilstrap LC III, Leveno KJ, Burris J, Little BB. Umbilical artery acid–base status in the preterm infant. Obstet Gynecol 1989;74:256–258
12. Dickinson JE, Eriksen NL, Meyer BA, Parisi VM. The effect of preterm birth on umbilical cord blood gases. Obstet Gynecol 1992;79:575–578
13. Winkler CL, Hauth JC, Tucker JM, Owen J, Brumfield CG. Neonatal complications at term as related to the degree of umbilical artery acidemia. Am J Obstet Gynecol 1991;164: 637–641
14. Ruth VJ, Raivio KO. Perinatal brain damage: predictive value of metabolic acidosis and the Apgar score. BMJ 1988;297:24–27
15. Sykes GS, Molloy PM, Johnson P, Gu W, Ashworth F, Stirrat GM, et al. Do Apgar scores indicate asphyxia? Lancet 1982;1:494–496
16. Gilstrap LC III, Leveno KJ, Burris J, Williams ML, Little BB. Diagnosis of birth asphyxia on the basis of fetal pH, Apgar score, and newborn cerebral dysfunction. Am J Obstet Gynecol 1989;161:825–830

17. Goodwin TM, Belai I, Hernandez P, Durand M, Paul RH. Asphyxial complications in the term newborn with severe umbilical acidemia. Am J Obstet Gynecol 1992;162: 1506–1512

18. Fee SC, Malee K, Deddish R, Minogue JP, Socol ML. Severe acidosis and subsequent neurologic status. Am J Obstet Gynecol 1990;162:802–806

19. Johnson JWC, Riley W. Cord blood gas studies: a survey. Clin Obstet Gynecol 1993;36:99–101

20. Catlin EA, Carpenter MW, Brann BS, Mayfield SR, Shaul PW, Goldstein M, et al. The Apgar score revisited: influence of gestational age. J Pediatr 1986;109:865–868

21. Goldenberg RL, Huddleston JF, Nelson KG. Apgar scores and umbilical artery pH in preterm infants. Am J Obstet Gynecol 1984;149:651–654

22. Gilstrap LC, Cunningham FG. Umbilical cord blood acid–base analysis. Williams obstetrics. 18th ed. (suppl 1). East Norwalk, Connecticut: Appleton and Lange, August/September 1989

This Technical Bulletin was developed under the direction of the Committee on Technical Bulletins of the American College of Obstetricians and Gynecologists as an educational aid to obstetricians and gynecologists. The committee wishes to thank Larry C. Gilstrap, MD, and Susan M. Ramin, MD, for their assistance in the development of this bulletin. This Technical Bulletin does not define a standard of care, nor is it intended to dictate an exclusive course of management. It presents recognized methods and techniques of clinical practice for consideration by obstetrician–gynecologists for incorporation into their practices. Variations of practice taking into account the needs of the individual patient, resources, and limitations unique to the institution or type of practice may be appropriate.

ISSN 1074-8628

THE AMERICAN COLLEGE OF OBSTETRICIANS AND GYNECOLOGISTS
409 12th Street, SW
Washington, DC 20024-2188

12345/98765

Number 213—October 1995
(Replaces #100, January 1987)

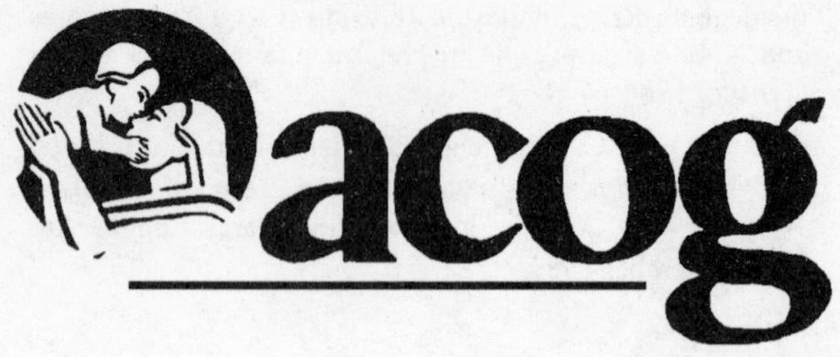

Technical Bulletin
An Educational Aid to Obstetrician–Gynecologists

Urinary Incontinence

Urinary incontinence is defined as the involuntary loss of urine which is objectively demonstrable and a social or hygienic problem (1). Urinary incontinence has been reported to affect 10–25% of women under age 65, 15–30% of noninstitutionalized women over age 60, and more than 50% of nursing home residents (2).

Estimates of the incidence of urinary incontinence vary, ranging from 8–10% of women developing incontinence over 3 years (3, 4) to 20% in 1 year according to another author (5). The rate of spontaneous remission has been reported to be 11–33%. Remissions are more common among the elderly, in whom one third of cases of incontinence may be due to transient factors such as urinary tract infections; drugs; delirium; depression; excess urine production due to excess intake, fluid mobilization, or endocrinologic problems; restricted mobility; or fecal impaction (2).

Urinary incontinence has been shown to affect a person's social, clinical, and psychologic well-being. It is estimated that less than one half of incontinent women seek medical care. Often, incontinent women rely on absorbent pads or changes in their life style to cope with the condition. These women may become socially isolated as a result of restricting their interactions with friends and family members and avoiding excursions outside their homes. Incontinent individuals have been reported to be more likely to be depressed; they may be fearful and embarrassed about their appearance or the odor of urine (2, 6). Sexual relationships are often affected. Recent estimates regarding the direct financial costs of urinary incontinence were $10.3 billion per year in 1987. Unfortunately, only 1% of this amount was spent on the diagnosis and treatment of this disorder, while 60% was spent on palliative measures (7).

Etiology

The obstetrician–gynecologist should recognize the factors that contribute to the development of urinary incontinence and pelvic organ prolapse. These include genetic factors; vaginal birth; aging; gynecologic surgery; smoking; underlying neurologic, gastrointestinal, or pulmonary diseases; and occupational and recreational factors (8). Gynecologists who treat urinary incontinence should also be knowledgeable regarding pelvic organ prolapse and fecal incontinence. These conditions may coexist or develop after surgical treatment of incontinence or prolapse. Thus, the evaluation of women with urinary incontinence should include assessment of the entire pelvic support system.

Stress Incontinence

Stress incontinence is the involuntary loss of urine during physical activity. One of the most important causes of genuine stress incontinence is loss of anatomic support of the urethra, bladder, and urethrovesical junction that allows the proximal urethra to be displaced outside the abdominal zone of pressure. This damage may be the result of pregnancy and vaginal delivery or due to tissue atrophy that results from advancing age. When there is hypermobility of the proximal continence mechanism (proximal urethral and urethrovesical junction), any increase in intraabdominal pressure generated by a stressful activity is transmitted to the bladder and, to a lesser extent, to the urethra. Thus, an increase in intravesical pressure occurs without an equivalent rise in intraurethral pressure. The normal gradient favoring continence is lost; intravesical pressure exceeds intraurethral pressure with resultant leakage of urine.

Stress incontinence may also be due to intrinsic urethral sphincter deficiency, regardless of abnormalities of the anatomic support of the urethra. Intrinsic sphincter deficiency can be found in women with scarring following pelvic surgery or bladder suspension operations or as a result of denervation injuries to the pelvic musculature. In some women, vaginal delivery has been reported to produce partial denervation of the urethra due to stretching of the distal portion of the pudendal nerve during the second stage of labor. Thus, vaginal delivery may be associated with direct and indirect injuries to the tissues and neuromuscular function of the pelvic floor (9, 10).

Hypoestrogenic changes of the genitourinary system following menopause may contribute to stress incontinence by a decrease in the periurethral vascularity and urethral mucosal atrophy, both of which contribute to a loss of coaptive forces of the urethra (11). In addition, atrophic changes within the urethral and periurethral muscular component and connective tissue may occur.

Urge Incontinence

Urge incontinence is the involuntary loss of urine associated with an abrupt and strong desire to void (urgency). Normal micturition is under voluntary control. The detrusor muscle, the smooth muscle wall of the bladder, contracts reflexively after voluntary relaxation of the pelvic floor and urethral musculature. Urge incontinence is due to overactivity of the detrusor muscle and is referred to as detrusor instability. In the presence of detrusor overactivity and a relevant neurologic disease (eg, stroke, Parkinson disease), the term *detrusor hyperreflexia* is commonly used. A paradoxical condition called detrusor hyperreflexia with impaired contractility (DHIC) may be encountered in the elderly. These individuals have inappropriate detrusor contractions (involuntary), yet the detrusor does not have sufficient strength to complete voluntary voiding. Thus, in these patients, urge incontinence due to detrusor overactivity exists in combination with urinary retention.

Other Conditions Causing Incontinence

Occasionally, patients may experience overflow incontinence due to underactivity of the detrusor muscle. This is less common than urge incontinence. In this clinical condition, the bladder fails to empty adequately, resulting in a large postvoid residual urine volume (usually over 300 ml). Leakage may be precipitated by small increases in intraabdominal pressure simulating stress incontinence or may be manifested by a relatively steady leakage of small volumes of urine resembling a fistula. A postvoid residual urine measurement will clarify the diagnosis.

Women with normally adequate bladder control may experience incontinence due to physical limitations, such as arthritis or mobility restrictions. This is called functional incontinence. Clinicians may significantly improve functional incontinence by focusing on factors other than the lower urinary tract, for example, by providing a bedside commode or treating arthritis. Psychogenic incontinence is a rare disorder and should be considered a diagnosis of exclusion. Systemic or traumatic nervous system disorders may affect lower urinary tract dysfunction. These include spinal cord lesions, diabetes, Parkinson disease, and stroke.

Extraurethral Causes of Incontinence

An uncommon cause for urinary incontinence is an anatomic bypass of the normal continence mechanisms due to the presence of a urinary fistula (ureterovaginal, vesicovaginal, or urethrovaginal), an ectopic ureter, or a urinary diverticulum. Fistulae or ectopic ureters usually cause continuous urinary leakage. Urethral diverticulum may produce postmicturition dribbling as the urine that is trapped within the diverticular sac subsequently empties on standing. A diverticulum may also be suspected when there is a painful suburethral mass; it may be a cause of recurrent urinary tract infections.

Diagnosis of Incontinence

Urinary incontinence may be a symptom, a sign, or a condition (1). The purpose of the clinical evaluation of incontinence is to 1) clarify the patient's symptoms, 2) demonstrate the loss of urine objectively, 3) determine the etiology of the incontinence using clinical testing, and 4) identify women who require more sophisticated urodynamic or imaging studies or consultation.

History

A detailed medical and surgical history should be obtained in all women with lower urinary tract symptoms. A history of diabetes mellitus, thyroid disease, multiple sclerosis, prior cerebrovascular accidents, back pain or injuries, or surgery raises the possibility that the patient's lower urinary tract symptoms may be due to an underlying neuromuscular or systemic disorder. The patient's parity, mode of deliveries, and previous pelvic surgical procedures must be ascertained to determine the possible effects of these factors on lower urinary tract function.

A drug history is important, as commonly prescribed drugs such as alpha methyldopa, prazosin, phenothiazines, or diazepam may precipitate stress incontinence by decreasing urethral smooth or skeletal muscle tone. Diuretics may cause incontinence transiently by overwhelming a marginal bladder control mechanism. Urinary retention with the development of overflow incontinence may be a side effect of antihistamine or anticholinergic therapy. Alterations in the dosage or type of drug administered may be all that is required to alleviate the symptoms.

The evaluation of incontinence may be facilitated by using a urogynecologic questionnaire. The questionnaire should be supplemented by a thorough discussion with the patient regarding the circumstances of her symptoms. Involuntary loss of urine as a result of coughing, laughing, sneezing, vigorous physical activity, or a change in position may occur with stress incontinence.

Symptoms of urgency, frequency, nocturia, or urge incontinence are usually associated with detrusor instability but may be reported in some women with a diagnosis of pure genuine stress incontinence or with a combination of both conditions. *Urgency* is defined as a strong desire to void that is accompanied by the fear of impending urinary leakage. The term *urinary frequency* is used when the patient voids more than seven times in 24 hours, assuming a normal fluid intake; the term *nocturia* is defined as being awakened from sleep by the urge to void two or more times per night (1). Leakage of large volumes of urine or a history of nocturnal enuresis (bed wetting) suggests the presence of detrusor instability. If the history reveals that the symptoms of urgency, frequency, nocturia, and urge incontinence are all present, the diagnosis of detrusor instability is accurate in up to 90% of cases. Constant urinary leakage implies a functionless urethra, fistula, ectopic ureter, or overflow incontinence.

Although an accurate history is helpful in guiding the physician's diagnostic evaluation, therapeutic decisions should not be based on history alone. Lower urinary tract symptoms are notoriously nonspecific and overlapping (12). Early reports stating that a history and physical examination alone constituted a sufficient workup in the majority of patients with stress incontinence have been contradicted by numerous recent investigators who found that the diagnosis of genuine stress incontinence based on history is correct in only 50–70% of cases (13). Surgery for stress urinary incontinence should not be undertaken if the diagnosis is based on historical information alone. Stress leakage should be demonstrated prior to surgical attempts to relieve incontinence.

Voiding Diary

A voiding diary is one of the most important aspects of a urogynecologic investigation. The patient is asked to record the time and volume of her spontaneous voids over a 24–72-hour period. Additional information regarding urgency prior to voiding, frequency of incontinent episodes, activity precipitating incontinence, and the type and volume of fluid intake may also be recorded.

From this diary, important information regarding the patient's normal voiding pattern, functional bladder capacity, and the severity of her incontinence episodes can be obtained. The findings from the voiding diary can be used to adjust the type, timing, or amount of fluid or medication intake or to alter the voiding schedule. Occasionally, the voiding pattern may alert the clinician to the possibility of diabetes insipidus in a patient with polydipsia and polyuria. Thus, a voiding diary is an inexpensive, noninvasive evaluation of lower urinary tract function that should be obtained early in the course of all urologic evaluations.

Physical Examination

Following a general physical examination, clinical evaluation of the lower urinary tract should begin with a screening neurologic examination of the lower thoracic, lumbar, and sacral nerves to detect sensory or motor nerve dysfunction of the pelvic muscles, bladder, or urethra. Examination of the lower extremity functions dependent on these nerves can provide indirect evidence regarding urinary function. Motor function can be assessed by flexion and extension maneuvers against resistance at the ankle, knee, and hip. Pelvic floor muscle tone can be determined by voluntary contraction of the anal sphincter and vagina. Normal sensation in the upper leg and perineal dermatomes implies intact sensory innervation of the lower urinary tract. Finally, a reflex contraction of the pelvic musculature in response to the anal sphincter and bulbocavernosus reflexes provides evidence of the integrity of the S2–S4 sacral reflexes. It should be noted that the anal sphincter reflex may be normally absent in up to 25% of older women. Findings suggestive of neurologic deficits may require more in-depth evaluation or consultation with a neurologist.

During the pelvic examination, the patient's estrogen status should be assessed, and the presence of any concomitant pelvic pathology or pelvic support defects should be detected. The urethra, trigone, and vagina are all hormonally responsive structures. Thus, hypoestrogenic atrophy of the vaginal mucosa indicates similar changes in the urethra. The possibility of a urethral diverticulum should be considered in the patient with a suburethral mass. A genitourinary fistula may be suggested by visualization of urine within the vagina (14).

Evaluation of defects in genitourinary support can be accomplished by inspection of the anterior and posterior vaginal walls using a Sims retractor or the lower blade of a bivalve vaginal speculum. This will facilitate identification of any cystocele, rectocele, or enterocele that should be taken into account if an operative approach to stress incontinence is considered.

Because anatomic genuine stress incontinence is due to hypermobility of the urethrovesical junction with displacement of the proximal urethra and urethrovesical junction outside the abdominal zone of pressure, an integral part of the workup for urinary incontinence is assessing the mobility of this tissue. A number of tests have been designed to ascertain the mobility of the proximal urethra and bladder base including direct observation during pelvic examination, the Q-tip test, beaded chain cystourethrography, straining cystography, and ultrasound evaluation.

These tests provide evidence of urethrovesical junction mobility but do not confirm a diagnosis of genuine stress incontinence; rather, they assist in surgical planning. The demonstration of urethral hypermobility is important in the preoperative evaluation of women with genuine stress incontinence, as most operations reposition the hypermobile urethra. While no data exist to clearly distinguish what constitutes hypermobility, there should be sufficient mobility on clinical examination to permit repositioning at the time of surgery. If no hypermobility is demonstrated in women with documented stress incontinence, alternative diagnostic and therapeutic approaches are needed.

Urine Culture

A urine culture should be obtained. One option is to obtain a clean catch midstream urine test. Because a postvoid residual should be measured to exclude urinary retention of any etiology, in lieu of a clean catch midstream urine test, the catheterized specimen may be sent for microscopic urinalysis and culture. Bacteriuria should be treated since the endotoxin produced by *Escherichia coli* may trigger abnormal detrusor activity resulting in detrusor instability or act as an alpha adrenergic blocker (15, 16). This latter action may result in loss of urethral pressure and the subsequent development of stress incontinence.

Stress Test

Since objective evidence of urinary leakage with stress is necessary to establish the diagnosis of genuine stress incontinence, the stress test is an important part of the evaluation of female urinary incontinence (17). The patient is asked to cough repetitively with a bladder volume of at least 300 ml or a subjectively full bladder in the lithotomy or standing position. Simultaneous loss of urine from the external urethral meatus during coughing is highly suggestive of genuine stress incontinence.

The stress test can easily be obtained at the beginning of the examination if the patient is asked to arrive at the office with a full bladder. Once the test is performed, the patient can void for a uroflow determination and a postvoid residual volume can be measured. Alternatively, while filling the bladder during cystometry, the stress test can be done at 50–100-ml intervals to determine the volume at which leakage occurs.

The Bonney and Marshall tests are modifications of the stress test. These were devised to predict the likelihood of surgical success in patients with stress incontinence. Although the reliability of these tests has been emphasized in the literature, other studies have since questioned their validity in selecting patients for surgical intervention (18). It appears that even in the most careful hands, these tests restore urinary continence by external compression and occlusion of the urethra. Because of these inaccuracies, most investigators have abandoned the use of these tests as prognostic tests in the preoperative evaluation of female incontinence.

A variant of the stress test may be indicated in women with genitourinary prolapse who may be paradoxically continent due to kinking, obstruction, or compression of the urethra by the prolapse. The stress test can be performed as previously outlined after reducing the prolapse by using a Sims retractor or placing the examining hand or a loose-fitting pessary in the posterior fornix (19). If the patient demonstrates involuntary urinary loss with coughing following reduction of the prolapse, additional anatomic support of the proximal urethra and urethrovesical junction may be required at the time of surgical correction of the genitourinary prolapse to prevent the development of postoperative stress incontinence.

Pad Test

The perineal pad test is occasionally useful to document urinary incontinence in women who have not demonstrated leakage during office testing. The test does not determine the cause of incontinence but simply verifies its presence. In the 1-hour test outlined by the International Continence Society, a preweighed pad is applied to the patient's perineum, and she is asked to complete a series of preset maneuvers (1). The pad is reweighed at the end of the hour, and any increase in pad weight of more than 2 g is indicative of urinary loss.

Cystometry

Cystometry indicates the pressure–volume relationship of the bladder during filling. The main diagnostic value of cystometry is its ability to detect detrusor overactivity.

A catheter may be inserted into the patient's bladder and attached to a catheter-tip syringe with the piston removed. Fluid is gradually poured into the syringe (no more than 100 ml/min) while a constant fluid level is maintained. A rise in the fluid level associated with urgency or leakage is suggestive of detrusor instability. Alternatively, a spinal manometer may be utilized to determine intravesical pressure. Commonly, a single pressure is recorded; however, additional pressures may be recorded at the clinician's discretion. In addition to the detection of detrusor overactivity, abnormal compliance or sensation or both may be diagnosed. These abnormalities of compliance or sensation generally require in-depth evaluation. The sensitivity of cystometry in detecting detrusor instability may be improved by performing the cystometrics 1) to maximum bladder capacity, 2) with the patient in the standing position, and 3) with the detrusor-provoking maneuvers of repetitive coughing, heel bounce, and hand washing performed intermittently during the test.

If electronic equipment is available, studies can be done using retrograde flow of sterile water or carbon dioxide at a flow rate of 50–100 ml/min. Although carbon dioxide cystometry may be easier to use and cleaner, it is less physiologic than water as a distention medium. Carbon dioxide may irritate the bladder mucosa and mix with urine to form carbonic acid. As a gas, carbon dioxide is compressible, which may lead to less reproducible results.

Approximately 10% of patients with urinary incontinence will require more extensive testing, such as multichannel urodynamics, to elucidate their diagnosis. These sophisticated urologic tests use specialized catheters to simultaneously record urethral, vesical, and intraabdominal (via a vaginal catheter) pressures and electromyographic activity of the pelvic musculature. Multichannel urodynamics can include subtracted urethrocystometry, urethral pressure profilometry, leak point pressure measurements, instrumented voiding studies, or electromyographic recordings of the urethral sphincter with or without fluoroscopy. Because of the expense, multichannel urodynamic studies should be used only when answers to specific clinical questions are sought. For example, such studies might be used to 1) confirm the type of incontinence in a patient with mixed incontinence symptoms or one for whom prior continence procedures have failed; 2) rule out the presence of detrusor instability in a woman with a suggestive history but negative simple cystometry; 3) identify risk factors for surgical failure, such as intrinsic sphincter dysfunction; or 4) determine the voiding mechanism in an attempt to predict which patients may experience postoperative urinary retention.

Cystourethroscopy

In incontinent women, cystourethroscopy is used to rule out intrinsic bladder pathology such as fistulae or diverticula, tumors, foreign bodies, or nonfunctioning ureters. The routine use of cystourethroscopy in the evaluation of urinary incontinence is under debate; however, this procedure should be performed in women with prior unsuccessful incontinence procedures or in older incontinent women to rule out neoplasia. Cystourethroscopy should be avoided in women with bacteriuria.

Examination of the urethra is best accomplished by using a 0° telescope with the filling medium running to facilitate distention of the urethra. The bladder trigone and ureteral function can be assessed with a 0° or, optimally, a 30° endoscope. Thorough examination of the entire bladder surface should be performed with a 30° or 70° telescope in a systematic fashion. During this procedure the bladder should be filled with a distention medium at a rate of no more than 100 ml/min to allow sufficient time for accommodation.

Treatment

Therapy for urinary incontinence consists of behavioral modification, pharmacologic treatment, and surgical management. Women with stress incontinence can be treated by using any of these methods, while those with urge incontinence respond best to behavioral techniques or medications. A treatment plan should offer the least invasive approach first; surgical options should be reserved for women who decline or do not improve following conservative management (2).

All incontinent women should be encouraged to avoid excess fluid intake, limiting their fluid to approximately 2 L/d. Consumption of caffeine-containing beverages should be eliminated or reduced to no more than 8 oz/d. Women should be instructed to void regularly. The recommended voiding interval can be determined after reviewing the woman's voiding patterns and frequency of incontinent episodes documented on her initial 24-hour voiding diary.

Palliative Measures

Protective perineal pads may be required by some women. Although panty liners or menstrual pads may suffice, women who experience significant leakage problems may need to wear specially designed absorbent products or garments, such as perineal shields, undergarments with pads held in place with waist straps, combination pad–pant systems, or adult diapers; they may also need to use absorbent bed pads. While these products may provide the patient with a measure of security against visible leakage, they are costly, may decrease a patient's motivation to seek medical care for incontinence, and may contribute to skin irritation and breakdown. Thus, long-term reliance on protective garments should be reserved for women who have exhausted alternative treatment options.

Internal or external collection devices may be required in some women. Clean, intermittent self-catheterization is useful for women with overflow incontinence due to acute or chronic urinary retention. No antiseptic urethral preparation is required. Antibiotic prophylaxis is discouraged except in symptomatic or high-risk women (ie, those with immunosuppression or vesicoureteral reflux) due to the emergence of resistant organisms. This technique is preferable to long-term indwelling catheterization. While indwelling catheters may be indicated for the treatment of short-term urinary retention (less than 2–4 weeks), they should be avoided in women with more chronic problems.

The efficacy of external collection devices in women is unclear. Women with an apical vesicovaginal fistula may wish to use a vaginal collection device similar to a diaphragm that collects urine and allows it to drain via a catheter into a collection bag.

Behavioral Therapy

Behavioral therapy includes bladder training (retraining), timed voiding, prompted voiding, and pelvic muscle exercises (2). The effectiveness of pelvic muscle exercises may be enhanced by biofeedback techniques either using pressure catheters in the bladder, vagina, or rectum that provide visual or auditory feedback concerning bladder function or using intravaginal weighted cones to aid in the performance of pelvic muscle exercises.

The key components of bladder retraining are education regarding the continence mechanism, urinary incontinence, and normal and abnormal voiding patterns; maintenance of a strict voiding schedule; and positive reinforcement. This technique attempts to reestablish the cortical inhibition of reflex bladder emptying that is lost in patients with detrusor instability.

With the patient's pretreatment voiding diary as a guide, a voiding interval that is more frequent than her incontinence episodes is designated. The patient is instructed to void regularly during the waking hours according to the preset interval, whether or not she has the urge to void. She is told to ignore other desires to void using distraction or relaxation techniques even if this results in urinary leakage. She records her micturition times on a preprinted card or sheet of paper. After 7–10 days, there should be fewer episodes of incontinence, and the scheduled voiding interval can be increased by 15–30 minutes. This process is continued until the desired voiding interval of every 2–3 hours is achieved. Positive reinforcement is essential. Success depends on the motivation of the patient and physician but can approach 80%.

Timed voiding and prompted voiding are generally reserved for the elderly, institutionalized patient. Timed voiding is scheduled voiding at preset intervals that are designed to match the patient's normal voiding frequency. No attempt is made to delay or suppress the urge to void or progressively alter the voiding interval. Prompted voiding is indicated in the dependent or cognitively impaired institutionalized resident. The patient is checked frequently by the caregivers and asked to determine whether she is wet or dry in an attempt to teach her to recognize her continence status. Patients are then asked (prompted) to use the toilet. Finally, she is given praise for maintaining continence and attempting to void. Success of these programs is dependent on the motivation of the institution staff and is inversely related to the number of baseline voiding episodes.

Pelvic Muscle Exercises

Pelvic muscle exercises (Kegel exercises) facilitate improved urinary control in 40–75% of patients (20); the patient performs the exercise by contracting the pubococcygeous muscle, thus improving the tone of the voluntary external urethral musculature. Exercises are indicated in patients with either stress or urge incontinence. The success of pelvic muscle exercises depends on the patient's ability to identify the correct muscles for the exercise and her commitment to performing the exercises. Simple written or verbal instructions may be insufficient to teach patients how to properly perform pelvic muscle exercises (21).

The correct method can be taught during a routine pelvic examination. While the examiner identifies the muscle by direct palpation, the patient is asked to contract the muscle, and verbal feedback can be provided to ensure appropriate performance of the exercise. Those women who are unable to isolate their pelvic muscles or who cannot contract these muscles may need biofeedback or electrical stimulation.

Patients should be instructed to perform 10–20 10-second pelvic floor contractions three or more times per day. A total of 40–80 contractions per day for at least 6 weeks is usually required to achieve a detectable beneficial effect. Older women may need a longer training period. These exercises should be performed indefinitely to prevent recurrence of incontinence.

Biofeedback

Biofeedback can be combined with behavioral therapy to improve the response to therapy. Biofeedback uses electrophysiologic (electromyographic) signals or pressure readings to provide visual or auditory feedback to the patient regarding the status of her lower urinary tract function or pelvic floor musculature. Home perineometer devices are one of the simplest forms of biofeedback. Multiple units are available; however, there are conflicting reports regarding the success rate of treatment.

Intravaginal, intraurethral, or intrarectal manometric devices can be used on a weekly or twice-weekly basis during office biofeedback sessions to augment pelvic floor tone in women with stress incontinence. Biofeedback can also facilitate the inhibition of abnormal detrusor contractions by using a pressure catheter in the bladder that provides an auditory or visual stimulus when bladder pressure rises. The patient is encouraged to relax her detrusor muscle to decrease the recorded signal and inhibit the involuntary detrusor contraction. The success of all biofeedback techniques relies on the experience and skill of the clinician and the motivation of the patient. When these techniques are properly performed, a combination of behavioral therapy and biofeedback may result in a 50–95% improvement in incontinence. Although advocates of both bladder retraining and biofeedback report excellent success rates without side effects, the time-consuming nature of these treatments may make them unacceptable for some women.

Devices

Weighted vaginal cones are tamponlike devices that are progressively weighted. These have been found to be effective in decreasing the number of episodes of incontinence in premenopausal women. A set of cones that are of the same shape and size but of gradually increasing weight is provided to the patient. She is instructed to begin by using the heaviest cone that she can retain in the vagina. The patient is asked to attempt to keep the cone in her vagina for 15 minutes twice daily. Cones are believed to improve the patient's awareness of the pelvic floor musculature. The sustained contraction required to maintain the cone in place strengthens the pelvic floor muscles, thereby improving continence. Some women have atrophy of the pelvic muscles from disuse and may be unable to hold the lightest cone. Such women should be treated with an alternative therapy.

Functional electrical stimulation is an alternative for treating stress or urge incontinence. A vaginal or rectal probe is inserted, usually twice daily for 15–30 minutes, to provide electrical stimulation to the pelvic viscera, pelvic muscles, or nerves to these structures. Stimulation of the afferent fibers of the pudendal nerve can produce contractions of the pelvic floor and periurethral skeletal muscles augmenting their tone in women with stress incontinence. Additionally, stimulation inhibits involuntary detrusor contractions. These devices may be efficacious in women in whom more traditional treatment approaches have failed. Further studies need to be undertaken to clarify the objective efficacy of this technique in treating urinary incontinence.

Vaginal pessaries or contraceptive diaphragms have been used to alleviate the symptoms of pelvic organ prolapse with or without concomitant urinary incontinence. By compressing the urethra between the pessary ring and the pubic symphysis, urethral resistance is increased, and the urethra and urethrovesical junction are stabilized in an appropriate anatomic position during episodes of stress (22). An appropriately fitted ring, Smith–Hodge, or Gelhorn pessary may result in continence in up to 75% of women. This form of therapy is particularly well suited for older women with prolapse and incontinence who are poor surgical candidates. In addition, younger women who experience stress incontinence only during intense exercise (eg, aerobics, tennis) may benefit from insertion of a pessary, diaphragm, or tampon temporarily just prior to exercise (23).

Pharmacotherapy

Pharmacotherapy for urinary incontinence is directed at either relaxing an overactive detrusor muscle in women with urge incontinence or augmenting intrinsic urethral tone in those patients who experience stress incontinence.

Several categories of drugs are available to treat detrusor instability. These medications provide an alternative to behavioral therapy, with cure rates of 20–30% and reduction in the frequency of incontinence episodes of 10–80% in placebo-controlled trials (24). Initial therapy may be with either oxybutynin hydrochloride, which is effective but carries a significant risk of side effects, or propantheline bromide, which appears to be associated with less adverse reactions. Other anticholinergic or antispasmodic products that have been marketed for detrusor instability do not appear to be any more efficacious than oxybutynin or propantheline and are more costly.

Imipramine hydrochloride, 50–150 mg/d, is advantageous in treating mixed stress incontinence and detrusor instability because of its combined alpha-adrenergic and anticholinergic properties. Imipramine may also be indicated in women with significant nocturnal frequency or urge incontinence due to its sedative effects. This medication should be used judiciously in the elderly since imipramine can occasionally raise blood pressure, cause orthostatic hypotension, or precipitate a dysphoric reaction at low dosages.

The side effects of drugs used for detrusor instability are typically anticholinergic symptoms—most prominently dry mouth, constipation, or blurred vision. These drugs are contraindicated in women with narrow-angle glaucoma and should be used cautiously in those with significant cardiovascular disease. In patients who experience troublesome side effects, the combination of low doses of more than one type of medication may produce an additive beneficial response while diminishing the reported side effects.

Alpha-adrenergic stimulation of the urethral smooth muscle with phenylpropanolamine, 75–150 mg/d, may improve urinary control in 20–60% of patients with mild to moderate stress incontinence. Many over-the-counter appetite suppressants contain phenylpropanolamine as the active ingredient, although the patient should be careful to avoid caffeine-containing products. Side effects can include nausea, restlessness, insomnia, dry mouth, and itching. These medications should be used with caution in women with hypertension, hyperthyroidism, cardiac arrhythmia, or coronary artery disease.

In postmenopausal women, estrogen replacement is recommended to treat either stress or urge incontinence. Estrogen appears to raise the sensory threshold for involuntary detrusor contractions (25), thus decreasing urinary urgency, frequency, and urge incontinence. Estrogen improves the urethral mucosal seal by its effect on the uroepithelium, submucosal vascular plexus, and submucosal elastic tissues (26). Following estrogen administration, there is also enhancement of the alpha-adrenergic contractile response of the urethral smooth muscle and an increase in pressure transmission ratios (27). Estrogen may be given systemically or as a topical vaginal cream. The use of the vaginal route (rather than oral administration) may diminish side effects (28) and prevent the need for progestin therapy in women with an intact uterus. The usual dosage of vaginal estrogen cream is one-half to one applicatorful (depending on the preparation), two to three times a week, for 6–12 weeks. A longer duration of therapy may be required in some women with markedly atrophic tissues. Up to 70% of patients with mild to moderate incontinence have reported a favorable clinical response following initiation of estrogen therapy.

Surgery

Unlike that of extirpative procedures, the success rate of surgery to restore urinary continence declines with repeated attempts. Therefore, precise preoperative diagnosis and careful planning and execution of the procedure are essential.

The surgical management of genuine stress incontinence can be divided into 1) procedures that restore the anatomic support of the proximal urethra and the urethrovesical junction in women with hypermobility and a normal intrinsic urethral sphincter and 2) procedures designed to compensate for a poorly functioning urethral sphincter. Several surgical principles should be emphasized when treating a patient with stress incontinence with or without significant pelvic prolapse:

- Surgical procedures for urinary incontinence may provide a chance for cure but are associated with more potential complications than nonsurgical approaches. Thus, operative procedures should be reserved for women who decline or do not improve following conservative therapies and, ideally, for women who have completed childbearing.
- Defects in pelvic support should be identified preoperatively, and the surgical procedure should be designed to correct current pelvic support defects as well as to prevent anatomic alterations that could cause pelvic organ prolapse postoperatively (eg, an enterocele or rectocele due to anterior displacement of the vaginal axis).
- There is no evidence to indicate that removal of a normal, well-supported uterus will improve the cure rate for operations designed to correct stress incontinence. Because there are no prospective, randomized, clinical trials addressing this issue, hysterectomy generally should be reserved for gynecologic indications alone.
- Paradoxically, patients with severe pelvic organ prolapse may be continent due to the obstructive or compressive effects or both of the prolapse on the urethra. Preoperative assessment of these women should include a stress test with the prolapse reduced to determine if additional surgical support of the urethrovesical junction should be performed at the time of the prolapse surgery.
- Unless there is proven obstruction or kinking of the urethra due to a severe cystocele that, in turn, produces urinary retention, correction of a cystocele will not improve a patient's retention or correct an elevated postvoid residual. At times, the increased urethral resistance following pelvic surgery may actually worsen a patient's urinary retention.

The operations for urethral hypermobility include anterior colporrhaphy, abdominal retropubic urethropexies, and vaginal needle suspension procedures. While the traditional vaginal approach to stress incontinence has been the Kelly–Kennedy plication, numerous recent studies have found that the standard anterior colporrhaphy may not provide adequate long-term support of the urethrovesical junction (29). The objective cure rate for stress incontinence following anterior colporrhaphy is only 40–70%.

The best treatment for stress urinary incontinence resulting from hypermobility of the urethrovesical junction appears to be an abdominal retropubic urethropexy such as the Marshall–Marchetti–Krantz or Burch procedure (29). These operations may be used in women with either primary or recurrent incontinence. Objective cure rates for primary incontinence operations range from 70% to 90%, while rates for recurrent incontinence are between 50% and 80%. A combined review of nearly 3,000 patients revealed an average cure rate of 78.2%.

In the Marshall–Marchetti–Krantz procedure, the periurethral tissue is sutured to the periosteum of the pubic symphysis or the symphyseal cartilage. The Burch operation involves securing the vaginal fascia to the iliopectineal line (Cooper's ligament) creating a hammocklike support of the urethra using the vaginal wall. With either operation there is a 7–19% risk of subsequent enterocele formation. Thus, the depth and size of the cul-de-sac must be assessed intraoperatively. Prophylactic obliteration of the cul-de-sac may be indicated. Between 15% and 20% of women may experience complications of colposuspension procedures including urinary retention, detrusor instability, urgency/frequency symptoms, bladder or urethral injury, recurrent urinary tract infections, and osteitis pubis (with the Marshall–Marchetti– Krantz procedure) and postcolposuspension pain syndrome (with the Burch procedure). While the Marshall–Marchetti–Krantz and Burch procedures are effective in women with hypermobility and a normal intrinsic urethra, their role in women with intrinsic sphincter dysfunction remains to be ascertained. Cure rates for these procedures have been reported between 55% and 85% in women with a poorly functioning intrinsic urethra and urethral hypermobility.

Recently, paravaginal defect repair has been advocated for the treatment of lateral detachment cystoceles and stress incontinence. In this operation, the anterolateral vaginal wall is reattached to the arcus tendineous fascia pelvis from just below the pubic symphysis to the ischial spines. Ongoing clinical trials are evaluating the success of this procedure in curing genuine stress incontinence.

Some studies have found good success with needle suspension procedures for the treatment of anatomic stress incontinence. In an evaluation of over 1,300 patients who had undergone such procedures, 84% were continent, 2% were "almost dry," 2% were improved, and 14% showed no improvement (2). These operations may be particularly beneficial for the patient with significant pelvic organ prolapse who requires additional vaginal surgery. Needle suspension procedures are probably inadequate for women with intrinsic urethral sphincter dysfunction. The choice of a needle suspension procedure should be made based on the experience of the surgeon. There is considerably more clinical experience with the Pereyra, Stamey, and Raz operations. Regardless of which technique is chosen, permanent suspending sutures are recommended due to the higher failure rate with absorbable sutures (30). The integrity of the lower urinary tract must be assessed by endoscopy at the time of the procedure. Complications from needle suspension procedures range from 2% to 60% (2). These include urinary retention or voiding problems; injury to the lower urinary tract; suture or bolster (with the Stamey operation) removal due to pain, infection, rejection, or erosion; detrusor instability; and pelvic prolapse.

Intrinsic urethral sphincter dysfunction may be treated by use of a suburethral sling procedure, periurethral bulking injections (with GAX-collagen or Teflon paste) to improve urethral coaptation, or placement of an artificial urinary sphincter, depending on whether coexisting urethral hypermobility is present. The best approach for intrinsic urethral sphincter dysfunction with hypermobility is the suburethral sling procedure; for intrinsic urethral sphincter dysfunction without hypermobility, use of injections or an artificial sphincter is recommended because sling procedures are less successful in these patients. These operations may be associated with a high risk of postoperative complications, especially urinary retention.

Suburethral slings may be performed using autologous material such as fascia lata or rectus fascia. Because of the difficulties associated with harvesting these tissues, synthetic materials have also been used. However, synthetic materials are more prone to infection or rejection. Once the sling has been secured beneath the urethra, it can be attached to the rectus fascia or iliopectineal line. Cure rates for suburethral sling procedures are reported to be 70–95%. However, complications are common, including urinary retention or voiding problems, recurrent bladder infections, trauma to the bladder or urethra, and rejection of synthetic graft material. Because of the significant risk of retention necessitating prolonged catheter use, women who are unwilling or unable to perform intermittent self-catheterization may not be good candidates for a sling procedure.

Periurethral injections of GAX-collagen may be a reasonable alternative to a suburethral sling procedure in women with a well-supported but poorly functioning intrinsic urethra, with short-term cure rates approaching 70–90% (31). Periurethral collagen injections are not indicated in women with urethral hypermobility because cure rates are only 20–50% in this group of women (2, 32). Artificial urinary sphincters should be reserved for use by specialists in this procedure. Regardless of which operation is selected for the treatment of intrinsic urethral dysfunction, adequate preoperative counseling is required prior to surgical intervention for this condition.

Surgical intervention for detrusor instability is associated with significant morbidity and should be reserved only for severely affected individuals. These procedures may include transvaginal resection or partial denervation of the hypogastric nerve plexus with phenol injections, selective sacral blockade or sacral neurectomy, implantation of a device to stimulate the sacral nerve root, augmentation cystoplasty, or, in extreme cases, urinary diversion (24).

Patient Education and Counseling

Numerous educational resources and nonprofit organizations are available that provide information for patients and health care practitioners regarding urinary incontinence. In 1992, the Agency for Health Care Policy and Research published *Clinical Practice Guidelines for Urinary Incontinence in Adults* with accompanying brochures for both patients and practitioners. Two other organizations that publish educational and product resource material may be helpful:

Help for Incontinent People (HIP)
PO Box 544
Union, SC 29379
1-800-252-2337

The Simon Foundation
PO Box 835
1-800-23-SIMON

Patients should be encouraged to learn about incontinence and to attend or form support groups as needed.

REFERENCES

1. International Continence Society Committee on Standardisation of Terminology. The standardisation of terminology of lower urinary tract function. Scand J Urol Nephrol 1988;114(suppl):5–19

2. Urinary Incontinence Guideline Panel. Urinary incontinence in adults: clinical practice guideline. Rockville, Maryland: Agency for Health Care Policy and Research, Public Health Service, U.S. Department of Health and Human Services, 1992; AHCPR publication no. 92-0038

3. Burgio KL, Matthews KA, Engel BT. Prevalence, incidence and correlates of urinary incontinence in healthy, middle-aged women. J Urol 1991;146:1255–1259

4. Campbell AJ, Reinken J, McCosh L. Incontinence in the elderly: prevalence and prognosis. Age Ageing 1985;14: 65–70

5. Herzog AR, Diokno AC, Brown MB, Normolle DP, Brock BM. Two-year incidence, remission and change patterns of urinary incontinence in noninstitutionalized older adults. J Gerontol 1990;45:M67–M74

6. Wyman JF, Harkins S, Choi SC, Taylor JR, Fantl JA. Psychosocial impact of urinary incontinence in women. Obstet Gynecol 1987;70:378–381

7. Consensus Conference. Urinary incontinence in adults. JAMA 1989;261:2685–2690

8. DeLancey JOL. Anatomic aspects of vaginal eversion after hysterectomy. Am J Obstet Gynzecol 1992;166:1717–1728

9. Allen RE, Hosker GL, Smith ARB, Warrell DW. Pelvic floor damage and childbirth: a neurophysiological study. Br J Obstet Gynaecol 1990;97:770–779

10. Smith ARB, Hosker GL, Warrell DW. The role of pudendal nerve damage in the aetiology of genuine stress incontinence in women. Br J Obstet Gynaecol 1989; 96:29–32

11. Staskin DR. Age-related physiologic and pathologic changes affecting lower urinary tract function. Clin Geriatr Med 1986;2:701–710

12. Cardozo LD, Stanton SL. Genuine stress incontinence and detrusor instability—a review of 200 patients. Br J Obstet Gynaecol 1980;87:184–190

13. Jensen JK, Nielsen FR, Ostergard DR. The role of patient history in the diagnosis of urinary incontinence. Obstet Gynecol 1994;83:904–910

14. American College of Obstetricians and Gynecologists. Genitourinary fistulas. ACOG Technical Bulletin 83. Washington, DC: ACOG, 1985

15. Nergardh A, Boreus L, Holme T. The inhibitory effect of coli-endotoxin on alpha-adrenergic receptor function in the lower urinary tract. An in vitro study in cats. Scand J Urol Nephrol 1977;11:219–224

16. Bhatia NN, Bergman A. Cystometry: unstable bladder and urinary tract infection. Br J Urol 1986;58:134–137

17. Fischer-Rasmussen W, Hansen RI, Stage P. Predictive values of diagnostic tests in the evaluation of female urinary stress incontinence. Acta Obstet Gynecol Scand 1986;65: 291–294

18. Migliorini GD, Glenning PP. Bonney's test—fact or fiction? Br J Obstet Gynaecol 1987;94:157–159

19. Richardson DA, Bent AE, Ostergard DR. The effect of uterovaginal prolapse on urethrovesical pressure dynamics. Am J Obstet Gynecol 1983;146:901–905

20. Tchou DCH, Adams C, Varner RE, Denton B. Pelvic floor musculature exercises in treatment of anatomical urinary stress incontinence. Phys Ther 1988;68:652–655

21. Bump RC, Hurt WG, Fantl JA, Wyman JF. Assessment of Kegel pelvic muscle exercise performance after brief verbal instruction. Am J Obstet Gynecol 1991;165:322–329

22. Bhatia NN, Bergman A, Gunning JE. Urodynamic effects of a vaginal pessary in women with stress urinary incontinence. Am J Obstet Gynecol 1983;147:876–884

23. Nygaard I. Prevention of exercise incontinence with mechanical devices. J Reprod Med 1995;40:89–94

24. Wall LL. Diagnosis and management of urinary incontinence due to detrusor instability. Obstet Gynecol Surv 1990;45(suppl):1S–47S

25. Fantl JA, Wyman JF, Anderson RL, Matt DW, Bump RC. Postmenopausal urinary incontinence: comparison between non-estrogen-supplemented and estrogen-supplemented women. Obstet Gynecol 1988;71:823–828

26. Bhatia NN, Bergman A, Karram MM. Effects of estrogen on urethral function in women with urinary incontinence. Am J Obstet Gynecol 1989;160:176–181

27. Kinn A-C, Lindskoy M. Estrogens and phenylpropanolamine in combination for stress urinary incontinence in postmenopausal women. Urology 1988;32:273–280

28. Elia G, Bergman A. Estrogen effects on the urethra: beneficial effects in women with genuine stress incontinence. Obstet Gynecol Surv 1993;48:509–517

29. Bergman A, Ballard CA, Koonings PP. Comparison of three different surgical procedures for genuine stress incontinence: prospective randomized study. Am J Obstet Gynecol 1989;160:1102–1106

30. Korn AP. Does use of permanent suture material affect outcome of the modified Pereyra procedure? Obstet Gynecol 1994;83:104–107

31. Eckford SD, Abrams P. Para-urethral collagen implantation for female stress incontinence. Br J Urol 1991;68: 586–589

32. Appell RA. Injectables for urethral incompetence. World J Urol 1990;89:208–211

This Technical Bulletin was developed under the direction of the Committee on Technical Bulletins of the American College of Obstetricians and Gynecologists as an educational aid to obstetricians and gynecologists. The committee wishes to thank Nicolette S. Horbach, MD, for her assistance in the development of this bulletin. This Technical Bulletin does not define a standard of care, nor is it intended to dictate an exclusive course of management. It presents recognized methods and techniques of clinical practice for consideration by obstetrician–gynecologists for incorporation into their practices. Variations of practice taking into account the needs of the individual patient, resources, and limitations unique to the institution or type of practice may be appropriate.
ISSN 1074-8628

THE AMERICAN COLLEGE OF OBSTETRICIANS AND GYNECOLOGISTS
409 12th Street, SW
Washington, DC 20024-2188

12345/98765

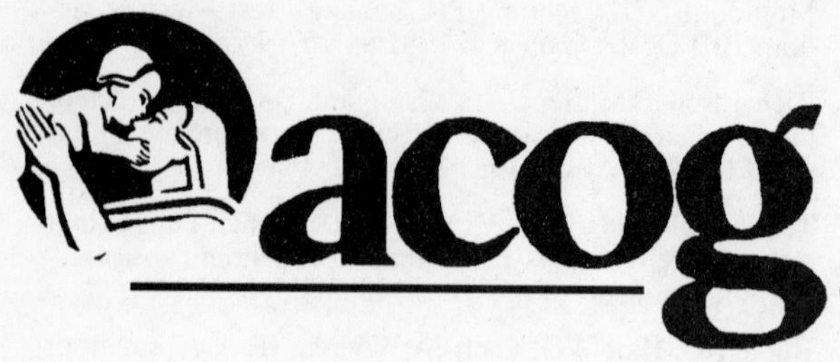

Number 226—July 1996
(Replaces #221, March 1996)

Technical Bulletin

An Educational Aid to Obstetrician–Gynecologists

Vaginitis

Vaginitis is the most common gynecologic problem encountered by physicians providing primary care to women. It affects all age groups and has a variety of causes. A first-time occurrence of vaginitis may be easily diagnosed and treated; recurrent episodes may be more difficult to manage. Therefore, it is important that an initial episode of vaginitis be properly evaluated, diagnosed, and treated.

Vaginitis can be a significant source of physical and emotional distress for the patient and frustration for the physician, especially if it is recurrent or chronic. Vaginitis may be difficult to establish because of the various causes. It may result from bacterial infections, fungal infection, protozoan infection, contact dermatitis, atrophic vaginitis, or allergic reaction. In some patients, the possibility of coexistent infections should be considered. Patients with vulvodynia may be misdiagnosed as having vaginitis. Management is complicated by the wide variety of vaginal preparations available (such as antifungal agents, sulfa preparations, douches, and antimicrobial agents), many of which are self-prescribed and self-administered.

Vaginal Ecosystem

The vaginal ecosystem is a complex environment that consists of interrelationships among the endogenous microflora, metabolic products of the microflora and host, estrogen, and the pH level. The dynamic equilibrium of this ecosystem is challenged constantly by endogenous and exogenous factors. The microflora is made up of numerous microorganisms, such as yeast and Gram-positive and Gram-negative aerobic, facultative, and obligate anaerobic bacteria. Some of these bacteria exist in a commensal state with the host, others act synergistically, and others are antagonistic.

Vaginitis occurs because the vaginal ecosystem has been altered, either by the introduction of an organism or by a disturbance that allows the pathogens normally residing in this environment to proliferate. An altered vaginal ecosystem usually results from a combination of factors, such as use of medications, repeated douching, or self-diagnosis and self-treatment. Among the medications and other factors that may alter the delicate equilibrium are the following:

- Antibiotics
- Hormones
- Contraceptive preparations (oral and topical)
- Douches
- Vaginal medication
- Sexual intercourse
- STDs
- Stress
- Change in partners

Antibiotics, for example, may allow for the overgrowth of yeast. They may also suppress the growth of commensal organisms and allow the pathogenic strains to dominate, giving rise to conditions such as bacterial vaginosis. Douching may alter the pH level or selectively suppress the growth of endogenous bacteria. Sexual intercourse may alter the vaginal pH or introduce microbes that can cause significant shifts in equilibrium. The presence of a foreign body, such as a tampon in prolonged use, can initiate an inflammatory reaction that can disturb the endogenous healthy microflora.

Maintaining a normal pH level—3.8–4.2—is considered vital to stabilizing the vaginal ecosystem. Normal pH levels are believed to be maintained, in part, by *Lactobacillus acidophilus*, which are the dominant bacteria in a healthy vaginal ecosystem (1, 2). Lactobacilli suppress the growth of the Gram-negative and Gram-positive facultative and obligate anaerobes and maintain normal pH through the production of lactic acid. In addition, these bacteria produce hydrogen peroxide, which is toxic to the anaerobes.

The normal vagina contains approximately 5–15 different species of bacteria (1, 2). When the pH level rises, lactobacilli growth is inhibited, while pathogen growth is facilitated. Hydrogen ion concentration is lowered as well, which favors adherence of pathogenic organisms to vaginal epithelial cells (3, 4, 5).

Decreased hydrogen ion concentration is accompanied by increased growth of *Gardnerella vaginalis* and decreased oxygen concentration, resulting in an increase in growth of anaerobic bacteria. The decrease in hydrogen ion concentration and alteration in the vaginal microflora produce a noticeable decrease in the growth of lactobacilli. A similar situation also occurs when trichomonads are introduced into the vaginal ecosystem, thus creating an environment conducive to their growth as well as the growth of facultative and obligate anaerobes.

Evaluation of the Vagina

Evaluation of the vagina begins with close inspection of the external genitalia for excoriations, ulcerations, blisters, papillary structures, erythema, edema, or thinning and pallor. To establish whether the problem arises from the vulva or vagina, or both, the patient should point to the area that is causing her discomfort.

If the vagina is involved, alterations in the ecosystem must be determined by identifying the gross and microscopic characteristics of the vaginal discharge, measuring the pH level, and establishing the presence or absence of amines. The clinical characteristics of various entities are listed in the box. Figure 1 presents a flow chart for diagnosing vaginitis.

The pH level can be determined by placing pH paper on the lateral vaginal wall or immersing the pH paper in the vaginal discharge. A pH level greater than 4.5 indicates an imbalance in the vaginal ecosystem that is most likely due to an increase in Gram-negative facultative anaerobes as well as Gram-positive and Gram-negative obligate anaerobic bacteria, and often signals the presence of bacterial vaginosis. A pH level greater than 4.5 may also indicate the presence of *Trichomonas vaginalis*.

The whiff test can detect the presence of amines; it is inexpensive and simple to perform. A drop of the vaginal discharge is placed on a glass slide, and a drop of 10% potassium hydroxide (KOH) is added. If anaerobic bacteria are present, a fishy odor will be noted due to the liberation of amines. Microscopic examination of the vaginal discharge should be performed to determine whether trichomonads or clue cells are present.

Evaluation of the vaginal ecosystem of a pregnant woman should be performed at the first prenatal visit if the patient reports an abnormal discharge or other symptoms of vaginitis. Infection with bacterial vaginosis, trichomonads, or group B streptococci has been associated with septic abortion, premature rupture of amniotic membranes, premature labor, and premature delivery (6, 7, 8).

Clinical Manifestations of Vaginitis

Candidal Vaginitis

Nonmalodorous, thick, white, "cottage cheese–like" discharge that adheres to vaginal walls

Presence of hyphal forms or budding yeast cells on wet-mount microscopic evaluation

Pruritus

Bacterial Vaginosis

Thin, dark or dull grey, homogeneous, malodorous discharge that adheres to the vaginal walls

Elevated pH level (> 4.5)

Positive KOH (whiff/amine test)

Presence of clue cells on wet-mount microscopic evaluation

Trichomonas vaginalis

Copious, yellow-gray or green, homogeneous or frothy, malodorous discharge

Elevated pH level (> 4.5)

Presence of mobile, flagellated organisms and leukocytes on wet-mount microscopic evaluation

Vulvovaginal irritation, dysuria

Atrophic Vaginitis

Vaginal dryness or burning

Patients with an altered vaginal ecosystem who undergo cesarean delivery are at risk for developing postpartum endometritis (9).

Patients also should be evaluated preoperatively if any symptoms of vaginitis are reported. Patients with an altered vaginal ecosystem who undergo pelvic surgery that involves the vaginal flora may be at risk for developing postoperative pelvic cellulitis (10).

Patients with a short history of vulvar irritation should be questioned about use of substances that commonly cause allergic or chemical irritation such as deodorant soaps, laundry detergent, vaginal contraceptives, bath oils, perfumed or dyed toilet paper, hot tub or swimming pool chemicals, and synthetic clothing. Almost any material can elicit an allergic reaction, and sometimes only dermatologic testing or a systematic elimination of potential contact irritants can identify the cause. Topical steroids can help alleviate the symptoms until the irritant can be identified.

Candidal Vaginitis

Approximately 30% of women with a healthy vaginal ecosystem harbor *Candida*, usually *Candida albicans*.

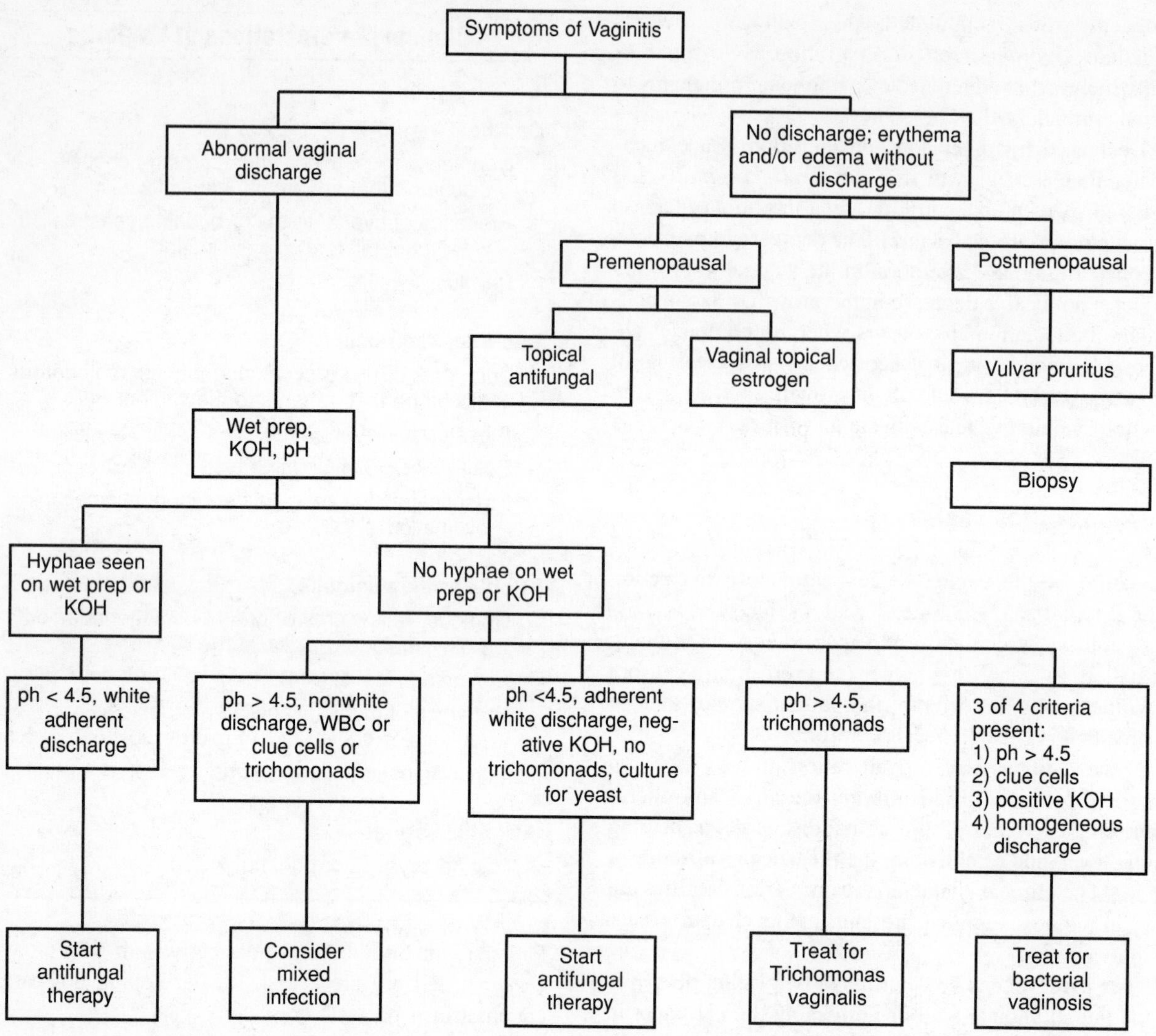

FIG. 1. Diagnostic flow chart for vaginitis. KOH indicates 10% potassium hydroxide (whiff test); WBC, white blood cells.

These patients are asymptomatic, and often yeast cannot be found on routine microscopic examination of the vaginal discharge. Several factors may trigger a change from colonization to proliferation and invasion and cause the patient to develop symptoms. Such factors include both phenotypic changes in the yeast and changes to the vaginal ecosystem. Vaginal isolation of yeast in an asymptomatic woman presumably represents colonization rather than infection. However, patients with diabetes mellitus or immunosuppressive conditions such as infection with the human immunodeficiency virus (HIV) are at increased risk for candidal vaginitis. If a previously asymptomatic individual experiences a sudden increase in these infections, the physician should consider that such diseases may exist.

Candidal vaginitis will occur in approximately 25%–70% of women after antibiotic therapy (11, 12, 13). Postantibiotic candidiasis has been reported with almost all systemically absorbed antimicrobial agents, with broad-spectrum antibiotics suspected to have the greatest effect. Most physicians are aware of this relationship but often overlook it. Therefore, patients should be counseled about the possibility of the development of candidal symptoms after the use of any antibiotic.

Diagnosis

Diagnosing an acute vulvovaginal candidiasis begins with a history focused on the duration, description, and factors related to the onset of symptoms. Candidal infections can occur with specific vulvar or vaginal symptoms and sometimes both. The most common symptom is pruritus. Vulvar burning may be noted, and this can be exacerbated with micturition or sexual intercourse. Also common is an increase or change in consistency of the vaginal discharge.

On physical examination, candidal vaginitis most often includes a nonmalodorous, thick, adherent, white vaginal discharge that appears "cottage cheese-like." Variations in the thickness, color, and odor of the discharge can occur, but care should be taken to rule out coexisting vaginal infections.

Often, the vagina is found to be hyperemic and edematous. Vulvar signs are similar, although erythema and excoriations may be present due to scratching or contact irritation.

The normal pH level is not usually altered with uncomplicated candidal vaginitis. Microscopic examination of vaginal discharge diluted with saline (wet-mount) and 10% KOH preparations will reveal hyphal forms or budding yeast cells in approximately 50%–70% of individuals with yeast infections (14, 15). Some yeast infections are not detected by direct microscopy because of several factors: there are relatively few numbers of organisms, the presence of nonalbicans species tend not to form pseudohyphae, and preparation and technique are inadequate. Confirmation of candidal vaginitis by culture is not recommended because of the specificity of the symptoms and the relatively inexpensive cost of microscopic screening.

Cytologic diagnosis of the presence of yeast has been reported to correlate with culture-confirmed studies in approximately 80% of cases (16). Clinical correlation is necessary to establish that infection, rather than colonization, exists because positive test results do not always indicate infection is present.

The growing use of over-the-counter (OTC) nonspecific and antifungal agents can result in confusing symptoms. The use of OTC antifungal agents may mask another cause of vaginitis or select for resistant yeast. Therefore, patients should be asked to discontinue use of OTC medications 72 hours before examination. In these cases, obtaining a culture for yeast may be helpful.

Patients often call their physicians to request prescriptions for antifungal agents. However, because of the inaccuracies of self-diagnosis, patients should be encouraged to come to the office for examination. This is especially important if self-treatment with OTC antifungal agents has not been effective, in which case the risk of misdiagnosis is high.

Recurrent infections always should be evaluated to confirm the presence of candidal infections. Cultures are helpful in determining, first, whether yeast is truly present and, second, whether a noncandidal and difficult-to-treat species is present. Repeated positive cultures of *C. albicans* suggest reinfection, not resistance. In these instances, the source of the reinfection needs to be ascertained (eg, gastrointestinal reservoir, sexual transmission).

Treatment

Uncomplicated, acute candidal infections can now be treated initially with one of a variety of products (Table 1). There is little evidence that patients who are asymptomatic but have evidence of yeast on a Pap test benefit from routine treatment.

Most *C. albicans* isolates are susceptible to either clotrimazole or miconazole. An increasing number of nonalbicans species are now being recognized in patients with vulvovaginitis, however (17). These nonalbicans species (for example, *Candida tropicalis* and *Torulopsis glabrata,* also known as *Candida glabrata*) may be resistant to several of the OTC antifungal agents and may require the use of prescription antifungal agents.

In vitro susceptibility testing is poorly standardized and difficult to correlate with in vivo vaginal antifungal efficacy. Greater in vitro or in vivo activity has been achieved using terconazole, butoconazole, tioconazole, ketoconazole, and fluconazole. Oral ketoconazole and fluconazole are effective treatment of vulvovaginal infections; however, only fluconazole currently is approved by the U.S. Food and Drug Administration for this use. Ketoconazole regimens of 200-mg oral tablets twice daily for 5 days, as well as 100-mg to 200-mg daily for 6 months, have been effective in treating resistant and recurrent candidal infections (18, 19). Their effectiveness is believed to be due to the elimination of the rectal reservoir of yeast. Ketoconazole and fluconazole cause significant liver toxicity and should be used with caution in patients with altered liver function tests. However, fluconazole appears to present a much lower risk of liver toxicity. Resistant infections also may respond to vaginal use of boric acid, 600 mg in size 0 gelatin capsules daily for 14 days.

Treatment of male partners is usually not necessary but may be considered if the partner has symptoms of yeast balanitis or is uncircumcised. Under these conditions, a reservoir of yeast in the man may serve as a source of reinfection of the woman.

Bacterial Vaginosis

The terminology for bacterial infections of the vagina has undergone several changes. In 1955, Gardner and Dukes described a clinical condition, originally termed *nonspecific vaginitis*, that they believed was caused by the organism *Haemophilus vaginalis* (20). The name *H. vaginalis* was later changed to *Corynebacterium vaginalis* in 1963 and again changed to *Gardnerella vaginalis,* in honor of Dr. Herman Gardner, in 1980. The name *G. vaginalis* vaginitis was used for almost a decade until several investigations showed that a variety of organisms

TABLE 1. FDA-APPROVED ANTIFUNGAL MEDICATIONS

Medication	How Supplied	Dosage
Prescription		
Oral agents		
Fluconazole	150-mg tablet	1 tablet orally 1 time
Topical agents		
Butoconazole	2% vaginal cream (5 g)	Nonpregnant: 1 applicatorful at bedtime for 3 days Pregnant: 1 applicatorful at bedtime for 6 days (2nd or 3rd trimester only)
Clotrimazole	100-mg tablet	1 tablet vaginally at bedtime for 7 days
	500-mg tablet	1 tablet vaginally 1 time
	1% vaginal cream	1 applicatorful at bedtime for 7 days
Miconazole suppositories	200-mg vaginal	1 suppository vaginally at bedtime for 3 days
Tioconazole	6.5% ointment (4.6 g)	1 applicatorful vaginally 1 time
Terconazole	0.8% cream (5 g)	1 applicatorful vaginally at bedtime for 3 days
	80-mg vaginal suppositories	1 suppository vaginally at bedtime for 3 days
Over-the-Counter		
Clotrimazole	1% vaginal cream (5 g)	1 applicatorful at bedtime for 7–14 days
	100-mg vaginal tablets	1 tablet vaginally at bedtime for 7–14 days
Miconazole	2% cream (5 g)	1 applicatorful vaginally at bedtime for 7 days
	100-mg vaginal suppository	1 suppository vaginally at bedtime for 7 days

appear to be associated with the condition. Thus, the name *bacterial vaginosis* has been introduced to describe the presence of an overgrowth of several bacterial species and the frequent absence of inflammatory cells. Although several new terms have been introduced to include the presence of leukocytes in the syndrome, such as *bacterial vaginitis* (21) and *vaginitis of undetermined etiology* (22), the term bacterial vaginosis has had the greatest use.

Bacterial vaginosis has been found in 10%–25% of patients in general gynecologic and obstetric clinics and in up to 64% of patients visiting STD clinics (23, 24, 25). Among women with bacterial vaginosis, 50% are asymptomatic (23).

Examination

Examination for bacterial vaginosis should include a detailed history, characterization of any discharge, and determination of the pH level. Women with symptomatic bacterial vaginosis have a malodorous fishy vaginal discharge. The odor, a result of metabolic by-products produced primarily by anaerobic bacteria, is exacerbated during menses and following intercourse due to the alkaline nature of blood and semen. The vaginal discharge is thin, dark or dull grey, and homogeneous. Vulvar pruritus is not a common feature of bacterial vaginosis but may be present if the discharge is profuse.

A whiff test should be performed. A wet-mount test can be performed to detect clue cells and to ascertain the makeup of the vaginal flora. An abundance of bacteria of various morphologies and the absence or decrease of homogeneous bacilli (presumed lactobacilli) is consistent with a diagnosis of bacterial vaginosis. There is a concomitant overgrowth of *Bacteroides* species, *Peptostreptococcus* species, *G. vaginalis*, *Mycoplasma hominis*, and members of the Enterobacteriaceae. The numbers of bacteria increase from 100-fold to 1,000-fold.

The diagnosis is made by finding three of the four signs outlined in the box. Using these criteria, more than 90% of patients with bacterial vaginosis will be diagnosed correctly, and the number of false-positive diagnoses will be less than 10% (26, 27). Pap tests cannot accurately identify *G. vaginalis*. Cultures of the vaginal bacteria are usually not necessary unless the discharge is recalcitrant to treatment, fungal and trichomonal etiologies have been ruled out, and overgrowth of a specific facultative organism is suspected.

Treatment

Treatment of bacterial vaginosis is focused on antimicrobial agents with anaerobic activity. Two topical (intravaginal) regimens are available: 0.75% metronidazole gel applied twice daily to the vagina for 5 days and 2% clindamycin cream applied daily for 7 days (28, 29). Oral regimens of these two antimicrobial agents appear to be equally as effective as the topical regimens.

Several 7-day regimens of oral metronidazole have shown greater than 90% efficacy, including dosages of 500 mg twice daily or 250 mg three times daily. Recently, a single 2-g dose has been demonstrated to be adequate and is listed as one of the appropriate treatment regimens in the guidelines provided by the Centers for Disease Control and Prevention (30). However, the single-dose regimen may be slightly less effective (69–72%) (31, 32, 33), and the single high dose may lead to greater gastrointestinal upset (34). Patient counseling must emphasize that all alcohol products should be avoided with any metronidazole regimen because profuse nausea and vomiting (disulfiram reaction) may occur. Oral clindamycin at a dosage of 300 mg twice daily for 7 days also appears to be effective but may be associated with a higher incidence of diarrhea.

Treatment of the partner remains controversial. Despite evidence that bacterial vaginosis is significantly more prevalent in sexually active patients and those with other concurrent STDs, most studies have not demonstrated an improved cure rate or lower reinfection rate with treatment of the partner with the first episode (35). However, if the patient has repeated episodes of bacterial vaginosis, treatment of her partner with an oral regimen may be helpful (36). Also, because the genital flora of men with female partners with bacterial vaginosis has been noted to harbor similar microorganisms, some investigators recommend that the couple abstain from intercourse or that the man wear a condom during intercourse while the woman completes her treatment regimen. However, few clinical data support the efficacy of this practice. Patients with recurrent episodes of bacterial vaginosis should also be screened for gonorrhea and chlamydial infection. If either of these conditions is present, the patient should also be tested for syphilis, hepatitis B, and HIV infection.

Treatment in Pregnancy

In the past, ampicillin was recommended for use in early pregnancy, with metronidazole reserved for failures or treatment in the later trimesters. It should be noted, however, that ampicillin is largely ineffective. Because recent data suggest that bacterial vaginosis is associated with maternal and fetal complications (37, 38, 39, 6), more efficacious therapy may be warranted. Therefore, in pregnancy, clindamycin should be considered, either intravaginally as a daily application of 2% cream or orally, 300 mg twice daily for 7 days. After the first trimester, oral or topical therapy with metronidazole would also be acceptable alternatives.

Association with Other Disorders

Recently, a variety of complications have been associated with bacterial vaginosis. These include pelvic inflammatory disease, posthysterectomy vaginal cuff cellulitis, postabortal infection, preterm delivery, premature rupture of membranes, amnionitis, chorioamnionitis, and postpartum endometritis (37, 38, 39, 6, 40, 41, 42, 43, 44). The effectiveness of bacterial vaginosis treatment in preventing these conditions remains unclear.

Trichomonas Vaginalis

Trichomoniasis causes approximately 25% of vulvovaginal infections. These infections have a wide range of symptoms, and 20%–50% of women with the organism are asymptomatic (45). Trichomoniasis is predominantly transmitted sexually. If questions about the patient's sexual practices reveal that she is at high risk for other STDs, a thorough evaluation for STDs should be performed. Transmission by fomites has been suspected. However, the infrequent nature of nonsexual transmission should alert the physician to the possibility of sexual abuse if trichomoniasis is diagnosed in a child.

Diagnosis

Symptomatic women most often have a copious, yellow-gray or green homogeneous discharge. They may also describe a foul odor, vulvovaginal irritation, and, occasionally, dysuria. The pH level is usually greater than 4.5. Frothy discharge is present in less than 35% of infected patients, and punctate lesions, or "strawberry cervix," are seen in less than 25% of cases (20, 45).

The diagnosis of trichomonal infection is made by examining a fresh wet-mount preparation for mobile, flagellated organisms. An abundance of leukocytes usually is also seen. Culture diagnosis studies suggest that 70% of trichomonal infections can be detected by Pap test. Approximately 75% of trichomonal infections can be detected by wet-mount examination. Cultures should be performed when a persistent leukocytic vaginal discharge is reported. If a documented trichomonal infection is recalcitrant to metronidazole therapy, cultures may be necessary to obtain the organism for sensitivity testing.

Occasionally, the diagnosis is determined based on the results of a Pap test without use of a wet-mount examination. Approximately 65% of cases will be interpreted as positive on the basis of Pap tests (46, 47). If the patient has not received antitrichomonad therapy for another indication, or if the patient reports symptoms of vaginitis, metronidazole treatment should be considered.

Treatment

The accepted treatment regimen for trichomoniasis is a single oral 2-g dose of metronidazole. Sexual partners must be treated simultaneously for treatment to be effective. Less than 10% of patients experience nausea and vomiting with the 2-g dose. An alternative regimen is 500 mg orally twice daily for 7 days.

If patients are compliant but develop recurrent infections, treatment of their sexual partners should be confirmed. Resistant trichomonal infections are rare; however, in patients with documented persistent infection despite compliance with treatment by the patient and her partner(s), a resistant trichomonad strain should be considered. The treatment of resistant trichomoniasis has not been established, but may require high dosages of metronidazole (more than 2.5 g/d), often combined with intravaginal metronidazole suppositories prepared by a pharmacist (500 mg once or twice daily) for at least 10 days. Metronidazole may also be given intravenously, which often requires hospitalization (48). Other causes for treatment failure include poor metronidazole absorption or delivery and interference by other drugs. In such cases, 500-mg doses of intravenous metronidazole every 8 hours are effective (49). Commercial preparations of currently available metronidazole gel have not been found to be effective either alone or in combination with oral therapy. Although metronidazole has been shown to be carcinogenic in mice at high doses, this effect has not been found in humans or other animal species.

Treatment in Pregnancy

The use of metronidazole is contraindicated during the first trimester of pregnancy. Patients may be treated after the first trimester with metronidazole in a single 2-g oral dose (30). One study reported a 48% cure rate of *T. vaginalis* with clotrimazole (50); however, clotrimazole is not approved by the U.S. Food and Drug Administration for this indication.

Other Conditions

Estrogen deficiency results in a thinning of vaginal epithelial mucosa. Some patients with thin epithelium develop vaginal dryness and burning, which is referred to as atrophic vaginitis. This can be treated with systemic or local estrogen. Daily doses of 0.625 mg oral or topical estrogen preparation should provide relief. Other regimens include:

- 0.01% estradiol vaginal cream: 2–4 g daily for 1–2 weeks, then decrease by 50% for 1–2 weeks; maintenance dosage is 1 g one to three times weekly
- Conjugated estrogen vaginal cream: 2–4 g daily (3 weeks on, 1 week off) for 3–6 months
- 0.01% dienestrol cream: One to two applicators full for 1–2 weeks, then decrease dosage and provide maintenance dosage similar to regimen for estradiol vaginal cream

Patients who cannot take estrogen may benefit from use of a lubricant. If hormonal therapy does not reduce symptoms, another cause should be investigated. Any postmenopausal patient with pruritus should have a vulvar biopsy of the affected area if symptoms persist after adequate antifungal treatment or if a yeast infection cannot be confirmed.

REFERENCES

1. McCue JD. Evaluation and management of vaginitis. An update for primary care practitioners. Arch Intern Med 1989;149:565–568
2. Hammill HA. Normal vaginal flora in relation to vaginitis. Obstet Gynecol Clin North Am 1989;16: 329–336
3. Mårdh P-A. The vaginal ecosystem. Am J Obstet Gynecol 1991;165:1163–1168
4. Skarin A, Sylwan F. Vaginal lactobacilli inhibiting growth of *Gardnerella vaginalis, Mobiluncus* and other bacterial species cultured from vaginal content of women with bacterial vaginosis. Acta Pathol Microbiol Immunol Scand 1986;94:399–403
5. Peeters M, Piot P. Adhesion of *Gardnerella vaginalis* to vaginal epithelial cells: variables affecting adhesion and inhibition by metronidazole. Genitourin Med 1985;61: 391–395
6. Gravett MG, Hummel D, Eschenbach DA, Holmes KK. Preterm labor associated with subclinical amniotic fluid infection and with bacterial vaginosis. Obstet Gynecol 1986;67:229–237
7. Minkoff H, Grunebaum AN, Schwarz RH, Feldman J, Cummings M, Crombleholme W, et al. Risk factors for prematurity and premature rupture of membranes: a prospective study of the vaginal flora in pregnancy. Am J Obstet Gynecol 1984; 150:965–972
8. Bobitt JR, Damato JD, Sakakini J Jr. Perinatal complications in group B streptococcal carriers: a longitudinal study of prenatal patients. Am J Obstet Gynecol 1985;151:711–717
9. Watts DH, Eschenbach DA, Kenny GE. Early postpartum endometritis: the role of bacteria, genital mycoplasmas, and *chlamydia trachomatis*. Obstet Gynecol 1989; 73:52–60
10. Faro S, Phillips LE, Martens MG. Perspectives on the bacteriology of postoperative obstetric–gynecologic infections. Am J Obstet Gynecol 1988;158: 694–700
11. O'Connor MI, Sobel JD. Epidemiology of recurrent vulvovaginal candidiasis: identification and strain differentiation of *Candida albicans*. J Infect Dis 1986;154: 358–363

12. Oriel JD, Waterworth PM. Effect of minocycline and tetracycline on the vaginal yeast flora. J Clin Pathol 1975;28: 403–406

13. Odds FC, ed. Iatrogenic factors that predispose to candidosis. In: Candida and candidosis. 2nd ed. London: Bailliere Tindall, 1988:104–114

14. Oriel JD, Partridge BM, Denny MJ, Coleman JC. Genital yeast infections. BMJ 1972;4:761–764

15. Pattman RS, Sprott MS, Moss TR. Evaluation of a culture slide in the diagnosis of vaginal candidosis. Br J Vener Dis 1981;57:67–69

16. Siapco BJ, Kaplan BJ, Bernstein GS, Moyer DL. Cytodiagnosis of Candida organisms in cervical smears. Acta Cytol 1986;30:477–480

17. Spinillo A, Pizzoli G, Colonna L, Nicola S, DeSeta F, Guaschino S. Epidemiologic characteristics of women with idiopathic recurrent vulvovaginal candidiasis. Obstet Gynecol 1993;81:721–727

18. Van Der Pas H, Peeters F, Janssens D, Snauwert E, Van Custem J. Treatment of vaginal candidosis with oral ketoconazole. Eur J Obstet Gynecol Reprod Biol 1983; 14:399–404

19. Sobel JD. Management of recurrent vulvovaginal candidiasis with intermittent ketoconazole prophylaxis. Obstet Gynecol 1985;65:435–440

20. Gardner HL, Dukes CD. *Haemophilus vaginalis* vaginitis. A newly defined specific infection previously classified "nonspecific" vaginitis. Am J Obstet Gynecol 1955;69: 962–976

21. Martens MG. Vulvovaginitis. In: Rakel RE, ed. Conn's current therapy. Philadelphia: WB Saunders and Co, 1993:1065–1069

22. Faro S, Phillips LE. Nonspecific vaginitis or vaginitis of undetermined aetiology. Int J Tiss Reac 1987;9:173–177

23. Eschenbach DA, Hillier S, Critchlow C, Stevens C, DeRouen T, Holmes KK. Diagnosis and clinical manifestations of bacterial vaginosis. Am J Obstet Gynecol 1988;158:819–828

24. Embree J, Caliando JJ, McCormack WM. Nonspecific vaginitis among women attending a sexually transmitted diseases clinic. Sex Transm Dis 1984;11:81–84

25. Hallén A, Påhlson C, Forsum U. Bacterial vaginosis in women attending STD clinics: diagnostic criteria and prevalence of *Mobiluncus* spp. Genitourin Med 1987;63: 386–389

26. Amsel R, Totten PA, Spiegel CA, Chen KCS, Eschenbach DA, Holmes KK. Nonspecific vaginitis. Diagnostic criteria and microbial and epidemiologic associations. Am J Med 1983;74:14–22

27. Thomason JL, Gelbart SM, Anderson RJ, Walt AK, Osypowski PJ, Broekhuizen FF. Statistical evaluation of diagnostic criteria for bacterial vaginosis. Am J Obstet Gynecol 1990;162:155–160

28. Hillier SL, Lipinski C, Briselden AM, Eschenbach DA. Efficacy of intravaginal 0.75% metronidazole gel for the treatment of bacterial vaginosis. Obstet Gynecol 1993; 81:963–967

29. Hillier S, Krohn MA, Watts DH, Wolner-Hanssen P, Eschenbach D. Microbiologic efficacy of intravaginal clindamycin cream for the treatment of bacterial vaginosis. Obstet Gynecol 1990;76:407–413

30. Centers for Disease Control and Prevention. 1993 Sexually transmitted diseases guidelines. MMWR 1993;42 (RR-14):1–102

31. Eschenbach DA, Critchlow CW, Watkins H, Smith K, Spiegel CA, Chen KCS, et al. A dose-duration study of metronidazole for the treatment of nonspecific vaginosis. Scand J Infect Dis 1983;Suppl 40:73–80

32. Swedberg J, Steiner JF, Deiss F, Steiner S, Driggers DA. Comparison of single-dose vs one-week course of metronidazole for symptomatic bacterial vaginosis. JAMA 1985; 254:1046–1049

33. Lugo-Miro VI, Green M, Mazur L. Comparison of different metronidazole therapeutic regimens for bacterial vaginosis. A meta-analysis. JAMA 1992;268: 92–95

34. Hager WD, Brown ST, Kraus SJ, Kleris GS, Perkins GJ, Henderson M. Metronidazole for vaginal trichomoniasis: Seven-day vs single-dose regimens. JAMA 1980;244: 1219–1220

35. Holmes KK. Lower genital tract infections in women: cystitis/urethritis, vulvovaginitis, and cervicitis. In: Holmes KK, Mårdh PA, Sparling PF, Wiesner PJ, eds. Sexually transmitted diseases. 2nd ed. New York, New York: McGraw Hill, 1990: 527–545

36. Pheifer TA, Forsyth PS, Durfee MA, Pollock HM, Holmes KK. Nonspecific vaginitis: role of *Haemophilus vaginalis* and treatment with metronidazole. N Engl J Med 1978; 298:1429–1434

37. Martius J, Krohn MA, Hillier SL, Stamm WE, Holmes KK, Eschenbach DA. Relationships of vaginal *Lactobacillus* species, cervical *Chlamydia trachomatis*, and bacterial vaginosis to preterm birth. Obstet Gynecol 1988;71:89–95

38. Gravett MG, Nelson HP, DeRouen T, Critchlow C, Eschenbach DA, Holmes KK. Independent associations of bacterial vaginosis and *Chlamydia trachomatis* infection with adverse pregnancy outcome. JAMA 1986;256: 1899–1903

39. Hill LVH, Luther ER, Young D, Pereira L, Embil JA. Prevalence of lower genital tract infections in pregnancy. Sex Transm Dis 1988;15:5–10

40. Soper DE, Bump RC, Hurt WG. Bacterial vaginosis and trichomoniasis vaginitis are risk factors for cuff cellulitis after abdominal hysterectomy. Am J Obstet Gynecol 1990;163:1016–1023

41. Larsson P-G, Platz-Christensen J-J, Forsum U, Påhlson C. Clue cells in predicting infections after abdominal hysterectomy. Obstet Gynecol 1991;77: 450–452

42. Osser S, Persson K. Postabortal pelvic infection associated with *Chlamydia trachomatis* and the influence of humoral immunity. Am J Obstet Gynecol 1984;150:699–703

43. Qvigstad E, Skaug K, Jerve F, Fylling P, Ulstrup JC. Pelvic inflammatory disease associated with Chlamydia trachomatis infection after therapeutic abortion. Br J Vener Dis 1983;59:189–192

44. Larsson P-G, Platz-Christensen J-J, Thejls H, Forsum U, Påhlson C. Incidence of pelvic inflammatory disease after first-trimester legal abortion in women with bacterial vaginosis after treatment with metronidazole: a double-blind, randomized study. Am J Obstet Gynecol 1992;166:100–103

45. McLellan R, Spence MR, Brockman M, Raffel L, Smith JL. The clinical diagnosis of trichomoniasis. Obstet Gynecol 1982;60:30–34

46. Krieger JN, Tam MR, Stevens CE, Nielsen IO, Hale J, Kiviat NB, et al. Diagnosis of trichomoniasis. Comparison of conventional wet-mount examination with cytologic studies, cultures, and monoclonal antibody staining of direct specimens. JAMA 1988;259:1223–1227

47. Clay JC, Veeravahu M, Smyth RW. Practical problems of diagnosing trichomoniasis in women. Genitourin Med 1988;64:115–117

48. Lossick JG, Müller M, Gorell TE. In vitro drug susceptibility and doses of metronidazole required for cure in cases of refractory vaginal trichomoniasis. J Infect Dis 1986;153: 948–955

49. Larsen B, Wilson AH, Glover DD, Charles D. Implications of metronidazole pharmacodynamics for therapy of trichomoniasis. Gynecol Obstet Invest 1986;21:12–18

50. Schnell JD. The incidence of vaginal candida and trichomonas infections and treatment of trichomonas vaginalis with clotrimazole. Postgrad Med J 1974;July Suppl: 79–81

This Technical Bulletin was developed under the direction of the Committee on Technical Bulletins of the American College of Obstetricians and Gynecologists as an educational aid to obstetricians and gynecologists. The committee wishes to thank Mark G. Martens, MD, for his assistance in the development of this bulletin. This Technical Bulletin does not define a standard of care, nor is it intended to dictate an exclusive course of management. It presents recognized methods and techniques of clinical practice for consideration by obstetrician–gynecologists for incorporation into their practices. Variations of practice taking into account the needs of the individual patient, resources, and limitations unique to the institution or type of practice may be appropriate.

ISSN 1074-8628

THE AMERICAN COLLEGE OF OBSTETRICIANS AND GYNECOLOGISTS
409 12th Street, SW
Washington, DC 20024-2188

12345/09876

ACOG EDUCATIONAL BULLETIN

Number 248, July 1998

Viral Hepatitis in Pregnancy

Viral hepatitis is one of the most serious infections that can occur in pregnant women. Six different forms of viral hepatitis have now been defined. This bulletin describes the various types of hepatitis, their implications during pregnancy, the risk of perinatal transmission, and treatment.

Etiology, Epidemiology, and Natural History

Hepatitis A

In the United States, approximately one third of cases of acute hepatitis are caused by hepatitis A virus. The virus usually is transmitted by person-to-person contact through fecal–oral contamination. Poor hygiene, poor sanitation, and intimate personal or sexual contact facilitate transmission. Epidemics frequently result from exposure to contaminated food and water. In obstetric populations in the United States, the patients at greatest risk for hepatitis A infection are those who recently have emigrated from, or traveled to, developing nations where hepatitis A is endemic, particularly in Southeast Asia, Africa, Central America, Greenland, Mexico, and the Middle East. In the United States, the incidence of acute hepatitis A in pregnancy is approximately 1/1,000.

Hepatitis A is caused by an RNA virus. Its incubation period ranges from 15 to 50 days; the mean is 28–30 days. Feces contain the highest concentration of virus particles, and virus excretion reaches its maximum late in the incubation period and early in the prodromal phase of the illness. The duration of viremia is short, and the virus normally is not excreted in urine or other body fluids.

Serious complications of hepatitis A are uncommon. Among all acutely ill patients who require hospitalization, the overall fatality rate does not exceed 2/1,000 cases in the United States. A chronic carrier state of hepatitis A does not exist. In addition, perinatal transmission of the virus has not been demonstrated (1). Hepatitis A immune globulin is recommended for household contacts and contacts in day care centers and custodial institutions. It should be given as soon as possible after exposure; it is ineffective if given more than 2 weeks after exposure. A vaccine is available, which may be taken during pregnancy (2).

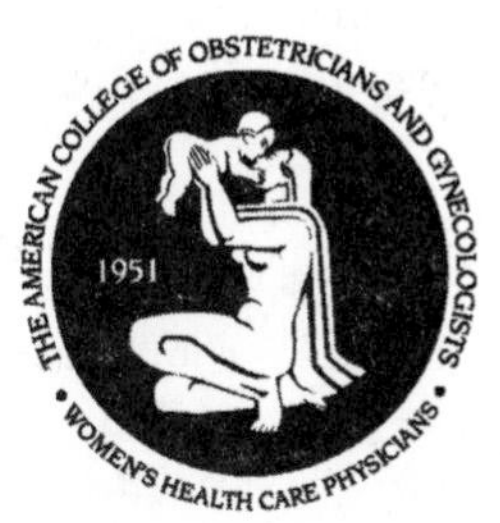

Replaces Number 174, November 1992

Hepatitis B

Hepatitis B is caused by a small DNA virus. The intact virus is termed the Dane particle. Hepatitis B virus contains three principal antigens. Hepatitis B surface antigen (HBsAg) is present on the surface of the virus and also circulates freely in the serum in spherical and filamentous forms. The middle portion of the Dane particle contains hepatitis B core antigen (HBcAg). The core antigen is present only in hepatocytes and does not circulate in the serum. Hepatitis B e antigen (HBeAg) is encoded by the same portion of the viral genome that codes for the core antigen. The presence of HBeAg indicates an extremely high viral inoculum and active virus replication (1, 3).

Hepatitis B infection occurs throughout the world. In the United States, it is responsible for 40–45% of all cases of hepatitis. Approximately 300,000 new cases of hepatitis B occur annually, and more than 1 million Americans are chronic carriers. Acute hepatitis B occurs in 1–2/1,000 pregnancies. Chronic infection is present in 5–15/1,000 pregnancies (3, 4), but is more prevalent among certain ethnic groups (ie, Asians, Inuits).

Hepatitis B virus is transmitted by parenteral and sexual contact. Individuals at greatest risk of becoming infected are those who have multiple sexual partners, inject drugs percutaneously, or have sexual partners who engage in these risk-taking behaviors. Other important risk factors are receipt of blood products and household or institutional contact.

All blood donors are screened routinely for HBsAg. Thus, transmission of hepatitis B virus by transfusion of blood or blood products is rare (1). Drug addiction is an important risk factor for horizontal transmission of hepatitis B virus. Sexual contact is an efficient mechanism for spreading the virus. Approximately 25% of the regular sexual contacts of infected individuals will themselves become seropositive.

The mortality associated with acute hepatitis B is approximately 1%. Of patients who become infected, 85–90% experience complete resolution of their physical findings and develop protective levels of the antibody. The other 10–15% of patients become chronically infected; they continue to have detectable serum levels of HBsAg but are asymptomatic and have no biochemical evidence of hepatic dysfunction. In 15–30% of those chronically infected, viral replication continues and is manifested by persistence of the e antigen and active viral DNA synthesis. These individuals are at risk for the subsequent development of chronic or persistent hepatitis and cirrhosis, and approximately 4,000–5,000 die annually of complications of chronic liver disease (5, 6), including hepatocellular carcinoma.

Because hepatitis B virus is highly pathogenic and infectious, perinatal transmission of infection occurs with disturbing regularity. Approximately 10–20% of women who are seropositive for HBsAg transmit the virus to their neonates in the absence of immunoprophylaxis. In women who are seropositive for both HBsAg and HBeAg, the frequency of vertical transmission increases to approximately 90%.

In patients with acute hepatitis B, the frequency of vertical transmission also depends on the time during gestation that maternal infection occurs. When maternal infection occurs in the first trimester, up to 10% of neonates will be seropositive for HBsAg (1, 3). In women acutely infected in the third trimester, 80–90% of offspring will be infected (3).

Between 85% and 95% of cases of perinatal transmission of hepatitis B virus occur as a consequence of intrapartum exposure of the infant to contaminated blood and genital tract secretions. The remaining cases result from hematogenous transplacental dissemination, breastfeeding, and close postnatal contact between the infant and the infected parent. Infants of women who are HBsAg positive at the time of delivery should receive both hepatitis B immune globulin (HBIG) and hepatitis B vaccine within 12 hours of birth, followed by two more injections of hepatitis B vaccine in the first 6 months of life.

Hepatitis C

Hepatitis C virus (previously termed nonA, nonB hepatitis) is a single-stranded RNA virus that appears to infect as much as 0.6% of the pregnant population (7, 8). The principal risk factors for acquiring hepatitis C virus are the same as for hepatitis B.

Approximately 50% of patients with acute hepatitis C develop biochemical evidence of chronic liver disease. Of these individuals, at least 20% subsequently have chronic active hepatitis or cirrhosis. Vertical transmission has been well documented and is proportional in likelihood to the titer of hepatitis C virus RNA present in the mother's blood (7, 9). Approximately 7–8% of hepatitis C virus-positive women transmit hepatitis C virus to their offspring (7, 8). Vertical transmission of hepatitis C may be more likely if the mother also is infected with human immunodeficiency virus (HIV) (8, 10). Currently, no method has been found to prevent prenatal transmission. Many experts believe that hepatitis C virus-positive women should not breastfeed because there is a 2–3% risk of vertical transmission. Unlike hepatitis B, antibodies to hepatitis C are not protective.

Hepatitis D

Hepatitis D requires hepatitis B virus for replication and expression and so occurs only in people already infected with hepatitis B. In acute hepatitis B, once HBsAg clears the bloodstream, so does hepatitis D. Approximately 20–25% of chronic hepatitis B virus carriers ultimately are coinfected with hepatitis D virus (11, 12). In acute hepatitis D, immunoglobulin M (IgM) antibodies against hepatitis D predominate, whereas IgG antibodies may be found in chronic infections.

Chronic hepatitis D produces severe disease more often than other forms of chronic hepatitis. Of patients with chronic hepatitis D, 70–80% ultimately develop cirrhosis and portal hypertension, 15% of whom suffer an unusually rapid progression to cirrhosis within 2 years of the initial onset of acute illness. Mortality due to hepatic failure approaches 25% (11–13). In contrast, only 15–30% of patients with chronic hepatitis B virus infection develop cirrhosis and portal hypertension, and the disease progression typically is much slower.

Vertical transmission of hepatitis D virus has been documented. Transmission is uncommon, however, because the measures used to prevent perinatal infection with hepatitis B virus are almost uniformly effective in preventing infection by hepatitis D.

Hepatitis E

The epidemiologic features of hepatitis E are similar to those of hepatitis A. Although the disease has been reported only rarely in the United States, it is endemic in several developing nations, similar to those mentioned for hepatitis A. In these regions, maternal mortality often has been alarmingly high. In the 1980s, India and Burma reported 10–18% of pregnant women with hepatitis E died as a complication of their infection (14). Most of these women lived under conditions of extreme poverty. Women who have a higher standard of living and greater access to medical care are unlikely to have the same high rate of mortality.

Although acute hepatitis E can be a serious disease, it usually is self-limited and does not result in a chronic carrier state (14, 15). As with hepatitis A, hepatitis E is transmitted via contaminated food or water, though less efficiently. Vertical transmission of hepatitis E has been reported (16).

Hepatitis G

Hepatitis G infection is more likely in people already infected with hepatitis B or C or who have a history of intravenous drug use (17). In a study of 47 women infected with HIV or hepatitis C virus, 9 of whom also were infected with the hepatitis G virus, the risk of vertical transmission was higher for hepatitis G than it was for the other two agents (18). Hepatitis G probably does not cause chronic active hepatitis or cirrhosis.

Clinical Manifestations

The usual subjective symptoms in patients with acute viral hepatitis are malaise, fatigue, anorexia, nausea, and right upper quadrant or epigastric pain. Typical physical findings include jaundice, upper abdominal tenderness, and hepatomegaly, although many cases of hepatitis are anicteric. The patient's urine usually is darkened, and the stool may be acholic. In cases of fulminant hepatitis, signs of coagulopathy and encephalopathy may be evident.

In patients with hepatitis A or E, these clinical manifestations usually are temporally related to recent travel to an endemic area or exposure to an infected person. Similarly, hepatitis B, C, D, or G typically ensues after parenteral exposure to contaminated blood or sexual contact with an infected partner. The evolution of acute clinical illness in patients with hepatitis D often follows a biphasic course. In the initial phase of infection, patients with hepatitis D are indistinguishable from individuals with acute hepatitis B. Two to four weeks after apparent resolution of symptoms, patients have a relapse, which usually is of a milder nature and is associated with a second episode of elevation in serum transaminases. At this time serologic assays for hepatitis D virus usually are positive.

As noted previously, among those patients originally infected with hepatitis B, C, or D virus whose acute symptoms resolve, some become chronic carriers of viral antigens. The same may be true for hepatitis G, although a carrier state has yet to be identified. Although most viral hepatitis carriers initially are asymptomatic, up to one third subsequently develop chronic active or persistent hepatitis or cirrhosis. Once cirrhosis ensues, patients demonstrate the typical signs of end-stage liver disease, such as jaundice, muscle wasting, ascites, spider angioma, palmar erythema, and, ultimately, hepatic encephalopathy. Hepatitis C is probably the leading cause of hepatocellular carcinoma in the United States, whereas hepatitis B virus is the leading cause worldwide.

Diagnosis

Jaundice, a primary symptom of hepatitis infection, also occurs with numerous other disorders. The principal disorders that should be considered in the differential diagnosis of jaundice in pregnancy are shown in Table 1. Testing strategies should be directed toward discriminating among clinically likely diagnoses.

General Tests

Coincident with the onset of symptoms, patients with acute hepatitis usually have a marked increase in the serum concentration of alanine aminotransferase (ALT, previously SGPT) and aspartate aminotransferase (AST, previously SGOT). In addition, the serum bilirubin concentration often is increased. In patients who are moderately to severely ill, coagulation abnormalities and hyperammonemia also may be present. Although liver

Table 1. Disorders to Consider in the Differential Diagnosis of Jaundice in Pregnancy

Condition	Distinguishing Characteristics
Viral hepatitis	Mild to marked elevation in serum transaminases Positive viral serology Prominent inflammatory infiltrate with hepatocellular disarray
Acute fatty liver of pregnancy	Minimal elevation in transaminases Little if any inflammatory infiltrate with prominent microvesicular fat deposition
Toxic injury	History of drug exposure (eg, tetracycline, isoniazid, erythromycin estolate, alpha methyldopa)
Cholestasis of pregnancy	Pruritus Elevation of bile salts Cholestasis with little inflammation
Severe preeclampsia	Hypertension, edema, proteinuria, oliguria Elevated blood urea nitrogen, creatinine, uric acid, transaminases, and lactate dehydrogenase Thrombocytopenia
Mononucleosis	Flulike illness Positive heterophile antibody Elevated transaminases
Cytomegalovirus (CMV) hepatitis	CMV antibodies Positive viral culture or polymerase chain reaction Elevated transaminases
Autoimmune hepatitis	Antinuclear antibodies, liver–kidney microsomal antibodies Elevated transaminases

biopsy is rarely indicated in pregnancy, viral hepatitis may be distinguished histologically from other causes of hepatic injury by its characteristic pattern of extensive hepatocellular injury and inflammatory infiltrate. Initial evaluation of the patient with suspected viral hepatitis should include tests for: anti-HA IgM, HBsAg, and HC PCR. In selected patients, additional testing can include anti-HBc IgM, HD PCR, anti-HE, and anti-HG.

Specific Tests

If hepatitis is suspected based on the initial evaluation and general tests, the type of virus is determined through laboratory analysis.

Hepatitis A

The diagnosis of acute hepatitis A is confirmed by detecting IgM antibodies to the virus. A chronic carrier state for this infection does not exist, but IgG antibodies to hepatitis A virus will persist in patients with previous exposure to the virus (1).

Hepatitis B

In the acute stage of hepatitis B virus infection, the diagnosis is confirmed by the identification of the surface antigen and the IgM antibody to the core antigen. The presence of e antigen is indicative of an exceptionally high viral inoculum and active virus replication, and implies a high degree of infectivity. Chronic hepatitis B virus infection is characterized by the persistence of the surface antigen in the liver and serum. The time of infection can be evaluated by measuring IgG and IgM antibodies to HBcAg. Typically, the IgG hepatitis B core antibody (HBcAb) appears 6 months or more after infection, with the IgM moiety being predominant prior to that time.

Occasionally patients with acute hepatitis B will demonstrate HBsAg only briefly and will develop anti-HBc (IgM) as their only marker of acute hepatitis B infection. Anti-HBc (IgM) may be helpful in HBsAg-negative patients in whom hepatitis B is strongly suspected (19).

Hepatitis C

The diagnosis of hepatitis C is confirmed by the identification of the antibody to hepatitis C virus. However, the antibody may not be present until 6–16 weeks after the onset of clinical illness. Hepatitis C viral RNA can be detected by polymerase chain reaction assay of serum soon after infection as well as in chronic disease.

Hepatitis D

Laboratory tests that may be used to confirm the diagnosis of acute hepatitis D are detection of D antigen in hepatic tissue or serum and identification of the IgM antibody to hepatitis D virus. D antigenemia usually persists in patients with chronic hepatitis D despite the appearance of the IgG antibody to the virus. Thus, as in hepatitis C and HIV infection, viremia and end-organ damage can continue despite the presence of the antibody to the virus (11, 12).

Hepatitis E and G

The diagnoses of infection with hepatitis E and hepatitis G are similar. In both cases, the infection is documented by the presence of virus-specific antibodies.

Management

General Supportive Measures

Patients with acute hepatitis should be hospitalized if they have encephalopathy, coagulopathy, or severe debilitation. Nutritional needs should be addressed within the context of the severity of the disease. Fluid and electrolyte abnormalities should be corrected. If a coagulopathy is present, administration of erythrocytes, platelets, and clotting factors such as fresh frozen plasma or cryoprecipitate may be necessary. Activity should be limited, and the patient should be protected from upper abdominal trauma.

Women who are less severely ill may be treated as outpatients. They should reduce their level of activity, avoid upper abdominal trauma, and maintain good nutrition as well. Infected women also should avoid intimate contact with household members and sexual partners until these individuals receive appropriate prophylaxis outlined as follows.

Specific Immunotherapy

Hepatitis A

Currently, no antiviral agent is available for treatment of acute hepatitis A. An inactivated-virus vaccine that is safe in pregnancy is available. Women at risk for infection with hepatitis A, such as those traveling to endemic areas, should be vaccinated (2).

Patients who have close personal or sexual contact with an individual who has hepatitis A should receive immune globulin if they have not been immunized. Immune globulin does not pose a risk to either a pregnant woman or her fetus, and therefore the preparation should be administered during pregnancy if indicated. For post-exposure prophylaxis, a single intramuscular dose of 1 mL should be administered as soon as possible after contact with the infected individual. Administration of immune globulin more than 2 weeks after exposure is not effective in preventing or ameliorating the severity of hepatitis A (1).

Hepatitis B

Although interferon alfa has been shown to alter the natural history of acute hepatitis B, C, and D virus infection, it has multiple side effects including myelosuppression, autoantibody formation, thyroid disturbances, and possible cardiotoxicity. Interferon alfa should be avoided during pregnancy because of its possible abortifacient effects. Accordingly, prevention of infection is of paramount importance. Specific immunotherapy with hepatitis B immune globulin (HBIG) has been effective (20).

Vaccination. Individuals who have risk factors should be vaccinated against infection. In general, it is cost-effective to screen for the antibody to hepatitis B virus in women who belong to groups with a high risk of infection. In most other risk groups, antibody screening prior to vaccination is probably not indicated.

Two vaccines for hepatitis B virus, Recombivax HB and Engerix-B, have been developed. The original vaccine (Heptavax-B), licensed in 1982 but not currently available, was prepared by purification of surface antigen extracted from the serum of hepatitis B virus carriers. Because of concerns, later disproven, that this vaccine might transmit HIV infection, many individuals who were appropriate candidates for the vaccine refused to receive it. Currently available vaccines prepared from yeast cultures by using recombinant DNA technology clearly pose no risk of transmission of HIV infection. They are highly immunogenic and result in seroconversion in more than 95% of recipients (1).

The vaccine should be administered into the deltoid muscle. Intragluteal and intradermal injections result in lower rates of seroconversion. Pregnancy is not a contraindication to vaccination. In fact, susceptible pregnant women who are at risk for hepatitis B infection should be specifically targeted for vaccination.

Individuals who have been exposed to hepatitis B virus before they are vaccinated should receive passive immunization with HBIG and undergo the immunization series—preferably in the contralateral arm. Hepatitis B immune globulin is prepared from pooled plasma that has an HBsAg antibody titer of at least 1/100,000, as determined by radioimmunoassay. The preparation is administered intramuscularly in a dose of 0.06 mL/kg. When exposure has occurred as a result of sexual contact, the patient should receive a single dose of HBIG within 14 days of contact. For prophylaxis after percutaneous or mucous membrane injury, treatment should include an initial injection of HBIG, followed by a second dose 1 month later. These regimens are approximately 75% effective in preventing hepatitis B virus infection. If an antibody response is documented, clinical hepatitis B virus infection is rare (1). However, because of the high rate of usually conferred protection, evaluation of immune status at any interval is not deemed necessary (1). Human immunodeficiency virus infection has not been transmitted by HBIG. In addition, pregnancy is not a contraindication to administration of HBIG (1).

Perinatal Management. The combination of passive and active immunization, as outlined here, has been particularly effective in reducing the frequency of perinatal transmission of hepatitis B virus. Several investigations conducted in Asian nations have shown that passive and active immunization of the newborn is 85–95% effective in preventing perinatal transmission of hepatitis B virus.

The Centers for Disease Control and Prevention and the American College of Obstetricians and Gynecologists recommend hepatitis B virus screening for all pregnant women. Pregnant women should be routinely tested for HBsAg during an early prenatal visit. If, at the time of admission to the hospital for delivery, the test has not been performed or the results are not available, the HBsAg test should be done. Women in high-risk groups who initially test negative for hepatitis B virus should be targeted for vaccination if they have not been vaccinated previously. Seropositive women should be encouraged to inform their children and sexual partners of the need for testing and vaccination. Serum transaminases should be measured in seropositive women to detect biochemical evidence of chronic active hepatitis. If the test results are abnormal or if the liver is palpable, the patient should be evaluated further to determine whether the disease is acute or chronic.

The Centers for Disease Control and Prevention recommends universal active immunization of all infants born in the United States (6). The immunization schedule for infants of women who have been screened and are negative should be started preferably before discharge, but by no later than 2 months of age. Infants of women who are known to be HBsAg positive or whose status is unknown should have both passive and active immunization treatment. It should be given simultaneously at different sites intramuscularly and started within 12 hours after birth. Such a strategy will prevent postnatal and neonatal acquisition of hepatitis B virus in most cases. The physician responsible for the care of a newborn delivered to a mother with chronic hepatitis B should be informed of the mother's carrier status so that the appropriate doses of hepatitis B virus vaccine and HBIG can be given as soon as possible following delivery.

Hepatitis C and D

Treatment with interferon alfa produced clinical improvement in 28–46% of patients with chronic hepatitis C. Unfortunately, however, approximately 50% of patients who initially improved suffered a relapse within 6 months of the cessation of therapy. In addition, pregnant women were specifically excluded from the investigation (21). Similar results are seen with hepatitis D.

Precautions for Health Care Workers

Each year, approximately 12,000 health care workers in the United States contract hepatitis B virus infection as a result of an occupational injury. Of these individuals, about 200 experience a fulminant course and die. Another 1,000–1,200 become chronic carriers of the surface antigen (22).

The principal mechanism of transmission of hepatitis B virus from patient to health care worker is through injury from a sharp object, such as a needle or scalpel, that is contaminated with infected blood. Of the individuals exposed in these ways, 10–20% subsequently become seropositive for HBsAg. Although most remain asymptomatic, they are still at increased risk for development of chronic liver disease (1, 22). Another important, but less frequent, mechanism of transmission is a splash injury, resulting in contact between skin or mucosal surfaces and contaminated secretions or blood.

Physicians and other health care workers should use standard precautions to reduce their risk of acquiring hepatitis B virus infection (23). The primary element of universal precautions is the use of appropriate barrier precautions by all health care personnel to prevent the exposure of their skin and mucous membranes to the blood or other body fluids of any patient. Most important, all health care workers who may have direct or indirect exposure to patients should be immunized.

Reports have been published documenting transmission of hepatitis B from infected health care workers, including obstetrician–gynecologists, to patients during invasive procedures (24). In each instance in which complete serologic testing has been performed, the health care workers were seropositive for both surface and e antigens.

Summary

Hepatitis A is an uncommon complication of pregnancy and is not associated with perinatal transmission. In contrast, hepatitis B virus infection is more common and clearly poses a serious risk to the household contacts and neonates of infected mothers. Accordingly, all pregnant women should be tested for hepatitis B virus. Universal vaccination of all neonates with hepatitis B vaccine is now recommended. Infants delivered to HBsAg seropositive mothers also should receive HBIG and vaccination immediately after birth. Hepatitis E is extremely rare in the United States and is quite similar to hepatitis A, although perinatal transmission does occur with hepatitis E. Hepatitis C and D, which are transmitted parenterally and by sexual contact, have been associated with vertical transmission. No immunoprophylaxis currently is available for neonates of mothers with hepatitis C or E virus. Immunization against hepatitis B is protective against vertical transmission of hepatitis D.

References

1. Centers for Disease Control. Protection against viral hepatitis. Recommendations of the Immunization Practices Advisory Committee (ACIP). MMWR 1990;39(RR-2):1–26
2. Totos G, Gizaris V, Papaevangelou G. Hepatitis A vaccine: persistence of antibodies 5 years after the first vaccination. Vaccine 1997;15:1252–1253
3. Sweet RL. Hepatitis B infection in pregnancy. Obstetrics/Gynecology Report 1990;2:128–139
4. Snydman DR. Hepatitis in pregnancy. N Engl J Med 1985; 313:1398–1401
5. Hoofnagle JH. Chronic hepatitis B. N Engl J Med 1990; 323:337–339
6. Centers for Disease Control. Hepatitis B virus: A comprehensive strategy for eliminating transmission in the United States through universal childhood vaccination: recommendations of the Immunization Practices Advisory Committee (ACIP). MMWR 1991;40(RR-13):1–25
7. Ohto H, Terazawa S, Sasaki N, Sasaki N, Hino K, Ishiwata C, et al. Transmission of hepatitis C virus from mothers to infants. N Engl J Med 1994;330:744–750
8. Silverman NS, Snyder M, Hodinka RL, McGillen P, Knee G. Detection of hepatitis C virus antibodies and specific hepatitis C virus ribonucleic acid sequences in cord bloods from a heterogeneous prenatal population. Am J Obstet Gynecol 1995;173:1396–1400
9. Matsubara T, Sumazaki R, Takita H. Mother-to-infant transmission of hepatitis C virus: a prospective study. Eur J Pediatr 1995;154:973–978
10. Zucotti GV, Ribero ML, Giovannini M, Fasola M, Riva E, Portera G, et al. Effect of hepatitis C genotype on mother-to-infant transmission of virus. J Pediatr 1995;127:278–280
11. Hoofnagle JH. Type D (delta) hepatitis. JAMA 1989;261: 1321–1325 [Erratum in JAMA 1989;261:3552]
12. Rizzetto M. The delta agent. Hepatology 1983;3:729–737
13. Shattock AG, Irwin FM, Morgan BM, Hillary IB, Kelly MG, Fielding JF, et al. Increased severity and morbidity of acute hepatitis in drug abusers with simultaneously acquired hepatitis B and hepatitis D virus infections. BMJ 1985;290:1377–1380
14. Bradley DW, Maynard JE. Etiology and natural history of post-transfusion and enterically-transmitted non-A, non-B hepatitis. Semin Liver Dis 1986;6:56–66
15. Velázquez O, Stetler HC, Avila C, Ornelas G, Alvarez C, Hadler SC, et al. Epidemic transmission of enterically transmitted non-A, non-B hepatitis in Mexico, 1986-1987. JAMA 1990;263:3281–3285
16. Khuroo MS, Kamill S, Jameel S. Vertical transmission of hepatitis E virus. Lancet 1995;345:1025–1026
17. Linnen J, Wages J Jr, Zhang-Keck Z-Y, Fry KE, Krawzynski KZ, Alter H, et al. Molecular cloning and disease association of hepatitis G virus: a transfusion-transmissible agent. Science 1996;271:505–508
18. Feucht HH, Zollner B, Polywka S, Laufs R. Vertical transmission of hepatitis G. Lancet 1996;347:615–616
19. Kryger P. Significance of anti-HBc IgM in the differential diagnosis of viral hepatitis. J Virol Methods 1985;10:283–289
20. Vassiliadis S, Athanassakis I. Type II interferon may be a potential hazardous therapeutic agent during pregnancy. Br J Haematol 1992;82:782–783
21. Davis GL, Balart LA, Schiff ER, Lindsay K, Bodenheimer HC Jr, Perillo RP, et al. Treatment of chronic hepatitis C with recombinant interferon alfa. N Engl J Med 1989; 321:1501–1506
22. Jagger J, Hunt EH, Brand-Elnaggar J, Pearson RD. Rates of needle-stick injury caused by various devices in a university hospital. N Engl J Med 1988;319:284–288
23. Occupational Safety and Health Administration. Bloodborne pathogens (29 CFR 1910.1030). Fed Regis. December 6, 1991; 56:64004–64182
24. Welch J, Webster M, Tilzey AJ, Noah ND, Banatvala JE. Hepatitis B infections after gynaecological surgery. Lancet 1989;1:205–206

ISSN 1074-8628

The American College of Obstetricians and Gynecologists
409 12th Street, SW
PO Box 96920
Washington, DC 20090-6920

12345/21098

Number 186—November 1993
(Replaces #77, June 1984)

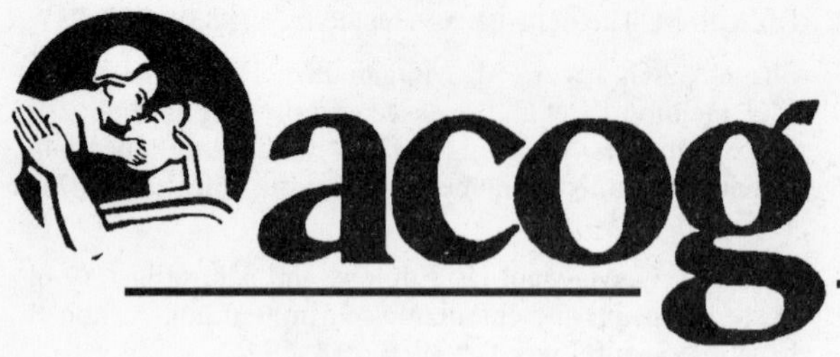

Technical Bulletin
An Educational Aid to Obstetrician–Gynecologists

Vulvar Cancer

Vulvar cancer is an uncommon tumor, accounting for 5% of all gynecologic malignancies. Ninety percent of vulvar tumors are squamous cell carcinomas, but less common vulvar malignancies include melanomas, Bartholin gland carcinomas, and a variety of sarcomas.

During the past decade, prognostic factors for vulvar cancer have been more clearly defined, and treatment has been individualized in many centers. The tendency has been toward conservative surgical approaches and rational utilization of preoperative or postoperative radiation in selected patients. The impetus to perform more conservative surgery has been the realization that radical vulvectomy is associated with marked psychosexual sequelae. When compared with healthy adult women, women who have undergone a vulvectomy report lower levels of sexual arousal (reduced to the eighth percentile) and poor body image (reduced to the fourth percentile) (1).

Squamous Cell Carcinoma

Clinical Considerations

The etiology of squamous cell carcinoma is uncertain but is most likely multifactorial. Younger women are more likely to have tumors containing human papillomavirus and to have associated vulvar intraepithelial neoplasia in the adjacent skin. Older women are more likely to have tumors without human papillomavirus infection and to have squamous hyperplasia in the adjacent skin (2). Although vulvar intraepithelial neoplasia may progress to invasive cancer, it may not have the same malignant potential as its counterpart in the cervix. Progression to invasion is most common in the elderly and the immunosuppressed (3).

The average age at diagnosis is 65 years. Late diagnosis is common due to both patient and physician delay. The most frequent symptom is a long history of vulvar itching; the most common sign is a vulvar mass. Less commonly, women present with symptoms such as bleeding, discharge, or dysuria. On physical examination, the lesion is usually raised and may appear fleshy, ulcerated, leukoplakic, or wartlike. Most squamous carcinomas are unifocal and occur on the labia majora; however, about 5% are multifocal.

Diagnosis

There are no gross or macroscopic features diagnostic of vulvar cancer. Diagnosis is based on biopsy. To avoid delay in diagnosis, biopsy should be performed when there is a grossly suspicious lesion; a confluent, wartlike mass; ulceration which persists for over a month; or vulvar intraepithelial neoplasia.

Staging

Vulvar cancer was staged clinically by the International Federation of Gynecologists and Obstetricians (FIGO) until 1989, when the Cancer Committee of FIGO approved a surgical staging classification for vulvar cancer (see the box). Because surgical staging relies on histopathologic classification of lymph nodes, it more accurately reflects the prognostic significance of the disease.

Patterns of Spread

Vulvar cancer spreads by the following routes:

- Direct extension to adjacent structures, including the vagina, urethra, and anus
- Lymphatic embolization to regional lymph nodes
- Hematogenous metastasis to distant organs such as the liver, lungs, and bone

The overall incidence of lymph node metastases in vulvar cancer about 30%. The incidence increases with size (4). For T1 lesions, the incidence also correlates well with depth of stromal invasion, as shown in Table 1. From the inguinal-femoral nodes, metastasis may reach the pelvic nodes, particularly the external iliac group.

Pelvic node metastases occur in about 5% of patients. Metastases usually occur when there are three or more positive groin nodes (5, 6). Although direct lymphatic pathways have been described from the clitoris and

FIGO Staging of Vulvar Carcinoma

Stage 0	
Tis	Carcinoma in situ, intraepithelial carcinoma
Stage 1	
T1 N0 M0	Tumor confined to the vulva and/or perineum—2 cm or less in greatest dimension, nodes are not palpable
Stage II	
T2 N0 M0	Tumor confined to the vulva and/or perineum—more than 2 cm in greatest dimension, nodes are not palpable
Stage III	
T3 N0 M0	Tumor of any size with...
T3 N1 M0	(1) Adjacent spread to the lower urethra and/or the vagina, or the anus, and/or...
T1 N1 M0	(2) Unilateral regional lymph node metastasis
T2 N1 M0	
Stage IVA	
T1 N2 M0	Tumor invades any of the following
T2 N2 M0	Upper urethra, bladder mucosa, rectal mucosa, Pelvic bone, and/or bilateral reginal node metasasis
T3 N2 M0	
T4 any N M0	
Stage IVB	
Any T	Any Distant metastasis including
Any N M1	Pelvic lymph nodes

TNM Classification of Carcinoma of the Vulva (FIGO)

T	Primary tumor
Tis	Preinvasive carcinoma (carcinoma in situ)
T1	Tumor confined to the vulva and/or perineum—≤2 cm in greatest dimension
T2	Tumor confined to the vulva and/or perineum—>2 cm in greatest dimension
T3	Tumor of any size with adjacent spread to the urethra and/or vagina and/or to the anus
T4	Tumor of any size infiltrating the bladder mucosa and/or the rectal mucosa, including the upper part of the urethral mucosa and/or fixed to the bone
N	Reginal lymph nodes
N0	No lymph node metastasis
N1	Unilateral regional lymph node metastasis
N2	Bilateral regional lymph node metastasis
M	Distant metastasis
M0	No clinical metastasis
M1	Distant metastasis (including pelvic lymph node metastasis)

(Adapted from Internatinal Federation of Gynecology and Obstetrics. Annual report on the results of treatment in gynecologic cancer. Int J Gynecol Obstet 1989;28:189–190)

TABLE 1. INCIDENCE OF LYMPH NODE METASTASES IN RELATION TO DEPTH OF INVASION IN T1 VULVAR CANCER

	No. of Nodes	
Depth of Invasion (mm)	Total	Positive (%)
<1	120	0 (0)
1.1-2	121	8 (6.6)
2.1-3	97	8 (8.2)
3.1-4	50	11 (22.0)
4.1-5	40	10 (25.0)
>5	32	12 (37.5)
Total	460	49 (10.7)

(Reproduced with permission from Hacker NF. Vulvar cancer. In: Berek JS, Hacker NF, eds. Practical gynecologic oncology. Baltimore, Maryland: Williams and Wilkins, 1989:39)

Bartholin gland to (Reproduced with permission from the pelvic nodes, these channels seem to be of minimal clinical significance.

Treatment

Over the past decade, a number of significant advances have occurred in the management of squamous cell vulvar cancer:

- Vulvar conservation for patients with unifocal lesions and an otherwise normal vulva (7-9)
- Elimination of routine pelvic lymphadenectomy (5, 10)
- Avoidance of groin dissection for patients with stage I tumors and less than 1 mm of stromal invasion (8, 9)
- Elimination of the contralateral groin dissection in patients with lateral T1 lesions and negative ipsilateral nodes (8, 11)

- Use of separate incisions for the groin dissections (12)
- Use of preoperative radiation therapy to reduce the need for exenteration in patients with advanced disease (13)
- Use of postoperative radiation to decrease the incidence of groin recurrence in patients with two or more positive groin nodes (14)

Modern treatment for vulvar cancer must be individualized. There is no longer a standard operation appropriate for all cases. Optimal management requires careful consideration of the most appropriate surgical procedure for both the primary tumor and the groins and the appropriate integration of surgery and radiation therapy.

Prior to any treatment, patients should have colposcopy of the cervix, vagina, and vulva. Preinvasive (and occasionally invasive) lesions are often present at other sites in the lower genital tract (15).

Management of T1 Lesions (Tumors 2 cm or smaller)

PRIMARY LESION. A biopsy should be taken from the primary tumor, and depth of invasion should be determined. If invasion is less than 1 mm, the entire lesion should be excised locally and analyzed histologically to allow a precise determination of the depth of invasion. If there is still no invasive focus greater than 1 mm, groin dissection is not necessary.

If the tumor is unifocal, there is more than 1 mm of invasion, and the remainder of the vulva is normal, radical local excision is the treatment of choice. There has been some uncertainty regarding the extent of excision required to prevent local recurrence, but a recent clinical-pathologic review has indicated that surgical margins should clear the tumor by at least 1 cm (16). Resection should extend down to the level of the inferior fascia of the urogenital diaphragm. The incidence of local invasive recurrence following radical local excision is not higher than that following radical vulvectomy (17).

GROIN LYMPH NODES. The risk for lymph node metastases with invasion of less than 1 mm is insignificant, and therefore a groin node dissection is not needed (Table 1). However, since patients who develop recurrent disease in an undissected groin have very high mortality, an accurate histologic assessment of the depth of invasion should be determined before this decision is made (17).

Those patients who have unilateral lesions with more than 1 mm of invasion should undergo ipsilateral groin node dissection. The classical inguinal-femoral node dissection includes removal of the nodes, both superficial and deep to the cribriform fascia with full exposure of the femoral vessels. Because of the morbidity of wound breakdown, cellulitis, lymphedema, and occasional femoral artery rupture, a more conservative groin node dissection has been proposed for patients with clinically nonsuspicious nodes (7). The cribriform fascia over the femoral vessels is left intact, and node tissue superficial to it is removed. The hospital stay, wound complication, and lymphedema are reduced when compared with historical controls (18). However, in this study, nine of 121 patients (7.3%) had a groin recurrence, and six of these patients had a recurrence in the dissected (node-negative) groin. Five of these nine had already died of the disease at the time of reporting. The authors concluded that the recurrence rate in the operated groin was of concern and may be attributable to the decision to leave the femoral nodes intact. Lymph node dissection of both groins is necessary for those women with bilateral lesions or lesions crossing the midline.

HISTOLOGICALLY POSITIVE GROIN NODES. Patients with one microscopically positive groin node require no additional treatment, provided both groins have had inguinal-femoral dissection. Patients with two or more positive ipsilateral groin nodes are best treated with adjuvant radiation to the pelvis and groin. A phase III study by the Gynecologic Oncology Group showed that for patients with positive groin nodes, survival following radiation was better than that following pelvic lymphadenectomy, because the risk of recurrence in the skin and subcutaneous tissues of the lower abdomen and upper thighs was significantly reduced (14). In this report, the addition of radiotherapy did not significantly increase lymphedema or impair healing, although lymphedema may have been underreported because its onset is often delayed.

T2 and Early T3 Tumors Without Clinically Suspicious Groin Nodes

SURGICAL OPTIONS. In general, patients with tumors that are larger than 2cm (T2) or that have minimal spread to the vagina, urethra, or anus (early T3) are treated with radical vulvectomy and bilateral inguinal-femoral lymphadenectomy, although more conservative vulvarresections are being used in a few centers for unifocal lesions, provided the remainder of the vulva appears normal (19). For radical vulvectomy and bilateral groin dissection, two basic surgical approaches can be used:

- The separate incision approach, using three separate incisions: one for the radical vulvectomy and one for each groin dissection. This approach ensures better primary healing, and, with appropriate use of postoperative radiation for patients with multiple positive groin nodes, survival is not compromised. In the absence of postoperative radiation, skin bridge recurrence is more likely in patients with multiple positive groin nodes or a macroscopically positive groin node.
- The en bloc approach, using a butterfly incision. The incision has a significant wound separation rate (50%).

COMPLICATIONS OF SURGERY. Acute complications include wound infection and breakdown, urinary tract infections, seromas in the femoral triangle, deep venous thrombosis, pulmonary embolism, and, rarely, osteitis pubis. The major late complication is chronic leg edema, which may be complicated by recurrent cellulitis. Urinary stress incontinence, with or without genital prolapse, occurs in about 10% of patients. Other potential problems are introital stenosis and femoral hernias.

Tumors with Clinically Suspicious Nodes

Patients with palpably suspicious nodes differ from those in the previous groups since they have a high likelihood of having histologically positive groin nodes. The treatment should be individualized and will depend on the resectability of the nodes. Patients with nonfixed or nonulcerated nodes should undergo a groin node dissection to remove all nodal tissue. This usually includes opening the femoral sheath and exposing the femoral vessels. Patients with two or more positive nodes should undergo external radiotherapy to the groin and pelvis with up to 5,000 cGy.

Routine dissection of the pelvic lymph nodes in patients with positive groin nodes has not been shown to improve survival (5, 10). Since the survival of patients with positive pelvic nodes is about 10%, it is reasonable to remove enlarged pelvic nodes detected by imaging techniques, followed by radiotherapy or chemoradiotherapy to the groin and pelvis if patients are medically fit.

For the rare patient with fixed or ulcerated groin nodes, a course of radiotherapy with chemotherapy may be indicated prior to attempted resection. If surgical resection is possible, then myocutaneous skin flaps may be helpful in subsequent healing.

Advanced Disease

When the disease involves the anus, rectum, rectovaginal septum, or proximal urethra, the standard radical vulvectomy will not encompass all of the disease. Early surgical attempts to encompass all gross disease by performing extended radical vulvectomy were associated with a high local failure rate, so pelvic exenteration, combined with radical vulvectomy and bilateral groin dissection, has become more popular in the last 30 years. Such radical surgery carries an operative mortality of about 10%, a high postoperative morbidity, and a high psychologic morbidity. Nevertheless, a 5-year survival rate of about 50% can be anticipated (20).

An alternative approach to these patients is preoperative radiotherapy (13), using external-beam therapy with or without intracavitary or interstitial irradiation, in order to shrink the primary tumor and allow a more conservative surgical resection. Chemotherapy using 5-fluorouracil, with or without mitomycin, in combination with radiotherapy is also effective (21), but whether it produces any greater benefit than radiation alone is not known. More recently, chemotherapy using 5-fluorouracil in combination with cisplatin has been given concurrently with radiotherapy (22). These approaches will usually obviate the need for exenteration, and cure rates are at least comparable to those obtained by exenteration, with significantly less physical and psychologic morbidity.

Prognosis for Vulvar Cancer

The 5-year survival rate for operable cases is about 70%. Patients with negative groin nodes have a 5-year survival rate of about 90%, but this falls to about 50% for patients with positive nodes (17). The number of positive groin nodes is the single most important prognostic variable. Patients with one microscopically positive node have a good prognosis regardless of the stage of disease, with survival rates of up to 94% at 5 years being reported (5). In a Gynecologic Oncology Group study, patients with one or two positive groin nodes had a 5-year survival rate of 75.2%, those with three or four positive nodes had a rate of 36.1%, and those with five or six positive nodes had a rate of 24% (4). There were no survivors among patients with seven or more positive nodes.

Follow-up

Patients should be seen every 3 months for 2 years and every 6 months for 5 years. Thereafter, visits should occur annually. A thorough pelvic examination and Pap test of the cervix and vagina should be performed at each visit.

Other Vulvar Carcinomas

Melanoma

Malignant melanomas are the second most common vulvar malignancy. They occur predominantly in white women between the ages of 50 and 80 years. Melanomas may arise de novo or from a preexisting junctional nevus and occur mainly on the labia minora and clitoris. Patients at increased risk for melanoma include those with a family history of melanoma and those with dysplastic nevi elsewhere on the body. Dysplastic melanocytic nevi occur in 2-5% of white adults and in one third of patients with cutaneous melanoma (23).

Most patients present because of a lump or tumor on the external genitalia, although complaints of itching, bleeding, or discharge are often volunteered. Change in a preexisting mole may also prompt some patients to seek attention. Because it is difficult to observe vulvar lesions adequately, most pigmented lesions in this location should be excised, unless they have been present and unchanged for some years.

The FIGO system used for staging squamous cell carcinomas is not applicable to melanomas because these lesions are usually much smaller, and prognosis is mainly related to depth of penetration of the tumor (24).

The treatment of vulvar melanoma may be patterned after that for cutaneous melanomas. The primary lesion should be removed, providing a margin of at least 2 cm (25). Tumors with invasion of less than 0.75 mm do not require regional node dissection since survival is virtually 100% (24). For more deeply penetrating lesions, en bloc resection with removal of the regional nodes is recommended. While the mean 5-year survival rate for reported cases of vulvar melanoma is about 32% (17), the prognosis is related to the thickness of the tumor and the status of the regional lymph nodes. Late recurrences are possible with melanomas.

Bartholin Gland Carcinoma

Primary carcinoma of the Bartholin gland accounts for about 5% of vulvar malignancies. Although transition from normal to malignant glandular tissue is the most diagnostic criterion, some cases will be appropriately diagnosed on the basis of their histology and anatomic location.

A history of inflammation of the gland may be obtained from about 10% of patients, and malignancies may be mistaken for benign cysts or abscesses. Physician and patient delay in diagnosis are common. Because the overlying skin will be intact until the tumor is advanced, biopsy of a mass in this area is often delayed because malignancy is not always suspected. Therefore, any persistent mass in this region, especially in patients over 40 years of age, should be biopsied.

Bartholin gland carcinoma traditionally has been treated by radical vulvectomy, with bilateral groin and pelvic node dissection. Because pelvic node metastases are rare in the absence of groin node metastases, a decision to perform pelvic node dissection should be based on the same criteria as previously outlined for squamous cell carcinomas.

Similarly, less radical excisions, such as hemivulvectomy or radical local excision, may be as effective as radical vulvectomy (26). Postoperative vulvar radiation may reduce the incidence of local recurrence.

Paget Disease of the Vulva

In contrast to Paget disease of the breast, which is always associated with an underlying ductal carcinoma, underlying adenocarcinoma occurs in only about 20% of patients with vulvar Paget disease. Invasive lesions may demonstrate local infiltration, without a discrete underlying mass.

Clinically, the disease predominantly affects postmenopausal Caucasian women. The presenting symptoms are usually pruritus and local soreness, and the lesion has an erythematous, scaly appearance. From the vulva, the disease may spread to the mons pubis, thighs, vagina, and buttocks, while extension to the mucosa of the rectum and urinary tract also has been described. A second synchronous or metachronous primary neoplasm is associated with extramammary Paget disease in about 30% of patients. Second primary tumors are particularly likely to occur in the genitourinary or gastrointestinal tract or in the breasts (27). If disease occurs in these organs, cytoscopy or sigmoidoscopy or both should be performed. When the anal mucosa is involved, there is usually an underlying rectal adenocarcinoma (28).

Treatment of Paget disease requires wide local excision, as the disease usually extends well beyond the gross lesion. It is helpful to obtain frozen sections of the surgical margins to ensure adequate excision. If there is an underlying adenocarcinoma or underlying stromal invasion, a more radical local excision or radical vulvectomy is required, which should be combined with at least an ipsilateral inguinal-femoral lymphadenectomy. Because of the possibility of underlying invasive disease, laser ablation is inappropriate for primary Paget disease. It may, however, have a role in recurrent cases.

Verrucous Carcinoma

Verrucous carcinomas are cauliflowerlike tumors. Adequate biopsy, to include the base of the lesion, is necessary to distinguish a verrucous carcinoma from a benign condyloma acuminatum or a squamous cell carcinoma with a verrucous growth pattern (29).

The lesions usually occur in postmenopausal women, and most patientspresent with a long-standing, slow-growing wartlike lesion. The tumors are locally destructive, and even bone may be invaded. Metastasis to regional lymph nodes has been reported but is rare (30).

Treatment should be by radical local excision. Local recurrences are common if the tumor is incompletely excised, and some type of radical resection may be necessary to excise recurrent disease. Radiation therapy is not useful.

Conclusion

Modern management of vulvar cancer requires an individualized approach, with careful determination of the most appropriate operation for the primary lesion and the regional lymph nodes. In addition, the possible integration of radiation therapy (and possibly chemotherapy) into the overall management should be taken into account before embarking on any surgery. Because of the large variety of histologic types, adequate biopsy and careful histologic review are necessary to guide treatment.

Radical vulvectomy should no longer be considered mandatory for most vulvar malignancies. Procedures which spare much of the vulva may be appropriate in many instances, thereby decreasing psychologic morbidity. When more conservative procedures are used, careful patient selection is critical to ensure that survival is not compromised.

REFERENCES

1. Andersen BL, Hacker NF. Psychosexual adjustment after vulvar surgery. Obstet Gynecol 1983;62:457–462
2. Toki T, Kurman RJ, Park JS, Kessis T, Daniel RW, Shah KV. Probable nonpapillomavirus etiology of squamous cell carcinoma of the vulva in older women: a clinicopathologic study using in situ hybridization and polymerase chain reaction. Int J Gynecol Pathol 1991;10:107–125
3. Buscema J, Woodruff JD, Parmley TH, Genadry R. Carcinoma in situ of the vulva. Obstet Gynecol 1980;55: 225–230
4. Homesley HD, Bundy BN, Sedlis A, Yordan E, Berek JS, Jahshan A, et al. Assessment of current International Federation of Gynecology and Obstetrics staging of vulvar carcinoma relative to prognostic factors for survival (a Gynecologic Oncology Group study). Am J Obstet Gynecol 1991;164:997–1004
5. Hacker NF, Berek JS, Lagasse LD, Leuchter RS, Moore JG. Mangement of regional lymph nodes and their prognostic influence in vulvar cancer. Obstet Gynecol 1983;61:408–412
6. Podratz KC, Symmonds RE, Taylor WF, Williams TJ. Carcinoma of the vulva: analysis of treatment and survival. Obstet Gynecol 1983;61:63–74
7. DiSaia PJ, Creasman WT, Rich WM. An alternative approach to early cancer of the vulva. Am J Obstet Gynecol 1979;133:825–832
8. Hacker NF, Berek JS, Lagasse LD, Nieberg RK, Leuchter RS. Individualization of treatment for stage I squamous cell vulvar carcinoma. Obstet Gynecol 1984;63:155–162
9. Iversen T, Abeler V, Aalders J. Individualized treatment of stage I carcinoma of the vulva. Obstet Gynecol 1981;57: 85–89
10. Curry SL, Wharton JT, Rutledge F. Positive lymph nodes in vulvar squamous carcinoma. Gynecol Oncol 1980;9:63–67
11. Figge DC, Tamimi HK, Greer BE. Lymphatic spread in carcinoma of the vulva. Am J Obstet Gynecol 1985;152: 387–394
12. Hacker NF, Leuchter RS, Berek JS, Castaldo TW, Lagasse LD. Radical vulvectomy and bilateral inguinal lymphadenectomy through separate groin incisions. Obstet Gynecol 1981;58:574–579
13. Boronow RC. Therapeutic altenative to primary exenteration for advanced vulvovaginal cancer. Gynecol Oncol 1973:1:223–255
14. Homesley HD, Bundy BN, Sedlis A, Adcock L. Radiation therapy versus pelvic node resection for carcinoma of the vulva with positive groin nodes. Obstet Gynecol 1986;68:733–740
15. Sherman KJ, Daling JR, Chu J, McKnight B, Weiss NS. Multiple primary tumours in women with vulvar neoplasms: a case-control study. Br J Cancer 1988;57:423–427
16. Heaps JM, Fu YS, Montz FJ, Hacker NF, Berek JS. Surgical-pathologic variables predictive of local recurrence in squamous cell carcinoma of the vulva. Gynecol Oncol 1990;38:309–314
17. Hacker NF. Vulvar cancer. In: Berek JS, Hacker NF, eds. Practical gynecologic oncology. Baltimore, Maryland: Williams and Wilkins, 1989
18. Stehman FB, Bundy BN, Dvoretsky PM, Creasman WT. Early stage I carcinoma of the vulva treated with ipsilateral superficial inguinal lymphadenectomy and modified radical hemivulvectomy: a prospective study of the Gynecologic Oncology Group. Obstet Gynecol 1992;79: 490–497
19. Burrell MO, Franklin EW III, Campion MJ, Crozier MA, Stacy DW. The modified radical vulvectomy with groin dissection: an eight-year experience. Am J Obstet Gynecol 1988;159:715–722
20. Cavanagh D, Roberts WS, Bryson SCP, Marsden DE, Ingram JM, Anderson WR. Changing trends in the surgical treatment of invasive carcinoma of the vulva. Surg Gynecol Obstet 1986;162:164–168
21. Thomas G, Dembo A, DePetrillo A, Pringle J, Ackerman I, Bryson P, et al. Concurrent radiation and chemotherapy in vulvar carcinoma. Gynecol Oncol 1989;34:263–267
22. Berek JS, Heaps JM, Fu YS, Juillard GJF, Hacker NF. Concurrent cisplatin and 5-fluorouracil chemotherapy and radiation therapy for advanced-stage squamous carcinoma of the vulva. Gynecol Oncol 1991;42:197–201
23. Fitzpatrick TB, Rhodes AR, Sober AJ. Prevention of melanoma by recognition of its precursors. N Engl J Med 1985;312:115–116
24. Podratz KC, Gaffey TA, Symmonds RE, Johansen KL, O'Brien PC. Melanoma of the vulva: an update. Gynecol Oncol 1983;16:153–168
25. Rose PG, Piver MS, Tsukada Y, Lau T. Conservative therapy for melanoma of the vulva. Am J Obstet Gynecol 1988;159:52–55
26. Copeland LJ, Sneige N, Gershenson DM, McGuffee VB, Abdul-Karin F, Rutledge FN. Bartholin gland carcinoma. Obstet Gynecol 1986;67:794–801
27. Jones RE Jr, Austin C, Ackerman AB. Extramammary Paget's disease. A critical reexamination. Am J Dermatopathol 1979;1:101–132
28. Stacy D, Burrell MO, Franklin EW III. Extramammary Paget's disease of the vulva and anus: use of intraoperative frozen-section margins. Am J Obstet Gynecol 1986;155: 519–523
29. Partridge EE, Murad T, Shingleton HM, Austin JM, Hatch KD. Verrucous lesions of the female genitalia. II. Verrucous carcinoma. Am J Obstet Gynecol 1980;137:419–424
30. Gallousis S. Verrucous carcinoma. Report of three vulvar cases and review of the literature. Obstet Gynecol 1972; 40:502–507

This Technical Bulletin was developed under the direction of the Committee on Technical Bulletins of the American College of Obstetricians and Gynecologists as an educational aid to obstetricians and gynecologists. The committee wishes to thank Neville F. Hacker, MD, for his assistance in the development of this bulletin. This Technical Bulletin does not define a standard of care, nor is it intended to dictate an exclusive course of management. It presents recognized methods and techniques of clinical practice for consideration by obstetrician-gynecologists for incorporation into their practices. Variations of practice taking into account the needs of the individual patient, resources, and limitations unique to the institution or type of practice may be appropriate.

THE AMERICAN COLLEGE OF OBSTETRICIANS AND GYNECOLOGISTS
409 12th Street, SW
Washington, DC 20024-2188

2345/7654

ACOG EDUCATIONAL BULLETIN

Number 241, October 1997

Vulvar Nonneoplastic Epithelial Disorders

The nomenclature and definitions of vulvovaginal disease have been evolving. In 1987, the International Society for the Study of Vulvovaginal Disease (ISSVD), in collaboration with the International Society of Gynecological Pathologists, proposed the following classification of vulvar nonneoplastic epithelial disorders (previously called vulvar dystrophies) (1, 2), which isaccepted by the World Health Organization:

- Lichen sclerosus
- Squamous cell hyperplasia
- Other dermatoses

The term *lichen sclerosus* was retained, as proposed by the ISSVD in 1976, with the "et atrophicus" portion of the term deleted. *Squamous cell hyperplasia* is a new term, introduced in the 1987 classification, which replaced the original term of *hyperplastic dystrophy* proposed by the ISSVD in 1976. The term *mixed dystrophy* used in the 1976 classification was also removed because it is currently recognized that hyperplastic changes of the epithelium are commonly observed concurrent with lichen sclerosus and are within the spectrum of epithelial changes seen with lichen sclerosus (2).

Other dermatoses are listed in the classification as a general inclusive term because the 1987 classification was not intended to introduce a comprehensive classification for all nonneoplastic dermatologic conditions, but rather to replace the 1976 ISSVD classification, remove the term *dystrophy* (which was considered ambiguous), and refine the general terminology relevant to conditions previously included under such terms as *dystrophy, kraurosis*, and *leukoplakia*.

This Educational Bulletin was developed under the direction of the Committee on Educational Bulletins of the American College of Obstetricians and Gynecologists as an aid to obstetricians and gynecologists. The College wishes to thank Edward J. Wilkinson, MD, for his assistance in the development of this bulletin. This document is not to be construed as establishing a standard of practice or dictating an exclusive course of treatment. Rather, it is intended as an educational tool that presents current information on obstetric–gynecologic issues.

Lichen Sclerosus

Lichen sclerosus is a benign epithelial disorder that can occur at any age, although it is most common in prepubertal and postmenopausal patients. It is characterized by epithelial thinning with edema and fibrosis of the dermis and associated shrinkage and agglutination of the labia and introital stenosis.

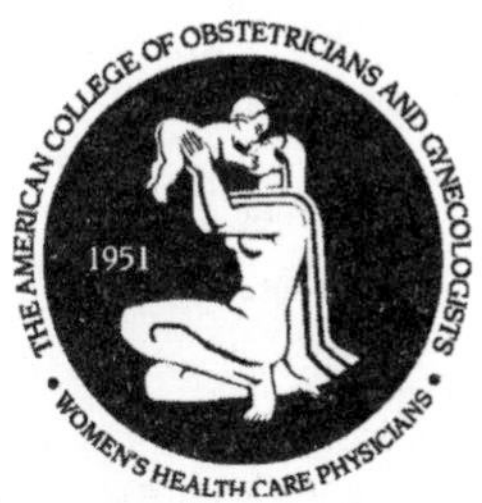

Replaces Number 139, January 1990

Vulvar lichen sclerosus accounts for approximately 10% of clinic visits related to vulvar symptoms.

Lichen sclerosus typically does not involve the vagina or urethra but may involve the vulvar vestibule, especially the lateral labia minora. The edematous skin has a white, thin, paperlike appearance. Subcutaneous bleeding with ecchymosis, subcutaneous hematomas, and fissures with superficial ulceration and erosion may be present. Early lesions are typically symmetrical and may extend about the vulva, excluding the mons pubis, and the rectum. The lesions often appear in an hourglass configuration but may not extend beyond the labia majora. Women with lichen sclerosus may have affected skin sites other than the vulva. There is a recognized familial association, and some human leukocyte antigen subtypes occur more often in individuals with lichen sclerosus. In affected children, painful defecation or voiding complaints such as interference with the urinary stream may occur as a result of stricture of the perianal skin or shrinkage and agglutination of the labia minora (3). The presence and severity of symptoms may decrease in adolescence; however, the process may persist in these individuals (3). Both children and adults often experience pruritus in the involved areas. Sexually active women may experience external or entry dyspareunia related to the labial changes and introital shrinkage. In adults, long-standing lichen sclerosus is commonly associated with hyperplastic changes and hyperkeratosis (4, 5). In addition, shrinkage of the labia, prepuce, and frenulum may occur with agglutination of the labia minora, as well as the prepuce. This can lead to severe introital stenosis and, in some cases, to perianal stenosis with the clitoris buried beneath the agglutinated labia minora.

Diagnosis

Diagnosis is confirmed by biopsy. Characteristic histopathologic features include thinning of the epithelium with loss of rete ridges; however, variations in histopathologic findings vary with the duration of the process. Hyperkeratosis may be present. Dermal changes include edema, fibrin deposition, and loss of vascularity (5). In the deeper dermis, immediately beneath the edematous area, a chronic inflammatory cell infiltrate is present composed predominantly of lymphocytes. Blood is often seen within the edematous dermis, reflected clinically as ecchymosis. Erosion and ulceration of the epithelium is often observed and may confuse the histopathologic picture, especially if there are long-standing ulcerated areas with chronic inflammatory changes. Epithelial thickening secondary to hyperplasia may be seen adjacent to areas of lichen sclerosus and as part of the spectrum of the disease. In severe cases, subepithelial vesicles and bullae may be observed. Such cases must be distinguished from bullous–vesicular diseases, including pemphigoid and pemphigus. In advanced cases, severe scarring and stenosis may be seen with marked epithelial thinning. In these cases, the differential diagnosis includes advanced scleroderma, morphea, lupus erythematosus, advanced lichen planus, and radiation fibrosis.

Management

The current treatment of lichen sclerosus includes very high-potency topical corticosteroids such as a cream containing 0.05% clobetasol propionate or a 0.05% preparation of halobetasol, applied twice daily for 2–3 weeks and then decreased to once daily, usually at night, until symptoms and findings begin to subside (4, 6, 7). Clinical response usually occurs in 1 month or less; however, the response may be limited to relief of symptoms, with physical changes of the involved areas observed over months. The dosage thereafter can be decreased to one or three times per week depending on response. High-potency topical corticosteroids for lichen sclerosus are appropriate for long-term maintenance, provided applications are limited to one to three times per week (7) (see Table 1).

Topical progesterone and topical testosterone have been commonly used for lichen sclerosus, with varying results. Testosterone is systemically absorbed and should not be used in children. Women may find such treatment objectionable because of testosterone effects such as acne, hair growth, and oiliness of the skin. The effectiveness of topical progesterone or testosterone may be no better than that of the carrier used without the steroid component (6). Topical estrogens have been attempted as therapy for lichen sclerosus but have no proven efficacy.

Nonmedical treatment for vulvar lichen sclerosus includes maintaining good personal hygiene, keeping the vulva dry, and protecting the skin from injury or irritating soaps, lotions, or deodorants. Simple emollients, includ-

Table 1. Representative Topical Corticosteriods Grouped According to Antiinflammatory Activity

Potency	Topical Corticosteroid	Strength % (cream)
Very high	Halobetasol propionate	0.05
	Clobetasol propionate	0.05
High	Betamethasone valerate	0.1*
Medium	Triamcinolone acetonide	0.1
Low	Fluocinolone acetonide	0.01
	Desonide	0.05
	Hydrocortisone acetate	1.0

* Ointment

ing lanolin and hydrogenated vegetable oil, often give relief and improve the involved skin. Antipruritic compounds and antibiotic ointments should be avoided because they can cause irritation. Soaks in Burow's solution and sitz baths may help relieve severe symptoms, but excessive use can cause dryness and should be avoided. Vaginal dilators may help reduce introital stenosis provided the lichen sclerosus is not fissured, ulcered, or ecchymotic. In general, dilation is useful only after topical medical management has relieved symptoms and reduced severe atrophy and edema.

Although appropriate biopsies of the involved vulvar areas are necessary to establish the diagnosis of lichen sclerosus (except in prepubertal patients), no evidence suggests that surgical excision of involved areas is of any benefit. Minor reconstructive surgery may be appropriate in treated cases in which the clitoris is buried by fused labia minora or the introitus is stenotic. Some women with vulvar lichen sclerosus will develop vulvar squamous cell carcinoma. The risk of vulvar carcinoma in these women cannot be predicted with certainty; however, retrospective analysis of women with vulvar squamous cell carcinoma reveals that more than 3–9% have lichen sclerosus (8, 9). There are few prospective studies; however, in a study of more than 350 women with vulvar lichen sclerosus, 3.5% subsequently developed squamous cell carcinoma (10). The subsequent incidence actually may be higher because this study is ongoing. A persistent ulcer or nodule in a field of lichen sclerosus is an indication for biopsy or local excision.

Squamous Cell Hyperplasia

Squamous cell hyperplasia is a benign epithelial disorder, which may be indistinguishable clinically from lichen simplex chronicus (5). The term was accepted for clinical use to describe patients who typically present with vulvar pruritus and have localized nonspecific thickening of the vulvar skin. The involved skin color may range from white to gray, primarily as a result of epithelial edema. The involved areas are typically not symmetrical, and the process may be localized to a small area on the vulva.

Diagnosis

The diagnosis is one of exclusion. On microscopic examination, the epithelium is thickened and acanthotic. The rete ridges are broadened and deepened without significant dermal inflammation or other features that would define the condition as another specific dermatosis. Hyperkeratosis and spongiosis may be present (5).

Although squamous cell hyperplasia has been equated with lichen simplex chronicus, a diagnosis of lichen simplex chronicus includes histopathologic evidence of some chronic inflammatory cells within the superficial dermis, as well as fibrosis and collagenization of the superficial dermis immediately beneath the epithelium. These findings are not evident in squamous cell hyperplasia. Lichen simplex chronicus has epithelial features like squamous cell hyperplasia but also has dermal changes.

Squamous cell hyperplasia must be distinguished from condyloma acuminatum. Condylomata are usually multiple and typically have koilocytes, a prominent granular layer, parabasal cell hyperplasia, and accentuated intracellular bridges—all of which are absent in squamous cell hyperplasia.

Psoriasis may be included in the differential diagnosis; however, it usually presents with red and white epithelial areas and typically is more diffuse and involves other sites beyond the vulva. Microscopically, psoriasis has acanthosis and inflammation within the epithelium and dermis.

Lichen planus may have hyperplastic features and be within the differential diagnosis. However, lichen planus also has a prominent inflammatory infiltrate that is immediately adjacent and below the epithelium. It may also involve the vagina and the oral mucosa and other dermatologic sites (11).

Seborrhea and chronic candidal infection can be associated with squamous hyperplastic features. Taking a thorough history and searching for fungal organisms (species causing candidiasis, *Trichophyton* species) are important in identifying fungal infection.

Vulvar intraepithelial neoplasia (also called dysplasia or carcinoma in situ) may be in the clinical differential diagnosis and typically presents with maculopapular lesions that are white, aceto-white, pigmented, or red; they are usually multifocal. Microscopically, vulvar intraepithelial neoplasia has epithelial nuclear pleomorphism and hyperchromasia, lacks keratinocyte maturation, and often has atypical mitotic figures. When such cellular atypia is present in a thickened epithelium, a diagnosis of vulvar intraepithelial neoplasia is appropriate, rather than the old term *hyperplastic dystrophy with atypia* (5).

Management

The treatment for squamous cell hyperplasia is topical, medium-strength corticosteroids applied twice daily, decreased to once daily when symptoms resolve (4) (see Table 1). Most patients respond to treatment with resolution of symptoms and evidence of clinical improvement within 2–3 weeks. Thereafter, the treatment can be discontinued. Continued treatment can cause allergic contact dermatitis to the carrier. Avoidance of contact with local irritants (eg, detergents, dyes, perfumes) and maintenance of good personal hygiene, with an emphasis on keeping the area dry, are beneficial. Treatment is generally curative.

Other Dermatoses

Lichen Simplex Chronicus

Lichen simplex chronicus is a dermatosis that can occur on the vulva. In some clinics, it may be the most commonly encountered dermatosis. The clinical presentation is usually vulvar pruritus; on examination, thickened white epitelium is identified, which is often unilateral and localized. Biopsy may be necessary to establish the diagnosis.

Aside from the presence of chronic inflammatory cells and fibrosis and collagenization of the superficial dermis, the histopathologic features of lichen simplex chronicus are the same as those of squamous cell hyperplasia, and the differential diagnosis is the same as for squamous cell hyperplasia (5). The condition is typically limited to the vulva, and topical, medium-strength corticosteroid treatment brings prompt response with resolution of both the lesion(s) and the symptoms. Symptoms usually subside within 2 weeks of beginning treatment; however, several weeks of treatment may be needed before the visible lesion completely resolves.

Lichen Planus

In vulvar referral clinics, lichen planus comprises approximately 5% of cases. It is a papulosquamous chronic inflammatory dermatosis of unknown etiology. When lichen planus involves the vulva, it commonly involves the vulvar vestibule as well as the vagina. Of the women with diagnosed vulvovaginal lichen planus, one third to two thirds will have cutaneous lichen planus. Oral lesions as well as involvement of extragenital cutaneous sites also may occur. One manifestation of lichen planus is a clinical complex of erosive lesions, termed the vulvovaginal gingival syndrome of lichen planus. Lichen planus can result in ulcers and synechiae within the vagina and around the vestibule. Scarring results in stenosis and loss of function. The initial clinical presentation of lichen planus in the vulva may vary from a severe erosive process to mild inflammatory changes involving the vagina and presenting as mild desquamative vaginitis. In such cases, the vestibular epithelium typically also is involved, which may help in making the diagnosis.

Diagnosis

The histopathologic findings in lichen planus vary from a mild, localized, lichenoid chronic inflammatory process involving the epithelial dermal junction, to an ulcerative and erosive process with fibrosis and scarring associated with severe acute and chronic inflammation. Clinical pathologic correlation is essential to establish the appropriate diagnosis. Immunofluorescent examination of slides for immunoglobulins and basement membrane should be performed to exclude pemphigus, cicatricial pemphigoid, and linear immunoglobulin A disease. Although such studies have relatively specific findings for these conditions, lichen planus typically shows no specific localization of immunoglobulins or antibasement membrane antibodies by fluorescence. Various infectious causes of vaginitis must also be excluded.

Management

The clinical behavior of genital lichen planus is one of progressive scarring and shrinkage of the vulva and vagina if treatment is not administered or is ineffective. Vaginal hydrocortisone suppositories are the treatment of choice (25 mg hydrocortisone suppositories). In acute cases, 0.1% betamethasone cream can be applied vaginally once daily at night for 2 weeks. The vaginal application of foaming cortisone enemas also has been used for acute symptoms. Vulvar involvement is usually initially treated with topical corticosteroids. In postmenopausal women with atrophic changes in the vagina and vestibule, vaginal estrogen therapy is recommended in addition to the vaginal hydrocortisone treatment. Commercially available estrogen creams containing alcohol can be irritating. Soaks in Burow's solution and sitz baths may be of value in acute cases. Lichen planus cannot be cured but usually can be controlled with long-term management (11). Treatment with topical vulvar and vaginal hydrocortisone can be tapered to three times per week but must be continued indefinitely. Vaginal dilators may be of value if vaginal stenosis or adhesions are observed.

Nonneoplastic Epithelial Disorders Confined to the Vulvar Vestibule

Vulvar Vestibulitis

Vulvar vestibulitis is a poorly understood inflammatory process involving the vulvar vestibule. It is associated with a constellation of symptoms and physical findings including vulvodynia (12–14). An association with interstitial cystitis has been reported (15). Patients with vulvar vestibulitis frequently experience dyspareunia with insertion as well as postcoital vulvar pain. These symptoms often are so severe as to preclude coitus. Less common symptoms include persistent vulvar burning and itching, a burning sensation within the vestibule, and urinary frequency or dysuria. In many patients, the onset of symptoms can be dated to a specific event, such as following vulvar–vaginal candidal infection or vulvar laser therapy. The excessive use of topical vulvar steroids; exposure to irritants such as topical 5-fluorouracil, gentian violet, trichloroacetic acid, or topical antibiotics; or overwashing using irritant soaps or deodorants also may cause symptoms. In some cases, the symptoms are related to sexual contact or a history of abuse.

Diagnosis

Physical examination may reveal clinical evidence of inflammation of the vulvar vestibule that may be localized about the minor vestibular glands as well as the Bartholin gland ducts (12, 16). The patient may experience exquisite pinpoint pressure tenderness within the vestibule when pressure is applied to the inflamed areas with a cotton swab. In some cases, deep palpation of the Bartholin gland areas also evokes pain. These findings, and the clinical history, are sufficient for diagnosis. Vulvar biopsy is not necessary in most cases.

The histopathologic features within the vestibule include superficial chronic inflammation with an inflammatory cell infiltrate composed predominantly of lymphocytes. Plasma cells are seen in about three fourths of the cases (17, 18). The inflammatory infiltrate extends to the minor vestibular glands and may extend to the superficial Bartholin duct and periurethral glands. Inflammation typically extends into the epithelium (inflammatory exocytosis), with thinning of the epithelium and epithelial erosion. Vestibular ulceration may be seen in severe cases. Spongiosis may occur within the epithelium, suggesting human papillomavirus (HPV) changes. However, multinucleation (bi-nucleation) of the keratinocytes, nuclear enlargement, nuclear atypia, dyskeratosis, and parabasal hyperplasia are typically not seen. In women of reproductive age, the epithelium of the vulvar vestibule is glycogen rich, like that of the vagina, and this must be distinguished from the HPV effect. In most studies, women with vestibulitis are no more likely to have HPV detected in the involved vestibular epithelium than is the general population (17, 19). Currently, HPV is not considered an etiologic factor in vulvar vestibulitis. Vulvar vestibulitis is clinically distinct from lichen planus in that it does notinvolve the vagina or vulvar epithelium beyond thevestibule.

Management

No curative therapy exists for vulvar vestibulitis. Treatment choices are summarized in the box. Conservative medical therapy is the initial treatment of choice, and surgical excision of the vestibule should be reserved only for intractable cases (13). Proposed medical treatments that have not been scrutinized by prospective controlled studies are numerous, and partial relief of symptoms has been claimed in 40–50% of cases regardless of treatment. Topical corticosteroids of medium or high potency may provide some relief. Interferon has been used with mixed results. Topical, physician-applied capsaicin, which reduces neural response, relieves symptoms in some patients (20). Low-dose antidepressants may be of some value but appear more appropriate for the treatment of dysesthetic "essential" vulvodynia (21).

Laser vaporization therapy is not indicated for the treatment of vestibulitis. Surgical treatment of vulvar vestibulitis can be classified into three techniques: vestibuloplasty, partial vestibulectomy with vaginal advancement, and total vestibulectomy with vaginal advancement. Vestibuloplasty is a conservative surgical technique used to enlarge the vaginal orifice using a vertical incision of the posterior vaginal introitus, which is then closed horizontally (13). Partial excision of the perineal body may be appropriate in cases in which recurrent or persist-

Treatments for Vulvar Vestibulitis

Local topical treatment
- Warm sitz baths
- Burow's solution
- Topical sorbitrate/glycerine cream

Topical medical treatment
- Topical corticosteroid cream
- Topical estrogen cream
- Topical lidocaine (2% gel or 5% ointment)

Oral medication
- Calcium citrate (2 tablets 3 times daily for at least 1 year with or without a low-oxalate diet)
- Oral corticosteroids (short-term with topical corticosteroids)
- Fluconazole (100–200 mg/d for 1–2 months; be aware of adverse drug reactions and side effects)

Injectable medical treatment
- Interferon therapy (30-gauge dental needle and 1 mL syringe–1 million IU per injection site [3 million IU/mL], with a total of 12 injection sites [12 million IU], given over the course of 4 weeks)

Neurophysiologic treatment
- Use of graduated vaginal dilators with creams
- Biofeedback techniques including electromyographic feedback methods
- Topical capsaicin to reduce sensitivity
- Tricyclic antidepressants to reduce neural feedback (eg, amitriptyline; start with a low dosage and increase dosage as tolerated to relieve symptoms [10–25 mg orally, three times daily])

Surgical techniques
- Vestibuloplasty
- Partial vestibulectomy with vaginal advancement
- Total vestibulectomy with vaginal advancement

ent perineal body fissures occur. Partial vestibulectomy, with vaginal advancement, includes excision of the posterior portion of the vulvar vestibule, with advancement of the vaginal epithelium over the vestibule. The third procedure, total vestibulectomy with vaginal advancement, involves excision of the entire vestibule with sparing of the periclitoral and periurethral epithelium and vaginal advancement to the labia minora laterally and perineal body posteriorly. These procedures give initial relief in approximately one half to three quarters of the cases (13). No long-term studies are available on the results of these surgical procedures. However, long-term follow-up shows symptoms recur in some patients; the recurrence may be as severe as the initial onset.

Vestibular Papillomatosis

Vulvar vestibular papillomatosis also may be present with vulvodynia. Although patients with the condition may have pruritus, in most cases they are asymptomatic (14, 16). On examination, tight clusters of small papillae, typically approximately 1 mm in diameter and 2–3 mm in length, are found on the medial aspects of the labia minora. The papillae typically occur in a focal patch, up to several centimeters in diameter. In some cases, they have a symmetrical distribution on the medial labia minora. These lesions should be distinguished from congenital vestibular papillae, which are of similar size but are usually not clustered and typically occur near, or attached to, the hymen and are asymptomatic.

Diagnosis

Pathologic features are distinctive, with small (usually 0.1×0.3 cm or less) epithelial-covered, squamous papillae having fibrovascular stalks. The epithelial surface is nonkeratinized squamous epithelium and may be glycogen rich. Although HPV epithelial changes have been described, they are usually not seen in these patients. Studies on the identification of HPV in these lesions do not suggest significant frequency of HPV in these cases; thus, based on current data, HPV cannot be considered a causal factor (16).

Management

The treatment of pruritic vestibular papillae is directed toward destroying or excising the papillae and promoting good perineal hygiene, including keeping the vulva clean and dry and avoiding irritating soaps, deodorants, or garments. These papillae and associated symptoms may be relatively refractory to treatment and can persist or recur.

Idiopathic Vulvodynia

Idiopathic vulvodynia also has been referred to as dysesthetic or essential vulvodynia (21). As with vestibulitis and vestibular papillomatosis, the cause of idiopathic vulvodynia is unknown. Patients with idiopathic vulvodynia have no specific physical findings within the vulva, and symptoms may wax and wane. When other causes of vulvodynia have been excluded, diagnosis of idiopathic vulvodynia is appropriate.

These patients are best treated with low-dose tricyclic antidepressants to reduce neural feedback. One regimen is to start with a low dosage of amitriptyline and increase the dosage slowly as tolerated to relieve symptoms (10–25 mg orally, three times daily) (21). As with the other patients with vulvodynia, long-term support and management are essential because medical treatment alone is not necessarily curative. In patients with essential vulvodynia, surgical excision of the vestibule has no proven value. The natural history of vulvodynia remains in question, and only long-term controlled prospective studies will address the many issues surrounding this complex subject.

References

1. Ridley CM, Frankman O, Jones ISC, Pincus SH, Wilkinson EJ. New nomenclature for vulvar disease. Am J Obstet Gynecol 1989;160:769–770 (Level III)
2. Wilkinson EJ. The 1989 presidential address: International Society for the Study of Vulvar Disease. J Reprod Med 1990;35:981–990 (Level III)
3. Berth-Jones J, Graham-Brown RAC, Burns DA. Lichen sclerosus et atrophicus—a review of 15 cases in young girls. Clin Exp Dermatol 1991;16:14–17 (Level III)
4. Cattaneo A, Bracco GL, Maestrini G, Carli P, Taddei GL, Colafranceschi M, et al. Lichen sclerosus and squamous hyperplasia of the vulva: a clinical study of medical treatment. J Reprod Med 1991;36:301–305 (Level III)
5. Lawrence WD. Non-neoplastic epithelial disorders of the vulva (vulvar dystrophies): historical and current perspectives. Pathol Annu 1993;28:23–51 (Level III)
6. Bracco GL, Carli P, Sonni L, Maestrini G, De Marco A, Taddei GL, et al. Clinical and histologic effects of topical treatments of vulval lichen sclerosus: a critical evaluation. J Reprod Med 1993;38:37–40 (Level II-3)
7. Dalziel KL, Wojnarowska F. Long-term control of vulval lichen sclerosus after treatment with a potent topical steroid cream. J Reprod Med 1993;38:25–27 (Level III)
8. Borgno G, Micheletti L, Barbero M, Preti M, Cavanna L, Ghiringhello B. Epithelial alterations adjacent to 111 vulvar carcinomas. J Reprod Med 1988;33:500–502 (Level II-3)
9. Gomez-Rueda N, Garcia A, Vighi S, Belardi MG, Cardinal L, di-Paola G. Epithelial alterations adjacent to invasive squamous carcinoma of the vulva. J Reprod Med 1994; 39:526–530 (Level II-3)
10. Thomas RHM, Ridley CM, McGibbon DH, Black MM. Lichen sclerosus et atrophicus and autoimmunity: a study of 350 women. Br J Dermatol 1988;118:41–46 (Level III)

11. Eisen D. The vulvovaginal-gingival syndrome of lichen planus: the clinical characteristics of 22 patients. Arch Dermatol 1994;130:1379–1382 (Level III)

12. Bazin S, Bouchard C, Brisson J, Morin C, Meisels A, Fortier M. Vulvar vestibulitis syndrome: an exploratory case-control study. Obstet Gynecol 1994;83:47–50 (Level II-2)

13. Marinoff SC, Turner MLC. Vulvar vestibulitis syndrome. Dermatol Clin 1992;10:435–444 (Level III)

14. McKay M, Frankman O, Horowitz BJ, Lecart C, Micheletti L, Ridley CM, et al. Vulvar vestibulitis and vestibular papillomatosis: report of the ISSVD Committee on Vulvodynia. J Reprod Med 1991;36:413–415 (Level III)

15. Fitzpatrick CC, DeLancey JOL, Elkins TE, McGuire EJ. Vulvar vestibulitis and interstitial cystitis: a disorder of urogenital sinus-derived epithelium? Obstet Gynecol 1993; 81:860–862 (Level III)

16. Bergeron C, Ferenczy A, Richart RM, Guralnick M. Micropapillomatosis labialis appears unrelated to human papillomavirus. Obstet Gynecol 1990;76:281–286 (Level II-2)

17. Prayson RA, Stoler MH, Hart WR. Vulvar vestibulitis: a histopathologic study of 36 cases, including human papillomavirus in situ hybridization analysis. Am J Surg Pathol 1995;19:154–160 (Level III)

18. Pyka RE, Wilkinson EJ, Friedrich EG Jr, Croker BP. The histopathology of vulvar vestibulitis syndrome. Int J Gynecol Pathol 1988;7:249–257 (Level III)

19. Wilkinson EJ, Guerrero E, Daniel R, Shah K, Stone IK, Hardt NS, et al. Vulvar vestibulitis is rarely associated with human papillomavirus infection types 6, 11, 16, or 18. Int J Gynecol Pathol 1993;12:344–349 (Level III)

20. Rumsfield JA, West DP. Topical capsaicin in dermatologic and peripheral pain disorders. Ann Pharmacother 1991;25:381–387 (Level III)

21. McKay M. Dysesthetic ("essential") vulvodynia: treatment with amitriptyline. J Reprod Med 1993;38:9–13 (Level III)

The references in this bulletin are graded according to the method outlined by the U.S. Preventive Services Task Force:

- I Evidence obtained from at least one properly designed randomized controlled trial
- II-1 Evidence obtained from well-designed controlled trials without randomization
- II-2 Evidence obtained from well-designed cohort or case–control analytic studies, preferably from more than one center or research group
- II-3 Evidence obtained from multiple time series, with or without intervention, or dramatic results in uncontrolled experiments
- III Opinions of respected authorities, based on clinical experience, descriptive studies, or reports of expert committees

ISSN 1074-8628

The American College of Obstetricians and Gynecologists
409 12th Street, SW
PO Box 96920
Washington, DC 20090-6920

12345/10987

Number 173—October 1992
(Replaces #87, September 1985)

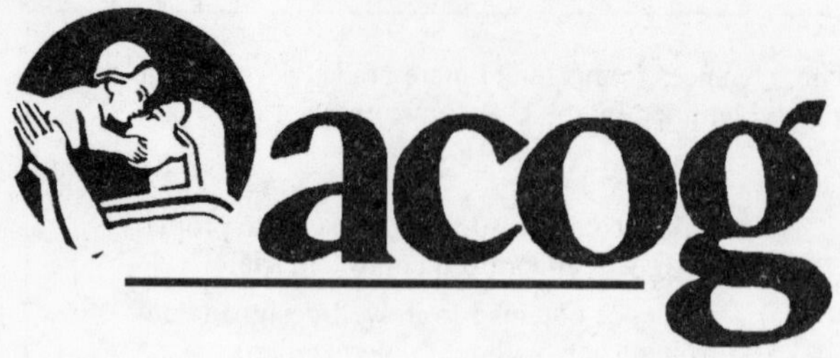

Technical Bulletin
An Educational Aid to Obstetrician–Gynecologists

Women and Exercise

During the 1980s, general awareness of the benefits of exercise and fitness as a way to attain better health markedly increased. Due in large part to requests from women and recommendations in the media, the need for exercise programs for women grew rapidly and were followed by numerous questions to physicians. This Technical Bulletin gives a general overview of the physiology of exercise and fitness, reviews some basic principles of safety, and describes the effects of exercise on female reproductive health. It is meant to provide information about exercise in nonpregnant women only.

Components of General Fitness

General fitness is a broad term that includes cardiovascular fitness, weight control, strength, flexibility, and coordination. Other factors related to prevention of bone loss, alteration of lipid profile, and the prevention of heart disease are also important by-products that appear to be related to fitness (1). Exercise has an impact on each of these areas, and programmed exercise is the single most useful means of attaining fitness.

Cardiovascular Fitness

Cardiovascular fitness should be the major goal of most exercise programs (2). Cardiovascular fitness is the total body response that results in the ability of the individual to maintain a prolonged period of physical activity. The usual format consists of a low-intensity program that lasts for 30–60 minutes three to four times a week. A variety of programs can accomplish this goal, but all are designed to build aerobic capacity, or the ability of the body to supply adequate oxygen to permit prolonged activity.

Repeated exercise that depletes cellular oxygen places the body in a state of stress. In response to this stress, the body gradually increases the oxygen storage capacity in cells by increasing the number of mitochondria. The more prolonged the program, the greater the response. In the laboratory, this is referred to as *aerobic capacity* and is measured by determining the maximum oxygen uptake (Vo_2max) (3). As the exercise progresses, the use of oxygen increases, and the oxygen available at the cellular level for continued metabolism is depleted.

By aerobic conditioning, the individual can increase her Vo_2max. This increased oxygen access allows the individual to prolong her exercise or other physical activity and to perform more efficiently. When exercise has continued long enough to deplete cellular oxygen, the anaerobic pathways begin to dominate, with a resultant buildup in lactic acid (1). Determination of lactic acid values is used to evaluate the effectiveness of aerobic training programs, just as Vo_2max is used by exercise physiologists to measure fitness. When lactic acid levels (measured as serum lactate) increase, it is an indication that the maximum level of aerobic fitness has been reached. In this situation, the individual has greater difficulty performing physical activity and exhaustion is imminent. As training progresses, the time needed to increase serum lactate will increase, and thus aerobic training time will increase. However, for the average physician, neither Vo_2max nor lactic acid determinations are readily available nor are they necessary in counseling patients. Other methods, such as heart rate, can be utilized effectively.

Measurement of the heart rate during exercise is an excellent method by which to evaluate cardiovascular fitness and estimate the Vo_2max (3). As conditioning, (ie, cardiovascular fitness) improves, the heart rate will stabilize at a fixed level of exercise. Since it is possible to establish the heart rate at which conditioning will develop, this value can be calculated to obtain the goal necessary to produce conditioning. The level of exercise that needs to be attained is determined by a simple formula:

$$(220 - \text{age}) \times 60\text{–}80\% = \text{target heart rate range}$$

By using this formula, a woman can determine her own target heart rate based on her age and then find a suitable program that will help her reach this goal (4). For instance, a 35-year-old woman will have a target heart rate of 111–148 beats per minute. The target rate must be maintained for a period of at least 20–30 minutes and repeated at least three times per week. By following this exercise program, the average woman will take 12 or more weeks to develop significant fitness.

Since any exercise program results in increased blood supply to the muscles, a cool-down period should be added to the end of each exercise program (2). During the cool-down period, light activity, such as walking, should be continued until the heart rate has returned to near-normal levels. The cool-down period allows the large quantities of blood diverted to the muscle and skin to gradually return to the central vasculature. This gradual decrease in activity level effects a more even return of the blood supply and prevents dizziness, fainting, and nausea. As conditioning occurs, this return will occur more rapidly, but the length of the cool-down period should remain unchanged. Hot tub baths, showers, and saunas should be avoided until the heart rate is back to the resting level; they will cause further shifting of blood to peripheral pooling and thus result in reduced blood flow to the heart and brain. It has been suggested that this may be part of the etiology of postexercise hypotension, with resultant cardiac and central nervous system ischemia.

Weight Control

Exercise can be successfully used by nonpregnant women for weight reduction and weight maintenance. A weight reduction program that combines both exercise and diet is more effective and results in maintaining weight loss longer than a program based on either one alone. It has also been reported that exercise alters the pattern of fat distribution by reducing the abdominal fat component to a greater extent than other body areas (5). Since abdominal fat has a more significant correlation with heart disease, this is a significant finding even if total weight loss is less than desired (6).

Weight loss from exercise is slow, and the woman who starts an exercise program to achieve rapid weight loss is likely to be disappointed. Depending upon the intensity, it takes an hour to utilize 300–600 calories. Table 1 indicates the average kilocalories utilized during exercise by an average 60–70-kg (132–154-lb) individual in various physical activities. If the woman weighs less, the utilization will be slightly less, and if she weighs more, the utilization will increase. In addition, utilization during the active exercise period will extend through the postexercise period; the elevated heart rate and metabolism may utilize an additional 50–100 kcal during the 10–20 minutes that it takes for the body to return to normal. As conditioning improves, however, this additional calorie expenditure will decline due to the decreased time required for the body to return to resting levels.

The expenditure of 3,500 calories is required to lose 1 pound of fat. This many calories will be burned by 5–10 exercise sessions, assuming the woman has no increase in caloric intake. In addition, muscle hypertrophy will occur in the early phases of exercise. Since muscle is twice the weight of fat per unit volume, a patient can lose fat without losing weight. This fact must be explained to any woman who is using exercise for weight loss. An excellent measure is the fit of her clothing. If it is becoming looser without appreciable weight loss, she is losing fat.

TABLE 1. AVERAGE CALORIE EXPENDITURE FOR COMMON ACTIVITIES*

Activity	Calories/Minute (kcal)
Canoeing, leisure	3.0
Climbing stairs	8.4
Gardening, weeding	5.6
Cycling, 9.4 mph	7.0
Dancing, waltz	5.7
Golf	5.0
Running	
9 minutes/mile	20.0
14 minutes/mile	9.0
Sitting, eating	1.5
Skiing, leisure	9.9
Swimming	
Slow	11.5
Fast	14.0
Tennis	7.1
Walking, 3 mph	4.0

*Approximate caloric expenditure based on an average 60–70-kg (132–154-lb) person

Adapted from: Passmore R, Durnin JVGA. Human energy expenditure. Physiol Rev 1955;35:801–840

Some women will attempt to lose weight by dieting strenuously while in an aerobic exercise program. While this may seem at first to be an ideal method of weight loss, it should be avoided since the resulting energy loss will make exercise difficult and may result in a feeling of exhaustion that prohibits further exercise. A better method is to slightly reduce caloric intake only after establishing an exercise habit; then, gradually increase that reduction over several weeks or until the sensation of being acutely tired no longer persists beyond 2 hours after exercise.

Muscle Strength

In order to strengthen a muscle, the muscle must be subjected to repeated contraction against resistance. As a result, the muscle will begin to hypertrophy and thus be capable of greater force or strength. Most exercise programs result in an increase in muscle strength. However, strength is restricted to those muscles that are actively involved in the exercise program. There is very little crossover of training benefits from one set of limbs to the other (7). Since many of the currently popular exercise programs predominantly involve the lower extremities, a woman will need to engage in a program involving the upper extremities if she wishes to develop arm strength

(7). Evidence is accumulating that individuals who participate in appropriately planned programs involving the upper arms can also develop some cardiovascular fitness. Most weight-training programs, however, do not accomplish a significant improvement in cardiovascular fitness, even with significant gains in strength. As a result, a woman who is seeking cardiovascular fitness should concentrate on an aerobic type of program and avoid those designed only to increase strength.

Bone Density

Recent studies have shown that women who engage in active fitness programs that include weight-bearing exercises have higher bone densities than sedentary women (8). These exercises include impact aerobics, resistance training, and other activities that involve the use of large muscle groups to resist counter pressures; in contrast, swimming and casual walking cause only minimal changes in bone density. The basis for the resulting bone increase is related to the stress placed on the bone by the muscles during the exercise; stress on the bone causes an increase in osteoblastic activity, which results in a buildup of bone density. It occurs regardless of the individual's calcium intake or her estrogen status, although the presence of estrogen certainly decreases bone resorption (9).

Even postmenopausal women can increase their bone density with a moderate exercise program. There are still questions as to how long the effect lasts and how much exercise is necessary to prevent osteoporosis. Until adequate long-term research becomes available, the current opinion is that continual exercise may be necessary to maintain the result.

Osteoporosis is also an important consideration for premenopausal women who have become amenorrheic due to an endocrine disorder. The presence of estrogen is essential to osteoblastic activity as well as reduced osteoclastic activity, and the lack of estrogen—regardless of the reason—is a major reason for calcium loss in these individuals. Therefore, they need the same counseling as postmenopausal women. An active program that includes weight-bearing exercises may be useful to prevent or reduce loss of bone density in any patient who has reduced or absent levels of estrogen (10). Even when the amenorrhea is secondary to exercise itself, bone loss will be minimal in those patients who are participating in weight-bearing exercise programs.

Flexibility

Flexibility depends on ligaments, muscles, and the bony skeleton. Since flexibility is measured by the movement that occurs at any joint or group of joints, any of these areas will be a factor in the flexibility of an individual. In most exercise programs, improved flexibility is accomplished through a routine of systematic stretching of the muscles and slowly warming up (2).

Disagreement exists over the appropriate time to stretch. Some researchers recommend that it be done before the exercise, while others recommend stretching afterwards. Although some of the most recent evidence appears to favor the latter approach (3), it is still recommended that stretching be performed before and after an exercise program. The type of stretching depends upon the anticipated exercise. Stretching is of most value to those muscles and joints that have just been or will be used. For any patient who has severe problems of flexibility, referral for therapy is indicated. Self-directed programs are usually unsatisfactory and can even be dangerous.

Coordination and Balance

The more a muscle repeats an activity, the more efficient the muscle becomes. The more a group of muscles or several groups of muscles perform an activity, the more efficient that activity becomes. As the same activity occurs repetitively over a prolonged time period, the neuromuscular pathways develop patterns that become reflex in nature. This same pattern is seen with any type of coordinative activity (eg, typing, throwing, hitting); as the individual becomes better trained, the ability to perform improves greatly. For this reason, exercises that are designed to improve a specific function and are used repeatedly will improve the individual's ability to perform that function. In the same fashion, any exercise program will improve the overall ability of the person to perform tasks that require similar or related activity.

Designing a General Fitness Program

Any successful exercise program should be designed to fit the needs of the individual by taking into consideration her desires and motivation. The goals of women who exercise vary according to individual preferences. Many women exercise for weight control, while others just wish to feel better. The physician should therefore carefully determine the individual's goals prior to recommending or encouraging any specific program and make necessary adjustments at periodic intervals as her goals change.

Activities to Promote Aerobic Endurance

Any exercise program that requires the body to utilize its oxygen stores for a prolonged period of time will result in an increase in the body's oxygen storage capacity. As the program continues over time, the capability to perform greater activity increases. Many exercises fall in this category, including swimming; running or jogging; bicycling; walking; skiing, especially cross-country; and aerobic dancing (3). Other activities, such as racquetball or tennis, can accomplish the same goal, but frequent periods of rest within the game diminish effectiveness. Golf is a poor exercise for conditioning unless it includes rapid, prolonged walking. Team sports such as volleyball and basketball are effective when there is prolonged activity.

Swimming is an ideal program for exercise of both upper and lower extremities. It is an excellent aerobic conditioner and has the added advantage of minimal impact. The water buoyancy can be very helpful for individuals with minor orthopedic problems. Because of its low impact and low risk of fractures, swimming is an activity that is especially well suited for elderly women with osteoporosis, although it is not weight bearing and has no effect on bone density. The rapid increase in the numbers of women of all ages participating in Masters swimming programs attests to its popularity and ability to satisfy a competitive spirit. Masters swimming programs are designed for individuals wishing to maintain an active fitness program, using competitive swimming as its basis. These programs for adults aged 19 to 95-plus provide active competition within 5-year age groups. (U.S. Masters Swimming may be contacted at Two Peter Avenue, Rutland, MA 01543.)

Bicycling can provide both an enjoyable activity and good aerobic exercise. While bicycling primarily uses the legs, riding at an active pace will exercise the abdomen, lower back, and parts of the upper body as well. Cross-country skiing and rowing are also effective exercise activities. The highest Vo_2max ever recorded was in a cross-country skier.

For most individuals, running or jogging and walking is the major exercise program. A walking or jogging program has the advantage that it can be done virtually anywhere and in any weather. Most current aerobic research has been performed on joggers. A 20–30-minute jog or 45–60-minute walk three to four times a week will accomplish aerobic fitness for almost any person.

A recent innovation has been circuit training. Now available in many public parks and recreation areas, circuit training offers running, jumping, climbing, pulling, and pushing exercises at regular intervals. Recommended levels or times are listed for each activity. By combining several types of exercise, the individual is able to develop muscular strength and aerobic fitness in a combined fashion. A major advantage of circuit training is that the change in activity helps to avoid the boredom of a single program and thus encourages continued participation. For the woman who is interested in increasing strength as well as fitness, circuit training is an appropriate format.

Indoor exercise machines that imitate outdoor activities offer another type of exercise program. These devices include rowing machines, stationary bicycles, machines that imitate cross-country skiing, a variety of treadmills, and combinations of these. They have been used for years in rehabilitation programs, so their aerobic and strength-building benefits are proven (11). An advantage of using exercise machines is that they allow the individual to exercise in a secure, protected environment. This becomes very important when inclement weather or personal safety is a factor. Another advantage is resistance features that allow exercising at the same speed but that require greater effort as conditioning improves. The disadvantage most often cited is boredom with the activity. Some have overcome this boredom by watching television, reading a book, or listening to music during the activity. Another disadvantage, ironically, is the concern for safety. The machines all come with manufacturer's advice for use. However, the individual should be aware that these machines can cause harm if used inappropriately. For example, by setting the tension too high on an exercise bicycle, muscle tears or ligament damage may occur; setting a treadmill too fast can result in injuries during attempted dismount; rowing machines used improperly can cause lower back problems. However, in most circumstances, the stationary exerciser will reach fitness goals as safely and efficiently as the exerciser following any other program.

Activities to Promote Muscle Strength and Toning

Since strength is muscle specific, any activity that is undertaken to develop a particular area of strength will require an exercise designed for that muscle or muscle group. All such exercises are based on the principle of resistance. A muscle must have a resistance to its action to stimulate it to hypertrophy. This can be accomplished by a number of methods. These include: free weights, isometric exercises, elastic resistance, body weight resistance (as with push-ups), or weight-training machines. All of these methods will accomplish the goal of increasing strength. For safety reasons, weight training should always be supervised by a trained instructor. Not only can the individual harm herself if she attempts to perform inappropriate exercises with weights, but she can also strengthen the wrong muscle groups. This can result in an outcome far different from her initial goal.

Toning or improving the appearance of the body by increasing muscle mass and shape is another reason some women undertake weight training. There are now contests for women body builders. However, for most women, participating in such contests is not a goal. They simply want to look better, usually with a flatter stomach, smaller hips and thighs, and firmer upper body. These women will use weight training to hypertrophy muscles in these areas and improve their perception of their appearance. This appearance is further enhanced if total body fat is also reduced, thus making the increased musculature more noticeable. Regardless of the effort, most women will not assume a masculine musculature appearance. An exception is with the use of anabolic steroids which have known and theoretic risks associated with their use.

Although weight training will increase strength and alter appearance, it is not an efficient method of increasing aerobic fitness. Most of these programs have only a slight aerobic component. An individual who wishes to develop aerobic fitness as well as strength needs to adopt a general fitness program in addition to weight training.

Prevention of Injury

The most important measures for preventing injuries are those of good common sense. Start gradually, don't overdo, maintain adequate hydration, avoid high impact, wear appropriate attire, and be aware of bodily responses. Specific safety guidelines for aerobic exercise, strengthening exercises, and stretching exercises should be noted (see the box: Safety Guidelines). It is extremely important to use proper footwear. In most exercise programs, the feet are a key component. Shoes are designed for specific purposes, such as running, walking, or aerobics; they are not transferable. Women should wear a shoe that is specifically designed for their form of exercise. Usually a moderately priced shoe will suffice; for strenuous programs and active competition, better-quality footwear may be necessary.

During any exercise program, certain warning signs that signal overexertion (4) should not be ignored (see the box: Warning Signs of Overexertion). If any of these signs occur, the exercise program should be stopped and then modified; if the symptom reoccurs or remains, an evaluation is required. Muscle pain is usually caused by a buildup of lactic acid in the muscle, resulting from excessive anaerobic metabolism, or by damage to the muscle fibers themselves. When a woman is exercising for fitness, pain has no place. The adage "no pain, no gain" is out of place in a well-designed exercise program for fitness.

Exercise can be overdone. Any activity that is practiced to the extreme can result in injury. For the average woman, attaining fitness is the only goal; once she reaches a satisfactory level, usually in 12–16 weeks, she can maintain her level of fitness without increasing the amount of exercise. The elite athlete (ie, one who is training for a competitive program) will require different counseling than the woman who is just attempting to acquire fitness. Elite athletes need to exercise strenuously over prolonged periods of time in order to accomplish their goals. Such women should be encouraged to seek the help of a competent coach for their sport and, if an injury occurs, be referred to a physician who has special interests not only in sports medicine but also in the problems related to their sport.

Any exercise program can result in an injury. Not only may this harm the individual, it can also interfere with the exercise program. Depending upon the seriousness of the injury, the patient could be permanently prevented from future exercise. However, a more likely result is failure to resume exercising. Individuals who are exercising regularly and then experience a prolonged period away from exercise may find it difficult to start again.

Warning Signs of Overexertion

- Sudden sharp pain
- Excessive fatigue
- Difficulty breathing
- Persistent lethargy
- Nausea
- Vomiting
- Faintness
- Dizziness
- Excessive muscle soreness or pain
- Any irregularity of the heartbeat

Effects on Reproduction

Strenuous exercise can have a major impact on the reproductive system. Reproductive complications were the first reported nonorthopedic problems related to exercise.

Menarche

It has been questioned whether exercise affects the timing of menarche. In studies of Olympic athletes, athletes had a later menarche relative to a comparable population for their country (12). Although this study appeared to indicate that vigorous exercise was related to a delayed onset of menses, many investigators questioned whether this finding was not so much a reflection of the effect of exercise as it was a finding that larger, stronger women were those who had later menarche. Very few studies have been performed that were designed to answer this question. In the few that have been reported, there appears to be a correlation between prepubertal exercise programs and a delayed onset of menses (13).

Attempts to study this phenomenon have concentrated on the hypothalamic–pituitary axis and the effect that exercise has on this hormonal relationship. Initial reports attempted to implicate fat loss secondary to exercise and establish a critical fat level which affected the pituitary hormones (14). Subsequent research has failed to support this theory (15). At this time, no one has been able to identify an etiology. Until further research can define an etiologic factor, the only advice that can be given to the patient or her parents is that the cause is unknown. However, they can be reassured that this delay does not appear to have any significant impact on the woman's future reproductive capacity (16).

Menstrual Irregularities

Exercise alters the amount and frequency of menstrual flow for many women (16). Although dysfunction in the hypothalamic–pituitary axis can affect menstrual function, the causative factor for irregularities related to exercise has not been found to date. In addition to the disproven fat loss theory, other proposed causes have included effects of elevated core temperature on the ovaries, stress reaction, altered central levels of endorphins and other neuropeptides, changes in energy levels, and modification of gonadotropin output (17–20).

Oligomenorrhea and amenorrhea are related to the amount of exercise. Menstrual changes occur when the woman exceeds a specific level of exercise, such as running 20 miles or more per week (21). Since this level varies from woman to woman and depends on her activity, it is impossible to develop a general formula for predicting at what intensity of exercise these irregularities will occur.

Data indicate that exercising women who become amenorrheic have a significant reduction in their circulating estrogen level and thus are at a greater risk for osteoporosis than women with regular cycles (22). Since the relationship between bone loss and reduced levels of estrogen is well established in postmenopausal women, there is little doubt that this same causative factor is at work in amenorrheic women who exercise (22, 23). The major question, as yet unanswered, is how low the estrogen levels must drop for bone loss to begin and whether amenorrhea itself is sufficient to constitute a potential problem. There is some evidence to indicate that women may vary widely in this regard and that not all women with amenorrhea or low estrogen levels will develop osteoporosis. If there is significant bone loss, fractures can become a health problem for women who become amenorrheic with exercise (24). However, most studies now show that once exercise is reduced or stopped, menses resume and bone loss is halted or even reversed.

Dysmenorrhea

Several studies (25) have shown that women who exercise have more, or at least a greater awareness of, dysmenorrhea. This is especially true of high-intensity exercise programs found at the intercollegiate or national level. Objective data to support these findings have not been readily available. It is known that exercise and, especially, the injuries occurring with exercise increase the amount of circulating prostaglandins (26). This is the basis of antiprostaglandin therapy for the minor pains and inflammations associated with exercise. Since prostaglandins are also released from the endometrium during the menstrual cycle, it is at least theoretically possible that the total amount of circulating prostaglandin would greatly increase uterine muscle contractions and thus result in significant ischemia and resultant pain. As a result, in exercising women who complain of severe dysmenorrhea that is not relieved by antiprostaglandin therapy, a prolonged suppressive regimen of one of the estrogen–progesterone combinations may be necessary to alleviate discomfort.

Infertility

Many women who develop amenorrhea or irregular cycles as the result of an exercise program become concerned about their ability to conceive. With the possible exception of oligomenorrhea and anovulation (27), there is currently no evidence to indicate that exercise is a cause of infertility. Since oligomenorrhea has been reported to occur with greater frequency in nulliparous women, as compared with multiparous women, there has been speculation that development of oligomenorrhea may also indicate that these women are more likely to have difficulty conceiving (28). Since there have been few studies of this potential problem, there is no conclusive evidence.

Regardless, any woman who is infertile requires a complete work-up of her problem. All known causes of infertility should be excluded before exercise is considered. If exercise is suspected after this evaluation, specific areas of investigation should include establishment of regular ovulation and determination of luteal phase adequacy, both of which can be affected by low estrogen levels as the result of exercise. Timing of intercourse is also important. A woman who is exercising strenuously may not be having adequate opportunities for intercourse during her ovulatory phase because of the demands of her training schedule.

Once it is established that there is a possibility that exercise may be a contributing factor, the initial therapy is to reduce the amount of exercise or stop it completely. If exercise is the only factor, this should allow pregnancy to occur. If conception has not occurred within 6 months, further evaluation or therapy or both are indicated.

Contraception

There are no contraindications to any of the currently approved contraceptive methods because a woman engages in exercise. Many physicians feel a hemoglobin level of 12 mg/dl should be the minimum in an exercising woman; therefore, the woman using an intrauterine device should be monitored closely. If hemoglobin concentration drops below this level, supplemental iron and folate are indicated. Oral contraceptives have been used by athletes at all levels of competition, and no reports have been published that indicate an adverse effect on performance (25).

Breast

There are no reports of any serious adverse effects of exercise on the breasts, although minor problems such as nipple abrasions may occur. Women should be advised to wear a sports bra while exercising.

Summary

Exercise programs for women can serve many purposes, including developing fitness; controlling weight; improving strength, flexibility, and coordination; enhancing competition with other athletes, and promoting general good health. Depending upon the goal, a realistic method of exercise should be chosen and a program should be developed and followed carefully. Most programs will require aerobic training, which is best maintained by using training heart rates.

Exercise is not without the potential for problems, and any warning signs should not be ignored. As the intensity of the program increases, it may have effects on the reproductive system varying from minor menstrual changes to amenorrhea. The physician needs to be aware of these occurrences, and evaluation is necessary to ensure that no other pathology has occurred. When carefully selected and appropriately followed, an exercise program will result in a healthier patient.

REFERENCES

1. Smith CW Jr. Exercise: a practical guide for helping the patient achieve a healthy lifestyle. J Am Board Fam Pract 1989;2:238–246
2. Wilmore JH. The Wilmore fitness program: a personalized guide to total fitness and health. New York: Simon & Schuster, 1981:75–83, 88–109, 111–123
3. Hanson P. Clinical guidelines for exercise testing. In: Strauss RH, ed. Sports medicine. Philadelphia: WB Saunders Co, 1984:45–56
4. Hartley LH. General principles of exercise prescription. In: Strauss RH, ed. Sports medicine. Philadelphia: WB Saunders Co, 1984:41–45
5. Larsson B, Svardsudd K, Welin L, Wilhelmsen L, Bjorntorp P, Tibblin G. Abdominal adipose tissue distribution, obesity, and risk of cardiovascular disease and death: 13 year follow up of participants in the study of men born in 1913. BMJ 1984;288:1401–1404
6. Tremblay A, Després JP, Leblanc C, Craig CL, Ferris B, Stephens T, et al. Effect of intensity of physical activity on body fatness and fat distribution. Am J Clin Nutr 1990;51:153–157
7. Franklin BA. Aerobic exercise training programs for the upper body. Med Sci Sports Exerc 1989;21:S141–S148
8. McCulloch RG, Bailey DA, Houston CS, Dodd BL. Effects of physical activity, dietary calcium intake and selected lifestyle factors on bone density in young women. Can Med Assoc J 1990;142:221–227
9. Birge SJ, Dalsky G. The role of exercise in preventing osteoporosis. Public Health Rep Suppl 1989;104:54–58
10. Dalsky GP, Stocke KS, Ehsani AA, Slatopolsky E, Lee WC, Birge SJ Jr. Weight-bearing exercise training and lumbar bone mineral content in postmenopausal women. Ann Intern Med 1988;108:824–828
11. Franklin BA, Buchal M, Hollingsworth V, Gordon S, Timmis GC. Exercise prescription. In: Strauss RH, ed. Sports medicine. 2nd ed. Philadelphia: WB Saunders Co, 1991:48–64
12. Malina RM, Bouchard C, Shoup RF, Demirjian A, Lariviere G. Age at menarche, family size, and birth order in athletes at the Montreal Olympic Games, 1976. Med Sci Sports 1979;11:354–358
13. Stager JM, Wigglesworth JK, Hatler LK. Interpreting the relationship between age of menarche and prepubertal training. Med Sci Sports Exerc 1990;22:54–58
14. Wentz AC. Body weight and amenorrhea. Obstet Gynecol 1980;56:482–487
15. Sanborn CF, Albrecht BH, Wagner WW Jr. Athletic amenorrhea: lack of association with body fat. Med Sci Sports Exerc 1987;19:207–212
16. Frisch RE, Gotz-Welbergen AV, McArthur JW, Albright T, Witschi J, Bullen B, et al. Delayed menarche and amenorrhea of college athletes in relation to age of onset of training. JAMA 1981;246:1559–1563
17. Fries H, Nillius SJ, Pettersson F. Epidemiology of secondary amenorrhea. II. A retrospective evaluation of etiology with special regard to psychogenic factors and weight loss. Am J Obstet Gynecol 1974;118:473–479
18. Ding JH, Sheckter CB, Drinkwater BL, Soules MR, Bremner WJ. High serum cortisol levels in exercise-associated amenorrhea. Ann Intern Med 1988;108:530–534
19. Russell JB, Mitchell D, Musey PI, Collins DC. The relationship of exercise to anovulatory cycles in female athletes: hormonal and physical characteristics. Obstet Gynecol 1984;63:452–456
20. Hohtari H, Elovainio R, Salminen K, Laatkainen T. Plasma corticotropin-releasing hormone, corticotropin, and endorphins at rest and during exercise in eumenorrheic and amenorrheic athletes. Fertil Steril 1988; 50:233–238
21. Hale RW, Kosasa T, Krieger J, Pepper S. A marathon: the immediate effect on female runners' luteinizing hormone, follicle-stimulating hormone, prolactin, testosterone, and cortisol levels. Am J Obstet Gynecol 1983;146:550–556
22. Marcus R, Cann C, Madvig P, Minkoff J, Goddard M, Bayer M, et al. Menstrual function and bone mass in elite women distance runners: endocrine and metabolic features. Ann Intern Med 1985;102:158–163
23. Lane NE, Bloch DA, Jones HH, Marshall WH Jr, Wood PD, Fries JF. Long-distance running, bone density and osteoarthritis. JAMA 1986;255:1147–1151
24. Wyshak G, Frisch RE, Albright TE, Albright NL, Schiff I. Bone fractures among former college athletes compared with nonathletes in menopausal and postmenopausal years. Obstet Gynecol 1987;69:121– 126
25. Hale RW. Exercise, sports, and menstrual dysfunction. Clin Obstet Gynecol 1983;26:728–735
26. Viinikka L, Vuori J, Ylikorkala O. Lipid peroxides, prostacyclin, and thromboxane A_2 in runners during acute exercise. Med Sci Sports Exerc 1984;16:275– 277
27. Speroff L, Redwine DB. Exercise and menstrual function. Phys Sportsmed 1980;8:41–52
28. Pepper SJ, Hale RW, Lally DA. Variable effects of strenuous physical training on female reproductive hormone levels. Trans Pac Coast Obstet Gynecol Soc 1984;52:150–156

Safety Guidelines

The following guidelines will help the ob-gyn counsel the average woman seeking to improve her physical fitness through exercise without incurring excessive risk of injury.

Guidelines for Aerobic Exercise

1. For impact activities, it is recommended that exercise routines involving repeated foot impacts be limited to 30 minutes in duration at intensities not exceeding 75% of maximal heart rate. There should be a day of rest between such sessions.
2. A resilient floor should be selected for exercise that involves repeated foot impacts. If such a surface is not available, the exercise routines should be modified to ensure that the feet remain close to the floor throughout the program.
3. Aerobic exercise should be preceded by a gentle warm-up routine that utilizes the full range of motion of the joints. This increases the elasticity of the muscles and will help prevent potentially injurious movements.
4. Muscles that are used repeatedly during aerobic exercise must be carefully stretched before and afterward.
5. To reduce the severity of impact shock on the lower extremities, repetitive jumping on the same foot should not exceed four consecutive jumps.
6. Extremes of joint flexion and extension (such as deep knee bends and ballistic hyperextension of the knee) should be avoided.
7. The feet should be moved repeatedly to prevent cramping in the intrinsic muscles of the foot.
8. Trunk rotation should be avoided while on the feet with hips or lower spine flexed. Rotational activity in this position subjects the intervertebral disks to very high mechanical stress.
9. Intense physical activity should always be followed by a cool-down period of at least 10 minutes of lighter activity to prevent pooling of blood in the extremities. Hot showers and baths should be avoided immediately after intense physical activity.
10. Participants should be given a specific means of assessing physical status and progress. Working heart rate should be measured during peak levels of exercise to ensure that the intensity of activity is within the desired range. Regular measurement of the recovery heart rate will motivate participants by documenting their progress. Failure to progress as measured by this method may indicate the need for more intense activity during the aerobic phase or may signal the presence of other problems.

Guidelines for Strengthening Exercises

1. Strengthening exercises should not be performed on the same muscles on consecutive days.
2. A general warm-up routine should be performed before muscles are made to work against resistance.
3. Muscle-strengthening exercises should be preceded and followed by stretching exercises that are specific for the muscles that are made to work against resistance.
4. All strengthening exercises should be performed in a slow and controlled manner. Ballistic (rapid or jerky) movements increase the risk of injury.
5. The most efficient way to improve strength is to allow brief rest periods between bouts of vigorous exercise. Repetitions should be limited to short sets (10 or fewer) that are repeated later.
6. When the strength of one muscle or muscle group is disproportionate to that of the antagonist(s) for that muscle or group, the weaker muscle should be strengthened to restore balance around the joint.
7. The breath should not be held during strength-training exercises. Exhalation should take place during the exertion phase of each repetition.

Guidelines for Stretching Exercises

1. Stretching exercises may be performed as often as desired, preferably at least once a day.
2. A general warm-up routine should be performed before muscles are stretched.
3. Stretching routines should be performed statically, without holding the breath. Rapid, jerky movements should be avoided.
4. Each stretch should be held long enough so that relaxation will occur sufficiently to achieve the maximum benefit of the stretch. This can vary from as little as 6 seconds in some individuals to 20 seconds in others.
5. Muscles should be stretched only to the point of tension. Pain should be regarded as a signal that a stretch has gone too far.

This Technical Bulletin was developed under the direction of the Committee on Technical Bulletins of the American College of Obstetricians and Gynecologists as an educational aid to obstetricians and gynecologists. The committee wishes to thank Ralph W. Hale, MD, for his assistance in the development of this bulletin. This Technical Bulletin does not define a standard of care, nor is it intended to dictate an exclusive course of management. It presents recognized methods and techniques of clinical practice for consideration by obstetrician–gynecologists for incorporation into their practices. Variations of practice taking into account the needs of the individual patient, resources, and limitations unique to the institution or type of practice may be appropriate.

THE AMERICAN COLLEGE OF OBSTETRICIANS AND GYNECOLOGISTS
409 12th Street, SW
Washington, DC 20024-2188

45678/21098

Lists of Titles

Committee Opinions

Educational and Technical Bulletins

Practice Bulletins

Practice Patterns

Policy Statements

Index

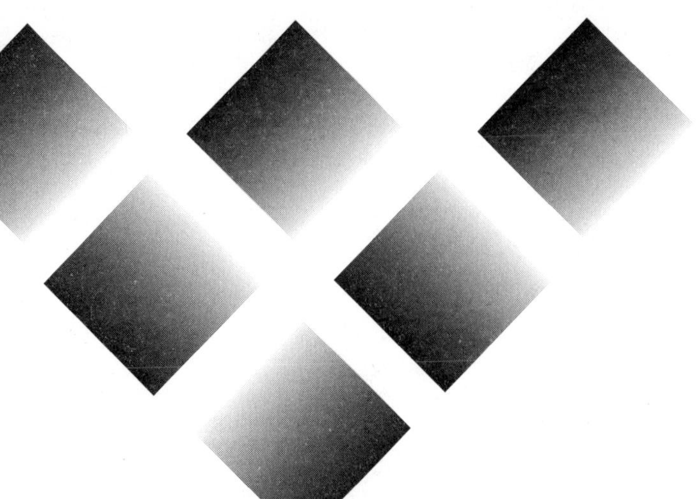

ACOG PRACTICE BULLETIN

CLINICAL MANAGEMENT GUIDELINES FOR OBSTETRICIAN–GYNECOLOGISTS

NUMBER 9, OCTOBER 1999

(Replaces Technical Bulletin Number 188, January 1994)

This Practice Bulletin was developed by the ACOG Committee on Practice Bulletins—Obstetrics with the assistance of Dwight J. Rouse, MD. The information is designed to aid practitioners in making decisions about appropriate obstetric and gynecologic care. These guidelines should not be construed as dictating an exclusive course of treatment or procedure. Variations in practice may be warranted based on the needs of the individual patient, resources, and limitations unique to the institution or type of practice.

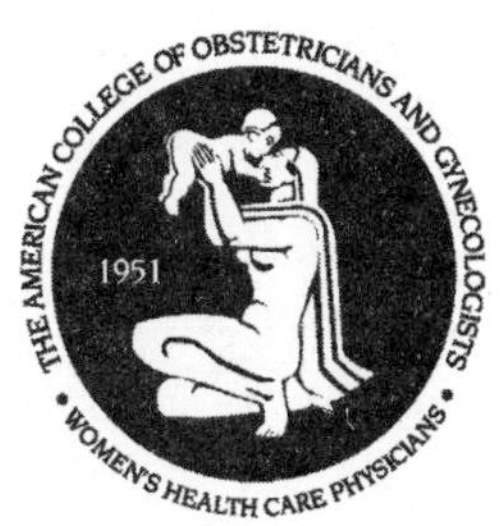

Antepartum Fetal Surveillance

The goal of antepartum fetal surveillance is to prevent fetal death. Antepartum fetal surveillance techniques based on assessment of fetal heart rate patterns have been in clinical use for almost three decades. More recently, real-time ultrasonography and Doppler velocimetry have been used to evaluate fetal well-being. Antepartum fetal surveillance techniques are now routinely used to assess the risk of fetal death in pregnancies complicated by preexisting maternal conditions (eg, type 1 diabetes mellitus) as well as those in which complications have developed (eg, intrauterine growth restriction). This document will review the current indications for and techniques of antepartum fetal surveillance and outline management guidelines for antepartum fetal surveillance, consistent with the best contemporary scientific evidence.

Background

Physiology of Fetal Heart Response and Fetal Behavioral State Alteration

In both animals and humans, fetal heart rate pattern, level of activity, and degree of muscular tone are sensitive to hypoxemia and acidemia (1–4). Redistribution of fetal blood flow in response to hypoxemia may result in diminished renal perfusion and oligohydramnios (5). Surveillance techniques such as cardiotocography, real-time ultrasonography, and maternal perception of fetal movement can identify the fetus that is either suboptimally oxygenated or, with increasing degrees of placental dysfunction, acidemic. Identification of suspected fetal compromise provides the opportunity to intervene before progressive metabolic acidosis can lead to fetal death. However, acute, catastrophic changes in fetal status, such as those that can occur with abruptio placentae or an umbilical cord accident, are generally not predicted by tests of fetal well-being. Therefore, fetal deaths from such events are not as amenable to prevention.

In humans, the range of normal umbilical blood gas parameters has been established by cordocentesis performed in pregnancies in which the fetus ultimately proved to be healthy, and ranges vary by gestational age (6). Although the degree of hypoxemia and acidemia at which various indices of fetal well-being become abnormal is not known with precision, it can be estimated, based on data from published studies. In one investigation, the fetal biophysical profile (BPP) was performed immediately before cordocentesis. Fetuses with a nonreactive nonstress test (NST) were found to have a mean (± standard deviation) umbilical vein pH of 7.28 ± 0.11. Cessation of fetal movement appears to occur at lower pH levels; fetuses with abnormal movement were found to have an umbilical vein pH of 7.16 ± 0.08 (7). Thus, a reasonable correlation between certain measurable aspects of fetal heart rate and behavior and evidence of fetal metabolic compromise can be inferred.

However, when abnormal antepartum fetal surveillance results are compared with evidence of hypoxia or acidemia, the degree of acid–base disturbance may range from mild to severe. Furthermore, factors other than acid–base and oxygenation status (eg, prematurity, fetal sleep–wake cycle, maternal medication exposure, and fetal central nervous system abnormalities) can adversely affect biophysical parameters. Finally, neither the degree nor the duration of intrauterine hypoxemia and acidemia necessary to adversely affect short- and long-term neonatal outcome has been established with any precision.

Antepartum Fetal Surveillance Techniques

Several antepartum fetal surveillance techniques (tests) are in use. These include fetal movement assessment, NST, contraction stress test (CST), BPP, modified BPP, and umbilical artery Doppler velocimetry.

Fetal Movement Assessment

A diminution in the maternal perception of fetal movement often but not invariably precedes fetal death, in some cases by several days (8). This observation provides the rationale for fetal movement assessment by the mother ("kick counts") as a means of antepartum fetal surveillance.

Although several counting protocols have been employed, neither the optimal number of movements nor the ideal duration for counting movements has been defined. Thus, numerous protocols have been reported and appear to be acceptable. In one approach, the woman lies on her side and counts distinct fetal movements (9). Perception of 10 distinct movements in a period of up to 2 hours is considered reassuring. Once 10 movements have been perceived, the count may be discontinued. In another approach, women are instructed to count fetal movements for 1 hour three times per week (10). The count is considered reassuring if it equals or exceeds the woman's previously established baseline count. In the absence of a reassuring count, further fetal assessment is recommended.

Contraction Stress Test

The CST is based on the response of the fetal heart rate to uterine contractions. It relies on the premise that fetal oxygenation will be transiently worsened by uterine contractions. In the suboptimally oxygenated fetus, the resultant intermittent worsening in oxygenation will, in turn, lead to the fetal heart rate pattern of late decelerations. Uterine contractions also may provoke or accentuate a pattern of variable decelerations caused by fetal umbilical cord compression, which in some cases is associated with oligohydramnios.

With the patient in the lateral recumbent position, the fetal heart rate and uterine contractions are simultaneously recorded with an external fetal monitor. If at least three spontaneous contractions of 40 seconds' duration each or longer are present in a 10-minute period, no uterine stimulation is necessary. If fewer than three contractions of at least 40 seconds' duration occur in 10 minutes, contractions are induced with either nipple stimulation or intravenous administration of dilute oxytocin.

Nipple stimulation usually is successful in inducing an adequate contraction pattern and allows completion of testing in approximately half the time required when intravenous oxytocin is given (11). In one nipple stimulation technique, the woman is instructed to rub one nipple through her clothing for 2 minutes or until a contraction begins (11). If by that time the contraction frequency has not become adequate (as defined previously), stimulation is stopped and restarted again after 5 minutes. If nipple stimulation is unsuccessful, or if the use of oxytocin is preferred, an intravenous infusion of dilute oxytocin may be initiated at a rate of 0.5 mU/min and doubled every 20 minutes until an adequate contraction pattern is achieved (12).

The CST is interpreted according to the presence or absence of late fetal heart rate decelerations (13), which are defined as decelerations that reach their nadir after the peak of the contraction and that usually persist beyond the end of the contraction. The results of the CST are categorized as follows:

- Negative: no late or significant variable decelerations

- Positive: late decelerations following 50% or more of contractions (even if the contraction frequency is fewer than three in 10 minutes)
- Equivocal–suspicious: intermittent late decelerations or significant variable decelerations
- Equivocal–hyperstimulatory: fetal heart rate decelerations that occur in the presence of contractions more frequent than every 2 minutes or lasting longer than 90 seconds
- Unsatisfactory: fewer than three contractions in 10 minutes or an uninterpretable tracing

Relative contraindications to the CST generally include conditions associated with an increased risk of preterm labor and delivery, uterine rupture, or uterine bleeding. These include the following (12):

- Preterm labor or certain patients at high risk of preterm labor
- Preterm membrane rupture
- History of extensive uterine surgery or classical cesarean delivery
- Known placenta previa

Nonstress Test

The NST is based on the premise that the heart rate of the fetus that is not acidotic or neurologically depressed will temporarily accelerate with fetal movement. Heart rate reactivity is thought to be a good indicator of normal fetal autonomic function. Loss of reactivity is associated most commonly with a fetal sleep cycle but may result from any cause of central nervous system depression, including fetal acidosis.

With the patient in the lateral tilt position, the fetal heart rate is monitored with an external transducer. Ideally, the patient should not have smoked recently, because this may adversely affect test results (14). The tracing is observed for fetal heart rate accelerations that peak (but do not necessarily remain) at least 15 beats per minute above the baseline and last 15 seconds from baseline to baseline. It may be necessary to continue the tracing for 40 minutes or longer to take into account the variations of the fetal sleep–wake cycle. Acoustic stimulation of the nonacidotic fetus may elicit fetal heart rate accelerations that appear to be valid in the prediction of fetal well-being. Such stimulation offers the advantage of safely reducing overall testing time without compromising detection of the acidotic fetus (15–17). To perform acoustic stimulation, an artificial larynx (ideally one of the commercially available models especially designed for this purpose) is positioned on the maternal abdomen and a stimulus of 1–2 seconds is applied. This may be repeated up to three times for progressively longer durations of up to 3 seconds to elicit fetal heart rate accelerations.

Nonstress test results are categorized as reactive or nonreactive. Various definitions of reactivity have been used. Using the most common definition, the NST is considered reactive (normal) if there are two or more fetal heart rate accelerations (as defined previously) within a 20-minute period, with or without fetal movement discernible by the woman (18). A nonreactive NST is one that lacks sufficient fetal heart rate accelerations over a 40-minute period. The NST of the noncompromised preterm fetus is frequently nonreactive: from 24 to 28 weeks of gestation, up to 50% of NSTs may not be reactive (19), and from 28 to 32 weeks of gestation, 15% of NSTs are not reactive (20, 21).

Variable decelerations may be observed in up to 50% of NSTs (22). If nonrepetitive and brief (<30 seconds), they indicate neither fetal compromise nor the need for obstetric intervention (22). Repetitive variable decelerations (at least 3 in 20 minutes), even if mild, have been associated with an increased risk of cesarean delivery for a nonreassuring intrapartum fetal heart rate pattern (23, 24). Fetal heart rate decelerations during an NST that persist for 1 minute or longer are associated with a markedly increased risk of both cesarean delivery for a nonreassuring fetal heart rate pattern and fetal demise (25–27).

Biophysical Profile

The BPP consists of an NST combined with four observations made by real-time ultrasonography (28). Thus, the BPP comprises five components:

1. Nonstress test (which, if all four ultrasound components are normal, may be omitted without compromising the validity of the test results) (28)
2. Fetal breathing movements (one or more episodes of rhythmic fetal breathing movements of 30 seconds or more within 30 minutes)
3. Fetal movement (three or more discrete body or limb movements within 30 minutes)
4. Fetal tone (one or more episodes of extension of a fetal extremity with return to flexion, or opening or closing of a hand)
5. Determination of the amniotic fluid volume (a single vertical pocket of amniotic fluid exceeding 2 cm is considered evidence of adequate amniotic fluid) (29, 30)

Each of the five components is assigned a score of either 2 (normal or present as defined previously) or 0 (abnormal, absent, or insufficient). A composite score of 8 or 10 is normal, a score of 6 is considered equivocal, and a score of 4 or less is abnormal. Regardless of the composite score, in the presence of oligohydramnios (largest vertical pocket of amniotic fluid volume ≤ 2 cm), further evaluation is warranted (30).

Modified Biophysical Profile

In the late second- or third-trimester fetus, amniotic fluid reflects fetal urine production. Placental dysfunction may result in diminished fetal renal perfusion, leading to oligohydramnios (5). Amniotic fluid volume assessment can therefore be used to evaluate long-term uteroplacental function. This observation fostered the development of what has come to be termed the "modified BPP" as a primary mode of antepartum fetal surveillance. The modified BPP combines the NST (with the option of acoustic stimulation), as a short-term indicator of fetal acid–base status, with the amniotic fluid index (AFI), which is the sum of measurements of the deepest cord-free amniotic fluid pocket in each of the abdominal quadrants, as an indicator of long-term placental function (15). An AFI greater than 5 cm generally is considered to represent an adequate volume of amniotic fluid (31). Thus, the modified BPP is considered normal if the NST is reactive and the AFI is more than 5, and abnormal if either the NST is nonreactive or the AFI is 5 or less.

Umbilical Artery Doppler Velocimetry

Doppler ultrasonography is a noninvasive technique used to assess the hemodynamic components of vascular impedance. Umbilical artery Doppler flow velocimetry has been adapted for use as a technique of fetal surveillance, based on the observation that flow velocity waveforms in the umbilical artery of normally growing fetuses differ from those of growth-restricted fetuses. Specifically, the umbilical flow velocity waveform of normally growing fetuses is characterized by high-velocity diastolic flow, whereas with intrauterine growth restriction, there is diminution of umbilical artery diastolic flow (32–34). In some cases of extreme intrauterine growth restriction, flow is absent or even reversed. The perinatal mortality rate in such pregnancies is quite high (35). Abnormal flow velocity waveforms have been correlated histopathologically with small-artery obliteration in placental tertiary villi (36) and functionally with fetal hypoxia and acidosis (37), as well as with perinatal morbidity and mortality (35). Commonly measured flow indices, based on the characteristics of peak systolic frequency shift (S), end-diastolic frequency shift (D), and mean peak frequency shift over the cardiac cycle (A), include the following:

- Systolic to diastolic ratio (S/D)
- Resistance index (S-D/S)
- Pulsatility index (S-D/A)

Randomized studies (38–44) of the utility of umbilical artery Doppler velocimetry generally have defined abnormal flow as either absent end diastolic flow, or a flow index greater than two standard deviations above the mean for gestational age. To maximize interpretability, multiple waveforms should be assessed, and wall-filter settings should be set low enough (typically <150 Hz) to avoid masking diastolic flow.

Clinical Considerations and Recommendations

▶ ***Is there compelling evidence that any form of antepartum fetal surveillance decreases the risk of fetal demise or otherwise improves perinatal outcome?***

There is a dearth of evidence from randomized controlled trials that antepartum fetal surveillance decreases the risk of fetal death (45). Moreover, in one comprehensive review, antepartum fetal surveillance was categorized as a form of care "likely to be ineffective or harmful" (46). In spite of its unproven value, antepartum fetal surveillance is widely integrated into clinical practice in the developed world. Therefore, a definitive evaluation of antepartum fetal surveillance (which would require the random allocation of gravidas to prenatal care that included some form of antepartum fetal surveillance versus prenatal care that did not include any form of antepartum fetal surveillance) is unlikely to be conducted in a setting that can be generalized to current U.S. obstetric practice. In the absence of a definitive, relevant randomized clinical trial, evidence for the value of antepartum fetal surveillance will remain circumstantial and rest principally on the observation that antepartum fetal surveillance has been consistently associated with rates of fetal death that are substantially lower than the rates of fetal death in both untested (and presumably lower-risk) contemporaneous pregnancies from the same institutions (15, 16, 47) and pregnancies with similar complicating factors that were managed before the advent of currently employed techniques of antepartum fetal surveillance (historic controls). However, these perceived benefits of antepartum fetal surveillance may be influenced by the low incidence of adverse fetal outcome in the general population. The lower the incidence of adverse outcomes, the more likely favorable outcomes will be achieved regardless of test performance.

▶ *What are the indications for antepartum fetal surveillance?*

Because antepartum fetal surveillance results have not been definitively demonstrated to improve perinatal outcome, all indications for antepartum testing must be considered somewhat relative. In general, antepartum fetal surveillance has been employed in pregnancies in which the risk of antepartum fetal demise is increased. Accordingly, some of the conditions under which testing may be appropriate include the following:

- Maternal conditions
  - —Antiphospholipid syndrome
  - —Hyperthyroidism (poorly controlled)
  - —Hemoglobinopathies (hemoglobin SS, SC, or S-thalassemia)
  - —Cyanotic heart disease
  - —Systemic lupus erythematosus
  - —Chronic renal disease
  - —Type 1 diabetes mellitus
  - —Hypertensive disorders
- Pregnancy-related conditions
  - —Pregnancy-induced hypertension
  - —Decreased fetal movement
  - —Oligohydramnios
  - —Polyhydramnios
  - —Intrauterine growth restriction
  - —Postterm pregnancy
  - —Isoimmunization (moderate to severe)
  - —Previous fetal demise (unexplained or recurrent risk)
  - —Multiple gestation (with significant growth discrepancy)

▶ *When during gestation should antepartum fetal surveillance be initiated?*

Choosing the appropriate point in gestation to begin antepartum testing depends on balancing several considerations, including the prognosis for neonatal survival, the severity of maternal disease, the risk of fetal death, and the potential for iatrogenic prematurity complications resulting from false-positive test results. The importance of the last consideration is illustrated by the experience of one large center, in which 60% of infants delivered because of an abnormal antepartum test result had no evidence of short-term or long-term fetal compromise (16). Both theoretic models (48) and large clinical studies (49, 50) confirm that initiating testing at 32–34 weeks of gestation is appropriate for most at-risk patients. However, in pregnancies with multiple or particularly worrisome high-risk conditions (eg, chronic hypertension with suspected intrauterine growth restriction), testing might begin as early as 26–28 weeks of gestation.

▶ *What is the proper frequency of testing?*

How frequently to perform fetal testing depends on several factors, including clinical judgment. If the indication for testing is not persistent (eg, a single episode of decreased fetal movement followed by reassuring testing in an otherwise uncomplicated pregnancy), it need not be repeated. When the clinical condition that prompted testing persists, the test should be repeated periodically until delivery to monitor for continued fetal well-being. If the maternal medical condition is stable and CST results are negative, the CST is typically repeated in 1 week (12). Other tests of fetal well-being (NST, BPP, or modified BPP) are typically repeated at weekly intervals (16), but in the presence of certain high-risk conditions, such as postterm pregnancy, type 1 diabetes, intrauterine growth restriction, or pregnancy-induced hypertension, some investigators have performed twice-weekly NST, BPP, or modified BPP testing. Any significant deterioration in the maternal medical status requires fetal reevaluation, as does any acute diminution in fetal activity, regardless of the amount of time that has elapsed since the last test.

▶ *How reassuring is a normal test result?*

In most cases, a normal test result is highly reassuring, as reflected in the false-negative rate of antepartum fetal surveillance, defined as the incidence of stillbirth occurring within 1 week of a normal test result. The stillbirth rate, corrected for lethal congenital anomalies and unpredictable causes of demise, was 1.9 per 1,000 in the largest series of NSTs (5,861) versus 0.3 per 1,000 in 12,656 CSTs (13), 0.8 per 1,000 in 44,828 BPPs (51), and 0.8 per 1,000 in 54,617 modified BPPs (16). Based on these data, the negative predictive value of the NST is 99.8%, and greater than 99.9% for the CST, BPP, and modified BPP. Although similar data from a large series are not available for umbilical artery Doppler velocimetry, in one randomized clinical trial among women with pregnancies complicated by intrauterine growth restriction (38), no stillbirths occurred in 214 pregnancies in which umbilical artery Doppler velocimetry was the primary means of antepartum fetal surveillance (negative predictive value of 100%). The low false-negative rate of these tests depends on an appropriate response to any significant deterioration in the maternal clinical status, including retesting of the fetal condition. As mentioned previously, these tests generally do not predict stillbirths related to acute changes in maternal–fetal status, such as those that occur with abruptio placentae or an umbilical cord accident. Moreover, recent, normal antepartum fetal test results should not preclude the use of intrapartum fetal monitoring.

▶ *How should one respond to an abnormal test result?*

An abnormal fetal test result should always be considered in the context of the overall clinical picture, taking into account the substantial possibility that the test result is falsely positive. Certain acute maternal conditions (eg, diabetic ketoacidosis, pneumonia with hypoxemia) can result in abnormal test results, which generally will become normal as the maternal condition improves. In these circumstances, stabilizing the maternal condition and retesting the fetus may be appropriate.

In cases where an abnormal test result is not associated with any clinical evidence of worsening in the maternal status, a sequenced approach to the investigation of the fetal condition should be undertaken. Such an approach takes advantage of the high negative predictive value generally exhibited by all commonly used antepartum tests (see above), and minimizes the potential for unnecessary delivery based on a false-positive (ie, abnormal) test result. False-positive rates, in contrast to false-negative rates, have typically not been calculated using the outcome of stillbirth. This is because most antepartum tests were introduced into clinical practice before an unbiased evaluation of their sensitivity and specificity. In clinical practice, abnormal test results usually are followed by another test or delivery is effected, which obscures the relationship between a positive test result and the subsequent risk of stillbirth. Therefore, in the absence of unbiased evaluations, the positive predictive value of antepartum tests has been estimated using surrogate markers, such as the rate of positive follow-up test results when the primary test result is positive. For example, it has been observed that up to 90% of nonreactive NSTs are followed by a negative CST result (18). Based on this observation, the positive predictive value of an NST is only 10%. Another way that the false-positive rate of fetal testing has been estimated is to calculate the incidence of abnormal test results that prompt delivery but are not associated with evidence of fetal compromise, as manifested by a nonreassuring intrapartum fetal heart rate, meconium-stained amniotic fluid, 5-minute Apgar scores of less than 7, or birth weight greater than the 10th percentile for gestational age. By this latter definition, in one large series, a testing scheme in which abnormal modified BPPs were followed by full BPPs had a false-positive rate of 60% (positive predictive value = 40%) (18). In another study in which the physicians were blinded to test results, a CST was found to have a positive predictive value of less than 35% (52).

Therefore, the response to an abnormal test result should be tailored to the clinical situation. Maternal reports of decreased fetal movement should be evaluated by an NST, CST, BPP, or modified BPP; these results, if normal, usually are sufficient to exclude imminent fetal jeopardy. A nonreactive NST or an abnormal modified BPP generally should be followed by additional testing (either a CST or a full BPP). A positive CST result suggests that NST nonreactivity is a consequence of hypoxia-induced acidosis, whereas a negative result implies that the NST nonreactivity exists for another reason, such as a premature fetus, maternal exposure to certain drugs or medications, a fetal sleep cycle, or preexisting neurologic damage. In many circumstances, a positive CST result generally indicates that delivery is warranted. However, the combination of a nonreactive NST and a positive CST result is associated frequently with serious fetal malformation and justifies ultrasonographic investigation for anomalies whenever possible (53). Indeed, evaluation for grossly abnormal fetal anatomy should precede any intervention for suspected fetal compromise whenever possible.

A BPP score of 6 is considered equivocal; in the term fetus, this score generally should prompt delivery, whereas in the preterm fetus, it should result in a repeat BPP in 24 hours (30). In the interim, maternal corticosteroid administration should be considered for pregnancies of less than 34 weeks of gestation. Repeat equivocal scores should result either in delivery or continued intensive surveillance. A BPP score of 4 usually indicates that delivery is warranted, although in extremely premature pregnancies, management should be individualized. Biophysical profiles less than 4 should result in expeditious delivery. Regardless of the overall score, oligohydramnios always requires further evaluation.

In the absence of obstetric contraindications, delivery of the fetus with an abnormal test result often may be attempted by induction of labor, with continuous monitoring of both the fetal heart rate and contractions.

▶ *Are there clinical circumstances in which one test is distinguished by its utility or lack thereof?*

A large-scale, definitive randomized trial comparing the relative efficacy of one technique of antepartum fetal testing to another has not yet been performed. Accordingly, in most clinical situations, no single antepartum fetal test can be considered superior to any other.

As mentioned previously, in certain clinical situations, the CST is considered relatively contraindicated (increased risk of preterm labor and delivery, uterine rupture, and uterine bleeding), although even in these situations the value of the information provided by the test may outweigh its potential risks.

▶ *When should oligohydramnios prompt delivery?*

Amniotic fluid volume is estimated using ultrasonography. One widely used definition of oligohydramnios is no measurable vertical pocket of amniotic fluid greater than 2 cm (29), and another is an AFI of 5 cm or less (31). Nevertheless, from a clinical standpoint, an ideal cutoff level for intervention using the AFI has yet to be established. Determining when to intervene for oligohydramnios depends on several factors, including gestational age, the maternal and fetal clinical condition as determined by other indices of fetal well-being, and the actual measured AFI value. Because rupture of the fetal membranes can cause diminished amniotic fluid volume, an evaluation for membrane rupture may be appropriate.

In postterm pregnancy, oligohydramnios is common and is associated with an increased risk of meconium staining of the amniotic fluid and cesarean delivery for nonreassuring fetal heart rate (54, 55). Thus, oligohydramnios has been considered an indication for delivery of the postterm pregnancy (15), although the effectiveness of this approach in improving perinatal outcome has not been established by randomized investigation.

In a term pregnancy complicated by oligohydramnios, delivery often is the most appropriate course of action. However, management should be individualized, and in certain situations, delivery may be safely postponed (eg, an uncomplicated pregnancy with an AFI of 5 cm but otherwise reassuring fetal testing and an unfavorable cervix at 37 weeks of gestation).

In the preterm fetus, depending on the maternal and fetal condition, expectant management may be the most appropriate course of action (eg, with preterm premature rupture of membranes or in the presence of fetal anomalies). Once oligohydramnios is diagnosed, if delivery is not undertaken, follow-up amniotic fluid volume and fetal growth assessments are indicated. If the oligohydramnios is persistent, close monitoring of the maternal condition and ongoing antepartum fetal surveillance should be performed to guide further management. If the oligohydramnios results from fetal membrane rupture, follow-up amniotic fluid volume assessment often may be safely omitted.

▶ *What is the role of Doppler velocimetry?*

At least three randomized trials (38, 56, 57) have evaluated the utility of umbilical artery Doppler velocimetry as a technique of antepartum fetal surveillance in pregnancies complicated by suspected intrauterine growth restriction. In the first and largest of these trials (38), 214 pregnancies were allocated to Doppler umbilical artery velocimetry as the primary technique of fetal surveillance, and 212 were allocated to cardiotocography (NST). Overall, women in the Doppler group were significantly less likely to undergo obstetric intervention, including antepartum hospital admission, labor induction, and emergency cesarean delivery for nonreassuring fetal status. On average, women in the Doppler group underwent antenatal testing less frequently (4 times) than women in the cardiotocography group (8 times). Other perinatal outcomes, such as gestational age at birth, birthweight, Apgar scores, and cesarean birth rates, did not differ between the groups.

Subsequent trials (56, 57) have supported the findings of less frequent antenatal monitoring (56) and shorter durations of maternal hospitalization (56, 57) in the Doppler group. However, rates of obstetric interventions, such as antepartum admission and labor induction, were not lower in the Doppler groups, and perinatal outcome was not improved. On balance, the available evidence suggests that primary antepartum surveillance of suspected intrauterine growth restriction with umbilical artery Doppler velocimetry can achieve at least equivalent (and possibly better) fetal and neonatal outcomes as primary antepartum surveillance based on results of the NST. Furthermore, frequency of antepartum testing and certain aspects of obstetric intervention are reduced with use of Doppler (58). If umbilical artery Doppler velocimetry is used, decisions regarding timing of delivery should be made using a combination of information from the Doppler ultrasonography and other tests of fetal well-being, such as amniotic fluid volume assessment, NST, CST, and BPP, along with careful monitoring of maternal status.

No benefit has been demonstrated for umbilical artery velocimetry for conditions other than suspected intrauterine growth restriction, such as postterm gestation, diabetes mellitus, systemic lupus erythematosus, or antiphospholipid syndrome. Doppler ultrasonography has not been shown to be of value as a screening test for detecting fetal compromise in the general obstetric population, and its use for this purpose cannot be recommended (59). In addition to the umbilical artery, it is possible to evaluate blood flow in major fetal vessels. Multiple investigators have observed a correlation between increased flow resistance (elevated S/D ratio) in the umbilical artery and decreased resistance to flow (reduced S/D ratio) in the middle cerebral artery. This phenomenon has been attributed to a "brain sparing" adaptive response to fetal hypoxemia, and it has been suggested that the ratio of middle cerebral artery S/D ratio to umbilical artery S/D ratio might serve as a useful predictor of fetal compromise (60). However, the only randomized clinical trial of middle cerebral artery Doppler velocimetry failed to demonstrate any clinical benefit to assessing this parameter (61). Moreover, women in this trial who were allocated to standard fetal evaluation plus assessment of the ratio of middle cerebral artery or umbilical artery Doppler flow, or both, were delivered on average 5.7 days earlier after the institution of fetal testing than women who were allocated to standard fetal evaluation without assessment of middle cerebral artery blood flow. This suggests that incorporation of middle cerebral artery Doppler flow assessment into clinical practice might increase unnecessary intervention. Therefore, at present, middle cerebral artery Doppler flow measurement should be considered investigational.

▶ *Should all women perform daily fetal movement assessment?*

Whether programs of fetal movement assessment actually can reduce the risk of stillbirth is not clear. Only two randomized trials have addressed this issue. The first was conducted in a mixed high-risk (39%) and low-risk (61%) population of 3,111 Danish women who, after 32 weeks of gestation, were randomly assigned to an experimental (counting) group or a control group (10). Women in the experimental group were asked to count fetal movements for 1 hour three times a week and to contact their hospital immediately if they detected fewer movements than their previously established baseline. The control group of women were given no special fetal movement assessment instructions but were asked about fetal movement at their prenatal visits. Of the 1,583 women in the counting group, three experienced stillbirths of normally formed infants weighing more than 1,500 g, versus 12 stillbirths among the 1,569 women in the control group ($P<0.05$). Of women allocated to the counting group, 80% complied well with the protocol for counting, and 4% were evaluated for decreased fetal movement. The rates of operative vaginal birth and cesarean delivery did not differ significantly between the groups.

The second randomized study to evaluate fetal movement allocated 68,000 women at 28–32 weeks of gestation to a counting policy (in which normal fetal movement was defined as the perception of 10 movements within 10 hours) or to routine care in which no special counting policies were employed (62). Women in the counting group with fewer than 10 movements in 10 hours for two successive days were instructed to alert their care provider, at whose discretion further evaluation was undertaken. Overall fetal death rates were low in this trial and did not differ significantly between the two groups (2.9/1,000 in the counting group versus 2.7/1,000 in the control group). More women in the counting group (7% versus 5%) underwent fetal heart rate testing, and more (5% versus 4%) were admitted antenatally to the hospital. However, the rates of labor induction and elective cesarean delivery did not differ significantly between the two groups. It should be noted that in the counting group, only 46% of women with decreased fetal movement alerted their care providers. Compliance for both recording fetal movements and reporting when they were diminished was even lower for women who experienced a stillbirth.

Consistent evidence that a formal program of fetal movement assessment will result in a reduction in fetal deaths is lacking. Moreover, whether fetal movement assessment adds benefit to an established program of regular fetal surveillance has not been evaluated. One of the two randomized studies of fetal movement assessment suggests that its use may reduce stillbirths; the other does not. Formal movement assessment may increase, by a small degree, the number of antepartum visits and fetal evaluations. In the randomized trials, however, this increased surveillance did not result in a higher rate of intervention (10, 62).

Summary

The following recommendations are based on limited or inconsistent scientific evidence (Level B):

- Women with high-risk factors for stillbirth should undergo antepartum fetal surveillance using the NST, CST, BPP, or modified BPP.
- Initiating testing at 32–34 weeks of gestation is appropriate for most pregnancies at increased risk of stillbirth, although in pregnancies with multiple or particularly worrisome high-risk conditions, testing may be initiated as early as 26–28 weeks of gestation.
- When the clinical condition that has prompted testing persists, a reassuring test should be repeated periodically (either weekly or, depending on the test used and the presence of certain high-risk conditions, twice weekly) until delivery. Any significant deterioration in the maternal medical status or any acute diminution in fetal activity requires fetal reevaluation, regardless of the amount of time that has elapsed since the last test.
- An abnormal NST or modified BPP usually should be further evaluated by either a CST or a full BPP. Subsequent management should then be predicated on the results of the CST or BPP, the gestational age, the degree of oligohydramnios (if assessed), and the maternal condition.

- Oligohydramnios, defined as either no ultrasonographically measurable vertical pocket of amniotic fluid greater than 2 cm or an AFI of 5 cm or less, requires (depending on the degree of oligohydramnios, the gestational age, and the maternal clinical condition) either delivery or close maternal or fetal surveillance.
- In the absence of obstetric contraindications, delivery of the fetus with an abnormal test result often may be attempted by induction of labor with continuous monitoring of the fetal heart rate and contractions. If repetitive late decelerations are observed, cesarean delivery generally is indicated.
- Recent, normal antepartum fetal test results should not preclude the use of intrapartum fetal monitoring.
- Umbilical artery Doppler velocimetry has been found to be of benefit only in pregnancies complicated by intrauterine growth restriction. If used in this setting, decisions regarding timing of delivery should be made using a combination of information from the Doppler ultrasonography and other tests of fetal well-being, along with careful monitoring of maternal status.
- Middle cerebral artery Doppler velocimetry should be considered an investigational approach to antepartum fetal surveillance.

References

1. Boddy K, Dawes GS, Fisher R, Pinter S, Robinson JS. Foetal respiratory movements, electrocortical and cardiovascular responses to hypoxaemia and hypercapnia in sheep. J Physiol 1974;243:599–618 (Level III)
2. Manning FA, Platt LD. Maternal hypoxemia and fetal breathing movements. Obstet Gynecol 1979;53:758–760 (Level III)
3. Murata Y, Martin CB Jr, Ikenoue T, Hashimoto T, Taira S, Sagawa T, et al. Fetal heart rate accelerations and late decelerations during the course of intrauterine death in chronically catheterized rhesus monkeys. Am J Obstet Gynecol 1982;144:218–223 (Level III)
4. Natale R, Clewlow F, Dawes GS. Measurement of fetal forelimb movements in the lamb in utero. Am J Obstet Gynecol 1981;140:545–551 (Level III)
5. Seeds AE. Current concepts of amniotic fluid dynamics. Am J Obstet Gynecol 1980;138:575–586 (Level III)
6. Weiner CP, Sipes SL, Wenstrom K. The effect of fetal age upon normal fetal laboratory values and venous pressure. Obstet Gynecol 1992;79:713–718 (Level III)
7. Manning FA, Snijders R, Harman CR, Nicolaides K, Menticoglou S, Morrison I. Fetal biophysical profile score. VI. Correlation with antepartum umbilical venous fetal pH. Am J Obstet Gynecol 1993;169:755–763 (Level II-2)
8. Pearson JF, Weaver JB. Fetal activity and fetal wellbeing: an evaluation. BMJ 1976;1(6021):1305–1307 (Level III)
9. Moore TR, Piacquadio K. A prospective evaluation of fetal movement screening to reduce the incidence of antepartum fetal death. Am J Obstet Gynecol 1989;160: 1075–1080 (Level II-2)
10. Neldam S. Fetal movements as an indicator of fetal wellbeing. Dan Med Bull 1983;30:274–278 (Level II-1)
11. Huddleston JF, Sutliff G, Robinson D. Contraction stress test by intermittent nipple stimulation. Obstet Gynecol 1984;63:669–673 (Level II-3)
12. Freeman RK. The use of the oxytocin challenge test for antepartum clinical evaluation of uteroplacental respiratory function. Am J Obstet Gynecol 1975;121:481–489 (Level III)
13. Freeman RK, Anderson G, Dorchester W. A prospective multi-institutional study of antepartum fetal heart rate monitoring. I. Risk of perinatal mortality and morbidity according to antepartum fetal heart rate test results. Am J Obstet Gynecol 1982;143:771–777 (Level II-3)
14. Graca LM, Cardoso CG, Clode N, Calhaz-Jorge C. Acute effects of maternal cigarette smoking on fetal heart rate and fetal body movements felt by the mother. J Perinat Med 1991;19:385–390 (Level III)
15. Clark SL, Sabey P, Jolley K. Nonstress testing with acoustic stimulation and amniotic fluid volume assessment: 5973 tests without unexpected fetal death. Am J Obstet Gynecol 1989;160:694–697 (Level II-3)
16. Miller DA, Rabello YA, Paul RH. The modified biophysical profile: antepartum testing in the 1990s. Am J Obstet Gynecol 1996;174:812–817 (Level II-3)
17. Smith CV, Phelan JP, Platt LD, Broussard P, Paul RH. Fetal acoustic stimulation testing. II. A randomized clinical comparison with the nonstress test. Am J Obstet Gynecol 1986;155:131–134 (Level I)
18. Evertson LR, Gauthier RJ, Schifrin BS, Paul RH. Antepartum fetal heart rate testing. I. Evolution of the nonstress test. Am J Obstet Gynecol 1979;133:29–33 (Level II-3)
19. Bishop EH. Fetal acceleration test. Am J Obstet Gynecol 1981;141:905–909 (Level II-2)
20. Lavin JP Jr, Miodovnik M, Barden TP. Relationship of nonstress test reactivity and gestational age. Obstet Gynecol 1984;63:338–344 (Level II-3)
21. Druzin ML, Fox A, Kogut E, Carlson C. The relationship of the nonstress test to gestational age. Am J Obstet Gynecol 1985;153:386–389 (Level III)
22. Meis PJ, Ureda JR, Swain M, Kelly RT, Penry M, Sharp P. Variable decelerations during nonstress tests are not a sign of fetal compromise. Am J Obstet Gynecol 1986;154: 586–590 (Level II-3)
23. Anyaegbunam A, Brustman L, Divon M, Langer O. The significance of antepartum variable decelerations. Am J Obstet Gynecol 1986;155:707–710 (Level II-2)
24. O'Leary JA, Andrinopoulos GC, Giordano PC. Variable decelerations and the nonstress test: an indication of cord compromise. Am J Obstet Gynecol 1980;137:704–706 (Level III)

25. Bourgeois FJ, Thiagarajah S, Harbert GM Jr. The significance of fetal heart rate decelerations during nonstress testing. Am J Obstet Gynecol 1984;150:213–216 (Level III)

26. Druzin ML, Gratacos J, Keegan KA, Paul RH. Antepartum fetal heart rate testing. VII. The significance of fetal bradycardia. Am J Obstet Gynecol 1981;139:194–198 (Level III)

27. Pazos R, Vuolo K, Aladjem S, Lueck J, Anderson C. Association of spontaneous fetal heart rate decelerations during antepartum nonstress testing and intrauterine growth retardation. Am J Obstet Gynecol 1982;144: 574–577 (Level II-2)

28. Manning FA, Morrison I, Lange IR, Harman CR, Chamberlain PF. Fetal biophysical profile scoring: selective use of the nonstress test. Am J Obstet Gynecol 1987;156:709–712 (Level II-3)

29. Chamberlain PF, Manning FA, Morrison I, Harman CR, Lange IR. Ultrasound evaluation of amniotic fluid volume. I. The relationship of marginal and decreased amniotic fluid volumes to perinatal outcome. Am J Obstet Gynecol 1984;150:245–249 (Level II-3)

30. Manning FA, Harman CR, Morrison I, Menticoglou SM, Lange IR, Johnson JM. Fetal assessment based on fetal biophysical profile scoring. IV. An analysis of perinatal morbidity and mortality. Am J Obstet Gynecol 1990;162:703–709 (Level II-3)

31. Rutherford SE, Phelan JP, Smith CV, Jacobs N. The four-quadrant assessment of amniotic fluid volume: an adjunct to antepartum fetal heart rate testing. Obstet Gynecol 1987;70:353–356 (Level III)

32. Erskine RL, Ritchie JW. Umbilical artery blood flow characteristics in normal and growth-retarded fetuses. Br J Obstet Gynaecol 1985;92:605–610 (Level II-2)

33. Gudmundsson S, Marsal K. Umbilical and uteroplacental blood flow velocity waveforms in pregnancies with fetal growth retardation. Eur J Obstet Gynecol Reprod Biol 1988;27:187–196 (Level III)

34. Reuwer PJ, Bruinse HW, Stoutenbeek P, Haspels AA. Doppler assessment of the fetoplacental circulation in normal and growth-retarded fetuses. Eur J Obstet Gynecol Reprod Biol 1984;18:199–205 (Level II-2)

35. Karsdorp VH, van Vugt JM, van Geijn HP, Kostense PJ, Arduini D, Montenegra N, et al. Clinical significance of absent or reversed end diastolic velocity waveforms in umbilical artery. Lancet 1994;344:1664–1668 (Level II-2)

36. Giles WB, Trudinger BJ, Baird PJ. Fetal umbilical artery flow velocity waveforms and placental resistance: pathological correlation. Br J Obstet Gynaecol 1985;92:31–38 (Level II-2)

37. Nicolaides KH, Bilardo CM, Soothill PW, Campbell S. Absence of end diastolic frequencies in umbilical artery: a sign of fetal hypoxia and acidosis. BMJ 1988;297: 1026–1027 (Level III)

38. Almstrom H, Axelsson O, Cnattingius S, Ekman G, Maesel A, Ulmsten U, et al. Comparison of umbilical-artery velocimetry and cardiotocography for surveillance of small-for-gestational-age fetuses. Lancet 1992;340: 936–940 (Level I)

39. Johnstone FD, Prescott R, Hoskins P, Greer IA, McGlew T, Compton M. The effect of introduction of umbilical Doppler recordings to obstetric practice. Br J Obstet Gynaecol 1993;100:733–741 (Level I)

40. Newnham JP, O'Dea MR, Reid KP, Diepeveen DA. Doppler flow velocity waveform analysis in high risk pregnancies: a randomized controlled trial. Br J Obstet Gynaecol 1991;98:956–963 (Level I)

41. Omtzigt AM, Reuwer PJ, Bruinse HW. A randomized controlled trial on the clinical value of umbilical Doppler velocimetry in antenatal care. Am J Obstet Gynecol 1994; 170:625–634 (Level I)

42. Pattinson RC, Norman K, Odendaal HJ. The role of Doppler velocimetry in the management of high risk pregnancies. Br J Obstet Gynaecol 1994;101:114–120 (Level I)

43. Trudinger BJ, Cook CM, Giles WB, Connelly A, Thompson RS. Umbilical artery flow velocity waveforms in high-risk pregnancy. Randomised controlled trial. Lancet 1987;1(8526):188–190 (Level I)

44. Tyrrell SN, Lilford RJ, Macdonald HN, Nelson EJ, Porter J, Gupta JK. Randomized comparison of routine vs highly selective use of Doppler ultrasound and biophysical scoring to investigate high risk pregnancies. Br J Obstet Gynaecol 1990;97:909–916 (Level I)

45. Thacker SB, Berkelman RL. Assessing the diagnostic accuracy and efficacy of selected antepartum fetal surveillance techniques. Obstet Gynecol Surv 1986;41:121–141 (Level III)

46. Enkin M, Keirse MJNC, Renfrew M, Neilson J. A guide to effective care in pregnancy and childbirth. 2nd ed. Oxford: Oxford University Press, 1995:410 (Level III)

47. Nageotte MP, Towers CV, Asrat T, Freeman RK. Perinatal outcome with the modified biophysical profile. Am J Obstet Gynecol 1994;170:1672–1676 (Level I)

48. Rouse DJ, Owen J, Goldenberg RL, Cliver SP. Determinants of the optimal time in gestation to initiate antenatal fetal testing: a decision-analytic approach. Am J Obstet Gynecol 1995;173:1357–1363 (Decision Analysis)

49. Lagrew DC, Pircon RA, Towers CV, Dorchester W, Freeman RK. Antepartum fetal surveillance in patients with diabetes: when to start? Am J Obstet Gynecol 1993;168:1820–1826 (Level III)

50. Pircon RA, Lagrew DC, Towers CV, Dorchester WL, Gocke SE, Freeman RK. Antepartum testing in the hypertensive patient: when to begin. Am J Obstet Gynecol 1991;164:1563–1570 (Level III)

51. Manning FA, Morrison I, Harman CR, Lange IR, Menticoglou S. Fetal assessment based on fetal biophysical profile scoring: experience in 19,221 referred high-risk pregnancies. II. An analysis of false-negative fetal deaths. Am J Obstet Gynecol 1987;157:880–884 (Level II-3)

52. Staisch KJ, Westlake JR, Bashore RA. Blind oxytocin challenge test and perinatal outcome. Am J Obstet Gynecol 1980;138:399–403 (Level II-2)

53. Garite TJ, Linzey EM, Freeman RK, Dorchester W. Fetal heart rate patterns and fetal distress in fetuses with congenital anomalies. Obstet Gynecol 1979;53:716–720 (Level II-2)

54. Leveno KJ, Quirk JG Jr, Cunningham FG, Nelson SD, Santos-Ramos R, Toofanian A, et al. Prolonged pregnancy. I. Observations concerning the causes of fetal distress. Am J Obstet Gynecol 1984;150:465–473 (Level III)

55. Phelan JP, Platt LD, Yeh SY, Broussard P, Paul RH. The role of ultrasound assessment of amniotic fluid volume in the management of the postdate pregnancy. Am J Obstet Gynecol 1985;151:304–308 (Level II-2)

56. Haley J, Tuffnell DJ, Johnson N. Randomised controlled trial of cardiotocography versus umbilical artery Doppler in the management of small for gestational age fetuses. Br J Obstet Gynaecol 1997;104:431–435 (Level I)

57. Nienhuis SJ, Vles JS, Gerver WJ, Hoogland HJ. Doppler ultrasonography in suspected intrauterine growth retardation: a randomized clinical trial. Ultrasound Obstet Gynecol 1997;9:6–13 (Level I)

58. Neilson JP, Alfirevic Z. Doppler ultrasound for fetal assessment in high risk pregnancies (Cochrane Review). In: The Cochrane Library, Issue 3, 1999. Oxford: Update Software (Meta-analysis)

59. Mason GC, Lilford RJ, Porter J, Nelson E, Tyrell S. Randomised comparison of routine versus highly selective use of Doppler ultrasound in low risk pregnancies. Br J Obstet Gynaecol 1993;100:130–133 (Level I)

60. Mari G, Deter RL. Middle cerebral artery flow velocity waveforms in normal and small-for-gestational-age fetuses. Am J Obstet Gynecol 1992;166:1262–1270 (Level II-2)

61. Ott WJ, Mora G, Arias F, Sunderji S, Sheldon G. Comparison of the modified biophysical profile to a "new" biophysical profile incorporating the middle cerebral artery to umbilical artery velocity flow systolic/diastolic ratio. Am J Obstet Gynecol 1998;178:1346–1353 (Level I)

62. Grant A, Elbourne D, Valentin L, Alexander S. Routine formal fetal movement counting and risk of antepartum late death in normally formed singletons. Lancet 1989;2(8659):345–349 (Level I)

The MEDLINE database, the Cochrane Library, and ACOG's own internal resources and documents were used to conduct a literature search to locate relevant articles published between January 1985 and February 1999. The search was restricted to articles published in the English language. Priority was given to articles reporting results of original research, although review articles and commentaries also were consulted. Abstracts of research presented at symposia and scientific conferences were not considered adequate for inclusion in this document. Guidelines published by organizations or institutions such as the National Institutes of Health and the American College of Obstetricians and Gynecologists were reviewed, and additional studies were located by reviewing bibliographies of identified articles. When reliable research was not available, expert opinions from obstetrician–gynecologists were used.

Studies were reviewed and evaluated for quality according to the method outlined by the U.S. Preventive Services Task Force:

- I Evidence obtained from at least one properly designed randomized controlled trial.
- II-1 Evidence obtained from well-designed controlled trials without randomization.
- II-2 Evidence obtained from well-designed cohort or case–control analytic studies, preferably from more than one center or research group.
- II-3 Evidence obtained from multiple time series with or without the intervention. Dramatic results in uncontrolled experiments also could be regarded as this type of evidence.
- III Opinions of respected authorities, based on clinical experience, descriptive studies, or reports of expert committees.

Based on the highest level of evidence found in the data, recommendations are provided and graded according to the following catetories:

Level A—Recommendations are based on good and consistent scientific evidence.

Level B—Recommendations are based on limited or inconsistent scientific evidence.

Level C—Recommendations are based primarily on consensus and expert opinion.

ISSN 1099-3630

The American College of Obstetricians and Gynecologists
409 12th Street, SW
PO Box 96920
Washington, DC 20090-6920

12345/32109

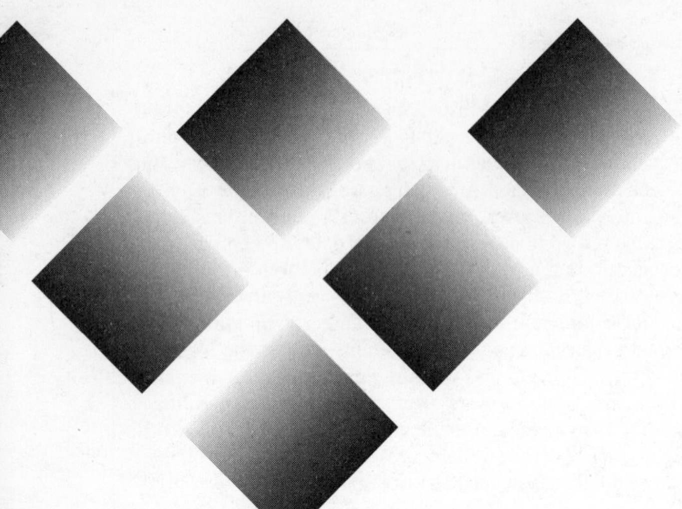

ACOG PRACTICE BULLETIN

CLINICAL MANAGEMENT GUIDELINES FOR OBSTETRICIAN–GYNECOLOGISTS

NUMBER 13, FEBRUARY 2000

(Replaces Practice Pattern Number 4, July 1997)

This Practice Bulletin was developed by the ACOG Committee on Practice Bulletins—Obstetrics. The information is designed to aid practitioners in making decisions about appropriate obstetric and gynecologic care. These guidelines should not be construed as dictating an exclusive course of treatment or procedure. Variations in practice may be warranted based on the needs of the individual patient, resources, and limitations unique to the institution or type of practice.

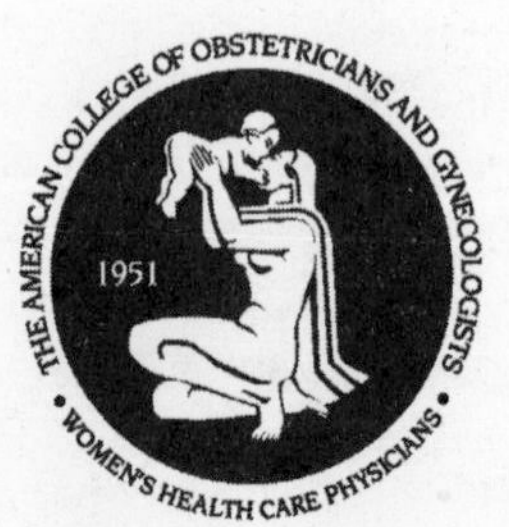

External Cephalic Version

In the United States, there is a widespread belief that the overall cesarean delivery rate is higher than necessary. Efforts are being directed toward decreasing the number of these procedures, in part by encouraging physicians to make changes in their management practices. Because breech presentations are associated with a high rate of cesarean delivery, there is renewed interest in techniques such as external cephalic version (ECV) and vaginal breech delivery. The purpose of this document is to provide information about ECV by summarizing the relevant evidence presented in published studies and to make recommendations regarding its use in obstetric practice.

Background

Breech presentation occurs in 3–4% of term pregnancies. In 1997, 84.5% of all malpresentations, including breech presentation, resulted in cesarean deliveries (1). External cephalic version involves applying pressure to the mother's abdomen to turn the fetus in either a forward or backward somersault to achieve a vertex presentation. The goal of ECV is to increase the proportion of vertex presentations among fetuses that were formerly in the breech position near term. Once a vertex presentation is achieved, the chances for a vaginal delivery increase.

Clinical Considerations and Recommendations

▶ ***Which patients are candidates for external cephalic version?***

Patients who have completed 36 weeks of gestation are preferred candidates for ECV for several reasons. First, if spontaneous version is going to occur, it is likely to have taken place by 36 completed weeks of gestation (2, 3). Second, risk of a spontaneous reversion is decreased after external cephalic version at term compared with earlier gestations. Preterm version attempts are associated with high initial success rates but also with higher reversion rates, necessitating additional procedures (4, 5). Third, if complications arise during an attempted version, emergency delivery of a term infant can be accomplished (6). Finally, most of the evidence pertaining to ECV comes from recent studies that selected patients near term.

There is scant information concerning ECV attempts among women who have a preexisting uterine scar or who undergo the procedure during the early stages of labor. For women with a previous cesarean delivery, compared with those who had not experienced cesarean delivery, results from one small randomized controlled trial indicate that they experience comparable success rates (7). Although no serious adverse events occurred in a small series (8), larger studies would be needed to establish the risk of uterine rupture. There are scattered reports of successful ECV performed during early labor; to date, however, no large study has been published (4, 5, 9, 10).

Contraindications to ECV are based on a commonsense approach designed to minimize the risks of an adverse outcome and to maximize the chances for success. Clearly any indication for a cesarean delivery in a patient, such as placenta previa, would be a contraindication to ECV (4, 9, 11–20), but there is insufficient evidence to construct a comprehensive list.

▶ *What are the benefits and risks of external cephalic version?*

The immediate benefit of successful version is an increased probability that the fetus will be in a vertex presentation for delivery. The ultimate goal is an uncomplicated vaginal delivery. Reports from published studies indicate there are fewer cesarean deliveries among women who have undergone successful version compared with women who have not undergone attempted version (4, 6, 18, 21–24). One randomized trial found no significant difference between the cesarean delivery rates of patients with an ECV attempt and controls who did not undergo ECV (25). In this study, however, the majority of patients undergoing ECV were between 33 and 36 weeks of gestation rather than closer to term as in the other reports. An additional randomized trial reported similar rates of cesarean delivery for women who underwent ECV and for those who did not, but the rate of breech vaginal deliveries was very high; approximately 80% of breech presentations in each group was delivered vaginally, resulting in an unusually low cesarean delivery rate (4).

Fetal heart rate changes during attempted versions are not uncommon but usually stabilize when the procedure is discontinued (4, 21, 23, 26, 27). Serious adverse effects associated with ECV do not occur often, but there have been a few reported cases of placental abruption and preterm labor. A report from Copenhagen described two cases of intrauterine death 2 and 5 weeks after version among 316 women and one instance of premature partial separation of the placenta 2 days following an unsuccessful version attempt, but the two deaths could not be causally linked to ECV with certainty (16). In the study including mothers at 36 weeks of gestation or less, two placental abruptions and one premature labor occurred shortly after version, resulting in one neonatal and two fetal deaths (25). Subsequently, there has been a follow-up study at the same institution, but changes in management practices and selection criteria had been made (18). Only term gestations were selected, and tocolytic agents as well as fetal monitoring were used during version attempts. There were no fetal deaths causally linked to ECV. The authors concluded that ECV can substantially decrease breech presentations and the cesarean delivery rate for these patients (18). A more recent study reported a placental abruption during an ECV attempt requiring emergency cesarean delivery of a viable but depressed infant (28). It was the only major complication attributed to ECV among 113 women. Although the incidence of serious complications associated with ECV is low, the potential is present, making it prudent to perform ECV in a facility that has ready access to cesarean delivery services.

▶ *What are the success rates for external cephalic version, and what factors are predictive of either success or failure?*

A review of 20 studies indicates that success rates for ECV range from 35% to 86%, with an average success rate of 58% (4, 6, 9, 12–14, 16–18, 21–25, 27, 29–31). Most authors report a positive association between parity and successful version (4, 6, 13, 21–25, 30, 31). A transverse or oblique lie is associated with higher immediate success rates (13, 29, 30). Opinion is divided about the predictiveness of other factors, including amniotic fluid volume, location of placenta, and maternal weight. Some reports indicate an association between normal or increased amounts of amniotic fluid and successful ECV (12, 13, 24, 32), whereas other reports do not (20). Two authors reported an association between successful ECV and placenta location (20, 24), whereas others failed to find an association (12, 13, 29). Two authors found obesity to be associated with a higher failure rate (23, 30), whereas others found maternal weight not to be a significant predictor of success (12, 13, 19, 20).

Although scoring systems have been developed to predict which candidates will have a successful version attempt, these have not been validated by multiple studies. One system considered parity, dilatation, estimated fetal weight, placenta location, and station. Nulliparity, advanced dilatation, fetal weight of less than 2,500 g, anterior placenta, and low station were less likely to be associated with success (20). Such variables may provide useful clinical information for obtaining informed consent from individuals for ECV; no single system, however, has been shown to have complete accuracy.

▶ *How does the use of tocolysis affect the success rate of external cephalic version?*

Two of six randomized controlled trials failed to find a significant advantage in using tocolytics during ECV attempts (19, 27). One third reported significantly greater success associated with hexoprenaline but not with ritodrine (33). An additional randomized study reported an initial advantage associated with the use of ritodrine, specifically among nulliparous women. However, as the physicians became proficient at the ECV technique, the advantage diminished (34). The largest randomized study using a ritodrine infusion found significant improvement only among nulliparous patients (35). Finally, a randomized study of terbutaline found the success rate of version associated with use of this tocolytic to be almost double the rate without its use (36). In the vast majority of published studies, a tocolytic agent was used routinely (6, 11–18, 20–23, 27–29, 37). Several studies used tocolytics selectively (5, 7, 9, 34), and some used no tocolytic agents (4, 25). Existing evidence may support the use of a tocolytic agent during ECV attempts, particularly in nulliparous patients.

▶ *Does successful version translate into lower cesarean delivery rates?*

Whether ECV results in a lower cesarean delivery rate for women with breech presentation who elect this procedure compared with those women who do not depends upon several factors. Obviously, the first factor is whether the version is successful. Clearly, women who have successful version have lower cesarean delivery rates than those who do not (6, 9, 12–14, 21–24, 26, 29, 30). Two randomized studies also have shown a significant decrease in cesarean delivery rates among patients assigned to version compared with those not assigned to version (18, 23). Factors that tend to lessen overall differences between version and nonversion groups include spontaneous conversion of presentation from breech to vertex or vice versa and the willingness of providers to perform vaginal breech deliveries. Clearly, cesarean delivery rates for version and nonversion groups will be less when there is a greater willingness to attempt a vaginal breech delivery. The need to perform a cesarean delivery for other indications in women who have had a successful version also may lessen the overall impact of version on the cesarean delivery rate. One author has reported that women who have had successful ECV have higher cesarean delivery rates due to fetal distress and dystocia compared with matched controls who never required the procedure (31).

Although ECV may not lead to a substantial reduction in the national cesarean delivery rate, it is nonetheless a valuable management technique. In a properly selected population, this procedure poses little risk to either mother or fetus. If successful, ECV provides a clear benefit to the individual woman by allowing her an opportunity for a successful vertex vaginal delivery.

▶ *How does the use of anesthesia affect the success rate of external cephalic version?*

A randomized study found a significantly greater success rate associated with the use of epidural anesthesia, although the success rate was unusually low for the women who did not receive epidural anesthesia (32%) (38). Two studies reported results for women in whom ECV was performed while using epidural anesthesia (10, 15). In one study, use of epidural anesthesia was associated with a significantly greater success rate compared with no use of epidural anesthesia (15). However, the procedure was administered selectively to patients according to physician preference, raising the potential for selection bias. The other study merely noted that ECV was performed without difficulty on three women undergoing epidural anesthesia (10). It also has been suggested that epidural anesthesia be considered for women who failed a previous version attempt (39). Another randomized trial addressed the use of spinal anesthesia before the version attempt and found no significant difference between treatment groups (40). Currently, there is not enough consistent evidence to make a recommendation favoring spinal or epidural anesthesia during ECV attempts.

▶ *What is an example of a standard protocol for performing an external cephalic version attempt?*

Prior to attempting ECV, patients must provide informed consent and should undergo an ultrasound examination. The ultrasound examination is necessary to confirm the breech position of the fetus and rule out the presence of any anomalies that would complicate a vaginal delivery.

Fetal well-being should be assessed by a prior nonstress test or concurrent biophysical profile (see Fig. 1).

Because there is a chance that an expedient delivery may become necessary, patients should have ready access to a facility that is equipped to perform emergency cesarean deliveries. One version technique involves lifting the breech upward from the pelvis with one hand and providing pressure on the head with the other hand to produce a forward roll. If the forward roll fails, a backward somersault may be attempted. Version may be performed by one person or two. A version attempt will be abandoned if there is significant fetal bradycardia, if there is discomfort to the patient, or if the attempt cannot be completed easily or is unsuccessful after a brief period. Following the attempt, fetal evaluation is repeated and the patient is monitored until stable. Rh-negative patients may receive anti-D im-mune globulin. There is no support for routine practice of immediate induction of labor to minimize reversion.

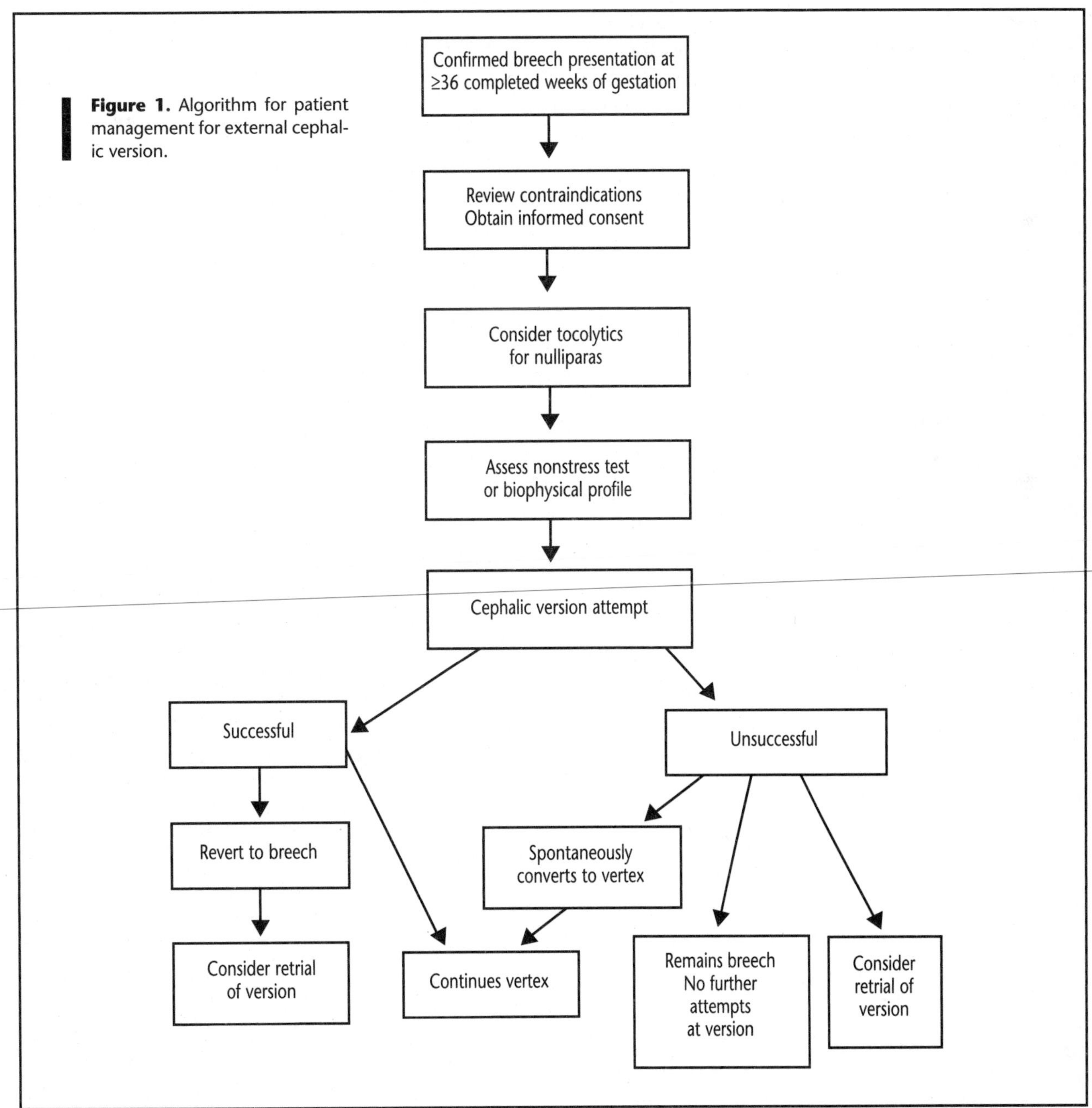

Figure 1. Algorithm for patient management for external cephalic version.

▶ *What are the cost implications of external cephalic version?*

A recent decision analysis measuring cost implications associated with four potential methods of managing term pregnancies with breech presentations predicted that use of ECV would result in fewer cesarean deliveries and lower costs than either scheduled cesarean delivery or trial of labor without an ECV attempt (41). Even if failed ECV attempts were followed by routine cesarean delivery, the overall cesarean delivery rate would be lower than that of a trial of labor without an ECV attempt. Sensitivity analysis revealed that as long as less than 52% of all breech presentations are eligible for a trial of labor, a policy of attempting ECV followed by either a trial of labor or routine cesarean delivery (for failed attempts) would be less expensive than a policy of routine cesarean delivery or trial of labor without ECV (41). It should be noted that the decision analysis included X-ray pelvimetry to assess eligibility for a trial of labor, a practice that may not be widely accepted.

Summary

The following recommendation is based on good and consistent scientific evidence (Level A):

- ▶ Because the risk of an adverse event occurring as a result of ECV is small and the cesarean delivery rate is significantly lower among women who have undergone successful version, all women near term with breech presentations should be offered a version attempt.

The following recommendations are based on limited or inconsistent scientific evidence (Level B):

- ▶ Patients should have completed 36 weeks of gestation before attempting ECV.
- ▶ Previous cesarean delivery is not associated with a lower rate of success; however, the magnitude of the risk of uterine rupture is not known.
- ▶ There is insufficient evidence to recommend routine tocolysis for ECV attempts for all patients, but it may particularly benefit nulliparous patients.
- ▶ Evidence is inconsistent regarding the benefits of anesthesia use during ECV attempts.
- ▶ Cost-effectiveness depends upon utilization of vaginal breech deliveries and costs of the version protocol at a particular institution, but at least one decision analysis suggests the policy is cost effective.

The following recommendations are based primarily on consensus and expert opinion (Level C):

- ▶ Fetal assessment before and after the procedure is recommended.
- ▶ External cephalic version should be attempted only in settings in which cesarean delivery services are readily available.

References

1. Ventura SJ, Martin JA, Curtin SC, Mathews TJ. Births: final data for 1997. Natl Vital Stat Rep 1999;47(18):1–96 (Level II-3)
2. Hickok DE, Gordon DC, Milberg JA, Williams MA, Daling JR. The frequency of breech presentation by gestational age at birth: a large population-based study. Am J Obstet Gynecol 1992;166:851–852 (Level II-2)
3. Westgren M, Edvall H, Nordstrom L, Svalenius E, Ranstam J. Spontaneous cephalic version of breech presentation in the last trimester. Br J Obstet Gynaecol 1985; 92:19–22 (Level II-3)
4. Van Veelen AJ, Van Cappellen AW, Flu PK, Straub MJ, Wallenburg HC. Effect of external cephalic version in late pregnancy on presentation at delivery: a randomized controlled trial. Br J Obstet Gynaecol 1989;96:916–921 (Level I)
5. Kornman MT, Kimball KT, Reeves KO. Preterm external cephalic version in an outpatient environment. Am J Obstet Gynecol 1995;172:1734–1738; discussion 1738–1741 (Level II-2)
6. Goh JT, Johnson CM, Gregora MG. External cephalic version at term. Aust N Z J Obstet Gynaecol 1993;33:364–366 (Level II-2)
7. Flamm BL, Fried MW, Lonky NM, Giles WS. External cephalic version after previous cesarean section. Am J Obstet Gynecol 1991;165;370–372 (Level I)
8. de Meeus JB, Ellia F, Magnin G. External cephalic version after previous cesarean section: a series of 38 cases. Eur J Obstet Gynecol Reprod Biol 1998;81:65–68 (Level III)
9. Cook HA. Experience with external cephalic version and selective vaginal breech delivery in private practice. Am J Obstet Gynecol 1993;168:1886–1889; discussion 1889–1890 (Level II-3)
10. Ferguson JE 2d, Dyson DC. Intrapartum external cephalic version. Am J Obstet Gynecol 1985;152:297–298 (Level II-3)
11. Lau TK, Stock A, Rogers M. Fetomaternal haemorrhage after external cephalic version at term. Aust N Z J Obstet Gynaecol 1995;35:173–174 (Level III)
12. Shalev E, Battino S, Giladi Y, Edelstein S. External cephalic version at term—using tocolysis. Acta Obstet Gynecol Scand 1993;72:455–457 (Level II-3)
13. Hellstrom AC, Nilsson B, Stange L, Nylund L. When does external cephalic version succeed? Acta Obstet Gynecol Scand 1990;69:281–285 (Level II-3)

14. Morrison JC, Myatt RE, Martin JN Jr, Meeks GR, Martin RW, Bucovaz ET, et al. External cephalic version of the breech presentation under tocolysis. Am J Obstet Gynecol 1986;154:900–903 (Level II-3)

15. Carlan SJ, Dent JM, Huckaby T, Whittington EC, Shaefer D. The effect of epidural anesthesia on safety and success of external cephalic version at term. Anesth Analg 1994;79:525–528 (Level II-3)

16. Thunedborg P, Fischer-Rasmussen W, Tollund L. The benefit of external cephalic version with tocolysis as a routine procedure in late pregnancy. Eur J Obstet Gynecol Reprod Biol 1991;42:23–27 (Level II-3)

17. Bewley S, Robson SC, Smith M, Glover A, Spencer JA. The introduction of external cephalic version at term into routine clinical practice. Eur J Obstet Gynecol Reprod Biol 1993;52:89–93 (Level II-3)

18. Mahomed K, Seeras R, Coulson R. External cephalic version at term. A randomized controlled trial using tocolysis. Br J Obstet Gynaecol 1991;98:8–13 (Level I)

19. Tan GW, Jen SW, Tan SL, Salmon YM. A prospective randomised controlled trial of external cephalic version comparing two methods of uterine tocolysis with a non-tocolysis group. Singapore Med J 1989;30:155–158 (Level I)

20. Newman RB, Peacock BS, VanDorsten JP, Hunt HH. Predicting success of external cephalic version. Am J Obstet Gynecol 1993;169:245–249; discussion 249–250 (Level II-3)

21. Dyson DC, Ferguson JE 2d, Hensleigh P. Antepartum external cephalic version under tocolysis. Obstet Gynecol 1986;67:63–68 (Level II-2)

22. Marchick R. Antepartum external cephalic version with tocolysis: a study of term singleton breech presentations. Am J Obstet Gynecol 1988;158:1339–1346 (Level II-2)

23. Brocks V, Philipsen T, Secher NJ. A randomized trial of external cephalic version with tocolysis in late pregnancy. Br J Obstet Gynaecol 1984;91:653–656 (Level II-1)

24. Hofmeyr GJ, Sadan O, Myer IG, Galal KC, Simko G. External cephalic version and spontaneous version rates: ethnic and other determinants. Br J Obstet Gynaecol 1986;93:13–16 (Level II-2)

25. Kasule J, Chimbira TH, Brown IM. Controlled trial of external cephalic version. Br J Obstet Gynaecol 1985; 92:14–18 (Level I)

26. Stine LE, Phelan JP, Wallace R, Eglinton GS, Van Dorsten JP, Schifrin BS. Update on external cephalic version performed at term. Obstet Gynecol 1985;65:642–646 (Level II-3)

27. Robertson AW, Kopelman JN, Read JA, Duff P, Magelssen DJ, Dashow EE. External cephalic version at term: is a tocolytic necessary? Obstet Gynecol 1987;70:896–899 (Level I)

28. Calhoun BC, Edgeworth D, Brehm W. External cephalic version at a military teaching hospital: predictors of success. Aust N Z J Obstet Gynaecol 1995;35:277–279 (Level II-3)

29. Donald WL, Barton JJ. Ultrasonography and external cephalic version at term. Am J Obstet Gynecol 1990;162: 1542–1545; discussion 1545–1547 (Level II-3)

30. Mauldin JG, Mauldin PD, Feng TI, Adams EK, Durkalski VL. Determining the clinical efficacy and cost savings of successful external cephalic version. Am J Obstet Gynecol 1996;175:1639–1644 (Level II-3)

31. Lau TK, Lo KW, Wan D, Rogers MS. Predictors of successful external cephalic version at term: a prospective study. Br J Obstet Gynaecol 1997;104:798–802 (Level II-3)

32. Healey M, Porter R, Galimberti A. Introducing external cephalic version at 36 weeks or more in a district general hospital: a review and an audit. Br J Obstet Gynaecol 1997;104:1073–1079 (Level II-3)

33. Stock A, Chung T, Rogers M, Ming WW. Randomized, double blind, placebo controlled comparison of ritodrine and hexoprenaline for tocolysis prior to external cephalic version at term. Aust N Z J Obstet Gynaecol 1993; 33:265–268 (Level I)

34. Chung T, Neale E, Lau TK, Rogers M. A randomized, double blind, controlled trial of tocolysis to assist external cephalic version in late pregnancy. Acta Obstet Gynecol Scand 1996;75:720–724 (Level I)

35. Marquette GP, Boucher M, Theriault D, Rinfret D. Does the use of a tocolytic agent affect the success rate of external cephalic version? Am J Obstet Gynecol 1996;175: 859–861 (Level I)

36. Fernandez CO, Bloom SL, Smulian JC, Ananth CV, Wendel GD Jr. A randomized placebo-controlled evaluation of terbutaline for external cephalic version. Obstet Gynecol 1997;90:775–779 (Level I)

37. Hanss JW Jr. The efficacy of external cephalic version and its impact on the breech experience. Am J Obstet Gynecol 1990;162:1459–1463; discussion 1463–1464 (Level II-3)

38. Schorr SJ, Speights SE, Ross EL, Bofill JA, Rust OA, Norman PF, et al. A randomized trial of epidural anesthesia to improve external cephalic version success. Am J Obstet Gynecol 1997;177:1133–1137 (Level I)

39. Neiger R, Hennessey MD, Patel M. Reattempting failed external cephalic version under epidural anesthesia. Am J Obstet Gynecol 1998;179:1136–1139 (Level III)

40. Dugoff L, Stamm CA, Jones OW 3rd, Mohling SI, Hawkins JL. The effect of spinal anesthesia on the success rate of external cephalic version: a randomized trial. Obstet Gynecol 1999;93:345–349 (Level I)

41. Gifford DS, Keeler E, Kahn KL. Reductions in cost and cesarean rate by routine use of external cephalic version: a decision analysis. Obstet Gynecol 1995;85:930–936 (Level III)

The MEDLINE database, the Cochrane Library, and ACOG's own internal resources and documents were used to conduct a literature search to locate relevant articles published between January 1981 and May 1999. The search was restricted to articles published in the English language. Priority was given to articles reporting results of original research, although review articles and commentaries also were consulted. Abstracts of research presented at symposia and scientific conferences were not considered adequate for inclusion in this document. Guidelines published by organizations or institutions such as the National Institutes of Health and the American College of Obstetricians and Gynecologists were reviewed, and additional studies were located by reviewing bibliographies of identified articles. When reliable research was not available, expert opinions from obstetrician–gynecologists were used.

Studies were reviewed and evaluated for quality according to the method outlined by the U.S. Preventive Services Task Force:

I Evidence obtained from at least one properly designed randomized controlled trial.

II-1 Evidence obtained from well-designed controlled trials without randomization.

II-2 Evidence obtained from well-designed cohort or case–control analytic studies, preferably from more than one center or research group.

II-3 Evidence obtained from multiple time series with or without the intervention. Dramatic results in uncontrolled experiments could also be regarded as this type of evidence.

III Opinions of respected authorities, based on clinical experience, descriptive studies, or reports of expert committees.

Based on the highest level of evidence found in the data, recommendations are provided and graded according to the following catetories:

Level A—Recommendations are based on good and consistent scientific evidence.

Level B—Recommendations are based on limited or inconsistent scientific evidence.

Level C—Recommendations are based primarily on consensus and expert opinion.

ISSN 1099-3630

The American College of
Obstetricians and Gynecologists
409 12th Street, SW
PO Box 96920
Washington, DC 20090-6920

12345/43210

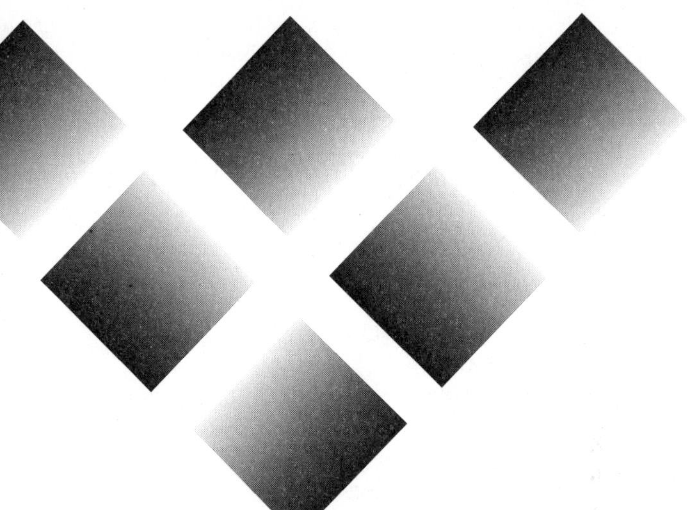

ACOG PRACTICE BULLETIN

CLINICAL MANAGEMENT GUIDELINES FOR OBSTETRICIAN–GYNECOLOGISTS

NUMBER 22, NOVEMBER 2000

(Replaces Technical Bulletin Number 159, September 1991)

This Practice Bulletin was developed by the ACOG Committee on Practice Bulletins—Obstetrics with the assistance of William H. Barth, Jr, MD. The information is designed to aid practitioners in making decisions about appropriate obstetric and gynecologic care. These guidelines should not be construed as dictating an exclusive course of treatment or procedure. Variations in practice may be warranted based on the needs of the individual patient, resources, and limitations unique to the institution or type of practice.

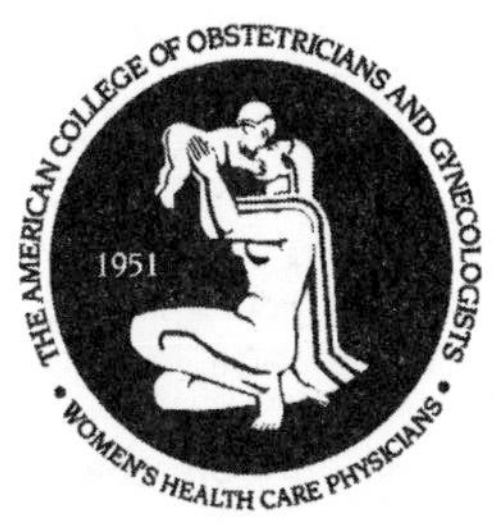

Fetal Macrosomia

Suspected fetal macrosomia is a common obstetric condition. As birth weight increases, the likelihood of labor abnormalities, shoulder dystocia, birth trauma, and permanent injury to the neonate increases. The purpose of this document is to quantify those risks, address the accuracy and limitations of methods for estimating fetal weight, and suggest clinical management for the pregnancy with suspected fetal macrosomia.

Background

Definition

Two terms identify excessive fetal growth: *large for gestational age* and *macrosomia*. The term large for gestational age generally implies a birth weight equal to or greater than the 90th percentile for a given gestational age. For years, clinicians have relied on popular fetal growth curves to identify weight cutoffs for the 90th percentile for a given gestational age (1–3). A national reference for fetal growth is now available. A study using the 1991 U.S. Live Birth File of the National Center for Health Statistics reported data for fetal growth based on more than 3.8 million births (4). The 50th, 90th, and 95th percentiles for birth weight from 37 to 42 completed weeks of gestation are shown in Table 1.

The term *fetal macrosomia* implies growth beyond a specific weight, usually 4,000 g or 4,500 g, regardless of the gestational age. Although the risks of morbidity for infants and mothers when birth weight is between 4,000 g and 4,500 g are greater than those of the general obstetric population, these risks increase sharply beyond 4,500 g (5–10). Recent large cohort studies (11–14) further support the continued use of 4,500 g as an appropriate estimated weight beyond which the fetus should be considered macrosomic.

Rather than assigning a different minimum estimated fetal weight for macrosomia among infants of women with diabetes, understanding that maternal diabetes is an independent predictor of fetal morbidity will help avoid confusion. Regardless of their birth weight, infants of women with diabetes have

Table 1. Percentiles for Birth Weight for Gestational Age: U.S. 1991 Single Live Births to Resident Mothers 37–42 Completed Weeks

	Birth Weight (g)		
Gestational Age	50th Percentile	90th Percentile	95th Percentile
37	3,117	3,755	3,956
38	3,263	3,867	4,027
39	3,400	3,980	4,107
40	3,495	4,060	4,185
41	3,527	4,094	4,217
42	3,522	4,098	4,213

Modified from Alexander GR, Himes JH, Kaufman RB, Mor J, Kogan M. A United States national reference for fetal growth. Obstet Gynecol 1996;87:163–168

an increased risk of shoulder dystocia, clavicular fracture, and brachial plexus injury (14, 15–17).

Frequency of Occurrence

Information from the National Center for Health Statistics shows that 10% of all liveborn infants in the United States weigh more than 4,000 g (18). In contrast, only 1.5% weigh more than 4,500 g. The most serious complication of fetal macrosomia is shoulder dystocia. Fortunately, shoulder dystocia is rare, complicating only 1.4% of all vaginal deliveries (19). When birth weight exceeds 4,500 g, however, the risk of shoulder dystocia is increased, with rates reported from 9.2% to 24% (8, 11–14). In the presence of maternal diabetes, birth weights greater than 4,500 g have been associated with rates of shoulder dystocia from 19.9% to 50% (8, 12, 14). Figure 1 shows the relationship between birth weight, maternal diabetes status, spontaneous or assisted vaginal delivery, and the mean frequency of shoulder dystocia based on a study of more than 175,000 deliveries in California in 1992 (14).

Several issues complicate attempts to define precisely the incidence of shoulder dystocia among macrosomic infants. First, clinicians tend to underreport the occurrence of shoulder dystocia (20, 21). Second, the incidence of shoulder dystocia and the likelihood of subsequent fetal injury vary depending on the criteria used to render a diagnosis of dystocia (22). Studies requiring the use of auxiliary maneuvers other than gentle downward traction and episiotomy to effect delivery (16) report a lower overall incidence of shoulder dystocia—but greater proportional fetal morbidity—than those studies with less precise definitions (11). Finally, although macrosomia clearly increases risk, it is important to note that most instances of shoulder dystocia occur unpredictably among infants of normal birth weight (19, 23).

Risk Factors for Macrosomia

A number of factors predispose to newborn macrosomia. A large case–control study examined the relative contributions of proposed risk factors for macrosomia, excluding preexisting diabetes (24). In decreasing order of importance, these risk factors included a prior history of macrosomia, maternal prepregnancy weight, weight gain during pregnancy, multiparity, male fetus, gestational age greater than 40 weeks, ethnicity, maternal birth weight, maternal height, maternal age younger than 17 years, and a positive 50-g glucose screen with a negative result on the 3-hour glucose tolerance test. Although maternal smoking decreases the likelihood of newborn macrosomia (25), it should not be recommended as a protective measure for obvious reasons.

Both pregestational diabetes and gestational diabetes are associated with fetal macrosomia. Even in patients without diabetes, observational cohort studies and case–control studies demonstrate that graded increases in the level of maternal glycemia are associated with increases in newborn birth weight (26, 27). A study reported that 6% of mothers with untreated borderline gestational diabetes delivered infants exceeding 4,500 g, compared with only 2% of women with normal glucose tolerance (28). If gestational diabetes is unrecognized and untreated, the risk of macrosomia may be as high as 20% (29).

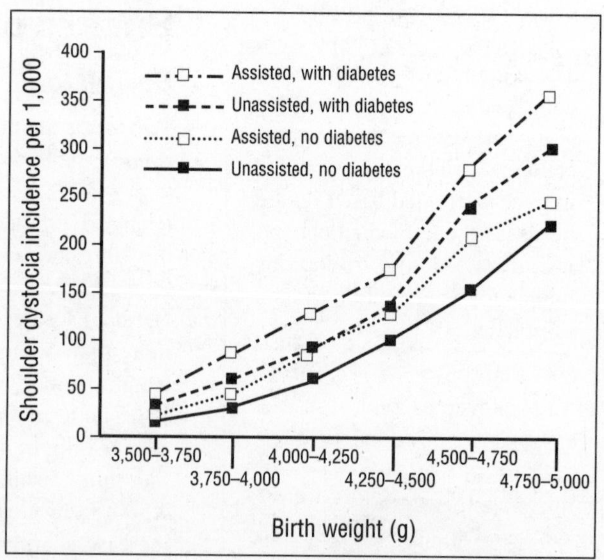

Figure 1. Frequency of shoulder dystocia for increasing birth weight by maternal diabetes status and method of vaginal delivery—spontaneous or assisted. (Nesbitt TS, Gilbert WM, Herrchen B. Shoulder dystocia and associated risk factors with macrosomic infants born in California. Am J Obstet Gynecol 1998;179:476–480)

Anthropometric studies suggest that the macrosomia produced by maternal glucose intolerance is different from that associated with other predisposing factors (30, 31). These macrosomic infants tend to have greater total body fat, greater shoulder and upper-extremity circumferences, greater upper-extremity skin-fold measurements, and smaller head-to-abdominal-circumference ratios than macrosomic infants of mothers without diabetes. Some have suggested that it is this altered fetal body shape that is responsible for the higher incidence of shoulder dystocia seen among infants of women with diabetes (31).

The relative contributions of maternal diabetes and obesity to fetal macrosomia remain controversial. One study reported that the risk for fetal macrosomia associated with unrecognized gestational diabetes persisted after controlling for both maternal body mass index and maternal weight gain (29). In a study among women with diet-controlled gestational diabetes, adjusting for maternal weight decreased the relative risk for large infants (greater than the 90th percentile) from 2.5 to 1.5 (32). Although both diabetes and maternal obesity increase the risk of fetal macrosomia, most agree that maternal obesity plays a greater role (7, 24, 33).

The interaction of maternal weight, weight gain during pregnancy, and newborn macrosomia is complex. There is little doubt that birth weight, in general, increases with maternal body mass index (34–36). Almost all authors report that obese women are more likely than women of normal weight to have large infants (35, 37). However, several issues confound this observation. First, obese women are more likely to have diabetes mellitus. One study demonstrated that morbidly obese women (>300 lb) are eight times more likely to deliver an infant exceeding 4,500 g (38). Second, high weight gain during pregnancy is itself a risk factor for excessive fetal growth (39). The risk of newborn macrosomia associated with excessive maternal weight gain is greater for obese women than for nonobese women (35, 37).

Understandably, gestational age influences birth weight and the risk of macrosomia. Among all races in the United States, the risk of macrosomia increases from 1.6% at term to 2.5% if gestational age exceeds 42 weeks (18). However, as Table 1 shows, there is little additional weight gain after 41 weeks of gestation.

A number of maternal historic factors and habits also influence infant birth weight. Women who have previously delivered an infant weighing more than 4,000 g are five to 10 times more likely to deliver an infant exceeding 4,500 g than women without such a history (5, 24, 40). To a degree, maternal birth weight may predict newborn weight. Women whose own birth weight exceeded 8 lb (approximately 3,600 g) are twice as likely to deliver infants greater than 4,000 g than are women whose birth weight was between 6 lb and 7.9 lb (approximately 2,700–3,500 g) (41). Finally, three cohort studies show that multiparity and grand-multiparity (≥ 5 deliveries) increase the risk of macrosomia (42–44).

Genetic, racial, and ethnic factors also influence birth weight and the risk of macrosomia. Male infants typically weigh more than female infants at any gestational age and, therefore, constitute a greater proportion of infants with birth weights exceeding 4,500 g (12, 45). The risk of macrosomia varies with race and ethnicity as well. Two reports, both of which controlled for diabetes, have demonstrated that Hispanic women have a higher risk of fetal macrosomia than do white, black, or Asian women (46, 47). Genetic factors such as parental height and race play a role in determining newborn birth weight, but these factors interact in a complex manner with environmental factors during pregnancy (48, 49). No combination of these risk factors predicts macrosomia well enough to be used clinically. Much of the variation in birth weights remains unexplained, and most infants greater than 4,500 g do not have identifiable risk factors (6).

Diagnosis

An accurate diagnosis of macrosomia can be made only by weighing the newborn after delivery. Unfortunately, the prenatal diagnosis of fetal macrosomia remains imprecise. Methods used to predict birth weight include assessment of maternal risk factors, clinical examination, and ultrasound measurement of the fetus. Although ultrasonography enables the direct measurement of various fetal body parts, its accuracy in predicting macrosomia has been unreliable (50–52). Furthermore, the superiority of ultrasound-derived estimates of fetal weight over clinical estimates has not been established (53–55). Indeed, parous women are able to predict the weight of their newborns as well as clinicians who use ultrasound measurements or Leopold's maneuvers (56).

Risks Associated with Macrosomia

Maternal Morbidity

The primary maternal risk associated with macrosomia is an increased risk of cesarean delivery. With birth weights greater than 4,500 g, cohort studies show that the risk of cesarean delivery for women attempting a vaginal delivery is at least double that of controls (5, 7, 13, 40). Almost all the increased risk is attributed to labor abnormalities

(5, 11). Not surprisingly, a study has demonstrated that the inaccurate ultrasonographic prediction of macrosomia predisposes to the diagnosis of labor abnormalities and cesarean delivery independent of actual birth weight (57). The risks of postpartum hemorrhage and significant vaginal lacerations also are elevated with macrosomia. A case–control study of risk factors for major obstetric hemorrhage (estimated blood loss >1 L) reported that a birth weight greater than 4,000 g doubled the odds of significant maternal blood loss (odds ratio [OR]: 1.9, 95% confidence interval [CI]: 1.38–2.6) (58). Although the risk of third- and fourth-degree lacerations is slightly increased with macrosomia (12), this is especially true if delivery is complicated by shoulder dystocia (59). Maternal infectious morbidity generally is limited to urinary tract infection in women undergoing elective cesarean delivery (60) and puerperal fever in women undergoing cesarean delivery after a trial of labor (12).

Fetal Morbidity and Mortality

The fetal injuries most commonly associated with macrosomia and shoulder dystocia are fracture of the clavicle and damage to the nerves of the brachial plexus, specifically C5 and C6, producing Erb-Duchenne paralysis. Fracture of the clavicle complicates 0.3–0.7% of all deliveries and usually resolves without permanent sequelae (61–63). For macrosomic infants, the risk of clavicular fracture is increased approximately 10-fold (63).

Brachial plexus injury is rare, with an incidence reported between 0.5 and 1.89 injuries per 1,000 vaginal deliveries (9, 15, 17, 63–65). Case–control studies demonstrate that the risk of brachial plexus injury among infants delivered vaginally is increased 18- to 21-fold when birth weight exceeds 4,500 g (9, 17, 63). Recent reports place the occurrence of brachial plexus injury for macrosomic infants delivered vaginally between 4% and 8% (12, 13, 65). Even though shoulder dystocia is underreported (20), the occurrence of brachial plexus injury in the absence of documented shoulder dystocia is well described (14, 21). Brachial plexus injury has been associated with cesarean delivery (66). As with clavicular fracture, most brachial plexus injuries resolve without permanent handicap. Among 59 confirmed brachial plexus injuries described in the Collaborative Perinatal Project, only 6 (12%) were still evident by age 4 months (64). By age 2 years, all but 4 (7%) had resolved. Other large case series confirm that 80–90% of brachial plexus injuries will resolve by age 1 year (23, 67). However, persistent injury may be more common with birth weights greater than 4,500 g (68). Nonetheless, as with shoulder dystocia, most brachial plexus injuries occur in nonmacrosomic infants (65).

Macrosomia is associated with a number of other risks to the newborn. These infants face an increased risk of depressed 5-minute Apgar scores and increased rates of admission to a neonatal intensive care unit (65). However, most of this risk likely is the result of complications of the birth process, because macrosomic infants do not have higher rates of fetal heart rate abnormalities in labor (5). Finally, overweight newborns are more likely to be overweight later in life than are normal-weight newborns (69).

Clinical Considerations and Recommendations

▶ ***How accurate are clinical estimates of fetal weight?***

The two primary methods for clinical estimation of fetal weight are Leopold's maneuvers (abdominal palpation) and measurement of the height of the uterine fundus above the maternal symphysis pubis. In a prospective study of 602 term patients, clinical palpation alone predicted macrosomia as accurately as any reported ultrasonographic method (53). A study of more than 1,700 women concluded that although ultrasound-derived estimates are more accurate for newborns weighing between 2,500 g and 4,000 g, above this level, ultrasound measurement and clinical palpation have similar accuracy (70).

Measurement of the symphysis–fundal height alone is a poor predictor of fetal macrosomia. Although the average fundal height measurement is greater for fetuses exceeding 4,500 g (71), the utility of this measurement alone is questionable (72). To be useful, measurement of the uterine fundal height must be combined with clinical palpation or Leopold's maneuvers. Prospective studies designed to evaluate Leopold's maneuvers with fundal height measurement for the detection of macrosomia report sensitivities of 10–43%, specificities of 99.0–99.8%, and positive predictive values between 28% and 53% (55, 73). Ultrasound measurements of those women with suspected fetal macrosomia on the basis of clinical examination alone decreased sensitivity and positive predictive value without measurably affecting specificity (73). Prospective studies among women with diabetes also have shown that clinical estimates of macrosomia are as predictive as those derived with ultrasonography (54).

Finally, simply asking a parous woman her estimate of the fetal weight may provide an estimate as accurate as any other. In one study, a parous woman's ability to predict birth weight greater than 4,000 g was as accurate as that of clinicians using Leopold's maneuvers alone (56).

▶ *How accurate is ultrasound measurement in determining fetal weight?*

Ultrasound-derived estimates of fetal weight are obtained by entering the measurements of various fetal body parts, usually including the abdominal circumference, into one of several popular regression equations (74, 75). Most commercially available ultrasound units have one or more of these equations already programmed into the software of the system, allowing immediate calculation of estimated fetal weights. Unfortunately, most of the regression formulas currently in use are associated with significant errors when the fetus is macrosomic. For example, Hadlock's formula to predict fetal weight has a mean absolute percent error of 13% for infants greater than 4,500 g, compared with 8% for nonmacrosomic infants (76).

Ultrasound-derived diagnosis of an estimated fetal weight exceeding 4,500 g is not as accurate as many believe it to be. Among women without diabetes, ultrasound biometry used to detect macrosomia has a sensitivity of 22–44%, a specificity of 99%, a positive predictive value of 30–44%, and a negative predictive value of 97–99% (77, 78). Reports demonstrating greater accuracy generally rely on less stringent criteria for macrosomia, such as birth weight greater than 4,000 g or that exceeding the 90th percentile for a given gestational age. However, when birth weight exceeds 4,500 g, only 50% of fetuses weigh within 10% of the ultrasound-derived estimate (79). Using existing formulas, an estimated fetal weight would have to exceed 4,800 g for the fetus to have more than a 50% chance of being macrosomic (77, 80). These observations suggest that the usefulness of ultrasonography for obtaining estimated weights is limited, and these limitations are neither operator-dependent nor equipment-dependent (79).

As with clinical estimates of fetal weight, the true value of ultrasonography in the management of expected fetal macrosomia may be its ability to rule out the diagnosis, which may help avoid maternal morbidity. One study revealed that clinicians who suspected fetal macrosomia on the basis of an ultrasonogram were more likely to diagnose labor abnormalities and were more likely to perform cesarean deliveries despite normal birth weights (57).

▶ *Are interventions for treating suspected macrosomia available?*

For mothers without diabetes, no clinical interventions designed to treat or curb fetal growth when macrosomia is suspected have been reported. For pregnancies that are complicated by diabetes mellitus, one clinical trial suggests that the addition of insulin to diet therapy may treat early macrosomia diagnosed between 29 and 33 weeks of gestation (81). This study randomized 98 women with a fetal abdominal circumference exceeding the 75th percentile for gestational age to either diet therapy alone or diet therapy with twice-daily insulin. The addition of insulin therapy decreased the likelihood of birth weight greater than the 90th percentile from 45% among those treated with diet only to 13% among those receiving insulin ($P < 0.01$) (81).

Three large cohort studies confirm that excessive weight gain during pregnancy is associated with fetal macrosomia, suggesting a possible role for caloric restriction (35, 37, 39). One of these studies demonstrated that for most women, excessive weight gain doubled the risk of delivering an infant weighing more than 4,500 g. Although this relationship held true for average, obese, and very obese women, the actual incidence of macrosomia was still low (between 2.7% and 5.6%). Although dietary regulation has long been a mainstay of therapy for gestational diabetes, a recent meta-analysis of four randomized clinical trials examining primary diet therapy for women with impaired glucose tolerance showed no significant reduction in the number of newborns weighing more than 4,000 g (OR: 0.73, 95% CI: 0.45–1.35) (82). Although maternal obesity and weight gain during pregnancy are two of the strongest birth weight predictors, no randomized clinical trials have investigated dietary intervention to prevent macrosomia among obese women without diabetes.

▶ *When is cesarean delivery appropriate for suspected macrosomia at a particular estimated fetal weight?*

Controversy surrounds the question of cesarean delivery for suspected fetal macrosomia. First, the risk of birth trauma associated with vaginal delivery increases with birth weight (9, 17, 63). Second, cesarean delivery reduces—but does not eliminate—the risk of birth trauma and brachial plexus injury associated with fetal macrosomia (7, 9, 17, 83). The protective effect of cesarean delivery is large. Using a multivariate analysis to investigate risk factors for brachial plexus injury, investigators reported an odds ratio for cesarean delivery of 0.01–0.20 (17). It thus seems logical that for each woman, there must be a fetal weight beyond which the risks of vaginal delivery to the fetus are high enough to warrant cesarean delivery.

Despite such reasoning, the clinical effectiveness of offering prophylactic cesarean delivery to women with any specific estimated fetal weight has not been established in randomized clinical trials. Currently, only one observational study has evaluated a policy of using ultrasound-derived fetal weight estimates to determine the route of delivery (84). The use of historic controls, the nonrandomized design of the study, the use of multiple interventions, and the small sample size severely limit the usefulness of conclusions from the study. In this study, 1,337 women with diabetes were offered elective cesarean delivery based on ultrasound-derived fetal weight estimates beyond 4,250 g and induction of labor if ultrasound measurements resulted in a prediction of a large-for-gestational-age infant with an estimated fetal weight less than 4,250 g (84). The study cohort was compared with a historic control group of 1,227 women with diabetes who were managed without intervention for accelerated fetal growth during the 3 years preceding implementation of the study protocol. Implementation of the study protocol was associated with a nonsignificant reduction in the risk of shoulder dystocia from 2.4% in controls to 1.1% in the intervention group. In addition, a significant increase in the institutional cesarean delivery rate from 21.7% in controls to 25.1% in the intervention group was reported. Although the sample size was insufficient for comparison, the risk of birth trauma was not eliminated (2 versus 1 brachial plexus injury, 12 versus 6 fractures).

Currently, no prospective studies have assessed the true risk of either shoulder dystocia or brachial plexus injury in conjunction with estimated fetal weight alone. Until well-designed randomized clinical trials of sufficient sample size are available, clinicians must rely on retrospective data to make clinical management decisions.

In addition, recent large cohort and case–control studies demonstrate the safety of allowing a trial of labor for estimated birth weights of more than 4,000 g (12, 13). Among the 2,924 infants previously identified with birth weights greater than 4,000 g in utero, only 48 injuries (1.6%) related to shoulder dystocia were noted. Among the 22 brachial plexus injuries with documented follow-up, only 5 (17%) were clinically evident at 6 months (68). A second study reported 27 episodes (11.4%) of shoulder dystocia and 3 instances (1.3%) of brachial plexus paralysis in a group of 236 neonates weighing at least 4,200 g (85). In an additional series of 87 infants with birth weights greater than 4,500 g who were delivered vaginally, investigators reported only 5 cases (5.7%) of Erb-Duchenne paralysis. By 3 months of age, all affected infants were without evidence of brachial plexus paralysis (13). A fourth study reported that of the 157 infants delivered vaginally with birth weights greater than 4,500 g, no permanent sequelae were identified by age 2 months (12). The risks of short-term morbidity associated with vaginal delivery in this group are low, and those of permanent injury are even lower.

In conjunction with published cost-effectiveness data, the sum of these reports does not support a policy of prophylactic cesarean delivery for suspected fetal macrosomia with estimated weights less than 5,000 g (86). Along with a description of the limitations of estimating fetal weight, the obstetrician should present accurate statistics for the short- and long-term risks of maternal and fetal morbidity for both vaginal and cesarean delivery as discussed previously.

Despite the poor predictive value of an estimated fetal weight beyond 5,000 g and a lack of evidence supporting cesarean delivery at any estimated fetal weight, most, but not all, authors agree that consideration should be given to cesarean delivery in this situation (7, 13, 65). Among infants with birth weights exceeding 5,000 g, there are reports of cesarean delivery rates of 35–60%, brachial paralysis rates of 7–11%, and a perinatal death rate as high as 2.4% (7). In contrast, despite reporting an OR of 45 (95% CI: 16–129) for brachial plexus injury among vaginally delivered infants exceeding 5,000 g, some investigators suggest that ultrasound-derived fetal weight estimates alone should not be used to determine the route of delivery (17, 52).

▶ *Is there a role for induction of labor in the management of term patients with suspected fetal macrosomia?*

Current evidence from cohort studies does not support a policy of early induction of labor in term patients with suspected fetal macrosomia. Three recent reports show that induction of labor at least doubles the risk of cesarean delivery without reducing shoulder dystocia or newborn morbidity (87–89). Although the increased risk of cesarean delivery with induction of labor is clear, on the basis of these reports, one cannot rule out the possibility of a small beneficial effect on fetal outcome. These studies, however, are affected by small sample size and possible bias introduced by their retrospective nature.

One randomized clinical trial of women without diabetes has addressed the role of induction of labor for suspected fetal macrosomia at term. A total of 273 women with ultrasound-derived estimated fetal weights between 4,000 g and 4,500 g were randomized to either planned induction of labor or expectant management (90). Inductions were performed with oxytocin or prostaglandins followed by oxytocin, depending on the condition of the cervix. The cesarean delivery rates were similar: 19.4% for the induction group and 21.6% for the expectant group. There were 11 cases of shoulder dystocia, 5 in the induction group and 6 in the expectant group. All were managed without brachial plexus injury or other trauma.

▶ *How many elective cesarean deliveries for suspected fetal macrosomia would have to be performed to prevent one case of brachial plexus injury?*

The cost-effectiveness of elective cesarean delivery for fetal macrosomia usually is expressed as the number of cesarean deliveries required to prevent one brachial plexus injury or the cost, in dollars, of each brachial plexus injury avoided. A case–control study of brachial plexus paralysis demonstrated that 51 cesarean deliveries would be needed to prevent one case of brachial plexus paralysis if the cutoff for cesarean delivery were 4,500 g among patients without diabetes (17). For a cutoff of 5,000 g, this number decreased to 19. Assuming persistent rates for brachial plexus impairment are between 5% and 22%, the authors suggested that to prevent a single permanent injury, the number of cesarean deliveries increases to between 233 and 1,026 for a birth weight cutoff of 4,500 g, and from 85 to 373 for a cutoff of 5,000 g. Another study using similar methods concluded that 155–588 cesarean deliveries are needed to prevent a single permanent injury using a cutoff of 4,500 g for infants of women without diabetes (65). However, because the authors did not consider the imperfect predictive values of ultrasonography for macrosomia, they underestimated the number of cesarean deliveries that would be needed to implement such a policy.

In two reports analyzing a policy of prophylactic cesarean delivery for macrosomia, which took into account the reported sensitivity and specificity of ultrasonography for the detection of macrosomia (4,500 g), it was calculated that 3,695 cesarean deliveries would be required to prevent one permanent injury at a cost of $8.7 million for each injury avoided (86, 91). For pregnancies complicated by diabetes, these figures were still high at 443 cesarean deliveries to prevent a single permanent injury. In summary, because of the lack of well-designed and well-executed randomized clinical trials, a policy of prophylactic cesarean delivery for suspected fetal macrosomia less than 5,000 g may not be effective for pregnancies without diabetes. Furthermore, even for pregnancies complicated by diabetes, the cost-effectiveness of such a policy is doubtful.

▶ *How should a diagnosis of suspected fetal macrosomia affect the management of labor and vaginal delivery?*

Perhaps the most important consideration for labor and delivery with suspected fetal macrosomia is the decision to conduct a midpelvic operative vaginal delivery. As depicted in Figure 1, the risk of shoulder dystocia is associated with assisted vaginal delivery. Case–control and cohort studies consistently demonstrate an increased risk of shoulder dystocia when the macrosomic fetus is delivered by forceps, especially midforceps for a prolonged second stage (8, 10, 14, 19, 92). Rates of shoulder dystocia with midforceps deliveries of infants greater than 4,500 g have been reported to be above 50%. Barring extreme emergencies, cesarean delivery should be performed for midpelvic arrest of the fetus with suspected macrosomia. If a decision is made to proceed with cesarean delivery in the presence of suspected macrosomia, the incision should be large enough to avoid a difficult abdominal delivery.

Suspected fetal macrosomia is not a contraindication to attempt vaginal birth after prior cesarean delivery. A cohort study compared maternal and fetal outcomes associated with a trial of labor for infants suspected to be macrosomic and with documented birth weights less than 4,000 g versus those greater than 4,000 g (93). The success rate for vaginal delivery was 58% for birth weights between 4,000 g and 4,499 g and 43% for birth weights of 4,500 g and higher. Maternal and newborn morbidities were equal. A case–control study examining risk factors for uterine rupture during a trial of labor found no association between rupture and birth weight greater than 4,000 g (94).

Summary

The following recommendation is based on good and consistent scientific evidence (Level A):

- ▶ The diagnosis of fetal macrosomia is imprecise. For suspected fetal macrosomia, the accuracy of estimated fetal weight using ultrasound biometry is no better than that obtained with clinical palpation (Leopold's maneuvers).

The following recommendations are based on limited or inconsistent scientific evidence (Level B):

- ▶ Suspected fetal macrosomia is not an indication for induction of labor, because induction does not improve maternal or fetal outcomes.

- Labor and vaginal delivery are not contraindicated for women with estimated fetal weights up to 5,000 g in the absence of maternal diabetes.
- With an estimated fetal weight greater than 4,500 g, a prolonged second stage of labor or arrest of descent in the second stage is an indication for cesarean delivery.

The following recommendations are based primarily on consensus and expert opinion (Level C):

- Although the diagnosis of fetal macrosomia is imprecise, prophylactic cesarean delivery may be considered for suspected fetal macrosomia with estimated fetal weights greater than 5,000 g in women without diabetes and greater than 4,500 g in women with diabetes.
- Suspected fetal macrosomia is not a contraindication to attempted vaginal birth after a previous cesarean delivery.

References

1. Lubchenco LO, Hansman C, Dressler M, Boyd E. Intrauterine growth as estimated from liveborn birthweight data at 24 to 42 weeks of gestation. Pediatrics 1963;32:793–800 (Level III)
2. Williams RL. Intrauterine growth curves: intra- and international comparisons with different ethnic groups in California. Prev Med 1975;4:163–172 (Level III)
3. Brenner WE, Edelman DA, Hendricks CH. A standard of fetal growth in the United States of America. Am J Obstet Gynecol 1976;126:555–564 (Level III)
4. Alexander GR, Himes JH, Kaufman RB, Mor J, Kogan M. A United States national reference for fetal growth. Obstet Gynecol 1996;87:163–168 (Level III)
5. Modanlou HD, Dorchester WL, Thorosian A, Freeman RK. Macrosomia—maternal, fetal and neonatal implications. Obstet Gynecol 1980;55:420–424 (Level II-2)
6. Boyd ME, Usher RH, McLean FH. Fetal macrosomia: prediction, risks, proposed management. Obstet Gynecol 1983;61:715–722 (Level II-2)
7. Spellacy WN, Miller S, Winegar A, Peterson PQ. Macrosomia—maternal characteristics and infant complications. Obstet Gynecol 1985;66:158–161 (Level II-2)
8. Acker DB, Sachs BP, Friedman EA. Risk factors for shoulder dystocia. Obstet Gynecol 1985;66:762–768 (Level II-3)
9. McFarland LV, Raskin M, Daling JR, Benedetti TJ. Erb/Duchenne's palsy: a consequence of fetal macrosomia and method of delivery. Obstet Gynecol 1986;68:784–788 (Level II-2)
10. Gross TL, Sokol RJ, Williams T, Thompson K. Shoulder dystocia: a fetal-physician risk. Am J Obstet Gynecol 1987;156:1408–1418 (Level II-2)
11. Menticoglou SM, Manning FA, Morrison I, Harman CR. Must macrosomic fetuses be delivered by a cesarean section? A review of outcome for 786 babies ≥ 4,500 g. Aust N Z J Obstet Gynaecol 1992;32:100–103 (Level III)
12. Lipscomb KR, Gregory K, Shaw K. The outcome of macrosomic infants weighing at least 4500 grams: Los Angeles county + University of Southern California experience. Obstet Gynecol 1995;85:558–564 (Level II-3)
13. Bérard J, Dufour P, Vinatier D, Subtil D, Vanderstichèle S, Monnier JC, et al. Fetal macrosomia: risk factors and outcome. A study of the outcome concerning 100 cases >4500 g. Eur J Obstet Gynecol Reprod Biol 1998; 77:51–59 (Level II-3)
14. Nesbitt TS, Gilbert WM, Herrchen B. Shoulder dystocia and associated risk factors with macrosomic infants born in California. Am J Obstet Gynecol 1998;179:476–480 (Level II-3)
15. Acker DB, Gregory KD, Sachs BP, Friedman EA. Risk factors for Erb-Duchenne palsy. Obstet Gynecol 1988; 71:389–392 (Level II-3)
16. Bahar AM. Risk factors and fetal outcome in cases of shoulder dystocia compared with normal deliveries of a similar birth weight. Br J Obstet Gynaecol 1996;103: 68–872 (Level II-2)
17. Ecker JL, Greenberg JA, Norwitz ER, Nadel AS, Repke JT. Birth weight as a predictor of brachial plexus injury. Obstet Gynecol 1997;89:643–647 (Level II-2)
18. Ventura SJ, Martin JA, Curtin SC, Mathews TJ, Park MM. Births: final data for 1998. Natl Vital Stat Rep 2000;48: 1–100 (Level II-3)
19. Nocon JJ, McKenzie DK, Thomas LJ, Hansell RS. Shoulder dystocia: an analysis of risks and obstetric maneuvers. Am J Obstet Gynecol 1993;168:1732–1739 (Level II-2)
20. Gonik B, Hollyer L, Allen R. Shoulder dystocia recognition: differences in neonatal risks for injury. Am J Perinatol 1991;8:31–34 (Level II-3)
21. Jennett RJ, Tarby TJ, Kreinick CJ. Brachial plexus palsy: an old problem revisited. Am J Obstet Gynecol 1992;166: 1673–1677 (Level II-2)
22. Gross SJ, Shime J, Farine D. Shoulder dystocia: predictors and outcome. A five-year review. Am J Obstet Gynecol 1987;156:334–336 (Level II-3)
23. Morrison JC, Sanders JR, Magann EF, Wiser WL. The diagnosis and management of dystocia of the shoulder. Surg Gynecol Obstet 1992;175:515–522 (Level II-3)
24. Okun N, Verma A, Mitchell BF, Flowerdew G. Relative importance of maternal constitutional factors and glucose intolerance of pregnancy in the development of newborn macrosomia. J Matern Fetal Med 1997;6:285–290 (Level II-2)
25. Hellerstedt WL, Himes JH, Story M, Alton IR, Edwards LE. The effects of cigarette smoking and gestational weight change on birth outcomes in obese and normal-

weight women. Am J Public Health 1997;87:591–596 (Level II-2)

26. Sermer M, Naylor CD, Gare DJ, Kenshole AB, Ritchie JW, Farine D, et al. Impact of increasing carbohydrate intolerance on maternal-fetal outcomes in 3637 women without gestational diabetes. The Toronto Tri-Hospital Gestational Diabetes Project. Am J Obstet Gynecol 1995; 173:146–156 (Level II-2)

27. Verma A, Mitchell BF, Demianczuk N, Flowerdew G, Okun NB. Relationship between plasma glucose levels in glucose-intolerant women and newborn macrosomia. J Matern Fetal Med 1997;6:187–193 (Level II-2)

28. Naylor CD, Sermer M, Chen E, Sykora K. Cesarean delivery in relation to birth weight and gestational glucose tolerance: pathophysiology or practice style? Toronto Trihospital Gestational Diabetes Investigators. JAMA 1996;275:1165–1170 (Level II-2)

29. Adams KM, Li H, Nelson RL, Ogburn PL Jr, Danilenko-Dixon DR. Sequelae of unrecognized gestational diabetes. Am J Obstet Gynecol 1998;178:1321–1332 (Level II-2)

30. Nasrat H, Abalkhail B, Fageeh W, Shabat A, el Zahrany F. Anthropometric measurements of newborns of gestational diabetic mothers: does it indicate disproportionate fetal growth? J Matern Fetal Med 1997;6:291–295 (Level II-2)

31. McFarland MB, Trylovich CG, Langer O. Anthropometric differences in macrosomic infants of diabetic and nondiabetic mothers. J Matern Fetal Med 1998;7:292–295 (Level II-2)

32. Casey BM, Lucas MJ, McIntire DD, Leveno KJ. Pregnancy outcomes in women with gestational diabetes compared with the general obstetric population. Obstet Gynecol 1997;90:869–873 (Level II-2)

33. Lucas MJ, Lowe TW, Bowe L, McIntire DD. Class A1 gestational diabetes: a meaningful diagnosis? Obstet Gynecol 1993;82:260–265 (Level II-2)

34. Larsen CE, Serdula MK, Sullivan KM. Macrosomia: Influence of maternal overweight among a low-income population. Am J Obstet Gynecol 1990;162:490–494 (Level II-3)

35. Cogswell ME, Serdula MK, Hungerford DW, Yip R. Gestational weight gain among average-weight and overweight women—what is excessive? Am J Obstet Gynecol 1995;172:705–712 (Level II-2)

36. Ogunyemi D, Hullett S, Leeper J, Risk A. Prepregnancy body mass index, weight gain during pregnancy, and perinatal outcome in a rural black population. J Matern Fetal Med 1998;7:190–193 (Level II-3)

37. Bianco AT, Smilen SW, Davis Y, Lopez S, Lapinski R, Lockwood CJ. Pregnancy outcome and weight gain recommendations for the morbidly obese woman. Obstet Gynecol 1998;91:97–102 (Level II-2)

38. Perlow JH, Morgan MA, Montgomery D, Towers CV, Porto M. Perinatal outcome in pregnancy complicated by massive obesity. Am J Obstet Gynecol 1992;167:958–962 (Level II-2)

39. Parker JD, Abrams B. Prenatal weight gain advice: an examination of the recent prenatal weight gain recommendations of the Institute of Medicine. Obstet Gynecol 1992;79:664–669 (Level II-3)

40. Lazer S, Biale Y, Mazor M, Lewenthal H, Insler V. Complications associated with the macrosomic fetus. J Repro Med 1986;31:501–505 (Level II-2)

41. Klebanoff MA, Mills JL, Berendes HW. Mother's birth weight as a predictor of macrosomia. Am J Obstet Gynecol 1985;153:253–257 (Level II-2)

42. Toohey JS, Keegan KA Jr, Morgan MA, Francis J, Task S, deVeciana M. The "dangerous multipara": fact or fiction? Am J Obstet Gynecol 1995;172:683–686 (Level II-2)

43. Juntunen K, Kirkinen P, Kauppila A. The clinical outcome in pregnancies of grand grand multiparous women. Acta Obstet Gynecol Scand 1997;76:755–759 (Level II-3)

44. Babinszki A, Kerenyi T, Torok O, Grazi V, Lapinski RH, Berkowitz RL. Perinatal outcome in grand and great-grand multiparity: effects of parity on obstetric risk factors. Am J Obstet Gynecol 1999;181:669–674 (Level II-3)

45. Brunskill AJ, Rossing MA, Connel FA, Daling J. Antecedents of macrosomia. Paediatr Perinat Epidemiol 1991;5:392–401 (Level II-2)

46. Dooley SL, Metzger BE, Cho NH. Gestational diabetes mellitus. Influence of race on disease prevalence and perinatal outcome in a U.S. population. Diabetes 1991;40:25–29 (Level II-3)

47. Homko CJ, Sivan E, Nyirjesy P, Reece EA. The interrelationship between ethnicity and gestational diabetes in fetal macrosomia. Diabetes Care 1995;18:1442–1445 (Level II-3)

48. Little RE, Sing CF. Genetic and environmental influences on human birth weight. Am J Hum Genet 1987;40: 512–526 (Level III)

49. Wilcox MA, Newton CS, Johnson IR. Paternal influences on birth weight. Acta Obstet Gynecol Scand 1995;74: 15–18 (Level II-3)

50. Deter RL, Hadlock FP. Use of ultrasound in the detection of macrosomia: a review. J Clin Ultrasound 1985;13: 519–524 (Level III)

51. Rossavik IK, Joslin GL. Macrosomatia and ultrasonography: what is the problem? South Med J 1993; 86:1129–1132 (Level II-3)

52. Sandmire HF. Whither ultrasonic prediction of fetal macrosomia? Obstet Gynecol 1993;82:860–862 (Level III)

53. Chauhan SP, Cowan BD, Magann EF, Bradford TH, Roberts WE, Morrison JC. Intrapartum detection of a macrosomic fetus: clinical versus 8 sonographic models. Aust N Z J Obstet Gynaecol 1995;35:3:266–270 (Level II-2)

54. Johnstone FD, Prescott RJ, Steel JM, Mao JH, Chambers S, Muir N. Clinical and ultrasound prediction of macrosomia in diabetic pregnancy. Br J Obstet Gynaecol 1996; 103:747–754 (Level II-3)

55. Chauhan SP, Hendrix NW, Magann EF, Morrison JC, Kenney SP, Devoe LD. Limitations of clinical and sonographic estimates of birth weight: experience with 1034 parturients. Obstet Gynecol 1998;91:72–77 (Level II-2)

56. Chauhan SP, Sullivan CA, Lutton TD, Magann EF, Morrison JC. Parous patients' estimate of birth weight in postterm pregnancy. J Perinatol 1995;15:192–194 (Level II-2)

57. Levine AB, Lockwood CJ, Brown B, Lapinski R, Berkowitz RL. Sonographic diagnosis of the large for gestational age fetus at term: does it make a difference? Obstet Gynecol 1992;79:55–58 (Level II-2)

58. Stones RW, Paterson CM, Saunders NJ. Risk factors for major obstetric haemorrhage. Eur J Obstet Gynecol Reprod Biol 1993;48:15–18 (Level II-2)

59. el Madany AA, Jallad KB, Radi FA, el Hamdan H, O'deh HM. Shoulder dystocia: anticipation and outcome. Int J Gynaecol Obstet 1990;34:7–12 (Level II-2)

60. Irion O, Hirsbrunner Almagbaly P, Morabia A. Planned vaginal delivery versus elective caesarean section: a study of 705 singleton term breech presentations. Br J Obstet Gynaecol 1998;105:710–717 (Meta-analysis)

61. Oppenheim WL, Davis A, Growdon WA, Dorey FJ, Davlin LB. Clavicle fractures in the newborn. Clin Orthop 1990;250:176–180 (Level II-2)

62. Chez RA, Carlan S, Greenberg SL, Spellacy WN. Fractured clavicle is an unavoidable event. Am J Obstet Gynecol 1994;171:797–798 (Level II-2)

63. Perlow JH, Wigton T, Hart J, Strassner HT, Nageotte MP, Wolk BM. Birth trauma. A five-year review of incidence and associated perinatal factors. J Reprod Med 1996;41: 754–760 (Level II-2)

64. Gordon M, Rich H, Deutschberger J, Green M. The immediate and long-term outcome of obstetric birth trauma. I. Brachial plexus paralysis. Am J Obstet Gynecol 1973; 117:51–56 (Level II-2)

65. Bryant DR, Leonardi MR, Landwehr JB, Bottoms SF. Limited usefulness of fetal weight in predicting neonatal brachial plexus injury. Am J Obstet Gynecol 1998; 179:686–689 (Level II-3)

66. Gherman RB, Goodwin TM, Ouzounian JG, Miller DA, Paul RH. Brachial plexus palsy associated with cesarean section: an in utero injury? Am J Obstet Gynecol 1997; 177:1162–1164 (Level III)

67. Hardy AE. Birth injuries of the brachial plexus: incidence and prognosis. J Bone Joint Surg Br 1981;63-B:98–101 (Level III)

68. Kolderup LB, Laros RK Jr, Musci TJ. Incidence of persistent birth injury in macrosomic infants: association with mode of delivery. Am J Obstet Gynecol 1997;177:37–41 (Level II-2)

69. Seidman DS, Laor A, Stevenson DK, Sivan E, Gale R, Shemer J. Macrosomia does not predict overweight in late adolescence in infants of diabetic mothers. Acta Obstet Gynecol Scand 1998;77:58–62 (Level II-2)

70. Sherman DJ, Arieli S, Tovbin J, Siegel G, Caspi E, Bukovsky I. A comparison of clinical and ultrasonic estimation of fetal weight. Obstet Gynecol 1998;91:212–217 (Level II-3)

71. Wikstrom I, Bergstrom R, Bakketeig L, Jacobsen G, Lindmark G. Prediction of high birth weight from maternal characteristics, symphysis fundal height and ultrasound biometry. Gynecol Obstet Invest 1993;35:27–33 (Level II-2)

72. Neilson JP. Symphysis-fundal height measurement in pregnancy. Cochrane Database Syst Rev 2000; 2: CD000944. Review (Meta-analysis)

73. Gonen R, Spiegel D, Abend M. Is macrosomia predictable, and are shoulder dystocia and birth trauma preventable? Obstet Gynecol 1996;88:526–529 (Level II-3)

74. Shepard MJ, Richards VA, Berkowitz RL, Warsof SL, Hobbins JC. An evaluation of two equations for predicting fetal weight by ultrasound. Am J Obstet Gynecol 1982; 142: 47–54 (Level II-3)

75. Hadlock FP, Harrist RB, Carpenter RJ, Deter RL, Park SK. Sonographic estimation of fetal weight. The value of femur length in addition to head and abdomen measurements. Radiology 1984;150:535–540 (Level II-3)

76. Alsulyman OM, Ouzounian JG, Kjos SL. The accuracy of intrapartum ultrasonographic fetal weight estimation in diabetic pregnancies. Am J Obstet Gynecol 1997;177: 503–506 (Level II-2)

77. Smith GC, Smith MF, McNay MB, Fleming JE. The relation between fetal abdominal circumference and birth weight: findings in 3512 pregnancies. Br J Obstet Gynaecol 1997;104:186–190 (Level II-3)

78. O'Reilly-Green CP, Divon MY. Receiver operating characteristic curves of sonographic estimated fetal weight for prediction of macrosomia in prolonged pregnancies. Ultrasound Obstet Gynecol 1997;9:403–408 (Level II-3)

79. Benacerraf BR, Gelman R, Frigoletto FD Jr. Sonographically estimated fetal weights: accuracy and limitation. Am J Obstet Gynecol 1988;159:1118–1121 (Level II-2)

80. McLaren RA, Puckett JL, Chauhan SP. Estimators of birth weight in pregnant women requiring insulin: a comparison of seven sonographic models. Obstet Gynecol 1995;85: 565–569 (Level II-2)

81. Buchanan TA, Kjos SL, Montoro MN, Wu PY, Madrilejo NG, Gonzalez M, et al. Use of fetal ultrasound to select metabolic therapy for pregnancies complicated by mild gestational diabetes. Diabetes Care 1994;17:275–283 (Level II-1)

82. Walkinshaw SA. Dietary regulation for 'gestational diabetes.' Cochrane Database Syst Rev 2000;2:CD000070. Review (Meta-analysis)

83. Gregory KD, Henry OA, Ramicone E, Chan LS, Platt LD. Maternal and infant complications in high and normal weight infants by method of delivery. Obstet Gynecol 1998;92:507–513 (Level II-2)

84. Conway DL, Langer O. Elective delivery of infants with macrosomia in diabetic women: reduced shoulder dystocia versus increased cesarean deliveries. Am J Obstet Gynecol 1998;178:922–925 (Level II-2)

85. Blickstein I, Ben-Arie A, Hagay ZJ. Antepartum risks of shoulder dystocia and brachial plexus injury for infants weighing 4,200 g or more. Gynecol Obstet Invest 1998;45:77–80 (Level II-2)

86. Rouse DJ, Owen J, Goldenberg RL, Cliver SP. The effectiveness and costs of elective cesarean delivery for fetal macrosomia diagnosed by ultrasound. JAMA 1996;276: 1480–1486 (Level III)

87. Combs CA, Singh NB, Khoury JC. Elective induction versus spontaneous labor after sonographic diagnosis of fetal macrosomia. Obstet Gynecol 1993;81:492–496 (Level II-2)

88. Friesen CD, Miller AM, Rayburn WF. Influence of spontaneous or induced labor on delivering the macrosomic fetus. Am J Perinatol 1995;12:63–66 (Level II-2)

89. Leaphart WL, Meyer MC, Capeless EL. Labor induction with a prenatal diagnosis of fetal macrosomia. J Matern Fetal Med 1997;6:99–102 (Level II-2)

90. Gonen O, Rosen DJ, Dolfin Z, Tepper R, Markow S, Fejgin MD. Induction of labor versus expectant management in macrosomia: a randomized study. Obstet Gynecol 1997;89:913–917 (Level I)

91. Rouse DJ, Owen J. Prophylactic cesarean delivery for fetal macrosomia diagnosed by means of ultrasonography—a Faustian bargain? Am J Obstet Gynecol 1999;181: 332–338 (Level III)

92. Benedetti TJ, Gabbe SG. Shoulder dystocia. A complication of fetal macrosomia and prolonged second stage of labor with midpelvic delivery. Obstet Gynecol 1978;52: 526–529 (Level III)

93. Flamm BL, Goings JR. Vaginal birth after cesarean section: is suspected fetal macrosomia a contraindication? Obstet Gynecol 1989;74:694–697 (Level II-2)

94. Leung AS, Farmer RM, Leung EK, Medearis AL, Paul RH. Risk factors associated with uterine rupture during trial of labor after cesarean delivery: a case-control study. Am J Obstet Gynecol 1993;168:1358–1363 (Level II-2)

The MEDLINE database, the Cochrane Library, and ACOG's own internal resources and documents were used to conduct a literature search to locate relevant articles published between January 1985 and May 1999. The search was restricted to articles published in the English language. Priority was given to articles reporting results of original research, although review articles and commentaries also were consulted. Abstracts of research presented at symposia and scientific conferences were not considered adequate for inclusion in this document. Guidelines published by organizations or institutions such as the National Institutes of Health and the American College of Obstetricians and Gynecologists were reviewed, and additional studies were located by reviewing bibliographies of identified articles. When reliable research was not available, expert opinions from obstetrician–gynecologists were used.

Studies were reviewed and evaluated for quality according to the method outlined by the U.S. Preventive Services Task Force:

- I Evidence obtained from at least one properly designed randomized controlled trial.
- II-1 Evidence obtained from well-designed controlled trials without randomization.
- II-2 Evidence obtained from well-designed cohort or case–control analytic studies, preferably from more than one center or research group.
- II-3 Evidence obtained from multiple time series with or without the intervention. Dramatic results in uncontrolled experiments also could be regarded as this type of evidence.
- III Opinions of respected authorities, based on clinical experience, descriptive studies, or reports of expert committees.

Based on the highest level of evidence found in the data, recommendations are provided and graded according to the following catetories:

Level A—Recommendations are based on good and consistent scientific evidence.

Level B—Recommendations are based on limited or inconsistent scientific evidence.

Level C—Recommendations are based primarily on consensus and expert opinion.

ISSN 1099-3630

The American College of Obstetricians and Gynecologists
409 12th Street, SW, PO Box 96920
Washington, DC 20090-6920

12345/43210

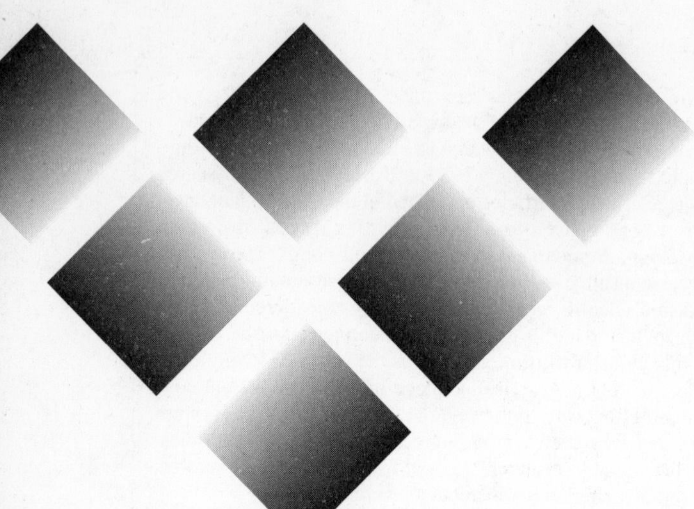

ACOG PRACTICE BULLETIN

CLINICAL MANAGEMENT GUIDELINES FOR OBSTETRICIAN–GYNECOLOGISTS

NUMBER 10, NOVEMBER 1999

(Replaces Technical Bulletin Number 217, December 1995)

This Practice Bulletin was developed by the ACOG Committee on Practice Bulletins—Obstetrics with the assistance of Susan M. Ramin, MD. The information is designed to aid practitioners in making decisions about appropriate obstetric and gynecologic care. These guidelines should not be construed as dictating an exclusive course of treatment or procedure. Variations in practice may be warranted based on the needs of the individual patient, resources, and limitations unique to the institution or type of practice.

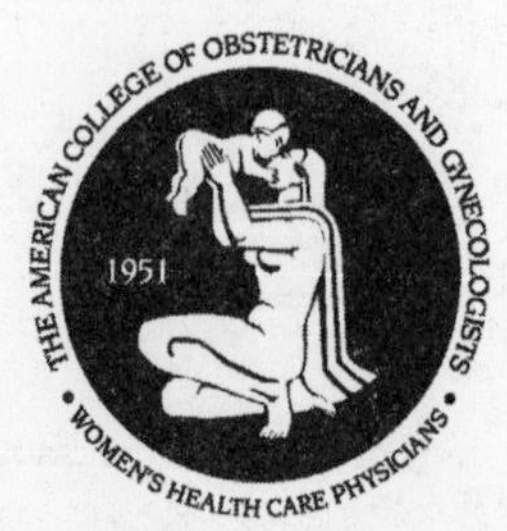

Induction of Labor

The goal of induction of labor is to achieve vaginal delivery by stimulating uterine contractions before the spontaneous onset of labor. According to the National Center for Health Statistics, the overall rate of induction of labor in the United States has increased from 90 per 1,000 live births in 1989 to 184 per 1,000 live births in 1997 (1). Generally, induction of labor has merit as a therapeutic option when the benefits of expeditious delivery outweigh the risks of continuing the pregnancy. The benefits of labor induction must be weighed against the potential maternal or fetal risks associated with this procedure. The purpose of this bulletin is to review current methods for cervical ripening and induction of labor and to summarize the effectiveness of these approaches based on appropriately conducted outcomes-based research. These practice guidelines classify the indications for and contraindications to induction of labor, describe the various agents used for cervical ripening, cite methods used to induce labor, and outline the requirements for the safe clinical use of the various methods of inducing labor.

Background

In 1948, Theobald and associates described their use of the posterior pituitary extract, oxytocin, by intravenous drip for labor induction (2). Five years later, oxytocin was the first polypeptide hormone synthesized by du Vigneaud and associates (3). This synthetic polypeptide hormone has since been used to stimulate uterine contractions. Other methods used for induction of labor include membrane stripping, amniotomy, and administering prostaglandin E (PGE) analogues.

Cervical Ripening

If induction is indicated and the status of the cervix is unfavorable, agents for cervical ripening may be used. The status of the cervix can be determined by the Bishop pelvic scoring system (Table 1) (4). If the total score is more than 8,

Table 1. Bishop Scoring System

Score	Factor				
	Dilation (cm)	Effacement (%)	Station*	Cervical Consistency	Position of Cervix
0	Closed	0–30	−3	Firm	Posterior
1	1–2	40–50	−2	Medium	Midposition
2	3–4	60–70	−1, 0	Soft	Anterior
3	5–6	80	+1, +2	—	—

*Station reflects a −3 to +3 scale.

Modified from Bishop EH. Pelvic scoring for elective induction. Obstet Gynecol 1964;24:267

the probability of vaginal delivery after labor induction is similar to that after spontaneous labor.

Acceptable methods for cervical ripening include mechanical cervical dilators and administration of synthetic prostaglandin E_1 (PGE_1) and prostaglandin E_2 (PGE_2) (5-9). Mechanical dilation methods are effective in ripening the cervix and include hygroscopic dilators, osmotic dilators (*Laminaria japonicum*), the 24-French Foley balloon, and the double balloon device (Atad Ripener Device) (10-15). Laminaria ripen the cervix but may be associated with increased peripartum infections (6, 16).

Misoprostol, a synthetic PGE_1 analogue, can be administered intravaginally or orally and is used for both cervical ripening and induction. It currently is available as a 100-mcg or 200-mcg tablet, and can be broken to provide 25-mcg or 50-mcg doses. Misoprostol currently is approved by the U.S. Food and Drug Administration (FDA) for the prevention of peptic ulcers, but not for cervical ripening or induction of labor.

Two PGE_2 preparations are commercially available: a gel available in a 2.5-mL syringe containing 0.5 mg of dinoprostone and a vaginal insert containing 10 mg of dinoprostone. Both are approved by the FDA for cervical ripening in women at or near term. The vaginal insert releases prostaglandin (PG) at a slower rate (0.3 mg/h) than the gel. Both the gel and the vaginal insert have been reported to increase the probability of successful initial induction, shorten the interval from induction to delivery, and decrease the total and maximal doses of oxytocin needed to induce contractions (17).

Other pharmacologic methods for cervical ripening include continuous intravenous oxytocin drip, extraamniotic saline infusion, vaginal recombinant human relaxin, and intracervical purified porcine relaxin. The safety and efficacy of these latter methods are unclear.

Methods of Labor Induction

In addition to oxytocin and misoprostol, other agents can be used for induction of labor. The progesterone antagonist mifepristone (RU 486) is one such suitable and effective induction agent (18). Nonpharmacologic methods of labor induction include stripping the amniotic membranes, amniotomy, and nipple stimulation.

Oxytocin

Oxytocin, an octapeptide, is one of the most commonly used drugs in the United States. The physiology of oxytocin-stimulated labor is similar to that of spontaneous labor, although individual patients vary in sensitivity and response to oxytocin. Based on pharmacokinetic studies of synthetic oxytocin, uterine response ensues after 3–5 minutes of infusion, and a steady state of oxytocin is achieved in plasma by 40 minutes (19). The uterine response to oxytocin depends on the duration of the pregnancy; there is a gradual increase in response from 20 to 30 weeks of gestation, followed by a plateau from 34 weeks of gestation until term, when sensitivity increases (20). Cervical dilation, parity, and gestational age are predictors of the dose response to oxytocin for labor stimulation (21).

Membrane Stripping

Stripping the amniotic membranes is commonly practiced to induce labor. However, several studies have yielded conflicting results regarding the efficacy of membrane stripping (22–24). Significant increases in phospholipase A_2 activity and prostaglandin $F_{2\alpha}$ ($PGF_{2\alpha}$) levels occur from membrane stripping (25). Stripping membranes appears to be associated with a greater frequency of spontaneous labor and fewer inductions for postterm pregnancy. In a randomized trial of 195 normal pregnancies beyond 40 weeks of gestation, two thirds of the patients who underwent membrane stripping labored spontaneously within 72 hours, compared with one third of the patients who underwent examination only (26).

Amniotomy

Artificial rupture of the membranes may be used as a method of labor induction, especially if the condition of the cervix is favorable. Used alone for inducing labor, amniotomy can be associated with unpredictable and sometimes long intervals before the onset of contractions. However, in a trial of amniotomy combined with early oxytocin infusion compared with amniotomy alone, the induction-to-delivery interval was shorter with the amniotomy-plus-oxytocin method (27).

Clinical Considerations and Recommendations

▶ *What are the indications and contraindications to induction of labor?*

Indications for induction of labor are not absolute but should take into account maternal and fetal conditions, gestational age, cervical status, and other factors. Following are examples of maternal or fetal conditions that may be indications for induction of labor:

- Abruptio placentae
- Chorioamnionitis
- Fetal demise
- Pregnancy-induced hypertension
- Premature rupture of membranes
- Postterm pregnancy
- Maternal medical conditions (eg, diabetes mellitus, renal disease, chronic pulmonary disease, chronic hypertension)
- Fetal compromise (eg, severe fetal growth restriction, isoimmunization)
- Preeclampsia, eclampsia

Labor also may be induced for logistic reasons, for example, risk of rapid labor, distance from hospital, or psychosocial indications. In such circumstances, at least one of the criteria in the box should be met or fetal lung maturity should be established (28).

Generally, the contraindications to labor induction are the same as those for spontaneous labor and vaginal delivery. They include, but are not limited to, the following situations:

- Vasa previa or complete placenta previa
- Transverse fetal lie
- Umbilical cord prolapse
- Previous transfundal uterine surgery

Confirmation of Term Gestation

- Fetal heart tones have been documented for 20 weeks by nonelectronic fetoscope or for 30 weeks by Doppler.
- It has been 36 weeks since a positive serum or urine human chorionic gonadotropin pregnancy test was performed by a reliable laboratory.
- An ultrasound measurement of the crown–rump length, obtained at 6–12 weeks, supports a gestational age of at least 39 weeks.
- An ultrasound obtained at 13–20 weeks confirms the gestational age of at least 39 weeks determined by clinical history and physical examination.

However, the individual patient and clinical situation should be considered in determining when induction of labor is contraindicated. Several obstetric situations are not contraindications to the induction of labor but do necessitate special attention. These include, but are not limited to, the following:

- One or more previous low-transverse cesarean deliveries
- Breech presentation
- Maternal heart disease
- Multifetal pregnancy
- Polyhydramnios
- Presenting part above the pelvic inlet
- Severe hypertension
- Abnormal fetal heart rate patterns not necessitating emergent delivery

▶ *What criteria should be met before the cervix is ripened or labor is induced?*

Assessment of gestational age and consideration of any potential risks to the mother or fetus are of paramount importance for appropriate evaluation and counseling before initiating cervical ripening or labor induction. The patient should be counseled regarding the indications for induction, the agents and methods of labor stimulation, and the possible need for repeat induction or cesarean delivery.

Additional requirements for cervical ripening and induction of labor include cervical assessment, pelvic assessment, assessment of fetal size and presentation, and personnel familiar with the effects of uterine stimulants on the mother and fetus because uterine hyperstimulation may occur with induction of labor. Monitoring fetal heart rate and uterine contractions is recommended as for any high-risk patient in active labor. Although trained nursing personnel can monitor labor induction, a physician capable of performing a cesarean delivery should be readily available.

▶ *What is the relative effectiveness of available pharmacologic methods for cervical ripening?*

Intracervical or intravaginal PGE_2 (dinoprostone) commonly is used and is superior to placebo or no therapy in promoting cervical ripening (29). Several prospective randomized clinical trials and a meta-analysis have demonstrated that PGE_1 (misoprostol) is an effective method for cervical ripening (30-34). Misoprostol administered intravaginally has been reported to be either superior to or as efficacious as dinoprostone gel (9, 32, 34, 35). It is difficult, however, to compare the results of studies on misoprostol because of differences in endpoints, including Bishop score, duration of labor, total oxytocin use, successful induction, and cesarean delivery rate. The rates of operative vaginal delivery and cesarean delivery are inconsistent between trials. The cesarean delivery rate has been reported to be higher with dinoprostone compared with misoprostol (31); however, further studies are needed. The results of cesarean delivery rate with dinoprostone use are inconsistent; some have shown a reduction but most have not shown a significant decrease.

▶ *How should prostaglandin be administered?*

If there is inadequate cervical change with minimal uterine activity after one dose of intracervical PGE_2, a second dose may be given 6–12 hours later. The manufacturers recommend a maximum cumulative dose of 1.5 mg of dinoprostone (three doses or 7.5 mL of gel) within a 24-hour period. A minimum safe time interval between PG administration and initiation of oxytocin has not been determined. According to the manufacturers' guidelines, after use of 1.5 mg of dinoprostone in the cervix or 2.5 mg in the vagina, oxytocin induction should be delayed for 6–12 hours because the effect of PG may be heightened with oxytocin. After use of dinoprostone in sustained-release form, delaying oxytocin induction for 30–60 minutes after removal is sufficient. One quarter of one 100-mcg tablet (approximately 25-mcg) of misoprostol should be considered for cervical ripening and labor induction.

▶ *What are the potential complications with each method of cervical ripening, and how are they managed?*

Hyperstimulation may occur with the use of the PGE analogues. There is no uniform definition of uterine hyperstimulation. In some studies hyperstimulation is never defined. In others, uterine hyperstimulation has been defined as either a series of single contractions lasting 2 minutes or more or a contraction frequency of five or more in 10 minutes (36). Another definition of hyperstimulation is uterine contractions lasting 2 minutes or more or a contraction frequency of 5 or more in 10 minutes with evidence that the fetus is not tolerating this contraction pattern, as demonstrated by late deceleration, or fetal bradycardia (37). Fortunately, most women and their fetuses tolerate uterine hyperstimulation without adverse outcome.

The intracervical PGE_2 gel (0.5 mg) has a 1% rate of uterine hyperstimulation, while the intravaginal PGE_2 gel (2–5 mg) or vaginal insert is associated with a 5% rate (29, 36–38). Uterine hyperstimulation typically begins within 1 hour after the gel or insert is placed but may occur up to 9 1/2 hours after the vaginal insert has been placed (36–38).

Removing the PGE_2 vaginal insert usually will help reverse the effect of hyperstimulation. Irrigation of the cervix and vagina is not beneficial. Maternal side effects from low-dose PGE_2 (fever, vomiting, and diarrhea) are quite uncommon (17). Prophylactic antiemetics, antipyretics, and antidiarrheal agents usually are not needed. The manufacturers recommend that caution be exercised when using PGE_2 in patients with glaucoma, severe hepatic or renal dysfunction, or asthma. However, PGE_2 is a bronchodilator, and there are no reports of bronchoconstriction or significant blood pressure changes after the administration of the low-dose gel.

In several studies of misoprostol, the term tachysystole was used to define hyperstimulation without corresponding fetal heart rate abnormalities in order to distinguish this complication from hyperstimulation with fetal heart rate changes. Data indicate that both tachysystole (defined in some studies as six or more uterine contractions in 10 minutes in consecutive 10-minute intervals) and hyperstimulation (with and without fetal heart rate changes) are increased with a 50-mcg or greater dose of misoprostol (9, 30, 39, 40). There seems to be a trend toward lower rates of uterine hyperstimulation with fetal heart rate changes with lower dosages of misoprostol (25 mcg every 6 hours versus every 3 hours) (40). Although in studies of misoprostol there were no differences in perinatal outcome, the studies have been insufficient in size to exclude the possibility of uncommon serious adverse effects (40). The use of misoprostol in women with prior cesarean birth has been associated with an increase in uterine rupture (41). Misoprostol use for second-trimester pregnancy termination also has been associated with uterine rupture, especially when used with oxytocin infusion (40). An increase in meconium-stained amniotic fluid also has been reported with misoprostol use (34). Although misoprostol appears to be safe and effective in inducing labor in women with unfavorable cervices, further studies are needed to determine the optimal dosage, timing interval, and pharmacokinetics of misoprostol. Moreover, data are needed on the management of complications related to misoprostol and when it should be discontinued. If uterine hyperstimulation and a nonreassuring fetal heart rate pattern occur with misoprostol use and there is no response to routine corrective measures (maternal repositioning and supplemental oxygen administration), cesarean delivery should be considered. Subcutaneous terbutaline also can be used in an attempt to correct the nonreassuring fetal heart rate tracing or the abnormal contraction pattern or both.

Increased maternal and neonatal infection have been reported in connection with the use of laminaria and hygroscopic dilators when compared with the PGE_2 analogues (6, 12, 16).

▶ *What are the recommended guidelines for fetal surveillance for each type of prostaglandin preparation?*

The PG preparations should be administered at or near the labor and delivery suite, where uterine activity and fetal heart rate can be monitored continuously. The patient should remain recumbent for at least 30 minutes. The fetal heart rate and uterine activity should be monitored continuously for a period of 30 minutes to 2 hours after administration of the PGE_2 gel (42). The patient may be transferred elsewhere if there is no increase in uterine activity and the fetal heart rate is unchanged after this period of observation. Uterine contractions usually are evident in the first hour and exhibit peak activity in the first 4 hours (42, 43). Fetal heart rate monitoring should be continued if regular uterine contractions persist; maternal vital signs should be recorded as well.

Because uterine hyperstimulation can occur as late as 9 1/2 hours after placement of the PGE_2 vaginal insert, fetal heart rate and uterine activity should be monitored electronically from the time the device is placed until at least 15 minutes after it is removed (44). This controlled-release PGE_2 vaginal pessary should be removed at the onset of labor (37).

Patients treated with misoprostol should receive fetal heart rate and uterine activity monitoring in a hospital setting until further studies evaluate the safety of outpatient therapy.

▶ *Are cervical ripening methods restricted to inpatient use only?*

One small, randomized trial found that sequential outpatient administration of low-dose (2-mg) PGE_2 gel was no better than placebo in ripening the cervix in postterm patients (45). Larger controlled studies are needed to establish an effective and safe dose and vehicle for PGE_2 before application on an outpatient basis can be recommended. However, outpatient use may be appropriate in carefully selected patients.

▶ *What are the potential complications of various methods of induction?*

The side effects of oxytocin use are principally dose related; uterine hyperstimulation and subsequent fetal heart rate deceleration are the most common side effects. Hyperstimulation may result in abruptio placentae or uterine rupture. Fortunately, uterine rupture secondary to oxytocin use is rare even in parous women (46). Water intoxication can occur with high concentrations of oxytocin infused with large quantities of hypotonic solutions. The antidiuretic effect usually is observed only after prolonged administration with at least 40mU of oxytocin per minute (47).

Misoprostol appears to be safe and beneficial for inducing labor in a woman with an unfavorable cervix. Although the exact incidence of uterine tachysystole is unknown and the criteria used to define this complication are not always clear in the various reports, there are reports of uterine tachysystole occurring more frequently in women given misoprostol (30–32). There does not appear to be a significant increase in adverse fetal outcomes from tachysystole (31, 35); however, one also must consider the possibility of uterine rupture as a rare complication of induction of labor with misoprostol (40). The occurrence of complications does appear to be dose-dependent (9, 40). Oral misoprostol administration is associated with fewer abnormal fetal heart rate patterns and episodes of uterine hyperstimulation when compared with vaginal administration (48), but there are not yet enough data to support oral administration as an alternative method.

The potential risks associated with amniotomy include prolapse of the umbilical cord, chorioamnionitis, significant umbilical cord compression, and rupture of vasa previa. The physician should palpate for an umbili-

Table 2. Labor Stimulation with Oxytocin: Examples of Low- and High-Dose Oxytocin

Regimen	Starting Dose	Incremental Increase (mU/min)	Dosage Interval (min)
Low-Dose	0.5–1	1	30–40
	1–2	2	15
High-Dose	~6	~6	15
	6	6*, 3, 1	20–40

*The incremental increase is reduced to 3 mU/min in presence of hyperstimulation and reduced to 1 mU/min with recurrent hyperstimulation.

cal cord and avoid dislodging the fetal head. The fetal heart rate should be assessed before and immediately after amniotomy.

Stripping the amniotic membranes is associated with bleeding from undiagnosed placenta previa or low-lying placenta, and accidental amniotomy. Uterine hyperactivity and fetal heart rate decelerations have been reported in association with nipple stimulation (49).

▶ *When oxytocin is used for induction of labor, what dosage should be used and what precautions should be taken?*

Any of the low- or high-dose oxytocin regimens outlined in Table 2 are appropriate for labor induction (50–56). Most women attain normal progression of labor with 150–350 Montevideo units of uterine activity (50). Low-dose regimens and less frequent increases in dose are associated with decreased uterine hyperstimulation (52). High-dose regimens and more frequent dose increases are associated with shorter labor and less frequent cases of chorioamnionitis and cesarean delivery for dystocia, but increased rates of uterine hyperstimulation (52).

Each hospital's obstetrics and gynecology department should develop guidelines for the preparation and administration of oxytocin. Synthetic oxytocin generally is diluted 10 U in 1,000 mL of an isotonic solution for an oxytocin concentration of 10 mU/mL. Oxytocin should be administered by infusion using a pump that allows precise control of the flow rate and permits accurate minute-to-minute control. Bolus administration of oxytocin can be avoided by piggybacking the infusion into the main intravenous line near the venipuncture site. Oxytocin also can be administered by pulsatile infusion, which may better simulate spontaneous labor (53). The total amount of oxytocin given may be decreased by administering oxytocin in 10-minute pulse infusions (53, 57).

A numeric value for the maximum dose of oxytocin has not been established. The fetal heart rate and uterine contractions should be monitored closely. Oxytocin should be administered by trained personnel who are familiar with its effects.

▶ *How should complications associated with oxytocin use be managed?*

If hyperstimulation with a nonreassuring fetal heart rate occurs, intravenous infusion of oxytocin should be decreased or discontinued to correct the pattern. Additional measures may include turning the woman on her side and administering oxygen or more intravenous fluid. If hyperstimulation persists, use of terbutaline or other tocolytics may be considered.

Hypotension may occur following a rapid intravenous injection of oxytocin; therefore, it is imperative that a dilute oxytocin infusion be used even in the immediate puerperium. Although amniotic fluid embolism was once thought to be associated with oxytocin-induced labor, there is no causal relationship between oxytocin use or antecedent hyperstimulation and amniotic fluid embolism (58, 59).

▶ *Are the various methods of labor induction equally applicable to patients with intact or ruptured membranes?*

The same precautions should be exercised when prostaglandins are used for induction of labor with ruptured membranes as for intact membranes. Intravaginal PGE_2 for induction of labor in women with premature rupture of membranes appears to be safe and effective, although it has not been approved by the FDA for this indication (60). In a meta-analysis of labor induction in women with premature rupture of membranes at term, only one dose of intravaginal misoprostol was necessary for successful labor induction in 86% of the patients (61). There is no evidence that use of either of these prostaglandins increases the risk of infection in women with ruptured membranes (60, 61).

▶ *What methods can be used for induction of labor with intrauterine fetal demise in the late second or third trimester?*

Intravenous oxytocin usually is a safe and effective method of inducing labor for a fetal death near term but is less effective remote from term (62). Laminaria or hygroscopic cervical dilators may be beneficial before the use of oxytocin or PGE for induction (63, 64). High-dose PGE_2 vaginal suppositories and more concentrated intravenous oxytocin are effective for achieving delivery, particularly when the gestational age is 28 weeks or less (62, 65, 66). Reported side-effects associated with higher doses of PGE_2 include nausea, vomiting, and diarrhea, which may be ameliorated with pretreatment medications. Although PGE_2 vaginal suppositories have been used safely in the third trimester (67), the risk of uterine rupture is increased. Vaginal misoprostol, intramuscular or extraamniotic infusion of $PGF_{2\alpha}$ and mifepristone also have been used safely and effectively; however, studies are few. In one study, mifepristone (600 mg per day for 48 hours) was effective in achieving delivery within 72 hours after the initial dose in 63% of women (68). In another study using intravaginal misoprostol, the mean time from induction to delivery was 12.6 hours, and all women delivered by 48 hours (69).

▶ *What is the cost effectiveness of these agents?*

There is a significant cost difference for induction of labor between misoprostol and dinoprostone. The approximate cost of a 100-mcg tablet of misoprostol ranges from $0.36 to $1.20, whereas a dinoprostone gel kit ranges from $65 to $75, and the dinoprostone vaginal insert is $165 (34, 35, 39, 70). The cost would be increased further if oxytocin augmentation were needed. Moreover, dinoprostone is an unstable compound that requires refrigeration to maintain its potency, whereas misoprostol is stable at room temperature.

Summary

The following recommendations are based on good and consistent scientific evidence (Level A):

- Prostaglandin E analogues are effective in promoting cervical ripening and inducing labor.
- Women in whom induction of labor is indicated may be appropriately managed with either a low- or high-dose oxytocin regimen.
- Fetal heart rate and uterine activity should be continuously monitored from the time the PGE_2 vaginal insert is placed until at least 15 minutes after it is removed.
- High-dose PGE_2 vaginal suppositories may be used in the management of intrauterine fetal demise in the second trimester of pregnancy.
- Although the optimal dose and timing interval of misoprostol is unknown, lower doses (25 mcg every 3–6 hours) are effective for cervical ripening and induction of labor.
- With term premature rupture of membranes, labor may be induced with prostaglandins.

The following recommendations are based on evidence that may be limited or inconsistent (Level B):

- Misoprostol use in women with prior cesarean birth should be avoided because of the possibility of uterine rupture.
- The use of higher doses of misoprostol (50 mcg every 6 hours) to induce labor may be appropriate in some situations, although there are reports of increased risk of complications, including uterine hyperstimulation.

The following recommendations are based primarily on consensus and expert opinion (Level C):

- For women with third-trimester intrauterine fetal demise, intravaginal misoprostol can be used to induce labor.
- Fetal heart rate and uterine activity should be continuously monitored from 30 minutes to 2 hours after administration of PGE_2 gel.

References

1. Ventura SJ, Martin JA, Curtin SC, Mathews TJ. Births: Final data for 1997. National Center for Health Statistics, National Vital Statistics Reports, 1999;47(18):1–96 (Level II-3)
2. Theobald GW, Graham A, Campbell J, Gange PD, Driscoll WJ. The use of post-pituitary extract in physiological amounts in obstetrics. BMJ 1948;2:123–127 (Level III)
3. du Vigneaud V, Ressler C, Swan JM, Roberts CW, Katsoyannis PG, Gordon S. The synthesis of an octapeptide amide with the hormonal activity of oxytocin. J Am Chem Soc 1953;75:4879–4880 (Level III)

4. Bishop EH. Pelvic scoring for elective induction. Obstet Gynecol 1964;24:266–268 (Level III)

5. Cross WG, Pitkin RM. Laminaria as an adjunct in induction of labor. Obstet Gynecol 1978;51:606–608 (Level I)

6. Krammer J, Williams MC, Sawai SK, O'Brien WF. Preinduction cervical ripening: a randomized comparison of two methods. Obstet Gynecol 1995;85:614–618 (Level I)

7. Fletcher HM, Mitchell S, Simeon D, Frederick J, Brown D. Intravaginal misoprostol as a cervical ripening agent. Br J Obstet Gynaecol 1993;100:641–644 (Level I)

8. Porto M. The unfavorable cervix: methods of cervical priming. Clin Obstet Gynecol 1989;32:262–268 (Level III)

9. Wing DA, Rahall A, Jones MM, Goodwin TM, Paul RH. Misoprostol: an effective agent for cervical ripening and labor induction. Am J Obstet Gynecol 1995;172:1811–1816 (Level I)

10. Atad J, Hallak M, Ben-David Y, Auslender R, Abramovici H. Ripening and dilatation of the unfavourable cervix for induction of labour by a double balloon device: experience with 250 cases. Br J Obstet Gynaecol 1997;104:29–32 (Level III)

11. Blumenthal PD, Ramanauskas R. Randomized trial of Dilapan and Laminaria as cervical ripening agents before induction of labor. Obstet Gynecol 1990;75:365–368 (Level I)

12. Chua S, Arulkumaran S, Vanja K, Ratnam SS. Preinduction cervical ripening: prostaglandin E_2 gel vs. hygroscopic mechanical dilator. J Obstet Gynaecol Res 1997;23:171–177 (Level I)

13. Gilson GJ, Russell DJ, Izquierdo LA, Qualls CR, Curet LB. A prospective randomized evaluation of a hygroscopic cervical dilator, Dilapan, in the preinduction ripening of patients undergoing induction of labor. Am J Obstet Gynecol 1996;175:145–149 (Level I)

14. Lin A, Kupferminc M, Dooley SL. A randomized trial of extra-amniotic saline infusion versus laminaria for cervical ripening. Obstet Gynecol 1995;86:545–549 (Level I)

15. Lyndrup J, Nickelsen C, Weber T, Molnitz E, Guldbaek E. Induction of labour by balloon catheter with extra-amniotic saline infusion (BCEAS): a randomized comparison with PGE_2 vaginal pessaries. Eur J Obstet Gynecol Reprod Biol 1994;53:189–197 (Level I)

16. Kazzi GM, Bottoms SF, Rosen MG. Efficacy and safety of laminaria digitata for preinduction ripening of the cervix. Obstet Gynecol 1982;60:440–443 (Level II-2)

17. Brindley BA, Sokol RJ. Induction and augmentation of labor: basis and methods for current practice. Obstet Gynecol Surv 1988;43:730–743 (Level III)

18. Frydman R, Lelaidier C, Baton-Saint-Mleux C, Fernandez H, Vial, M, Bourget P. Labor induction in women at term with mifepristone (RU 486): a double-blind, randomized, placebo-controlled study. Obstet Gynecol 1992;80:972–975 (Level I)

19. Seitchik J, Amico J, Robinson AG, Castillo M. Oxytocin augmentation of dysfunctional labor. IV. Oxytocin pharmacokinetics. Am J Obstet Gynecol 1984;150:225–228 (Level III)

20. Caldeyro-Barcia R, Poseiro JJ. Physiology of the uterine contraction. Clin Obstet Gynecol 1960;3:386–408 (Level III)

21. Satin AJ, Leveno KJ, Sherman ML, McIntire DD. Factors affecting the dose response to oxytocin for labor stimulation. Am J Obstet Gynecol 1992;166:1260–1261 (Level II-3)

22. Crane J, Bennett K, Young D, Windrim R, Kravitz H. The effectiveness of sweeping membranes at term: a randomized trial. Obstet Gynecol 1997;89:586–590 (Level I)

23. Goldenberg M, Dulitzky M, Feldman B, Zolti M, Bider D. Stretching of the cervix and stripping of the membranes at term: a randomised controlled study. Eur J Obstet Gynecol Reprod Biol 1996;66:129–132 (Level I)

24. Wiriyasirivaj B, Vutyavanich T, Ruangsri RA. A randomized controlled trial of membrane stripping at term to promote labor. Obstet Gynecol 1996;87:767–770 (Level I)

25. McColgin SW, Bennett WA, Roach H, Cowan BD, Martin JN Jr, Morrison JC. Parturitional factors associated with membrane stripping. Am J Obstet Gynecol 1993;169:71–77 (Level I)

26. Allott HA, Palmer CR. Sweeping the membranes: a valid procedure in stimulating the onset of labour? Br J Obstet Gynaecol 1993;100:898–903 (Level I)

27. Moldin PG, Sundell G. Induction of labour: a randomised clinical trial of amniotomy versus amniotomy with oxytocin infusion. Br J Obstet Gynaecol 1996;103:306–312 (Level I)

28. American College of Obstetricians and Gynecologists. Assessment of fetal lung maturity. ACOG Educational Bulletin 230. Washington DC: ACOG, 1996 (Level III)

29. Rayburn WF. Prostaglandin E_2 gel for cervical ripening and induction of labor: a critical analysis. Am J Obstet Gynecol 1989;160:529–534 (Level III)

30. Buser D, Mora G, Arias F. A randomized comparison between misoprostol and dinoprostone for cervical ripening and labor induction in patients with unfavorable cervices. Obstet Gynecol 1997;89:581–585 (Level I)

31. Sanchez-Ramos L, Kaunitz AM, Wears RL, Delke I, Gaudier FL. Misoprostol for cervical ripening and labor induction: a meta-analysis. Obstet Gynecol 1997;89:633–642 (Meta-analysis)

32. Sanchez-Ramos L, Peterson DE, Delke I, Gaudier FL, Kaunitz AM. Labor induction with prostaglandin E_1 misoprostol compared with dinoprostone vaginal insert: a randomized trial. Obstet Gynecol 1998;91:401–405 (Level I)

33. Srisomboon J, Piyamongkol W, Aiewsakul P. Comparison of intracervical and intravaginal misoprostol for cervical ripening and labour induction in patients with an unfavorable cervix. J Med Assoc Thai 1997;80:189–194 (Level I)

34. Wing DA, Jones MM, Rahall A, Goodwin TM, Paul RH. A comparison of misoprostol and prostaglandin E_2 gel for preinduction cervical ripening and labor induction. Am J Obstet Gynecol 1995;172:1804–1810 (Level I)

35. Wing DA, Ortiz-Omphroy G, Paul RH. A comparison of intermittent vaginal administration of misoprostol with continuous dinoprostone for cervical ripening and labor induction. Am J Obstet Gynecol 1997;177:612–618 (Level I)

36. Rayburn WF, Wapner RJ, Barss VA, Spitzberg E, Molina RD, Mandsageer N, Yonekura ML. An intravaginal controlled-release prostaglandin E_2 pessary for cervical ripening and initiation of labor at term. Obstet Gynecol 1992;79:374–379 (Level I)

37. Witter FR, Rocco LE, Johnson TR. A randomized trial of prostaglandin E_2 in a controlled-release vaginal pessary for cervical ripening at term. Am J Obstet Gynecol 1992; 166:830–834 (Level I)

38. Witter FR, Mercer BM. Improved intravaginal controlled-release prostaglandin E_2 insert for cervical ripening at term. The Prostaglandin E_2 Insert Study Group. J Matern Fetal Med 1996;5:64–69 (Level I)

39. Magtibay PM, Ramin KD, Harris DY, Ramsey PS, Ogburn PL Jr. Misoprostol as a labor induction agent. J Matern Fetal Med 1998;7:15–18 (Level I)

40. Hofmeyr GJ. Vaginal misoprostol for cervical ripening and labour induction in late pregnancy. The Cochrane Library 1999; Issue 2:1–18 (Meta-analysis)

41. Wing DA, Lovett K, Paul RH. Disruption of prior uterine incision following misoprostol for labor induction in women with previous cesarean section. Obstet Gynecol 1998;91:828–830 (Level III)

42. Bernstein P. Prostaglandin E_2 gel for cervical ripening and labour induction: a multicentre placebo-controlled trial. CMAJ 1991;145:1249–1254 (Level I)

43. Miller AM, Rayburn WF, Smith CV. Patterns of uterine activity after intravaginal prostaglandin E_2 during preinduction cervical ripening. Am J Obstet Gynecol 1991; 165:1006–1009 (Level II-1)

44. American College of Obstetricians and Gynecologists. Monitoring during induction of labor with dinoprostone. ACOG Committee Opinion 209. Washington DC: ACOG, 1998 (Level III)

45. Sawai SK, Williams MC, O'Brien WF, Angel JL, Mastrogiannis DS, Johnson L. Sequential outpatient application of intravaginal prostaglandin E_2 gel in the management of postdates pregnancies. Obstet Gynecol 1991;78: 19–23 (Level I)

46. Flannelly GM, Turner MJ, Rassmussen MJ, Stronge JM. Rupture of the uterus in Dublin; An update. J Obstet Gynaecol 1993;13:440–443 (Level II-3)

47. Whalley PJ, Pritchard JA. Oxytocin and water intoxication. JAMA 1963:186;601–603

48. Toppozada MK, Anwar MY, Hassan HA, El-Gazaerly WS. Oral or vaginal misoprostol for induction of labor. Int J Gynaecol Obstet 1997;56:135–139 (Level I)

49. Schellpfeffer MA, Hoyle D, Johnson JWC. Antepartal uterine hypercontractility secondary to nipple stimulation. Obstet Gynecol 1985;65:588–591 (Level III)

50. Hauth JC, Hankins GD, Gilstrap LC III, Strickland DM, Vance P. Uterine contraction pressures with oxytocin induction/augmentation. Obstet Gynecol 1986;68: 305–309 (Level II-2)

51. Satin AJ, Leveno KJ, Sherman ML, Brewster DS, Cunningham FG. High- versus low-dose oxytocin for labor stimulation. Obstet Gynecol 1992;80:111–116 (Level II-1)

52. Crane JM, Young DC. Meta-analysis of low-dose versus high-dose oxytocin for labour induction. J Soc Obstet Gynaecol Can 1998;20:1215–1223 (Meta-analysis)

53. Cummiskey KC, Dawood MY. Induction of labor with pulsatile oxytocin. Am J Obstet Gynecol 1990;163: 1868–1874 (Level I)

54. Blakemore KJ, Qin NG, Petrie RH, Paine LL. A prospective comparison of hourly and quarter-hourly oxytocin dose increase intervals for the induction of labor at term. Obstet Gynecol 1990;75:757–761 (Level I)

55. Mercer B, Pilgrim P, Sibai B. Labor induction with continuous low-dose oxytocin infusion: a randomized trial. Obstet Gynecol 1991;77:659–663 (Level I)

56. Muller PR, Stubbs TM, Laurent SL. A prospective randomized clinical trial comparing two oxytocin induction protocols. Am J Obstet Gynecol 1992;167:373–380; discussion 380–381 (Level I)

57. Willcourt RJ, Pager D, Wendel J, Hale RW. Induction of labor with pulsatile oxytocin by a computer-controlled pump. Am J Obstet Gynecol 1994;170:603–608 (Level I)

58. Clark SL, Hankins GD, Dudley DA, Dildy GA, Porter TF. Amniotic fluid embolism: analysis of the national registry. Am J Obstet Gynecol 1995;172:1158–1169 (Level III)

59. Morgan M. Amniotic fluid embolism. Anaesthesia 1979; 34:20–32 (Level III)

60. Ray DA, Garite TJ. Prostaglandin E_2 for induction of labor in patients with premature rupture of membranes at term. Am J Obstet Gynecol 1992;166:836–843 (Level I)

61. Sanchez-Ramos L, Chen AH, Kaunitz AM, Gaudier FL, Delke I. Labor induction with intravaginal misoprostol in term premature rupture of the membranes: a randomized study. Obstet Gynecol 1997;89:909–912 (Level I)

62. Pitkin RM. Fetal death: diagnosis and management. Am J Obstet Gynecol 1987;157:583–589 (Level III)

63. Berkus MD, Laufe LE, Castillo M. Lamicel for induction of labor. J Reprod Med 1990;35:219–221 (Level II-2)

64. Sanchez-Ramos L, Kaunitz AM, Connor PM. Hygroscopic cervical dilators and prostaglandin E_2 gel for preinduction cervical ripening. A randomized, prospective comparison. J Reprod Med 1992;37:355–359 (Level I)

65. Kochenour NK. Management of fetal demise. Clin Obstet Gynecol 1987;30:322–330 (Level III)

66. American College of Obstetricians and Gynecologists. Diagnosis and management of fetal death. ACOG Technical Bulletin 176. Washington DC: ACOG, 1993 (Level III)

67. Kent DR, Goldstein AI, Linzey EM. Safety and efficacy of vaginal prostaglandin E_2 suppositories in the management of third-trimester fetal demise. J Reprod Med 1984;29: 101–102 (Level III)

68. Cabrol D, Dubois C, Cronje H, Gonnet JM, Guillot M, Maria B, et al. Induction of labor with mifepristone (RU 486) in intrauterine fetal death. Am J Obstet Gynecol 1990;163:540–542 (Level I)

69. Bugalho A, Bique C, Machungo F, Faaundes A. Induction of labor with intravaginal misoprostol in intrauterine fetal death. Am J Obstet Gynecol 1994;171:538–541 (Level III)

70. Chuck FJ, Huffaker BJ. Labor induction with intravaginal misoprostol versus intracervical prostaglandin E_2 gel (Prepidil gel): randomized comparison. Am J Obstet Gynecol 1995;173:1137–1142 (Level I)

The MEDLINE database, the Cochrane Library, and ACOG's own internal resources and documents were used to conduct a literature search to locate relevant articles published between January 1985 and February 1999. The search was restricted to articles published in the English language. Priority was given to articles reporting results of original research, although review articles and commentaries also were consulted. Abstracts of research presented at symposia and scientific conferences were not considered adequate for inclusion in this document. Guidelines published by organizations or institutions such as the National Institutes of Health and the American College of Obstetricians and Gynecologists were reviewed, and additional studies were located by reviewing bibliographies of identified articles. When reliable research was not available, expert opinions from obstetrician–gynecologists were used.

Studies were reviewed and evaluated for quality according to the method outlined by the U.S. Preventive Services Task Force:

- I Evidence obtained from at least one properly designed randomized controlled trial.
- II-1 Evidence obtained from well-designed controlled trials without randomization.
- II-2 Evidence obtained from well-designed cohort or case–control analytic studies, preferably from more than one center or research group.
- II-3 Evidence obtained from multiple time series with or without the intervention. Dramatic results in uncontrolled experiments could also be regarded as this type of evidence.
- III Opinions of respected authorities, based on clinical experience, descriptive studies, or reports of expert committees.

Based on the highest level of evidence found in the data, recommendations are provided and graded according to the following catetories:

Level A—Recommendations are based on good and consistent scientific evidence.

Level B—Recommendations are based on limited or inconsistent scientific evidence.

Level C—Recommendations are based primarily on consensus and expert opinion.

ISSN 1099-3630

The American College of
Obstetricians and Gynecologists
409 12th Street, SW
PO Box 96920
Washington, DC 20090-6920

12345/32109

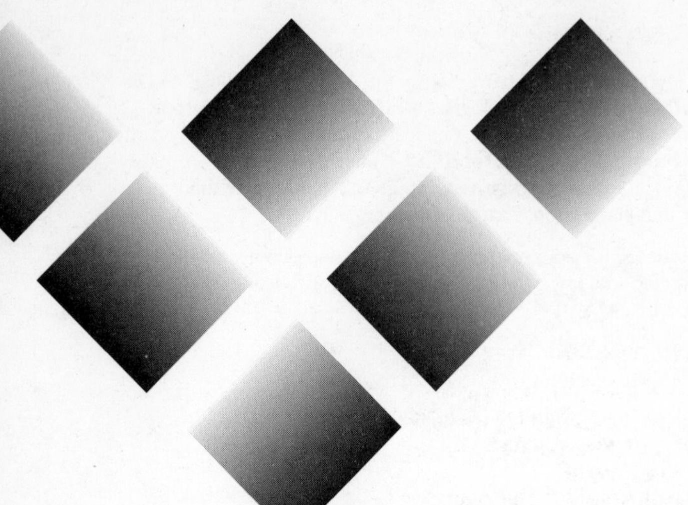

ACOG PRACTICE BULLETIN

CLINICAL MANAGEMENT GUIDELINES FOR OBSTETRICIAN–GYNECOLOGISTS
NUMBER 12, JANUARY 2000

This Practice Bulletin was developed by the ACOG Committee on Practice Bulletins—Obstetrics with the assistance of Susan M. Cox, MD. The information is designed to aid practitioners in making decisions about appropriate obstetric and gynecologic care. These guidelines should not be construed as dictating an exclusive course of treatment or procedure. Variations in practice may be warranted based on the needs of the individual patient, resources, and limitations unique to the institution or type of practice.

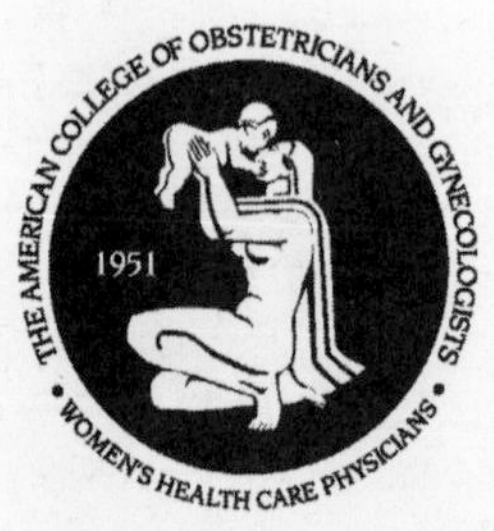

Intrauterine Growth Restriction

Intrauterine growth restriction (IUGR) is one of the most common and complex problems in modern obstetrics. Diagnosis and management are complicated by the use of ambiguous terminology and a lack of uniform diagnostic criteria. In addition, some authors do not make a clear distinction between suspected prenatal growth restriction and confirmed IUGR in the perinatal period. Furthermore, size alone is not an indication of a complication. As a result of this confusion, underintervention and overintervention can occur. This bulletin will focus on the etiology, diagnosis, and management of intrauterine growth restriction.

Background

Definitions

Several factors have contributed to the confusion in terminology associated with IUGR:

- By definition, 10% of infants in any population will have birth weights at or below the 10th percentile. Intrauterine growth restriction could be manifest at a weight above the population determined at the 10th percentile (eg, an undernourished infant born at the 15th percentile whose genetic makeup would have placed it at the 90th percentile). Distinctions between normal and pathologic growth often cannot reliably be made in clinical practice, especially prior to birth.
- Although defining a pathologic condition using a 10th percentile cutoff makes statistical sense, it may not be clinically relevant. One study suggests that adverse perinatal outcome generally is confined to those infants with birth weights below the 5th percentile, and in most cases below the 3rd percentile (1).

- Although specific ethnic- and geographic-based growth curves are increasingly used to evaluate birth weight, it remains unclear whether this is appropriate. These distinctions become even more difficult in ethnically heterogeneous and geographically mobile populations, such as those in the United States. Birth weight also is related to maternal height, parity, paternal height, and the fetus' sex.

The use of the terms "small for gestational age" (SGA) and "intrauterine growth restriction" has been confusing, and the terms often are used interchangeably. For the purpose of this document, SGA will be used only in reference to the infant and IUGR to the fetus.

Small for Gestational Age

Infants with a birth weight at the lower extreme of the normal birth weight distribution are termed SGA. In the United States, the most commonly used definition of SGA is a birth weight below the 10th percentile for gestational age (2, 3).

Intrauterine Growth Restriction

Intrauterine growth restriction is a term used to describe a fetus whose estimated weight appears to be less than expected, usually less than the 10th percentile, which is the convention this document will adopt. The term IUGR includes normal fetuses at the lower end of the growth spectrum, as well as those with specific clinical conditions in which the fetus fails to achieve its inherent growth potential as a consequence of either pathologic extrinsic influences (such as maternal smoking) or intrinsic genetic defects (such as aneuploidy).

Etiology

Several conditions have been found to be associated with IUGR (see the box). These antecedents can be divided into several broad categories: maternal, fetal, or placental. Maternal behavioral conditions include substance use (including smoking and alcohol use) (4–6), extremes of reproductive age (younger than 16 years and older than 35 years), little maternal weight gain (7), malnutrition, and low prepregnancy weight (7). In addition, low socioeconomic status is associated with IUGR (7).

Risk Factors for Intrauterine Growth Restriction

- Maternal medical conditions
  - –Hypertension
  - –Renal disease
  - –Restrictive lung disease
  - –Diabetes (with microvascular disease)
  - –Cyanotic heart disease
  - –Antiphospholipid syndrome
  - –Collagen-vascular disease
  - –Hemoglobinopathies
- Smoking and substance use and abuse
- Severe malnutrition
- Primary placental disease
- Multiple gestation
- Infections (viral, protozoal)
- Genetic disorders
- Exposure to teratogens

Maternal Medical Conditions

Medical complications that affect the microcirculation causing fetal hypoxemia or vasoconstriction or a reduction in fetal perfusion also are significantly associated with IUGR (8). These include hypertension, both chronic and acute (as in preeclampsia) (9), and severe chronic diseases, such as renal insufficiency (10), systemic lupus erythematosus, antiphospholipid antibody syndrome, chronic anemia, and pregestational diabetes (especially White's classifications C, D, F, and R). Growth restriction may be preceded by defective maternal volume adaptation in early pregnancy (11, 12).

Placental association with IUGR is unique in that it can be the primary cause (eg, mosaicism) or merely involved in an adaptive process of a pregnancy complication. The placenta and impaired placental perfusion are the most common cause of SGA in nonanomalous infants (13), as seen in early-onset preeclampsia, which produces the most severe IUGR (14). Intrauterine growth restriction also is related to other placental abnormalities, including partial abruptions, previa, infarcts, and hematomas (15). In unexplained IUGR, placental mosaicism may be identified in up to 25% of patients (16). Factors not associated with IUGR include caffeine use in nonsmokers (6, 17) and passive smoking (18).

Substance Use and Abuse

Maternal alcohol abuse is associated with impaired fetal growth; virtually all neonates with fetal alcohol syndrome will exhibit significant growth restriction (6, 19). It is unknown whether a threshold effect exists for alcohol, but effects on the fetus are related to the amount consumed.

Women who smoke have a 3.5-fold increase of SGA infants, compared with nonsmokers (9). Newborns of smokers are smaller at every gestational age. Women who stop smoking before 16 weeks of gestation have infants with birth weights similar to those of babies of women who never smoked (20), and women who quit as late as the seventh month have mean birth weights higher than those who smoked during the entire pregnancy (21).

The incidence of IUGR is markedly increased in pregnant women who use illicit drugs, but it is difficult to differentiate the drug effect from the effects of other behaviors associated with drug use. The incidence of SGA infants in mothers with heroin addiction is as high as 50% (22) and is reported to be as high as 35% in patients managed with methadone (23). Cocaine abuse in pregnancy is associated with delivery of an SGA neonate in 30% or more of cases (24).

Malnutrition

There is a common belief that severe maternal malnutrition will result in fetal growth restriction. The data from studies of the Siege of Leningrad during World War II (25) and the Dutch famine of the same period (26) suggest that maternal intake must be reduced to below 1,500 kilocalories per day before a measurable effect on birth weight becomes evident. In these studies, it is not entirely clear, however, how much of the effect on birth weight was the result of IUGR and how much the result of preterm delivery.

Although low prepregnancy weight and low maternal weight gain have been positively associated with an increase in IUGR (7, 27, 28), and increased weight gain has been associated with decreased IUGR in some populations (29), there is as yet no demonstration that altering dietary recommendations or habits can affect birth weight in a positive manner. Rather, although there are associations between maternal prepregnancy weight, maternal weight gain, and birth weight, there has been no trial showing that any intervention to alter pregnancy weight gain has a beneficial effect on fetal weight gain.

Placental Disease

Primary placental disease (such as chorioangioma) is a rare but recognized cause of growth restriction (30). Placenta previa has been associated with an increase in growth restriction, presumably secondary to abnormal placental implantation. Confined placental mosaicism has been identified three times more frequently from placentas of SGA infants than in infants of normal growth (16).

Multiple Gestation

Intrauterine growth restriction is a common complication of multiple gestation. It is more pronounced in higher order multiple gestations when compared with twin gestations (31). Investigators have reported a greater likelihood of IUGR among surviving fetuses after multifetal reduction (32, 33). The growth restriction is a result of placental reserve inadequate to sustain the normal growth of more than one fetus. Growth restriction can occur in dizygotic twin gestations but is more common and severe in monozygotic twins. It is evident that equal sharing of functional placental mass is not the norm; rather, one twin is more likely to have a larger share of functional placental mass than the other (31).

Infections

Viral infections have been estimated to be etiologic in less than 5% of all growth-restricted fetuses (34). However, when evaluated in documented cases of in utero viral infection, the frequency of IUGR can be strikingly high. Fetal rubella infection is associated with growth restriction in up to 60% of cases (35). Cytomegalovirus also is a recognized cause of growth restriction (36). In one study, approximately 40% of fetuses with varicella syndrome exhibited growth restriction (37). Bacterial infections have not been shown to cause growth restriction. Some protozoal infections, such as *Toxoplasma gondii, Trypanosoma cruzi* (Chagas disease), and syphilis, are associated with growth restriction (38, 39).

Genetic Disorders

Chromosome anomalies are a major cause of IUGR (40, 41). Many fetal structural anomalies also are associated with an increased risk of growth restriction, with a relative risk ranging from as high as 24.7 with anencephaly to as low as 1.2 with pyloric stenosis (42).

Exposure to Teratogens

Maternal ingestion of certain medications is a recognized cause of growth restriction; the incidence and severity vary by substance, gestational age at exposure, duration of exposure, and dosage. Therapeutic agents known to be associated with growth restriction include anticonvulsants (eg, trimethadione, phenytoin) (43–45), folic acid antagonists (eg, methotrexate) (46), and warfarin (47, 48).

Morbidity and Mortality

Fetal Morbidity and Mortality

Perinatal morbidity and mortality is significantly increased in the presence of low birth weight for gestational age, especially with weights below the 3rd percentile for gestational age (1). One study found that 26% of all stillbirths were SGA (49). The risk of death in the presence of IUGR also is affected by gestational age and the primary etiology and may be further modified by the severity and progression of associated maternal etiologic factors (eg, hypertension) (50) (see Table 1).

Both intrapartum and neonatal complications are increased in the presence of IUGR. During labor, up to 50% of growth-restricted fetuses exhibit abnormal heart rate patterns, most often variable decelerations, and such fetuses have an increased cesarean delivery rate (51, 52). Oligohydramnios is a common finding in growth-restricted fetuses and may render the umbilical cord vulnerable to compression (53–55). Sustained antepartum cord compression in growth-restricted fetuses is a presumed cause of sudden fetal death (51, 55). Incidences of low Apgar scores and cord blood acidemia increase significantly in SGA neonates (56).

Neonatal Morbidity

Neonatal complications in the SGA infant include polycythemia, hyperbilirubinemia, hypoglycemia, hypothermia, and apneic episodes (57, 58), as well as low Apgar scores, umbilical artery pH less than 7.0, need for intubation in the delivery room, seizures, sepsis, and neonatal death (1). It is uncertain whether IUGR accelerates fetal pulmonary maturity. One study found a decreased incidence of both respiratory distress syndrome and intraventricular hemorrhage in infants with SGA compared with a control group of infants of appropriate size for their gestational age (59). In contrast, other studies failed to document a difference in lung profile in a matched series (60) and found no difference in the need for ventilatory support in newborns with SGA when compared with controls. The use of glucocorticoids in fetuses with IUGR has not been studied, but current recommendations are to give glucocorticoids to women with complicated pregnancies who are likely to deliver before 34 weeks of gestation (61).

Long-term development of infants born with SGA depends in part on the cause of the growth failure. In infants with karyotype abnormalities or viral infection, the etiology rather than the weight percentile ultimately will determine the outcome. There are conflicting data on whether infants catch up in growth. Most otherwise normal infants with SGA secondary to placental insufficiency will exhibit normal catch-up growth by the age of 2 years, although this pattern may not be seen universally in severely affected infants (58, 62–64) or in preterm growth-restricted infants (65). A comparison of 714 neonates of appropriate size for age with 347 SGA neonates, derived from several studies, indicated a twofold increase of major neurologic sequelae among SGA infants (54). There is no evidence to suggest that any specific management scheme or delivery route prevents neurologic injury in such fetuses. Long-term follow-up of infants with SGA shows that they are more prone to develop adult-onset hypertension and cardiovascular complications (66). It is important to note that IUGR and SGA both have a multitude of etiologies, and there is a danger in grouping them. There may be no consequences of low birth weight under some circumstances; under others, it may be devastating.

Table 1. Corrected Perinatal Mortality Rates (Excluding Lethal Anomaly) Among Low-risk and High-risk (Screened/Unscreened) Pregnancies and Among SGA Fetuses (Screened/Unscreened), Manitoba Experience

Category	Number of Cases	Corrected Perinatal Mortality Rates (per 1,000 live births)
All cases	144,786	5.6
All low risk	101,350	3.8
All high risk	43,436	9.8
Screened high risk	31,740	2.2
All SGA (7% total population)	10,135	17.8
Unscreened SGA	7,460	21.3
Screened SGA*	2,675	8.4

* Serial fetal assessment management by fetal biophysical profile score.

Manning FA. Intrauterine growth retardation, etiology, pathophysiology, diagnosis, and treatment. In: Fetal medicine: principles and practice. Norwalk, Connecticut: Appleton & Lange, 1995:372

Antenatal Diagnosis of Intrauterine Growth Restriction

There are two essential steps involved in the antenatal recognition of growth restriction. The first step involves the elucidation of maternal risk factors associated with growth restriction and the clinical assessment of uterine size in relation to gestational age. The second step involves the ultrasonographic assessment of fetal size and growth, supplemented by invasive fetal testing for aneuploidy or viral infection in select cases.

Clinical Evaluation

The key physical finding in IUGR is a uterine size that is smaller than expected for gestational age. Several methods are available for clinical determination of uterine size, the most common of which is an objective measurement of fundal height. Such techniques, however, are prone to considerable inaccuracy and should be used for screening only, not as a sole guide to obstetric management in the presence of risk factors for or suspicions of IUGR. These inaccuracies are revealed in clinical studies suggesting that growth restriction is undetected in about one third of cases and is incorrectly diagnosed about 50% of the time (3, 67).

Prior to birth, the diagnosis of IUGR is not precise. Currently, the use of ultrasonographically estimated fetal weight, head- or femur-to-abdomen ratios, or serial observation of biometric growth patterns (growth velocity) are all acceptable and widely used methods to diagnose IUGR (68–72). This document does not address the concept of asymmetrical versus symmetrical IUGR, because it is unclear whether the distinction is important with respect to etiology or neonatal outcome.

Four standard fetal measurements generally are obtained as part of any complete obstetric ultrasound examination after the first trimester: 1) fetal abdominal circumference, 2) head circumference, 3) biparietal diameter, and 4) femur length (73). Fetal morphologic parameters can be converted to fetal weight estimates using published formulas and tables (74). An abdominal circumference within the normal range reliably excludes growth restriction with a false-negative rate of less than 10% (71). A small abdominal circumference or fetal weight estimate below the 10th percentile suggests the possibility of growth restriction, with the likelihood increasing as the percentile rank decreases (71). When IUGR is suspected, serial measurements of fetal biometric parameters provide an estimated growth rate. Such serial measurements are of considerable clinical value in confirming or excluding the diagnosis and assessing the progression and severity of growth restriction. Given the high incidence of genetic and structural defects associated with IUGR, a detailed ultrasound survey for the presence of fetal structural and functional defects may be indicated.

Amniotic fluid volume is an important diagnostic and prognostic parameter in fetuses with IUGR (75, 76). Oligohydramnios is highly suggestive of growth failure and indicates an increased risk of fetal death. Oligohydramnios is diagnosed ultrasonographically in approximately 77–83% of pregnancies with growth-restricted fetuses (75–77). In contrast, amniotic fluid volume often is normal even in a fetus with significant growth restriction; thus, the absence of oligohydramnios should not detract from the diagnosis of IUGR.

Although Doppler velocimetry of the umbilical arteries is not useful as a screening technique for IUGR (78, 79), it has been demonstrated to be useful once IUGR has been diagnosed. Not only are Doppler velocimetry findings normal in growth-restricted fetuses with chromosomal or other structural etiologies (80) but Doppler velocimetry has been shown to both reduce interventions and improve fetal outcome in pregnancies at risk for IUGR (81). Thus, once IUGR is suspected or diagnosed, Doppler velocimetry may be useful as a part of fetal evaluation. Fetuses with normal flow patterns seem less likely to benefit from consideration of early delivery than do their counterparts with abnormal studies.

Clinical Considerations and Recommendations

▶ ***Which pregnancies should be screened for intrauterine growth restriction, and how is screening accomplished?***

Unfortunately, approximately one half of growth-restricted fetuses are not diagnosed until delivery. In essence, all pregnancies are screened for IUGR using serial fundal height measurements. A single measurement at 32–34 weeks of gestation is approximately 70–85% sensitive and 96% specific for detecting the growth-restricted fetus (82). A third-trimester ultrasound examination, with a single measurement of abdominal circumference, detects about 80% of IUGR fetuses (70). Even so, this does not justify ultrasonography as a screening tool, because fundal height measurement performs comparably (70). All pregnancies should be screened with serial fundal height assessments, reserving ultrasonography for those with risk factors, lagging growth, or no growth (69, 83, 84).

Women who have previously given birth to an SGA infant are at an increased risk for this condition in subsequent pregnancies (9). Physicians should consider an early ultrasound examination to confirm gestational age, as well as subsequent ultrasonography to evaluate sequential fetal growth, in women with significant risk factors.

▶ ***What are the best ways to evaluate and monitor a pregnancy complicated by suspected intrauterine growth restriction?***

Once IUGR is suspected (ie, lagging fundal height), it should be confirmed using multiple ultrasonographic parameters, such as estimated weight percentile, amniotic fluid volume, elevated head circumference and abdominal circumference ratio, and possibly Doppler criteria (ie, elevated systolic–diastolic ratio or reversed or absent end-diastolic flow) (85). Identification of IUGR is improved by recording growth velocity or through two sets of examinations generally 2–4 weeks apart.

The diagnosis of IUGR as the fetus approaches term may be an indication for delivery (86). If pregnancy is remote from term or if delivery is not elected, the optimal mode of monitoring has not been established. Periodic fetal assessment (approximately weekly) using Doppler velocimetry, contraction stress test, traditional biophysical profile (BPP), modified BPP, or nonstress test (NST) are all accepted monitoring techniques. Randomized controlled trials have demonstrated that monitoring with Doppler velocimetry reduces the risk of perinatal morbidity (81). Comparable studies for the other methods have not been done.

Serial ultrasonograms to determine the rate of growth should be obtained approximately every 2–4 weeks. Measurements at shorter intervals (<2 weeks) may overlap with measurement errors. If any test result is abnormal (decreased amniotic fluid volume or low BPP scores), more frequent testing, possibly daily, may be indicated. An abnormal result from fetal heart rate testing (decreased variability) coupled with abnormal results from Doppler velocimetry suggests poor fetal well-being and a potential need for delivery, despite prematurity (72).

▶ *What interventions improve pregnancy outcome in cases of intrauterine growth restriction or suspected intrauterine growth restriction?*

Evidence from randomized controlled trials finds few interventions beneficial in preventing or treating IUGR. Avoidance of smoking during pregnancy has been shown to have a positive effect on birth weight (20). Treatment of infections such as malaria in endemic areas has been shown to be of some benefit (87, 88).

A number of interventions have been suggested for which there is insufficient evidence from randomized clinical trials to conclude either benefit or harm. Among them are bed rest, which demonstrated no benefit in one small study (89), and early delivery in the presence of pulsatile flow in waveforms from the umbilical vein, which remains to be assessed in a randomized control trial. Other interventions of questionable efficacy and safety include nutrient treatment or supplementation (90), zinc supplementation (91), calcium supplementation (92), plasma volume expansion (93), maternal oxygen therapy (94), heparin (47), and low-dose aspirin (95–99). Thus, such interventions should be used only in experimental protocols.

▶ *Is there any evidence that prenatal diagnosis or suspicion of intrauterine growth restriction with antenatal surveillance alters outcome?*

The nonanomalous fetus with IUGR should be monitored serially for risk of perinatal mortality and morbidity. Risk to the fetus can be determined by several methods: traditional or modified BPP, contraction stress test, NST, amniotic fluid volume, or Doppler velocimetry of fetal vessels. Unfortunately, these tests are performed to determine the optimal time for delivery and are not predictive of individual fetuses at greatest risk for a complicated neonatal course (100).

There are no randomized trials of interventions in a fetus with abnormal heart rate tracings. Thus, in the case of a very premature infant, delivery or expectant management are the usual courses of action at present. Overall experience with the NST confirms that with a reactive NST the fetus is not likely to die in utero immediately. In several studies, nonreactive or abnormal NSTs were found in fetuses with acidosis, hypoxemia, or both (101, 102). In four randomized clinical trials comparing BPP with conventional fetal monitoring in high-risk pregnancies (including those with IUGR), there was no obvious benefit for pregnancy outcome using BPP for surveillance (103), although different results might have been obtained in an IUGR-only population.

Doppler ultrasound has been shown to be useful in the assessment of the growth-restricted fetus (104). Absent or reversed end-diastolic flow velocities in the umbilical arteries have a poor positive predictive value but are associated with poor perinatal outcome and high perinatal mortality (105–107). In contrast, a normal systolic–diastolic ratio in a growth-restricted fetus has excellent negative predictive value and may be used as a rationale to delay delivery with some reassurance. Currently, there are not enough data to warrant cordocentesis in the management of IUGR.

With the exception of Manning's data, which includes IUGR among other high-risk conditions, there is no evidence that antenatal surveillance in fetuses with suspected IUGR alters perinatal outcome. Instead, it is used to predict which fetuses are at risk for in utero demise and thus may potentially benefit from preterm delivery. Currently, there are no intrauterine therapies available for affected fetuses; therefore, delivery is the optimal treatment in the mature fetus, but must be weighed against gestational age for the immature fetus.

▶ *How does knowledge of the etiology of intrauterine growth restriction alter management?*

If maternal medical conditions are thought to be the cause of IUGR, there is no evidence that changes in maternal medical management other than delivery alter outcome. For example, antihypertensive therapy has not been shown to have a benefit with respect to IUGR (108). However, it is still important to optimize maternal treatment.

Although the etiology and manifestations of IUGR are numerous, a concerted effort should be made to determine the underlying cause. If a lethal anomaly is identified, one would not usually undertake antepartum surveillance.

A detailed ultrasound survey should be performed to detect fetal structural defects. Fetal karyotype determinations are not routinely indicated in the assessment of growth-restricted fetuses, but should be considered when early or severe IUGR is detected or when the fetus has a recognized structural anomaly. It is estimated that about 10% of structurally abnormal fetuses with fetal growth restriction will have a karyotype anomaly.

Prenatal diagnosis of in utero infections also can be accomplished via amniotic fluid or fetal blood analyses. Viral infections associated with IUGR, such as rubella, cytomegalovirus, or varicella, can be diagnosed by polymerase chain reaction or by measuring viral-specific immunoglobulin M antibodies. There are, however, no in utero treatments for these infections. However, if toxoplasmosis is identified, medication taken by the mother may prevent the spread of maternal infection to the fetus (38).

▶ *When should a growth-restricted fetus be delivered?*

The fetus should be delivered if the risk of fetal death exceeds that of neonatal death, although in many cases these risks are difficult to assess. The timing of delivery in the growth-restricted fetus should be individualized. Early delivery may yield an infant with all the serious sequelae of prematurity, whereas delaying delivery may yield a hypoxic, acidotic infant with long-term neurologic sequelae. Gestational age and the findings of antenatal surveillance should be taken into account. The decision to deliver is based often on nonreassuring fetal assessment or a complete cessation of fetal growth assessed ultrasonographically over a 2–4-week interval. When extrauterine survival is likely despite significantly abnormal antenatal testing, delivery should be seriously considered.

Summary

The general approach to management of the fetus with ultrasonographically suspected IUGR involves risk factor modification when possible and the initiation of antepartum fetal surveillance, ultrasonography, and delivery when the risks of continued in utero development outweigh the benefits.

The risks to the growth-impaired fetus are well documented. Currently, although the incidence of IUGR has not changed appreciably, the prognosis for SGA infants has improved dramatically. It must be emphasized, however, that perinatal morbidity and mortality will continue to occur despite optimal management of the fetus with suspected IUGR. In those fetuses managed expectantly, antepartum injury or death may occur because current methods of fetal surveillance are less than perfect in the prediction of fetal outcome.

The following recommendations are based on good and consistent scientific evidence (Level A):

- ▶ The use of Doppler ultrasonography to measure umbilical artery waveforms in the management of IUGR is associated with a reduction in perinatal death, and may be considered a part of fetal evaluation once IUGR is suspected or diagnosed.
- ▶ Nutrient treatment or supplementation, zinc or calcium supplementation, plasma volume expansion, maternal oxygen therapy, antihypertensive therapy, heparin, and aspirin therapy have not been shown to be effective for prevention or treatment of IUGR.

The following recommendations are based primarily on consensus and expert opinion (Level C):

- ▶ Antepartum surveillance should be instituted once the possibility of extrauterine survival for the growth-restricted fetus has been determined. This may include Doppler velocimetry, contraction stress testing, NST with amniotic fluid volume assessment, and BPP.
- ▶ Routine screening for IUGR in low-risk patients should comprise classical clinical monitoring techniques. Ultrasound evaluation of the fetus is appropriate in patients determined to be at high risk.

References

1. McIntire DD, Bloom SL, Casey BM, Leveno KJ. Birth weight in relation to morbidity and mortality among newborn infants. N Engl J Med 1999;340:1234–1238 (Level II-2)
2. Battaglia FC, Lubchenco LO. A practical classification of newborn infants by weight and gestational age. J Pediatr 1967;71:159–163 (Level III)
3. Jahn A, Razum O, Berle P. Routine screening for intrauterine growth retardation in Germany: low sensitivity and questionable benefit for diagnosed cases. Acta Obstet Gynecol Scand 1998;77:643–648 (Level II-2)
4. Spinillo A, Capuzzo E, Nicola SE, Colonna L, Egbe TO, Zara C. Factors potentiating the smoking-related risk of fetal growth retardation. Br J Obstet Gynaecol 1994;101: 954–958 (Level II-2)
5. Lieberman E, Gremy I, Lang JM, Cohen AP. Low birth weight at term and the timing of fetal exposure to maternal smoking. Am J Public Health 1994;84:1127–1131 (Level II-2)
6. Shu XO, Hatch MC, Mills J, Clemens J, Susser M. Maternal smoking, alcohol drinking, caffeine consumption, and fetal growth: results from a prospective study. Epidemiology 1995;6:115–120 (Level II-3)
7. Nieto A, Matorras R, Serra M, Valenzuela P, Molero J. Multivariate analysis of determinants of fetal growth retardation. Eur J Obstet Gynecol Reprod Biol 1994;53:107–113 (Level II-2)

8. Rotmensch S, Liberati M, Luo JS, Kliman HJ, Gollin Y, Bellati U, et al. Color Doppler flow patterns and flow velocity waveforms of the intraplacental fetal circulation in growth-retarded fetuses. Am J Obstet Gynecol 1994; 171:1257–1264 (Level II-2)

9. Ounsted M, Moar VA, Scott A. Risk factors associated with small-for-dates and large-for-dates infants. Br J Obstet Gynaecol 1985;92:226–232 (Level II-2)

10. Cunningham FG, Cox SM, Harstad TW, Mason RA, Pritchard JA. Chronic renal disease and pregnancy outcome. Am J Obstet Gynecol 1990;163:453–459 (Level II-3)

11. Duvekot JJ, Cheriex EC, Pieters FA, Menheere PP, Schouten HJ, Peeters LL. Maternal volume homeostasis in early pregnancy in relation to fetal growth restriction. Obstet Gynecol 1995;85:361–367 (Level III)

12. Duvekot JJ, Cheriex EC, Pieters FA, Peeters LL. Severely impaired fetal growth is preceded by maternal hemodynamic maladaptation in very early pregnancy. Acta Obstet Gynecol Scand 1995;74:693–697 (Level III)

13. Salafia CM, Minior VK, Pezzullo JC, Popek EJ, Rosenkrantz TS, Vintzileos AM. Intrauterine growth restriction in infants of less than thirty-two weeks' gestation: associated placental pathologic features. Am J Obstet Gynecol 1995;173:1049–1057 (Level III)

14. Ounsted M, Moar V, Scott WA. Perinatal morbidity and mortality in small-for-dates babies: the relative importance of some maternal factors. Early Hum Dev 1981;5:367–375 (Level II-2)

15. Laurini R, Laurin J, Marsal K. Placental histology and fetal blood flow in intrauterine growth retardation. Acta Obstet Gynecol Scand 1994;73:529–534 (Level II-3)

16. Wilkins-Haug L, Roberts DJ, Morton CC. Confined placental mosaicism and intrauterine growth retardation: a case-control analysis of placentas at delivery. Am J Obstet Gynecol 1995;172:44–50 (Level II-2)

17. Cook DG, Peacock JL, Feyerabend C, Carey IM, Jarvis MJ, Anderson HR, et al. Relation of caffeine intake and blood caffeine concentrations during pregnancy to fetal growth: prospective population based study. BMJ 1996; 313:1358–1362 (Level II-3)

18. Fortier I, Marcoux S, Brisson J. Passive smoking during pregnancy and the risk of delivering a small-for-gestational-age infant. Am J Epidemiol 1994;139:294–301 (Level II-3)

19. Virji SK. The relationship between alcohol consumption during pregnancy and infant birthweight. An epidemiologic study. Acta Obstet Gynecol Scand 1991;70:303–308 (Level II-3)

20. MacArthur C, Knox EG. Smoking in pregnancy: effects of stopping at different stages. Br J Obstet Gynaecol 1988; 95:551–555 (Level II-2)

21. Rush D, Cassano P. Relationship of cigarette smoking and social class to birth weight and perinatal mortality among all births in Britain, 5-11 April 1970. J Epidemiol Community Health 1983;37:249–255 (Level II-2)

22. Naeye RL, Blanc W, Leblanc W, Khatamee MA. Fetal complications of maternal heroin addiction: abnormal growth, infections and episodes of stress. J Pediatr 1973;83:1055–1061 (Level III)

23. Newman RG, Bashkow S, Calko D. Results of 313 consecutive live births of infants delivered to patients in the New York City Methadone Maintenance Treatment Program. Am J Obstet Gynecol 1975;121:233–237 (Level III)

24. Fulroth R, Phillips B, Durand DJ. Perinatal outcome of infants exposed to cocaine and/or heroin in utero. Am J Dis Child 1989;143:905–910 (Level II-3)

25. Anatov AN. Children born during the siege of Leningrad in 1942. J Pediatr 1947;30:250–259 (Level III)

26. Smith CA. Effect of maternal undernutrition upon the newborn infant in Holland (1944-1945). J Pediatr 1947; 30:229–243 (Level III)

27. Neggers YH, Goldenberg RL, Tamura T, Cliver SP, Hoffman HJ. The relationship between maternal dietary intake and infant birthweight. Acta Obstet Gynecol Scand 1997;165:71–75 (Level II-3)

28. Wen SW, Goldenberg RL, Cutter GR, Hoffman HJ, Cliver SP. Intrauterine growth retardation and preterm delivery: prenatal risk factors in an indigent population. Am J Obstet Gynecol 1990;162:213–218 (Level II-3)

29. Hickey CA, Cliver SP, Goldenberg RL, Kohatsu J, Hoffman HJ. Prenatal weight gain, term birth weight, and fetal growth retardation among high-risk multiparous black and white women. Obstet Gynecol 1993;81: 529–535 (Level II-2)

30. Pollack RN, Divon MY. Intrauterine growth retardation: definition, classification, and etiology. Clin Obstet Gynecol 1992;35:99–107 (Level III)

31. Sassoon DA, Castro LC, Davis JL, Hobel CJ. Perinatal outcome in triplet versus twin gestations. Obstet Gynecol 1990;75:817–820 (Level II-2)

32. Alexander JM, Hammond KR, Steinkampf MP. Multifetal reduction of high-order multiple pregnancy: comparison of obstetrical outcome with nonreduced twin gestations. Fertil Steril 1995;64:1201–1203 (Level II-2)

33. Silver RK, Helfand BT, Russell TL, Ragin A, Sholl JS, MacGregor SN. Multifetal reduction increases the risk of preterm delivery and fetal growth restriction in twins: a case-control study. Fertil Steril 1997;67:30–33 (Level II-2)

34. Klein JO, Remington JS. Current concepts of infections of the fetus and newborn infant. In: Remington JS, Klein JO, eds. Infectious diseases of the fetus & newborn infant. 4th ed. Philadelphia: W.B. Saunders, 1995:1–19 (Level III)

35. Peckham CS. Clinical and laboratory study of children exposed in utero to maternal rubella. Arch Dis Child 1972;47:571–577 (Level II-3)

36. Donner C, Liesnard C, Content J, Busine A, Aderca J, Rodesch F. Prenatal diagnosis of 52 pregnancies at risk for congenital cytomegalovirus infection. Obstet Gynecol 1993;82:481–486

37. Alkalay AL, Pomerance JJ, Rimoin DL. Fetal varicella syndrome. J Pediatr 1987;111:320–323 (Level III)

38. Daffos F, Forestier F, Capella-Pavlovsky M, Thulliez P, Aufrant C, Valenti D, et al. Prenatal management of 746 pregnancies at risk for congenital toxoplasmosis. N Engl J Med 1988;318:271–275 (Level III)

39. Ricci JM, Fojaco RM, O'Sullivan MJ. Congenital syphilis: The University of Miami/Jackson Memorial Medical Center experience, 1986-1988. Obstet Gynecol 1989;74:687–693 (Level II-2)

40. Nicolaides KH, Economides DL, Soothill PW. Blood gases, pH, and lactate in appropriate- and small-for-gestational-age fetuses. Am J Obstet Gynecol 1989;161: 996–1001 (Level II-3)

41. van Vugt JM, Karsdorp VH, van Zalen-Sprock RM, van Geijn HP. Fetal growth retardation and structural anomalies. Eur J Obstet Gynecol Reprod Biol 1991;42 Suppl: S79–S83 (Level III)

42. Khoury MJ, Erickson JD, Cordero JF, McCarthy BJ. Congenital malformations and intrauterine growth retardation: a population study. Pediatrics 1988;82:83–90 (Level II-3)

43. Battino D, Granata T, Binelli S, Caccamo ML, Canevini MP, Canger R, et al. Intrauterine growth in the offspring of epileptic mothers. Acta Neurol Scand 1992;86:555–557 (Level III)

44. Hiilesmaa VK, Teramo K, Granstrom ML, Bardy AH. Fetal head growth retardation associated with maternal antiepileptic drugs. Lancet 1981;2:165–167 (Level II-2)

45. Mastroiacovo P, Bertollini R, Licata D. Fetal growth in the offspring of epileptic women: results of an Italian multicentric cohort study. Acta Neurol Scand 1988;78:110–114 (Level II-2)

46. Aviles A, Diaz-Maqueo JC, Talavera A, Guzman R, Garcia EL. Growth and development of children of mothers treated with chemotherapy during pregnancy: current status of 43 children. Am J Hematol 1991;36:243–248 (Level III)

47. Hall JG, Pauli RM, Wilson KM. Maternal and fetal sequelae of anticoagulation during pregnancy. Am J Med 1980;68:122–140 (Level III)

48. Stevenson RE, Burton OM, Ferlauto GJ, Taylor HA. Hazards of oral anticogulants during pregnancy. JAMA 1980;243:1549–1551 (Level III)

49. Morrison I, Olsen J. Weight-specific stillbirths and associated causes of death: an analysis of 765 stillbirths. Am J Obstet Gynecol 1985;152:975–980 (Level III)

50. Piper JM, Langer O, Xenakis EM, McFarland M, Elliott BD, Berkus MD. Perinatal outcome in growth-restricted fetuses: do hypertensive and normotensive pregnancies differ? Obstet Gynecol 1996;88:194–199 (Level II-2)

51. Druzin ML, Gratacos J, Keegan KA, Paul RH. Antepartum fetal heart rate testing. VII. The significance of fetal bradycardia. Am J Obstet Gynecol 1981;139:194–198 (Level III)

52. Bekedam DJ, Visser GH. Effects of hypoxemic events on breathing, body movements, and heart rate variation: a study in growth-retarded human fetuses. Am J Obstet Gynecol 1985;153:52–56 (Level III)

53. Magann EF, Bass JD, Chauham SP, Young RA, Whitworth NS, Morrison JC. Amniotic fluid volume in normal singleton pregnancies. Obstet Gynecol 1997;90:524–528 (Level III)

54. Manning FA, Morrison I, Harman CR, Lange IR, Menticoglou S. Fetal assessment based on the fetal biophysical profile scoring: experience in 19,221 referred high-risk pregnancies. II. An analysis of false-negative fetal deaths. Am J Obstet Gynecol 1987;157:880–884 (Level III)

55. Peipert JF, Donnenfeld AE. Oligohydramnios: a review. Obstet Gynecol Surv 1991;46:325–339 (Level III)

56. Kramer MS, Olivier M, McLean FH, Willis DM, Usher RH. Impact of intrauterine growth retardation and body proportionality on fetal and neonatal outcome. Pediatrics 1990;86:707–713 (Level II-3)

57. Jones RA, Robertson NR. Problems of the small-for-dates baby. Clin Obstet Gynaecol 1984;11:499–524 (Level III)

58. Alkalay AL, Graham JM Jr, Pomerance JJ. Evaluation of neonates born with intrauterine growth retardation: review and practice guidelines. J Perinatol 1998;18:142–151 (Level III)

59. Procianoy RS, Garcia-Prats JA, Adams JM, Silvers A, Rudolph AJ. Hyaline membrane disease and intraventricular haemorrhage in small for gestational age infants. Arch Dis Child 1980;55:502–505 (Level II-2)

60. Piper JM, Langer O. Is lung maturation related to fetal growth in diabetic or hypertensive pregnancies? Eur J Obstet Gynecol Reprod Biol 1993;51:15–19 (Level II-3)

61. Effect of cortiscosteroids for fetal maturation on perinatal outcomes. NIH Consens Statement 1994;12:1–24 (Level III)

62. Fay RA, Ellwood DA. Categories of intrauterine growth retardation. Fetal Matern Med Rev 1993;5:203–212 (Level III)

63. Bergsjo P. Why are some children stunted at birth, and do they catch up with their peers in infancy? Acta Obstet Gynecol Scand Suppl 1997;165:1–2 (Level III)

64. Hadders-Algra M, Touwen BC. Body measurements, neurological and behavioural development in six-year-old children born preterm and/or small-for-gestational-age. Early Hum Dev 1990;22:1–13 (Level II-2)

65. Smedler C, Faxelius G, Bremme K, Lagerstrom M. Psychological development in children born with very low birth weight after severe intrauterine growth retardation: a 10-year follow-up study. Acta Paediatr 1992;81:197–203 (Level III)

66. Barker DJ, Osmond C, Golding J, Kuh D, Wadsworth ME. Growth in utero, blood pressure in childhood and adult life, and mortality from cardiovascular diseases. BMJ 1989;298:564–567 (Level II-3)

67. Kean LH, Liu DT. Antenatal care as a screening tool for the detection of small for gestational age babies in the low risk population. J Obstet Gynaecol 1996;16:77–82 (Level III)

68. Harding K, Evans S, Newnham J. Screening for the small fetus: a study of the relative efficacies of ultrasound biometry and symphysiofundal height. Aust N Z J Obstet Gynaecol 1995;35:160–164 (Level I)

69. Neilson JP, Munjanja SP, Whitfield CR. Screening for small for dates fetuses: a controlled trial. BMJ 1984; 289:1179–1182 (Level II-2)

70. Pearce JM, Campbell S. A comparison of symphysis-fundal height and ultrasound as screening tests for light-for-gestational age infants. Br J Obstet Gynaecol 1987;94: 100–104 (Level II-3)

71. Warsof SL, Cooper DJ, Little D, Campbell R. Routine ultrasound screen for antenatal detection of intrauterine growth restriction. Obstet Gynecol 1986;67:33–39 (Level II-2)

72. Weiner Z, Farmakides G, Schulman H, Lopresti S, Schneider E. Surveillance of growth-retarded fetuses with computerized fetal heart rate monitoring combined with Doppler velocimetry of the umbilical and uterine arteries. J Reprod Med 1996;41:112–118 (Level III)

73. Hadlock FP, Deter RL, Harrist RB, Park SK. Estimating fetal age: computer-assisted analysis of multiple fetal growth parameters. Radiology 1984;152:497–501 (Level II-3)

74. Shepard MJ, Richards VA, Berkowitz RL, Warsof SL, Hobbins JC. An evaluation of two equations for predicting fetal weight by ultrasound. Am J Obstet Gynecol 1982; 142:47–54 (Level III)

75. Chamberlain PF, Manning FA, Morrison I, Harman CR, Lange IR. Ultrasound evaluation of amniotic fluid volume. I. The relationship of marginal and decreased amniotic fluid volumes to perinatal outcome. Am J Obstet Gynecol 1984:150:245–249 (Level II-3)

76. Varma TR. Bateman S, Patel RH, Chamberlain GV, Pillai U. Ultrasound evaluation of amniotic fluid: outcome of pregnancies with severe oligohydramnios. Int J Gynaecol Obstet 1988;27:185–192 (Level II-2)

77. Philipson EH, Sokol RJ, Williams T. Oligohydraminios: clinical associations and predictive value for intrauterine growth retardation. Am J Obstet Gynecol 1983;146: 271–278 (Level II-2)

78. Davies JA, Gallivan S, Spencer JA. Randomised con- trolled trial of Doppler ultrasound screening of placental perfusion during pregnancy. Lancet 1992;340:1299–1303 (Level I)

79. Low JA. The current status of maternal and fetal blood flow velocimetry. Am J Obstet Gynecol 1991;164: 1049–1063 (Level III)

80. Wladimiroff JW, v.d.Wijngaard JA, Degani S, Noordam MJ, van Eyck J, Tonge HM. Cerebral and umbilical arterial blood flow velocity waveforms in normal and growth-retarded pregnancies. Obstet Gynecol 1987;69:705–709 (Level II-2)

81. Alfirevic Z, Neilson JP. Doppler ultrasonography in high-risk pregnancies: systemic review with meta-analysis. Am J Obstet Gynecol 1995;172:1379–1387 (Meta-analysis)

82. Leeson S, Aziz N. Customised fetal growth assessment. Br J Obstet Gynaecol 1997;104:648–651 (Level III)

83. Ewigman BG, Crane JP, Frigoletto FD, LeFevre ML, Bain RP, McNellis D. Effect of prenatal ultrasound screening on perinatal outcome. RADIUS Study Group. N Engl J Med 1993;329:821–827 (Level I)

84. Newnham JP, Evans SF, Michael CA, Stanley FJ, Landau LI. Effect of frequent ultrasound during pregnancy: a randomised conrolled trial. Lancet 1993;342:887–891 (Level I)

85. Doubilet PM, Benson CB. Sonographic evaluation of intrauterine growth retardation. AJR Am J Roentgenol 1995;164:709–717 (Level III)

86. Snijders R, Hyett J. Fetal testing in intra-uterine growth retardation. Curr Opin Obstet Gynecol 1997;9:91–95 (Level III)

87. Garner P, Brabin B. A review of randomized controlled trials of routine antimalarial drug prophylaxis during pregnancy in endemic malarious areas. Bull World Health Organ 1994;72:89–99 (Level III)

88. Taha Tel T, Gray RH, Mohamedani AA. Malaria and low birth weight in central Sudan. Am J Epidemiol 1993; 138:318–325 (Level II-2)

89. Laurin J, Persson PH. The effect of bedrest in hospital on fetal outcome in pregnancies complicated by intra-uterine growth retardation. Acta Obstet Gynecol Scand 1987; 66:407–411 (Level II-1)

90. Gulmezoglu AM, Hofmeyr GJ. Maternal nutrient supplementation for suspected impaired fetal growth (Cochrane Review). In: The Cochrane Library, Issue 2, 1999. Oxford: Update Software (Meta-analysis)

91. Mahomed K. Zinc supplementation in pregnancy (Cochrane Review). In: The Cochrane Library, Issue 2, 1999. Oxford: Update Software (Meta-analysis)

92. Carroli G, Duley L, Belizan JM, Villar J. Calcium supplementation during pregnancy: a systematic review of randomised controlled trials. Br J Obstet Gynaecol 1994; 101:753–758 (Meta-analysis)

93. Gulmezoglu AM, Hofmeyr GJ. Plasma volume expansion for suspected impaired fetal growth (Cochrane Review). In: The Cochrane Library, Issue 2, 1999. Oxford: Update Software (Level III)

94. Gulmezoglu AM, Hofmeyr GJ. Maternal oxygen administration for suspected impaired fetal growth. (Cochrane Review). In: The Cochrane Library, Issue 2, 1999. Oxford: Update Software (Level III)

95. Bar J, Hod M, Pardo J, Fisch B, Rabinerson D, Kaplan B, et al. Effect on fetal circulation of low-dose aspirin for prevention and treatment of pre-eclampsia and intrauterine growth restriction: Doppler flow study. Ultrasound Obstet Gynecol 1997;9:262–265

96. CLASP: a randomised trial of low-dose aspirin for the prevention and treatment of pre-eclampsia among 9364 pregnant women. CLASP (Collaborative Low-Dose Aspirin Study in Pregnancy) Collaborative Group. Lancet 1994; 343:619–629 (Level I)

97. Golding J. A randomised trial of low dose aspirin for primiparae in pregnancy. The Jamaica Low Dose Aspirin Study Group. Br J Obstet Gynaecol 1998;105:293–299 (Level I)

98. Leitich H, Egarter C, Husslein P, Kaider A, Schemper M. A meta-analysis of low dose aspirin for the prevention of intrauterine growth retardation. Br J Obstet Gynaecol 1997;104:450–459 (Meta-analysis)

99. Newnham JP, Godfrey M, Walters BJ, Phillips J, Evans SF. Low dose aspirin for the treatment of fetal growth restriction: a randomized controlled trial. Aust N Z J Obstet Gynaecol 1995;35:370–374 (Level I)

100. Craigo SD, Beach ML, Harvey-Wilkes KB, D'Alton ME. Ultrasound predictors of neonatal outcome in intrauterine growth restriction. Am J Perinatol 1996;13:465–471 (Level II-3)

101. Visser GH, Sandovsky G, Nicolaides KH. Antepartum fetal heart rate patterns in small-for-gestational-age third-trimester fetuses: correlations with blood gas values obtained at cordocentesis. Am J Obstet Gynecol 1990; 162:698–703 (Level II-2)

102. Donner C, Vermeylen D, Kirkpatrick C, de Maertelaer V, Rodesch F. Management of the growth-restricted fetus: the role of noninvasive tests and fetal blood sampling. Obstet Gynecol 1995;85:965–970 (Level II-3)

103. Alfirevic Z, Neilson JP. Biophysical profile for fetal assessment in high risk pregnancies (Cochrane review). In: The Cochrane Library, Issue 2, 1999. Oxford: Update Software (Meta-analysis)

104. Arduini D, Rizzo G. Doppler studies of deteriorating growth-retarded fetuses. Curr Opin Obstet Gynecol 1993;5:195–203 (Level III)

105. Kingdom JC, Burrell SJ, Kaufmann P. Pathology and clinical implications of abnormal umbilical artery Doppler waveforms. Ultrasound Obstet Gynecol 1997;9:271–286 (Level III)

106. Karsdorp VH, van Vugt JM, van Geijn HP, Kostense PJ, Arduini D, Montenegro N, et al. Clinical significance of absent or reversed end diastolic velocity waveforms in umbilical artery. Lancet 1994;344:1664–1668 (Level II-3)

107. Pardi G, Cetin I, Marconi AM, Lanfranchi A, Bozzetti P, Ferrazzi E, et al. Diagnostic value of blood sampling in fetuses with growth retardation. N Engl J Med 1993; 328:692–696 (Level III)

108. Redman CW. Fetal outcome in trial of antihypertensive treatment in pregnancy. Lancet 1976;2:753–756 (Level II-1)

The MEDLINE database, the Cochrane Library, and ACOG's own internal resources were used to conduct a literature search to locate relevant articles published between January 1985 and March 1999. The search was restricted to articles published in the English language. Priority was given to articles reporting results of original research, although review articles and commentaries also were consulted. Abstracts of research presented at symposia and scientific conferences were not considered adequate for inclusion in this document. Guidelines published by organizations or institutions such as the National Institutes of Health and the American College of Obstetricians and Gynecologists were reviewed, and additional studies were located by reviewing bibliographies of identified articles. When reliable research was not available, expert opinions from obstetrician–gynecologists were used.

Studies were reviewed and evaluated for quality according to the method outlined by the U.S. Preventive Services Task Force:

I Evidence obtained from at least one properly designed randomized controlled trial.

II-1 Evidence obtained from well-designed controlled trials without randomization.

II-2 Evidence obtained from well-designed cohort or case–control analytic studies, preferably from more than one center or research group.

II-3 Evidence obtained from multiple time series with or without the intervention. Dramatic results in uncontrolled experiments could also be regarded as this type of evidence.

III Opinions of respected authorities, based on clinical experience, descriptive studies, or reports of expert committees.

Based on the highest level of evidence found in the data, recommendations are provided and graded according to the following catetories:

Level A—Recommendations are based on good and consistent scientific evidence.

Level B—Recommendations are based on limited or inconsistent scientific evidence.

Level C—Recommendations are based primarily on consensus and expert opinion.

ISSN 1099-3630

The American College of Obstetricians and Gynecologists
409 12th Street, SW
PO Box 96920
Washington, DC 20090-6920

12345/43210

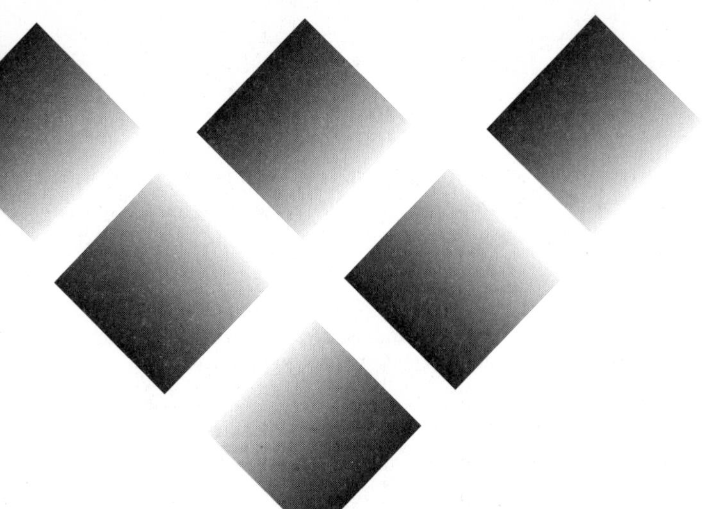

ACOG PRACTICE BULLETIN

CLINICAL MANAGEMENT GUIDELINES FOR OBSTETRICIAN–GYNECOLOGISTS

NUMBER 14, MARCH 2000

This Practice Bulletin was developed by the ACOG Committee on Practice Bulletins—Gynecology with the assistance of Dale Stovall, MD. The information is designed to aid practitioners in making decisions about appropriate obstetric and gynecologic care. These guidelines should not be construed as dictating an exclusive course of treatment or procedure. Variations in practice may be warranted based on the needs of the individual patient, resources, and limitations unique to the institution or type of practice.

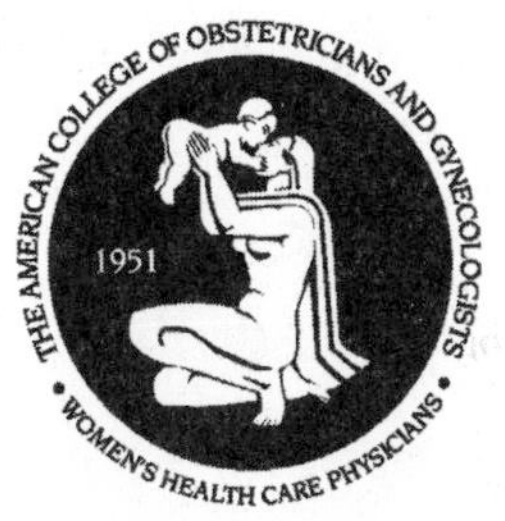

Management of Anovulatory Bleeding

Anovulatory bleeding, the most common form of noncyclic uterine bleeding, is a condition for which women frequently seek gynecologic care and accounts for considerable patient anxiety and inconvenience. Over the past decade, significant advances have been made in the evaluation and management of women with anovulatory bleeding. The choice of treatment for anovulatory bleeding depends on several factors, including the woman's age, the severity of her bleeding, and her desire for future fertility. The purpose of this document is to provide management guidelines for the treatment of patients with menstrual irregularities associated with anovulation based on the best available evidence.

Background

Definition and Nomenclature

The terms menses, menstrual flow, and menstruation will be used in this document interchangeably, and each of these terms simply refer to the presence of menstrual effluent irrespective of whether the effluent is normal or abnormal. Anovulatory uterine bleeding is defined as noncyclic menstrual blood flow that may range from spotty to excessive, is derived from the uterine endometrium, and is due to anovulatory sex steroid production specifically excluding an anatomic lesion. Several terms have been used to describe anovulatory bleeding, including dysfunctional, irregular, and abnormal. In this bulletin, the term *anovulatory uterine bleeding* will be used as the standard terminology to describe menstrual bleeding arising from anovulation or oligo-ovulation.

Several descriptive terms also are used to describe menstrual bleeding patterns, including menorrhagia, metrorrhagia, polymenorrhea, and menometrorrhagia. Menorrhagia is defined as prolonged or excessive uterine bleeding that occurs at regular intervals, or more strictly, the loss of 80 mL or more of blood per menstrual cycle or bleeding that lasts for more than 7 days (1). Metrorrhagia is defined as irregular menstrual bleeding or bleeding between periods. Polymenorrhea is defined as frequent menstrual bleeding or, more strictly, menstrual bleeding that occurs every 21 days or less. Menometrorrhagia is defined as frequent menstrual bleeding that is excessive and irregular in amount and duration.

Ovulatory Cycle

During a normal ovulatory cycle—including follicular development, ovulation, corpus luteal function, and luteolysis—the endometrium is sequentially exposed to ovarian production of estrogen alone, followed by a combination of estrogen and progesterone; the cycle is culminated by estrogen and progesterone withdrawal. Ovulation is associated with a cyclic pattern of endometrial histology commencing with proliferation followed by secretion change, desquamation, and repair. Normal ovarian steroid production is important for nidation and pregnancy. From a clinical perspective, the result is cyclic, predictable, and relatively consistent menstrual blood loss (2).

Pathophysiology

With anovulation, a corpus luteum is not produced, and the ovary fails to secrete progesterone, although estrogen production continues. This condition results in continual endometrial proliferation without progesterone-induced desquamation and bleeding. The clinical result is bleeding that is noncyclic, unpredictable, and inconsistent in volume.

Continuous, unopposed estrogen stimulation of the endometrium results in unsustainable endometrial growth. The endometrium becomes excessively vascular without sufficient stromal support and becomes fragile, resulting in variable endometrial bleeding. Unlike the uniform, synchronized endometrial sloughing and bleeding that occurs with normal cyclic estrogen and progesterone stimulation, endometrial loss during continuous estrogen stimulation is irregular. As one area of bleeding begins to heal, another area begins to slough, resulting in irregular and prolonged menstrual flow.

Alterations in endometrial prostaglandin (PG) synthesis and release appear to occur in women with anovulatory uterine bleeding. In particular, lower concentrations of $PGF_{2\alpha}$ have been found in the endometrium of women with anovulatory bleeding as compared with women with ovulatory menstrual cycles (3). Furthermore, these investigators found a reverse correlation between the endometrial $PGF_{2\alpha}/PGE_2$ ratio and the amount of menstrual blood lost. Therefore, abnormal vasoconstriction produced by altered endometrial prostaglandins may enhance blood loss in women with chronic anovulation.

Establishing the Diagnosis

The diagnosis of anovulatory uterine bleeding is made after the exclusion of anatomic pathology. Diagnostic techniques to exclude anatomic pathology include physical examination supplemented by endometrial sampling, transvaginal ultrasonography, sonohysterography, hysterosalpingography, hysteroscopy, curettage, endometrial cultures, and timed tests for determining progesterone levels in serum. Recognized causes of anovulation are given in the box below and should be considered when evaluating the medical history and results of the physical examination. There are numerous other causes of noncyclic vaginal bleeding. The differential diagnosis of abnormal bleeding is listed in the box on the next page. In this document, recommendations are based on the assumption that the diagnosis of anovulatory bleeding has been firmly established.

The physical examination should include an assessment for obesity and hirsutism, because these findings are associated with chronic anovulation (4, 5). Thyroid disease may cause anovulation as well as hyperprolactinemia. Approximately one third of all women with hyperprolactinemia will have galactorrhea (6). In women of reproductive age with noncyclic uterine bleeding, pregnancy must be ruled out. If medical therapy fails to resolve bleeding thought to be the result of anovulation, an anatomic cause, including a malignant or premalignant lesion or a coagulopathy, should be reconsidered and the patient reevaluated.

Causes of Anovulation

Physiologic
- Adolescence
- Perimenopause
- Lactation
- Pregnancy

Pathologic
- Hyperandrogenic anovulation (eg, polycystic ovary syndrome, congenital adrenal hyperplasia, androgen-producing tumors)
- Hypothalamic dysfunction (eg, secondary to anorexia nervosa)
- Hyperprolactinemia
- Hypothyroidism
- Primary pituitary disease
- Premature ovarian failure
- Iatrogenic (eg, secondary to radiation or chemotherapy)

Differential Diagnosis of Noncyclic Uterine Bleeding

- Anovulation
- Uterine leiomyoma
- Endometrial polyp
- Endometrial hyperplasia or carcinoma
- Cervical or vaginal neoplasia
- Endometritis
- Adenomyosis
- Bleeding associated with pregnancy
  - –threatened or incomplete abortion
  - –trophoblastic disease
  - –ectopic pregnancy
- Bleeding associated with the puerperium
  - –retained products of conception
  - –placental polyp
  - –subinvolution of the uterus
- Coagulopathies (von Willebrand's disease, platelet abnormalities, thrombocytopenic purpura)
- Iatrogenic causes and medications
- Systemic diseases

Age Considerations of Anovulatory Bleeding

Adolescents (13–18 Years)

Anovulatory bleeding is a normal physiologic process in the perimenarchal years of the reproductive cycle. Ovulatory menstrual cycles may not be established until a year or more after menarche. This phenomenon is attributed to the immaturity of the hypothalamic–pituitary– gonadal axis. Anovulatory bleeding at this age can be excessive, resulting in anemia and requiring emergency care. Occasionally, adolescents with blood dyscrasias, including von Willebrand's disease and prothrombin deficiency, have heavy vaginal bleeding beginning at menarche. Disorders such as leukemia, idiopathic thrombocytopenic purpura, and hypersplenism can all produce platelet dysfunction and cause excessive bleeding. Studies have demonstrated a wide variation in the prevalence of blood dyscrasias ranging from 5% to 20% of hospitalized adolescents (7, 8). Because the prevalence of blood dyscrasias in the adolescent population is significant, routine screening for coagulation disorders is warranted in these patients, including a partial thromboplastin time, prothrombin time, and assessment of platelet function. Physical examination should include an assessment for petechiae or ecchymoses.

Women of Reproductive Age (19–39 Years)

Between 6% and 10% of women have hyperandrogenic chronic anovulation (eg, polycystic ovary syndrome), which includes noncyclic menstrual bleeding, hirsutism, and obesity (body mass index ≥25 kg/m^2). As many as 65% of hirsute, chronically anovulatory women are obese (4). Numerous underlying biochemical abnormalities exist, including noncyclic estrogen production, elevated serum testosterone levels, hypersecretion of luteinizing hormone, and hyperinsulinemia (9). A history of rapidly progressing hirsutism accompanied by virilization suggests a tumor. In most cases, tumors can be ruled out by testing testosterone and dehydroepiandrosterone sulfate levels in serum.

Although anovulation may be considered physiologic in adolescents, adult women of reproductive age who have menorrhagia, metrorrhagia, or amenorrhea require evaluation for a specific cause. The laboratory assessment of these women should include a pregnancy test, a fasting serum prolactin level, and determination of levels of thyroid-stimulating hormone (TSH). When the diagnosis of ovarian failure is suspected, levels of follicle-stimulating hormone (FSH) also should be determined. Anovulation was found to be the most common cause of amenorrhea in a series of 262 women who experienced adult-onset amenorrhea (10). Chronic anovulation that results from hypothalamic dysfunction, as diagnosed by a low FSH level, may be the result of excessive psychologic stress, exercise, or weight loss (10). Both hyperthyroidism and hypothyroidism can be excluded using the sensitive TSH assay. In patients with amenorrhea who have a negative pregnancy test result and normal FSH, TSH, and prolactin levels, the diagnosis of anovulation can be made.

Women of Later Reproductive Age (40 Years to Menopause)

The incidence of anovulatory uterine bleeding increases as women approach the end of their reproductive years. In this regard, perimenopausal women are not unlike their perimenarchal counterparts. In perimenopausal women, the onset of anovulatory cycles represents a continuation of declining ovarian function. These patients need to be educated regarding the specific health risks associated with menopause so that an early proactive approach toward the prevention of menopause-associated conditions, such as osteoporosis, can be initiated. In addition to the use of hormone replacement therapy for cycle control, important lifestyle changes include exercise, dietary modification, and smoking cessation.

Clinical Considerations and Recommendations

▶ ***In women of each age group with anovulatory bleeding, when is endometrial evaluation indicated?***

Adolescents (13–18 Years). In 1995, the incidence of endometrial cancer in women between the ages of 15 and 19 years was 0.1 per 100,000 (11). In one report of endometrial carcinoma in adolescents, the patients experienced 2–3 years of anovulatory uterine bleeding (12). One patient experienced precocious puberty, which extended the number of years of unopposed estrogen exposure for someone of her age. All of the adolescents were obese. Because obesity is associated with conversion of androgens to estrogens and chronic anovulation, obese patients may be at an increased risk for developing endometrial hyperplasia and carcinoma. Therefore, one should consider endometrial assessment particularly for those adolescents who have a history of 2–3 years of untreated anovulatory bleeding and especially for those who are obese.

Women of Reproductive Age (19–39 Years). The incidence of endometrial carcinoma increases with age. However, the incidence of endometrial carcinoma is still very low in women between the ages of 19 and 39 years, reported as 9.5 per 100,000 in 1995 (11). However, there is a distinct increase in the incidence of endometrial carcinoma from ages 30–34 years (2.3/100,000 in 1995) to ages 35–39 years (6.1/100,000 in 1995) (11). Therefore, based on age alone, endometrial assessment to exclude cancer is indicated in any woman older than 35 years who is suspected of having anovulatory uterine bleeding.

Although endometrial carcinoma is rare in women younger than 35 years, patients between the ages of 19 and 35 years who do not respond to medical therapy or have prolonged periods of unopposed estrogen stimulation secondary to chronic anovulation are candidates for endometrial assessment.

Women of Later Reproductive Age (40 Years to Menopause). The incidence of endometrial carcinoma in women ages 40–49 years was 36.2 per 100,000 in 1995 (11). Therefore, all women older than 40 years who present with suspected anovulatory uterine bleeding should be evaluated with endometrial assessment (after pregnancy has been excluded).

▶ ***What medical therapies are most appropriate for each age group?***

Because anovulatory uterine bleeding is by definition an endocrinologic abnormality, medical management is the preferred method of therapy. The goals of medical treatment for anovulatory bleeding are to alleviate acute bleeding, prevent future episodes of noncyclic bleeding, decrease the patient's risk of long-term complications from anovulation, and improve the patient's overall quality of life. To encourage compliance with medical therapy, it is important to counsel patients that treatment may cause initial heavy menstrual bleeding secondary to endometrial buildup, but will lighten over time (within three cycles).

Adolescents (13–18 Years). Most adolescents who experience anovulatory bleeding can be treated with medical therapy. Occasionally, adolescents may have acute, profuse menstrual bleeding. High-dose estrogen therapy is an appropriate treatment to control acute bleeding episodes because it promotes rapid endometrial growth to cover denuded endometrial surfaces. Patients with blood dyscrasias need to be treated for their specific disease, and leukemia needs to be ruled out in this population. Conjugated equine estrogens can be administered orally up to 10 mg/d in four divided doses or intravenously at 25 mg every 4 hours for up to 24 hours (13). In a retrospective study, most adolescent patients with acute bleeding (93%) responded to medical therapy (8). After acute bleeding has been treated, recurrent anovulatory bleeding should be prevented with either a cyclic progestogen or an oral contraceptive.

Women with chronic anovulation can be treated successfully using either a cyclic progestogen or an oral contraceptive. Oral contraceptives suppress both ovarian and adrenal androgen production and increase sex hormone binding globulin, further reducing bioavailable androgens (14, 15). They also may inhibit 5α-reductase activity in the skin of adults (16). Treatment with a low-dose combination oral contraceptive (≤35 μg ethinyl estradiol) is appropriate, and maintenance oral contraceptives are the treatment of choice in women with chronic anovulation, especially if they are hyperandrogenic and hirsute (17).

Women of Reproductive Age (19–39 Years). Adult women of reproductive age with anovulatory uterine bleeding can be treated safely with either a cyclic progestogen or oral contraceptives similar to those prescribed for adolescent patients. However, estrogen-containing oral contraceptives are relatively contraindicated in some women (eg, those with hypertension or diabetes). Estrogen-containing oral contraceptives are contraindicated for women older than 35 years who smoke or have a history of thromboembolic disease.

If pregnancy is desired, induction of ovulation with clomiphene citrate is the initial treatment of choice (18). Patients can have withdrawal bleeding induced with progestogen followed by initiation of therapy with clomiphene citrate, 50 mg/d for 5 days, beginning between days 3 and 5 of the menstrual cycle.

Women of Later Reproductive Age (40 Years to Menopause). Women who are older than 40 years and who have anovulatory uterine bleeding can be treated with cyclic progestogen, low-dose oral contraceptives, or cyclic hormone replacement therapy. Not unlike younger women, these patients usually have adequate estrogen production. However, women older than 40 years with oligomenorrhea may have reduced estrogen production. Women with hot flashes secondary to declining estrogen production can obtain symptomatic relief with estrogen replacement therapy in combination with continuous or cyclic progestogen. Up to 90% of perimenopausal women receiving continuous estrogen and cyclic progestogen therapy will respond with predictable progesterone withdrawal bleeding (19).

▶ *In patients who have completed childbearing, what is the benefit of treating anovulatory bleeding surgically rather than medically?*

Currently, there are few randomized trials comparing medical versus surgical therapy for anovulatory uterine bleeding. One randomized trial that compared endometrial resection with medical management for women with menorrhagia found that women who underwent medical therapy were less likely to be satisfied with their therapy (20). However, because of its reduced cost and risks, medical therapy should be offered before surgical intervention unless it is otherwise contraindicated. Surgical therapy is indicated for women with excessive anovulatory bleeding in whom medical management has failed and who have completed their childbearing. Avoidance of anemia, reduction of excessively heavy bleeding, and increased, though imperfect, predictability of bleeding are appropriate goals to attempt to achieve with medical therapy. Success and failure of medical therapy should be defined in partnership with the patient, to better achieve the therapeutic goal.

▶ *In women who have completed childbearing, what is the evidence of efficacy among surgical techniques?*

The surgical options include hysterectomy and endometrial ablation. Recent studies have reported morbidity rates of 7% (21) and 15% (22) for women undergoing hysterectomy for various indications. The overall mortality rate for hysterectomy is 12 deaths per 10,000 procedures, for all surgical indications (23). A surgical alternative to hysterectomy is endometrial ablation. Endometrial ablation can be performed with or without the assistance of hysteroscopy.

Hysteroscopic-assisted endometrial ablation can be performed with the resectoscope. Using the resectoscope, the endometrium can be removed or resected with an electrocautery loop or ablated with the rollerball. Endometrial ablation also can be accomplished with the YAG laser. An alternative to hysteroscopic-assisted endometrial ablation is thermal balloon ablation in which the endometrium is ablated by heating saline inside an intrauterine balloon to approximately 85°C. The most frequently reported complications of hysteroscopy are uterine perforation, which occurs in approximately 14 per 1,000 procedures (24) and fluid overload, which occurs in approximately 2 per 1,000 cases.

Studies evaluating the effectiveness of endometrial ablation have been performed in a group of women who were diagnosed with menorrhagia and who were not necessarily anovulatory. However, women with anovulatory uterine bleeding are candidates for endometrial ablation if they have failed medical therapy and have completed their childbearing. The proportion of women who are amenorrheic after undergoing an endometrial resection using the resectoscope or endometrial laser ablation is approximately 45%, and the percentage of women at 12 months postoperatively who are satisfied with their therapy approaches 90% (25, 26). This high degree of satisfaction indicates that reduction of flow is adequate symptom control for most women, and achievement of amenorrhea is not as important. Endometrial ablation with the thermal balloon yields an amenorrhea rate of approximately 15% and a 12-month postoperative satisfaction rate of approximately 90% (27, 28).

Patient satisfaction with hysterectomy and endometrial ablation performed for dysfunctional uterine bleeding has been compared. One study demonstrated a higher satisfaction rate in women who underwent hysterectomy as compared with women who underwent hysteroscopic-assisted endometrial ablation (29). Furthermore, the long-term satisfaction of women who have undergone endometrial ablation has been questioned. In a 3-year follow-up study, 8.5% of women who had undergone endometrial ablation later underwent repeat ablation, and an additional 8.5% had undergone hysterectomy (30). In a 5-year follow-up study, 34% of women who had undergone hysteroscopic ablation subsequently had a hysterectomy (31). Because women who undergo endometrial ablation can have residual active endometrium, these women should receive progestogen if they are prescribed estrogen replacement therapy.

Numerous studies have compared costs and surgical outcomes between endometrial resection or ablation and hysterectomy. The evidence suggests that hysteroscopic endometrial ablation results in less morbidity and shorter recovery periods and is more cost-effective than hysterectomy (32–37). However, if as many as one third of women who undergo endometrial ablation undergo hysterectomy within the following 5 years, that would have a significant impact on these cost analyses.

Evidence from randomized trials supports the use of either a gonadotropin-releasing hormone agonist or danazol prior to endometrial ablation or resection with regard to improved intrauterine operating environment and short-term postoperative outcome (38). The choice of agents should be based on cost, efficacy, and side effects. There are insufficient data to assess the value of progestogen therapy prior to endometrial ablation.

▶ *What is the role of high-dose estrogen in acute vaginal bleeding?*

Women who experience acute, profuse anovulatory bleeding are candidates for estrogen therapy. In approximately 90% of cases, acute bleeding does not require surgical intervention, but it can be treated with medical therapy (8). In a large series of 61 adolescents (mean age, 13.8 ± 2.1 years) with acute anovulatory uterine bleeding, only five (8.2%) failed medical therapy and required dilation and curettage to stop their bleeding. Conjugated equine estrogen therapy can be administered intravenously (25 mg every 4 hours for 24 hours). However, oral conjugated estrogen therapy at 10–20 mg per day in four divided doses can be substituted for intravenous estrogen administration. In a randomized trial of intravenous conjugated equine estrogen therapy versus placebo, conjugated estrogens were effective in stopping vaginal bleeding in a significantly greater proportion of women (72%) than those who received a placebo (38%) (13). Although this study included women with biopsy-proven pathology, it is one of the few studies performed to assess the efficacy of intravenous estrogen therapy for the treatment of women with anovulatory uterine bleeding. Patients who do not respond to 1–2 doses of estrogen with a significant decline in blood loss or are not hemodynamically stable should undergo dilation and curettage. Furthermore, as high-dose estrogen therapy is commonly associated with nausea, concomitant medical therapy with antiemetics should be considered.

After the acute episode of bleeding has been controlled, amenorrhea should be maintained for several weeks to allow for resolution of anemia. The best method of therapy is a combination oral contraceptive. To extend the interval before the next menses, continuous oral contraceptives (without the use of placebo pills) can be given for several months; however, over time the patient will be susceptible again to breakthrough bleeding. Once the patient's anemia has resolved, cyclic oral contraceptives can be prescribed. All anemic patients should be given iron therapy.

Summary

The following recommendations are based on good and consistent scientific evidence (Level A):

- ▶ The treatment of choice for anovulatory uterine bleeding is medical therapy with oral contraceptives. Cyclic progestins also are effective.
- ▶ Women who have failed medical therapy and no longer desire future childbearing are candidates for endometrial ablation, which appears to be an efficient and cost-effective alternative treatment to hysterectomy for anovulatory uterine bleeding. However, endometrial ablation may not be definitive therapy.

The following recommendations are based primarily on consensus and expert opinion (Level C):

- ▶ An underlying coagulopathy, such as von Willebrand's disease, should be considered in all patients (particularly adolescents) with abnormal uterine bleeding, especially when bleeding is not otherwise easily explained or does not respond to medical therapy.
- ▶ Although there is limited evidence evaluating the efficacy of conjugated equine estrogen therapy in anovulatory bleeding, it is effective in controlling abnormal uterine bleeding.

References

1. Hallberg L, Hogdahl AM, Nilsson L, Rybo G. Menstrual blood loss—a population study. Variation at different ages and attempts to define normality. Acta Obstet Gynecol Scand 1966;45:320–351 (Level III)
2. Hallberg L, Nilsson L. Constancy of individual menstrual blood loss. Acta Obstet Gynecol Scand 1964;43:352–359 (Level III)
3. Smith SK, Abel MH, Kelly RW, Baird DT. The synthesis of prostaglandins from persistent proliferative endometrium. J Clin Endocrinol Metab 1982;55:284–289 (Level II-2)
4. Singh KB, Mahajan DK, Wortsman J. Effect of obesity on the clinical and hormonal characteristics of the polycystic ovary syndrome. J Reprod Med 1994;39:805–808 (Level II-2)
5. Falsetti L, Eleftheriou G. Hyperinsulinemia in the polycystic ovary syndrome: a clinical, endocrine and echographic study in 240 patients. Gynecol Endocrinol 1996;10:319–326 (Level II-2)
6. Schlechte J, Sherman B, Halmi N, VanGilder J, Chapler F, Dolan K, et al. Prolactin-secreting pituitary tumors in amenorrheic women: a comprehensive study. Endocr Rev 1980;1:295–308
7. Claessens EA, Cowell CL. Acute adolescent menorrhagia. Am J Obstet Gynecol 1981;139:277–280 (Level III)
8. Falcone T, Desjardins C, Bourque J, Granger L, Hemmings R, Quiros E. Dysfunctional uterine bleeding in adolescents. J Reprod Med 1994;39:761–764 (Level II-2)
9. Goudas VT, Dumesic DA. Polycystic ovary syndrome. Endocrinol Metab Clin North Am 1997;26:893–912 (Level III)
10. Reindollar RH, Novak M, Tho SP, McDonough PG. Adult-onset amenorrhea: a study of 262 patients. Am J Obstet Gynecol 1986;155:531–543 (Level III)
11. SEER cancer statistics review, 1973–1996 [serial online]. Available at <http://www-seer.ims.nci.nih.gov/Publications/CSR1973_1996>. Retrieved February 1, 2000 (Level II-3)
12. Stovall DW, Anderson RJ, De Leon FD. Endometrial adenocarcinoma in teenagers. Adolesc Pediatr Gynecol 1989; 2:157–159 (Level III)
13. DeVore GR, Owens O, Kase N. Use of intravenous Premarin in the treatment of dysfunctional uterine bleeding—a double-blind randomized controlled study. Obstet Gynecol 1982;59:285–291 (Level I)
14. Wild RA, Umstot ES, Andersen RN, Givens JR. Adrenal function in hirsutism. II. Effect of an oral contraceptive. J Clin Endocrinol Metab 1982;54:676–681 (Level III)
15. Wiebe RH, Morris CV. Effect of an oral contraceptive on adrenal and ovarian androgenic steroids. Obstet Gynecol 1984;63:12–14 (Level III)
16. Cassidenti DL, Paulson RJ, Serafini P, Stanczyk FZ, Lobo RA. Effects of sex steroids on skin 5 alpha-reductase activity in vitro. Obstet Gynecol 1991;78:103–107 (Level III)
17. Rittmaster RS. Clinical review 73: Medical treatment of androgen-dependent hirsutism. J Clin Endocrinol Metab 1995;80:2559–2563 (Level III)
18. Hughes E, Collins J, Vandekerckhove P. Clomiphene citrate for unexplained subfertility in women (Cochrane review). In: The Cochrane Library, Issue 4, 1999. Oxford: Update Software. (Meta-analysis)
19. Strickland DM, Hammond TL. Postmenopausal estrogen replacement in a large gynecologic practice. Am J Gynecol Health 1988;2(1):26–31 (Level III)
20. Cooper KG, Parkin DE, Garratt AM, Grant AM. Two-year follow up of women randomised to medical management or transcervical resection of the endometrium for heavy menstrual loss: clinical and quality of life outcomes. Br J Obstet Gynaecol 1999;106:258–265 (Level I)
21. Carlson KJ, Miller BA, Fowler FJ Jr. The Maine Women's Health Study: I. Outcomes of hysterectomy. Obstet Gynecol 1994;83:556–565 (Level II-3)
22. Summitt RL Jr, Stovall TG, Steege JF, Lipscomb GH. A multicenter randomized comparison of laparoscopically assisted vaginal hysterectomy and abdominal hysterectomy in abdominal hysterectomy candidates. Obstet Gynecol 1998;92:321–326 (Level I)
23. Bachmann GA. Hysterectomy: A critical review. J Reprod Med 1990;35:839–862 (Level III)
24. Hulka JF, Peterson HA, Phillips JM, Surrey MW. Operative hysteroscopy: American Association of Gynecologic Laparoscopists' 1993 membership survey. J Am Assoc Gynecol Laparosc 1995;2:131–132 (Level II-3)
25. Bhattacharya S, Cameron IM, Parkin DE, Abramovich DR, Mollison J, Pinion SB, et al. A pragmatic randomised comparison of transcervical resection of the endometrium with endometrial laser ablation for the treatment of menorrhagia. Br J Obstet Gynaecol 1997;104:601–607 (Level I)
26. A randomized trial of endometrial ablation versus hysterectomy for the treatment of dysfunctional uterine bleeding: outcome at four years. Aberdeen Endometrial Ablation Trials Group. Br J Obstet Gynaecol 1999;106: 360–366 (Level I)
27. Amso NN, Stabinsky SA, McFaul P, Blanc B, Pendley L, Neuwirth R. Uterine thermal balloon therapy for the treatment of menorrhagia: the first 300 patients from a multicentre study. International Collaborative Uterine Thermal Balloon Working Group. Br J Obstet Gynaecol 1998;105: 517–523 (Level 1)
28. Meyer WR, Walsh BW, Grainger DA, Peacock LM, Loffer FD, Steege JF. Thermal balloon and rollerball ablation to treat menorrhagia: a multicenter comparison. Obstet Gynecol 1998;92:98–103 (Level I)
29. Pinion SB, Parkin DE, Abramovich DR, Naji A, Alexander DA, Russell IT, et al. Randomised trial of hysterectomy, endometrial laser ablation, and transcervical endometrial resection for dysfunctional uterine bleeding. BMJ 1994; 309:979–983 (Level I)
30. Chullapram T, Song JY, Fraser IS. Medium-term follow-up of women with menorrhagia treated by rollerball

endometrial ablation. Obstet Gynecol 1996;88:71–76 (Level II-3)

31. Unger JB, Meeks GR. Hysterectomy after endometrial ablation. Am J Obstet Gynecol 1996;175:1432–1436; discussions 1436–1437 (Level II-3)

32. Gannon MJ, Holt EM, Fairbank J, Fitzgerald M, Milne MA, Crystal AM, et al. A randomised trial comparing endometrial resection and abdominal hysterectomy for the treatment of menorrhagia. BMJ 1991;303:1362–1364 (Level I)

33. Brooks PG, Clouse J, Morris LS. Hysterectomy vs. resectoscopic endometrial ablation for the control of abnormal uterine bleeding. A cost-comparative study. J Reprod Med 1994;39:755–760 (Level II-2)

34. Goldenberg M, Sivan E, Bider D, Mashiach S, Seidman DS. Endometrial resection vs. abdominal hysterectomy for menorrhagia. Correlated sample analysis. J Reprod Med 1996;41:333–336 (Level II-2)

35. Cameron IM, Mollison J, Pinion SB, Atherton-Naji A, Buckingham K, Torgerson D. A cost comparison of hysterectomy and hysteroscopic surgery for the treatment of menorrhagia. Eur J Obstet Gynecol Reprod Biol 1996;70:87–92 (Level I)

36. Vilos GA, Pispidikis JT, Botz CK. Economic evaluation of hysteroscopic endometrial ablation versus vaginal hysterectomy for menorrhagia. Obstet Gynecol 1996;88:241–245 (Level II-2)

37. Brumsted JR, Blackman JA, Badger GJ, Riddick DH. Hysteroscopy versus hysterectomy for the treatment of abnormal uterine bleeding: a comparison of cost. Fertil Steril 1996;65:310–316 (Level II-2)

38. Fraser IS, Healy DL, Torode H, Song JY, Mamers P, Wilde F. Depot goserelin and danazol pre-treatment before rollerball endometrial ablation for menorrhagia. Obstet Gynecol 1996;87:544–550 (Level I)

The MEDLINE database, the Cochrane Library, and ACOG's own internal resources and documents were used to conduct a literature search to locate relevant articles published between January 1985 and May 1999. The search was restricted to articles published in the English language. Priority was given to articles reporting results of original research, although review articles and commentaries also were consulted. Abstracts of research presented at symposia and scientific conferences were not considered adequate for inclusion in this document. Guidelines published by organizations or institutions such as the National Institutes of Health and the American College of Obstetricians and Gynecologists were reviewed, and additional studies were located by reviewing bibliographies of identified articles. When reliable research was not available, expert opinions from obstetrician–gynecologists were used.

Studies were reviewed and evaluated for quality according to the method outlined by the U.S. Preventive Services Task Force:

I Evidence obtained from at least one properly designed randomized controlled trial.

II-1 Evidence obtained from well-designed controlled trials without randomization.

II-2 Evidence obtained from well-designed cohort or case–control analytic studies, preferably from more than one center or research group.

II-3 Evidence obtained from multiple time series with or without the intervention. Dramatic results in uncontrolled experiments could also be regarded as this type of evidence.

III Opinions of respected authorities, based on clinical experience, descriptive studies, or reports of expert committees.

Based on the highest level of evidence found in the data, recommendations are provided and graded according to the following catetories:

Level A—Recommendations are based on good and consistent scientific evidence.

Level B—Recommendations are based on limited or inconsistent scientific evidence.

Level C—Recommendations are based primarily on consensus and expert opinion.

The American College of Obstetricians and Gynecologists
409 12th Street, SW
PO Box 96920
Washington, DC 20090-6920

12345/43210

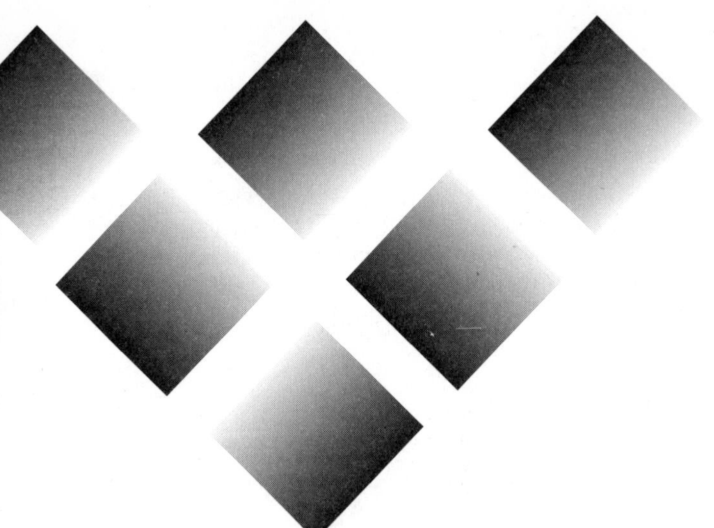

ACOG PRACTICE BULLETIN

CLINICAL MANAGEMENT GUIDELINES FOR OBSTETRICIAN–GYNECOLOGISTS

NUMBER 8, OCTOBER 1999

This Practice Bulletin was developed by the ACOG Committee on Practice Bulletins—Obstetrics with the assistance of David A. Baker, MD. The information is designed to aid practitioners in making decisions about appropriate obstetric and gynecologic care. These guidelines should not be construed as dictating an exclusive course of treatment or procedure. Variations in practice may be warranted based on the needs of the individual patient, resources, and limitations unique to the institution or type of practice.

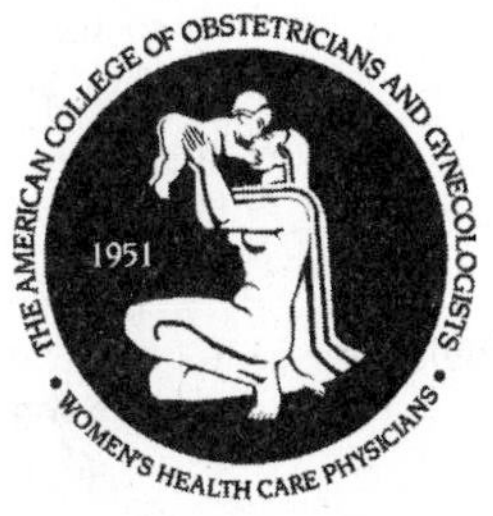

Management of Herpes in Pregnancy

Genital herpes simplex virus (HSV) infection during pregnancy poses a significant risk to the developing fetus and newborn. In the United States, the incidence of this sexually transmitted disease (STD) has increased significantly since 1970 (1). Because many women of childbearing age are infected or are becoming infected, the risk of maternal transmission of this virus to the fetus or newborn is a major health concern. The purpose of this document is to define the stages of herpetic infection, outline the spectrum of maternal and neonatal infection, including rates of transmission and risks, and provide management guidelines that have been validated by appropriately conducted outcome-based research. Additional guidelines based on consensus and expert opinion also are presented to permit a review of most clinical aspects of HSV.

Background

Etiology

Two types of HSV, herpes simplex virus type 1 (HSV-1) and herpes simplex virus type 2 (HSV-2), can be identified on the basis of divergent biologic properties. They also can be differentiated by minor differences in antigenic composition and biochemical characteristics. Although they are distinct types, the degree of sharing of antigenic determinants between HSV-1 and HSV-2 results in cross-reacting antibodies capable of neutralizing the other virus type (2).

Initial contact with HSV usually occurs early in childhood and involves HSV-1. Less than 10% of primary infections with HSV-1 are clinically overt. Herpes simplex virus type 1 causes most nongenital herpetic lesions: eg, herpes labialis, gingivostomatitis, and keratoconjunctivitis. The female genital tract can be infected with HSV-1 or HSV-2. In the United States, most genital infection is from HSV-2.

Incidence

Herpes simplex virus infection of the genital tract is one of the most common viral STDs. Approximately 45 million adolescent and adult Americans have been infected with genital herpes based on positive serology test results for HSV-2 and estimates of genital HSV-1 infection (1). The greatest incidence of overt HSV-2 infection occurs in women in their late teens and early twenties. In one study, 5% of reproductive-aged women indicated a history of genital herpes virus infection (3). However, approximately 30% of the female population in the United States have antibodies to HSV-2 (1). Factors that influence the incidence of genital infection with HSV are age of the patient, duration of sexual activity, race, previous genital infections, family income, and number of sex partners (4). The number of initial visits to physicians' offices as a result of genital HSV infection increased from approximately 75,000 per year in 1978 to more than 150,000 per year in the early 1990s (1).

The last available data from the mid-1980s indicated that, in the United States, approximately 1,500–2,000 newborns contracted neonatal herpes each year (5). Most infections occur in the perinatal period from contact with infected maternal secretions. Most newborns acquire the virus from asymptomatic mothers without identified lesions (3, 6).

Presentation of Infection

There are three stages of HSV infection based on clinical presentation and serology (see the box). Primary infections are those in which no HSV-1 or HSV-2 antibodies are present. In nonprimary first-episode disease, HSV-1 antibodies are present in the woman who has HSV-2 infection or HSV-2 antibodies are present in the woman who has HSV-1 infection. In recurrent infections, homologous antibodies are present.

Clinical Designation of HSV Infection

Primary genital HSV: Antibodies to both HSV-1 and HSV-2 are absent at the time the patient acquires genital HSV due to HSV-1 or HSV-2.

Nonprimary first-episode genital HSV: Acquisition of genital HSV (due to HSV-1) with preexisting antibodies to HSV-2 or acquisition of genital HSV (due to HSV-2) with preexisting antibodies to HSV-1.

Recurrent genital HSV: Reactivation of genital HSV where the HSV type recovered from the lesion is the same type as the antibody in the sera.

Riley LE. Herpes simplex virus. Sem Perinatol 1998;22:284–292.

In the absence of systemic symptoms, the distinction between first-episode and recurrent herpetic infections is difficult. In one study, women with severe first-recognized clinical outbreaks of genital herpes in the second and third trimesters of pregnancy were evaluated serologically and virologically (7). Of these 23 women with clinical illnesses consistent with primary genital HSV infections, only one had serologically verified primary infection. This primary infection was caused by HSV-1. Three women had nonprimary HSV-2 infections, and 19 women had recurrent infections.

Primary Infection

Initial genital infection due to herpes may be either asymptomatic or associated with severe symptoms. With symptomatic primary infection, lesions may occur on the vulva, vagina, or cervix, or on all three between 2 and 14 days following exposure to infectious virus. These lesions are larger in number and size than those observed in patients with recurrent disease and patients who have had prior infection with HSV-1. The initial vesicles rupture and subsequently appear as shallow and eroded ulcers. Inguinal lymphadenopathy is demonstrated readily as the consequence of virus replication in the sites of lymphatic drainage (2).

When systemic symptoms (malaise, myalgia, and fever) occur, they are most commonly restricted to presumed primary herpetic infections. These symptoms reflect the viremia that occurs more likely with primary infection. Local symptoms of pain, dysuria, and soreness of the vulva and vagina are common in both primary and recurrent infections. The lesions of primary infection tends to resolve within 3 weeks without therapy. However, when secondary bacterial or mycotic infection is present and not treated, the lesions may persist up to 6 weeks.

Increased symptomatic and subclinical shedding from the lower genital tract of women occurs during the first 3 months after primary genital HSV-2 lesions have healed. Subclinical cervical and vulvar shedding occur at a rate of approximately 2.3% in women with HSV-2 infection and 0.65% in women with HSV-1 infection (8).

Nonprimary First Episode

Prior infection with HSV-1 does not fully protect a patient from initial infection with HSV-2 in the genital tract. It may be difficult for a physician to differentiate primary disease from nonprimary first-episode disease based only on clinical findings and patient symptoms (9); serologic confirmation would be required for definitive diagnosis.

A nonprimary first episode can be identified as a first clinically recognized genital HSV infection that does not behave clinically like a symptomatic primary infection. There are fewer systemic manifestations, less pain, a briefer duration of viral shedding, and a more rapid resolution of the clinical lesions in the nonprimary infection. These episodes usually are thought to be the result of an initial HSV-2 infection in the presence of partially protective HSV-1 antibodies.

Recurrent Infection

Recurrences of genital HSV infection can be symptomatic or subclinical, and there is significant variation from patient to patient in the frequency, severity, and duration of symptoms and amount of viral shedding (8, 10–12). Confinement of the ulcers to the genital area is more common in recurrent forms of the disease. The ulcers tend to be limited in size, number, and duration. Local symptoms predominate over systemic symptoms, with many patients indicating increased vaginal discharge or pain (13).

Shedding of the virus from the genital tract without symptoms or signs of clinical lesions (subclinical shedding) is episodic and lasts an average of 1.5 days (11). During this time, the virus quantity is lower than when a lesion is present; however, a susceptible partner can acquire the infection. Subclinical shedding makes this viral STD difficult to control and prevent.

Neonatal Herpes

Most neonatal HSV infection is the consequence of delivery of a neonate through an infected birth canal. There are three categories of neonatal disease: localized disease of the skin, eye, and mouth; central nervous system (CNS) disease with or without skin, eye, and mouth disease; or disseminated disease. Most infected neonates have localized skin, eye, and mouth disease, which generally is a mild illness. Localized disease may progress to encephalitis or disseminated disease. Subtle signs, such as poor feeding, listlessness, and irritability, may indicate CNS disease. One study of the predictors of mortality and morbidity of neonatal HSV showed no mortality with skin, eye, and mouth disease, 15% mortality with CNS disease, and 57% mortality with disseminated disease (14).

Transmission

Sexual and Direct Contact

Herpes simplex virus is transmitted via direct contact with an individual who is infected. Genital-to-genital contact or contact of the genital tract with an area that is infected with HSV, such as oral-to-genital contact, can result in transmission. One study showed that among sexual partners who were discordant for HSV infection, the annual risk of acquisition of genital HSV infection was 31.9% among women who were HSV-1-negative and HSV-2-negative versus 9.1% among women who were HSV-1-positive (4). Furthermore, most of the transmission between discordant couples occurs when there is no evidence of active lesions, which suggests that asymptomatic shedding is the source of more than half of all cases of transmission (15). In one study, about 10% of pregnant women were at risk of contracting primary HSV-2 infection from their HSV-2-seropositive husbands (16).

Maternal–Fetal Transmission

The vertical transmission of HSV appears to be related to gestational age and whether the disease is primary, nonprimary first episode, or recurrent. Investigators prospectively obtained HSV cultures on 15,923 women in early labor who were without signs or symptoms of genital HSV infection (17). Herpes simplex virus was isolated from 56 women (0.35%) with serum samples for HSV antibody testing available from 52 women. Eighteen women (35%) had serologic evidence of recently acquired, subclinical first-episode HSV, and 34 (65%) had asymptomatic recurrent disease. Herpes simplex virus infection developed in six (33%) of 18 neonates born to women with subclinical first-episode disease and in one (3%) of 34 infants born to women with recurrent HSV. This study also showed that preexisting antibody to HSV-2 but not to HSV-1 reduced the vertical transmission of HSV-2. In a more recent study, 8,538 women were prospectively evaluated during pregnancy and at delivery with HSV cultures. Investigators found that 94 (1.3%) of 7,046 women who were susceptible to either HSV-1 or HSV-2 seroconverted during pregnancy. Nine women acquired HSV at or near the time of delivery. Of these nine women, four delivered neonates who developed HSV (one died, and one had developmental delay). In this cohort, there were no cases of neonates with HSV-2 born to women with recurrent HSV (18). Vertical transmission rates at the time of vaginal delivery based on the type of maternal disease may be summarized as follows: primary HSV resulted in approximately 50% transmission; nonprimary first-episode HSV resulted in approximately 33% transmission; and recurrent HSV resulted in 0–3% transmission (17).

During Pregnancy

A threefold increase in the rate of spontaneous abortion following primary maternal genital infection with HSV early in pregnancy has been reported (17). However, this finding was not confirmed in a more recent study (18).

Primary infection in the second or third trimesters increases the risk for preterm delivery as well as the risk of HSV transmission to the newborn (17). Asymptomatic genital shedding of herpes from a subclinical primary genital infection may be associated with preterm delivery (18).

During pregnancy, primary maternal herpetic infection, in the absence of cross-protecting antibodies, theoretically may result in hematogenous dissemination of the virus to the fetus. Isolated case reports have associated in utero infection during the first 12–14 weeks of gestation with a variety of anomalies, such as microcephaly, microphthalmia, intracranial calcifications, and chorioretinitis (19–21).

Clinical Considerations and Recommendations

▶ *How can the diagnosis of HSV be confirmed?*

Herpes simplex virus infection may be documented in several ways. The standard and most sensitive test for detecting HSV from clinical specimens continues to be isolation of the virus by cell culture. Because HSV is a DNA virus, it produces cytopathic effects in cells indicative of virus replication. However, the sensitivity of this technique is affected by numerous factors related to sampling and transporting the specimen. Cytologic tests have a maximum sensitivity of 60–70% when dealing with overt clinical disease (22); thus, both the Papanicolaou and Tzanck tests are poor HSV screening procedures. Newer, more sensitive techniques are increasingly available, such as polymerase chain reaction and hybridization methods (23–25).

Early primary and nonprimary first-episode ulcers yield the virus in 80% of patients, whereas ulcers from recurrent infections are less likely to be culture-positive; only 40% of crusted lesions contain recoverable virus (26). When testing for HSV, overt lesions that are not in the ulcerated state should be unroofed and the fluid sampled.

Commercially available serologic tests designed to detect antibodies to genital herpes infection cannot reliably distinguish between HSV-1 and HSV-2. Serologic diagnosis of primary infection is possible by documenting seroconversion from a negative to a positive antibody titer. The usual time for obtaining a second specimen is 2–3 weeks after the onset of infection. The presence of an antibody titer in the initial specimen, obtained at the onset of disease, strongly suggests nonprimary first-episode or recurrent infection. Newer tests to differentiate between HSV-1 and HSV-2 antibodies are currently in development.

▶ *What is the optimal medical management of women with primary HSV infection during pregnancy?*

Antiviral therapy for primary infection is recommended for women with primary HSV infection during pregnancy to reduce viral shedding and enhance lesion healing. It is important to recognize that primary HSV cannot be distinguished from nonprimary first-episode disease unless serology is performed. Primary infection during pregnancy constitutes a higher risk for vertical transmission than does recurrent infection. The absence of episodes of symptomatic genital HSV infection throughout pregnancy does not eliminate the risk of asymptomatic shedding at delivery (27). Furthermore, suppressive therapy for the duration of the pregnancy needs to be considered to reduce the potential of continued viral shedding (8) and the likelihood of recurrent episodes (28).

Data are limited concerning prevention of disease in the fetus with maternal antiviral therapy. In one randomized study, 21 women received acyclovir and 25 did not to determine whether suppressive therapy started at 36 weeks of gestation could decrease viral shedding, prevent neonatal herpes, and reduce the need for cesarean delivery (29). Although the study did not differentiate between primary and nonprimary first episodes, it did show a significant reduction in cesarean delivery. There were no cases of neonatal herpes in either group, a finding that is compatible with a maximum 14% risk of infection with either therapy.

Significant benefits of acyclovir antiviral therapy using acyclovir have been shown in cases of pregnant women with disseminated HSV, herpes pneumonitis, herpes hepatitis, and herpes encephalitis (30–32).

▶ *What is the optimal medical management of women with recurrent HSV infection during pregnancy?*

A randomized trial of acyclovir given after 36 weeks of gestation in women with recurrent genital herpes infection demonstrated a significant decrease in clinical recurrences. The trial also showed a reduction in the number of cesarean deliveries performed for active infection, although this finding was not statistically significant (33).

▶ *What medications are available for treatment of HSV infection during pregnancy?*

Numerous compounds are available for the treatment of genital herpes (34), although none of these antiviral compounds has received approval for use in pregnancy by the U.S. Food and Drug Administration. These compounds are nucleoside analogues that selectively inhibit viral replication and produce minimal effect on the cell. Research in antiviral therapy has focused on improving bioavailability, which improves absorption and increases plasma levels of the compound while decreasing the number of daily doses of medication.

Acyclovir, a class-C medication, has selective activity against HSV-1 and HSV-2. In the treatment of primary genital herpes infections, oral acyclovir reduces viral shedding, reduces pain, and heals lesions faster when compared with a placebo (35). Acyclovir has been shown to be safe and has minimal side effects (36). However, only approximately 20% of each oral dose is absorbed.

The newer antiherpetic drugs valacyclovir and famciclovir are class-B medications. Their increased bioavailability means that they may require less frequent dosing to achieve the same therapeutic benefits as acyclovir. The U.S. Food and Drug Administration has approved both valacyclovir and famciclovir for the treatment of primary genital herpes, the treatment of episodes of recurrent disease, and the daily treatment for suppression of outbreaks of recurrent genital herpes.

Daily treatment with oral acyclovir significantly reduces symptomatic recurrences and suppresses subclinical viral shedding (28, 37). One study showed that 6 years of continuous daily acyclovir suppressive therapy did not produce the emergence of acyclovir-resistant isolates in immunocompetent patients (36). Valacyclovir therapy, 500 mg once daily, is effective in suppressing recurrent genital herpes (38). Suppressive famciclovir therapy requires a twice daily, 250 mg dosage (38). See Table 1.

Numerous studies have demonstrated the safety of acyclovir use during pregnancy (29, 32, 39). Neither medically indicated nor inadvertent use in the first trimester of pregnancy demonstrated any increased risk to the developing fetus. When acyclovir is given orally or intravenously, it crosses the placenta, concentrates in amniotic fluid and breast milk, and reaches therapeutic levels in the fetus (40). An acyclovir pregnancy registry has been maintained since 1984. In 1993, the Centers for Disease Control and Prevention published data showing no increase in fetal problems in women who received acyclovir during the first trimester of pregnancy (39).

▶ *Is there a role for universal screening during pregnancy or at delivery?*

Viral cultures are costly and imprecise. The correlation between asymptomatic viral shedding and ensuing neonatally acquired disease is poor. Negative cultures do not preclude the possibility of subsequent neonatal infection because the culture sensitivity is well below 100%, and infection may occur in the interim. Virologic monitoring is not recommended for pregnant women whose onset of disease antedated pregnancy or for those whose sexual partners have had herpetic lesions (27). Similarly, there are no data to support the value of culturing asymptomatic patients with a history of recurrent disease (11).

Table 1. Antiviral Treatment for Herpes Simplex Virus

Indication	Valacyclovir	Acyclovir	Famciclovir
First clinical episode	1,000 mg twice a day for 7–14 days	200 mg five times a day or 400 mg three times a day for 7–14 days	250 mg three times a day for 7–14 days
Recurrent episodes	500 mg twice a day for 5 days	200 mg five times a day or 400 mg three times a day for 5 days	125 mg twice a day for 5 days
Daily suppressive therapy	500 mg once a day (≤9 recurrences per year) or 1,000 mg once a day or 250 mg twice a day (>9 recurrences per year)	400 mg twice a day	250 mg twice a day

Baker DA. Antiviral therapy for genital herpes in nonpregnant and pregnant women. Int J Fertil 1998;43:243–248

▶ *In which situations should cesarean delivery be considered?*

Cesarean delivery is indicated in women with active genital lesions or symptoms of vulvar pain or burning, which may indicate an impending outbreak. The incidence of infection in infants whose mothers have recurrent infections is low, but cesarean delivery is warranted because of the potentially serious nature of the disease. The low incidence of neonatal HSV has raised concern that cesarean delivery is unwarranted for recurrent genital herpes (41). The extent to which maternal antibodies will protect a neonate from infection during a recurrence has not been determined with certainty. Cesarean delivery is not warranted in women with a history of HSV infection but with no active genital disease during labor (42).

▶ *Is cesarean delivery recommended for women with recurrent HSV lesions on areas distant from the vulva, vagina, or cervix (eg, thigh or buttock)?*

Among women with recurrent HSV and genital lesions at the time of labor, the risk of neonatal HSV infection associated with vaginal birth is low, estimated to be no more than 3% (17). In part, this low risk is probably attributable to preexisting maternal type-specific antibodies. When infection occurs among neonates of women with recurrent HSV, it is due either to shedding of the virus from the genital lesion itself or to shedding from the cervix. In patients with recurrent genital HSV and nongenital lesions at the time of labor, the only viral exposure faced by the infant during vaginal delivery is that of cervical shedding, which occurs in approximately 2% of such cases (43). Thus, the risk of neonatal HSV associated with vaginal delivery in a woman with recurrent HSV and nongenital lesions would appear to be very low. Cesarean delivery is not recommended for these women. Nongenital lesions should be covered with an occlusive dressing; the patient then can deliver vaginally.

▶ *In a patient with active HSV infection and ruptured membranes, is there any length of time at which vaginal delivery remains appropriate?*

In patients with active HSV infection and ruptured membranes at or near term, a cesarean delivery should be performed as soon as the necessary personnel and equipment can be readied. There is no evidence that there is a duration of premature rupture of membranes beyond which the fetus does not benefit from cesarean delivery (44).

▶ *How should a woman with active HSV and preterm premature rupture of membranes be managed?*

In the decision to deliver a patient with preterm premature rupture of membranes and active HSV, the risk of prematurity versus the potential risk of neonatal disease should be considered. In pregnancies remote from term, especially in women with recurrent disease, there is increasing support for continuing the pregnancy to gain benefit from time and glucocorticoids (45). If this expectant management plan is followed, treatment with an antiviral agent is indicated. Concern has been raised about the potential effects of glucocorticoids on patients with viral infection, but there is no conclusive evidence that this is a concern in this setting. The decision to perform a cesarean delivery depends on whether active lesions are present at the time of delivery.

The utility of suppressive antiviral therapy to prevent ascending infection has not been proven. The lack of evidence complicates the situation, because it is clear that premature neonates are at the greatest risk of infection. In such situations, it may be appropriate to consult personnel well versed in the management of such complicated cases.

▶ *Are invasive procedures contraindicated in women with HSV?*

In patients with recurrent HSV, invasive procedures, such as amniocentesis, percutaneous umbilical cord blood sampling, or transabdominal chorionic villus sampling may be performed; however, transcervical procedures should be delayed until lesions appear to have resolved. In a patient with primary HSV and systemic symptoms, it seems prudent to delay invasive procedures until symptoms appear to resolve.

Local neonatal infection may result from the use of fetal scalp electrode monitoring in patients with a history of herpes, even when lesions are not present (46–48). However, if there are indications for fetal scalp monitoring, it may be appropriate in a woman who has a history of recurrent HSV and no active lesions. If vesicular or vesiculopustular lesions develop at the site of the electrode, it is important to make a quick and accurate diagnosis and start systemic antiviral therapy.

▶ *Should women with active HSV breastfeed or handle their infants?*

Postnatally acquired disease can be as lethal as that acquired during delivery through an infected birth canal. Oropharyngeal or cutaneous lesions can be an effective source of virus. It is unlikely that breastfeeding will lead to neonatal infection; however, if the mother has an obvious lesion on the breast, breastfeeding is contraindicated. Because the herpes virus is transmitted through direct contact (eg, hand-to-mouth), neonatal infection may be acquired from family members other than the mother and from sites other than the genital tract (49, 50). Most strains of HSV responsible for nosocomial neonatal disease are HSV-1 rather than HSV-2. Mothers with active lesions should use caution when handling their babies.

Summary

The following recommendations are based on limited or inconsistent scientific evidence (Level B):

- Women with primary HSV during pregnancy should be treated with antiviral therapy.
- Cesarean delivery should be performed on women with first-episode HSV who have active genital lesions at delivery.
- For women at or beyond 36 weeks of gestation with a first episode of HSV occurring during the current pregnancy, antiviral therapy should be considered.

The following recommendations are based primarily on consensus and expert opinion (Level C):

- Cesarean delivery should be performed on women with recurrent HSV infection who have active genital lesions or prodromal symptoms at delivery.
- Expectant management of patients with preterm labor or preterm premature rupture of membranes and active HSV may be warranted.
- For women at or beyond 36 weeks of gestation who are at risk for recurrent HSV, antiviral therapy also may be considered, although such therapy may not reduce the likelihood of cesarean delivery.
- In women with no active lesions or prodromal symptoms during labor, cesarean delivery should not be performed on the basis of a history of recurrent disease.

References

1. Fleming DT, McQuillan GM, Johnson RE, Nahmias AJ, Aral SO, Lee FK. Herpes simplex virus type 2 in the United States, 1976 to 1994. N Engl J Med 1997;337: 1105–1111 (Level II-3)
2. Corey L, Spear PG. Infections with herpes simplex viruses. N Engl J Med 1986;314:686–691 (Level III)
3. Prober C, Corey L, Brown ZA, Hensleigh PA, Frenkel LM, Bryson YJ. The management of pregnancies complicated by genital infections with herpes simplex virus. Clin Infect Dis 1992;15:1031–1038 (Level III)
4. Mertz GL, Benedetti J, Ashley R, Selke SA, Corey L. Risk factors for the sexual transmission of genital herpes. Ann Intern Med 1992;116:197–202 (Level II-3)
5. Whitley RJ, Hutto C. Neonatal herpes simplex virus infections. Pediatr Rev 1985;7:119–126 (Level III)
6. Frenkel LM, Garratty EM, Shen JP, Wheeler N, Clark O, Bryson YJ. Clinical reactivation of herpes simplex virus type 2 infection in seropositive pregnant women with no history of genital herpes. Ann Intern Med 1993;118: 414–418 (Level II-3)
7. Hensleigh PA, Andrews WW, Brown Z, Greenspoon J, Yasukawa L, Prober CG. Genital herpes during pregnancy: inability to distinguish primary and recurrent infections clinically. Obstet Gynecol 1997;89:891–895 (Level III)
8. Koelle DM, Benedetti J, Langenberg A, Corey L. Asymptomatic reactivation of herpes simplex virus in women after the first episode of genital herpes. Ann Intern Med 1992;116:433–437 (Level II-3)
9. Mertz GL. Epidemiology of genital herpes infections. Infect Dis Clin North Am 1993;7:825–839 (Level III)
10. Brock BV, Selke S, Benedetti J, Douglas JM Jr, Corey L. Frequency of asymptomatic shedding of herpes simplex virus in women with genital herpes. JAMA 1990;263:418–420 (Level III)
11. Prober CG. Herpetic vaginitis in 1993. Clin Obstet Gynecol 1993;36:177–187 (Level III)
12. Wald A, Zeh J, Selke S, Ashley RL, Corey L. Virologic characteristics of subclinical and symptomatic genital herpes infections. N Engl J Med 1995;333:770–775 (Level II-3)
13. Hirsch MS. Herpes simplex virus. In: Mandell GL, Bennett JE, Dolin R, eds. Mandell, Douglas and Bennett's principles and practice of infectious diseases. 4th ed. New York: Churchill Livingstone, 1995:1336–1345 (Level III)
14. Whitley R, Arvin A, Prober C, Corey L, Burchett S, Plotkin S. Predictors of morbidity and mortality in neonates with herpes simplex infections. The National Institute of Allergy and infectious Diseases Collaborative Antiviral Study Group. N Engl J Med 1991;324:450–454 (Level III)
15. Mertz GJ, Schmidt O, Jourden JL, Guinan ME, Remington ML, Fahnlander A. Frequency of acquisition of first-episode genital infection with herpes simplex virus from symptomatic and asymptomatic source contacts. Sex Transm Dis 1985;12:33–39 (Level III)
16. Kulhanjian JA, Soroush V, Au DS, Bronzan RN, Yasukawa LL, Weylman LE. Identification of women at unsuspected risk of primary infection with herpes simplex virus type 2 during pregnancy. N Engl J Med 1992;326: 916–920 (Level II-3)

17. Brown ZA, Benedetti J, Ashley R, Burchett S, Selke S, Berry S. Neonatal herpes simplex virus infection in relation to asymptomatic maternal infection at the time of labor. N Engl J Med 1991;324:1247–1252 (Level II-3)

18. Brown ZA, Selke S, Zeh J, Kopelman J, Maslow A, Ashley RL. The acquisition of herpes simplex virus during pregnancy. N Engl J Med 1997;337:509–515 (Level II-3)

19. Altshuler G. Pathogenesis of congenital herpesvirus infection: case report including a description of the placenta. Am J Dis Child 1974;127:427–429 (Level III)

20. Chalhub EG, Baenziger J, Feigen RD, Middlekamp JN, Shackelford GD. Congenital herpes simplex type II infection with extensive hepatic calcification bone lesions and cataracts: complete postmortem examination. Dev Med Child Neurol 1977;19:527–534 (Level III)

21. Monif GR, Kellner KR, Donnelly WH Jr. Congenital herpes simplex type II infection. Am J Obstet Gynecol 1985;152:1000–1002 (Level III)

22. Woods GL. Update on laboratory diagnosis of sexually transmitted diseases. Clin Lab Med 1995;15:665–684 (Level III)

23. Hardy DA, Arvin AM, Yasukawa LL, Bronzan RN, Lewinsohn DM, Hensleigh PA. Use of polymerase chain reaction for successful identification of asymptomatic genital infection with herpes simplex virus in pregnant women at delivery. J Infect Dis 1990;162:1031–1035 (Level III)

24. Boggess KA, Watts DH, Hobson AC, Ashley RL, Brown ZA, Corey L. Herpes simplex type 2 detection by culture and polymerase chain reaction and relationship to genital symptoms and cervical antibody status during the third trimester of pregnancy. Am J Obstet Gynecol 1997;176: 443–451 (Level III)

25. Cone RW, Hobson AC, Palmer J, Remington M, Corey L. Extended duration of herpes simplex virus DNA in genital lesions detected by the polymerase chain reaction. J Infect Dis 1991;164:757–760 (Level III)

26. Mosely RC, Corey L, Benjamin D, Winter C, Remington ML. Comparison of viral isolation, direct immunofluorescence, and indirect immunoperoxidase techniques for detection of genital herpes simplex virus infection. J Clin Microbiol 1981;13:913–918 (Level II-2)

27. Arvin AM, Hensleigh PA, Prober CG, Au DS, Yasukawa LL, Wittek AE. Failure of antepartum maternal cultures to predict the infant's risk of exposure to herpes simplex virus at delivery. N Engl J Med 1986;315:796–800 (Level II-3)

28. Goldberg LK, Kaufman R, Kurtz TO, Conant MA, Eron LJ, Batenhorst RL. Long-term suppression of recurrent genital herpes with acyclovir. A 5-year benchmark. Acyclovir Study Group. Arch Dermatol 1993;129:582–587 (Level I)

29. Scott LL, Sanchez PJ, Jackson GL, Zeray F, Wendel GD Jr. Acyclovir suppression to prevent cesarean delivery after first-episode genital herpes. Obstet Gynecol 1996;87: 69–73 (Level I)

30. Grover L, Kane J, Kravitz J, Cruz A. Systemic acyclovir in pregnancy: a case report. Obstet Gynecol 1985;65:284–287 (Level III)

31. Lagrew DC Jr, Furlow TG, Hager WD, Yarrish RL. Disseminated herpes simplex virus infection in pregnancy. Successful treatment with acyclovir. JAMA 1984;252: 2058–2059 (Level III)

32. Brown ZA, Baker DA. Acyclovir therapy during pregnancy. Obstet Gynecol 1989;3:526–531 (Level III)

33. Brockelhurst P, Kinghorn G, Carney O, Helsen K, Ross E, Ellis E, et al. A randomised placebo controlled trial of suppressive acyclovir in late pregnancy in women with recurrent genital herpes infection. Br J Obstet Gynaecol 1998; 105:275–280 (Level I)

34. Lavoie SR, Kaplowitz LG. Management of genital herpes infection. Semin Dermatol 1994;13:248–255 (Level III)

35. Mertz GJ, Critchlow CW, Benedetti J, Reichman RC, Dolin R, Connor J. Double-blind placebo-controlled trial of oral acyclovir in first-episode genital herpes simplex virus infections. JAMA 1984;252:1147–1151 (Level I)

36. Fife KH, Crumpacker CS, Mertz GJ, Hill EL, Boone GS. Recurrence and resistance patterns of herpes simplex virus following cessation of > or = 6 years of chronic suppression with acyclovir. Acyclovir Study Group. J Infect Dis 1994;169:1338–1341 (Level II-3)

37. Wald A, Zeh J, Barnum G, Davis LG, Corey L. Suppression of subclinical shedding of herpes simplex virus type 2 with acyclovir. Ann Intern Med 1996;124: 8–15 (Level I)

38. Centers for Disease Control and Prevention. 1998 guidelines for treatment of sexually transmitted diseases. MMWR Morb Mortal Wkly Rep 1998;47(RR-1):20–24 (Level III)

39. Pregnancy outcomes following systemic acyclovir exposure. June 1, 1984–June 30, 1993. MMWR Morb Mortal Wkly Rep 1993;42:806–809 (Level III)

40. Frenkel LM, Brown ZA, Bryson YJ, Corey L, Unadkat JD, Hensleigh PA, et al. Pharmacokinetics of acyclovir in the term human pregnancy and neonate. Am J Obstet Gynecol 1991;164:569–576 (Level II-2)

41. Randolph AG, Washington E, Prober CG. Cesarean delivery for women presenting with genital herpes lesions. Efficacy, risks, and costs. JAMA 1993;270:77–82 (Decision Analysis)

42. Roberts SW, Cox SM, Dax J, Wendel GD Jr, Leveno KJ. Genital herpes during pregnancy: no lesions, no cesarean. Obstet Gynecol 1995;85:261–264 (Level II-2)

43. Wittek AE, Yeager AS, Au DS, Hensleigh PA. Asymptomatic shedding of herpes simplex virus from the cervix and lesion site during pregnancy. Correlation of antepartum shedding with shedding at delivery. Am J Dis Child 1984;138:439–442 (Level II-3)

44. Nahmias AJ, Josey WE, Naib ZM, Freeman MG, Fernandez RJ, Wheeler JH. Perinatal risk associated with maternal genital herpes simplex virus infection. Am J Obstet Gynecol 1971;110:825–837 (Level II-3)

45. National Institutes of Health. Consensus Development Conference Statement. Effect of corticoids for fetal maturation on perinatal outcomes, February 28–March 2, 1994. Am J Obstet Gynecol 1995;173:246–252 (Level III)

46. Amann ST, Fagnant RJ, Chartrand SA, Monif GR. Herpes simplex infection with short-term use of a fetal scalp electrode. A case report. J Reprod Med 1992;37:372–374 (Level III)

47. Golden SM, Merenstein GB, Todd WA, Hill JM. Disseminated herpes simplex neonatorum: a complication of fetal monitoring. Am J Obstet Gynecol 1977;129:917–918 (Level III)

48. Goldkrand JW. Intrapartum inoculation of herpes simplex virus by fetal scalp electrode. Obstet Gynecol 1982;59: 263–265 (Level III)

49. Douglas J, Schmidt O, Corey L. Acquisition of neonatal HSV-1 infection from a paternal source contact. J Pediatr 1983;103:908–910 (Level III)

50. Hammerberg O, Watts J, Chernesky M, Luchsinger I, Rawls W. An outbreak of herpes simplex virus type 1 in an intensive care nursery. Pediatr Infect Dis J 1983;2:290–294 (Level III)

The MEDLINE database was used to conduct a literature search to locate relevant articles published between January 1985 and December 1998. The search was restricted to articles published in the English language. Priority was given to articles reporting results of original research, although review articles and commentaries also were consulted. Abstracts of research presented at symposia and scientific conferences were not considered adequate for inclusion in this document. Guidelines published by organizations or institutions such as the National Institutes of Health and the American College of Obstetricians and Gynecologists were reviewed, and additional studies were located by reviewing bibliographies of identified articles. When reliable research was not available, expert opinions from obstetrician–gynecologists were used.

Studies were reviewed and evaluated for quality according to the method outlined by the U.S. Preventive Services Task Force:

- I Evidence obtained from at least one properly designed randomized controlled trial.
- II-1 Evidence obtained from well-designed controlled trials without randomization.
- II-2 Evidence obtained from well-designed cohort or case–control analytic studies, preferably from more than one center or research group.
- II-3 Evidence obtained from multiple time series with or without the intervention. Dramatic results in uncontrolled experiments also could be regarded as this type of evidence.
- III Opinions of respected authorities, based on clinical experience, descriptive studies, or reports of expert committees.

Based on the highest level of evidence found in the data, recommendations are provided and graded according to the following catetories:

Level A—Recommendations are based on good and consistent scientific evidence.

Level B—Recommendations are based on limited or inconsistent scientific evidence.

Level C—Recommendations are based primarily on consensus and expert opinion.

ISSN 1099-3630

The American College of
Obstetricians and Gynecologists
409 12th Street, SW
PO Box 96920
Washington, DC 20090-6920

12345/32109

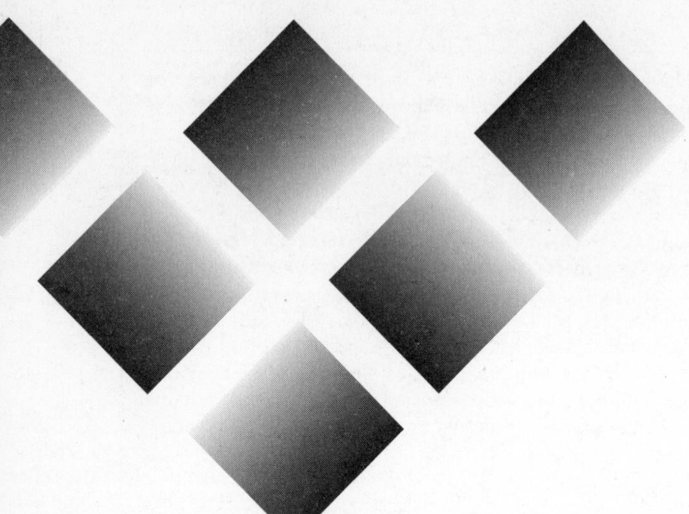

ACOG PRACTICE BULLETIN

CLINICAL MANAGEMENT GUIDELINES FOR OBSTETRICIAN–GYNECOLOGISTS

NUMBER 11, DECEMBER 1999

(Replaces Technical Bulletin Number 184, September 1993)

This Practice Bulletin was developed by the ACOG Committee on Practice Bulletins—Gynecology with the assistance of Kamran S. Moghissi, MD and Craig A. Winkel, MD. The information is designed to aid practitioners in making decisions about appropriate obstetric and gynecologic care. These guidelines should not be construed as dictating an exclusive course of treatment or procedure. Variations in practice may be warranted based on the needs of the individual patient, resources, and limitations unique to the institution or type of practice.

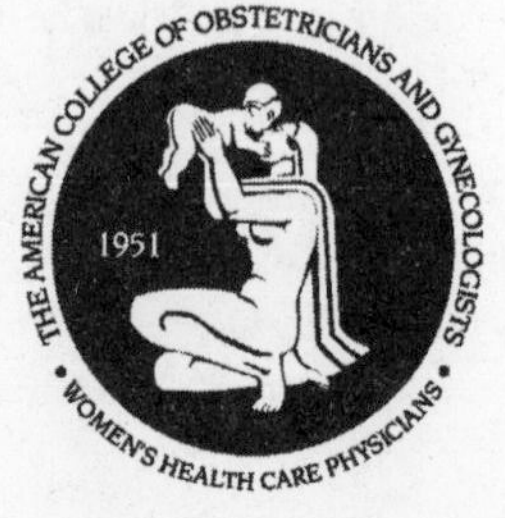

Medical Management of Endometriosis

Endometriosis represents a significant health problem for women of reproductive age. Defined as the presence of endometrial-like glands and stroma in any extrauterine site, endometriosis continues to defy our complete understanding regarding etiology, the relationship between extent of disease and the degree of symptoms, its relationship to fertility, and the most appropriate means of therapy. The purpose of this document is to present the evidence, including risks and benefits, for the effectiveness of medical therapy for women who experience symptoms and problems believed to be secondary to endometriosis.

Background

Incidence

Endometriosis is a gynecologic condition that occurs in 7–10% of women in the general population and up to 50% of premenopausal women (1), with a prevalence of 38% (range, 20–50%) (2–4) in infertile women, and in 71–87% of women with chronic pelvic pain (5–7). Contrary to much speculation, there are no data to support the view that the incidence of endometriosis is increasing, although improved recognition of endometriosis lesions (8) may have led to an increase in the rate of detection. There also appears to be no particular racial predisposition to endometriosis.

A familial association of endometriosis has been documented (9), and patients with an affected first-degree relative have nearly a 10-fold increased risk of developing endometriosis. The proposed inheritance is characteristic of a polygenic-multifactorial mechanism.

Etiology

Although the pathogenesis of endometriosis remains unclear, leading theories include retrograde menstruation, hematogenous or lymphatogenous transport, and coelomic metaplasia. It has been suggested that virtually all women are potentially vulnerable to the development of the lesions of endometriosis, but appropriate immunocompetency in most eradicates such lesions in a timely fashion, preventing clinical sequelae (10). Menstrual flow that produces a greater volume of retrograde menstruation may increase the risk of developing endometriosis. Cervical or vaginal atresia with outflow obstruction also is linked with the development of endometriosis (11). Early menarche, regular cycles (especially without intervening pregnancy-induced amenorrhea), and a longer and heavier than normal flow are associated with this disease (12). Because endometriosis is an estrogen-dependent disease, factors that reduce estrogen levels, such as exercise-induced menstrual disorders, decreased body-fat content, and tobacco smoking, are associated with reduced risk of developing endometriosis (12).

Clinical Manifestations

The clinical manifestations of endometriosis are variable and unpredictable in both presentation and course. Dysmenorrhea, chronic pelvic pain, dyspareunia, uterosacral ligament nodularity, and adnexal mass (either symptomatic or asymptomatic) are among the most well-recognized manifestations (13–16). A significant number of women with endometriosis remain asymptomatic.

The association between endometriosis and infertility remains the subject of considerable debate. It is clear that endometriosis may induce infertility as a result of anatomic distortion secondary to invasive endometriosis and related adhesions. Although it was previously believed that patients with minimal and mild endometriosis displayed reduced monthly fecundity rates (17), a cause-and-effect relationship has not been proven, and more recent prospective controlled trials suggest that minimal to mild endometriosis is not associated with reduced fecundity (18) and may not be a direct cause of infertility (19).

Pelvic pain that is typical of endometriosis is characteristically described as secondary dysmenorrhea (with pain frequently commencing prior to the onset of menses), deep dyspareunia (exaggerated during menses), or sacral backache with menses. Endometriosis that involves specific organs may result in pain or physiologic dysfunction of those organs, such as perimenstrual tenesmus or diarrhea in cases of bowel involvement or dysuria and hematuria in cases of bladder involvement.

The pain associated with endometriosis has little relationship to the type or location of the lesions that are visible at laparoscopy (20). Surgical assessment is complicated by the varying, and subtle appearances of endometriosis (21, 22), and may be demonstrated histologically in a normal-appearing peritoneum (23, 24). It has been shown that the depth of infiltration of endometriosis lesions correlates best with pain severity (6, 25, 26). Systematic analysis of the source of pain in awake patients undergoing laparoscopy (sometimes referred to as "pain mapping") demonstrates that pain arises from stimulation of adjacent normal peritoneal surfaces that extend well beyond the visible lesions of endometriosis. This suggests that painful lesions are those involving peritoneal surfaces innervated by peripheral spinal nerves, rather than those innervated by the autonomic nervous system (20).

Diagnosis

Direct visualization confirmed by histologic examination, especially of lesions with nonclassical appearance (21, 22, 27), remains the standard for diagnosing endometriosis. The presence of two or more of the following histologic features is used as the threshold criteria for the diagnosis by a pathologist (28):

- Endometrial epithelium
- Endometrial glands
- Endometrial stroma
- Hemosiderin-laden macrophages

Visual inspection as the sole means for making the diagnosis of endometriosis requires an experienced surgeon who is familiar with the protean appearances of endometriosis. Experience is associated with increased diagnostic accuracy (8, 21, 22), but the correlation between visual inspection and histologic confirmation of the presence of endometriosis in biopsy specimens is imperfect (22). The finding of microscopic endometriosis in normal-appearing peritoneum (23, 24) exemplifies the inaccuracy of diagnosis by visualization alone. Peritoneal biopsy may be used for diagnosing questionable peritoneal lesions (22).

Because tissue confirmation of the diagnosis of endometriosis requires a surgical procedure, investigators have searched for a noninvasive alternative. The correlation between the presence of moderate and severe endometriosis and an increased concentration of CA 125 in serum has been known for more than 10 years (29). Although the specificity of CA 125 measurements had been reported to be greater than 85%, with sensitivities between 20% and 50% (30–33), the clinical utility of measuring CA 125 as a diagnostic marker for endometriosis appears to be limited. Determining the level of CA 125 in serum appears to be useful in detecting women with severe endometriosis but is of questionable value in detecting women with minimal or mild disease (34, 35).

Measurement of peritoneal fluid levels, however, appears to be better for detecting minimal and moderate disease (34).

Concentrations of CA 125 in serum also have been studied as a marker to determine the response to medical therapy for endometriosis. Although CA 125 levels may decrease during treatment when compared with pretreatment values (36–38), posttreatment values that are normal do not confirm the absence of endometriosis (36, 38), nor are they useful for predicting disease recurrence (37).

Imaging studies, such as ultrasonography, magnetic resonance imaging, and computed tomography, appear to be useful only in the presence of a pelvic or adnexal mass. Ovarian endometriomas, visualized ultrasonographically, typically appear as cysts that contain low-level, homogeneous internal echoes consistent with old blood. Imaging studies alone appear to have greater predictive accuracy in differentiating ovarian endometriomas from other adnexal masses than when used in combination with measurement of CA 125 levels in plasma (39). Magnetic resonance imaging may detect deeply infiltrating endometriosis that involves the uterosacral ligaments and the cul-de-sac, but lacks sensitivity in detecting rectal involvement (40).

American Society for Reproductive Medicine
Revised Classification of Endometriosis

Patient's name ______________ Date ______________

Stage I (minimal) — 1–5
Stage II (mild) — 6–15
Stage III (moderate) — 16–40
Stage IV (severe) — >40

Laparoscopy_____ Laparotomy _____ Photography _____
Recommended treatment ______________

Total ______________

Prognosis ______________

		<1 cm	1–3 cm	>3 cm
Peritoneum	Endometriosis			
	Superficial	1	2	4
	Deep	2	4	6
Ovary	R Superficial	1	2	4
	Deep	4	16	20
	L Superficial	1	2	4
	Deep	4	16	20

	Partial	Complete
Posterior cul-de-sac obliteration	4	40

		<1/3 Enclosure	1/3–2/3 Enclosure	>2/3 Enclosure
	Adhesions			
Ovary	R Filmy	1	2	4
	Dense	4	8	16
	L Filmy	1	2	4
	Dense	4	8	16
Tube	R Filmy	1	2	4
	Dense	4*	8*	16
	L Filmy	1	2	4
	Dense	4*	8*	16

*If the fimbriated end of the fallopian tube is completely enclosed, change the point assignment to 16. Denote appearance of superficial implant types as red [(R), red, red-pink, flamelike, vesicular blobs, clear vesicles], white [(W), opacifications, peritoneal defects, yellow-brown], or black [(B), black, hemosiderin deposits, blue]. Denote percent of total described as R__%, W__%, and B__%. Total should equal 100%.

Figure 1. Modified from the revised American Fertility Society classification of endometriosis. (Reprinted with permission from the American Society for Reproductive Medicine. Fertility and Sterility 1996;67(5):819–820)

Classification

Numerous classification schemas have been proposed to describe endometriosis by anatomic location and severity of disease. The American Society for Reproductive Medicine (ASRM [formerly the American Fertility Society]) classification, which is the most commonly used system, was revised for the third time in 1996 (41) (see Figure 1) but still has limitations and inherent defects. The system is not a good predictor of pregnancy following treatment despite adjustments to the point scores and cut-points for disease stage. The ASRM system does not correlate well with the symptoms of pain and dyspareunia (6). The true value of the ASRM 1996 revised system is in uniform recording of operative findings and perhaps for comparing the results of various therapies.

Clinical Considerations and Recommendations

▶ ***In women with endometriosis-related pain who desire future fertility, how does medical therapy compare with no therapy for the treatment of pain and long-term preservation of fertility potential?***

Deeply infiltrating endometriosis, rather than surface noninfiltrating endometriosis, is commonly associated with pelvic pain (6). At present, evidence suggests that pain associated with endometriosis can be reduced with the use of a variety of medications (progestins, danazol, oral contraceptives, nonsteroidal antiinflammatory drugs, and gonadotropin-releasing hormone [GnRH] agonists) (42–47). There is also evidence that such medical therapies are likely to reduce the size of endometriosis lesions and, thus, the stage of disease (42, 48, 49). There are no data, however, showing that medical therapy eradicates the lesions. Although medical treatment may eliminate the symptoms associated with endometriosis, there is no evidence that such treatment has an impact on the future fertility of women with endometriosis. Because early-stage endometriosis is more likely to be associated with pain symptoms without associated alterations in fecundity, it is unlikely that such data will be forthcoming. Furthermore, whereas infiltrating lesions of endometriosis are associated with pain, studies are lacking that suggest the absence of treatment is associated with a progressive or future decline in fertility.

In a woman with normal or minor gynecologic findings suggesting mild disease (pelvic tenderness, uterosacral nodularity), ovarian suppression with a combination oral contraceptive may be effective in reducing pain (50). The efficacy of continuous administration of oral contraceptives compared with cyclic administration has not been tested in a prospective fashion. Oral contraceptives probably should not be used for more than 3 months if the patient experiences no relief of symptoms. Furthermore, there is no reason to suspect that one oral contraceptive is better than another for suppression of pain symptoms. If recurrent symptoms do not respond to oral contraceptives, then therapy with medroxyprogesterone acetate (MPA), danazol, or a GnRH agonist may be appropriate.

Danazol, when used in doses of 600–800 mg per day appears to as effective as GnRH agonists for pain relief in most patients, but is associated with a significantly greater incidence of side effects (51). The cost of treatment with danazol is about one third less than treatment with a GnRH agonist but nearly twice as costly as treatment with oral contraceptives and oral or depot MPA.

▶ ***In women with endometriosis-related pain who desire future fertility, how does medical therapy compare with surgical therapy alone for the management of pain and long-term preservation of fertility potential?***

The debate regarding medical treatment versus surgical treatment for the management of pain related to endometriosis continues despite of the lack of substantive data on either side of the argument. Surgical therapy for women with endometriosis is associated with a significant reduction in pain symptoms during the first 6 months following surgery (52). With continued follow-up, however, a substantial portion (44%) of women experience recurrence of symptoms within 1 year postoperatively (53). The cumulative recurrence rate of pain symptoms during the initial 5 years following discontinuation of therapy with a GnRH agonist is 53% (54). No evidence exists regarding the effectiveness of adjunctive treatment with danazol, oral contraceptives, or progestins in comparison with surgical treatment alone in the management of endometriosis-related pelvic pain. A major issue in considering comparisons of surgical treatment with medical treatment is the experience and expertise of the surgeon.

Likewise, debate continues over the best means of surgical therapy. One opinion considers vaporization or cautery of peritoneal implants adequate, whereas the other recommends surgical excision as necessary for adequate treatment (55). Currently, there are limited data to show that one method is better than the other. Moreover, there are no data regarding whether surgical therapy influences long-term fertility. Also, no data exist to indicate whether medical or surgical treatments result in the best fertility outcomes.

▶ *Following surgical diagnosis of endometriosis, what is the role of surgical destruction of lesions, or medical therapy in conjunction with surgery, for long-term pain relief in patients with minimal to moderate endometriosis that has been completely resected?*

It is probably impossible to completely resect all endometriosis lesions, if for no other reason than in up to 25% of biopsies of normal-appearing peritoneum one will find histologic evidence of endometriosis (23, 24). In addition, even when experienced surgeons attempt to resect completely a deeply infiltrating lesion, histologic study often reveals that the lesion is incompletely resected (26).

Operative laparoscopy for surgical treatment of pelvic pain related to endometriosis appears to have numerous advantages over laparotomy. These include more rapid recovery, the potential to decrease postoperative adhesion formation (56), and complication rates of 10% with laparoscopy (57). Although technical difficulties can be overcome partially through skill and experience, the efficacy of surgical therapy still depends heavily on the surgeon. Regardless of the technique employed—excision, endocoagulation, electrocautery, or laser vaporization—no study demonstrates the superiority of any one method, and recurrence rates average 19% (58). For successful surgical treatment, considering the varied appearances of endometriosis, the challenge lies in the surgeon's ability to recognize all visible lesions.

The only prospective, double-blind, randomized, controlled trial designed to evaluate the effectiveness of laparoscopic surgery for women with pelvic pain was reported in 1994 (52). Of the women who underwent laser ablation of endometriosis and laser uterosacral nerve ablation, 62% experienced pain relief 6 months after surgery, compared with 22% who underwent laparoscopic visualization only (52). If one considers the results of this study and a number of retrospective analyses, it appears that surgical treatment alone will confer pain relief in approximately two thirds of women for up to 1 year.

Postoperative medical treatment could be useful when residual disease is expected, when pain is not relieved, or to extend the pain-free interval following surgery. Although not demonstrated on the basis of clinical studies available at present, postoperative treatment should minimize the risk of recurrence. Two studies support the use of postoperative GnRH agonists to extend the period of pain relief. In a randomized, controlled trial of an intranasal GnRH agonist, 31% of women who received the GnRH agonist following laparoscopy needed additional medical treatment 18 months following surgery, whereas 57% of the women who received placebo required additional medical suppression (59).

The efficacy of other hormonal therapy in conjunction with surgery for treating women with endometriosis remains unclear. Oral MPA has been shown to induce regression of endometriosis lesions. One study has demonstrated that depot MPA is safe and effective in reducing pain associated with endometriosis (45). Importantly, depot MPA confers contraception during therapy while the use of low-dose danazol (200–400 mg) to reduce the dose-related side effects may not prevent conception and thus exposes the patient to the potential for teratogenesis. A combination of low-dose danazol and oral contraceptives appears to offer a similar degree of efficacy while providing effective contraception (45).

Few reports have examined the use of danazol as an adjunct to surgical therapy. It appears that danazol treatment for 3 months following laparoscopic surgery for women with Stage III and Stage IV endometriosis offers no advantage over expectant management with regard to pain recurrence (60).

▶ *Following surgical diagnosis of endometriosis, what is the role of surgical destruction of lesions, or medical therapy in conjunction with surgery, for long-term pain relief in patients with severe endometriosis with residual disease present?*

The recurrence rates for endometriosis appear to correlate with severity of disease (54), with a recurrence rate over a 7-year period following medical treatment of 37% for women with mild disease and 74% for women with severe disease. Although one might conclude that postoperative medical treatment would make sense for the woman with severe endometriosis with residual disease, there are no data documenting the efficacy of this therapy. In most cases, studies of the efficacy of postoperative medical treatment specifically address those patients with minimal to moderate disease, excluding those with severe endometriosis. Treatment with a GnRH agonist prior to laparoscopic surgery was associated with a higher fecundity rate within the first year following surgery than with preoperative danazol or gestrinone (61). However, such therapy was not associated with a reduction in operating time or any decrease in recurrence rate 1 year after surgery for ovarian endometriomata (62). For women with severe endometriosis, with or without suspected residual disease, the efficacy of either preoperative or postoperative medical therapy has yet to be established.

▶ *In women receiving a 3–6-month regimen of GnRH analog therapy for treatment of endometriosis-related pelvic pain, what are the advantages and disadvantages of an "add-back" regimen?*

Gonadotropin-releasing hormone agonists have been shown to be efficacious and safe for treating women with endometriosis-related pelvic pain (47, 49, 63–66). However, because these agents create a state of relative estrogen deficiency, their use has been limited generally to a 6-month course of therapy, particularly because of the potential effects on bone density, as well as the side effects, most notably vasomotor symptoms.

To minimize both the loss of bone and side effects, add-back regimens (using either sex-steroid hormones or other specific bone-sparing agents) have been advocated for use in women undergoing long-term therapy (ie, >6 months). Such treatment strategies have included progestins alone (67–69), progestins and organic bisphosphonates (70), low-dose progestins and estrogens (71,72), pulsatile parathyroid hormone (73), and nasal calcitonin (74). Although there are no published studies specifically designed to compare the various add-back regimens, virtually all add-back regimens (except nasal calcitonin) have considerable efficacy in reducing the loss of bone mineral density associated with GnRH agonist treatment. Some regimens appear to reduce vasomotor symptoms better than others; parathyroid hormone therapy has little effect on such symptoms.

The potential advantages of add-back therapy for women undergoing short-term (3–6 months) GnRH agonist therapy are twofold. First, while it has been shown that the bone loss after 3 months of treatment with a GnRH agonist is less than that after 6 months of treatment (69, 70, 72), add-back therapy does reduce the bone loss observed after only 3 months of GnRH agonist therapy (72). Add-back treatment does not diminish the efficacy of pain relief observed during 3 months or 6 months of GnRH agonist therapy. Second, add-back regimens that employ progestins alone (67–72) or in combination with estrogens (71, 72, 75) reduce significantly the vasomotor symptoms associated with GnRH agonist treatment. There appear to be no disadvantages to the use of an add-back regimen in combination with a GnRH agonist other than the incremental cost associated with the additional medication.

▶ *In women who have had a good response to GnRH therapy and who may benefit from an extended duration of therapy with add-back therapy (>6 months), what is the safety and efficacy of such long-term treatment?*

There are few data available on the use of GnRH agonists for more than 6 months. The major concern with prolonged use of GnRH agonists is the loss of bone mineral density that is observed during 6 months of therapy with these drugs (76). The mean loss of bone mineral density during a 6-month course of therapy with GnRH agonists ranges from 5.9% to 15% and may depend on the dose, route, and particular agonist being used (77). Marked individual differences in susceptibility to bone loss have been noted. Bone loss during a 6-month course of intranasal GnRH agonist was less than that observed with the intramuscular form (3% versus 5%) (78). Gonadotropin-releasing hormone agonists do not have adverse effects on triglyceride or cholesterol metabolism (79), as may be seen with danazol (80) or MPA (81).

A 12-month course of GnRH agonist therapy was associated with approximately a 6% decrease in bone density. The addition of norethindrone acetate alone or in combination with conjugated equine estrogens had no adverse impact on pain relief but did prevent bone mineral loss (44); there was also an associated increase in low-density lipoprotein cholesterol, a decrease in high-density lipoprotein cholesterol, and an increase in triglycerides. The clinical significance of these latter changes is unclear. Currently, there are no data regarding extended treatment with GnRH agonists beyond 1 year. Patients receiving this treatment should be monitored regularly for physical findings, bone density, and serum lipid parameters.

If the woman has previously undergone therapy with a GnRH agonist, it appears safe to retreat with a GnRH agonist alone provided there has been suitable time for recovery of bone mineral density since the previous course of treatment (82). If bone mineral density has not recovered fully, or if bone density has not been evaluated, the use of either a potent progestin or danazol is recommended. No studies have been reported to evaluate bone density after progestin administration following initial GnRH agonist therapy. Finally, a GnRH agonist in combination with add-back treatment may be considered, especially if the add-back regimen is commenced coincidentally with the reinitiation of therapy with the GnRH agonist. The long-term effects of multiple courses of treatment with a GnRH agonist have yet to be assessed.

▶ *In a woman with symptoms consistent with endometriosis, is empiric medical therapy (without definitive surgical diagnosis) an efficacious and cost-effective approach to pain relief?*

The need for laparoscopy (or any other surgical procedure) for diagnosis or treatment of pelvic pain secondary to suspected endometriosis has been the subject of debate (83). Arguments against the requirement to perform surgery to definitively diagnose endometriosis include the imprecision of surgical diagnosis as well as the inherent risks of surgery. "Empiric" therapy is used commonly in clinical gynecology when the signs and symptoms support the particular diagnosis being entertained and the consequences of an inaccurate diagnosis are likely to be minimal (eg, mild cystitis, suspected pelvic infection, and bacterial vaginosis).

In a woman with pelvic pain, diagnostic evaluation should include a thorough history and physical examination to rule out other gynecologic causes of pain, such as chronic pelvic inflammatory disease, leiomyomata uteri, and ovarian cysts. Nongynecologic causes of pain, such as gastrointestinal and urinary tract problems, may be ruled out by appropriate testing. Consideration also should be given to pelvic ultrasonography, complete blood count, urinalysis, and endocervical sampling for gonococcal and chlamydial infection if signs and symptoms warrant.

Based on a well-designed, prospective, randomized, controlled, double-blind clinical trial, the following statement can be made (7). After an appropriate pretreatment evaluation (to exclude other conditions) and failure of initial treatment with oral contraceptives and nonsteroidal antiinflammatory drugs, empiric therapy with a 3-month course of a GnRH agonist is appropriate. This approach is associated with clinically and statistically significant improvement in dysmenorrhea, pelvic pain, and pelvic tenderness. Furthermore, if the diagnostic algorithm described is employed prior to the initiation of empiric GnRH therapy, the likelihood of endometriosis being present on posttreatment laparoscopy is 78–87%. Thus, it appears that empiric treatment with a GnRH agonist (ie, without surgical diagnosis) is efficacious.

Comparing costs of empiric medical management versus definitive surgical diagnosis is more difficult to address. Although there are a lack of well-designed studies that compare the actual costs between the two approaches, it has been estimated that the cost of 3 months of empiric therapy is less than that of a laparoscopic procedure. No trials comparing primary medical and surgical therapies have been reported, nor have data been reported regarding the percentage of women who will still require surgical therapy following satisfactory empiric treatment.

▶ *In asymptomatic women in whom endometriosis is discovered incidentally, how does medical therapy compare with no intervention for long-term pain relief and preservation of fertility?*

The pathophysiology of endometriosis remains poorly understood. Largely because of failure to identify a suitable animal model, there is little systematic research regarding either the progression of the disease or the prediction of clinical outcomes. The presence of endometriosis among asymptomatic infertility patients varies between 20% and 50%, suggesting that it may not always be pathologic. In biopsies of apparently normal peritoneum, one can demonstrate the presence of endometrial glands and stroma in 25%, thus confirming the presence of endometriosis (23). In 50% of cases, endometriosis regresses spontaneously or remains constant (84). There are a number of obstacles, therefore, to predicting what the presence of endometriosis holds for a given woman. There are no data available regarding medical therapy for prevention of disease progression or for prevention of future pain.

Although preliminary data suggest that the destruction of all apparent lesions is associated with improved fecundity during the next 36 months (85), there are no data available on which to make a recommendation regarding medical therapy to prevent progression of disease or to prevent pain symptoms.

Endometriosis frequently is associated with infertility, although a cause-and-effect relationship between the two remains controversial. Essential steps in the development of endometriosis require a series of complex interactions between peritoneal leukocytes and endometrial cells, but the exact etiologic factor(s) remains unknown. In addition, both specific and nonspecific immunologic alterations are likely required. Whether these are the result or the cause of the disease also remains unclear. Although the pathophysiology of infertility arising from endometriosis that results in distortion of normal anatomy is relatively easy to understand, the mechanisms by which nonadhesive disease leads to infertility are still not clear.

There are no data to support the suggestion that medical treatment to prevent the progression of the disease will result in successful fertility in the future. It is not even clear whether fertility can be predicted based on the presence of endometriosis unless there is gross distortion of tubal and ovarian anatomy.

▶ ***In women with endometriosis-related pain who have completed childbearing, how does medical management compare with no therapy for long-term pain relief?***

The rates for recurrence of pain symptoms following medical or surgical treatment for endometriosis do not differ greatly. Following surgical therapy, about two thirds of patients experience recurrence of pain symptoms within 2 years of surgery (52, 56). However, the recurrence of pain symptoms may be delayed by the addition of 3 months of treatment with a GnRH agonist (59).

Medical therapy alone is likely to result in a significant pain-free interval following treatment with a GnRH agonist (54, 86) in the absence of surgical treatment. In addition, treatment with either oral contraceptives, danazol, or progestins has been shown to reduce, at least in the short term, pain symptoms associated with endometriosis (43, 45, 46). Currently, there are no follow-up data beyond 7 years after medical treatment. The long-term impact of medical therapy on pain recurrence beyond this period remains unclear.

▶ ***In a woman with pelvic pain arising from known endometriosis, does the presence of an ovarian endometrioma on ultrasound influence the efficacy or safety of employing medical therapy for pain relief?***

The reliability of ultrasonography for diagnosing endometriosis depends on the nature of the lesions. The endovaginal ultrasonographic approach appears to be superior to the transvesical approach for the evaluation of an ovarian mass. For the diagnosis of ovarian endometriomas, ultrasonography is reliable, with sensitivity up to 83% and specificity of 98% (87). Scattered internal echoes that tend to appear homogeneous are characteristic of endometriomas.

Gonadotropin-releasing hormone agonist treatment resulted in a greater than 25% reduction in the diameter of endometriomas for more than 80% of the women observed, compared with 30% of those treated with danazol (61). These authors did not report on the reduction in pain symptoms. Although it is theorized that preoperative medical treatment of the woman with an ovarian endometrioma might facilitate surgery by reducing inflammation and vascularity, there are no studies that address this practice. A 3-month preoperative course of a GnRH agonist has been reported to produce decreased cyst wall thickness and inflammation (88), but was not associated with either reduced operating time or reduced incidence of recurrence 1 year later (62). There is only anecdotal information regarding responses of suspected ovarian endometriomas to therapy with oral contraceptives or MPA. When medical treatment is used in a woman with an ovarian mass that is assumed to be an endometrioma, the potential for missed diagnosis or delay in diagnosis of a more serious condition (such as a malignant or borderline tumor) must always be kept in mind.

Because it is likely that the pain associated with endometriosis is most closely related to deeply infiltrating peritoneal disease rather than the ovarian endometrioma, medical therapy aimed at suppressing ovarian function is likely to result in a similar reduction in pain symptoms, whether or not there is a coincident ovarian endometrioma. There are no studies, however, of the efficacy of medical therapy for pain in the presence or absence of an endometrioma.

▶ ***In patients with pain or bleeding arising from known endometriosis affecting nonreproductive organs, what is the evidence for the efficacy of medical therapy for these symptoms?***

Extrapelvic endometriosis has been reported in a variety of sites, including the upper abdomen, the diaphragm, the abdominal wall (particularly the umbilicus), the perineum (episiotomy scar), and the thorax (89, 90). In addition, endometriosis may invade the full thickness of the rectum, large and small bowel, ureters, or bladder. The symptoms that are associated with endometriosis at these sites vary depending on location and depths of infiltration, including women who experience cyclic episodes of gross hematuria, hematochezia, and hemoptysis. Although a number of therapeutic approaches have been employed for women with presumed extrapelvic endometriosis (91), the efficacy of ovarian suppression with a GnRH agonist appears to support it as the first line of therapy (92, 93). Based on current available evidence, medical treatment appears to be efficacious for women with signs and symptoms of extrapelvic endometriosis provided other, potentially serious diseases have been excluded.

▶ ***In a woman who has undergone a total abdominal hysterectomy for definitive therapy for endometriosis, what is the risk of symptomatic recurrence with estrogen replacement therapy, and is there a role for suppressive therapy after total abdominal hysterectomy with bilateral salpingo-oophorectomy if there is residual disease?***

The rates of recurrence of endometriosis after initial conservative surgery tend to vary based on stage or extent of disease at the time of surgery. It is particularly difficult, however, to distinguish between recurrence and persistence of endometriosis. Recurrence rates range between 20% and 40% within 5 years after surgery for endometriosis (52, 53, 55, 94).

Hysterectomy, with or without bilateral oophorectomy, is often regarded as "definitive" therapy for the treatment of endometriosis associated with intractable pelvic pain, adnexal masses, or multiple previous conservative surgical procedures. Based on the results of a recently published retrospective analysis of women monitored for a mean duration of 58 months after hysterectomy, ovarian conservation was associated with a 62% likelihood of recurrent symptoms and a 31% chance of requiring additional surgical treatment (95). In women who underwent bilateral adnexectomy, there was a 10% chance of recurrence of symptoms with only a 4% likelihood of additional surgery (95). The relative risk for pain recurrence after total abdominal hysterectomy was found to be 6.1 (95% confidence interval: 2.5–14.6) with ovarian preservation when compared with women who have their ovaries removed. The relative risk of additional surgery was 8.1 (95% confidence interval: 2.1–31.3) with ovarian conservation (95).

Symptoms may recur in women even after hysterectomy and oophorectomy. Endometriosis may recur in up to 15% of women whether or not the patients are treated with estrogen replacement therapy following bilateral oophorectomy (96). Although the true rate of recurrence is unknown, among those patients in whom recurrent symptoms result in an additional surgical procedure, endometriosis lesions may be demonstrated. The most common site of recurrent lesions is the large and small bowel. It is not clear whether such lesions were present at the time of the oophorectomy and were overlooked or were not visualized because they were present only as microscopic disease in normal-appearing peritoneum.

After total abdominal hysterectomy with bilateral salpingo-oophorectomy, delayed initiation of estrogen replacement therapy has been thought to decrease the risk of recurrent symptoms. Furthermore, the possibility does exist that estrogen replacement therapy may support infiltration of endometriosis lesions and result in continued progression of the disease (97). Currently, there are limited data on which to base a recommendation. It appears there is no advantage, in terms of recurrence rate, in delaying introduction of estrogen treatment following surgery (96, 98). There is also a concern about the possibility of estrogen induced malignant transformation in residual endometriosis implants (99), which has led some to recommend the routine addition of a progestin to the estrogen therapy, although there are no outcomes-based evidence to support this recommendation.

Although limited data indicate hormone replacement therapy may stimulate the growth of residual ovarian or endometrial tissue after total abdominal hysterectomy, the overall benefits of hormone replacement (cardiovascular benefits, reduced risk of osteoporosis, relief of vasomotor symptoms) may outweigh these risks, and the decision should be individualized.

Summary

The following recommendations are based on good and consistent scientific evidence (Level A):

- For pain relief, treatment with a GnRH agonist for at least 3 months or with danazol for at least 6 months appears to be equally effective in most patients.
- When relief of pain from treatment with a GnRH agonist supports continued therapy, the addition of add-back therapy reduces or eliminates GnRH-induced bone mineral loss without reducing the efficacy of pain relief.

The following recommendations are based on limited or inconsistent scientific evidence (Level B):

- Therapy with a GnRH agonist is an appropriate approach to the management of the woman with chronic pelvic pain, even in the absence of surgical confirmation of endometriosis, provided that a detailed initial evaluation fails to demonstrate some other cause of pelvic pain.
- For pain relief, oral contraceptives and oral or depot MPA are effective in comparison with placebo and may be equivalent to other more costly regimens.
- Hormone replacement therapy with estrogen is not contraindicated following hysterectomy and bilateral salpingo-oophorectomy for endometriosis.

The following recommendations are based primarily on consensus and expert opinion (Level C):

- For severe endometriosis, medical treatment alone may not be sufficient.
- Because endometriosis often is unpredictable and may regress, expectant management may be appropriate in asymptomatic patients.

References

1. Wheeler JM. Epidemiology of endometriosis-associated infertility. J Reprod Med 1989;34:41–46 (Level III)
2. Rawson JM. Prevalence of endometriosis in asymptomatic women. J Reprod Med 1991;36:513–515 (Level III)
3. Strathy JH, Molgaard CA, Coulam CB, Melton LJ 3d. Endometriosis and infertility: a laparoscopic study of endometriosis among fertile and infertile women. Fertil Steril 1982;38:667–672 (Level II-2)
4. Verkauf BS. Incidence, symptoms, and signs of endometriosis in fertile and infertile women. J Fla Med Assoc 1987;74:671–675 (Level II-2)
5. Carter JE. Combined hysteroscopic and laparoscopic findings in patients with chronic pelvic pain. J Am Assoc Gynecol Laparosc 1994;2:43–47 (Level III)
6. Koninckx PR, Meuleman C, Demeyere S, Lesaffre E, Cornillie FJ. Suggestive evidence that pelvic endometriosis is a progressive disease, whereas deeply infiltrating endometriosis is associated with pelvic pain. Fertil Steril 1991;55:759–765 (Level III)
7. Ling FW. Randomized controlled trial of depot leuprolide in patients with chronic pelvic pain and clinically suspected endometriosis. Pelvic Pain Study Group. Obstet Gynecol 1999;93:51–58 (Level I)
8. Ripps BA, Martin DC. Endometriosis and chronic pelvic pain. Obstet Gynecol Clin North Am 1993;20:709–717 (Level III)
9. Cramer DW. Epidemiology of endometriosis. In: Wilson EA, ed. Endometriosis. New York: Alan R. Liss Inc, 1987:5–22 (Level III)
10. Vigano P, Vercellini P, Di Blasio AM, Colombo A, Candiani GB, Vignali M. Deficient antiendometrium lymphocyte-mediated cytotoxicity in patients with endometriosis. Fertil Steril 1991;56:894–899 (Level II-2)
11. Keltz MD, Berger SB, Comite F, Olive DL. Duplicated cervix and vagina associated with infertility, endometriosis, and chronic pelvic pain. Obstet Gynecol 1994;84: 701–703 (Level III)
12. Cramer DW, Wilson E, Stillman RJ, Berger MJ, Belisle S, Schiff I, et al. The relation of endometriosis to menstrual characteristics, smoking and exercise. JAMA 1986;255: 1904–1908 (Level II-2)
13. Adamson GD. Diagnosis and clinical presentation of endometriosis. Am J Obstet Gynecol 1990;162:568–569 (Level III)
14. Management of endometriosis in the presence of pelvic pain. The American Fertility Society. Fertil Steril 1993; 60:952–955 (Level III)
15. Luciano AA, Pitkin RM. Endometriosis: approaches to diagnosis and treatment. Surg Annu 1984;16:297–312 (Level III)
16. Muse K. Clinical manifestations and classification of endometriosis. Clin Obstet Gynecol 1988;31:813–822 (Level III)
17. Candiani GB, Vercellini P, Fedele L, Colombo A, Candiani M. Mild endometriosis and infertility: a critical review of epidemiologic data, diagnostic pitfalls, and classification limits. Obstet Gynecol Surv 1991;46:374–382 (Level III)
18. Berube S, Marcoux S, Langevin M, Maheux R. Fecundity of infertile women with minimal or mild endometriosis and women with unexplained infertility. Canadian Collaborative Group on Endometriosis. Fertil Steril 1998; 69:1034–1041 (Level II-2)
19. Ronnberg L. Endometriosis and infertility. Ann Med 1990;22:91–96 (Level III)
20. Demco L. Mapping the source and character of pain due to endometriosis by patient-assisted laparoscopy. J Am Assoc Gynecol Laparosc 1998;5:241–245 (Level III)
21. Martin DC, Hubert GD, Vander Zwaag R, el-Zeky FA. Laparoscopic appearances of peritoneal endometriosis. Fertil Steril 1989;51:63–67 (Level III)
22. Stripling MC, Martin DC, Chatman DL, Zwaag RV, Poston WM. Subtle appearance of pelvic endometriosis. Fertil Steril 1988;49:427–431 (Level III)
23. Murphy AA, Green WR, Bobbie D, dela Cruz ZC, Rock JA. Unsuspected endometriosis documented by scanning electron microscopy in visually normal peritoneum. Fertil Steril 1986;46:522–524 (Level III)
24. Redwine DB, Yocum LB. A serial section study of visually normal pelvic peritoneum in patients with endometriosis. Fertil Steril 1990;54:648–651 (Level III)
25. Koninckx PR, Martin DC. Deep endometriosis: a consequence of infiltration or retraction or possibly adenomyosis externa? Fertil Steril 1992;58:924–928 (Level III)
26. Koninckx PR, Oosterlynck D, D'Hooghe T, Meuleman C. Deeply infiltrating endometriosis is a disease whereas mild endometriosis could be considered a non-disease. Ann NY Acad Sci 1994;734:333–341 (Level III)
27. Jansen RP, Russell P. Nonpigmented endometriosis: clinical, laparoscopic, and pathologic definition. Am J Obstet Gynecol 1986;155:1154–1159 (Level III)
28. Pittaway DE. CA-125 in women with endometriosis. Obstet Gynecol Clin North Am 1989;16:237–252 (Level II-1)
29. Barbieri RL, Niloff JM, Bast RC Jr, Scaetzl E, Kistner RW, Knapp RC. Elevated serum concentrations of CA-125 in patients with advanced endometriosis. Fertil Steril 1986;45:630–634 (Level II-2)
30. Barbati A, Cosmi EV, Spaziani R, Ventura R, Montanino G. Serum and peritoneal fluid CA-125 in patients with endometriosis. Fertil Steril 1994;61:438–442 (Level II-2)
31. Franchi M, Beretta P, Zanaboni F, Donadello N, Ghezzi F. Use of serum CA125 measurement in patients with endometriosis. Ital J Gynaecol Obstet 1993;5:149–152 (Level III)
32. Moretuzzo RW, DiLauro S, Jenison E, Chen SL, Reindollar RH, McDonough PG. Serum and peritoneal lavage fluid CA-125 levels in endometriosis. Fertil Steril 1988;50:430–433 (Level II-2)

33. Pittaway DE, Fayez JA. The use of CA-125 in the diagnosis and management of endometriosis. Fertil Steril 1986; 46:790–795 (Level II-2)

34. Colacurci N, Fortunato N, DeFranciscis P, Fratta M, Cioffi M, Zarcone R, et al. A. Serum and peritoneal CA-125 levels as diagnostic test for endometriosis. Eur J Obstet Gynecol Reprod Biol 1996;66:41–43 (Level III)

35. Mol BW, Bayram N, Lijmer JG, Wiegerinck MA, Bongers MY, van der Veen F, Bossuyt PM. The performance of CA-125 measurement in the detection of endometriosis: a meta-analysis. Fertil Steril 1998;70:1101–1108 (Meta-analysis)

36. Chen FP, Soong YK, Lee N, Lo SK. The use of serum CA-125 as a marker for endometriosis in patients with dysmenorrhea for monitoring therapy and for recurrence of endometriosis. Acta Obstet Gynecol Scand 1998;77: 665–670 (Level III)

37. Ozaksit G, Caglar T, Cicek N, Kuscu E, Batioglu S, Gokmen O. Serum CA 125 levels before, during and after treatment for endometriosis. Int J Gynaecol Obstet 1995; 50:269–273 (Level III)

38. Takahashi K, Kijima S, Yoshino K, Shibukawa T, Kitao M. Serum CA 125 as a marker for patients with external endometriosis. Int J Fertil 1989;34:143–148 (Level II-2)

39. Guerriero S, Mais V, Ajossa S, Paoletti AM, Angiolucci M, Melis GB. Transvaginal ultrasonography combined with CA-125 plasma levels in the diagnosis of endometrioma. Fertil Steril 1996;65:293–298 (Level II-2)

40. Kinkel K, Chapron C, Balleyguier C, Fritel X, Dubuisson JB, Moreau JF. Magnetic resonance imaging characteristics of deep endometriosis. Hum Reprod 1999;14: 1080–1086 (Level III)

41. Revised American Society for Reproductive Medicine classification of endometriosis: 1996. Fertil Steril 1997; 67:817–821 (Level III)

42. Bergqvist A, Bergh T, Hogstrom L, Mattson S, Nordenskjold F, Rasmussen C. Effects of triptorelin versus placebo on the symptoms of endometriosis. Fertil Steril 1998;69:702–708 (Level I)

43. Bulletti C, Flamigni C, Polli V, Giacomucci E, Albonetti A, Negrini V, et al. The efficacy of drugs in the management of endometriosis. J Am Assoc Gynecol Laprosc 1996;3:495–501 (Level II-2)

44. Hornstein MD, Surrey ES, Weisberg GW, Casino LA. Leuprolide acetate depot and hormonal add-back in endometriosis: a 12-month study. Lupron Add-Back Study Group Obstet Gynecol 1998;91:16–24 (Level I)

45. Vercellini P, De Giorgi O, Oldani S, Cortesi I, Panazza S, Crosignani PG. Depot medroxyprogesterone acetate versus an oral contraceptive combined with very-low-dose danazol for long-term treatment of pelvic pain associated with endometriosis. Am J Obstet Gynecol 1996;175: 396–401 (Level I)

46. Vercellini P, Cortesi I, Crosignani PG. Progestins for symptomatic endometriosis: a critical analysis of the evidence. Fertil Steril 1997;68:393–401 (Critical Analysis)

47. Rock JA, Truglia JA, Caplan RJ. Zoladex (goserelin acetate implant) in the treatment of endometriosis: a randomized comparison with danazol. The Zoladex Endometriosis Study Group Obstet Gynecol 1993;82: 198–205 (Level I)

48. Wheeler JM, Knittle JD, Miller JD. Depot leuprolide acetate versus danazol in the treatment of women with symptomatic endometriosis: a multicenter, double-blind, randomized clinical trial. II. Assessment of safety. The Lupron Endometriosis Study Group. Am J Obstet Gynecol 1993;169:26–33 (Level I)

49. Zorn JR, Mathieson J, Risquez F, Comaru-Schally AM, Schally AV. Treatment of endometriosis with delayed release preparation of the agonist D-Trp6-luteinizing hormone-releasing hormone: long-term follow-up in a series of 50 patients. Fertil Steril 1990;53:401–406 (Level II-3)

50. Vercellini P, Trespidi L, Colombo A,Vendola N, Marchini M, Crosignani PG. A gonadotropin-releasing hormone agonist versus a low-dose oral contraceptive for pelvic pain associated with endometriosis. Fertil Steril 1993; 60:75–79 (Level I)

51. Telimaa S, Puolakka J, Ronnberg L, Kauppila A. Placebo-controlled comparison of danazol and high-dose medroxprogesterone acetate in the treatment of endometriosis. Gynecol Endocrinol 1987;1:13–23 (Level I)

52. Sutton CJ, Ewen SP, Whitelaw N, Haines P. Prospective, randomized, double-blind, controlled trial of laser laparoscopy in the treatment of pelvic pain associated with minimal, mild, and moderate endometriosis. Fertil Steril 1994;62:696–700 (Level I)

53. Sutton CJ, Pooley AS, Ewen SP, Haines P. Follow-up report on a randomized controlled trial of laser laparoscopy in the treatment of pelvic pain associated with minimal to moderate endometriosis. Fertil Steril 1997; 68:1070–1074 (Level I)

54. Waller KG, Shaw RW. Gonadotropin-releasing hormone analogues for the treatment of endometriosis: long-term follow-up. Fertil Steril 1993;59:511–515 (Level I)

55. Redwine DB. Conservative laparoscopic excision of endometriosis by sharp dissection: life table analysis of reoperation and persistent or recurrent disease. Fertil Steril 1991;56:628–634 (Level II-3)

56. Cook AS, Rock JA. The role of laparoscopy in the treatment of endometriosis. Fertil Steril 1991;55:663–680 (Level III)

57. Saidi MH, Vancaillie TG, White AJ, Sadler RK, Akright BD, Farhardt SA. Complications of major operative laparoscopy. A review of 452 cases. J Reprod Med 1996; 41:471–476 (Level III)

58. Revelli A, Modottii M, Ansaldi C, Massobrio M. Recurrent endometriosis: a review of biological and clinical aspects. Obstet Gynecol Surv 1995;50:747–754 (Level III)

59. Hornstein MD, Hemmings J, Yuzpe AA, Heinrichs WL. Use of nafarelin versus placebo after reductive laparoscopic surgery for endometriosis. Fertil Steril 1997;68: 860–864 (Level I)

60. Bianchi S, Busacca M, Agnoli B, Candiani M, Calia C, Vignali M. Effects of 3 month therapy with danazol after laparoscopic surgery for stage III/IV endometriosis: a randomized study. Hum Reprod 1999;14:1335–1337 (Level I)

61. Donnez J, Nisolle M, Clerckx F. Evaluation of preoperative use of danazol, gestrinone, lynestrenol, buserelin spray and buserelin implant, in the treatment of endometriosis associated infertility. In: Chadha DR, Buttram VC Jr eds. Current concepts in endometriosis. New York: Alan R. Liss, Inc, 1990:427–442 (Level II-2)

62. Muzii L, Marana R, Caruana P, Mancuso S. The impact of preoperative gonadotropin-releasing hormone agonist treatment in laparoscopic excision of ovarian endometriotic cysts. Fertil Steril 1996;65:1235–1237 (Level II-1)

63. Dlugi AM, Miller JD, Knittle J, Lupron Depot (leuprolide acetate for depot suspension) in the treatment of endometriosis: A randomized, placebo-controlled, double-blind study. Lupron Study Group. Fertil Steril 1990; 54:419–427 (Level I)

64. Henzl MR, Corson SL, Moghissi K, Buttram VC, Berqvist C, Jacobson J. Administration of nasal nafarelin as compared with oral danazol for endometriosis. A multicenter double-blind comparative clinical trial. N Engl J Med 1988;318:485–489 (Level I)

65. Hornstein MD, Yuzpe AA, Burry KA, Heinrichs LR, Buttram VC Jr, Orwoll ES. Prospective randomized double-blind trial of 3 versus 6 months of nafarelin therapy for endometriosis associated with pelvic pain. Fertil Steril 1995;63:955–962 (Level I)

66. Tummon IS, Pepping ME, Binor Z, Radwanska E, Dmowski WP. A randomized, prospective comparison of endocrine changes induced with intranasal leuprolide or danazol for treatment of endometriosis. Fertil Steril 1989;51:390–394 (Level I)

67. Cedars MI, Lu JK, Meldrum DR, Judd HL. Treatment of endometriosis with a long-acting gonadotropin-releasing hormone agonist plus medroxyprogesterone acetate. Obstet Gynecol 1990;75:641–645 (Level III)

68. Makarainen L, Ronnberg L, Kauppila A. Medroxyprogesterone acetate supplementation diminishes the hypoestrogenic side effects of gonadotropin-releasing hormone agonist without changing its efficacy in endometriosis. Fertil Steril 1996;65:29–34 (Level I)

69. Surrey ES, Judd HL. Reduction of vasomotor symptoms and bone mineral density loss with combined norethindrone and long-acting gonadotropin-releasing hormone agonist therapy of symptomatic endometriosis: a prospective randomized trial. J Clin Endocrinol Metab 1992; 75:558–563 (Level I)

70. Surrey ES, Fournet N, Voigt B, Judd HL. Effects of sodium etidronate in combination with low-dose norethindrone in patients administered a long-acting GnRH agonist. a preliminary report. Obstet Gynecol 1993;81: 581–586 (Level I)

71. Kiilholma P, Tuimala R, Kivinen S, Korhonen M, Hagman E. Comparison of the gonadotropin-releasing hormone agonist goserelin acetate alone versus goserelin combined with estrogen-progestin add-back therapy in the treatment of endometriosis. Fertil Steril 1995;64:903–908 (Level I)

72. Moghissi KS, Schlaff WD, Olive DL, Skinner MA, Yin H. Goserelin acetate (Zoladex) with or without hormone replacement therapy for the treatment of endometriosis. Fertil Steril 1998;69:1056–1062 (Level I)

73. Finkelstein JS, Klibanski A, Schaefer EH, Hornstein MD, Schiff I, Neer RM. Parathyroid hormone for the prevention of bone loss induced by estrogen deficiency. N Engl J Med 1994;331:1618–1623 (Level I)

74. Roux C, Pelissier C, Listrat V, Kolta S, Simonetta C, Guignard M, et al. Bone loss during gonadotropin releasing hormone agonist treatment and use of nasal calcitonin. Osteoporos Int 1995;5:185–190 (Level I)

75. Howell R, Edmonds DK, Dowsett M, Crook D, Lees B, Stevenson JC. Gonadotropin-releasing hormone analogue (goserelin) plus hormone replacement therapy for the treatment of endometriosis: a randomized controlled trial. Fertil Steril 1995;64:474–481 (Level I)

76. Fogelman I. Gonadotropin-releasing hormone agonists and the skeleton. Fertil Steril 1992;57:715–724 (Level III)

77. Dawood MY. Hormonal therapies for endometriosis: implications for bone metabolism. Acta Obstet Gynecol Scand 1994;159:22–34 (Level III)

78. Agarwal SK, Harmrang C, Henzl MR, Judd HL. Nafarelin vs. leuprolide acetate depot for endometriosis. Changes in bone mineral density and vasomotor symptoms. Nafarelin Study Group. J Reprod Med 1997;42:413–423 (Level I)

79. Lemay A, Brideau NA, Forest JC, Dodin S, Maheux R. Cholesterol fractions and apolipoproteins during endometriosis treatment by a gonadotrophin releasing hormone (GnRH) agonist implant or by danazol. Clin Endocrinol (Oxf)1991;35:305–310 (Level II-3)

80. Fahraeus L, Larsson-Cohn U, Ljungberg S, Wallentin L. Profound alterations of the lipoprotein metabolism during danazol treatment in premenopausal women. Fertil Steril 1984;42:52–57 (Level III)

81. Fahraeus L, Sydsjo A, Wallentin L. Lipoprotein changes during treatment of pelvic endometriosis with medroxyprogesterone acetate. Fertil Steril 1986;45:503–506 (Level III)

82. Hornstein MD, Yuzpe AA, Burry K, Buttram VC Jr, Heinrichs LR, Soderstrom RM, et al. Retreatment with nafarelin for recurrent endometriosis symptoms: efficacy, safety and bone mineral density. Fertil Steril 1997; 67:1013–1018 (Level III)

83. Howard FM. The role of laparoscopy in chronic pelvic pain: promises and pitfalls. Obstet Gynecol Surv 1993; 48:357–387 (Level III)

84. Wardle PG, Hull MG. Is endometriosis a disease? Baillieres Clin Obstet Gynaecol 1993;7:673–685 (Level III)

85. Marcoux S, Maheux R, Berube S. Laparoscopic surgery in infertile women with minimal or mild endometriosis. Canadian Collaborative Group on Endometriosis. N Engl J Med 1997;337:217–222 (Level I)

86. Canadian Consensus Conference on Endometriosis Chapter 2 Consensus Statements. J SOGC 1999;21: 471–473 (Level III)

87. Guerriero S, Mais V, Ajossa S, Paoletti AM, Angiolucci M, Labate F, et al. The role of endovaginal ultrasound in differentiating endometriomas from other ovarian cysts. Clin Exp Obstet Gynecol 1995;22:20–22 (Level III)

88. Donnez J, Nisolle M, Clerckx F, Casanas-Roux F, Saussoy P, Gillerot S. Advanced endoscopic techniques used in dysfunctional bleeding, fibroids and endometriosis, and the role of gonadotropin-releasing hormone agonist treatment. Br J Gynaecol 1994;101(Suppl 10):2–9 (Level III)

89. Shimizu I, Nakanishi R, Yoshino I, Yasumoto K. An endometrial nodule in the lung without pelvic endometriosis. J Cardiovasc Surg (Torino) 1998;39:867–868 (Level III)

90. Hughes ML, Bartholomew D, Paluzzi M. Abdominal wall endometriosis after amniocentesis. A case report. J Reprod Med 1997;42:597–599 (Level III)

91. Shek Y, De Lia JE, Pattillo RA. Endometriosis with a pleural effusion and ascites. Report of a case treated with nafarelin acetate. J Reprod Med 1995;40:540–542 (Level III)

92. Espaulella J, Armengol J, Bella F, Lain JM, Calaf J. Pulmonary endometriosis: conservative treatment with GnRH agonists. Obstet Gynecol 1991;78:535-537 (Level III)

93. Johnson WM 3d, Tyndal CM. Pulmonary endometriosis: treatment with danazol. Obstet Gynecol 1987;69:506–507 (Level III)

94. Wheeler JH, Malinak LR. Recurrent endometriosis: incidence, management, and prognosis. Am J Obstet Gynecol 1983;146:247–253 (Level III)

95. Namnoun AB, Hickman TN, Goodman SB, Gehlbach DL, Rock JA. Incidence of symptom recurrence after hysterectomy for endometriosis. Fertil Steril 1995;64:898–902 (Level III)

96. Redwine DB. Endometriosis persisting after castration: clinical characteristics and results of surgical management. Obstet Gynecol 1994;83:405–413 (Level III)

97. Lam AM, French M, Charnock FM. Bilateral ureteric obstruction due to recurrent endometriosis associated with hormone replacement therapy. Aust N Z J Obstet Gynaecol 1992;32:83–84 (Level III)

98. Hickman TN, Namnoun AB, Hinton EL, Zacur HA, Rock JA Timing of estrogen replacement therapy following hysterectomy with oophorectomy for endometriosis. Obstet Gynecol 1998;91:673–677 (Level II-3)

99. Gucer F, Pieber D, Arikan MG. Malignancy arising in extraovarian endometriosis during estrogen stimulation. Eur J Gynaecol Oncol 1998;19:39–41 (Level III)

The MEDLINE database, the Cochrane Library, and ACOG's own internal resources were used to conduct a literature search to locate relevant articles published between January 1985 and May 1999. The search was restricted to articles published in the English language. Priority was given to articles reporting results of original research, although review articles and commentaries also were consulted. Abstracts of research presented at symposia and scientific conferences were not considered adequate for inclusion in this document. Guidelines published by organizations or institutions such as the National Institutes of Health and the American College of Obstetricians and Gynecologists were reviewed, and additional studies were located by reviewing bibliographies of identified articles. When reliable research was not available, expert opinions from obstetrician–gynecologists were used.

Studies were reviewed and evaluated for quality according to the method outlined by the U.S. Preventive Services Task Force:

- I Evidence obtained from at least one properly designed randomized controlled trial.
- II-1 Evidence obtained from well-designed controlled trials without randomization.
- II-2 Evidence obtained from well-designed cohort or case–control analytic studies, preferably from more than one center or research group.
- II-3 Evidence obtained from multiple time series with or without the intervention. Dramatic results in uncontrolled experiments could also be regarded as this type of evidence.
- III Opinions of respected authorities, based on clinical experience, descriptive studies, or reports of expert committees.

Based on the highest level of evidence found in the data, recommendations are provided and graded according to the following catetories:

Level A—Recommendations are based on good and consistent scientific evidence.

Level B—Recommendations are based on limited or inconsistent scientific evidence.

Level C—Recommendations are based primarily on consensus and expert opinion.

ISSN 1099-3630

The American College of
Obstetricians and Gynecologists
409 12th Street, SW
PO Box 96920
Washington, DC 20090-6920

12345/32109

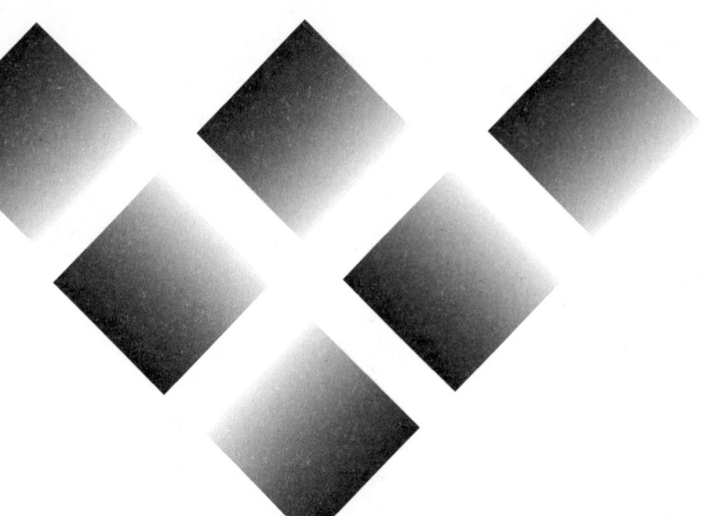

ACOG PRACTICE BULLETIN

CLINICAL MANAGEMENT GUIDELINES FOR OBSTETRICIAN–GYNECOLOGISTS

NUMBER 3, December 1998

(Replaces Technical Bulletin Number 150, December 1990)

This Practice Bulletin was developed by the ACOG Committee on Practice Bulletins—Gynecology with the assistance of Steven J. Ory, MD. The information is designed to aid practitioners in making decisions about appropriate obstetric and gynecologic care. These guidelines should not be construed as dictating an exclusive course of treatment or procedure. Variations in practice may be warranted based on the needs of the individual patient, resources, and limitations unique to the institution or type of practice.

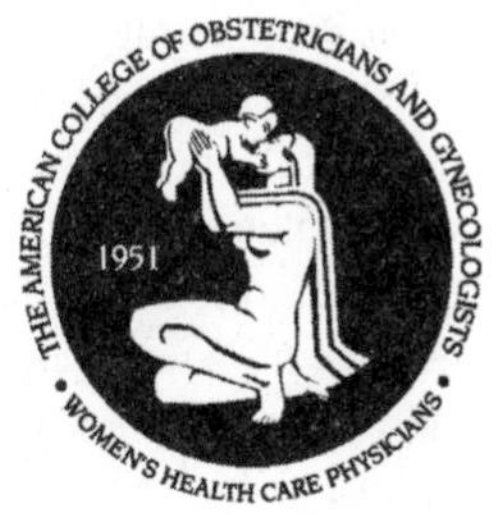

Medical Management of Tubal Pregnancy

Ectopic pregnancy is a major health problem for women of reproductive age and, in the United States, is the leading cause of pregnancy-related death during the first trimester. Diagnosis and treatment of tubal pregnancy before tubal rupture occurs decreases the risk of death. Early detection may make it possible for some patients to receive medical therapy instead of surgery. Methotrexate, a folinic acid antagonist, has been used to treat patients with small unruptured tubal pregnancies. The purpose of this document is to present evidence, including risks and benefits, about methotrexate as an alternative treatment for selected ectopic pregnancies.

Background

Incidence

The incidence of ectopic pregnancy has increased in the United States since 1970, the year the Centers for Disease Control (CDC; now the Centers for Disease Control and Prevention) first began collecting data, when the rate was 4.5 per 1,000 reported pregnancies. In 1992, there were an estimated 108,800 ectopic pregnancies, accounting for about 20 per 1,000 pregnancies and about 9% of all pregnancy-related deaths (1). Current data do not include conditions diagnosed and treated in physicians' offices; therefore, the true incidence of ectopic pregnancy is probably underestimated.

Etiology

Prior pelvic inflammatory disease, especially that caused by *Chlamydia trachomatis*, is the most important risk factor for ectopic pregnancy; observed odds ratios range from 2.0 to 7.5 (2). Other factors that appear to be associated with an increased risk of ectopic pregnancy include prior ectopic pregnancy, cigarette smoking, prior tubal surgery (especially for distal tubal disease), diethylstilbestrol exposure, and increasing age.

A history of infertility, independent of tubal disease, and ovulation induction also appear to be risk factors for ectopic pregnancy. Ectopic pregnancy is more likely to be diagnosed early in patients being treated for infertility. Such patients may be good candidates for medical therapy.

Effects of Therapy

Methotrexate is a folinic acid antagonist that inhibits dihydrofolic acid reductase, interfering with DNA synthesis, repair, and cellular replication. Actively proliferating tissue such as malignant cells, bone marrow, fetal cells, buccal and intestinal mucosa, and cells of the urinary bladder generally are more sensitive to these effects of methotrexate. Methotrexate has the potential for serious toxicity. Toxic effects usually are related to the amount and duration of therapy, but toxicity has been seen even with low doses. When methotrexate is used as a treatment for ectopic pregnancy, most reported side effects have been mild and self-limiting (3–12). This is probably a reflection of the lower dosage and shortened duration of treatment compared with dosages used in treating malignancies.

Diagnosis

Serial quantitative levels of the beta subunit of human chorionic gonadotropin (β-hCG) can be used in combination with transvaginal ultrasonography and, in some cases, suction curettage and serum progesterone measurements to differentiate failed intrauterine pregnancy, threatened abortion, and intrauterine or ectopic pregnancies. A presumptive diagnosis of unruptured tubal ectopic pregnancy is required before medical management can be considered.

Beta Subunit of Human Chorionic Gonadotropin

The mean plasma concentration of human chorionic gonadotropin (hCG) is significantly lower for an ectopic pregnancy than for a viable intrauterine pregnancy, but there is no definitive laboratory level permitting distinction between the two. A consistently declining hCG level indicates a nonviable pregnancy.

Conventionally, serial hCG testing to diagnose suspected ectopic pregnancy is performed at 48-hour intervals; a 66% or greater increase should be observed in a normal pregnancy. Approximately 15% of normal intrauterine pregnancies are associated with less than a 66% increase in hCG, and 17% of ectopic pregnancies have normal doubling times (13). Limitations of serial hCG testing include its inability to distinguish a failing intrauterine pregnancy from an ectopic pregnancy and the inherent 48-hour delay. A prospective study of asymptomatic patients described a 36% sensitivity and a 63–71% specificity (14). However, most reports and clinicians have found serial hCG testing useful in the early diagnosis of ectopic pregnancy. The rate of hCG doubling decreases from every 1.4–1.5 days in early pregnancy to every 3.3–3.5 days at 6–7 weeks of gestation, at which point the reliability of serial testing may be diminished.

The elimination of hCG after treatment of ectopic pregnancy follows a two-phase distribution. The major elimination has a half-life of 5–9 hours and a second, longer phase has a half-life of 22–32 hours.

The quantitation of hCG has been complicated by the existence of three different reference standards for hCG assays, the existence of multiple antibodies in commercial assays, and confusing nomenclature. These complicating factors can cause varying and inconsistent results, both from one laboratory to another and within the same laboratory, and affect interpretation of the results and clinical management.

Ultrasonography

Transvaginal ultrasonography often can detect intrauterine pregnancy within 5 weeks of the last menstrual period. The concept of the discriminatory hCG zone, originally applied to transabdominal ultrasonography, is the range of serum hCG concentration above which a normal intrauterine gestation can be visualized consistently. When the hCG level exceeds the discriminatory zone, the absence of an intrauterine gestational sac is suggestive of ectopic pregnancy, but this also can occur with multiple gestation or failed intrauterine pregnancy. The specific discriminatory zone varies with the hCG assay chosen, the reference standard with which it is calibrated, and the available ultrasound resolution. Findings also may be compromised by obesity, fibroids, and the axis of the uterus. An intrauterine gestational sac in a normal uterus usually can be seen with transvaginal ultrasonography when the hCG level is between 1,000 to 2,000 mIU/mL (1st and 2nd International Reference Preparation or IRP) (15, 16). If the precise gestational age is known, as in the case of patients receiving hCG for ovulation induction or oocyte retrieval, the failure to detect a gestational sac 24 days or later after conception is presumptive evidence of an abnormal pregnancy (13).

Historically, detection of an intrauterine sac has led to the presumptive exclusion of ectopic pregnancy, based on the estimate of the incidence of heterotopic pregnancy of 1 in 30,000. This figure was calculated almost 50 years ago by multiplying the incidence of ectopic pregnancy by that of dizygotic twinning, thus producing a hypothetical estimate. The incidence of heterotopic pregnancy appears to have increased with the use of assisted reproductive techniques. It has been reported to be as high as 1% in some series (17), although the overall incidence of heterotopic pregnancy is probably much lower.

The identification of an ectopic gestational sac is diagnostic of ectopic pregnancy, but it is not seen in all cases. Sensitivity and specificity of transvaginal ultrasonography to identify ectopic pregnancy vary according to criteria used for diagnosis. Reported sensitivity of transvaginal ultrasonography ranges from 20.1% to 84% and specificity from 98.9% to 100%, depending on the criteria applied (18). Color flow Doppler may aid in the diagnosis of ectopic pregnancy; however, it requires considerably greater technical expertise (19, 20).

Serum Progesterone

Some clinicians maintain that measurement of serum progesterone levels may be useful for distinguishing viable intrauterine pregnancies from spontaneous abortions and ectopic pregnancies, but serum progesterone levels cannot distinguish ectopic pregnancy from spontaneous abortion (21). There is no single progesterone value that will definitively confirm the viability or nonviability of an intrauterine pregnancy or the presence of an ectopic pregnancy. Serum progesterone levels increase during pregnancy (22). If the duration of the pregnancy is unknown, interpretation of the test results is less reliable. The use of ovulation-induction agents is associated with higher serum progesterone levels in intrauterine and ectopic pregnancies.

Of pregnant patients with serum progesterone values of less than 5 ng/mL, 85% have spontaneous abortions, 0.16% have viable intrauterine pregnancies, and 14% have ectopic pregnancies (23). Pregnant patients with serum progesterone levels between 20.0 and 24.9 ng/mL have ectopic pregnancies in 4% of cases; 2% of ectopic pregnancies occur with serum progesterone levels greater than 25 ng/mL. Most ectopic pregnancies (52%) are associated with serum progesterone levels between 10 and 20 ng/mL, thus limiting the clinical utility of this assessment (24).

The absence of products of conception on curettage in the presence of an elevated β-hCG level is evidence of a presumptive diagnosis of ectopic pregnancy. More rarely, gestational trophoblastic disease, nongestational choriocarcinoma, or an embryonal cell tumor may be the cause.

Success Rates

Success is defined as resolution of the ectopic pregnancy without surgical intervention. Reported success rates range from 67% to 100%, with a median of 84% for the single-dose methotrexate regimen (3–12). The largest study involved 120 women and had an overall success rate of 94.1% (10). Variation in success rates may be affected by the selection criteria and differences in management. Of those cases with successful outcome, as many as 25% required more than one dose of methotrexate (3, 6, 8, 25).

Clinical Considerations and Recommendations

▶ ***Who are candidates for medical management?***

General factors to consider in determining candidates for medical therapy include the size of the ectopic mass, whether it has ruptured, and the desire for future fertility. Patients should be hemodynamically stable without active bleeding or signs of hemoperitoneum. Furthermore, they should be willing and able to return for follow-up care.

Criteria for Receiving Methotrexate

Absolute indications
- Hemodynamically stable without active bleeding or signs of hemoperitoneum
- Nonlaparoscopic diagnosis
- Patient desires future fertility
- General anesthesia poses a significant risk
- Patient is able to return for follow-up care
- Patient has no contraindications to methotrexate

Relative indications
- Unruptured mass ≤3.5 cm at its greatest dimension
- No fetal cardiac motion detected
- Patients whose β-hCG level does not exceed a predetermined value (6,000–15,000 mIU/mL)

Contraindications to Medical Therapy

Absolute contraindications
- Breastfeeding
- Overt or laboratory evidence of immunodeficiency
- Alcoholism, alcoholic liver disease, or other chronic liver disease
- Preexisting blood dyscrasias, such as bone marrow hypoplasia, leukopenia, thrombocytopenia, or significant anemia
- Known sensitivity to methotrexate
- Active pulmonary disease
- Peptic ulcer disease
- Hepatic, renal, or hematologic dysfunction

Relative contraindications
- Gestational sac ≥3.5 cm
- Embryonic cardiac motion

Absolute and relative indications and contraindications to medical therapy are shown in the boxes.

▶ *How is methotrexate used in the medical management of tubal ectopic pregnancy?*

Because injected methotrexate is a relatively new treatment for ectopic pregnancy, a standardized protocol has yet to be defined. There are small variations among the published protocols, but all share a basic strategy. The differences are in the amount of methotrexate given, the frequency of follow-up visits, and the types of tests and procedures routinely used to monitor treatment response.

Before methotrexate is injected, blood is drawn to determine baseline laboratory values for renal, liver, and bone marrow function, as well as to measure the β-hCG level. Progesterone also may be measured. Blood type, Rh factor, and the presence of antibodies should be determined. Patients who are Rh negative receive Rh immune globulin. The methotrexate dose usually is calculated according to estimated body surface area (50 mg/m^2) and is given in one dose. Treatment with a standard 75 mg dose (11) and multiple serial doses with a folinic acid rescue on alternate days (four doses of methotrexate [1.0 mg/kg] on days 0, 2, 4, and 6 and four doses of leucovorin [0.1 mg/kg] on days 1, 3, 5, and 7) (26, 27) also have been successful. Methotrexate is given either in divided doses, half into each buttock, or in one intramuscular injection (3–12).

Follow-up care continues until β-hCG levels are nondetectable. Time to resolution is variable and can be protracted, taking a month or longer (3, 5, 6, 9, 10, 12). With the single-dose regimen, levels of β-hCG usually increase during the first several days following methotrexate injection and peak 4 days after injection. If a treatment response is observed, hCG levels should decline by 7 days after injection (4, 10, 11). If the β-hCG level does not decline by at least 15% from day 4 to day 7, the patient may require either surgery (4), or a second dose of methotrexate if no contraindications exist (3, 5, 10–12). If there is an adequate treatment response, hCG determinations are reduced to once a week. An additional dose of methotrexate may be given if β-hCG levels plateau or increase in 7 days (6–10). Surgical intervention may be required for patients who do not respond to medical therapy. Ultrasound examination may be repeated to evaluate significant changes in clinical status, such as increased pelvic pain, bleeding, or inadequate declines of β-hCG levels (5, 6, 9, 10).

Side Effects Associated with Methotrexate Treatment

Drug side effects
- Nausea
- Vomiting
- Stomatitis
- Diarrhea
- Gastric distress
- Dizziness
- Severe neutropenia (rare)
- Reversible alopecia (rare)
- Pneumonitis

Treatment effects
- Increase in abdominal pain (occurs in up to two thirds of patients)
- Increase in β-hCG levels during first 1–3 days of treatment
- Vaginal bleeding or spotting

Signs of treatment failure and tubal rupture
- Significantly worsening abdominal pain, regardless of change in β-hCG levels
- Hemodynamic instability
- Levels of β-hCG that do not decline by at least 15% between day 4 and day 7 postinjection
- Increasing or plateauing β-hCG levels after the first week of treatment

▶ *What are the potential problems associated with medical management of ectopic pregnancy?*

Potential problems can be divided into three categories: 1) drug-related side effects, 2) treatment-related complications, and 3) treatment failure (see the box). If medical therapy fails, additional treatment is required; in case of tubal rupture, rapid surgical intervention is necessary. It is important, therefore, to monitor patients for signs and symptoms of tubal rupture and treatment failure.

During treatment, patients should be counseled to discontinue folinic acid supplements, including prenatal vitamins. Because of its potential toxicity, patients receiving methotrexate should be monitored carefully. Physicians using this drug should be aware of potential side effects and signs of toxicity and be advised to avoid the use of nonsteroidal antiinflammatory drugs.

An initial increase in β-hCG levels often occurs by the third day and is not a cause for alarm (4, 10, 11). Most patients experience at least one episode of increased abdominal pain sometime during treatment (5, 6, 9–11). Because abdominal pain also is suggestive of tubal rupture, care should be taken to evaluate any significant change in discomfort. The pain associated with resolution of tubal pregnancy usually can be distinguished from tubal rupture. It generally is milder, of limited duration (24–48 hours), and not associated with signs of an acute abdomen or hemodynamic instability.

Medical treatment has failed when β-hCG levels either increase or plateau by day 7 postinjection, indicating a continuing ectopic pregnancy, or when the tube ruptures. Tubal rupture may occur despite declining β-hCG levels (6, 9, 10).

▶ *How should patients be counseled about immediate and long-term effects of medical therapy?*

Patients should receive information about the types of side effects they may experience and about activity restrictions during treatment. They should be informed of the ongoing risk of tubal rupture during treatment; it is important to educate patients about symptoms of tubal rupture and emphasize the need to seek immediate medical attention if these symptoms occur (see the box).

It is difficult to assess the impact of methotrexate treatment for ectopic pregnancy on a woman's ability to conceive. Published evidence regarding conception rates following methotrexate administration is limited. One study reported a 20% conception rate among 15 women, with a mean follow-up time of 11.8 months (5). Another study reported a significantly greater conception rate of 79.6%, with a mean time to conception of 3.2 months (10); 12.8% of the conceptions were recurrent ectopic pregnancies. The impact of methotrexate on future fertility requires further study.

▶ *How cost-effective is methotrexate treatment?*

There is evidence that methotrexate therapy is a cost-effective treatment for small unruptured ectopic pregnancies when compared with laparoscopic salpingostomy. The direct cost advantages are due to elimination of operating room use, anesthesia services, and surgical fees. Indirect costs decrease as a result of quicker recovery times; however, the amount of savings depends on the proportion of patients eligible to receive medical therapy and the overall success rate. A study comparing direct costs of methotrexate with laparoscopic salpingostomy found there are significant savings if methotrexate is used as the primary therapy (28). An additional study looked retrospectively at patients treated for ectopic pregnancy and also found methotrexate was cost-effective (29).

Counseling Patients

Patients should be instructed on the following points:

- To expect to experience one or more side effects, including abdominal pain, vaginal bleeding or spotting, or medication side effects
- To contact the physician in the presence of sudden onset of severe abdominal pain; substantial increase in abdominal pain; heavy vaginal bleeding; or dizziness, syncope, or tachycardia
- To avoid alcoholic beverages, vitamins containing folic acid, nonsteroidal antiinflammatory drugs, and sexual intercourse until advised otherwise

▶ *Is there ever a role for expectant management?*

Distinguishing patients who are experiencing spontaneous resolution of their ectopic pregnancies from patients who have proliferating ectopic pregnancies and require active intervention is a clinical dilemma. In patients who are suspected to be undergoing spontaneous clinical resolution, expectant management is an option that has been used in the hope of avoiding therapy that might otherwise be unnecessary. Candidates for successful expectant management must be willing to accept the potential risks of tubal rupture and hemorrhage; they should be asymptomatic and have objective evidence of resolution (generally manifested by declining hCG levels). In general, patients with early, small tubal gestations with lower hCG levels are the best candidates for observant management. Approximately 20–30% of ectopic pregnancies are associated with declining hCG levels at the time of presentation (30). If the initial hCG level is less than 200 mIU/mL, 88% of patients experience spontaneous resolution. Lower success rates can be anticipated with higher hCG levels (31). Reasons for abandoning expectant management include intractable or significant increase in pain, failure of hCG levels to decrease, and tubal rupture with hemoperitoneum.

Summary

The following recommendations are based on limited or inconsistent scientific evidence (Level B):

- ▶ Intramuscular methotrexate is an appropriate method for treating selected patients with small, unruptured tubal pregnancies.*
- ▶ Successful treatment with methotrexate may require more than one dose of methotrexate.*
- ▶ Failure of β-hCG levels to decrease by at least 15% from day 4 to day 7 after methotrexate administration indicates the need for an additional dose of methotrexate or surgery.*

* Evidence is limited but consistent.

The following recommendation is based primarily on consensus and expert opinion (Level C):

▶ There may be a role for expectant management of hemodynamically stable patients with presumptive ectopic pregnancy in whom β-hCG levels are low (<200 mIU/mL) and declining.

References

1. Centers for Disease Control and Prevention. Ectopic pregnancy—United States, 1990–1992. MMWR Morb Mortal Wkly Rep 1995;44:46–48 (Level II-3)
2. Chow WH, Daling JR, Cates W Jr, Greenberg RS. Epidemiology of ectopic pregnancy. Epidemiol Rev 1987;9:70–94 (Level III)
3. Corsan GH, Karacan M, Qasim S, Bohrer MK, Ransom MX, Kemmann E. Identification of hormonal parameters for successful systemic single-dose methotrexate therapy in ectopic pregnancy. Hum Reprod 1995;10:2719–2722 (Level II-3)
4. Fernandez H, Bourget P, Ville Y, Lelaidier C, Frydman R. Treatment of unruptured tubal pregnancy with methotrexate: pharmacokinetic analysis of local versus intramuscular administration. Fertil Steril 1994;62:943–947 (Level I)
5. Glock JL, Johnson JV, Brumsted JR. Efficacy and safety of single-dose systemic methotrexate in the treatment of ectopic pregnancy. Fertil Steril 1994;62:716–721 (Level II-3)
6. Gross Z, Rodriguez JJ, Stalnaker BL. Ectopic pregnancy: nonsurgical, outpatient evaluation and single-dose methotrexate treatment. J Reprod Med 1995;40:371–374 (Level III)
7. Henry MA, Gentry WL. Single injection of methotrexate for treatment of ectopic pregnancies. Am J Obstet Gynecol 1994;171:1584–1587 (Level II-3)
8. Ransom MX, Garcia AJ, Bohrer M, Corsan GH, Kemmann E. Serum progesterone as a predictor of methotrexate success in the treatment of ectopic pregnancy. Obstet Gynecol 1994;83:1033–1037 (Level II-3)
9. Stika CS, Anderson L, Frederiksen MC. Single-dose methotrexate for the treatment of ectopic pregnancy: Northwestern Memorial Hospital three-year experience. Am J Obstet Gynecol 1996;174:1840–1846; discussion 1846–1848 (Level II-3)
10. Stovall TG, Ling FW. Single-dose methotrexate: an expanded clinical trial. Am J Obstet Gynecol 1993;168:1759–1765 (Level II-3)
11. Wolf GC, Nickisch SA, George KE, Teicher JR, Simms TD. Completely nonsurgical management of ectopic pregnancies. Gynecol Obstet Invest 1994;37:232–235 (Level II-3)
12. Yao M, Tulandi T, Falcone T. Treatment of ectopic pregnancy by systemic methotrexate, transvaginal methotrexate, and operative laparoscopy. Int J Fertil 1996;41:470–475 (Level II-3)
13. Kadar N, Caldwell BV, Romero R. A method of screening for ectopic pregnancy and its indications. Obstet Gynecol 1981;58:162–166 (Level II-2)
14. Shepherd RW, Patton PE, Novy MJ, Burry KA. Serial beta-hCG measurements in the early detection of ectopic pregnancy. Obstet Gynecol 1990;75:417–420 (Level III)
15. Fossum GT, Davajan V, Kletzky OA. Early detection of pregnancy with transvaginal ultrasound. Fertil Steril 1988;49:788–791 (Level II-3)
16. Goldstein SR, Snyder JR, Watson C, Danon M. Very early pregnancy detection with endovaginal ultrasound. Obstet Gynecol 1988;72:200–204 (Level II-3)
17. Svare J, Norup P, Grove Thomsen S, Hornnes P, Maigaard S, Helm P, et al. Heterotopic pregnancies after in-vitro fertilization and embryo transfer—a Danish survey. Hum Reprod 1993;8:116–118 (Level III)
18. Brown DL, Doubilet PM. Transvaginal sonography for diagnosing ectopic pregnancy: positivity criteria and performance characteristics. J Ultrasound Med 1994;13:259–266 (Level III)
19. Kirchler HC, Seebacher S, Alge AA, Muller-Holzner E, Fessler S, Kolle D. Early diagnosis of tubal pregnancy: changes in tubal blood flow evaluated by endovaginal color Doppler sonography. Obstet Gynecol 1993;82:561– 565 (Level II-2)
20. Pellerito JS, Troiano RN, Quedens-Case C, Taylor KJ. Common pitfalls of endovaginal color Doppler flow imaging. Radiographics 1995;15:37–47 (Level III)
21. Stovall TG, Ling FW, Carson SA, Buster JE. Serum progesterone and uterine curettage in differential diagnosis of ectopic pregnancy. Fertil Steril 1992;57:456–457 (Level III)
22. Stern JJ, Voss F, Coulam CB. Early diagnosis of ectopic pregnancy using receiver-operator characteristic curves of serum progesterone concentrations. Hum Reprod 1993;8:775–779 (Level III)
23. McCord ML, Muram D, Buster JE, Arheart KL, Stovall TG, Carson SA. Single serum progesterone as a screen for ectopic pregnancy: exchanging specificity and sensitivity to obtain optimal test performance. Fertil Steril 1996;66:513–516 (Level II-3)
24. Gelder MS, Boots LR, Younger JB. Use of a single random serum progesterone value as a diagnostic aid for ectopic pregnancy. Fertil Steril 1991;55:497–500 (Level II-2)
25. Lipscomb GH, Bran D, McCord ML, Portera JC, Ling FW. Analysis of three hundred fifteen ectopic pregnancies treated with single-dose methotrexate. Am J Obstet Gynecol 1998;178:1354–1358 (Level II-3)
26. Hajenius PJ, Engelsbel S, Mol BW, Van der Veen F, Ankum WM, Bossuyt PM, et al. Randomised trial of systemic methotrexate versus laparoscopic salpingostomy in tubal pregnancy. Lancet 1997;350:774–779 (Level I)
27. Stovall TG, Ling FW, Gray LA, Carson SA, Buster JE. Methotrexate treatment of unruptured ectopic pregnancy: a report of 100 cases. Obstet Gynecol 1991;77:749–753 (Level II-3)
28. Alexander JM, Rouse DJ, Varner E, Austin JM Jr. Treatment of the small unruptured ectopic pregnancy: a

cost analysis of methotrexate versus laparoscopy. Obstet Gynecol 1996;88:123–127 (Level III)

29. Creinin MD, Washington AE. Cost of ectopic pregnancy management: surgery versus methotrexate. Fertil Steril 1993;60:963–969 (Level II-2)

30. Shalev E, Peleg D, Tsabari A, Romano S, Bustan M. Spontaneous resolution of ectopic tubal pregnancy: natural history. Fertil Steril 1995;63:15–19 (Level II-3)

31. Korhonen J, Stenman UH, Ylöstalo P. Serum human chorionic gonadotropin dynamics during spontaneous resolution of ectopic pregnancy. Fertil Steril 1994;61:632–636 (Level III)

The MEDLINE database, the Cochrane Library, and ACOG's own internal resources and documents were used to conduct a literature search to locate relevant articles published between January 1985 and June 1998. The search was restricted to articles published in the English language. Priority was given to articles reporting results of original research, although review articles and commentaries also were consulted. Abstracts of research presented at symposia and scientific conferences were not considered adequate for inclusion in this document. Guidelines published by organizations or institutions such as the National Institutes of Health and the American College of Obstetricians and Gynecologists were reviewed, and additional studies were located by reviewing bibliographies of identified articles. When reliable research was not available, expert opinions from obstetrician–gynecologists were used.

Studies were reviewed and evaluated for quality according to the method outlined by the U.S. Preventive Services Task Force:

I Evidence obtained from at least one properly designed randomized controlled trial

II-1 Evidence obtained from well-designed controlled trials without randomization

II-2 Evidence obtained from well-designed cohort or case–control analytic studies, preferably from more than one center or research group

II-3 Evidence obtained from multiple time series with or without the intervention. Dramatic results in uncontrolled experiments could also be regarded as this type of evidence.

III Opinions of respected authorities, based on clinical experience, descriptive studies, or reports of expert committees

Based on the highest level of evidence found in the data, recommendations are provided and graded according to the following catetories:

Level A—Recommendations are based on good and consistent scientific evidence.

Level B—Recommendations are based on limited or inconsistent scientific evidence.

Level C—Recommendations are based primarily on consensus and expert opinion.

ISSN 1099-3630 12345/21098

The American College of Obstetricians and Gynecologists
409 12th Street, SW
PO Box 96920
Washington, DC 20090-6920

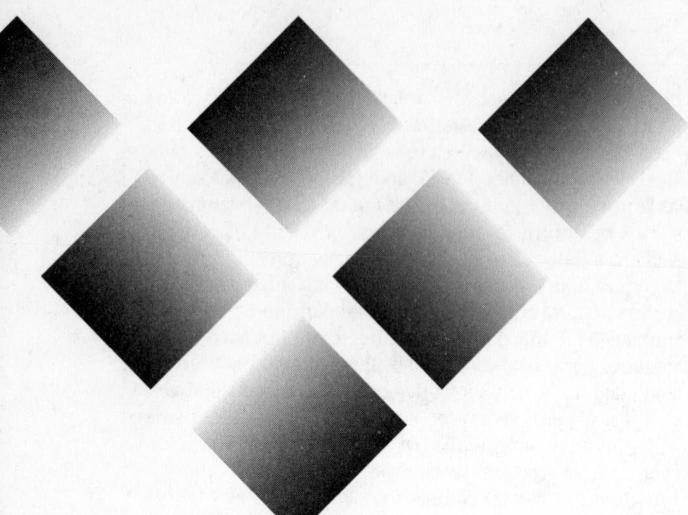

ACOG PRACTICE BULLETIN

CLINICAL MANAGEMENT GUIDELINES FOR OBSTETRICIAN–GYNECOLOGISTS

NUMBER 17, JUNE 2000

(Replaces Technical Bulletin Number 196, August 1994)

This Practice Bulletin was developed by the ACOG Committee on Practice Bulletins—Obstetrics with the assistance of Michael Belfort, MD. The information is designed to aid practitioners in making decisions about appropriate obstetric and gynecologic care. These guidelines should not be construed as dictating an exclusive course of treatment or procedure. Variations in practice may be warranted based on the needs of the individual patient, resources, and limitations unique to the institution or type of practice.

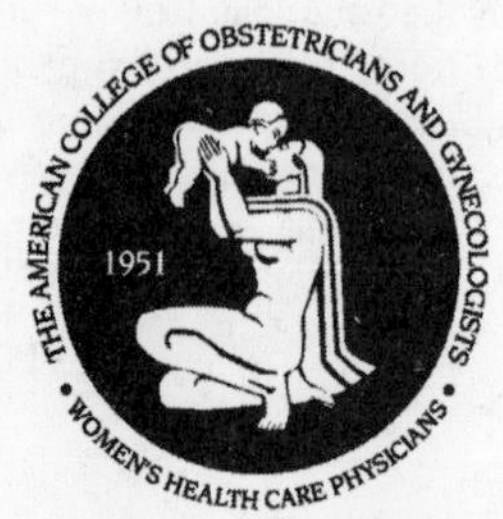

Operative Vaginal Delivery

The incidence of operative vaginal delivery in the United States is estimated to be 10–15% (1), and although these procedures are safe in appropriate circumstances, controversy about them persists. Recent reports have highlighted the potential for maternal and neonatal complications associated with operative vaginal delivery, although the risks associated with alternative procedures also must be considered. This document will address specific controversial issues about the use of forceps and vacuum extractors for operative vaginal delivery and present the available information on which to base decisions concerning their use. The technical aspects of the use of forceps and vacuum extractors are beyond the scope of this publication.

Background

Clinical studies performed before the 1970s suggested that the risk of fetal morbidity and mortality was higher when the second stage of labor exceeded 2 hours. Currently, more intensive intrapartum surveillance provides the ability to identify the fetus that may not be tolerating labor well. Thus, the length of the second stage of labor is not in itself an absolute or even strong indication for operative termination of labor. When other obstetric factors prevail, however, there is a place for forceps or vacuum-assisted operations.

Operative vaginal deliveries are accomplished by applying direct traction on the fetal skull with forceps, or by applying traction to the fetal scalp by means of a vacuum extractor. The indications for operative vaginal delivery performed with either the vacuum extractor or forceps are the same (see the box, "Indications for Operative Vaginal Delivery").

The rate of cesarean deliveries in the United States has declined from 22.8% in 1987 to 20.8% in 1997 (2). During the same period, the percentage of births delivered by forceps or vacuum extraction increased slightly, from 9.0% to 9.4% (2). Of this number, the percentage of forceps deliveries has decreased

Indications for Operative Vaginal Delivery

No indication for operative vaginal delivery is absolute. The following indications apply when the fetal head is engaged and the cervix is fully dilated.

- Prolonged second stage:
  - –Nulliparous women: lack of continuing progress for 3 hours with regional anesthesia, or 2 hours without regional anesthesia
  - –Multiparous women: lack of continuing progress for 2 hours with regional anesthesia, or 1 hour without regional anesthesia
- Suspicion of immediate or potential fetal compromise.
- Shortening of the second stage for maternal benefit.

and the percentage of vacuum extraction deliveries has increased. Although some authors have suggested that operative vaginal deliveries have been replaced by cesarean deliveries, the relationship remains unclear. Geographic differences in operative delivery rates have been reported, with the lowest rate in the northeast United States and the highest rate in the South.

In 1988, ACOG redefined the classification of station and types of forceps deliveries. The revised classification uses the level of the leading bony point of the fetal head in centimeters at or below the level of the maternal ischial spines to define station (0–5 cm), instead of the previously used method of describing the birth canal in terms of thirds (0–3+).

The definitions of types of forceps deliveries also were refined to avoid the inclusion of either trivial or extremely difficult deliveries under the category of midforceps (see the box, "Criteria for Types of Forceps Deliveries"). Before this reclassification, a rotational delivery from occiput posterior at 0 station was classified the same as a delivery from left occiput anterior on the perineum. In a validation of ACOG's reclassification, investigators demonstrated that the lower the fetal head and the less rotation required, the less the risk of injury to the mother and the child (3). Assessment of clinical pelvimetry and fetal position is important in predelivery evaluation (see the box, "Predelivery Considerations").

Clinical Issues

Complications of Operative Vaginal Delivery

General statements about the applicability of operative vaginal delivery and the procedures for implementation in a particular situation are difficult. Selection of the appropriate instrument and decisions about the potential maternal and fetal consequences should be based on clinical findings at the time of delivery. Research into the complications of operative vaginal delivery is hampered by a number of potential biases, including the level of experience of the operators, the small numbers of patients studied under similar circumstances, changes in practice and definition, and the inability to achieve statistical power to answer relevant questions. The following discussion is based on currently available evidence and attempts to address maternal and fetal complications associated with operative vaginal delivery.

In a randomized trial comparing elective low-forceps delivery with spontaneous vaginal delivery in 50 term patients, there were no significant immediate differences in maternal or neonatal outcome variables. The researchers did show that in the forceps group, the mean time to delivery was shorter (10.2 minutes versus 18 minutes) and the cord arterial pH was higher (7.27 versus 7.23) (4). However, a larger randomized study comparing outlet forceps delivery with spontaneous vaginal delivery in 333 women at term showed that, although the use of forceps had no immediate adverse effects on the neonate, there was no significant shortening of the second stage of labor. However, the incidence of maternal perineal trauma increased in primiparous women (5).

Criteria for Types of Forceps Deliveries

Outlet forceps

1. Scalp is visible at the introitus without separating labia.
2. Fetal skull has reached pelvic floor.
3. Sagittal suture is in anteroposterior diameter or right or left occiput anterior or posterior position.
4. Fetal head is at or on perineum.
5. Rotation does not exceed 45°.

Low forceps

Leading point of fetal skull is at station ≥ +2 cm and not on the pelvic floor.

Rotation is 45° or less (left or right occiput anterior to occiput anterior, or left or right occiput posterior to occiput posterior).

Rotation is greater than 45°.

Midforceps

Station is above +2 cm but head is engaged.

High forceps

Not included in classification.

Predelivery Considerations

Position: the relationship of the fetal presenting part to the maternal pelvis. In a cephalic presentation the designated point is the occiput, while in a breech presentation it is the sacrum. The position always is described in relation to the maternal left and right sides of the pelvis.

Presentation: the relationship between the leading fetal part and the maternal pelvic inlet. The fetus may have a cephalic, breech, or shoulder presentation.

Lie: the relationship between the fetal and maternal longitudinal axes, which may be longitudinal, oblique, or transverse.

Engagement: the relationship that is present when the widest diameter of the fetal presenting part (biparietal diameter in a cephalic presentation, and bitrochanteric diameter in a breech presentation) has passed beyond the plane of the maternal pelvic brim. In a cephalic presentation the head usually is engaged when the leading point of the skull is at or below the maternal ischial spines.

Asynclitism: the relationship between the anterior and posterior parietal bones and the sagittal suture with the maternal pelvis. When neither of the parietal bones precedes the sagittal suture, the head is synclitic; if the anterior parietal bone precedes the sagittal suture, there is anterior asynclitism; and when the posterior parietal bone precedes the sagittal suture, there is posterior asynclitism.

Clinical Pelvimetry: assessment of the maternal pelvis before performing midpelvic delivery.

A meta-analysis comparing vacuum extraction to forceps delivery showed that vacuum extraction was associated with significantly less maternal trauma and less need for general and regional anesthesia. Overall, fewer cesarean deliveries were carried out in the vacuum extractor group (6). Other studies comparing vacuum extraction to forceps delivery indicate that more maternal morbidity (soft tissue injury, discomfort) occurs with forceps delivery (7, 8).

Both forceps delivery and vacuum extraction have been associated with the development of maternal hematomas, (9) and possibly linked to pelvic floor injury. However, other factors associated with pelvic floor injury include normal spontaneous vaginal delivery, episiotomy, prolonged second stage of labor, and increased fetal size (10).

To evaluate the risk of operative vaginal delivery with suspected fetal macrosomia, one study compared 2,924 macrosomic infants (birth weight >4,000 g) to those with a birth weight between 3,000 g and 3,999 g. Macrosomic infants delivered by forceps had a sixfold higher rate of significant injury (relative risk = 6.7; confidence interval, 6.5–6.9). Forceps delivery in this situation also was associated with a fourfold risk of clinically persistent neurologic abnormalities when compared with spontaneous vaginal delivery or cesarean delivery. The overall incidence of persistent injury was low (0.3%), and the authors calculated that as many as 258 elective cesarean deliveries would have to be performed for macrosomia to prevent a single case of persistent injury (11). In addition, a randomized study of forceps and vacuum-assisted vaginal delivery identified three factors associated with the development of shoulder dystocia: use of vacuum device ($P = 0.04$), time required for delivery ($P = 0.03$), and birth weight ($P = 0.0001$) (12). Therefore, a trial of labor and judicious use of operative vaginal delivery techniques for macrosomic infants are not contraindicated, although caution should be used given the possibility of shoulder dystocia.

Potential Newborn Complications of Vacuum-Assisted Deliveries

With forceps, almost unlimited compression and traction can be applied to the fetal head and cervical spine. Vacuum extractors are designed to limit the amount of traction on the fetal skull because detachment can occur. Nevertheless, traction achieved with vacuum extraction is substantial (up to 50 lb) (13) and can result in significant fetal injury if misused. The vacuum cup can cause scalp lacerations if torsion is excessive. In addition, separation of the scalp from the underlying structures can lead to cephalohematoma, which is more common in infants delivered by vacuum extractor (14–16%) than in those delivered with forceps (2%) (6, 7). The incidence of subgaleal hematomas (collections of blood occurring in the potential space between the cranial periosteum and the epicranial aponeurosis) following vacuum deliveries is estimated to range from 26 to 45 per 1,000 vacuum deliveries (14, 15).

Other potential neonatal complications associated with vacuum deliveries include intracranial hemorrhage, hyperbilirubinemia, and retinal hemorrhage. The higher rates of neonatal jaundice associated with vacuum delivery may be related to the higher rate of cephalohematoma (16). There is a higher rate of retinal hemorrhages (38%) with vacuum delivery than with forceps delivery (17%) (6, 7, 17, 18). However, corneal abrasions and external ocular trauma are more common with forceps delivery than with normal spontaneous delivery and are rare with vacuum extraction unless the cup is inadvertently placed over the eye. Long-term sequelae are extremely rare, and ophthalmologic screening should be reserved for specific cases (18). Overall, the incidence of serious complications with vacuum extraction is approximately 5% (19). Given the maternal and neonatal risks associated with operative vaginal delivery, it is important that the patient be made aware of the potential complications of the proposed procedure.

In 1998, the U.S. Food and Drug Administration (FDA) released a Public Health Advisory to alert individuals that vacuum extractors may cause serious or fatal complications, including subgaleal (subaponeurotic) hematoma and intracranial hemorrhage (20). The FDA indicated that between 1994 and 1998, 12 deaths and nine serious injuries were reported among neonates on whom vacuum-assisted devices had been used. This rate was greater than five times the rate for the preceding 11 years. According to the advisory, data collected from 1989 to 1995 showed that use of the vacuum cup had increased from 3.5% to 5.9% of all deliveries. Among the FDA recommendations for use of the vacuum device, two are particularly useful:

1. Rocking movements or torque should not be applied to the device; only steady traction in the line of the birth canal should be used.
2. Clinicians caring for the neonate should be alerted that a vacuum device has been used so that they can adequately monitor the neonate for the signs and symptoms of device-related injuries.

A recent study evaluating the incidence of severe birth trauma following operative deliveries assessed the outcome of 83,340 singleton infants born to nulliparous women between 1992 and 1994 in California (21). A database was created linking birth and death certificates with hospital discharge records of maternal and neonatal outcomes. The lowest risk of fetal injury was found in infants delivered spontaneously. An intermediate risk was observed for those infants delivered by forceps or vacuum alone or by cesarean delivery during labor. The highest risk of fetal injury was reported for those infants who were delivered with combined forceps and vacuum extraction or who were delivered by cesarean following failed operative vaginal delivery. There was no difference in outcome between vacuum and forceps delivery versus cesarean delivery during labor (Table 1). The morbidity that previously had been thought to be due to operative vaginal delivery actually may have resulted from the process of abnormal labor that led to the need for intervention. The study population was large, but data were collected retrospectively from medical records and hospital discharge reports. Therefore, detailed information on the operative vaginal delivery, frequency of congenital anomalies, or number of infants readmitted following the initial discharge was not available. Despite its limitations, this study confirms that injury can occur before operative delivery as a result of abnormal labor forces and that not all neonatal injuries are the result of poor operative technique.

Table 1. Effect of Delivery on Neonatal Injury

Delivery Method	Death	Intracranial Hemorrhage	Other*
Spontaneous vaginal delivery	1/5,000	1/1,900	1/216
Cesarean delivery during labor	1/1,250	1/952	1/71
Cesarean delivery after vacuum/forceps	N/R	1/333	1/38
Cesarean delivery with no labor	1/1,250	1/2,040	1/105
Vacuum alone	1/3,333	1/860	1/122
Forceps alone	1/2,000	1/664	1/76
Vacuum and forceps	1/1,666	1/280	1/58

Abbreviation: N/R indicates not reported.

*Facial nerve/brachial plexus injury, convulsions, central nervous system depression, mechanical ventilation

Data from Towner D, Castro MA, Eby-Wilkens E, Gilbert WM. Effect of mode of delivery in nulliparous women on neonatal intracranial injury. N Engl J Med 1999;341:1709–1714

Long-Term Infant Consequences

One randomized comparison of vacuum versus forceps delivery that evaluated children at 9 months of age found no statistically significant differences between the two groups regarding head circumference, weight, head-circumference-to-weight ratio, hearing, or vision (22). The study did note that infants delivered with the vacuum device were more likely to have been readmitted with jaundice than were those delivered with forceps.

In another study, the effects of forceps delivery on cognitive development were examined in a cohort of 3,413 children. No significant differences were seen in the 1,192 children delivered with forceps (114 were midforceps), compared with the 1,499 delivered spontaneously (23). A 10-year matched follow-up evaluation of 295 children delivered by vacuum extractor and 302 control patients who had been delivered spontaneously at the same hospital revealed no differences between the two groups in terms of scholastic performance, speech, ability of self-care, or neurologic abnormality (24).

Clinical Considerations and Recommendations

▶ ***What are contraindications to operative vaginal delivery?***

Under certain circumstances, operative vaginal delivery should be avoided or, at the least, carefully considered in terms of relative maternal and fetal risk. Most authorities consider vacuum extraction inappropriate in pregnancies before 34 weeks of gestation because of the risk of fetal intraventricular hemorrhage. Operative delivery also is contraindicated if a live fetus is known to have a bone demineralization condition (eg, osteogenesis imperfecta), a bleeding disorder (eg, alloimmune thrombocytopenia, hemophilia, or von Willebrand's disease) is present, the fetal head is unengaged, or the position of the fetal head is unknown.

Operative vaginal delivery should be performed only by individuals with privileges for such procedures and in settings in which personnel are readily available to perform a cesarean delivery in the event the operative vaginal delivery is unsuccessful. One study showed that in cases in which the vacuum extractor was used to deliver fetuses with nonreassuring fetal heart rate patterns, blood gas parameters did not differ from those in cases with normal spontaneous deliveries. The authors concluded that the use of vacuum extraction is not contraindicated in cases of nonreassuring fetal heart rate patterns (25).

▶ ***Is there a role for a trial of operative vaginal delivery?***

Few studies address the issue of maternal and neonatal outcome after an unsuccessful attempt at operative delivery. Earlier published reports were small retrospective studies that suggested outcome was no worse after failed operative delivery (26, 27). In a recent report of 102 cases of failed instrument delivery, almost half (43%) of cases where a trial of operative vaginal delivery was attempted resulted in the need for cesarean delivery. Of those where success was expected, only 3% went on to cesarean delivery (28). In addition, the California study previously discussed demonstrated significantly higher incidences of intracranial hemorrhage and other birth trauma following a failed operative vaginal delivery (21). Unless the preoperative assessment is highly suggestive of a successful outcome, trial of operative vaginal delivery is best avoided.

▶ ***Is there a role for the use of alternative instruments after a failed attempt?***

Persistent efforts to obtain a vaginal delivery using different instruments may increase the potential for maternal and fetal injury and often indicates cephalopelvic disproportion. Although studies are limited, the weight of available evidence appears to be against attempting multiple efforts at operative vaginal delivery with different instruments, unless there is a compelling and justifiable reason (28). The California study reported that the incidence of intracranial hemorrhage was highest in infants delivered by combined vacuum and forceps compared with other reported methods of delivery (21). The incidences of other injuries also were increased with combined methods of operative vaginal delivery.

▶ ***What special equipment and techniques should be considered with the use of a vacuum extractor?***

Vacuum extractors differ substantially from the original metal cup and currently vary by material, cup size and shape, and the method of vacuum application to the fetal scalp (manual or automatic). The proliferation and increased use of these instruments have resulted in the development of a number of different techniques. Randomized trials comparing soft vacuum cups to the original metal cup indicate that the pliable cup is associated with decreased fetal scalp trauma but increased rates of detachment from the fetal head (29–32). However, there are no differences between Apgar scores, cord pH, neurologic outcome, retinal hemorrhage, maternal trauma, and blood loss (32). These findings support those of another study, which found a 22% incidence of significant fetal scalp trauma with the soft cup, as opposed to a 37% incidence with the metal cup. This study also concluded the soft cup was more likely to fail than the metal cup when excessive caput was present (29).

Data show that the use of rapid vacuum application leads to a reduction in time to delivery (33, 34). No differences in detachment from the fetal scalp or in maternal or neonatal morbidity between the two techniques have been noted (33, 34). Specifically, one randomized study of 94 women comparing a one-step rapid application of vacuum with conventional stepwise application of vacuum found a significant reduction in the time from application to delivery (6 minutes) in the rapid application group without any differences in maternal or neonatal morbidity (33).

Cephalohematoma has been shown to be more likely to develop as the duration of vacuum application increases. One study demonstrated that 28% of neonates in whom the application-to-delivery time exceeded 5 minutes developed cephalohematoma (35). A further technical issue that has raised questions is whether the vacuum should be reduced between contractions to prevent fetal scalp injury. A randomized controlled trial involving 322 patients at 34 weeks or more of gestation highlighted factors involved in the development of fetal cephalohematoma from vacuum extraction using the M-cup (a semirigid plastic cup, modeled after the Malmstrom cup). To prevent fetal loss of station, 164 patients had continuous vacuum application (600 mm Hg) during and between contractions as well as during active efforts at delivery. In the comparison group, 158 patients had intermittent suction (reduction of vacuum application to 100 mm Hg between contractions) and no effort to prevent loss of station between contractions. Time to delivery, method failure, maternal lacerations, episiotomy extension, incidence of cephalohematoma, and neonatal outcome were similar between the two groups. Overall, the efficacy of the vacuum cup was 93.5%, and the cephalohematoma rate was 11.5%. The authors concluded that there are no differences in maternal or fetal outcome with intermittent reduction in vacuum or attempts to prevent loss of station. They also concluded that the results obtained with the M-cup are comparable to those reported with the stainless-steel Malmstrom cup (36).

▶ ***Is there a role for midforceps rotational deliveries in current practice?***

The decrease in experienced teachers and the increase in medical–legal concerns have reduced the number of current practitioners skilled in the art of midcavity rotational delivery. Studies comparing midforceps and cesarean deliveries indicate that midforceps delivery is not associated with worse neonatal outcome (Apgar score, cord blood gas, neonatal intensive care admissions, birth trauma) than is cesarean delivery (37, 38). In addition, outcome appeared no worse for those infants in whom Kielland's forceps rotation was attempted but was unsuccessful (38). One retrospective analysis compared 358 midforceps deliveries with 486 cesarean deliveries and found maternal morbidity (intraoperative and postoperative complications, blood loss, and length of stay) to be higher in the cesarean delivery group (37). Another study reported similar findings in a 5-year retrospective study involving 253 patients (38).

A retrospective study compared 552 deliveries with Kielland's forceps rotation, 95 cases using Scanzoni maneuver with a different type of forceps, and 160 cases using manual rotation and forceps. Investigators found no significant differences in maternal or neonatal outcomes between the groups regardless of whether the indication was relative dystocia or nonreassuring fetal status (39). An earlier study found that Kielland's forceps rotation was associated with a higher incidence of neonatal trauma, although the analysis did not specify the indications for operative delivery (40).

There are no randomized controlled studies of long-term follow-up from which to draw conclusions. However, retrospective case–control analyses seem to indicate no differences in outcome between midforceps delivery and cesarean delivery or vacuum extraction (41, 42). A matched-pairs analysis of patients 2 years after a midforceps delivery compared with a group delivered via cesarean delivery (matched for the immediate indication for operative delivery, birth weight, gestational age, sex, and race) found no difference in abnormal outcomes between the groups (41). An 18-year follow-up study of males delivered by midcavity Kielland's forceps rotation did not show any late adverse effects when subjects were compared with males delivered by vacuum extractor (42). Thus, there appears to be a role for midforceps rotational deliveries in current practice. However, given the potential complications, this procedure is only for practitioners skilled in midforceps delivery and for cases where maternal and fetal assessment prior to the operation suggest a high chance of success.

Summary

The following recommendations are based on good and consistent scientific evidence (Level A):

- ▶ Both forceps and vacuum extractors are acceptable and safe instruments for operative vaginal delivery. Operator experience should determine which instrument should be used in a particular situation.
- ▶ The vacuum extractor is associated with an increased incidence of neonatal cephalohematomata, retinal hemorrhages, and jaundice when compared with forceps delivery.

The following recommendations are based on limited or inconsistent scientific evidence (Level B):

- ▶ Operators should attempt to minimize the duration of vacuum application, because cephalohematoma is more likely to occur as the interval increases.
- ▶ Midforceps operations should be considered an appropriate procedure to teach and to use under the correct circumstances by an adequately trained individual.
- ▶ The incidence of intracranial hemorrhage is highest among infants delivered by cesarean following a failed vacuum or forceps delivery. The combination of vacuum and forceps has a similar incidence of intracranial hemorrhage. Therefore, an operative vaginal delivery should not be attempted when the probability of success is very low.

The following recommendations are based primarily on consensus and expert opinion (Level C):

- Operative vaginal delivery is not contraindicated in cases of suspected macrosomia or prolonged labor; however, caution should be used because the risk of shoulder dystocia increases with these conditions.
- Neonatal care providers should be made aware of the mode of delivery in order to observe for potential complications associated with operative vaginal delivery.

References

1. Bofill JA, Rust OA, Perry KG, Roberts WE, Martin RW, Morrison JC. Operative vaginal delivery: a survey of fellows of ACOG. Obstet Gynecol 1996;88:1007–1010 (Level III)
2. Ventura SJ, Martin JA, Curtin SC, Mathews TJ. Births: final data for 1997. Natl Vital Stat Rep 1999;47(18):1–96 (Level II-3)
3. Hagadorn-Freathy AS, Yeomans ER, Hankins GD. Validation of the 1988 ACOG forceps classification system. Obstet Gynecol 1991;77:356–360 (Level II-2)
4. Carmona F, Martinez-Roman S, Manau D, Cararach V, Iglesias X. Immediate maternal and neonatal effects of low-forceps delivery according to the new criteria of The American College of Obstetricians and Gynecologists compared with spontaneous vaginal delivery in term pregnancies. Am J Obstet Gynecol 1995;173:55–59 (Level I)
5. Yancey MK, Herpolsheimer A, Jordan GD, Benson WL, Brady K. Maternal and neonatal effects of outlet forceps delivery compared with spontaneous vaginal delivery in term pregnancies. Obstet Gynecol 1991;78:646–650 (Level I)
6. Johanson RB, Menon BKV. Vacuum extraction versus forceps for assisted vaginal delivery (Cochrane Review). In: The Cochrane Library, Issue 4, 1999. Oxford: Update Software (Meta-analysis)
7. Dell DL, Sightler SE, Plauche WC. Soft cup vacuum extraction: a comparison of outlet delivery. Obstet Gynecol 1985;66:624–628 (Level I)
8. Johanson R, Pusey J, Livera N, Jones P. North Staffordshire/Wigan assisted delivery trial. Br J Obstet Gynaecol 1989;96:537–544 (Level I)
9. Gei AF, Belfort MA. Forceps-assisted vaginal delivery. Obstet Gynecol Clin North Am 1999;26:345–370 (Level III)
10. Handa VL, Harris TA, Ostergard DR. Protecting the pelvic floor: obstetric management to prevent incontinence and pelvic organ prolapse. Obstet Gynecol 1996;88:470–478 (Level III)
11. Kolderup LB, Laros RK Jr, Musci TJ. Incidence of persistent birth injury in macrosomic infants: association with mode of delivery. Am J Obstet Gynecol 1997;177:37–41 (Level II-2)
12. Bofill JA, Rust OA, Devidas M, Roberts WE, Morrison JC, Martin JN Jr. Shoulder dystocia and operative vaginal delivery. J Matern Fetal Med 1997;6:220–224 (Level I)
13. Moolgaoker AS, Ahamed SOS, Payne PR. A comparison of different methods of instrumental delivery based on electronic measurements of compression and traction. Obstet Gynecol 1979;54:299–309 (Level II-3)
14. Boo NY. Subaponeurotic haemorrhage in Malaysian neonates. Singapore Med J 1990;31:207–210 (Level II-3)
15. Govaert P, Defoort P, Wigglesworth JS. Cranial haemorrhage in the term newborn infant. Clin Dev Med 1993;129: 1–223 (Level III)
16. Vacca A, Grant A, Wyatt G, Chalmers I. Portsmouth operative delivery trial: a comparison of vacuum extraction and forceps delivery. Br J Obstet Gynaecol 1983;90: 1107–1112 (Level I)
17. Williams MC, Knuppel RA, O'Brien WF, Weiss A, Kanarek KS. A randomized comparison of assisted vaginal delivery by obstetric forceps and polyethylene vacuum cup. Obstet Gynecol 1991;78:789–794 (Level I)
18. Holden R, Morsman DG, Davidek GM, O'Connor GM, Coles EC, Dawson AJ. External ocular trauma in instrumental and normal deliveries. Br J Obstet Gynaecol 1992; 99:132–134 (Level II-2)
19. Robertson PA, Laros RK Jr, Zhao RL. Neonatal and maternal outcome in low-pelvic and midpelvic operative deliveries. Am J Obstet Gynecol 1990;162:1436–1442; discussion 1442–1444 (Level II-2)
20. Center for Devices and Radiological Health. FDA Public Health Advisory: need for caution when using vacuum assisted delivery devices. May 21, 1998. Available at http://www.fda.gov/cdrh/fetal598.html. Retrieved December 31, 1999 (Level III)
21. Towner D, Castro MA, Eby-Wilkens E, Gilbert WM. Effect of mode of delivery in nulliparous women on neonatal intracranial injury. N Engl J Med 1999; 341:1709–1714 (Level II-2)
22. Carmody F, Grant A, Mutch L, Vacca A, Chalmers I. Follow up of babies delivered in a randomized controlled comparison of vacuum extraction and forceps delivery. Acta Obstet Gynecol Scand 1986;65:763–766 (Level I)
23. Wesley BD, van den Berg BJ, Reece EA. The effect of forceps delivery on cognitive development. Am J Obstet Gynecol 1993;169:1091–1095 (Level II-2)
24. Ngan HY, Miu P, Ko L, Ma HK. Long-term neurological sequelae following vacuum extractor delivery. Aust N Z J Obstet Gynaecol 1990;30:111–114 (Level II-2)
25. Vintzileos AM, Nochimson DJ, Antsaklis A, Varvarigos I, Guzman ER, Knuppel RA. Effect of vacuum extraction on umbilical cord blood acid-base measurements. J Matern Fetal Med 1996;5:11–17 (Level II-2)
26. Revah A, Ezra Y, Farine D, Ritchie K. Failed trial of vacuum or forceps—maternal and fetal outcome. Am J Obstet Gynecol 1997;176:200–204 (Level II-3)
27. Boyd ME, Usher RH, McLean FH, Norman BE. Failed forceps. Obstet Gynecol 1986;68:779–783 (Level II-3)
28. Edozien LC, Williams JL, Chattopadhyay I, Hirsch PJ. Failed instrumental delivery: how safe is the use of a second instrument? J Obstet Gynaecol 1999;19:460–462 (Level III)

29. Chenoy R, Johanson R. A randomized prospective study comparing delivery with metal and silicone rubber vacuum extractor cups. Br J Obstet Gynaecol 1992;99:360–363 (Level I)

30. Cohn M, Barclay C, Fraser R, Zaklama M, Johanson R, Anderson D, et al. A mulitcentre randomized trial comparing delivery with a silicone rubber cup and rigid metal vacuum extractor cups. Br J Obstet Gynaecol 1989;96: 545–551 (Level I)

31. Hofmeyr GJ, Gobetz L, Sonnendecker EW, Turner MJ. New design rigid and soft vacuum extractor cups: a preliminary comparison of traction forces. Br J Obstet Gynaecol 1990;97:681–685 (Level I)

32. Kuit JA, Eppinga HG, Wallenburg HC, Huikeshoven FJ. A randomized comparison of vacuum extraction delivery with a rigid and a pliable cup. Obstet Gynecol 1993; 82:280–284 (Level I)

33. Lim FT, Holm JP, Schuitemaker NW, Jansen FH, Hermans J. Stepwise compared with rapid application of vacuum in ventouse extraction procedures. Br J Obstet Gynaecol 1997;104:33–36 (Level I)

34. Svenningsen L. Birth progression and traction forces developed under vacuum extraction after slow or rapid application of suction. Eur J Obstet Gynecol Reprod Biol 1987;26:105–112 (Level II-2)

35. Bofill JA, Rust OA, Devidas M, Roberts WE, Morrison JC, Martin JN Jr. Neonatal cephalohematoma from vacuum extraction. J Reprod Med 1997;42:565–569 (Level I)

36. Bofill JA, Rust OA, Schorr SJ, Brown RC, Roberts WE, Morrison JC. A randomized trial of two vacuum extraction techniques. Obstet Gynecol 1997;89:758–762 (Level I)

37. Bashore RA, Phillips WH Jr, Brinkman CR 3rd. A comparison of the morbidity of midforceps and cesarean delivery. Am J Obstet Gynecol 1990;162:1428–1434; discussion 1434–1435 (Level II-2)

38. Traub AI, Morrow RJ, Ritchie JW, Dornan KJ. A continuing use for Kielland's forceps? Br J Obstet Gynaecol 1984;91:894–898 (Level II-2)

39. Healy DL, Quinn MA, Pepperell RJ. Rotational delivery of the fetus: Kielland's forceps and two other methods compared. Br J Obstet Gynaecol 1982;89:501–506 (Level II-2)

40. Chiswick ML, James DK. Kielland's forceps: association with neonatal morbidity and mortality. Br Med J 1979; 1:7–9 (Level II-3).

41. Dierker LJ Jr, Rosen MG, Thompson K, Lynn P. Midforceps deliveries: long-term outcome of infants. Am J Obstet Gynecol 1986;154:764–768 (Level II-2)

42. Nilsen ST. Boys born by forceps and vacuum extraction examined at 18 years of age. Acta Obstet Gynecol Scand 1984;63:549–554 (Level II-2)

The MEDLINE database, the Cochrane Library, and ACOG's own internal resources and documents were used to conduct a literature search to locate relevant articles published between January 1985 and November 1999. The search was restricted to articles published in the English language. Priority was given to articles reporting results of original research, although review articles and commentaries also were consulted. Abstracts of research presented at symposia and scientific conferences were not considered adequate for inclusion in this document. Guidelines published by organizations or institutions such as the National Institutes of Health and the American College of Obstetricians and Gynecologists were reviewed, and additional studies were located by reviewing bibliographies of identified articles. When reliable research was not available, expert opinions from obstetrician–gynecologists were used.

Studies were reviewed and evaluated for quality according to the method outlined by the U.S. Preventive Services Task Force:

- I Evidence obtained from at least one properly designed randomized controlled trial.
- II-1 Evidence obtained from well-designed controlled trials without randomization.
- II-2 Evidence obtained from well-designed cohort or case–control analytic studies, preferably from more than one center or research group.
- II-3 Evidence obtained from multiple time series with or without the intervention. Dramatic results in uncontrolled experiments also could be regarded as this type of evidence.
- III Opinions of respected authorities, based on clinical experience, descriptive studies, or reports of expert committees.

Based on the highest level of evidence found in the data, recommendations are provided and graded according to the following catetories:

Level A—Recommendations are based on good and consistent scientific evidence.

Level B—Recommendations are based on limited or inconsistent scientific evidence.

Level C—Recommendations are based primarily on consensus and expert opinion.

ISSN 1099-3630

The American College of Obstetricians and Gynecologists
409 12th Street, SW
PO Box 96920
Washington, DC 20090-6920

12345/43210

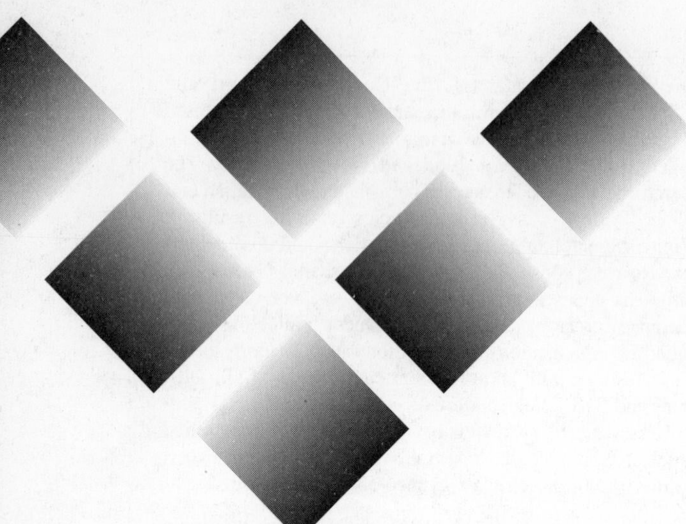

ACOG PRACTICE BULLETIN

CLINICAL MANAGEMENT GUIDELINES FOR OBSTETRICIAN–GYNECOLOGISTS

NUMBER 20, SEPTEMBER 2000

(Replaces Educational Bulletin Number 177, February 1993)

This Practice Bulletin was developed by the ACOG Committee on Practice Bulletins—Obstetrics with the assistance of Kim Boggess, MD. The information is designed to aid practitioners in making decisions about appropriate obstetric and gynecologic care. These guidelines should not be construed as dictating an exclusive course of treatment or procedure. Variations in practice may be warranted based on the needs of the individual patient, resources, and limitations unique to the institution or type of practice.

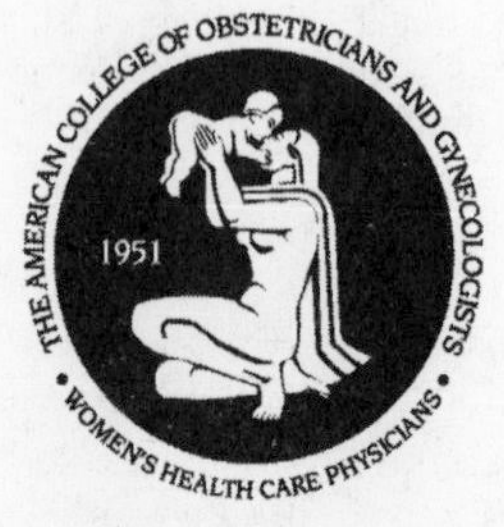

Perinatal Viral and Parasitic Infections

Many viral and parasitic infections are associated with significant maternal and fetal consequences if acquired during pregnancy. In the United States, some of the most commonly encountered infections with subsequent perinatal effects include cytomegalovirus (CMV), parvovirus B19, varicella zoster virus (VZV), and toxoplasmosis. The purpose of this document is to describe these infections, their modes of transmission, and their maternal and fetal effects, and to offer guidelines for counseling about and management of these infections during pregnancy.

Background

In general, perinatal infections have more severe fetal consequences when they occur early in gestation, because first-trimester infections may disrupt organogenesis. Second- and third-trimester infections can cause neurologic impairment or growth disturbances. In utero infection may be associated with certain ultrasound findings, including intrauterine growth restriction, echogenic bowel, intracranial or intrahepatic calcifications, hydrocephalus, microcephaly, isolated ascites, pericardial or pleural effusions, or nonimmune hydrops, although congenital infections also can be asymptomatic.

Cytomegalovirus

Cytomegalovirus is a double-stranded DNA herpesvirus that is transmitted by contact with infected blood, saliva, or urine, or by sexual contact. The incubation period of CMV is 28–60 days, with a mean of 40 days. Infection induces an immunoglobulin M (IgM) antibody response that disappears within 30–60 days. Viremia can be detected 2–3 weeks following primary infection. Primary CMV infection in adults generally is asymptomatic. Occasionally, patients experience a mononucleosislike syndrome, with leukocytosis, lymphocytosis, abnormal liver function tests, fever, malaise, myalgias, and chills (1). After the initial infection, CMV remains latent in host cells; recurrent infection can occur following reactivation of latent virus. In rare cases, recurrent CMV infection can occur by infection with a new strain of virus.

Prevalence of both primary and recurrent infection in pregnant women varies regionally from 0.7% to 4% for primary infection and up to 13.5% for recurrent infection (2). Vertical transmission of CMV may occur as a result of transplacental infection after primary or recurrent CMV infection, exposure to contaminated genital tract secretions at parturition, or breastfeeding. Most infants with congenital CMV are asymptomatic at birth. Clinical findings of symptomatic congenital CMV infection include jaundice, petechiae, thrombocytopenia, hepatospleno-megaly, growth restriction, and nonimmune hydrops (3, 4). The annual cost of treating the complications of CMV infections in the United States is estimated to be approximately $2 billion (2), which reflects the 50–80% seropositivity rate of pregnant women.

Cytomegalovirus is the most common congenital infection, occurring in 0.2–2.2% of all neonates (5), and is the leading cause of congenital hearing loss. Vertical transmission may occur at any stage of pregnancy, with the overall risk of infection greatest when the infection occurs during the third trimester. However, more serious fetal sequelae occur after maternal CMV infection during the first trimester. With primary maternal CMV infection, the risk of transmission to the fetus is 30–40% (6). Of those infected in utero following a primary infection, 10% will have signs and symptoms of CMV infection at birth and develop sequelae (7). Approximately 30% of severely infected infants die, and 80% of survivors have severe neurologic morbidity (5, 8). The incidence of severe fetal infection is much lower after recurrent maternal infection than after primary infection. Vertical transmission after a recurrent infection is 0.15–2% (8, 9). Infants infected after maternal CMV reactivation generally are asymptomatic at birth. Congenital hearing loss is typically the most severe sequela of secondary infection, and congenital infection following recurrent infection is unlikely to produce multiple sequelae (9). Cytomegalovirus infection acquired as a result of exposure to infected cervical secretions or breast milk is typically asymptomatic and is not associated with severe neonatal sequelae.

Parvovirus B19

Parvovirus B19 is a single-stranded DNA virus that causes the childhood exanthem erythema infectiosum, also known as fifth disease. In immunocompetent adults, the most common symptoms of parvovirus B19 infection are a reticular rash on the trunk and peripheral arthropathy, although approximately 33% of infections are asymptomatic (10). Another manifestation of parvovirus B19 infection is transient aplastic crisis, which is more common in those with an underlying hemoglobinopathy. Most infections are mild; most individuals recover completely from parvovirus B19 infection and require only supportive care.

Transmission of parvovirus B19 most commonly occurs through respiratory secretions and hand-to-mouth contact. The infected person generally is infectious 5–10 days after exposure prior to the onset of the rash or other symptoms and is no longer infectious with the onset of the rash (11). Both IgM and IgG are produced in response to infection. The IgM response, which persists for 1 to several months, is indicative of a recent infection. IgG antibodies persist indefinitely and, in the absence of IgM, indicate prior infection and immunity. Prevalence of seropositivity to parvovirus B19 increases with age and is greater than 60% in adolescents and adults (11). The risk of maternal infection of parvovirus B19 varies with level of exposure to the infected individual. Exposure to a household member infected with parvovirus B19 is associated with an approximate 50% risk of seroconversion (12–15). The risk of transmission in a child care setting or classroom is lower, ranging from approximately 20% to 50% (15–17).

Recent maternal infection with parvovirus B19 constitutes a low risk for fetal morbidity (18), although some cases have been associated with adverse fetal effects. Transplacental transmission has been reported to be as high as 33% (19), and fetal infection with parvovirus B19 has been associated with spontaneous abortion, hydrops fetalis, and stillbirth. The rate of fetal loss among women with serologically proven parvovirus B19 infection ranges from 2% to 9% (20–22). In utero, parvovirus B19 infection is responsible for up to 18% of cases of nonimmune hydrops fetalis in some series (23, 24). Hydrops fetalis results from aplastic anemia, myocarditis, or chronic fetal hepatitis. Severe effects are seen most frequently among fetuses when maternal parvovirus B19 infection occurs at less than 20 weeks of gestation (20). Stillbirth resulting from maternal infection has occurred from 1 to 11 weeks after maternal infection. However, hydrops is unlikely to develop if it has not occurred by 8 weeks after maternal infection (23). Long-term development appears to be normal in fetuses with congenital parvovirus B19 infection that do not succumb to the disease (25, 26).

Varicella Zoster Virus

Varicella zoster virus is a DNA herpesvirus that is highly contagious and is transmitted by respiratory droplets or close contact. The attack rate among susceptible contacts is 60–90% after exposure. The incubation period after infection is 10–20 days, with a mean of 14 days (27). The period of infectivity begins 48 hours before the rash appears and lasts until the vesicles crust over. The primary infection causes chickenpox, which is characterized by fever, malaise, and a maculopapular pruritic rash that becomes vesicular. After the primary infection, VZV remains dormant in sensory ganglia and can be reactivated to cause a vesicular erythematous skin rash known as herpes zoster. The antibody to VZV develops within a few days after the onset of infection, and prior infection with VZV confers lifelong immunity.

Varicella infection is uncommon in pregnancy (occurring in 0.4–0.7 per 1,000 patients), because of the high prevalence of natural immunity (28). Pregnancy complicated by maternal varicella infection is associated with untoward maternal, fetal, and neonatal effects. The disease usually is a benign and self-limited illness in children; however, varicella national mortality data indicate that although less than 5% of varicella cases occur among adults 20 years of age or older, that group contributes to 55% of varicella-related deaths (29). Severe complications, such as encephalitis and pneumonia, are more common in adults than in children; VZV pneumonia in pregnancy is a risk factor for maternal mortality (30, 31).

In pregnancy, varicella may be transmitted across the placenta, resulting in congenital or neonatal chickenpox. The risk of congenital varicella syndrome is limited to exposure during the first 20 weeks of gestation, occurs uncommonly (up to 2%), and is characterized by skin scarring, limb hypoplasia, chorioretinitis, and microcephaly (32–34). Neonatal VZV infection is associated with a high neonatal death rate when maternal disease develops from 5 days before delivery up to 48 hours postpartum as a result of the relative immaturity of the neonatal immune system and the lack of protective maternal antibody (35, 36).

Toxoplasmosis

Toxoplasmosis is caused by the intracellular parasite *Toxoplasma gondii*. *T gondii* exists in several forms: a trophozoite, which is the invasive form, and a cyst or an oocyst, which are latent forms. Human infection is acquired by consuming cysts in undercooked meat of infected animals, by insect contamination of food, by contact with oocysts from the feces of infected cats (the only definitive hosts), or by contact with infected materials or insects in soil. Infection with *T gondii* usually is asymptomatic, although after an incubation of 5–18 days, some nonspecific symptoms may occur. Most often, toxoplasmosis presents as asymptomatic cervical lymphadenopathy, with symptoms occurring in only 10–20% of adult cases. Other symptoms include fever, malaise, night sweats, myalgias, and hepatosplenomegaly. Parasitemia can occur after infection, which, in pregnant women, can seed the placenta and cause subsequent fetal infection. Congenital transmission of *T gondii* from an infected woman was the first form of transmission to be recognized, and transmission depends on the time of acquisition of maternal infection. The later in gestation that the infection occurs, the more likely transmission is to occur. The rate of vertical transmission increases from 10% to 15% in the first trimester, to 25% in the second trimester, and to more than 60% in the third trimester (37, 38). The severity of infection depends on gestational age at the time of transmission. The earlier the fetus is infected, the more severe the disease. Most infected infants do not have clinical signs of infection at birth, but 55–85% will develop sequelae, including chorioretinitis (leading to severe impairment of vision), hearing loss, or mental retardation (39–41). Other clinical manifestations of congenital toxoplasmosis include rash, hepatosplenomegaly, ascites, fever, periventricular calcifications, ventriculomegaly, and seizures (42–44).

After an acute infection, IgM antibodies appear early and reach maximum levels in 1 month. IgG antibodies appear after IgM antibodies, are detectable within a few weeks after infection, and confer immunity. High titers of both IgG and IgM may persist for years. In the immunocompetent adult, the clinical course is benign and self-limited.

Clinical Considerations and Recommendations

Cytomegalovirus

▶ ***How is maternal CMV infection diagnosed?***

The majority of adult CMV infections are asymptomatic, which makes diagnosis of primary infection difficult. Cytomegalovirus may be detected by culture or polymerase chain reaction (PCR) of infected blood, urine, saliva, cervical secretions, or breast milk, although diagnosis of CMV infection in adults usually is confirmed by serologic testing. Serum samples collected 3–4 weeks apart, tested in parallel for anti-CMV IgG, are essential for the diagnosis of primary infection. Seroconversion from negative to positive or a significant increase (greater than fourfold, eg, from 1:4 to 1:16) in anti-CMV IgG titers is evidence of infection. The presence of CMV-specific IgM is a useful but not completely reliable indication of a primary infection. IgM titers may not be positive during an acute infection, or they may persist for months after the primary infection (45). A small proportion of women with recurrent infection will demonstrate anti-CMV IgM (7). The reported sensitivity of CMV IgM serologic assays ranges from 50% to 90% (45).

▶ *How is fetal CMV infection diagnosed?*

Congenital CMV may be suspected prenatally after a documented maternal primary infection or, more typically, after detection of ultrasound findings suggestive of infection (46). These include abdominal and liver calcifications, calcification of the lateral border of the lateral ventricles, hydrops, echogenic bowel, ascites, hepatosplenomegaly, and ventriculomegaly (46–53). Fetuses that demonstrate abnormalities, particularly if they involve the central nervous system, generally have a much poorer prognosis (46, 54).

Cytomegalovirus has been diagnosed prenatally by detection of anti-CMV IgM in fetal blood (55–57), although this test has a high false-positive rate (58). In addition, IgM is not detectable in the first half of pregnancy, presumably because of the immaturity of the fetal immune system, limiting the usefulness of fetal serologic testing. Testing for fetal thrombocytopenia or abnormal liver function has been suggested as a method to diagnose congenital CMV. However, these tests are not specific for CMV, and normal results do not preclude severe infection.

Cytomegalovirus can be detected in the amniotic fluid of infected fetuses by either culture or PCR. The sensitivity of CMV culture ranges from 50% to 69%, compared with a sensitivity of 77–100% for PCR. Negative and positive predictive values are comparable between amniotic fluid culture and PCR (55–57, 59–64). The sensitivity of amniotic fluid testing for prenatal diagnosis of congenital CMV infection is markedly lower if performed before 21 weeks of gestation (65), and the time interval between maternal infection and testing may influence the reliability (62). Although these tests are promising, neither amniotic fluid culture nor PCR can detect all cases of congenital CMV infection. In addition, the detection of CMV in amniotic fluid does not predict the severity of congenital CMV infection. A combination of amniotic fluid culture and PCR has been suggested to have a sensitivity of 80–100% in identifying infected fetuses (56). Fetal blood sampling is less sensitive than amniotic fluid testing (64). Specific ultrasonographic findings may further assist in the accurate diagnosis of a congenitally infected infant with a poor prognosis.

▶ *How are maternal, fetal, and congenital neonatal infections with cytomegalovirus treated?*

Currently, no therapies are available for the treatment of maternal or fetal CMV infection. Antiviral treatment with ganciclovir or foscarnet is approved only for treatment of CMV retinitis in patients with acquired immunodeficiency syndrome (AIDS). However, ganciclovir has been shown in vitro to cross the placenta by simple diffusion (66), and there are reports of its postnatal use for the treatment of congenital CMV (67–69). Ganciclovir and CMV hyperimmune gamma globulin have shown promise for the treatment of neonates with congenital CMV infection (70–72). The effectiveness of treatment in the prevention of long-term neurologic sequelae has not been proven.

A live attenuated vaccine using the Towne 125 strain has been developed, and appears to be safe, somewhat protective (73–76), and economically beneficial (77). There is reluctance to embrace vaccination because of concerns about the ability of the vaccine strain to reactivate and potentially infect the host, the potential for viral shedding from the cervix or breast milk, and the possible oncogenic potential of vaccine virus (78). However, the science in this area is advancing rapidly, and new treatment options may become available.

▶ *How should women at high risk be counseled about prevention of CMV?*

Factors associated with an increased risk of CMV infection include history of abnormal cervical cytology, lower socioeconomic status, birth outside North America, first pregnancy at younger than 15 years, and infection with other sexually transmitted diseases. The greatest impact obstetrician–gynecologists can have on reducing CMV disease is by educating patients about preventive measures. Counseling should cover careful handling of potentially infected articles, such as diapers, and thorough hand-washing when around young children or immunocompromised individuals, explaining that careful attention to hygiene is effective in helping to prevent transmission (3, 12, 79). In addition, women should be counseled, when appropriate, about the avoidance of high-risk behaviors, such as intravenous drug use and sharing of needles. Condom use should be encouraged as a method of contraception.

▶ *Should women at high risk be screened before or during pregnancy?*

Currently, routine serologic testing for CMV during pregnancy is not recommended (4, 7, 80, 81). Maternal IgM antibody screening is limited for differentiating primary from recurrent infection, which makes it difficult to use such results in counseling patients about fetal risk. In addition, maternal immunity does not eliminate the possibility of fetal infection.

Although the virus is not highly contagious, some groups of women are at higher risk for the acquisition of CMV infection. Eleven percent of seronegative child care workers demonstrate seroconversion within 10 months of hire (82), and 53% of families of young children have one or more family members seroconvert within a year (83, 84). In two cross-sectional studies, increasing parity had an independent effect on increasing CMV seroprevalence, demonstrating the possibility of child-to-mother transmission (85). Therefore, women with young children or those who work with young children should be advised that the risk of infection can be reduced significantly by safe-handling techniques, such as the use of latex gloves and rigorous hand-washing after handling diapers or after exposure to respiratory secretions (3, 12, 86).

Parvovirus B19

▶ *Which methods are available to diagnose maternal parvovirus B19 infection?*

Maternal serology is the most commonly used test to diagnose acute infection with parvovirus B19. Enzyme-linked immunosorbent assay (ELISA), radioimmunoassay, and Western blot tests can measure the antibody to parvovirus B19 (20). The sensitivity of IgM and IgG assays is generally 79% (10, 87). Identification of parvovirus-specific IgM in maternal serum is diagnostic of a primary infection, although a laboratory with experience should measure titers, because false-positive results can occur. Previous exposure and infection with parvovirus B19 is indicated by the presence of antiparvovirus B19 IgG in the absence of IgM and has not been associated with adverse perinatal outcome.

Parvovirus B19 can be identified by direct visualization of viral particles in infected tissues or serum by electron microscopy or by identification of characteristic intranuclear inclusions within erythroblasts (88).

▶ *What methods are available for diagnosing fetal parvovirus B19 infection?*

Diagnosis of fetal parvovirus B19 infection can be accomplished by isolation of viral particles in abortuses or placental specimens (89, 90). Polymerase chain reaction also has been used to detect parvovirus B19 in fetal specimens, including autopsy tissue, serum, amniotic fluid, and placenta (91–95).

Sensitivity of PCR for detection of parvovirus may be as high as 100%, although data are limited by small sample sizes (94, 96). Reliable serologic tests for specific IgM antibodies in the fetus are not available. As with other intrauterine infections, IgM antibodies appear in the fetal circulation after 22 weeks of gestation, limiting the usefulness of such tests.

Ultrasonography has been the mainstay for diagnosing fetal parvovirus infection. Severely infected fetuses typically have evidence of hydrops fetalis. Serial ultrasound examinations for up to 10 weeks after maternal infection are indicated. If the fetus shows no signs of hydrops fetalis, additional tests are unnecessary.

▶ *How are maternal, fetal, and congenital neonatal infections with parvovirus B19 managed?*

After documented exposure to parvovirus B19, the woman should have serologic testing to determine if she is immune with evidence of antiparvovirus IgG. If nonimmune, the test should be repeated in 3–4 weeks and paired samples tested to document whether the woman is seropositive for parvovirus. If seroconversion does not occur, the fetus is not at risk for in utero infection. If seroconversion does occur, the fetus should be monitored for 10 weeks by serial ultrasound examination to evaluate for presence of hydrops fetalis, placentomegaly, and growth disturbances (9).

In a series of 618 pregnant women exposed to parvovirus, only 311 (50.3%) were susceptible to infection. Of those susceptible, only 52 contracted parvovirus. None of the 52 infants exposed to maternal parvovirus developed hydrops fetalis (14). However, if hydrops fetalis develops, percutaneous umbilical blood sampling should be performed to determine the fetal hematocrit, leukocyte and platelet count, and viral DNA in preparation for supportive care using transfusion (97, 98). Intrauterine transfusion should be considered if anemia is present (21, 99).

▶ *Should seronegative women with work-related exposure be taken out of work?*

When outbreaks of parvovirus B19 infection occur in situations in which prolonged, close-contact exposure occurs, as in schools, homes, or child care centers, options for prevention of transmission are limited (20). Exposure cannot be eliminated by identifying and excluding persons with acute parvovirus B19 infection; up to 20% are asymptomatic, and those with infection are infectious before they develop symptoms. Exclusion of pregnant women from the workplace during endemic periods is controversial, and a policy to routinely exclude members of high-risk groups from work during an outbreak of parvovirus B19 is not recommended (14, 20).

Varicella Zoster Virus

▶ *How is maternal VZV infection diagnosed?*

Usually, this diagnosis is based on clinical findings, and laboratory testing is not needed, especially if a rash occurs after known exposure. If laboratory diagnosis is required, the VZV antigen can be demonstrated within skin lesions or vesicular fluid by immunofluorescence. Varicella infection also can be documented by the detection of the fluorescence antibody to the membrane antigen or of the VZV antibody by ELISA (28).

▶ *How is fetal VZV infection diagnosed?*

Although two small studies estimate the rate of congenital varicella syndrome after maternal infection with VZV to be 1–2% (32, 34), these studies were subject to bias, and these rates may be overestimated. The risk of congenital varicella syndrome is small; however, the outcome for the affected infant is serious enough that a reliable method of prenatal diagnosis would be valuable.

Fetal varicella can be suspected by the presence of ultrasonographic abnormalities. Ultrasound findings suggestive of congenital varicella include hydrops, hyperechogenic foci in the liver and bowel, cardiac malformations, limb deformities, microcephaly, and intrauterine growth restriction. In one series, five fetuses with congenital VZV demonstrated some ultrasound findings that suggested infection, and all the infants died by 4 months of age (100). However, not all fetuses with congenital VZV that have ultrasound abnormalities do poorly (101). Although the sensitivity of ultrasonography is unknown, it is the preferred method of diagnosis of congenital VZV.

Invasive prenatal diagnosis in women who acquire VZV in the first half of pregnancy may serve to provide reassurance if test results are negative (102). However, if the virus is present, identifying it by culture or viral DNA by PCR in chorionic villi, amniotic fluid or fetal blood, or the viral-specific antibody does not accurately predict the severity of fetal infection (101, 103).

▶ *What therapies are available and effective for maternal, fetal, and congenital neonatal infections with varicella?*

Oral acyclovir, if instituted within 24 hours of the rash, has been shown to reduce the duration of new lesion formation and the total number of new lesions and to improve constitutional symptoms in children, adolescents, and adults (104–106). Oral acyclovir appears to be safe and can be prescribed for pregnant women if lesions develop (107). Maternal varicella complicated by pneumonia should be treated with intravenous acyclovir, because intravenous acyclovir may reduce maternal morbidity and mortality associated with varicella pneumonia (31, 108).

Maternal treatment with acyclovir has not been shown to ameliorate or prevent the fetal effects of congenital varicella syndrome (109). Varicella-zoster immune globulin (VZIG) should be given to infants born to women who develop varicella between 5 days before and 2 days after delivery, although this does not universally prevent neonatal varicella (110). Infants who develop varicella within the first 2 weeks of life should be treated with intravenous acyclovir (107, 111).

▶ *What preventive strategies are effective for varicella?*

Nonpregnant women of childbearing age should be questioned about previous infection with varicella preconceptionally and offered vaccination if no report of chickenpox is elicited. Varicella vaccine has been available since March 1995 and is approved for use in healthy susceptible persons 12 months or older (112). Conception should be delayed until 1 month after the second vaccination dose is given.

Among women who do not recall a history of varicella, 70–90% have detectable antibodies (112). Antenatal VZV screening of all pregnant women with negative or indeterminate varicella histories is not believed to be cost-effective by some (113). However, others argue that from a cost-effectiveness/cost-benefit standpoint, management based on immune testing is preferable to universal VZIG administration when caring for pregnant women exposed to VZV with a negative or indeterminate infection history (114). Patients known to be nonimmune to VZV should be counseled to avoid contact with individuals who have chickenpox. If exposure does occur, prophylactic intervention with VZIG early in the incubation period can prevent or attenuate the disease manifestations of VZV in susceptible contacts at high risk from this infection (106). Expeditious determination of the VZV membrane antigen or equivalent anti-VZV antibody status in pregnant women exposed to VZV appears to be a rapid, satisfactory method for determining who should promptly receive VZIG passive immunization (115). Although VZIG is effective in reducing the severity of maternal varicella when administered up to 72 hours after exposure, it should be given as soon as possible (116, 117). Maternal administration of VZIG does not ameliorate or prevent fetal infection.

Toxoplasmosis

▶ *How is maternal toxoplasmosis infection diagnosed?*

Isolation of *T gondii* from blood or body fluids establishes that the infection is acute; however, serologic testing for the detection of the specific antibody to *T gondii* is the primary method of diagnosis. Numerous antibody assays are available. The Sabin-Feldman dye test is the IgG test with which all others are compared, but it is performed at only a few reference laboratories. Indirect fluorescent antibody, indirect hemagglutination and agglutination tests, and ELISA also are available to detect the antitoxoplasma antibody. However, serologic assays for toxoplasmosis are not well standardized and have a high false-positive rate. IgM titers may persist at high levels (eg, ≥1:512) for years in healthy individuals (118). Both IgG and IgM testing should be used for the initial evaluation of patients suspected to have toxoplasmosis. Testing of serial specimens 3 weeks apart in parallel gives the most accurate assessment if the initial test results are equivocal. In cases in which clinical suspicion is high, specimens should be saved for repeat testing because of the wide variation between laboratories. Repeat testing in a well-recognized reference laboratory should be performed if there is evidence of a primary infection.

▶ *Which methods are available for diagnosing and monitoring fetal infection?*

Ultrasonography can demonstrate severe congenital toxoplasmosis; suggestive findings include ventriculomegaly, intracranial calcifications, microcephaly, ascites, hepatosplenomegaly, and intrauterine growth restriction. Testing fetal blood samples after 20 weeks of gestation for the presence of specific IgM is the most sensitive test in diagnosing congenital toxoplasmosis (119). Using fetal blood for antibody testing or mouse inoculation, amniotic fluid for PCR, or fetal ultrasonography to detect ventriculomegaly, 77–93% of infected infants were identified prenatally, although no single test was very sensitive (43, 120). Successful identification of *T gondii* intrauterine infection with PCR testing of amniotic fluid allows for earlier testing than fetal blood sampling, with high sensitivity (37, 121–124), although false-positive and false-negative findings do occur (125).

▶ *How are maternal, fetal, and congenital neonatal infections with toxoplasmosis treated?*

Treatment of the pregnant woman with acute toxoplasmosis reduces but does not eliminate the risk of congenital infection (42, 43). Identification of acute maternal infection necessitates immediate institution of treatment until results of fetal testing are known. Spiramycin, which concentrates in the placenta, may reduce the risk of fetal transmission by 60% (126), but as a single agent, it does not treat established fetal infection. Spiramycin is available only through the U.S. Food and Drug Administration after serologic confirmation at a reference laboratory; it is recommended for pregnant women at risk unless fetal infection is documented. If fetal infection is established, pyrimethamine, sulfonamides, and folinic acid are added to the regimen because they more effectively eradicate parasites in the placenta and in the fetus than spiramycin alone (127). With treatment, even early fetal infection with toxoplasmosis can result in successful pregnancy outcomes (128).

Treatment of infants with symptomatic congenital toxoplasmosis consists of pyrimethamine and sulfadiazine, alternating monthly with spiramycin, for 1 year (127). Treatment will diminish or resolve intracranial calcifications if present, suggesting improved neurologic function (129).

▶ *Should women be screened for toxoplasmosis during pregnancy?*

A multicenter study in the United States found that approximately 38% of pregnant women have evidence of prior toxoplasmosis infection (130). Evidence of previous infection signifies that the future mother is not at risk of giving birth to a child with congenital toxoplasmosis. Serologic screening as a way to prevent congenital toxoplasmosis would have the most impact in countries with a high frequency of seropositivity, and routine prenatal screening is performed in France and Austria (39). However, in the United States, routine screening during pregnancy currently is not recommended, except in women infected with human immunodeficiency virus (HIV). Serologic screening during pregnancy may yield equivocal results, because IgM antibodies can persist for long periods (131). Exceptional circumstances may justify toxoplasmosis titer screening for pregnant women who are cat owners. One study in Belgium demonstrated a 63% reduction in the rate of maternal toxoplasmosis infection after institution of an educational program that recommended avoiding eating undercooked or raw meat, wearing gloves when working with soil, and avoiding caring for cats unless they are strictly "indoor cats" whose food is rigidly controlled (131).

Summary

The following recommendations are based on limited and inconsistent scientific data (Level B):

- Pregnant women who are seronegative for VZV and exposed to chickenpox should receive VZIG.
- Pregnant women who develop chickenpox should be treated with oral acyclovir to minimize maternal symptoms; if pneumonia develops, they should be treated with intravenous acyclovir.
- Pregnant women who have acute parvovirus B19 infection during pregnancy should be monitored with serial ultrasound examinations for at least 10 weeks following infection for the presence of hydrops fetalis.
- Fetuses with evidence of hydrops should undergo fetal blood sampling and transfusion as needed.
- Pregnant women who acquire toxoplasmosis should be treated with spiramycin. When diagnosed, fetal toxoplasmosis should be treated with a combination of pyrimethamine, sulfadiazine, and folinic acid, alternating with spiramycin.

The following recommendations are based primarily on consensus and expert opinion (Level C):

- Routine serologic screening of all pregnant women for CMV and toxoplasmosis is not recommended.
- Nonpregnant women of reproductive age who have no history of varicella infection should be offered varicella vaccine.
- The diagnosis of toxoplasmosis should be confirmed by a reliable reference laboratory.
- Pregnant women exposed to parvovirus B19 should have serologic screening performed to determine if they are at risk for seroconversion.
- Pregnant women should be counseled about methods to prevent acquisition of CMV or toxoplasmosis during pregnancy.

References

1. Klemola E, Kaariainen L. Cytomegalovirus as a possible cause of a disease resembling infectious mononucleosis. Br Med J 1965;5470:1099–1102 (Level III)
2. Fowler KB, Stagno S, Pass RF. Maternal age and congenital cytomegalovirus infection: screening of two diverse newborn populations, 1980–1990. J Infect Dis 1993;168:552–556 (Level II-3)
3. Adler SP, Finney JW, Manganello AM, Best AM. Prevention of child-to-mother transmission of cytomegalovirus by changing behaviors: a randomized controlled trial. Pediatr Infect Dis J 1996;15:240–246 (Level II-1)
4. Daniel Y, Gull I, Peyser MR, Lessing JB. Congenital cytomegalovirus infection. Eur J Obstet Gynecol Reprod Biol 1995;63:7–16 (Level III)
5. Stagno S, Pass RF, Dworsky ME, Alford CA Jr. Maternal cytomegalovirus infection and perinatal transmission. Clin Obstet Gynecol 1982;25:563–576 (Level III)
6. Stagno S, Pass RF, Cloud G, Britt WJ, Henderson RE, Walton PD, et al. Primary cytomegalovirus infection in pregnancy. Incidence, transmission to fetus, and clinical outcome. JAMA 1986;256:1904–1908 (Level II-2)
7. Hagay ZJ, Biran G, Ornoy A, Reece EA. Congenital cytomegalovirus infection: a long-standing problem still seeking a solution. Am J Obstet Gynecol 1996;174:241–245 (Level III)
8. Stagno S, Whitley RJ. Herpesvirus infections of pregnancy. Part 1: Cytomegalovirus and Epstein-Barr virus infections. N Engl J Med 1985;313:1270–1274 (Level II-3)
9. Fowler KB, Stagno S, Pass RF, Britt WJ, Boll TJ, Alford CA. The outcome of congenital cytomegalovirus infection in relation to maternal antibody status. N Engl J Med 1992;326:663–667 (Level II-2)
10. Chorba T, Coccia P, Holman RC, Tattersall P, Anderson LJ, Sudman J, et al. The role of parvovirus B19 in aplastic crisis and erythema infectiosum (fifth disease). J Infect Dis 1986;154:383–393 (Level II-2)
11. Thurn J. Human parvovirus B19: historical and clinical review. Rev Infect Dis 1988;10:1005–1011 (Level III)
12. Cytomegalovirus (CMV) infection and prevention. Atlanta, Georgia: Centers for Disease Control and Prevention, 1998 (Level III)
13. Rice PS, Cohen BJ. A school outbreak of parvovirus B19 infection investigated using salivary antibody assays. Epidemiol Infect 1996;116:331–338 (Level II-3)
14. Harger JH, Adler SP, Koch WC, Harger GF. Prospective evaluation of 618 pregnant women exposed to parvovirus B19: risks and symptoms. Obstet Gynecol 1998;91:413–420 (Level II-3)
15. Valeur-Jensen AK, Pedersen CB, Westergaard T, Jensen IP, Lebech M, Andersen PK, et al. Risk factors for parvovirus B19 infection in pregnancy. JAMA 1999; 281:1099–1105 (Level II-2)
16. Gillespie SM, Cartter ML, Asch S, Rokos JB, Gary GW, Tsou CJ, et al. Occupational risk of human parvovirus B19 infection for school and day-care personnel during an outbreak of erythema infectiosum. JAMA 1990;263: 2061–2065 (Level II-3)
17. Cartter ML, Farley TA, Rosengren S, Quinn DL, Gillespie SM, Gary GW, et al. Occupational risk factors for infection with parvovirus B19 among pregnant women. J Infect Dis 1991;163:282–285 (Level II-2)

18. Guidozzi F, Ballot D, Rothberg AD. Human B19 parvovirus infection in an obstetric population. A prospective study determining fetal outcome. J Reprod Med 1994;39:36–38 (Level III)

19. Public Health Laboratory Service Working Party on Fifth Disease. Prospective study of human parvovirus (B19) infection in pregnancy. BMJ 1990;300:1166–1170 (Level II-3)

20. Risks associated with human parvovirus B19 infection. MMWR Morbid Mortal Wkly Rep 1989;38:81–88, 93–97 (Level III)

21. Rodis JF, Quinn DL, Gary GW Jr, Anderson LJ, Rosengren S, Cartter ML, et al. Management and outcomes of pregnancies complicated by human B19 parvovirus infection: a prospective study. Am J Obstet Gynecol 1990;163:1168–1171 (Level III)

22. Gratacos E, Torres PJ, Vidal J, Antolin E, Costa J, Jimenez de Anta MT, et al. The incidence of human parvovirus B19 infection during pregnancy and its impact on perinatal outcome. J Infect Dis 1995;171:1360–1363 (Level II-2)

23. Yaegashi N, Okamura K, Yajima A, Murai C, Sugamura K. The frequency of human parvovirus B19 infection in nonimmune hydrops fetalis. J Perinat Med 1994;22: 159–163 (Level III)

24. Jordan JA. Identification of human parvovirus B19 infection in idiopathic nonimmune hydrops fetalis. Am J Obstet Gynecol 1996;174:37–42 (Level II-3)

25. Miller E, Fairley CK, Cohen BJ, Seng C. Immediate and long term outcome of human parvovirus B19 infection in pregnancy. Br J Obstet Gynaecol 1998;105:174–178 (Level II-3)

26. Rodis JF, Rodner C, Hansen AA, Borgida AF, Deoliveira I, Shulman Rosengren S, et al. Long-term outcome of children following maternal human parvovirus B19 infection. Obstet Gynecol 1998;91:125–128 (Level II-2)

27. Preblud SR, Orenstein WA, Bart KJ. Varicella: clinical manifestations, epidemiology and health impact in children. Pediatr Infect Dis 1984;3:505–509 (Level III)

28. Enders G. Serodiagnosis of Varicella-Zoster virus infection in pregnancy and standardization of the ELISA IgG and IgM antibody tests. Dev Biol Stand 1982;52: 221–236 (Level III)

29. Varicella-related deaths among adults—United States, 1997. MMWR Morb Mortal Wkly Rep 1997;46: 409–412 (Level III)

30. Paryani SG, Arvin AM. Intrauterine infection with varicella-zoster virus after maternal varicella. N Engl J Med 1986;314:1542–1546 (Level II-3)

31. Smego RA Jr, Asperilla MO. Use of acyclovir for varicella pneumonia during pregnancy. Obstet Gynecol 1991;78:1112–1116 (Level III)

32. Enders G, Miller E, Cradock-Watson J, Bolley I, Ridehalgh M. Consequences of varicella and herpes zoster in pregnancy: prospective study of 1739 cases. Lancet 1994;343:1548–1551 (Level II-2)

33. Jones KL, Johnson KA, Chambers CD. Offspring of women infected with varicella during pregnancy: a prospective study. Teratology 1994;49:29–32 (Level II-2)

34. Pastuszak AL, Levy M, Schick B, Zuber C, Feldkamp M, Gladstone J, et al. Outcome after maternal varicella infection in the first 20 weeks of pregnancy. N Engl J Med 1994;330:901–905 (Level II-2)

35. Brunell PA. Placental transfer of varicella-zoster antibody. Pediatrics 1966;38:1034–1038 (Level III)

36. Brunell PA. Fetal and neonatal varicella-zoster infections. Semin Perinatol 1983;7:47–56 (Level III)

37. Hohlfeld P, Daffos F, Costa JM, Thulliez P, Forestier F, Vidaud M. Prenatal diagnosis of congenital toxoplasmosis with a polymerase-chain-reaction test on amniotic fluid. N Engl J Med 1994;331:695–699 (Level II-2)

38. Foulon W, Villena I, Stray-Pedersen B, Decoster A, Lappalainen M, Pinon JM, et al. Treatment of toxoplasmosis during pregnancy: a multicenter study of impact on fetal transmission and children's sequelae at age 1 year. Am J Obstet Gynecol 1999;180:410–415 (Level II-3)

39. Stray-Pedersen B. Toxoplasmosis in pregnancy. Baillieres Clin Obstet Gynaecol 1993;7:107–137 (Level III)

40. Wilson CB, Remington JS, Stagno S, Reynolds DW. Development of adverse sequelae in children born with subclinical congenital Toxoplasma infection. Pediatrics 1980;66:767–774 (Level II-3)

41. de Roever-Bonnet H, Koppe JG, Loewer-Seger DH. Follow-up of children with congenital toxoplasma infection and children who became serologically negative after 1 year of age, all born in 1964–1965. In: Thalhammer O, Baumgarten K, Pollak A, eds. Perinatal medicine: Sixth European Congress, Vienna. Littleton, Massachusetts: PSG Publishing Company, 1979:61–75 (Level III)

42. Desmonts G, Couvreur J. Congenital toxoplasmosis. A prospective study of 378 pregnancies. N Engl J Med 1974;290:1110–1116 (Level II-3)

43. Daffos F, Forestier F, Capella-Pavlovsky M, Thulliez P, Aufrant C, Valenti D, et al. Prenatal management of 746 pregnancies at risk for congenital toxoplasmosis. N Engl J Med 1988;318:271–275 (Level II-3)

44. Remington JS, McLeod R, Desmonts G. Toxoplasmosis. In: Remington JS, Klein JO, eds. Infectious disease of the fetus and newborn infant. 4th ed. Philadelphia: WB Saunders, 1995:140–267 (Level III)

45. Stagno S, Tinker MK, Elrod C, Fuccillo DA, Cloud G, O'Beirne AJ. Immunoglobulin M antibodies detected by enzyme-linked immunosorbent assay and radioimmunoassay in the diagnosis of cytomegalovirus infections in pregnant women and newborn infants. J Clin Microbiol 1985;21:930–935 (Level II-3)

46. Drose JA, Dennis MA, Thickman D. Infection in utero: US findings in 19 cases. Radiology 1991;178:369–374 (Level III)

47. Stein B, Bromley B, Michlewitz H, Miller WA, Benacerraf BR. Fetal liver calcifications: sonographic appearance and postnatal outcome. Radiology 1995; 197:489–492 (Level III)

48. Ghidini A, Sirtori M, Vergani P, Mariani S, Tucci E, Scola GC. Fetal intracranial calcifications. Am J Obstet Gynecol 1989;160:86–87 (Level III)

49. Yamashita Y, Iwanaga R, Goto A, Kaneko S, Yamashita F, Wasedna N, et al. Congenital cytomegalovirus infection associated with fetal ascites and intrahepatic calcifications. Acta Paediatr Scand 1989;78:965–967 (Level III)

50. Forouzan I. Fetal abdominal echogenic mass: an early sign of intrauterine cytomegalovirus infection. Obstet Gynecol 1992;80:535–537 (Level III)

51. Twickler DM, Perlman J, Maberry MC. Congenital cytomegalovirus infection presenting as cerebral ventriculomegaly on antenatal sonography. Am J Perinatol 1993;10:404–406 (Level III)

52. Weiner Z. Congenital cytomegalovirus infection with oligohydramnios and echogenic bowel at 14 weeks' gestation. J Ultrasound Med 1995;14:617–618 (Level III)

53. Yaron Y, Hassan S, Geva E, Kupferminc MJ, Yavetz H, Evans MI, et al. Evaluation of fetal echogenic bowel in the second trimester. Fetal Diagn Ther 1999;14:176–180 (Level II-3)

54. Bale JF Jr, Blackman JA, Sato Y. Outcome in children with symptomatic congenital cytomegalovirus infection. J Child Neurol 1990;5:131–136 (Level III)

55. Lynch L, Daffos F, Emanuel D, Giovangrandi Y, Meisel R, Forestier F, et al. Prenatal diagnosis of fetal cytomegalovirus infection. Am J Obstet Gynecol 1991;165: 714–718 (Level III)

56. Donner C, Liesnard C, Content J, Busine A, Aderca J, Rodesch F. Prenatal diagnosis of 52 pregnancies at risk for congenital cytomegalovirus infection. Obstet Gynecol 1993;82:481–486 (Level III)

57. Nicolini U, Kustermann A, Tassis B, Fogliani R, Galimberti A, Percivalle E, et al. Prenatal diagnosis of congenital human cytomegalovirus infection. Prenat Diagn 1994;14:903–906 (Level III)

58. Stango S. Cytomegalovirus. In: Remington JS, Klein JO, eds. Infectious disease of the fetus and newborn infant. 4th ed. Philadelphia: WB Saunders, 1995:312–353 (Level III)

59. Hohlfeld P, Vial Y, Maillard-Brignon C, Vaudaux B, Fawer CL. Cytomegalovirus fetal infection: prenatal diagnosis. Obstet Gynecol 1991;78:615–618 (Level III)

60. Lamy ME, Mulongo KN, Gadisseux JF, Lyon G, Gaudy V, Van Lierde M. Prenatal diagnosis of fetal cytomegalovirus infection. Am J Obstet Gynecol 1992;166:91–94 (Level III)

61. Hogge WA, Buffone GJ, Hogge JS. Prenatal diagnosis of cytomegalovirus (CMV) infection: a preliminary report. Prenat Diagn 1993;13:131–136 (Level III)

62. Revello MG, Baldanti F, Furione M, Sarasini A, Percivalle E, Zavattoni M, et al. Polymerase chain reaction for prenatal diagnosis of congenital human cytomegalovirus infection. J Med Virol 1995;47:462–466 (Level II-3)

63. Lipitz S, Yagel S, Shalev E, Achiron R, Mashiach S, Schiff E. Prenatal diagnosis of fetal primary cytomegalovirus infection. Obstet Gynecol 1997;89: 763–767 (Level II-3)

64. Lazzarotto T, Guerra B, Spezzacatena P, Varani S, Gabrielli L, Pradelli P, et al. Prenatal diagnosis of congenital cytomegalovirus infection. J Clin Microbiol 1998;36:3540–3544 (Level II-3)

65. Donner C, Liesnard C, Brancart F, Rodesch F. Accuracy of amniotic fluid testing before 21 weeks' gestation in prenatal diagnosis of congenital cytomegalovirus infection. Prenat Diagn 1994;14:1055–1059 (Level II-3)

66. Gilstrap LC, Bawdon RE, Roberts SW, Sobhi S. The transfer of the nucleoside analog ganciclovir across the perfused human placenta. Am J Obstet Gynecol 1994;170:967–972; discussion 972–973 (Level III)

67. Attard-Montalto SP, English MC, Stimmler L, Snodgrass GJ. Ganciclovir treatment of congenital cytomegalovirus infection: a report of two cases. Scand J Infect Dis 1993;25:385–388 (Level III)

68. Fukuda S, Miyachi M, Sugimoto S, Goshima A, Futamura M, Morishima T. A female infant successfully treated by ganciclovir for congenital cytomegalovirus infection. Acta Paediatr Jpn 1995;37:206–210 (Level III)

69. Stronati M, Revello MG, Cerbo RM, Furione M, Rondini G, Gerna G. Ganciclovir therapy of congenital human cytomegalovirus hepatitis. Acta Paediatr 1995;84: 340–341 (Level III)

70. Nigro G, Scholz H, Bartmann U. Ganciclovir therapy for symptomatic congenital cytomegalovirus infection in infants: a two-regimen experience. J Pediatr 1994;124: 318–322 (Level II-3)

71. Barbi M, Binda S, Primache V, Novelli C. Cytomegalovirus in peripheral blood leukocytes of infants with congenital or postnatal infection. Pediatr Infect Dis J 1996;15:898–903 (Level II-3)

72. Whitley RJ, Cloud G, Gruber W, Storch GA, Demmler GJ, Jacobs RF, et al. Ganciclovir treatment of symptomatic congenital cytomegalovirus infection: results of a phase II study. National Institute of Allergy and Infectious Diseases Collaborative Antiviral Study Group. J Infect Dis 1997;175:1080–1086 (Level II-3)

73. Plotkin SA, Starr SE, Friedman HM, Gonczol E, Brayman K. Vaccines for the prevention of human cytomegalovirus infection. Rev Infect Dis 1990;12 (Suppl 7):S827–S838 (Level III)

74. Plotkin SA, Starr SE, Friedman HM, Brayman K, Harris S, Jackson S, et al. Effect of Towne live virus vaccine on cytomegalovirus disease after renal transplant. A controlled trial. Ann Intern Med 1991;114:525–531 (Level I)

75. Plotkin SA, Higgins R, Kurtz JB, Morris PJ, Campbell DA Jr, Shope TC, et al. Multicenter trial of Towne strain attenuated virus vaccine in seronegative renal transplant recipients. Transplantation 1994;58:1176–1178 (Level I)

76. Adler SP, Hempfling SH, Starr SE, Plotkin SA, Riddell S. Safety and immunogenicity of the Towne strain cytomegalovirus vaccine. Pediatr Infect Dis J 1998; 17:200–206 (Level II-3)

77. Porath A, McNutt RA, Smiley LM, Weigle KA. Effectiveness and cost benefit of a proposed live cytomegalovirus vaccine in the prevention of congenital disease. Rev Infect Dis 1990;12:31–40 (Level III)

78. Scott LL, Hollier LM, Dias K. Perinatal herpesvirus infections. Herpes simplex, varicella, and cytomegalovirus. Infect Dis Clin North Am 1997;11:27–53 (Level III)

79. Raynor BD. Cytomegalovirus infection in pregnancy. Semin Perinatol 1993;17:394–402 (Level III)

80. Adler SP. Cytomegalovirus and pregnancy. Curr Opin Obstet Gynecol 1992;4:670–675 (Level III)

81. Grangeot-Keros L, Simon B, Audibert F, Vial M. Should we routinely screen for cytomegalovirus antibody during pregnancy? Intervirology 1998;41:158–162 (Level III)

82. Pass RF, August AM, Dworsky M, Reynolds DW. Cytomegalovirus infection in day-care center. N Engl J Med 1982;307:477–479 (Level II-2)

83. Olson LC, Ketusinha R, Mansuwan P, Snitbhan R. Respiratory tract excretion of cytomegalovirus in Thai children. J Pediatr 1970;77:499–504 (Level II-3)

84. Yeager AS. Transmission of cytomegalovirus to mothers by infected infants: another reason to prevent transfusion-acquired infections. Pediatr Infect Dis 1983;2: 295–297 (Level III)

85. Tookey PA, Ades AE, Peckham CS. Cytomegalovirus prevalence in pregnant women: the influence of parity. Arch Dis Child 1992;67:779–783 (Level II-3)

86. Biomedical Research Institute. CMV: diagnosis, prevention, and treatment. 2nd ed. St. Paul, Minnesota: Children's Hospital of St. Paul & Children's Biomedical Research Institute, 1989 (Level III)

87. Anderson LJ, Tsou C, Parker RA, Chorba TL, Wulff H, Tattersall P, et al. Detection of antibodies and antigens of human parvovirus B19 by enzyme-linked immunosorbent assay. J Clin Microbiol 1986;24:522–526 (Level II-2)

88. Schwarz TF, Nerlich A, Hottentrager B, Jager G, Wiest I, Kantimm S, et al. Parvovirus B19 infection of the fetus. Histology and in situ hybridization. Am J Clin Pathol 1991;96:121–126 (Level III)

89. Schwarz TF, Nerlich A, Hillemanns P. Detection of parvovirus B19 in fetal autopsies. Arch Gynecol Obstet 1993;253:207–213 (Level III)

90. Sifakis S, Ergazaki M, Sourvinos G, Koffa M, Koumantakis E, Spandidos DA. Evaluation of Parvo B19, CMV and HPV viruses in human aborted material using the polymerase chain reaction technique. Eur J Obstet Gynecol Reprod Biol 1998;76:169–173 (Level II-3)

91. Clewley JP. Polymerase chain reaction assay of parvovirus B19 DNA in clinical specimens. J Clin Microbiol 1989;27:2647–2651 (Level II-3)

92. Salimans MM, van de Rijke FM, Raap AK, van Elsacker-Niele AM. Detection of parvovirus B19 DNA in fetal tissues by in situ hybridisation and polymerase chain reaction. J Clin Pathol 1989;42:525–530 (Level III)

93. Kovacs BW, Carlson DE, Shahbahrami B, Platt LD. Prenatal diagnosis of human parvovirus B19 in nonimmune hydrops fetalis by polymerase chain reaction. Am J Obstet Gynecol 1992;167:461–466 (Level III)

94. Torok TJ, Wang QY, Gary GW Jr, Yang CF, Finch TM, Anderson LJ, et al. Prenatal diagnosis of intrauterine infection with parvovirus B19 by the polymerase chain reaction technique. Clin Infect Dis 1992;14:149–155 (Level III)

95. Rogers BB, Mak SK, Dailey JV, Saller DN Jr, Buffone GJ. Detection of parvovirus B19 DNA in amniotic fluid by PCR DNA amplification. Biotechniques 1993;15: 406–408, 410 (Level III)

96. Torok TJ. Human parvovirus B19. In: Remington JS, Klein JO, eds. Infectious disease of the fetus and newborn infant. 4th ed. Philadelphia: WB Saunders, 1995:668–702 (Level III)

97. Peters MT, Nicolaides KH. Cordocentesis for the diagnosis and treatment of human fetal parvovirus infection. Obstet Gynecol 1990;75:501–504 (Level III)

98. Levy R, Weissman A, Blomberg G, Hagay ZJ. Infection by parvovirus B 19 during pregnancy: a review. Obstet Gynecol Surv 1997;52:254–259 (Level III)

99. Fairley CK, Smoleniec JS, Caul OE, Miller E. Observational study of effect of intrauterine transfusions on outcome of fetal hydrops after parvovirus B19 infection. Lancet 1995;346:1335–1337 (Level II-3)

100. Pretorius DH, Hayward I, Jones KL, Stamm E. Sonographic evaluation of pregnancies with maternal varicella infection. J Ultrasound Med 1992;11:459–463 (Level III)

101. Lecuru F, Taurelle R, Bernard JP, Parrat S, Lafay-pillet MC, Rozenberg F, et al. Varicella zoster virus infection during pregnancy: the limits of prenatal diagnosis. Eur J Obstet Gynecol Reprod Biol 1994;56:67–68 (Level III)

102. Kustermann A, Zoppini C, Tassis B, Della Morte M, Colucci G, Nicolini U. Prenatal diagnosis of congenital varicella infection. Prenat Diagn 1996;16:71–74 (Level III)

103. Isada NB, Paar DP, Johnson MP, Evans MI, Holzgreve W, Qureshi F, et al. In utero diagnosis of congenital varicella zoster virus infection by chorionic villus sampling and polymerase chain reaction. Am J Obstet Gynecol 1991;165:1727–1730 (Level III)

104. Balfour HH Jr, Rotbart HA, Feldman S, Dunkle LM, Feder HM Jr, Prober CG, et al. Acyclovir treatment of varicella in otherwise healthy adolescents. The Collaborative Acyclovir Varicella Study Group. J Pediatr 1992;120:627–633 (Level I)

105. Wallace MR, Bowler WA, Murray NB, Brodine SK, Oldfield EC 3d. Treatment of adult varicella with oral acyclovir. A randomized, placebo-controlled trial. Ann Intern Med 1992;117:358–363 (Level I)

106. Ogilvie MM. Antiviral prophylaxis and treatment in chickenpox. A review prepared for the UK Advisory Group on Chickenpox on behalf of the British Society for the Study of Infection. J Infect 1998;36(Suppl 1):31–38 (Level III)

107. Kesson AM, Grimwood K, Burgess MA, Ferson MJ, Gilbert GL, Hogg G, et al. Acyclovir for the prevention and treatment of varicella zoster in children, adolescents and pregnancy. J Paediatr Child Health 1996;32:211–217 (Level III)

108. Cox SM, Cunningham FG, Luby J. Management of varicella pneumonia complicating pregnancy. Am J Perinatol 1990;7:300–301 (Level III)

109. American Academy of Pediatrics Committee on Infectious Diseases: the use of oral acyclovir in otherwise healthy children with varicella. Pediatrics 1993;91:674–676 (Level III) [erratum Pediatrics 1993;91:858]

110. Miller E, Cradock-Watson JE, Ridehalgh MK. Outcome in newborn babies given anti-varicella-zoster immunoglobulin after perinatal maternal infection with varicella-zoster virus. Lancet 1989;8659:371–373 (Level II-3)

111. Williams H, Latif A, Morgan J, Ansari BM. Acyclovir in the treatment of neonatal varicella. J Infect 1987;15:65–67 (Level III)

112. Centers for Disease Control and Prevention. Prevention of varicella: recommendations of the Advisory Committee on Immunization Practices (ACIP). MMWR Morb Mortal Wkly Rep 1996;45(RR-11):1–36 (Level III)

113. Glantz JC, Mushlin AI. Cost-effectiveness of routine antenatal varicella screening. Obstet Gynecol 1998;91:519–528 (Level III)

114. Rouse DJ, Gardner M, Allen SJ, Goldenberg RL. Management of the presumed susceptible varicella (chickenpox)-exposed gravida: a cost-effectiveness/cost-benefit analysis. Obstet Gynecol 1996;87:932–936 (Level III)

115. McGregor JA, Mark S, Crawford GP, Levin MJ. Varicella zoster antibody testing in the care of pregnant women exposed to varicella. Am J Obstet Gynecol 1987;157:281–284 (Level II-3)

116. Brunell PA, Ross A, Miller LH, Kuo B. Prevention of varicella by zoster immune globulin. N Engl J Med 1969;280:1191–1194 (Level II-1)

117. Varicella-zoster immune globulin for the prevention of chickenpox. Recommendations of the Immunization Practices Advisory Committee, Centers for Disease Control. Ann Intern Med 1984;100:859–865 (Level III)

118. Montoya JG, Remington JS. Toxoplasma gondii. In: Mandell GL, Bennett JE, Dolin R, eds. Principles and practices in infectious disease. 5th ed. New York: Churchill Livingstone, 2000:2858–2888 (Level III)

119. Fricker-Hidalgo H, Pelloux H, Racinet C, Grefenstette I, Bost-Bru C, Goullier-Fleuret A, et al. Detection of Toxoplasma gondii in 94 placentae from infected women by polymerase chain reaction, in vivo, and in vitro cultures. Placenta 1998;19:545–549 (Level II-3)

120. Hezard N, Marx-Chemla C, Foudrinier F, Villena I, Quereux C, Leroux B, et al. Prenatal diagnosis of congenital toxoplasmosis in 261 pregnancies. Prenat Diagn 1997;17:1047–1054 (Level II-3)

121. Grover CM, Thulliez P, Remington JS, Boothroyd JC. Rapid prenatal diagnosis of congenital Toxoplasma infection by using polymerase chain reaction and amniotic fluid. J Clin Microbiol 1990;28:2297–2301 (Level II-2)

122. van de Ven E, Melchers W, Galama J, Camps W, Meuwissen J. Identification of Toxoplasma gondii infections by BI gene amplification. J Clin Microbiol 1991;29:2120–2124 (Level III)

123. Cazenave J, Forestier F, Bessieres MH, Broussin B, Begueret J. Contribution of a new PCR assay to the prenatal diagnosis of congenital toxoplasmosis. Prenat Diagn 1992;12:119–127 (Level II-2)

124. Jenum PA, Holberg-Petersen M, Melby KK, Stray-Pedersen B. Diagnosis of congenital Toxoplasma gondii infection by polymerase chain reaction (PCR) on amniotic fluid samples. The Norwegian experience. APMIS 1998;106:680–686 (Level II-3)

125. Guy EC, Pelloux H, Lappalainen M, Aspock H, Hassl A, Melby KK, et al. Interlaboratory comparison of polymerase chain reaction for the detection of Toxoplasma gondii DNA added to samples of amniotic fluid. Eur J Clin Microbiol Infect Dis 1996;15:836–839 (Level III)

126. Mombro M, Perathoner C, Leone A, Nicocia M, Moiraghi Ruggenini A, et al. Congenital toxoplasmosis: 10-year follow up. Eur J Pediatr 1995;154:635–639 (Level II-3)

127. Stray-Pedersen B. Treatment of toxoplasmosis in the pregnant mother and newborn child. Scand J Infect Dis Suppl 1992;84:23–31 (Level III)

128. Berrebi A, Kobuch WE, Bessieres MH, Bloom MC, Rolland M, Sarramon MF, et al. Termination of pregnancy for maternal toxoplasmosis. Lancet 1994;344:36–39 (Level II-3)

129. Patel DV, Holfels EM, Vogel NP, Boyer KM, Mets MB, Swisher CN, et al. Resolution of intracranial calcifications in infants with treated congenital toxoplasmosis. Radiology 1996;199:433–440 (Level II-3)

130. Sever JL, Ellenberg JH, Ley AC, Madden DL, Fuccillo DA, Tzan NR, et al. Toxoplasmosis: maternal and pediatric findings in 23,000 pregnancies. Pediatrics 1988;82:181–192 (Level II-3)

131. Foulon W. Congenital toxoplasmosis: is screening desirable? Scand J Infect Dis Suppl 1992;84:11–17 (Level II-3)

The MEDLINE database, the Cochrane Library, and ACOG's own internal resources and documents were used to conduct a literature search to locate relevant articles published between January 1985 and January 2000. The search was restricted to articles published in the English language. Priority was given to articles reporting results of original research, although review articles and commentaries also were consulted. Abstracts of research presented at symposia and scientific conferences were not considered adequate for inclusion in this document. Guidelines published by organizations or institutions such as the National Institutes of Health and the American College of Obstetricians and Gynecologists were reviewed, and additional studies were located by reviewing bibliographies of identified articles. When reliable research was not available, expert opinions from obstetrician–gynecologists were used.

Studies were reviewed and evaluated for quality according to the method outlined by the U.S. Preventive Services Task Force:

- I Evidence obtained from at least one properly designed randomized controlled trial.
- II-1 Evidence obtained from well-designed controlled trials without randomization.
- II-2 Evidence obtained from well-designed cohort or case–control analytic studies, preferably from more than one center or research group.
- II-3 Evidence obtained from multiple time series with or without the intervention. Dramatic results in uncontrolled experiments also could be regarded as this type of evidence.
- III Opinions of respected authorities, based on clinical experience, descriptive studies, or reports of expert committees.

Based on the highest level of evidence found in the data, recommendations are provided and graded according to the following catetories:

Level A—Recommendations are based on good and consistent scientific evidence.

Level B—Recommendations are based on limited or inconsistent scientific evidence.

Level C—Recommendations are based primarily on consensus and expert opinion.

ISSN 1099-3630

The American College of
Obstetricians and Gynecologists
409 12th Street, SW
PO Box 96920
Washington, DC 20090-6920 12345/43210

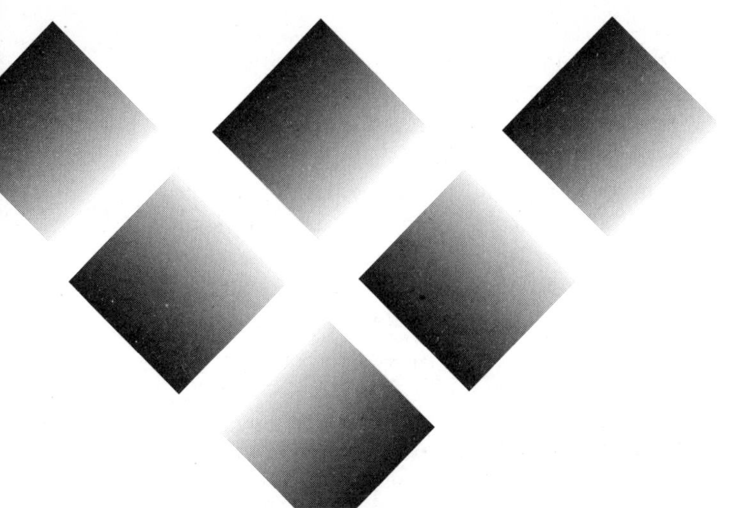

ACOG PRACTICE BULLETIN

CLINICAL MANAGEMENT GUIDELINES FOR OBSTETRICIAN–GYNECOLOGISTS

NUMBER 1, JUNE 1998

This Practice Bulletin was developed by the ACOG Committees on Practice Bulletins—Obstetrics and Gynecology with the assistance of Brian M. Mercer, MD. The information is designed to aid practitioners in making decisions about appropriate obstetric and gynecologic care. These guidelines should not be construed as dictating an exclusive course of treatment or procedure. Variations in practice may be warranted based on the needs of the individual patient, resources, and limitations unique to the institution or type of practice.

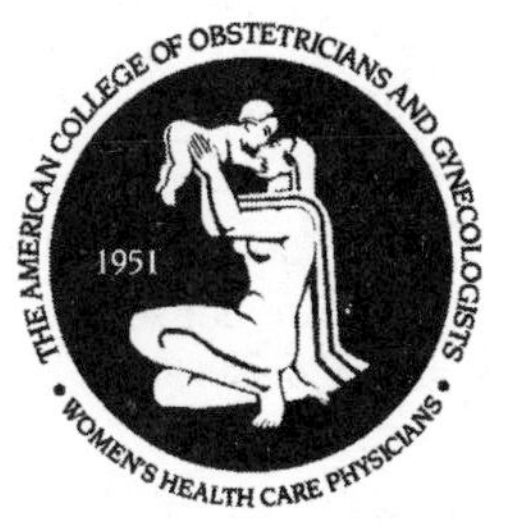

Premature Rupture of Membranes

Preterm delivery occurs in approximately 11% of all births in the United States and is a major factor contributing to perinatal morbidity and mortality. Despite extensive research in this area, the rate of preterm birth has increased by 17% over the past 15 years (1). Premature rupture of membranes (PROM) is a complication in one quarter to one third of preterm births. In both term and preterm births, numerous controversies exist regarding optimal methods of clinical assessment and treatment of PROM. Management hinges on evaluation of the relative risks of infection, cord accident, operative delivery, and of the gestational age in patients not in labor. The purpose of this document is to review the current understanding of this condition and to provide management guidelines that have been validated by appropriately conducted outcome-based research. Additional guidelines based on consensus and expert opinion also are presented to permit a review of most clinical aspects of PROM.

Background

The definition of PROM is rupture of membranes before the onset of labor. When membrane rupture occurs before 37 weeks of gestation, it is referred to as preterm PROM. Premature rupture of membranes can result from a wide array of pathologic mechanisms acting individually or in concert (2). The gestational age at membrane rupture has significant implications regarding the etiology and consequences of PROM. Management may be dictated by the presence of overt intrauterine infection, advanced labor, or fetal compromise. When such factors are not present, especially with preterm PROM, other interventions may have a significant impact on maternal and infant morbidity. An accurate assessment of gestational age and knowledge of the maternal, fetal, and neonatal risks are essential to appropriate evaluation, counseling, and management of patients with PROM.

Etiology

Membrane rupture may occur for a variety of reasons. At term, weakening of the membranes may result from physiologic changes combined with shearing forces created by uterine contractions (2, 3). Intrauterine infection has been shown to play an important role in preterm PROM, especially at earlier gestational ages (4). Factors associated with an increase in PROM include lower socioeconomic status, sexually transmissible infections, prior preterm delivery (especially due to PROM), vaginal bleeding, cervical conization, and cigarette smoking during pregnancy (2, 5–7). Uterine distention (hydramnios, twins), emergency cervical cerclage, prior antepartum antibiotic treatment, and preterm labor also may be associated with PROM (2, 6, 8). In many cases, however, PROM may occur in the absence of recognized risk factors.

Term Premature Rupture of Membranes

At term, PROM complicates approximately 8% of pregnancies and is generally followed by the onset of labor and delivery. In a large randomized trial, half of women with PROM who were managed expectantly delivered within 5 hours, and 95% delivered within 28 hours of membrane rupture (9). Other studies have reported similar rates (10).

The most significant maternal risk of term PROM is intrauterine infection, a risk that increases with the duration of membrane rupture (6, 9–12). Fetal risks associated with PROM include umbilical cord compression and ascending infection.

Preterm Premature Rupture of Membranes

Regardless of management or clinical presentation, birth within 1 week is the most likely outcome of any patient with PROM prior to term. A review of 13 randomized trials reported that approximately 75% of patients with preterm PROM who were managed expectantly delivered within 1 week (13). The earlier in gestation that PROM occurs, the greater the potential for pregnancy prolongation. With expectant management, 2.8–13% of women can anticipate cessation of fluid leakage (12, 14).

Of women with preterm PROM, clinically evident intraamniotic infection occurs in 13–60% and postpartum infection occurs in 2–13% (14–18). The incidence of infection increases with decreasing gestational age at membrane rupture (19, 20) and increases with digital vaginal examination (21). With appropriate management, however, serious maternal sequelae are uncommon (13, 16). Fetal malpresentation is increased with preterm PROM. Abruptio placentae affects 4–12% of pregnancies with preterm PROM (22, 23).

The most significant risks to the fetus after preterm PROM are complications of prematurity. At all gestational ages prior to term, respiratory distress has been reported to be the most common complication (15, 24). Other serious forms of morbidity, including necrotizing enterocolitis and intraventricular hemorrhage, also are associated with prematurity but are less common nearer to term. The presence of maternal infection poses the additional risk of neonatal infection. Infection, cord accident, and other factors contribute to the 1–2% risk of antenatal fetal demise after preterm PROM (13).

Midtrimester Premature Rupture of Membranes

Premature rupture of membranes occurring before and around the time of neonatal viability often is referred to as midtrimester PROM. Premature rupture of membranes at 16–26 weeks of gestation complicates almost 1% of pregnancies (7, 25). Before the 1970s, delivery in the second trimester was generally associated with neonatal death resulting from complications of prematurity. Primarily because of advances in neonatal intensive care over the past two decades, neonates are surviving at increasingly younger gestational ages. Currently, overall infant survival after delivery at 24–26 weeks of gestation is reported to be between 50% and 75% (24, 26, 27). Survival rates in pregnancies complicated by PROM are comparable (28–30) but decreased in the presence of infection or deformations.

A small number of patients with midtrimester PROM will have an extended latency period. In a review of 12 studies evaluating patients with midtrimester PROM, the mean latency period ranged from 10.6 to 21.5 days (25). Although delivery occurred within 1 week of membrane rupture in 57% of patients, in 22% of patients pregnancy continued for 1 month. Most studies of midtrimester PROM have been retrospective and include only those patients amenable to expectant management. Patients usually are excluded from analysis in the presence of labor, infection, prolapsed membranes, and fetal demise, thus potentially exaggerating the latency period to delivery and deceptively decreasing the apparent maternal and infant morbidity.

Reported maternal complications of midtrimester PROM include intraamniotic infection, endometritis, abruptio placentae, retained placentae, and postpartum hemorrhage. Maternal sepsis is a rare but serious complication reported to affect approximately 1% of cases (25, 29).

The incidence of stillbirth subsequent to PROM at 16–25 weeks of gestation ranges from 3.8% to 21.7% (7, 15, 31) compared with 0–2% with PROM at 30–36 weeks of gestation (32, 33). This increased rate of death may be explained by increased susceptibility of the umbilical cord to compression or of the fetus to hypoxia and intrauterine infection. Alternatively, this finding may reflect the lack of intervention for fetal compromise prior to neonatal viability. The fetal survival rate subsequent to PROM at less than 24 weeks of gestation has been reported to be about 30%, compared with a 57% survival rate with rupture at 24–26 weeks of gestation (25).

Several trials have described outcomes of survivors after PROM at 16–26 weeks of gestation (7, 29–31, 34, 35). Although up to 69% of these neonates were reported as having normal neurologic development, these results may be biased by a lack of follow-up. Generalized developmental delay, delayed motor development, and other less frequent complications, including cerebral palsy, chronic lung disease, blindness, hydrocephalus, and mental retardation, also were reported to occur.

A variety of conditions that are associated with fetal lung compression or oligohydramnios or both can result in pulmonary hypoplasia. Reported risks of pulmonary hypoplasia after PROM at 16–26 weeks of gestation vary from less than 1% to 27% (18, 29). Pulmonary hypoplasia rarely occurs with membrane rupture subsequent to 26 weeks of gestation, presumably because alveolar growth adequate to support postnatal development already has occurred (36, 37). Prolonged oligohydramnios also is associated with in utero deformation including abnormal facies (ie, low-set ears and epicanthal folds) and limb positioning abnormalities.

When leakage of amniotic fluid occurs after amniocentesis, the outcome is better than after spontaneous preterm PROM. In one study of 603 women who had second-trimester amniocentesis for prenatal diagnosis of genetic disorders, seven women (1.2%) experienced PROM, and leakage stopped in all with conservative management (8).

Clinical Considerations and Recommendations

▶ *How is premature rupture of membranes diagnosed?*

An accurate diagnosis is crucial to the management of suspected membrane rupture. Most cases can be diagnosed on the basis of the history and physical examination (38). Other causes of discharge include urinary leakage, excess vaginal discharge with advanced dilatation or membrane prolapse, cervicitis, bloody show, semen, and vaginal douches. Symptoms suggestive of PROM should be confirmed. Delay in evaluation may result in a missed opportunity for intervention.

Examination should be performed in a manner that minimizes the risk of introducing infection, particularly prior to term. Digital cervical examinations increase the risk of infection and add little information to that available with speculum examination (21, 39). Thus, digital examinations should be avoided unless prompt labor and delivery are anticipated. Sterile speculum examination can confirm the diagnosis of PROM as well as provide an opportunity to inspect for cervicitis or umbilical cord or fetal prolapse, assess cervical dilatation and effacement, and obtain cultures as appropriate (40).

The diagnosis of membrane rupture is confirmed by the visualization of amniotic fluid in the posterior vaginal fornix or clear fluid passing from the cervical canal. If the diagnosis remains in question, the pH of the vaginal sidewalls or fluid pool can be assessed.

The pH of the vaginal secretions is generally 4.5–6.0 whereas amniotic fluid usually has a pH of 7.1–7.3. Nitrazine paper will turn blue with a pH above 6.0–6.5. False-positive results may occur in the presence of blood or semen contamination, alkaline antiseptics, or bacterial vaginosis. Alternatively, false-negative results may occur with prolonged leakage and minimal residual fluid. More information can be obtained by swabbing the posterior fornix (avoiding cervical mucus) and allowing the vaginal fluid to dry on a microscope slide. The presence of arborization (ferning) under microscopic visualization further suggests membrane rupture.

When the clinical history or physical examination is unclear, ultrasound examination may be useful to document oligohydramnios, which in the absence of fetal urinary tract malformations or significant growth restriction is suggestive of membrane rupture. Membrane rupture can be diagnosed unequivocally with ultrasonographically guided transabdominal instillation of indigo carmine dye (1 mL in 9 mL sterile normal saline), followed by observation for passage of blue fluid from the vagina within 30 minutes of amniocentesis.

▶ *What is the optimal method of initial management for a patient with PROM at term?*

Fetal heart rate monitoring may be used to assess fetal status. Dating criteria should be reviewed to assign gestational age because virtually all aspects of subsequent care will hinge on that information. Group B streptococcal status and the need for intrapartum prophylaxis should be determined (41).

▶ *When should labor be induced in patients with term PROM?*

Fetal presentation, gestational age, and status should be established before determining whether labor should be induced. The decision to induce labor involves an assessment of the relative risks of infection or fetal compromise (which may increase with the duration of PROM) versus the risks of failed induction and operative vaginal delivery (which may increase with induced as opposed to spontaneous labor).

If the condition of the cervix is unfavorable, there is little difference in outcome when comparing induction to expectant management. Options evaluated ranged from immediate induction to observation for up to 24–72 hours prior to induction (9, 42–45). While time from admission to delivery is shortened with induction, time in labor is longer, and the need for operative vaginal delivery seems to be higher (44, 46).

Risk of cesarean delivery and risk of neonatal infectious complications do not appear to depend on the mode of management (expectant versus induction), although the risks of maternal infection may increase with expectant management (9, 43, 45). Thus, it is reasonable for consideration of the patient's wishes and hospitalization costs to influence management.

▶ *What does the initial evaluation involve once PROM has been confirmed?*

Fetal presentation, gestational age, and status should be determined. The gravida with evident intrauterine infection, abruptio placentae, or evidence of fetal compromise is best cared for by expeditious delivery. In the absence of an indication for immediate delivery, swabs for diagnosis of *Chlamydia trachomatis* and *Neisseria gonorrhoeae* may be obtained from the cervix if appropriate. The need for group B streptococcal intrapartum prophylaxis should be determined (41).

▶ *When should one elect delivery for the fetus near term in the presence of premature rupture of membranes?*

After initial assessment, relative maternal and fetal risks with expectant management, neonatal risks with early delivery, and the potential neonatal benefit from expectant management can then be determined. Because serious neonatal morbidity is uncommon with demonstrated pulmonary maturity and delivery after 32–36 weeks of gestation (33), amniotic fluid may be collected from the vaginal pool or by amniocentesis for assessment of fetal pulmonary maturity.

If pulmonary maturity has been documented after PROM at 32–36 weeks of gestation, labor induction may be considered. Available clinical trial data concerning expectant management versus immediate induction at 30–34 weeks of gestation (32) and at 32–36 weeks of gestation (33) show increased risks of chorioamnionitis and prolonged hospitalization with expectant management but equal risks of respiratory distress syndrome, intraventricular hemorrhage, necrotizing enterocolitis, and neonatal death. It is noteworthy that in the studies cited (32, 33), which were conducted in major centers with neonatal intensive care units, antibiotics (32, 33) or antenatal corticosteroids (32) were not utilized. Although it is uncertain whether the use of prophylactic antibiotics and antenatal corticosteroids will improve the outcome of expectant management at these gestational ages, it is clear that delivery of a preterm infant should take place in a facility with experience in the management of such infants.

The gravida who experiences PROM before 30–32 weeks of gestation and whose condition is stable is generally best served by expectant management. The prophylactic use of antibiotics and antenatal corticosteroids can help reduce the risks of gestational age-dependent neonatal morbidity.

▶ *What general approaches are utilized in patients with preterm PROM managed expectantly?*

Expectant management of preterm PROM generally consists of modified bed rest to potentially enhance amniotic fluid reaccumulation and complete pelvic rest to avoid infection. Patients should be assessed periodically for evidence of infection or labor. In a patient with preterm PROM, a temperature exceeding 38.0°C (100.4°F) may be indicative of infection, although some investigators have suggested that fever, with additional factors such as uterine tenderness and maternal or fetal tachycardia, is a more accurate indicator of maternal infection (15, 47). Leukocyte counts are nonspecific in the absence of clinical evidence of infection, especially if antenatal corticosteroids have been administered.

If the presence of intraamniotic infection is suspected and additional diagnostic confirmation is required, amniocentesis may be considered (48). The diagnosis of intraamniotic infection may be suggested by an amniotic fluid glucose concentration of less than 20 mg/dL, by a positive Gram stain, or a positive amniotic fluid culture (49–51). The presence of amniotic fluid leukocytes alone is not diagnostic of infection. In a case-control study comparing amniotic fluid tests used to predict infection, investigators concluded interleukin-6 was the only test that had significant clinical value in predicting neonatal complications (51). Other investigators have rejected amniocentesis because of a low success rate and the need for repeat procedures (52).

▶ *Should tocolytics be considered in patients with preterm PROM in labor?*

Prophylactic tocolysis after preterm PROM has been shown to prolong latency in the short term (53–55), while therapeutic tocolysis (ie, instituting tocolysis only after contractions have ensued) has not been shown to prolong latency (56). No study to date has demonstrated that tocolytics benefit neonatal outcome, but none has utilized antibiotics or antenatal corticosteroids. As detailed below, use of both antibiotics and antenatal corticosteroids improves outcome in patients with preterm PROM who are not having contractions. The effect of tocolysis to permit antibiotic and antenatal corticosteroid administration in the patient with preterm PROM who is having contractions has yet to be investigated.

▶ *Should antenatal corticosteroids be administered to patients with preterm PROM?*

Two meta-analyses have evaluated the impact of corticosteroid use after preterm PROM on respiratory distress syndrome. These studies produced somewhat conflicting results. While both found significant reduction in respiratory distress syndrome with antenatal corticosteroid administration, one found the opposite result after deleting the study with the lowest quality score after having accepted it based on predetermined criteria (57). The other meta-analysis demonstrated a significant benefit with corticosteroids (58), including reduced rates of neonatal periventricular hemorrhage, necrotizing enterocolitis, and death.

A more recent trial of corticosteroid use after preterm PROM demonstrated a significant reduction in respiratory distress syndrome with corticosteroid administration (18% versus 44%) (59). All patients in this study also received prophylactic antibiotics. Further, multivariate analysis of prospective observational trials also has suggested a benefit of antenatal corticosteroid use regardless of membrane rupture (60).

The National Institutes of Health Consensus Development Panel recommends corticosteroid use for women with PROM prior to 30–32 weeks of gestation in the absence of intraamniotic infection (61). The available data indicate that the benefit of antenatal corticosteroids may outweigh the risk in these patients between 24 and 32 weeks of gestation. Should the pregnancy extend beyond the week that antenatal corticosteroids have known benefit, it is unclear if repeat therapy is efficacious.

Because of the possible adverse fetal effects and possible effects on maternal immune status of repeated weekly courses of antenatal corticosteroids, it would seem reasonable to adopt a rescue approach to therapy in the treatment of perterm labor rather than a routine readministration regimen. Following the initial course of antenatal corticosteroids, repeated doses should only be given on an as-needed basis (ie, if the woman is retreated for threatened preterm birth).

▶ *Should antibiotics be administered to patients with preterm PROM in an effort to prolong the latency period?*

A large number of randomized prospective clinical trials assessing the utility of adjunctive antibiotic therapy during expectant management of preterm PROM have been published over the past 10 years and are summarized in two meta-analyses. One meta-analysis demonstrated significant prolongation of pregnancy and reduced chorioamnionitis, postpartum endometritis, neonatal sepsis, pneumonia, and intraventricular hemorrhage with antibiotic treatment compared with expectant management alone (13). The other meta-analysis indicated significant reduction in neonatal sepsis and intraventricular hemorrhage (62). An additional large, multicenter trial utilizing antibiotics but no antenatal corticosteroids or tocolytics demonstrated a significant reduction in perinatal morbidity, including respiratory distress syndrome and necrotizing enterocolitis (47). In that same study, patients negative for group B streptococci also experienced longer pregnancies and less neonatal sepsis and pneumonia. A recent prospective, double-blinded trial that did utilize antenatal corticosteroids for all patients found similar perinatal benefits associated with the use of antibiotics (63).

A number of regimens appear to be effective in prolonging the latency period. Investigators in the National Institute of Child Health and Human Development trial (47) demonstrated significant perinatal benefit with a combination of ampicillin and erythromycin administered intravenously for the first 48 hours, followed by oral amoxicillin and erythromycin for an additional 5 days if delivery did not occur. The other clinical trial utilized intravenous ampicillin followed by oral amoxicillin or intravenous ampicillin/sulbactam followed by oral amoxicillin/clavulanate (63). The available clinical data provide no basis for selecting one of the prophylactic regimens over the other. The administration of antibiotics to prolong the latency period must be distinguished from well-established protocols directed at prevention of group B streptococcal infection in term and preterm patients (41). Either of the prophylactic antibiotic regimens utilized by the aforementioned clinical trials would appropriately treat group B streptococcal infections. Once labor begins, however, the need for group B streptococcal prophylaxis needs to be determined.

▶ *Can women with preterm PROM be managed at home?*

Generally, hospitalization for bed rest and pelvic rest is indicated after preterm PROM. Recognizing that latency is frequently brief, that intrauterine and fetal infection may occur suddenly, and that the fetus is at risk for umbilical cord compression, ongoing surveillance of both mother and fetus is necessary.

One clinical trial of discharge after preterm PROM suggested that gravidas can be discharged before delivery to reduce health care costs (64). Those with preterm PROM and no evidence of intrauterine infection, labor, or fetal compromise were evaluated in hospital for 72 hours. Those with negative cervical cultures and no evident labor, intrauterine infection, or fetal compromise were then randomly assigned to either continued inpatient management or discharge. Only 67 of 349 women (18%) were eligible for discharge after 72 hours. There were no identifiable differences in latency, or in the incidences of intraamniotic infection, variable decelerations, or cesarean delivery. Infant outcomes also were similar.

While the potential for a reduction in health care costs with antepartum discharge is enticing, it is important to ensure that such management will not be associated with increased risks and costs related to perinatal morbidity and mortality. Any cost savings from antenatal discharge may be rapidly lost with a small increase in neonatal intensive care unit stay. Further study regarding the risks and benefits of home care after preterm PROM is warranted.

▶ *What is the optimal form of antepartum fetal surveillance for patients with preterm PROM managed expectantly?*

Fetal testing offers the opportunity to identify occult umbilical cord compression. One study demonstrated a 32% incidence of variable decelerations after preterm PROM (38). In addition, nonreactive nonstress tests have been associated with perinatal infection. With daily fetal evaluation, one study demonstrated the last test before delivery to be nonreactive in 78% of patients who subsequently developed infection (versus 14% for those with a reactive test) (65). Biophysical profile test scores of 6 or less within 24 hours of delivery also have been demonstrated to correlate with positive amniotic fluid cultures and perinatal infection. At least eight studies have confirmed this association (66). Most of these studies have included daily fetal assessment after preterm PROM. An abnormal test should lead to reassessment of the clinical circumstances and may lead to a decision to proceed to delivery. However, no evidence exists that any specific form or frequency of fetal surveillance directly improves perinatal outcome.

▶ *What is the optimal management for a patient with preterm PROM and a cervical cerclage?*

A retrospective comparative study demonstrated prolongation of pregnancy but increased maternal and perinatal morbidity and perinatal mortality when the cerclage was left in place following PROM (67). Two additional studies found no significant increase in maternal or perinatal morbidity in patients with cerclage removal when compared with patients with PROM and no cerclage (68, 69).

There are limited data to suggest removal of cerclage after PROM, but management with antibiotics or antenatal corticosteroids has not been addressed. The optimal management of preterm PROM in the presence of a cerclage is yet to be determined.

▶ *How does management differ in patients with second-trimester PROM?*

Initial management of gravidas with midtrimester PROM should reflect the potential for neonatal survival. Those presenting at 24–26 weeks of gestation may be considered viable (24, 70) and treated with expectant management. Given the lack of clinical trial data regarding optimal management of these patients, the recommendations reflect general clinical practice.

Women presenting with PROM before presumed viability should be counseled regarding the impact of immediate delivery and the potential risks and benefits of expectant management. Counseling should include a realistic appraisal of neonatal outcomes, including the availability of obstetric monitoring and neonatal intensive care facilities. Because of advances in perinatal care, morbidity and mortality rates continue to improve rapidly (24). An attempt should be made to provide parents with the most up-to-date information possible.

Although no evidence or consensus exists regarding the benefit of an initial period of inpatient observation in these patients, evaluation for the confirmation of PROM, evidence of infection, and the presence of associated fetal anomalies is essential if expectant management is to be considered. In addition to clinical follow-up, it may be useful to instruct patients to abstain from intercourse, limit their activities, and monitor their temperatures. Hospitalization for the duration of amniotic fluid leakage also may be appropriate.

Summary

Reports of patient care and outcome use ranges of gestational age. These ranges may be arbitrary. The recommendations that follow are based on available published data supplemented by consensus and expert opinion, with the recognition that the recommendations may not apply uniformly to patients at the extremes of gestational age.

The following recommendations are based on good and consistent scientific evidence (Level A):

- ▶ With term PROM, labor may be induced at the time of presentation or patients may be observed for up to 24–72 hours for the onset of spontaneous labor.
- ▶ Antibiotics prolong the latency period and improve perinatal outcome in patients with preterm PROM and should be administered according to one of several published protocols if expectant management is to be pursued prior to 35 weeks of gestation.
- ▶ Antenatal corticosteroids should be administered to gravidas with PROM before 32 weeks of gestation to reduce the risks of respiratory distress syndrome, neonatal intraventricular hemorrhage, necrotizing enterocolitis, and neonatal death.
- ▶ Digital cervical examinations should not be performed in patients with PROM who are not in labor and in whom immediate induction of labor is not planned.
- ▶ Patients with PROM prior to 30–32 weeks of gestation should be managed conservatively if no maternal or fetal contraindications exist.

The following recommendations are based primarily on consensus and expert opinion (Level C):

- ▶ Tocolysis may be utilized in patients with preterm PROM to permit administration of antenatal corticosteroids and antibiotics.
- ▶ Antenatal corticosteroids may be administered to gravidas with PROM up to 34 weeks of gestation.

References

1. Ventura SJ, Martin JA, Curtin SC, Mathews TJ. Report of final natality statistics, 1995. Monthly vital statistics report; vol 45, no. 11, supp. Hyattsville, Maryland: National Center for Health Statistics, 1997 (Level III)
2. French JI, McGregor JA. The pathobiology of premature rupture of membranes. Semin Perinatol 1996;20:344–368 (Level III)
3. Lavery JP, Miller CE, Knight RD. The effect of labor on the rheologic response of chorioamniotic membranes. Obstet Gynecol 1982;60:87–92 (Level II-3)
4. McGregor JA, French JI. Evidence-based prevention of preterm birth and rupture of membranes: infection and inflammation. J SOGC 1997;19:835–852 (Level III)
5. Harger JH, Hsing AW, Tuomala RE, Gibbs RS, Mead PB, Eschenbach DA, et al. Risk factors for preterm premature rupture of fetal membranes: a multicenter case-control study. Am J Obstet Gynecol 1990;163:130–137 (Level II-2)
6. Novak-Antolic Z, Pajntar M, Verdenik I. Rupture of the membranes and postpartum infection. Eur J Obstet Gynecol Reprod Biol 1997;71:141–146 (Level II-3)
7. Taylor J, Garite TJ. Premature rupture of the membranes before fetal viability. Obstet Gynecol 1984;64:615–620 (Level II-3)
8. Gold RB, Goyert GL, Schwartz DB, Evans MI, Seabolt LA. Conservative management of second trimester post-amniocentesis fluid leakage. Obstet Gynecol 1989;74:745–747 (Level III)
9. Hannah ME, Ohlsson A, Farine D, Hewson SA, Hodnett ED, Myhr TL, et al. Induction of labor compared with expectant management for prelabor rupture of the membranes at term. N Engl J Med 1996;334:1005–1010 (Level I)
10. Wagner MV, Chin VP, Peters CJ, Drexler B, Newman LA. A comparison of early and delayed induction of labor with spontaneous rupture of membranes at term. Obstet Gynecol 1989;74:93–97 (Level II-1)
11. Guise JM, Duff P, Christian JS. Management of term patients with premature rupture of membranes and an unfavorable cervix. Am J Perinatol 1992;9:56–60 (Level II-2)
12. Johnson JWC, Egerman RS, Moorhead J. Cases with ruptured membranes that "reseal." Am J Obstet Gynecol 1990;163:1024–1032 (Level II-2)
13. Mercer BM, Arheart KL. Antimicrobial therapy in expectant management of preterm premature rupture of the membranes. Lancet 1995;346:1271–1279 (Meta-analysis)
14. Mercer BM. Management of premature rupture of membranes before 26 weeks' gestation. Obstet Gynecol Clin North Am 1992;19:339–351 (Level III)
15. Beydoun SN, Yasin SY. Premature rupture of the membranes before 28 weeks: conservative management. Am J Obstet Gynecol 1986;155:471–479 (Level II-3)
16. Garite TJ, Freeman RK. Chorioamnionitis in the preterm gestation. Obstet Gynecol 1982;59:539–545 (Level II-3)
17. Simpson GF, Harbert GM Jr. Use of β-methasone in management of preterm gestation with premature rupture of membranes. Obstet Gynecol 1985;66:168–175 (Level II-2)
18. Vergani P, Ghidini A, Locatelli A, Cavallone M, Ciarla I, Cappellini A, et al. Risk factors for pulmonary hypoplasia in second-trimester premature rupture of membranes. Am J Obstet Gynecol 1994;170:1359–1364 (Level II-3)
19. Hillier SL, Martius J, Krohn M, Kiviat N, Holmes KK, Eschenbach DA. A case-control study of chorioamnionic infection and histologic chorioamnionitis in prematurity. N Engl J Med 1988;319:972–978 (Level II-3)

20. Morales WJ. The effect of chorioamnionitis on the developmental outcome of preterm infants at one year. Obstet Gynecol 1987;70:183–186 (Level II-3)

21. Schutte MF, Treffers PE, Kloosterman GJ, Soepatmi S. Management of premature rupture of membranes: the risk of vaginal examination to the infant. Am J Obstet Gynecol 1983;146:395–400 (Level II-3)

22. Ananth CV, Savitz DA, Williams MA. Placental abruption and its association with hypertension and prolonged rupture of membranes: a methodologic review and meta-analysis. Obstet Gynecol 1996;88:309–318 (Meta-analysis)

23. Gonen R, Hannah ME, Milligan JE. Does prolonged preterm premature rupture of the membranes predispose to abruptio placentae? Obstet Gynecol 1989;74:347–350 (Level II-2)

24. Fanaroff AA, Wright LL, Stevenson DK, Shankaran S, Donovan EF, Ehrenkranz RA, et al. Very-low-birth-weight outcomes of the National Institute of Child Health and Human Development Neonatal Research Network, May 1991 through December 1992. Am J Obstet Gynecol 1995; 173:1423–1431 (Level II-3)

25. Schucker JL, Mercer BM. Midtrimester premature rupture of the membranes. Semin Perinatol 1996;20:389–400 (Level III)

26. Hack M, Taylor HG, Klein N, Eiben R, Schatschneider C, Mercuri-Minich N. School-age outcomes in children with birth weights under 750 g. N Engl J Med 1994;331:753–759 (Level II-2)

27. Kilpatrick SJ, Schlueter MA, Piecuch R, Leonard CH, Rogido M, Sola A. Outcome of infants born at 24-26 weeks' gestation: I. Survival and cost. Obstet Gynecol 1997;90:803–808 (Level II-3)

28. Bottoms SF, Paul RH, Iams JD, Mercer BM, Thom EA, Roberts JM, et al. Obstetric determinants of neonatal survival: influence of willingness to perform cesarean delivery on survival of extremely low-birth-weight infants. Am J Obstet Gynecol 1997;176:960–966 (Level II-3)

29. Moretti M, Sibai BM. Maternal and perinatal outcome of expectant management of premature rupture of the membranes in midtrimester. Am J Obstet Gynecol 1988;159: 390–396 (Level II-3)

30. Rib DM, Sherer DM, Woods JR Jr. Maternal and neonatal outcome associated with prolonged premature rupture of membranes below 26 weeks' gestation. Am J Perinatol 1993;10:369–373 (Level II-3)

31. Bengtson JM, VanMarter LJ, Barss VA, Greene MF, Tuomala RE, Epstein MF. Pregnancy outcome after premature rupture of the membranes at or before 26 weeks' gestation. Obstet Gynecol 1989;73:921–926 (Level II-3)

32. Cox SM, Leveno KJ. Intentional delivery versus expectant management with preterm ruptured membranes at 30–34 weeks' gestation. Obstet Gynecol 1995;86:875–879 (Level I)

33. Mercer BM, Crocker LG, Boe NM, Sibai BM. Induction versus expectant management in premature rupture of the membranes with mature amniotic fluid at 32 to 36 weeks: a randomized trial. Am J Obstet Gynecol 1993;169:775–782 (Level I)

34. Major CA, Kitzmiller JL. Perinatal survival with expectant management of midtrimester rupture of membranes. Am J Obstet Gynecol 1990;163:838–844 (Level II-3)

35. Morales WJ, Talley T. Premature rupture of membranes at <25 weeks: a management dilemma. Am J Obstet Gynecol 1993;168:503–507 (Level II-3)

36. Rotschild A, Ling EW, Puterman ML, Farquharson D. Neonatal outcome after prolonged preterm rupture of the membranes. Am J Obstet Gynecol 1990;162:46–52 (Level II-3)

37. van Eyck J, van der Mooren K, Wladimiroff JW. Ductus arteriosus flow velocity modulation by fetal breathing movements as a measure of fetal lung development. Am J Obstet Gynecol 1990;163:558–566 (Level II-3)

38. Smith CV, Greenspoon J, Phelan JP, Platt LD. Clinical utility of the nonstress test in the conservative management of women with preterm spontaneous premature rupture of the membranes. J Reprod Med 1987;32:1–4 (Level II-3)

39. Lenihan JP Jr. Relationship of antepartum pelvic examinations to premature rupture of the membranes. Obstet Gynecol 1984;83:33–37 (Level II-1)

40. Munson LA, Graham A, Koos BJ, Valenzuela GJ. Is there a need for digital examination in patients with spontaneous rupture of the membranes? Am J Obstet Gynecol 1985; 153:562–563 (Level II-3)

41. American College of Obstetricians and Gynecologists. Prevention of early-onset group B streptococcal disease in newborns. ACOG Committee Opinion 173. Washington, DC: ACOG, 1996 (Level III)

42. Ingemarsson I. Controversies: premature rupture of membranes at term—no advantage of delaying induction >24 hours. J Perinat Med 1996;24:573–579 (Level III)

43. Mozurkewich EL, Wolf FM. Premature rupture of membranes at term: a meta-analysis of three management schemes. Obstet Gynecol 1997;89:1035–1043 (Meta-analysis)

44. Ottervanger HP, Keirse MJ, Smit W, Holm JP. Controlled comparison of induction versus expectant care for prelabor rupture of the membranes at term. J Perinatol Med 1996;24: 237–242 (Level I-1)

45. Sanchez-Ramos L, Chen AH, Kaunitz AM, Gaudier FL, Delke I. Labor induction with intravaginal misoprostol in term premature rupture of membranes: a randomized study. Obstet Gynecol 1997;89:909–912 (Level I)

46. Alcalay M, Hourvitz A, Reichman B, Luski A, Quint J, Barkai G, et al. Prelabour rupture of membranes at term: early induction of labour versus expectant management. Eur J Obstet Gynecol Reprod Biol 1996;70:129–133 (Level I)

47. Mercer BM, Miodovnik M, Thurnau GR, Goldenberg RL, Das AF, Ramsey RD, et al. Antibiotic therapy for reduction of infant morbidity after preterm premature rupture of the membranes: a randomized controlled trial. JAMA 1997;278: 989–995 (Level I)

48. Gomez R, Romero R, Edwin SS, David C. Pathogenesis of preterm labor and preterm premature rupture of membranes associated with intraamniotic infection. Infect Dis Clin North Am 1997;11:135–176 (Level III)

49. Belady PH, Farkouh LJ, Gibbs RS. Intra-amniotic infection and premature rupture of the membranes. Clin Perinatol 1997;24:43–57 (Level III)

50. Broekhuizen FF, Gilman M, Hamilton PR. Amniocentesis for gram stain and culture in preterm premature rupture of the membranes. Obstet Gynecol 1985;66:316–321 (Level II-3)

51. Romero R, Yoon BH, Mazor M, Gomez R, Gonzalez R, Diamond MP, et al. A comparative study of the diagnostic performance of amniotic fluid glucose, white blood cell count, interleukin-6, and Gram stain in the detection of microbial invasion in patients with preterm premature rupture of membranes. Am J Obstet Gynecol 1993;169:839–851 (Level II-2)

52. Ohlsson A, Wang E. An analysis of antenatal tests to detect infection in preterm premature rupture of the membranes. Am J Obstet Gynecol 1990;162:809–818 (Level III)

53. Christensen KK, Ingemarsson I, Leideman T, Solum H, Svenningsen N. Effect of ritodrine on labor after premature rupture of the membranes. Obstet Gynecol 1980;55:187–190 (Level I)

54. Levy DL, Warsof SL. Oral ritodrine and preterm premature rupture of membranes. Obstet Gynecol 1985;66:621–623 (Level II-1)

55. Weiner CP, Renk K, Klugman M. The therapeutic efficacy and cost-effectiveness of aggressive tocolysis for premature labor associated with premature rupture of the membranes. Am J Obstet Gynecol 1988;159:216–222 (Level I)

56. Garite TJ, Keegan KA, Freeman RK, Nageotte MP. A randomized trial of ritodrine tocolysis versus expectant management in patients with premature rupture of membranes at 25 to 30 weeks of gestation. Am J Obstet Gynecol 1987;157:388–393 (Level II-1)

57. Ohlsson A. Treatments of preterm premature rupture of the membranes: a meta-analysis. Am J Obstet Gynecol 1989; 160:890–906 (Meta-analysis)

58. Crowley PA. Antenatal corticosteroid therapy: a meta-analysis of the randomized trials, 1972 to 1994. Am J Obstet Gynecol 1995;173:322–335 (Meta-analysis)

59. Lewis DF, Brody K, Edwards MS, Brouillette RM, Burlison S, London SN. Preterm premature ruptured membranes: a randomized trial of steroids after treatment with antibiotics. Obstet Gynecol 1996;88:801–805 (Level I)

60. Wright LL, Verter J, Younes N, Stevenson D, Fanaroff AA, Shankaran S, et al. Antenatal corticosteroid administration and neonatal outcome in very low birth weight infants: the NICHD Neonatal Research Network. Am J Obstet Gynecol 1995;173:269–274 (Level II-3)

61. National Institutes of Health. National Institutes of Health Consensus Development Conference Statement: Effect of corticosteroids for fetal maturation on perinatal outcomes, February 28–March 2, 1994. Am J Obstet Gynecol 1995;173:246–252 (Level III)

62. Egarter C, Leitich H, Karas H, Wieser F, Husslein P, Kaider A, et al. Antibiotic treatment in preterm premature rupture of membranes and neonatal morbidity: a meta-analysis. Am J Obstet Gynecol 1996;174:589–597 (Meta-analysis)

63. Lovett SM, Weiss JD, Diogo MJ, Williams PT, Garite TJ. A prospective double-blind, randomized, controlled clinical trial of ampicillin-sulbactam for preterm premature rupture of membranes in women receiving antenatal corticosteroid therapy. Am J Obstet Gynecol 1997;176:1030–1038 (Level I)

64. Carlan SJ, O'Brien WF, Parsons MT, Lense JJ. Preterm premature rupture of membranes: a randomized study of home versus hospital management. Obstet Gynecol 1993; 81:61–64 (Level I)

65. Vintzileos AM, Campbell WA, Nochimson DJ, Weinbaum PJ. The use of the nonstress test in patients with premature rupture of the membranes. Am J Obstet Gynecol 1986; 155:149–153 (Level II-3)

66. Hanley ML, Vintzileos AM. Biophysical testing in premature rupture of the membranes. Semin Perinatol 1996; 20:418–425 (Level III)

67. Ludmir J, Bader T, Chen L, Lindenbaum C, Wong G. Poor perinatal outcome associated with retained cerclage in patients with premature rupture of membranes. Obstet Gynecol 1994;84:823–826 (Level II-2)

68. Yeast JD, Garite TR. The role of cervical cerclage in the management of preterm premature rupture of the membranes. Am J Obstet Gynecol 1988;158:106–110 (Level II-2)

69. Blickstein I, Katz Z, Lancet M, Molgilner BM. The outcome of pregnancies complicated by preterm rupture of the membranes with and without cerclage. Int J Gynecol Obstet 1989;28:237–242 (Level II-2)

70. American College of Obstetricians and Gynecologists. Perinatal care at the threshold of viability. ACOG Committee Opinion 163. Washington, DC: ACOG, 1995 (Level III)

The MEDLINE database, the Cochrane Library, and ACOG's own internal resources and documents were used to conduct a literature search to locate relevant articles published between 1980 and August 1997. The search was restricted to articles published in the English language. Priority was given to articles reporting results of original research although review articles and commentaries also were consulted. Abstracts of research presented at symposiums and scientific conferences were not considered adequate for inclusion in this document. Guidelines published by organizations or institutions such as the National Institutes of Health and ACOG were reviewed, and additional studies were located by reviewing bibliographies of identified articles. When reliable research was not available, expert opinions from obstetrician–gynecologists were used. Studies were reviewed and evaluated for quality according to the method outlined by the U.S. Preventive Services Task Force.

I Evidence obtained from at least one properly designed randomized controlled trial.

II-1 Evidence obtained from well-designed controlled trials without randomization.

II-2 Evidence obtained from well-designed cohort or case-control analytic studies, preferably from more than one center or research group.

II-3 Evidence obtained from multiple time series with or without the intervention. Dramatic results in uncontrolled experiments also could be regarded as this type of evidence.

III Opinions of respected authorities, based on clinical experience, descriptive studies, or reports of expert committees.

Based on the highest level of evidence found in the data, the recommendations are graded according to the following categories:

A The recommendation is based on good and consistent scientific evidence

B The recommendation is based on limited or inconsistent scientific evidence

C The recommendation is based primarily on consensus and expert opinion

ISSN 1099-3630 12345/21098

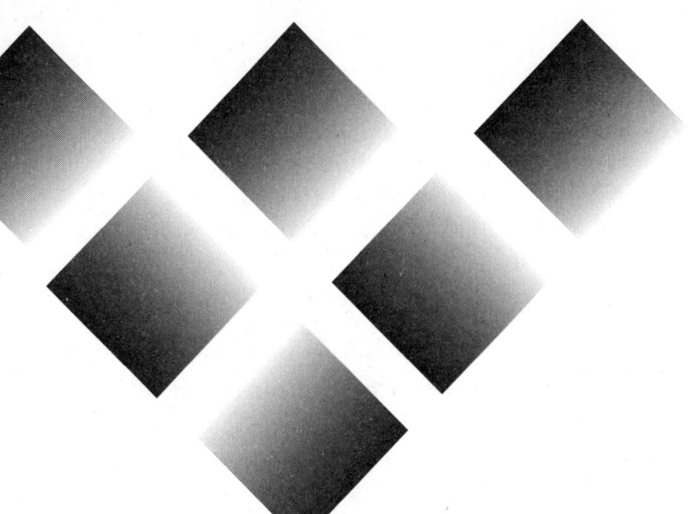

ACOG PRACTICE BULLETIN

CLINICAL MANAGEMENT GUIDELINES FOR OBSTETRICIAN–GYNECOLOGISTS

NUMBER 15, APRIL 2000

This Practice Bulletin was developed by the ACOG Committee on Practice Bulletins—Gynecology with the assistance of Ann J. Davis, MD and Susan R. Johnson, MD, MS. The information is designed to aid practitioners in making decisions about appropriate obstetric and gynecologic care. These guidelines should not be construed as dictating an exclusive course of treatment or procedure. Variations in practice may be warranted based on the needs of the individual patient, resources, and limitations unique to the institution or type of practice.

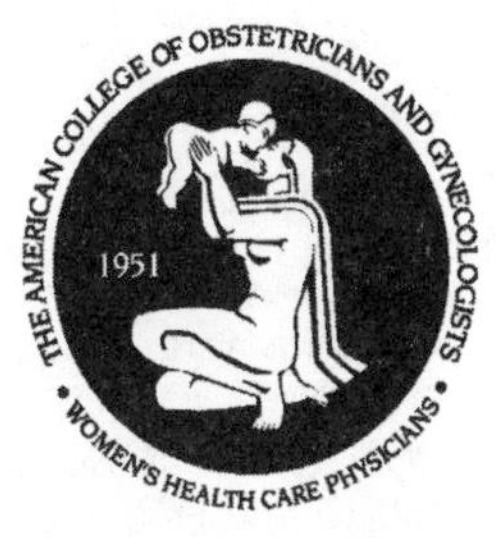

Premenstrual Syndrome

Premenstrual syndrome (PMS) is a common problem for many women. Determining the appropriate clinical management of this condition often creates frustration for both physicians and patients. Until recently, the difficulty in managing PMS was largely attributed to imprecise diagnostic criteria, poorly designed clinical trials, and the promotion of treatment options for which there was no scientific support. In the mid-1980s, however, rigorous criteria for the diagnosis of PMS were defined. Since then, most studies of pathophysiology and treatment have met recognized standards of scientific design. This document will examine the evidence for commonly used approaches in the treatment of PMS and identify those that are effective.

Background

Premenstrual syndrome has been defined as "the cyclic occurrence of symptoms that are of sufficient severity to interfere with some aspects of life and that appear with consistent and predictable relationship to the menses" (1). Although the symptoms themselves are not unique, the restriction of the symptoms to the luteal phase of the menstrual cycle is pathognomonic of PMS (2).

Epidemiology

Premenstrual symptoms are common and are considered a normal aspect of ovulatory cycles. Most surveys have found that as many as 85% of menstruating women report one or more premenstrual symptoms. Severe symptoms that meet the criteria for PMS, however, are much less common, with only 5–10% of women reporting significant impairment in their lifestyles because of PMS (3, 4).

Risk Factors

Advancing age often is cited as a risk factor for PMS, based on surveys that find women are most likely to seek treatment after age 30 years. However, this syndrome can occur in menstruating women of any age. Genetics appears to play a role in PMS; the concordance rate of PMS is twice as high among monozygotic twins as among dizygotic twins (5, 6). Although women with PMS have a high rate of affective disorders, a causal relationship has not yet been demonstrated (7, 8).

There are no significant personality profile differences between women with PMS and asymptomatic women (9). Furthermore, PMS is not more likely to be diagnosed in women with higher levels of stress (10). However, women who have PMS may not tolerate stress as well as women who do not have PMS. Premenstrual symptoms seem to affect women irrespective of culture or socioeconomic status, although specific symptoms may vary in frequency by culture (11–13).

Etiology

The etiology of PMS is incompletely understood, but considerable progress has been made in the past decade in understanding some facets of the pathophysiology. Circulating sex steroid levels (progesterone, estrogen, and testosterone) are normal, although there may be an underlying neurobiologic vulnerability to normal fluctuations of one or more of these hormones (14, 15). Most likely, the biochemical changes involve central-nervous-system–mediated neurotransmitter interactions with sex steroids. Serotoninergic dysregulation is currently the most plausible theory. Among the several studies supporting this theory is a well-designed study in which women with severe PMS responded better to selective serotonin reuptake inhibitors (SSRIs) than to noradrenergic antidepressants such as maprotiline (16). Because not all women with PMS respond to SSRIs, other etiologic factors probably are involved.

Clinical Considerations and Recommendations

Establishing evidenced-based recommendations for PMS is difficult for many reasons. Definitions and inclusion criteria for PMS vary significantly among studies. In addition, the PMS patient populations studied in rigorous trials also may be different from the patient population of a given practitioner. For example, many recent PMS trials have properly included only women with the full-blown syndrome, including mood-related symptoms, whereas many women seek care from their practitioners for a less severe condition, with primarily somatic symptoms.

▶ *How is the diagnosis of PMS established?*

The key elements of the diagnosis are a) symptoms consistent with PMS; b) restriction of these symptoms to the luteal phase of the menstrual cycle assessed prospectively; c) impairment of some facet of the woman's life; and d) exclusion of other diagnoses that may better explain the symptoms.

The National Institute of Mental Health criteria for diagnosis are 1) a marked change of about 30% in the intensity of symptoms measured instrumentally, from cycle days 5 to 10 (as compared with those premenstrually), within the 6-day interval prior to menses and 2) documentation of these changes for at least two consecutive cycles (17). Another definition of PMS developed for research purposes by the University of California at San Diego is based on women's prospective self-reports. Their definition requires that patients have the cyclic manifestation of at least 1 of 6 behavioral symptoms and 1 of 4 somatic symptoms (see the box). Dysfunction in social or economic performance is included in this definition. Finally, the *Diagnostic and Statistical Manual of Mental Disorders*, fourth edition, includes similar criteria for the diagnosis of premenstrual dysphoric disorder, which identifies women with PMS who have more severe emotional symptoms (18).

The diagnosis of PMS should be based on prospective symptom diaries, because as many as half of the

Diagnostic Criteria for Premenstrual Syndrome

Premenstrual syndrome can be diagnosed if the patient reports at least one of the following affective and somatic symptoms during the 5 days before menses in each of the three prior menstrual cycles*:

Affective
- Depression
- Angry outbursts
- Irritability
- Anxiety
- Confusion
- Social withdrawal

Somatic
- Breast tenderness
- Abdominal bloating
- Headache
- Swelling of extremities

*These symptoms are relieved within 4 days of the onset of menses, without recurrence until at least cycle day 13. The symptoms are present in the absence of any pharmacologic therapy, hormone ingestion, or drug or alcohol use. The symptoms occur reproducibly during two cycles of prospective recording. The patient suffers from identifiable dysfunction in social or economic performance.

Adapted from Mortola JF, Girton L, Yen SC. Depressive episodes in premenstrual syndrome. Am J Obstet Gynecol 1989;161:1682–1687

women reporting a luteal phase pattern will be found to have some other pattern when such diaries are examined. Because some women experience cycle-to-cycle variability in symptoms, reviewing 2–3 months of prospective charting is preferable to reviewing a single cycle (19).

In the clinical setting, a simple system in which the woman records the dates of her menstrual periods and notes her symptoms on a daily basis is usually sufficient (20). However, a variety of standardized instruments and diaries developed for research purposes are also available. The most commonly used are the Calendar of Premenstrual Experiences (COPE) (21) and the Prospective Record of the Impact and Severity of Menstruation (PRISM) (22). Another type of instrument, the Visual Analogue Scales (VAS), may be especially appropriate in non-English-reading populations (23).

A careful medical and psychologic history and physical examination in conjunction with the prospective symptom diary usually will direct the clinician toward the correct diagnosis. Laboratory testing should be restricted to the identification of other disorders suggested by the evaluation, such as measuring levels of thyroid-stimulating hormone when hypothyroidism is suspected. Routine measurement of steroid hormones or gonadotropins is not useful.

▶ *How is PMS objectively differentiated from similar conditions?*

Only a small portion of women presenting for evaluation and treatment of PMS are likely to have PMS. For example, in a sample of women who responded to a newspaper recruitment for a PMS study, the most common symptoms reported were consistent with PMS: irritability, depression, mood swings, anxiety, mastalgia, abdominal bloating, weight gain, fatigue, aggression, headache, tension, muscle aches, food cravings, and breast swelling (24). However, individuals who respond to such recruitment may not be representative of the general population. In this study, after a complete evaluation, 60% of the women also were found to have psychiatric disorders.

The phenomenon of *menstrual magnification* (sometimes called premenstrual or perimenstrual exacerbation) helps explain this situation. Many medical and psychiatric conditions are exacerbated in the late luteal or menstrual phase of the cycle, leading a woman to believe that she must be experiencing PMS. The underlying mechanism of this increase in symptoms is not understood.

The differential diagnosis of PMS therefore includes any medical and psychiatric condition that either has some of the many symptoms associated with PMS or is subject to menstrual magnification. Depressive disorders, which share a similar set of symptoms, are the most common consideration (25). Depressive disorders also are subject to the magnification effect, making the distinction from PMS even more difficult. A key feature of depressive disorders, however, is that symptoms are almost always present every day of the cycle. Other psychiatric conditions that may be magnified are panic disorder and generalized anxiety disorder.

The most common medical disorders subject to menstrual magnification are migraines, seizure disorders, irritable bowel syndrome, asthma, chronic fatigue syndrome, and allergies. Endocrine abnormalities such as thyroid and adrenal disorders also should be considered. The diagnosis of these conditions usually is straightforward because the key symptoms are not part of the typical PMS symptom set, and emotional symptoms are not prominent, as they are in PMS.

Finally, women in the period of transition to menopause may have symptoms typical of PMS, especially mood disturbance, fatigue, and hot flashes. Because menstrual periods often are less predictable, these women may be less aware of the relationship of the symptoms to the menstrual cycle. The correct diagnosis usually can be made by considering the patient's age, a history of recent menstrual cycle changes, and a symptom diary showing sporadic or daily occurrence of symptoms.

▶ *Which patients require therapeutic intervention for PMS?*

Premenstrual syndrome, by definition, is associated with symptoms that interfere with some part of the patient's normal life, but there are usually no medical sequelae if the disorder is not treated. Therefore, the decision to treat the disorder should be based on the patient's desire for an improvement in her symptoms. Furthermore, because there is a wide range of symptom severity, the treatment approach should match the patient's needs.

▶ *What is the evidence supporting the effectiveness of the following common treatments for PMS?*

A wide variety of supportive, lifestyle, and dietary supplementation approaches to PMS have been recommended over the years, and a few of these have been demonstrated to have real benefit. Therefore, these strategies can be recommended to women with mild to moderate symptoms as a primary therapy and to women with severe symptoms as adjunctive therapy.

Women with severe symptoms or with symptoms resistant to nonmedical approaches should be considered for drug therapy. Although no drugs currently are specifically approved by the U.S. Food and Drug Administration for the treatment of PMS, several available drugs have been found to be effective for PMS and can be prescribed.

Supportive Therapy. Supportive therapy has been employed as a central component in PMS management, although it has not been studied rigorously. Reassurance and informational counseling may relieve many anxieties and increase the patient's sense of control. Women anecdotally report relief when they are informed that PMS is a common medical problem with a physiologic basis. Supportive therapy may contribute in part to the high response rate to placebos for virtually every form of treatment used for PMS.

The value of more formal psychologic interventions has not been conclusively demonstrated. The best evidence is for relaxation therapy. In one small comparative study, relaxation therapy had its greatest effects in women with the most severe symptoms (26). In a study of cognitive behavior therapy, the comparison group who received information about PMS, relaxation training, and lifestyle and nutrition guidelines fared nearly as well as the study group who received cognitive restructuring training (27).

Aerobic Exercise. Aerobic exercise has been found in epidemiologic studies to be associated with fewer reported PMS symptoms, and exercise has been found to reduce symptoms among people with depressive disorders. Limited evidence supports a similar role for this intervention in PMS. In a 3-month randomized trial of 23 women with prospectively diagnosed PMS, the group taking regular moderate aerobic exercise reported more improvement than the control group who did nonaerobic exercise (28). In another small prospective but not randomized study, two groups of women who exercised aerobically reported fewer PMS symptoms at the end of a 6-month trial than did a nonexercising comparison group (29). Although the evidence base is modest at this time, aerobic exercise can be recommended to all women with PMS because of its numerous other health benefits.

Dietary Supplementation. Calcium and magnesium have each been shown to be effective in the treatment of PMS. However, most of these trials have tested small numbers of patients and must be validated in larger trials before strong evidence-based recommendations can be made. One large well-designed multicenter trial of 466 women with PMS reported that 1,200 mg/d of calcium carbonate was efficacious in reducing total symptom scores (30). Two small trials have found that 200–400 mg of magnesium may be somewhat effective (31, 32).

Minimal data are available on the effectiveness of vitamin E and the treatment of premenstrual syndrome. Vitamin E has been recommended as a treatment for mastalgia. In one randomized, double-blind, controlled study comparing vitamin E 400 IU/d during the luteal phase with placebo, vitamin E was found to improve significantly affective and somatic symptoms in PMS patients (33). Although effectiveness probably is minimal, no serious side effects are reported with vitamin E 400 IU/d, and as an antioxidant it has other beneficial effects.

In one study, mood symptomatology and carbohydrate food cravings were shown to be improved by carbohydrate-rich beverages (34). This small, well-designed study should be repeated with larger numbers of subjects before evidence-based recommendations can be made. One hypothesis to explain these benefits is that diets rich in carbohydrates increase levels of tryptophan, the precursor to serotonin.

Well-designed scientific studies have not demonstrated that primrose oil is effective in the treatment of PMS. However, it may be useful in treating breast tenderness (35).

On the basis of a recent systematic review of several weak clinical studies, vitamin B_6 is considered to be of limited clinical benefit in the treatment of PMS (36). Dosages in excess of 100 mg/d may cause medical harm, including peripheral neuropathy (36).

Selective Serotonin Reuptake Inhibitors. The SSRIs are the initial drugs of choice for severe PMS. Fluoxetine is the most studied drug of this group. Its use has been studied in almost 1,000 women in rigorous trials. The largest, a 6-month, multicenter trial, evaluated 313 women with PMS who were prescribed dosages of 20–60 mg/d (37). Investigators observed 44% dropouts at dosages of 60 mg/d and 11% at dosages of 20 mg/d. This study, along with several smaller, shorter-duration placebo-controlled trials, have consistently reported the efficacy of fluoxetine. The dosage in these trials generally was 20 mg/d throughout the menstrual cycle administered as a single morning dose to avoid insomnia. One study reported efficacy in 64 women with PMS over a mean treatment time of 18 months (38). In this 18-month study, symptoms recurred in most of the women not taking fluoxetine and resolved when treatment was restarted.

Other SSRI drugs that have had a beneficial effect similar to that of fluoxetine are sertraline, paroxetine, clomipramine, fluvoxamine, and nefaxazone. In the largest study of sertraline, in which there were 233 subjects, dosages ranged from 50 to 150 mg/d (39).

Intermittent therapy, with an SSRI given only during the symptomatic phase, also has been efficacious in several small, randomized, double-blind, placebo-controlled trials (40–42). This method of administration has many advantages: it is less expensive, reduces the overall rate of side effects, and is more acceptable to many women. The drug is started between 7 and 14 days before the next menstrual period, with the start day individualized to begin the medication at or just before the expected onset of symptoms.

Side effects associated with fluoxetine include headaches, nausea, and jitteriness. Insomnia often can be avoided by early-morning dosing or, if appropriate, by lowering the dosage. Decreased libido also is problematic in some patients. In cases in which improvement of libido is not seen after dosage changes, alternative therapies may be considered (4).

Other Pharmacologic Approaches. Some placebo-controlled trials have shown alprazolam, an anxiolytic medication, to be effective as a treatment for PMS (43–45), and some have not (46). There is a potential for dependency and development of tolerance with this medication, especially if dosing is not limited to the luteal phase. Sedation also can be a bothersome side effect in some patients, and withdrawals can be problematic. Alprazolam may potentially be useful for PMS patients who are not relieved by other interventions. It may be especially useful if agitation and anxiety are the primary symptoms.

Because complaints of fluid retention are common in the luteal phase, diuretic therapy has been advocated. No evidence exists that thiazide diuretics are of benefit. Spironolactone, an aldosterone antagonist with antiandrogenic properties, is the only diuretic that has been shown to be of benefit in PMS. Several randomized, double-blind, placebo-controlled trials have shown a significant reduction in somatic and affective complaints (47–51). Usual dosage in most studies is 100 mg/d in the morning during the 14-day luteal phase. However, not all reports evaluating spironolactone for PMS have shown benefit.

Historically, natural progesterone has been one of the most commonly employed therapies in women with PMS, but careful scientific scrutiny has not supported an overall benefit of this hormone when compared with placebo, whether administered as a vaginal suppository (52) or as oral micronized progesterone (45). Progesterone may be helpful for specific symptoms, such as breast tenderness and bloating, or specific psychologic symptoms, such as worrying (53).

▶ ***What is the role of hormonal suppression in the treatment of PMS?***

Oral Contraceptives. Although oral contraceptives are widely prescribed for the treatment of PMS, few data support their effectiveness. In one randomized trial, a triphasic formulation reduced physical symptoms but not mood alterations (54). In another study comparing triphasic and monophasic regimens, the monophasic formulation was less likely to cause mood alterations (55). Many patients experience breast tenderness, nausea, mood alterations, and other side effects the first few months of oral contraceptive use. The evidence suggests that oral contraceptives should be considered if symptoms are primarily physical, but may not be effective if mood symptoms are more prevalent.

Gonadotropin-Releasing Hormone Agonists. Improvement in PMS symptoms with gonadotropin-releasing hormone (GnRH) agonists has been reported in the majority of well-designed studies (56–57) but not in all of them (58). The hypoestrogenic side effects and cost of GnRH agonists limit the usefulness of this method except in severe cases of PMS unresponsive to other treatment.

If this therapy is to be used for more than a few months, bone loss becomes a concern. The most commonly used approach is add-back estrogen therapy (with progestin if indicated). Add-back therapy also may result in a return of symptoms, although studies are limited and sometimes confusing. In a double-blind, placebo-controlled study of 10 women, both estrogen add-back therapy alone and progesterone therapy alone were associated with a significant recurrence of symptoms (15). Another small rigorous study evaluated eight women with PMS. Administration of the GnRH agonist resulted in an improvement of approximately 75% in luteal phase symptom scores. The addition of estrogen as well as progesterone was associated with worsening symptoms, but a similar worsening also was seen with placebo (59). If hormone therapy results in a return of symptoms, alendronate should be considered for osteoporosis prevention.

Bilateral Salpingo-Oophorectomy. Surgery for PMS is controversial because it is irreversible, it is associated with morbidity and mortality, and the resulting hypoestrogenemia must be addressed to prevent long-term complications. If employed, this approach should be reserved for those severely affected patients who meet strict diagnostic criteria and who do not respond to any potentially effective therapy other than GnRH agonists (60). These limitations are critical, because a major cause of therapeutic failure with any of the described treatments is an incorrect diagnosis of PMS. It is advisable to perform a diagnostic trial with an agonist for a minimum of 3 months to determine if oophorectomy will be effective. An additional advantage to an extended trial with an agonist is the opportunity to assess the woman's tolerance for estrogen replacement therapy.

Summary

The following recommendations are based on good and consistent scientific evidence (Level A):

- Women in whom PMS has been diagnosed should meet standard diagnostic criteria and should have the timing of their symptoms confirmed using a prospective symptom calendar.
- Risk factors such as increased imposed stress and specific personality profiles are not helpful in differentiating women with PMS from those without PMS.
- The SSRIs, particularly fluoxetine and sertraline, have been shown to be effective in treating PMS.
- The bulk of scientific evidence does not support the usefulness of natural progesterone or primrose oil in the treatment of PMS.

The following recommendations are based on limited or inconsistent scientific evidence (Level B):

- The use of GnRH agonists and surgical oophorectomy have been shown to be effective in PMS. However, the side effects of GnRH agonists and oophorectomy limit their usefulness in most patients.
- Treatment with the anxiolytic alprazolam is effective in some patients. Its side effects limit its use as a first-line approach.
- Carbohydrate-rich foods and beverages may improve mood symptoms and food cravings in women with PMS and are a reasonable first-line approach in many patients.
- Calcium supplements have been shown to be effective in the treatment of PMS.
- Magnesium, vitamin B_6, and vitamin E may have minimal effectiveness in the treatment of PMS.
- Oral contraceptives may improve physical symptoms of PMS.

The following recommendations are based primarily on consensus and expert opinion (Level C):

- Supportive therapy is central to the management of all PMS patients.
- Aerobic exercise can be recommended to PMS patients.
- As an overall clinical approach, treatments should be employed in increasing orders of complexity. Using this principle, in most cases, the therapies should be used in the following order:

Step 1. Supportive therapy, complex carbohydrate diet, aerobic exercise, nutritional supplements (calcium, magnesium, vitamin E), spironolactone

Step 2. The SSRIs (fluoxetine or sertraline as the initial choice); for women who do not respond, consider an anxiolytic for specific symptoms

Step 3. Hormonal ovulation suppression (oral contraceptives or GnRH agonists)

References

1. Gise LH, Kase NG, Berkowitz RL, eds. Contemporary issues in obstetrics and gynecology. Vol 2. The premenstrual syndromes. New York: Churchill Livingstone, 1988 (Level III)
2. Mortola JF. Issues in the diagnosis and research of premenstrual syndrome. Clin Obstet Gynecol 1992;35: 587–598 (Level III)
3. Stout AL, Steege JF. Psychosocial assessment of women seeking treatment for premenstrual syndrome. J Psychosom Res 1985;29:621–629 (Level III)
4. Steiner M. Premenstrual syndromes. Annu Rev Med 1997;48:447–455 (Level III)
5. Kendler KS, Silberg JL, Neale MC, Kessler RC, Heath AC, Eaves LJ. Genetic and environmental factors in the aetiology of menstrual, premenstrual and neurotic symptoms: a population-based twin study. Psychol Med 1992;22: 85–100 (Level II-3)
6. Condon JT. The premenstrual syndrome: a twin study. Br J Psychiatry 1993;162:481–486 (Level II-3)
7. Halbreich U, Endicott J. Relationship of dysphoric premenstrual changes to depressive disorders. Acta Psychiatr Scand 1985;71:331–338 (Level III)
8. DeJong R, Rubinow DR, Roy-Byrne P, Hoban MC, Grover GN, Post RM. Premenstrual mood disorder and psychiatric illness. Am J Psychiatry 1985:142:1359–1361 (Level III)
9. Trunnell EP, Turner CW, Keye WR. A comparison of the psychological and hormonal factors in women with and without premenstrual syndrome. J Abnorm Psychol 1988;97:429–436 (Level II-2)
10. Beck LE, Girvertz R, Mortola JF. The predictive role of psychosocial stress on symptom severity in premenstrual syndrome. Psychosom Med 1990;52:536–543 (Level III)
11. Adenaike OC, Abidoye RO. A study of the incidence of premenstrual syndrome in a group of Nigerian women. Public Health 1987;101:49–58 (Level III)

12. Hasin M, Dennerstein L, Gotts G. Menstrual cycle related complaints: a cross-cultural study. J Psychosom Obstet Gynaecol 1988;9:35–42 (Level II-3)

13. Stout AL, Grady TA, Steege JF, Blazer DG, George LK, Melville ML. Premenstrual symptoms in black and white community samples. Am J Psychiatry 1986;143; 1436–1439 (Level III)

14. Freeman EW. Premenstrual syndrome: current perspectives on treatment and etiology. Curr Opin Obstet Gynecol 1997;9:147–153 (Level III)

15. Schmidt PJ, Nieman LK, Danaceau MA, Adams LF, Rubinow DR. Differential behavioral effects of gonadal steroids in women with and in those without premenstrual syndrome. N Engl J Med 1998;338:209–216 (Level I)

16. Eriksson E, Hedberg MA, Andersch B, Sundblad C. The serotonin reuptake inhibitor paroxetin is superior to the noradrenaline reuptake inhibitor maprotiline in the treatment of premenstrual syndrome. Neuropsychopharmacology 1995;12:167–176 (Level II-2)

17. Hamilton JA, Parry BL, Alagna S, Blumenthal S, Herz E. Premenstrual mood changes: a guide to evaluation and treatment. Psychiatr Ann 1984;14:426-435 (Level III)

18. American Psychiatric Association. Diagnostic and statistical manual of mental disorders: DSM-IV. 4th ed. Washington, DC: APA, 1994:714–718 (Level III)

19. Hart WG, Coleman GJ, Russell JW. Assessment of premenstrual symptomatology: a re-evaluation of the predictive validity of self-report. J Psychosom Res 1987;31: 185–190 (Level III)

20. Johnson SR. Clinician's approach to the diagnosis and management of premenstrual syndrome. Clin Obstet Gynecol 1992;35:637–657 (Level III)

21. Mortola JF, Girton L, Beck L, Yen SS. Diagnosis of premenstrual syndrome by a simple, prospective, and reliable instrument: the calendar of premenstrual experiences. Obstet Gynecol 1990;76:302–307 (Level II-2)

22. Reid RL. Premenstrual syndrome. Curr Probl Obstet Gynecol Fertil 1985;8(2):1–57 (Level III)

23. McCormack HM, Horne DJ, Sheather S. Clinical applications of visual analogue scales: a critical review. Psychol Med 1988;18:1007–1019 (Level I)

24. Corney RH, Stanton R. A survey of 658 women who report symptoms of premenstrual syndrome. J Psychosom Res 1991;35:471–482 (Level III)

25. Plouffe L Jr, Stewart KS, Craft KS, Maddox MS, Rausch JL. Diagnostic and treatment results from a southeastern academic center-based premenstrual syndrome clinic: the first year. Am J Obstet Gynecol 1993;169:295–303; discussion 303–307 (Level III)

26. Goodale IL, Domar AD, Benson H. Alleviation of premenstrual syndrome symptoms with the relaxation response. Obstet Gynecol 1990;75:649–655 (Level I)

27. Christensen AP, Oei TP. The efficacy of cognitive behaviour therapy in treating premenstrual dysphoric changes. J Affect Disord 1995;33:57–63 (Level II-3)

28. Steege JF, Blumenthal JA. The effects of aerobic exercise on premenstrual symptoms in middle-aged women: a preliminary study. J Psychosom Res 1993;37:127–133 (Level II-1)

29. Prior JC, Vigna Y, Sciarretta D, Alojado N, Schulzer M. Conditioning exercise decreases premenstrual symptoms: a prospective, controlled 6-month trial. Fertil Steril 1987;47:402–408 (Level II-2)

30. Thys-Jacobs, Starkey P, Bernstein D, Tian J. Calcium carbonate and the premenstrual syndrome: effects on premenstrual and menstrual symptoms. Premenstrual Syndrome Study Group. Am J Obstet Gynecol 1998;179:444–452 (Level I)

31. Facchinetti F, Borella P, Sances G, Fioroni L, Nappi RE, Genazzani AR. Oral magnesium successfully relieves premenstrual mood changes. Obstet Gynecol 1991;78: 177–181 (Level I)

32. Walker AF, De Souza MC, Vickers MF, Abeyasekera S, Collins ML, Trinca LA. Magnesium supplementation alleviates premenstrual symptoms of fluid retention. J Womens Health 1998;7:1157–1165 (Level I)

33. London RS, Murphy L, Kitlowski KE, Reynolds MA. Efficacy of alpha-tocopherol in the treatment of the premenstrual syndrome. J Reprod Med 1987;32:400–404 (Level I)

34. Sayegh R, Schiff I, Wurtman J, Spiers P, McDermott J, Wurtman R. The effect of a carbohydrate-rich beverage on mood, appetite, and cognitive function in women with premenstrual syndrome. Obstet Gynecol 1995,86:520–528 (Level II-2)

35. Budeiri D, Li Wan Po A, Dorman JC. Is evening primrose oil of value in the treatment of premenstrual syndrome? Control Clin Trials 1996;17:60–68 (Level III)

36. Wyatt KM, Dimmock PW, Jones PW, Shaughn O'Brien PM. Efficacy of vitamin B-6 in the treatment of premenstrual syndrome: systematic review. BMJ. 1999;318: 1375–1381 (Level III)

37. Steiner M, Steinberg S, Stewart D, Carter D, Berger C, Reid R, et al. Fluoxetine in the treatment of premenstrual dysphoria. Canadian Fluoxetine/Premenstrual Dysphoria Collaborative Study Group. N Engl J Med 1995;332: 1529–1534 (Level I)

38. Pearlstein TB, Stone AB. Long-term fluoxetine treatment of late luteal phase dysphoric disorder. J Clin Psychiatry 1994;55:332–335 (Level II-2)

39. Yonkers KA, Halbreich U, Freeman E, Brown C, Endicott J, Frank E, et al. Symptomatic improvement of premenstrual dysphoric disorder with sertraline treatment. A randomized controlled trial. Sertraline Premenstrual Dysphoric Collaborative Study Group. JAMA 1997; 278:983–988 (Level I)

40. Steiner M, Korzekwa M, Lamont J, Wilkins A. Intermittent fluoxetine dosing in the treatment of women with premenstrual dysphoria. Psychopharmacol Bull 1997;33:771–774 (Level II-3)

41. Young SA, Hurt PH, Benedek DM, Howard RS. Treatment of premenstrual dysphoric disorder with sertraline during the

luteal phase: a randomized, double-blind, placebo-controlled crossover trial. J Clin Psychiatry 1998;59:76–80 (Level II-1)

42. Wikander I, Sundblad C, Andersch B, Dagnell I, Zylberstein D, Bengtsson F, et al. Citalopram in premenstrual dysphoria: is intermittent treatment during luteal phases more effective than continuous medication throughout the menstrual cycle? J Clin Psychopharmacol 1998;18:390–398 (Level I)

43. Harrison WM, Endicott J, Nee J. Treatment of premenstrual dysphoria with alprazolam. A controlled study. Arch Gen Psychiatry 1990;47:270–275 (Level I)

44. Smith S, Rinehart JS, Ruddock VE, Schiff I. Treatment of premenstrual syndrome with alprazolam: results of a double-blind, placebo-controlled, randomized crossover clinical trial. Obstet Gynecol 1987;70:37–43 (Level I)

45. Freeman EW, Rickels K, Sondheimer SJ, Polansky M. A double-blind trial of oral progesterone, alprazolam, and placebo in treatment of severe premenstrual syndrome. JAMA 1995;274:51–57 (Level I)

46. Schmidt PJ, Grover GN, Rubinow DR. Alprazolam in the treatment of premenstrual syndrome: a double-blind, placebo-controlled trial. Arch Gen Psychiatry 1993;50: 467–473 (Level I)

47. O'Brien PM, Craven D, Selby C, Symonds EM. Treatment of premenstrual syndrome by spironolactone. Br J Obstet Gynaecol 1979;86:142–147 (Level I)

48. Vellacott ID, Shroff NE, Pearce MY, Stratford ME, Akbar FA. A double-blind, placebo-controlled evaluation of spironolactone in the premenstrual syndrome. Curr Med Res Opin 1987;10:450–456 (Level I)

49. Wang M, Hammarback S, Lindhe BA, Backstrom T. Treatment of premenstrual syndrome by spironolactone: a double-blind, placebo controlled study. Acta Obstet Gynecol Scand 1995;74:803–808 (Level I)

50. Burnet RB, Radden HS, Easterbrook EG, McKinnon RA. Premenstrual syndrome and spironolactone. Aust N Z J Obstet Gynaecol 1991;31:366–368 (Level I)

51. Hellberg D, Claesson B, Nilsson S. Premenstrual tension: a placebo-controlled efficacy study with spironolactone and medroxyprogesterone acetate. Int J Gynaecol Obstet 1991;34:243–248 (Level II-1)

52. Freeman E, Rickels K, Sondheimer SJ, Polansky M. Ineffectiveness of progesterone suppository treatment for premenstrual syndrome. JAMA 1990;264:349–353 (Level I)

53. Baker ER, Best RG, Manfredi RL, Demers LM, Wolf GC. Efficacy of progesterone vaginal suppositories in alleviation of nervous symptoms in patients with premenstrual syndrome. J Assist Reprod Genet 1995;12:205–209 (Level II-1)

54. Graham CA. Sherwin BB. A prospective treatment study of premenstrual symptoms using a triphasic oral contraceptive. Psychosom Res 1992;36:257–266 (Level II-2)

55. Backstrom T, Hansson-Malmstrom Y, Lindhe BA, Cavilli-Bjorkman B, Nordenstrom S. Oral contraceptives in premenstrual syndrome: a randomized comparison of triphasic and monophasic preparations. Contraception 1992;46:253–268 (Level II-1)

56. Johnson SR. Premenstrual syndrome therapy. Clin Obstet Gynecol 1998;41:405–421 (Level III)

57. Freeman EW, Sondheimer SJ, Rickels K. Gonadotropin-releasing hormone agonist in treatment of premenstrual symptoms with and without ongoing dysphoria: a controlled study. Psychopharmacol Bull 1997;33:303–309 (Level I)

58. West CP, Hillier H. Ovarian suppression with the gonadotrophin-releasing hormone agonist goserelin (Zoladex) in management of the premenstrual tension syndrome. Hum Reprod 1994;9:1058–1063 (Level I)

59. Mortola JF, Girton L, Fischer U. Successful treatment of severe premenstrual syndrome by combined use of gonadotropin-releasing hormone agonist and estrogen/ progestin. J Clin Endocrinol Metab 1991;72:252A–252F (Level III)

60. Casson P, Hahn PM, Van Vugt DA, Reid RL. Lasting response to ovariectomy in severe intractable premenstrual syndrome. Am J Obstet Gynecol 1990;162:99–105 (Level II-3)

The MEDLINE database, the Cochrane Library, and ACOG's own internal resources and documents were used to conduct a literature search to locate relevant articles published between January 1985 and May 1999. The search was restricted to articles published in the English language. Priority was given to articles reporting results of original research, although review articles and commentaries also were consulted. Abstracts of research presented at symposia and scientific conferences were not considered adequate for inclusion in this document. Guidelines published by organizations or institutions such as the National Institutes of Health and the American College of Obstetricians and Gynecologists were reviewed, and additional studies were located by reviewing bibliographies of identified articles. When reliable research was not available, expert opinions from obstetrician–gynecologists were used.

Studies were reviewed and evaluated for quality according to the method outlined by the U.S. Preventive Services Task Force:

- I Evidence obtained from at least one properly designed randomized controlled trial.
- II-1 Evidence obtained from well-designed controlled trials without randomization.
- II-2 Evidence obtained from well-designed cohort or case–control analytic studies, preferably from more than one center or research group.
- II-3 Evidence obtained from multiple time series with or without the intervention. Dramatic results in uncontrolled experiments also could be regarded as this type of evidence.
- III Opinions of respected authorities, based on clinical experience, descriptive studies, or reports of expert committees.

Based on the highest level of evidence found in the data, recommendations are provided and graded according to the following catetories:

Level A—Recommendations are based on good and consistent scientific evidence.

Level B—Recommendations are based on limited or inconsistent scientific evidence.

Level C—Recommendations are based primarily on consensus and expert opinion.

ISSN 1099-3630

The American College of Obstetricians and Gynecologists
409 12th Street, SW
PO Box 96920
Washington, DC 20090-6920

12345/43210

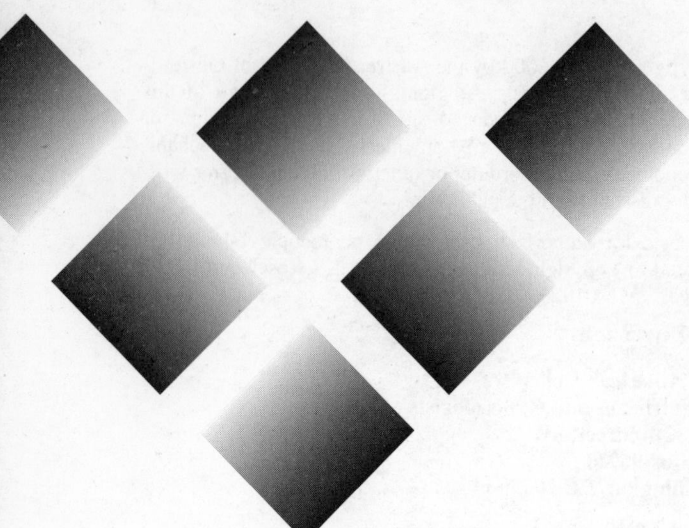

ACOG PRACTICE BULLETIN

CLINICAL MANAGEMENT GUIDELINES FOR OBSTETRICIAN–GYNECOLOGISTS
NUMBER 21, OCTOBER 2000

This Practice Bulletin was developed by the ACOG Committee on Practice Bulletins—Gynecology with the assistance of Linda A. Barbour, MD and Kathryn L. Hassell, MD. The information is designed to aid practitioners in making decisions about appropriate obstetric and gynecologic care. These guidelines should not be construed as dictating an exclusive course of treatment or procedure. Variations in practice may be warranted based on the needs of the individual patient, resources, and limitations unique to the institution or type of practice.

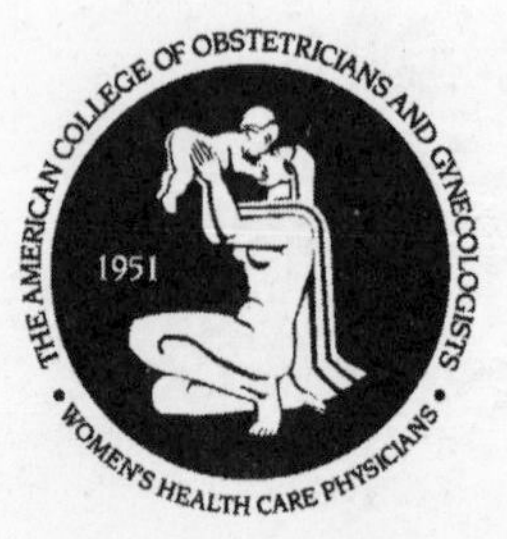

Prevention of Deep Vein Thrombosis and Pulmonary Embolism

In the United States, venous thromboembolism remains a leading cause of death and morbidity among hospitalized patients. Overall, approximately 60,000 deaths per year are attributed to venous thromboembolism and the subsequent complications, including postthrombotic syndrome, venous insufficiency, pulmonary hypertension, and pulmonary dysfunction (1). Venous thromboembolism often has no symptoms, and pulmonary embolism is not suspected clinically in 70–80% of patients in whom it is detected postmortem. Most patients who die from pulmonary embolism do so within 30 minutes of the event, reinforcing the need for rapid and accurate diagnosis. Fatal pulmonary embolism is a common preventable cause of death in hospitalized patients. Venous thromboembolism also predisposes patients to long-term morbidity from postthrombotic syndrome. The purpose of this document is to review the current literature on the prevention of thromboembolism in gynecologic patients, discuss the rationale behind sometimes conflicting guidelines, and offer evidence-based recommendations to address the most clinically relevant issues in the management of these patients.

Background

Detection of Deep Vein Thrombosis

Detection of deep vein thrombosis (DVT) is difficult, especially when patients are asymptomatic. Thus, the occurrence of venous thromboembolism in surgical patients varies from one study to another. Most trials examining the efficacy of DVT prophylaxis in general surgical and gynecologic patients have used the fibrinogen I-125 uptake test to diagnose DVT. This technique is sensitive for detecting DVT only distally (calf) and is poor at detecting DVT in the upper thigh (2, 3). Because of concerns about the transmission of blood-borne diseases, the fibrinogen I-125 uptake test is no longer commercially available in the United States or in many European countries. Equally inhibiting is the limited sensitivity and predictive value of duplex compression ultrasonography and impedance plethysmography to detect asymptomatic proximal vein thrombosis (4–8). Compression ultrasound examination of the femoral and popliteal veins and calf trifurcation has been found to be a highly sensitive (>90%) and specific (>99%) method of detecting proximal vein DVT, but less reliable (50%) for detecting calf vein DVT (6, 8).

Diagnosis of pelvic vein thrombosis and internal iliac thrombosis is exceedingly difficult even with magnetic resonance imaging, which is considered the imaging modality of choice (9). Fatal pulmonary emboli have been reported at postmortem examination to be from internal iliac or pelvic veins, for which there is no highly sensitive diagnostic imaging technique. Because diagnosis is difficult, perioperative prophylaxis has become the mainstay of management.

Prophylaxis in Gynecologic Surgery

The prevalence of venous thromboembolism after surgery varies and depends on multiple risk factors. Most events occur within 7 days postoperatively in gynecologic surgical patients; however, patients continue to be at risk for the first 3 weeks after discharge, probably secondary to decreased ambulation. Patients undergoing surgery for cancer or orthopedic surgery are at the highest risk for later complications from venous thromboembolism; the risk of pulmonary embolism continues for 30 days after surgery (10). Postoperative venous thromboembolism, as diagnosed by the fibrinogen I-125 uptake test, ranges from 7% to 29% in general gynecologic surgery and up to 45% in patients with malignant disease (11–13). Pulmonary embolism occurs in 0.1–5% of cases depending on the level of risk. Unfortunately, pulmonary embolism occurs without clinical evidence of DVT in 50–80% of cases and is fatal in approximately 10–20% of cases (14).

In a univariate analysis of all characteristics identified to be statistically significantly related to venous thromboembolism, significant variables included recurrent malignant disease, a prior history of DVT, duration of anesthesia greater than 5 hours, prior pelvic radiation, venous stasis changes or venous varicosities, and age older than 45 years (11). The same analysis concluded that the type of surgery, specifically radical vulvectomy with inguinal lymphadenopathy or pelvic exenteration (ie, surgeries that result in extensive periods of immobilization), was a significant variable in determining risk.

Hypercoagulable States

It is now estimated that nearly half of patients with thrombosis have an identifiable thrombotic disorder (15, 16) as a result of the discovery of the factor V Leiden mutation (resistance to activated protein C) and the prothrombin gene mutation G20210A. The most commonly identified hypercoagulable states are listed in Table 1. It has been observed that approximately 50–60% of patients with a hereditary form of thrombosis will not experience a thrombotic event until an environmental risk factor such as oral contraceptive use, pregnancy, orthopedic trauma, immobilization, or surgery is present (17, 18). Currently, the coexistence of multiple inherited risk factors has been acknowledged, which markedly increases the risk of thrombosis (16). Antiphospholipid antibody syndrome is an acquired hypercoagulable state that often manifests as venous or arterial thrombosis, thrombocytopenia, recurrent fetal loss, intrauterine growth restriction, or early preeclampsia (19, 20). Hyperhomocystinemia may be acquired or inherited and is associated with an increased risk of venous thromboembolism and early atherosclerotic disease with arterial thrombosis.

Preoperative patients should be classified according to levels of risk of thrombosis to determine the benefits and risks of pharmacologic and physical methods of preventing venous thromboembolism. Table 2 summarizes the classification of risk level based on published data.

Prophylaxis Alternatives

Graduated Compression Stockings

The use of graduated compression stockings, which reduce stasis, is by far the simplest of the prophylactic approaches and has the advantages of being inexpensive, easy to use, and free of side effects if properly fitted (21). Graduated compression stockings reduce the prevalence of DVT (especially calf) in medium-risk patients when compared with placebo according to a meta-analysis of all randomized controlled trials (21), including one study of gynecologic surgery (22). However, patients with malignant disease and other high-risk conditions have not been evaluated in sufficient numbers to reach conclusions about the use of graduated compression stockings in these settings (23).

Pneumatic Compression

If used at induction of anesthesia and continued until patients are fully ambulatory, pneumatic compression

Table 1. Common Hypercoagulable States

Abnormality	Prevalence in Patients with Thrombosis	Testing Methods	Can patients be tested during pregnancy?	Is the test reliable during acute thrombosis?	Is the test reliable while on anti-coagulation?
Factor V Leiden	40–70%*	APC resistance assay	No	Yes	Yes
		DNA analysis	Yes	Yes	Yes
Prothrombin gene mutation G20210A	8–30%†	DNA analysis	Yes	Yes	Yes
Antiphospholipid antibody	10–15%‡	Functional assay (eg, dilute Russell viper venom time)	Yes	Yes	Yes
		Anticardiolipin antibodies	Yes	Yes	Yes
		β_2-Glycoprotein-1 antibodies	Yes	Yes	Yes
Protein C deficiency	—	Protein C activity	Yes	No	No
Protein S deficiency	10–15%§	Protein S total and free antigen	Yes	No	No
AT-III deficiency	—	AT-III activity	Yes	No	No
Hyperhomocystinemia	8–25%	Fasting plasma homocystine	Yes	Unclear	Yes

* Bokarewa MI, Bremme K, Blombäck M. Arg[506]-Gln mutation in factor V and risk of thrombosis during pregnancy. Br J Haematol 1996;92:473–478; Hellgren M, Svensson PJ, Dahlbäck B. Resistance to activated protein C as a basis for venous thromboembolism associated with pregnancy and oral contraceptives. Am J Obstet Gynecol 1995;173:210–213; Faioni EM, Razzari C, Martinelli I, Panzeri D, Franchi F, Mannucci PM. Resistance to activated protein C in unselected patients with arterial and venous thrombosis. Am J Hematol 1997;55:59–64

† Grandone E, Margaglione M, Colaizzo D, D'Andrea G, Cappucci G, Brancaccio V, et al. Genetic susceptibility to pregnancy-related venous thromboembolism: roles of factor V Leiden, prothrombin G20210A, and methylenetetrahydrofolate reductase C677T mutations. Am J Obstet Gynecol 1998;179:1324–1328; Martinelli I, Taioli E, Bucciarelli P, Akhavan S, Mannucci PM. Interaction between the G20210A mutation of the prothrombin gene and oral contraceptive use in deep vein thrombosis. Arterioscler Thromb Vasc Biol 1999;19:700–703; Salomon O, Steinberg DM, Zivelin A, Gitel S, Dardik R, Rosenberg N, et al. Single and combined prothrombotic factors in patients with idiopathic venous thromboembolism: prevalence and risk assessment. Arterioscler Thromb Vasc Biol 1999;19:511–518

‡ Ginsberg JS, Wells PS, Brill-Edwards P, Donovan D, Moffat K, Johnston M, et al. Antiphospholipid antibodies and venous thromboembolism. Blood 1995;86:3685–3691

§ Aiach M, Borgel D, Gaussem P, Emmerich J, Alhenc-Gelas M, Gandrille S. Protein C and protein S deficiencies. Semin Hematol 1997;34:205–216; De Stefano V, Leone G, Mastrangelo S, Tripodi A, Rodeghiero F, Castaman G, et al. Clinical manifestations and management of inherited thrombophilia: retrospective analysis and follow-up after diagnosis of 238 patients with congenital deficiency of antithrombin III, protein C, protein S. Thromb Haemost 1994;72:352–358; Pabinger I, Schneider B. Thrombotic risk in hereditary antithrombin III, protein C, or protein S deficiency. A cooperative, retrospective study. Gesellschaft fur Thrombose- und Hamostaseforschung (GTH) Study Group on Natural Inhibitors. Arterioscler Thromb Vasc Biol 1996;16:742–748

appears to be effective in reducing DVT in medium-risk and high-risk patients (21, 23–25). Pneumatic compression may be useful in reducing leg DVT in high-risk patients with malignant disease; however, its efficacy in preventing pulmonary embolism is unknown because of limited sample sizes (26). Patient compliance is essential for the effectiveness of pneumatic compression.

Low-Dose Heparin

Low-dose unfractionated heparin has been shown to be effective as prophylaxis for DVT and pulmonary embolism in moderate-risk patients without underlying malignancy or other clinical risk factors. A review of randomized trials published before 1988, which included gynecologic patients, showed that low-dose heparin decreased DVT by nearly 70% and pulmonary embolism by 40–50% (27). Unfractionated heparin, 5,000 U administered every 8 hours postoperatively, does appear to be effective prophylaxis for DVT in patients undergoing gynecologic oncologic surgery, as demonstrated in a randomized unblinded trial (28). Although the efficacy in reducing postoperative venous thrombosis was similar between low-dose heparin and intermittent pneumatic calf compression, patients receiving low-dose heparin required significantly more postoperative transfusions (25). In a randomized, multicenter, double-blinded trial

Table 2. Classification of Risk Levels for Venous Thromboembolism Among Gynecologic Surgery Patients

Classification	Definition
Low risk (<3% risk of DVT*)	Age ≤40 y and Surgery lasting <30 min
Moderate risk (10–40% risk of DVT)	Age >40 y and Surgery of any duration No other clinical risk factors
High risk (40–70% risk of DVT; 1–5% risk of pulmonary embolism)	Age >40 y plus risk factors: • Prior DVT or pulmonary embolism • Varicose veins • Infection • Malignancy • Estrogen therapy • Obesity • Prolonged surgery

*DVT indicates deep vein thrombosis.

Data from NIH Consensus Conference. Prevention of venous thrombosis and pulmonary embolism. JAMA 1986;256:744–749

of 631 patients with evaluable venograms who were undergoing abdominal or pelvic surgery for cancer, low-dose heparin, 5,000 U every 8 hours, was as good as low-molecular-weight heparin (LMWH) (enoxaparin, 40 mg once a day) in the prevention of DVT (29). A trial of patients undergoing gynecologic surgery, in which 84% of the patients had underlying malignancy, used two different preoperative regimens of unfractionated heparin and compared them with no perioperative prophylaxis. The findings of this study suggest that two to nine doses of heparin preoperatively were not statistically better in preventing DVT than only one preoperative dose of 5,000 U administered 2 hours before the surgery (28). Both regimens used heparin every 8 hours postoperatively until discharge.

Low-Molecular-Weight Heparin

Low-molecular-weight heparin has been used in numerous trials for prophylaxis in abdominal surgery with at least the same efficacy as unfractionated heparin in preventing DVT. This finding has been substantiated in a meta-analysis of 36 double-blinded randomized controlled trials, 25 of which were in the general surgery population (30, 31). Some data suggest there is a lower bleeding risk with LMWH compared with unfractionated heparin (30). Once-daily administration and a lower rate of heparin-induced thrombocytopenia are additional advantages of LMWH over unfractionated heparin (23). A randomized, double-blinded multicenter trial that used the fibrinogen I-125 uptake test compared two different doses of dalteparin (2,500 antifactor-Xa U versus 5,000 antifactor-Xa U) in the general surgery population in which 66% of patients had malignant disease (32). It found the efficacy overall was better in the high-dose LMWH group than in the low-dose LMWH group (6.6% DVT and 12.7% DVT, respectively) in preventing DVT, but bleeding complications were higher in the high-dose group (4.7% versus 2.7%). However, in the subgroup with malignant disease, efficacy remained better in the high-dose group than the low-dose group (8.5% DVT versus 14.9% DVT) but bleeding complications were no different (4.6% versus 3.6%). In a randomized study of 80 patients undergoing pelvic or abdominal surgery for malignancy that used the fibrinogen I-125 uptake test, dalteparin (5,000 antifactor-Xa U) was equally effective as unfractionated heparin, 5,000 U administered every 8 hours. Seventy-five percent of the patients had gynecologic cancers, and there was no difference in blood loss between the groups (33).

Anesthesia Concerns

The use of major conduction anesthesia (spinal or epidural) in patients receiving heparin or LMWH thromboembolic prophylaxis is controversial (34). Intraoperative or postoperative anticoagulation after regional anesthesia is thought to be safe; however, the safety of LMWH, unfractionated heparin, or oral anticoagulants administered before the procedure is unclear. In a retrospective review of 61 reported cases of spinal hematoma associated with epidural or spinal anesthesia, 42 (61%) were associated with a hemostatic abnormality (35). At least 25 patients received heparin intravenously or subcutaneously, and in 15 of 32 patients with indwelling catheters, the spinal hematomas occurred immediately after the removal of the epidural catheter. Unfractionated low-dose heparin appeared not to pose a significant risk for spinal hematoma in over 5,000 patients who received it in combination with a single-dose spinal or epidural anesthesia, nor did antiplatelet prophylaxis (36). Low-molecular-weight heparin, however, may pose a risk if it is used preoperatively, intraoperatively, or within 3 hours postoperatively in patients receiving continuous epidural analgesia. In 1997, the U.S. Food and Drug Administration issued a public health advisory regarding reported cases of epidural or spinal hematomas with concurrent use of enoxaparin and spinal or epidural anesthesia or spinal puncture (37). Many of the epidural or spinal hematomas caused neurologic injury, including long-term or permanent paralysis, and approximately 75% of the patients were elderly women undergoing orthopedic surgery.

Clinical Considerations and Recommendations

▶ *Who are candidates for perioperative DVT thromboprophylaxis?*

Candidates for surgical prophylaxis include patients who are found to have deficiencies of protein C, protein S, or antithrombin III (AT-III), who have the factor V Leiden or prothrombin gene mutation G20210A without a personal history of thrombosis, or who experience orthopedic trauma (15, 18, 38–40), especially if they have a strong family history of thrombosis.

In addition, Table 2 outlines a risk stratification adopted from the 1986 National Institutes of Health Consensus Conference (41). Most of the evidence for determining risk status was obtained from the control arms of more than 100 trials conducted primarily among patients older than 40 years who were undergoing general surgery.

▶ *Which prophylactic methods should be considered for low-, medium-, and high-risk patients undergoing gynecologic surgery?*

Patients in the low-risk category (as defined in Table 2) who are undergoing gynecologic surgery probably do not need any thromboprophylactic agent as long as they are quickly mobilized.

Patients in the moderate-risk category would likely benefit from prophylaxis with either graduated compression stockings, pneumatic compression, low-dose unfractionated heparin (5,000 U every 8 hours) in which the first dose is given before surgery, or low-dose LMWH (dalteparin, 2,500 U once a day, or enoxaparin, 40 mg once a day). However, the need for prophylaxis should include consideration of the length and complexity of surgery, the patient's age, and the evaluation of other risk factors. In the United States, dalteparin and enoxaparin are considerably more expensive alternatives to standard heparin and have not been shown to be significantly more efficacious or associated with less bleeding risks in comparison with low-dose unfractionated heparin in moderate-risk patients. Prophylaxis with thigh-high graduated compression stockings has not been as extensively studied for moderate-risk patients compared with standard heparin.

High-risk patients should be offered standard heparin, 5,000 U every 8 hours (28). A more expensive alternative for high-risk patients is LMWH given as either dalteparin, 5,000 antifactor-Xa U once a day, or enoxaparin, 40 mg once a day (the first dose given the evening before surgery). However, it is not clear that the latter approach offers any advantage or is significantly more efficacious (29, 32). Pneumatic compression appears to be as effective (23) but has not been as well studied as heparin and LMWH.

Adding graduated compression stockings or pneumatic compression to anticoagulant therapy may be a good alternative for high-risk patients, especially those undergoing radical vulvectomy with inguinal lymphadenectomy or pelvic exenteration for malignancy (23, 25), although no clinical trials have confirmed this approach.

▶ *Should patients discontinue oral contraceptives or hormone replacement therapy before surgery?*

There are no studies to confirm the clinical benefit of stopping oral contraceptives preoperatively (42). The hypercoagulable changes induced by oral contraceptives do not return to normal for 4–6 weeks after discontinuation of therapy (43). The risk of postoperative thromboembolism has been reported to be 0.96% for oral contraceptive users and 0.5% for nonusers (44). However, the risk of stopping oral contraceptives 4–6 weeks before major surgery must be balanced against the risks of pregnancy (which carries a much higher risk of DVT and pulmonary embolism than does oral contraceptive use), the effects of surgery and anesthesia on pregnancy, and the possibility of subsequent termination of pregnancy with its associated physical and psychologic risks.

Discontinuation of hormone replacement therapy (HRT) before major gynecologic surgery to prevent deep vein thrombosis or pulmonary embolism has not been evaluated in randomized clinical trials. However, three retrospective case-control studies have evaluated the risk of hospital admission for deep vein thrombosis in HRT users (45–47). These studies reported that the current users of HRT had an increased risk of VTE (odds ratio 2.1 to 3.6) when compared with matched HRT nonusers, and that past use did not affect this risk. However, the absolute risk for both users and nonusers of HRT was low. One analysis of nearly 350,000 women aged 50–79 years reported that of these, 292 women were admitted to the hospital with DVT or pulmonary embolism, which represents only a modest increase in morbidity (risk of 1.3 per 10,000 per year for nonusers; risk of less than 2 additional cases per 10,000 women per year in HRT users) (47). For women with other risk factors who are undergoing gynecologic surgery, the benefit of stopping HRT has not yet been established.

▶ *Which patients should be tested for clotting abnormalities, and which tests should be ordered?*

Because of its high prevalence in the Caucasian population, all patients who are not Hispanic, Asian, or African American who have a history of DVT may be tested for the factor V Leiden mutation (16, 48–54). In non-Caucasian patients, the decision to test should be individualized. Patients with histories of extensive or recurrent thrombosis or family histories of thrombosis may have the factor V Leiden mutation in combination with another congenital or acquired disorder (55). Patients with a strong family history of thrombosis who are negative for the factor V Leiden mutation may benefit from testing for the prothrombin gene mutation G20210A and deficiencies in the natural inhibitors, including protein C, protein S, and AT-III. Patients with a history of thrombosis, recurrent fetal loss, early or severe preeclampsia, severe unexplained intrauterine growth restriction, or unexplained thrombocytopenia may be tested for antiphospholipid antibodies. Fasting plasma homocystine levels may be assessed, especially in women of childbearing age who have had venous or arterial thrombosis, because elevated levels can be treated with vitamins (folic acid, vitamin B_{12}, and vitamin B_6). The specific tests and optimal timing for testing are described in Table 1.

▶ *Should women on prolonged heparin be evaluated for heparin-induced osteoporosis or heparin-induced thrombocytopenia?*

Heparin-induced osteoporosis appears to occur predominantly in patients taking heparin for 7 weeks or longer (56, 57) and is not an issue for those taking prophylactic or short-term doses.

Heparin-induced thrombocytopenia is uncommon with the use of porcine heparin (1–3%) and is less common with LMWH (<1%), but immune-related thrombocytopenia can have severe thrombotic consequences (58). Platelet counts should be monitored at the initiation of standard heparin therapy and periodically up to 15 days after starting heparin (59). If the platelet count is unchanged at that time, further platelet counts are not needed because the vast majority of immune, heparin-induced thrombocytopenia occurs within 15 days of starting standard heparin therapy. If confirmed, heparin therapy should be stopped immediately. A low-molecular-weight heparinoid (danaparoid sodium) is available in the United States and was shown to be efficacious in 93% of 88 patients with heparin-induced thrombocytopenia and thrombosis not related to pregnancy (60). Lepirudin (recombinant hirudin), a direct thrombin inhibitor, also is available for intravenous use in patients with heparin-induced thrombocytopenia (59).

▶ *What special considerations should be given when using low-molecular-weight heparin in patients undergoing regional anesthesia?*

Low-molecular-weight heparin has a longer half-life than standard heparin, and its anticoagulant activity cannot be measured using an activated partial thromboplastin time. If used in low doses as a once-a-day regimen, at least 12 hours should lapse after administration before offering central neural blockade. No regional anesthesia should be employed within 12 hours of an injection of LMWH, and LMWH should be withheld for at least 2 hours after removal of an epidural catheter (35, 36, 61). The safety of a twice-daily dose of LMWH in patients receiving epidural anesthesia has not been studied sufficiently, and it is not known whether 24 hours is an adequate amount of time to wait after the last injection. In institutions in which an antifactor-Xa level can be obtained in a timely manner, it may be reasonable to offer spinal or epidural anesthesia as long as the antifactor-Xa levels are not above the prophylactic range. However, the safety of this practice has not been evaluated prospectively.

▶ *Which prophylactic methods are considered cost-effective?*

It is estimated that half of patients with proximal DVT and one third of patients with distal DVT develop a postthrombotic syndrome characterized by pain, swelling, and occasional ulceration of the skin and legs (62). Prophylaxis with either graduated compression stockings, pneumatic compression, low-dose standard heparin, or LMWH is less expensive than no prophylaxis in patients undergoing general abdominal surgery (63, 64). Routine surveillance is the most expensive strategy because of the lack of sensitivity of noninvasive tests to diagnose DVT (63). Although a cost analysis in Europe determined LMWH to be more cost-effective than unfractionated heparin (63), LMWH is substantially more expensive in the United States than in Europe. A cost-analysis in the United States determined that pneumatic compression was more cost-effective than either LMWH or unfractionated heparin (65).

Summary

The following recommendations are based on good and consistent scientific evidence (Level A):

- Alternatives for thromboprophylaxis for moderate-risk patients undergoing gynecologic surgery include the following:
  1. Thigh-high graduated compression stockings placed intraoperatively and continued until the patient is fully ambulatory
  2. Pneumatic compression placed intraoperatively and continued until the patient is fully ambulatory
  3. Unfractionated heparin (5,000 U) administered 2 hours before surgery and continued postoperatively every 8 hours until discharge
  4. Low-molecular-weight heparin (dalteparin, 2,500 antifactor-Xa U, or enoxaparin, 40 mg) administered 12 hours before surgery and once a day postoperatively until discharge
- Alternatives for prophylaxis for high-risk patients undergoing gynecologic surgery, especially for malignancy, include:
  1. Pneumatic compression placed intraoperatively and continued until the patient is fully ambulatory
  2. Unfractionated heparin (5,000 U) administered 8 hours before surgery and continued postoperatively until discharge
  3. Dalteparin (5,000 antifactor-Xa U) administered 12 hours before surgery and then once a day thereafter
  4. Enoxaparin (40 mg) administered 12 hours before surgery and then once a day thereafter

The following recommendations are based primarily on consensus and expert opinion (Level C):

- Low-risk patients who are undergoing gynecologic surgery do not require specific prophylaxis other than early ambulation.
- Postoperative prophylaxis should be continued for 7 days or until discharge.

References

1. Hirsh J, Hoak J. Management of deep vein thrombosis and pulmonary embolism. A statement for healthcare professionals. Council on Thrombosis (in consultation with the Council on Cardiovascular Radiology), American Heart Association. Circulation 1996;93:2212–2245 (Level III)
2. Lensing AW, Hirsh J. 125I-fibrinogen leg scanning: reassessment of its role for the diagnosis of venous thrombosis in post-operative patients. Thromb Haemost 1993;69:2–7 (Level III)
3. Weinmann EE, Salzman EW. Deep vein thrombosis. N Engl J Med 1994;331:1630–1641 (Level III)
4. Agnelli G, Cosmi B, Ranucci V, Renga C, Mosca S, Lupattelli L, et al. Impedance plethysmography in the diagnosis of asymptomatic deep vein thrombosis in hip surgery. A venography-controlled study. Arch Intern Med 1991;151:2167–2171 (Level II-2)
5. Borris LC, Christiansen HM, Lassen MR, Olsen AD, Schøtt P. Comparison of real-time B-mode ultrasonography and bilateral ascending phlebography for detection of postoperative deep vein thrombosis following elective hip surgery. The Venous Thrombosis Group. Thromb Haemost 1989;61:363–365 (Level II-2)
6. Jongbloets LM, Lensing AW, Koopman MM, Büller HR, ten Cate JW. Limitations of compression ultrasound for the detection of symptomless postoperative deep vein thrombosis. Lancet 1994;343:1142–1144 (Level II-2)
7. Lensing AW, Doris CI, McGrath FP, Cogo A, Sabine MJ, Ginsberg J, et al. A comparison of compression ultrasound with color Doppler ultrasound for the diagnosis of symptomless postoperative deep vein thrombosis. Arch Intern Med 1997;157:765–768 (Level II-2)
8. Wells PS, Lensing AW, Davidson BL, Prins MH, Hirsh J. Accuracy of ultrasound for the diagnosis of deep venous thrombosis in asymptomatic patients after orthopedic surgery. A meta-analysis. Ann Intern Med 1995;122:47–53 (Meta-analysis)
9. Spritzer CE, Evans AC, Kay HH. Magnetic resonance imaging of deep venous thrombosis in pregnant women with lower extremity edema. Obstet Gynecol 1995; 85:603–607 (Level III)
10. Bergqvist D. Prolonged prophylaxis against postoperative venous thromboembolism. Haemostasis 1996;26(suppl 4):379–387 (Level III)
11. Clarke-Pearson DL, DeLong ER, Synan IS, Coleman RE, Creasman WT. Variables associated with postoperative deep venous thrombosis: a prospective study of 411 gynecology patients and creation of a prognostic model. Obstet Gynecol 1987;69:146–150 (Level III)
12. Clarke-Pearson DL, Jelovsek FR, Creasman WT. Thromboembolism complicating surgery for cervical and uterine malignancy: incidence, risk factors, and prophylaxis. Obstet Gynecol 1983;61:87–94 (Level II-2)

13. Crandon AJ, Koutts J. Incidence of post-operative deep vein thrombosis in gynaecological oncology. Aust NZ J Obstet Gynaecol 1983;23:216–219 (Level III)

14. Farquharson DI, Orr JW Jr. Prophylaxis against thromboembolism in gynecologic patients. J Reprod Med 1984;29:845–862 (Level III)

15. Bauer KA. Management of patients with hereditary defects predisposing to thrombosis including pregnant women. Thromb Haemost 1995;74:94–100 (Level III)

16. Florell SR, Rodgers GM. Inherited thrombotic disorders: an update. Am J Hematol 1997;54:53–60 (Level III)

17. De Stefano V, Leone G, Mastrangelo S, Tripodi A, Rodeghiero F, Castaman G, et al. Clinical manifestations and management of inherited thrombophilia: retrospective analysis and follow-up after diagnosis of 238 patients with congenital deficiency of antithrombin III, protein C, protein S. Thromb Haemost 1994;72:352–358 (Level III)

18. Middledorp S, Henkens CM, Koopman MM, van Pampus EC, Hamulyák K, van der Meer J, et al. The incidence of venous thromboembolism in family members of patients with factor V Leiden mutation and venous thrombosis. Ann Intern Med 1998;128:15–20 (Level II-2)

19. Petri M. Pathogenesis and treatment of the antiphospholipid antibody syndrome. Med Clin North Am 1997; 81:151–177 (Level III)

20. Shapiro GA. Antiphospholipid syndrome in obstetrics and gynecology. Semin Thromb Hemost 1994;20:64–70 (Level III)

21. Wells PS, Lensing AW, Hirsh J. Graduated compression stockings in the prevention of postoperative venous thromboembolism. A meta-analysis. Arch Intern Med 1994; 154:67–72 (Meta-analysis)

22. Turner GM, Cole SE, Brooks JH. The efficacy of graduated compression stockings in the prevention of deep vein thrombosis after major gynaecological surgery. Br J Obstet Gynaecol 1984;91:588–591 (Level I)

23. Clagett GP, Anderson FA Jr, Heit J, Levine MN, Wheeler HB. Prevention of venous thromboembolism. Chest 1995;108 (suppl 4):312S–334S (Level III)

24. Clarke-Pearson DL, Synan IS, Hinshaw WM, Coleman RE, Creasman WT. Prevention of postoperative venous thromboembolism by external pneumatic calf compression in patients with gynecologic malignancy. Obstet Gynecol 1984;63:92–98 (Level I)

25. Clarke-Pearson DL, Synan IS, Dodge R, Soper JT, Berchuck A, Coleman RE. A randomized trial of low-dose heparin and intermittent pneumatic calf compression for the prevention of deep venous thrombosis after gynecologic oncology surgery. Am J Obstet Gynecol 1993; 168:1146–1153; discussion 1153–1154 (Level I)

26. Clagett GP, Reisch JS. Prevention of venous thromboembolism in general surgical patients. Results of meta-analysis. Ann Surg 1988;208:227–240 (Meta-analysis)

27. Collins R, Scrimgeour A, Yusuf S, Peto R. Reduction in fatal pulmonary embolism and venous thrombosis by perioperative administration of subcutaneous heparin. Overview of results of randomized trials in general orthopedic and urologic surgery. N Engl J Med 1988;318: 1162–1173 (Level III)

28. Clarke-Pearson DL, DeLong E, Synan IS, Soper JT, Creasman WT, Coleman RE. A controlled trial of two low-dose-heparin regimens for the prevention of postoperative deep vein thrombosis. Obstet Gynecol 1990;75:684–689 (Level I)

29. Enoxacan Study Group. Efficacy and safety of enoxaparin versus unfractionated heparin for prevention of deep vein thrombosis in elective cancer surgery: a double-blind randomized multicentre trial with venographic assessment. Br J Surg 1997;84:1099–1103 (Level I)

30. Kakkar VV, Boeckl O, Boneu B, Bordenave L, Brehm OA, Brücke P, et al. Efficacy and safety of a low-molecular-weight heparin and standard unfractionated heparin for prophylaxis of postoperative venous thromboembolism: European multicenter trial. World J Surg 1997;21:2–8; discussion 8–9 (Level I)

31. Koch A, Bouges S, Ziegler S, Dinkel H, Daures JP, Victor N. Low molecular weight heparin and unfractionated heparin in thrombosis prophylaxis after major surgical intervention: update of previous meta-analyses. Br J Surg 1997;84:750–759 (Meta-analysis)

32. Bergqvist D, Burmark US, Flordal PA, Frisell J, Hallböök T, Hedberg M, et al. Low molecular weight heparin started before surgery as prophylaxis against deep vein thrombosis: 2500 versus 5000 XaI units in 2070 patients. Br J Surg 1995;82:496–501 (Level I)

33. Fricker JP, Vergnes Y, Schach R, Heitz A, Eber M, Grunebaum L, et al. Low dose heparin versus low molecular weight heparin (Kabi 2165, Fragmin) in the prophylaxis of thromboembolic complications of abdominal oncological surgery. Eur J Clin Invest 1988;18:561–567 (Level I)

34. Haljamäe H. Thromboprophylaxis, coagulation disorders, and regional anesthesia. Acta Anaesthesiol Scand 1996; 40:1024–1040 (Level III)

35. Vandermeulen EP, Van Aken H, Vermylen J. Anticoagulants and spinal-epidural anesthesia. Anesth Analg 1994; 79:1165–1177 (Level III)

36. Horlocker TT. Regional anesthesia and analgesia in the patient receiving thromboprophylaxis. Reg Anesth 1996;21:503–507 (Level III)

37. U.S. Department of Health and Human Services. FDA Public Health Advisory. Subject: Reports of epidural or spinal hematomas with the concurrent use of low molecular weight heparin and spinal/epidural anesthesia or spinal puncture. Rockville, Maryland: Food and Drug Administration, December 1997 (Level III)

38. Friederich PW, Sanson BJ, Simioni P, Zanardi S, Huisman MV, Kindt I, et al. Frequency of pregnancy-related venous thromboembolism in anticoagulant factor-deficient

women: implications for prophylaxis. Ann Intern Med 1996;125:955–960 (Level III)

39. Pabinger I, Schneider B. Thrombotic risk in hereditary antithrombin III, protein C, or protein S deficiency. A cooperative, retrospective study. Gesellschaft fur Thrombose- und Hamostaseforschung (GTH) Study Group on Natural Inhibitors. Arterioscler Thromb Vasc Biol 1996;16:742–748 (Level III)

40. Thomas DP, Roberts HR. Hypercoagulability in venous and arterial thrombosis. Ann Intern Med 1997;126: 638–644 (Level III)

41. Prevention of venous thrombosis and pulmonary embolism. NIH Consensus Development. JAMA 1986; 256:744–749 (Level III)

42. Hutchison GL. Oral contraception and post-operative thromboembolism: an epidemiological review. Scott Med J 1989;34:547–549 (Level III)

43. Robinson GE, Burren T, Mackie IJ, Bounds W, Walshe K, Faint R, et al. Changes in hemostasis after stopping the combined contraceptive pill: implications for major surgery. BMJ 1991;302:269–271 (Level III)

44. Vessey M, Mant D, Smith A, Yeates D. Oral contraceptives and venous thromboembolism: findings in a large prospective study. Br Med J (Clin Res Ed) 1986;292:526 (Level II-2)

45. Daly E, Vessey MP, Hawkins MM, Carson JL, Gough P, Marsh S. Risk of venous thromboembolism in users of hormone replacement therapy. Lancet 1996;348:977–980 (Level II-2)

46. Jick H, Derby LE, Myers MW, Vasilakis C, Newton KM. Risk of hospital admission for idiopathic venous thromboembolism among users of postmenopausal oestrogens. Lancet 1996;348:981–983 (Level II-2)

47. Perez Gutthann S, Garcia Rodríguez LA, Castellsague J, Duque Oliart A. Hormone replacement therapy and risk of venous thromboembolism: population based case-control study. BMJ 1997;314:796–800 (Level II-2)

48. Bokarewa MI, Bremme K, Blombäck M. Arg506-Gln mutation in factor V and risk of thrombosis during pregnancy. Br J Haematol 1996;92:473–478 (Level II-3)

49. Dahlbäck B. Resistance to activated protein C as risk factor for thrombosis: molecular mechanisms, laboratory investigation, and clinical management. Semin Hematol 1997;34:217–234 (Level III)

50. Dizon-Townson DS, Nelson LM, Jang H, Varner MW, Ward K. The incidence of the factor V Leiden mutation in an obstetric population and its relationship to deep vein thrombosis. Am J Obstet Gynecol 1997;176:883–886 (Level III)

51. Faioni EM, Razzari C, Martinelli I, Panzeri D, Franchi F, Mannucci PM. Resistance to activated protein C in unselected patients with arterial and venous thrombosis. Am J Haematol 1997;55:59–64 (Level II-2)

52. Hellgren M, Svensson PJ, Dahlbäck B. Resistance to activated protein C as a basis for venous thromboembolism associated with pregnancy and oral contraceptives. Am J Obstet Gynecol 1995;173:210–213 (Level II-2)

53. Rintelen C, Mannhalter C, Ireland H, Lane DA, Knöbl P, Lechner K, et al. Oral contraceptives enhance the risk of clinical manifestation of venous thrombosis at a young age in females homozygous for factor V Leiden. Br J Haematol 1996;93:487–490 (Level III)

54. Vandenbroucke JP, Koster T, Briët E, Reitsma PH, Bertina RM, Rosendaal FR. Increased risk of venous thrombosis in oral-contraceptive users who are carriers of factor V Leiden mutation. Lancet 1994;344:1453–1457 (Level II-2)

55. Rosendaal FR. Thrombosis in the young: epidemiology and risk factors. A focus on venous thrombosis. Thromb Haemost 1997;78:1–6 (Level III)

56. Barbour LA. Current concepts of anticoagulant therapy in pregnancy. Obstet Gynecol Clin North Am 1997;24: 499–521 (Level III)

57. Dahlman TC. Osteoporotic fractures and the recurrence of thromboembolism during pregnancy and the puerperium in 184 women undergoing thromboprophylaxis with heparin. Am J Obstet Gynecol 1993;168:1265–1270 (Level III)

58. Warkentin TE, Levine MN, Hirsh J, Horsewood P, Roberts RS, Gent M, et al. Heparin-induced thrombocytopenia in patients treated with low-molecular weight heparin or unfractionated heparin. N Engl J Med 1995;332: 1330–1335 (Level II-2)

59. Hirsh J, Warkentin TE, Raschke R, Granger C, Ohman EM, Dalen JE. Heparin and low-molecular-weight heparin: mechanism of action, pharmacokinetics, dosing considerations, monitoring, efficacy and safety. Chest 1998;114 (suppl 5):489S–510S (Level III)

60. Magnani HN. Heparin-induced thrombocytopenia (HIT): an overview of 230 patients treated with Orgaran (Org 10172). Thromb Haemost 1993;70:554–561 (Level II-3)

61. Hynson JM, Katz JA, Bueff HU. Epidural hematoma associated with enoxaparin. Anesth Analg 1996;82:1072–1075 (Level III)

62. Prandoni P, Lensing AW, Cogo A, Cuppini S, Villalta S, Carta M. The long-term clinical course of acute deep venous thrombosis. Ann Intern Med 1996;125:1–7 (Level III)

63. Bergqvist D, Lindgren B, Mätzsch T. Comparison of the cost of preventing postoperative deep vein thrombosis with either unfractionated or low molecular weight heparin. Br J Surg 1996;83:1548–1152 (Level II-2)

64. Bergqvist D, Jendteg S, Johansen L, Persson U, Ödegaard K. Cost of long-term complications of deep venous thrombosis of the lower extremities: an analysis of a defined patient population in Sweden. Ann Intern Med 1997;126:454–457 (Level II-2)

65. Maxwell GL, Myers ER, Clarke-Pearson DL. Cost-effectiveness of deep venous thrombosis prophylaxis in gynecologic oncology surgery. Obstet Gynecol 2000;95:206– 214 (Level III)

The MEDLINE database, the Cochrane Library, and ACOG's own internal resources and documents were used to conduct a literature search to locate relevant articles published between January 1985 and April 2000. The search was restricted to articles published in the English language. Priority was given to articles reporting results of original research, although review articles and commentaries also were consulted. Abstracts of research presented at symposia and scientific conferences were not considered adequate for inclusion in this document. Guidelines published by organizations or institutions such as the National Institutes of Health and the American College of Obstetricians and Gynecologists were reviewed, and additional studies were located by reviewing bibliographies of identified articles. When reliable research was not available, expert opinions from obstetrician–gynecologists were used.

Studies were reviewed and evaluated for quality according to the method outlined by the U.S. Preventive Services Task Force:

- I Evidence obtained from at least one properly designed randomized controlled trial.
- II-1 Evidence obtained from well-designed controlled trials without randomization.
- II-2 Evidence obtained from well-designed cohort or case–control analytic studies, preferably from more than one center or research group.
- II-3 Evidence obtained from multiple time series with or without the intervention. Dramatic results in uncontrolled experiments also could be regarded as this type of evidence.
- III Opinions of respected authorities, based on clinical experience, descriptive studies, or reports of expert committees.

Based on the highest level of evidence found in the data, recommendations are provided and graded according to the following catetories:

Level A—Recommendations are based on good and consistent scientific evidence.

Level B—Recommendations are based on limited or inconsistent scientific evidence.

Level C—Recommendations are based primarily on consensus and expert opinion.

ISSN 1099-3630

The American College of
Obstetricians and Gynecologists
409 12th Street, SW
PO Box 96920
Washington, DC 20090-6920

12345/43210

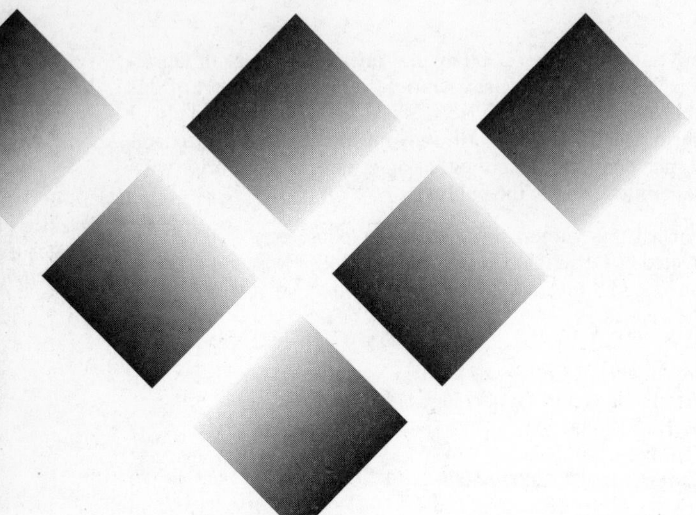

ACOG PRACTICE BULLETIN

CLINICAL MANAGEMENT GUIDELINES FOR OBSTETRICIAN–GYNECOLOGISTS

NUMBER 4, MAY 1999

(Replaces Educational Bulletin Number 147, October 1990)

This Practice Bulletin was developed by the ACOG Committee on Practice Bulletins—Obstetrics with the assistance of Michael L. Socol, MD, and T. Flint Porter, MD, MPH. The information is designed to aid practitioners in making decisions about appropriate obstetric and gynecologic care. These guidelines should not be construed as dictating an exclusive course of treatment or procedure. Variations in practice may be warranted based on the needs of the individual patient, resources, and limitations unique to the institution or type of practice.

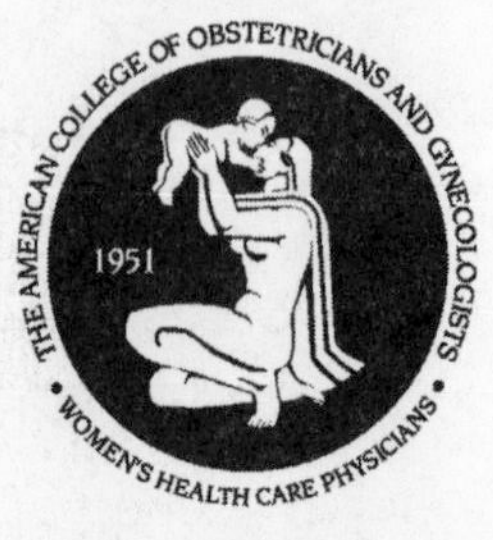

Prevention of Rh D Alloimmunization

Before the introduction of anti-D immune globulin (formerly referred to as Rho[D] immune globulin), hemolytic disease of the fetus and newborn affected 9–10% of pregnancies and was a major cause of perinatal morbidity and mortality (1, 2). Among Rh D-alloimmunized pregnancies, mild-to-moderate hemolytic anemia and hyperbilirubinemia occur in 25–30% of fetuses/neonates, and hydrops fetalis occurs in another 25% of such cases (3). The administration of anti-D immune globulin is successful in reducing the rate of developing antibodies to the D antigen. Protocols for the antenatal and postpartum administration of anti-D immune globulin have been responsible for the dramatic decrease in alloimmunization and subsequent hemolytic disease in the past two decades. However, Rh D alloimmunization remains a clinical concern, with many cases due to failure to follow established protocols. Finally, there is concern that overuse of anti-D immune globulin may lead to a worldwide shortage. The purpose of this document is to provide direction for the appropriate and efficient management of patients at risk in order to further decrease the frequency of Rh D alloimmunization.

Background

Nomenclature

Nomenclature of blood group systems, including the Rh system, may appear confusing to the clinician. According to the *American Medical Association Manual of Style*, erythrocyte antigen and phenotype terminology should use single letters or dual letters depending on the antigen in question (eg, O, AB, Le, Rh) (4). A second designation should be used for specific subtypes (eg, Rh D, Rh C). This publication uses the designation Rh D to signify the erythrocyte antigen.

Women who carry the Rh D antigen are identified as Rh D positive, and those who do not carry the Rh D antigen are identified as Rh D negative. The use of immune globulin to counter the Rh D antigen is referred to as anti-D immune globulin.

Causes of Rh D Alloimmunization

One study indicates that 17% of Rh D-negative women who do not receive anti-D immune globulin prophylaxis during pregnancy will become alloimmunized (5). Nearly 90% of these cases result from fetomaternal hemorrhage at delivery. Approximately 10% of cases result from spontaneous antenatal fetomaternal hemorrhage, and most of these cases occur in the third trimester. The amount of Rh D-positive blood required to cause alloimmunization is small. Most women who become alloimmunized do so as a result of fetomaternal hemorrhage of less than 0.1 mL (6).

Several first- and second-trimester clinical events may cause Rh D alloimmunization. Therapeutic and spontaneous abortions are associated respectively with a 4–5% and a 1.5–2% risk of alloimmunization in susceptible (nonalloimmunized) women (6–8). Ectopic pregnancy also is associated with alloimmunization in susceptible women. Threatened abortion infrequently causes alloimmunization, although approximately 10% of women with threatened abortion have evidence of fetomaternal hemorrhage (9).

Clinical procedures, which may breach the integrity of the choriodecidual space, also may cause Rh D alloimmunization. Chorionic villus sampling is associated with a 14% risk of fetomaternal hemorrhage (10) of more than 0.6 mL (11), and amniocentesis is associated with a 7–15% risk of fetomaternal hemorrhage, even if the placenta is not traversed (5, 12). Likewise, cordocentesis and other percutaneous fetal procedures pose a risk for fetomaternal hemorrhage, although the actual risk of alloimmunization has not been quantified (13, 14). External cephalic version, whether or not it is successful, results in fetomaternal hemorrhage in 2–6% of cases (15, 16).

Anti-D Immune Globulin to Prevent Alloimmunization

The correct administration of anti-D immune globulin dramatically reduces the rate of alloimmunization. Initial studies proved that the postpartum administration of a single dose of anti-D immune globulin to susceptible Rh D-negative women within 72 hours of delivery reduced the alloimmunization rate by 90% (17). It was subsequently recognized that third-trimester antenatal alloimmunization posed a lingering and significant problem; later it was shown that the routine antenatal administration of anti-D immune globulin to Rh D-negative women at 28–29 weeks of gestation reduced the rate of third-trimester alloimmunization from nearly 2% to 0.1% (6). With the effectiveness of anti-D immune globulin clearly demonstrated, authorities recommended its administration to Rh D-negative women who were undergoing clinical events or procedures associated with potential fetomaternal hemorrhage.

In the United States, recommendations for the administration of anti-D immune globulin were introduced in the 1970s. The current antenatal immunoprophylaxis regimen of a single dose of 300 μg at 28 weeks of gestation was based on recommendations from the 1977 McMaster Conference, and is associated with a low failure rate (18). The efficacy of the single antenatal dose of 300 μg at 28 weeks of gestation is comparable to the same dose given at both 28 weeks and 34 weeks of gestation (6). In one study of antenatal prophylaxis, three women who delivered more than 12 weeks after their antenatal dose was administered became alloimmunized. Based on these limited data, some authorities recommend that if delivery has not occurred within 12 weeks of the injection, at 28 weeks of gestation, a second 300 μg dose of anti-D immune globulin should be given (5).

In the United Kingdom, recommendations (19, 20) differ somewhat from those in the United States in that antenatal prophylaxis is given at both 28 weeks and 34 weeks of gestation, and the dose for each antenatal administration, as well as the dose given after delivery, is 100 μg. These recommendations are based on two studies (21, 22) that demonstrated the superiority of a regimen of 100 μg of anti-D immune globulin at 28 weeks and 34 weeks of gestation and postpartum compared with a regimen of only postpartum administration. The British regimen uses less anti-D immune globulin (300 μg versus 600 μg) to achieve similarly low rates of alloimmunization (7, 20), but requires a third injection at 34 weeks of gestation.

Anti-D immune globulin is extracted by cold alcohol fractionation from plasma donated by individuals with high-titer D immune globulin G antibodies. It has been shown experimentally that one prophylactic dose of 300 μg of anti-D immune globulin can prevent Rh D alloimmunization after an exposure to up to 30 mL of Rh D-positive blood or 15 mL of fetal cells (23). For exposure to larger volumes of Rh D-positive blood, more anti-D immune globulin is required. Accordingly, the American Association of Blood Banks and the National Blood Transfusion Service of the United Kingdom recommend that Rh D-negative mothers delivering Rh D-positive infants undergo a test to screen for fetomaternal hemorrhage in excess of the amount covered by the standard dose of anti-D immune globulin. This test will determine if additional anti-D immune globulin is necessary (24, 25). In the past, the American College of Obstetricians and Gynecologists recommended that only women with certain high-risk conditions, such as those experiencing abruptio placenta or manual removal of the placenta, be screened for excess fetomaternal hemorrhage. However, this policy has been shown to miss 50% of cases requiring more than the standard postpartum dose of anti-D immune globulin (26).

The risk of transmission of viral infections (human immunodeficiency virus [HIV] and hepatitis B and hepatitis C viruses) through anti-D immune globulin is minimal to absent (27). All plasma lots used for the production of anti-D immune globulin have been tested for viral infection since 1985. Moreover, the fractionation process used to prepare anti-D immune globulin effectively removes any viral particles that may be present.

Failure to Prevent Rh D Alloimmunization

In spite of recommendations for immunoprophylaxis, 0.1–0.2% of susceptible Rh D-negative women still become alloimmunized (21). There are two primary reasons for the continuing problem.

One reason women become alloimmunized is failure to implement recommended immunoprophylaxis protocols, resulting in preventable Rh D alloimmunizations. Two recent studies from the United Kingdom emphasize the scope of the problem. One study of more than 900 Rh D-negative women reported that only 59% received recommended treatment with anti-D immune globulin after potentially alloimmunizing clinical events (8). Another study showed that 16% of 63 cases of Rh D alloimmunization occurred because of failure to follow recommendations for administration of anti-D immune globulin (28). Preventable Rh D alloimmunization occurs in susceptible Rh D-negative women for the following three reasons:

1. Failure to administer an antenatal dose of anti-D immune globulin at 28–29 weeks of gestation
2. Failure to recognize clinical events that place patients at risk for alloimmunization and failure to administer anti-D immune globulin appropriately
3. Failure to administer or failure to administer timely anti-D immune globulin postnatally to women who have given birth to an Rh D-positive or untyped fetus

The second reason for the continuing problem of Rh D alloimmunization is the small rate (0.1–0.2%) of spontaneous immunization despite the recommended prophylaxis protocol. These cases most often occur in pregnancies during which there have been no prior overt sensitizing events. This problem may become the largest single cause of new Rh D alloimmunization, because alloimmunization from other causes has decreased proportionally (28).

Potential Shortage of Anti-D Immune Globulin

Anti-D immune globulin is collected by apheresis from volunteer donors who have high titers of circulating anti-Rh D antibodies. The donated plasma is pooled and fractionated by commercial manufacturers, and anti-D immune globulin is prepared in varying doses. The number of potential donors may be dwindling worldwide, raising concern about future supplies of anti-D immune globulin (29, 30). Experts in the United Kingdom estimate that supplies of anti-D immune globulin are inadequate for immunoprophylaxis of all susceptible Rh D-negative women, both primigravidas and multiparas, if standard recommendations are followed (19). In Australia, a shortage prompted importation of anti-D immune globulin. Subsequently, some physicians proposed strictly limiting the dose given for first-trimester indications and discontinuing administration of anti-D immune globulin after external cephalic version (unless fetomaternal hemorrhage is documented), ectopic pregnancy, or threatened miscarriage (31). Others disagreed, considering it unethical to withhold anti-D immune globulin in any situation. Estimates regarding future needs compared with potential supply in the United States have not been published; however, limiting doses for first-trimester indications and using lower doses of Rh D immune globulin for antenatal prophylaxis may be necessary.

Cost-Effectiveness of Rh D Prophylaxis Programs

The cost-effectiveness of preventing perinatal mortality and morbidity secondary to Rh D hemolytic disease of the newborn is an important consideration. Economic analysis of anti-D immune globulin prophylaxis is based on the cost of anti-D immune globulin and the number of alloimmunizations that would be prevented. In 1977, the McMaster Conference concluded that routine postnatal prophylaxis was cost-effective but that routine antenatal treatment should be undertaken only if supplies of anti-D immune globulin were adequate and if cases of hemolytic disease of the newborns occurred that might have been prevented by antenatal treatment (7). Some experts concluded that antenatal prophylaxis is effective only in primigravidas (32), and the debate regarding the cost-effectiveness of antenatal prophylaxis of all pregnant women remains unsettled (20, 32–37). The Scottish National Blood Transfusion Service has concluded that the administration of 100 μg of anti-D immune globulin at 28 weeks and 34 weeks of gestation is cost-effective only in primigravidas (38). Others estimate that the most cost-effective antenatal regimen is a single dose of 250 μg of anti-D immune globulin at 28 weeks of gestation (39).

The use of anti-D prophylaxis in the case of certain clinical events is even more controversial. For example, the risk of Rh D alloimmunization from threatened abortion in the first trimester is uncertain, though probably very small. The cost-effectiveness of anti-D immune globulin for threatened abortion, which has never been studied, is questionable (19).

In summary, the cost-effectiveness of antenatal Rh D immune globulin to all Rh D-negative pregnant women and in all circumstances wherein fetomaternal hemorrhage might occur has not been proved. Available data support that third-trimester antenatal prophylaxis is cost-effective in primigravidas. As long as the supply of anti-D immune globulin is adequate and data do not exist to support other recommendations, most experts believe that it is unethical to withhold anti-D immune globulin from any patient at risk of Rh D alloimmunization (19). Recommendations for the use of anti-D immune globulin in this document will be made accordingly.

Clinical Considerations and Recommendations

▶ *Should anti-D immune globulin ever be withheld from a woman undergoing sterilization?*

The use of anti-D immune globulin following postpartum and postabortal sterilization should be guided by the patient's desire for protection against any chance of alloimmunization. Proponents of its use maintain that anti-D immune globulin administration will preserve the future option of transfusing Rh D-positive blood in times of emergency (40). Opponents of this view cite the low probability of sensitization with the previous pregnancy and the improbability of receiving Rh D-incompatible blood (41).

▶ *How should one deal with the issue of paternity?*

If the father is known to be Rh D negative, antenatal prophylaxis is unnecessary. If there is doubt about the father's identity or his blood type, anti-D immune globulin prophylaxis should be given.

▶ *Is it necessary to repeat antibody screening in patients at 28 weeks of gestation prior to the administration of anti-D immune globulin?*

The American Association of Blood Banks recommends that the physician should consider a repeat antibody screen prior to the administration of antenatal anti-D immune globulin if the patient was screened for antibodies prior to 28 weeks of gestation (24). The primary rationale for repeating the antibody screen is to identify women who have become alloimmunized before 28 weeks of gestation in order to manage their pregnancies properly. However, the incidence of Rh D alloimmunization occurring prior to 28 weeks of gestation is reported to be as low as 0.18% (18), and the cost-effectiveness of routinely repeating the antibody test has not been studied. The consequences of antenatal Rh D alloimmunization can be severe, but the decision to obtain a repeat antibody screen should be dictated by individual circumstances and left to the judgment of the physician.

▶ *Is anti-D immune globulin indicated in a sensitized pregnancy?*

If Rh D antibodies are present, anti-D immune globulin is not beneficial, and management should proceed in accordance with protocols for Rh D-alloimmunized pregnancies.

▶ *How should a D^u blood type be interpreted, and what management should be undertaken?*

In the past, a woman whose blood was typed as D^u was thought to have blood cells positive for a variant of the Rh D antigen. Nomenclature and practice have changed in recent years, and currently the D^u designation has been changed to "weak D positive" (24). Patients with this designation are considered Rh D positive and should not receive anti-D immune globulin. In some centers, the D^u antigen is not assessed, and women may unnecessarily receive anti-D immune globulin. In the rare circumstance of delivery by a woman whose antenatal Rh status is negative or unknown and whose postpartum screen reveals a D^u-positive or weak D-positive result, anti-D immune globulin should be given, and the possibility of fetomaternal hemorrhage should be investigated (24).

▶ *Is threatened abortion an indication for anti-D immune globulin prophylaxis?*

Whether to administer anti-D immune globulin to a patient with threatened abortion and a live embryo or fetus at or before 12 weeks of gestation is controversial, and no evidence-based recommendation can be made. The Rh D antigen has been reported on fetal erythrocytes as early as 38 days of gestation (42), and fetomaternal hemorrhage has been documented in women with threatened abortion from 7 to 13 weeks of gestation (9). However, Rh D alloimmunization apparently attributable to threatened abortion is exceedingly rare. Experts have compared the overall benefit with the cost of the widespread use of anti-D immune globulin for a condition as common as threatened abortion (19, 43), and, thus, many physicians do not routinely administer anti-D immune globulin to women with threatened abortion and a live embryo or fetus up to 12 weeks of gestation.

▶ ***How much anti-D immune globulin should be given for first-trimester events and procedures?***

Because the red cell mass of the first-trimester fetus is small, the dose of anti-D immune globulin necessary for first-trimester events is 50 μg to protect against sensitization by 2.5 mL of red blood cells (5, 44). If therapeutic or spontaneous abortion occurs after the first trimester, the standard 300 μg dose is recommended (5).

▶ ***Should anti-D immune globulin be given in cases of molar pregnancy?***

Although reported (45), the risk of Rh D alloimmunization in cases of hydatidiform mole is unknown. In theory, Rh D alloimmunization would not occur in cases of classic complete molar pregnancy because organogenesis does not occur, and Rh D antigens are probably not present on trophoblast cells, although this theory has been disputed (46–48). In partial and transitional molar pregnancies, however, the embryo may not die until after erythrocyte production has begun, making maternal exposure to the Rh D antigen possible (49). Given that the diagnosis of partial versus complete molar pregnancy depends on pathologic and cytogenetic evaluations, it seems reasonable to administer anti-D immune globulin to Rh D-negative women who are suspected of molar pregnancy and who undergo uterine evacuation.

▶ ***Should anti-D immune globulin be given in cases of intrauterine fetal death occurring in the second or third trimester?***

Fetal death is due to fetomaternal hemorrhage in 11–13% of cases in which no obvious other cause (eg, maternal hypertensive disease, fetal anomalies) is found (50, 51). Rh D alloimmunization has been reported in cases of fetal death from massive fetomaternal hemorrhage (52), although the influence of this cause on the overall problem of Rh D alloimmunization is unknown. The efficacy of anti-D immune globulin in this clinical situation has not been tested in properly designed trials. However, authorities agree that anti-D immune globulin should be administered to Rh D-negative women who experience fetal death in the second or third trimester. All such cases should be screened for excessive fetomaternal hemorrhage to determine if additional anti-D immune globulin is required (25, 53).

▶ ***Is second- or third-trimester antenatal hemorrhage an indication for anti-D immune globulin prophylaxis?***

In patients with second- or third-trimester antenatal hemorrhage, the risk of Rh D alloimmunization is uncertain. Although the efficacy of anti-D immune globulin in this clinical situation has not been tested in properly designed trials, authorities agree that anti-D immune globulin should be administered to Rh D-negative women with second- or third-trimester hemorrhage (25, 53). Man-agement of the patient with persistent or intermittent antenatal bleeding is complex. Though unproven, one commonly used strategy is to monitor the Rh D-negative patient with continuing antenatal hemorrhage with serial indirect Coombs testing approximately every 3 weeks. If the result is positive, indicating the persistence of anti-D immune globulin, no additional treatment is necessary. If the Coombs test is negative, excessive fetomaternal hemorrhage may have occurred, and a Kleihauer-Betke test should be performed in order to determine the amount of additional anti-D immune globulin necessary.

▶ ***Is anti-D immune globulin prophylaxis indicated after abdominal trauma in susceptible pregnant women?***

Although the exact risk of Rh D alloimmunization is unknown, abdominal trauma may be associated with fetomaternal hemorrhage, which may lead to alloimmunization (54–57). The efficacy of anti-D immune globulin in this clinical situation has not been tested in properly designed trials. However, authorities agree that anti-D immune globulin should be administered to Rh D-negative women who have experienced abdominal trauma (25, 53). Also, all of these patients should be screened for excessive fetomaternal hemorrhage.

▶ ***What should be done if an Rh D-negative patient is discharged without receiving anti-D immune globulin after a potentially sensitizing event?***

Volunteers have been shown to receive partial protection if anti-D immune globulin was given as late as 13 days after exposure (58). The longer prophylaxis is delayed the less likely it is that the patient will be protected, but it has been recommended that a patient may still receive some benefit from anti-D immune globulin as late as 28 days postpartum (5).

▶ ***How long does the effect of anti-D immune globulin last?***

The half-life of anti-D immune globulin is 24 days, although titers decrease over time. If delivery occurs within 3 weeks of the standard antenatal anti-D immune globulin administration, the postnatal dose may be withheld in the absence of excessive fetomaternal hemorrhage (53). The same is true when anti-D immune globulin is given for antenatal procedures, such as external cephalic version or amniocentesis, or for third-trimester bleeding. An excessive amount of fetal erythrocytes not covered by anti-D immune globulin administration can be assumed to have entered maternal blood if either the results of the Kleihauer-Betke test are positive or the results of the indirect Coombs test are negative.

▶ ***Should administration of anti-D immune globulin be repeated in patients with a postdate pregnancy?***

One study found that three patients became alloimmunized to the Rh D antigen when delivery occurred more than 12 weeks after the standard prophylaxis at 28 weeks of gestation (5). Based on these limited data, some experts have recommended that if delivery has not occurred within 12 weeks after injection at 28 weeks of gestation, a second antenatal dose should be given (5). Because this recommendation is based on so few cases, the final decision whether to administer a second dose should be left to the physician's judgment.

▶ ***Should all Rh D-negative women be screened for excessive fetomaternal hemorrhage after delivery of an Rh D-positive infant?***

The risk of excessive fetomaternal hemorrhage exceeding 30 mL (the amount covered by the standard 300 μg dose of anti-D immune globulin) at the time of delivery is approximately 1 in 1,250 (5). Previous American College of Obstetricians and Gynecologists documents have recommended that only pregnancies designated as high risk be screened for excessive fetomaternal hemorrhage, including cases of abdominal trauma, abruptio placentae, placenta previa, intrauterine manipulation, multiple gestation, or manual removal of the placenta. However, such a screening program has been reported to detect only 50% of patients who required additional anti-D immune globulin (26). Based on this finding, the American Association of Blood Banks has recommended that all Rh D-negative women who deliver Rh D-positive infants be screened using the Kleihauer-Betke or rosette test (24).

Summary

The reduction in the incidence of Rh D alloimmunization is a prototype for the effectiveness of preventive medicine. Some controversies remain, however, such as the use of anti-D immune globulin in patients with either threatened abortion or antenatal hemorrhage. Similarly, it may not be cost-effective either to screen all Rh D-negative patients with an indirect Coombs test at 24–28 weeks of gestation or to screen all postpartum patients for excessive fetomaternal hemorrhage.

The following recommendations are based on good and consistent scientific evidence (Level A):

The Rh D-negative woman who is not Rh D-alloimmunized should receive anti-D immune globulin:

- ▶ At approximately 28 weeks of gestation, unless the father of the baby is also known to be Rh D negative
- ▶ Within 72 hours after the delivery of an Rh D-positive infant
- ▶ After a first-trimester pregnancy loss
- ▶ After invasive procedures, such as chorionic villus sampling, amniocentesis, or fetal blood sampling

The following recommendations are based primarily on consensus and expert opinion (Level C):

Anti-D immune globulin prophylaxis should be considered if the patient has experienced:

- ▶ Threatened abortion
- ▶ Second- or third-trimester antenatal bleeding
- ▶ External cephalic version
- ▶ Abdominal trauma

References

1. Mollison PL, Engelfreit CP, Contreras M. Haemolytic disease of the newborn in blood. In: Transfusion in clinical medicine. 8th ed. Oxford: Blackwell Scientific Publications, 1987:637–687 (Level III)
2. Huchcroft S, Gunton P, Bowen T. Compliance with postpartum Rh isoimmunization prophylaxis in Alberta. Can Med Assoc J 1985;133:871–875 (Level II-3)
3. Tannirandorn Y, Rodeck CH. New approaches in the treatment of haemolytic disease of the fetus. Baillieres Clin Haematol 1990;3:289–320 (Level III)
4. Iverson C, Flanagin A, Fontanarosa PB, Glass RM, Glitman P, Lantz JC, et al. American Medical Association manual of style. 9th ed. Baltimore: Williams and Wilkins, 1998 (Level III)
5. Bowman JM. Controversies in Rh prophylaxis. Who needs Rh immune globulin and when should it be given? Am J Obstet Gynecol 1985;151:289–294 (Level III)
6. Bowman JM. The prevention of Rh immunization. Transfus Med Rev 1988;2:129–150 (Level III)
7. McMaster conference on prevention of Rh immunization. 28–30 September, 1977. Vox Sang 1979;36:50–64 (Level III)
8. Howard HL, Martlew VJ, McFadyen IR, Clarke CA. Preventing Rhesus D haemolytic disease of the newborn by giving anti-D immunoglobulin: are the guidelines being adequately followed? Br J Obstet Gynaecol 1997;104: 37–41 (Level II-3)
9. Von Stein GA, Munsick RA, Stiver K, Ryder K. Fetomaternal hemorrhage in threatened abortion. Obstet Gynecol 1992;79:383–386 (Level II-2)
10. Brambati B, Guercilena S, Bonnachi I, Oldrini A, Lanzani A, Piceni L. Feto-maternal transfusion after chorionic villus sampling: clinical implications. Hum Reprod 1986;1:37–40 (Level II-3)
11. Blakemore KJ, Baumgarten A, Schoenfeld-Dimaio M, Hobbins JC, Mason EA, Mahoney MJ. Rise in maternal

serum alpha-fetoprotein concentration after chorionic villus sampling and the possibility of isoimmunization. Am J Obstet Gynecol 1986;155:988–993 (Level III)

12. Blajchman MA, Maudsley RF, Uchida I, Zipursky A. Letter: Diagnostic amniocentesis and fetal-maternal bleeding. Lancet 1974;1:993–994 (Level III)

13. Daffos F, Capella-Pavlovsky M, Forestier F. Fetal blood sampling during pregnancy with use of a needle guided by ultrasound: a study of 606 consecutive cases. Am J Obstet Gynecol 1985;153:655–660 (Level II-3)

14. Pielet BW, Socol ML, MacGregor SN, Ney JA, Dooley SL. Cordocentesis: an appraisal of risks. Am J Obstet Gynecol 1988;159:1497–1500 (Level III)

15. Lau TK, Stock A, Rogers M. Fetomaternal hemorrhage after external cephalic version at term. Aust N Z J Obstet Gynaecol 1995;35:173–174 (Level II-3)

16. Marcus RG, Crewe-Brown H, Krawitz S, Katz J. Fetomaternal haemorrhage following successful and unsuccessful attempts at external cephalic version. Br J Obstet Gynaecol 1975;82:578–580 (Level III)

17. Freda VJ, Gorman JG, Pollack W, Bowe E. Prevention of Rh hemolytic disease—ten years' clinical experience with Rh immune globulin. N Engl J Med 1975;292:1014–1016 (Level III)

18. Bowman JM, Chown B, Lewis M, Pollock JM. Rh isoimmunization during pregnancy: antenatal prophylaxis. Can Med Assoc J 1978;118:623–627 (Level III)

19. Robson SC, Lee D, Urbaniak S. Anti-D immunoglobulin in RhD prophylaxis. Br J Obstet Gynaecol 1998;105:129–134 (Level III)

20. Statement from the consensus conference on anti-D prophylaxis. 7 and 8 April 1997. The Royal College of Physicians of Edinburgh. The Royal College of Obstetricians and Gynaecologists, UK. Vox Sang 1998;74:127–128 (Level III)

21. Tovey LA, Townley A, Stevenson BJ, Taverner J. The Yorkshire antenatal anti-D immunoglobulin trial in primigravidae. Lancet 1983;2:244–246 (Level II-2)

22. Huchet J, Dallemagne S, Huchet C, Brossard Y, Larsen M, Parnet-Mathieu F. Antepartum administration of preventive treatment of Rh-D immunization in rhesus-negative women. Parallel evaluation of transplacental passage of fetal blood cells. Results of a multicenter study carried out in the Paris region. J Gynecol Obstet Biol Reprod (Paris) 1987;16:101–111 (Level II-2)

23. Pollack W, Ascari WQ, Kochesky RJ, O'Connor RR, Ho TY, Tripodi D. Studies on Rh prophylaxis. 1. Relationship between doses of anti-Rh and size of antigenic stimulus. Transfusion 1971;11:333–339 (Level II-1)

24. Snyder EL. Prevention of hemolytic disease of the newborn due to anti-D. Prenatal/perinatal testing and Rh immune globulin administration. American Association of Blood Banks Association Bulletin 1998;98(2):1–6 (Level III)

25. National Blood Transfusion Service Immunoglobulin Working Party. Recommendations for the use of anti-D immunoglobulin. 1991;137–145 (Level III)

26. Ness PM, Baldwin ML, Niebyl JR. Clinical high-risk designation does not predict excess fetal-maternal hemorrhage. Am J Obstet Gynecol 1987;156:154–158 (Level II-3)

27. Centers for Disease Control and Prevention. Lack of transmission of human immunodeficiency virus through Rho (D) immune globulin (human). MMWR 1987;36:728–729 (Level II-3)

28. Hughes RG, Craig JI, Murphy WG, Greer IA. Causes and clinical consequences of Rhesus (D) haemolytic disease of the newborn: a study of a Scottish population, 1985–1990. Br J Obstet Gynaecol 1994;101:297–300 (Level III)

29. Beveridge HE. Dwindling supplies of anti-D. Med J Aust 1997;167:509–510 (Level III)

30. Nelson M, Popp HJ, Kronenberg H. Dwindling supplies of anti-D. Med J Aust 1998;168:311 (Level III)

31. de Crespigny L, Davison G. Anti-D administration in early pregnancy—time for a new protocol. Aust N Z J Obstet Gynaecol 1995;35:385–387 (Level III)

32. Tovey LA, Taverner JM. A case for the antenatal administration of anti-D immunoglobulin to primigravidae. Lancet 1981;1:878–881 (Level III)

33. Clarke C, Whitfield AG. Rhesus immunization during pregnancy: the cause for antenatal anti-D. BMJ 1980;280:903–904 (Level III)

34. Tovey GH. Should anti-D immunoglobulin be given antenatally? Lancet 1980;2:466–468 (Level II-3)

35. Bowman JM, Friesen AD, Pollack JM, Taylor WE. WinRho: Rh immune globulin prepared by ion exchange for intravenous use. Can Med Assoc J 1980;123:1121–1127 (Level II-3)

36. Bowman JM, Pollock JM. Failures of intravenous Rh immune globulin prophylaxis: an analysis of the reasons for such failures. Transfus Med Rev 1987;1:101–112 (Level III)

37. Torrance GW, Zipursky A. Cost-effectiveness of antepartum prevention of Rh immunization. Clin Perinatol 1984;11:267–281 (Level III)

38. Cairns JA. Economics of antenatal prophylaxis. Br J Obstet Gynaecol 1998;105(suppl 18):19–22 (Level III)

39. Vick S, Cairns J, Urbaniak S, Whitfield C, Raafat A. Cost-effectiveness of antenatal anti-D prophylaxis. Health Econ 1996;5:319–328 (Cost-effectiveness analysis)

40. Gorman JG, Freda VJ. Rh immune globulin is indicated for Rh-negative mothers undergoing sterilization. Am J Obstet Gynecol 1972;112:868–869 (Level III)

41. Scott JR, Guy LR. Is Rh immunoglobulin indicated in patients having puerperal sterilization? Obstet Gynecol 1975;46:178–180 (Level II-3)

42. Bergstrom H, Nillson L, Ryttinger L. Demonstration of Rh antigens in a 38-day old fetus. Am J Obstet Gynecol 1967;1:130–133 (Level III)

43. Haines P. An overview from a panel member. Br J Obstet Gynaecol 1998;105(suppl 18):5–6 (Level III)

44. Stewart FH, Burnhill MS, Bozorgi N. Reduced dose of Rh immunoglobulin following first trimester pregnancy termination. Obstet Gynecol 1978;51:318–322 (Level II-1)

45. Price JR. RH sensitization by hydatiform mole. N Engl J Med 1968;278:1021 (Level III)

46. Fischer HE, Lichtiger B, Cox I. Expression of Rh0(D) antigen in choriocarcinoma of the uterus in an Rh0(D)-negative patient: report of a case. Hum Pathol 1985;16: 1165–1167 (Level III)

47. van't Veer MB, Overbeeke MA, Geertzen HG, van der Lans SM. The expression of Rh-D factor in human trophoblast. Am J Obstet Gynecol 1984;150:1008–1010 (Level III)

48. Goto S, Nishi H, Tomoda Y. Blood group Rh-D factor in human trophoblast determined by immunofluorescent method. Am J Obstet Gynecol 1980;137:707–712 (Level III)

49. Morrow CP, Curtin JP. Tumors of the placental trophoblast. In: Synopsis of gynecologic oncology. 5th ed. New York: Churchill Livingstone, 1998:315–351 (Level III)

50. Laube DW, Schauberger CW. Fetomaternal bleeding as a cause for "unexplained" fetal death. Obstet Gynecol 1982;60:649–651 (Level III)

51. Owen J, Stedman CM, Tucker TL. Comparison of predelivery versus postdelivery Kleihauer-Betke stains in cases of fetal death. Am J Obstet Gynecol 1989;161:663–666 (Level III)

52. Stedman CM, Quinlan RW, Huddleston JF, Cruz AC, Kellner KR. Rh sensitization after third-trimester fetal death. Obstet Gynecol 1988;71:461–463 (Level III)

53. American Association of Blood Banks. Technical Manual. 12th ed. Bethesda, Maryland: American Association of Blood Banks, 1996 (Level III)

54. Rose PG, Strohm PL, Zuspan FP. Fetomaternal hemorrhage following trauma. Am J Obstet Gynecol 1985;153:844–847 (Level II-2)

55. Chhibber G, Zacher M, Cohen AW, Kline AJ. Rh isoimmunization following abdominal trauma: a case report. Am J Obstet Gynecol 1984;149:692 (Level III)

56. Kettel LM, Branch DW, Scott JR. Occult placental abruption after maternal trauma. Obstet Gynecol 1988;71: 449–453 (Level III)

57. Dahmus MA, Sibai BM. Blunt abdominal trauma: are there any predictive factors for abruptio placentae or maternal-fetal distress? Am J Obstet Gynecol 1993; 169:1054–1059 (Level III)

58. Samson D, Mollison PL. Effect on primary Rh immunization of delayed administration of anti-Rh. Immunology 1975;28:349–357 (Level II-1)

The MEDLINE database, the Cochrane Library, and ACOG's own internal resources and documents were used to conduct a literature search to locate relevant articles published between January 1980 and December 1998. The search was restricted to articles published in the English language. Priority was given to articles reporting results of original research, although review articles and commentaries also were consulted. Abstracts of research presented at symposia and scientific conferences were not considered adequate for inclusion in this document. Guidelines published by organizations or institutions such as the National Institutes of Health and the American College of Obstetricians and Gynecologists were reviewed, and additional studies were located by reviewing bibliographies of identified articles. When reliable research was not available, expert opinions from obstetrician–gynecologists were used.

Studies were reviewed and evaluated for quality according to the method outlined by the U.S. Preventive Services Task Force:

- I Evidence obtained from at least one properly designed randomized controlled trial.
- II-1 Evidence obtained from well-designed controlled trials without randomization.
- II-2 Evidence obtained from well-designed cohort or case–control analytic studies, preferably from more than one center or research group.
- II-3 Evidence obtained from multiple time series with or without the intervention. Dramatic results in uncontrolled experiments could also be regarded as this type of evidence.
- III Opinions of respected authorities, based on clinical experience, descriptive studies, or reports of expert committees.

Based on the highest level of evidence found in the data, recommendations are provided and graded according to the following catetories:

Level A—Recommendations are based on good and consistent scientific evidence.

Level B—Recommendations are based on limited or inconsistent scientific evidence.

Level C—Recommendations are based primarily on consensus and expert opinion.

ISSN 1099-3630 12345/32109

The American College of Obstetricians and Gynecologists
409 12th Street, SW
PO Box 96920
Washington, DC 20090-6920

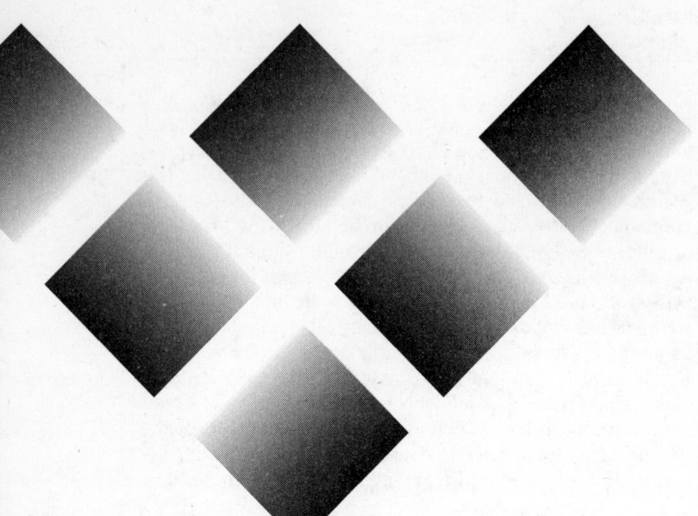

ACOG PRACTICE BULLETIN

CLINICAL MANAGEMENT GUIDELINES FOR OBSTETRICIAN–GYNECOLOGISTS
NUMBER 7, SEPTEMBER 1999
(Replaces Technical Bulletin Number 111, December 1987)

This Practice Bulletin was developed by the ACOG Committee on Practice Bulletins—Gynecology with the assistance of Douglas W. Laube, MD. The information is designed to aid practitioners in making decisions about appropriate obstetric and gynecologic care. These guidelines should not be construed as an exclusive course of treatment or procedure. Variations in practice may be warranted based on the needs of the individual patient, resources, and limitations unique to the institution or type of practice.

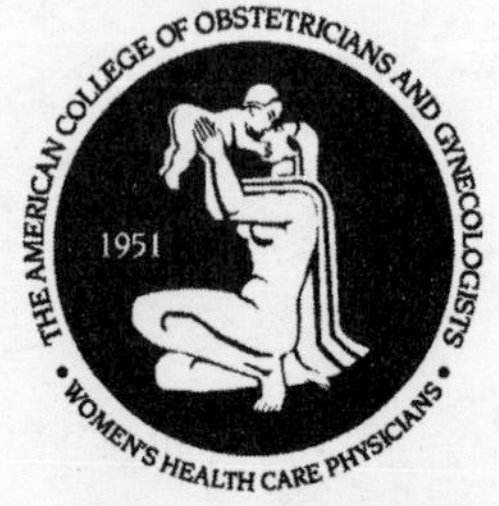

Prophylactic Oophorectomy

In the United States, approximately 600,000 hysterectomies are performed each year, one half of which involve oophorectomy (1). Historically, the putative benefits of prophylactic oophorectomy have included the alleviation of symptoms related to retained ovaries and the prevention of cancer. These benefits are countered by arguments favoring the retention of ovaries, which allows continued hormone production in both premenopausal and postmenopausal women. This document will weigh the risks and benefits of prophylactic oophorectomy and provide a framework for the evaluation and counseling of patients who would be candidates for this procedure.

Background

Prophylactic oophorectomy is the removal of the ovaries for the potential benefit of preventing long-term morbidity and mortality. The term *prophylactic* implies that the ovaries are normal at the time of removal. Oophorectomy can be performed either alone as a planned surgical procedure or in conjunction with other planned surgical procedures such as hysterectomy or colectomy. *Incidental oophorectomy* is a term commonly used when the ovaries are removed at the time of another indicated surgery, and this term should not be used interchangeably with *prophylactic oophorectomy*. The term *incidental* implies that the surgery occurs by chance or without consequence. There are obvious consequences associated with oophorectomy; therefore, when oophorectomy is performed for future benefit, the surgery should be termed *prophylactic*.

Ovarian Physiology

The ovary is a complex metabolic organ consisting of follicular and stromal compartments. Follicles produce both androgens and estrogen, and stromal tissue synthesizes androgens. With the loss of all follicles around menopause, both androgen and estrogen levels decrease, but the ovary remains a source of androgens that are peripherally converted to estrogen. The role of endogenous androgens and the consequences of their removal may be significant but have not yet been clarified.

The positive effects of estrogen production on lipid metabolism and bone remodeling remain the primary argument for retention of the ovaries in premenopausal women. The benefits of estrogen are well documented (2–4), but any benefits of ovarian androgen production remain to be documented.

Cancer Prevention

In the United States, one in 70 women will develop ovarian cancer in her lifetime. Between 4% and 14% of these women will have had antecedent hysterectomies in which the ovaries were retained (5). Current screening techniques for ovarian cancer, including the use of ultrasonography and tumor markers, are neither sensitive nor specific enough to detect early cancer as part of a screening program for the general population. A high proportion of ovarian cancer is detected when it is in advanced stages. Prevention of ovarian cancer is the primary reason for prophylactic oophorectomy. Although oophorectomy does not eliminate the risk of cancer (patients still can develop peritoneal carcinoma, which acts like ovarian cancer), reported cases are rare (6).

The literature has recorded elective oophorectomy rates of between 50% and 66% in women 40–64 years of age undergoing hysterectomy (7, 8). Data from the Centers for Disease Control and Prevention collected between 1988 and 1993 concur that ovarian retention occurs in approximately 40–50% of patients undergoing hysterectomy at 40 years of age or older (1). It has been suggested that, in the United States, approximately 1,000 cases of ovarian cancer can be prevented if prophylactic oophorectomy is practiced in all women older than 40 years of age who undergo hysterectomy. This assumes an annual incidence of 24,000 new ovarian cancer cases and does not take into account the incidence of peritoneal carcinoma. The dilemma for the patient and the clinician is whether the estimated number of cancer cases prevented (1,000) is worth the number of oophorectomies performed (approximately 300,000) (9). The benefit of prophylactic oophorectomy may be offset by the consequence of estrogen loss early in life.

Factors to Consider for Prophylactic Oophorectomy

The potential risks and benefits of this procedure need to be considered within the context of the potential risks and benefits of extended hormone production or prescribed hormone replacement. The potential for alleviation of symptoms related to ovarian function should be considered, especially in patients with documented premenstrual syndrome. New developments in genetic testing, early diagnosis, refinements in diagnostic imaging, knowledge of hormone interactions with the cardiovascular and central nervous systems, and refined surgical techniques must all be considered with the individual patient.

Risk Factors for Ovarian Cancer

There is no consensus regarding the benefits of oophorectomy performed at the time of hysterectomy. Patients at greater risk for developing ovarian cancer are those with low parity, decreased fertility, and delayed childbearing if they did not use oral contraceptives (6, 10–12).

Women who have used oral contraceptives have a lower risk for invasive epithelial ovarian cancer than nonusers do. Both hospital and population studies revealed that, among those who have used oral contraceptives, the risk continues to decrease as years of use increase, although there is little additional protection conferred by oral contraceptives beyond 6 years of use. The protective benefits of higher parity, as well as longer duration of breastfeeding, also have been reported. Use of fertility drugs may be associated with a higher risk of ovarian cancer, as is a history of longer premenopausal sexual activity without contraception. There are no consistent data linking age at menarche, age at menopause, or duration of estrogen replacement therapy with development of epithelial ovarian cancer (10).

Operative Risk at the Time of Hysterectomy

There are no studies evaluating increased operative risk or morbidity at the time of abdominal hysterectomy when prophylactic oophorectomy is included. Retrospective studies looking at prophylactic oophorectomy at the time of vaginal hysterectomy have shown that the ovaries can be removed successfully in 65–97% of patients (13, 14). One study found no significant increase in operating time, estimated blood loss, length of hospital stay, or postoperative morbidity between patients who had their ovaries removed and those who did not (13). Another study found that oophorectomy added 23.4 minutes to the total operating time compared with vaginal hysterectomy alone (14).

Genetic Factors

The emergence of data suggesting the close link of ovarian cancer with familial breast–ovarian cancer syndromes has contributed to arguments favoring oophorectomy in subsets of patients identified with genetic risk factors.

The role of *BRCA1* mutations in ovarian cancer indicates that these tumors have unique biologic clinical and pathologic features (15). Recent evidence identifies the significant contribution of *BRCA1* mutations to the development of ovarian cancer, revealing that this mutation occurs in approximately 5% of women in whom cancer is diagnosed before 70 years of age (16). Although screening for *BRCA1* mutations has been suggested, it is difficult to define those women at risk based only on the number of family members affected. Because of the relatively small number (5%) of all ovarian cancers related to inherited mutations in the *BRCA1* gene, the optimal strategy for decreasing cancer mortality in these patients has yet to be determined.

BRCA2 mutations increase the risk of ovarian cancer but to a lesser degree than *BRCA1* mutations (17). The risk of ovarian cancer in families with Lynch syndrome II is reported to be 3.5 times higher than expected, with the estimated cumulative risk by 70 years of age still less than 10% (18). The mean age at diagnosis for ovarian cancer in women with Lynch syndrome II is approximately 45 years of age, roughly 20 years earlier than in the general population (19).

Patient Factors to Consider in Prophylactic Oophorectomy

Age
Parity
Previous abdominal surgery
Risk of ovarian cancer
Menopausal status
Family and personal history
Desire and willingness to use hormone replacement therapy
Risk for osteoporosis
Risk for coronary heart disease
Effect on self-image

Clinical Considerations and Recommendations

▶ *Who are candidates for prophylactic oophorectomy?*

In determining candidates who would benefit from prophylactic oophorectomy, the advantages and disadvantages of prophylactic oophorectomy need to be evaluated (11, 20). The decision to perform prophylactic oophorectomy should be based not only on the patient's age but also on other factors that weigh individual risk for developing ovarian cancer against loss of ovarian function (see the box).

▶ *With ovary retention, what is the risk of needing a future oophorectomy for benign disease?*

The retention of ovaries following prior hysterectomy has been reported to contribute to reoperation in up to 5% of patients (21, 22), with pain in the retained ovary or ovaries the most commonly cited reason. In a retrospective study of more than 1,200 women who had at least one ovary retained after undergoing hysterectomy for benign indications, there was an approximate 4% reoperation rate (23). The author noted that the risk of having pathology in retained ovaries after hysterectomy was significantly higher in women who had only one ovary retained, compared with those who had both ovaries retained. In addition, the mean age at the time of hysterectomy was significantly lower in women who developed ovarian disorders following hysterectomy than in those who did not develop subsequent ovarian disorders. These findings suggest that the removal of one ovary at the time of hysterectomy in premenopausal women indicates the suspicion of clinical disease. The likelihood of future pathology in the retained ovary is therefore greater. Also, the younger the woman is at the time of hysterectomy, the more years there are for her to develop nonmalignant ovarian disorders that will require oophorectomy. In another study that followed a group of 84 premenopausal women undergoing radical hysterectomy, 27% experienced early loss of hormonal function or required subsequent oophorectomy (24).

▶ *Is prophylactic oophorectomy associated with increased morbidity?*

The morbidity associated with prophylactic oophorectomy is primarily related to the loss of estrogen. It is unclear whether exogenous estrogen fully compensates for the lost function of the ovaries, but it appears that estrogen replacement therapy is adequate compensation. However, there may be underlying advantages of ovarian function that have not yet been identified, particularly postmenopausal androgen production. Also, patients who do not take hormone replacement therapy will experience symptoms of early menopause, such as vasomotor hot flashes and vaginal atrophy (25), and are at a higher risk for osteoporosis (3, 26).

▶ *Should hormone replacement therapy be recommended for women undergoing prophylactic oophorectomy?*

Hormone replacement therapy should be recommended for women undergoing prophylactic oophorectomy just as it is for women undergoing natural menopause. The benefit of estrogen replacement therapy appears to be the same in natural or surgical menopause (3, 27), and the same risks and benefits should be discussed with the patient. If the patient is premenopausal, her need for estrogen replacement may be even greater because of her age and potential life span.

The favorable effects of estrogen replacement on bone metabolism have been well documented since the first reports of randomized trials. Additionally, in an evaluation of 27 premenopausal women undergoing oophorectomy, levels of lipoprotein A and cholesterol, along with other hemostatic factors, were found to be lower or not statistically different from preoperative levels, when estrogen replacement therapy was given (28). These observations are consistent with the beneficial effects of estrogen on cardiovascular hemodynamics and cardiovascular disease.

Despite the potentially favorable effects of estrogen replacement and the development of a number of promising synthetic hormone replacement medications, current estrogen replacement usage rates in postmenopausal women are low, and compliance with hormone replacement therapy is poor (29). Therefore, an unwillingness to accept hormone replacement therapy represents a potentially serious health problem, making the decision for elective oophorectomy more difficult.

▶ *What is the risk–benefit relationship associated with oophorectomy?*

The risk–benefit relationship for an individual woman is difficult to calculate. Compliance with estrogen replacement therapy and the risks of coronary artery disease and osteoporosis versus the risk of reoperation or ovarian cancer must be considered. Speroff and colleagues used Markov cohort modeling to evaluate prophylactic oophorectomy considering the influence of estrogen on coronary heart disease, breast cancer, and osteoporotic fractures (30). When compliance with estrogen replacement therapy was perfect, oophorectomy yielded longer life expectancy. When actual drug-taking behavior is considered, retaining the ovaries resulted in longer survival. While only a theoretical model, this analysis emphasizes the need to consider patient compliance with estrogen replacement therapy in decision making.

▶ *When is prophylactic oophorectomy indicated as adjunctive treatment for premenopausal women with breast cancer?*

Prophylactic oophorectomy as adjunctive treatment in the management of premenopausal breast cancer has been practiced for more than 40 years. The efficacy of this procedure has been assumed as part of an accepted endocrine management strategy for breast cancer. Today, with the use of multiagent chemotherapy, tamoxifen, and GnRH agonists, the role for oophorectomy is unclear. Large, prospective trials are currently underway to evaluate the efficacy of oophorectomy for node-positive, estrogen-sensitive breast tumors in premenopausal women.

▶ *Are there genetic risks that should be considered in the decision to perform prophylactic oophorectomy?*

Women with *BRCA1* have a 45% lifetime risk of ovarian cancer, and *BRCA2* conveys a 25% risk (12). Although large-scale prospective data are lacking, most clinicians agree that prophylactic oophorectomy in select women at high risk of inherited ovarian cancer *(BRCA1 and BRCA2)* should be considered (11, 31, 32). Multicenter studies are currently ongoing to assess the assumed benefit of prophylactic oophorectomy in this subset of patients. Because the average age of ovarian cancer in women with these genetic mutations is mid 40s, prophylactic oophorectomy should be performed at completion of childbearing or at 35 years of age.

Contemporary recommendations for women with Lynch syndrome II include at least an annual physical examination with bimanual rectovaginal examination, determinations of CA 125 levels, and transvaginal ultrasonography, with consideration of laparoscopic prophylactic bilateral oophorectomy upon completion of childbirth or by 35 years of age (11). The role of oophorectomy at the time of surgery for primary nonhereditary (sporadic) colorectal cancer is not clear. Some contemporary literature suggests that removing ovaries in this group of women decreases the likelihood of metastatic disease to the ovary (18). Prior to surgical intervention, a familial syndrome should be established by a full pedigree analysis, and the patient should be counseled as to the ethical and medical implications of this testing.

▶ *Are there other considerations in assessing the risks and benefits of prophylactic oophorectomy?*

The decision to perform prophylactic oophorectomy should be individual to the patient. Ovarian retention or removal in some patients may have a distinct bearing on their self-image. In addition to the ovarian contribution to the hormonal milieu, questions regarding the patient's self-image, reproductive function, and sexuality should be considered. Intact reproductive organs may be linked to self-perception of sexuality. Body image also may be related to the occurrence of posthysterectomy depression, although other factors, including preoperative depression, prior psychiatric disturbances, age younger than 35 years, nulliparity, and fewer than 12 years of formal education, also may serve as risk factors (33).

Summary

The following recommendations are based primarily on consensus and expert opinion (Level C):

- The decision to perform prophylactic oophorectomy should not be based only on age; it should be a highly individualized decision that takes into account several patient factors and choices.
- Removal of one ovary at the time of hysterectomy in premenopausal women may indicate the suspicion of clinical disease. The likelihood of future pathology in the retained ovary is therefore greater. The patient should be counseled before surgery that if ovarian pathology is found, bilateral oophorectomy may be indicated.
- Hormone replacement therapy should be considered for women undergoing prophylactic oophorectomy, and patients should be counseled about the risks and benefits of hormone replacement therapy prior to undergoing surgery.
- Compliance with hormone replacement therapy is important in women undergoing prophylactic oophorectomy to reduce the risk of future morbidity.
- Prophylactic oophorectomy should be considered for select women at high risk of inherited ovarian cancer.
- In addition to health risks and benefits, patient counseling should include consideration of how oophorectomy may relate to the individual patient's body image, perceptions concerning sexuality, and personal feelings.

References

1. Lepine LA, Hillis SD, Marchbanks PA, Koonin LM, Morrow B, Kieke BA, et al. Hysterectomy surveillance—United States 1980–1993. MMWR Morb Mortal Wkly Rep 1997;46:1–15 (Level II-3)
2. Bush TL, Barrett-Connor E, Cowan LD, Criqui MH, Wallace RB, Suchindran CM, et al. Cardiovascular mortality and noncontraceptive use of estrogen in women: results from the Lipid Research Clinics Program Follow-up Study. Circulation 1987;75;1102–1109 (Level II-2)
3. Ettinger B, Genant HK, Cann CE. Postmenopausal bone loss is prevented by treatment with low-dosage estrogen with calcium. Ann Intern Med 1987;106:40–45 (Level II-1)
4. Effects of estrogen or estrogen/progestin regimens on heart disease risk factors in postmenopausal women: The Postmenopausal Estrogen/Progestin Interventions (PEPI) Trial. The Writing Group of the PEPI Trial. JAMA 1995;273:199–208 (Level I)
5. Sightler SE, Boike GM, Estape RE, Averette HE. Ovarian cancer in women with prior hysterectomy: a 14-year experience at the University of Miami. Obstet Gynecol 1991;78:681–684 (Level II-3)
6. Piver MS, Jishi MF, Tsukada Y, Nava G. Primary peritoneal carcinoma after prophylactic oophorectomy in women with a family history of ovarian cancer. Cancer 1993;71:2751–2755 (Level III)
7. Dicker RC, Scally MJ, Greenspan JR, Layde PM, Ory HW, Maze JM, et al. Hysterectomy among women of reproductive age. JAMA 1982;248:323–327 (Level II-3)
8. Pokras R, Hufnagel VG. Hysterectomy in the United States, 1965–84. Am J Public Health 1988;78:852–853 (Level II-3)
9. Averette HE, Nguyen HN. The role of prophylactic oophorectomy in cancer prevention. Gynecol Oncol 1994;55:S38–S41 (Level III)
10. Whittemore AS, Harris R, Itnyre J. Characteristics relating to ovarian cancer risk: collaborative analysis of 12 US case-control studies. II. Invasive epithelial ovarian cancers in white women. Collaborative Ovarian Cancer Group. Am J Epidemiol 1992;136:1184–1203 (Level II-2)
11. NIH consensus conference. Ovarian cancer: screening, treatment, and follow-up. NIH Consensus Development Panel on Ovarian Cancer. JAMA 1995;273:491–497 (Level III)
12. Narod SA, Risch H, Moslehi R, Dorum A, Neuhausen S, Olsson H, et al. Oral contraceptives and the risk of hereditary ovarian cancer. Hereditary Ovarian Cancer Clinical Study Group. N Engl J Med 1998;339:424–428 (Level II-2)
13. Ballard LA, Walters MD. Transvaginal mobilization and removal of ovaries and fallopian tubes after vaginal hysterectomy. Obstet Gynecol 1996;87:35–39 (Level II-2)
14. Davies A, O'Connor H, Magos AL. A prospective study to evaluate oophorectomy at the time of vaginal hysterectomy. Br J Obstet Gynaecol 1996;103:915–920 (Level II-2)
15. Rubin SC, Benjamin I, Behbakht K, Takahashi H, Morgan MA, LiVolsi VA, et al. Clinical and pathological features of ovarian cancer in women with germ-line mutations of *BRCA1*. N Engl J Med 1996;335:1413–1416 (Level II-2)
16. Stratton JF, Gayther SA, Russell P, Dearden J, Gore M, Blake P, et al. Contribution of *BRCA1* mutations to ovarian cancer. N Engl J Med 1997;336:1125–1130 (Level II-3)
17. Ford D, Easton DF. The genetics of breast and ovarian cancer. Br J Cancer 1995;72:805–812 (Level III)

18. Burke W, Petersen G, Lynch P, Botkin J, Daly M, Garber J, et al. Recommendations for follow-up care of individuals with an inherited predisposition to cancer. I. Hereditary nonpolyposis colon cancer. JAMA 1997;277:915–919 (Level III)

19. Watson P, Lynch HT. Extracolonic cancer in hereditary nonpolyposis colorectal cancer. Cancer 1993;71:677–685 (Level II-3)

20. Irwin KL, Weiss NS, Lee NC, Peterson HB. Tubal sterilization, hysterectomy, and the subsequent occurrence of epithelial ovarian cancer. Am J Epidemiol 1991;134: 362–369 (Level II-2)

21. Christ JE, Lotze EC. The residual ovary syndrome. Obstet Gynecol 1975;46:551–556 (Level II-3)

22. Grogan RH, Duncan CJ. Ovarian salvage in routine abdominal hysterectomy. Am J Obstet Gynecol 1955;70: 1277–1283 (Level III)

23. Plockinger B, Kolbl H. Development of ovarian pathology after hysterectomy without oophorectomy. J Am Coll Surg 1994;178:581–585 (Level II-2)

24. Parker M, Bosscher J, Barnhill D, Park R. Ovarian management during radical hysterectomy in the premenopausal patient. Obstet Gynecol 1993;82:187–190 (Level II-3)

25. American College of Obstetricians and Gynecologists. Hormone replacement therapy. ACOG Educational Bulletin 247. Washington, DC: ACOG, 1998 (Level III)

26. Lindsay R, Tohme JF. Estrogen treatment of patients with established postmenopausal osteoporosis. Obstet Gynecol 1990;76:290–295 (Level II-1)

27. Lindsay R. Estrogen/progestogen therapy: prevention and treatment of postmenopausal osteoporosis. Proc Soc Exp Biol Med 1989;191:275–277 (Level III)

28. Lip GY, Blann AD, Jones AF, Beevers DG. Effects of hormone-replacement therapy on hemostatic factors, lipid factors, and endothelial function in women undergoing surgical menopause: implications for prevention of atherosclerosis. Am Heart J 1997;134:764–771 (Level II-3)

29. Ravnikar VA. Compliance with hormone therapy. Am J Obstet Gynecol 1987;156:1332–1334 (Level III)

30. Speroff T, Dawson NV, Speroff L, Haber RJ. A risk-benefit-analysis of elective bilateral oophorectomy: effect of changes in compliance with estrogen therapy on outcome. Am J Obstet Gynecol 1991;164:165–174 (Level III)

31. Struewing JP, Watson P, Easton DF, Ponder BA, Lynch HT, Tucker MA. Prophylactic oophorectomy in inherited breast/ovarian cancer families. J Natl Cancer Inst Monogr 1995;17:33–35 (Level II-2)

32. Burke W, Daly M, Garber J, Botkin J, Kahn MJ, Lynch P, et al. Recommendations for follow-up care of individuals with an inherited predisposition to cancer. II. BRCA1 and BRCA2. JAMA 1997;277:997–1003 (Level III)

33. Moore JT, Tolley DH: Depression following hysterectomy. Psychosomatics 1976;17:86–89 (Level II-3)

The MEDLINE database, the Cochrane Library, and ACOG's own internal resources were used to conduct a literature search to locate relevant articles published between January 1985 and January 1999. The search was restricted to articles published in the English language. Priority was given to articles reporting results of original research, although review articles and commentaries also were consulted. Abstracts of research presented at symposiums and scientific conferences were not considered adequate for inclusion in this document. Guidelines published by organizations or institutions such as the National Institutes of Health and ACOG were reviewed, and additional studies were located by reviewing bibliographies of identified articles. When reliable research was not available, expert opinions from obstetrician–gynecologists were used.

Studies were reviewed and evaluated for quality according to the method outlined by the U.S. Preventive Services Task Force:

I Evidence obtained from at least one properly designed randomized controlled trial.

II-1 Evidence obtained from well-designed controlled trials without randomization.

II-2 Evidence obtained from well-designed cohort or case–control analytic studies, preferably from more than one center or research group.

II-3 Evidence obtained from multiple time series with or without the intervention. Dramatic results in uncontrolled experiments also could be regarded as this type of evidence.

III Opinions of respected authorities, based on clinical experience, descriptive studies, or reports of expert committees.

Based on the highest level of evidence found in the data, recommendations are provided and graded according to the following categories:

Level A—Recommendations are based on good and consistent scientific evidence.

Level B—Recommendations are based on limited or inconsistent scientific evidence.

Level C—Recommendations are based primarily on consensus and expert opinion.

ISSN 1099-3630

The American College of
Obstetricians and Gynecologists
409 12th Street, SW
PO Box 96920
Washington, DC 20090-6920

12345/32109

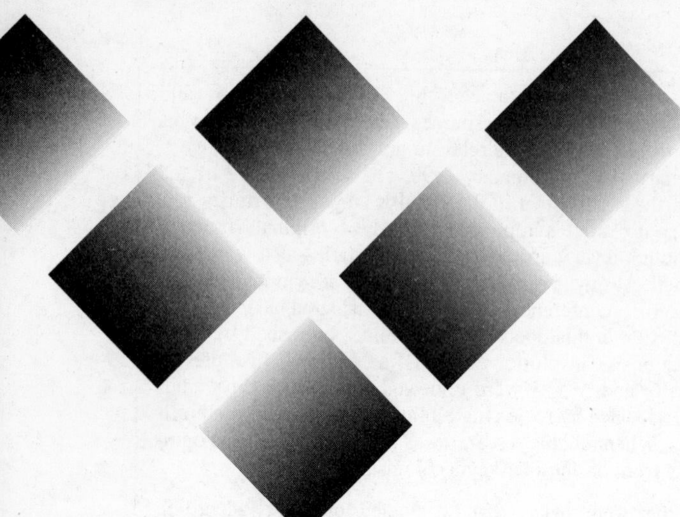

ACOG
PRACTICE
BULLETIN

CLINICAL MANAGEMENT GUIDELINES FOR
OBSTETRICIAN–GYNECOLOGISTS

NUMBER 16, MAY 2000

(Replaces Educational Bulletin Number 192, May 1994)

This Practice Bulletin was developed by the ACOG Committee on Practice Bulletins—Gynecology with the assistance of Elizabeth A. Stewart, MD. The information is designed to aid practitioners in making decisions about appropriate obstetric and gynecologic care. These guidelines should not be construed as dictating an exclusive course of treatment or procedure. Variations in practice may be warranted based on the needs of the individual patient, resources, and limitations unique to the institution or type of practice.

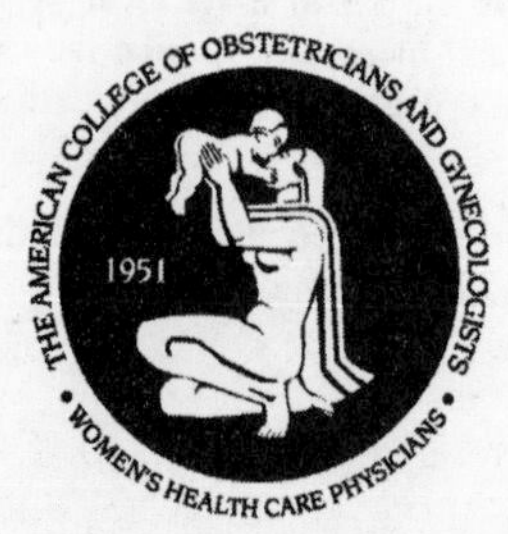

Surgical Alternatives to Hysterectomy in the Management of Leiomyomas

Uterine leiomyomas (also called fibroids) are the most common solid pelvic tumors in women and the leading indication for hysterectomy. Although most women with uterine leiomyomas are asymptomatic and can be followed without treatment, some will require more active measures. Hysterectomy remains the most common treatment for leiomyomas because it is the only treatment that provides a cure and eliminates the possibility of recurrence. Many women seek an alternative to hysterectomy because they desire future childbearing or wish to retain their uteri even if they have completed childbearing. As alternatives to hysterectomy become increasingly available, the efficacies of these treatments and the risk of potential problems are important to delineate. The purpose of this bulletin is to review the literature about surgical alternatives to hysterectomy and to offer treatment recommendations.

Background

As benign neoplasms, uterine leiomyomas usually require treatment only when they cause symptoms. The two most common symptoms for which women seek treatment are abnormal uterine bleeding and pelvic pressure or pain. However, not all bleeding is caused by leiomyomas; therefore, other causes of abnormal bleeding should be ruled out. The most common kind of abnormal uterine bleeding associated with leiomyomas is menorrhagia. Often, menses last 7 days or more, frequently resulting in iron deficiency anemia. This heavy flow also may require frequent changes of sanitary protection, causing significant interruptions in a woman's work or social schedule.

Uterine leiomyomas are clinically apparent in 25–50% of women (1), although studies in which careful pathologic examination of the uterus is carried out suggest the prevalence may be as high as 80% (2). The lack of a simple, inexpensive, and safe long-term medical treatment means that most symptomatic leiomyomas are still managed surgically.

Leiomyomas range greatly in size. Both size and location can play a role in symptoms and potential treatments. Leiomyomas may be subserosal, submucosal, or intramural; however, some types may be combined, for example, largely intramural with a submucosal extension.

The pelvic and abdominal discomfort that women experience with leiomyomas often is referred to as pressure and often is analogous to the discomforts women experience during pregnancy due to the enlarging of the uterus. In addition to pelvic pressure, the leiomyomas may press on adjacent structures, leading to difficulty with urination or defecation or dyspareunia.

Surgical Alternatives to Hysterectomy

In choosing a surgical alternative to hysterectomy, both safety and efficacy need to be established for each procedure. It must be recognized that all surgical alternatives to hysterectomy allow the possibility for new leiomyomas to form, and preexisting leiomyomas that were too small to be detected or were intentionally not removed may exhibit significant growth, necessitating another procedure. Complications of other surgical procedures may lead to an unanticipated hysterectomy.

Myomectomy

For women who desire future childbearing or who prefer to retain their uteri, myomectomy may be an option. Myomectomy removes only the visible and accessible leiomyomas, and the uterus is reconstructed. Most myomectomies traditionally have been performed by laparotomy.

Laparoscopic Myomectomy

Endoscopic myomectomy is now a treatment option for many women. Laparoscopic myomectomy minimizes the size of the abdominal incision, although it usually requires a minimum of three small incisions. Because the laparoscope usually is inserted at the umbilicus, the uterus must be small enough to be well-visualized with this approach; thus, this technique would not be appropriate for large uteri.

Hysteroscopic Procedures

Hysteroscopic procedures are primarily efficacious for the control of leiomyoma-related bleeding and do not significantly reduce uterine size. Only if a leiomyoma is submucosal or has a submucosal component can it be removed through the vagina (ie, hysteroscopic myomectomy).

For women with primarily intramural leiomyomas or women who have simultaneous hysteroscopic myomectomies, destruction of the endometrium by endometrial ablation can decrease bleeding. Endometrial ablation can be performed for a variety of indications, and it also can be useful in the control of leiomyoma-related menorrhagia. Endometrial ablation can utilize a variety of techniques, including laser ablation, thermal ablation, physical resection, or chemical destruction. Theoretically, even if leiomyomas remain, menstrual bleeding cannot occur because there is no endometrium. These procedures require hysteroscopic expertise.

Procedures Under Development

Several innovative options are being studied as possible alternative treatments for leiomyomas. Although all of these procedures may prove to be effective treatments for leiomyomas compared with current options, the number of patients treated have been small, the follow-up periods have been relatively short, and the safety of the procedures in women desiring pregnancy has not been demonstrated.

Uterine artery embolization is a radiologic alternative to surgery that involves partial blockage of the uterine arteries and, thus, decreased blood flow to the leiomyomatous uterus. Several case series of embolizations have been reported, with 8–53 patients monitored for intervals of 3–20 months (3–5). These reports suggest that most patients have a significant decrease in bleeding symptoms, as well as a reduction in uterine size. However, uterine artery embolization may have serious consequences including infection, massive uterine bleeding, and uterine necrosis, requiring emergency surgery (6). Patients can experience significant uterine pain, ischemia, and hypoxic changes following embolization of the myoma. Therefore, uterine artery embolization is regarded as investigational. Myolysis involves delivering electric current with needles or the use of lasers to coagulate myomas at the time of laparoscopy. A large series of cases have been reported from a single center (7).

As the biology of leiomyomas is better understood, new medical treatment options may become available. Both the progesterone antagonist mifepristone (RU 486) and gonadotropin-releasing hormone (GnRH) antagonists have been shown in small studies to produce equivalent levels of uterine shrinkage and rates of amenorrhea to GnRH agonists (8–10), with the attendant advantages of normal follicular levels of estradiol (mifepristone) and rapidity of action (antagonists). Understanding the derangements of growth factors and genes that lead to leiomyoma formation and growth also may lead to new medical therapies aimed at these underlying mechanisms (11).

Clinical Considerations and Recommendations

▶ ***In symptomatic women with leiomyomas and an indication for surgery, does hysterectomy produce a better outcome than myomectomy in relation to long-term morbidity (eg, pain, bleeding, recurrence, operative complications, and patient satisfaction)?***

Randomized studies are difficult to perform on this subject for which patient preference often is strong. However, reports of retrospective series have provided some information on this topic.

Abdominal Myomectomy. Although early studies suggested the morbidity associated with myomectomy was increased compared with hysterectomy, more recent studies suggest that the risks of the two procedures are similar (12–14). However, women choosing myomectomy face the additional risks of recurrence of leiomyomas and the possibility of having to proceed with hysterectomy because of intraoperative complications.

There is less outcomes research available for myomectomy than there is for hysterectomy (15). However, clinical experience and pooled results of numerous small studies suggest that there is excellent resolution of menorrhagia symptoms (overall 81% resolution; range, 40–93%) with similar results for resolution of pelvic pressure with abdominal myomectomy (1).

In the long term, however, the risk of formation of new leiomyomas limits the efficacy of myomectomy. There are a number of studies that have examined the use of ultrasonography to assess the recurrence risk of leiomyomas after abdominal myomectomy (16–19). Clearly, an estimate depends on the detection power of the measuring instrument. Thus, later studies using transvaginal ultrasonography tend to give higher estimates of recurrence (51% at 5 years) compared with earlier transabdominal ultrasound studies (27% at 10 years) but, presumably, are more accurate (16, 17). Studies have indicated that women who experience childbirth after a myomectomy appear to have a decreased recurrence risk (16, 17). There have been conflicting reports over whether the preoperative use of GnRH agonists affects recurrence risk (18, 19).

The clinically relevant endpoint is whether a second surgical procedure is needed after conservative surgery. A summary of a small case series conducted since the 1920s suggests the risk of follow-up treatment (in this instance, defined as hysterectomy, second myomectomy, or radiation therapy) varied from 3% to 32%, with a mean risk of 15%, although no information on the length of follow-up was given (1). In a relatively large series (125 patients followed at least 5 years and up to 23 years), there was evidence that recurrence depended on the number of leiomyomas present, with a recurrence risk of 11% for a single myoma and a recurrence risk of 26% with multiple myomas (20). A more recent study of 80 patients found a similar reoperation rate of 18% after 10 years (21).

The risk of undergoing an unexpected hysterectomy at the time of myomectomy appears to be low with skilled surgical technique (<1%), even when uterine size is substantial (14, 22–24). There may, however, be higher rates of hysterectomy for surgeons inexperienced in the procedure. Blood loss and the risk of transfusion may be increased in women with larger uteri (14, 25).

Laparoscopic Myomectomy. There are a number of case series of laparoscopic myomectomies, the largest of them reporting on more than 200 patients covering a period in excess of 5 years (26–28). The two major concerns with laparoscopic myomectomy versus hysterectomy are the removal of large myomas through small abdominal incisions and the repair of the uterus. The introduction of more efficient morcellators has made the removal easier, although skilled operative technique is necessary because injury to other organs is possible. Although there are multiple techniques available for laparoscopic suturing, there is controversy as to whether the closure techniques available are equal to those achieved at laparotomy. This is most relevant to women contemplating a future pregnancy.

Recommendations differ regarding cases amenable to a laparoscopic approach; most recommend a laparotomy or a laparoscopically assisted approach with leiomyomas in excess of 5–8 cm, multiple leiomyomas, or the presence of deep intramural leiomyomas (26–28). In addition to routine surgical complications, reported complications include a 2–8% conversion rate to a more open procedure, the formation of uteroperitoneal fistulas, and the possibility of uterine rupture during a subsequent pregnancy (26–28). It appears that the risk of recurrent leiomyomas may be higher after a laparoscopic myomectomy than after a traditional myomectomy, with a 33% recurrence risk at 27 months (29).

Hysteroscopic Myomectomy. Several series of between 100 and 200 patients undergoing hysteroscopic myomectomies with good results have been published. In a series in which almost all patients were treated for menorrhagia, 16% of the submucosal resection group ultimately underwent a second surgery after a mean follow-up of 9 years (30). In the same series, women undergoing ablation with or without submucosal myomectomy had an 8% chance of undergoing a second surgery after a mean of 6 years of follow-up (30). In a series of 167 patients who were followed for 3 years after hysteroscopic myomectomy plus myolysis, approximately 5% underwent a second surgery (31). For women desiring pregnancy, fertility rates appear good: 59% of patients with submucosal leiomyomas conceived after hysteroscopic myomectomy (32).

Endometrial Ablation. Endometrial ablation appears to be an effective therapy for the control of menstrual bleeding in women with abnormal bleeding only. For leiomyomas, one study suggested endometrial ablation had a failure rate of 40%, compared with a failure rate of 5% in women with a normal uterus (33). Thus, ablation for women with clinically significant leiomyomas may prove to be a less desirable course of action than for women with idiopathic menorrhagia. Currently, there is no evidence to support the use of this procedure for women with leiomyomas; however, new techniques are being explored.

Complications with all techniques involving operative hysteroscopy include the risk of injury to intraabdominal structures either by uterine perforation or secondary to electrical or thermal injury (34). In addition, there can be significant complications as a consequence of the distending medium used. The uterine vasculature can rapidly absorb the substance distending the uterus. Fatal events have been reported with air embolism using an Nd-YAG laser with saline as the distending medium, as well as with hyponatremic encephalopathy with sorbitol as the distending medium (35, 36). Many newer technologies have been designed to minimize this risk, including systems that accurately measure inflow and outflow of hysteroscopic fluids and devices that use physiologic saline as the uterine distending medium.

▶ *In women with leiomyomas who are candidates for surgery, does the use of adjunctive medical treatment result in better outcomes?*

Preoperative Adjuvants. Gonadotropin-releasing hormone agonists have been used widely for preoperative treatment of uterine leiomyomas, both for myomectomy and hysterectomy. These medications are very effective in inducing amenorrhea and causing uterine shrinkage in a large proportion of women who take them. However, they are expensive and have significant side effects for most women in the short term and significant effects on bone density if taken over longer periods.

Currently, GnRH agonists are the only drugs available that result in clinically significant uterine shrinkage and amenorrhea. When a significant reduction in uterine volume is necessary to achieve surgical goals (eg, when the patient prefers a low-transverse incision instead of a vertical incision or an endoscopic procedure), GnRH agonists may be useful.

By inducing amenorrhea, GnRH agonists have been shown to improve hematologic parameters, shorten hospital stay, and decrease blood loss, operating time, and postoperative pain when given for 2–3 months preoperatively (37–39). However, because no study has shown a significant decrease in transfusion risk or improvement in quality of life, and the cost of these medications is substantial, the decision to use GnRH agonists preoperatively remains complex. It also is worth noting that in a study that achieved hematologic improvement with GnRH agonist treatment in 74% of women, there was a 46% improvement rate in the placebo group with iron supplementation alone (38). One surgical disadvantage to preoperative GnRH agonist therapy is that it may make the leiomyomas softer and the surgical planes less distinct. Although many studies find the operative time equivalent for laparotomies, one study of laparoscopic myomectomies found that overall operating time decreased after GnRH agonist treatment. However, in the subgroup in which the largest leiomyoma was hypoechoic, operative time was longer because of the difficulty in dissection (39).

Intraoperative Adjuvants. Several studies suggest that the infiltration of vasopressin into the myometrium decreases blood loss at the time of myomectomy. A study of 20 patients demonstrated that vasopressin significantly decreased blood loss compared with saline injection in a randomized myomectomy study (40). Two studies compared the use of physical vascular compression, primarily a tourniquet around the lower uterine segment, with pharmacologic vasoconstriction (vasopressin administration). In one study using a Penrose drain tourniquet and vascular clamps, there was no significant difference between the two techniques (25). A more recent study using a Foley catheter as a tourniquet found blood loss to be significantly greater in the tourniquet group (41). There are no studies comparing tourniquet with placebo. Additionally, one study demonstrated that injection of vasopressin into the cervix at the time of operative hysteroscopy decreased blood loss, fluid intravasation, and operative time (42).

▶ *In pregnant women who have undergone a myomectomy, does a planned cesarean delivery versus a trial of labor help prevent uterine rupture?*

No study directly addresses the issue of cesarean delivery versus a trial of labor after myomectomy. The widely quoted clinical dictum is that if the endometrial cavity is entered at the time of myomectomy, then cesarean delivery is recommended. This appears to arise from a 3-year collaborative trial of data reporting a rate of uterine rupture of approximately 0.1% (43). Most of these ruptures had cesarean deliveries as antecedents, and because myomectomy also can produce a transmural incision in the uterus, it appears to have been treated in an analogous way. However, in the original study, the incidence of uterine rupture after myomectomy was only 0.002% (43). There are rare case reports of rupture remote from term after traditional abdominal myomectomy (44, 45). Uterine rupture can carry significant consequences for both mother and fetus.

However, several case reports have demonstrated uterine rupture at 33–34 weeks of gestation following laparoscopic myomectomy (46–48) and myolysis (49, 50). Although most of the case reports detail ruptures with intramural leiomyomas, one describes a case in which the 5-cm leiomyoma was subserosal; however, in this case no suturing was performed (48). Clearly long-term follow-up is necessary to determine the safety of innovative approaches to leiomyomas in women attempting pregnancy, and patients should be counseled preoperatively regarding these issues.

▶ *In women with leiomyomas who desire to become pregnant, does removal of leiomyomas versus expectant management increase the pregnancy rate?*

It is difficult to assess the contributions of leiomyomas to infertility for several reasons. First, there is a high prevalence of leiomyomas in the population, and the incidence of leiomyomas increases with age, as does infertility. Because not all leiomyomas are symptomatic, many women may conceive without even knowing that they have them. Finally, studies to date have been case series; randomized trials have not been conducted.

It appears that distortion of the uterine cavity may cause infertility and lead to pregnancy complications (51, 52). One study examining women attempting in vitro fertilization showed a decreased implantation rate in women with distortion of the cavity (53). When myomectomies have been performed on infertile patients with no other infertility factor, pregnancy rates have been reported in the range of 40–60% after 1–2 years (54–56). However, the use of additional fertility treatments in these studies was not excluded and may have contributed to the increase as well.

Two recent studies have examined the effect of leiomyomas on the outcome of assisted reproduction when there is no distortion of the uterine cavity. Using age-matched patients with similar embryo characteristics, the first study found significant decreases in both clinical pregnancies (53% versus 37%) and delivery rates (48% versus 33%) in patients with leiomyomas (57). The second study showed both significantly decreased pregnancy rates and implantation rates with both intramural and submucosal leiomyomas but not with subserosal leiomyomas (58). Although a general problem with the myomatous uterus or other associated factors may play a role in this process, indications for myomectomy in women undergoing assisted reproductive techniques remain to be clarified.

Some surgeons feel that a prophylactic myomectomy for women with large fibroids who want to preserve future fertility may be appropriate in some circumstances. The evidence that the complication rate is low in skilled surgical hands, even with substantial uterine size, suggests myomectomy may be indicated (14, 22–24); however, the risk of recurrent myomas is high, which may make myomectomy a less effective treatment (16, 17). Consideration of multiple factors is important, including size and location of myomas, previous fertility, and the woman's age.

▶ *In menopausal women with leiomyomas, what is the effect of hormone replacement therapy on leiomyoma growth, bleeding, and pain?*

For many years, health care providers have counseled patients that leiomyomas are a self-limiting problem that will resolve when a woman completes the transition to menopause. Because leiomyomas are responsive to estrogen, the hypoestrogenism of menopause most women experience results in uterine shrinkage, and all women have cessation of physiologic menses. However, as more women elect hormone replacement therapy, there is the possibility that problems with leiomyomas may persist into menopause.

There is some evidence that women with leiomyomas who take hormone replacement therapy are more likely to have abnormal bleeding. In a study using hysteroscopy to evaluate women with abnormal bleeding who were taking hormone replacement therapy (using women with no abnormal bleeding as controls), women with structural abnormalities of the cavity, including endometrial polyps and submucosal leiomyomas, had an increased likelihood of abnormal bleeding (59).

A small pilot study examined whether hormone replacement therapy during menopause caused an increase in size of asymptomatic leiomyomas (60). This study showed a significant increase in leiomyoma dimension after 1 year of transdermal hormone replacement therapy but no increase with oral conjugated estrogens. Because the clinical magnitude of the increase associated with the transdermal route is small (14.3–19.7 mm) and the follow-up time short, it is not clear whether this will result in clinically significant changes.

▶ ***In asymptomatic women with leiomyomas, does expectant management produce a better outcome than surgical treatment in relation to long-term morbidity?***

Expectant management in an asymptomatic patient should be the norm; however, in some instances an asymptomatic leiomyomatous uterus might require treatment. If there is concern that the mass is not a leiomyoma but instead a sarcoma, further evaluation is warranted. Traditionally, the major clinical sign used to make this distinction was rapid growth in uterine size. However, in a study of 1,332 hysterectomy specimens for which the preoperative diagnosis was uterine leiomyomas, sarcomas were not only rare (2–3 per 1,000) but no more common in the subgroup of women who had experienced rapidly enlarging uterine size (61). If a comparison is made between the prevalence of leiomyosarcomas discovered incidentally (1:2,000) and the mortality rate for hysterectomy for benign disease (1.0–1.6 per 1,000 for premenopausal women), the decision to proceed to hysterectomy to find potential sarcomas should be made cautiously (62). Other risk factors for sarcomas, including increasing age or a history of prior pelvic radiation, may influence this decision. Alternatively, both endometrial biopsy and magnetic resonance imaging appear to be useful in diagnosing sarcomas and differentiating them from other intrauterine lesions (63, 64).

In rare circumstances, the uterus will cause significant compression of the ureters that can lead to the compromise of renal function, which requires further evaluation. Finally, in a woman contemplating pregnancy or experiencing recurrent miscarriage, significant distortion of the uterine cavity may require intervention in an asymptomatic patient (51, 52). Proximity of the leiomyoma to the placental implantation site and large size of the leiomyoma appear to increase obstetric risk, including placental abruption and premature labor. However, no consensus exists for when myomectomy should be recommended in women desiring pregnancy but with no history of infertility (52).

Historically, it has been argued that uterine size alone should be an indication for hysterectomy. The argument has usually been twofold. The first issue was that a large leiomyomatous uterus made assessment of the ovaries and early surveillance for ovarian cancer impossible. However, the National Institutes of Health and National Cancer Institute Consensus Conference acknowledge the futility of routine pelvic examinations in the identification of early ovarian cancer. Second, the argument is made that because of increased morbidity during surgery for a large uterus, surgery is a safer option when the uterus is smaller. Although some studies have shown increased morbidity, others show no differences in perioperative complications (13, 14, 62). This currently does not appear to be a cogent argument for intervention.

▶ ***In women with leiomyomas planning future pregnancies who are candidates for surgery, what is the impact on future fertility (pregnancy rate) of surgery versus expectant management?***

As with any woman with leiomyomas, asymptomatic women with leiomyomas who desire future fertility should be managed expectantly because they have no indication for surgery. For mildly symptomatic women, given the risk of recurrence, intervening as close to the desired pregnancy as practical is desirable. The consequences of postoperative adhesions after myomectomy are unclear and should be avoided, despite the availability of assisted reproductive technology. Finally, although the risk of hysterectomy appears low for most surgical alternatives to hysterectomy, it is never eliminated. This risk should be considered in determining the appropriate treatment for women planning future pregnancies.

Summary

The following recommendations are based on good and consistent scientific evidence (Level A):

- ▶ In women with symptomatic leiomyomas, hysterectomy provides a definitive cure.
- ▶ In women with symptomatic leiomyomas, abdominal myomectomy is a safe and effective option for women who wish to retain their uterus. If this option is selected, women should be counseled preoperatively about the relatively high risk of reoperation.

- Use of GnRH agonists preoperatively is beneficial, especially when improvement of hematologic status and uterine shrinkage are important goals. Benefits of the use of GnRH agonists should be weighed against their cost and side effects for individual patients.
- The use of vasopressin at the time of myomectomy appears to limit blood loss.

The following recommendation is based on limited or inconsistent scientific evidence (Level B):

- The clinical diagnosis of rapidly growing leiomyomas has not been shown to predict uterine sarcoma and thus should not be used as the sole indication for myomectomy or hysterectomy.

The following recommendations are based primarily on consensus and expert opinion (Level C):

- Laparoscopic myomectomy appears to be a safe and effective option for women with a small number of moderately sized uterine leiomyomas who do not desire future fertility. Further studies are necessary to evaluate the safety of this procedure for women planning pregnancy.
- Hysteroscopic myomectomy is an effective option for controlling menorrhagia in women with submucosal leiomyomas.
- Although endometrial ablation appears to be an effective option in controlling menorrhagia in women without leiomyomas, further studies are needed in women who have clinically significant leiomyomas.
- Because leiomyomas may be a factor in infertility for some patients, the issues are complex, and myomectomy should not be performed without first completing a comprehensive fertility evaluation.
- Although postmenopausal women with leiomyomas may have more bleeding problems and some increase in leiomyoma size while taking hormone replacement therapy, there appears to be no reason to withhold this treatment option from women who desire or need such therapy.

References

1. Buttram VC Jr, Reiter RC. Uterine leiomyomata: etiology, symptomatology, and management. Fertil Steril 1981;36:433–445 (Level III)
2. Cramer SF, Patel A. The frequency of uterine leiomyomas. Am J Clin Pathol 1990;94:435–438 (Level II-3)
3. Bradley EA, Reidy JF, Forman RG, Jarosz J, Braude PR. Transcatheter uterine artery embolisation to treat large uterine fibroids. Br J Obstet Gynaecol 1998;105:235–240 (Level III)
4. Goodwin SC, Vedantham S, McLucas B, Forno AE, Perrella R. Preliminary experience with uterine artery embolization for uterine fibroids. J Vasc Interv Radiol 1997;8:517–526 (Level III)
5. Ravina JH, Herbreteau D, Ciraru-Vigneron N, Bouret JM, Houdart E, Aymard A, et al. Arterial embolisation to treat uterine myomata. Lancet 1995;346:671–672 (Level III)
6. Barbieri RL. Ambulatory management of uterine leiomyomata. Clin Obstet Gynecol 1999;42:196–205 (Level III)
7. Goldfarb HA. Bipolar laparoscopic needles for myoma coagulation. J Am Assoc Gynecol Laparosc 1995;2:175–179 (Level II-2)
8. Kettel LM, Murphy AA, Morales AJ, Rivier J, Vale W, Yen SS. Rapid regression of uterine leiomyomas in response to daily administration of gonadotropin-releasing hormone antagonist. Fertil Steril 1993;60:642–646 (Level III)
9. Murphy AA, Kettel LM, Morales AJ, Roberts VJ, Yen SS. Regression of uterine leiomyomata in response to the antiprogesterone RU 486. J Clin Endocrinol Metab 1993;76:513–517 (Level III)
10. Murphy AA, Morales AJ, Kettel LM, Yen SS. Regression of uterine leiomyomata to the antiprogesterone RU486: dose-response effect. Fertil Steril 1995;64:187–190 (Level III)
11. Stewart EA, Nowak RA. Leiomyoma-related bleeding: a classic hypothesis updated for the molecular era. Hum Reprod Update 1996;2:295–306 (Level III)
12. Hillis SD, Marchbanks PA, Peterson HB. Uterine size and risk of complications among women undergoing abdominal hysterectomy for leiomyomas. Obstet Gynecol 1996;87:539–543 (Level II-2)
13. Iverson RE Jr, Chelmow D, Strohbehn K, Waldman L, Evantash EG. Relative morbidity of abdominal hysterectomy and myomectomy for management of uterine leiomyomas. Obstet Gynecol 1996;88:415–419 (Level II-2)
14. Ecker JL, Foster JT, Friedman AJ. Abdominal hysterectomy or abdominal myomectomy for symptomatic leiomyoma: a comparison of preoperative demography and postoperative morbidity. J Gynecol Surg 1995;11:11–18 (Level II-2)
15. Carlson KJ, Miller BA, Fowler FJ Jr. The Maine Women's Health Study: I. Outcomes of hysterectomy. Obstet Gynecol 1994;83:556–565 (Level II-3)
16. Candiani GB, Fedele L, Parazzini F, Villa L. Risk of recurrence after myomectomy. Br J Obstet Gynaecol 1991;98:385–389 (Level II-3)
17. Fedele L, Parazzini F, Luchini L, Mezzopane R, Tozzi L, Villa L. Recurrence of fibroids after myomectomy: a transvaginal ultrasonographic study. Hum Reprod 1995;10:1795–1796 (Level II-3)
18. Fedele L, Vercellini P, Bianchi S, Brioschi D, Dorta M. Treatment with GnRH agonists before myomectomy and

the risk of short-term myoma recurrence. Br J Obstet Gynaecol 1990;97:393–396 (Level I)

19. Friedman AJ, Daly M, Juneau-Norcross M, Fine C, Rein MS. Recurrence of myomas after myomectomy in women pretreated with leuprolide acetate depot or placebo. Fertil Steril 1992;58:205–208 (Level I)
20. Malone LJ. Myomectomy: recurrence after removal of solitary and multiple myomas. Obstet Gynecol 1969;34:200–203 (Level II-3)
21. Acien P, Quereda F. Abdominal myomectomy: results of a simple operative technique. Fertil Steril 1996;65:41–51 (Level II-3)
22. Smith DC, Uhlir JK. Myomectomy as a reproductive procedure. Am J Obstet Gynecol 1990;162:1476–1479; discussion 1479–1482 (Level III)
23. Chong RK, Thong PH, Tan SL, Thong PW, Salmon YM. Myomectomy: indications, results of surgery and relation to fertility. Singapore Med J 1988;29:35–37 (Level III)
24. LaMorte AI, Lalwani S, Diamond MP. Morbidity associated with abdominal myomectomy. Obstet Gynecol 1993; 82:897–900 (Level III)
25. Ginsburg ES, Benson CB, Garfield JM, Gleason RE, Friedman AJ. The effect of operative technique and uterine size on blood loss during myomectomy: a prospective randomized study. Fertil Steril 1993;60:956–962 (Level I)
26. Dubuisson JB, Chapron C, Levy L. Difficulties and complications of laparoscopic myomectomy. J Gynecol Surg 1996;12:159–165 (Level II-3)
27. Nezhat C, Nezhat F, Silfen SL, Schaffer N, Evans D. Laparoscopic myomectomy. Int J Fertil 1991;36:275–280 (Level II-3)
28. Seinera P, Arisio R, Decko A, Farina C, Crana F. Laparoscopic myomectomy: indications, surgical technique and complications. Hum Reprod 1997;12:1927–1930 (Level II-3)
29. Nezhat FR, Roemisch M, Nezhat CH, Seidman DS, Nezhat CR. Recurrence rate after laparoscopic myomectomy. J Am Assoc Gynecol Laparosc 1998;5:237–240 (Level III)
30. Derman SG, Rehnstrom J, Neuwirth RS. The long-term effectiveness of hysteroscopic treatment of menorrhagia and leiomyomas. Obstet Gynecol 1991;77:591–594 (Level II-3)
31. Phillips DR, Milim SJ, Nathanson HG, Haselkorn JS. Experience with laparoscopic leiomyoma coagulation and concomitant operative hysteroscopy. J Am Assoc Gynecol Laparosc 1997;4:425–433 (Level II-3)
32. Ubaldi F, Tournaye H, Camus M, Van der Pas H, Gepts E, Devroey P. Fertility after hysteroscopic myomectomy. Hum Reprod Update 1995;1:81–90 (Level III)
33. Yin CS, Wei RY, Chao TC, Chan CC. Hysteroscopic endometrial ablation without endometrial preparation. Int J Gynaecol Obstet 1998;62:167–172 (Level II-3)
34. Kivnick S, Kanter MH. Bowel injury from rollerball ablation of the endometrium. Obstet Gynecol 1992;79: 833–835 (Level III)
35. Arieff AI, Ayus JC. Endometrial ablation complicated by fatal hyponatremic encephalopathy. JAMA 1993;270: 1230–1232 (Level III)
36. Challener RC, Kaufman B. Fatal venous air embolism following sequential unsheathed (bare) and sheathed quartz fiber Nd:YAG laser endometrial ablation. Anesthesiology 1990;73:548–551 (Level III)
37. Gerris J, Degueldre M, Peters AA, Romao F, Stjernquist M, al-Taher H. The place of Zoladex in deferred surgery for uterine fibroids. Zoladex Myoma Study Group. Horm Res 1996;45:279–284 (Level I)
38. Stovall TG, Muneyyirci-Delale O, Summitt RL Jr, Scialli AR. GnRH agonist and iron versus placebo and iron in the anemic patient before surgery for leiomyomas: a randomized controlled trial. Leuprolide Acetate Study Group. Obstet Gynecol 1995;86:65–71 (Level I)
39. Zullo F, Pellicano M, De Stefano R, Zupi E, Mastrantonio P. A prospective randomized study to evaluate leuprolide acetate treatment before laparoscopic myomectomy: efficacy and ultrasonographic predictors. Am J Obstet Gynecol 1998;178:108–112 (Level I)
40. Frederick J, Fletcher H, Simeon D, Mullings A, Hardie M. Intramyometrial vasopressin as a haemostatic agent during myomectomy. Br J Obstet Gynaecol 1994;101:435–437 (Level I)
41. Fletcher H, Frederick J, Hardie M, Simeon D. A randomized comparison of vasopressin and tourniquet as hemostatic agents during myomectomy. Obstet Gynecol 1996;87:1014–1018 (Level I)
42. Phillips DR, Nathanson HG, Milim SJ, Haselkorn JS, Khapra A, Ross PL. The effect of dilute vasopressin solution on blood loss during operative hysteroscopy: a randomized controlled trial. Obstet Gynecol 1996;88:761–766 (Level I)
43. Garnet JD. Uterine rupture during pregnancy: an analysis of 133 patients. Obstet Gynecol 1964;23:898–905 (Level II-3)
44. Golan D, Aharoni A, Gonen R, Boss Y, Sharf M. Early spontaneous rupture of the post myomectomy gravid uterus. Int J Gynaecol Obstet 1990;31:167–170 (Level III)
45. Ozeren M, Ulusoy M, Uyanik E. First-trimester spontaneous uterine rupture after traditional myomectomy: case report. Isr J Med Sci 1997;33:752–753 (Level III)
46. Dubuisson JB, Chavet X, Chapron C, Gregorakis SS, Morice P. Uterine rupture during pregnancy after laparoscopic myomectomy. Hum Reprod 1995;10:1475–1477 (Level III)
47. Harris WJ. Uterine dehiscence following laparoscopic myomectomy. Obstet Gynecol 1992;80:545–546 (Level III)
48. Pelosi MA 3rd, Pelosi MA. Spontaneous uterine rupture at thirty-three weeks subsequent to previous superficial laparoscopic myomectomy. Am J Obstet Gynecol 1997; 177:1547–1549 (Level III)
49. Arcangeli S, Pasquarette MM. Gravid uterine rupture after myolysis. Obstet Gynecol 1997;89:857 (Level III)
50. Vilos GA, Pispidikis JT, Botz CK. Economic evaluation of hysteroscopic endometrial ablation versus vaginal hys-

terectomy for menorrhagia. Obstet Gynecol 1996;88: 241–245 (Level II-2)

51. Garcia CR, Tureck RW. Submucosal leiomyomas and infertility. Fertil Steril 1984;42:16–19 (Level III)
52. Rice JP, Kay HH, Mahony BS. The clinical significance of uterine leiomyomas in pregnancy. Am J Obstet Gynecol 1989;160:1212–1216 (Level II-2)
53. Farhi J, Ashkenazi J, Feldberg D, Dicker D, Orvieto R, Ben Rafael Z. Effect of uterine leiomyomata on the results of in-vitro fertilization treatment. Hum Reprod 1995;10: 2576–2578 (Level II-2)
54. Babaknia A, Rock JA, Jones HW Jr. Pregnancy success following abdominal myomectomy for infertility. Fertil Steril 1978;30:644–647 (Level III)
55. Gehlbach DL, Sousa RC, Carpenter SE, Rock JA. Abdominal myomectomy in the treatment of infertility. Int J Gynaecol Obstet 1993;40:45–50 (Level III)
56. Sudik R, Husch K, Steller J, Daume E. Fertility and pregnancy outcome after myomectomy in sterility patients. Eur J Obstet Gynecol Reprod Biol 1996;65:209–214 (Level II-2)
57. Stovall DW, Parrish SB, Van Voorhis BJ, Hahn SJ, Sparks AE, Syrop CH. Uterine leiomyomas reduce the efficacy of assisted reproduction cycles: results of a matched follow-up study. Hum Reprod 1998;13:192–197 (Level II-2)
58. Eldar-Geva T, Meagher S, Healy DL, MacLachlan V, Breheny S, Wood C. Effect of intramural, subserosal, and submucosal uterine fibroids on the outcome of assisted reproductive technology treatment. Fertil Steril 1998;70: 687–691 (Level II-2)
59. Akkad AA, Habiba MA, Ismail N, Abrams K, al-Azzawi F. Abnormal uterine bleeding on hormone replacement: the importance of intrauterine structural abnormalities. Obstet Gynecol 1995;86:330–334 (Level II-2)
60. Sener AB, Seckin NC, Ozmen S, Gokmen O, Dogu N, Ekici E. The effects of hormone replacement therapy on uterine fibroids in postmenopausal women. Fertil Steril 1996;65:354–357 (Level II-1)
61. Parker WH, Fu YS, Berek JS. Uterine sarcoma in patients operated on for presumed leiomyoma and rapidly growing leiomyoma. Obstet Gynecol 1994;83:414–418 (Level II-3)
62. Reiter RC, Wagner PL, Gambone JC. Routine hysterectomy for large asymptomatic uterine leiomyomata: a reappraisal. Obstet Gynecol 1992;79:481–484 (Level II-3)
63. Schwartz LB, Diamond MP, Schwartz PE. Leiomyosarcomas: clinical presentation. Am J Obstet Gynecol 1993;168:180–183 (Level II-3)
64. Schwartz LB, Zawin M, Carcangiu ML, Lange R, McCarthy S. Does pelvic magnetic resonance imaging differentiate among the histologic subtypes of uterine leiomyomata? Fertil Steril 1998;70:580–587 (Level II-3)

The MEDLINE database, the Cochrane Library, and ACOG's own internal resources and documents were used to conduct a literature search to locate relevant articles published between January 1985 and May 1999. The search was restricted to articles published in the English language. Priority was given to articles reporting results of original research, although review articles and commentaries also were consulted. Abstracts of research presented at symposia and scientific conferences were not considered adequate for inclusion in this document. Guidelines published by organizations or institutions such as the National Institutes of Health and the American College of Obstetricians and Gynecologists were reviewed, and additional studies were located by reviewing bibliographies of identified articles. When reliable research was not available, expert opinions from obstetrician–gynecologists were used.

Studies were reviewed and evaluated for quality according to the method outlined by the U.S. Preventive Services Task Force:

- I Evidence obtained from at least one properly designed randomized controlled trial.
- II-1 Evidence obtained from well-designed controlled trials without randomization.
- II-2 Evidence obtained from well-designed cohort or case–control analytic studies, preferably from more than one center or research group.
- II-3 Evidence obtained from multiple time series with or without the intervention. Dramatic results in uncontrolled experiments also could be regarded as this type of evidence.
- III Opinions of respected authorities, based on clinical experience, descriptive studies, or reports of expert committees.

Based on the highest level of evidence found in the data, recommendations are provided and graded according to the following catetories:

Level A—Recommendations are based on good and consistent scientific evidence.

Level B—Recommendations are based on limited or inconsistent scientific evidence.

Level C—Recommendations are based primarily on consensus and expert opinion.

ISSN 1099-3630

The American College of Obstetricians and Gynecologists
409 12th Street, SW
PO Box 96920
Washington, DC 20090-6920

12345/43210

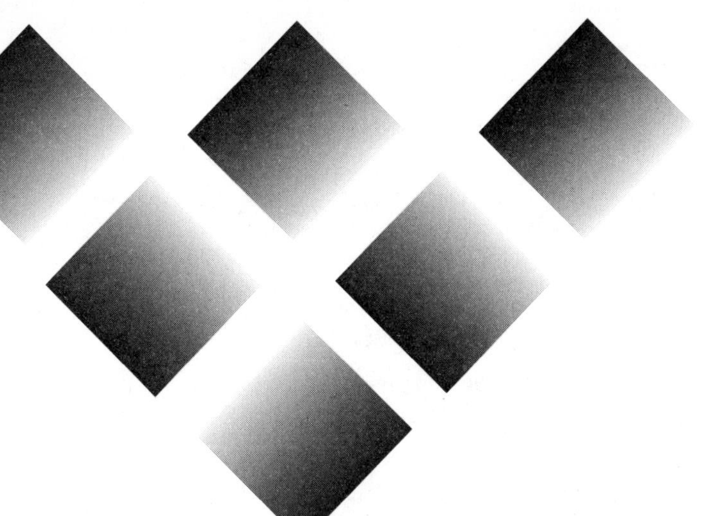

ACOG PRACTICE BULLETIN

CLINICAL MANAGEMENT GUIDELINES FOR OBSTETRICIAN–GYNECOLOGISTS

NUMBER 18, JULY 2000

This Practice Bulletin was developed by the ACOG Committee on Practice Bulletins—Gynecology with the assistance of Andrew M. Kaunitz, MD. The information is designed to aid practitioners in making decisions about appropriate obstetric and gynecologic care. These guidelines should not be construed as dictating an exclusive course of treatment or procedure. Variations in practice may be warranted based on the needs of the individual patient, resources, and limitations unique to the institution or type of practice.

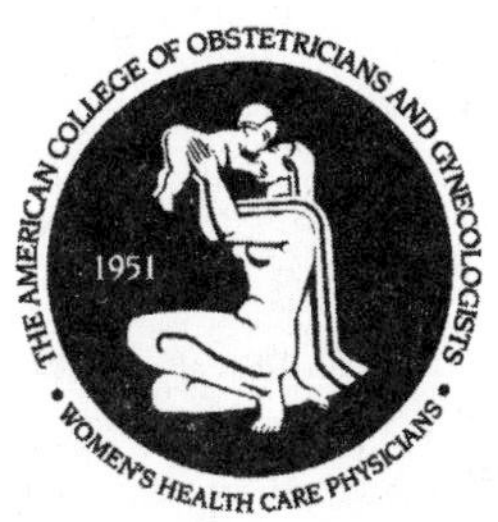

The Use of Hormonal Contraception in Women with Coexisting Medical Conditions

Although numerous studies have addressed the safety and effectiveness of hormonal contraceptive use in healthy women, data are far less complete for women with underlying medical problems or other special circumstances. Because recommendations vary widely, substantial confusion exists with respect to contraceptive guidelines for women with coexisting medical conditions or other concerns. Using available scientific evidence, this Practice Bulletin will provide information to facilitate contraceptive counseling and selection for women with coexisting medical conditions.

Background

Decisions regarding contraception for women with coexisting medical problems may be complicated. In some cases, medications taken for certain chronic conditions may alter the effectiveness of hormonal contraception, and pregnancy in these cases may pose substantial risks to the mother as well as her fetus. Package labeling approved by the U.S. Food and Drug Administration for progestin-only oral contraceptives (OCs) is occasionally the same as that for combined estrogen-progestin preparations. For instance, current labeling for norethindrone progestin-only OCs no longer lists a history of thromboembolism as a contraindication (1). Such a history, however, remains listed as a contraindication in package labeling for norgestrel progestin-only pills and for depot medroxyprogesterone acetate (DMPA) injections.

Sometimes, simultaneous use of two contraceptive methods is appropriate. For instance, although hormonal contraception provides effective birth control for women at risk for human immunodeficiency virus or other sexually transmitted diseases (or those currently infected), such patients also should be encouraged to use male or female condoms correctly and consistently to prevent disease. For women concomitantly using major teratogens, such as isotretinoin or thalidomide, simultaneous use of two methods of contraception (eg, OCs and condoms) also may be appropriate.

This Practice Bulletin will focus on selection of hormonal contraceptives for women with coexisting medical problems. However, practitioners should recognize that the use of other nonhormonal forms of contraception, such as intrauterine devices, represent a safe, effective choice for many women.

Clinical Considerations and Recommendations

This document will address the use of combination OCs in women who have the following conditions and risk factors:

- Older than 35 years
- Smoke tobacco products
- Hypertension
- Diabetes
- Migraine headaches
- Fibrocystic breast changes, fibroadenoma, or family history of breast cancer
- Uterine fibroids
- Lipid disorders
- Breastfeeding/postpartum
- Take concomitant medication
- Anticipate surgery
- Venous thromboembolism (VTE)
- Systemic lupus erythematosus (SLE)
- Sickle cell disease

In addition, the document will review clinical settings in which the use of progestin-only contraceptives represent safe alternatives for women with contraindications to combination OCs (see the box). The effect of DMPA use on bone mineral density (BMD) will be reviewed, particularly with respect to adolescent candidates. Practitioners should be aware that patients who have any of the previously mentioned conditions or risk factors and use OCs require close monitoring and follow-up evaluation.

Indications for Contraception Methods Other Than Oral Contraceptives

In women with the following conditions, use of progestin-only oral contraceptives, depot medroxyprogesterone acetate,* or implants may be safer than combination oral contraceptives. An intrauterine device also represents an appropriate contraceptive choice for women with these conditions.

Migraine headaches

Older than 35 years and smoke cigarettes

History of thromboembolic disease

Coronary artery disease

Congestive heart failure

Cerebrovascular disease

Less than 2 weeks postpartum†

Hypertension with vascular disease or older than 35 years

Diabetes with vascular disease or older than 35 years

Systemic lupus erythematosus with vascular disease, nephritis, or antiphospholipid antibodies

Hypertriglyceridemia

* Because of its long duration of action and potential for hypoestrogenic effects, depot medroxyprogesterone acetate may be less appropriate than other progestin-only contraceptives for some women with these listed conditions.

†Use of an intrauterine device may not be an appropriate contraceptive choice.

▶ *Is combination OC use safe for women older than 35 years?*

Use of combination OCs is safe in healthy, nonsmoking women older than 35 years. Recent large U.S. population-based case–control studies found no increased risk of myocardial infarction (2) or stroke (3) among healthy, nonsmoking women older than 35 years who use OCs formulated with less than 50 μg of estrogen.

Perimenopausal women benefit from the more regular menses and positive effect on BMD (4, 5) offered by combination OCs. In addition, use of combination OCs may reduce vasomotor symptoms in perimenopausal women (6). Furthermore, the reduced risk of endometrial and ovarian cancers associated with OC use is of particular importance to older women of reproductive age.

As increasing numbers of women in their late 40s and early 50s use combination OCs, the question of when women no longer need contraception and can consider transitioning to hormone replacement therapy will arise more frequently. Assessment of follicle-stimulating hormone levels to determine when older OC users have become menopausal and thus no longer need contraception is expensive and may be misleading (7–10). Until a well-validated tool to confirm menopause is available, an alternative approach is for healthy, nonsmoking women doing well on combination OCs to discontinue OCs routinely between the ages of 50 and 55 years. By age 55, the likelihood that a woman has reached menopausal status is at least 85% (11, 12).

▶ *Is combination OC use safe for women who smoke cigarettes?*

Smoking represents the single most important preventable cause of death and disability in U.S. women (13). At every opportunity, women should be encouraged to quit smoking, regardless of hormonal contraception use.

Numerous epidemiologic studies conducted from the 1960s through the 1980s observed high relative risks of myocardial infarction among women who used OCs formulated with 50 μg or more of estrogen and smoked cigarettes, compared with women who neither smoked nor used OCs (14). The absolute rates of myocardial infarction in this study increased substantially among OC users who smoked and were in their mid-30s or older. Accordingly, package labeling for combination OCs was modified to warn clinicians and OC users of the risks associated with smoking among OC users in general and particularly among those aged 35 years and older.

Data are sparse on U.S. women older than 35 years who smoke and use OCs. Recently, epidemiologic studies assessing the risk of arterial events among U.S. women using contemporary OCs formulated with less than 50 μg of estrogen have been published. These large case–control studies found no evidence that use of these lower-dose contemporary formulations increased risks of myocardial infarction (2) or stroke (3) in nonsmokers or in women who smoked, regardless of their age. Reflecting current U.S. clinical practice, these studies included few OC users who were older than 35 years or who smoked. Therefore, unless other studies confirm the safety of contemporary combination OCs in older women who smoke, practitioners should prescribe combination OCs to such women with caution, if at all. Nonetheless, the recent U.S. studies provide evidence that combination OCs should not be denied to women younger than 30 years who smoke cigarettes (15). When considering OCs for women who are between the ages of 30 and 35 years and are smokers, the number of cigarettes smoked and the competing risk of pregnancy should be taken into account. In women who are older than 35 years and are smokers, the risk of using OCs is likely to exceed the risk of pregnancy.

▶ *Is combination OC use safe for women with chronic hypertension?*

Hypertension is a common condition associated with increased maternal and fetal risks should pregnancy occur, which emphasizes the importance of effective contraception for women with chronic hypertension.

Use of OCs appears to increase blood pressure, even with contemporary OC preparations. A small clinical trial found that an OC containing 30 μg of ethinyl estradiol and 150 μg of progestin increased the ambulatory blood pressure of normotensive women (approximately 8 mm Hg systolic and 6 mm Hg diastolic) (16). A small cross-sectional study of Italian women with mild hypertension found that those using combination OCs (most with 30 μg of estrogen) had ambulatory systolic blood pressures approximately 7 mm Hg higher than those not using OCs (17).

It is unclear if the use of contemporary OCs in women with hypertension increases the risk of vascular events. A large Danish case–control study of women with cerebral thromboembolism found that the risk of stroke was increased threefold in hypertensive women whether or not they used OCs (18). A large World Health Organization study conducted in developing and European countries observed that combination OC users with a history of hypertension had an increased risk of myocardial infarction and stroke (19). A pooled analysis of two U.S. population-based, case–control studies on OC use and myocardial infarction (2) and stroke (3) suggests that current OC use may not substantially increase the risk of stroke or myocardial infarction in women with hypertension. However, the studies included too few women who were hypertensive or older than 35 years to draw firm conclusions.

In healthy women of reproductive age, the incidence of myocardial infarction or stroke with use of low-dose OCs is extremely low. Although the relative risk of these conditions is increased in women with hypertension, the absolute risk remains low. In view of the increased risk of myocardial infarction and stroke associated with hypertension and uncertainty regarding additional risks of OCs, the decision to use OCs in these patients should be weighed against the risk of pregnancy associated with hypertension, and the noncontraceptive benefits of OCs should be taken into account. Women with well-controlled and monitored hypertension who are aged 35 years or younger are appropriate candidates for a trial of combination OCs formulated with 35 μg or less of estrogen, provided they are otherwise healthy, show no evidence of end-organ vascular disease, and do not smoke cigarettes. If blood pressure remains well-controlled with careful monitoring several months after initiating OCs, use can be continued.

Although coronary artery disease, congestive heart failure, and cerebrovascular disease are uncommon in women of reproductive age, the risk of pregnancy and delivery in these women can be substantial, making effective contraception important. Inadequate data are available to address the use of OCs in women with these conditions; therefore, given the increased risk of venous thromboembolism with combined OCs, their use is contraindicated. However, progestin-only contraceptives such as DMPA, progestin-only OCs, or levonorgestrel implants may be appropriate.

▶ *Is combination OC use safe for women with diabetes?*

Pregnancy in women with diabetes is associated with an array of serious maternal and perinatal complications, which emphasizes the importance of effective contraception in this patient population. In theory, the steroids in combination OCs might impair carbohydrate metabolism and accelerate the occurrence of vascular disease in diabetic women. Fortunately, current combination OCs do not appear to have this effect. In a cross-sectional U.S. study, 43 women with type 1 (formerly insulin-dependent) diabetes who used combination OCs for 1–7 years (mean duration, 3.4 years) were compared with a similar number of women with type 1 diabetes who were not using OCs. The overall mean age and duration of diabetes was 23 and 14 years, respectively, in this study group. Hemoglobin A_{1c} values were similar in the OC users and nonusers, which suggests that OC use did not affect control of diabetes. Likewise, the degree of nephropathy and retinopathy was similar in both groups, which suggests that OC use did not accelerate the development of diabetic vascular disease (20).

Although studies of OC use in women with type 2 (formerly non–insulin-dependent) diabetes have not been reported, two recent papers offer reassurance that combination OC use does not precipitate this disease. A prospective cohort study, which followed more than 98,000 U.S. women nurses, found that use of combination OCs did not significantly increase the risk of developing type 2 diabetes over a 4-year follow-up period; likewise, past use did not appear to increase risk (21). In a California population of Hispanic women with gestational diabetes followed for up to 7 years postpartum, use of combination OCs did not accelerate the development of type 2 diabetes. The use of progestin-only pills by the relatively small subgroup of women who nursed their infants was associated with a significantly increased risk of developing type 2 diabetes (22), an unexpected finding that is difficult to interpret.

Although the above data support the use of combination OCs in women with diabetes, based on theoretical concerns, such use should be limited to nonsmoking, otherwise healthy women with diabetes who are younger than 35 years and show no evidence of hypertension, nephropathy, retinopathy, or other vascular disease. Practitioners who provide contraception to women with diabetes should coordinate care with the physician treating the diabetes and follow such patients closely. Appropriate follow-up includes monitoring blood pressure, weight, and lipid status. Regardless of hormonal contraception use, women with the following risk factors should undergo blood glucose screening every 3 years: history of gestational diabetes, family history of diabetes in parents or siblings, obesity (body weight greater than 120% of ideal) or hypertension, and member of high-risk ethnic groups (African American, Hispanic, Native American).

▶ *Is combination OC use safe for women with migraine headaches?*

Headaches are a frequent occurrence in women of reproductive age. Most of these headaches are tension headaches, not migraines (23). Some women with migraines experience improvement in their symptoms with the use of OCs, while some women's symptoms worsen. However, in women using OCs, most migraines occur during the hormone-free interval. Because the presence of true migraine headaches affects the decision to use OCs, careful consideration of the diagnosis is important.

A large hospital-based case–control study performed at five European centers found that women with classic migraines (with aura) had a statistically significant fourfold increased risk of ischemic stroke; women with simple migraine (without aura) had a threefold increased risk that was not statistically significant (24). Women with a history of migraines using OCs (<50 μg of estrogen) had a greater than sixfold increased risk of ischemic stroke (not statistically significant [OR 6.6; 95% CI, 0.8–55]) when compared with women who were not using OCs and who had no migraine headaches. Compared with women who did not smoke, did not use OCs, and had no history of migraines, women who smoked, were using OCs, and had a history of migraines had a 34-fold increased risk of ischemic stroke (OR 34.4; 95% CI, 3.3–361).

A pooled analysis of two large, U.S. population-based case–control studies also observed a statistically significant twofold elevated risk of ischemic stroke, as well as hemorrhagic stroke (not statistically significant) among current users of OCs who reported migraine headaches compared with women with migraines who did not use OCs (3). A large Danish population-based case–control study found that among women with a history of migraine headaches, the risk of stroke was elevated approximately threefold ($P< 0.01$) (18). Neither study categorized migraines by type. The additional risk of thrombotic stroke attributable to women with migraines using OCs has been estimated as 8 per 100,000 women at age 20 years, and 80 per 100,000 women at age 40 years (25).

Although cerebrovascular events rarely occur among women with migraines who use combination OCs, the impact of a stroke on a woman of reproductive age is so devastating that clinicians should consider the use of progestin-only, intrauterine, or barrier contraceptives in this setting. Concerns remain that all women with migraines are at increased risk of stroke. However, because absolute risk remains low, the use of combination OCs may be considered for women with migraine headaches if they do not have focal neurologic signs, do not smoke, are otherwise healthy, and are younger than 35 years.

▶ *Does the use of combination OCs increase the risk of breast cancer in women with fibrocystic breast changes, fibroadenoma, or a family history of breast cancer?*

Women with fibroadenoma, benign breast disease with epithelial hyperplasia with or without atypia, or a family history of breast cancer have an increased risk of breast cancer (26). A recently published massive reanalysis of 54 studies assessing the association of OC use and breast cancer risk, however, provides reassurance to these women and to their clinicians regarding OC use. Overall, this reanalysis found that 10 years or more after discontinuing OC use, the risk of breast cancer was identical among these former OC users and those who never used OCs. Small but significantly increased relative risks (RR) were observed in current OC users (RR, 1.24) and those who had used OCs in the previous 1–4 years (RR, 1.16) or 5–9 years earlier (RR, 1.07). The increase in risk was restricted to women with localized disease; there was an associated reduced risk of metastatic disease, which suggests that much if not all of the risk can be attributed to early diagnosis of existing disease (27).

A positive family history of breast cancer in a mother or sister, or both, or a history of benign breast disease should not be regarded as contraindications to OC use. Use of OCs has an identical effect on the risk of breast cancer for women with and without each of these two risk categories (27).

▶ *What are the effects of combination OC use in women with uterine leiomyomata?*

Use of combination OCs reduces menstrual blood loss in women with normal menses as well as in those with menorrhagia (28). A Swedish study conducted in the 1960s using high-dose oral contraceptives, which are not currently used, noted OC use significantly reduced bleeding in women with menorrhagia associated with uterine fibroids (29). Oral contraceptive use also reduces dysmenorrhea (28). Some practitioners routinely employ the use of combination OCs as first-line medical management in women with menorrhagia or dysmenorrhea associated with uterine leiomyomata. Several large epidemiologic studies have observed that OC use does not induce the growth of uterine fibroids and may decrease bleeding disorders in these women (30–32).

▶ *Is combination OC use safe for women with lipid disorders?*

The term "dyslipidemia" includes disorders of lipoprotein metabolism that lead to atherosclerosis. These abnormalities arise from genetic and secondary factors and are caused by excessive entry of lipoproteins into the bloodstream, an impairment in their removal, or both.

The estrogen component of combination OCs enhances removal of low-density lipoprotein (LDL) and increases levels of high-density lipoprotein (HDL) cholesterol. Both of these actions can have a favorable effect on a woman's risk of coronary artery disease. Oral estrogen also increases triglyceride levels; however, in the setting of concomitantly increased HDL and decreased LDL levels, the moderate triglyceride elevations caused by oral estrogen use do not appear to increase the risk of atherogenesis. Numerous epidemiologic studies of past use of OCs find no increased risk of cardiovascular disease, arguing against any adverse long-term effect of OCs on the risk of atherogenesis (33). The progestin component of combination OCs antagonizes these estrogen-induced lipid changes, which increases LDL levels and decreases HDL and triglyceride levels. Accordingly, among women taking combination OCs with an identical dose of estrogen, the choice (and dose) of the progestin component affects net lipid changes. It is not known whether the differential lipid effects of distinct OC formulations have any clinical significance in women with normal baseline lipid levels or those with lipid disorders.

Using guidelines from the National Cholesterol Education Program (34), experts have recommended that most women with controlled dyslipidemia can use combination OCs formulated with 35 μg or less of estrogen. In contrast, in women with uncontrolled LDL cholesterol greater than 160 mg/dL or multiple additional risk factors for coronary artery disease (including smoking, diabetes, obesity, hypertension, family history of premature coronary artery disease, HDL level <35 mg/dL, or triglyceride level >250 mg/dL), use of alternative contraceptives should be considered (35). Fasting serum lipid levels should be monitored as frequently as each month after initiating combination OC use in dyslipidemic women; less frequent monitoring is appropriate once stabilization of lipid parameters has been observed.

Ongoing communication with the patient's primary care physician (or internist) is appropriate, and the importance of a low-fat diet, daily exercise, and the achievement of ideal body weight should be emphasized (22). Concomitant hormonal contraception and lipid-lowering therapy may be appropriate in some women.

▶ *What hormonal contraceptive options are available for postpartum and lactating women?*

Postpartum women remain in a hypercoagulable state for weeks after childbirth. Product labeling for combination OCs advises deferring use until 4 weeks postpartum in nonbreastfeeding women. Because first ovulation after delivery can occur in as little as 25 days (36), some practitioners initiate the use of combination OCs in nonbreastfeeding women as early as 2 weeks after childbirth, although no data support or refute the safety of this approach. Because progestin-only OCs, DMPA, and implants do not contain estrogen, these methods may be safely initiated immediately postpartum (37).

Combination OCs are not recommended as the first choice for breastfeeding mothers because of the negative effect of contraceptive doses of estrogen on lactation. The estrogenic component of combination OCs can reduce the volume of milk production and the caloric and mineral content of breast milk in lactating women (38). However, use of combination OCs by well-nourished breastfeeding women does not appear to result in infant development problems (38). Their use can be considered once milk flow is well established.

Progestin-only contraceptives do not impair lactation and, in fact, may increase the quality and duration of lactation (39). In nursing women using progestin-only OCs, very small amounts of progestin are passed into the breast milk, and no adverse effects on infant growth have been observed (40). Product labeling for progestin-only pills may suggest that fully breastfeeding women begin tablets 6 weeks postpartum and advise partially breastfeeding women to begin at 3 weeks.

Like other progestin-only methods, DMPA use does not adversely affect breastfeeding (38). Product labeling for DMPA advises initiation of use within the first 5 days postpartum if not breastfeeding and, if exclusively breastfeeding, at 6 weeks postpartum. When initiated immediately postpartum, however, use of DMPA does not adversely affect lactation (38) or infant development (41).

Product labeling for progestin subdermal implants indicates that insertion should be deferred until 6 weeks postpartum in lactating women. Studies of the effects of implant use on lactation and infant development investigated outcomes of insertion at least 30 days postpartum (42, 43). Although the results of these studies have been reassuring, data assessing immediate postpartum implant insertion in breastfeeding women are needed. Given the lack of procoagulation effect and the apparent safety in nursing mothers with DMPA and implants, their immediate postpartum use in both lactating and nonlactating women appears reasonable.

▶ *What hormonal contraceptive options are available for women taking concomitant medications?*

For women with seizure disorders, the frequency of seizures may increase during pregnancy (44). In addition, the risk of birth defects is intrinsically increased in these women (44). Finally, many anticonvulsants are teratogens (44). Each of these observations emphasizes the importance of providing effective contraception for women with seizure disorders.

Anticonvulsants that induce hepatic enzymes can decrease serum concentrations of the estrogen or progestin component of OCs, or both (45) (see the box, "Interaction of Anticonvulsants and Combination Oral Contraceptives"). This effect has been observed with phenobarbital (46), phenytoin, carbamazepine (47), felbamate (48), and topiramate (49). Therapeutic doses of vigabatrin do not induce hepatic enzymes. Nonetheless, a small clinical trial found ethinyl estradiol levels lower than during placebo use in two of 13 volunteers taking this anticonvulsant (50). Although each of these studies demonstrated reduced serum levels of OC steroids during anticonvulsant use, and many of them demonstrated associated breakthrough bleeding, investigators did not observe ovulation or accidental pregnancy during anticonvulsant use. Although some clinicians prescribe OCs containing 50 μg of ethinyl estradiol to women taking these anticonvulsants, no published data support the enhanced contraceptive efficacy of this practice. Use of condoms in conjunction with OCs or use of DMPA or an intrauterine device may be considered for such women (see the box).

In contrast to the above anticonvulsants, use of valproic acid (51), gabapentin (52), and tiagabine (53) does not appear to decrease serum levels of contraceptive steroids in women using combination OCs. Practitioners should be aware, however, that studies of the latter agents were performed using anticonvulsant doses lower than those used in clinical practice (54).

Interaction of Anticonvulsants and Combination Oral Contraceptives

Anticonvulsants that decrease steroid levels in women taking combination oral contraceptives

- Barbiturates (including phenobarbital and primidone)
- Phenytoin
- Carbamazepine
- Felbamate
- Topiramate
- Vigabatrin

Anticonvulsants that do not decrease steroid levels in women taking combination oral contraceptives

- Valproic acid
- Gabapentin*
- Lamotrigine*
- Tiagabine*

*Pharmacokinetic study used anticonvulsant dose lower than that usedin clinical practice.

Although there have been many anecdotal reports of OC failure in women taking concomitant antibiotics, pharmacokinetic evidence of lower serum steroid levels exists only for rifampin (55) and griseofulvin (56) (see the box, "Interaction of Antiinfective Agents and Combination Oral Contraceptives"). Because OC steroids are strikingly reduced in women concomitantly taking rifampin, such women should not rely on combination OCs, progestin-only OCs, or implants for contraceptive protection. Pharmacokinetic studies have not demonstrated lowered OC steroid levels with concomitant use of tetracycline (57), doxycycline (58), ampicillin or metronidazole (59), or quinolone antibiotics (60–62).

Interaction of Antiinfective Agents and Combination Oral Contraceptives

Antiinfective agents that decrease steroid levels in women taking combination oral contraceptives

- Rifampin
- Griseofulvin

Antiinfective agents that do not decrease steroid levels in women taking combination oral contraceptives

- Tetracycline
- Doxycycline
- Ampicillin
- Metronidazole
- Quinolone antibiotics

Serum progestin levels during use of progestin-only OCs and implants are lower than during combined OC use. Accordingly, these low-dose progestin-only contraceptives are not appropriate choices for women using concomitant liver enzyme inducers (40, 63). The contraceptive efficacy of DMPA in women taking hepatic enzyme inducers has not been explicitly studied. A potential advantage of using DMPA in women with seizure disorders is DMPA's intrinsic anticonvulsant effect (23).

▶ *Is hormonal contraceptive use safe for women with a history of thromboembolism?*

The estrogenic component of combination OCs, which increases hepatic production of serum globulins involved in coagulation (including factor VII, factor X, and fibrinogen), increases the risk of VTE in users. Beginning in 1995, European studies clarified that, compared with nonusers, current users of OCs formulated with 35 μg or less of estrogen experience a threefold to fourfold increased risk of VTE. This risk, in absolute terms, remains lower than the increased risk of VTE during pregnancy.

The goal of screening OC candidates with respect to VTE risk is to identify those women for whom the VTE risk associated with OC use outweighs OC benefits. In addition to current use of exogenous estrogens, risk factors for VTE include pregnancy and the puerperium, personal or family history of VTE, obesity, surgery, and certain familial coagulation disorders. Although cigarette smoking, hypertension, and diabetes represent risk factors for arterial disease, including myocardial infarction and stroke, they do not increase VTE risk (64). Likewise, the presence of superficial varicose veins does not increase VTE risk (64). Health risks (including VTE) associated with pregnancy, noncontraceptive OC benefits, and the potential for effective use of contraceptives that do not increase VTE risk (eg, progestin-only OCs and intrauterine and barrier methods) should all be factored into risk–benefit considerations. Practitioners should be aware that package labeling for DMPA and for certain brands of progestin-only OCs inappropriately indicates that a history of VTE contraindicates the use of these progestin-only methods.

Women with a documented history of unexplained VTE or VTE associated with pregnancy or exogenous estrogen use should not use combination OCs unless they are currently taking anticoagulants. An OC candidate who had experienced a single episode of VTE years earlier associated with a nonrecurring risk factor (eg, VTE occurring after immobilization following a motor vehicle accident) may not currently be at increased risk for VTE. Accordingly, the decision to initiate combination OCs in such a candidate can be individualized.

▶ *Should women awaiting surgery discontinue combination OC use?*

Venous thromboembolism with pulmonary embolism remains a major cause of fatalities associated with surgical (including gynecologic) procedures. Findings of a large British prospective cohort study suggested that the risk of postoperative VTE was approximately twice as high ($P>0.05$) in OC users as in nonusers (65). A prospective study found that, among women taking OCs formulated with 30 μg of estrogen, OC-induced procoagulant changes did not substantially resolve until 6 or more weeks after OC discontinuation (66). Accordingly, the risks associated with stopping OCs 1 month or more before major surgery should be balanced against the risks of an unintended pregnancy (67). In current OC users having major surgical procedures, heparin prophylaxis should be considered (67). Because of the low perioperative risk of VTE, it currently is not considered necessary to discontinue combination OCs before laparoscopic tubal sterilization or other brief surgical procedures.

▶ *Is OC use safe in women with hypercoagulable states?*

Women with factor V Leiden mutation who use OCs experience a risk of VTE 30 times higher than non-OC users who are not carriers of the mutation (68). A clotting assay can determine activated protein C resistance, and a polymerase chain reaction test can identify the presence of factor V Leiden mutation. Such screening would identify approximately 5% of U.S. OC candidates as having factor V Leiden mutation; however, the great majority of these women will never experience VTE, even if they use combination OCs (69). Given the rarity of fatal VTE, one group of investigators concluded that screening more than 1 million combination OC candidates for thrombophilic markers would, at best, prevent two OC-associated deaths (70). Some practitioners may choose to test for factor V Leiden mutation in women with a positive family history of VTE who are considering OC use or pregnancy. In this setting, the clinician should weigh factors including age of onset of thrombosis in affected family members, the clinical setting, and severity of thrombotic episodes. The risks, benefits, and financial implications of such selective testing, however, are unknown.

Women using warfarin for chronic anticoagulation may experience menorrhagia and, rarely, hemoperitoneum following rupture of ovarian cysts. In addition, warfarin is a teratogen. Because use of combination OCs can reduce menstrual blood loss (28) and does not increase the risk of recurrent thrombosis in well-anticoagulated women (69, 71), some authorities recommend their use in such patients. Because intramuscular injection of DMPA consistently suppresses ovulation (72), DMPA represents another potential contraceptive choice in anticoagulated women.

▶ *Does the use of emergency contraception increase the risk of VTE?*

Use of postcoital (emergency) contraception may increase in the United States with the recent availability of a dedicated product. A recent retrospective cohort analysis from Britain found no cases of thromboembolism in more than 100,000 episodes of postcoital contraception use with the Yuzpe regimen (73).

▶ *Are hormonal contraceptives safe for women with SLE?*

Because the risks of maternal and perinatal morbidity as well as mortality can be high in pregnancies complicated by SLE, effective contraception is an important component of the care of such women. Particular concerns about hormonal contraception use in women with SLE relate to the increased risk of venous and arterial thrombosis in women with this disease. A small retrospective cohort study noted that while combination OC use was associated with flare-ups in SLE patients with renal disease, progestin-only OC use was not associated with increased disease activity (74). One retrospective cohort study of 85 women with SLE noted that among 31 patients using combination OCs, increased disease activity was not precipitated by OC use. However, deep vein thrombosis was diagnosed in two OC users; both of these women had antiphospholipid antibodies (75). A small prospective cohort study found that use of progestin-only OCs or contraceptive injections was not associated with increased SLE activity (76).

Existing data from observational studies suggest that combination OC use should be avoided in SLE patients with a history of vascular disease, nephritis, or antiphospholipid antibodies, although progestin-only methods are safe alternatives. Data are insufficient to address the use of combination OCs among women with stable or inactive disease who have no history of thrombosis, nephropathy, or antiphospholipid antibodies (77). If such women do not wish to use progestin-only methods, use of combination OCs with close monitoring can be considered in selected cases.

▶ *Is hormonal contraceptive use safe for women with sickle cell disease?*

In persons with sickle cell disease, abnormal hemoglobin precipitates and becomes rigid when subjected to oxygen deprivation. Vasoocclusive episodes in those with sickle cell disease, however, differ from intravascular thrombosis (78). Pregnancy in women with sickle cell disease carries increased risks of maternal complications and is associated with elevated rates of spontaneous abortion, intrauterine growth restriction, and neonatal mortality.

No well-controlled study has assessed whether VTE risk in OC users with sickle cell disease is higher than in other combination OC users. Accordingly, recommendations regarding use of combination OCs in this patient population vary widely. On the basis of studies of pregnant women with sickle cell disease, small observational studies of women with sickle cell disease who use combination OCs, and theoretical considerations, the consensus is that pregnancy carries a greater risk than combination OC use.

Two controlled studies have assessed the use of DMPA in women with sickle cell disease (79, 80). Both of these found that use of DMPA reduced the incidence of painful crises. Accordingly, DMPA may be a particularly appropriate contraceptive for women with sickle cell disease.

▶ *What are the effects of DMPA on bone density?*

Use of DMPA in contraceptive doses suppresses ovarian production of estradiol. Thus, there has been concern that women using DMPA for contraception might develop osteopenia. A New Zealand study of women who used DMPA for at least 5 years found significantly reduced bone density in the lumbar spine and femoral neck compared with premenopausal controls (81). A subsequent study performed by the same investigator noted that among women who had used DMPA for at least 3 years, deficits in BMD of the lumbar spine were reversible following DMPA discontinuation (82). Five recent cross-sectional studies suggest that DMPA use decreases BMD of the spine (83–87). In the largest of these studies, the median duration of DMPA use was 12 years. In this study, initiation of DMPA use before age 21 years and use for more than 15 years were identified as risk factors for osteopenia (84). None of these cross-sectional studies found evidence of osteoporosis or fractures in DMPA users.

Information on the effects of DMPA use on BMD during adolescence is limited. However, a small study compared BMD of the lumbar spine in females aged 12–21 years. In this prospective cohort study, BMD in those using no hormones was compared with those using DMPA, OCs, or implants. After 1 year of use, bone density in DMPA users decreased 1.5%, whereas it increased 1.5% in OC users, 2.5% in levonorgestrel implant users, and 2.9% in those using no hormones. None of those who initially selected an OC continued after 2 years. However, follow-up BMD measurements at 2 years showed a total decrease of 3.1% in DMPA users and total increases of 9.5% in nonhormone users and 9.3% in implant users (88).

The rate-of-loss trends in BMD seen with DMPA seem to be similar to those noted during lactation (89, 90) in that no long-term decrease occurs. Two recent cross-sectional studies of menopausal women found no long-term BMD declines in former DMPA users. In these reports, BMD in former DMPA users was not significantly different from never-users (91, 92). Estrogen supplementation (eg, conjugated estrogen, 1.25 mg daily, or equivalent doses of other estrogens) can be considered for long-term users of DMPA, including adolescents. However, no data address the effect of such an add-back regimen on BMD in women using DMPA. Caution should be exercised in prescribing DMPA for adolescents, women known to be at high risk for low BMD, and perimenopausal women.

Summary

The following recommendations are based on good and consistent scientific evidence (Level A):

- Women with fibroadenoma, benign breast disease with epithelial hyperplasia with or without atypia, or a family history of breast cancer are at little or no additional risk of breast cancer because of OC use. Therefore, OCs can be prescribed for such women if they are otherwise appropriate candidates.
- Progestin-only preparations are safe and preferable forms of hormonal contraception for lactating women. Combination OCs are not recommended as the first choice for breastfeeding mothers because of the negative impact of contraceptive doses of estrogen on lactation. However, use of combination OCs by well-nourished breastfeeding women does not appear to result in infant development problems; therefore, their use can be considered once milk flow is well established.
- Hormonal contraceptive effectiveness is compromised by the use of the antibiotics rifampin and griseofulvin; thus, women taking these antibiotics should use nonhormonal contraceptives.
- Progestin-only preparations are appropriate for women at increased risk for VTE. Combination OCs

are not recommended for women with a documented history of unexplained VTE or VTE associated with pregnancy or exogenous estrogen use, unless they are taking anticoagulants.

- Combination OCs should be prescribed with caution, if ever, to women who are older than 35 years and are smokers. Women younger than 30 years who smoke and are otherwise healthy generally can be prescribed combination OCs.
- If desired, healthy, nonsmoking women doing well on combination OCs may continue their use until menopause.

The following recommendations are based on limited or inconsistent scientific evidence (Level B):

- Women with well-controlled and monitored hypertension aged 35 years and younger are appropriate candidates for a trial of combination OCs formulated with 35 μg or less of estrogen, provided they are otherwise healthy with no evidence of end-organ vascular disease and do not smoke cigarettes. If blood pressure remains well-controlled several months after initiating OCs, use can be continued.
- The use of combination OCs by women with diabetes should be limited to such women who do not smoke, are younger than 35 years, and are otherwise healthy with no evidence of hypertension, nephropathy, retinopathy, or other vascular disease.
- Women with migraine headaches who have focal neurologic signs are not appropriate candidates for OC use. Combination OCs can be used by women with simple migraine headaches (ie, no focal neurologic signs) if they do not smoke, are younger than 35 years, and are otherwise healthy. If such women experience increased frequency or severity of headaches or develop headaches with focal neurologic signs or symptoms, they should discontinue OC use.
- Combination OCs may be beneficial in treating dysmenorrhea and menorrhagia in women with uterine fibroids.
- The risks associated with stopping OCs 1 month or more before major surgery should be balanced against the risks of an unintended pregnancy. In current OC users undergoing major surgical procedures, heparin prophylaxis should be considered. Because of the low perioperative risk of VTE, it generally is considered unnecessary to discontinue combination OCs before laparoscopic tubal sterilization or other brief surgical procedures.
- Progestin-only OCs and contraceptive injections appear to be the hormonal contraception methods of choice for women with SLE. Use of combination OCs in women with SLE can be considered if the women have stable or inactive disease and no history of thrombosis, nephropathy, or antiphospholipid antibodies.

The following recommendations are based primarily on consensus and expert opinion (Level C):

- Most women with controlled dyslipidemia can use combination OCs formulated with 35 μg or less of estrogen. In women with uncontrolled LDL cholesterol greater than 160 mg/dL, a triglyceride level greater than 250 mg/dL, or multiple additional risk factors for coronary artery disease, alternative contraceptives should be considered.
- DMPA has noncontraceptive benefits and is the contraceptive method of choice for many women with sickle cell disease.
- Progestin-only contraceptives may be appropriate for women with coronary artery disease, congestive heart failure, or cerebrovascular disease. However, combination oral contraceptives are contraindicated in these women.

References

1. Corfman P. Labeling guidance text for progestin-only oral contraceptives. Contraception 1995;52:71–76 (Level III)
2. Sidney S, Siscovick DS, Petitti DB, Schwartz SM, Quesenberry CP, Psaty BM, et al. Myocardial infarction and use of low-dose oral contraceptives: a pooled analysis of 2 US studies. Circulation 1998;98:1058–1063 (Level II-2)
3. Schwartz SM, Petitti DB, Siscovick DS, Longstreth WT Jr, Sidney S, Raghunathan TE, et al. Stroke and use of low-dose oral contraceptives in young women: a pooled analysis of two US studies. Stroke 1998;29:2277–2284 (Level II-2)
4. Gambacciani M, Spinetti A, Taponeco F, Cappagli B, Piaggesi L, Fioretti P. Longitudinal evaluation of perimenopausal vertebral bone loss: effects of a low-dose oral contraceptive preparation on bone mineral density and metabolism. Obstet Gynecol 1994;83:392–396 (Level I)
5. Sulak PJ. Oral contraceptives: therapeutic uses and quality-of-life benefits—case presentations. Contraception 1999;59(suppl):35S–38S (Level III)
6. Casper RF, Dodin S, Reid RL. The effect of 20 μg ethinyl estradiol/1 mg norethindrone acetate (Minestrin), a low-dose oral contraceptive, on vaginal bleeding patterns, hot flashes, and quality of life in symptomatic perimenopausal women. Menopause 1997;4:139–147 (Level I)
7. Gebbie AE, Glasier A, Sweeting V. Incidence of ovulation in perimenopausal women before and during hormone replacement therapy. Contraception 1995;52:221–222 (Level II-3)

8. Burger HG. Diagnostic role of follicle-stimulating hormone (FSH) measurements during the menopausal transition—an analysis of FSH, oestradiol and inhibin. Eur J Endocrinol 1994;130:38–42 (Level III)

9. Castracane VD, Gimpel T, Goldzieher JW. When is it safe to switch from oral contraceptives to hormonal replacement therapy? Contraception 1995;52:371–376 (Level II-2)

10. Creinin MD. Laboratory criteria for menopause in women using oral contraceptives. Fertil Steril 1996;66:101–104 (Level II-3)

11. Stanford JL, Hartge P, Brinton LA, Hoover RN, Brookmeyer R. Factors influencing the age at natural menopause. J Chronic Dis 1987;40:995–1002 (Level II-3)

12. McKinlay SM, Bifano NL, McKinlay JB. Smoking and age at menopause in women. Ann Intern Med 1985;103: 350–356 (Level II)

13. American College of Obstetricians and Gynecologists. Smoking and women's health. ACOG Educational Bulletin 240. Washington, DC: ACOG, 1997 (Level III)

14. Croft P, Hannaford PC. Risk factors for acute myocardial infarction in women: evidence from the Royal College of General Practitioners' oral contraception study. BMJ 1989;298:165–168 (Level II-2)

15. Schwingl PJ, Ory HW, Visness CM. Estimates of the risk of cardiovascular death attributable to low-dose oral contraceptives in the United States. Am J Obstet Gynecol 1999;180:241–249 (Level III)

16. Cardoso F, Polonia J, Santos A, Silva-Carvalho J, Ferreira-de-Almeida J. Low-dose oral contraceptives and 24-hour ambulatory blood pressure. Int J Gynaecol Obstet 1997;59:237–243 (Level II-3)

17. Narkiewicz K, Graniero GR, D'Este D, Mattarei M, Zonzin P, Palatini P. Ambulatory blood pressure in mild hypertensive women taking oral contraceptives. A case-control study. Am J Hyperten 1995;8:249–253 (Level II-2)

18. Lidegaard O. Oral contraceptives, pregnancy and the risk of cerebral thromboembolism: the influence of diabetes, hypertension, migraine and previous thrombotic disease. Br J Obstet Gynaecol 1996;102:153–159 (Level II-2)

19. WHO Collaborative Study of Cardiovascular Disease and Steroid Hormone Contraception. Ischemic stroke and combined oral contraceptives: results of an international, multicentre, case-control study. Lancet 1996;348:498–505 (Level II-2)

20. Garg SK, Chase HP, Marshall G, Hoops SL, Holmes DL, Jackson WE. Oral contraceptives and renal and retinal complications in young women with insulin-dependent diabetes mellitus. JAMA 1994;271:1099–1102 (Level II-2)

21. Chasan-Taber L, Willett WC, Stampfer MJ, Hunter DJ, Colditz GA, Spiegelman D, et al. A prospective study of oral contraceptives and NIDDM among U.S. women. Diabetes Care 1997;20:330–335 (Level II-2)

22. Kjos SL, Peters RK, Xiang A, Thomas D, Schaefer U, Buchanan T. Contraception and the risk of type 2 diabetes mellitus in Latina women with prior gestational diabetes mellitus. JAMA 1998;28:533–538 (Level II-3)

23. Mattson RH, Rebar RW. Contraceptive methods for women with neurologic disorders. Am J Obstet Gynecol 1993;168(6 Pt 2):2027–2032 (Level II-3)

24. Chang CL, Donaghy M, Poulter N. Migraine and stroke in young women: case control study. The World Health Organisation Collaborative Study of Cardiovascular Disease and Steroid Hormone Contraception. BMJ 1999;318:13–18 (Level II-2)

25. MacGregor EA, Guillebaud J. Combined oral contraceptives, migraine and ischaemic stroke. Clinical and Scientific Committee of the Faculty of Family Planning and Reproductive Health Care and the Family Planning Association. Br J Fam Plann 1998;24:53–60 (Level III)

26. Dupont WD, Page DL. Risk factors for breast cancer in women with proliferative breast disease. N Engl J Med 1985;312:146–151 (Level II-2)

27. Collaborative Group on Hormonal Factors in Breast Cancer. Breast cancer and hormonal contraceptives: collaborative reanalysis of individual data on 53,297 women with breast cancer and 100,239 women without breast cancer from 54 epidimiological studies. Lancet 1996;347: 1713–1727 (Level III)

28. Larsson G, Milsom I, Lindstedt G, Rybo G. The influence of a low-dose combined oral contraceptive on menstrual blood loss and iron status. Contraception 1992;46: 327–334 (Level III)

29. Nilsson L, Rybo G. Treatment of menorrhagia. Am J Obstet Gynecol 1971;110:713–720 (Level II-2)

30. Ross RK, Pike MC, Vessey MP, Bull D, Yeates D, Casagrande JT. Risk factors for uterine fibroids: reduced risk associated with oral contraceptives. BMJ (Clin Res Ed) 1986;293:359–362 (Level II-2)

31. Marshall LM, Spiegelman D, Goldman MB, Manson JE, Colditz GA, Barbieri RL, et al. A prospective study of reproductive factors and oral contraceptive use in relation to the risk of uterine leiomyomata. Fertil Steril 1998;70: 432–439 (Level II-2)

32. Parazzini F, Negri E, LaVecchia C, Fedele L, Rabaiotti M, Luchini L. Oral contraceptive use and risk of uterine fibroids. Obstet Gynecol 1992;79:430–433 (Level II-2)

33. Chasen-Taber L, Stampfer MJ. Epidemiology of oral contraceptives and cardiovascular disease. Ann Intern Med 1998;128:467–477 (Level III)

34. National Cholesterol Education Program Expert Panel on Detection, Evaluation, and Treatment of High Blood Cholesterol in Adults. Report of the National Cholesterol Education Program Expert Panel on Detection, Evaluation, and Treatment of High Blood Cholesterol in Adults. Arch Intern Med 1988;148:36–69 (Level III)

35. Knopp RH, LaRosa JC, Burkman RT Jr. Contraception and dyslipidemia. Am J Obstet Gynecol 1993;168: 1994–2005 (Level III)

36. Campbell OM, Gray RH. Characteristics and determinants of postpartum ovarian function in women in the United States. Am J Obstet Gynecol 1993;169:55–60 (Level II-2)

37. American College of Obstetricians and Gynecologists. Hormonal contraception. ACOG Technical Bulletin 198. Washington, DC: ACOG, 1994 (Level III)

38. World Health Organization (WHO) Task Force on Oral Contraceptives. Effects of hormonal contraceptives on breast milk composition and infant growth. Stud Fam Plann 1988;19(6 Pt 1):361–369 (Level II-2)

39. Koetsawang S. The effects of contraceptive methods on the quality and quantity of breast milk. Int J Gynaecol Obstet 1987;25(suppl):115–127 (Level III)

40. McCann MF, Potter LS. Progestin-only oral contraception: a comprehensive review. Contraception 1994;50(suppl 1): S1–S195 (Level III)

41. Karim M, Ammar R, el-Mahgoub S, el-Ganzoury B, Fikri F, Abdou I. Injected progestogen and lactation. BMJ 1971;1:200–203 (Level II-2)

42. Shaaban MM, Salem HT, Abdullah KA. Influence of levonorgestrel contraceptive implants, Norplant, initiated early postpartum upon lactation and infant growth. Contraception 1985;32:623–635 (Level II-2)

43. Abdulla KA, Elwan SI, Salem HS, Shaaban MM. Effect of early postpartum use of the contraceptive implants, NORPLANT, on the serum levels of immunoglobulins of the mothers and their breastfed infants. Contraception 1985;32:261–266 (Level II-2)

44. O'Brien MD, Gilmour-White S. Epilepsy and pregnancy. BMJ 1993;307:492–495 (Level III)

45. Back DJ, Orme ML. Pharmacokinetic drug interactions with oral contraceptives. Clin Pharmacokinet 1990;18: 472–484 (Level III)

46. Back DJ, Bates M, Bowden A, Breckenridge AM, Hall MJ, Jones H, et al. The interaction of phenobarbital and other anticonvulsants with oral contraceptive steroid therapy. Contraception 1980;22:495–503 (Level II-3)

47. Crawford P, Chadwick DJ, Martin C, Tjia J, Back DJ, Orme M. The interaction of phenytoin and carbamazepine with combined oral contraceptive steroids. Br J Clin Pharmacol 1990;30:892–896 (Level II-3)

48. Saano V, Glue P, Banfield CR, Reidenberg P, Colucci RD, Meehan JW, et al. Effects of felbamate on the pharmacokinetics of a low-dose combination oral contraceptive. Clin Pharmacol Ther 1995;58:523–531 (Level I)

49. Rosenfeld WE, Doose DR, Walker SA, Nayak RK. Effect of topiramate on the pharmacokinetics of an oral contraceptive containing norethindrone and ethinyl estradiol in patients with epilepsy. Epilepsia 1997;38:317–323 (Level II-3)

50. Bartoli A, Gatti G, Cipolla G, Barzaghi N, Veliz G, Fattore C, et al. A double-blind, placebo-controlled study on the effect of vigabatrin on in vivo parameters of hepatic microsomal enzyme induction and on the kinetics of steroid oral contraceptives in healthy female volunteers. Epilepsia 1997;38:702–707 (Level I)

51. Crawford P, Chadwick D, Cleland P, Tjia J, Cowie A, Back DJ, et al. The lack of effect of sodium valproate on the pharmacokinetics of oral contraceptive steroids. Contraception 1986;33:23–29 (Level II-3)

52. Eldon MA, Underwood BA, Randinitis EJ, Sedman AJ. Gabapentin does not interact with a contraceptive regimen of norethindrone acetate and ethinyl estradiol. Neurology 1998;50:1146–1148 (Level II-3)

53. Mengel HB, Houston A, Back DJ. An evaluation of the interaction between tiagabine and oral contraceptives in female volunteers. J Pharm Med 1994;4:141–150 (Level II-3)

54. Natsch S, Hekster YA, Keyser A, Deckers CL, Meinardi H, Renier WO. Newer anticonvulsant drugs: role of pharmacology, drug interactions and adverse reactions in drug choice. Drug Saf 1997;17:228–240 (Level III)

55. Back DJ, Breckenridge AM, Crawford F, MacIver M, Orme ML, Park BK, et al. The effect of rifampicin on norethisterone pharmacokinetics. Euro J Clin Pharmacol 1979;15:193–197 (Level III)

56. Geurts TB, Goorissen EM, Sitsen JM. Summary of drug interactions with oral contraceptives. Pearl River, New York: Parthenon Publishing, 1993:27–124 (Level III)

57. Murphy AA, Zacur HA, Charache P, Burkman RT. The effect of tetracycline on levels of oral contraceptives. Am J Obstet Gynecol 1991;164(1 Pt 1):28–33 (Level II-3)

58. Neely JL, Abate M, Swinker M, D'Angio R. The effect of doxycycline on serum levels of ethinyl estradiol, norethindrone, and endogenous progesterone. Obstet Gynecol 1991;77:416–420 (Level II-2)

59. Joshi JV, Joshi UM, Sankholi GM, Krishna U, Mandlekar A, Chowdhury V, et al. A study of interaction of low-dose combination oral contraceptive with ampicillin and metronidazole. Contraception 1980;22:643–652 (Level II-2)

60. Maggiolo F, Puricelli G, Dottorini M, Caprioli S, Bianchi W, Suter F. The effect of ciprofloxacin on oral contraceptive steroid treatments. Drugs Exp Clin Res 1991;17: 451–454 (Level II-1)

61. Back DJ, Tjia J, Martin C, Millar E, Mant T, Morrison P, et al. The lack of interaction between temafloxacin and combined oral contraceptive steroids. Contraception 1991;43:317–323 (Level II-2)

62. Csemiczky G, Alvendal C, Landgren BM. Risk for ovulation in women taking a low-dose oral contraceptive (Microgynon) when receiving antibacterial treatment with a fluoroquinolone (ofloxacin). Adv Contracep 1996;12: 101–109 (Level II-1)

63. Haukkamaa M. Contraception by Norplant subdermal capsules is not reliable in epileptic patients on anticonvulsant treatment. Contraception 1986;33:559–565 (Level II-3)

64. World Health Organization. Cardiovascular disease and steroid hormone contraception. Report of a WHO Scientific Group. World Health Organ Tech Rep Ser 1998;877:i-vii,1–89 (Level III)

65. Vessey M, Mant D, Smith A, Yeates D. Oral contraceptives and venous thromboembolism: findings in a large prospective study. BMJ (Clin Res Ed) 1986;292:526 (Level II-2)

66. Robinson GE, Burren T, Mackie IJ, Bounds W, Walshe K, Faint R, et al. Changes in haemostasis after stopping the combined contraceptive pill: implications for major surgery. BMJ 1991;302:269–271 (Level II-3)

67. Bonnar J. Can more be done in obstetric and gynecologic practice to reduce morbidity and mortality associated with venous thromboembolism? Am J Obstet Gynecol 1999; 180:784–791(Level III)

68. Vandenbroucke JP, Koster T, Briet E, Reitsma PH, Bertina RM, Rosendaal FR. Increased risk of venous thrombosis in oral-contraceptive users who are carriers of factor V Leiden mutation. Lancet 1994;344:1453–1457 (Level II-2)

69. Comp PC. Thrombophilic mechanisms of OCs. Int J Fertil Womens Med 1997;42 (suppl 1):170–176 (Level III)

70. Price DT, Ridker PM. Factor V Leiden mutation and the risks for thromboembolic disease: a clinical perspective. Ann Intern Med 1997;127:895–903 (Level III)

71. Comp PC, Zacur HA. Contraceptive choices in women with coagulation disorders. Am J Obtset Gynecol 1993;168:1990–1993 (Level III)

72. Mishell DR Jr. Pharmacokinetics of depot medroxyprogesterone acetate contraception. J Reprod Med 1996; 41(suppl):381–390 (Level III)

73. Vasilakis C, Jick SS, Jick H. The risk of venous thromboembolism in users of postcoital contraceptive pills. Contraception 1999;59:79–83 (Level II-2)

74. Jungers P, Dougados M, Pelissier C, Kuttenn F, Tron F, Lesavre P, et al. Influence of oral contraceptive therapy on the activity of systemic lupus erythematosus. Arthritis Rheum 1982:25:618–623 (Level III)

75. Julkunen HA. Oral contraceptives in systemic lupus erythematosus: side-effects and influence on the activity of SLE. Scand J Rheumatol 1991;20:427–433 (Level III)

76. Mintz G, Gutierrez G, Deleze M, Rodriguez E. Contraception with progestagens in systemic lupus erythematosus. Contraception 1984;30:29–58 (Level II-2)

77. Petri M, Robinson C. Oral contraceptives and systemic lupus erythematosus. Arthritis Rheum 1997;40:797–803 (Level III)

78. Charache S, Niebyl JR. Pregnancy in sickle cell disease. Clin Haematol 1985;14:729–746 (Level III)

79. De Ceulaer K, Gruber C, Hayes R, Serjeant GR. Medroxyprogesterone acetate and homozygous sickle-cell disease. Lancet 1982;2:229–231 (Level II-2)

80. de Abood M, de Castillo Z, Guerrero F, Espino M, Austin KL. Effect of Depo-Provera or Microgynon on the painful crises of sickle cell anemia patients. Contraception 1997;56:313–316 (Level I)

81. Cundy T, Evans M, Roberts H, Wattie D, Ames R, Reid IR. Bone density in women receiving depot medroxyprogesterone acetate for contraception. BMJ 1991;303:13–16 (Level II-2)

82. Cundy T, Cornish J, Evans M, Roberts H, Reid IR. Recovery of bone density in women who stop using medroxyprogesterone acetate. BMJ 1994;308:247–248 (Level II-2)

83. Gbolade B, Ellis S, Murby B, Randall S, Kirkman R. Bone density in the long term users of depot medroxyprogesterone acetate. Br J Obstet Gynaecol 1998;105:790–794 (Level II-3)

84. Cundy T, Cornish J, Roberts H, Elder H, Reid IR. Spinal bone density in women using depot medroxyprogesterone contraception. Obstet Gynecol 1998;92:569–573 (Level II-2)

85. Paiva LC, Pinto-Neto AM, Faundes A. Bone density among long-term users of medroxyprogesterone acetate as a contraceptive. Contraception 1998;58:351–355 (Level II-2)

86. Scholes D, Lacroix AZ, Ott SM, Ichikawa LE, Barlow WE. Bone mineral density in women using depot medroxyprogesterone acetate for contraception. Obstet Gynecol 1999;93:233–238 (Level II-2)

87. Tang OS, Tang G, Yip P, Li B, Fan S. Long-term depot-medroxyprogesterone acetate and bone mineral density. Contraception 1999;59:25–29 (Level II-2)

88. Cromer BA, Blair JM, Mahan JD, Zibners L, Naumovski Z. A prospective comparison of bone density in adolescent girls receiving depot medroxyprogesterone acetate (Depo-Provera), levonorgestrel (Norplant), or oral contraceptives. J Pediatr 1996;129:671–676 (Level II-2)

89. Kolthoff N, Eiken P, Kristensen B, Nielsen SP. Bone mineral changes during pregnancy and lactation: a longitudinal cohort study. Clin Sci (Colch) 1998;94:405–412 (Level II-3)

90. Kalkwarf HJ, Specker BL, Bianchi DC, Ranz J, Ho M. The effect of calcium supplementation on bone density during lactation and after weaning. N Engl J Med 1997;337:523–528 (Level I)

91. Orr-Walker BJ, Evans MC, Ames RW, Clearwater JM, Cundy TR, Reid IR. The effect of past use of the injectable contraceptive depot medroxyprogesterone acetate on bone mineral density in normal post-menopausal women. Clin Endocrinol (Oxf) 1998;49:615–618 (Level II-3)

92. Petitti DB, Piaggio G, Mehta S, Cravioto MC, Meirik O. Steroid hormone contraception and bone mineral density: a cross sectional study in an international population. Obstet Gynecol 2000;95:736–744 (Level II-3)

The MEDLINE database, the Cochrane Library, and ACOG's own internal resources and documents were used to conduct a literature search to locate relevant articles published between January 1985 and March 1998. The search was restricted to articles published in the English language. Priority was given to articles reporting results of original research, although review articles and commentaries also were consulted. Abstracts of research presented at symposia and scientific conferences were not considered adequate for inclusion in this document. Guidelines published by organizations or institutions such as the National Institutes of Health and the American College of Obstetricians and Gynecologists were reviewed, and additional studies were located by reviewing bibliographies of identified articles. When reliable research was not available, expert opinions from obstetrician–gynecologists were used.

Studies were reviewed and evaluated for quality according to the method outlined by the U.S. Preventive Services Task Force:

- I Evidence obtained from at least one properly designed randomized controlled trial.
- II-1 Evidence obtained from well-designed controlled trials without randomization.
- II-2 Evidence obtained from well-designed cohort or case–control analytic studies, preferably from more than one center or research group.
- II-3 Evidence obtained from multiple time series with or without the intervention. Dramatic results in uncontrolled experiments also could be regarded as this type of evidence.
- III Opinions of respected authorities, based on clinical experience, descriptive studies, or reports of expert committees.

Based on the highest level of evidence found in the data, recommendations are provided and graded according to the following catetories:

Level A—Recommendations are based on good and consistent scientific evidence.

Level B—Recommendations are based on limited or inconsistent scientific evidence.

Level C—Recommendations are based primarily on consensus and expert opinion.

ISSN 1099-3630

The American College of Obstetricians and Gynecologists
409 12th Street, SW
PO Box 96920
Washington, DC 20090-6920

12345/32109

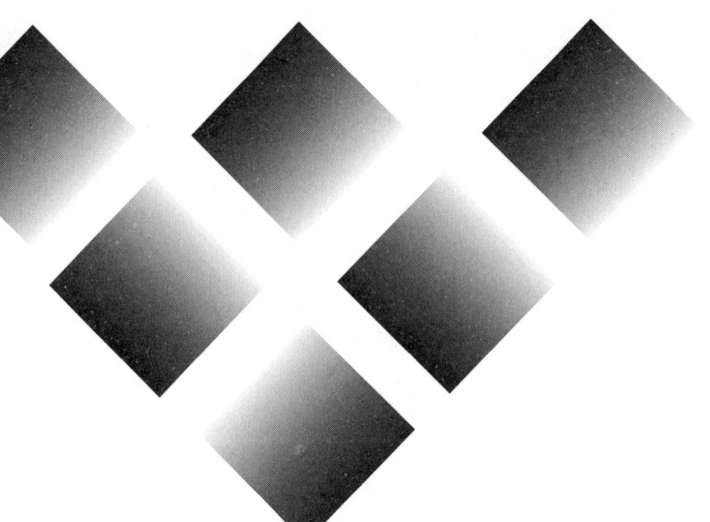

ACOG PRACTICE BULLETIN

CLINICAL MANAGEMENT GUIDELINES FOR OBSTETRICIAN–GYNECOLOGISTS
NUMBER 6, SEPTEMBER 1999

This Practice Bulletin was developed by the ACOG Committee on Practice Bulletins—Obstetrics with the assistance of Robert M. Silver, MD, Richard L. Berkowitz, MD, and James Bussel, MD. The information is designed to aid practitioners in making decisions about appropriate obstetric and gynecologic care. These guidelines should not be construed as dictating an exclusive course of treatment or procedure. Variations in practice may be warranted based on the needs of the individual patient, resources, and limitations unique to the institution or type of practice.

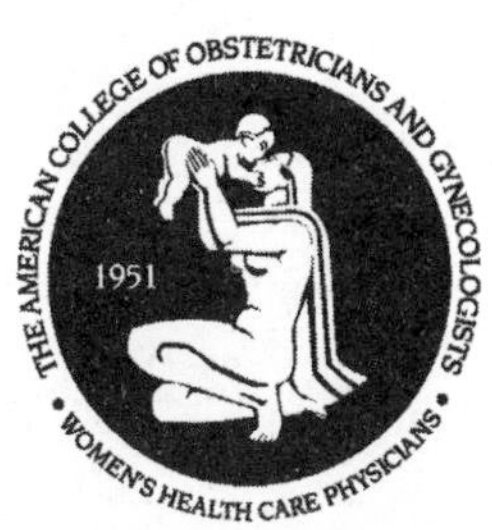

Thrombocytopenia in Pregnancy

Thrombocytopenia in pregnant women is diagnosed frequently by obstetricians because platelet counts are now included with automated complete blood cell counts (CBCs) obtained during routine prenatal screening (1). The condition is common, occurring in 7–8% of pregnancies (2). Thrombocytopenia can result from a variety of physiologic or pathologic conditions, several of which are unique to pregnancy. Some causes of thrombocytopenia are serious medical disorders that have the potential for profound maternal and fetal morbidity. In contrast, other conditions, such as gestational thrombocytopenia, are benign and pose no maternal or fetal risks. Because of the increased recognition of maternal and fetal thrombocytopenia, there are numerous controversies regarding obstetric management. Clinicians must weigh the risks of maternal and fetal bleeding complications against the costs and morbidity of diagnostic tests and invasive interventions.

Background

Platelet Function

Unlike other bleeding disorders in which bruising often is the initial clinical manifestation, platelet disorders, such as thrombocytopenia, usually result in bleeding into mucous membranes. Although bruising can occur, the most common manifestations of thrombocytopenia are petechiae, ecchymoses, epistaxis, gingival bleeding, and menometrorrhagia. In contrast to hemophilia, bleeding into joints usually does not occur; life-threatening bleeding is less common but can occur, resulting in hematuria, gastrointestinal bleeding, and, although rare, intracranial hemorrhage.

Definition of Thrombocytopenia

The normal range of the platelet count in nonpregnant individuals is 150,000–400,000/μL. In this population, thrombocytopenia is defined as any platelet value less than 150,000/μL, with counts of 100,000–150,000/μL indicative of mild thrombocytopenia, 50,000–100,000/μL indicative of moderate thrombocytopenia, and less than 50,000/μL indicative of severe thrombocytopenia. The definition of thrombocytopenia is somewhat arbitrary and not necessarily clinically relevant. Clinically significant bleeding usually is limited to patients with platelet counts less than 10,000/μL. Serious bleeding complications are rare, even in those with severe thrombocytopenia (3). Excessive bleeding associated with trauma or surgery is uncommon unless the patient's platelet count is less than 50,000/μL. The mean platelet count in pregnant women is lower than in nonpregnant individuals (4, 5).

Differential Diagnosis of Thrombocytopenia

Thrombocytopenia is due to either increased platelet destruction or decreased platelet production. In pregnancy, the former is responsible for most cases (2). Increased platelet destruction can be caused by an immunologic destruction, abnormal platelet activation, or platelet consumption resulting from excessive bleeding or exposure to abnormal vessels. Decreased platelet production is less common, and usually is associated with either leukemia, aplastic anemia, or folate deficiency (6, 7).

The most common cause of thrombocytopenia during pregnancy is gestational thrombocytopenia, which accounts for about two thirds of cases (2) (see the box).

Causes of Thrombocytopenia in Pregnancy

- Gestational thrombocytopenia
- Pregnancy-induced hypertension
- HELLP syndrome
- Pseudothrombocytopenia (laboratory artifact)
- Human immunodeficiency virus (HIV) infection
- Immune thrombocytopenic purpura
- Systemic lupus erythematosus
- Antiphospholipid syndrome
- Hypersplenism
- Disseminated intravascular coagulation
- Thrombotic thrombocytopenic purpura
- Hemolytic uremic syndrome
- Congenital thrombocytopenias
- Medications (heparin, quinine, quinidine, zidovudine, sulfonamides)

Gestational Thrombocytopenia

Gestational thrombocytopenia, also termed essential thrombocytopenia or benign or incidental thrombocytopenia of pregnancy, is by far the most common cause of mild thrombocytopenia during pregnancy, affecting up to 8% of gestations (2). There are several characteristics of this condition (2). First, the thrombocytopenia is relatively mild with platelet counts usually remaining greater than 70,000/μL. However, a lower threshold for gestational thrombocytopenia has never been established. Second, women are asymptomatic with no history of bleeding. The thrombocytopenia usually is detected as part of routine prenatal screening. Third, women have no history of thrombocytopenia prior to pregnancy (except in previous pregnancies). Although gestational thrombocytopenia may recur in subsequent pregnancies (8), the recurrence risk is unknown. Fourth, platelet counts usually return to normal within 2–12 weeks following delivery. Finally, there is an extremely low risk of fetal or neonatal thrombocytopenia. In a large, prospectively evaluated cohort study of 756 women with gestational thrombocytopenia, only one woman's infant had a platelet count of less than 50,000/μL (9). However, this infant had thrombocytopenia due to congenital bone marrow dysfunction. Another study confirmed the extremely low risk of fetal thrombocytopenia in women with gestational thrombocytopenia (10). Thus, women with gestational thrombocytopenia are not at risk for maternal or fetal hemorrhage or bleeding complications.

Although its cause is uncertain, gestational thrombocytopenia may be due to accelerated platelet consumption (4). Antiplatelet antibodies often are detectable in women with gestational thrombocytopenia, but neither their presence nor their absence can be used to diagnose the disorder or differentiate it from immune thrombocytopenic purpura (ITP) (11). Indeed, there are no specific diagnostic tests to definitively distinguish gestational thrombocytopenia from mild ITP (1). The primary means of differentiation is to monitor platelet counts closely, to look for levels that decrease below the 50,000–70,000/μL range, and to document a normal neonatal platelet count and a restoration of normal maternal platelet values after delivery.

Thrombocytopenia with an Immunologic Basis

Thrombocytopenia with an immunologic basis during pregnancy can be broadly classified as two disorders: neonatal alloimmune thrombocytopenia and ITP, an autoimmune condition. Neonatal alloimmune thrombocytopenia has no effect on the mother but probably is responsible for more intracranial hemorrhage due to thrombocytopenia than all the other primary thrombocytopenic conditions combined. In contrast, ITP may affect both mothers and fetuses, but with appropriate management the outcome for both is excellent.

Neonatal Alloimmune Thrombocytopenia

Neonatal alloimmune thrombocytopenia is the platelet equivalent of hemolytic (Rh) disease of the newborn, developing as a result of maternal alloimmunization to fetal platelet antigens. It affects one in 1,000–2,000 live births and can be a serious and potentially life-threatening condition (12, 13). Unlike Rh disease, neonatal alloimmune thrombocytopenia can occur during a first pregnancy. Almost half of the clinically evident cases of neonatal alloimmune thrombocytopenia are discovered in the first live-born infant (14).

In typical cases of unanticipated neonatal alloimmune thrombocytopenia, the mother is healthy and has a normal platelet count, and her pregnancy, labor, and delivery are indistinguishable from those of other low-risk obstetric patients. The neonates, however, are either born with evidence of profound thrombocytopenia or develop symptomatic thrombocytopenia within hours after birth. Affected infants often manifest generalized petechiae or ecchymoses over the presenting fetal part. Hemorrhage into viscera and bleeding following circumcision or venipuncture also may ensue. The most serious complication of neonatal alloimmune thrombocytopenia is intracranial hemorrhage, which occurs in 10–20% of infants (14, 15). Fetal intracranial hemorrhage due to neonatal alloimmune thrombocytopenia can occur in utero, and 25–50% of fetal intracranial hemorrhage in untreated mothers may be detected by ultrasonography before the onset of labor (16). Ultrasonographic findings may include intracranial hemorrhage, porencephalic cysts, and obstructive hydrocephalus. These observations are in contrast to neonatal intracranial hemorrhage due to ITP, which is exceedingly rare and usually occurs during the neonatal period.

Several polymorphic, diallelic antigen systems residing on platelet membrane glycoproteins are responsible for neonatal alloimmune thrombocytopenia. Many of these antigen systems have several names because they were identified in different parts of the world concurrently. Recently, a uniform nomenclature has been adopted that describes these antigens as human platelet antigens (HPA-1 and HPA-2), with alleles designated as "a" or "b" (17). Although there are at least 10 officially recognized platelet-specific antigens at this time, more than 50% of the reported cases in Caucasians and most of the severe cases have occurred as a result of sensitization against HPA-1a, also known as Pl^{A1} and Zw^{a}.

Fetal thrombocytopenia due to HPA-1a sensitization tends to be severe and can occur early in gestation. In a cohort study of 107 fetuses with neonatal alloimmune thrombocytopenia (97 with HPA-1a incompatibility) studied in utero before receiving any therapy, 50% had initial platelet counts of less than 20,000/μL (13). This percentage included 21 of 46 fetuses tested before 24 weeks of gestation. Furthermore, this series documented that the fetal platelet count decreases at a rate of more than 15,000/μL per week in the absence of therapy.

The recurrence risk of neonatal alloimmune thrombocytopenia is extremely high and approaches 100% in cases involving HPA-1a if the subsequent sibling carries the pertinent antigen (13). Thus, the recurrence risk is related to the zygosity of the father. As with red cell alloimmunization, the disease tends to be equally severe or progressively worse in subsequent pregnancies.

Immune Thrombocytopenic Purpura

Acute ITP is a self-limited disorder that usually occurs in childhood. It may follow a viral infection and rarely persists. Chronic ITP typically occurs in the second or third decade of life and has a female to male ratio of 3:1 (18). Estimates of the frequency of ITP during pregnancy vary widely, affecting one in 1,000–10,000 pregnancies (19).

Immune thrombocytopenic purpura is characterized by immunologically mediated platelet destruction. The patient produces IgG antiplatelet antibodies that recognize platelet membrane glycoproteins. This process leads to increased platelet destruction by cells of the reticuloendothelial system (18). The rate of destruction exceeds the compensatory ability of the bone marrow to produce new platelets, which leads to thrombocytopenia. Most of the platelet destruction occurs in the spleen, although other sites also are involved.

There are no pathognomonic signs, symptoms, or diagnostic tests for ITP; it is a diagnosis of exclusion. However, four findings have been traditionally associated with the condition: 1) persistent thrombocytopenia (platelet count <100,000/μL with or without accompanying megathrombocytes on the peripheral smear), 2) normal or increased numbers of megakaryocytes determined from bone marrow, 3) exclusion of other systemic disorders or drugs that are known to be associated with thrombocytopenia, and 4) absence of splenomegaly.

Most women with ITP have a history of bruising easily and petechiae, or of possible epistaxis and gingival bleeding, which precedes their pregnancy, but some women are completely asymptomatic. Important hemorrhagic symptoms rarely occur unless the platelet count is less than 20,000/μL. It is believed that the course of ITP usually is not affected by pregnancy, although there have been anecdotal reports of patients' conditions worsening during pregnancy and improving postpartum (20, 21). Pregnancy may be adversely affected by severe thrombocytopenia, and the primary risk to the mother is hemorrhage during the peripartum period.

Maternal IgG antiplatelet antibodies can cross the placenta, placing the fetus and neonate at risk for the development of thrombocytopenia. Retrospective case series of ITP in pregnancy indicate that 12–15% of infants born to mothers with ITP will develop platelet counts less than 50,000/μL (22, 23). Sometimes, this results in minor clinical bleeding such as purpura, ecchymoses, or melena. On rare occasions, fetal thrombocytopenia associated with ITP leads to intracranial hemorrhage unrelated to the mode of delivery. When it occurs, intracranial hemorrhage can result in severe neurologic impairment and even death. Serious bleeding complications are estimated to occur in 3% of infants born to women with ITP, and the rate of intracranial hemorrhage is less than 1% (22, 23). These data may overestimate the risk, as a result of publication bias. In a prospective, population-based study of almost 16,000 pregnancies delivered at a single center, no infant born to a mother with ITP suffered intracranial hemorrhage (9). The only three infants with intracranial hemorrhage had neonatal alloimmune thrombocytopenia, not ITP. The platelet count of the affected newborn usually will decrease after delivery, and the nadir may not be reached for several days (20).

Pregnancy-Induced Hypertension

Pregnancy-induced hypertension (PIH) is reported to be the cause of 21% of cases of maternal thrombocytopenia (9). The thrombocytopenia usually is moderate, and platelet counts rarely decrease below 20,000/μL. Clinical hemorrhage is uncommon unless the patient develops disseminated intravascular coagulopathy, but a decreasing maternal platelet count generally is considered a sign of worsening disease and is an indication for delivery.

In some cases, microangiopathic hemolytic anemia and elevated liver function tests are associated with thrombocytopenia in individuals with PIH. Such individuals are considered to have HELLP syndrome.

The cause of thrombocytopenia in women with severe PIH is unknown. The disease is associated with a state of accelerated platelet destruction, platelet activation, increased platelet volume, and increased megakaryocyte activity (21). Increased levels of platelet-associated IgG have been detected in patients with PIH (24). However, this finding is nonspecific and does not necessarily imply an immunologic basis for the thrombocytopenia. Platelet function also may be impaired in women with PIH, even if their platelet count is normal. It is noteworthy that the platelet count may decrease before the other clinical manifestations of PIH are apparent (25).

The neonates of mothers with PIH are at increased risk of neonatal thrombocytopenia (2). However, this is true only for infants born prematurely, and especially those with growth restriction. Term infants of mothers with PIH are no more likely to have thrombocytopenia than are controls. In a study of 1,414 mothers with hypertension, neonatal thrombocytopenia associated with PIH rarely decreased below 20,000/μL and caused no fetal bleeding complications (9).

Clinical Considerations and Recommendations

▶ ***What is the appropriate workup for maternal thrombocytopenia?***

When thrombocytopenia is diagnosed in a pregnant woman, it is important that the diagnosis be as precise as possible. The differential diagnosis of thrombocytopenia in pregnancy includes gestational thrombocytopenia, pseudothrombocytopenia, HIV infection, drug-induced thrombocytopenia, PIH, HELLP syndrome, thrombotic thrombocytopenic purpura, hemolytic uremic syndrome, disseminated intravascular coagulation, systemic lupus erythematosus, antiphospholipid syndrome, and congenital thrombocytopenias. These disorders usually can be determined on the basis of a detailed medical and family history and a physical examination, with attention to blood pressure, splenomegaly, HIV serology, and adjunctive laboratory studies as appropriate.

A CBC and examination of the peripheral blood smear generally are indicated in the evaluation of maternal thrombocytopenia. A CBC is helpful to exclude pancytopenia. Evaluation of the peripheral smear serves to rule out platelet clumping that may be associated with pseudothrombocytopenia. Bone marrow biopsy rarely is needed to distinguish between inadequate platelet production and increased platelet turnover. Numerous assays have been developed for both platelet-associated (direct) antibodies and circulating (indirect) antiplatelet antibodies. Although many individuals with ITP will have elevated levels of platelet-associated antibodies and sometimes circulating antiplatelet antibodies, these assays are not recommended for the routine evaluation of maternal thrombocytopenia (26). Tests for antiplatelet antibodies are nonspecific, poorly standardized, and subject to a large degree of interlaboratory variation (1). Also, gestational thrombocytopenia and ITP cannot be differentiated on the basis of antiplatelet antibody testing (11).

If drugs and other medical disorders are excluded, the primary differential diagnosis in the first and second trimesters will be either gestational thrombocytopenia or ITP. It should be noted that although gestational thrombocytopenia can occur in the first trimester, it typically becomes manifest later in pregnancy. In general, in a woman with no history of thrombocytopenia or the milder the thrombocytopenia, the more likely she is to have gestational thrombocytopenia. If the platelet count is less than 70,000/μL, ITP is more likely to be present, and if the platelet count is less than 50,000/μL, ITP is almost certainly present. During the third trimester or postpartum period, the sudden onset of significant maternal thrombocytopenia should lead to consideration of PIH, thrombotic thrombocytopenic purpura, hemolytic uremic syndrome, acute fatty liver, or disseminated intravascular coagulation, although ITP can present this way as well.

▶ *When should women with ITP receive medical therapy?*

The goal of medical therapy during pregnancy in women with ITP is to minimize the risk of bleeding complications associated with severe thrombocytopenia. Because the platelet function of these patients usually is normal, it is not necessary to maintain their counts in the normal range. There is general agreement that asymptomatic pregnant women with platelet counts greater than 50,000/μL do not require treatment. Also, most authorities recommend treatment in the presence of a platelet count significantly less than 50,000/μL or in the presence of bleeding. However, the degree of thrombocytopenia in asymptomatic pregnant women that requires treatment is somewhat controversial, and consultation from a physician experienced in these matters should be considered. Higher counts (eg, >50,000/μL) are desirable for invasive procedures and delivery, which may be associated with hemorrhage, the need for surgery, or the desire to use regional anesthesia. Bleeding times are not useful in assessing platelet function in patients with ITP.

▶ *What therapy should be used to treat ITP during pregnancy?*

The first line of treatment for ITP is prednisone, usually initiated in a dosage of 1–2 mg/kg/d. A response to antenatal corticosteroids usually occurs within 3–7 days and reaches a maximum within 2–3 weeks. Once platelet counts reach acceptable levels, the dosage can be tapered by 10–20% per week until the lowest dosage required to maintain a platelet count greater than 50,000/μL is reached. An increase in the platelet count occurs in about 70% of patients, and up to 25% will achieve complete remission (27).

Intravenous immune globulin (IVIG) is appropriate therapy for cases refractory to steroids as well as in circumstances such as platelet counts less than 10,000/μL in the third trimester, or platelet counts less than 30,000/μL associated with bleeding or with preoperative or predelivery status. A response to therapy can be expected in as few as 6 hours or in as many as 72 hours. In 70% of cases, the platelet count will return to pretreatment levels within 30 days after treatment (26, 28). Intravenous immune globulin is costly and of limited availability. When considering use of IVIG, it is prudent to seek consultation from a physician experienced in such cases.

Splenectomy is associated with complete remission in approximately 66% of patients with ITP (18); however, it often is not successful in patients who do not respond to intravenous immunoglobulin (29). The procedure usually is avoided during pregnancy because of fetal risks and technical difficulties late in gestation. However, splenectomy can be accomplished safely during pregnancy, ideally in the second trimester. It is appropriate for severe cases (platelet counts of less than 10,000/μL) that have failed treatment with antenatal corticosteroids and IVIG (26).

Platelet transfusions should be used only as a temporary measure to control life-threatening hemorrhage or to prepare a patient for surgery. The usual increase in platelets of approximately 10,000/μL per unit of platelets transfused is not achieved in patients with ITP because of the decreased survival of donor platelets. Thus, 6–10 U of platelet concentrate should be transfused. Other drugs used to treat ITP such as colchicine, azathioprine, vinca alkaloids, cyclophosphamide, and danazol have potential adverse fetal effects.

▶ *What additional specialized care should women with ITP receive?*

Other than serial assessment of the maternal platelet count (every trimester in asymptomatic women in remission and more frequently in thrombocytopenic individuals), little specialized care is required. Pregnant women with ITP should be instructed to avoid nonsteroidal anti-inflammatory agents, salicylates, and trauma. Individuals with splenectomies should be immunized against pneumococcus, *Hemophilus influenzae,* and meningococcus. If the diagnosis of ITP is made, consultation and ongoing evaluation with a physician experienced in such matters is appropriate.

▶ *Can fetal or neonatal intracranial hemorrhage be prevented in pregnancies complicated by ITP?*

It is logical to assume that therapies known to increase the maternal platelet count in patients with ITP also would improve the fetal platelet count. However, medical therapies such as IVIG (30) and steroids (22, 30–32) do not reliably prevent fetal thrombocytopenia or improve fetal outcome. Because some of these therapies (eg, IVIG) have not been adequately tested in appropriate trials, there are insufficient data to recommend maternal medical therapy for fetal indications.

Some investigators have recommended cesarean delivery to decrease the risk of intracranial hemorrhage by avoiding the potential trauma associated with vaginal birth (33). This strategy was based on anecdotal reports of intracranial hemorrhage associated with vaginal delivery (34) as well as the biologic plausibility of the hypothesis. Others have proposed that cesarean delivery be reserved for fetuses with platelet counts less than 50,000/μL (35, 36). This tactic was prompted by the observation that the risk of fetal bleeding is inversely proportional to the platelet count, and bleeding problems are extremely rare in fetuses with platelet counts more than 50,000/μL (31, 37).

Cesarean delivery has never been proven to prevent intracranial hemorrhage reliably. Several reports indicate that hemorrhagic complications in infants with thrombocytopenia are unrelated to the mode of delivery (22, 31, 37, 38). In a review of 474 neonates born to mothers with ITP, 29% of infants born vaginally with thrombocytopenia had a bleeding complication, compared with 30% delivered by cesarean birth (31). In this study, the rate of intracranial hemorrhage also was similar for both modes of delivery: 4% after vaginal delivery and 3% after cesarean delivery. In addition, it is unclear that intracranial hemorrhage is an intrapartum phenomenon. The neonatal platelet count often dramatically decreases after delivery. Thus, intracranial hemorrhage during the neonatal period could be mistakenly attributed to intrapartum events. No case of intracranial hemorrhage has been proven definitively to have occurred during labor (22, 23). Because cesarean delivery does not clearly prevent intraventricular hemorrhage, many obstetricians choose the mode of delivery in ITP based on obstetric considerations alone.

▶ *What tests or characteristics can be used to predict fetal thrombocytopenia in pregnancies complicated by ITP?*

No maternal test or characteristic can reliably predict the severity of thrombocytopenia in all cases of infants born to mothers with ITP. Maternal characteristics and serology, including prior splenectomy, platelet count, and the presence of platelet-associated antibodies, all correlate poorly with neonatal thrombocytopenia (39, 40). Fetal thrombocytopenia is rare in the absence of circulating antiplatelet antibodies (10), but exceptional cases have been reported (41). Also, these assays are difficult to perform and have a low positive predictive value (10).

▶ *Is there any role for fetal platelet count determination in ITP?*

At this time, most obstetricians do not obtain fetal platelet counts (42). Scalp sampling is fraught with inaccuracies and technical difficulties, and cordocentesis carries a 1–2% risk of necessitating an emergent cesarean delivery for fetal indications (43). The low incidence of intracranial hemorrhage and the lack of demonstrated difference in neonatal outcome between vaginal and cesarean deliveries also supports the opinion that the determination of fetal platelet count is unwarranted for ITP (22, 23, 31, 37, 44). A substantial minority of perinatologists (42) feel that the 5% risk of fetal thrombocytopenia of less than 20,000/μL and the attendant theoretically increased risk of an intracranial hemorrhage warrant informing patients of the availability of cordocentesis or scalp sampling during labor when choosing mode of delivery (45–47).

▶ *What is the appropriate neonatal care for infants born of pregnancies complicated by ITP?*

Regardless of the mode, delivery should be accomplished in a setting where an available clinician familiar with the disorder can treat any neonatal complications and have access to the medications needed for treatment.

▶ *Can a patient with thrombocytopenia be given regional anesthesia?*

The literature offers only limited and retrospective data to address this issue. However, two studies (48, 49) reported on a total of 184 patients with platelet counts less than 150,000/μL. Of these, 113 patients received epidural anesthesia without neurologic complication or sequelae. In all of these patients, the diagnosis was gestational thrombocytopenia. Another study of patients with platelet counts less than 100,000/μL due to preeclampsia, ITP, or infection also received epidural anesthesia without complication (50). Although the complication of greatest concern is that of epidural hematoma, there are only two cases in the literature of parturients who developed an epidural hematoma after regional anesthesia. One patient had preeclampsia and a lupus anticoagulant (51) and the other had an ependymoma (52). Cases reported in nonparturients have almost always been associated with anticoagulant therapy.

Although limited, data support the safety of epidural anesthesia in patients with platelet counts greater than 100,000/μL. In women with gestational thrombocytopenia with platelet counts less than 99,000/μL but greater than 50,000/μL, epidural anesthesia also may be safe, but its use in such patients will require a consensus among the obstetrician, anesthesiologist, and patient. When platelet counts are less than 50,000/μL, epidural anesthesia should not be given.

▶ *When should an evaluation for possible neonatal alloimmune thrombocytopenia be initiated, and what tests are useful in making the diagnosis?*

The most appropriate screening program incorporates evaluation of patients with a history of infants with otherwise unexplained bleeding or thrombocytopenia. Neonatal alloimmune thrombocytopenia should be suspected in cases of otherwise unexplained fetal or neonatal thrombocytopenia, porencephaly, or intracranial hemorrhage (either in utero or after birth). The laboratory diagnosis includes determination of platelet type and zygosity of both parents and the confirmation of maternal antiplatelet antibodies with specificity for paternal (or fetal–neonatal) platelets and the incompatible antigen. Platelet typing may be determined serologically or by genotyping because the genes and polymorphisms responsible for most cases of neonatal alloimmune thrombocytopenia have been identified. This is helpful when the father is heterozygous for the pertinent antigen because fetal platelet antigen typing can be performed using amniocytes (53). Chorionic villus sampling should not be performed because of its potential increased sensitization to antiplatelet antibodies. The laboratory evaluation of neonatal alloimmune thrombocytopenia can be complex, results may be ambiguous, and an antigen incompatibility cannot always be identified. Accordingly, testing for this disorder should be performed in an experienced regional laboratory that has special interest and expertise in neonatal alloimmune thrombocytopenia.

There is a theoretical benefit from population-based screening for platelet antigen incompatibility. However, such a program has not been shown to be clinically useful or cost-effective and is not currently recommended. Another area of controversy is the patient whose sister has had a pregnancy complicated by neonatal alloimmune thrombocytopenia. It may be worthwhile to evaluate these patients for platelet antigen incompatibility or human leukocyte antigen phenotype. However, the theoretical advantages of testing these women must be weighed against the potential for anxiety, cost, and morbidity without proven benefit.

▶ *How can one determine the fetal platelet count in pregnancies complicated by neonatal alloimmune thrombocytopenia?*

Unfortunately, as with ITP, there are no good indirect methods to determine the fetal platelet count. Maternal antiplatelet antibody titers correlate poorly with the severity of the disease. Also, characteristics such as the outcome of previously affected siblings (eg, birth platelet count or intracranial hemorrhage recognized after delivery) do not reliably predict the severity of fetal thrombocytopenia (13). Currently, the only accurate means of estimating the fetal platelet count is to sample the fetal blood directly, although this may increase the risk of fetal exsanguination.

▶ *What is the appropriate obstetric management of neonatal alloimmune thrombocytopenia?*

The primary goal of the obstetric management of pregnancies complicated by neonatal alloimmune thrombocytopenia is to prevent intracranial hemorrhage and its associated complications. In contrast to ITP, however, the higher frequency of intracranial hemorrhage associated with neonatal alloimmune thrombocytopenia justifies more aggressive interventions. Also, strategies intended to avoid intracranial hemorrhage must be initiated antenatally because of the risk of in utero intracranial hemorrhage.

The optimal management of fetuses at risk for neonatal alloimmune thrombocytopenia (those testing positive for the incompatible antigen or those whose fathers are homozygous for the antigen) remains controversial. The management decisions for these cases should be individualized and are best made after consultation with obstetric and pediatric specialists familiar with the disorder as soon as the diagnosis is made. Several therapies have been used in an attempt to increase the fetal platelet count and to avoid intracranial hemorrhage, including maternal treatment with IVIG, with or without steroids (15, 54–60), and fetal platelet transfusions (59, 61, 62). Intravenous immune globulin administered to the mother appears to be the most consistently effective antepartum therapy for neonatal alloimmune thrombocytopenia (15). However, none of these therapies is effective in all cases. Direct fetal administration of IVIG does not reliably improve the fetal platelet count, although only a few cases have been reported. Platelet transfusions with maternal platelets are consistently effective in raising the fetal platelet count. However, the short half-life of transfused platelets requires weekly procedures and may worsen the alloimmunization.

It is unknown whether it is necessary to determine the fetal platelet count before initiating therapy. The risks of cordocentesis in the setting of neonatal alloimmune thrombocytopenia must be weighed against the ability to determine the need for and the effectiveness of therapy. Although unproven, the benefit of transfusing maternal platelets at the time of cordocentesis may reduce the risk of bleeding complications from the procedure (63). The optimal time during gestation to first assess the fetal platelet count also is controversial. When fetal blood sampling is indicated, performance at 22–24 weeks of gestation may optimize medical therapy.

Most investigators recommend determination of the fetal platelet count once fetal pulmonary maturity is achieved, but before the onset of labor (eg, 37 weeks of gestation). A trial of labor is permitted for fetuses with platelet counts greater than 50,000/μL, while those with severe thrombocytopenia are delivered by cesarean birth. Although this strategy is of unproven efficacy, the high rate of intracranial hemorrhage in neonatal alloimmune thrombocytopenia is considered to warrant these interventions. Delivery should be accomplished in a setting equipped to handle a neonate with severe thrombocytopenia.

▶ ***What is appropriate obstetric management for gestational thrombocytopenia?***

Pregnancies with gestational thrombocytopenia are not at risk for maternal bleeding complications or fetal thrombocytopenia (4, 9). Thus, such interventions as the determination of the fetal platelet count or cesarean delivery are not indicated in patients with this condition. Women with gestational thrombocytopenia do not require any additional testing or specialized care, except follow-up platelet counts.

▶ ***Is it necessary to treat thrombocytopenia associated with PIH?***

The primary treatment of maternal thrombocytopenia in the setting of PIH or HELLP syndrome is delivery. Although antepartum reversal of thrombocytopenia has been reported with medical therapy (64), this course of treatment is not usual (65, 66). More importantly, the underlying pathophysiology of PIH will only resolve following birth. Thus, other than to allow for medical stabilization, the effect of betamethasone on fetal pulmonary maturity, or in special cases at preterm gestations, severe thrombocytopenia due to PIH is an indication for delivery (66).

Major hemorrhage is infrequent in patients with PIH but minor bleeding such as operative site oozing during cesarean delivery is common. Platelet transfusions occasionally are needed to improve hemostasis in patients with severe thrombocytopenia or DIC. However, transfusions are less effective in these women because of accelerated platelet destruction. Therefore, platelet transfusions are best reserved for patients with severe thrombocytopenia and active bleeding. An exception is the patient undergoing cesarean delivery. Although of uncertain benefit, many authorities recommend platelet transfusions to increase the platelet count to more than 50,000/μL before cesarean delivery (66).

Platelet counts often decrease for 24–48 hours after birth, followed by a rapid recovery (67–69). Most patients will achieve normal platelet counts within a few days to a week postpartum (67, 69). However, although rare, thrombocytopenia may continue for a prolonged period, which often is associated with persistent multisystem dysfunction (68). Plasma exchange has been reported to improve the platelet count in women with HELLP syndrome (70), but the efficacy remains unproven. Although thrombocytopenia associated with PIH or HELLP syndrome may improve after treatment with steroids or uterine curettage (71, 72), the clinical benefit of these therapies also is uncertain.

Summary

The following recommendation is based on good and consistent scientific evidence (Level A):

- ▶ Neonatal alloimmune thrombocytopenia should be treated with IVIG as the initial approach when fetal thrombocytopenia is documented.

The following recommendations are based on limited or inconsistent scientific evidence (Level B):

- ▶ The mode of delivery in pregnancies complicated by ITP should be chosen based on obstetric considerations alone. Prophylactic cesarean delivery does not appear to reduce the risk of fetal or neonatal hemorrhage.
- ▶ Epidural anesthesia is safe in patients with platelet counts greater than 100,000/μL.
- ▶ Mild maternal thrombocytopenia (≥ 70,000/μL) in asymptomatic pregnant women with no history of bleeding problems is usually benign gestational thrombocytopenia. These women should receive routine prenatal care with periodic repeat platelet counts (monthly to bimonthly).

The following recommendations are based primarily on consensus and expert opinion (Level C):

- Platelet counts of at least 50,000/μL rarely require treatment.
- Neonatal alloimmune thrombocytopenia should be suspected in cases of otherwise unexplained fetal or neonatal thrombocytopenia, hemorrhage, or porencephaly.
- Prior to initiating any plan of treatment for a woman based on thrombocytopenia in her fetus, consultation should be sought from a physician with experience dealing with that problem.
- Laboratory testing for neonatal alloimmune thrombocytopenia should be performed in a regional laboratory with special interest and expertise in dealing with the problem.

References

1. Rouse DJ, Owen J, Goldenberg RL. Routine maternal platelet count: an assessment of technologically driven practice. Am J Obstet Gynecol 1998;179:573–576 (Level III)
2. Burrows RF, Kelton JG. Thrombocytopenia at delivery: a prospective survey of 6,715 deliveries. Am J Obstet Gynecol 1990;162:731–734 (Level II-3)
3. Lacey JV, Penner JA. Management of idiopathic thrombocytopenic purpura in the adult. Semin Thromb Hemost 1977;3:160–174 (Level III)
4. Burrows RF, Kelton JG. Incidentally detected thrombocytopenia in healthy mothers and their infants. N Engl J Med 1988;319:142–145 (Level II-3)
5. Nagey DA, Alger LS, Edelman BB, Heyman MR, Pupkin MJ, Crenshaw C Jr. Reacting appropriately to thrombocytopenia in pregnancy. South Med J 1986;79:1385–1388 (Level III)
6. Jih DM, Werth VP. Thrombocytopenia after a single dose of methotrexate. J Am Acad Dermatol 1998;39:349–351 (Level III)
7. Mant MJ, Connolly T, Gordon PA, King EG. Severe thrombocytopenia probably due to acute folic acid deficiency. Crit Care Med 1979;7:297–300 (Level III)
8. Ruggeri M, Schiavotto C, Castaman G, Tosetto A, Rodeghiero F. Gestational thrombocytopenia: a prospective study. Haematologica 1997;82:341–342 (Level II-3)
9. Burrows RF, Kelton JG. Fetal thrombocytopenia and its relation to maternal thrombocytopenia. N Engl J Med 1993;329:1463–1466 (Level II-3)
10. Samuels P, Bussel JB, Braitman LE, Tomaski A, Druzin ML, Mennuti MT, et al. Estimation of the risk of thrombocytopenia in the offspring of pregnant women with presumed immune thrombocytopenic purpura. N Engl J Med 1990;323:229–235 (Level II-3)
11. Lescale KB, Eddleman KA, Cines DB, Samuels P, Lesser ML, McFarland JG, et al. Antiplatelet antibody testing in thrombocytopenic pregnant women. Am J Obstet Gynecol 1996;174:1014–1018 (Level II-2)
12. Blanchette VS, Chen L, de Friedberg ZS, Hogan VA, Trudel E, Decary F. Alloimmunization to the PlA1 platelet antigen: results of a prospective study. Br J Haematol 1990;74:209–215 (Level II-3)
13. Bussel JB, Zabusky MR, Berkowitz RL, McFarland JG. Fetal alloimmune thrombocytopenia. N Engl J Med 1997; 337:22–26 (Level II-2)
14. Mueller-Eckhardt C, Kiefel V, Grubert A, Kroll H, Weisheit M, Schmidt S, et al. 348 cases of suspected neonatal alloimmune thrombocytopenia. Lancet 1989; 1:363–366 (Level II-3)
15. Bussel JB, Berkowitz RL, Lynch L, Lesser ML, Paidas MJ, Huang CL, et al. Antenatal management of alloimmune thrombocytopenia with intravenous gamma-globulin: a randomized trial of the addition of low-dose steroid to intravenous gamma-globulin. Am J Obstet Gynecol 1996;174:1414–1423 (Level I)
16. Herman JH, Jumbelic MI, Ancona RJ, Kickler TS. In utero cerebral hemorrhage in alloimmune thrombocytopenia. Am J Pediatr Hematol Oncol 1986;8:312–317 (Level III)
17. von dem Borne AE, Decary F. Nomenclature of platelet-specific antigens. Transfusion 1990;30:477 (Level III)
18. George JN, el-Harake MA, Raskob GE. Chronic idiopathic thrombocytopenic purpura. N Engl J Med 1994;331: 1207–1211 (Level III)
19. Sainio S, Joutsi L, Jarvenpaa AL, Kekomaki R, Koistinen E, Riikonen S, et al. Idiopathic thrombocytopenic purpura in pregnancy. Acta Obstet Gynecol Scand 1998; 77: 272–277 (Level III)
20. Kelton JG, Inwood MJ, Barr RM, Effer SB, Hunter D, Wilson WE, et al. The prenatal prediction of thrombocytopenia in infants of mothers with clinically diagnosed immune thrombocytopenia. Am J Obstet Gynecol 1982;144:449–454 (Level II-3)
21. McCrae KR, Samuels P, Schreiber AD. Pregnancy-associated thrombocytopenia: pathogenesis and management. Blood 1992;80:2697–2714 (Level III)
22. Payne SD, Resnik R, Moore TR, Hedriana HL, Kelly TF. Maternal characteristics and risk of severe neonatal thrombocytopenia and intracranial hemorrhage in pregnancies complicated by autoimmune thrombocytopenia. Am J Obstet Gynecol 1997;177:149–155 (Level II-3)
23. Silver RM, Branch DW, Scott JR. Maternal thrombocytopenia in pregnancy: time for a reassessment. Am J Obstet Gynecol 1995;173:479–482 (Level III)
24. Burrows RF, Hunter DJ, Andrew M, Kelton JG. A prospective study investigating the mechanism of thrombocytopenia in preeclampsia. Obstet Gynecol 1987;70:334–338 (Level II-2)
25. Redman CW, Bonnar J, Beilin L. Early platelet consumption in pre-eclampsia. BMJ 1978;1:467–469 (Level II-2)
26. George JN, Woolf SH, Raskob GE, Wasser JS, Aledort LM, Ballem PJ, et al. Idiopathic thrombocytopenic purpura: a practice guideline developed by explicit methods for the American Society of Hematology. Blood 1996;88: 3–40 (Level III)
27. Karpatkin S. Autoimmune thrombocytopenic purpura. Am J Med Sci 1971;261:127–138 (Level III)
28. Bussel JB, Pham LC. Intravenous treatment with gamma globulin in adults with immune thrombocytopenic purpu-

ra: review of the literature. Vox Sang 1987;52:206–211 (Level III)

29. Law C, Marcaccio M, Tam P, Heddle N, Kelton JG. High-dose intravenous immune globulin and the response to splenectomy in patients with idiopathic thrombocytopenic purpura. N Engl J Med 1997;336:1494–1498 (Level III)

30. Kaplan C, Daffos F, Forestier F, Tertian G, Catherine N, Pous JC, et al. Fetal platelet counts in thrombocytopenic pregnancy. Lancet 1990;336:979–982 (Level II-3)

31. Cook RL, Miller RC, Katz VL, Cefalo RC. Immune thrombocytopenic purpura in pregnancy: a reappraisal of management. Obstet Gynecol 1991;78:578–583 (Level II-3)

32. Christiaens GC, Nieuwenhuis HK, von dem Borne AE, Ouwehand WH, Helmerhorst FM, Van Dalen CM, et al. Idiopathic thrombocytopenic purpura in pregnancy: a randomized trial on the effect of antenatal low dose corticosteroids on neonatal platelet count. Br J Obstet Gynaecol 1990;97:893–898 (Level I)

33. Carloss HW, McMillan R, Crosby WH. Management of pregnancy in women with immune thrombocytopenic purpura. JAMA 1980;224:2756–2758 (Level III)

34. Jones RW, Asher MI, Rutherford CJ, Munro HM. Autoimmune (idiopathic) thrombocytopenic purpura in pregnancy and the newborn. Br J Obstet Gynaecol 1977;84:679–683 (Level III)

35. Ayromlooi J. A new approach to the management of immunologic thrombocytopenic purpura in pregnancy. Am J Obstet Gynecol 1978;130:235–236 (Level III)

36. Scott JR, Cruikshank DP, Kochenour NK, Pitkin RM, Warenski JC. Fetal platelet counts in the obstetric management of immunologic thrombocytopenic purpura. Am J Obstet Gynecol 1980;136:495–499 (Level III)

37. Burrows RF, Kelton JG. Pregnancy in patients with idiopathic thrombocytopenic purpura: assessing the risks for the infant at delivery. Obstet Gynecol Surv 1993;48:781–788 (Level III)

38. Laros RK Jr, Kagan R. Route of delivery for patients with immune thrombocytopenic purpura. Am J Obstet Gynecol 1984;148:901–908 (Level III)

39. Scott JR, Rote NS, Cruikshank DP. Antiplatelet antibodies and platelet counts in pregnancies complicated by autoimmune thrombocytopenic purpura. Am J Obstet Gynecol 1983;145:932–939 (Level II-3)

40. Burrows RF, Kelton JG. Low fetal risks in pregnancies associated with idiopathic thrombocytopenic purpura. Am J Obstet Gynecol 1990;163:1147–1150 (Level II-3)

41. Risk of thrombocytopenia in offspring of mothers with presumed immune thrombocytopenic purpura. N Engl J Med 1990;323:1841–1843 (Level III)

42. Peleg D, Hunter SK. Perinatal management of women with immune thrombocytopenic purpura: survey of United States perinatologists. Am J Obstet Gynecol 1999;180:645–649 (Level II-3)

43. Ghidini A, Sepulveda W, Lockwood CJ, Romero R. Complications of fetal blood sampling. Am J Obstet Gynecol 1993;168:1339–1344 (Level III)

44. Berry SM, Leonardi MR, Wolfe HM, Dombrowski MP, Lanouette JM, Cotton DB. Maternal thrombocytopenia. Predicting neonatal thrombocytopenia with cordocentesis. J Reprod Med 1997;42:276–280 (Level III)

45. Garmel SH, Craigo SD, Morin LM, Crowley JM, D'Alton ME. The role of percutaneous umbilical blood sampling in the management of immune thrombocytopenic purpura. Prenat Diagn 1995;15:439–445 (Level III)

46. De Carolis S, Noia G, DeSantis M, Trivellini C, Mastromarino C, De Carolis MP, et al. Immune thrombocytopenic purpura and percutaneous umbilical blood sampling: an open question. Fetal Diagn Ther 1993;8:154–160 (Level II-2)

47. Scioscia AL, Grannum PA, Copel JA, Hobbins JC. The use of percutaneous umbilical blood sampling in immune thrombocytopenic purpura. Am J Obstet Gynecol 1988;159:1066–1068 (Level II-3)

48. Beilin Y, Zahn J, Comerford M. Safe epidural analgesia in thirty parturients with platelet counts between 69,000 and 98,000 mm^{-3}. Anesth Analg 1997;85:385–388 (Level III)

49. Rolbin SH, Abbott D, Musclow E, Papsin F, Lie LM, Freedman J. Epidural anesthesia in pregnant patients with low platelet counts. Obstet Gynecol 1988;71:918–920 (Level III)

50. Rasmus KT, Rottman RL, Kotelko DM, Wright WC, Stone JJ, Rosenblatt RM. Unrecognized thrombocytopenia and regional anesthesia in parturients: a retrospective review. Obstet Gynecol 1989;73:943–946 (Level III)

51. Lao TT, Halpern SH, MacDonald D, Huh C. Spinal subdural haematoma in a parturient after attempted epidural anaesthesia. Can J Anaesth 1993;40:340–345 (Level III)

52. Roscoe MWA, Barrington TW. Acute spinal subdural hematoma. A case report and review of literature. Spine 1984;9:672–675 (Level III)

53. McFarland JG, Aster RH, Bussel JB, Gianopoulos JG, Derbes RS, Newman PJ. Prenatal diagnosis of neonatal alloimmune thrombocytopenia using allele-specific oligonucleotide probes. Blood 1991;78:2276–2282 (Level III)

54. Bussel JB, Berkowitz RL, McFarland JG, Lynch L, Chitkara U. Antenatal treatment of neonatal alloimmune thrombocytopenia. N Engl J Med 1988:319:1374–1378 (Level II-2)

55. Lynch L, Bussel JB, McFarland JG, Chitkara U, Berkowitz RL. Antenatal treatment of alloimmune thrombocytopenia. Obstet Gynecol 1992;80:67–71 (Level II-2)

56. Marzusch K, Schnaidt M, Dietl J, Weist E, Hofstaetter C, Golz R. High-dose immunoglobulin in the antenatal treatment of neonatal alloimmune thrombocytopenia: case report and review. Br J Obstet Gynaecol 1992;99:260–262 (Level III)

57. Mir N, Samson D, House MJ, Kovar IZ. Failure of antenatal high-dose immunoglobulin to improve fetal platelet count in neonatal alloimmune thrombocytopenia. Vox Sang 1988;55:188–189 (Level III)

58. Bowman J, Harman C, Mentigolou S, Pollack J. Intravenous fetal transfusion of immunoglobulin for alloimmune thrombocytopenia. Lancet 1992;340:1034–1035 (Level III)

59. Nicolini U, Tannirandorn Y, Gonzalez P, Fisk NM, Beacham J, Letsky EA, et al. Continuing controversy in

alloimmune thrombocytopenia: fetal hyperimmunoglobulinemia fails to prevent thrombocytopenia. Am J Obstet Gynecol 1990;163:1144–1146 (Level III)

60. Zimmermann R, Huch A. In-utero fetal therapy with immunoglobulin for alloimmune thrombocytopenia. Lancet 1992;340:606 (Level III)

61. Kaplan C, Daffos F, Forestier F, Cox WL, Lyon-Caen D, Dupuy-Montbrun MC, et al. Management of alloimmune thrombocytopenia: antenatal diagnosis and in utero transfusion of maternal platelets. Blood 1988;72:340–343 (Level III)

62. Murphy MF, Pullon HW, Metcalfe P, Chapman JF, Jenkins E, Waters AH, et al. Management of fetal alloimmune thrombocytopenia by weekly in utero platelet transfusions. Vox Sang 1990;58:45–49 (Level III)

63. Paidas MJ, Berkowitz RL, Lynch L, Lockwood CJ, Lapinski R, McFarland JG, et al. Alloimmune thrombocytopenia: fetal and neonatal losses related to cordocentesis. Am J Obstet Gynecol 1995;172:475–479 (Level II-2)

64. Clark SL, Phelan JR, Allen SH, Golde SR. Antepartum reversal of hematologic abnormalities associated with the HELLP syndrome. A report of three cases. J Reprod Med 1986;31:70–72 (Level III)

65. Weinstein L. Syndrome of hemolysis, elevated liver enzymes, and low platelet count: a severe consequence of hypertension in pregnancy. Am J Obstet Gynecol 1982;142:159–167 (Level III)

66. Sibai BM. The HELLP syndrome (hemolysis, elevated liver enzymes, and low platelets): much ado about nothing? Am J Obstet Gynecol 1990;162:311–316 (Level III)

67. Katz VL, Thorp JM Jr, Rozas L, Bowes WA Jr. The natural history of thrombocytopenia associated with preeclampsia. Am J Obstet Gynecol 1990;163:1142–1143 (Level II-3)

68. Martin JN Jr, Blake PG, Lowry SL, Perry KG Jr, Files JC, Morrison JC. Pregnancy complicated by preeclampsia-eclampsia with the syndrome of hemolysis, elevated liver enzymes, and low platelet count: how rapid is postpartum recovery? Obstet Gynecol 1990;76:737–741 (Level II-3)

69. Neiger R, Contag SA, Coustan DR. The resolution of preeclampsia-related thrombocytopenia. Obstet Gynecol 1991;77:692–695 (Level II-3)

70. Martin JN Jr, Files JC, Blake PG, Norman PH, Martin RW, Hess LW, et al. Plasma exchange for preeclampsia. I. Postpartum use for persistently severe preeclampsia-eclampsia with HELLP syndrome. Am J Obstet Gynecol 1990;162:126–137 (Level III)

71. Magann EF, Martin JN Jr, Isaacs JD, Perry KG Jr, Martin RW, Meydrech EF. Immediate postpartum curettage: accelerated recovery from severe preeclampsia. Obstet Gynecol 1993;81:502–506 (Level I)

72. Magann EF, Bass D, Chauhan SP, Sullivan DL, Martin RW, Martin JN Jr. Antepartum corticosteroids: disease stabilization in patients with the syndrome of hemolysis, elevated liver enzymes, and low platelets (HELLP). Am J Obstet Gynecol 1994;171:1148–1153 (Level I)

The MEDLINE database, the Cochrane Library, and ACOG's own internal resources were used to conduct a literature search to locate relevant articles published between January 1985 and January 1999. The search was restricted to articles published in the English language. Priority was given to articles reporting results of original research, although review articles and commentaries also were consulted. Abstracts of research presented at symposiums and scientific conferences were not considered adequate for inclusion in this document. Guidelines published by organizations or institutions such as the National Institutes of Health and ACOG were reviewed, and additional studies were located by reviewing bibliographies of identified articles. When reliable research was not available, expert opinions from obstetrician–gynecologists were used.

Studies were reviewed and evaluated for quality according to the method outlined by the U.S. Preventive Services Task Force:

I Evidence obtained from at least one properly designed randomized controlled trial.

II-1 Evidence obtained from well-designed controlled trials without randomization.

II-2 Evidence obtained from well-designed cohort or case–control analytic studies, preferably from more than one center or research group.

II-3 Evidence obtained from multiple time series with or without the intervention. Dramatic results in uncontrolled experiments also could be regarded as this type of evidence.

III Opinions of respected authorities, based on clinical experience, descriptive studies, or reports of expert committees.

Based on the highest level of evidence found in the data, recommendations are provided and graded according to the following categories:

Level A—Recommendations are based on good and consistent scientific evidence.

Level B—Recommendations are based on limited or inconsistent scientific evidence.

Level C—Recommendations are based primarily on consensus and expert opinion.

ISSN 1099-3630

The American College of Obstetricians and Gynecologists
409 12th Street, SW
PO Box 96920
Washington, DC 20090-6920

12345/32109

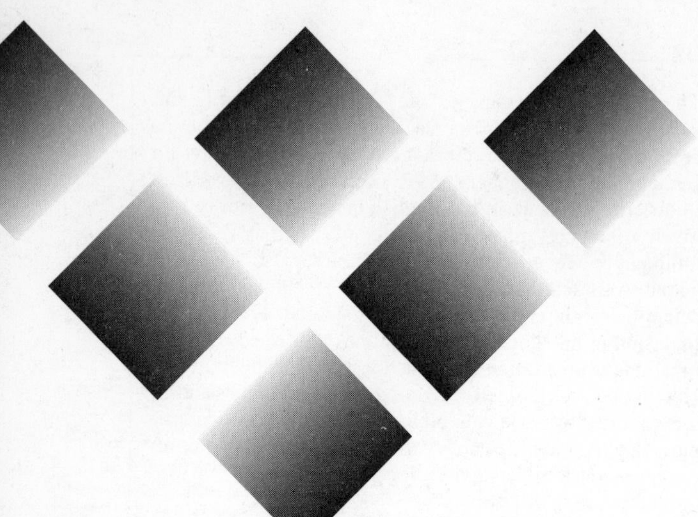

ACOG PRACTICE BULLETIN

CLINICAL MANAGEMENT GUIDELINES FOR OBSTETRICIAN–GYNECOLOGISTS
NUMBER 19, AUGUST 2000

(Replaces Educational Bulletin Number 234, March 1997)

This Practice Bulletin was developed by the ACOG Committee on Practice Bulletins—Obstetrics with the assistance of Linda A. Barbour, MD, MSPH. The information is designed to aid practitioners in making decisions about appropriate obstetric and gynecologic care. These guidelines should not be construed as dictating an exclusive course of treatment or procedure. Variations in practice may be warranted based on the needs of the individual patient, resources, and limitations unique to the institution or type of practice.

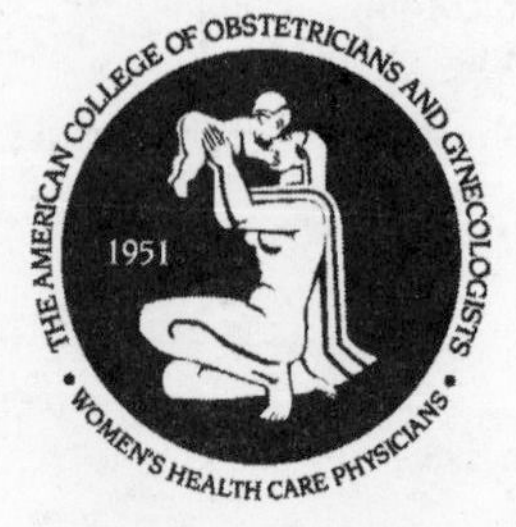

Thromboembolism in Pregnancy

During pregnancy, women have a fivefold increased risk of venous thromboembolism (VTE), compared with nonpregnant women. The absolute risk of symptomatic venous thrombosis during pregnancy is between 0.5 and 3.0 per 1,000 women based on studies using radiographic documentation (1–3). Pulmonary embolism (PE) is a leading cause of maternal death in the United States (4). The prevalence and severity of this condition warrant consideration of anticoagulant therapy in pregnancy for women at risk for VTE. Such therapy includes the treatment of acute thrombotic events, prophylaxis for patients with a history of thrombotic events or identified acquired or congenital thrombophilias, and prevention and treatment of systemic embolization in women with valvular heart disease. The purpose of this document is to review the current literature on the prevention and management of thromboembolism in obstetric patients, discuss the data behind sometimes conflicting guidelines from expert panels, and offer evidence-based recommendations to address the most clinically relevant issues in the management of these patients.

Background

Numerous changes in the coagulation system account for the hypercoagulable state associated with pregnancy (see the box). Recently, it has been recognized that up to half of women who have thrombotic events during pregnancy possess an underlying congenital or acquired thrombophilia (5). The most common thrombophilias in the Caucasian population are the factor V Leiden mutation, which has a prevalence of 5% in this population, and the prothrombin gene mutation G20210A, which has a prevalence of 2% in this population (5, 6). In approximately 50% of patients with a hereditary thrombophilia, the initial thrombotic event occurs in the presence of an additional risk factor such as pregnancy, oral contraceptive use, orthopedic trauma, immobilization, or surgery (7, 8).

Pregnancy-Associated Changes in Coagulation

Increases in clotting factors (I, VII, VIII, IX, X)
Decreases in protein S
Decreases in fibrinolytic activity
Increased venous stasis
Vascular injury associated with delivery
Increased activation of platelets
Resistance to activated protein C

Risk of Thromboembolism During Pregnancy

Traditionally, it was believed that the risk of venous thrombosis was greatest in the third trimester and immediately postpartum. More recent studies using objective criteria for diagnosis have found that antepartum deep vein thrombosis (DVT) is at least as common as postpartum thrombosis and occurs with equal frequency in all three trimesters (1). However, PE is more common postpartum.

Women with a history of thromboembolism have an increased risk of recurrence when they become pregnant; however, the estimates of recurrence are based primarily on two retrospective studies and range from 7.5% to 12% (9, 10). No studies differentiated the risk of recurrence based on underlying factors such as acquired or congenital thrombophilias, use of oral contraceptives, pregnancy, orthopedic trauma, recent surgery, or the occurrence of the event in the antepartum versus postpartum period. Most of the estimates of recurrence are based on women who had their initial event during oral contraceptive use or pregnancy. Risk factors for thromboembolic disorders are noted in the box.

Anticoagulation Medications in Pregnancy

Although many terms have been used to classify anticoagulant regimens, the following terminology will be used in this document:

- Low-dose prophylaxis—a fixed dose of anticoagulant given 1–2 times per day without use of routine monitoring to verify a therapeutic prolongation of the activated partial thromboplastin time (APTT).
- Adjusted-dose prophylaxis—anticoagulant administered for prophylaxis to achieve traditional therapeutic effects, given 2–3 times per day with frequent laboratory testing to verify adequate APTT prolongation of at least 1.5 to 2.5.

Heparin

There is considerable clinical experience with heparin use in pregnancy (11). Heparin requirements appear to increase during pregnancy because of increases in heparin-binding proteins, plasma volume, renal clearance, and heparin degradation by the placenta, which reduces the bioavailability of heparin (12). There are no prospective trials that have determined adequate prophylactic doses in pregnancy. The major concerns with heparin use during pregnancy are not fetal but maternal and include heparin-induced osteoporosis and heparin-induced thrombocytopenia (HIT).

Two prospective trials of pregnant women exposed to heparin confirmed a mean bone loss of 5% (13, 14), with approximately one third sustaining a 10% or greater decrease in bone density (13). The complete reversibility of this process has not been clearly established, nor does there appear to be a clear dose-response relationship (15). In selected patients, such as those who have a strong family history of osteoporosis or are smokers, postpartum evaluation of bone density may have prognostic and therapeutic implications (13, 14).

There are two types of heparin-induced thrombocytopenia. The more common type is the benign, reversible nonimmune form, which occurs in patients within the first few days of therapy and typically resolves by 5 days. This

Risk Factors for Deep Vein Thrombosis and Thromboembolic Disorders

Hereditary Thrombophilia (prevalence in general population)
- Factor V Leiden mutation (5–9%)*
- AT-III deficiency (0.02–0.2%)
- Protein C deficiency (0.2–0.5%)
- Protein S deficiency (0.08%)
- Hyperhomocystinemia (1–11%)
- Prothrombin gene mutation (2–4%)

Prior history of deep vein thrombosis
Mechanical heart valve
Atrial fibrillation
Trauma/prolonged immobilization/major surgery
Other familial hypercoagulable states
Antiphospholipid syndrome

*For African Americans, about 1%; for Caucasians, 6–11%.

Data from Lockwood CJ. Heritable coagulopathies in pregnancy. Obstet Gynecol Surv 1999;54:754–765

condition does not require cessation of heparin therapy. The less common but more severe type is the immune form of HIT, which occurs within 5–14 days of full-dose heparin therapy in as many as 3% of patients (16) and may result in widespread thrombosis (17, 18). The occurrence of autoimmune thrombocytopenia from prophylactic doses of heparin has been reported, but is rare. Deep vein thrombosis and PE are the most frequent clinical presentations of the immune form of HIT. It has been recommended, therefore, that platelet counts be checked on day 5 and then periodically for the first 2 weeks of heparin therapy. If the HIT is severe, heparin therapy must be stopped and alternative anticoagulation therapy initiated; low-molecular-weight heparin (LMWH) may not be a safe alternative because it has a low cross reactivity with heparin. In such situations, consultation with someone with expertise in the field may be needed (17, 18).

Low-Molecular-Weight Heparin

Low-molecular-weight heparin may reduce three of the complications caused by standard heparin: bleeding, osteoporosis, and thrombocytopenia (16, 18, 19). However, virtually all data on LMWH come from nonpregnant patients. It has been conclusively demonstrated that LMWH does not cross the placenta into the fetal circulation (20, 21). Although the bioavailability of LMWH should be improved over standard heparin because of the reduction of heparin binding, the increases in renal clearance and volume of distribution of the drug may necessitate dosage increases in pregnancy (22, 23). Another advantage of LMWH is that dosing can be limited to once or twice daily (22, 24). If laboratory monitoring is used, monitoring peak antifactor Xa levels every 4–6 weeks should be utilized particularly when twice daily dosing is given. The APTT does not correlate well with the anticoagulant effect of LMWH.

Warfarin

Warfarin derivatives cross the placenta and in most cases are relatively contraindicated in pregnancy; therefore, they primarily are used postpartum or in patients with certain types of mechanical heart valves (25–29). Warfarin use should be restricted to the second or early third trimester in selected patients in whom prolonged high-dose heparin therapy is relatively contraindicated. A skeletal embryopathy resulting in stippled epiphyses and nasal and limb hypoplasia can occur when warfarin is given between 6 and 12 weeks of gestation (30). Midtrimester exposure may result in optic atrophy, microcephaly, and developmental delay. Bleeding can occur in the fetus at any time, resulting in a high fetal loss rate (30).

Clinical Considerations and Recommendations

▶ *Who are candidates for thromboprophylaxis in pregnancy?*

Thromboprophylaxis is defined as administration of anticoagulants because of an increased risk of VTE during pregnancy rather than treatment for an acute event. Often this can be accomplished using relatively low doses, which have a minimal effect on laboratory measures of coagulation. Such low-dose prophylaxis carries fewer risks than full therapeutic anticoagulation. There are certain high-risk conditions that require dosage adjustments to achieve higher therapeutic levels of anticoagulation (adjusted-dose heparin prophylaxis). Each patient's regimen should be individualized once the risks of heparin therapy are weighed against the benefits (31).

Patients with the following conditions are at highest risk and should have adjusted-dose heparin prophylaxis (12):

- Artificial heart valves (some investigators recommend warfarin therapy after the first trimester in certain circumstances) (26–29)
- Antithrombin-III (AT-III) deficiency (with or without a history of thrombosis; also referred to as "antithrombin deficiency") (32, 33)
- Antiphospholipid syndrome (some investigators recommend low-dose prophylaxis for this condition if there is no history of DVT) (34, 35)
- History of rheumatic heart disease with current atrial fibrillation (36)
- Homozygous factor V Leiden mutation, homozygous prothrombin G20210A mutation
- Patients receiving chronic anticoagulation for recurrent thromboembolism

Patients who are identified carriers of other inherited thrombophilias who do not have a history of thrombosis but have a strong family history of thrombosis (36) and noncarriers with a history of thromboembolic events before the current pregnancy (34) appear to be at lower risk and may be candidates for low-dose prophylaxis. However, no data exist to support or refute this approach.

It is not clear whether patients with a history of thrombosis identified with a protein C or protein S deficiency should receive low-dose or adjusted-dose heparin prophylaxis during pregnancy. It is also not known whether asymptomatic women who have been identified as carriers of inherited thrombophilia (except AT-III or homozygosity to the factor V Leiden or prothrombin G20210A mutation) and who are without a personal or family history of thromboembolism should receive heparin prophylaxis because there is marked variation in the penetrance of the thrombotic trait.

Patients with a history of idiopathic thrombosis, extensive or life-threatening thrombosis, recurrent thrombosis, thrombosis related to a high estrogen state, or who have an underlying thrombophilia or postthrombotic syndrome are likely to be at a higher risk of recurrence in pregnancy than patients with a definite transient provocation (orthopedic trauma or surgery) without any of these risk factors. The former group should consider antepartum thromboprophylaxis beginning in the first trimester and continuing until 6 weeks postpartum. It is unclear whether patients who have sustained VTE from a transient and highly thrombogenic provocation (eg, orthopedic trauma) and who have no other risk factors may benefit from antepartum prophylaxis. Their risk of recurrence is likely higher than the baseline population, and an increasing number of thrombophilic states are being identified in patients who sustain thromboses in the setting of recognized transient provocations (37). Although data are limited, some experts recommend that, at minimum, such patients be given postpartum prophylaxis with warfarin.

▶ *How should a prophylactic heparin regimen be administered during pregnancy?*

Because of the absence of adequate prospective trials, a number of different prophylactic regimens have been offered by varying consensus panels, often based on nonpregnant patient studies (34, 38, 39) (see the box).

One study determined that during pregnancy, a doubling of the dose of heparin was required to achieve the same anticoagulant response of a nonpregnant patient taking 5,000 U of heparin twice daily for low-dose prophylaxis (12). Some patients who are AT-III deficient will not respond to heparin and may require AT-III factor therapy (40).

Pregnant patients who require adjusted-dose heparin for anticoagulation for long-term prophylaxis may theoretically benefit from the higher bioavailability and more consistent therapeutic anticoagulation with LMWH (41, 42).

Prophylactic Heparin Regimens in Pregnancy

Unfractionated Heparin

Low–dose prophylaxis:

1. 5,000–7,500 U every 12 hours during the first trimester
   7,500–10,000 U every 12 hours during the second trimester
   10,000 U every 12 hours during the third trimester unless the APTT* is elevated. The APTT may be checked near term and the heparin dose reduced if prolonged

OR

2. 5,000–10,000 U every 12 hours throughout pregnancy

Adjusted-dose prophylaxis:

≥10,000 U twice a day to three times a day to achieve APTT of 1.5–2.5

Low-Molecular-Weight Heparin

Low-dose prophylaxis:

Dalteparin, 5,000 U once or twice daily, or enoxaparin, 40 mg once or twice daily

Adjusted-dose prophylaxis:

Dalteparin, 5,000–10,000 U every 12 hours, or enoxaparin, 30–80 mg every 12 hours

*APTT indicates activated partial thromboplastin time.

Data from Colvin BT, Barrowcliffe TW. The British Society for Haematology guidelines on the use and monitoring of heparin 1992: second revision. J Clin Pathol 1993;46:97–103. Ginsberg JS, Hirsh J. Use of antithrombotic agents during pregnancy. Chest 1998;114: 524S–530S. Maternal and Neonatal Haemostasis Working Party of the Haemostasis and Thrombosis Task. Guidelines on the presentation, investigation and management of thrombosis associated with pregnancy. J Clin Pathol 1993;46:489–496

▶ *Who should be tested for inherited or acquired thrombophilias?*

Women who have a history of thrombosis should be offered testing, especially if such testing would affect management. It is controversial whether to test women who do not have a history of thrombosis but have a family history of thrombosis. Women who have a first-degree relative with an AT-III deficiency or homozygous factor V Leiden or prothrombin G20210A mutation may benefit from testing. Individuals with a strong family history of thrombophilias may be more likely to have multiple inherited risk factors with an increased risk of thrombosis (4–40%) during pregnancy (32, 43, 44). The coexistence of multiple inherited risk factors has been demonstrated. In one study, 15% of patients with protein C deficiency and 39% with protein S deficiency also were positive for factor V Leiden mutations, which markedly increased the risk of thrombosis for the patient (45).

Patients with a history of thrombosis, recurrent fetal loss, early or severe preeclampsia, or severe unexplained intrauterine growth restriction may be tested for antiphospholipid antibodies. Prophylactic anticoagulation for patients with antiphospholipid syndrome has been shown to improve pregnancy outcome (35, 46).

Deficiencies in protein C, protein S, and AT-III and mutations, including factor V Leiden, prothrombin G20210A, and C677T in the methylenetetrahydrofolate reductase (MTHFR) gene associated with hyperhomocystinemia, also have been associated with severe early preeclampsia, unexplained fetal loss or stillbirth, and placental abruption (47–49). However, there are no randomized clinical trials supporting the efficacy of anticoagulation therapy in preventing these conditions. It is important to discuss with the patient the implications of a positive test result for one of these thrombophilias and to determine whether patient management would be altered during the pregnancy or in the future if the test results are positive.

▶ *Which tests should be ordered?*

The following tests may be ordered to evaluate the risk for thromboembolic events in women with a history of thrombosis, a family history of thrombosis, or a first-degree relative with a specific mutation:

- Lupus anticoagulant (for women with a personal history of VTE)
- Anticardiolipin antibodies (for women with a personal history of VTE)
- Factor V Leiden mutation
- Prothrombin G20210A mutation
- AT-III antigen activity levels
- Fasting homocysteine levels or the MTHFR mutation
- Protein C antigen activity levels
- Protein S antigen activity levels (free and total)

Given the low prevalence of AT-III and the variable pathogenicity of protein C and protein S, consideration should be given to testing only when all other studies have yielded negative results. It is important to note that physiologic changes in normal pregnancy result in marked alterations in protein S and activated protein C resistance, which is associated with the factor V Leiden mutation; therefore, deferral of testing until after pregnancy may be warranted. For example, protein S levels decline by 40% in pregnancy (50, 51). Also, testing for AT-III, protein C, and protein S in the setting of extensive clotting, warfarin use, or heparin administration may result in falsely low values (33, 52, 53). DNA testing for the factor V Leiden, prothrombin G20210A mutation, and the MTHFR mutation are reliable in pregnancy.

▶ *How is deep vein thrombosis detected in pregnancy?*

A high index of suspicion is required for the diagnosis of DVT in pregnancy because some of the symptoms of DVT are similar to the common symptoms of pregnancy. Noninvasive testing for DVT includes compression ultrasound (CUS), which uses firm compression with the ultrasound transducer probe to detect an intraluminal filling defect and impedance plethysmography (IPG), which measures impedance flow with pneumatic cuff inflation around the thigh. In the symptomatic nonpregnant patient, IPG has a sensitivity of 83% and specificity of 92% of detecting proximal DVT. Compression ultrasound has a sensitivity of 95% for proximal DVT (73% for distal DVT) and specificity of 96% for detecting all DVT (54), with a negative predictive value of 98% and a positive predictive value of 97% in the nonpregnant symptomatic patient. It has been shown that if serial (3 or more follow-up tests over 7–14 days) IPGs have normal results in a symptomatic pregnant patient with a suspected DVT, it appears safe to withhold anticoagulation (55).

If the clinical suspicion is high and noninvasive test results are negative, limited venography with abdominal shielding that results in fetal exposure less than 0.05 rads should be considered (56). If iliac or pelvic thrombosis is suspected, full venography can be performed (bilateral venography without shielding results in fetal exposure <1.0 rads) (56). Diagnosis of pelvic vein thrombosis and internal iliac thrombosis is difficult. Although the use of venography is widespread, MRI may become the imaging modality of choice in these circumstances, but its role still is not well defined in the pregnant patient (57).

▶ *How is the diagnosis of pulmonary embolism made if suspected clinically?*

The diagnosis of PE has traditionally been evaluated initially with ventilation–perfusion scanning (V/Q). A V/Q scan results in minimal radiation exposure to the fetus (<0.1 rads). However, any outcome other than high probability or normal requires further testing because of insufficient accuracy to rule out PE in patients for which there is a high clinical suspicion (58). Unfortunately, about 40–60% of V/Q scans are nondiagnostic in the nonpregnant population (neither high probability nor normal), and further evaluation becomes necessary. If noninvasive testing (IPG, CUS) reveals a proximal DVT, then anticoagulation therapy can be initiated. If the results of these tests are negative, but clinical suspicion is high, then pulmonary angiography should be considered (54).

Spiral computed tomography (CT) may be useful for diagnosing PE; however, there is still difficulty reliably identifying emboli below the segmental level (59). Both sensitivity and specificity of spiral CT in nonpregnant patients for central pulmonary artery embolus are approximately 94%. It also may detect abnormalities other than PE responsible for symptoms (pleural effusions, consolidation, emphysema, pulmonary masses) and may be more specific in patients with underlying cardiopulmonary disease (60–62). Magnetic resonance angiography also may be promising, but current technology limits adequate visualization of subsegmental defects (63, 64). Both techniques are unstudied in pregnancy.

▶ *How should heparin be administered to women with acute thrombosis or embolism during pregnancy?*

Acute thromboembolism associated with pregnancy requires an intravenous heparin bolus of 5,000 U (80 IU/kg) followed by continuous infusion of at least 30,000 IU for 24 hours titrated to achieve full anticoagulation (3, 65). Intravenous anticoagulation should be maintained for at least 5–7 days. The patient can then be changed to subcutaneous adjusted-dose heparin therapy. Subcutaneous injections should be given to pregnant patients every 8 hours to prolong the APTT at least 1.5–2.5 times control throughout the dosing interval, similar to patients who are not pregnant (58, 66). The APTT cannot gauge the adequacy of anticoagulation with therapeutic heparin in patients with antiphospholipid syndrome for which small amounts of heparin may markedly increase the APTT. Levels of antifactor Xa may be used instead.

Therapeutic heparinization with subcutaneous dosing every 8–12 hours should be continued for at least 3 months after the acute event. After 3 months of therapeutic heparinization, experts differ as to what should be done for the remainder of the pregnancy. Some recommend using a lower dose of subcutaneous heparin. Others recommend continuing therapeutic anticoagulation for the remainder of the pregnancy (34).

Low-molecular-weight heparin may be an alternative treatment for acute thromboembolism. Although the actual dosing is unclear in pregnancy, dosage should be adjusted based on maternal weight. Although laboratory testing appears not to be essential in the nonpregnant patient, the role of monitoring antifactor Xa levels is not clear in the pregnant patient. The effectiveness of LMWH is less affected by changes in maternal physiology than is heparin, but there are still changes as pregnancy progresses. Therefore, it may be warranted to periodically reevaluate antifactor Xa levels during pregnancy in a woman on adjusted-dose or full anticoagulation. Ideally, dosing should be enough to achieve a peak antifactor Xa level of 0.5–1.2 U/mL (22, 34). Some experts also check trough levels to ensure that they remain in the lower limits of the anticoagulation range. Pending further informative data, the clinician may either use peak or trough levels, or both, to assess anticoagulation.

▶ *How is anticoagulation managed in the intrapartum and postpartum period?*

Intrapartum care is complicated, and treatment approaches vary. In such situations, it may be helpful to consult with personnel who have expertise in the intrapartum management of such patients. Patients requiring therapeutic adjusted-dose heparin during pregnancy, including those with recent thromboembolism, and patients with mechanical heart valves may be switched to intravenous heparin at the time of labor and delivery to take advantage of its short half-life (1½ hours). Patients can then be switched to warfarin postpartum. Heparin and warfarin therapy should be overlapped for the first 5–7 days postpartum until an international normalized ratio (INR) of approximately 2.0–3.0 has been achieved (67).

Patients receiving prophylactic anticoagulation with heparin should be instructed to withhold their injections at the onset of labor. Patients requiring adjusted-dose, prophylactic anticoagulation for high-risk conditions can resume their heparin injections 4–8 hours after an uncomplicated delivery, and warfarin can be administered the following morning. Postpartum dosing for women on low-dose prophylactic heparin varies widely, although all concur that the postpartum period is one of high risk. There are no definitive studies to guide one's approach in such situations.

▶ *Can regional anesthesia be administered to patients receiving anticoagulants?*

The use of major conduction anesthesia (spinal or epidural) in patients receiving thromboembolic prophylaxis is controversial (68, 69). Intraoperative or postoperative anticoagulation after regional anesthesia is thought to be safe; however, the safety of LMWH, unfractionated heparin, or oral anticoagulants administered before the procedure is unclear. Because there are no studies addressing anticoagulation in pregnancy relative to the use of conduction anesthesia, data from nonpregnant patients must be used.

Unfractionated low-dose heparin (≤5,000 IU twice daily) appeared not to pose a significant risk for spinal hematoma in over 5,000 nonpregnant patients who received it in combination with spinal or epidural anesthesia (70).

Although extensive clinical testing in Europe during the past decade suggested that there was no increased risk in patients receiving perioperative LMWH thromboprophylaxis, the U.S. Food and Drug Administration reported cases of epidural or spinal hematomas in nonpregnant patients with concurrent use of enoxaparin (a low-molecular-weight heparin) and spinal or epidural anesthesia or spinal puncture (71). Many of the epidural or spinal hematomas caused neurologic injury, including long-term or permanent paralysis. The discrepancy in the incidence of epidural or spinal hematomas in the European versus the United States literature may be related to higher dosing and preference in the United States of continuous epidurals rather than single shot spinals (70, 72). In one British study of pregnant women, there were no spinal hematomas in the 43 women receiving LMWH thromboprophylaxis who also received epidural analgesia (22). However, the doses given were lower than are currently employed and usually administered once a day.

The American Society of Regional Anesthesia has recommended that patients receiving higher doses of LMWH (specifically enoxaparin, 1 mg/kg twice daily) should not receive neuraxial blocks for 24 hours from the last dose (73). Also, obtaining an antifactor Xa level before placing the block was not recommended because it was believed not to be adequately predictive of the risk of bleeding. Needle placement in patients receiving low-dose, once daily LMWH should occur at least 10–12 hours after the LMWH dose. No specific recommendations were made for patients using an intermediate dose of 30–40 mg of enoxaparin twice daily. However, given that twice daily dosing may maintain antifactor Xa levels between 0.1 and 0.2 IU/mL 12 hours after injection, it would seem prudent to delay epidural anesthesia for 24 hours after the last injection. Alternatively, patients could be switched to standard heparin at term because a normal APTT usually is sufficient to ensure the safety of epidural anesthesia in a heparin anticoagulated patient as long as the platelet count also is normal.

Summary

The following recommendations are based primarily on consensus and expert opinion (Level C):

- Pregnant patients with a history of isolated venous thrombosis directly related to a transient, highly thrombogenic event (orthopedic trauma, complicated surgery) in whom an underlying thrombophilia has been excluded may be offered heparin prophylaxis or no prophylaxis during the antepartum period. However, they should be counseled that their risk of thromboembolism is likely to be higher than the normal population. Prophylactic warfarin should be offered for 6 weeks postpartum.
- Pregnant patients with a history of idiopathic thrombosis, thrombosis related to pregnancy or oral contraceptive use, or a history of thrombosis accompanied by an underlying thrombophilia other than homozygous for the factor V Leiden mutation, heterozygous for both the factor V Leiden and the prothrombin G20210A mutation, or AT-III deficiency should be offered antepartum and postpartum low-dose heparin prophylaxis.
- Patients without a history of thrombosis but who have an underlying thrombophilia and have a strong family history of thrombosis also are candidates for antepartum and postpartum prophylaxis. At the minimum, postpartum prophylaxis should be offered.
- Pregnant patients with a history of life-threatening thrombosis, with recent thrombosis, with recurrent thrombosis, receiving chronic anticoagulation, or patients with thrombosis found to be AT-III deficient, homozygous for the factor V Leiden mutation or prothrombin G20210A mutation, heterozygous for both the factor V Leiden and the prothrombin G20210A mutation should be given adjusted-dose heparin every 8 hours to maintain the APTT at least 1.5 times control throughout the dosing interval. Low-molecular-weight heparin administered twice daily also is an alternative.
- Patients at risk for thrombosis should receive warfarin postpartum for 6 weeks to achieve an INR of approximately 2.0–3.0. Heparin should be given immediately postpartum with warfarin for at least 5 days until the INR is therapeutic.
- Patients with antiphospholipid syndrome and a history of thrombosis require adjusted-dose prophylactic anticoagulation.
- Patients who are candidates for either prophylactic or therapeutic heparin may be given enoxaparin or dalteparin during pregnancy. However, because of the lack of data regarding adequate dosing during pregnancy, antifactor Xa levels may be monitored.
- The safety of epidural anesthesia with twice-daily dosing of LMWH is of concern and should be withheld until 24 hours after the last injection.

- Epidural anesthesia appears to be safe in women taking unfractionated low-dose heparin if the APTT is normal.

References

1. Gherman RB, Goodwin TM, Leung B, Byrne JD, Hethumumi R, Montoro M. Incidence, clinical characteristics, and timing of objectively diagnosed venous thromboembolism during pregnancy. Obstet Gynecol 1999;94:730–734 (Level II-3)
2. Lindqvist P, Dahlback B, Marsal K. Thrombotic risk during pregnancy: a population study. Obstet Gynecol 1999;94:595–599 (Level II-2)
3. Toglia MR, Weg JG. Venous thromboembolism during pregnancy. N Engl J Med 1996;335:108–114 (Level III)
4. Berg CJ, Atrash HK, Koonin LM, Tucker M. Pregnancy-related mortality in the United States, 1987–1990. Obstet Gynecol 1996;88:161–167 (Level II-3)
5. Grandone E, Margaglione M, Colaizzo D, D'Andrea G, Cappucci G, Brancaccio V, et al. Genetic susceptibility to pregnancy-related venous thromboembolism: roles of factor V Leiden, prothrombin G20210A, and methylenetetrahydrofolate reductase C677T mutations. Am J Obstet Gynecol 1998;179:1324–1328 (Level II-2)
6. Dizon-Townson DS, Nelson LM, Jang H, Varner MW, Ward K. The incidence of the factor V Leiden mutation in an obstetric population and its relationship to deep vein thrombosis. Am J Obstet Gynecol 1997;176:883–886 (Level III)
7. De Stefano V, Leone G, Mastrangelo S, Tripodi A, Rodeghiero F, Castaman G, et al. Clinical manifestations and management of inherited thrombophilia: retrospective analysis and follow-up after diagnosis of 238 patients with congenital deficiency of antithrombin III, protein C, protein S. Thromb Haemost 1994;72:352–358 (Level III)
8. Middledorp S, Henkens CM, Koopman MM, van Pampus EC, Hamulyák K, van der Meer J, et al. The incidence of venous thromboembolism in family members of patients with factor V Leiden mutation and venous thrombosis. Ann Intern Med 1998;128:15–20 (Level II-2)
9. Badaracco MA, Vessey MP. Recurrence of venous thromboembolic disease and use of oral contraceptives. Br Med J 1974;1:215–217 (Level II-2)
10. Tengborn L, Bergqvist D, Mätzsch T, Bergqvist A, Hedner U. Recurrent thromboembolism in pregnancy and puerperium. Is there a need for thromboprophylaxis? Am J Obstet Gynecol 1989:160(1);90–94 (Level II-2)
11. Ginsberg JS, Kowalchuk G, Hirsh J, Brill-Edwards P, Burrows R. Heparin therapy during pregnancy. Risks to the fetus and mother. Arch Intern Med 1989;149: 2233–2236 (Level II-3)
12. Barbour LA, Smith JM, Marlar RA. Heparin levels to guide thromboembolism prophylaxis during pregnancy. Am J Obstet Gynecol 1995;173:1869–1873 (Level III)
13. Barbour LA, Kick SD, Steiner JF, LoVerde ME, Heddleston LN, Lear JL, et al. A prospective study of heparin-induced osteoporosis in pregnancy using bone densitometry. Am J Obstet Gynecol 1994;170:862–869 (Level II-2)
14. Dahlman TC, Sjöberg HE, Ringertz H. Bone mineral density during long-term prophylaxis with heparin in pregnancy. Am J Obstet Gynecol 1994;170:1315–1320 (Level II-2)
15. Dahlman TC. Osteoporotic fractures and the recurrence of thromboembolism during pregnancy and the puerperium in 184 women undergoing thromboprophylaxis with heparin. Am J Obstet Gynecol 1993;168:1265–1270 (Level III)
16. Warkentin TE, Levine MN, Hirsh J, Horsewood P, Roberts RS, Gent M, et al. Heparin-induced thrombocytopenia in patients treated with low-molecular-weight heparin or unfractionated heparin. N Engl J Med 1995;332: 1330–1335 (Level II-2)
17. Kelton JG. The clinical management of heparin-induced thrombocytopenia. Semin Hematol 1999;36(suppl 1):17–21 (Level III)
18. Hirsh J, Warkentin TE, Raschke R, Granger C, Ohman EM, Dalen JE. Heparin and low-molecular-weight heparin: mechanisms of action, pharmacokinetics, dosing considerations, monitoring, efficacy, and safety. Chest 1998;114:489S–510S (Level III)
19. Bergqvist D. Low molecular weight heparins. J Intern Med 1996:240;63–72 (Level III)
20. Forestier F, Solé Y, Aiach M, Alhenc Gelás M, Daffos F. Absence of transplacental fragmin (Kabi) during second and third trimesters of pregnancy. Thromb Haemost 1992;67:180–181 (Level III)
21. Omri A, Delaloye JF, Andersen H, Bachmann F. Low molecular weight heparin Novo (LHN-1) does not cross the placenta during the second trimester of pregnancy. Thromb Haemost 1989;61:55–56 (Level II-2)
22. Nelson-Piercy C, Letsky EA, de Swiet M. Low-molecular-weight heparin for obstetric thromboprophylaxis: experience of sixty-nine pregnancies in sixty-one women at risk. Am J Obstet Gynecol 1997;176:1062–1068 (Level III)
23. Dulitzki M, Pauzner R, Langevitz P, Pras M, Many A, Schiff E. Low-molecular-weight heparin during pregnancy and delivery: preliminary experience with 41 pregnancies. Obstet Gynecol 1996;87:380–383 (Level III)
24. Rasmussen C, Wadt B, Jacobsen B. Thromboembolic prophylaxis with low molecular weight heparin during pregnancy. Int J Gynaecol Obstet 1994;47:121–125 (Level III)
25. Orme ML, Lewis PJ, de Swiet M, Serlin MJ, Sibeon R, Baty JD, et al. May mothers given warfarin breast-feed their infants? BMJ 1977;1(6076):1564–1565 (Level III)
26. Chan WS, Anand S, Ginsberg JS. Anticoagulation of pregnant women with mechanical heart valves. Arch Intern Med 2000;160:191–196 (Level III)
27. Iturbe-Alessio I, Fonseca M, Mutchinik O, Santos MA, Zajarías A, Salazar E. Risks of anticoagulant therapy in pregnant women with artificial heart valves. N Engl J Med 1986;315:1390–1393 (Level II-2)

28. Born D, Martinez EE, Almeida PAM, Santos DV, Carvalho AC, Moron AF, et al. Pregnancy in patients with prosthetic heart valves: the effects of anticoagulation on mother, fetus, and neonate. Am Heart J 1992;124:413–417 (Level II-2)

29. Salazar E, Izaguirre R, Verdejo J, Mutchinick O. Failure of adjusted doses of subcutaneous heparin to prevent thromboembolic phenomena in pregnant patients with mechanical cardiac valve prostheses. J Am Coll Cardiol 1996;27:1698–1703 (Level III)

30. Hall JG, Pauli RM, Wilson KM. Maternal and fetal sequelae of anticoagulation during pregnancy. Am J Med 1980;68:122–140 (Level III)

31. McColl MD, Ramsay JE, Tait RC, Walker ID, McCall F, Conkie JA, et al. Risk factors for pregnancy associated venous thromboembolism. Thromb Haemost 1997;78:1183–1188 (Level III)

32. Conard J, Horellou MH, Van Dredan P, Lecompte T, Samama M. Thrombosis and pregnancy in congenital deficiencies in AT III, protein C or protein S: study of 78 women. Thromb Haemost 1990;63:319–320 (Level III)

33. Van Boven HH, Lane DA. Antithrombin and its inherited deficiency states. Semin Hematol 1997;34:188–204 (Level III)

34. Ginsberg JS, Hirsh J. Use of antithrombotic agents during pregnancy. Chest 1998;114:524S–530S (Level III)

35. Branch DW, Silver RM, Blackwell JL, Reading JC, Scott JR. Outcome of treated pregnancies in women with antiphospholipid syndrome: an update of the Utah experience. Obstet Gynecol 1992;80:614–620 (Level II-2)

36. Barbour LA, Pickard J. Controversies in thromboembolic disease during pregnancy: a critical review. Obstet Gynecol 1995;86:621–633 (Level III)

37. Gerhardt A, Scharf RE, Beckmann MW, Struve S, Bender HG, Pillny M, et al. Prothrombin and factor V mutations in women with a history of thrombosis during pregnancy and the puerperium. N Engl J Med 2000;342:374–380 (Level II-2)

38. Colvin BT, Barrowcliffe TW. The British Society for Haematology Guidelines on the use and monitoring of heparin 1992: second revision. BCSH Haemostasis and Thrombosis Task Force. J Clin Pathol 1993;46:97–103 (Level III)

39. Maternal and Neonatal Haemostasis Working Party of the Haemostasis and Thrombosis Task. Guidelines on the prevention, investigation and management of thrombosis associated with pregnancy. J Clin Pathol 1993;46:489–496 (Level III)

40. Lechner K, Kyrle PA. Antithrombin III concentrates—are they clinically useful? Thromb Haemost 1995;73:340–348 (Level III)

41. Barbour LA. Current concepts of anticoagulant therapy in pregnancy. Obstet Gynecol Clin North Am 1997;24:499–521 (Level III)

42. Weitz JI. Drug therapy: low molecular weight heparin. N Engl J Med 1997;337:688–698 (Level III)

43. Miletich JP. Thrombophilia as a multigenic disorder. Semin Thromb Hemost 1998;24(suppl 1):13–20 (Level III)

44. Friederich PW, Sanson BJ, Simioni P, Zanardi S, Huisman MV, Kindt I, et al. Frequency of pregnancy-related venous thromboembolism in anticoagulant factor-deficient women: implications for prophylaxis. Ann Intern Med 1996;125:955–960 (Level III)

45. Florell SR, Rodgers GM. Inherited thrombotic disorders: an update. Am J Hematol 1997;54:53–60 (Level III)

46. Rai R, Cohen H, Dave M, Regan L. Randomised controlled trial of aspirin and aspirin plus heparin in pregnant women with recurrent miscarriage associated with phospholipid antibodies (or antiphospholipid antibodies). BMJ 1997;314:253–257 (Level I)

47. Brenner B, Mandel H, Lanir N, Younis J, Rothbart H, Ohel G, et al. Activated protein C resistance can be associated with recurrent fetal loss. Br J Haematol 1997;97:551–554 (Level II-2)

48. Dizon-Townson D, Meline L, Nelson LM, Varner M, Ward K. Fetal carriers of the factor V Leiden mutation are prone to miscarriage or placental infarction. Am J Obstet Gynecol 1997;177:402–405 (Level II-2)

49. Kupferminc MJ, Eldor A, Steinman N, Many A, Bar-Am A, Jaffa A, et al. Increased frequency of genetic thrombophilia in women with complications of pregnancy. N Engl J Med 1999;340:9–13 (Level II-2)

50. Faught W, Garner P, Jones C, Ivey B. Changes in protein C and protein S levels in normal pregnancy. Am J Obstet Gynecol 1995;172:147–150 (Level II-3)

51. Lefkowitz JB, Clarke SH, Barbour LA. Comparison of protein S functional and antigenic assays in normal pregnancy. Am J Obstet Gynecol 1996;175:657–650 (Level II-3)

52. Rao AK, Kaplan R, Sheth S. Inherited thrombophilic states. Semin Thromb Hemost 1998;24(suppl 1):3–12 (Level III)

53. Reiter W, Ehrensberger H, Steinbrückner B, Keller F. Parameters of haemostasis during acute venous thrombosis. Thromb Haemost 1995;74:596–601 (Level III)

54. Douketis JD, Ginsberg JS. Diagnostic problems with venous thromboembolic disease in pregnancy. Haemostasis 1995;25:58–71 (Level III)

55. Hull RD, Raskob GE, Carter CJ. Serial impedance plethysmography in pregnant patients with clinically suspected deep-vein thrombosis. Clinical validity of negative findings. Ann Intern Med 1990;112:663–667 (Level II-3)

56. Ginsberg JS, Hirsh J, Rainbow AJ, Coates G. Risks to the fetus of radiologic procedures used in the diagnosis of maternal venous thromboembolic disease. Thromb Haemost 1989;61:189–196 (Level III)

57. Spritzer CE, Evans AC, Kay HH. Magnetic resonance imaging of deep venous thrombosis in pregnant women with lower extremity edema. Obstet Gynecol 1995;85:603–607 (Level III)

58. Ginsberg JS. Management of venous thromboembolism. N Engl J Med 1996;335(24):1816–1828 (Level III)

59. Hansell DM. Spiral computed tomography and pulmonary embolism: current state. Clin Radiol 1997;52:575–581 (Level III)

60. Cross JJ, Kemp PM, Walsh CG, Flower CD, Dixon AK. A randomized trial of spiral CT and ventilation perfusion

scintigraphy for the diagnosis of pulmonary embolism. Clin Radiol 1998;53:177–182 (Level I)

61. Lipchik RJ, Goodman LR. Spiral computed tomography in the evaluation of pulmonary embolism. Clin Chest Med 1999;20:731–738 (Level III)
62. Kim KI, Muller NL, Mayo JR. Clinically suspected pulmonary embolism: utility of spiral CT. Radiology 1999;210:693–697 (Level III)
63. Meaney JF, Weg JG, Chenevert TL, Stafford-Johnson D, Hamilton BH, Prince MR. Diagnosis of pulmonary embolism with magnetic resonance angiography. N Engl J Med 1997;336:1422–1427 (Level II-2)
64. Woodard PK, Yusen RD. Diagnosis of pulmonary embolism with spiral computed tomography and magnetic resonance angiography. Curr Opin Cardiol 1999;14: 442–447 (Level III)
65. Bates SM, Ginsberg JS. Thrombosis in pregnancy. Curr Opin Hematol 1997;4:335–343 (Level III)
66. Ramin SM, Ramin KD, Gilstrap LC. Anticoagulants and thrombolytics during pregnancy. Semin Perinatol 1997;21: 149–153 (Level III)
67. Hyers TM, Agnelli G, Hull RD, Weg JG, Morris TA, Samama M, et al. Antithrombotic therapy for venous thromboembolic disease. Chest 1998;114:561S–578S (Level III)
68. Haljamäe H. Thromboprophylaxis, coagulation disorders, and regional anesthesia. Acta Anaesthesiol Scand 1996;40:1024–1040 (Level III)
69. Hynson JM, Katz JA, Bueff HU. Epidural hematoma associated with enoxaparin. Anesth Analg 1996;82:1072–1075 (Level III)
70. Horlocker TT, Wedel DJ. Neuraxial block and low-molecular-weight heparin: balancing perioperative analgesia and thromboprophylaxis. Reg Anesth Pain Med 1998;23(6 Suppl 2);164–177 (Level III)
71. U.S. Department of Health and Human Services. FDA Public Health Advisory, Subject: reports of epidural or spinal hematomas with the concurrent use of low molecular weight heparin and spinal/epidural anesthesia or spinal puuncture. Rockville, Maryland: Food and Drug Administration, December 1997 (Level III)
72. Tryba M. European practice guidelines: thromboembolism prophylaxis and regional anesthesia. Reg Anesth Pain Med 1998;23(6 Suppl 2):178–182 (Level III)
73. American Society of Regional Anesthesia (ASRA). Recommendations for neuraxial anesthesia and anticoagulation. Richmond, VA: ASRA, 1998 (Level III

The MEDLINE database, the Cochrane Library, and ACOG's own internal resources and documents were used to conduct a literature search to locate relevant articles published between January 1985 and March 1998. The search was restricted to articles published in the English language. Priority was given to articles reporting results of original research, although review articles and commentaries also were consulted. Abstracts of research presented at symposia and scientific conferences were not considered adequate for inclusion in this document. Guidelines published by organizations or institutions such as the National Institutes of Health and the American College of Obstetricians and Gynecologists were reviewed, and additional studies were located by reviewing bibliographies of identified articles. When reliable research was not available, expert opinions from obstetrician–gynecologists were used.

Studies were reviewed and evaluated for quality according to the method outlined by the U.S. Preventive Services Task Force:

- I Evidence obtained from at least one properly designed randomized controlled trial.
- II-1 Evidence obtained from well-designed controlled trials without randomization.
- II-2 Evidence obtained from well-designed cohort or case–control analytic studies, preferably from more than one center or research group.
- II-3 Evidence obtained from multiple time series with or without the intervention. Dramatic results in uncontrolled experiments could also be regarded as this type of evidence.
- III Opinions of respected authorities, based on clinical experience, descriptive studies, or reports of expert committees.

Based on the highest level of evidence found in the data, recommendations are provided and graded according to the following catetories:

Level A—Recommendations are based on good and consistent scientific evidence.

Level B—Recommendations are based on limited or inconsistent scientific evidence.

Level C—Recommendations are based primarily on consensus and expert opinion.

ISSN 1099-3630

**The American College of
Obstetricians and Gynecologists
409 12th Street, SW
PO Box 96920
Washington, DC 20090-6920**

12345/43210

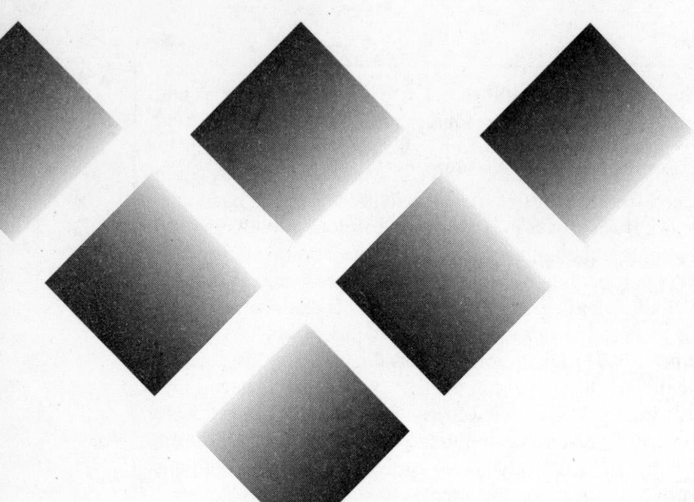

ACOG PRACTICE BULLETIN

CLINICAL MANAGEMENT GUIDELINES FOR OBSTETRICIAN–GYNECOLOGISTS

NUMBER 5, JULY 1999

(Replaces Practice Bulletin Number 2, October 1998)

This Practice Bulletin was developed by the ACOG Committee on Practice Bulletins—Obstetrics with the assistance of James R. Scott, MD. The information is designed to aid practitioners in making decisions about appropriate obstetric and gynecologic care. These guidelines should not be construed as dictating an exclusive course of treatment or procedure. Variations in practice may be warranted based on the needs of the individual patient, resources, and limitations unique to the institution or type of practice.

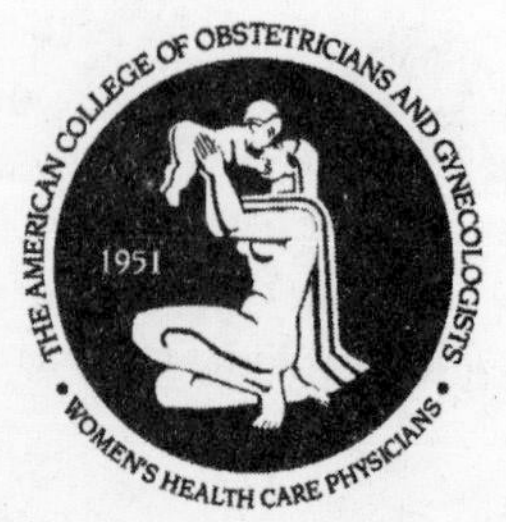

Vaginal Birth After Previous Cesarean Delivery

A trial of labor after previous cesarean delivery has been accepted as a way to lower the overall cesarean delivery rate. In 1995, 27.5% of women who had a previous cesarean delivery attempted vaginal birth; some clinicians believe that an even higher percentage is possible (1). Although there is a strong consensus that trial of labor is appropriate for most women who have had a previous low-transverse cesarean delivery, increased experience with vaginal birth after cesarean delivery (VBAC) indicates there are several potential problems. This document will review the current risks and benefits of VBAC in various situations and provide practical management guidelines.

Background

Beginning in the 1970s, the marked reduction in the maternal death rate focused obstetricians' attention on fetal morbidity and mortality. Physicians in the United States, facing increased medical–legal pressures, performed fewer vaginal breech deliveries and fewer midpelvic forceps deliveries. In addition, nonreassuring fetal status was diagnosed more frequently because of wide variations in the interpretation of continuous electronic fetal monitoring. Finally, dystocia, as an indication for cesarean delivery, was diagnosed more frequently. Consequently, the cesarean delivery rate in the United States increased from 5% to 20.8% between 1970 and 1995 (1) and reached 24.7% in 1988 (2, 3).

With few exceptions, major improvements in newborn outcome from the increased cesarean delivery rate are yet to be proven (4). It generally is agreed that the current rate is high. The overall number of cesarean deliveries can be reduced safely and effectively when the indications for primary cesarean birth are reviewed and audited (5–7). However, most efforts have focused on decreasing the number of elective repeat cesarean births because they account for one third of all cesarean deliveries.

Changing Concepts

The dictum "once a cesarean, always a cesarean" dominated obstetric practice in the United States for nearly 70 years (8). This concept began changing gradually about 30 years ago as improvements in obstetric care made trial of labor safer for both mother and infant. In 1981, when the VBAC rate was only 3%, the National Institutes of Health began to encourage trial of labor. The American College of Obstetricians and Gynecologists also was a leader in this effort (9), and a number of reports have documented the relative safety of trial of labor (10–14). Some third-party payers and managed care organizations have mandated that all women who had previous cesarean deliveries must undergo trial of labor. Consequently, physicians may find themselves pressured to attempt trial of labor either in situations that they consider to be unsuitable or with patients who do not desire the procedure.

Recent Issues

Despite more than 800 citations in the literature, there are no randomized trials to prove that maternal and neonatal outcomes are better with VBAC than with repeat cesarean delivery. Published evidence suggests that the benefits of VBAC outweigh the risks in most women with a prior low-transverse cesarean delivery. Nevertheless, most studies of VBAC have been conducted in university or tertiary-level centers with in-house staff coverage and anesthesia. The safety of trial of labor is less well documented in smaller community hospitals or facilities where resources may be more limited (15–18). It has become apparent that VBAC is associated with a small but significant risk of uterine rupture with poor outcome for both mother and infant (19–22). Reports indicate that maternal and infant complications also are associated with an unsuccessful trial of labor. Increasingly, these adverse events during trial of labor have led to malpractice suits (22–24). These developments, which have led to a more circumspect approach to trial of labor by even the most ardent supporters of VBAC, illustrate the need to reevaluate VBAC recommendations (23, 25).

Clinical Considerations and Recommendations

▶ ***Who are candidates for a trial of labor?***

Most patients who have had a low-transverse uterine incision from a previous cesarean delivery and who have no contraindications for vaginal birth are candidates for a trial of labor. Women who have had two previous low-transverse cesarean deliveries also may be considered for a trial of labor, but the risk of uterine rupture increases with the number of previous uterine incisions (13). Following are selection criteria useful in identifying candidates for VBAC:

- One or two prior low-transverse cesarean deliveries
- Clinically adequate pelvis
- No other uterine scars or previous rupture
- Physician immediately available throughout active labor capable of monitoring labor and performing an emergency cesarean delivery
- Availability of anesthesia and personnel for emergency cesarean delivery

There has been a tendency to expand the list of obstetric circumstances under which VBAC may be appropriate. These include multiple previous cesarean deliveries (26, 27), unknown uterine scar (13, 28), breech presentation (29, 30), twin gestation (31, 32), postterm pregnancy (33), and suspected macrosomia (34, 35). Whether trial of labor should be encouraged for patients with these obstetric circumstances and a low-vertical uterine incision is controversial (18, 36, 37). Although success has been reported in some series, continuing analysis of the risk of adverse outcome is necessary before VBAC is routinely adopted in these circumstances.

▶ ***What is the success rate for trials of labor?***

Most published series indicate that approximately 60–80% of trials of labor after a previous cesarean delivery result in successful vaginal births (14, 38, 39). However, these success rates often apply to a selected population. Patients thought to be inappropriate candidates for a trial of labor usually have been excluded, and the exact percentage of women undergoing trial of labor is not consistently stated.

Although a number of scoring systems have been used, there is no completely reliable way to predict whether a trial of labor will be successful in an individual patient (40–44). The success rates of VBAC in women whose first cesarean delivery was performed for a nonrecurring indication are similar to those of patients who have not undergone previous cesarean delivery (45). A woman who has undergone vaginal delivery at least once before or after her previous cesarean birth also is more likely to have a successful trial of labor than the woman who has not undergone vaginal delivery (45, 46).

Many patients with a previous diagnosis of dystocia successfully deliver vaginally, but the percentage is consistently lower (50–70%) than for those with nonrecurring indications (12, 14, 47, 48). The lower rate is most likely related to the accuracy of the original diagnosis of dystocia.

▶ *What are the risks and benefits associated with VBAC?*

Neither repeat cesarean delivery nor trial of labor is risk free. When VBAC is successful, it is associated with less morbidity than repeat cesarean delivery. The advantages include fewer blood transfusions, fewer postpartum infections, and shorter hospital stays, usually with no increased perinatal morbidity (11, 12, 14).

It often is stated that the cost of VBAC is less than that of repeat cesarean delivery. However, for a true analysis of all the costs one has to include the costs to the hospital, the method of reimbursement (ie, per diem diagnosis-related group or capitation), and medical malpractice payments. Higher costs may be incurred by a hospital if a woman has a prolonged labor or has significant complications, or if the newborn is admitted to a neonatal intensive care unit. Furthermore, 20–40% of women will fail the trial of labor, which will incur surgical costs. Increased time or attendance for a woman undergoing a trial of labor results in increased cost to the physician. The difficulty in assessing the cost-benefit of VBAC is that the costs are not all incurred by one entity.

Those patients who fail a trial of labor are at increased risk for infection and morbidity (49–52). Infants born by repeat cesarean delivery after a failed trial of labor also have increased rates of infection (53). In contrast to previous reports, the most recent series showed that major maternal complications such as uterine rupture, hysterectomy, and operative injury were more likely for women who underwent a trial of labor than for those who elected repeat cesarean delivery (50).

Rupture of the uterine scar can be life-threatening for both mother and infant (19–22). When catastrophic uterine rupture occurs, some patients will require hysterectomy and some infants will die or will be neurologically impaired (22, 50). In most cases, the cause of uterine rupture in a patient who has undergone VBAC is unknown, but poor outcomes can result even in appropriate candidates.

The occurrence of uterine rupture is dependent on the type and location of the previous incision. Estimated occurrence based on the literature is as follows (18, 39):

- Classical uterine scar (4–9%)
- T-shaped incision (4–9%)
- Low-vertical incision (1–7%)
- Low-transverse incision (0.2–1.5%)

The most common sign of uterine rupture is a nonreassuring fetal heart rate pattern with variable decelerations that may evolve into late decelerations, bradycardia, and undetectable fetal heart rate. Other findings are more variable and include uterine or abdominal pain, loss of station of the presenting part, vaginal bleeding, and hypovolemia.

▶ *What are contraindications for VBAC?*

A trial of labor is not recommended in patients at high risk for uterine rupture. Circumstances under which a trial of labor should not be attempted are as follows:

- Prior classical or T-shaped incision or other transfundal uterine surgery (54)
- Contracted pelvis (18)
- Medical or obstetric complication that precludes vaginal delivery
- Inability to perform emergency cesarean delivery because of unavailable surgeon, anesthesia, sufficient staff, or facility

A combination of factors, which singly may not be compelling for cesarean delivery in a patient without a uterine scar, may influence the decision to forego VBAC and recommend repeat cesarean delivery.

▶ *How should patients be counseled?*

The enthusiasm for VBAC varies greatly among patients and physicians. It is reasonable for women to undergo a trial of labor in a safe setting, but the potential complications should be discussed thoroughly and documented (55). If the type of previous incision is in doubt, attempts should be made to obtain medical records. After thorough counseling that weighs the individual benefits and risks of VBAC, the ultimate decision to attempt this procedure or undergo a repeat cesarean delivery should be made by the patient and her physician (see Fig. 1). Global mandates for a trial of labor after a previous cesarean delivery are inappropriate because individual risk factors are not considered. It should be recognized that there are repeat elective cesarean deliveries that are clinically indicated (56). The informed consent process and the plan of management should be documented in the prenatal record.

▶ *How does management of labor differ for patients undergoing VBAC?*

Despite extensive data on VBAC, there is relatively little information on how labor should be conducted. Management of labor varies in different situations.

External Cephalic Version. Limited data suggest that external cephalic version for breech presentation may be as successful for VBAC candidates as for women who have not undergone previous cesarean delivery (57).

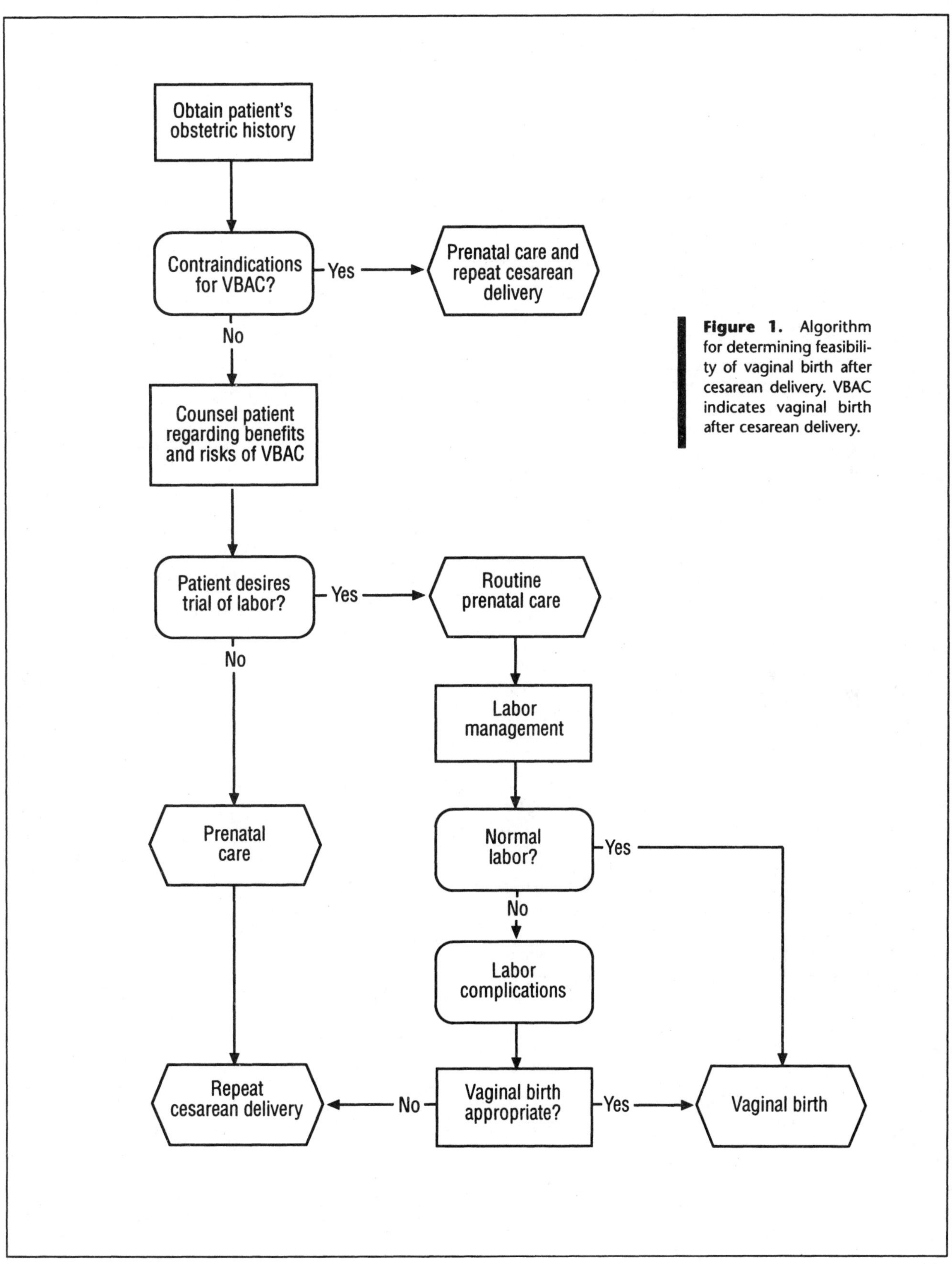

Figure 1. Algorithm for determining feasibility of vaginal birth after cesarean delivery. VBAC indicates vaginal birth after cesarean delivery.

Analgesia. Vaginal birth after cesarean delivery is not a contraindication to epidural anesthesia, and adequate pain relief may encourage more women to choose a trial of labor (58, 59). Success rates for VBAC are similar in women who do and those who do not receive epidural analgesia, as well as in those women who receive other types of pain relief (60–62). Epidural analgesia rarely masks the signs and symptoms of uterine rupture.

Intrapartum Management. Once labor has begun, the patient should be evaluated promptly. Most authorities recommend continuous electronic monitoring. Personnel who are familiar with the potential complications of VBAC should be present to watch for nonreassuring fetal heart rate patterns and inadequate progress in labor.

Induction. Induction or augmentation with oxytocin has been suspected as a factor responsible for uterine rupture. A meta-analysis found no relationship between the use of oxytocin and rupture of the uterine scar (14). However, other studies indicate that high infusion rates of oxytocin place women at greater risk (63, 64). Although there are studies that suggest that prostaglandin gel applied to the cervix or vagina appears to be safe (65–67), there are occasional reports of uterine rupture with prostaglandin preparations (68, 69).

Delivery. There is nothing unique about delivery of the infant after a trial of labor. The need to explore the uterus after successful vaginal delivery is controversial. Most asymptomatic scar dehiscences heal well, and there are no data to suggest that future pregnancy outcome is better if the dehiscence is surgically repaired. Excessive vaginal bleeding or signs of hypovolemia at delivery require prompt and complete assessment of the previous scar and the entire genital tract.

▶ ***How should future pregnancies be managed after uterine rupture?***

If the site of the ruptured scar is confined to the lower segment, the rate of repeat rupture or dehiscence in labor is 6% (70). If the scar includes the upper segment of the uterus, the repeat rupture rate is 32% (70, 71). Therefore, women who have had a prior uterine rupture should undergo repeat cesarean delivery as soon as the fetus is mature.

Summary

The following recommendations are based on good and consistent scientific evidence (Level A):

- Most women with one previous cesarean delivery with a low-transverse incision are candidates for VBAC and should be counseled about VBAC and offered a trial of labor.
- Epidural anesthesia may be used for VBAC.
- A previous uterine incision extending into the fundus is a contraindication for VBAC.

The following recommendations are based on limited or inconsistent scientific evidence (Level B):

- Women with two previous low-transverse cesarean deliveries and no contraindications who wish to attempt VBAC may be allowed a trial of labor. They should be advised that the risk of uterine rupture increases as the number of cesarean deliveries increases.
- Use of oxytocin or prostaglandin gel for VBAC requires close patient monitoring.
- Women with a vertical incision within the lower uterine segment that does not extend into the fundus are candidates for VBAC.

The following recommendations are based primarily on consensus and expert opinion (Level C):

- Because uterine rupture may be catastrophic, VBAC should be attempted in institutions equipped to respond to emergencies with physicians immediately available to provide emergency care.
- After thorough counseling that weighs the individual benefits and risks of VBAC, the ultimate decision to attempt this procedure or undergo a repeat cesarean delivery should be made by the patient and her physician.

References

1. Curtin SC. Rates of cesarean birth and vaginal birth after previous cesarean, 1991–95. Monthly vital statistics report; vol 45, no. 11 (suppl 3). Hyattsville, Maryland: National Center for Health Statistics, 1997 (Level II-3)
2. Centers for Disease Control. Rates of cesarean delivery—United States, 1991. MMWR Morb Mortal Wkly Rep 1993;42:285–289 (Level II-3)
3. Stafford RS. Alternative strategies for controlling rising cesarean section rates. JAMA 1990; 263:683–687 (Level III)
4. Scheller JM, Nelson KB. Does cesarean delivery prevent cerebral palsy or other neurologic problems of childhood? Obstet Gynecol 1994;83:624–630 (Level III)
5. Lagrew DC Jr, Morgan MA. Decreasing the cesarean section rate in a private hospital: success without mandated clinical changes. Am J Obstet Gynecol 1996;174:184–191 (Level II-3)
6. Myers SA, Gleicher N. A successful program to lower cesarean-section rates. N Engl J Med 1988;319:1511–1516 (Level II-3)

7. Robson MS, Scudamore IW, Walsh SM. Using the medical audit cycle to reduce cesarean section rates. Am J Obstet Gynecol 1996;174:199–205 (Level II-2)

8. Cragin EB. Conservatism in obstetrics. N Y Med J 1916; 104:1–3 (Level III)

9. American College of Obstetricians and Gynecologists. Vaginal delivery after previous cesarean birth. ACOG Practice Patterns 1. Washington, DC: ACOG, 1995 (Level III)

10. Cowan RK, Kinch RA, Ellis B, Anderson R. Trial of labor following cesarean delivery. Obstet Gynecol 1994;83: 933–936 (Level II-3)

11. Flamm BL, Newman LA, Thomas SJ, Fallon D, Yoshida MM. Vaginal birth after cesarean delivery: results of a 5-year multicenter collaborative study. Obstet Gynecol 1990;76:750–754 (Level II-3)

12. Flamm BL, Goings JR, Liu Y, Wolde-Tsadik G. Elective repeat cesarean delivery versus trial of labor: a prospective multicenter study. Obstet Gynecol 1994;83:927–932 (Level II-2)

13. Miller DA, Diaz FG, Paul RH. Vaginal birth after cesarean: a 10-year experience. Obstet Gynecol 1994;84:255–258 (Level III)

14. Rosen MG, Dickinson JC, Westhoff CL. Vaginal birth after cesarean: a meta-analysis of morbidity and mortality. Obstet Gynecol 1991;77:465–470 (Meta-analysis)

15. Hawkins JL, Gibbs CP, Orleans M, Martin-Salvaj G, Beaty B. Obstetric anesthesia work force survey, 1981 versus 1992. Anesthesiology 1997;87:135–143 (Level II-3)

16. Holland JG, Dupre AR, Blake PG, Martin RW, Martin JN Jr. Trial of labor after cesarean delivery: experience in the non-university level II regional hospital setting. Obstet Gynecol 1992;79:936–939 (Level II-3)

17. Raynor BD. The experience with vaginal birth after cesarean delivery in a small rural community practice. Am J Obstet Gynecol 1993;168:60–62 (Level III)

18. Scott JR. Avoiding labor problems during vaginal birth after cesarean delivery. Clin Obstet Gynecol 1997;40:533–541 (Level III)

19. Farmer RM, Kirschbaum T, Potter D, Strong TH, Medearis AL. Uterine rupture during trial of labor after previous cesarean section. Am J Obstet Gynecol 1991; 165:996–1001 (Level II-2)

20. Jones RO, Nagashima AW, Hartnett-Goodman MM, Goodlin RC. Rupture of low transverse cesarean scars during trial of labor. Obstet Gynecol 1991;77:815–817 (Level III)

21. Leung AS, Farmer RM, Leung EK, Medearis AL, Paul RH. Risk factors associated with uterine rupture during trial of labor after cesarean delivery: a case-control study. Am J Obstet Gynecol 1993;168:1358–1363 (Level II-2)

22. Scott JR. Mandatory trial of labor after cesarean delivery: an alternative viewpoint. Obstet Gynecol 1991;77:811–814 (Level III)

23. Phelan JP. VBAC: time to reconsider? OBG Manage 1996: 62–68 (Level III)

24. Stalnaker BL, Maher JE, Kleinman GE, Macksey JM, Fishman LA, Bernard JM. Characteristics of successful claims for payment by the Florida Neurologic Injury Compensation Association Fund. Am J Obstet Gynecol 1997; 177:268–271 (Level III)

25. Flamm BL. Once a cesarean, always a controversy. Obstet Gynecol 1997;90:312–315 (Level III)

26. Granovsky-Grisaru S, Shaya M, Diamant YZ. The management of labor in women with more than one uterine scar: is a repeat cesarean section really the only "safe" option? J Perinat Med 1994;22:13–17 (Level II-2)

27. Pruett KM, Kirshon B, Cotton DB, Poindexter AN 3rd. Is vaginal birth after two or more cesarean sections safe? Obstet Gynecol 1988;72:163–165 (Level III)

28. Beall M, Eglinton GS, Clark SL, Phelan JP. Vaginal delivery after cesarean section in women with unknown types of uterine scar. J Reprod Med 1984;29:31–35 (Level II-2)

29. Ophir E, Oettinger M, Yagoda A, Markovits Y, Rojansky N, Shapiro H. Breech presentation after cesarean section: always a section? Am J Obstet Gynecol 1989;161:25–28 (Level III)

30. Sarno AP Jr, Phelan JP, Ahn MO, Strong TH Jr. Vaginal birth after cesarean delivery. Trial of labor in women with breech presentation. J Reprod Med 1989;34:831–833 (Level III)

31. Miller DA, Mullin P, Hou D, Paul RH. Vaginal birth after cesarean section in twin gestation. Am J Obstet Gynecol 1996;175:194–198 (Level II-2)

32. Strong TH Jr, Phelan JP, Ahn MO, Sarno AP Jr. Vaginal birth after cesarean delivery in the twin gestation. Am J Obstet Gynecol 1989;161:29–32 (Level III)

33. Yeh S, Huang X, Phelan JP. Postterm pregnancy after previous cesarean section. J Reprod Med 1984;29:41–44 (Level II-2)

34. Flamm BL, Goings JR. Vaginal birth after cesarean section: is suspected fetal macrosomia a contraindication? Obstet Gynecol 1989;74:694–697 (Level II-2)

35. Phelan JP, Eglinton GS, Horenstein JM, Clark SL, Yeh S. Previous cesarean birth. Trial of labor in women with macrosomic infants. J Reprod Med 1984;29:36–40 (Level II-2)

36. Martin JN Jr, Perry KG Jr, Roberts WE, Meydrech EF. The case for trial of labor in the patient with a prior low-segment vertical cesarean incision. Am J Obstet Gynecol 1997;177:144–148 (Level III)

37. Naef RW 3rd, Ray MA, Chauhan SP, Roach H, Blake PG, Martin JN Jr. Trial of labor after cesarean delivery with a lower-segment, vertical uterine incision: is it safe? Am J Obstet Gynecol 1995;172:1666–1673; discussion 1673–1674 (Level II-2)

38. Flamm BL. Vaginal birth after cesarean section. In: Flamm BL, Quilligan EJ, eds. Cesarean section: guidelines for appropriate utilization. New York: Springer-Verlag, 1995: 51–64 (Level III)

39. Pridjian G. Labor after prior cesarean section. Clin Obstet Gynecol 1992;35:445–456 (Level III)

40. Abitbol MM, Taylor UB, Castillo I, Rochelson BL. The cephalopelvic disproportion index. Combined fetal sonography and x-ray pelvimetry for early detection of cephalopelvic disproportion. J Reprod Med 1991;36:369–373 (Level II-3)

41. Krishnamurthy S, Fairlie F, Cameron AD, Walker JJ, Mackenzie JR. The role of postnatal x-ray pelvimetry after caesarean section in the management of subsequent delivery. Br J Obstet Gynaecol 1991;98:716–718 (Level III)

42. Pickhardt MG, Martin JN Jr, Meydrech EF, Blake PG, Martin RW, Perry KG Jr, et al. Vaginal birth after cesarean delivery: are there useful and valid predictors of success or failure? Am J Obstet Gynecol 1992;166:1811–1815; discussion 1815–1819 (Level II-3)

43. Thurnau GR, Scates DH, Morgan MA. The fetal–pelvic index: a method of identifying fetal–pelvic disproportion in women attempting vaginal birth after previous cesarean delivery. Am J Obstet Gynecol 1991;165:353–358 (Level II-2)

44. Troyer LR, Parisi VM. Obstetric parameters affecting success in a trial of labor: designation of a scoring system. Am J Obstet Gynecol 1992;167:1099–1104 (Level II-3)

45. Bedoya C, Bartha JL, Rodriguez I, Fontan I, Bedoya JM, Sanchez-Ramos J. A trial of labor after cesarean section in patients with or without a prior vaginal delivery. Int J Gynecol Obstet 1992;39:285–289 (Level II-2)

46. Eglinton GS. Effect of previous indications for cesarean on subsequent outcome. In: Phelan JP, Clark SL, eds. Cesarean delivery. New York: Elsevier, 1988:476–483 (Level III)

47. Demianczuk NN, Hunter DJ, Taylor DW. Trial of labor after previous cesarean section: prognostic indicators of outcome. Am J Obstet Gynecol 1982;142:640–642 (Level II-3)

48. Hoskins IA, Gomez JL. Correlation between maximum cervical dilatation at cesarean delivery and subsequent vaginal birth after cesarean delivery. Obstet Gynecol 1997;89:591–593 (Level II-2)

49. Hadley CB, Mennuti MT, Gabbe SG. An evaluation of the relative risks of a trial of labor versus elective repeat cesarean section. Am J Perinatol 1986;3:107–114 (Level II-2)

50. McMahon MJ, Luther ER, Bowes WA Jr, Olshan AF. Comparison of a trial of labor with an elective second cesarean section. N Engl J Med 1996;335:689–695 (Level II-2)

51. Mootabar H, Dwyer JF, Surur F, Dillon TF. Vaginal delivery following previous cesarean section in 1983. Int J Gynaecol Obstet 1984;22:155–160 (Level II-2)

52. Yetman TJ, Nolan TE. Vaginal birth after cesarean section: a reappraisal of risk. Am J Obstet Gynecol 1989;161: 1119–1123 (Level II-3)

53. Hook B, Kiwi R, Amini SB, Fanaroff A, Hack M. Neonatal morbidity after elective repeat cesarean section and trial of labor. Pediatrics 1997;100:348–353 (Level II-2)

54. Pelosi MA 3rd, Pelosi MA. Spontaneous uterine rupture at thirty-three weeks subsequent to previous superficial laparo-scopic myomectomy. Am J Obstet Gynecol 1997;177:1547–1549 (Level III)

55. American College of Obstetricians and Gynecologists. Informed consent. ACOG Assistant 4. Washington, DC: ACOG, 1998 (Level III)

56. Gregory KD, Henry OA, Gellens AJ, Hobel CJ, Platt LD. Repeat cesareans: how many are elective? Obstet Gynecol 1994;84:574–578 (Level II-3)

57. Flamm BL, Fried MW, Lonky NM, Giles WS. External cephalic version after previous cesarean section. Am J Obstet Gynecol 1991;165:370–372 (Level II-2)

58. Johnson C, Oriol N. The role of epidural anesthesia in trial of labor. Reg Anesth 1990;15:304–308 (Level III)

59. Sakala EP, Kaye S, Murray RD, Munson LJ. Epidural analgesia. Effect on the likelihood of a successful trial of labor after cesarean section. J Reprod Med 1990;35:886–890 (Level II-2)

60. Flamm BL, Lim OW, Jones C, Fallon D, Newman LA, Mantis JK. Vaginal birth after cesarean section: results of a multicenter study. Am J Obstet Gynecol 1988;158:1079–1084 (Level II-2)

61. Meehan FP, Burke G, Kehoe JT. Update on delivery following prior cesarean section: a 15-year review 1972– 1987. Int J Gynaecol Obstet 1989;30:205–212 (Level III)

62. Stovall TG, Shaver DC, Solomon SK, Anderson GD. Trial of labor in previous cesarean section patients, excluding classical cesarean sections. Obstet Gynecol 1987;70:713–717 (Level II-3)

63. Grubb DK, Kjos SL, Paul RH. Latent labor with an unknown uterine scar. Obstet Gynecol 1996;88:351–355 (Level I)

64. Johnson C, Oriol N, Flood K. Trial of labor: a study of 110 patients. J Clin Anesth 1991;3:216–218 (Level III)

65. Stone JL, Lockwood CJ, Berkowitz G, Alvarez M, Lapinski R, Valcamonico A, et al. Use of cervical prostaglandin E_2 gel in patients with previous cesarean section. Am J Perinatol 1994;11:309–312 (Level II-2)

66. Blanco JD, Collins M, Willis D, Prien S. Prostaglandin E_2 gel induction of patients with a prior low transverse cesarean section. Am J Perinatol 1992;9:80–83 (Level II-2)

67. Norman M, Ekman G. Preinductive cervical ripening with prostaglandin E_2 in women with one previous cesarean section. Acta Obstet Gynecol Scand 1992;71:351–355 (Level II-2)

68. Bennett BB. Uterine rupture during induction of labor at term with intravaginal misoprostol. Obstet Gynecol 1997;89:832–833 (Level III)

69. Wing DA, Lovett K, Paul RH. Disruption of uterine incision following misoprostol for labor induction in women with previous cesarean delivery. Obstet Gynecol 1998;91:828–830 (Level III)

70. Ritchie EH. Pregnancy after rupture of the pregnant uterus. A report of 36 pregnancies and a study of cases reported since 1932. J Obstet Gynaecol Br Commonw 1971;78:642–648 (Level III)

71. Reyes-Ceja L, Cabrera R, Insfran E, Herrera-Lasso F. Pregnancy following previous uterine rupture. Study of 19 patients. Obstet Gynecol 1969;34:387–389 (Level III)

The MEDLINE database, the Cochrane Library, and ACOG's own internal resources a nd documents were used to conduct a literature search to locate relevant articles published between January 1985 and March 1998. The search was restricted to articles published in the English language. Priority was given to articles reporting results of original research, although review articles and commentaries also were consulted. Abstracts of research presented at symposiums and scientific conferences were not considered adequate for inclusion in this document. Guidelines published by organizations or institutions such as the National Institutes of Health and ACOG were reviewed, and additional studies were located by reviewing bibliographies of identified articles. When reliable research was not available, expert opinions from obstetrician–gynecologists were used.

Studies were reviewed and evaluated for quality according to the method outlined by the U.S. Preventive Services Task Force:

I Evidence obtained from at least one properly designed randomized controlled trial.

II-1 Evidence obtained from well-designed controlled trials without randomization.

II-2 Evidence obtained from well-designed cohort or case–control analytic studies, preferably from more than one center or research group.

II-3 Evidence obtained from multiple time series with or without the intervention. Dramatic results in uncontrolled experiments also could be regarded as this type of evidence.

III Opinions of respected authorities, based on clinical experience, descriptive studies, or reports of expert committees.

Based on the highest level of evidence found in the data, the recommendations are graded according to the following categories:

Level A—The recommendation is based on good and consistent scientific evidence.

Level B—The recommendation is based on limited or inconsistent scientific evidence.

Level C—The recommendation is based primarily on consensus and expert opinion.

ISSN 1099-3630 12345/32109

The American College of Obstetricians and Gynecologists
409 12th Street, SW
PO Box 96920
Washington, DC 20090-6920

Lists of Titles

Committee Opinions

Educational and Technical Bulletins

Practice Bulletins

Practice Patterns

Policy Statements

Index

Number 3, December 1996 *(Replaces #2, October 1996)*

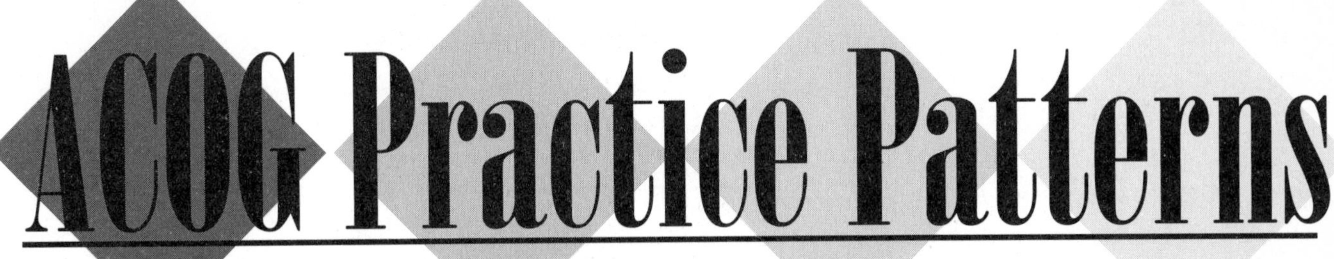

Evidence-Based Guidelines for Clinical Issues in Obstetrics and Gynecology

Emergency Oral Contraception

Purpose

Emergency contraception is a therapy for women who experience an act of unprotected sexual intercourse. It has also been called the "morning-after pill," interception, and postcoital contraception. Methods to achieve emergency contraception include use of combination oral contraceptives (the Yuzpe method), danazol, synthetic estrogens and conjugated estrogens, or antiprogestins and the insertion of an intrauterine device. This document addresses only combination oral contraceptives since this is the most frequently studied method.

The purpose of this Practice Pattern is to present evidence regarding safety, efficacy, risks, and benefits of the use of combination oral contraceptives for emergency contraception. The challenges to the more frequent use of this therapy include physician awareness of the method, public awareness of the method's availability, and access by the patient to a physician who will prescribe the method.

Objectives

These practice guidelines will enable physicians to:

- Identify patients who are candidates for emergency contraception
- Administer emergency contraception
- Estimate the efficacy of emergency contraception
- Determine the benefits and risks of emergency contraception

Methods

The MEDLINE database was used to conduct a literature search to locate relevant articles published between 1974 and 1996. The search was restricted to articles published in the English language. Articles reporting results of original research were given priority, although review articles, metaanalyses, and commentaries were consulted as well. Abstracts of research presented at symposia and scientific conferences were not considered adequate for inclusion in this document.

Studies were reviewed and evaluated for quality according to the method outlined by the U.S. Preventive Services Task Force:

I Evidence obtained from at least one properly designed randomized controlled trial

II-1 Evidence obtained from well-designed controlled trials without randomization

II-2 Evidence obtained from well-designed cohort or case–control analytic studies, preferably from more than one center or research group

II-3 Evidence obtained from multiple time series with or without the intervention. Dramatic results in uncontrolled experiments could also be regarded as this type of evidence.

III Opinions of respected authorities, based on clinical experience, descriptive studies, or reports of expert committees

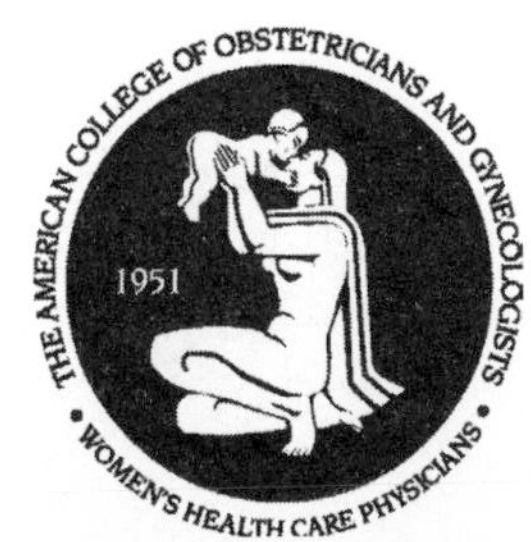

Results

Who are candidates for emergency contraception?

A potential candidate for emergency contraception is a reproductive-age woman who has unprotected sexual intercourse within 72 hours of presenting herself for medical care, independent of the time in the menstrual cycle (Level II-3) (1). From a demographic perspective, most women seeking postcoital contraception are less than 25 years old, have never been pregnant, have been sexually active for an average of 2 years, and have used some form of contraception in the past (Level II-3) (2, 3). The two most common reasons given for seeking the treatment are failure of a barrier method of contraception (usually condoms) and failure to use any method (Level II-3) (1, 4–19).

How is the Yuzpe method prescribed?

In the Yuzpe method, two tablets each containing ethinyl estradiol, 0.05 mg, and DL-norgestrel, 0.5 mg, (Ovral) are ingested 12 hours apart for a total of four tablets. Because levonorgestrel is the active ingredient in DL-norgestrel,approximately equivalent dosing can be obtained by using the prescriptive medications shown in Table 1.

Although emergency contraception is not an indication for use of combination oral contraceptives approved by the U.S. Food and Drug Administration, the method nevertheless can be prescribed appropriately. It is true that a drug approved for marketing may be labeled, promoted, and advertised by the manufacturer only for those uses for which the drug's safety and effectiveness have been established in the manufacturer's own studies and for which the U.S. Food and Drug Administration has approved (20). That is, the U.S. Food and Drug Administration cannot approve an indication that has not been brought to it by the manufacturer. Once a product has been approved and marketed, however, a physician may prescribe it for use in treatment regimens or patient populations that are not included in approved labeling. Such "off-label" uses (the term *unapproved* is, to some extent, misleading) may reflect approaches to medical therapy that have been extensively reported in the medical literature. Accepted medical practice in obstetrics and gynecology often includes medication use that is not reflected in approved drug labeling (21).

TABLE 1. Prescriptive Equivalents for the Yuzpe Method of Emergency Contraception*

Trade Name	Formulation	Number of Pills Taken With Each Dose
Ovral	0.05 mg of ethinyl estradiol 0.50 mg of norgestrel	2
Lo-Ovral	0.03 mg of ethinyl estradiol 0.30 mg of norgestrel	4
Nordette	0.03 mg of ethinyl estradiol 0.15 mg of levonorgestrel	4
Levlen	0.03 mg of ethinyl estradiol 0.15 mg of levonorgestrel	4
Triphasil	(Yellow pills only) 0.03 mg of ethinyl estradiol 0.125 mg of levonorgestrel	4
Trilevlen	(Yellow pills only) 0.03 mg of ethinyl estradiol 0.125 mg of levonorgestrel	4

* Treatment consists of two doses taken 12 hours apart. Use of an antiemetic agent before taking the medication will lessen the risk of nausea, a common side effect.

What are the most common side effects?

Nausea occurs in 30–66% of patients who receive emergency contraception (Level II-3) (11). It may occur after either dose of medication and tends to last for 2 days or less. Emesis occurs in 12–22% of patients. There is evidence that the incidence of nausea and vomiting is decreased when antiemetic agents are taken 1 hour before the dose (Level II-3) (1, 14). Such medications do not seem to be effective if taken after the onset of symptoms (Level II-3) (10). The likelihood of breast tenderness has varied from 1% to 47% (Level II-3) (1, 4, 6–19).

There is no evidence that emesis within 3 hours of ingesting the dose is associated with an increased failure rate; however, none of the studies was designed specifically to measure this effect. There is no evidence on which to base a recommendation for repeating the dose if emesis occurs. However, it seems reasonable to infer that if gastrointestinal symptoms are estrogen mediated secondary to an effect on the central nervous system, absorption of the dose should have occurred by the time of emesis.

How does the treatment affect the next menstrual cycle?

Up to 98% of patients will menstruate by 21 days after the treatment; the mean is 7–9 days (Level II-2) (1, 8, 16–18). In more than 90% of cases, menses will be of normal duration for that patient (Level II-3) (11, 14, 18). Whether the patient has a history of regular or irregular menstrual cycles does not appear to be a factor (Level II-3) (17, 18).

If the treatment is given prior to ovulation, the onset of menstrual bleeding may be 3–7 days earlier than expected. If the treatment is given after ovulation, the onset of menstrual bleeding may be on time or delayed (Level II-3) (6, 7, 10–12, 14–16).

How effective is the combination of norgestrel and ethinyl estradiol in preventing pregnancy?

At least 17 studies (Level II-3) published between 1974 and 1993 have examined the failure rate of emergency contraception with combination pills containing ethinyl estradiol and DL-norgestrel or levonorgestrel after a single act of unprotected sexual intercourse. However, a formal control group with randomization is not available for comparison in any study (1, 4–13, 15–19).

Several factors complicate the calculation of a failure rate for this method of emergency contraception. The day of ovulation for a particular menstrual cycle relative to the day of exposure can be determined only in retrospect when menses occurs. Moreover, emergency contraception with the combination pill can modify the time of onset of menses.

Other factors include dependence on the patient's history as to the time of the last menstrual period and day of exposure; the effect of regular and irregular menstrual cycles on the calculation of midcycle exposure in a patient; the possibility that the patient is already pregnant at the time of treatment; the possibility that more than one unprotected coitus has occurred in this cycle and the timing of coitus prior to, within, or after the 72-hour window; whether both doses of medicine were taken and at the proper time 12 hours apart; and the general fertility of the woman and her partner and the woman's ovulation status in this menstrual cycle (22–24).

Another consideration is that most studies included patients who were lost to follow-up. There is no consistent approach from one study to another as to including or excluding these patients from estimates of failure rates. It is not consistently known which of these patients did not conceive or conceived and had a spontaneous abortion, underwent termination of pregnancy, or carried to term.

Therefore, the method's ability to prevent an individual patient's chance of conceiving from a specific unprotected act of sexual intercourse can only be estimated. Authors have estimated the failure rate of emergency contraception with two approaches (24, 25). The most frequently used method compares the probability of conception on each day of the cycle before and after the day of ovulation to the actual number of pregnancies conceived on those days (26).

A recent study has shown that conception can occur each of the 5 days prior to and on the day of ovulation (22). There is a 0.37 probability (95% confidence interval, 0.31–0.48) of conception when daily coitus occurs in an ovulatory cycle. However, with a single exposure, the daily estimated conception rate in this 6-day window varies from 0.10 to 0.33 (Level II-2) (22). The conception probabilities based on this study have not been used to date.

A review of 10 studies finds effectiveness rates of 55–94%, with a weighted average of effectiveness of 74% (24). Because the observed number of pregnancies in these 10 studies is likely to be overestimated and the expected number of pregnancies is likely to be underestimated, the true effectiveness rate is likely to be at least 75% (24). It is important to communicate to patients that this 75% reduction in risk of pregnancy does not translate into a pregnancy rate of 25%. Rather, if 100 women have intercourse in the middle 2 weeks of their cycle, approximately 8 will become pregnant. Use of emergency contraceptive pills would reduce this number to 2 women (a 75% reduction). Even though this method of contraception reduces the risk of pregnancy substantially, patients should understand that it is still less effective than consistent use of other contraceptive methods. Therefore, this treatment should only be used in emergency situations.

What is the method of action of the treatment?

Although the mechanism of action has not been established, the only consistently reported changes are within the endometrium. This apparently results in failure of nidation (Level II-2) (27, 28). There is no evidence that emergency contraception increases the incidence of ectopic pregnancy; however, no studies specifically focused on this issue.

Are there contraindications to the use of the method?

No published studies have reported evidence-based criteria contraindicating use of this treatment. Some studies, however, excluded women from participating if they had an absolute contraindication to taking oral contraceptives. Results from all studies indicate no reports of major cardiovascular or neurologic side effects. However, studies have not specifically investigated outcomes among patients with preexisting contraindications to oral contraceptives and compared them with those among women without contraindications. In other words, there is neither evidence of increased risk nor evidence of safety among women who have contraindications to oral contraceptives.

The daily dose of steroid hormones in the Yuzpe method is greater than that used for oral contraception but the duration of use is quite short (29). Some contraindications to use of combination oral contraceptives are based on a presumption of long-term use (eg, use among women older than age 35 who smoke) and are not likely to pertain to the short duration of use required for emergency contraception (29).

Is there a time limit for initiating the treatment?

In almost all studies, the first dose was administered within 72 hours after unprotected sexual intercourse. A small number of patients in two studies received the two doses between 72 hours and 120 hours after exposure. There was a low rate of conception (Level II-3) (11, 16). Some authors have suggested that emergency contraception can be effective up to 120 hours after unprotected coitus (Level III) (30, 31).

There are conflicting reports regarding the amount of elapsed time after exposure to treatment within the 72-hour time limit and its effect on the success rate of treatment. Two studies found significant differences in the raw pregnancy rate associated with the amount of time elapsed before beginning treatment (Level II-3) (7, 8). An analysis of nine studies, however, found no difference in failure rates when treatment was started within 24, 48, or 72 hours. Therefore, the first dose can be taken at a time that will be convenient for taking the second dose (Level II-3) (31).

Is there evidence of a teratologic effect?

There are reports from 48 cases in which treatment failed and the women elected to continue the pregnancy. All delivered normal infants except for one whose infant was born with an absent left kidney and two who had infants with minor anomalies (Level II-3) (15, 19, 32). It is important to acknowledge that no studies have investigated teratologic effects associated with the use of oral emergency contraception. However, numerous studies of the teratologic risk of conception during regular use of oral contraceptives (including use of older, higher-dose preparations) found no increase in risk (33).

Cost Considerations

The purpose of emergency contraception is to avoid unintended pregnancy. Many of these pregnancies are also unwanted. The therapy described herein will prevent most pregnancies resulting from a single act of unprotected intercourse. This means that the treatment costs of any subsequent induced abortions, spontaneous abortions, ectopic pregnancies, and pregnancies carried to fetal viability will be avoided (Level III) (34). Separately, a cost savings can be calculated when a course of emergency contraception is provided routinely at a woman's annual visit for potential later use if unprotected coitus should occur (Level III) (34).

Summary and Recommendations

Based on the highest level of evidence found in the data, the following recommendations are provided and graded according to the following categories:

A There is good evidence to support the recommendation.
B There is fair evidence to support the recommendation.
C There is insufficient evidence to support the recommendation; however, the recommendation may be made on other grounds.

Efficacy

The Yuzpe method of emergency contraception (emergency contraceptive pills) consists of the ingestion of 0.1 mg of ethinyl estradiol and 1.0 mg of DL-norgestrel or its equivalent in two doses 12 hours apart within 72 hours of unprotected sexual intercourse. The following statements can be made in regard to the efficacy of this method:

- Based on published studies, this treatment can be offered with the assurance that it will be at least 75% effective. The estimate of efficacy may be affected by revised calculations based on new information reported concerning the probability of conception (22), but published data were not available at the time this document was published (A: II-3).

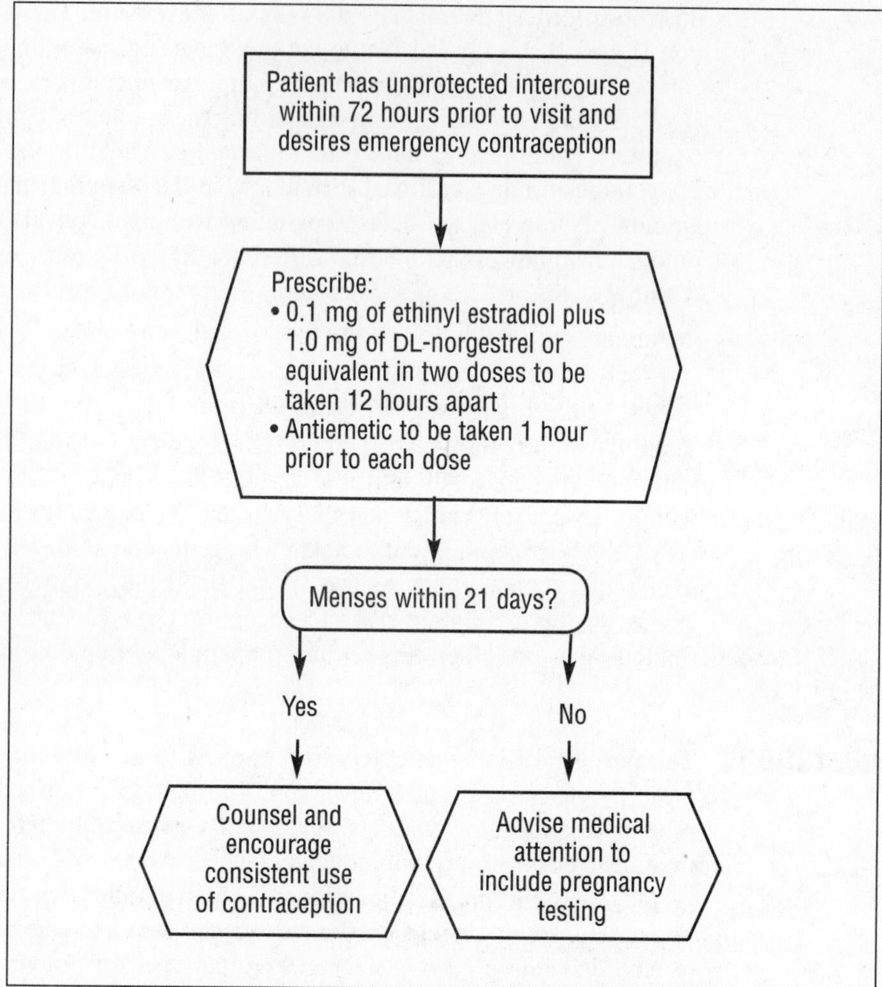

FIG. 1. Algorithm for patient management for emergency contraception.

- There appears to be no difference in efficacy relative to when in the 72 hours after exposure to unprotected sexual intercourse the regimen of two doses, 12 hours apart is administered (B: II-3).
- There are insufficient data to evaluate the effectiveness of the treatment when initiated more than 72 and up to 120 hours after a single act of unprotected sexual intercourse (C).

Risks and Benefits

- There is a substantial risk of nausea and vomiting associated with this treatment (A: II-3). There is limited evidence that providing an antiemetic agent prior to administration of each dose will decrease the risk of nausea and vomiting (A: II-3).
- There are insufficient data to evaluate the teratologic risk to pregnancy if the treatment fails. While no studies have specifically addressed the issue of teratogenesis, it may be reassuring that no adverse impact on the incidence or type of congenital anomalies has been found in pregnancies in which combination birth control pills of varying dose have been ingested daily during the first trimester (A: II-2).

Contraindications

There are no data providing information about the risk of using combination oral contraceptives for emergency contraception among women with contraindications to use of such preparations for ongoing contraception.

Management

- Patients should be advised to take an antiemetic agent 1 hour before each dose to prevent nausea and vomiting (A: II-3).
- Patients should be advised to seek medical attention including evaluation for pregnancy if menses has not begun within 21 days after the treatment (A: II-3).
- At the time emergency contraception is prescribed, the clinician should provide counseling to motivated patients regarding effective contraceptive methods, sexually transmissible diseases, and safer sex practice (C: III).

References

1. Bagshaw SN, Edwards D, Tucker AK. Ethinyl oestradiol and D-norgestrel is an effective emergency postcoital contraceptive: a report of its use in 1,200 patients in a family planning clinic. Aust N Z J Obstet Gynaecol 1988;28:137–140
2. Percival-Smith RK, Abercrombie B. Postcoital contraception: some characteristics of women who use this method. Contraception 1988;37:425–429
3. Rowlands S, Booth M, Guillebaud J. Behavioural patterns in women requesting postcoital contraception. J Biosoc Sci 1983;15:145–152
4. Buttermore S, Nolan C. Six years of clinical experience using postcoital contraception in college women. J Am Coll Health 1993;42:61–63
5. Friedman EH, Rowley DE. Post-coital contraception—a two year evaluation of a service. Br J Fam Plann 1987;13:139–144
6. Glasier A, Thong KJ, Dewar M, Mackie M, Baird DT. Mifepristone (RU 486) compared with high-dose estrogen and progestogen for emergency postcoital contraception. N Engl J Med 1992;327:1041–1044
7. Ho PC, Kwan MS. A prospective randomized comparison of levonorgestrel with the Yuzpe regimen in post-coital contraception. Hum Reprod 1993;8:389–392
8. Kane LA, Sparrow MJ. Postcoital contraception: a family planning study. N Z Med J 1989;102:151–153
9. Luerti M, Tonta A, Ferla P, Molla R, Santini F. Post-coital contrception by estrogen/progestagen combination or IUD insertion. Contraception 1986;33:61–68
10. Percival-Smith RK, Abercrombie B. Postcoital contraception with dl-norgestrel/ethinyl estradiol combination: six years experience in a student medical clinic. Contraception 1987;36:287–293
11. Rowlands S, Guillebaud J, Bounds W, Booth M. Side effects of danazol compared with an ethinyl-oestradiol/norgestrel combination when used for postcoital contraception. Contraception 1983;27: 39–49
12. Schilling LH. An alternative to the use of high-dose estrogens for postcoital contraception. J Am Coll Health Assoc 1979;27:247–249
13. Tully B. Post coital contraception—a study. Br J Fam Plann 1983;8:119–124
14. Van Santen MR, Haspels AA. Interception II. Postcoital low-dose estrogens and norgestrel combination in 633 women. Contraception 1985;31:275–293
15. Webb AM, Russell J, Elstein M. Comparison of Yuzpe regimen, danazol, and mifepristone (RU486) in oral postcoital contraception. BMJ 1992;305:927–931
16. Yuzpe AA, Thurlow HJ, Ramzy I, Leyshon JI. Post coital contraception—A pilot study. J Reprod Med 1974;13:53–58
17. Yuzpe AA, Lancee WJ. Ethinylestradiol and dl-norgestrel as a postcoital contraceptive. Fertil Steril 1977;28:932–936
18. Yuzpe AA, Smith RP, Rademaker AW. A multicenter clinical investigation employing ethinyl estradiol combined with dl-norgestrel as a postcoital contraceptive agent. Fertil Steril 1982;37:508–513
19. Zuliani G, Colombo UF, Molla R. Hormonal postcoital contraception with an ethinylestradiol-norgestrel combination and two danazol regimens. Eur J Obstet Gynecol Reprod Biol 1990;37:253–260

20. Use of approved drugs for unlabeled indications. FDA Drug Bull 1982;12:4–5
21. Rayburn WF. A physician's prerogative to prescribe drugs for off-label uses during pregnancy. Obstet Gynecol 1993;81:1052–1055
22. Wilcox AJ, Weinberg CR, Baird DD. Timing of sexual intercourse in relation to ovulation. Effects on the probability of conception, survival of the pregnancy, and sex of the baby. N Engl J Med 1995;333:1517–1521
23. Yuzpe AA. Postcoital hormonal contraception: uses, risks, and abuses. Int J Gynaecol Obstet 1977; 15:133–136
24. Trussell J, Ellertson C, Steward F. The effectiveness of the Yuzpe regimen of emergency contraception. Fam Plann Perspect 1996;28:58–64
25. Trussell J, Ellertson C. The efficacy of emergency contraception. Fertil Control Rev 1995;4:8–11
26. Dixon GW, Schlesselman JJ, Ory HW, Blye RP. Ethinyl estradiol and conjugated estrogens as postcoital contraceptives. JAMA 1980;244:1336–1339
27. Ling WY, Robichaud A, Zayid I, Wrixon W, MacLeod SC. Mode of action of DL-norgestrel and ethinylestradiol combination in postcoital contraception. Fertil Steril 1979;32:297–302
28. Ling WY, Wrixon W, Acorn T, Wilson E, Collins J. Mode of action of dl-norgestrel and ethinylestradiol combination in postcoital contraception. III. Effect of preovulatory administration following the luteininzing hormone surge on ovarian steroidogenesis. Fertil Steril 1983;40:631–636
29. Webb A. How safe is the Yuzpe method of emergency contraception? Fertil Control Rev 1995;4:16–18
30. Grou F, Rodrigues I. The morning-after pill—how long after? Am J Obstet Gynecol 1994;171: 1529–1534
31. Trussell J, Ellertson C, Rodriquez G. The Yuzpe regimen of emergency contraception: how long after the morning after? Obstet Gynecol 1996;88:150–154
32. Chez R, Rowlands S. Emergency postcoital contraception. Contemporary Ob/Gyn 1994;39:78–88
33. Bracken MB. Oral contraception and congenital malformations in offspring: a review and meta-analysis of the prospective studies. Obstet Gynecol 1990;76:552–557
34. Trussell J, Koenig J, Ellertson C, Steward F. Emergency contraception: a cost-effective approach to reducing unintended pregnancy. Princeton, New Jersey: Office of Population Research, Princeton University, 1995

Practice Patterns are clinical practice guidelines developed by The American College of Obstetricians and Gynecologists (ACOG) to assist practitioners and patients in making decisions about appropriate obstetric and gynecologic care. The assistance of Ronald A. Chez, MD, in the development of this document is gratefully acknowledged. Each Practice Pattern focuses on a clinical issue and is based on a review and analysis of the scientific literature. The information and recommendations reflect scientific and clinical knowledge current as of the publication date and are subject to change as advances in diagnostic techniques and treatments emerge. In addition, variations of practice, taking into account the needs of the individual patient, resources, and limitations unique to the institution or type of practice, may warrant alternative treatment or procedures to the recommendations outlined in this document. Therefore, these guidelines should not be construed as dictating an exclusive course of treatment or procedure.

ISSN 1083-3331 12345/09876

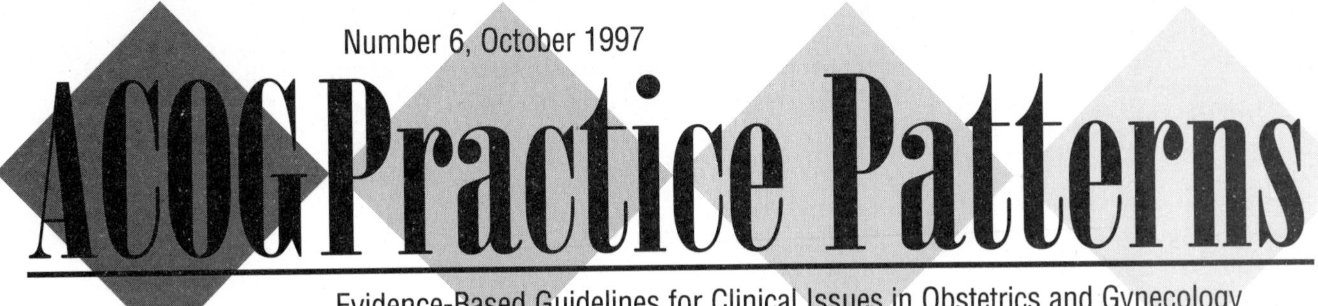

Number 6, October 1997
ACOG Practice Patterns
Evidence-Based Guidelines for Clinical Issues in Obstetrics and Gynecology

Management of Postterm Pregnancy

Purpose

Postterm pregnancy is one of the more common high-risk problems confronting many obstetricians. In the 1950s, attention in the United States became focused on prolonged pregnancy when it was recognized that some postterm infants exhibited dysmaturity that led to significant morbidity and mortality (1).

Postterm pregnancy, by definition, is a gestation of 42 weeks or more (294 days or more from the first day of the last menstrual period). The reported frequency is 3–12%. About 80% of all pregnancies last 38–42 weeks, 10% are delivered preterm, and the remaining 10% extend beyond the start of the 43rd week and are considered postterm. Although many apparent cases of postterm pregnancy are the result of an inability to define the date of conception, some cases clearly progress to excessively long gestations. Accurate assessment of gestational age and diagnosis of postterm gestation, as well as recognition and management of risk factors, can reduce the risk of adverse sequelae in most of these cases.

Antenatal surveillance and induction of labor are two widely used strategies that theoretically diminish fetal risk of an adverse outcome. The purpose of this document is to examine the evidence and make recommendations about these two management strategies.

Objectives

These practice guidelines will enable physicians to

- Determine whether there is an optimal time to begin antenatal surveillance in postterm pregnancies
- Determine which strategy—induction or surveillance—is appropriate for patients experiencing postterm pregnancies
- Determine whether prostaglandin gel can be used for induction of labor in patients with postterm pregnancy

Methods

The MEDLINE database was used to conduct a literature search to locate relevant articles published between 1985 and 1995 specifically comparing expectant monitoring to induction of labor in postterm pregnancies. The search was restricted to articles published in the English language. Articles reporting results of original research were given priority, although review articles, meta-analyses, and commentaries were also consulted. Abstracts of research presented at symposia and scientific conferences were not considered adequate for inclusion in this document.

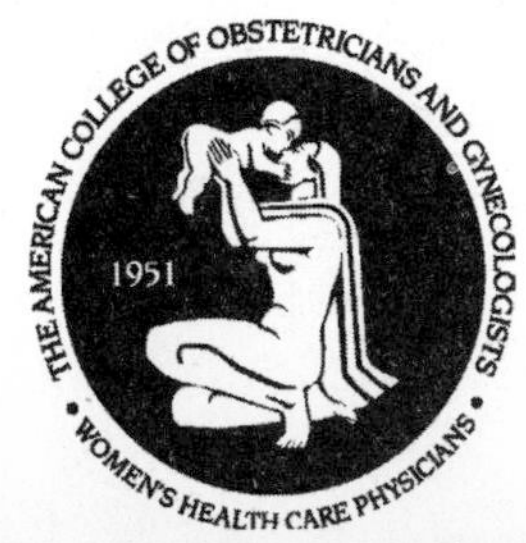

Studies were reviewed and evaluated for quality according to the method outlined by the U.S. Preventive Services Task Force:

- I Evidence obtained from at least one properly designed randomized controlled trial
- II-1 Evidence obtained from well-designed controlled trials without randomization
- II-2 Evidence obtained from well-designed cohort or case-control analytic studies, preferably from more than one center or research group
- II-3 Evidence obtained from multiple time series with or without the intervention. Dramatic results in uncontrolled experiments could also be regarded as this type of evidence.
- III Opinions of respected authorities, based on clinical expertise, descriptive studies, or reports of expert committees

Background

Etiologic Factors

The most frequent cause of apparently prolonged gestation is error in determining the time of ovulation and conception according to the time of the last menstrual period (1). Frequently encountered problems are the patient's failure to recall accurately the last menstrual dates and the variable length of the proliferative phase of the cycle, which allows the ovulation date to vary by days to weeks. When postterm pregnancy actually exists, the cause is usually unknown. In rare instances, postterm pregnancy is associated with fetal conditions such as anencephaly and placental sulfatase deficiency.

Assessment of Gestational Age

The accurate determination of the time of conception is extremely important in reducing the false diagnosis of postterm pregnancy and in ascertaining precisely the point at which the pregnancy becomes high risk. The estimated date of delivery (EDD) is most reliably and accurately determined early in pregnancy. Consistency between historical and physical data is important in establishing the reliability of dating. Regularity and length of menstrual cycles and the first day of the last spontaneous menses should be recorded. An EDD can be calculated by subtracting 3 months from the first day of the last menses and adding 7 days (Naegele's rule). Other clinical data should be consistent with the EDD:

- The mother usually feels the fetus move (quickening) at about 16–20 weeks.
- The fetal heart can be heard with a nonelectronic fetal stethoscope by 18–20 weeks in most patients.
- The size of the uterus at early examination (in the first trimester) should be consistent with dates.
- At 20 weeks, the fundal height should be about 20 cm above the symphysis pubis, which usually corresponds with the umbilicus.

Inconsistencies or concern about the accuracy of the dating requires further assessment with ultrasonography. Useful measurements include the crown–rump length of the fetus during the first trimester and the biparietal diameter or head circumference and the femur length during the second trimester. Because of the normal variationsin size of infants in the third trimester, dating the pregnancy at that time is unreliable (±3 weeks) (1).

Results

When should antenatal monitoring of a postterm pregnancy begin?

It is generally accepted that all postterm patients receive some form of antenatal monitoring, despite a lack of evidence that it improves the outcome. The literature search failed to locate any studies involving postterm patients who were not monitored. Due to ethical and medicolegal concerns, it is highly unlikely that any subsequent studies will include a no-monitoring group. Conversely, for the same reasons previously stated, there is no evidence that antenatal monitoring adversely affects patients experiencing postterm pregnancies. Therefore, even though evidence of either a positive or negative effect is lacking, antenatal surveillance has become a standard practice on the basis of universal acceptance.

Patients who have passed their EDD but who have not yet completed 42 weeks of gestation constitute another group for whom antenatal surveillance has been proposed. Some studies report a greater complication rate among women giving birth during the latter week of this 2-week period (Level II-2: 2, 3). However, no randomized controlled trial has demonstrated a benefit attributable to earlier testing (Level II-2: 4). Although complications may occur more frequently, there is no evidence that antenatal monitoring, commencing at the completion of 40 weeks of gestation, improves fetal outcome.

In most studies of postterm pregnancies, women are recruited and monitoring begins prior to 42 completed weeks of gestation (Level I: 5–10), further complicating matters. As with postterm patients, there is no demonstrable evidence that any form of antenatal testing is beneficial for patients between 40 and 42 completed weeks; however, monitoring is often performed during this time frame. From a scientific viewpoint, it is unknown whether routine antenatal surveillance of patients between 40 and 42 completed weeks of gestation improves the outcome of delivery.

What form of antenatal surveillance should be performed, and how frequently should a postterm patient be reevaluated?

There is no consistency in the literature regarding either the form or frequency of antenatal surveillance among postterm patients (Level I: 5–14) (Level II-2: 15) (Level II-3: 16). Generally, patients receive some combination of ultrasonography, cervical examination, and nonstress testing, but there are wide variations of practice. Frequency of testing varies; often, individual tests are administered according to different schedules. No recommendation based on published research can be made regarding the indicated form or frequency of antenatal surveillance among postterm patients.

Postterm patient with a favorable cervix: Induction or expectant management?

Among postterm patients who are otherwise at low risk for complications, labor is usually induced if the cervix is favorable. Recent studies of postterm pregnancies comparing outcomes of labor induction with those of expectant management excluded women with favorable cervices (Level I: 5–7, 9, 11, 12) (Level II-3: 16). Often, when women allocated to expectant management experienced a change in cervical status, expectant management ceased and an induction of labor was initiated (Level I: 5, 7, 9, 11, 14). In studies where women with favorable cervices were managed expectantly, there was no indication that expectant management had a deleterious effect on the outcome, but results were not stratified according to the condition of the cervix (Level I: 8, 10, 13) (Level II-2: 15). Thus, for women who are experiencing postterm pregnancies and who have favorable cervices, there is not enough information to determine whether either labor induction or expectant management results in the best outcome. According to current obstetric practice, labor is induced in most of these women.

Postterm patient with an unfavorable cervix: Induction or expectant management?

Among women with otherwise low-risk pregnancies who are postterm and have unfavorable cervices, studies confirm that either expectant management or immediate induction is associated with a very low complication rate and good outcomes (Level I: 5–7, 11, 12). One recent study was stopped because the primary measurements, perinatal mortality and morbidity, were so rare that recruiting enough women to calculate a statistical difference in management strategies was deemed impractical (Level I: 5).

The largest study to date, the Canadian Post-Term Pregnancy Trial, reported a significant increase in the cesarean birth rate for fetal distress among women managed expectantly (Level I: 6). However, the authors could not identify a particular cause related to postterm status. Smaller studies report mixed results regarding cesarean birth rates (increased: Level I: 9, 13) (no statistically significant difference: Level I: 5, 7, 10–12, 14). Two studies reported an increase in cesarean delivery rates only among certain subgroups of patients (Level I: 8) (Level II-2: 15). The evidence is inconsistent regarding how the selection of one strategy over another affects the cesarean birth rate.

What is the role of prostaglandin gel (PGE_2) in managing a postterm pregnancy?

Most studies conclude that PGE_2 gel is a valuable tool for improving cervical ripeness and inducing labor. A double-blind, placebo-controlled trial reported significant changes in Bishop scores, shorter durations of labor, lower maximum doses of oxytocin, and a reduced incidence of cesarean deliveries among postterm patients who received PGE_2 gel (Level I: 17). Another study, using outpatient-administered PGE_2 gel, confirmed these findings (Level I: 18). Compared with oxytocin for induction, PGE_2 gel has been associated with a lower failure rate and, consequently, a reduced cesarean delivery rate (Level I: 19). In contrast, the National Institute of Child Health and Human Development study reported no reduction in the cesarean delivery rate or the induction-to-delivery interval among postterm patients who were induced with PGE_2, although the gel was more effective than placebo in initiating persistent contractions in nulliparous women (Level I: 5).

Many studies used PGE_2 gel to induce labor, but there does not appear to be a standardized dose (5, 6, 9, 10, 15, 20). Postapplication monitoring was carried out in all studies to ensure fetal well-being; the medication was well tolerated, with few reported side effects.

Which method is more cost-effective?

A formal cost analysis based on results from the Canadian study concluded that expectant management costs slightly more than routine induction, assuming a slightly higher rate of cesarean delivery and more antenatal testing in the expectant group (Level III: 21). Expectant management cost $193 (in 1992 Canadian dollars) more than routine induction at 41 weeks. In contrast, a study reported higher costs associated with immediate induction, based on longer hospitalizations for patients undergoing inductions compared with patients managed expectantly (Level I: 14).

Summary and Recommendations

Based on the highest level of evidence found in the data, the following recommendations are provided and graded according to the following categories:

A There is good evidence to support the recommendation.
B There is fair evidence to support the recommendation.
C There is insufficient evidence to support the recommendation; however, the recommendation may be made on other grounds.

Evaluation of a Postterm Patient

- Antenatal surveillance of postterm pregnancies should be initiated by 42 weeks of gestation despite a lack of evidence that monitoring improves outcomes (C: III).
- There is insufficient evidence that initiating antenatal surveillance between 40–42 completed weeks of gestation improves outcomes.
- No single antenatal surveillance protocol for monitoring fetal well-being in a postterm pregnancy appears superior to another.

Managing a Postterm Pregnancy

- It is unknown whether induction or expectant management is preferable to manage an otherwise uncomplicated postterm patient with a favorable cervix (A:I).
- There is good evidence that either induction or expectant management will result in good outcomes among postterm patients with unfavorable cervices and without additional complications (A: I).

Prostaglandin Gel

Prostaglandin gel can be used safely in postterm pregnancies to promote cervical changes and induce labor (A: I).

Cost-Effectiveness

There is mixed evidence regarding which strategy is more cost-effective. No recommendation can be made.

References

1. American College of Obstetricians and Gynecologists. Ultrasongraphy in pregnancy. ACOG Technical Bulletin 187. Washington, DC: ACOG, 1993
2. Bochner CJ, Williams J, Castro L, Medearis A, Hobel CJ, Wade M. The efficacy of starting post-term antenatal testing at 41 weeks as compared with 42 weeks of gestational age. Am J Obstet Gynecol 1988;159:550–554
3. Guidetti DA, Divon MY, Langer O. Postdate fetal surveillance: is 41 weeks too early? Am J Obstet Gynecol 1989;161:91–93
4. Usher RH, Boyd ME, McLean FH, Kramer MS. Assessment of fetal risk in postdate pregnancies. Am J Obstet Gynecol 1988;158:259–264
5. A clinical trial of induction of labor versus expectant management in post-term pregnancy. The National Institute of Child Health and Human Development Network of Maternal–Fetal Medicine Units. Am J Obstet Gynecol 1994;170:716–723
6. Hannah ME, Hannah WJ, Hellmann J, Hewson S, Milner R, Willan A. Induction of labor as compared with serial antenatal monitoring in post-term pregnancy. A randomized controlled trial. The Canadian Multicenter Post-Term Pregnancy Trial Group. N Engl J Med 1992;326:1587–1592
7. Martin JN Jr, Sessums JK, Howard P, Martin RW, Morrision JC. Alternative approaches to the management of gravidas with prolonged-postterm-postdate pregnancies. J Miss State Med Assoc 1989; 30:105–111

8. Augensen K, Bergsjø, Eikeland T, Askvik K, Carlsen J. Randomised comparison of early versus late induction of labour in post-term pregnancy. Br Med J 1987;294:1192–1195
9. Dyson DC, Miller PD, Armstrong MA. Management of prolonged pregnancy: induction of labor versus antepartum fetal testing. Am J Obstet Gynecol 1987;156:928–934
10. Cardozo L, Fysh J, Pearce JM. Prolonged pregnancy: the management debate. Br Med J 1986;293:1059–1063
11. Herabutya Y, Prasertsawat PO, Tongyai T, Isarangura NA, Ayudthya N. Prolonged pregnancy: the management dilemma. Int J Gynecol Obstet 1992;37:253–258
12. Hedèn L, Ingemarsson I, Ahlström H, Solum T. Induction of labor versus conservative management in prolonged pregnancy: controlled study. Int J Feto-Maternal Med 1991;4:231–236
13. Bergsjø P, Huang GD, Yu SQ, Gao ZZ, Bakketeig LS. Comparison of induced versus non-induced labor in post-term pregnancy. A randomized prospective study. Acta Obstet Gynecol Scand 1989;68:683–687
14. Witter FR, Weitz CM. A randomized trial of induction at 42 weeks gestation versus expectant management for postdates pregnancies. Am J Perinat 1987;4:206–211
15. Almström H, Granström L, Ekman G. Serial antenatal monitoring compared with labor induction in post-term pregnancies. Acta Obstet Gynecol Scand 1995;74:599–603
16. Shaw KJ, Medearis AL, Horenstein J, Walla CA, Paul RH. Selective labor induction in postterm patients: observations and outcomes. J Reprod Med 1992;37:157–161
17. Rayburn W, Gosen R, Ramadei C, Woods R, Scott J Jr. Outpatient cervical ripening with prostaglandin E_2 gel in uncomplicated postdate pregnancies. Am J Obstet Gynecol 1988;158:1417–1423
18. Sawai SK, O'Brien WF, Mastrogiannis DS, Krammer J, Mastry MG, Porter GW. Patient-administered outpatient intravaginal prostaglandin E_2 suppositories in post-date pregnancies: a double-blind, randomized, placebo-controlled study. Obstet Gynecol 1994;84:807–810
19. Papageorgiou I, Tsionou C, Minaretzis D, Michalas S, Aravantinos D. Labor characteristics of uncomplicated prolonged pregnancies after induction with intracervical prostaglandin E2 gel versus intravenous oxytocin. Gynecol Obstet Invest 1992;34:92–96
20. Egarter C, Kofler E, Fitz R, Husslein P. Is induction of labor indicated in prolonged pregnancy? Gynecol Obstet Invest 1989:27:6–9
21. Goeree R, Hannah M, Hewson S. Cost-effectiveness of induction of labour versus serial antenatal monitoring in the Canadian Multicentre Postterm Pregnancy Trial. Can Med Assoc J 1995;152:1445–1450

Practice Patterns are clinical practice guidelines developed by The American College of Obstetricians and Gynecologists (ACOG) to assist practitioners and patients in making decisions about appropriate obstetric and gynecologic care. Each Practice Pattern focuses on a clinical issue and is based on a review and analysis of the scientific literature. The information and recommendations reflect scientific and clinical knowledge current as of the publication date and are subject to change as advances in diagnostic techniques and treatments emerge. In addition, variations of practice, taking into account the needs of the individual patient, resources, and limitations unique to the institution or type of practice, may warrant alternative treatment or procedures to the recommendations outlined in this document. Therefore, these guidelines should not be construed as dictating an exclusive course of treatment or procedure.

ISSN 1083-3331

12345/10987

Number 5, August 1997

ACOG Practice Patterns

Evidence-Based Guidelines for Clinical Issues in Obstetrics and Gynecology

Routine Ultrasound in Low-Risk Pregnancy

Purpose

The accepted indications for ultrasound during pregnancy are numerous (1). Approximately 60% to 70% of pregnant women in the United States undergo ultrasound at various times in gestation (1, 2). The purpose of this document is to present evidence regarding benefit or lack of benefit of routine ultrasound in women with low-risk pregnancy who do not already have an indication for ultrasound use.

Objectives

These practice guidelines will enable physicians to:

- Estimate the sensitivity and specificity of ultrasound in detecting fetal anomalies in low-risk pregnancy
- Describe the potential benefit, if any, from routine ultrasound in low-risk pregnancies, specifically for
  - — improving the survival rates of anomalous fetuses
  - — improving overall perinatal morbidity and mortality
  - — reducing the rate of unnecessary interventions

Methods

The MEDLINE database was used to conduct a literature search, which was restricted to articles published in the English language. Only studies conducted since 1985 were included because of implicit limitations in ultrasound technology prior to that time. For the purpose of assessing benefit of routine ultrasound in low-risk pregnancy, the evidence was limited to randomized clinical trials with a priori hypotheses appropriate to the stated purposes of this document. For the purpose of estimating the sensitivity of ultrasound in detecting fetal anomalies, evidence of any level was considered as long as the following were provided: a description of the study population, the rate of anomalies detected in infants at birth, and the numbers of fetuses representing true positives, true negatives, false positives, and false negatives. Studies that reported data by numbers of anomalies rather than fetuses were not considered because of overestimation of sensitivity.

Studies were reviewed and evaluated for quality according to the method outlined by the U.S. Preventive Services Task Force:

I Evidence obtained from at least one properly designed randomized controlled trial

II-1 Evidence obtained from well-designed controlled trials without randomization

II-2 Evidence obtained from well-designed cohort or case–control analytic studies, preferably from more than one center or research group

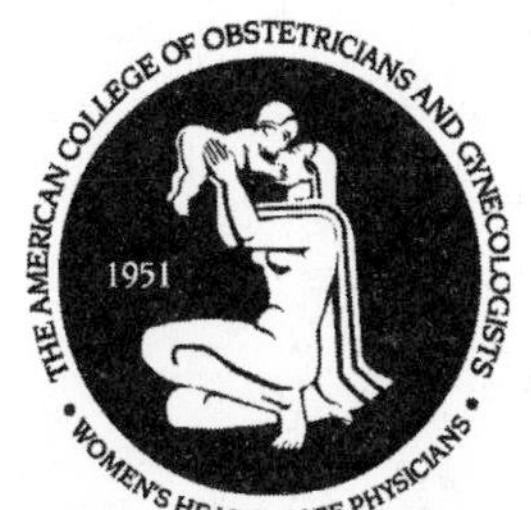

II-3 Evidence obtained from multiple time series with or without the intervention. Dramatic results in uncontrolled experiments could also be regarded as this type of evidence.

III Opinions of respected authorities, based on clinical experience, descriptive studies, or reports of expert committees

Results

What is the proportion of correctly identified fetal anomalies (sensitivity) and the proportion of correctly identified fetuses without anomalies (specificity) detected by ultrasound in low-risk pregnancy?

Estimates of the sensitivity of a fetal anatomic survey to detect fetal anomalies are shown in Table 1 (Level I: 3) (Level II-3: 4–6). Estimated sensitivity varies widely from 17% to 74%.

Some of the variation in reported sensitivity across studies may be accounted for by biases. For the two studies reporting the highest sensitivity (Level II-3: 4, 6), the overall rate of anomalies detected at birth was substantially below the reported rate of 3%, suggesting underdetection of anomalies at birth (7). The bias would tend to result in an overestimation of sensitivity. The lowest sensitivity is reported by the only study (Level I: 3) in which patient recruitment was practice based, rather than hospital based. A community-based population is the least likely to have an inadvertent selection bias. Although practice-based recruitment is not as optimal as that which is community based, the utilization of a large number of general obstetric practices in that study likely improved the chance that the study population was representative of low-risk women. Another potential bias is variation in the skill of individuals performing the ultrasound examination. In the Helsinki study, which included patient populations from two hospitals, sensitivity was more than twofold higher in the university hospital (77%) than in the city hospital (36%) (Level I: 8). A similar order of advantage was seen in the Routine Antenatal Diagnostic Imaging with Ultrasound (RADIUS) study, which reported a relative detection rate of 2.7 (confidence interval [CI] 1.3–5.8) in tertiary versus nontertiary ultrasound units (Level I: 3).

Thus, there is insufficient evidence to indicate a single estimate of the sensitivity of routine ultrasound screening for fetal anomalies. Instead, it should be acknowledged that there is a range of sensitivity, depending on the clinical setting and skill of those performing the examinations. Evidence does indicate that specificity

Table 1. Estimated Sensitivity of Second-Trimester Ultrasound to Detect Anomalies

Study	Study Design	Patient Source	Study (n)	Gestational Age at Ultrasound	Anomalies Detected at Birth	Anomalies Detected by Ultrasound	Sensitivity
Chitty et al 1991[4]	1988–89 series (retrospective)	Hospital based	8,342	<24 weeks	1.5%	93/125	74%
Crane et al 1994[3]	Randomized clinical trial	Practice based	7,575*	18–20 weeks 31–33 weeks	2.3%	31/187	17%
Levi et al 1995[5]	1990–92 series (prospective)	Hospital based	9,601	<23 weeks	2.4%	120/235	51%
Shirley et al 1992[6]	1989–90 series (prospective)	Hospital based	6,183	<22 weeks	1.4%	51/84	61%

*Number of women having ultrasound in the routine-ultrasound arm of the trial.

of a fetal anatomic survey exceeds 99% (Level I: 3) (Level II-3: 4–6). This suggests that, in low-risk populations, ultrasound may be helpful in ruling out anomalies, but it is not particularly reliable in detecting them.

The evidence for the following results was assessed from publications of three trials: the Helsinki study (Level I: 8), the Stockholm study (Level I: 9), and the RADIUS study (Level I: 2, 3, 10). For these trials, the timing of routine ultrasound was early to midsecond trimester; for the RADIUS study, an additional ultrasound was performed in the early third trimester. One additional trial was used to judge evidence for potential benefit unrelated to the ascertainment of fetal anomalies because this study used routine first-trimester ultrasound (Level I: 11). Indicated ultrasound examinations were permitted in the usual-care arm of each study.

Does routine ultrasound improve the survival rates of anomalous infants?

A potential benefit of the antenatal detection of anomalies, particularly life-threatening ones, is the delivery of these infants in tertiary centers capable of providing immediate, risk-appropriate care. Only one randomized clinical trial specifically addressed this question (Level I: 3). In a subgroup analysis of infants with life-threatening anomalies, 75% (21/28) in the routinely screened group survived versus 52% (11/21) in the routine-care group. This difference did not reach statistical significance (relative survival rate 1.4 [CI 0.9–2.3]), although this may in part be attributed to the relatively small sample size. Thus, there is insufficient evidence to support or refute benefit of routine ultrasound in reducing the mortality of infants with life-threatening anomalies.

Does routine ultrasound improve overall perinatal morbidity and mortality?

A benefit of routine diagnostic ultrasound in reducing perinatal morbidity and mortality might be anticipated by ameliorating the perinatal risk associated with inaccurate gestational age and undiagnosed conditions (eg, multiple gestation). In two of the trials, the perinatal mortality rate was similar between the routine-ultrasound and usual-care groups (Level I: 2, 9). In one trial, the perinatal mortality rate was significantly improved (4.2/1,000 versus 8.4/1,000; $P < 0.05$) (Level I: 8). The improvement was largely attributable to pregnancy termination of anomalous fetuses.

Perinatal morbidity as measured by admission to a neonatal unit was no different between the study groups in two trials (Level I: 8, 9). In the RADIUS study, rates of both moderate morbidity (eg, presumed neonatal sepsis, grade I or II intraventricular hemorrhage, stay of >5 days in the neonatal unit) and severe morbidity (eg, mechanical ventilation for >48 hours, stay of >30 days in the neonatal unit) were similar between the routine-ultrasound and usual-care groups (Level I: 2).

In one trial, there were fewer births of less than 2,500 g in the routine-ultrasound group (2.5% versus 4.0%; $P = 0.005$) (Level I: 9). In addition, for those women who reported smoking, the mean birth weight was greater in the routine-ultrasound group than in the usual-care group (3,413 g versus 3,354 g; $P = 0.047$). For infants of nonsmoking women, mean birth weight was also higher in the routine-ultrasound group compared with those of nonsmokers in the usual-care group, although this was not significantly different between groups. The investigators speculated that this improvement in birth weight of reported smokers receiving routine ultrasound may be attributed to healthier maternal behaviors after these women saw their fetuses on ultrasound. A similar birth weight distribution among all women was reported between the routine-ultrasound and usual-care groups in two other trials (Level I: 2, 8).

There is evidence from all trials to indicate that more twin gestations are diagnosed earlier with routine ultrasound. Subgroup analyses of twins, although showing no difference in perinatal mortality with routine ultrasound versus usual care, do not permit definitive conclusions because of limited power. In the RADIUS study, subgroup analyses also were performed for small-for-gestational-age infants and those born at 42 weeks or more. The data from this trial do not support an improvement in overall outcome for these conditions with routine ultrasound (Level I: 2).

In summary, evidence indicates that routine ultrasound does not significantly alter perinatal outcome, except for lowering perinatal mortality as the result of induced abortions following the detection of abnormalities.

Does routine ultrasound reduce the rate of obstetric interventions?

The evidence does not support any benefit from routine ultrasound in reducing the number of maternal hospital days or the cesarean delivery rate (Level I: 8–10). The evidence also does not demonstrate an overall reduction in the rate of induction of labor; these rates were similar between the routine-ultrasound and usual-care groups in all four trials (Level I: 8–11). The rate of induction specifically for postterm pregnancy was reduced in two trials (Level I: 9, 10) but not in the other two (Level I: 8, 11). However, for the trial finding the greatest reduction in induction for postterm pregnancy (3.7% to 1.7%, $P < 0.0001$), the study protocol did not permit correction of gestational age by indicated ultrasound in the usual-care arm (Level I: 9).

Only one trial examined the rate of induction for suspected small-for-gestational-age fetuses (Level I: 10). There was an increased rate of induction for this indication: 0.74% with routine ultrasound versus 0.28% in the usual-care arm. However, a similar proportion of induced pregnancies in each group resulted in infant birth weights at less than the 10th percentile (39% routine ultrasound, 43% usual care).

Only one trial examined other interventions (eg, tests for fetal well-being, performance of amniocentesis, recommendation for bed rest, version). It found no difference except for a decrease in the overall use of tocolysis (3.4% versus 4.2%, $P = 0.01$) (Level I: 10).

Cost Considerations

No cost–benefit analysis of routine versus selective ultrasound has been performed. Because the evidence supports neither an improvement in perinatal morbidity or mortality nor an overall reduction in unnecessary interventions with routine ultrasound, the cost of obstetric care would likely be increased in proportion to the excess number of ultrasound examinations in women having routine use versus selective (indicated) use. In one study, it was estimated that routine ultrasound added, on average, 1.6 scans per pregnancy. If more than 4 million pregnant women were screened annually in the United States at $200 per scan, costs would increase by more than $1 billion (2). However, this estimate includes a percentage of women who would have undergone ultrasound examination for medical indications as well. If estimates were confined to women who would not have had ultrasound examinations, the incremental cost has been calculated to be below $350 million (Level III: 12). If interventions were to be developed that improve outcome in obstetric complications such as twin gestation, or if a larger proportion of women ascertained to have fetuses with major anomalies chose pregnancy termination, then a cost advantage of routine ultrasound in low-risk pregnancy is plausible.

Summary and Recommendations

Based on the highest level of evidence found in the data, the following recommendations are provided and graded according to the following categories:

A There is good evidence to support the recommendation.
B There is fair evidence to support the recommendation.
C There is insufficient evidence to support the recommendation; however, the recommendation may be made on other grounds.

- The specificity of a fetal anatomic survey in detecting fetal anomalies can be anticipated to exceed 99% (A: I; II-3).
- The sensitivity of a fetal anatomic survey in detecting fetal anomalies cannot be estimated with precision; rather, it should be acknowledged that sensitivity may vary in different clinical settings and with different levels of skill of professionals performing the examination (A: I; II-3).
- It is uncertain whether an improvement in the survival of fetuses with life-threatening anomalies can be expected from routine ultrasound in low-risk pregnancy (C: I).
- In a population of women with low-risk pregnancy, neither a reduction in perinatal morbidity and mortality nor a lower rate of unnecessary interventions can be expected from routine diagnostic ultrasound. Thus ultrasound should be performed for specific indications in low-risk pregnancy (A: I).

References

1. American College of Obstetricians and Gynecologists. Ultrasonography in pregnancy. ACOG Technical Bulletin 187. Washington, DC: ACOG, 1993
2. Ewigman BG, Crane JP, Frigoletto FD, LeFevre ML, Bain RP, McNellis D. Effect of prenatal ultrasound screening on perinatal outcome. RADIUS Study Group. N Engl J Med 1993;329:821–827
3. Crane JP, LeFevre ML, Winborn RC, Evans JK, Ewigman BG, Bain RP, et al. A randomized trial of prenatal ultrasonographic screening: impact on the detection, management, and outcome of anomalous fetuses. The RADIUS Study Group. Am J Obstet Gynecol 1994;171:392–399
4. Chitty LS, Hunt GH, Moore J, Lobb MO. Effectiveness of routine ultrasonography in detecting fetal structural abnormalities in a low risk population. BMJ 1991;303:1165–1169
5. Levi S, Schaaps JP, De Havay P, Coulon R, Defoort P. End-result of routine ultrasound screening for congenital anomalies: the Belgium Multicentric Study 1984–92. Ultrasound Obstet Gynecol 1995; 5:366–371
6. Shirley IM, Bottomley F, Robinson VP. Routine radiographer screening for fetal abnormalities by ultrasound in an unselected low risk population. Br J Radiol 1992;65:564–569
7. Watkins ML, Edmonds L, McClearn A, Mullins L, Mulinare J, Khoury M. The surveillance of birth defects: the usefulness of the revised US standard birth certificate. Am J Public Health 1996;86:731–734
8. Saari-Kemppainen A, Karjalainen O, Ylostalo P, Heinonen OP. Ultrasound screening and perinatal mortality: controlled trial systematic one-stage screening in pregnancy. The Helsinki Ultrasound Trial. Lancet 1990;336:387–391
9. Waldenstrom U, Axelsson O, Nilsson S, Eklund G, Fall O, Lindeberg S, et al. Effects of routine one-stage ultrasound screening in pregnancy: a randomised controlled trial. Lancet 1988;2:585–588
10. LeFevre ML, Bain RP, Ewigman BG, Frigoletto FD, Crane JP, McNellis D. A randomized trial of prenatal ultrasonographic screening: impact on maternal management and outcome. RADIUS (Routine Antenatal Diagnostic Imaging with Ultrasound) Study Group. Am J Obstet Gynecol 1993; 169:483–489
11. Ewigman B, LeFevre M, Hesser J. A randomized trial of routine prenatal ultrasound. Obstet Gynecol 1990;76:189–194
12. Copel JA, Platt LD, Campbell S. Prenatal ultrasound screening and perinatal outcome [letter]. N J Med 1994;330:571–572

Practice Patterns are clinical practice guidelines developed by The American College of Obstetricians and Gynecologists (ACOG) to assist practitioners and patients in making decisions about appropriate obstetric and gynecologic care. Each Practice Pattern focuses on a clinical issue and is based on a review and analysis of the scientific literature. The information and recommendations reflect scientific and clinical knowledge current as of the publication date and are subject to change as advances in diagnostic techniques and treatments emerge. In addition, variations of practice, taking into account the needs of the individual patient, resources, and limitations unique to the institution or type of practice, may warrant alternative treatment or procedures to the recommendations outlined in this document. Therefore, these guidelines should not be construed as dictating an exclusive course of treatment or procedure.

ISSN 1083-3331 12345/10987

Number 7, October 1997

ACOG Practice Patterns

Evidence-Based Guidelines for Clinical Issues in Obstetrics and Gynecology

Shoulder Dystocia

Purpose

Shoulder dystocia is an obstetric emergency. Failure of the shoulders to deliver spontaneously immediately places both the pregnant woman and fetus at risk for injury. Reported incidence ranges from less than 1% to slightly more than 4% among vaginal cephalic deliveries. Differences in reported rates are partly due to clinical variation in describing shoulder dystocia. The diagnosis of shoulder dystocia has a subjective component. Although severe cases are readily apparent, milder forms may be over- or underestimated. As a result, researchers differ in their approaches to defining shoulder dystocia. Some accept a clinician's judgment, noted in the chart, that shoulder dystocia occurred. Others require documentation of specific release maneuvers or other procedures to substantiate a diagnosis of shoulder dystocia. As a result, incidence figures vary. Over time, several maneuvers to release impacted shoulders have been developed, but the rarity and urgency of this event makes prospective studies to compare them impractical. Prevention is largely confined to planned cesarean delivery for pregnancies considered to be most at risk for shoulder dystocia.

The purpose of this document is to provide information based on published studies regarding the prediction, prevention, and management of deliveries complicated by shoulder dystocia to assist obstetrician–gynecologists in providing care to their patients.

Objectives

These practice guidelines will enable physicians to:

- Determine whether shoulder dystocia can be predicted
- Identify strategies to manage shoulder dystocia
- Determine whether elective cesarean delivery is an effective strategy to prevent shoulder dystocia

Methods

The MEDLINE database was used to conduct a literature search to locate relevant articles published between 1985 and 1997. The search was restricted to articles published in the English language. Articles reporting results of original research were given priority, although review articles and commentaries were consulted as well. Abstracts of research presented at symposia and scientific conferences were not considered adequate for inclusion in this document. Guidelines published by organizations or institutions such as the National Institutes of Health and the American College of Obstetricians and Gynecologists were reviewed, and additional studies were located by reviewing bibliographies of articles located via MEDLINE. Studies were collected and grouped according to topic. In most cases, studies involving fewer than 50 subjects were not evaluated. When reliable research was not available, expert opinions from obstetrician–gynecologists were used.

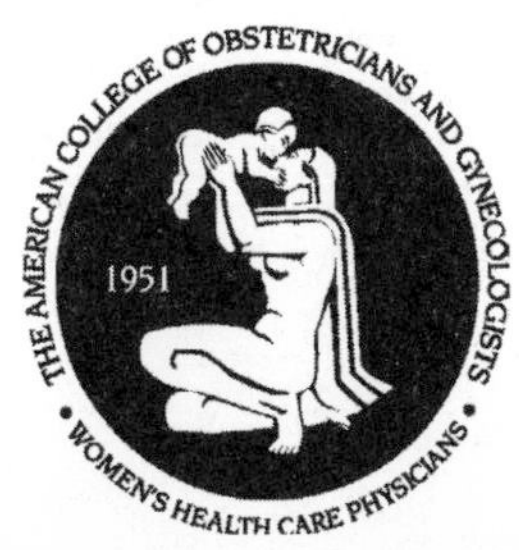

Studies were reviewed and evaluated for quality according to the method outlined by the U.S. Preventive Services Task Force:

- I Evidence obtained from at least one properly designed randomized controlled trial
- II-1 Evidence obtained from well-designed controlled trials without randomization
- II-2 Evidence obtained from well-designed cohort or case-control analytic studies, preferably from more than one center or research group
- II-3 Evidence obtained from multiple time series with or without the intervention. Dramatic results in uncontrolled experiments could also be regarded as this type of evidence
- III Opinions of respected authorities, based on clinical experience, descriptive studies, or reports of expert committees

Results

Can shoulder dystocia be accurately predicted and prevented?

The ideal management strategy for shoulder dystocia is prevention. Theoretically, most cases of shoulder dystocia could be avoided if fetuses at risk were identified before labor and selected for elective cesarean delivery. However, this strategy relies on several underlying assumptions that, in reality, are not true. These erroneous assumptions are

- Risk factors for shoulder dystocia can always be identified prior to labor.
- The presence of risk factors is highly predictive of shoulder dystocia.
- Risks associated with shoulder dystocia are greater than risks associated with planned cesarean deliveries to avoid shoulder dystocia.
- Costs associated with planned cesarean deliveries to avoid shoulder dystocia are less than the costs associated with shoulder dystocia-related injuries.

Predictors of shoulder dystocia

There have been many efforts to identify risk factors. Macrosomia and maternal diabetes consistently appear across many studies as the two risk factors most strongly associated with shoulder dystocia (Level II-2: 1–5) (Level II-3: 6). Pregnant women who have diabetes are two to six times more likely to experience shoulder dystocia than women who do not have diabetes (Level II-2: 1, 3, 5). The incidence of shoulder dystocia increases in direct proportion to infant birth weight whether or not the woman has diabetes, although women who have diabetes experience significantly greater rates of shoulder dystocia in each weight group (Level II-2: 2, 4, 5, 7–9) (see Tables 1 and 2).

TABLE 1. Risk of Shoulder Dystocia According to Diabetic Status

Author	Increase in Risk Associated with Diabetic Status
Acker et al 1985[1]	Rate ratio 5.2
Bahar 1996[3]	Odds ratio 4.3; 95% CI 2.2–8.3
Langer et al 1991[5]	Relative risk <4,000 g 2.6; 95% CI 1.29–5.34
	Relative risk >4,000 g 3.6; 95% CI 2.37–4.76
Sandmire et al 1988[4]	Relative risk 6.5; 95% CI 1.5–27.1

TABLE 2. Rate of Shoulder Dystocia Related to Birth Weight and Diabetic Status

Birth Weight (g)	Women Without Diabetes (%)	Women with Diabetes (%)
<4,000	0.1–1.1	0.6–3.7
4,000–4,449	1.1–10.0	4.9–23.1
≥4,500	4.1–22.6	20.0–50.0

Sources: Acker DB, Sachs BP, Friedman EA. Risk factors for shoulder dystocia. Obstet Gynecol 1985;66:762–768; al-Najashi S, al-Suleiman SA, el-Yahia A, Rahman MS, Rahman J. Shoulder dystocia: a clinical study of 56 cases. Aust N Z J Obstet Gynaecol 1989;29:129–132; Langer O, Berkus MD, Huff RW, Samueloff A. Shoulder dystocia: should the fetus weighing ≥4,000 grams be delivered by cesarean section? Am J Obstet Gynecol 1991;165:831–837.

Although risk increases with birth weight and diabetic status, a substantial proportion of cases occur among women who do not have diabetes and among infants with birth weights of less than 4,000 g. Predicting which patients are likely to experience shoulder dystocia based on the presence of risk factors has been unsuccessful. Acker et al reported a low sensitivity when diabetes mellitus and macrosomia were used to predict cases of shoulder dystocia; the presence of these risk factors accurately predicted only 55% of cases (Level II-2: 1). Additional studies failed to find any combination of risk factors that could predict which pregnancies would be complicated by shoulder dystocia (Level II-2: 3, 4, 7, 8, 10). In each case, risk factors could be identified, but their predictive value was not high enough to be useful in a clinical setting.

Planned cesarean delivery

Because identification of antenatal risk factors has not proved useful in preventing shoulder dystocia, a broad policy of planned cesarean delivery for macrosomic fetuses has been suggested. This strategy seeks to prevent shoulder dystocia by identifying a subgroup with a known risk factor, macrosomia, and selecting those fetuses for cesarean delivery. To be successful, several elements must exist. There must be a high correlation between macrosomia and shoulder dystocia, as well as a reliable method for identifying fetal macrosomia. In addition, the risks associated with shoulder dystocia must be greater than the risks associated with the additional cesarean deliveries resulting from the policy.

For women who do not have diabetes, the policy is unfeasible. Although there is a greater incidence of shoulder dystocia among macrosomic infants, most do not experience this complication. Consequently, if all fetuses suspected of being macrosomic underwent cesarean delivery, there would be a disproportionate impact on the increased cesarean rate compared with the reduction in rate of shoulder dystocia (Level II-2: 5, 8) (Level II-3: 11). For example, Gross et al projected a 27% increase in the total cesarean rate (rising from 15.1% to 19.1%) if cesarean deliveries were performed for all patients with fetuses that weighed 4,000 g or more; unfortunately, the number of shoulder dystocia cases would be reduced by only 42% (Level II-2: 8). Delpapa et al reported similar results among fetuses with estimated birth weights of 4,000 g or more; in their study, an additional 76 cesarean deliveries would have prevented only five cases of shoulder dystocia, none of which resulted in permanent injury (Level II-3: 11). A recently published decision analysis estimated an additional 2,345 cesarean deliveries would be required, at a cost of $4.9 million annually, to prevent one permanent injury resulting from shoulder dystocia if all fetuses suspected of weighing 4,000 g or more underwent cesarean delivery (Level III: 12).

Even if the weight threshold were increased to 4,500 g, the policy remains questionable. Opinion is divided over whether the benefits outweigh the risks. More cases of shoulder dystocia would be prevented, but the impact on the cesarean delivery rate would also be greater. Depending on the distribution of shoulder dystocia cases within a given population, planned cesarean delivery may provide more benefits than risks. Two investigators reported more than 50% of their cases occurred among infants weighing 4,500 g or more, but this finding was unusual (Level II-3: 6, 13). Others report that 20% or less of shoulder dystocia cases could be prevented by cesarean delivery for infants with birth weights of 4,500 g or more (Level II-2: 1, 5, 7) (Level II-3:14).

Gross et al argued that despite preventing fewer cases overall, infants weighing 4,500 g or more could benefit from planned cesarean delivery without adversely affecting the cesarean delivery rate; within the population studied, 20 cases of shoulder dystocia would have been prevented among 42 spontaneous vaginal deliveries with birth weights of 4,500 g or greater, and the cesarean delivery rate would only have increased from 15.1% to 15.7% (Level II-2: 8). Another investigator supporting routine cesarean delivery for birth weights greater than 4,500 g calculated the policy would reduce the incidence of shoulder dystocia by more than 50% while increasing the cesarean rate by only 1.7% (Level II-3: 6). At the other end of the spectrum, Baskett et al projected that implementing the policy within their study population would have resulted in an additional 817 cesarean deliveries while preventing only 69 cases of shoulder dystocia and 15 cases of brachial plexus palsy (Level II-2: 7). A separate study of 590 vaginal deliveries of infants weighing 4,500 g or more found only 54 cases of shoulder dystocia, with five brachial palsies, three fractured clavicles, and no permanent injuries (Level II-3: 15). According to a decision analysis, the national impact of this policy would be $8.7 million annually, with an additional 3,695 cesarean deliveries required to prevent one permanent injury (Level III: 12). The cesarean delivery rate would be projected to rise from 19.1% to 27.6% (Level III: 12). According to the evidence, the costs associated with routine cesarean delivery for estimated fetal weights of 4,500 g or more would be costly without commensurate benefits.

Among women with diabetes, shoulder dystocia cases are more concentrated within the heavier birth weight classes (Level II-2: 1, 2, 5). Approximately 70% of cases among women with diabetes occur at infant birth weights of 4,000 g or more, compared with 50% among those of women without diabetes. Therefore, a policy of planned cesarean delivery is more likely to prevent shoulder dystocia cases among pregnant women with diabetes. The evidence confirms this finding. Acker et al reported that almost 55% of shoulder dystocia among women with diabetes could be prevented if fetuses that weighed 4,000 g or more underwent cesarean delivery (Level II-2: 1). Langer et al found that 76% of shoulder dystocia cases among pregnant women with diabetes could be prevented if fetuses weighing 4,250 g or more underwent cesarean delivery (Level II-2: 5). In contrast, Keller et al found no justification for a 4,000-g threshold among women with gestational diabetes because more than half the cases occurred in infants weighing less than 4,000 g and the ultrasound estimates of fetal weight were inaccurate (Level II-2: 9). A decision analysis projected that a 4,500-g threshold for fetuses of women with diabetes would require an additional 443 procedures to prevent one permanent brachial plexus injury, at a cost of $930,000 (Level III: 12). The studies indicate that for pregnant women with diabetes who are suspected of carrying macrosomic fetuses, a planned cesarean delivery may be a reasonable course of action, depending on the incidence of shoulder dystocia, the accuracy of predicting macrosomia, and the cesarean delivery rate within a specific population.

The policy of planned cesarean delivery relies also on accurate estimates of fetal weight. Fetal weights are calculated from measurements taken during ultrasound examinations. Ultrasonography is an inaccurate predictor of macrosomia. Among the general population, ultrasonography could correctly identify macrosomia only about 60% of the time, according to a pooled estimate of 13 studies (Level III: 12). Within the diabetic population, ultrasonography has provided mixed results. There is evidence of accelerated fetal growth, most notably in the abdominal circumference and chest-to-head ratio (Level II-2: 16–18). However, the clinical usefulness of this information has been limited. One study correctly predicted 88.8% of macrosomia cases among pregnant women with diabetes, based on measurements of abdominal circumference and estimated fetal weight (Level II-2: 17). However, there are no studies documenting the usefulness of identifying macrosomic fetuses for planned cesarean delivery among women with diabetes.

How often does shoulder dystocia result in an injury to the newborn?

Brachial plexus injuries and fractures of the clavicle and humerus are associated with shoulder dystocia. The most potentially serious, brachial plexus injuries, can be caused by extreme amounts of traction and flexion exerted on the infant's neck. These injuries may result in permanent disability. The reported incidence of brachial plexus injuries following a delivery complicated by shoulder dystocia varies widely from 4% to 40% (1, 2, 6–9, 13, 14, 19–22). Fortunately, most cases resolve without permanent disability. Reports indicate between 9% and 25% of brachial plexus injuries persist (2, 7, 9, 14). Placed in perspective, fewer than 10% of all shoulder dystocia cases result in a persistent brachial plexus injury (2, 7, 9, 14). Moreover, brachial plexus injuries can occur without shoulder dystocia and at birth weights of less than 4,000 g (23).

Are any of the maneuvers used to release impacted shoulders either more likely to cause injuries or more likely to be successful?

Because of the rarity and urgency of shoulder dystocia, only a limited amount of data exists comparing management techniques. Two separate studies confirm that the combination of traction and fundal pressure is associated with brachial plexus injuries as well as with fractures of the humerus and clavicle (Level II-2: 7) (Level II-3: 20). There is no indication, however, that any particular management technique is superior to another once shoulder dystocia occurs.

There is evidence that injuries might and do occur despite application of appropriate obstetric maneuvers (Level II-3: 24). During a series of deliveries, the obstetrician wore a tactile-sensing device that recorded the peak and duration of forces applied to the head and neck of the fetus. During the study, two cases of shoulder dystocia occurred to infants with similar birth weights and obstetric protocols. One infant sustained a shoulder dystocia-related injury and the other did not (Level II-3: 24).

The McRoberts maneuver relies on maternal manipulation and is reported to be effective (Level II-2: 7, 19) (Level II-3: 25). Successful use of the McRoberts maneuver is documented in the scientific literature. The maneuver involves sharply flexing the patient's legs against her abdomen. Results from a laboratory study using models of the maternal pelvis, fetal head, and fetal shoulders demonstrated that less force was required to deliver fetuses using the McRoberts maneuver compared with the standard lithotomy position (26).

Summary and Recommendations

Based on this highest level of evidence found in the data, the following recommendations are provided and graded according to the following categories:

A There is good evidence to support the recommendation.
B There is fair evidence to support the recommendation.
C There is insufficient evidence to support the recommendation; however, the recommendation may be made on other grounds.

Prediction and prevention of shoulder dystocia

- Most cases of shoulder dystocia cannot be predicted or prevented because accurate methods for identifying which fetuses will experience this complication do not exist, and performing cesarean deliveries for all women suspected of carrying a macrosomic fetus is not appropriate (B: II-2).
- Ultrasonographic measurements to estimate macrosomia have limited accuracy (B: II-2).
- Planned cesarean delivery on the basis of suspected macrosomia in the general population is not a reasonable strategy because the number and cost of additional cesarean deliveries required to prevent one permanent injury is excessive (B: II-2).
- Planned cesarean delivery may be a reasonable strategy for diabetic pregnant women with estimated fetal weights exceeding 4,250–4,500 g (B: II-2).

Shoulder dystocia as a cause of injury to newborns

- Injuries are a common outcome associated with shoulder dystocia and may occur despite use of appropriate standard obstetric maneuvers (B: II-3). Brachial plexus injuries, fractures of the humerus, and fractures of the clavicle are the most commonly reported injuries associated with shoulder dystocia (A: II-2).
- Fewer than 10% of all deliveries complicated by shoulder dystocia will result in a persistent brachial plexus injury (A:II-2).

Release techniques

- There is no evidence that any one maneuver is superior to another in releasing an impacted shoulder or reducing the chance of injury. However, the McRoberts maneuver is easily facilitated and has a high success rate without an associated increase in risk of injury to the newborn (B: II-2).
- Traction combined with fundal pressure has been associated with a high rate of brachial plexus injuries and fractures (B: II-2).

References

1. Acker DB, Sachs BP, Friedman EA. Risk factors for shoulder dystocia. Obstet Gynecol 1985;66:762–768
2. al-Najashi S, al-Suleiman SA, el-Yahia A, Rahman MS, Rahman J. Shoulder dystocia: a clinical study of 56 cases. Aust N Z J Obstet Gynaecol 1989;29:129–132
3. Bahar AM. Risk factors and fetal outcome in cases of shoulder dystocia compared with normal deliveries of a similar birthweight. Br J Obstet Gynaecol 1996;103:868–872
4. Sandmire HF, O'Halloin TJ. Shoulder dystocia: its incidence and associated risk factors. Int J Gynaecol Obstet 1988;26:65–73
5. Langer O, Berkus MD, Huff RW, Samueloff A. Shoulder dystocia: should the fetus weighing ≥ 4000 grams be delivered by cesarean section? Am J Obstet Gynecol 1991; 165:831–837
6. el Madany AA, Jallad KB, Radi FA, el Hamdan H, O'deh HM. Shoulder dystocia: anticipation and outcome. Int J Gynecol Obstet 1990;34:7–12
7. Baskett TF, Allen AC. Perinatal implications of shoulder dystocia. Obstet Gynecol 1995;86:14–17

8. Gross TL, Sokol RJ, Williams T, Thompson K. Shoulder dystocia: a fetal–physician risk. Am J Obstet Gynecol 1987;156:1408–1418
9. Keller JD, Lopez-Zeno JA, Dooley SL, Socol ML. Shoulder dystocia and birth trauma in gestational diabetes: a five-year experience. Am J Obstet Gynecol 1991;165:928–930
10. Nocon JJ, McKenzie DK, Thomas LJ, Hansell RS. Shoulder dystocia: an analysis of risks and obstetric maneuvers. Am J Obstet Gynecol 1993;168:1732–1739
11. Delpapa EH, Mueller-Heubach E. Pregnancy outcome following ultrasound diagnosis of macrosomia. Obstet Gynecol 1991;78:340–343
12. Rouse DJ, Owen J, Goldenberg RL, Cliver SP. The effectiveness and costs of elective cesarean delivery for fetal macrosomia diagnosed by ultrasound. JAMA 1996;276:1480–1486
13. Hassan AA. Shoulder dystocia: risk factors and prevention. Aust N Z J Obstet Gynaecol 1988;28:107–109
14. Morrison JC, Sanders JR, Magann EF, Wiser WL. The diagnosis and management of dystocia of the shoulder. Surg Gynecol Obstet 1992;175:515–522
15. Menticoglou SM, Manning FA, Morrison I, Harman CR. Must macrosomic fetuses be delivered by a cesarean section? A review of outcome for 786 babies greater than or equal to 4,500 g. Aust N Z J Obstet Gynaecol 1992;32:100–103
16. Bracero LA, Baxi LV, Rey HR, Yeh MN. Use of ultrasound in antenatal diagnosis of large-for-gestational age infants in diabetic gravid patients. Am J Obstet Gynecol 1985;152:43–47
17. Tamura RK, Sabbagha RE, Depp R, Dooley SL, Socol ML. Diabetic macrosomia: accuracy of third trimester ultrasound. Obstet Gynecol 1986;67:828–832
18. Modanlou HD, Komatsu G, Dorchester W, Freeman RK, Bosu SK. Large-for-gestational-age neonates: anthropometric reasons for shoulder dystocia. Obstet Gynecol 1982;60:417–423
19. Gonik B, Hollyer L, Allen R. Shoulder dystocia recognition: differences in neonatal risks for injury. Am J Perinatol 1991;8:31–34
20. Gross SJ, Shime J, Farine D. Shoulder dystocia: predictors and outcome. A five-year review. Am J Obstet Gynecol 1987;156:334–336
21. Hopwood HG Jr. Shoulder dystocia: fifteen years' experience in a community hospital. Am J Obstet Gynecol 1982;144:162–166
22. Lurie S, Insler V, Hagay ZJ. Induction of labor at 38 to 39 weeks of gestation reduces the incidence of shoulder dystocia in gestational diabetic patients class A2. Am J Perinatol 1996;13:293–296
23. Graham EM, Forouzan I, Morgan MA. A retrospective analysis of Erb's palsy cases and their relation to birth weight and trauma at delivery. J Matern Fetal Med 1997;6:1–5
24. Allen R, Sorab J, Gonik B. Risk factors for shoulder dystocia: an engineering study of clinician-applied forces. Obstet Gynecol 1991;77:352–355
25. Smeltzer JS. Prevention and management of shoulder dystocia. Clin Obstet Gynecol 1986;29:299–308
26. Gonik B, Allen R, Sorab J. Objective evaluation of the shoulder dystocia phenomenon: effect of maternal pelvic orientation on force reduction. Obstet Gynecol 1989;74:44–48

Practice Patterns are clinical practice guidelines developed by The American College of Obstetricians and Gynecologists (ACOG) to assist practitioners and patients in making decisions about appropriate obstetric and gynecologic care. Each Practice Pattern focuses on a clinical issue and is based on a review and analysis of the scientific literature. The information and recommendations reflect scientific and clinical knowledge current as of the publication date and are subject to change as advances in diagnostic techniques and treatments emerge. In addition, variations of practice, taking into account the needs of the individual patient, resources, and limitations unique to the institution or type of practice, may warrant alternative treatment or procedures to the recommendations outlined in this document. Therefore, these guidelines should not be construed as dictating an exclusive course of treatment or procedure.

ISSN 1083-3331 12345/10987

Lists of Titles

Committee Opinions

Educational and Technical Bulletins

Practice Bulletins

Practice Patterns

Policy Statements

Index

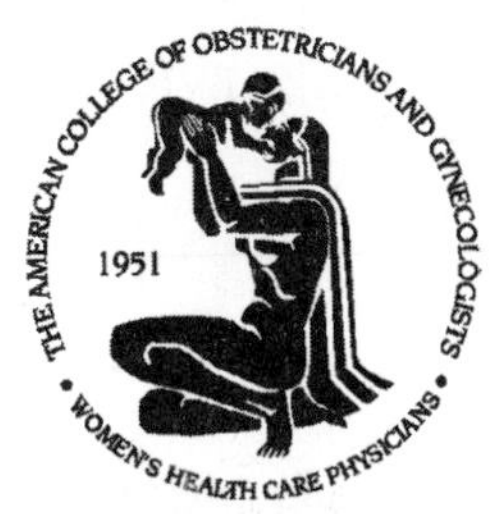

ACOG *Statement of Policy*

As issued by the ACOG Executive Board

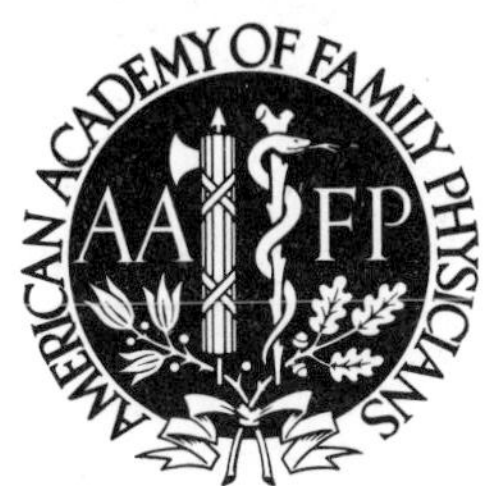

This document was developed by a joint task force of the American Academy of Family Physicians and the American College of Obstetricians and Gynecologists.

AAFP--ACOG JOINT STATEMENT ON COOPERATIVE PRACTICE AND HOSPITAL PRIVILEGES

Access to maternity care is an important public health concern in the United States. Providing comprehensive perinatal services to a diverse population requires a cooperative relationship among a variety of health professionals, including social workers, health educators, nurses and physicians. Prenatal care, labor and delivery, and postpartum care have historically been provided by midwives, family physicians and obstetricians. All three remain the major caregivers today. A cooperative and collaborative relationship among obstetricians, family physicians and nurse midwives is essential for provision of consistent, high-quality care to pregnant women.

Regardless of specialty, there should be shared common standards of perinatal care. This requires a cooperative working environment and shared decision making. Clear guidelines for consultation and referral for complications should be developed jointly. When appropriate, early and ongoing consultation regarding a woman's care is necessary for the best possible outcome and is an important part of risk management and prevention of professional liability problems. All family physicians and obstetricians on the medical staff of the obstetric unit should agree to such guidelines and be willing to work together for the best care of patients. This includes a willingness on the part of obstetricians to provide consultation and back-up for family physicians who provide maternity care. The family physician should have knowledge, skills and judgment to determine when timely consultation and/or referral may be appropriate.

The most important objective of the physician must be the provision of the highest standards of care, regardless of specialty. Quality patient care requires that all providers should practice within their degree of ability as determined by training, experience and current competence. A joint practice committee with obstetricians and family physicians should be established in health care organizations to determine and monitor standards of care and to determine proctoring guidelines. A collegial working relationship between family physicians and obstetricians is essential if we are to provide access to quality care for pregnant women in this country.

The American College of Obstetricians and Gynecologists
409 12th Street, SW, PO Box 96920 • Washington, DC 20090-6920 Telephone 202 638 5577

AAFP--ACOG JOINT STATEMENT ON COOPERATIVE PRACTICE AND HOSPITAL PRIVILEGES
Page 2

A. Practice privileges

The assignment of hospital privileges is a local responsibility and privileges should be granted on the basis of training, experience and demonstrated current competence. All physicians should be held to thesame standards for granting of privileges, regardless of specialty, in order to assure the provision of high-quality patient care. Prearranged, collaborative relationships should be established to ensure ongoing consultations, as well as consultations needed for emergencies.

The standard of training should allow any physician who receives training in a cognitive or surgical skill to meet the criteria for privileges in that area of practice. Provisional privileges in primary care, obstetric care and cesarean delivery should be granted regardless of specialty as long as training criteria and experience are documented. All physicians should be subject to a proctorship period to allow demonstration of ability and current competence. These principles should apply to all health care systems.

B. Interdepartmental relationships

Privileges recommended by the department of family practice shall be the responsibility of the department of family practice. Similarly, privileges recommended by the department of obstetrics-gynecology shall be the responsibility of the department of obstetrics-gynecology. When privileges are recommended jointly by the departments of family practice and obstetrics-gynecology, they shall be the joint responsibility of the two departments.

Published July 1980
Reformatted July 1988
Revised and Retitled March 1998

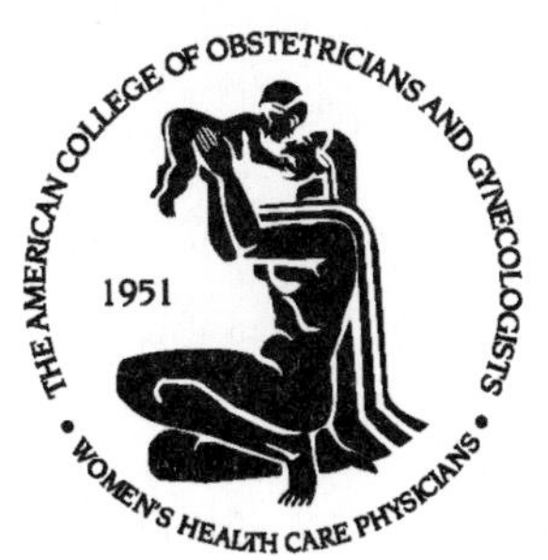

ACOG *Statement of Policy*

As issued by the ACOG Executive Board

ABORTION POLICY

The following statement is the American College of Obstetricians and Gynecologists' (ACOG) general policy related to abortion, with specific reference to the procedure referred to as "intact dilatation and extraction" (intact D & X).

1. The abortion debate in this country is marked by serious moral pluralism. Different positions in the debate represent different but important values. The diversity of beliefs should be respected.

2. ACOG recognizes that the issue of support of or opposition to abortion is a matter of profound moral conviction to its members. ACOG, therefore, respects the need and responsibility of its members to determine their individual positions based on personal values or beliefs.

3. Termination of pregnancy before viability is a medical matter between the patient and physician, subject to the physician's clinical judgment, the patient's informed consent and the availability of appropriate facilities.

4. The need for abortions, other than those indicated by serious fetal anomalies or conditions which threaten maternal welfare, represents failures in the social environment and the educational system.

The most effective way to reduce the number of abortions is to prevent unwanted and unintended pregnancies. This can be accomplished by open and honest education, beginning in the home, religious institutions and the primary schools. This education should stress the biology of reproduction and the responsibilities involved by boys, girls, men and women in creating life and the desirability of delaying pregnancies until circumstances are appropriate and pregnancies are planned.

In addition, everyone should be made aware of the dangers of sexually transmitted diseases and the means of protecting each other from their transmission. To accomplish these aims, support of the community and the school system is essential.

The medical curriculum should be expanded to include a focus on the components of reproductive biology which pertain to conception control. Physicians should be encouraged to apply these principles in their own practices and to support them at the community level.

Society also has a responsibility to support research leading to improved methods of contraception for men and women.

The American College of Obstetricians and Gynecologists
409 12th Street, SW, PO Box 96920 • Washington, DC 20090-6920 Telephone 202 638 5577

ABORTION POLICY
Page 2

5. Informed consent is an expression of respect for the patient as a person; it particularly respects a patient's moral right to bodily integrity, to self-determination regarding sexuality and reproductive capacities, and to the support of the patient's freedom within caring relationships.

   A pregnant woman should be fully informed in a balanced manner about all options, including raising the child herself, placing the child for adoption, and abortion. The information conveyed should be appropriate to the duration of the pregnancy. The professional should make every effort to avoid introducing personal bias.

6. ACOG supports access to care for all individuals, irrespective of financial status, and supports the availability of all reproductive options. ACOG opposes unnecessary regulations that limit or delay access to care.

7. If abortion is to be performed, it should be performed safely and as early as possible.

8. ACOG opposes the harassment of abortion providers and patients.

9. ACOG strongly supports those activities which prevent unintended pregnancy.

The College continues to affirm the legal right of a woman to obtain an abortion prior to fetal viability. ACOG is opposed to abortion of the healthy fetus that has attained viability in a healthy woman. Viability is the capacity of the fetus to survive outside the mother's uterus. Whether or not this capacity exists is a medical determination, may vary with each pregnancy and is a matter for the judgment of the responsible attending physician.

Intact Dilatation and Extraction

The debate regarding legislation to prohibit a method of abortion, such as the legislation banning "partial birth abortion," and "brain sucking abortions," has prompted questions regarding these procedures. It is difficult to respond to these questions because the descriptions are vague and do not delineate a specific procedure recognized in the medical literature. Moreover, the definitions could be interpreted to include elements of many recognized abortion and operative obstetric techniques.

ACOG believes the intent of such legislative proposals is to prohibit a procedure referred to as "intact dilatation and extraction" (Intact D & X). This procedure has been described as containing all of the following four elements:

1. deliberate dilatation of the cervix, usually over a sequence of days;
2. instrumental conversion of the fetus to a footling breech;
3. breech extraction of the body excepting the head; and
4. partial evacuation of the intracranial contents of a living fetus to effect vaginal delivery of a dead but otherwise intact fetus.

Because these elements are part of established obstetric techniques, it must be emphasized that unless all four elements are present in sequence, the procedure is not an intact D & X. Abortion intends to terminate a pregnancy while preserving the life and health of the mother. When abortion is performed after 16 weeks, intact D & X is one method of terminating a pregnancy.

ABORTION POLICY
Page 3

The physician, in consultation with the patient, must choose the most appropriate method based upon the patient's individual circumstances.
According to the Centers for Disease Control and Prevention (CDC), only 5.3% of abortions performed in the United States in 1993, the most recent data available, were performed after the 16th week of pregnancy. A preliminary figure published by the CDC for 1994 is 5.6%. The CDC does not collect data on the specific method of abortion, so it is unknown how many of these were performed using intact D & X. Other data show that second trimester transvaginal instrumental abortion is a safe procedure.

Terminating a pregnancy is performed in some circumstances to save the life or preserve the health of the mother.

Intact D & X is one of the methods available in some of these situations. A select panel convened by ACOG could identify no circumstances under which this procedure, as defined above, would be the only option to save the life or preserve the health of the woman. An intact D & X, however, may be the best or most appropriate procedure in a particular circumstance to save the life or preserve the health of a woman, and only the doctor, in consultation with the patient, based upon the woman's particular circumstances can make this decision. The potential exists that legislation prohibiting specific medical practices, such as intact D & X, may outlaw techniques that are critical to the lives and health of American women. **The intervention of legislative bodies into medical decision making is inappropriate, ill advised, and dangerous.**

Approval by the Executive Board
General policy: January 1993
Reaffirmed and revised July 1997
Intact D & X statement: January 1997
Combined: September 2000

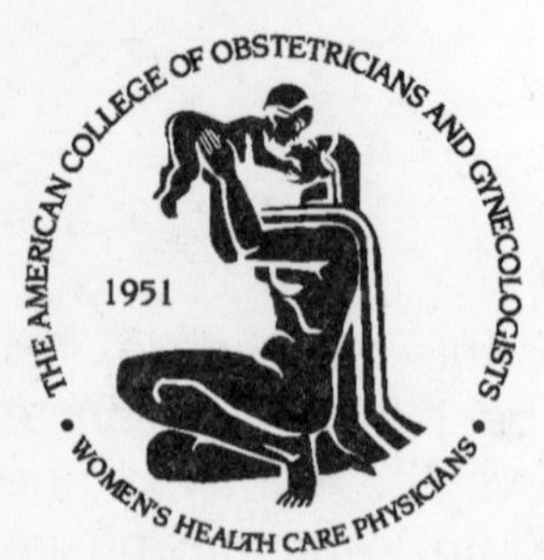

ACOG *Statement of Policy*

As issued by the ACOG Executive Board

ACCESS TO REPRODUCTIVE HEALTH CARE FOR ADOLESCENTS

Adolescence is a time of psychosocial, cognitive, and physical development as young people make the transition from childhood to adulthood. This transition includes sexual development and often entails behaviors that put young women at risk for pregnancy and sexually transmitted diseases. Guidance from a physician, as well as needed reproductive health screening and care, can greatly facilitate young peoples' healthy transition to adulthood.

Health professionals have an obligation to provide the best possible care to respond to the needs of their adolescent patients. This care should, at a minimum, include comprehensive reproductive health services, such as sexuality education, counseling, mental health assessment, diagnosis and treatment regarding pubertal development, access to contraceptives and abortion, pregnancy-related care, prenatal and delivery care, and diagnosis and treatment of sexually transmitted diseases. Every effort should be made to include male partners in such services and counseling.

Comprehensive services may be delivered to adolescents in a variety of sites, including schools, physician offices, and community-based and other health care facilities. Legal barriers that restrict the freedom of health care providers to provide these services should be removed. Institutional policies should be developed to require providers with views on confidentiality that restrict the provision of services to a minor to refer the patient to another provider.

Since the involvement of a concerned adult can contribute to the health and success of an adolescent, policies in health care settings should encourage and facilitate communication between a minor and her parent(s), when appropriate. However, concerns about confidentiality, as well as economic considerations, can be significant barriers to reproductive healthcare for some adolescents. The potential health risks to adolescents if they are unable to obtain reproductive health services are so compelling that legal barriers and deference to parental involvement should not stand in the way of needed health care for patients who request confidentiality. Therefore, laws and regulations that are unduly restrictive of adolescents' confidential access to reproductive health care should be revised. Institutional procedures that safeguard the rights of their adolescent patients, including confidentiality during initial and subsequent visits and in billing, should be established.

Billing mechanisms for services and procedures for insurance and other third-party reimbursement should ensure adolescent confidentiality. When these mechanisms and procedures compromise a patient's request for confidentiality, policies should be implemented allowing (1) payment alternatives such as reduced fees, sliding scales, and time installment payments and/or (2) patient referral to a practice or agency where subsidized care is offered.

Approved by the Executive Board July 2000

The American College of Obstetricians and Gynecologists
409 12th Street, SW, PO Box 96920 • Washington, DC 20090-6920 Telephone 202 638 5577

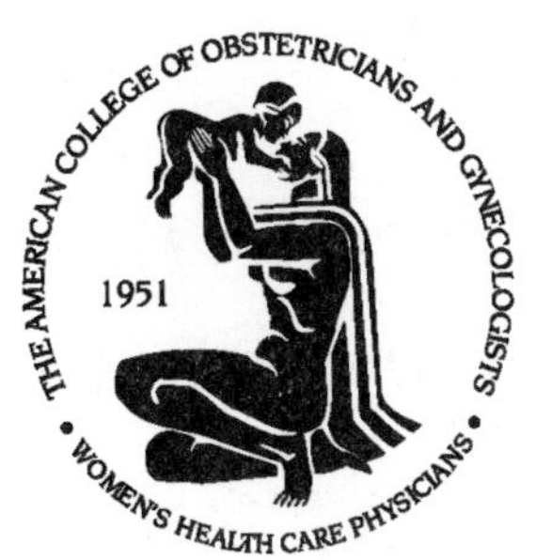

ACOG *Statement of Policy*

As issued by the ACOG Executive Board

ACCESS TO WOMEN'S HEALTH CARE

Excellence in women's health care is an essential element of the long-term physical, intellectual, social and economic well-being of any society. It is a basic determinant of the health of future generations.

The American College of Obstetricians and Gynecologists is the representative organization of physicians who are qualified specialists in providing health services unique to women. ACOG calls for quality health care appropriate to every woman's needs throughout her life and for assuring that a full array of clinical services be available to women without costly delays or the imposition of geographic, financial, attitudinal or legal barriers.

The College and its membership are committed to facilitating both access to and quality of women's health care. Fellows should exercise their responsibility to improve the health status of women and their offspring both in the traditional patient-physician relationships and by working within their community and at the state and national levels to assure access to high-quality programs meeting the health needs of all women.

In addition, it is critical that all Americans be provided with adequate and affordable health coverage. Despite economic prosperity and substantial job creation during the 1990s, there remains a considerable and increasing portion of the American population that does not have health insurance coverage. As a result, those individuals often defer obtaining preventive and medical services, jeopardizing the health and well being of themselves and their families. The College supports universal coverage that is designed to improve the individual and collective health of society. Expanding health coverage to all Americans must become a high priority.

Approved by the Executive Board July 1988
Amended September 1999

The American College of Obstetricians and Gynecologists
409 12th Street, SW, PO Box 96920 • Washington, DC 20090-6920 Telephone 202 638 5577

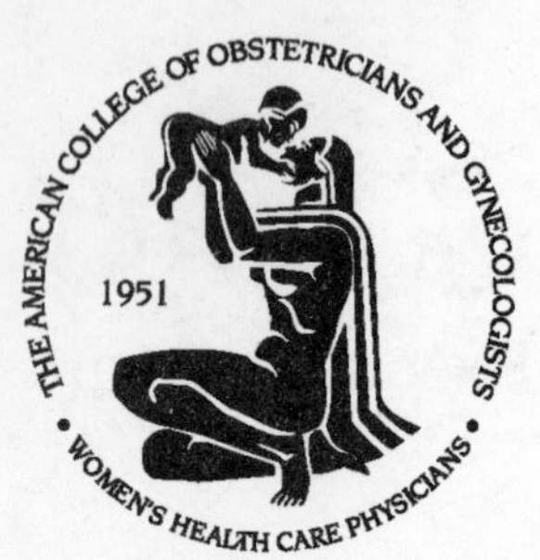

ACOG *Statement of Policy*

As issued by the ACOG Executive Board

HOME DELIVERY

Labor and delivery, while a physiologic process, clearly presents potential hazards to both mother and fetus before and after birth. These hazards require standards of safety which are provided in the hospital setting and cannot be matched in the home situation.

We support those actions that improve the experience of the family while continuing to provide the mother and her infant with accepted standards of safety available only in hospitals which conform to standards as outlined by the American Academy of Pediatrics and the American College of Obstetricians and Gynecologists.

Approved by the Executive Board May 1975
Amended March 1979
Reaffirmed September 1999

The American College of Obstetricians and Gynecologists
409 12th Street, SW, PO Box 96920 • Washington, DC 20090-6920 Telephone 202 638 5577

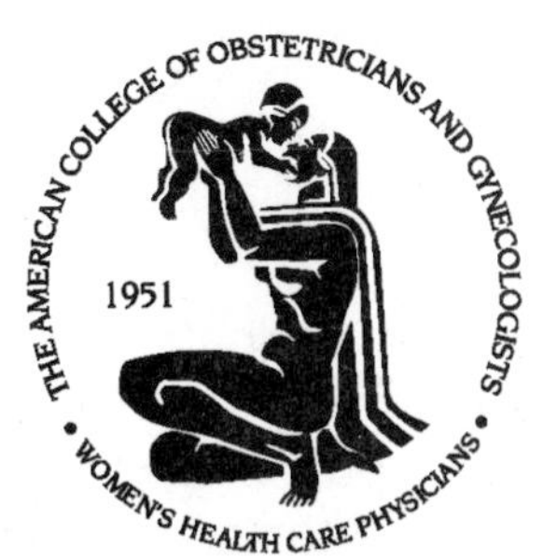

ACOG *Statement of Policy*

As issued by the ACOG Executive Board

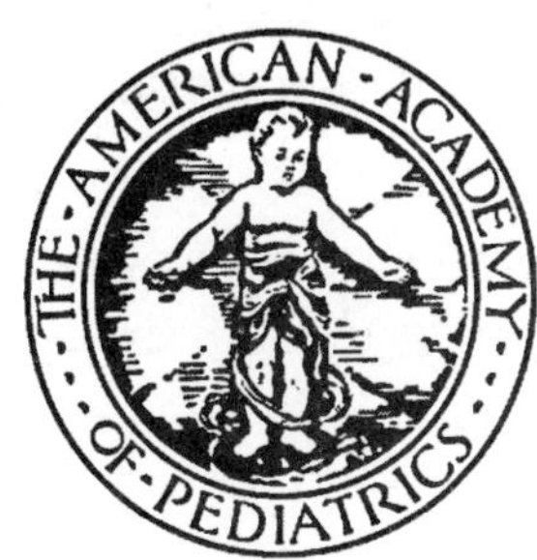

This document was developed jointly by the American Academy of Pediatrics and the American College of Obstetricians and Gynecologists.

JOINT STATEMENT ON HUMAN IMMUNODEFICIENCY VIRUS SCREENING

The problem of perinatal transmission of HIV infection was first appreciated in 1982. In 1991, the Institute of Medicine (IOM) recommended a policy of routine counseling and offering testing (with specific informed consent) for HIV infection to all pregnant women. Since 1991, there have been major advances in the treatment of HIV infection, including demonstration in 1994 of the efficacy of zidovudine to reduce perinatal transmission. The U.S. Public Health Service subsequently issued guidelines for use of zidovudine to reduce perinatal transmission and for counseling and voluntary testing for pregnant women. Dramatic declines in reported pediatric AIDS cases have been observed as a consequence of implementation of these guidelines. However, for a variety of reasons, screening pregnant women in the United States has been far from universal and infected babies continue to be born to undiagnosed infected women. Further reduction in the rate of perinatal HIV infection will require wider application of both screening to identify infected women, and treatments, which have demonstrated efficacy in reducing vertical transmission.

The IOM recently completed a study of interventions that would be helpful to further HIV infection in the United States (Reducing the Odds). They have recommended that "the United States should adopt a national policy of universal HIV testing, with patient notification, as a routine component of prenatal care". Early diagnosis of HIV infection in pregnant women allows them to institute effective antiretroviral therapy for their own health and to reduce the risk of HIV transmission to their infants. The use of "patient notification" provides women the opportunity to decline to be tested but eliminates the obligation to provide extensive pretest counseling, which has been a barrier to testing in many settings. Care providers would be charged with responsibility for the details of how the notification would take place. The IOM has recommended universal testing for two reasons. First, attempts to identify those "at risk" for infection inevitably fail to identify some infected individuals. Second, universal testing of all pregnant women avoids stereotyping and stigmatizing any social or ethnic group. The IOM recognizes in its report that many states now have laws requiring a formal, and in many cases written informed consent process prior to testing. They recommend that the Federal government adopt policies that will encourage these states to change their laws.

The American College of Obstetricians and Gynecologists
409 12th Street, SW, PO Box 96920 • Washington, DC 20090-6920 Telephone 202 638 5577

JOINT STATEMENT ON HUMAN IMMUNODEFICIENCY VIRUS SCREENING
Page 2

The AAP and the ACOG strongly support efforts to further reduce the rate of perinatal transmission of HIV in the United States. We therefore support the recommendation of the IOM for universal HIV testing with patient notification as a routine component of prenatal care. If a patient declines testing, this should be noted in the medical record. We recognize that current laws in some states may prevent implementation of this recommendation at this time. We encourage our members and Fellows to include counseling as a routine part of care, but not as a prerequisite for, and barrier to, prenatal HIV testing.

Approved by the ACOG Executive Board
Approved by the AAP Executive Board
May 1999

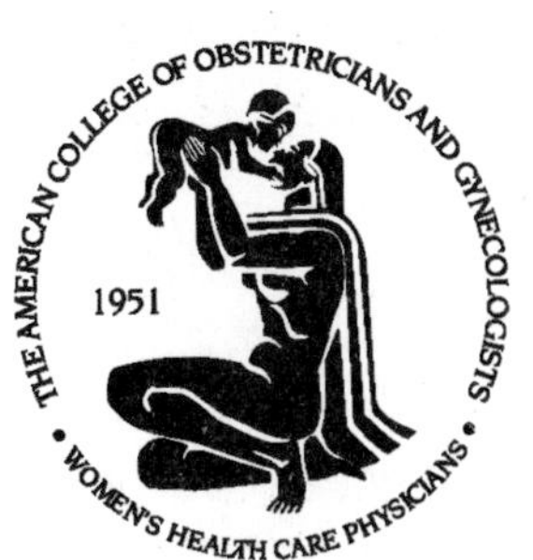

ACOG *Statement of Policy*

As issued by the ACOG Executive Board

JOINT STATEMENT OF PRACTICE RELATIONSHIPS BETWEEN OBSTETRICIAN-GYNECOLOGISTS AND CERTIFIED NURSE-MIDWIVES*

It is critical that obstetrician-gynecologists and certified nurse-midwives have a clear understanding of their individual, collaborative and interdependent responsibilities. As agreed upon in previous Joint Statements by the American College of Nurse-Midwives, the American College of Obstetricians and Gynecologists, and the Nurses Association of the American College of Obstetricians and Gynecologists, the maternity care team should be directed by a qualified obstetrician-gynecologist. The American College of Obstetricians and Gynecologists and the American College of Nurse-Midwives believe that the appropriate practice of the certified nurse-midwife includes the participation and involvement of the obstetrician-gynecologist as mutually agreed upon in written medical guideline/protocol. The American College of Obstetricians and Gynecologists and the American College of Nurse-Midwives also believe that the obstetrician-gynecologist should be responsive to the desire of certified nurse-midwives for the participation and involvement of the obstetrician-gynecologist. The following principles represent a joint statement of the American College of Obstetricians and Gynecologists and the American College of Nurse-Midwives and are recommended for consideration in all practice relationships and agreements.

1. Clinical practice relationship between the obstetrician-gynecologist and the certified nurse-midwife should provide for:
   a. mutually agreed upon written medical guidelines/protocols for clinical practice which define the individual and shared responsibilities of the certified nurse-midwife and the obstetrician-gynecologist in the delivery of health care services;
   b. mutually agreed upon written medical guidelines/protocols for ongoing communication which provide for and define appropriate consultation between the obstetrician-gynecologist and certified nurse-midwife; and other health care providers in the services offered;
   c. informed consent about the involvement of the obstetrician-gynecologist, certified nurse-midwife, and other health care providers in the services offered;
   d. periodic and joint evaluation of services rendered, e.g., chart review, case review, patient evaluation, review of outcome statistics; and
   e. periodic and joint review and updating of the written medical guidelines/protocols.

The American College of Obstetricians and Gynecologists
409 12th Street, SW, PO Box 96920 • Washington, DC 20090-6920 Telephone 202 638 5577

JOINT STATEMENT OF PRACTICE RELATIONSHIPS BETWEEN OBSTETRICIAN-GYNECOLOGISTS AND CERTIFIED NURSE-MIDWIVES*
Page 2

2. Quality of care is enhanced by the interdependent practice of the obstetrician-gynecologist and the certified nurse-midwife working in a relationship of mutual respect, trust and professional responsibility. This does not necessarily imply the physical presence of the physician when care is being given by the certified nurse-midwife.

3. Administrative relationships, including employment agreements, reimbursement mechanisms, and corporate structures, should be mutually agreed upon by the participating parties.

4. Access to practice within the hospital setting for the obstetrician-gynecologist and the certified midwife who have a practice relationship in concurrence with these principles is strongly urged by the respective professional organizations.

The American College of Obstetricians and Gynecologists and the American College of Nurse-Midwives strongly urge the implementation of these principles in all practice relationships between obstetrician-gynecologists and certified nurse-midwives, and consider the preceding an ideal model of practice.

* This statement supersedes previous Joint Statements of Maternity Care by the American College of Obstetricians and Gynecologists, the American College of Nurse-Midwives, and the Nurses Association of the American College of Obstetricians and Gynecologists dated 1971 and 1975.

The American College of Nurse-Midwives
The American College of Obstetricians and Gynecologists
November 1, 1982
Reaffirmed by ACOG September 1999

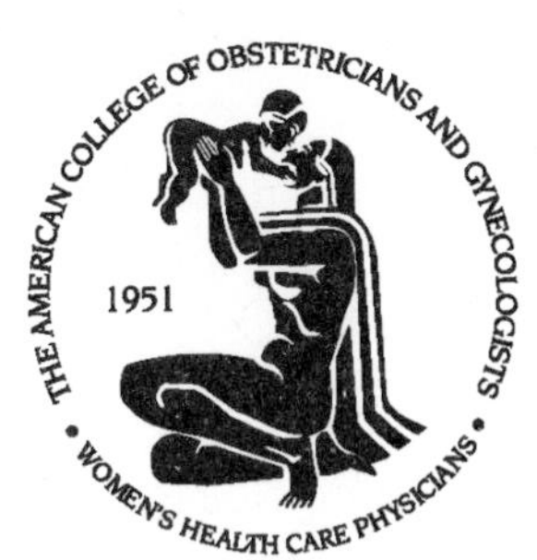

ACOG *Statement of Policy*

As issued by the ACOG Executive Board

LIMITATIONS OF ABSTINENCE-ONLY SEXUALITY EDUCATION

The American College of Obstetricians and Gynecologists has a long-standing commitment to comprehensive health and educational services for adolescents, including sexuality education (1). Recent federal welfare reformlaw describes a particular form of sexuality education often called "abstinence-only" sex education. This federal law, along with other factors, has led to a growing emphasis by some on this narrowly defined form of sexuality education (2).

Definitions

There are a variety of terms used to describe sexuality education programs, including, among others, "abstinence-only," "abstinence-based," "abstinence-plus," and "abstinence-centered." One particular form of "abstinence-only" education is characterized by a federal definition of abstinence that narrowly describes its contents and purposes. (2) Abstinence "based/plus/centered" programs, by contrast, not only promote abstinence but also incorporate reproductive health information, including materials on both the risks and benefits of various methods of contraception, STD prevention, and on forms of sexual expression alternative to intercourse.

Sexuality education programs in general have not been well evaluated. Although some "abstinence-based" programs have shown modest success in delaying the initiation of sexual activity and increasing the use of contraception, the impact of "abstinence-only" programs on behavior has not yet been determined through careful research. Accordingly, "abstinence-only" education should not be adopted as the sole curriculum until such appropriate evaluation has been completed (3).

In the absence of compelling data, communities planning appropriate sexuality education for adolescents should consider the following four points:

1. ACOG reaffirms its support for comprehensive age-appropriate sexuality education for grades K-12 (4).
2. ACOG affirms the goal of promoting healthy lifestyles for adolescents and their families. This includes the following objectives: (5)
   a. Promote abstinence from sexual intercourse as the preferred responsible behavior for adolescents;

The American College of Obstetricians and Gynecologists
409 12th Street, SW, PO Box 96920 • Washington, DC 20090-6920 Telephone 202 638 5577

LIMITATIONS OF ABSTINENCE-ONLY SEXUALITY EDUCATION
Page 2

b. Increase the use of contraceptives by sexually active adolescents;

c. Support increased availability of family planning services and services for the prevention and/or treatment of sexually transmitted diseases.

3. ACOG affirms that all sexuality education programs should provide scientifically accurate information about sexuality, STDs, contraception, and preventive health care.

4. ACOG encourages ongoing rigorous evaluation of the effectiveness of a variety of forms of sexuality education.

REFERENCES

1. ACOG Statements of Policy: Statement on Sexuality Education; Providing Effective Contraception to Minors; Reproductive Health Services for Adolescents.

2. Public Law 104-193, 104th Congress, August 22, 1996

"(2) For purposes of this section, the term "abstinence education" means an educational or motivational program which --

A. has as its exclusive purpose, teaching the social, psychological, and health gains to be realized by abstaining from sexual activity;
B. teaches abstinence from sexual activity outside marriage as the expected standard for all school age children;
C. teaches that abstinence from sexual activity is the only certain way to avoid out-of-wedlock pregnancy, sexually transmitted diseases, and other associated health problems;
D. teaches that a mutually faithful monogamous relationship in context of marriage is the expected standard of human sexual activity;
E. teaches that sexual activity outside of the context of marriage is likely to have harmful psychological and physical effects;
F. teaches that bearing children out-of-wedlock is likely to have harmful consequences for the child, the child's parents, and society;
G. teaches young people how to reject sexual advances and how alcohol and drug use increases vulnerability to sexual advances; and
H. teaches the importance of attaining self-sufficiency before engaging in sexual activity."

3. Kirby, D, No Easy Answers. Research findings on programs to reduce teen pregnancy, National Campaign to Prevent Teen Pregnancy, Washington, DC, 1997.

4. ACOG Statement of Policy, Statement on Sexuality Education, Washington, DC, 1996.

5. American Academy of Pediatrics, Goals and Objectives, July 1997-June 1998.

Approved by the Executive Board May 1998

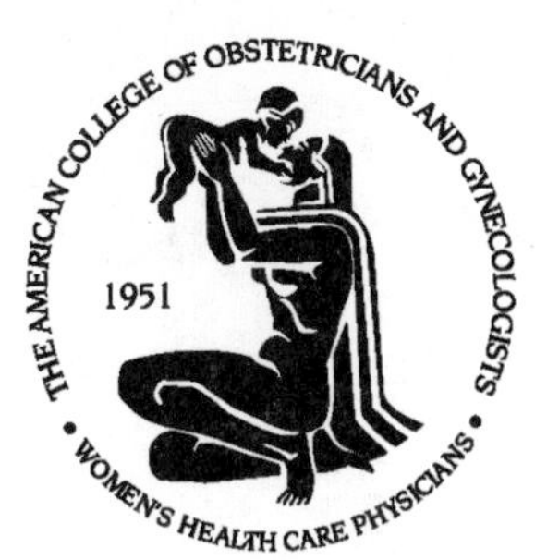

ACOG *Statement of Policy*

As issued by the ACOG Executive Board

LIPOSUCTION

Liposuction is not a gynecologic procedure and, therefore, is not standard in gynecologic training programs. Since liposuction is not a gynecologic procedure, it would be inappropriate for the College to establish guidelines for training. As with any other surgical procedure, credentialing for liposuction should be based on education, training, experience and demonstrated competence.

Approved by the Executive Board January 1988

The American College of Obstetricians and Gynecologists
409 12th Street, SW, PO Box 96920 • Washington, DC 20090-6920 Telephone 202 638 5577

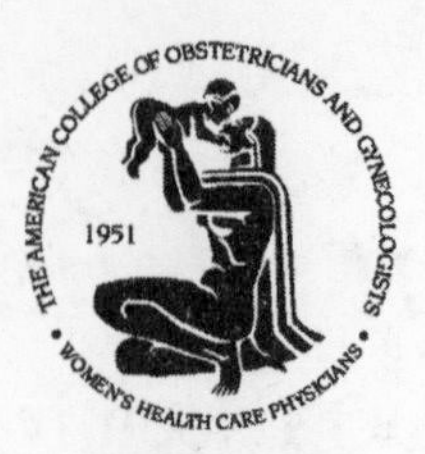

ACOG *Statement of Policy*

As issued by the ACOG Executive Board

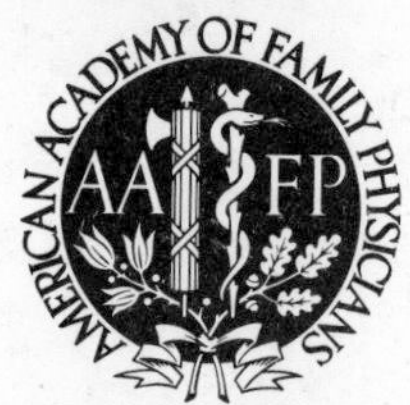

This document was developed by a joint task force of the American Academy of Family Physicians and the American College of Obstetricians and Gynecologists.

MATERNITY AND GYNECOLOGIC CARE -- RECOMMENDED CORE EDUCATIONAL GUIDELINES FOR FAMILY PRACTICE RESIDENTS

These core educational guidelines in maternity and gynecologic care for family practice residents are intended to aid residency directors in developing curricula and to assist residents in identifying areas of necessary training. Following these recommendations, which are designed as curricular guidelines rather than as residency program requirements, should result in graduates of family practice residency programs who are well-prepared to provide quality medical care in the areas of maternity care, labor and delivery, and the female reproductive system. These curricular guidelines are not intended to serve as criteria for hospital privileging or credentialling. The assignment of hospital privileges is a local responsibility and is based on training, experience and current competence.

Curriculum

Core knowledge and skills should require a minimum of three months of experience in a structured obstetric-gynecologic educational program, with adequate emphasis on ambulatory and hospital care. Residents will obtain substantial additional obstetric-gynecologic experience throughout the three years of their experience in family practice centers and in their continuity practices. Residents will return to the family practice centers for their scheduled continuity clinics.

The most important objective in family practice residency training should be to provide consistent, quality, evidence-based care. While there may be different approaches to patient care, in all cases, social and psychologic aspects of care, as well as an appropriate history and physical examination, must be an integral part of training. The knowledge, skills and judgment required in residency training are a necessary base, although they might not necessarily translate into the practice of every family physician.

Programs for family practice residents should have a joint training committee composed of obstetricians-gynecologists and family physicians, with members of the committee approved by the chairs of the respective departments in the sponsoring educational institution. It shall be the responsibility of the joint training committee to develop objectives commensurate with the goals of the training program, to monitor resident's experience and to assist in the evaluation of faculty teaching skills. Educational institutions sponsoring graduate medical education should assume corporate responsibility for the overall program.

Family physicians and obstetricians should collaborate in the design, implementation and evaluation of the training of family practice residents in obstetrics-gynecology. A curriculum in obstetrics-gynecology for family practice residents should incorporate knowledge of diagnosis and management, core skills and advanced skills. In this document, management implies responsibility for and provision of care and, when necessary, consultation and/or referral.

The American College of Obstetricians and Gynecologists
409 12th Street, SW, PO Box 96920 • Washington, DC 20090-6920 Telephone 202 638 5577

MATERNITY AND GYNECOLOGIC CARE -- RECOMMENDED CORE EDUCATIONAL GUIDELINES FOR FAMILY PRACTICE RESIDENTS
Page 2

A. Knowledge of diagnosis and management
   1. Normal female growth and development, and variants
   2. Appropriate history and physical examination for all age groups
   3. Gynecology
      a. Disease prevention/health promotion and periodic health evaluation
      b. Physiology of menstruation
      c. Abnormal uterine bleeding
      d. Gynecologic problems of children
      e. Infections and diseases of the female reproductive and urinary systems
      f. Breast health and diseases of the breast
      g. Sexual assault
      h. Domestic violence
      i. Trauma to the reproductive system
      j. Pelvic pain
      k. Benign and malignant neoplasms of the female reproductive system
      l. Menopause and geriatric gynecology
      m. Indications for surgical intervention
      n. Cervical lesions and abnormal cytology
      o. Ectopic pregnancy
   4. Obstetrics
      a. Pre-pregnancy planning and counseling
      b. Prenatal care, including risk assessment
      c. Labor and delivery
      d. Postpartum care
      e. Care of the normal newborn
      f. Common neonatal problems
      g. Analgesia and anesthesia for labor and delivery
      h. Indications for cesarean delivery
      i. Obstetric complications and emergencies
      j. Lactation
   5. Family life education
      a. Family planning
      b. Fertility problems
      c. Interconceptional care
      d. Family and sexual counseling
   6. Consultation and referral
      a. The role of the obstetrician, gynecologist and subspecialist
      b. Women's health care delivery systems
      c. Regionalized perinatal care for high-risk pregnancies
      d. Collaboration with other health care providers (i.e., nutritionist, dietitian, childbirth educator, lactation consultant, certified nurse midwife, nurse practitioner, etc.)

B. Core skills

   Emotional preparation for, and sensitive, thorough performance of, the gynecologic examination in patients of all ages.
   1. Gynecology
      a. Appropriate screening examination of the female, including breast examination
      b. Obtaining vaginal and cervical cytology
      c. Colposcopy
      d. Cervical biopsy, polypectomy
      e. Endometrial biopsy
      f. Culdocentesis
      g. Cryosurgery/cautery for benign disease

MATERNITY AND GYNECOLOGIC CARE -- RECOMMENDED CORE EDUCATIONAL GUIDELINES FOR FAMILY PRACTICE RESIDENTS
Page 3

h. Microscopic diagnosis of urine and vaginal smears
i. Bartholin duct cyst drainage or marsupialization
j. Dilation and curettage for incomplete abortion

2. Family planning and contraception
   a. Oral contraceptive counseling and prescribing
   b. Intrauterine contraceptive device counseling, insertion and removal
   c. Diaphragm fitting and counseling
   d. Insertion and removal of subcutaneous contraceptive implants and counseling
   e. Injectable long-term contraceptives and counseling
3. Pregnancy
   a. Pre-pregnancy evaluation
   b. Initial pregnancy visit
   c. Risk assessment
   d. History, physical examination, laboratory monitoring, and counseling throughout pregnancy
   e. Noninvasive evaluation of fetal gestational age and fetoplacental adequacy, including limited obstetric ultrasound examination
   f. Management of labor
   g. Pudendal and local block anesthesia
   h. Fetal assessment, antepartum and intrapartum, including limited obstetric ultrasound examination
   i. Induction of labor
   j. Internal fetal monitoring
   k. Normal cephalic delivery including use of vacuum extraction and outlet forceps
   l. Episiotomy and repair, including third-degree lacerations
   m. Management of common intrapartum problems (e.g., hypertension, mild pre-eclampsia, fever, infection, nonreassuring fetal status, unanticipated shoulder dystocia, manual removal of placenta)
   n. Exploration of vagina, cervix, uterus
   o. Emergency breech delivery
   p. Neonatal resuscitation
   q. Management of common postpartum problems (e.g., hemorrhage, endometritis)
   r. First-assist at cesarean delivery
   s. Vaginal delivery after previous cesarean delivery
4. Surgery
   a. Assist at common major surgical procedures

C. Advanced skills

For family practice residents who are planning to practice in communities without readily available obstetric-gynecologic consultation and who need to provide a more complete level of obstetric-gynecologic services for the proper care of patients, additional, intensified experience is recommended. This experience should be agreed on by the joint training committee and tailored to the needs of the resident's intended practice; it may occur within the three-year family practice residency.

Family practice residents planning to include the following in their practices should obtain additional intensified experience taught by or in collaboration with obstetrician-gynecologists. In programs where obstetrician-gynecologists are not available, these skills should be taught by appropriately skilled family physicians.

1. Gynecology
   a. Loop electrosurgical excision procedures
2. Family planning and contraception
   a. Voluntary interruption of pregnancy up to 10 weeks of gestation

MATERNITY AND GYNECOLOGIC CARE -- RECOMMENDED CORE EDUCATIONAL GUIDELINES FOR FAMILY PRACTICE RESIDENTS
Page 4

3. Pregnancy
   a. Ultrasound-guided amniocentesis, mid- and third-trimester
   b. Conduction anesthesia and analgesia (not routinely taught by obstetrician-gynecologists)
   c. Management of preterm labor
   d. Management of multiple gestation
   e. Management of breech delivery
   f. External cephalic version
   g. Amnioinfusion
   h. Use of low forceps
   i. Fourth-degree lacerations
   j. Severe pre-eclampsia
   k. Performance of cesarean delivery
   l. Management of complications of vaginal birth after previous cesarean delivery
4. Surgery
   a. Tubal ligation, postpartum and with cesarean delivery

Published July 1980
Reformatted July 1988
Revised and Retitled March 1998

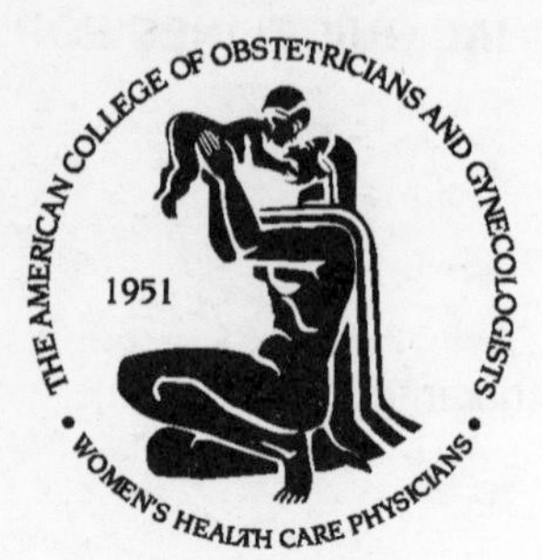

ACOG *Statement of Policy*

As issued by the ACOG Executive Board

PREGNANCY DISABILITY

Pregnancy is a physiologic process. All pregnant patients, however, have a variable degree of disability, on an individual basis, as indicated below, during which time they are unable to perform their usual activities.

1. In an uncomplicated pregnancy, disability occurs near the termination of pregnancy, during labor, delivery and the puerperium. The process of labor and puerperium is disabling in itself. The usual duration of such disability is approximately six to eight weeks.

2. Complications of pregnancy may occur which give rise to other disability. Examples of such complications include toxemia, infection, hemorrhage, ectopic pregnancy and abortion.

3. A woman with pre-existing disease, which in itself is not disabling, may become disabled with the addition of pregnancy. Certain patients with heart disease, diabetes, hypertensive cardiovascular disease, renal disease and other systemic conditions may become disabled during their pregnancy because of the adverse effect pregnancy has upon these conditions.

The onset, termination and cause of the disability as related to pregnancy can only be determined by a physician.

Approved by the Executive Committee March 1974
Reaffirmed September 1999

The American College of Obstetricians and Gynecologists
409 12th Street, SW, PO Box 96920 • Washington, DC 20090-6920 Telephone 202 638 5577

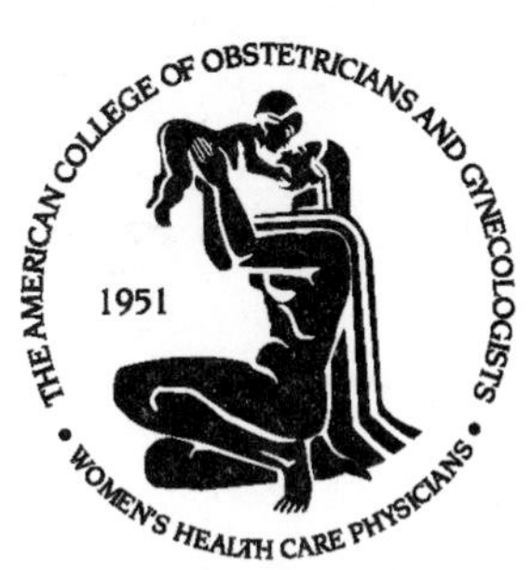

ACOG *Statement of Policy*

As issued by the ACOG Executive Board

SEXUALITY EDUCATION

The American College of Obstetricians and Gynecologists supports the inclusion of age-appropriate sexuality education from grades kindergarten through 12th grade as an integral part of comprehensive health education in schools and communities. ACOG encourages its members to advocate for and participate in such education.

Approved by the Executive Board July 1996

The American College of Obstetricians and Gynecologists
409 12th Street, SW, PO Box 96920 • Washington, DC 20090-6920 Telephone 202 638 5577

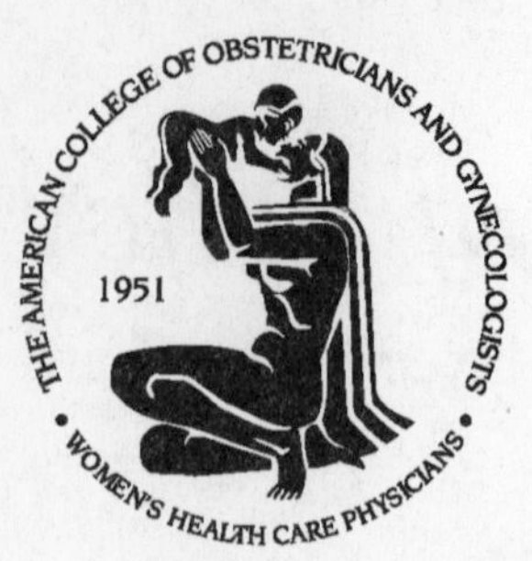

ACOG *Statement of Policy*

As issued by the ACOG Executive Board

TOBACCO ADVERTISING AIMED AT WOMEN

The American College of Obstetricians and Gynecologists opposes the unconscionable targeting of women by the tobacco industry.

The health risks of tobacco use to women are well documented. It also is well known that smoking by a pregnant woman may be harmful to her fetus. It is unnecessary to catalogue all of these risks here. Because of these well known dangers, it is irresponsible for tobacco companies to single out women, especially educationally or otherwise disadvantaged women, and encourage them to smoke.

Tobacco companies must stop encouraging young women to smoke cigarettes. The health of women and of our future generations demand at least that much consideration.

Approved by the Executive Board July 1990
Reaffirmed July 2000

The American College of Obstetricians and Gynecologists
409 12th Street, SW, PO Box 96920 • Washington, DC 20090-6920 Telephone 202 638 5577

Lists of Titles

Committee Opinions

Educational and Technical Bulletins

Practice Bulletins

Practice Patterns

Policy Statements

Index

Lists of Titles

Committee Opinions

Educational and Technical Bulletins

Practice Bulletins

Practice Patterns

Policy Statements

Index

Index

Note: Italicized letters *f* and *t* following page numbers indicate figures and tables, respectively.

F

M

N

P

Q

R

S

T

W

X

Y

Z